# NEUROPATHOLOGY
## The Diagnostic Approach

# NEUROPATHOLOGY
## The Diagnostic Approach

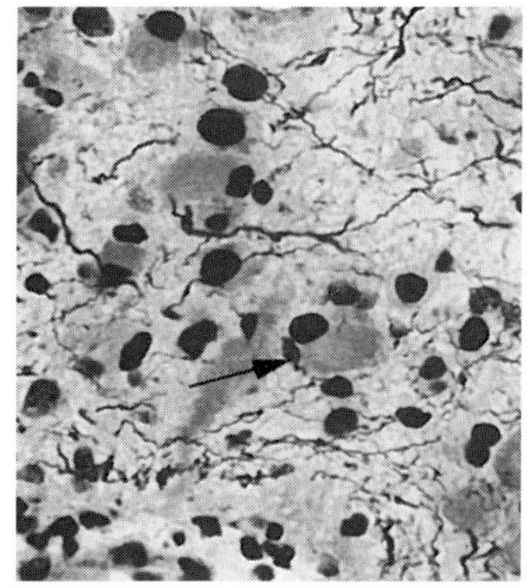

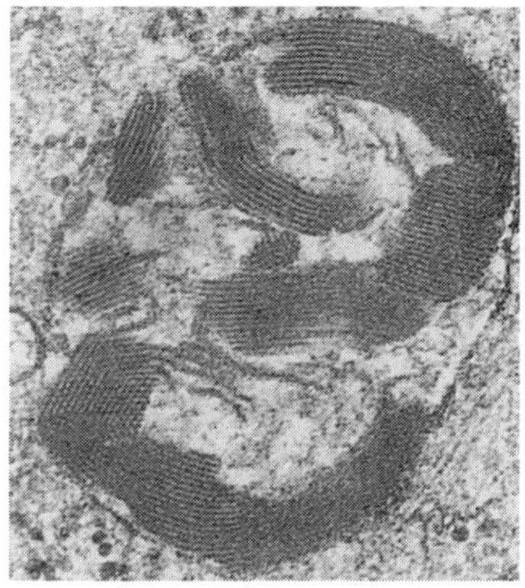

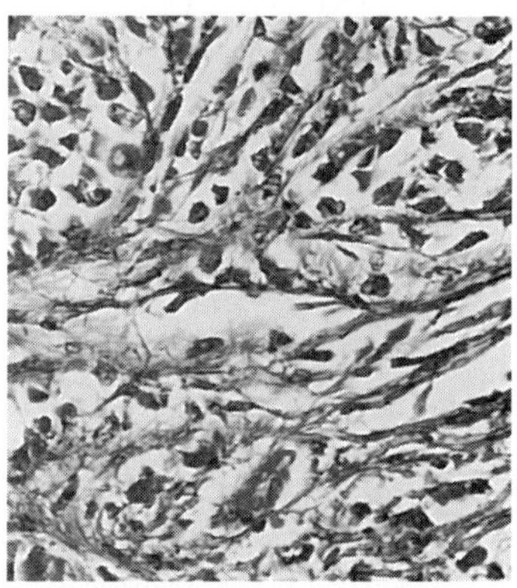

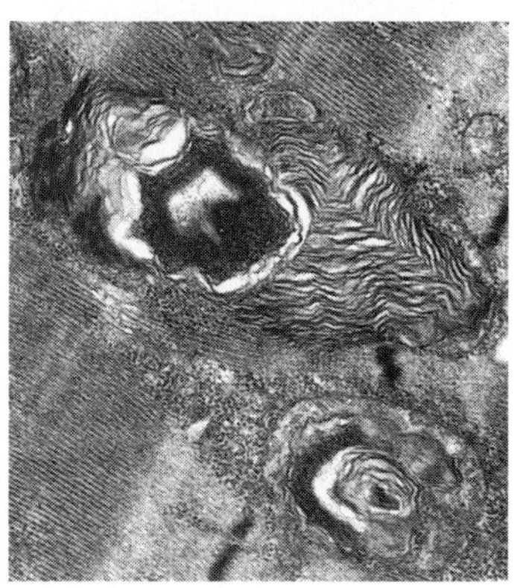


Editor

**JULIO H. GARCIA, MD**
Director, Neuropathology Division
Henry Ford Hospital
Detroit, Michigan
Professor of Pathology
Case Western Reserve University School of Medicine
Cleveland, Ohio

Associate Editors

**HERBERT BUDKA, MD**
Professor of Clinical Neuropathology
Klinisches Institut für Neurologie der Universität
Vienna, Austria

**PAUL E. MCKEEVER, MD, PhD**
Associate Professor and Chief
Section of Neuropathology
Department of Pathology
University of Michigan Medical School
Ann Arbor, Michigan

**HARVEY B. SARNAT, MD, FRCPC**
Professor of Neurology, Pediatrics, and Pathology (Neuropathology)
University of Washington School of Medicine
Seattle, Washington

**ANDERS A.F. SIMA, MD, PhD**
Professor of Pathology and Neurology
Wayne State University School of Medicine
Detroit, Michigan



Mosby

St. Louis Baltimore Boston Carlsbad Chicago Minneapolis New York Philadelphia Portland
London Milan Sydney Tokyo Toronto

Mosby
Dedicated to Publishing Excellence

A Times Mirror Company

*Vice President and Publisher:* Anne S. Patterson
*Senior Managing Editor:* Lynne Gery
*Developmental Editor:* Rebecca Gruliow
*Project Manager:* Chris Baumle
*Production Editor:* Susie Coladonato
*Design Manager:* Nancy J. McDonald
*Manufacturing Manager:* William Winneberger, Jr.



Printed in the United States of America
Composition by Maryland Composition
Printing/binding by R.R. Donnelley & Sons

Mosby–Year Book, Inc.
11830 Westline Industrial Drive
St. Louis, Missouri 63146

**Library of Congress Cataloging-in-Publication Data**

Neuropathology : the diagnostic approach / editor, Julio H. Garcia : associate editors, Herbert Budka . . . [et al.].
p. cm.
Includes bibliographical references and index.
ISBN 0-8151-5562-X
1. Nervous system—Diseases—Diagnosis. I. Garcia, Julio H., 1933– . II. Budka, H. (Herbert)
[DNLM: 1. Nervous System Diseases—diagnosis. 2. Nervous System Diseases—pathology. WL 141 N4934 1997]
RC348.N488 1997
616.8′0475—dc21
DNLM/DLC
for Library of Congress 96-48279
CIP

97 98 99 00 01 / 9 8 7 6 5 4 3 2 1

# CONTRIBUTORS

**Mila Blaivas, MD, PhD**
Clinical Associate Professor of Pathology
University of Michigan Medical School
Ann Arbor, Michigan

**Herbert Budka, MD**
Professor of Clinical Neuropathology
Klinisches Institut für Neurologie der Universität Wien
Abteilung für Neuropathologie und Neurochemie
Vienna, Austria

**Dario V. Cáccamo, MD**
Senior Staff, Department of Pathology
Henry Ford Hospital
Detroit, Michigan
Clinical Assistant Professor
Department of Pathology
Medical College of Ohio
Toledo, Ohio

**Constance D'Amato, BS**
Assistant Professor, Department of Pathology
University of Michigan
Ann Arbor, Michigan

**Julio H. Garcia, MD**
Director, Neuropathology Division
Henry Ford Hospital
Detroit, Michigan
Professor of Pathology
Case Western Reserve University School of Medicine
Cleveland, Ohio
Adjunct Professor of Pathology
Medical College of Ohio
Toledo, Ohio

**Umberto De Girolami, MD**
Associate Professor of Pathology
Harvard Medical School
Chief, Neuropathology Division, Department of Pathology
Brigham and Women's Hospital
Boston, Massachusetts

**Hans H. Goebel, MD**
Professor, Division of Neuropathology
Johannes Gutenberg-University
Mainz, Germany

**Jan E. Leestma, MD, MM**
Associate Medical Director and Neuropathologist
The Chicago Institute of Neurosurgery and Neuroresearch
Chicago, Illinois

**Ricardo V. Lloyd, MD, PhD**
Professor of Pathology
Consultant, Mayo Clinic
Rochester, Minnesota

**Paul E. McKeever, MD, PhD**
Associate Professor and Chief, Section of Neuropathology
Department of Pathology
University of Michigan Medical Center
Ann Arbor, Michigan

**Hernando Mena, MD, Col, MC, USA**
Chair, Department of Neuropathology
Armed Forces Institute of Pathology
Washington, DC

**Robert E. Mrak, MD, PhD**
Professor of Pathology (Neuropathology)
University of Arkansas College of Medicine
Staff, Pathologist (Neuropathology) and Chief Electron Microscopy Section
John L. McClellan Memorial Veterans' Hospital
Consulting Neuropathologist
Arkansas Children's Hospital and Arkansas State Crime Laboratory
Member, Arkansas Cancer Research Center
Little Rock, Arkansas

**Dara B. Nachmanoff, MD**
Clinical Fellow in Neuropathology
Harvard Medical School
Boston, Massachusetts

**James S. Nelson, MD**
Professor of Pathology, Department of Pathology
Louisiana State University Medical Center
New Orleans, Louisiana

**Roy H. Rhodes, MD, PhD**
Former Associate Professor of Pathology and Neurology
Case Western Reserve University School of Medicine
Head, Neuropathology MetroHealth Medical Center
Cleveland, Ohio

**Lucien J. Rubinstein, MD (Deceased)**
Director, Division of Neuropathology
University of Virginia School of Medicine
Charlottesville, Virginia

**Harvey B. Sarnat, MD, FRCPC**
Professor of Neurology, Pediatrics, and Pathology (Neuropathology)
University of Washington School of Medicine
Seattle, Washington

**Anders A.F. Sima, MD, PhD**
Professor of Pathology and Neurology
Wayne State University School of Medicine
Detroit, Michigan
Visiting Professor of Pathology
University of Michigan
Ann Arbor, Michigan
Staff Neuropathologist
Harper Hospital and Detroit Medical Center
Detroit, Michigan

**Linda A. Specht, MD, PhD**
Director of Neurology
Franciscan Children's Hospital
Associate Professor of Pediatrics
Boston University School of Medicine
Boston, Massachusetts

**Michael W. Stanley, MD**
Professor of Pathology and Director of Cytopathology
University of Arkansas College of Medicine
Little Rock, Arkansas

**Kinuko Suzuki, MD**
Professor, Department of Pathology and Laboratory Medicine
University of North Carolina at Chapel Hill School of Medicine
Attending Neuropathologist, University of North Carolina Hospital
Chapel Hill, North Carolina

**Ana Lia Taratuto, MD, PhD**
Assistant Professor of Pathology
University of Buenos Aires
Head, Department of Neuropathology
Instituto de Investigaciones Neurologicas Raul Carrea-FLENI
Neuropathologist, Hospital Nacional de Pediatria Juan P. Garrahan
Buenos Aires, Argentina

# FOREWORD

Neuropathology, once the sole domain of a few specialists concerned with those structural changes encountered in rare degenerative diseases of the nervous system, has lately been transformed into a subject of increasing relevance to the general pathologist and, indeed, to the general physician.

Where once determining the cause of a neurological disorder had been a leisurely intellectual exercise reserved for those trained in the arcane, it now represents a diagnostic challenge of critical importance to the living patient, and one demanding great accuracy. In past years *cure* was not a commonly heard word in neurology; but more recently many central nervous system ailments—including certain intracranial neoplasms, movement disorders, metabolic diseases, and even stroke—have become increasingly amenable to rational therapies. Rapid and accurate histopathological diagnosis, in conjunction with the newer neuro-imaging procedures, serves to identify the biological nature of the offending lesion and becomes the essential first step leading to realistic medical intervention.

The textbooks that lie open by their microscopes and are repeatedly used by the practicing pathologists should therefore reflect this dramatic transition in the mission and therapeutic capabilities of the clinical neurosciences.

Julio H. Garcia, MD, Chief of Neuropathology at Henry Ford Hospital and Professor of Pathology at Case Western Reserve University School of Medicine, is an internationally recognized authority in the field of experimental and clinical stroke and a gifted teacher who has been in the forefront of neuropathology since his early training years, some 35 years ago, at the State University of New York, Downstate Medical Center. He has now undertaken a heavy responsibility: to gather a transnational assemblage of knowledgable neuropathologists, all authorities in their fields, who collectively provide a new kind of neuropathology textbook, one that emphasizes the diagnostic imperatives confronting the hospital pathologist.

The practicing pathologist is certainly committed to lifelong learning about the obscure as well as the common components of human disease. More than any other medical discipline, however, pathology requires practitioners to be teachers as well as laboratory physicians; and indeed the bulk of hospital pathologists hold faculty posts in one medical school or another. But these same pathologists bear yet another responsibility: the task of supplying practical and prompt answers to the multitude of compelling questions raised by their clinical colleagues. The pediatricians, for example, submit a spinal fluid specimen for cytologic evaluation. Can laboratory tests possibly provide insights into the ill-defined but progressive neurological deficits seen in the eight-year-old child who is their patient? How should the specimen be processed? What should be looked for? What artifacts might be anticipated? Should virological studies be undertaken? Or the neurosurgeon's request for a frozen section on a biopsy derived from a poorly circumscribed supratentorial mass: What preliminary steps should be undertaken before the biopsy arrives? What staining procedures should be employed? What light microscopy findings [or unusual clinical features] call for parallel ultrastructural studies? When should the more sophisticated immunocytochemical procedures be utilized?

In truth, most neuropathology textbooks of enduring merit are assembled in encyclopedic fashion, offering the interested reader a consciously didactic, exhaustive tome best suited for the unhurried preparation of a lecture. These excellent sources are typically erudite and comprehensive but are essentially indifferent to the practical needs of the hospital pathologists who, beyond their professorial duties, must also answer the urgent demands of the here and now. A scholarly textbook of neuropathology that recognizes a sense of immediacy is necessary, an erudite book that will not sacrifice comprehensiveness but will nonetheless reorder the manner and content of its information so as to be responsive to that atmosphere of urgency that characterizes the average day of the hospital-based pathologist.

Give us a utilitarian text, the hospital-based pathologists say, one that is abundantly illustrated, pragmatic, meticulously edited, and one which will also provide us with clear, convincing information; present us with a guide that is practical but that does not sacrifice elaborate descriptions and reliable documentation for the sake of mere clarity.

And to these challenges, Garcia and his colleagues from United States, Austria, Germany and Argentina have been truly responsive. They now offer in these pages a masterful text and a dependable laboratory companion for the practicing pathologist.

*Stanley M. Aronson, MD*
*Dean of Medicine Emeritus*
*Brown University School of Medicine*
*Providence, Rhode Island*
*April, 1997*

# FOREWORD

Is Neuropathology that difficult or changing so rapidly that another book is necessary? And is it for the beginning student, who will undoubtedly be overwhelmed by the mass of minute details presented by the many different authors? Or is it for the already experienced and practicing teacher, who will find it difficult to change his mind about what the facts are?

To appreciate the answers to these questions one must remember how we got this far and realize how much farther we have to go. Neuropathology is not for the faint of heart or for the 90-day wonders of yesteryear but for those who are willing to correlate, not just staple together, all of the basic and clinical sciences that have contributed to the development of the specialty.

It is obvious that diseases are of many types and that each has its many variations from its classical definition. Nowhere is this more true than in the nervous system with its almost infinite mosaic of cells, both neurones and glia, new varieties of which appear with increasing frequency as new techniques are applied with bewildering success. If any one ever could, no one person can now even hope to see all of the possible varieties of disease. We all can only admire the giants of the last two centuries who were able to see the forests for the trees and to make enduring—even if subsequently slightly or even markedly modified—conributions to the classification of diseases of the nervous system. These began with the magnificent Atlas of Cruveilhier of the 1830s and extended to the gigantic Handbuch of Henke and Lubarsch in the 1930s. The hidden nature of the nervous system, hidden beneath skin and muscle and bone, made the autopsy (correlated, of course, with careful clinical examination) virtually the only source of accurate evidence of what *had been* wrong with the patient.

Increasingly, however, as more was learned from the autopsy, the question arose: what *is* wrong with the still-living patient? And does it matter? During the early 1990s positive answer came from increasingly brave neurosurgical explorations and diagnostic techniques, such as examination of the cerebrospinal fluid, pneumoencephalography, electroencephalography, and arteriography. These provided glimpses of premortem stages of many diseases, especially neoplasms and strokes, to the point where we might have imagined that we were beginning to understand at least these two major classes of diseases.

Then the question arose: *why* is the patient sick? What *was* wrong *before* he became sick? A whole new field arose, experimental neuropathology, opening up newer and newer models of the pathogeneses of diseases. Eventually we had to ask whether our patients more resembled guinea pigs, rats, rabbits, or monkeys, each of which was found to have its own unique little differences in reactions. Of course, humans have their own patterns of reactions, but the models have been very useful in pointing the ways to study humans. Advances in morphology (electronmicroscopy, immunocytochemistry, computerized tomography, and magnetic resonance imaging), chemistry (including immunology and genetics), and physiology have continued to push experimental neuropathology to the point that now almost every month we have another treatment for multiple sclerosis! And how much more of the early stages of strokes and neoplasia still remains for the future to reveal!

Not only has it become logistically impossible for one person to see all the varieties of all the diseases in their classical formats but also it has remained a challenge even to categorize all the atypical presentations and courses. Multi-authored texts have become the rule—but the reader must remain aware that each author probably still sees only a fraction of the subject! Only by comparison of one such text with another can the reader approach an understanding of the whole. Texts are notoriously out of date the day they are published and their useful life may be only a few more years, but the inter-observer comparisons are increasingly important. Such comparisons may be facilitated by further development of the "information super highway." Soon we may, with the stroke of a key, be able to compare pictures and text from one after another authority—temporary as he or she may prove to be—and to see at a glance whether the case at hand matches any or all of the many descriptions available.

Not only is the information becoming more detailed as we probe with newer and more powerful techniques, but also the environments are changing: the external environment with its many potential toxins and the internal environment with its circulation of increasingly powerful new therapies. Looking back 50 years, when penicillin had just been added to the sulfas and dilantin to phenobarbital, we can see that the limits of aspirin and morphine had hardly affected the natural history of many diseases so that the autopsy was still a source of much information. From a situation where only the surgeons could be accused by "spoiling our specimens" we pathologists have for the past decade or two been in a new pattern of non-learning, where the failure to follow patients to the end is becoming a national scandal, not even obtaining the specimen to see what the autopsy will reveal to "one who would see for oneself," to see what we therapists have wrought.

This failure, coupled with the increasing effectiveness of our current therapies greatly magnifies our problems in recognizing just what we are studying, increasing the need for tables of differential diagnosis and for decision trees, branching logical schemes to guide us. The beauty of the current text is just that: at last we have a text not merely describing diseases and their variations but providing a basic framework for differentiating one diseases (and its variations) from another disease (and its variations), defining how much or how little these variations overlap. From this approach, emphasizing the practical and diagnostic aspects of Neuropathology, much can be gained that should be helpful to both the neophyte and the expert. Just how practical the suggestions will prove in the actual practice of the reader may determine how soon the second edition is prepared.

*Ellsworth C. Alvord, Jr., MD*
*Professor of Pathology*
*University of Washington*
*School of Medicine*
*Seattle, WA*
*29 April 1997*

# PREFACE

The material contained in this book has been assembled as a source of information that may facilitate the undertaking of making diagnoses based on the interpretation of neuropathologic methods. Most authors who contributed to the completion of this book endeavored to present the information contained in their respective chapters in a succinct and tabular fashion that directs the reader through a logical and direct, almost algorithmic, process of differential diagnosis. Moreover, the applications of diverse methods currently used in neuropathology ranging from the evaluation of neoplasms by light microscopy, electron microscopy, and immunocytochemistry, to the molecular biological means of detecting prions are discussed in detail and the results of these applications are profusely illustrated.

In most instances, the process of arriving at a diagnosis, by neuropathologic means, can be greatly enhanced by integrating the interpretation of neuroimaging abnormalities with the educated analysis of the microscopic changes affecting the brain. As an example, the chapter dealing with leukoencephalopathies includes several illustrations of various brain abnormalities (primarily confined to the cerebral white matter) that are demonstrable by computed tomography and magnetic resonance imaging. The significance of these abnormalities is integrated with the corresponding description of the changes detectable at the microscopic level.

A determined effort was made to support most every important assertion with appropriate citations of judiciously chosen references to publications that appeared within the past 10 to 15 years. This decision was based on the assumption that in most recent publications the authors refer to previously published, classical papers on the subject; moreover, these recent publications are more likely to be readily available (through electronic data banks or similar facilities) to readers who lack access to large library facilities.

*Julio H. Garcia, M.D.*
*Detroit, Michigan*
*May 8, 1997*

# CONTENTS

# NEUROPATHOLOGY
## The Diagnostic Approach

CHAPTER

# 1

# *Cerebrospinal Fluid: Cytology*

**Michael W. Stanley**



## NON-NEOPLASTIC CYTOLOGY

Clinical indications for lumbar puncture include the following: presentation of a new seizure disorder; subtle neurologic change in a cancer patient; a change in the pattern of a chronic seizure disorder; sudden severe headache; fever associated with a headache of moderate severity; decreased level of consciousness; and weakness. The conditions necessitating examination of the cerebrospinal fluid (CSF) are a group of nonspecific signs and symptoms generally referable to the central nervous system (CNS). These may be vague or episodic, and may be difficult to document objectively.

Evaluation of cellular and biochemical alterations in the CSF plays an important role in the diagnosis or monitoring of numerous clinical conditions. Furthermore, several therapeutic maneuvers require access to the subarachnoid space (SAS), and may incidentally yield a fluid sample useful in monitoring a therapeutic response or complication. Clinical, historical, and technical considerations are all important in our efforts to optimize the results of CSF studies. Although the details of laboratory methodology are beyond the scope of our concerns here, this chapter will offer comments regarding specimen requirements for specific tests and will outline key cytopreparatory methods.

Our emphasis will be on the interpretation of cytologic findings. Cell counts will be discussed in areas where quantitative data affect diagnostic criteria. Chief among these will be low cell count CSF in children with acute lymphoblastic leukemia. Rather than offering a précis of cell count information readily available in standard references, we will highlight important cytopathologic issues. Biochemical analysis will be discussed from the point of view of its impact on cytologic diagnosis and classification of malignancy.

## PREPARATION AND STAINING OF CSF FOR CYTOLOGIC EXAMINATION

Three problems attend the preparation of CSF specimens for cytologic examination. The first is preservation of fragile cells sent in a fluid medium that is ill-equipped to support their metabolic requirements. The second difficulty is the need to achieve a concentration of cells that are frequently present in very low numbers. The final problem relates to contamination with cells from other specimens being processed in the cytology laboratory. Once these issues have been addressed, one must select either air drying for Romanowsky stain or fixation of the slides for Papanicolaou stain. The initial selection of a preparatory method restricts the staining options that are available.

Adequate preservation is best achieved by the simple expedient of immediate transport combined with rapid preparation. It has been suggested that optimal results are achieved if the fluid is prepared within 30 minutes of procurement.[72] With greater delay, many cells quickly undergo severe damage and may appear as "smudges" that take up various types of stain but show no details. Unlike fluids from other body cavities, prefixation and transport of CSF by dilution with alcohol or other solutions cannot be recommended. Such methods can result in decreased adherence of cells to glass slides, limitations in preparatory (staining) options, and poor staining.[46]

Many CSF specimens are sparsely cellular, and diagnostic accuracy is improved by concentration. Methods include membrane filtration, cytocentrifugation, and semiautomated filtration devices. All are acceptable methods that offer both concentration and high quality cytomorphology. Membrane filtration lyses red blood cells. This limits interpretation of specimens from leukemia and lymphoma patients, whose peripheral blood contains circulating tumor cells. Cytocentrifugation is widely available and is probably the most commonly used technique. Specific suggestions for instrument settings are offered by those seeking to critically evaluate certain types of specimens. These will be discussed subsequently, primarily during our consideration of the leukemias and lymphomas.

We have consistently noted that the cytocentrifuge imparts a "flattened" appearance to many cells, with slight increases in cell size, nuclear size, and nucleolar prominence. Nonetheless, there is good morphologic correlation between leukemic cells in CSF prepared by this method and the appearance of these cells in bone marrow aspirates prepared by traditional methods.[22] Others have reported cell loss and morphologic alteration following cytocentrifugation.[34] Both filtration and cytocentrifugation have a small false-negative rate, especially when CSF specimens contain very few neoplastic cells.[4,22] As discussed below, filtration methods place important limitations on staining options. These limitations are most important when hematopoietic cells are studied. In addition to these technical considerations, the pathologist of record must favor the type of material he or she is best able to interpret. (The recent flowering of fine-needle aspiration means that many more pathologists are now at home with both Papanicolaou-stained and Romanowsky-stained cytology. These individuals can combine these complementary methods to maximum diagnostic advantage.)

Normal CSF specimens are sparely cellular and show only a small number of readily identifiable lymphocytes and monocytes. Thus, any other type of cell may seem so out of context as to strongly suggest malignancy, regardless of its cytomorphologic constitution. A common example would be contamination of CSF slides with benign mesothelial cells that represent "floaters" from simultaneously processed fluids from other body cavities. Seen against the expected background of normal CSF, such cells are very striking; their large size and nucleoli closely resemble a common pattern of breast carcinoma involvement of the CSF (see below). Thus the danger of false-positive diagnoses of malignancy is very great, unless attention is given to the details of cytopreparatory standards. Most workers prefer to process CSF specimens separately from all other samples brought to the laboratory.[46,72] A separate stain line is often maintained for this purpose. At the very least, all stains and other solutions should be completely filtered before CSF samples are prepared.

A number of stains can be applied to cytologic material, including CSF samples. However, only the Romanowsky or blood-film stains and the method of Papanicolaou are in common use for this purpose. The former group of stains is applied to air-dried slides;[92] the latter is based on fixed cells. Numerous fixatives are available, but most laboratories employ immediate wet fixation with 95% ethanol. These approaches to slide preparation and staining yield several differences in final cytologic outcome. These have been reviewed in the context of fine-needle aspiration cytology.[78]

The two staining methods are distinguished by certain advantages when specific pathologic processes or types of tumors are considered. In the CSF, most epithelial malignancies can be readily diagnosed using either type of preparation; historical and contextual factors aid considerably in reaching this goal. However, for hematologic malignancies many workers strongly prefer air-dried, Romanowsky-stained slides to those that have been alcohol-fixed and stained according to Papanicolaou. The former approach results in cells that closely resemble their counterparts in blood and bone marrow smears, thus permitting identification and classification of even occasional cells by criteria imported from the hematopathology literature.

Since these malignancies are relatively common in CSF material, we prepare both fixed and dried slides in the majority of cases. Cytocentrifuge slides are amenable to this approach. Laboratories that rely on filtration methods will not have the opportunity to study Romanowsky-stained CSF slides. We consider this an important limitation of such methods. Some have suggested that combined use of both cytocentrifugation and filtration would lower the incidence of false-negative diagnoses;[4] it would also alleviate this limitation in staining options.

## NON-NEOPLASTIC ELEMENTS AND CONTAMINANTS

Normal CSF is clear and sparsely cellular. The latter contrasts with fluids aspirated from the body cavities into which mesothelial cells normally exfoliate in large numbers; the cells that line the SAS and the cerebral ventricles are rarely exfoliated into the CSF.

The cell types normally seen in CSF are limited to mature-appearing lymphocytes and monocytes that lack reactive changes. Rare neutrophils are acceptable when specimens are concentrated. As noted previously, this spartan background renders "foreign" cells so out of context as to strongly imply malignancy. However, a number of non-neoplastic cells and noncellular elements may be encountered, and it is important that these be recognized and not overinterpreted as evidence of malignancy or infection. These are summarized in Table 1-1.

In practice, cells of the choroid plexus and ependymal cells are difficult to distinguish confidently. They should be recognized as small clusters of cells that may be columnar or may seem to form a syncytium with indistinct cell borders. Both flat sheets and small papillary clusters may be encountered. These small cells have uniform nuclei and granular cytoplasm. Nucleoli are small or inapparent. Thus, cytologic features of malignancy are absent (Fig. 1-1). Rare examples of choroid plexus papilloma have been associated with ventricular CSF containing numerous papillary cell clusters.[16] Such tumors usually occur in children and are associated with suggestive radiographic findings. Pia-arachnoid cells are rarely present in CSF but can be seen as clusters of small, bland spindle cells.

Primitive (blastlike) cells can be seen in the CSF of neonates,[30] where they frequently are associated with intraventricular hemorrhage or hydrocephalus. This clinical association, coupled with immunohistochemical staining for neuron-specific enolase and lack of staining for leukocyte common antigen, led Fischer and co-authors[30] to suggest that such cells may originate in the subependymal germinal matrix. These cells feature scanty cytoplasm, delicate chromatin, and small nucleoli. These cells are distinguished from acute lymphoblastic leukemia by their cohesive groupings, and from choroid plexus/ependymal cells by their relatively high nucleocytoplasmic ratio. They can closely resemble cells derived from medulloblastoma. Accurate clinical and radiographic correlation is needed if an inappropriate diagnosis of malignancy is to be avoided.

**Table 1-1.** Contaminants that can be seen in cerebrospinal fluid cytology

| Uncommon types of cells | Noncellular contaminants |
|---|---|
| Central Nervous System Components<br>• choroid plexus cells*<br>• ependymal cells*<br>• primitive (blastlike) cell clusters*<br>• pia-arachnoid cells<br>Peripheral Blood Cells<br>• red blood cells<br>• leukocytes<br>Bone Marrow Elements<br>• megakaryocytes*<br>• other marrow cells*<br>Tissue Introduced into the Fluid by the Aspirating Needle<br>• chondrocytes*<br>• cutaneous squamous cells<br>• soft tissues (muscles or adipose tissue)<br>• brain tissue*<br>Non-Neural Contaminants Introduced Via Skull Fracture<br>• respiratory-type epithelial cells<br>• organisms (bacteria, *Candida*) | Corpora Amylacea†<br>Acellular Fragments of Bone or Cartilage<br>Talc |

* These contaminants can be mistaken for evidence of malignancy.
† These contaminants can be mistaken for fungal organisms and are positive when special stains used to identify fungi (PAS, silver) are applied.

The normal-appearing leukocytes in peripheral blood-contaminated fluids may initially suggest meningitis. The association of these cells with red blood cells in a normal ratio should alleviate this concern. Since some lysis or depigmentation of red cells can occur in fixed preparations or during membrane filtration, this type of assessment may be facilitated by examination of air-dried cytocentrifuge slides.

Bone marrow cells can be admitted to a CSF sample when the aspirating needle comes into contact with bone (Fig. 1-2).[24,48] Such cells are small and lie singly, so that their hematopoietic nature is usually apparent. Their polymorphism may suggest an inflammatory process (see below), while their immaturity may lead to an incorrect diagnosis of leukemia or lymphoma. Megakaryocytes can be interpreted by the unwary as suggesting malignancy of many possible types. These

A 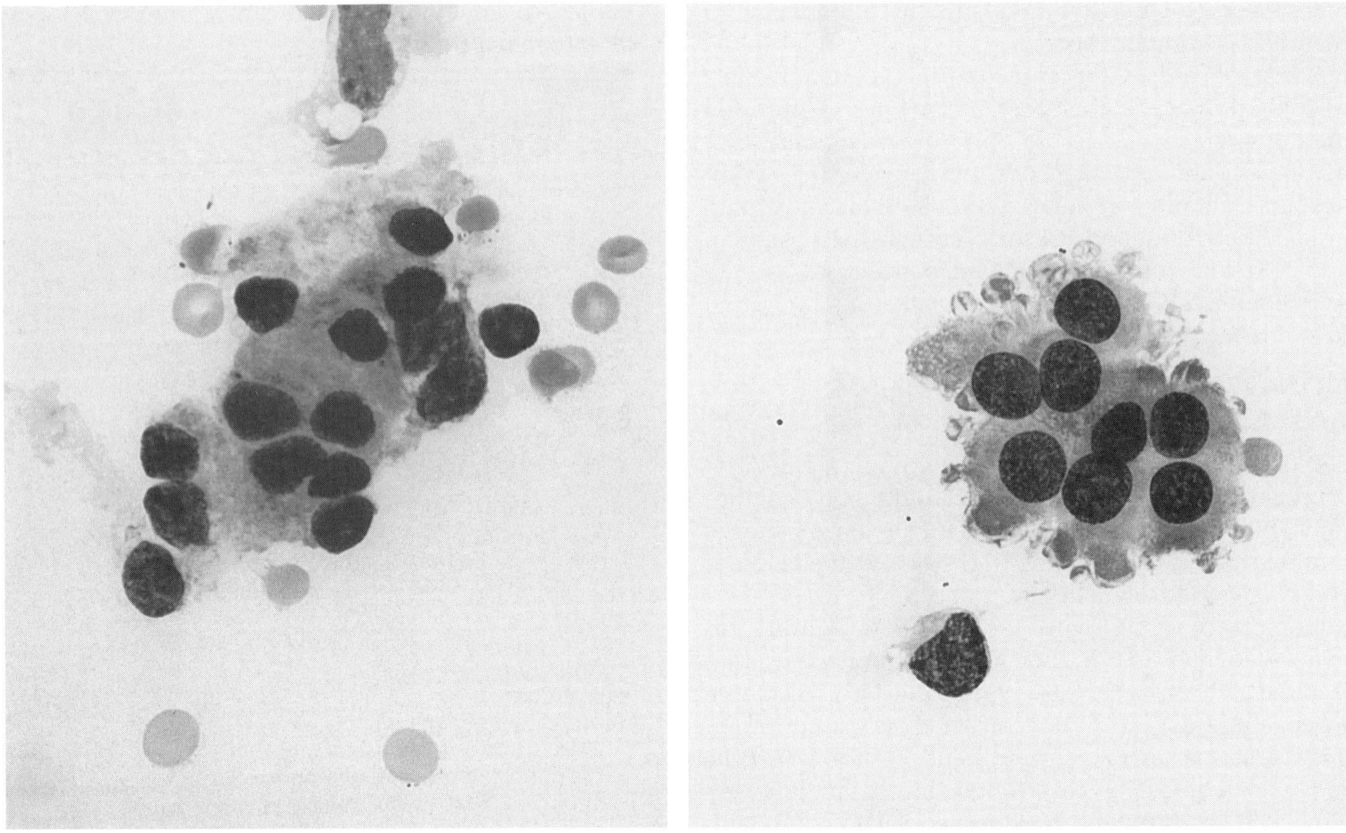 B

**Fig. 1-1.** Cuboidal to columnar ependymal-choroid plexus cells are seen in small syncytial clusters. These examples are arranged as flat sheets, but three-dimensional papillary groups also may be encountered. The uniform nuclei, inapparent nucleoli, and granular cytoplasm illustrated here are typical of ependyma. (**A**, Papanicolaou stain; ×600; **B**, Diff-Quik stain; ×600.)

problems are compounded when only fixed, Papanicolaou-stained slides are available, because most pathologists are not accustomed to the appearance of bone marrow elements prepared in this fashion. Study of air-dried slides is very helpful, as the characteristic appearance of normal bone marrow usually will be apparent. True extramedullary hematopoiesis can involve the meninges but is associated with various combinations of bone-marrow disease, anemia, and hemorrhage.[2,24]

As is the case with fine-needle aspiration cytology, cells from any tissue traversed by the needle can be introduced into the specimen. Most, including adipose tissue, skeletal muscle, and cutaneous squamous cells, are readily identified and discounted. Chondrocytes, on the other hand, may appear as large foreign cells, and since they are rare in most pathologists' cytology experience, they may be mistaken for evidence of malignancy. These cells probably originate in the intervertebral disks.[18,50] Seen singly or in clusters they show a shrunken nucleus with very little apparent substructure. Their abundant cytoplasm often features a prominent perinuclear halo (Fig. 1-3). Acellular fragments of bone or cartilage matrix may occasionally be seen (Fig. 1-4).

Corpora amylacea and talc can be present in CSF specimens. The primary significance of both is that these small rounded objects may be mistaken for fungal yeast. This difficulty is compounded by the fact that both are positive with PAS and silver stains. Corpora amylacea are laminated, whereas talc grains often show a central clearing. Starch shows a characteristic Maltese-cross configuration when viewed under polarized light. These and other pseudomicrobes, as well as silver staining artifacts in cytologic specimens, have been reviewed.[77]

When CSF is drawn from the ventricles or from an Ommaya reservoir, it may contain large numbers of choroid/ependymal cells. Fragments of brain tissue also may be encountered. These show various combinations of glial cells and neurons, and capillaries are often prominent (Fig. 1-5). Such tissues should not be mistaken for evidence of primary CNS malignancy.

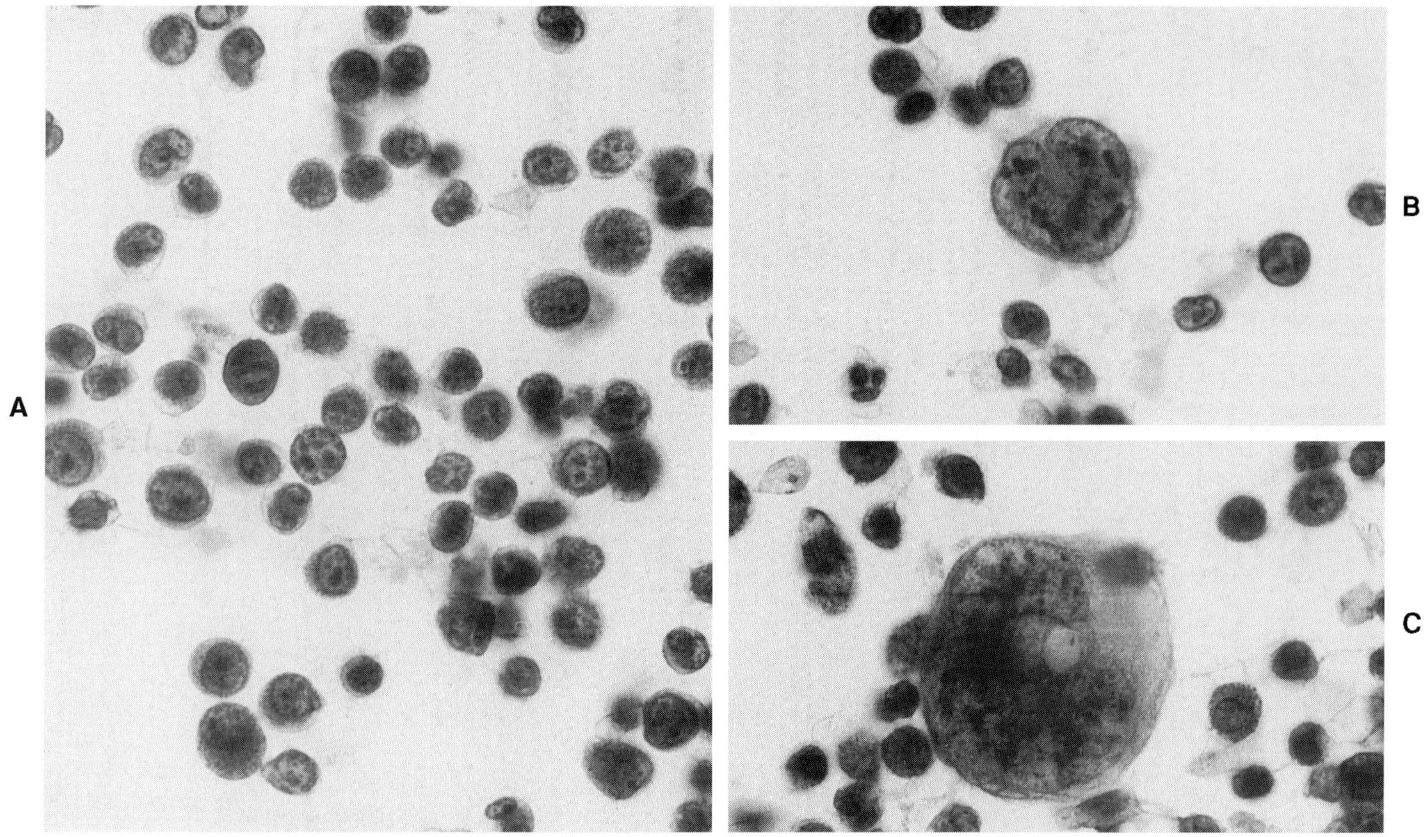


**Fig. 1-2.** This fluid is contaminated by normal bone marrow elements. The nature of these cells is clear when air-dried Romanowsky-stained slides are available. When encountered in fixed Papanicolaou-stained material, however, they can present diagnostic difficulties. In **A,** the granulocytic and erythroid precursors mimic the cells of malignant lymphoma or leukemia; they lie singly and feature clumped chromatin, prominent nucleoli, and scanty cytoplasm. The megakaryocytes shown in **B** and **C** may suggest a diagnosis of metastatic carcinoma. The nuclear lobulation, chromatin clumping, and hyperchromasia are characteristic. (Papanicolaou stain; ×600.)

## CELL COUNTS, DIFFERENTIALS, AND REACTIVE CHANGES

In adults, normal CSF contains up to five cells per μL, with lymphocytes predominating over monocytes. Fluid obtained from infants shows a slightly higher cell count (up to 10 cells per μL) and a reversal of this differential.

The diagnostic considerations that arise from increased numbers of a given cell type may be numerous. Neutrophils typify bacterial infections but can be associated with the early stage of other infections (viral, tuberculous, fungal) or with tissue damage due to hemorrhage, neoplastic meningitis, or various diagnostic maneuvers directed toward the CNS. Acute inflammation can be accompanied by obvious fibrin deposition (Fig. 1-6).

Lymphocytes may be numerous in a wide range of nonbacterial infections but also are seen in degenerative or demyelinating disorders, as well as other subacute or chronic processes. The latter group of conditions frequently features mixed inflammation, with various contributions from neutrophils, lymphocytes, macrophages, and even a few plasma cells. Eosinophilic reactions can be seen in parasitic infections more commonly than in other infections, and may be prominent in the meninges' reaction to foreign materials or drugs introduced into the SAS for diagnostic or therapeutic purposes, including shunt placement.[84] Eosinophils may rarely be associated with leukemia or carcinoma.[19,20] Macrophages may be numerous and very large following hemorrhage or infarcts. Lipid released by CNS tissue damage due to trauma or infarction can lead to striking cytoplasmic vacuoles in some macrophages. Myelography may bring about similar alterations. Transformation to multinucleated giant cells is common in such settings (Fig. 1-7). These cells can also

A

B

C

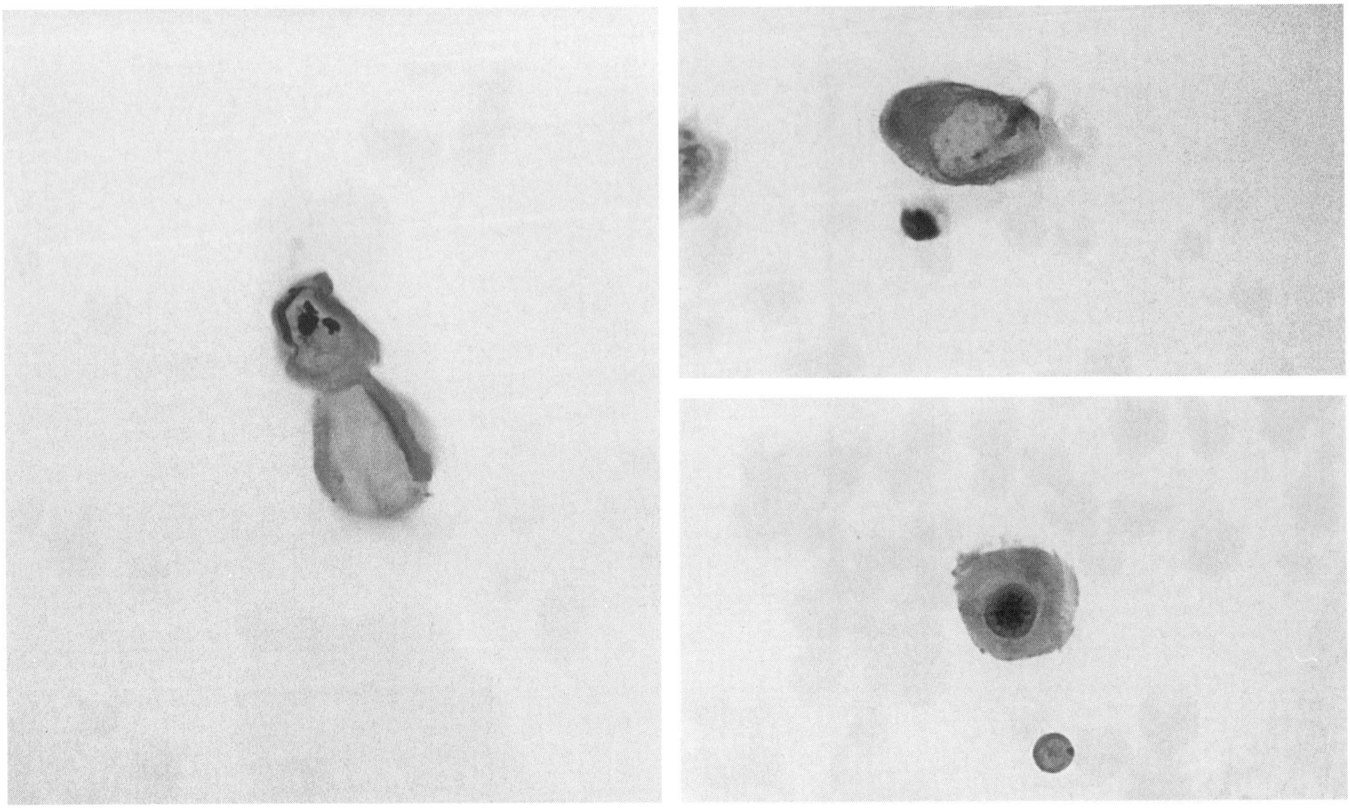

**Fig. 1-3.** These chondrocytes appear foreign to the expected CSF picture and can be mistaken for evidence of malignancy. The nuclear area appears cavitary. **A** and **C** show severely degenerated nuclei, while in **B,** the nuclear cavity is empty. (Papanicolaou stain; ×600.)

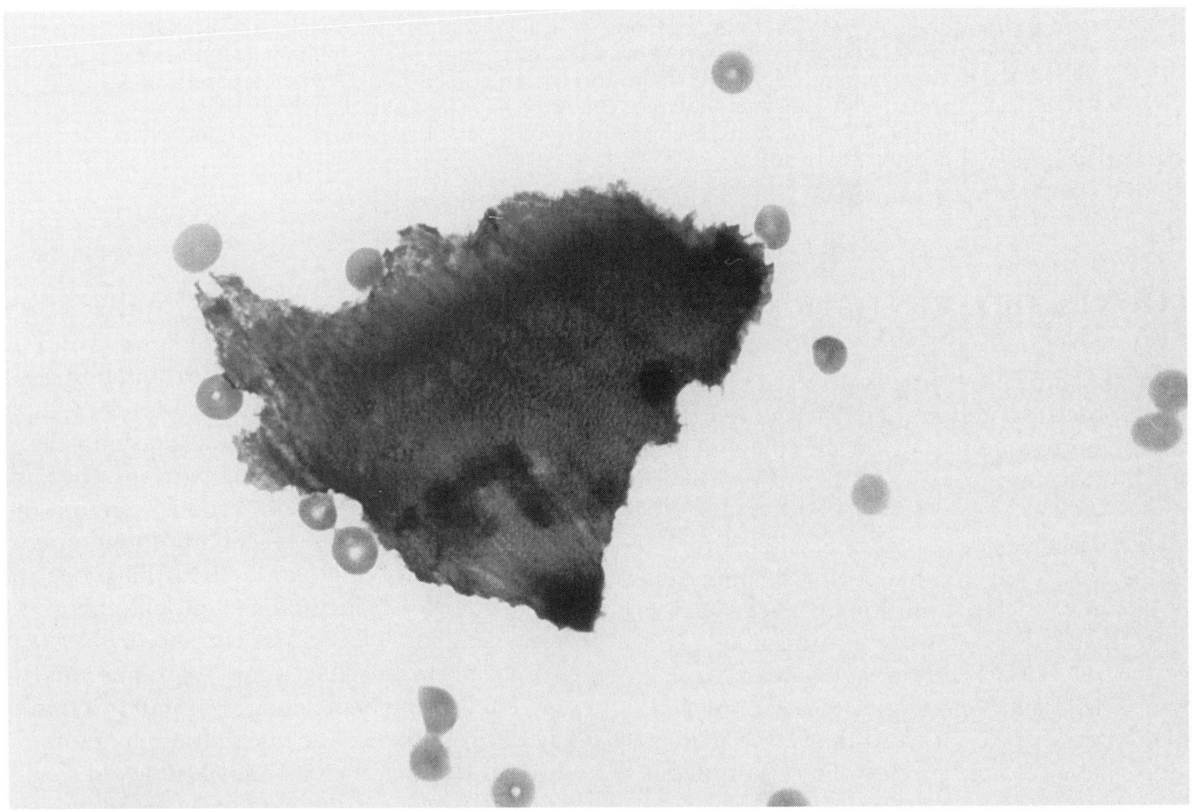

**Fig. 1-4.** This acellular, densely stained fragment of bone shows a fibrillar structure. (Diff-Quik stain; ×400.)

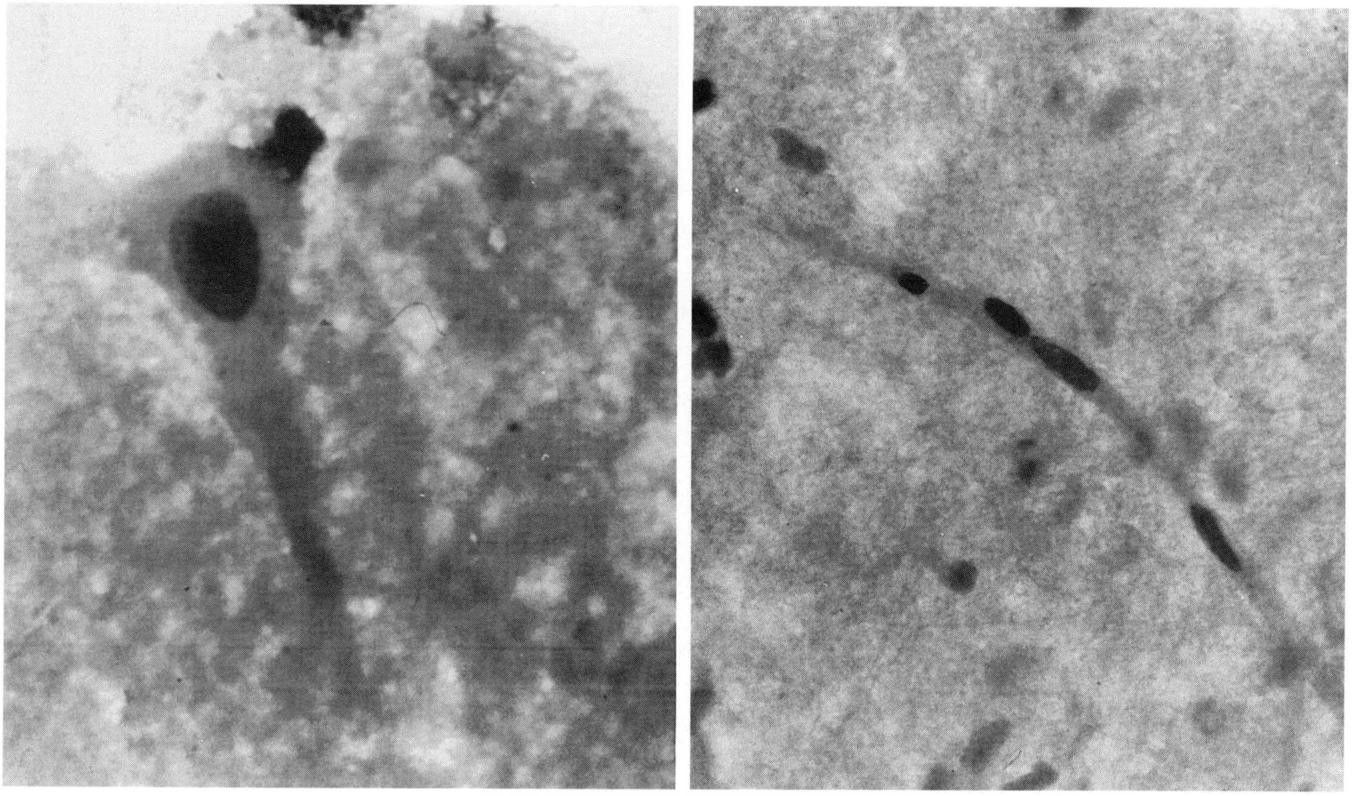

A B

**Fig. 1-5.** These fragments of brain tissue were identified in a ventricular CSF specimen. Both feature the smudgy appearance typical of coagulation necrosis. In **A,** a large neuron also shows degenerative changes, with blurring of cell borders and chromatin smudging. A capillary is prominent in **B.** (Papanicolaou stain; ×400.)

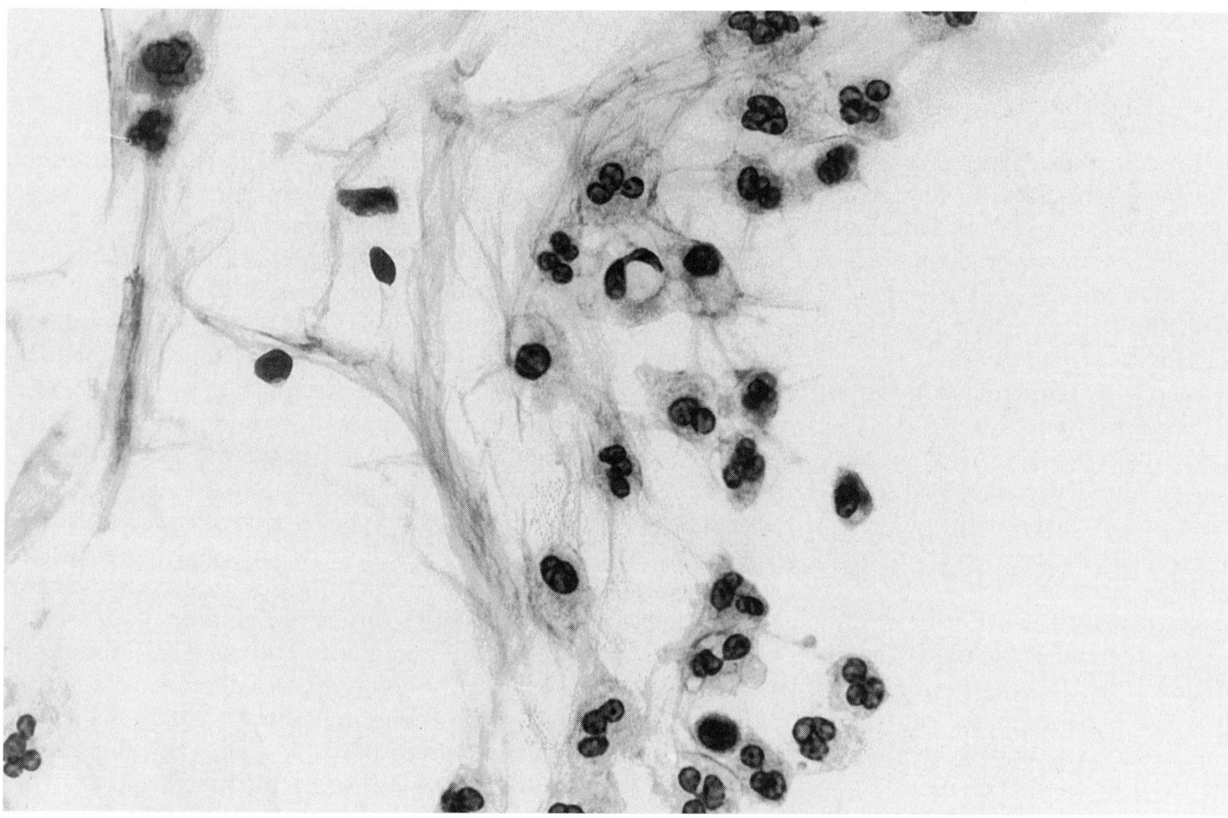

**Fig. 1-6.** In this example of acute meningitis, numerous neutrophils are associated with a web of fibrin strands. (Papanicolaou stain; ×600.)

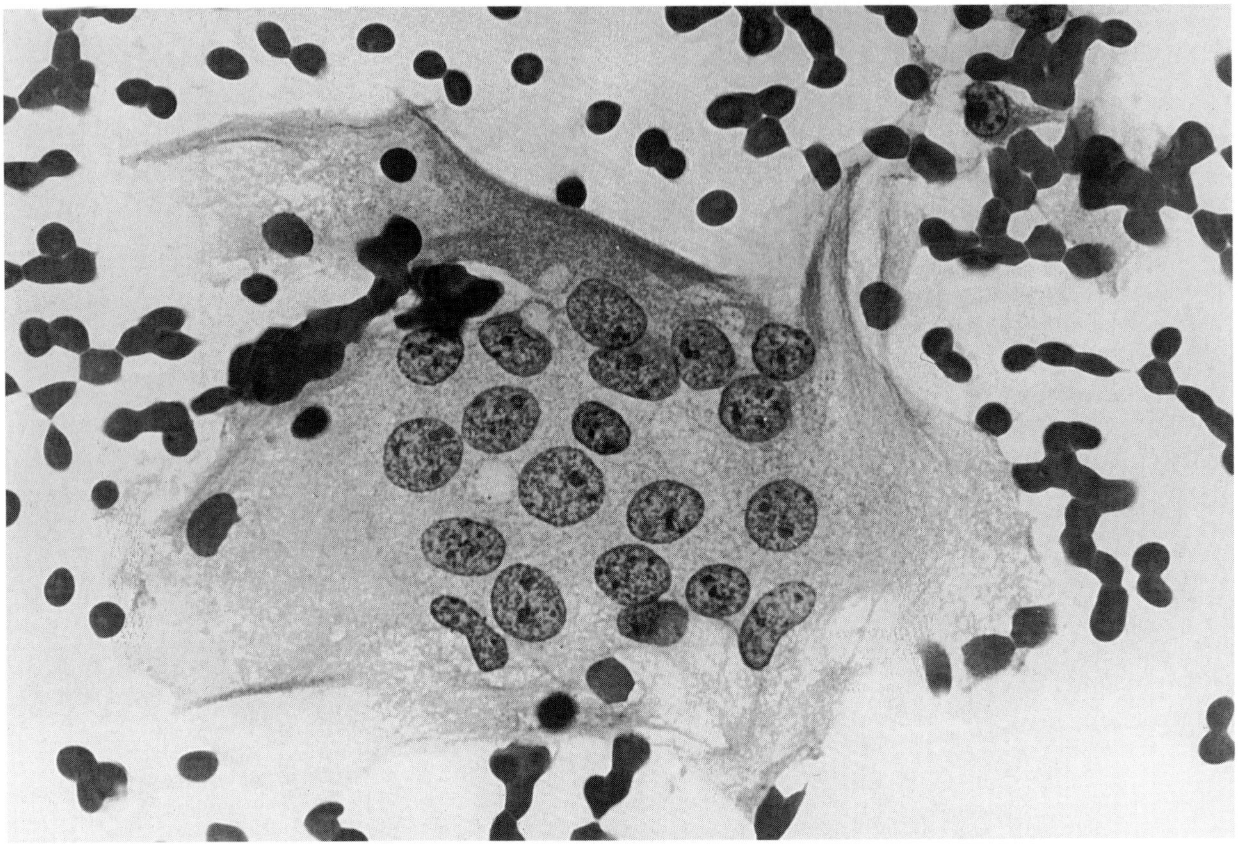

**Fig. 1-7.** Striking multinucleated giant cell. The abundant finely vacuolated cytoplasm betrays its histiocytic nature. The uniform nuclei show benign features, including finely stippled chromatin, smooth contours, and small nucleoli. (Papanicolaou stain; ×600.)

be seen in specimens collected during surgery, where they can be associated with foreign material,[20] or in patients with sarcoidosis[11] or ventricular shunts.[10]

Macrophages are important in processing blood that gains access to the CSF and are often accompanied by neutrophils following a hemorrhagic event. At different times following hemorrhage, one can see red blood cells (RBCs) pass sequentially through the following stages: numerous free RBCs; RBCs within macrophage cytoplasm; depigmentation of intracellular RBCs to leave large, round vacuoles; and green-brown hemosiderin or yellow hematoidin pigment within macrophage cytoplasm. The latter can persist for many months after hemorrhage. Similar cytologic changes have been described in other sites.[77] It is not possible to ascertain the cause of hemorrhage by observation of RBCs and their breakdown sequence in the CSF. Identical cytologic findings can be seen following bleeding associated with cerebrovascular accidents (Chapter 6) or trauma (Chapter 11).

The most important differential diagnostic considerations arising from increased numbers of inflammatory cells are the hematopoietic neoplasms. Although these will be discussed and illustrated in more detail subsequently, some general guidelines are in order at this point. One can be alarmed by the presence of lymphocytes in different stages of what is variously known as stimulation, transformation, or activation. In this setting, one sees various degrees of cell enlargement, nuclear enlargement, opening (and thus pallor) of the normally compact chromatin, and nucleolar prominence. Similar statements could be made about the cytologic features of all but the most well-differentiated malignant lymphomas. A useful analogy can be drawn with interpretation of lymphocytes recovered through fine-needle aspiration of enlarged lymph nodes. The cells of most common types of malignant lymphoma in both settings appear to be arrested at some stage of the "transformation" process. The cytomorphologic result is a monotonous population of identical cells. Reactive processes, in contrast, yield cells showing all possible degrees of "activation" and therefore give a polymorphous cytologic picture (Fig. 1-8). Thus, the diagnosis of malignant lymphoma is not based on any degree of "atypia" shown by a small number of cells. Rather the characteristics of the entire cell population

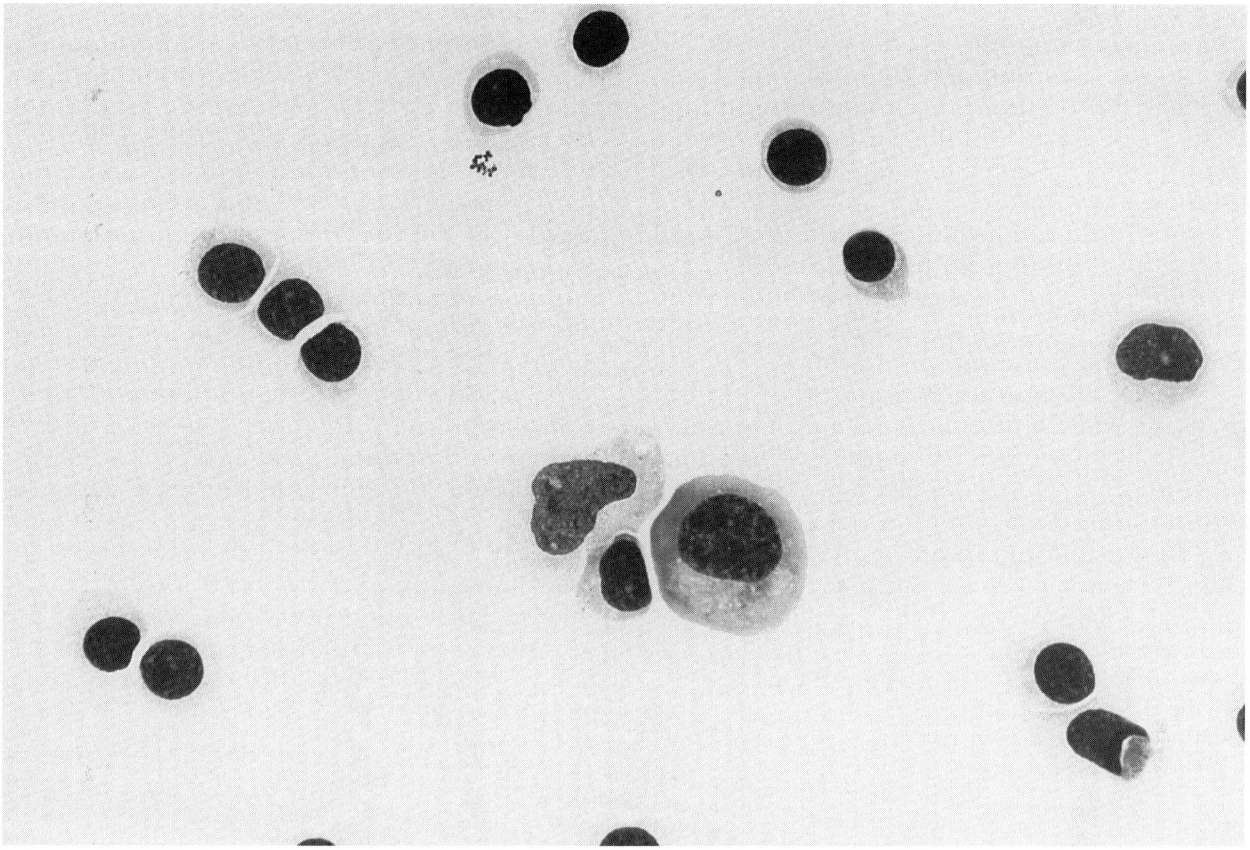

**Fig. 1-8.** The lymphocytes in this fluid are polymorphous. A large plasmacytoid form is noted in the center of the illustration, where it is accompanied by a monocyte. The other lymphocytes vary slightly in size, degree of chromatin clumping, and cytoplasmic volume. (Diff-Quik stain; ×600.)

must be evaluated. Mixed large and small cell malignant lymphomas obviously violate this diagnostic scheme; cell markers are often required for confident diagnosis of these neoplasms.

It is also important that vacuolated macrophages or clusters of monocytes not be mistaken for adenocarcinoma. In all these situations, the history and clinical findings often shed considerable light on the diagnosis. A thoughtful recital of the nuclear features of malignancy will usually suffice to prevent an inappropriate diagnosis of carcinoma.

## INFECTIONS

Despite the cytopathologist's observation of the above-captioned alterations in cell count and differential data, specific cytologic diagnosis of infections depends on direct visualization of the organism or its cytopathic effect. Alternatively, diagnosis must await culture or immunologic analysis. Broader issues in the diagnosis of CNS infections are addressed in Chapters 7 and 8.

As noted previously, a neutrophilic response suggests bacterial meningitis but actually can have several other etiologies. Microbiologic culture remains the cornerstone of such diagnoses, but one occasionally sees bacterial organisms in routine cytologic preparations. These small forms are more readily identified using Romanowsky-stained preparations than Papanicolaou-stained material. Bacteria stain darkly on both types of slide. It is important to note that this dark staining bears no relationship to the gram-positive or gram-negative nature of the organism. Thus, in routine cytologic studies of CSF from individuals suffering from bacterial meningitis, one can note the presence of neutrophils. If bacteria are identified, they can be described as few or numerous, and as bacilli or cocci. Further classification is not possible without intervention of the diagnostic microbiology laboratory. Intracellular organisms in a fresh specimen are evidence that the bacteria do not represent a contaminant. If cutaneous squamous cells are present, these will often be covered by bacteria that are of no diagnostic significance. Most pathologists will have encountered this finding in fine-needle aspiration specimens, where their interpretation is less problematic.

Fungal meningitis is most often due to *Cryptococcus*,

but rarely is caused by blastomycosis, histoplasmosis, aspergillosis, mucormycosis, coccidioidomycosis, or candidiasis. The latter disorders are more common in AIDS patients.[27,81] Much has been written regarding morphologic classification of fungi in cytologic preparations, particularly in pulmonary samples, where this is a common and very important problem. However, only *Cryptococcus* is routinely studied in CSF by cytologic means. The other organisms tend to result in parenchymal disease. Although this may be reflected in CSF inflammation, microbiologic diagnosis is usually not possible without tissue biopsy or culture.[27]

The cytomorphology of *Cryptococcus* is distinctive.[6,73] The yeast itself is round, with a diameter of 7 to 10 $\mu$m. It is surrounded by a mucoid capsule that can measure as much as 20 $\mu$m in diameter. Its buds have a teardrop shape and are connected to the parent organism by a thin or constricted neck. The capsule is pale and translucent in Papanicolaou-stained samples. In Romanowsky preparations, the capsule is so intensely basophilic as to obscure the underlying yeast and shows an ill-defined border. The yeast may be extracellular (Fig. 1-9) or intracellular. In the latter state, the capsule often stains faintly or not at all, and thus resembles a large cytoplasmic vacuole. The capsule stains positively with mucicarmine or with the Fontana-Masson and alcian blue methods. Silver stains will emphasize the yeast with their characteristic pattern of budding. The India ink method is rapid and simple but does not result in a permanent slide for the laboratory's archive. In this preparation, the yeasts appear as nonstaining, round clearings in the homogeneously black background. The cellular reaction associated with *Cryptococcus* is usually lymphocytic, with variable contributions from neutrophils, plasma cells, and macrophages. However, we have seen several cases in AIDS patients that showed abundant organisms without any cellular inflammatory response (Fig. 1-9).

The pale-staining yeast forms of *Cryptococcus* can be easily missed in routine cytologic preparations unless they are numerous and well preserved. They can also be mistaken for talc granules. Furthermore, the degenerated nuclei of senescent or damaged inflammatory

A 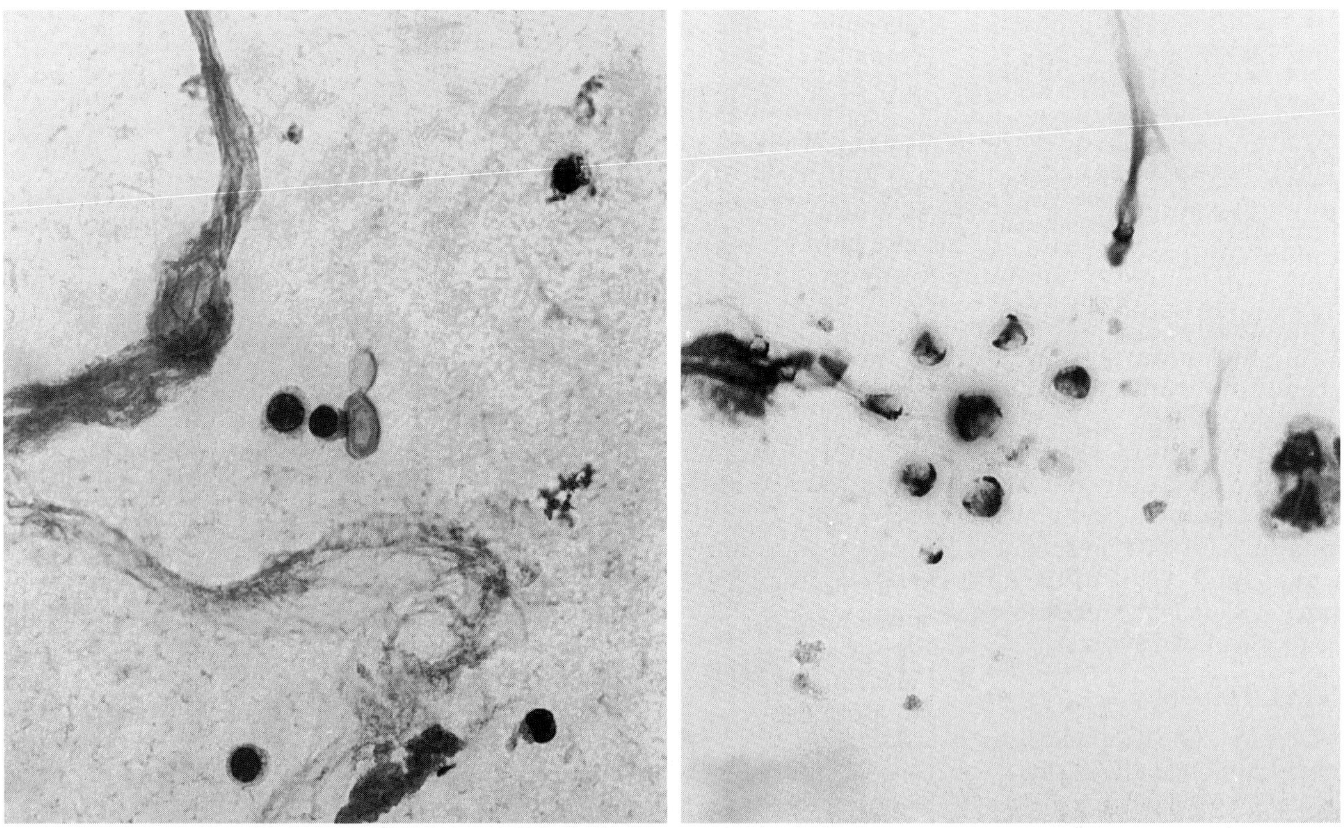 B

**Fig. 1-9. A,** Occasional small lymphocytes are noted in this fixed fluid. A single budding yeast of similar size is also present. The laminated appearance of the parent yeast suggests that a capsule is present. The daughter yeast is connected by a thin base. These features are typical of *Cryptococcus.* **B,** A cluster of cryptococcal yeast forms is depicted here in an air-dried preparation. The yeast is less distinctly rendered than in **A,** and the basophilic capsular material imparts a fuzzy appearance to the yeast. (**A,** Papanicolaou stain; ×600; **B,** Diff-Quik stain; ×600.)

cells can strongly resemble yeast of several forms.[77] The various staining methods listed previously are useful in difficult cases. The opposite problem occurs when macrophage vacuoles are mistaken for fungal organisms. This is especially likely to occur when large, round, uniform vacuoles that represent depigmented red blood cells are numerous following hemorrhage. These problems related to "pseudomicrobes" in cytology have received more detailed treatment elsewhere.[19,20]

A greater diagnostic dilemma is the capsule-deficient form of *Cryptococcus* seen most commonly in AIDS patients.[32,69] These small yeasts (mean diameter = 2.4 μm in Reference 32) are easily mistaken for those of *Candida* or *Histoplasma*. However they are usually positive in India ink or Fontana-Masson preparations. The degree of encapsulation is not related to cryptococcal antigen titer. These diagnostic clues, as well as the fact that other yeasts are uncommonly encountered in CSF cytology, should point toward the correct diagnosis.

Mycobacterial meningitis is most often marked by a lymphocytic reaction. Special stains are usually negative, so that diagnosis must await culture results. Early cases may show neutrophils, and tuberculosis is one cause of "persistent neutrophilic meningitis."[62]

Viral infections with a wide variety of agents can lead to meningoencephalitis, usually associated with a lymphocytic reaction. Diagnostic inclusions, however, are rarely encountered in CSF material studied by cytologic techniques.[37,45] Diagnosis is based on clinical, serologic, culture, and biopsy findings. Immunocytochemical analysis has occasionally been reported to be helpful when applied to cells in CSF.[53] The morphology of cytomegalovirus (CMV) inclusion-bearing cells is as described in detail for other sites.[77] A number of additional infections of the CNS may lead to reactive cell patterns but rarely give up diagnostic organisms or inclusions detectable by cytologic evaluation of CSF. Among these are cysticercosis, Lyme disease, infectious mononucleosis, *Cryptosporidium*, and *Pneumocystis carinii*.[26,66,81]

Toxoplasmosis is a common CNS infection in AIDS patients. Free-lying tachyzoites and encysted bradyzoites can be detected in tissue biopsies or in samples aspirated from the mass lesions. Inflammatory cells may harbor several cytoplasmic organisms to yield a pseudocyst. The organism is rarely seen in CSF cytology,[23] where it resembles the same organisms more commonly seen in pulmonary cytology material.[90] AIDS patients with CNS toxoplasmosis often have mass lesions, and in many instances this means that they are not candidates for lumbar puncture.

Mollaret meningitis (recurrent aseptic meningitis) is an uncommon condition that features fever, headache, nausea, vomiting, and signs of meningeal inflammation. As reviewed by Evans,[36] the illness progresses rapidly toward more severe neurologic dysfunction that may include coma and seizures. These difficulties resolve over a few days, and the patient is symptom-free until the next episode. Numerous attacks may occur over a period of years. The CSF rapidly acquires very high cell counts and passes from neutrophils to lymphocytes. The latter are accompanied by Mollaret cells, which are large monocytes that appear very active because of their abundant, vacuolated cytoplasm. Their existence during attacks of recurrent aseptic meningitis is ephemeral at best. The fragile nature of such cells also makes them difficult to identify. Cells similar to Mollaret cells can be seen in other types of meningitis (Fig. 1-10), but this fact does not detract from the unique clinical nature of this illness. When such cells are encountered, the term "Mollaret-like" cells seems appropriate. It should be noted that they are considered incidental; the designation "Mollaret meningitis" should remain a clinical diagnosis.

Both herpes simplex I and Epstein-Barr viruses have been associated with this disorder. The former agent was recovered by culture in one case,[80] and seems the most likely of the possible infectious etiologies.

## ADDITIONAL NON-NEOPLASTIC CONDITIONS

An extensive catalog of AIDS-associated CNS lesions has developed[68]; these lesions are more fully discussed in Chapter 9. Unfortunately CSF examination in most AIDS patients usually shows only nonspecific cellular alterations[45,52] and is insufficient for specific diagnosis of most entities. AIDS encephalopathy may feature seizures, headache, hallucinations, and altered mental status. Its only representation in CSF cytology may be an increase in mononucleated or multinucleated macrophages.[45] These may reflect the HIV-containing macrophages that have been described in the brains of AIDS patients.

Cytopathologists are familiar with the cytopathic effects of human polyoma virus infection as it affects genitourinary cells seen in urine samples from immunosuppressed patients. In that setting, the large nuclear inclusions must be distinguished from the abnormal nuclei of transitional cell carcinoma. The CNS can also harbor polyoma virus, where it causes progressive multifocal leukoencephalopathy (PML). This condition is usually not represented by CSF cytologic alterations.

Other conditions that feature demyelinization, including multiple sclerosis (MS), may eventuate in CSF T-cell lymphocytosis, especially during disease exacerbations (Chapter 16). The diagnostic significance of lymphocyte subclassification in this setting is controversial, but at least some workers find little to distinguish the CSF cellular content in MS from that seen in some infections, or in Guillain-Barré syndrome.[64] A lymphocytic reaction can also be seen in sarcoidosis

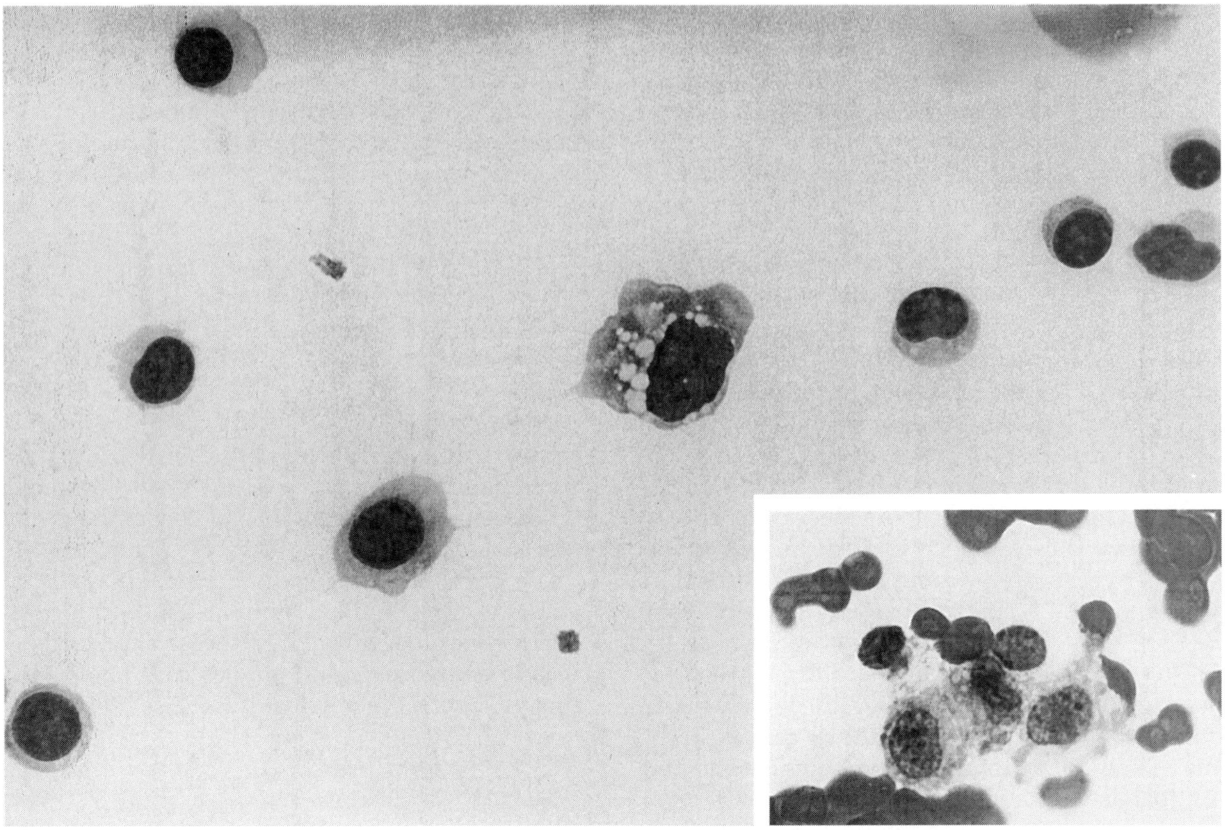

**Fig. 1-10.** Mollaret-type monocytes show abundant highly vacuolated cytoplasm. (Diff-Quik stain; ×600; **Inset,** Papanicolaou stain; ×600.)

and may be accompanied by multinucleated giant cells, as noted previously.[11] Other conditions that may lead to nonspecific increases in mononuclear cells in the CSF include pneumoencephalography and seizures of various types.[25]

## NEOPLASTIC CYTOLOGY

### GENERAL CONSIDERATIONS

Meningeal involvement by malignancy can be reflected in tumor cell shedding into the CSF; the extent to which purely intraparenchymal lesions are encountered in such material is unclear and has been the subject of controversy. Thus, hematologic malignancies,* metastases from melanoma or carcinoma,† germ cell malignancies,[26,89] and primary CNS neoplasms‡ can all be represented in CSF cytology. Some tumors are seen in these specimens only rarely, as reviewed by Bigner and Johnston[48] and may gain access to the SAS by direct extension from adjacent sites in the head and neck, retroperitoneum, or pelvis. The majority of positive diagnoses reflect either metastases from common epithelial malignancies of the breast, lung, and melanocytes, or the CNS manifestations of systemic hematopoietic neoplasms. A more complete catalog of these neoplasms is summarized in Table 1-2.

To some extent an institution's referral pattern will influence the frequency with which each type of malignancy is encountered. Tertiary care centers will study and follow most cases of malignant lymphoma and leukemia. Children's centers will find more cases of acute lymphoblastic leukemia (ALL), while those caring mostly for adult patients will study acute myelogenous leukemia (AML). Chronic leukemias and primary brain tumors are not commonly seen in CSF material but may be evaluated by institutions to which large numbers of patients with these conditions are referred. Primary CNS neoplasms are noted much less often in fluids than are tumors that involve these sites secondarily.

Most patients in whom malignancy is apparent in the CSF will have a previous history of malignancy or a synchronous manifestation of malignancy in some other site. In the former instance, recognition of malig-

* Refs. 3, 7, 9, 12, 13, 15, 17, 33, 36, 39, 40, 42–44, 47, 49, 51, 54–56, 58, 59, 63, 65, 67, 70, 76, 82, 85, 86, 93, 94.

† Refs. 1, 3, 8, 9, 14, 24, 28, 33, 35, 59, 74, 83, 85, 86, 88, 89.

‡ Refs. 3, 8, 9, 41, 60, 61, 85, 89.

**Table 1-2.** Malignant neoplasms in cerebrospinal fluid cytology

| Type of neoplasm | References |
|---|---|
| Hematopoietic | |
| Acute Lymphoblastic Leukemia | 3, 7, 9, 12, 13, 15, 17, 42–44, 47, 49, 54, 58, 63, 65, 67, 70, 93 |
| Acute Myelogenous Leukemia | 3, 9, 12, 15, 44, 56, 70, 85 |
| Chronic Leukemias | 3, 9, 15, 47 |
| Non-Hodgkin's Lymphoma | 3, 7, 9, 15, 47, 59, 93 |
| Hodgkin's Disease | 7, 9, 33, 59 |
| Not Otherwise Specified | 33, 51, 76, 85, 86 |
| Multiple Myeloma | 7, 9, 33, 47 |
| Metastatic or Direct Extension | |
| Carcinoma | 3, 8, 9, 14, 24, 28, 33, 35, 59, 85, 86, 88, 89 |
| Malignant Melanoma | 1, 3, 8, 9, 28, 33, 59, 74, 85, 86, 88 |
| Sarcoma | 8, 33, 85 |
| Unknown Primary Site | 8, 9, 59 |
| Rare Tumors | 8 |
| Germ Cell Tumors | 26, 89 |
| Primary CNS Lymphoma | 36, 39, 51 |
| Other Primary CNS Neoplasms | 3, 8, 9, 33, 41, 57, 60, 61, 85, 89 |

nant cells and confirmation that they are compatible with spread of the previously diagnosed process will often be relatively straightforward. Those in whom these conditions do not present special diagnostic problems will be discussed subsequently. Historical considerations are very important and can render certain interpretational difficulties trivial. For example, medulloblastoma and metastatic small cell pulmonary carcinoma look very much alike but occur in different clinical settings. Reactive lymphocytoses can be difficult to distinguish from malignant lymphoma or even acute leukemia; ependymal cells may mimic metastatic carcinoma, and amelanotic malignant melanoma can be mistaken for adenocarcinoma.

Some of these differential diagnostic dilemmas can be resolved with a variety of special studies, including flow cytometry, immunocytochemistry (ICC), and electron microscopy. The technical aspects of these procedures are beyond the scope of this chapter. Application of these methods to fluid cytology has recently been reviewed in detail,[5] and key problem-solving strategies will be discussed where appropriate. Immunocytochemistry and electron microscopy of brain tumors are discussed in Chapters 4 and 3, respectively.

The clinical manifestations of leptomeningeal malignancy are varied and may include headache, nausea and vomiting, vertigo, vision or hearing changes, radicular signs, mental status changes, weakness, and gait disturbances.[35,59,88] These may exist in diverse combinations that fail to localize disease to a particular point in the CNS.[59] It is this combination of neurologic dysfunctions that simultaneously implicates several levels of the neuraxis that is most typical of neoplastic meningitis.[52] For many patients with a history of malignancy, such signs and symptoms lead to lumbar puncture and CSF examination. The clinical differential diagnosis includes infections, metabolic encephalopathy, drug toxicity, extrinsic compression of the spinal cord, and other conditions not related to the malignancy or its treatment. As reviewed subsequently, cytologic examination of CSF for evidence of meningeal malignancy has a finite false-negative rate.[28,33,59,88] Therefore, a negative fluid study in a patient with compelling clinical findings may not be reassuring; other investigative maneuvers, including repeat lumbar punctures, may be needed.[33]

The pathology of neoplastic meningitis may reveal microscopic infiltrates in the absence of grossly detectable masses or thickenings. Furthermore, focal involvement may be confined to the spinal meninges.[28,59] Microscopic disease may lead to clinical symptoms.[59] Given these patterns of disease, it is not surprising that histologic confirmation of cytologically diagnosed infiltration may not be forthcoming, even at autopsy.[28] Furthermore, effective treatment may lead to negative findings at repeat lumbar puncture or at autopsy.[33]

Meningeal infiltration by malignant cells can be isolated or may be associated with parenchymal involvement of the CNS. The routes by which neoplastic cells reach the leptomeninges will be discussed subsequently, when systemic leukemia and metastases from solid tumors are considered. Multifocal microscopic disease is more likely to give positive CSF cytology than is less extensive involvement.[33] Describing autopsy findings in 363 cancer patients (carcinoma, melanoma, hematologic malignancies, and primary brain tumors were all included), Glass and associates noted 18 in whom leptomeningeal tumor was not accompanied by either parenchymal or dural disease.[33] Seventeen of 50 with dural involvement also showed leptomeningeal tumor. Of 142 with parenchymal tumor, 44 had leptomeningeal infiltrates. In another study, only 18 of 306 autopsied carcinoma patients with CNS metastases showed spread limited to the leptomeninges without parenchymal involvement.[35] These were among a total of 2227 carcinoma autopsies. Glass and associates suggest that some reports that purely parenchymal disease can be reflected in positive CSF cytology are based on inadequate autopsy examination of meninges (including those of the spinal cord).[33]

The diagnostic yield of CSF cytology compared to all patients with meningeal disease is difficult to fix accurately. Reasons for this include the following:

(1) as noted above, not all cases will be confirmed, even at autopsy[28]; (2) treatment may eradicate recognizable tumor[33]; (3) many cytologic diagnoses are not followed by any sort of antemortem tissue diagnosis; and (4) multiple examinations may be needed to detect tumor infiltration.[28,59,88] Reported rates for positive CSF cytology in patients with systemic malignancy are up to 30%. These rates depend heavily on patient selection criteria, the mix of tumor types in a given study, the cytopreparatory methods involved, and the autopsy rate at the reporting institution (reviewed in Reference 8).

False-positive and false-suspicious diagnoses that may adversely affect therapeutic decisions are discussed when metastatic solid tumors and systemic hematologic neoplasms are considered in detail.* False-negative diagnoses usually occur in low-grade tumors that are difficult to distinguish from normally-encountered cellular elements (Table 1-1; References 2, 8, 18, 21, 30, 48, 50), when a low cell count with abnormal cells is noted in patients with leukemia or lymphoma[3,33] or when only therapy-damaged tumor cells remain.[15,55,83] Several investigators have shown that the positive rate increases with multiple CSF examinations.[28,59,88] In one investigation, the positive rate increased from 45% to 80% as multiple studies were conducted. When lumbar punctures are paired with ventricular taps, the latter test is more likely to be positive; negative ventricular fluid in the face of a positive lumbar puncture occurs less often.[88]

## POSITIVE CSF CYTOLOGY WITHOUT A HISTORY OF MALIGNANCY

CSFs that show malignant cells in the absence of any history of malignancy represent a special dilemma.[9,15,28] Bigner and Johnston observed 25 (11.4%) such cases among 220 patients with positive CSF cytology.[9] Some of their findings are summarized in Table 1-3. In these authors' experience, most occult carcinomas with leptomeningeal manifestations were in the lung or the stomach. Breast carcinoma commonly involves this site but usually is clinically apparent prior to meningeal spread. Hematopoietic malignancies uncommonly present in this fashion (2% of 108 cases). Moreover, when atypical lymphoid cells have been interpreted as de novo malignancy, some false-positive diagnoses have been described.[15] Some of the reactive conditions discussed previously are much more common than this unusual presentation of lymphoma or leukemia. Furthermore, reactive lymphoid cells can resemble their neoplastic counterparts very closely.[3,33] Thus, in most instances it is advisable to offer such interpretations with circumspection and to await supporting evidence. Such evidence may be clinical or may

* Refs. 3, 7, 15, 33, 49, 70.

**Table 1-3.** Origin of malignancies initially identified as positive CSF cytology in patients without a previous history of malignancy

| Type of malignancy | Number (%) first diagnosed by positive CSF cytology |
|---|---|
| Unknown Primary Site* | 5 (70) |
| Gastric Adenocarcinoma | 2 (67) |
| Primary CNS Neoplasm† | 7 (5) |
| Pulmonary Carcinoma‡ | 8 (18) |
| Malignant Melanoma§ | 1 (8) |
| Malignant Lymphoma | 2 (2) |
| Breast Carcinoma | 0 (0) |

* Four cases of adenocarcinoma and one of "undifferentiated malignant neoplasm."

† Medulloblastoma, glioblastoma multiforme, as well as one case each designated as microgliomatosis, primary cerebral histiocytosis, and primary meningeal gliomatosis.

‡ Three cases each of adenocarcinoma and undifferentiated large cell carcinoma, as well as two cases of small cell anaplastic carcinoma.

§ Probably of cutaneous origin.

Data from Bigner SH, and Johnston WW: The diagnostic challenge of tumors manifested initially by the shedding of cells into cerebrospinal fluid, Acta Cytol 28:29-36, 1984.

be provided when marker studies are applied to the cells in question.

The diagnosis and classification of malignancy that presents initially in the CSF should proceed in a stepwise fashion. After the above-cited possibilities for a false-positive diagnosis have been explored, one begins by application of basic cytopathologic principles. It is usually possible to determine that the cells in question are hematopoietic or nonhematopoietic. Concerted study of both Papanicolaou-stained and Romanowsky-stained material may help in this distinction. Then, the carcinomas can be divided into adenocarcinoma, squamous cell carcinoma, small cell carcinoma, or undifferentiated (non-small cell) carcinoma. If these efforts are unsuccessful, or if additional certainty or nosologic precision is required, well established electron microscopic protocols or ICC panels can be applied.[5] These methods may be of limited utility unless an adequate volume of a richly cellular fluid is at hand. The diagnostic problem that is most likely to be resolved by this type of analysis is the distinction between amelanotic malignant melanoma and adenocarcinoma.

Once this level of morphologic explication has been achieved, only clinical and radiographic investigation can further illuminate the patient's problem. Most small cell carcinomas will have originated in the lung. Most squamous cell carcinomas involve the CSF by direct extension from a primary lesion in the head and neck or in the pelvis (cervical carcinoma). Occult adenocarcinomas may be found in the lung or the stomach.

Other types of adenocarcinoma may metastasize to the brain, but are rarely encountered in CSF samples. These include tumors of the colon and the kidney. Although ICC can be used to distinguish between malignant melanoma and adenocarcinoma, either of these entities may disseminate widely in the absence of an identifiable primary tumor.

## METASTATIC NEOPLASMS

Diagnosis of meningeal carcinomatosis is an important clinical issue. As with involvement of other body fluids by disseminated malignancy, it is attended by a grave outlook in most patients. The usual course is marked by continued and progressive neurologic deficits of the type previously discussed. Death typically follows within weeks or months.[14,88] CSF involvement may be the herald of recurrent disease after a long disease-free interval, and many patients with this finding will be shown to harbor active disease in non-CNS sites.[88] The period of latency between diagnosis of the primary tumor and positive CSF cytology ranged from 9 or 11 months (bladder carcinoma and lung carcinoma, respectively) to 52 months for breast carcinoma patients.[28] This tumor behavior may explain why positive CSF samples in the absence of a carcinoma history are much more common in pulmonary cancer patients than in those suffering from breast carcinoma.

As summarized in Table 1-2, a wide variety of solid neoplasms can lead to positive CSF cytology. The most common are adenocarcinomas of the breast and the lung, followed by malignant melanoma. Small cell pulmonary carcinomas are also encountered frequently. The many uncommon tumors occasionally seen in this site have been reviewed.[8] Squamous cell carcinomas are much less common in CSF than are adenocarcinomas.

Several investigators have considered the routes by which carcinoma cells would be able to reach the CSF.[8,33,35] An older theory holding that most arrive via the choroid plexus vasculature has been replaced by the concept that choroidal involvement is secondary to leptomeningeal carcinomatosis and takes place through the sheaths of choroid vessels.[35] Cells can arrive at the meninges by direct extension from sites adjacent to the CNS or from superficial parenchymal nodules. Intervertebral or cranial foramina may provide access points. In the former, spread from paravertebral lymph node metastases may initiate this type of CNS involvement. Available lymphatic paths include vessels of the perineurium, the endoneurium, and the perivascular sheaths (reviewed in Reference 8). Lymphatic dissemination of this sort can explain metastases confined to the meninges, without parenchymal involvement. Gonzalez-Vitale and Garcia-Bunuel reviewed their experience with tumors that showed "pure" leptomeningeal involvement as their only manifestation of spread beyond regional lymph nodes.[35] As discussed previously, the possibility that parenchymal metastases unassociated with leptomeningeal spread can lead to positive CSF cytology has been considered.[33,35] Those wishing to support this hypothesis must bear the burden of demonstrating that adequate examination of the meninges has been performed.

The cytology of adenocarcinomas metastatic to body fluids is well known to those who examine cytologic material with any frequency. In other body cavities, the great difficulty that often attends these cases is due to the morphologic similarity between carcinoma cells and reactive mesothelial cells. Our comments on specimen preparation indicated that as long as CSF material is relieved of any contaminants (Table 1-1), carcinoma cells are so clearly out of context as to be straightforward in most instances. This observation also applies to sparsely cellular samples and to well-differentiated tumor cells.

In other body cavity fluids, one can rely in part on the three-dimensional and intercellular features of carcinoma cell group morphology as useful guides to recognition of malignancy. These are then supplemented by study of nuclear details and comparisons with nearby mesothelial cells. In the CSF many adenocarcinomas shed primarily single cells, and cohesive groups may be difficult to find.[8] In this setting one must pursue four lines of evidence in reaching a realization that these cells represent carcinoma: (1) the cells are out of context in the usually almost acellular setting of CSF; (2) in all but the most well-differentiated examples, adenocarcinomas will show at least some nuclear features of malignancy; (3) most patients will have a history of malignancy that either will or will not be compatible with the diagnosis one is contemplating; (4) previous surgical or cytologic material can be compared with the CSF being evaluated. The need for high-quality cytomorphology that attains the standards of cell preservation and cytopreparation discussed previously is obvious.

Figure 1-11 shows the single-cell pattern of breast adenocarcinoma in a CSF specimen. This contrasts sharply with the cell groups and balls (so-called proliferation spheres) one commonly sees when breast carcinoma involves the pleural space. These cells are distinctly out of context in the CSF. Their large size is apparent when we consider the background red blood cells. That this sample represents spread of breast carcinoma to the CSF is straightforward. As noted previously, most of these cases follow recognition of breast carcinoma in its primary site. A similar tumor without a prior history of malignancy should lead at once to investigation of the lung and other potential primary sites.

This case also provides an opportunity to study a well-differentiated adenocarcinoma in which the cyto-

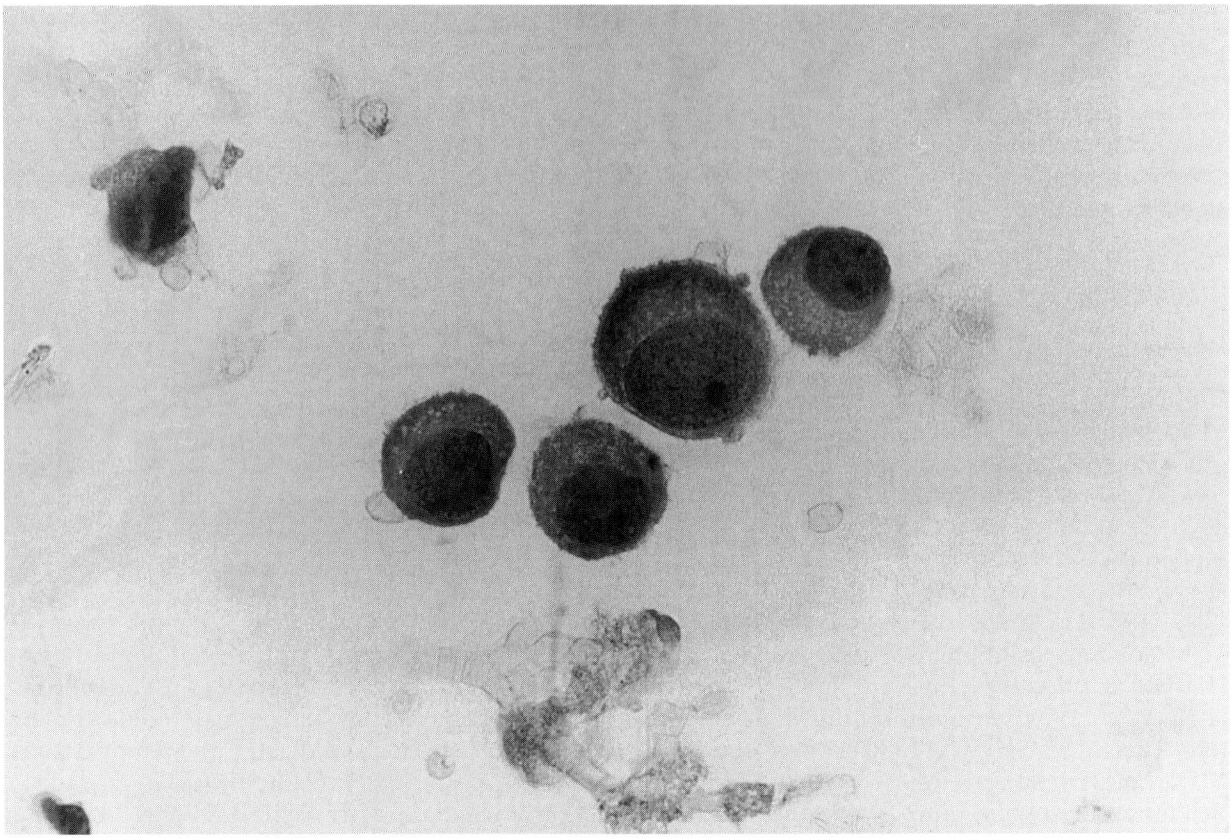

**Fig. 1-11.** These cells illustrate a common pattern of breast carcinoma in the CSF. They lie singly and are distinctly out of context. Despite some vacuolization, the dense cytoplasm and sharp cell borders indicate that they are not histiocytes. These features are very useful, because the nuclei lack striking evidence of malignancy. (Papanicolaou stain; ×600.)

logic features of malignancy are subtle. Lack of cohesion has already been mentioned. Indeed, if these same cells were set against a background of reactive mesothelial cells in a pleural specimen, the diagnosis would be exceedingly difficult without ICC support. These cells show striking nuclear pallor and feature only small nucleoli. Except for their large size and relatively high nucleocytoplasmic size (area) ratio, one might interpret them as macrophages. Their dense cytoplasm and sharp cell borders also militate against such an interpretation. (Compare these cells with those depicted in Figs. 1-7 and 1-10.) Nuclear pallor of this degree can cause one to hesitate to make the diagnosis of malignancy; the other criteria in this case are thus very important. Pulmonary adenocarcinomas may also feature very pale nuclei without the malignant features of prominent chromatin clumping and clearing.

Cytoplasmic vacuolization is also a feature of some adenocarcinomas. Figure 1-12 shows another example of the single-cell pattern of adenocarcinoma in a CSF and features one cell with a large signet-ring vacuole. Necrotic tumor cells are also present and offer compelling supportive evidence of malignancy. (Necrosis alone is never diagnostic of malignancy.) False signet rings can occur in benign CSF samples.[8] As cells degenerate, their membranes' metabolic integrity is quickly lost, and they imbibe fluid from their medium. The resulting cytoplasmic lakes can mimic signet-ring cells very closely. Thus, the mere presence of large vacuoles without other evidence of malignancy is nondiagnostic. Furthermore, other types of malignant cells can show vacuoles. We have observed this numerous times in the cytology of malignant melanoma.

Squamous cell carcinomas are seen in CSF samples much less often than are adenocarcinomas. Figure 1-13 shows an example. Poorly differentiated tumors may be difficult to recognize as squamous, and one must search for the occasional more mature cell, in which its dense cytoplasm and sharp cell borders betray its nature. Keratinized cytoplasm may be dense and concentrically laminated and lack the organophilia that is definitive (Papanicolaou stain). Most squamous cell carcinomas arrive at the CSF by direct extension; the example in Fig. 1-13 is from a head and neck tumor. These locally aggressive growths often are accompa-

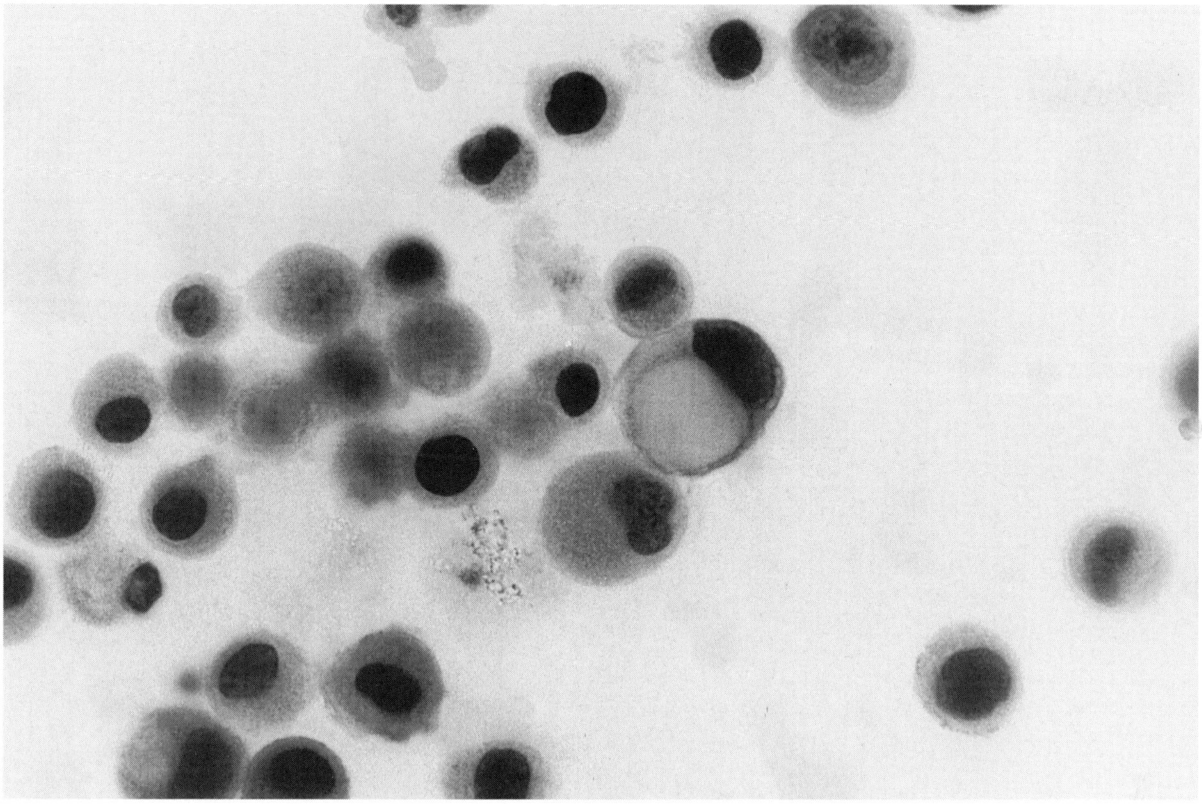

**Fig. 1-12.** Many cells of this metastatic adenocarcinoma are necrotic and appear ghostlike. One cell shows a prominent signet-ring configuration; the vacuole displaces a large nucleus with cytologic features of malignancy. (Papanicolaou stain; ×600.)

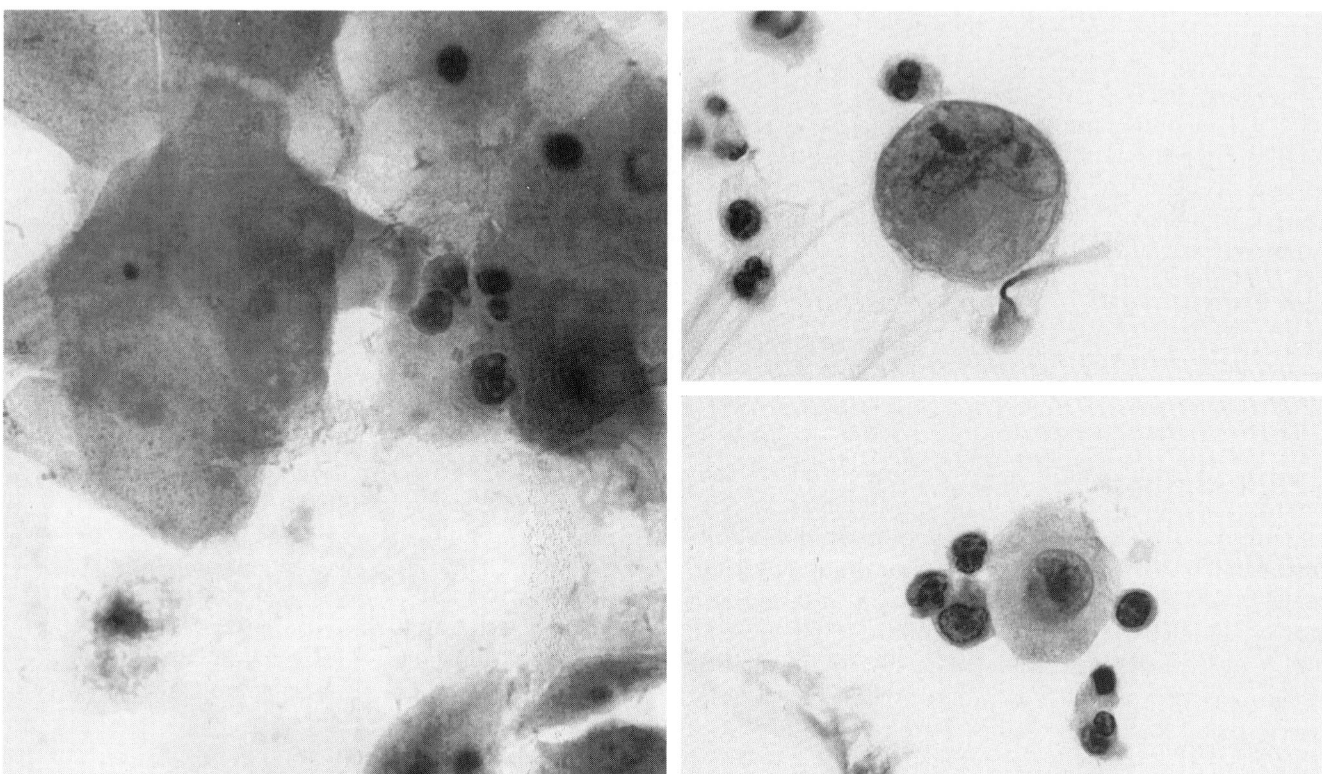

A

B

C

**Fig. 1-13.** **A,** This squamous cell carcinoma features both large, mature, anucleate squames. **B** and **C,** Single more clearly malignant-appearing cells. (Papanicolaou stain; ×600.)

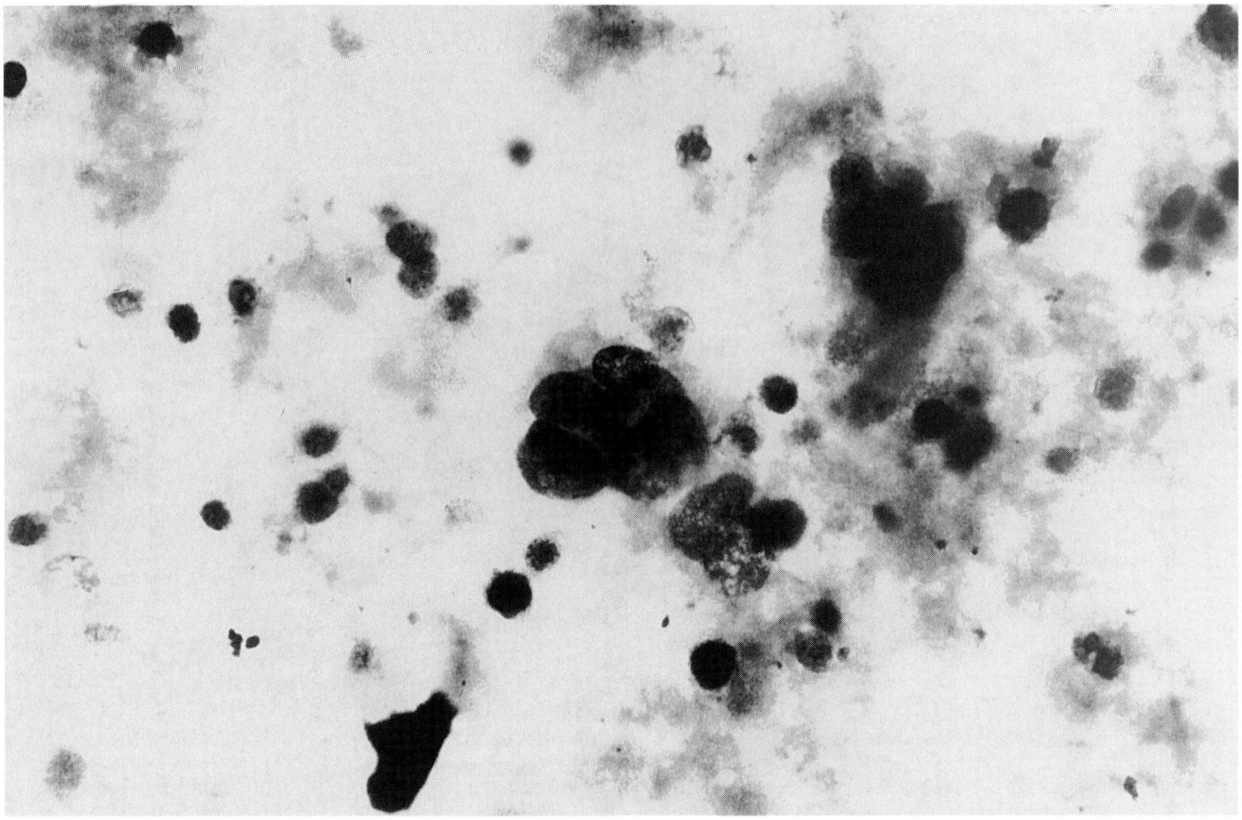

**Fig. 1-14.** The CSF involved by this pulmonary small-cell anaplastic carcinoma ("oat cell carcinoma") shows extensive necrosis with a few groups of intact tumor cells. The group in the center of this illustration features small cohesive cells with intense nuclear hyperchromasia and prominent nuclear molding. (Papanicolaou stain; ×600.)

nied by an inflammatory reaction that may be augmented by a foreign body reaction to keratin.

Small cell anaplastic carcinoma (SCAC) (oat cell carcinoma) can be seen in CSF material and usually is of pulmonary origin (Fig. 1-14). In a manner analogous to acute lymphoblastic leukemia, recurrent SCAC can present in the CSF following chemotherapy.[49] The older descriptions of this tumor's cytology were based on sputum. The dense nuclear hyperchromasia, the near total lack of chromatin substructure within the nucleus, the absence of apparent nucleoli, the extreme cytoplasmic contraction, and the advanced nuclear molding seen in such specimens are due in part to degeneration of exfoliated cells. In other preparations (bronchial brushings, fine-needle aspirations, and CSF) the cells are better preserved. They appear larger and feature distinctly particulate chromatin, small nucleoli, and scanty but visible cytoplasm. Furthermore, nuclear molding is more subtle than in sputum. Those to whom this appearance is new will hesitate to recognize it in the CSF.

SCAC may shed groups of various sizes, including linear arrangements of cells in single file. When single cells are numerous, one may be tempted to diagnose leukemia or malignant lymphoma. Searching for a few cohesive groups will aid in diagnosis. In our experience, necrosis and single necrotic tumor cells are present in all but the most sparsely cellular SCAC-containing samples. These findings are not usually expected in fluids showing one of the hematologic malignancies.

Malignant melanoma commonly spreads to the leptomeninges. The cells in Fig. 1-15 are typical of this entity. CSFs showing cells of this neoplasm are usually straightforward. Problems can occur when the primary tumor has not been previously diagnosed, especially if the cells are amelanotic. The cytopathology of malignant melanoma is as variable as its capricious clinical behavior. The typical case shows mostly single cells, moderate amounts of cytoplasm, one or two eccentric nuclei, a single prominent nucleolus per nucleus, and frequent intranuclear cytoplasmic inclusions.[8] When pigment is present, it completes the expected picture. Variable combinations of this cell type with spindle cells, large bizarre tumor cells, vacuolated tumor cells, and inflammatory cells impart ample cytologic diversity to any group of cases. Rare cases in which the melanoma cells closely resemble large lymphocytes are

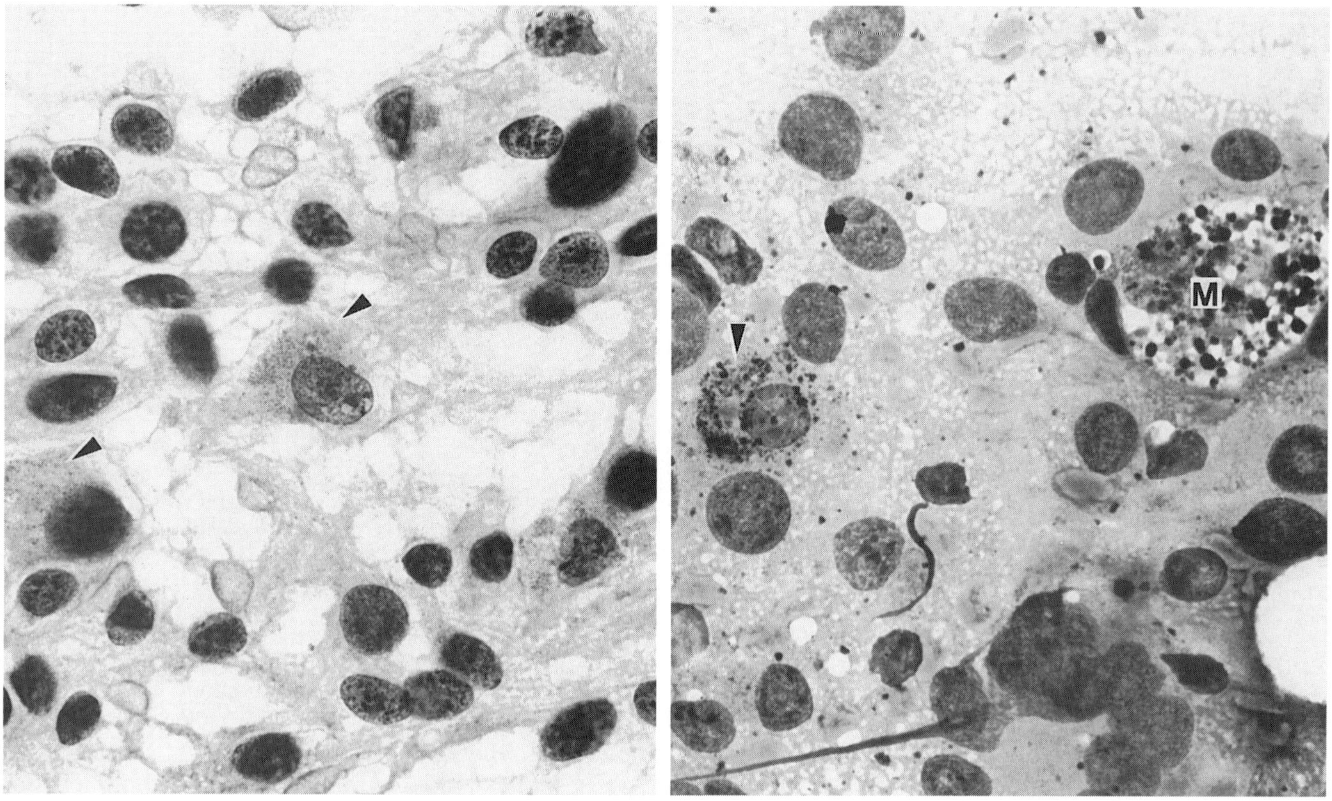


**Fig. 1-15.** Numerous cells of malignant melanoma are shown here. Pigment is identified in both fixed **(A)** and air-dried **(B)** material (*arrowheads*). The most obvious melanin accumulations are not in tumor cells, however, but within the cytoplasm of histiocytic melanophages (*M*). (**A,** Papanicolaou stain; ×600; **B,** Diff-Quik stain; ×600.)

vexing in fine-needle aspiration but have not been described in the CSF. Amelanotic malignant melanoma is difficult to distinguish from adenocarcinoma without ICC. However, rare cases of malignant lymphoma and adenocarcinoma may be positive with antimelanoma monoclonal antibody HMB-45.[31,38] While this reagent remains the most sensitive and specific identifier of this tumor, its use outside a panel of several antibodies can be misleading.

Primary malignant melanoma of the meninges should be considered only after a careful search reveals no cutaneous or mucosal primary lesion. Many cases arise in the setting of a neurocutaneous melanosis.[86] Even so, this neoplasm is less common than metastatic melanoma from an obstinately occult primary. Meningeal melanoma can spread diffusely over the meninges in a two-dimensional manner without tumefaction.[74] Once established, it can give rise to extracranial metastases that may further obfuscate the clinical picture.

In most instances, melanin and hemosiderin pigment are readily differentiated by application of criteria that are well known to most pathologists. Hemosiderin produces large greenish-brown granules that appear refractile when the microscope's condenser is lowered. In occasional cases an iron stain may be helpful. However, a greater problem is identifying melanin that may originate in conditions other than malignant melanoma. Other CNS tumors can occasionally produce melanin (reviewed in Reference 71). Leptomeningeal melanosis is a common condition frequently encountered in autopsy material. Benign melanin-containing meningeal cells may occur singly or in small aggregates but are uncommon in CSF samples. Regardless of its origin, melanin in the fluid will be ingested by macrophages that are then termed melanophages. Their pigment burden may be so great as to obscure the nucleus from view. Most pathologists are familiar with this problem in other settings and are accustomed to using a melanin–bleach preparation to better visualize the nuclei in highly pigmented cutaneous melanocytic lesions. Melanophages sometimes can be distinguished from tumor cells by electron microscopy. The former show only pigmented phagolysosomes, whereas the latter feature true melanosomes, albeit occasionally in small numbers.

The term "meningeal sarcoma" has previously been employed somewhat indiscriminately.[8,33] In some instances, it has even been applied to cases that we would currently consider examples of meningeal carcinomatosis.[8] Most cases that have been called meningeal sarcomas seem to have been medulloblastomas. Glass and co-workers specifically describe two cases of osteosarcoma with brain metastases and negative CSF cytology.[33] In general, most would now agree that the term meningeal sarcoma is to be avoided.

The strategy outlined above for classification of malignant cells detected by CSF cytology is applicable to the majority of cases; historical considerations are paramount. Biochemical markers of malignancy will be discussed in the next section, but most are applicable to the leukemias rather than metastases from solid tumors. The common finding of increased CSF protein and decreased glucose[88] is nonspecific, being seen not only in carcinomatous meningitis but also in tuberculosis, fungal infections, and sarcoidosis.[41] Furthermore, while approximately 80% of cases have increased protein, hypoglycorrhachia is limited to 20% or fewer.[39]

ICC can be useful in selected cases and has been applied to CSF samples in the study of carcinomas, malignant lymphoma, malignant melanoma, acute leukemias, primary CNS neoplasms, small cell carcinoma, and embryonal rhabdomyosarcoma.[14,85] As is always the case with such methods, their ultimate utility is directly proportional to the quality of the initial morphologic interpretation of routinely-stained slides. Selection and interpretation of these tests must be informed by complete understanding and cogent expression of the diagnostic dilemma one wishes to address.

Boogerd and colleagues concluded that ICC provided "minor help" in a few instances.[14] Most of these were from previously treated tumors or in fluids with low cellularity. These authors also pointed out the efficacy of staining for the cytokeratins when numerous reactive lymphoid cells obscure a small number of carcinoma cells. In practical terms, many potential applications of ICC or electron microscopy to CSF are severely limited by the fact that small specimen volumes are the rule and that many fluids are sparsely cellular. Furthermore, the number of specimens that benefit from special studies of this type is limited if one uses all clinical information and cytologic findings to best advantage.

In many surgical pathology laboratories it is now routine to prepare imprint cytology slides of most malignancies. These can provide valuable study materials for all of us, especially when interesting tumors are excised without antecedent fine-needle aspiration or other cytologic investigations. We have found these preparations to be very useful after surgery, when a recurrence is studied in cytologic samples. This is also true when the CSF shows tumor cells. Reviewing archival imprints of a patient's original material can enhance our confidence in cytologic diagnosis of recurrent disease.

## PRIMARY CNS NEOPLASMS

Referral patterns are a strong determinant of the extent to which primary CNS neoplasms are evaluated in a given institution or pathology practice. For most pathologists opportunities to study these tumors in CSF samples remain uncommon. Furthermore, our ability to recognize and classify these entities in CSF cytology is limited. The degree of CSF seeding depends on the tumor type and the extent of leptomeningeal involvement in a given case.[33] Furthermore, the actual rate of detection by the cytology laboratory is influenced by CSF collection and processing, as well as by patient selection.[8] In some circumstances there is a clinical prohibition against lumbar puncture in patients with a CNS mass lesion. This also decreases our opportunities to examine this type of material.[26]

Medulloblastomas shed tumor cells into the CSF more frequently than do well-differentiated glial neoplasms (astrocytoma, oligodendroglioma, ependymoma), or glioblastoma multiforme.[3,9] Meningiomas, in contrast, although propitiously situated are rarely reported in the CSF. In their tertiary-care institution Bigner and Johnston noted that 3.1% of primary CNS neoplasms were manifest in the CSF, but these cases represented 24% of tumors presenting initially in the CSF without an antecedent history of malignancy.[9] Some investigations have indicated that seeding of the CSF is much less common in patients without previous neurosurgery (reviewed in Reference 8). Primary CNS malignant lymphoma, for example, is rarely encountered in CSF samples prior to biopsy.[39]

When medulloblastoma presents initially in the CSF, it may clinically mimic meningitis.[8,9] The differential diagnosis of medulloblastoma centers around other small blue cell tumors, including neuroblastoma, retinoblastoma, and other primary CNS neoplasms (ependymoblastoma and pineoblastoma).[8,9,61] The location of tumor within the CNS, as well as the presence or absence of extracranial disease, can point toward the correct diagnosis. Metastatic tumors in the CNS are usually associated with demonstrable extracranial disease, whereas primary CNS neoplasms are not.

Cytologically, medulloblastoma resembles small cell carcinoma when cell groups are encountered, while its single cells can mimic leukemia or lymphoma. As noted previously, the location of the tumor, the patient's age, and other clinical and radiographic findings usually will point to the correct diagnosis, in spite of this seemingly nonspecific cytologic picture. In many patients precraniotomy lumbar puncture cannot be performed; therefore, the actual rate of CSF seeding by unoperated medulloblastomas is difficult to determine.[26]

In adults, the high grade primary CNS neoplasm most likely to be seen in CSF samples is glioblastoma multiforme (GBM).[8,85,86] These high-grade malignant

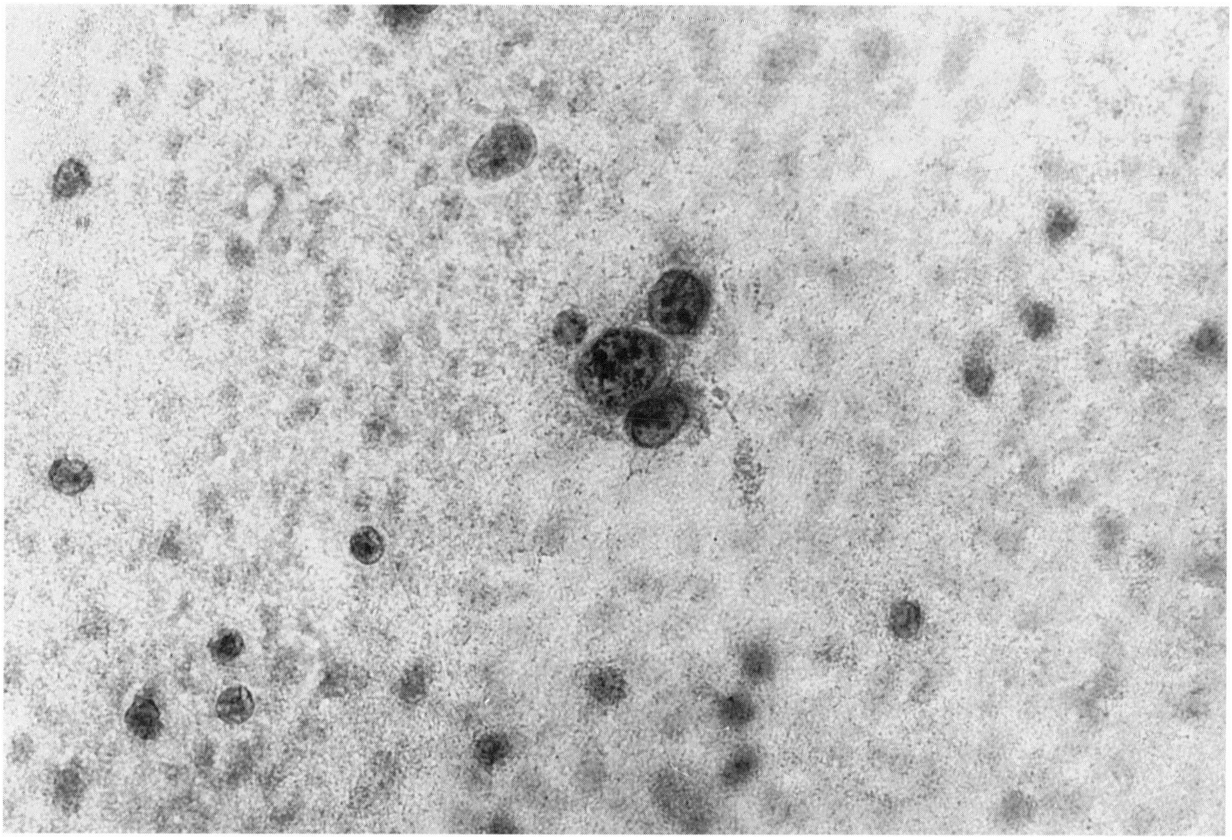

**Fig. 1-16.** When encountered in cytologic material including the CSF, the cells of glioblastoma multiforme are indistinguishable from those of other nonhematopoietic large-cell malignancies. This preparation also shows a background of necrosis. (Papanicolaou stain; ×600.)

cells are often set in a background of necrosis and resemble the cells of poorly differentiated non-small cell carcinoma.[85,86] (Fig. 1-16). The malignant nuclei are sometimes decorated by a thin rim of wispy cytoplasm. The latter cytologic characteristic is reminiscent of the macrophage-like cytoplasm associated with the cells of low-grade astrocytomas in fluid specimens. Most examples of GBM are positive with ICC for glial fibrillary acidic protein (GFAP), provided adequate sampling is achieved. Regardless of the results of immunostaining for GFAP, GBM is negative for cytokeratins in contrast to most of the carcinoma from which it must be cytologically distinguished.

Lower-grade glial neoplasms shed cells that closely resemble the macrophages seen in many non-neoplastic conditions.[8] Thus, while a significant portion of these tumors may shed cells into the CNS, these cells are without distinctive cytologic features in CSF samples. Cells or tissue fragments from these tumors resemble those extracted from the normal brain tissue (Table 1-1) and share GFAP positivity with such contaminants.[33] Gliomatosis cerebri, a rare manifestation of glial neoplasia, is often clinically enigmatic until autopsy, but CSF-positive cases have been described.[57] Primary meningeal gliomatosis may clinically mimic meningitis. The CSF is negative in these cases, as reviewed by Ho and associates.[41]

Choroid plexus neoplasms are propitiously located to shed cells into the CSF and have been discussed previously.[16] Choroid plexus carcinomas are cytologically indistinguishable from adenocarcinoma. When such a tumor is encountered in the CSF of a child, one should reflect on the rarity of adenocarcinoma in these patients and then consider choroid plexus carcinoma.

In summary, primary CNS neoplasms that can be reflected in the CSF usually fit into one of the following patterns: (1) high-grade, clinically aggressive, and difficult to confidently classify; (2) low-grade and hard to recognize as malignant; or (3) rare (choroid plexus papilloma or carcinoma).

## HEMATOPOIETIC NEOPLASMS

### Introduction and Technical Factors

As noted previously, CSF leukocytosis is more often reactive than neoplastic. Conditions such as the demyelinating disorders, encephalitis, and other infections enter the differential diagnosis of individuals with unexplained CNS findings.[3,15,33] In these patients, or in patients with a history of hematologic malignancy, one must carefully consider the possibility that even "atypical" cells are reactive rather than a reflection of systemic malignancy.[86] In some instances, no clinical explanation for provocative cells is forthcoming.[49]

The cytologic similarity between neoplastic and reactive lymphocytes means that the risk of false-positive diagnoses of leukemia or lymphoma is much greater than the risk of false-positive diagnoses of carcinoma.[33] Contaminants are the only elements that may resemble carcinoma cells (Table 1-1). Indeed, false-positive diagnoses have been described in patients with acute lymphoblastic leukemia (ALL), chronic lymphocytic leukemia (CLL), and other hematologic conditions, and in some with no evidence of any hematologic neoplasm.[15] Reactive lymphocytes may also mimic the cells of higher-grade non-Hodgkin's malignant lymphoma.[15] In our experience, some of the most provocative reactions are those associated with cryptococcal meningitis. As discussed earlier, the yeast may be difficult to identify in cytologic preparations.

We have previously indicated that polymorphous lymphocytoses are usually reactive, while those that are monomorphous are much more likely to represent a neoplasm. Such subjective distinctions serve us well as first approximations and may be quite reliable in areas like lymph node fine-needle aspiration. In sparsely cellular CSF samples, however, it may be difficult or impossible to apply this approach. Furthermore, the fact that reactive processes may be so monomorphous as to be mistaken for CLL indicates additional limitations of this approach.

Repeat lumbar punctures may not improve the situation, as the procedure itself can give rise to reactive lymphocytes that may resemble leukemic blasts or the cells of malignant lymphoma.[62] Intrathecal chemotherapy for malignancy can also initiate reactive lymphocytosis that may persist for months and cause diagnostic difficulties.[55] Overall, up to 30% of ALL patients may show nonleukemic CSF lymphocytosis that can be mistaken for CNS leukemia.[55] A variety of special studies have been applied to the distinction of neoplastic from reactive lymphoid cells; these studies are discussed in the next section.

Since the cells of malignant lymphoma so closely resemble reactive lymphocytes, false-negative diagnoses also occur.[15] In leukemia patients, CNS therapy may induce cell damage that renders residual blasts unidentifiable.[15,55,83] The cells in cases of acute myelogenous leukemia (AML) with monocytic differentiation may resemble small, benign monocytes.

In patients with a history of hematologic malignancy, the cornerstone of diagnosis remains comparison of cells in the CSF with those in the peripheral blood, bone marrow, or lymph nodes. Imprints prepared from fresh surgical specimens are especially valuable in the latter circumstance. We have previously discussed our preference for air-dried, Romanowsky-stained slides when evaluating hematopoietic cells in the CSF.[78,92] The commercially available Diff-Quik method is convenient and gives good results in the cytology laboratory.[78] Even pathologists who do not yet use these methods for fine-needle aspiration smears are comfortable with their application to blood and bone marrow. When confronted with a difficult interpretation regarding hematopoietic cells in the CSF, we have found that comparisons of Diff-Quik-stained slides with archival smears from the hematology laboratory can be very helpful. Comparisons between fixed, Papanicolaou-stained CSF slides and hematology material have been substantially less useful in our hands.

The foregoing indicates the importance of high quality preparations in the diagnosis of hematologic conditions. When the procedure is performed, the sample may be contaminated with blood or bone marrow, either of which may contain the cells of leukemia or malignant lymphoma. When these are introduced into the CSF, the opportunity to diagnose CNS involvement is lost.[7,15,76] A repeat puncture can be helpful, but several days or even weeks may be required to resolve the hemorrhage and reactive changes induced by the initial procedure.[7]

The primary evidence that blood or bone marrow contamination has occurred is the presence of RBCs. The mixing experiments performed by Rohlfing and co-workers demonstrated that if the blood (or bone marrow) blast count is high, minute amounts of contamination will suffice to admit tumor cells to a filter preparation.[70] The required level of contamination is far below that needed to result in a visually detectable "bloody tap." Furthermore, red blood cells are usually lysed during preparation of membrane filters. These observations indicate that tumor cells seen in this type of preparation may be considered evidence of CNS disease, whereas in reality they represent unrecognized contamination.[15] Furthermore, small numbers of RBCs are much more easily overlooked in fixed, Papanicolaou-stained preparations than in air-dried, Romanowsky-stained slides.

The foregoing discussion lends credence to our preference for air-dried, Diff-Quik-stained cytocentrifuge preparations for study of CSF from patients who have, or who are thought to have, a hematologic malignancy. Others have found this approach useful. The 1985 Rome Conference on Poor-Prognosis ALL defined CNS involvement with this type of leukemia in terms of lymphoblasts identified "from a cytocentrifuged sample."[54] This method is rapid, inexpensive, and technically simple. Cell recovery has improved with more modern versions of this instrument and has been compared to the yield obtained by filtration.[7,22,34] Preconcentration by whole-sample centrifugation prior to final slide preparation in the cytocentrifuge has been recommended for dilute fluids.[58]

We have described the morphologic alterations in cells that have been cytocentrifuged. The effect is primarily one of apparent flattening and thus of enlargement.[47] Problems associated with these changes and with cell damage can be minimized by careful adjustment of the instrument.[44,58,93] Yam and associates have indicated that at low centrifuge speeds cell recovery is poor, and the cells are not well distributed over the pellet area. At speeds that are too great, cells are damaged and tend to be clustered near the edge of the pellet area. These authors recommend speeds of 500 to 800 RPM applied for periods of 5 to 7 minutes.[93] Others have suggested 1200 RPM for 5 minutes.[58] We use a speed of 1000 RPM for 4 minutes with good results. Cell recovery is also reduced if too much sample volume is placed in the funnel.

### Cytology of the Acute Leukemias

When effective chemotherapy for ALL became available in the 1960s, patient survival increased to the point that relapse in such sanctuary sites as the testis and the CNS raised major therapeutic issues.[49,88] Prophylactic treatment of the CNS with radiation and intrathecal chemotherapy decreased the rate of relapse in this site from 50 to 80% to the current rate of approximately 10%.[13,49,58] Among the factors that have driven continued investigation of ALL in the CNS, two are of concern to the cytology laboratory. First, treatment of the CNS is not entirely benign and has been associated with important neuropsychologic impairment;[12] diagnostic accuracy is therefore imperative. Second, newer diagnostic techniques have resulted in ongoing modifications in our definition of CNS relapse and in our understanding of what constitutes adequate monitoring of the CSF in these patients. These newer ancillary techniques can significantly influence the number of CSF samples that are interpreted as positive for ALL.

Up to 10% of children with ALL relapse in the CNS despite prophylaxis, and most of these patients go on to develop bone marrow relapse and death.[13,58,63] Once overt CNS leukemia is established, it is usually refractory to chemotherapy. In contrast, when CNS disease is detected earlier, ALL is associated with a lower risk of simultaneous bone marrow relapse.[12,58] It is possible that the CNS disease reseeds the treated bone marrow. Alternatively, subclinical bone marrow involvement may be responsible for CNS relapse.[13] Since recrudescence in either site may initially be asymptomatic, these possibilities are usually difficult to distinguish.[58] In rare instances CNS leukemia may be a patient's initial mode of presentation. Cells from both sites will share identifying cell-surface and cytogenetic markers.[13]

The possible routes by which ALL cells enter the CNS have been considered by Bleyer.[13] These cells may enter via veins or may extend directly from adjacent cranial bone marrow. Very high peripheral blood blast counts with consequent leukostasis might facilitate the former mode of spread. Low platelet counts have been associated with a high risk of CNS involvement, perhaps mediated by small hemorrhages.

The cells of ALL are small, with scant basophilic cytoplasm and a high nucleocytoplasmic ratio. The nuclear chromatin is finely stippled or lacy, and small nucleoli are common (Fig. 1-17).[49] Their cytomorphology in air-dried cytocentrifuge slides corresponds closely to that noted in smears of blood or bone marrow.[22] We have noted slight alterations in this appearance that can be attributed to the effects of cytocentrifugation.

The progressive honing of the definition of CNS involvement by ALL has paralleled technical advances in cytologic diagnosis. The cytocentrifuge improved our ability to detect cells that are present in low numbers and to look in detail at their cytomorphology.[58] High cell counts in the absence of blasts may not constitute an indication for treatment.[55] The significance of blasts in low cell count fluids is continually reevaluated as ancillary techniques improve detection of even rare abnormal cells. Increased CSF protein or an increased cell count in the absence of identifiable blasts can be associated with a decreased probability of "event-free," 2-year survival, suggesting that undetectable CNS leukemia may be a problem in some patients.[65]

The 1985 Rome Conference on Poor-Prognosis ALL defined extramedullary disease in the CNS at diagnosis as more than five leukocytes per $\mu$L and "morphologically unequivocal blasts from a cytocentrifuged sample."[54] Other definitions have been used, therefore it is sometimes difficult to compare the results of different studies.[43,49,55,58] This problem is under almost continual reevaluation, as the ability to detect very low levels of involvement based on immunostains for cell surface markers and terminal deoxynucleotidyl transferase (TdT) improves. While the ultimate significance of these developments is not yet clear, some patients with low cell counts and rare blasts will experience CNS relapse.[43,49,58] It is important that the cytopathology laboratory work is in concert with the clinical laboratory to ensure accurate cell count and cytomorphologic data.

Acute myelogenous leukemia (AML) is less frequently encountered in CSF samples than ALL, perhaps because of the shorter overall survival of patients with AML.[7] However, our many experiences with ALL in extramedullary sites have framed our concepts about the cytology of acute leukemias in general.[12] In

A 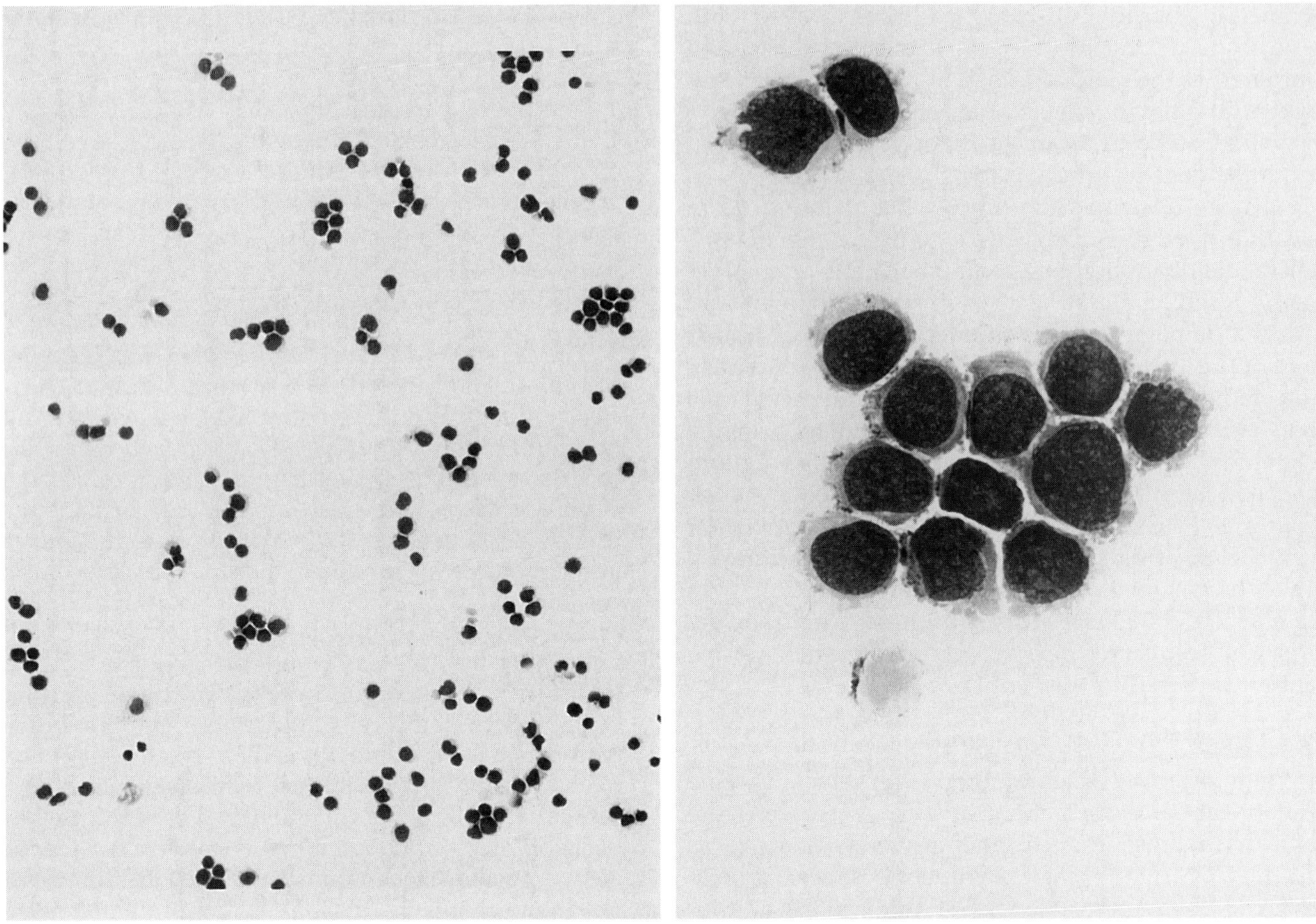 B

**Fig. 1-17. A,** Acute lymphoblastic leukemia (ALL) may lead to highly cellular CSF specimens such as that shown here. **B,** The leukemic cells may be thrown together by the cytocentrifuge but do not form true tissue fragments; this is a cytologic feature of hematologic cells in general. These cells closely resemble their counterparts in the bone marrow and feature scanty cytoplasm, small nucleoli, and stippled chromatin. (**A,** Diff-Quik stain; ×40; **B,** Diff-Quik stain; ×600.)

their study of AML, Meyer and colleagues found CSF involvement at the time of initial diagnosis in 7 of 39 cases.[56] All seven positive cases showed monocytic differentiation (acute myelomonocytic leukemia). Clinical findings associated with CNS disease included a high peripheral white blood cell count (6:7), splenomegaly (6:7), and skin or gingival involvement (4:7). Other studies support the observation that cases with a monocytic component are more likely than other AMLs to show positive CSF cytology (Fig. 1-18).[79]

Issues related to the morphologic subclassification of AML are beyond the scope of this chapter, but some findings are sufficiently characteristic to improve our accuracy and confidence in recognizing these cells. When seen in fixed Papanicolaou-stained material, the cells of ALL, AML, and many malignant lymphomas are virtually indistinguishable (Fig. 1-19). Such cases will usually be said to show "lymphoma/leukemia." Since reactive cells can have a similar appearance, additional morphologic clues are welcome, especially in those cases in which malignant cells are present in low numbers. This is important, since progressive disease can be seen even in patients with low CSF blast counts.[56] Many of the AMLs afford abundant diagnostic clues, as long as they are depicted in air-dried preparations. Both Auer rods and cytoplasmic granules can be identified.[7] The cytochemical stains used to diagnose and classify AML in smear material can also be applied to air-dried slides of CSF (myeloperoxidase, Sudan black).

Chronic myelogenous leukemia is usually not represented in the CSF. However, those cases in blast transformation may yield positive fluid studies. The phenotype of such cases varies widely.

### Cytology of Malignant Lymphoma and Related Conditions

Herman and co-workers described CNS disease in 5% of 1039 patients with malignant lymphoma.[40] Most

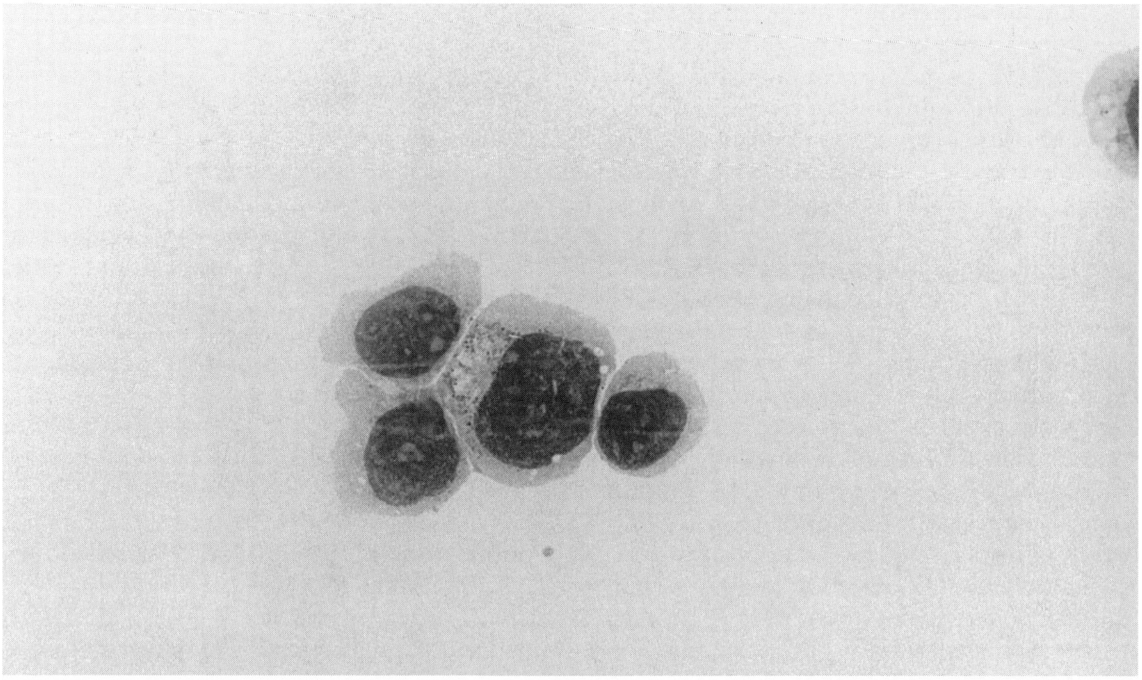

**Fig. 1-18.** This CSF shows involvement with the monoblastic type of acute myelogenous leukemia. The leukemic cells have been thrown together by the cytocentrifuge but do not form a true tissue fragment. The moderately abundant cytoplasm features vacuoles and tiny granules. The nuclei are oval and contain small nucleoli. (Diff-Quik stain; ×600.)

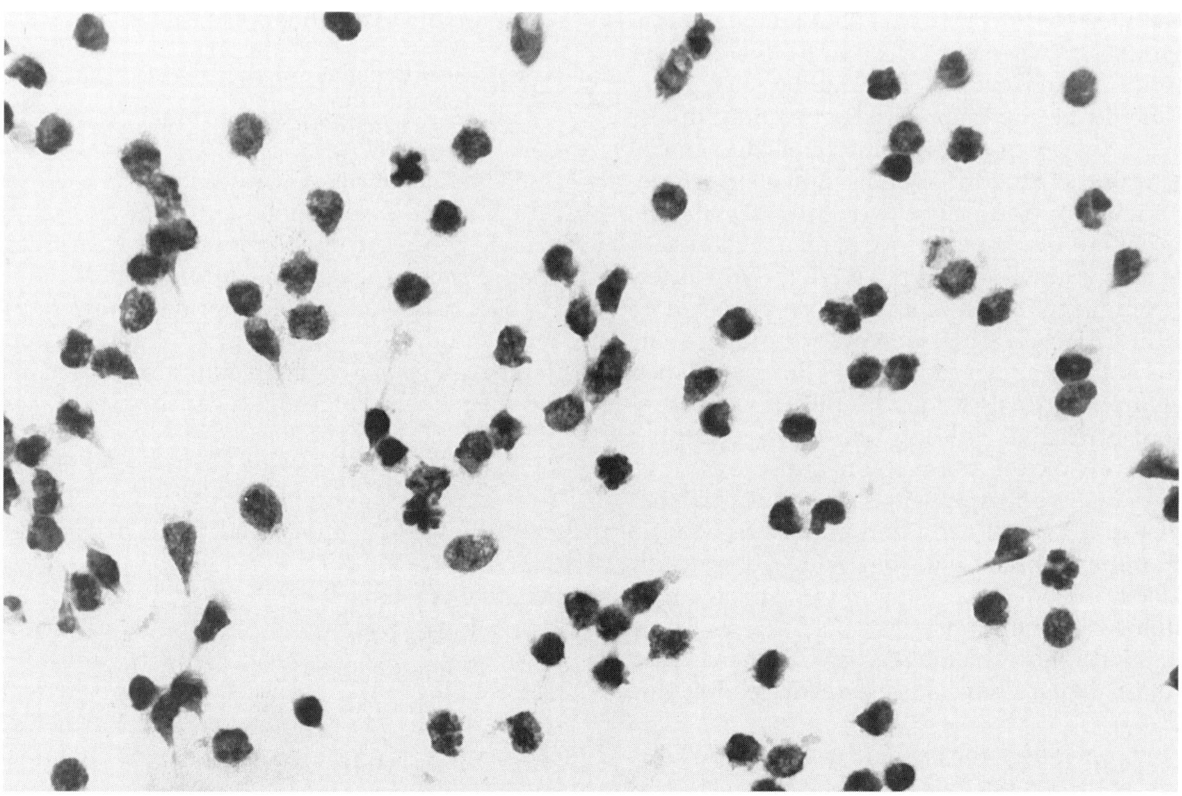

**Fig. 1-19.** When fixed and stained by the method of Papanicolaou, many cases of acute leukemia and malignant lymphoma of various types are cytologically indistinguishable from one another. (Papanicolaou stain; ×100.)

of these would now be classified as intermediate or high-grade non-Hodgkin's lymphomas (NHL). Meningeal involvement (3.7%) was more common than either focal cerebral disease (1%) or cord compression (0.1%). In most cases CNS disease was accompanied by other extranodal involvement (bone marrow, gastrointestinal tract, skin, and lung). CSF cytology was the most reliable diagnostic test.

Among immunocompetent patients, primary NHL of the CNS is usually associated with negative CSF cytology prior to surgery, but up to 40% may show a non-neoplastic lymphocytosis.[36,39] This malignancy occurs in older patients and is more common in males; most will not show systemic disease at presentation. When the immunosuppressed are considered, primary CNS lymphoma is more common; up to 40% of NHL in renal allograft recipients are confined to the CNS.[36] In AIDS, approximately 6% of 400 autopsied cases showed primary CNS lymphoma.[38] In another study, 20% of AIDS-associated lymphomas were limited to this site.[36] The percentage of cases confined to the CNS was higher (43%) in the series of Ziegler and co-workers.[94] Most involve only the brain and lead to negative CSF studies.[81] As noted previously, CSF from AIDS patients may show reactive changes, but in light of the data just summarized, one should resist the diagnosis of NHL in this setting unless the evidence is compelling.[45]

Chronic lymphocytic leukemia (CLL) is rarely seen in CSF samples.[15] When these very well-differentiated cells are encountered, even in large numbers, a reactive process should be the favored interpretation, unless contradicted by the patient's clinical history or cell marker studies. Furthermore, CLL patients have decreased immunity; thus, even with this history one must search carefully for evidence of an infection such as *Cryptococcus.* Small cleaved cell NHL (poorly differentiated lymphocytic lymphoma) is somewhat more common in CSF than CLL. However, the diagnostic approach outlined above for CLL should be pursued for this lymphoma,[15] as it may be difficult to distinguish from a reactive process unless highly cellular material is available for examination. Those low-grade lymphomas that are beginning to show transformation to a higher grade B cell neoplasm may be difficult to interpret properly, because the beginnings of transformation deprive them of the monomorphism on which their cytologic recognition is based. Three to 5% of large-cell NHL show meningeal involvement,[7] and most of these patients have other evidence of systemic disease.[15]

As noted previously, the Papanicolaou stain reduces most cases of acute leukemia and large-cell NHL to a common appearance. As shown in Fig. 1-20, air-dried slides reveal an appearance similar to that expected in bone marrow smears. It is sometimes very helpful to compare these cells to the same tumor seen in lymph node imprints.[7]

The primary differential diagnostic consideration in the NHL is reactive lymphocytosis. Cytologic factors and application of lymphocyte marker studies in difficult cases have been previously discussed.[81] The morphologic spectrum of B cell maturation has been well characterized through study of germinal center cells and forms part of the basis for our classification of B cell NHL. The cytology of reactive T cells is less clearly delineated.[49] Since most reactions seen in CSF cytology consist largely of T cells, the risk of false-positive diagnoses is considerable.

Evidence of Hodgkin's disease is rarely reported in CSF samples; we have never seen an example. One usually encounters plasma cells as part of a reactive lymphocytosis, where they are accompanied by numerous lymphocytes of various types. We most often encounter this picture in the setting of cryptococcal meningitis. We have also seen plasma cells in a single instance of systemic Castleman's disease with CNS symptoms.[75] Multiple myeloma is rarely seen in CSF specimens.[86] A large number of myeloma patients are cared for in our institution, and we have seen positive CSF on several occasions (Fig. 1-21). In contrast to reactive processes, the cells of multiple myeloma are relatively monomorphic in a given sample. Their cytology is somewhat variable, depending on the tumor's differentiation and the patient's treatment.

### Ancillary Studies Applied to ALL

When ICC stains for terminal deoxynucleotidyl transferase (TdT) or CD 10 (CALLA) are applied to CSF, the rate of involved samples increases.* The clinical relevance of minimal "occult" CNS disease identified by these means is not always clear because the relapse rate varies among studies.

TdT is a nuclear enzyme normally present in thymocytes and detected in 90% of ALL and 10% of AML.[49] Rapid, inexpensive immunofluorescence stains (IF) give good technical results, even in very low cell counts (<5 cells/$\mu$L) and show as positive cases that are cytologically normal.[17] In a study of 1661 CSF samples from $TdT^+$, ALL, and lymphoma patients by Hooijkaas and colleagues, the cytology and the TdT IF were concordant in 1511 (91.9%).[44] Patients who were cytologically negative or suspicious but that were $TdT^-$ ($n = 47$) showed no evidence of relapse after follow-up of up to 58 months. However, when negative or suspicious cytology was coupled with positive TdT IF, relapse occurred in 40 of 54 children. Furthermore, two consecutive $TdT^+$ samples always heralded CNS leukemia.

* Refs. 17, 43, 44, 49, 93.

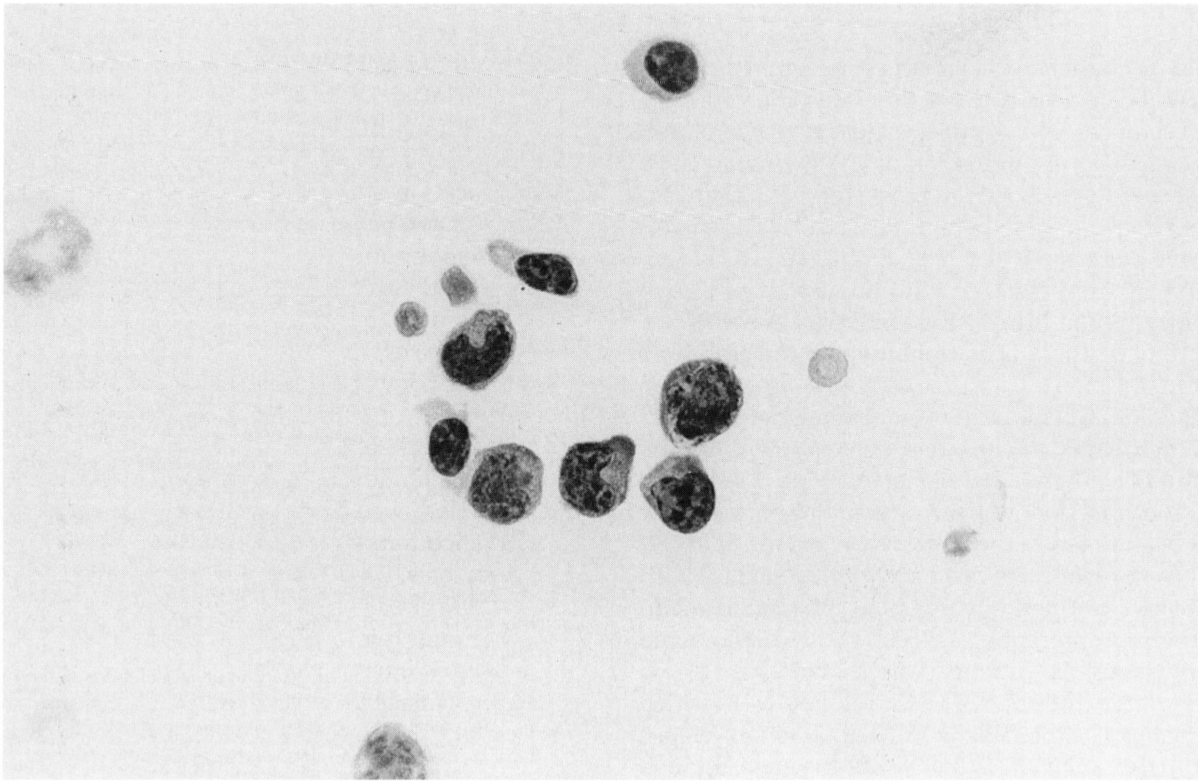

**Fig. 1-20.** The cells of this large-cell malignant lymphoma lie singly. They feature scanty cytoplasm and clumped chromatin. Some cells show small nucleoli. (Papanicolaou stain; ×600.)

**A** **B**

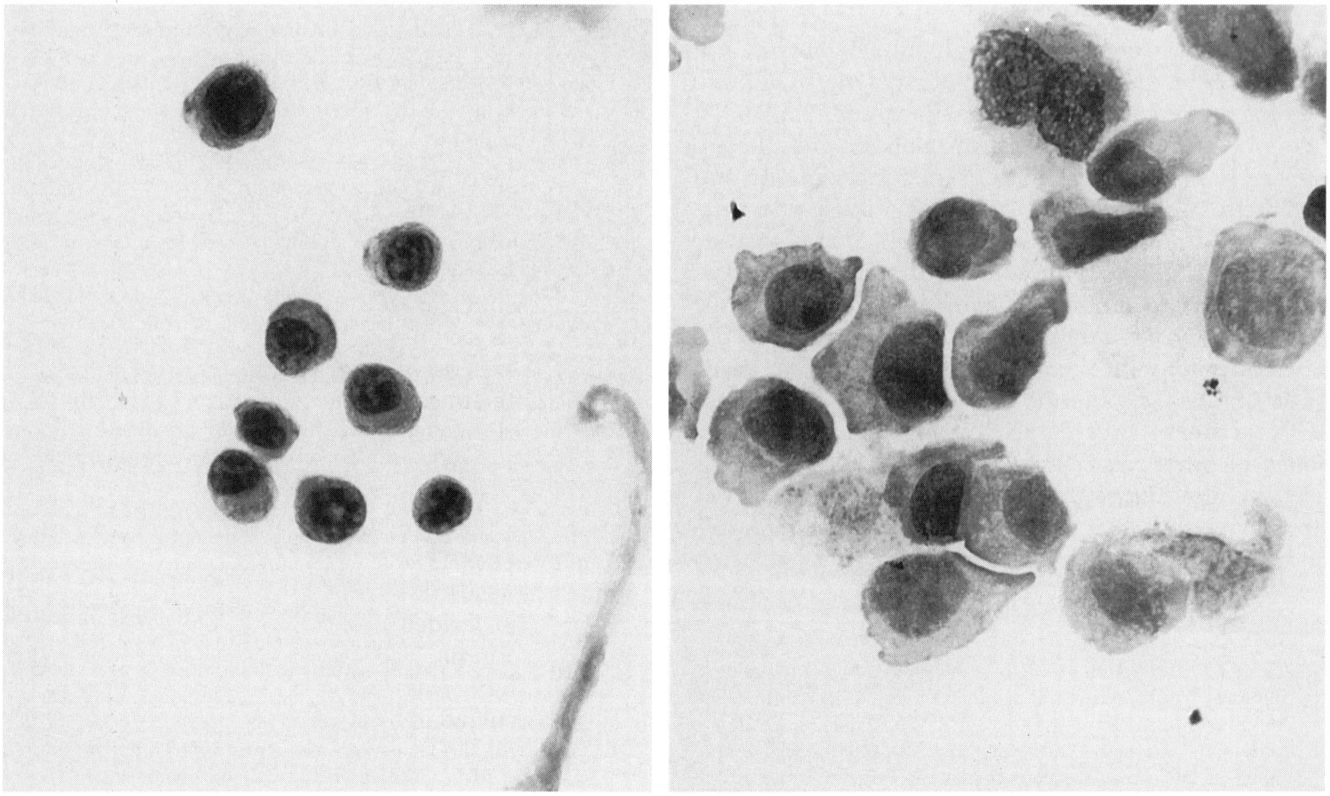

**Fig. 1-21.** Multiple myeloma is not commonly encountered in CSF specimens, but we have seen several examples in patients known to suffer from this malignancy. The plasma cell nature is usually obvious. (**A,** Papanicolaou stain; ×600; **B,** Diff-Quik stain; ×600.)

Problems and technical aspects of ICC in childhood ALL have been described.[44,47,49,93] It is important to note that samples for TdT studies must be free of blood. Issues related to contamination of CSF by blood have been discussed previously. In most studies TdT immunostains are negative in benign disease.[44,49] However, some have suggested that rare $TdT^+$ cells can be detected in CSF from children with no history of a $TdT^+$ malignancy. When the sensitive microspheres method is used, few of these cells double-label for both TdT and CALLA.[43] Rare CALLA-positive cells have also been described in children without malignancy.[42,43,47]

Flow cytometry (FCM) has been applied to the study of ALL. When bone marrow samples are evaluated, 40% of cases show DNA aneuploidy;[82] a similar rate has been noted in the CSF.[67] Abnormalities in cellular DNA content have been shown to correlate with cytologically detected involvement.[49,67] Increases in RNA and in proliferation rates can be identified, even when the sample is diploid.[67] Such studies require a relatively large number of cells for analysis, which means that cases amenable to FCM are often in relapse at the time of analysis. Thus, while the investigative aspects of FCM are very interesting, its diagnostic utility as applied to the CSF is limited. The potential application of image analysis to these issues remains incompletely explored.

## TUMOR MARKERS IN CSF CYTOLOGY

Despite early enthusiasm, evaluation of biochemical tumor markers in the CSF of patients with malignancies has proved to be of limited clinical utility. Ferritin, acid phosphatase, and $\beta2$ microglobulin may be increased in many such samples but lack sensitivity and specificity; thus they add little to cytologic examinations.[49] $\beta2$ microglobulin and $\beta$-glucuronidase can be increased in a variety of non-neoplastic conditions as well.[88,89] Carcinoembryonic antigen is increased in the CSF of many patients with metastatic carcinoma but is nonspecific with regard to tumor type.[26,88,89] Some cases of CNS germinoma show elevated levels of $\beta$-hCG, whereas increased $\alpha$ fetoprotein (AFP) is associated with other germ cell tumors. These markers can be used to monitor treatment response or for recurrence surveillance but do not obviate the requirement for histologic diagnoses at the time of initial presentation.[26]

### REFERENCES


1. Aichner F, and Schuler G: Primary leptomeningeal melanoma: diagnosis by ultrastructural cytology of cerebrospinal fluid and cranial computed tomography, Cancer 50:1751-1756, 1982.
2. Anderson C, Duggan C, and Kealy WF: Extramedullary hematopoiesis in the central nervous system: an unusual cause of epilepsy, J Neurol Neurosurg Psychiatry 50:640-641, 1987.
3. An-Foraker SH: Cytodiagnosis of malignant lesions in cerebrospinal fluid: review and cytohistologic correlation, Acta Cytol 29:286-290, 1985.
4. Barrett DL, and King EB: Comparison of cellular recovery rates and morphologic detail obtained using membrane filter and cytocentrifuge techniques, Acta Cytol 20:174-180, 1976.
5. Bedrossian CWM: Malignant effusions: a multimodal approach to cytologic diagnosis, New York and Tokyo, 1994, Igaku-Shoin.
6. Bernad PG, and others: Diagnosis of cryptococcal meningitis by cytologic methods: an old technique revisited, Neurology 30:102-105, 1980.
7. Bigner SH, and Johnston WW: The cytopathology of cerebrospinal fluid I: nonneoplastic conditions, lymphoma and leukemia, Acta Cytol 25:335-353, 1981.
8. Bigner SH, and Johnston WW: The cytopathology of cerebrospinal fluid II: meningeal carcinomatosis and primary central nervous system neoplasms, Acta Cytol 25:461-479, 1981.
9. Bigner SH, and Johnston WW: The diagnostic challenge of tumors manifested initially by the shedding of cells into cerebrospinal fluid, Acta Cytol 28:29-36, 1984.
10. Bigner SH, and others: The cytopathology of reactions to ventricular shunts, Acta Cytol 29:391-396, 1985.
11. Bigner SH, and others: Unusual presentations of inflammatory conditions in cerebrospinal fluid, Acta Cytol 29:291-296, 1985.
12. Bleyer WA: Central nervous system leukemia, Pediatr Clin North Am 35:789-814, 1988.
13. Bleyer WA: Biology and pathogenesis of CNS leukemia, Am J Pediatr Hematol Oncol 11:57-63, 1989.
14. Boogerd W, and others: CSF cytology versus immunocytochemistry in meningeal carcinomatosis, J Neurol Neurosurg Psychiatry 51:142-145, 1988.
15. Borowitz M, Bigner SH, and Johnston WW: Diagnostic problems in evaluation of cerebrospinal fluid for lymphoma and leukemia, Acta Cytol 25:665-674, 1981.
16. Buchino JJ, and Mason KG: Choroid plexus papilloma: report of a case with cytologic differential diagnosis, Acta Cytol 36:95-99, 1992.
17. Casper JT, and others: Evaluation of cerebrospinal fluid mononuclear cells obtained from children with acute lymphoblastic leukemia: Advantages of combining cytomorphology and terminal deoxynucleotidyl transferase, Am J Clin Pathol 80:666-670, 1983.
18. Chen KTK, and Moseley D: Cartilage cells in cerebrospinal fluid, Arch Pathol Lab Med 114:212, 1990.
19. Coleman A, and Schumann GB: Cytodiagnosis of acute lymphocytic leukemia and eosinophilia in cerebrospinal fluid, Diagn Cytopathol 3:330-334, 1987.
20. Conrad KA, Gross JL, and Trojanowski JQ: Leptomeningeal carcinomatosis presenting as eosinophilic meningitis, Acta Cytol 30:29-31, 1986.
21. Craver RD, and Carson TH: Hematopoietic elements in cerebrospinal fluid in children, Am J Clin Pathol 95:532-535, 1991.
22. Davey DD, Foucar K, and Giller R: Millipore filter vs cytocentrifuge for detection of childhood central nervous system leukemia, Arch Pathol Lab Med 110:705-708, 1986.
23. DeMent SH, Cox MC, and Gupta PK: Diagnosis of central nervous system Toxoplasma gondii from the cerebrospinal fluid in a patient with acquired immunodeficiency syndrome, Diagn Cytopathol 3:148-157, 1987.
24. de Reuck J, and others: Mitotic activity in cerebrospinal fluid cells, Clin Neurol Neurosurg 90:1117-1119, 1988.
25. Devinsky O, and others: Cerebrospinal fluid pleocytosis following simple, complex partial, and generalized tonic-clonic seizures, Ann Neurol 23:402-403, 1988.
26. Edwards MSB, Davis RL, and Laurent JP: Tumor markers and cytologic features of cerebrospinal fluid, Cancer 56:1773-1777, 1985.
27. Ehni WF, and Ellison RT: Spontaneous Candida albicans meningitis in a patient with the acquired immune deficiency syndrome, Am J Med 83:806-807, 1987.

28. Ehya H, Hajdu SI, and Melamed MR: Cytopathology of nonlymphoreticular neoplasms metastatic to the central nervous system, Acta Cytol 25:599-610, 1981.
29. Evans H: Cytology of Mollaret meningitis, Diagn Cytopathol 9: 373-376, 1993.
30. Fischer JR, and others: Blast-like cells in cerebrospinal fluid of neonates: Possible germinal matrix origin, Am J Clin Pathol 91: 255-258, 1989.
31. Friedman HD, and Tatum AH: HMB-45-positive malignant lymphoma: a case report with literature review of aberrant HMB-45 reactivity, Arch Pathol Lab Med 115:826-830, 1991.
32. Gal AA, Evan S, and Meyer PR: The clinical evaluation of cryptococcal infections in the acquired immunodeficiency syndrome, Diagn Microbiol Infect Dis 7:249-254, 1987.
33. Glass JP, and others: Malignant cells in cerebrospinal fluid (CSF): the meaning of a positive CSF cytology, Neurology 29:1369-1375, 1979.
34. Gondos B: Millipore filter vs cytocentrifuge for evaluation of cerebrospinal fluid, Arch Pathol Lab Med 110:687-688, 1986.
35. Gonzalez-Vitale JC, and Garcia-Bunuel R: Meningeal carcinomatosis, Cancer 37:2906-2911, 1976.
36. Grote TH, and others: Primary lymphoma of the central nervous system: a report of 20 cases and a review of the literature, Am J Clin Oncol 12:93-100, 1989.
37. Gupta PK, and others: Herpes simplex encephalitis cerebrospinal fluid cytology studies. Two case reports, Acta Cytol 16:563-565, 1972.
38. Hancock C, Allen BC, and Herrera GA: HMB-45 detection in adenocarcinomas, Arch Pathol Lab Med 115:886-890, 1991.
39. Helle TL, Britt RH, and Colby TV: Primary lymphoma of the central nervous system: clinicopathologic study of experience at Stanford, J Neurosurg 60:94-103, 1984.
40. Herman TS, and others: Involvement of the central nervous system by non-Hodgkin's lymphoma: the southwest oncology group experience, Cancer 43:390-397, 1979.
41. Ho K-L, Hoschner JA, and Wolfe DE: Primary leptomeningeal gliomatosis: symptoms suggestive of meningitis, Arch Neurol 38:662-666, 1981.
42. Homans AC, Forman EN, and Barker BE: Use of monoclonal antibodies to identify cerebrospinal fluid lymphoblasts in children with acute lymphoblastic leukemia, Blood 66:1321-1325, 1985.
43. Homans AC, and others: Immunophenotypic characteristics of cerebrospinal fluid cells in children with acute lymphoblastic leukemia at diagnosis, Blood 76:1807-1811, 1990.
44. Hooijkaas H, and others: Terminal deoxynucleotidyl transferase (TdT)-positive cells in cerebrospinal fluid and development of overt CNS leukemia: a 5-year follow-up study of 113 children with a TdT-positive leukemia or non-Hodgkin's lymphoma, Blood 74:416-422, 1989.
45. Katz RL, and others: Cerebrospinal fluid manifestations of the neurologic complications of human immunodefidiency virus infection, Acta Cytol 33:233-244, 1989.
46. Keebler CM: Cytopreparatory techniques. In Bibbo M, editor: Comprehensive Cytopathology, Philadelphia, 1991, WB Saunders.
47. Kranz BR, Thiel E, and Thierfelder S: Immunocytochemical identification of meningeal leukemia and lymphoma: poly-L-lysine-coated slides permit multimarker analysis even with minute cerebrospinal fluid cell specimens, Blood 73:1942-1950, 1989.
48. Kruskall MS, Carter SR, and Ritz LP: Contamination of cerebrospinal fluid by vertebral bone-marrow cells during lumbar puncture, N Engl J Med 308:697-700, 1983.
49. Lauer SJ, Kirchner PA, and Camitta BM: Identification of leukemic cells in the cerebrospinal fluid from children with acute lymphoblastic leukema: advances and dilemmas, Am J Pediatr Hematol Oncol 11:64-73, 1989.
50. Leiman G, Klein C, and Berry AV: Cells of the nucleus pulposus in cerebrospinal fluid: a case report, Acta Cytol 24:347-349, 1980.
51. Li C-Y, and others: Diagnosis of B-cell non-Hodgkin's lymphoma of the central nervous system by immunocytochemical analysis of cerebrospinal fluid lymphocytes, Cancer 57:737-744, 1986.
52. Lobenthal SW, Hajdu SI, and Urmacher C: Cytologic findings in homosexual males with acquired immunodeficiency, Acta Cytol 27:597-604, 1983.
53. Marmaduke DP, Brandt JT, and Theil KS: Rapid diagnosis of cytomegalovirus in the cerebrospinal fluid of a patient with AIDS-associated polyradiculopathy, Arch Pathol Lab Med 115: 1154-1157, 1991.
54. Mastrangelo R, and others: Report and recommendations of the Rome workshop concerning poor-prognosis acute lymphoblastic leukemia in children: biologic bases for staging, stratification, and treatment, Med Pediatr Oncol 14:191-194, 1986.
55. McIntosh S, and Ritchey K: Diagnostic problems in cerebrospinal fluid of children with lymphoid malignancies, Am J Pediatr Hematol Oncol 8:28-31, 1986.
56. Meyer RJ, and others: Central nervous system involvement at presentation in acute granulocytic leukemia, Am J Med 68:691-694, 1980.
57. Miller RR, Lin F, and Mallonee MM: Cytologic diagnosis of gliomatosis cerebri, Acta Cytol 25:37-39, 1981.
58. Odom LF, and others: Significance of blasts in low-cell-count cerebrospinal fluid specimens from children with acute lymphoblastic leukemia, Cancer 66:1748-1754, 1990.
59. Olson ME, Chernik NL, and Posner JB: Infiltration of the leptomeninges by systemic cancer, Arch Neurol 30:122-137, 1974.
60. Onda K, and others: Cerebral glioblastoma with cerebrospinal fluid dissemination: a clinicopathological study of 14 cases examined by complete autopsy, Neurosurgery 25:533-540, 1989.
61. Packer RJ, and others: Leptomeningeal dissemination of primary central nervous system tumors of childhood, Ann Neurol 18: 217-221, 1985.
62. Peacock JR, McGinnis MR, and Cohen MS: Persistent neutrophilic meningitis: report of four cases and review of the literature, Medicine 63:379-395, 1984.
63. Pochedly C: Meningeal leukemia: current concepts in biology and treatment (introduction to seminar) Am J Pediatr Hematol Oncol 11:55-56, 1989.
64. Polman CH, and others: Cerebrospinal fluid cells in multiple sclerosis and other neurological diseases: an immunohistochemical study, J Neurol 234:19-22, 1987.
65. Rautonen J: Elevated cerebrospinal fluid leukocyte count and protein concentration at diagnosis: independent risk factors in children with acute lymphoblastic leukemia, Blut 56:265-267, 1988.
66. Razavi-Encha R, and others: Cytologic features of cerebrospinal fluid in Lyme disease, Acta Cytol 31:439-440, 1987.
67. Redner A, Melamed M, and Andreeff M: Detection of central nervous system relapse in acute leukemia by multiparameter flow cytometry of DNA, RNA, and CALLA, Ann NY Acad Sci 468:241-255, 1986.
68. Rhodes RH: Histologic features in the central nervous system of 400 acquired immunodeficiency syndrome cases: implications of rates of occurrence, Hum Pathol 24:1189-1198, 1993.
69. Ro JY, Lee SS, and Ayala AG: Advantages of Fontana-Masson stain in capsule-deficient cryptococcal infection, Arch Pathol Lab Med 111:53-57, 1987.
70. Rohlfing MB, and others: Contamination of cerebrospinal fluid specimens with hematogenous blasts in patients with leukemia, Acta Cytol 25:611-615, 1981.

71. Rosenblum MK, and others: Melanotic ependymoma and subependymoma, Am J Surg Pathol 14:729-736, 1990.
72. Rosenthal DL, and Mandell DB: Central nervous system. In Keebler CM, Somrak TM, editors: The manual of cytotechnology, ed 7, Chicago, 1993, American Society of Clinical Pathologists Press.
73. Saigo P, and others: Identification of *Cryptococcus neoformans* in cytologic preparations of cerebrospinal fluid, Am J Clin Pathol 67:141-145, 1977.
74. Schmidt P, and others: Primary malignant melanoblastosis of the meninges: clinical, cytologic and neuropathologic findings in a case, Acta Cytol 32:713-718, 1988.
75. Stanley MW, Frizzera G, and Dehner LP: Castleman's disease, plasma-cell type: diagnosis of central nervous system involvement by cerebrospinal fluid cytology, Acta Cytol 30:481-486, 1986.
76. Stanley MW, and Henry MJ: The significance of leukemia and lymphoma cells in cerebrospinal fluid contaminated by blood containing malignant cells: a probabilistic approach based on the Poisson frequency distribution, Diagn Cytopathol 4:193-195, 1988.
77. Stanley MW, Henry-Stanley MJ, and Iber C: Bronchoalveolar lavage: Cytology and Clinical Applications, New York, 1991, Igaku-Shoin.
78. Stanley MW, Lōwhagen T: Fine needle aspiration of palpable masses, Boston, 1993, Butterworth-Heinemann.
79. Stanley MW, and others: Classification of 358 cases of acute myeloid leukemia by FAB criteria: analysis of clinical and morphologic features. In Bloomfield C, editor: Chronic and acute leukemias in adults, 1985, Martinus-Nijhoff.
80. Steel JG, Dix RD, and Baringer JR: Isolation of herpes simplex virus type I in recurrent (Mollaret) meningitis Ann Neurol 11: 17-21, 1982.
81. Strigle SM, and Gal AA: Review of the central nervous system cytopathology in human immunodeficiency virus infection, Diagn Cytopathol 7:387-401, 1991.
82. Suarez C, and others: DNA and RNA determination in 111 cases of childhood acute lymphoblastic leukaemia (ALL) by flow cytometry: correlation of FAB classification with DNA stemline and proliferation, Br J Haematol 60:677-686, 1985.
83. Takeda M, and others: Diagnostic pitfalls in cerebrospinal fluid cytology, Acta Cytol 25:245-250, 1981.
84. Tzvetanova EM, and Tzekov CT: Eosinophilia in the cerebrospinal fluid of children with shunts implanted for the treatment of internal hydrocephalus, Acta Cytol 30:277-280, 1986.
85. Vick WW, and others: The use of a panel of monoclonal antibodies in the evaluation of cytologic specimens from the central nervous system, Acta Cytol 31:815-824, 1987.
86. Walts AE: Cerebrospinal fluid cytology: selected issues, Diagn Cytopathol 8:394-408, 1992.
87. Wasdahl DA, Goellner JR, and Scheithauer BW: Red blood cell "ghosts" as look-alikes for infectious organisms: a report of two cases, Acta Cytol 37:100-102, 1993.
88. Wasserstrom WR, Glass JP, and Posner JB: Diagnosis and treatment of leptomeningeal metastases from solid tumors: experience with 90 patients, Cancer 49:759-772, 1982.
89. Wasserstrom WR, and others: Cerebrospinal fluid biochemical markers in central nervous system tumors: a review, Ann Clin Lab Sci 11:239-251, 1981.
90. Wheeler RR, and others: Toxoplasma pneumonia: cytologic diagnosis by bronchoalveolar lavage, Diagn Cytopathol: 11:52-55, 1994.
91. Wilbur RR, King EB, and Howes EL: Cerebrospinal fluid cytology in five patients with cerebral cysticercosis, Acta Cytol 24: 421-426, 1980.
92. Wittekind DH, and Gehring T: On the nature of Romanowsky-Giemsa staining and the Romanowsky-Giemsa effect: I. Model experiments on the specificity of Azure B-Eosin Y stain as compared with other thiazine dye-Eosin Y combinations, Histochem J 17:263-289, 1985.
93. Yam LT, and others: Immunocytochemistry of cerebrospinal fluid, Acta Cytol 31:825-833, 1987.
94. Ziegler JL, and others: Non-Hodgkin's lymphoma in 90 homosexual men: relation to generalized lymphadenopathy and the acquired immunodeficiency syndrome, N Engl J Med 311:565-570, 1984.

C • H • A • P • T • E • R

# 2

# *Tumors: Applications of Light Microscopic Methods*

**Paul E. McKeever**
**Mila Blaivas**
**James S. Nelson**

This chapter focuses on the diagnosis of brain tumor specimens by H&E and tinctorial histologic stains alone. When a tumor diagnosis requires ultrastructural or immunocytochemical confirmation, a reference is given to the appropriate chapter in this book. Headings in this chapter are organized by specific categories of brain tumors, such as gliomas, neuronal tumors, multipotential neuroectodermal tumors, and others. The grade after the name of the tumor agrees with the grade from the most recent meeting of neuropathologists sponsored by the World Health Organization (WHO) when a grade was assigned by WHO.[81] Tumors of the pituitary region are described in Chapter 5.

Summary Tables 2–4 through 2–8 give concise information that should provide quick assistance in diagnosis. A specific tumor can be checked directly on the individual table where the structural and topographic features of tumors are listed. These tables also should help with unknown tumors that are characterized by some distinguishing features, such as fibrillar cells (Table 2-4), epithelioid cells (Table 2-6), more than one type of cell (Table 2-5), small malignant cells (Table 2-7), or "syncytial" cells (Table 2-8).

## PERTINENT CLINICAL HISTORY

Knowledge of the clinical history is necessary when dealing with brain tumors.[100] One should know the precise location of the lesion as well as the age and sex of the patient because certain tumors predominate in pediatric, adult, or geriatric age categories. The pathologist also should be familiar with available neuroimaging information, since images often substitute for direct macroscopic examination of the brain. An appropriate communication system between the surgical suite and the pathology diagnostic room is especially important so that clinical and pathologic observations on tumors interpreted intraoperatively can be shared.

## SURGICAL PROCEDURES

Knowing the purpose of the surgery helps the pathologist provide optimal interpretation of the specimens. There are three major reasons for operative procedures on brain tumors: diagnostic, assessment of therapy, and therapeutic resection. In some cases more than one goal is accomplished at a single operation. For example, biopsy for diagnosis of an eighth cranial nerve tumor will include therapeutic resection if the diagnosis is schwannoma.

### Biopsy for Diagnosis

Clinically suspected gliomas often are biopsied with no intention of further resection unless they are cerebellar pilocytic astrocytoma or ependymoma. It helps pathologists to be aware of macroscopic findings in situ, especially of the margin, and the precise point of attachment of a tumor. Brain tumor biopsies are inspected by frozen sections and cytologic preparations such as smears or touch preparations.[13] In addition to a diagnosis, the examination may provide confirmation that a representative biopsy has been obtained for later diagnosis, grading on permanent sections, and that any special tissue processing is done (Table 2-1). The principal objective of intraoperative monitoring is to avoid yet another biopsy for diagnosis. This means that tissue should be obtained and properly preserved for confirmation of diagnosis. Rebiopsy of the brain is costly, hazardous, and plagued by reactive changes from the previous intervention.

**Table 2-1.** Special procedures best accomplished during neurosurgical biopsy

| |
|---|
| Proper surgical sampling of the lesion itself |
| Special tissue processing |
| Culture for microorganisms |
| Fixation for electron microscopy |
| Fixation or extra frozen sections for immunohistochemistry |
| Fresh tissue for cytogenetics or DNA analysis |
| Precise diagnosis, if it affects the current surgical procedure |

One cannot expect to diagnose and grade every tumor precisely during surgery. For example, oligodendrogliomas and astrocytomas can be difficult to distinguish intraoperatively. Glioblastomas contain regions of lower grade, and this may be the only region biopsied initially. Further sampling for permanent sections can reveal neoplastic cells with a higher grade of malignancy.[127] Table 2-2 shows a list of interim diagnoses of brain tumors before the permanent sections are completed.

### Stereotactic Biopsy

Radiographically guided stereotactic needle biopsies are becoming standard for nonresectable tumors in clinically sensitive neuroanatomic regions of brain.[63,64] Gliomas involving the speech and motor cortex, thalamus, basal ganglia, and brainstem are the lesions most frequently approached by stereotactic biopsy. In less clinically sensitive regions, open biopsy is preferable because it provides a better tissue sample than does needle biopsy. Lesions firmer than gliomas frequently resist aspiration and may be sampled only by using biopsy needles especially made for these firm specimens. Most gliomas tend to be easily aspirated, whereas most nonglial neoplasms are difficult to aspirate.

Stereotactic needle biopsy specimens usually are taken with the guidance of radiographic coordinates. Understandably, lack of direct visualization of the lesion in situ makes sampling rather precarious. Differ-

**Table 2-2.** Descriptive terms useful on frozen section when precise diagnosis is not yet known

| Term | Appropriate use of term |
|---|---|
| Nondiagnostic biopsy | Pathologist suspects improper sampling; sole presence of hemorrhage, necrosis, and gliosis where a more specific diagnosis had been anticipated; margin of glioma, gray matter, white matter, or meninges |
| Encephalomalacia | A nonneoplastic lesion of gray or white matter of unknown etiology |
| Vascular malformation | Abnormal collection of vessels of unknown type |
| Gliosis versus glioma (glial proliferation) | Minimal glial hypercellularity in gray or white matter with features insufficient to diagnose glioma |
| Glioma | A glial neoplasm with no distinctive differential features |
| Glioma with treatment effects | A glial neoplasm with changes consistent with radiation or chemotherapy |
| Epithelioid neoplasm | A neoplasm with distinct cytoplasm and nonfibrillar cell margins with no distinctive differential features |
| Small cell neoplasm | A neoplasm crowded with small cells |
| Nerve sheath tumor | A schwannoma or neurofibroma |
| Germ cell tumor | A germinoma, choriocarcinoma, embryonal carcinoma, endodermal sinus tumor, teratoma, or some combination of these neoplasms |

From McKeever PE, and Blaivas M: Surgical pathology of the brain, spinal cord and meninges, In Sternberg S, and others, editors: Diagnostic Surgical Pathology, ed 2, New York, 1994, Raven.

ent samples of the same tumor may produce gliotic or totally necrotic, and thus nondiagnostic, tissue. For these reasons, stereotactic biopsies should be monitored during surgery. We prefer combining frozen sections with a separate cytologic preparation of a fraction of the biopsy when this can be done without drying of the tissue. To avoid drying, the tissue should be kept moist on saline-soaked gauze until the moment it is frozen or squeezed between glass slides.[13] The pathologist should ask the neurosurgeon to take an additional sample for permanent section from the diagnostically optimal region and to place it directly into fixative or onto saline-soaked gauze in a container. Needle biopsy specimens for electron microscopy are preferably extruded directly from the needle into glutaraldehyde to assure proper fixation.

We do not recommend stereotactic biopsies of cysts or of tumors that resemble normal tissue, like pineocytoma or choroid plexus papilloma. Of these, pineocytoma in the pineal region is the most problematic, since the location is difficult for an open biopsy approach, and well-differentiated pineocytoma resembles pineal gland. Retrospective radiography of the needle track may help to assess the "purity" of the tumor sample in equivocal cases.

### Biopsy to Assess Response to Therapy

Months or years following radiotherapy of a glioma, the declining clinical status of the patient may necessitate another biopsy to differentiate between recurrence of tumor and radiation necrosis. Current neuroimaging techniques do not reliably distinguish these entities. Necrosis is common in such biopsies. The most useful indicator of a good therapeutic response is scarcity of neoplastic cells. Positron emission tomographic (PET) scans may help in the future to differentiate radiation effects from recurrent neoplasia.

### Therapeutic Resection

Categories of therapeutic resection include gross total (100% removal of visible mass), radical subtotal (95% to 99% removal), subtotal (75% to 94% removal), and partial (10% to 74% removal).[100] Gross total resection is frequently performed for meningiomas, schwannomas, pituitary adenomas, solitary metastases, cysts, ependymomas, hemangioblastomas, and cerebellar pilocytic astrocytomas.

Caution should be used in interpreting tumors removed with a Cavitron ultrasonic aspirator (CUSA). Blue-tinged "necrosis" and linear streaks of nuclear material suggest artifact that must be distinguished from pinker and less distorted spontaneous tumor necrosis.

Table 2-3 shows the relative frequency of the most common brain tumors. Pediatric tumors predominate in the posterior fossa, whereas adult tumors are more frequent in the anterior fossa. The remainder of this chapter describes these and the less common brain tumors. It is organized by type of neoplastic cell, beginning with neoplastic glia.

## GLIOMAS

This term includes astrocytoma, ependymoma, oligodendroglioma, and glioblastoma. Unusual variants like the gliofibroma that transgress standard classifications are also included among gliomas (Figs. 2-1, 2-2). "Glioma" is too vague for a final diagnosis of properly sampled paraffin histologic sections; however, in frozen sections where the subtype of glioma is obscured or when the center of the tumor is missing, "glioma"

**Table 2-3.** Relative frequency of most common pediatric and adult brain neoplasms

| Children | | | Adults | | |
|---|---|---|---|---|---|
| **Location** | **Diagnosis and frequency (%)** | | **Location** | **Diagnosis and frequency (%)** | |
| Anterior fossa | Miscellaneous | 33 | Anterior fossa | Gliomas (cerebrum) | 33 |
| | | | | Meningiomas (dura) | 13 |
| | | | | Metastases (cerebrum) | 12 |
| | | | | Pituitary adenomas (sella) | 5 |
| | | | | Miscellaneous | 4 |
| | | | Total | | 67 |
| Posterior fossa | Astrocytomas (cerebellum)* | 26 | Posterior fossa | Schwannomas (8th nerve) | 8 |
| | | | | Miscellaneous | 25 |
| | Medulloblastomas/PNET† (cerebellum) | 24 | Total | | 33 |
| | Ependymomas (4th ventricle) | 14 | | | |
| | Miscellaneous | 3 | | | |
| Total | | 67 | | | |

From McKeever PE, and Blaivas M: Surgical pathology of the brain, spinal cord and meninges, In Sternberg S, and others, editors: Diagnostic Surgical Pathology, ed 2, New York, 1994, Raven.

* Most common site in parentheses. See text for other locations.

† PNET: primitive neuroectodermal tumor.

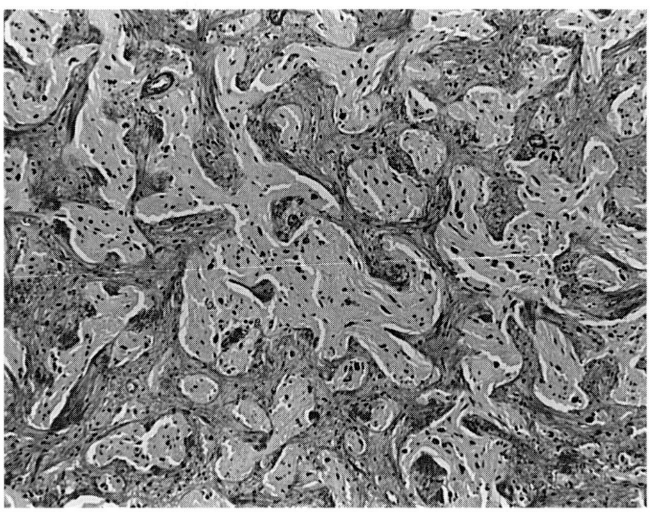

2-1

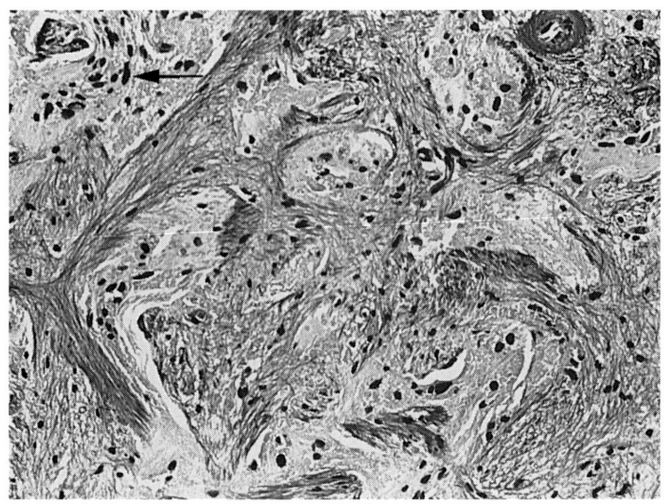

2-2

**Figs. 2-1, 2-2.** Gliofibroma. The 17-year-old man had a 2-cm tumor in his left parietal lobe. **Fig. 2-1,** This very firm tumor is a marbled mixture of collagenous bands and islands of astrocytes. (×100.) **Fig. 2-2,** A closer look at the islands of astrocytes reveals pleomorphic nuclei (*arrow*), low cellular density, and no mitoses. (×250.)

may be the best diagnosis (Table 2-2). Gliomas that involve the sella are described in Chapter 5.

The term "low-grade," applied to gliomas means low grade of malignancy and not that the glioma is a benign neoplasm. The designation "benign" implies that once removed the neoplasm will not recur, and this should not be confused with "low grade." Pilocytic astrocytomas and ependymomas are sometimes considered benign, but even these tumors need to be in favorable locations for there to be a good chance for cure.[1,26]

## Tumor and Margin

There are two types of glioma specimens. The first comes from the core of the tumor and has a cellular density exceeding that of cerebral white matter or neocortex (Fig. 2-3). A precise diagnosis and grade number can be assigned to this specimen using a particular grading system (i.e., 1993 World Health Organization (WHO),[81] Ringertz[113]). The highest grade found in the specimen is the grade to be reported. Some gliomas are exceedingly diffuse lacking a distinct mass (gliomatosis cerebri) (Fig. 2-4) and some others are multicentric.[91,129]

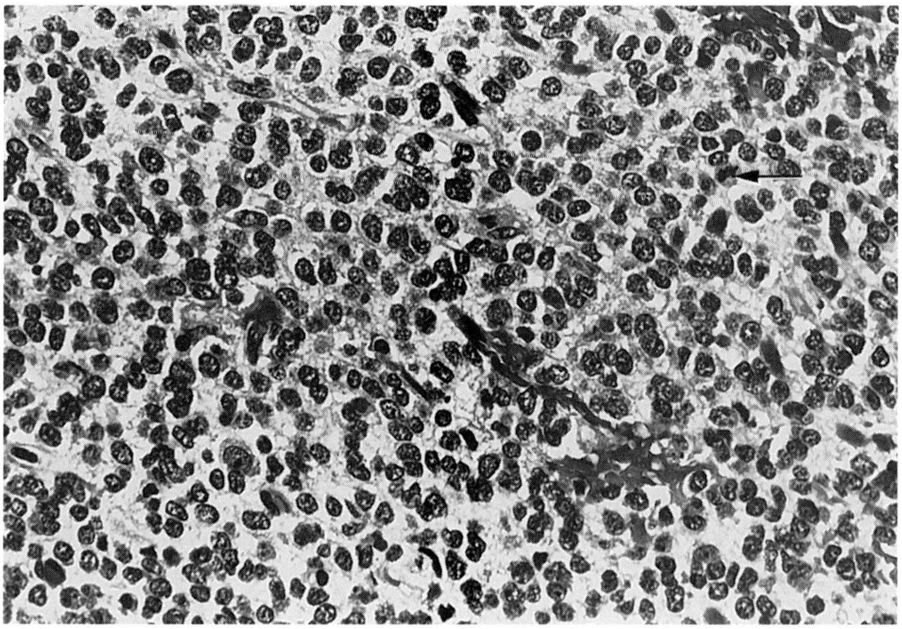

**Fig. 2-3.** Center of a glioma. Crowded cells with round and pleomorphic nuclei, perinuclear halos, and mitoses (*arrow*) comprise this tumor. Anaplastic oligodendroglioma. (×400.)

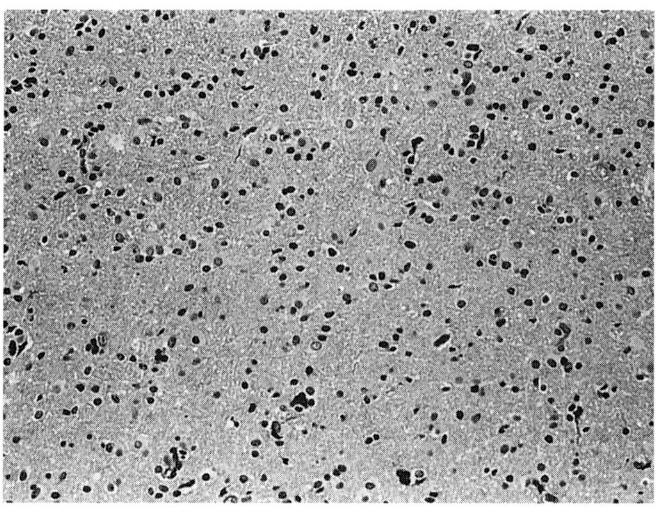

**Fig. 2-4.** Gliomatosis cerebri. Slight hypercellularity of the white matter is due to diffuse proliferation of small pleomorphic glial nuclei without visible cytoplasm. They form small clusters of satellites around rare neurons and small vessels. There is no necrosis, no significant mitotic activity, and no endothelial proliferation. The 56-year-old patient had right facial weakness followed by decreased right hand strength and mobility. (×165.)

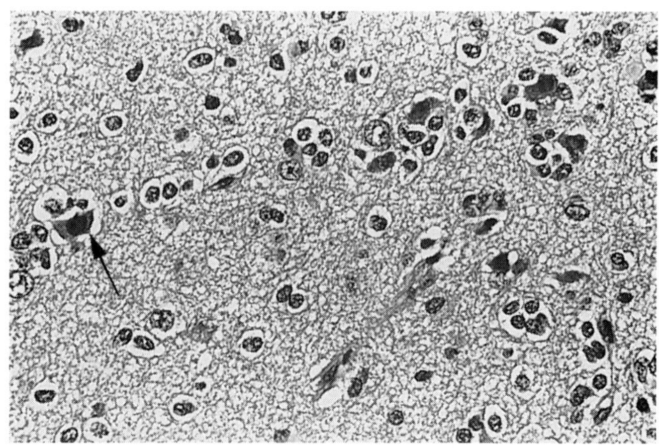

**Fig. 2-5.** Neoplastic cells cluster around shrunken neurons (*arrow*), forming perineuronal gliomatosis secondary structures. Perinuclear halos around round nuclei reflect the oligodendroglial origin of these neoplastic cells. While this tumor margin is from the anaplastic oligodendroglioma in Fig. 2-3, its precise diagnosis and grade are not revealed in this marginal sample. (×400.)

The second type of specimen is brain infiltrated by neoplastic glia that reflects the infiltrative margin of many gliomas (Fig. 2-5).[30,100] The histologic grade and type of the core of a glioma generating an infiltrative margin of neoplastic glia are moot when only the margin is available for examination.[127] The surgeon should be alerted to this during the procedure, thus providing the opportunity to obtain a better specimen. For this reason, monitoring each glioma biopsy with frozen sections is recommended. Unless glioblastoma is the unequivocal diagnosis at the time of biopsy, grading of the malignancy is best reserved until all tissue specimens have been collected and processed for paraffin sections.

Neoplastic glia infiltrating brain parenchyma frequently are difficult to distinguish from reactive gliosis. Mitoses, among other features mentioned below, suggest that the distant tumor could be a glioma of high grade.

### Gliosis Versus Glioma

Gliosis is sometimes difficult to differentiate from an incomplete sample of a glioma. Cellular density can provide valuable information. Gliosis is either even in distribution or has a subtly increasing cellularity from one side of the section to the other; gliomas may produce uneven hypercellularity and obscure the junction between gray and white matter.[100] Gliomas also *secondary structures of Scherer* (Fig. 2-6), the most diagnostic being subpial and perineuronal accumulations of neoplastic glia (Figs. 2-5, 2-7).

Nuclear spacing is different in gliosis and in a glioma. Glial nuclei in gliotic brain avoid touching one another (Fig. 2-8), whereas glioma nuclei touch and indent each other, producing so-called nuclear molding (Fig. 2-7).

Nuclear *hyperchromasia* and *pleomorphism* are additional features that help to differentiate gliomas from gliosis. The nuclei of neoplastic glia are darker and more pleomorphic than those of gliosis (Figs. 2-7, 2-8).

Radiographically, gliomas are expanding lesions, whereas gliosis is a contracting one. Serial radiographs and in situ observation provide valuable information.

### Astrocytomas

Most astrocytomas are fibrillar brain tumors (Table 2-4). The only gliomas to rival their fibrillarity are subependymomas and tanycytic ependymomas. Astrocytomas express GFAP.[103] The use of GFAP in their diagnosis is discussed in Chapter 4.

There are many subtypes of astrocytomas and their definition may be confusing because some classifications emphasize grade of malignancy whereas others emphasize structural differences. The most valuable structural features are those that indicate a different prognosis.[102] Those features are emphasized in a recent classification.[81] For example, the lowest grade of astrocytoma is reserved for the pilocytic astrocytoma, which frequently can be cured by surgical removal when it occurs in a clinically resectable region such as the cerebellum.

**Pilocytic astrocytoma—grade I.** Most pilocytic astrocytomas occur in children. These tumors are frequent in the posterior fossa, where they represent the astrocytomas most common in pediatric age (Fig. 2-9; Tables 2-3, 2-4). Pilocytic astrocytomas also can arise in the third

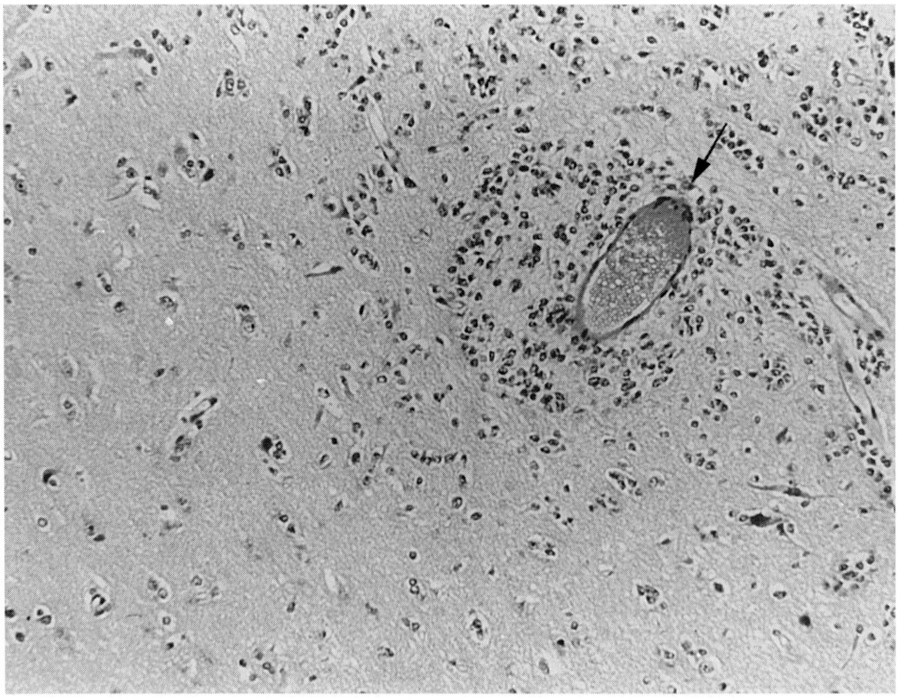

**Fig. 2-6.** Perivascular secondary structures of Scherer (*arrow*) are produced at the distant margin of an oligoastrocytoma. The 43-year-old man had partial complex seizures and a right temporal lobe mass. (×125.)

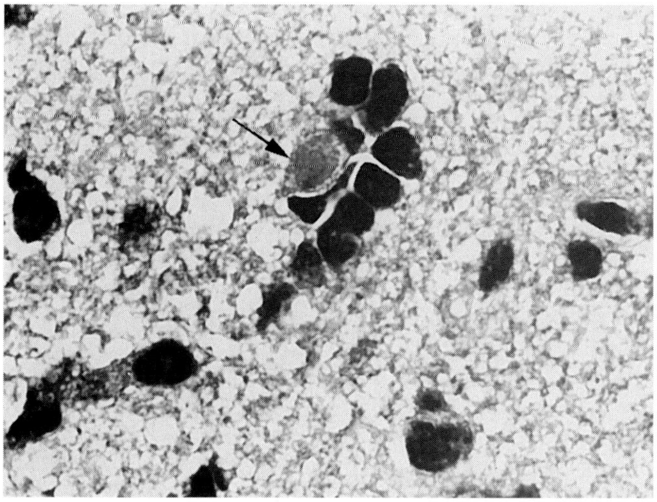

**Fig. 2-7.** Perineuronal gliomatosis. More than eight hyperchromatic and pleomorphic nuclei surround this neuron (*arrow*). The diagnosis and grade of the nearby glioma cannot be determined from this marginal sample. (×1600.)

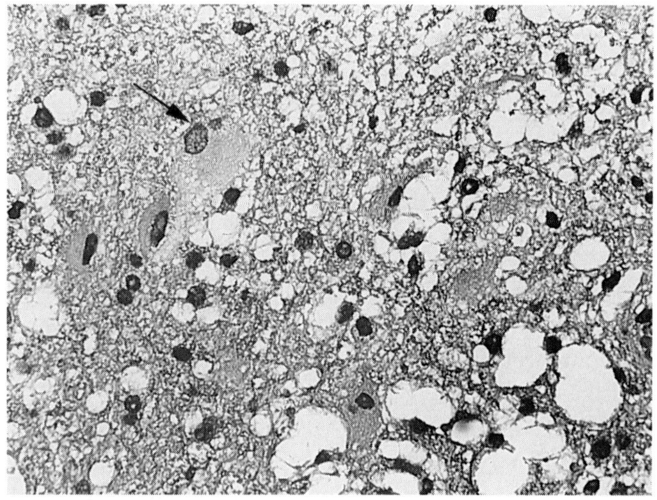

**Fig. 2-8.** Gliosis and edema. This brain tissue is busy with reactive astrocytes (*arrow*) and glia. Some astrocytes show nuclear and nucleolar enlargement as well as hypertrophic, pink cytoplasm. However, their chromatin is dispersed and finely granular, and their nuclei do not indent one another. Vacuolization is due to edema. (×400.)

**Table 2-4.** Features of different brain tumors with fibrillar cells

| | Features | |
|---|---|---|
| **Diagnosis*** | **Structures** | **Locations†** |
| Pilocytic astrocytoma | Hypercellularity; hairlike fibrillarity; Rosenthal fibers; microcysts | Cerebellum; thalamus/hypothalamus; optic nerve; CNS |
| Astrocytoma | Hypercellularity; angular nuclei cluster and indent each other; infiltrates CNS | Cerebrum; brainstem; spinal cord; CNS |
| Anaplastic astrocytoma | Increase in above features; mitoses; endothelial proliferation | Cerebrum; brainstem; CNS |
| Gemistocytic astrocytoma | Hypercellularity; cells swollen with hyaline pink cytoplasm and eccentric pleomorphic nuclei; infiltrates CNS | Cerebrum |
| Giant cell astrocytoma | Giant astrocytes with thick fibrils; large round/oval nuclei | Lateral ventricle; subependymal |
| Astroblastoma | Perivascular rosettes with expanded glial cell processes | Cerebrum; CNS |
| Pleomorphic xanthoastrocytoma | Pleomorphic cells often are vacuolated | Leptomeninges; cerebral cortex |
| Ependymoma | Hypercellularity; ependymal and/or perivascular rosettes; round/oval nuclei; cilia; basal bodies | Cerebrum; cerebellum; spinal cord; CNS |
| Anaplastic ependymoma | Above features with mitoses; necrosis; endothelial proliferation | Cerebrum; cerebellum |
| Tanycytic ependymoma/ subependymoma | Clusters of cells and fibrils; round/oval nuclei cluster among fibrillar mats | Spinal cord; 4th ventricle; subependymal; CNS |
| Glioblastoma multiforme | Regions of coagulation necrosis; mitoses; pleomorphism; endothelial proliferation | Cerebrum; CNS |
| Gliosarcoma | Glioblastoma plus fibrosarcoma intermixed | Cerebrum |
| Ganglion-cell tumors | Pleomorphic and binucleated neurons; diagnosis depends on gliomatous and neuroblastic elements | Cerebrum; CNS |
| Central neurocytoma | Round cells and nuclei; perinuclear halos; thin fibrils near vessels | Septum pellucidum; lateral ventricles |
| Pineocytoma | Resembles pineal structures | Pineal body |

*Continued.*

**Table 2-4.** Features of different brain tumors with fibrillar cells—cont'd

| Diagnosis* | Features | |
|---|---|---|
| | **Structures** | **Locations†** |
| Polar spongioblastoma | Rhythmic pallisades of fibrillary cells | Cerebrum; CNS |
| Fibroblastic meningioma | Spindle cells; interdigitating cell processes and desmosomes; (thick collagen); (whorls)‡ | Falx, tentorium; meninges; choroid plexus |
| Fibrosarcoma/malignant fibrous histiocytoma | Hypercellular; pleomorphic spindle cells and nuclei; mitoses; necrosis | Meninges; CNS |
| Schwannoma | Verocay bodies; Antoni A and B; thin pericellular basement membrane | 8th cranial nerve; spinal roots; PNS |
| Neurofibroma | Multiple cell types spread axons | Spinal root; PNS; cranial nerve |
| Histiocytosis | Sheetlike pattern of macrophages, fibroblasts, and leukocytes | Parasellar; CNS; systemic |
| Hemangioblastoma | Multivacuolated stromal cells between many capillaries; hypervascularity; (fibrillarity is frozen section artifact) | Cerebellum; spinal cord; CNS |
| Melanoma | Anaplasia, mitoses, necrosis, melanin | CNS/meninges; frequent multiple metastases; systemic |

* Adapted from McKeever PE, and Blaivas M: The brain, spinal cord and meninges, In Sternberg S, and others: Diagnostic Surgical Pathology, ed 2, New York, 1994, Raven Press.
† Most common or most specific craniospinal location is listed first.
‡ Parentheses around a differential feature indicate an uncommon feature very useful in differential diagnosis when found. CNS = central nervous system; PNS = peripheral nervous system.

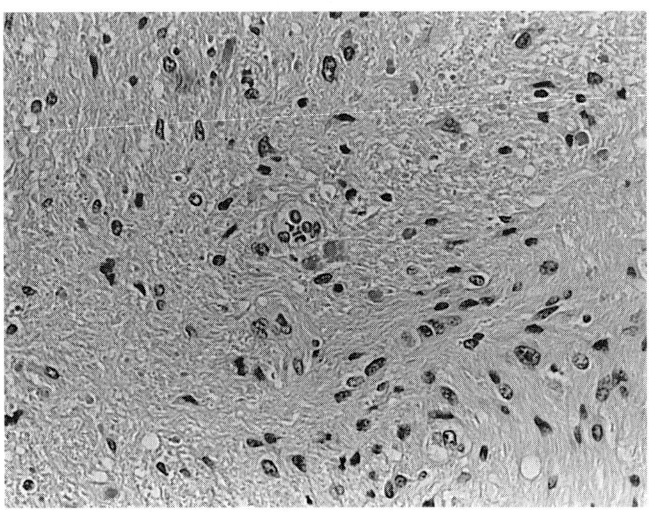

**Fig. 2-9.** Pilocytic astrocytoma. Vast bundles of fibrillary cellular processes are produced by these neoplastic astrocytes with pleomorphic nuclei and no mitoses. The 9-year-old girl had a cystic tumor with a mural nodule in her cerebellum. (×400.)

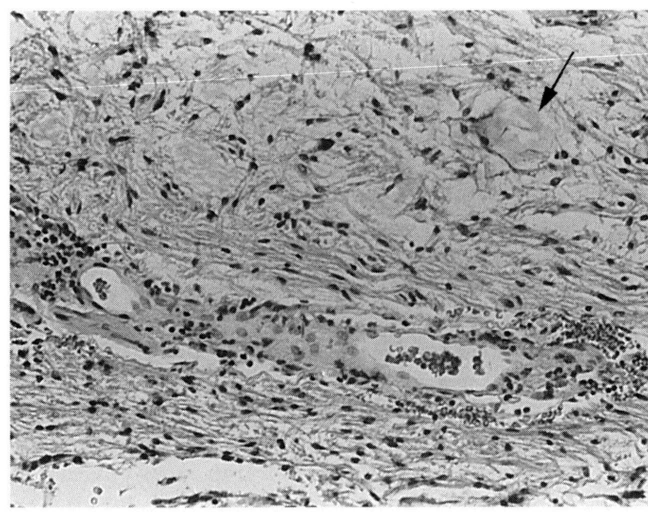

**Fig. 2-10.** Optic nerve glioma. Typically these are pilocytic astrocytomas. Numerous fibrillar cellular processes extend from widely-separated neoplastic astrocytes. Scattered small microcysts contain faintly hematoxylinophilic mucin (*arrow*). The 7-year-old girl had a tumor involving her optic chiasm. (×200.)

ventricle, thalamus, hypothalamus, optic chiasm (Fig. 2-10), and neurohypophysis. Cerebral pilocytic astrocytomas are less common than those in the cerebellum.[24] Radiographically and macroscopically, these astrocytomas are well demarcated from brain, but local microscopic infiltration may be encountered.[25]

It is important to identify the pilocytic astrocytoma because its prognosis is much better than that of infiltrative astrocytomas.[58] The 10-year survival is 100% after gross total resection and 74% after subtotal resection or biopsy.[40]

"Pilocytic" means "hair cell," and refers to parallel

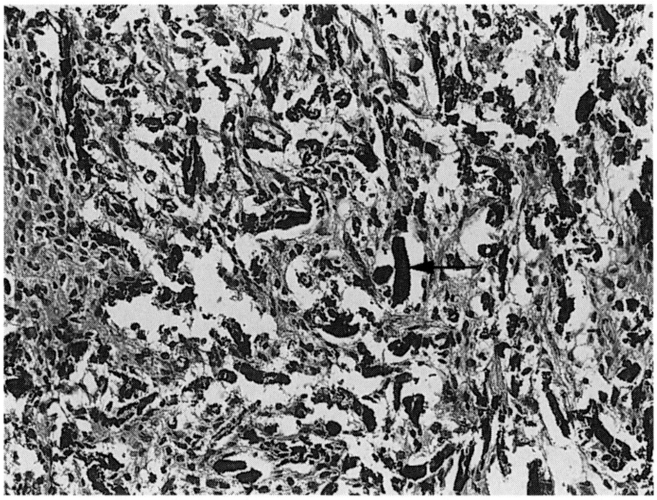

**Fig. 2-11.** Pilocytic astrocytoma. The vessels are calcified (*arrow*), causing the fibrillary astrocytic cells of this astrocytoma to break apart upon sectioning. The 30-year-old woman has had headaches for 18 years, increasing over the last 2 years, and a cyst with this nodule in her right basal ganglia. (×200.)

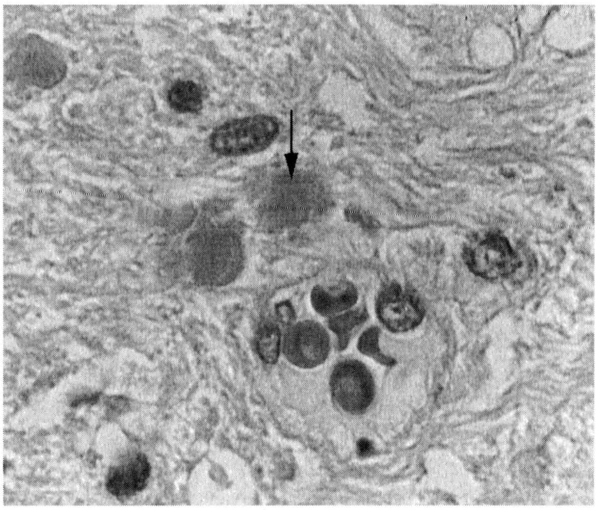

**Fig. 2-12.** Rosenthal fibers. The Rosenthal fibers (*arrow*) in this pilocytic astrocytoma are more pink and more heterogeneous in size and shape than the orange, biconcave erythrocytes in the vessel below them. (×1600.) (See Plate 1A.)

bundles of elongated fibrillar cytoplasmic processes, a characteristic feature of this neoplasm. These hairlike processes contain large amounts of glial fibrils (see Chapters 3 and 4). As is true of many low-grade gliomas, pilocytic astrocytomas may calcify[100] (Fig. 2-11).

Another characteristic feature of pilocytic astrocytomas, *Rosenthal fibers* are bright pink hyaline structures in H&E stained sections (Fig. 2-12, Plate 1A). These fibers are round, oval, or beaded, with slightly irregular margins.[24] Rosenthal fibers are formed within glial processes and often are confused with erythrocytes, even though they are pink rather than orange and vary in size and shape more than erythrocytes. Rosenthal fibers help distinguish the pilocytic astrocytoma from other astrocytomas; however, Rosenthal fibers also occur at sites of gliosis. This is particularly confusing in cases of gliosis around a craniopharyngioma, an ependymoma, a multiple sclerosis plaque, or a syrinx, where Rosenthal fibers can be abundant and inadequate sampling may not identify the actual tumor.

Eosinophilic intracellular protein droplets are commonly seen in pilocytic astrocytomas. These droplets are more pink than the lipid droplets seen within reactive macrophages and are highly variable in size, usually from 1 to 10 $\mu$m. Oligodendroglioma-like foci of cells with perinuclear halos also can be present in these neoplasms.

Macroscopic cavities or cysts occur frequently in pilocytic astrocytomas of the cerebellum, in which case they must be distinguished from cavitary hemangioblastomas.[17] Both of these tumors may exist as a nodule in the wall of the cavity; however, in pilocytic astrocytoma the nodule is formed by fibrillar astrocytes that lack the lipid droplets detectable in the stroma cells of a hemangioblastoma.

The pilocytic astrocytoma is the most "benign" astrocytoma. Nonetheless, adequate surgical removal of a pilocytic astrocytoma depends on its location. Many pilocytic astrocytomas have discrete margins that allow total resection.

Features such as vascular proliferation, necrosis, and invasion of the subarachnoid space in pilocytic astrocytomas lack the ominous significance that these features imply in other astrocytomas.

**Astrocytoma (low-grade astrocytoma)—grade II.** The designation "low-grade" is often dropped, and this group of gliomas is described simply as "astrocytomas." These astrocytomas are most prevalent in the cerebrum in adults and the brainstem in children. The diffuse astrocytoma margin gradually diminishes in cellularity as neoplastic cells intermingle with brain tissue. These astrocytomas are difficult to distinguish from gliosis in small tissue samples.[155]

Fibrillary astrocytomas are a mixture of fibrils and nuclei with greater angularity and density than those seen in normal glia (Fig. 2-13). Most important to their diagnosis are pleomorphic and hyperchromatic nuclei, as described in the section on gliosis versus glioma. Their nuclei are more elongated than those of oligodendrogliomas and they have fibrillary cellular processes that extend from the neoplastic cells.

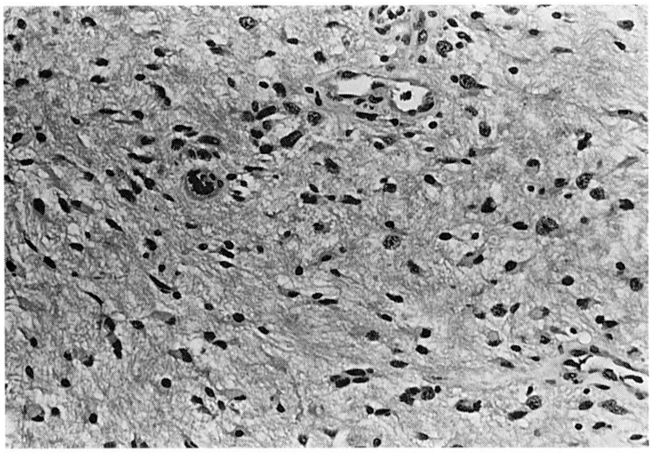

**Fig. 2-13.** Fibrillary astrocytoma. Cells with slightly hyperchromatic and pleomorphic nuclei infiltrate spinal cord parenchyma, and are mixed with gliosis. This diffuse astrocytoma is grade II. The 22-year-old woman had an intrinsic spinal cord tumor expanding her conus medullaris. (×250.)

Protoplasmic astrocytomas are less common than fibrillary astrocytomas. They have fewer and shorter cellular processes than fibrillary or pilocytic astrocytomas (Fig. 2-14). Patients with diffuse cerebral astrocytomas are seldom cured despite the relatively benign course of these neoplasms. Postoperative survival averages 7 years, ranging between 1 and 20 years. As expected from their critical location, brainstem astrocytomas have a poorer prognosis than do those involving the cerebrum; this is particularly true of pontine tumors not associated with neurofibromatosis.[112] Dedifferentiation to a more malignant astrocytoma was a more common cause of death than the growth of the original low-grade tumor in at least one study.[162]

**Anaplastic astrocytoma—grade III.** "Anaplastic" corresponds to the grade of malignancy. Mitoses are an important feature of anaplastic astrocytomas (Fig. 2-15). The following are increased compared with low-grade astrocytoma: cellular density, nuclear pleomorphism, and nuclear hyperchromatism (Fig. 2-16). Most of these features are subjective and difficult to quantitate. Nonetheless, astrocytomas of grade III or higher usually have regions where the average distance between two nuclei that are not actually touching is less than the average nuclear diameter.[100] Anaplastic astrocytomas rarely undergo granular cell change that could confuse these tumors with reactive processes.[47]

Absence of regions of coagulation necrosis in astroglial tumors with increased cell density, mitoses, and pleomorphism distinguishes anaplastic astrocytomas from glioblastomas[118]; however, individual degenerative cells with pyknotic nuclei are found in anaplastic astrocytomas.[147] A recent classification considers the presence of prominent vascular cell proliferation to be sufficient reason to classify an anaplastic astrocytoma as a glioblastoma.[81] This change will affect clinical studies of survival rate that use this new grading system as compared with previous ones.[16,71,100,118,172]

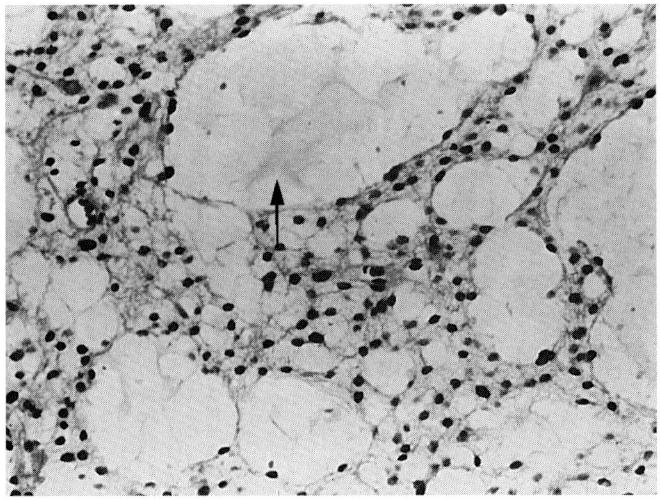

**Fig. 2-14.** Protoplasmic astrocytoma. Neoplastic astrocytes extend short cytoplasmic processes from their small cell bodies. Microcysts are filled with pale, eosinophilic material (*arrow*). Cellular fibrils are less prominent than fibrils of fibrillary astrocytomas. The 14-year-old girl had a 10-month history of seizures, and a parietal mass. (×200.)

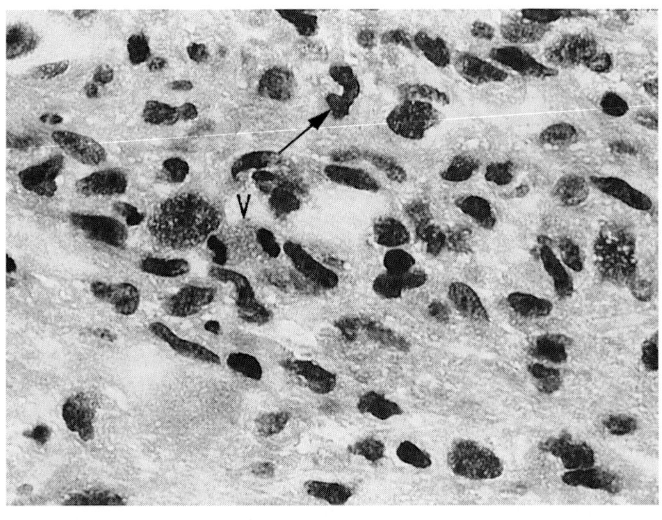

**Fig. 2-15.** Anaplastic astrocytoma. Mitotic activity (*arrowhead*) and considerable nuclear pleomorphism (*arrow*) characterize this left frontal fibrillary astrocytoma as grade III. The 80-year-old woman recently developed progressive right facial paralysis. She had a large left frontal and parietal tumor. (×1000.) (Courtesy of Dr. Roger A. Hawkins, Greenville, PA.)

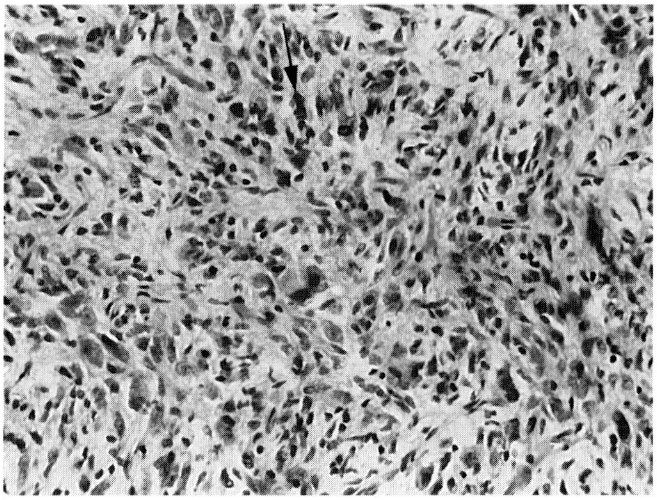

**Fig. 2-16.** Anaplastic astrocytoma. Pleomorphic cells and nuclei crowd together. Nuclear pleomorphism and hyperchromasia (*arrow*) and mitoses are present. The 38-year-old man had progressive headaches, recent memory problems, and a mass in his frontal lobe. (×200.)

Patients with anaplastic astrocytomas survive an average of slightly more than 2 years.[118] Rare anaplastic astrocytomas occur in the clinical context of hereditary colonic polyposis[119] and neurofibromatosis.[32]

**Gemistocytic astrocytoma—grade II with poor prognosis.** These astrocytomas are formed by gemistocytes, which are cells with swollen, plump, hyaline, pink cytoplasm (Fig. 2-17). Their hyperchromatic pleomorphic nuclei are at the periphery, producing a bizarre caricature of a reactive astrocyte.[100] (Non-neoplastic highly reactive astrocytes are also called gemistocytes.) Many gemistocytic astrocytomas have perivascular cuffs of polyclonal lymphocytes.

The grade of these astrocytomas is controversial. Pure or predominantly gemistocytic astrocytomas frequently behave aggressively and have a poorer prognosis than suggested by their histologic grade. Even grade II astrocytomas that contain as few as 20% gemistocytes, according to Krouwer and associates,[84] had shorter average 5-year survival. These authors recommended that gemistocytic astrocytomas be considered anaplastic astrocytomas.

Gemistocytic astrocytomas may resemble gangliogliomas, but their gemistocytes are not neoplastic neurons since they lack Nissl substance, neuronal proteins, and axons (Fig. 2-18, Plate 1B) (Chapter 4). They also resemble subependymal giant cell tumors but compared to these, gemistocytic astrocytomas have smaller nuclei and a greater tendency to infiltrate CNS.

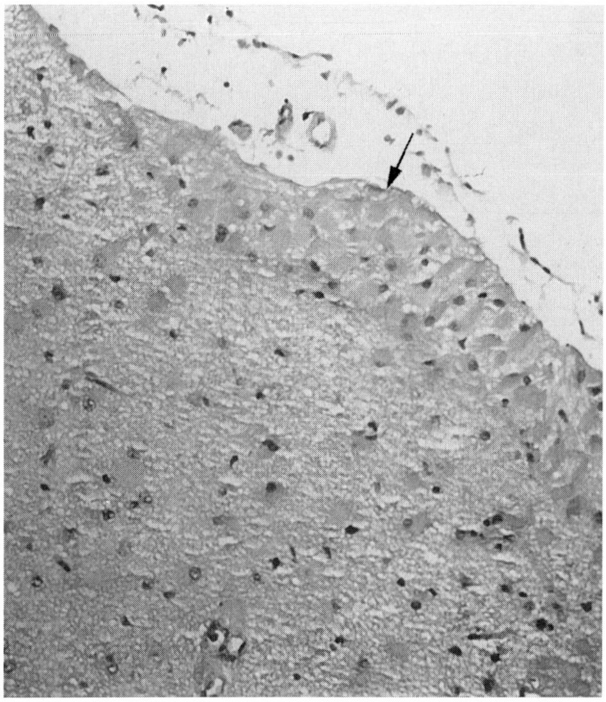

**Fig. 2-17.** Gemistocytic astrocytoma: subpial secondary structure of Scherer. Neoplastic gemistocytes cluster beneath the pia (*arrow*) at this margin of a gemistocytic astrocytoma. (×125.)

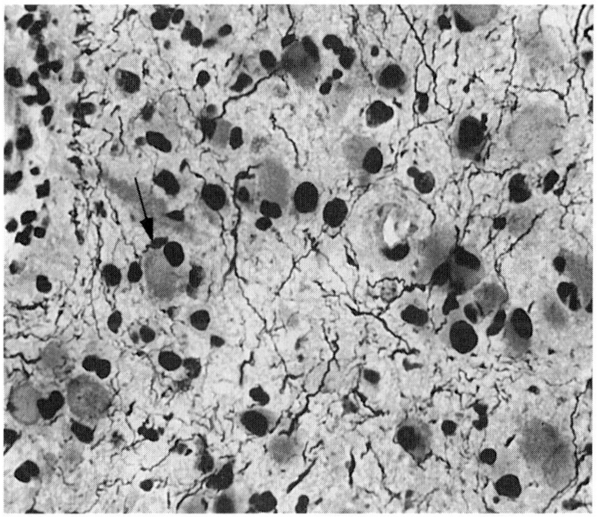

**Fig. 2-18.** Gemistocytic astrocytoma. Black axons of cerebral white matter are infiltrated and spread apart by neoplastic gemistocytes (*arrow*) of a gemistocytic astrocytoma. Axons do not originate in neoplastic cells. Similar infiltration is common among gliomas of grade II and higher, such as fibrillary astrocytomas. (LFB/Homes Stain; ×400.) (See Plate 1B.)

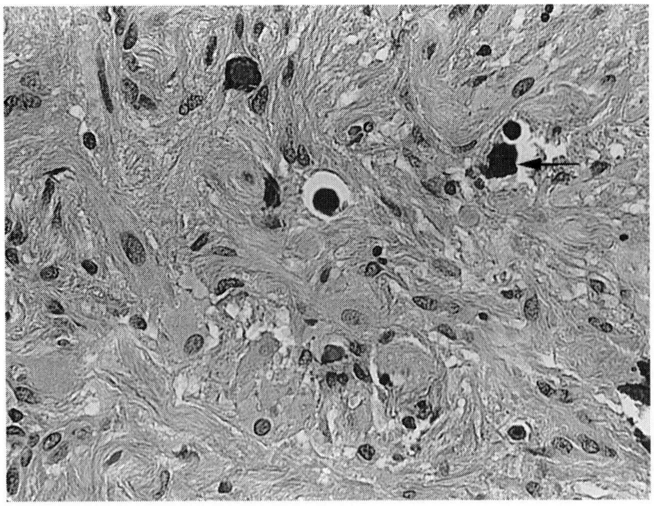

**Fig. 2-19.** Subependymal giant cell astrocytoma. Large astrocytes extend numerous fibrils that separate cells to low density. Microscopic calcifications (*arrow*) are present, but mitoses are not. The 18-year-old man with tuberous sclerosis had headaches, visual impairment, and a large mass protruding into his third ventricle. (×400.)

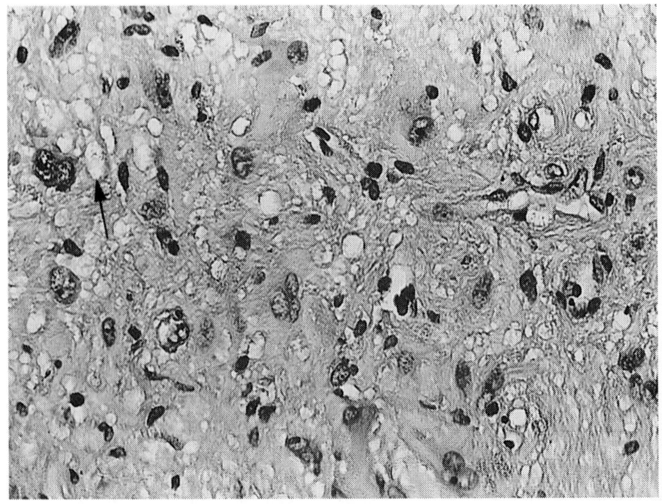

**Fig. 2-20.** Pleomorphic xanthoastrocytoma. Some of these pleomorphic astrocytes have pink cytoplasm and others are filled with cytoplasmic vacuoles (*arrow*). (×400.)

**Subependymal giant-cell astrocytoma—grade I.** This tumor often is associated with tuberous sclerosis and has a characteristic location and histology.[32] The tumor usually is attached to the medial portion of the floor of a lateral ventricle, but it may involve a different site. In the context of tuberous sclerosis, nearby subependymal nodules of giant astrocytes, called "candle gutterings," can be found. The tumor is exophytic and may cause obstructive hydrocephalus by blocking the foramen of Monro.

Giant astrocytes with large nuclei and prominent nucleoli can frighten the unwary diagnostician (Fig. 2-19). However, these large oval nuclei lack sharp angular features of malignancy. The giant astrocytes form disoriented fascicles composed of characteristically thick cytoplasmic processes. The immunocytochemistry of these cells is both characteristic and fascinating (Chapter 4).

It is very important to recognize the giant-cell astrocytoma because it is less aggressive than its histologic appearance suggests. The neoplasm is associated with tuberous sclerosis, and features considered high-grade in diffuse fibrillary astrocytomas are not as worrisome here. Mitoses are neither as common nor as ominous as in diffuse cerebral astrocytomas.

**Pleomorphic xanthoastrocytoma—grade II.** The pleomorphic xanthoastrocytoma is a superficial cerebral astrocytoma of young people that often involves the meninges.[89] It is formed by fibrillary, pleomorphic, hyaline, lipid-laden, and multinucleated cells that distinguish it from other astrocytomas, but can cause confusion with nonastrocytic tumors (Fig. 2-20). Immunocytochemical confirmation of neoplastic astrocytes is recommended (Chapter 4); cells of this astrocytoma have odd features suggestive of histiocytes, and some cells express neuronal antigens.[83,131] Intracellular lipid content varies among individual tumors. The presence of pericellular reticulin fibers is an exception to the general rule that glioma cells lack reticulin (Fig. 2-21).[51,76] Some tumors have more reticulin in their superficial margins than in their deep margins. Rare xanthoastrocytomas are overtly malignant (Figs. 2-22 to 2-24).

**Astroblastoma.** This tumor is rare. Its relation to astrocytoma, its grade, and even its existence as a pure pathologic entity remain controversial.[62,81,145] Astroblastic "rosettes" differ subtly from perivascular pseudorosettes of ependymomas in that their cellular processes remain thick the entire distance from cell body to adventitia of the vessel.[100,145] Foot processes may form near the adventitia (Fig. 2-25).

### Ependymomas

Ependymomas vary by their subtype between fibrillar and epithelial (Tables 2-4 and 2-5). Subependymomas are more fibrillar and resemble astrocytomas, whereas myxopapillary and clear cell ependymomas are more epithelioid and resemble meningiomas and oligodendrogliomas. In specimens of sufficient size, focal fibrillarity is often present in these epithelioid ependymomas (Table 2-5).

In cases of suspected ependymoma, finding rosettes and specific ultrastructural features (Chapter 3) will help confirm the diagnosis. The luminal rosette or true

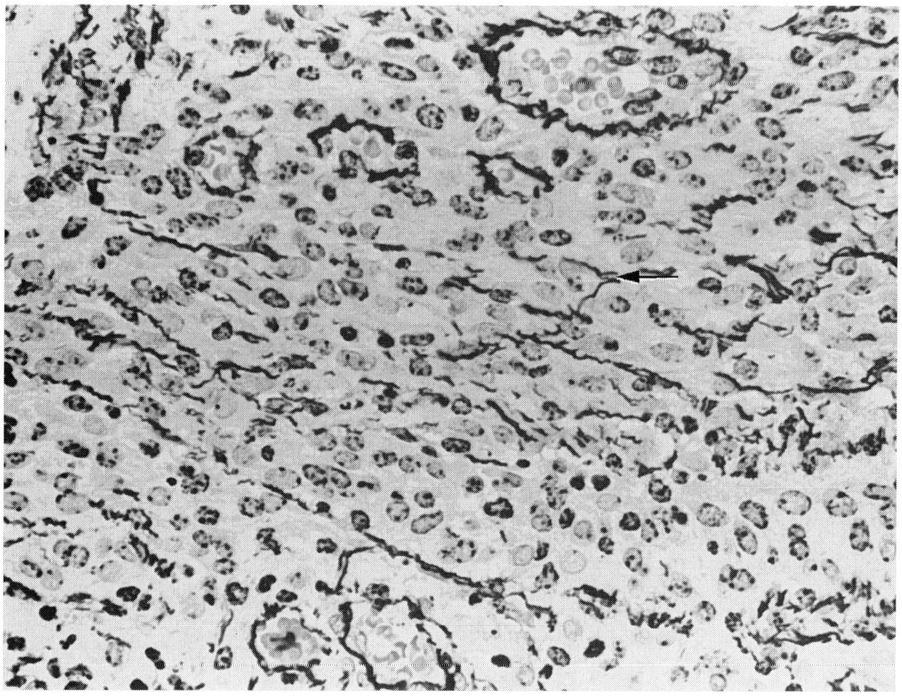

**Fig. 2-21.** Pleomorphic xanthoastrocytoma. Reticulin is present not only around vessels, but also between tumor cells (*arrow*). The 13-year-old patient had a slow onset of headaches and seizures and a partially cystic mass within the superficial right temporal and parietal lobes. Snook's silver stain for reticulin with nuclear fast red counterstain. (×400.) (Courtesy of Dr. George K. Tong, Saginaw, MI.)

**Table 2-5.** Features of brain tumors composed of conspicuously different cells

| Diagnosis | Features: Structure* | Features: Location† |
|---|---|---|
| Ependymoma/malignant ependymoma | Ependymoma or malignant ependymoma plus epithelioid cells | Cerebellum; cerebrum; spinal cord; CNS |
| Myxopapillary ependymoma | Cuboidal/columnar epithelium on hyaline fibrovascular papillae; variable fibrillarity; mucin | Region of the filum terminale |
| Oligoastrocytoma | Mixture of astrocytoma and oligodendroglioma | Cerebrum; CNS |
| Anaplastic oligoastrocytoma | Above features with mitoses and pleomorphism | Cerebrum; CNS |
| Glioblastoma/gliosarcoma with epithelial metaplasia | Glioblastoma/gliosarcoma plus epithelial regions | Cerebrum; CNS |
| Ganglion cell tumors | Binucleated and pleomorphic neurons ± glioma plus fibrosis ± inflammation | Cerebrum; CNS |
| Desmoplastic medulloblastoma | Regions of medulloblastoma and fibrosis | Lateral cerebellum; CNS; meninges; (extraaxial)‡ |
| Transitional meningioma | Regions of fibrous and syncytial meningioma | Falx; tentorium; meninges; choroid plexus |
| Germinoma | Regions of large epithelioid cells and small lymphocytes | Pineal; parasellar; CNS |
| Teratoma | Well-differentiated tissues from more than one germinal layer; may contain another germ-cell-tumor component; mucin; collagen | Pineal; suprasellar; sacrococcygeal |
| Choriocarcinoma | Syncytial and cytotrophoblast | Pineal; parasellar; CNS§ |
| Desmoplastic carcinoma | Regions of carcinoma and fibrosis ± inflammation; mucin | Cerebrum; cerebellum; meninges; CNS; frequent multiple masses; systemic |
| Melanoma | Regions of fibrillar and epithelioid melanoma; melanin | Cerebrum; cerebellum; meninges; CNS; frequently multiple masses; systemic |

* Adapted from McKeever PE, and Blaivas M: The brain, spinal cord and meninges, In Sternberg S, and others, editors: Diagnostic Surgical Pathology, ed 2, New York, 1994, Raven Press. Refer to primary entry in Tables 2-4, 2-6, 2-8 for further description of structures.

† Most common or most specific craniospinal location is listed first.

‡ Parentheses around a differential feature indicate an uncommon feature very useful in differential diagnosis when found.

§ As a primary midline tumor or metastasis to CNS from pelvic or gonadal primary.

**Figs. 2-22 to 2-24.** Malignant pleomorphic xanthoastrocytoma. The 44-year-old woman had several months' history of headaches diagnosed as a cavernous malformation in the superficial left temporal region associated with the dura. She developed right arm numbness, more severe sudden headaches, and aphasia. MRI was still consistent with a cavernous malformation; however, the lesion tripled in size within the last 3 months. **Fig. 2-22,** Markedly pleomorphic hypercellular neoplasm is composed of astrocytes with hyperchromatic bizarre shaped nuclei, mitoses (*arrow*) and abundant vacuolated cytoplasm. (×330.) **Fig. 2-23,** Mitotic figures are abundant and lymphocytic inflammation (*arrow*) is common. (×165.) **Fig. 2-24,** Reticulin fibers are scattered throughout the clusters of neoplastic cells as in the more common benign variant. (×165.)

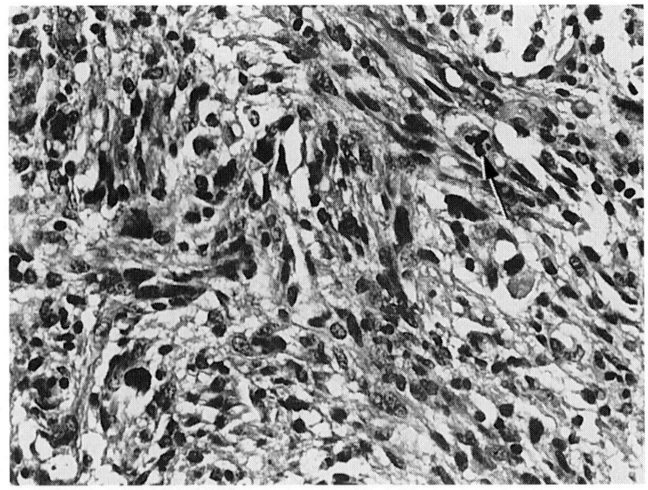

2-22

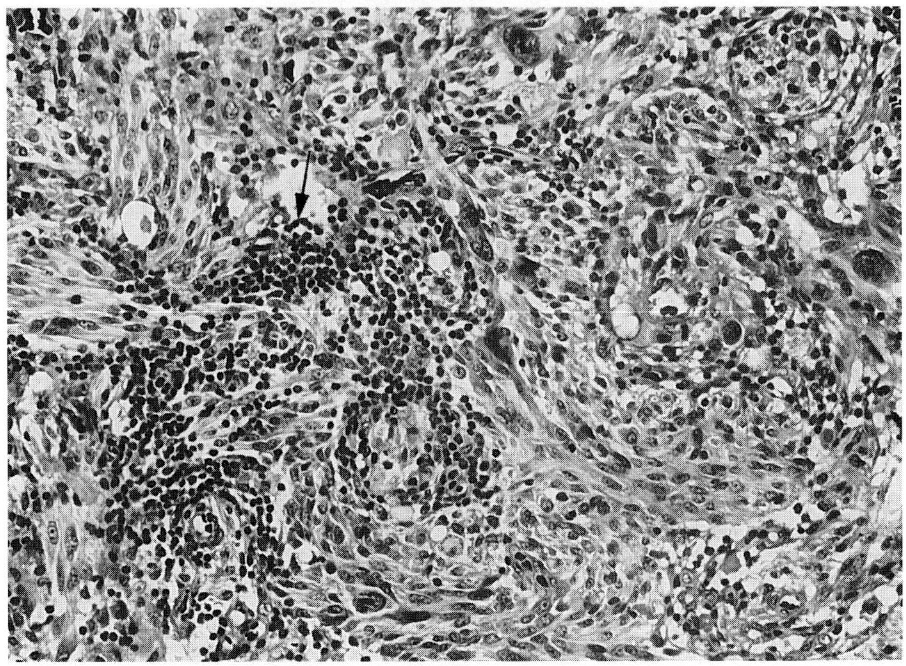

2-23

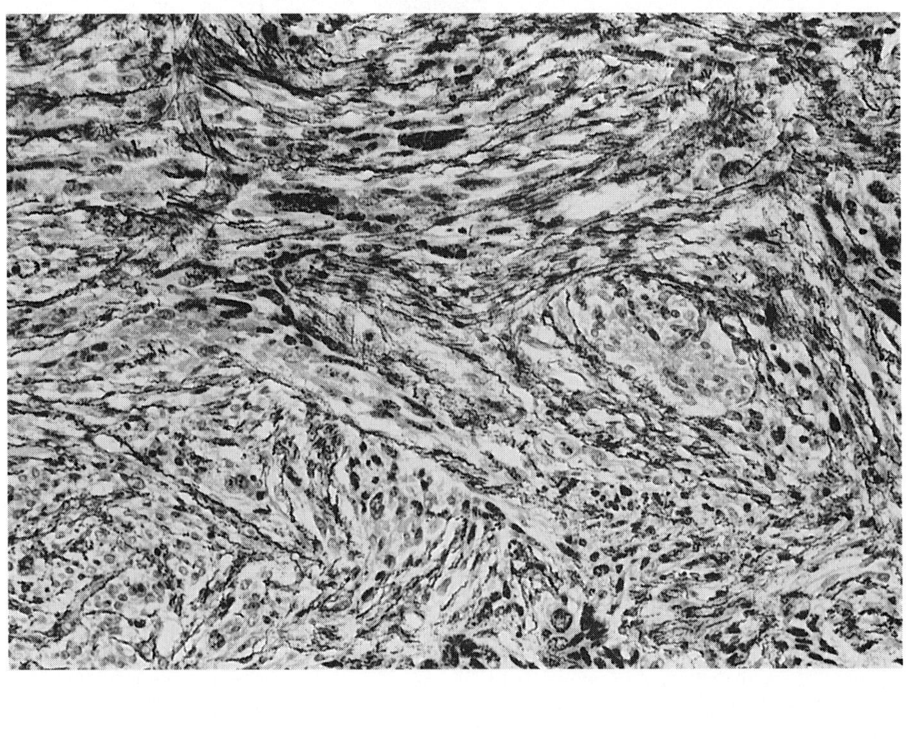

2-24

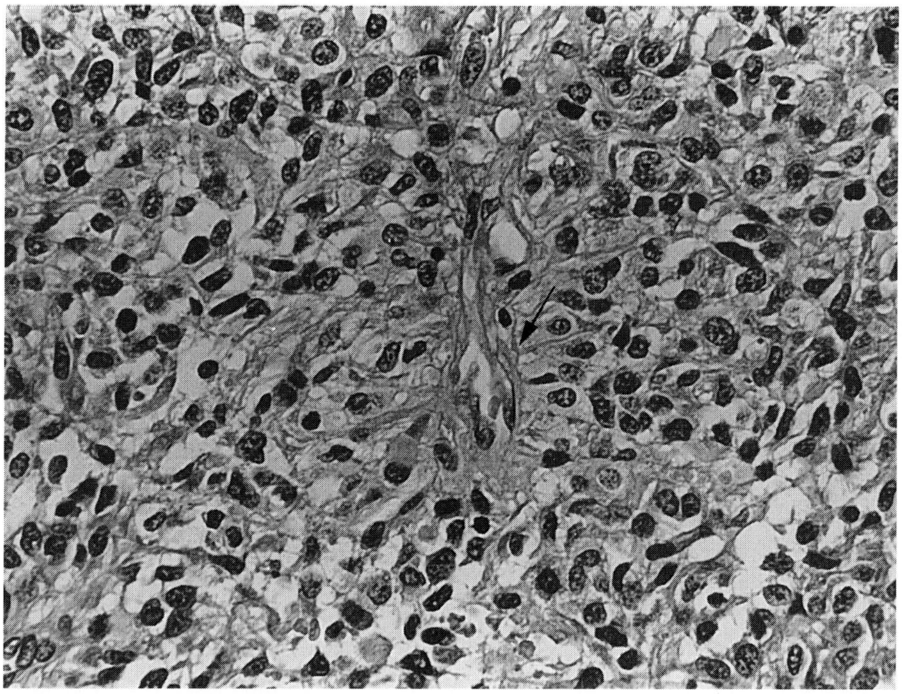

**Fig. 2-25.** Astroblastoma. Neoplastic fibrillar cells extend processes toward vessels. These processes thicken near the vascular adventitia (*arrow*). (×500.)

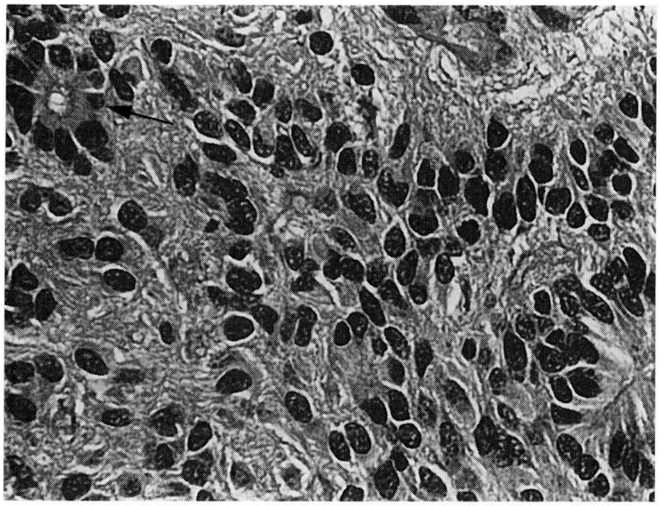

**Fig. 2-26.** Ependymoma. This true ependymal rosette (*arrow*) has a small lumen formed by encircling neoplastic ependymoma cells. Cells are fibrillar with oval nuclei. The 1-year-old infant had a large mass in her cerebellum. (×650.) (Reprinted from McKeever PE, and Blaivas M: The brain, spinal cord, and meninges, In Sternberg SS, and others, editors: Diagnostic Surgical Pathology, ed 2, New York, 1994, Raven Press.)

ependymal rosette consists of neoplastic ependymal cells evenly spaced around a lumen that resembles the central canal of the spinal cord (Fig. 2-26). At the outer portion of the rosettes, cells blend into the tumor itself. Occasionally, the tumors also contain so-called ependymal lining structures or linear strands of ependymoma cells.

While true ependymal rosettes are highly characteristic of ependymomas, they are not seen in each of them. Perivascular pseudorosettes are more common and can be numerous (Fig. 2-27). They show a fibrillar zone that is at least 20 $\mu$m (three erythrocyte diameters) wide around central vessels. The processes decrease in diameter as they radiate from the cells to the vascular adventitia, distinguishing them from thick astroblastic processes. The features described above when they are present are useful to identify ependymomas of any type. Unfortunately, such features are not present in every specimen.

The nuclear features of grade I and II ependymomas are consistent regardless of subtype. Nuclei are round or oval with prominent light and dark regions stained with hematoxylin that give a speckled pattern (Fig. 2-26). Pleomorphism obscures but does not abolish these features in higher grade tumors.

**Ependymoma (low-grade ependymoma)—grade II.** "Low-grade" is implied when a tumor of this group is referred to simply as "ependymoma." Ependymomas are more densely cellular than grade II astrocytomas and contain the cytologic features and characteristic rosettes that were described above (Fig. 2-27). Histologic grade is less prognostic in ependymoma than in astrocytoma.[59,148] Features like

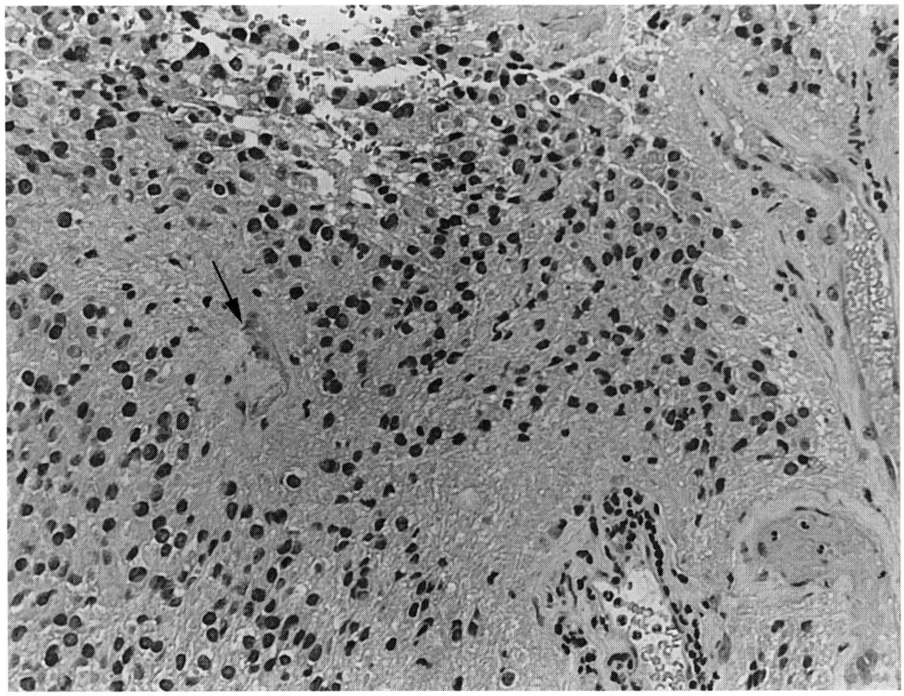

**Fig. 2-27.** Ependymoma. Cells with round and oval nuclei form perivascular rosettes around vessels (*arrow*) by encircling them with a zone of fibrillary cellular processes. The 20-year-old woman had a 2-year history of cervical and thoracic spine pain and stiffness followed by insidious lower extremity numbness and weakness. Her intramedullary spinal cord tumor extended from C3 to T7. (×200.)

spontaneous tumor necrosis do not necessarily predict poor outcome.[81] Recognition of ependymoma during the operative procedure is important because the surgeon frequently will attempt gross total excision of the tumor.

**Papillary ependymomas—grade II.** Papillae are the distinguishing feature of these tumors (Fig. 2-28). A reason for recognizing these as a subgroup is that they resemble choroid plexus papillomas. Immunocytochemistry (Chapter 4) and reticulin staining distinguish most of them. Solid regions of ependymoma where neoplastic cells grow upon one another in papillary ependymomas are negative for reticulin. Choroid plexus papillomas lack these.

**Clear-cell ependymoma—grade II.** These uncommon gliomas are noteworthy because their appearance by conventional light microscopy mimics other tumors (Fig. 2-29). They look like central neurocytoma, oligodendroglioma, or renal cell carcinoma. Cells have round nuclei, sometimes with prominent nucleoli, and perinuclear halos.[100] Nuclear chromatin is ependymal, and rosettes may or may not be present in surgical material. Their ultrastructural features are ependymal, and electron microscopy is helpful in their diagnosis (Chapter 3).

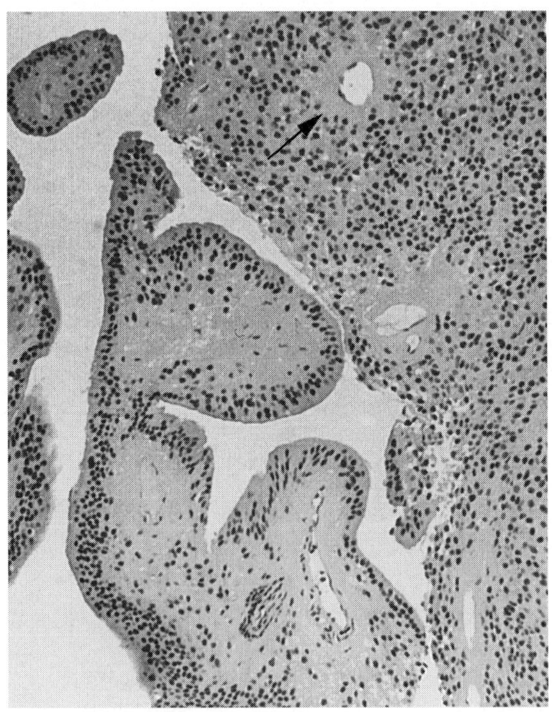

**Fig. 2-28.** Papillary ependymoma. The papillae are lined by neoplastic ependymoma cells. Vessels are surrounded by zones of fibrillar cell processes, producing perivascular rosettes (*arrow*). (×100.)

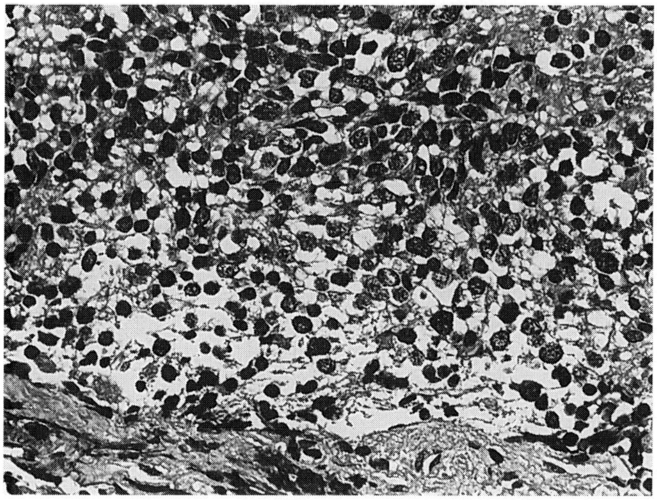

**Fig. 2-29.** Clear cell ependymoma. This ependymoma has cells with round nuclei and perinuclear halos that resemble those of an oligodendroglioma. It can be diagnosed ultrastructurally (Chapter 4). The 40-year-old patient developed pain and numbness in his extremities and third ventricular and posterior fossa lesions. (×400.)

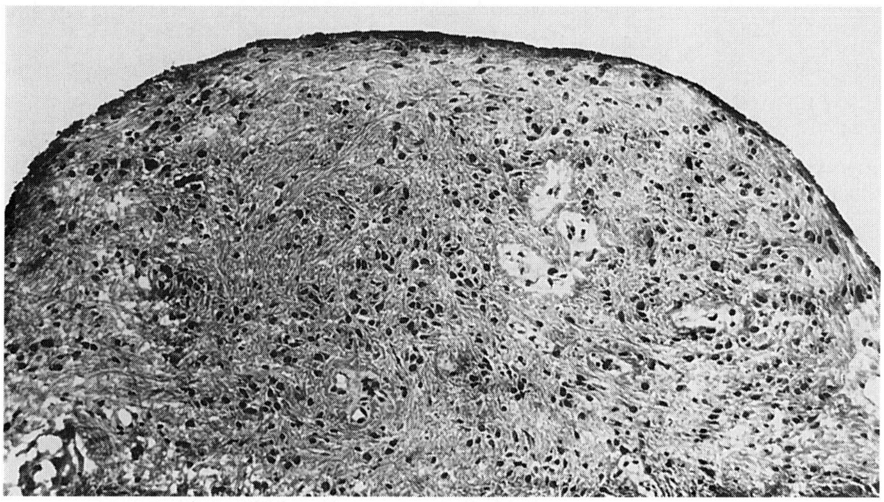

**Fig. 2-30.** Subependymoma. This mixture of clusters of cells and fibrils protrudes from its subependymal attachment. The 57-year-old woman had a mass protruding into her fourth ventricle. (×125.) (Reprinted from McKeever PE, and Blaivas M: The brain, spinal cord, and meninges, In Sternberg SS, and others, editors: Diagnostic Surgical Pathology, ed 2, New York, 1994, Raven Press.)

**Subependymoma and tanycytic ependymoma—grade I.** These highly fibrillar ependymomas look alike, but occur in different locations. Subependymomas protrude into the ventricular space from beneath the ependymal lining.[100] They are composed of groups of ependymal cells separated from one another by regions of fibrillary glial cell processes (Fig. 2-30).

Tanycytic ependymomas are frequent in the spinal cord parenchyma and show ependymal and astrocytic features (Fig. 2-27). However, their nuclei are ependymal and round to oval, with distinct light and dark speckles of chromatin.

These ependymomas are highly fibrillar and resemble astrocytomas. Characteristically they display regions filled with nuclei alternating with regions formed by fibrillar cellular processes. The fibrils are not limited to the vessels as in perivascular rosettes of other ependymomas. Tumor margins tend to be discrete and potentially resectable, which is a compelling reason to distinguish them from astrocytomas. To ensure appropriate surgical consideration of resection, it is best to identify the lesion as an ependymoma rather than an astrocytoma at the time of the intraoperative consultation.

Some tanycytic ependymomas and subependymomas are mixed with classic ependymoma. The reactive astrocytosis around classic ependymomas mimics the tanycytic pattern. Some neuropathologists do not recognize tanycytic ependymoma as a distinct entity, but instead classify these tumors as either ependymoma or subependymoma.

**Myxopapillary ependymoma—grade I.** This type of ependymoma almost always occurs in the region of the filum terminale and cauda equina, and its location is a critical diagnostic feature.

Variants of myxopapillary ependymoma can be nearly all myxoid or epithelial. The myxoid variety shows papillae of epithelioid cells in a mucoid matrix (Fig. 2-31). Chordoma, a neoplasm found in the same

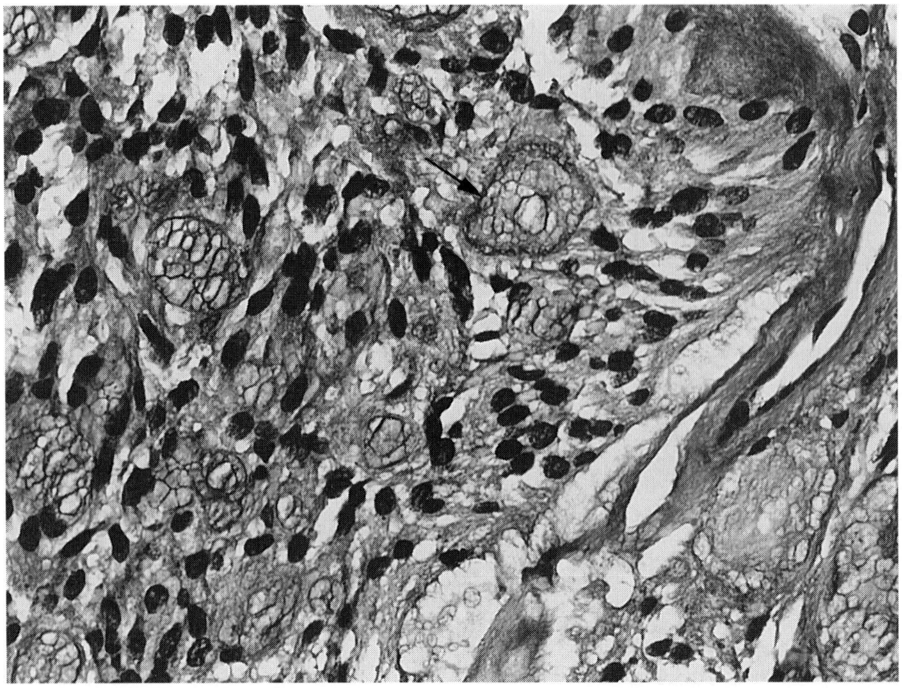

**Fig. 2-31.** Myxopapillary ependymoma. PAS stain highlights the mucin (*arrow*) in this tumor composed of neoplastic ependymal cells with round, oval, and pleomorphic nuclei. (×400.)

location, can be identified by its large cytoplasmic vacuoles. Immunocytochemistry distinguishes myxopapillary ependymoma from both chordoma and paraganglioma (Chapter 4).

Fibrillary myxopapillary ependymomas look more glial than do other ependymomas (Fig. 2-32). However, they may be confused with meningioma and schwannoma, the other two tumors that grow in this region. Light microscopic features that distinguish the ependymoma include ependymal rosettes and perivascular rosettes. The distinctive ultrastructural features of each of these neoplasms can prove helpful for diagnosis when light microscopy does not distinguish them (Chapter 3).

**Anaplastic ependymoma (malignant ependymoma)—grade III.** Anaplastic ependymomas are uncommon.[145] These are ependymomas with conspicuous mitotic activity, variable nuclear pleomorphism and hyperchromasia, high cellular density, and often marked vascular cell proliferation (Figs. 2-33 and 2-34). Nuclear pleomorphism and hyperchromasia may obscure typical ependymal nuclear features, but careful scrutiny will reveal them. Necrosis alone does not make the ependymoma anaplastic. The pseudorosettes may be obscured by sheets of cells or may remain intact. While many histopathologic features were not reliable prognostic features, the mitotic index was a predictor of poor prognosis in a large series of supratentorial ependymomas.[148]

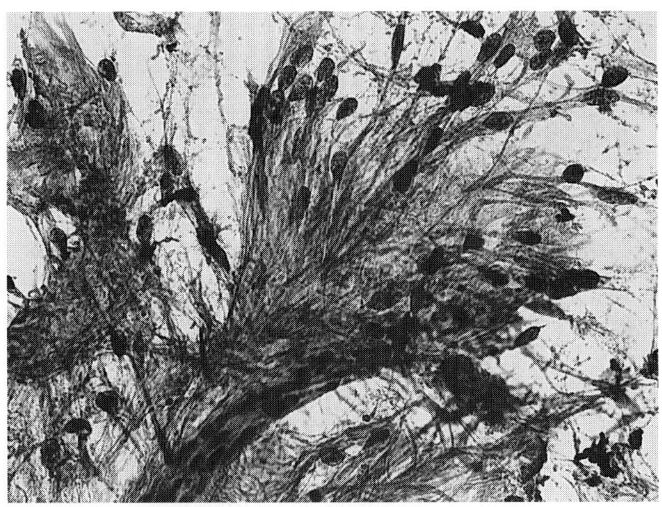

**Fig. 2-32.** Cytologic preparation of myxopapillary ependymoma. This preparation emphasizes the fibrillarity of these ependymoma cells and their oval nuclei. The 40-year-old woman had lower extremity pain for years. An intradural tumor was resected from her cauda equina. (×400.)

**Ependymoblastoma—grade IV.** This is a rare tumor classified as embryonal by some. It has conspic-

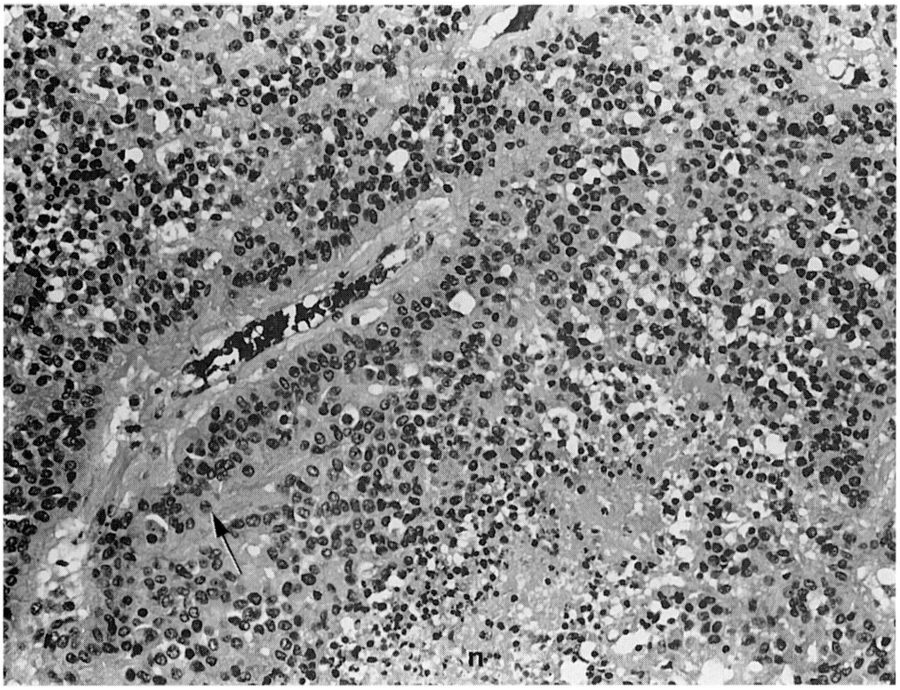

2-33

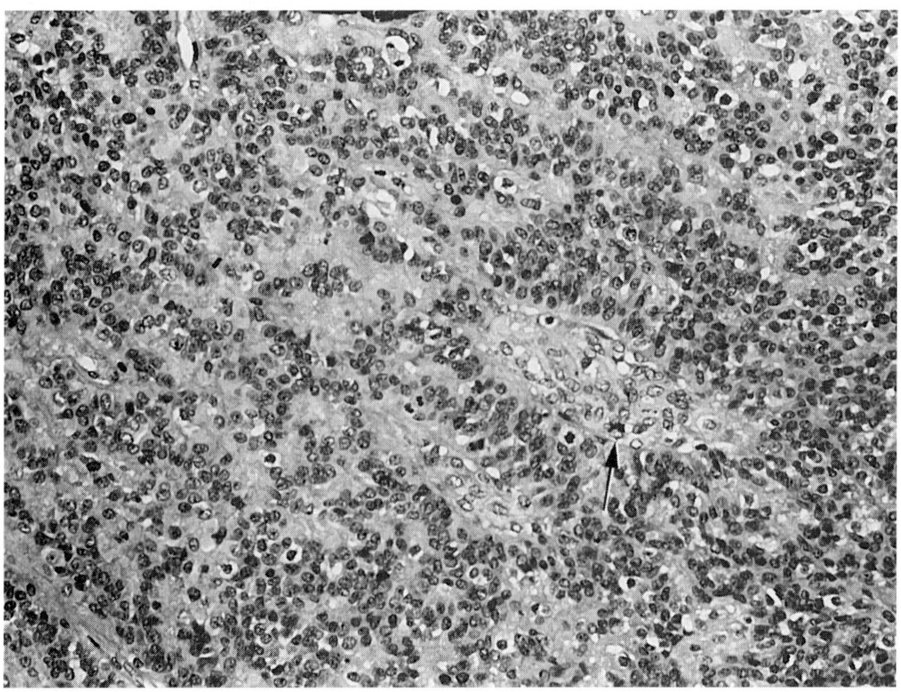

2-34

**Figs. 2-33, 2-34.** Anaplastic ependymoma. The 1-year-old boy had an enhancing posterior fossa mass. (×165.) **Fig. 2-33,** With small round nuclei, the anaplastic ependymoma retains a few indistinct perivascular rosettes (*arrow*). Tumor necrosis (*n*) is a common occurrence. **Fig. 2-34,** Mitotic figures and endothelial proliferation (*arrow*) are prominent.

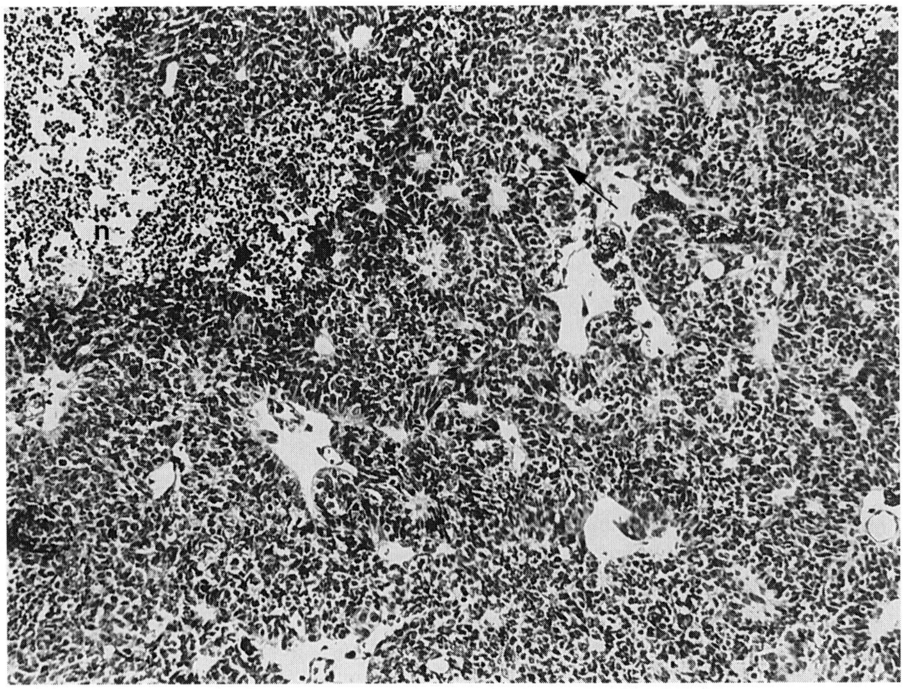


**Fig. 2-35.** Ependymoblastoma. This highly cellular neoplasm has spontaneous necrosis (*n*) and numerous true ependymal rosettes (*arrow*). (Reprinted from McKeever PE, and Blaivas M: The brain, spinal cord, and meninges, In Sternberg SS, and others, editors: Diagnostic Surgical Pathology, ed 2, New York, 1994, Raven Press.)

**Table 2-6.** Features of different brain tumors with epithelioid cells

| Diagnosis* | Features: Structures | Features: Locations† |
|---|---|---|
| Oligodendroglioma | Round cells and nuclei with prominent perinuclear halos; nests of cells between delicate vessels | Cerebrum; CNS |
| Anaplastic oligodendroglioma | Above features with mitoses and pleomorphism | Cerebrum; CNS |
| Choroid plexus papilloma | Large mass with structure of choroid plexus | Fourth ventricle; lateral ventricle; CP angle; choroid plexus |
| Choroid plexus carcinoma | Above features with anaplasia and mitoses; (necrosis)‡ | Above lesions |
| Medulloepithelioma | Columnar epithelium with "basement membrane" on both surfaces; fibrovascular base for papillae and tubules | Deep cerebrum; cauda equina; CNS |
| Meningioma | Whorls; psammoma bodies; interdigitating cell processes and desmosomes; (thick collagen) | Falx, tentorium; meninges; choroid plexus; (extracranial) |
| Chordoma | Masses or cords of physaliphorous cells | Sacrococcygeal tissues; cauda equina; clivus; spinal canal |
| Paraganglioma | Nests of clear or granular cells surrounded by many capillaries | Petrous ridge; spinal cord; epidural |
| Pituitary adenoma | Secretory granules | Sellar; suprasellar |
| Endodermal sinus tumor | Schiller-Duvall bodies | Pineal; parasellar |
| Embryonal carcinoma | Anaplasia; mitoses | Pineal; parasellar |
| Hemangioblastoma | Multivacuolated stromal cells between many capillaries; hypervascularity | Cerebellum; spinal cord; CNS |
| Craniopharyngioma | Squamous; adamantinomatous | Suprasellar; sellar |
| Carcinoma | Distinct margin with CNS; anaplasia; mitoses; necrosis | Cerebrum; cerebellum; meninges; CNS; frequent multiple masses; systemic |
| Melanoma | Anaplasia; mitoses, necrosis | Above locations |

* Adapted from McKeever PE, and Blaivas M: The brain, spinal cord and meninges, In Sternberg S, and others, editors: Diagnostic Surgical Pathology, ed 2, New York, 1994, Raven Press.

† Most common or most specific craniospinal location is listed first.

‡ Parentheses around a differential feature indicate an uncommon feature very useful in differential diagnosis when found.

uous hypercellularity equal to that of a medulloblastoma. It is placed with ependymomas here because it has true ependymal rosettes (Fig. 2-35). Most ependymoblastomas occur in infants and children.

The tumor shows numerous mitoses and regions of coagulation necrosis as well as frequent individual necrotic cells. Ependymoblastoma lacks multinucleation and giant cells and has virtually no vascular proliferation.[116] This tumor frequently infiltrates the leptomeninges and spreads along cerebrospinal fluid pathways.[151]

### Oligodendroglioma—Grade II

This tumor primarily, but not exclusively, afflicts the cerebrum of adults. Most oligodendrogliomas contain foci of calcification.

The pure oligodendroglioma is more epithelioid than fibrillar in both frozen and permanent sections (Table 2-6). *Perinuclear halos* are an important diagnostic feature (Figs. 2-36 to 2-38). The clear halo in the cytoplasm around each nucleus is a constant effect of delayed fixation. One may benefit from postponing the interpretation of oligodendroglioma until the permanent sections bring out typical cells with halos that resemble "fried eggs." Among the features visible on frozen sections that help identify these tumors are remarkable round and regular nuclei centrally placed within the cytoplasm. Another feature is provided by thin vessels that criss-cross the neoplastic cell groups (Fig. 2-37). These vessels sometimes segregate the parenchyma into small lobules.[11]

Oligodendrogliomas resemble central neurocyto-

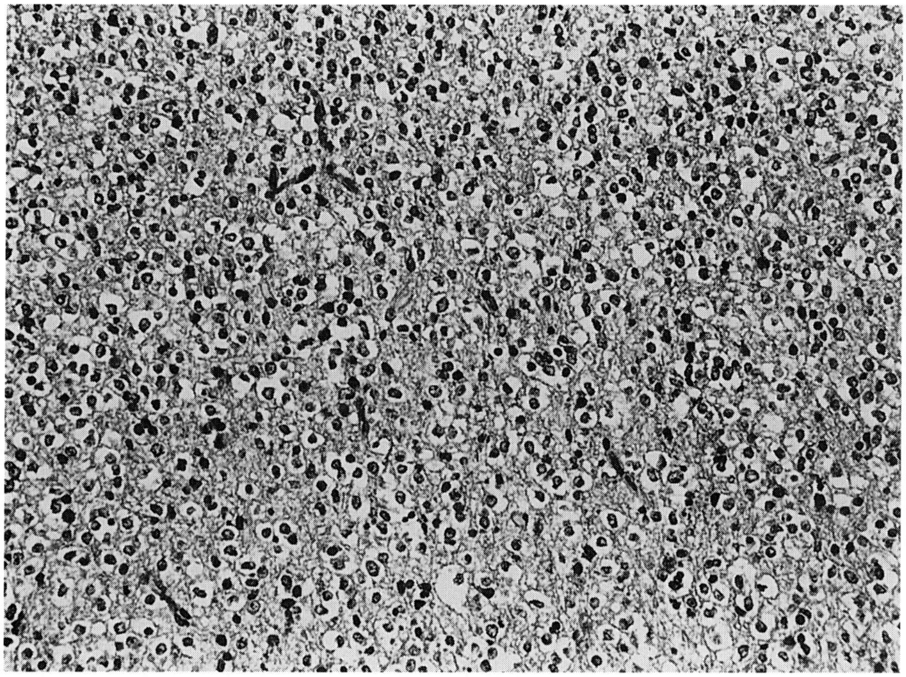

2-36

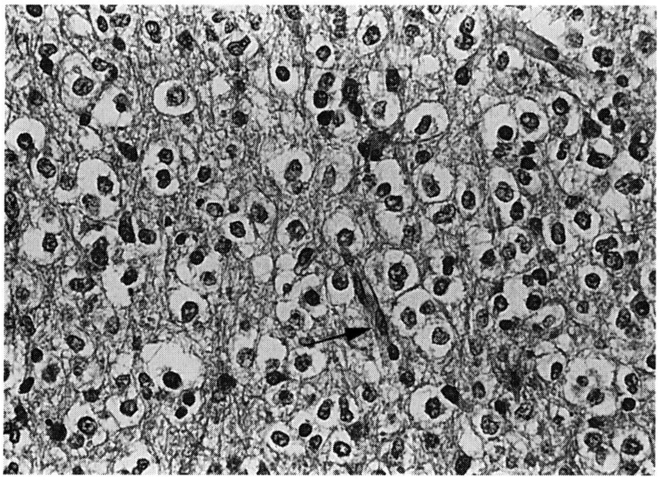

2-37

**Figs. 2-36, 2-37.** Oligodendroglioma. The 55-year-old patient had a 4-cm diameter right frontal mass that did not enhance with contrast media. **Fig. 2-36,** Round nuclei, low cellular density, and perinuclear halos characterize this tumor. (×200.) **Fig. 2-37,** Oligodendroglioma cells resemble fried eggs. Perinuclear halos are an artifact of processing paraffin sections consistent enough to be diagnostically useful. Vessels (*arrow*) are small with thin walls. (×400.)

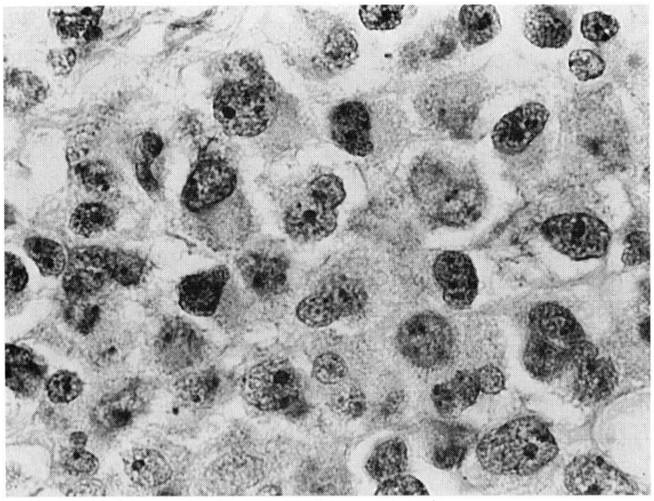

**Fig. 2-38.** Neoplastic oligodendroglia. Nuclei tend to be round, although they become more pleomorphic in anaplastic tumors. (×1250.)

mas, meningiomas, pituitary adenomas, and renal cell carcinomas. Location in brain parenchyma without ventricular, meningeal, or sellar involvement favors oligodendroglioma over the first three diagnoses. Calcifications, present in over 50% of all oligodendrogliomas, suggest a diagnosis of oligodendroglioma over carcinoma.[53] Electron microscopy is characteristic for each of these alternative tumors (Chapter 3).

Its infiltrative margin distinguishes oligodendroglioma from all of the above tumors except for central neurocytoma. Individual neoplastic glia infiltrate the brain parenchyma around even grossly discrete oligodendrogliomas. Secondary structures of Scherer, especially perineuronal gliomatosis (Fig. 2-5), indicate oligodendroglioma in the context of this differential diagnosis; however, these features are not always visible on stereotactic biopsies.

Neoplastic oligodendroglial cells occasionally are reminiscent of macrophages laden with lipid droplets. Their round nuclei, of variable size and showing a heterochromatin pattern, are more centrally placed within the cytoplasm than are the slightly smaller and more regular nuclei of lipid-laden macrophages. Oligodendroglia have a single large perinuclear halo rather than the multiple smaller phagocytic vacuoles of macrophages.

Minigemistocytes in oligodendrogliomas are cells with eccentric nuclei and eosinophilic hyaline cytoplasmic inclusions. Although these cells resemble the cells seen in gemistocytic astrocytomas, they have round oligodendroglial nuclei.[15,61,82]

**Anaplastic oligodendroglioma (malignant oligodendroglioma)—grade III.** The features of anaplastic transformation in oligodendroglioma consist of in-

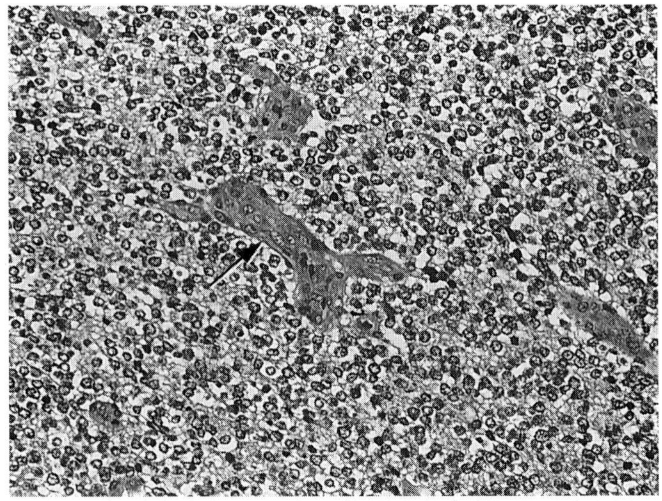

**Fig. 2-39.** Anaplastic oligodendroglioma. Cells with round nuclei and perinuclear halos are crowded together. Vascular cell proliferation (*arrow*) and mitoses are evident. The 35-year-old man had a 5-cm diameter mass in his right parietal region. (×200.)

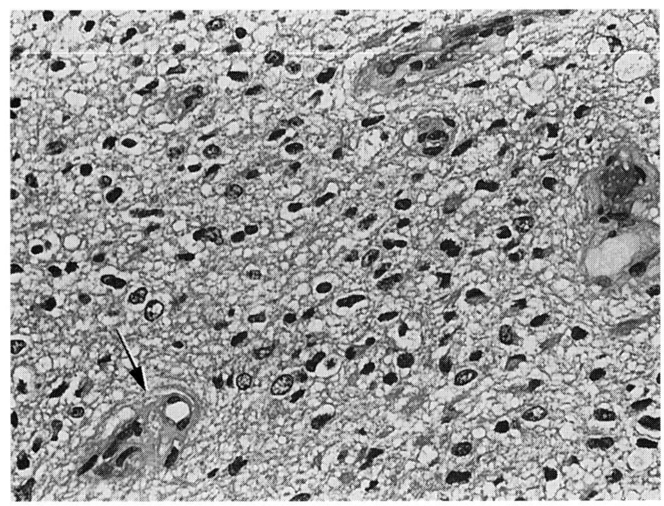

**Fig. 2-40.** Anaplastic oligodendroglioma margin. Nuclear pleomorphism, hyperchromasia, mitotic figures, and minimal vascular cell proliferation (*arrow*) are present in the margin of this anaplastic oligodendroglioma. The 51-year-old man had a left frontal craniotomy for his enhancing neoplasm that was resected 2 years previously. (×330.)

creased cellular density, nuclear pleomorphism, hyperchromasia, and vascular cell proliferation (Figs. 2-39 to 2-41).[14] Most important, mitotic activity is sufficient to be easily recognized on H&E sections (Fig. 2-3). Distinguishing very malignant oligodendrogliomas from glioblastomas is difficult. Glioblastomas are more pleomorphic and fibrillar, and have a poorer prognosis than malignant oligodendrogliomas.

Anaplastic oligodendrogliomas recur more quickly than grade II oligodendrogliomas. After treatment,

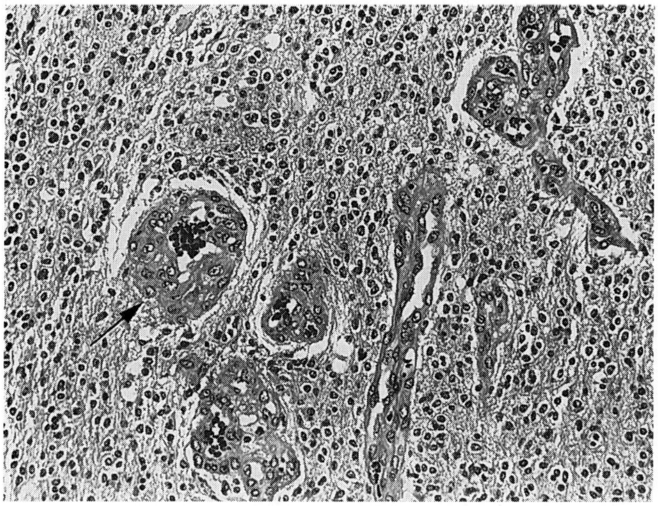

**Fig. 2-41.** Anaplastic oligodendroglioma. Cells are enlarged and abundant in the vascular walls, forming vascular cell proliferations (*arrow*). The 35-year-old patient had this recurrence of a left frontal oligodendroglioma 3 years after it was 90% removed and irradiated. (×200.)

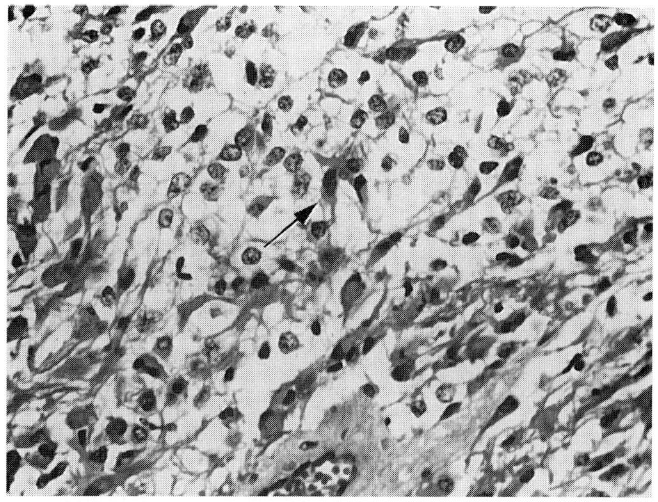

**Fig. 2-42.** Oligoastrocytoma. Neoplastic astrocytes (*arrow*) have elongated nuclei and extend fibrillar cytoplasmic processes from their pink cell bodies. Neoplastic oligodendroglia with round nuclei and perinuclear halos are more prominent near the top of the illustration. The 39-year-old man had recent memory difficulties, 2 weeks of headaches, and a cerebral mass in his right frontal lobe. (×300.)

high cellular density, mitoses, and vascular cell proliferation all suggest a poor outcome (Fig. 2-41).

### Oligoastrocytoma (Mixed Oligodendroglioma-Astrocytoma)—Grade II

This is a mixed glioma composed of astrocytoma and oligodendroglioma (Fig. 2-42). The frequency of its diagnosis varies between medical centers; this is probably because of individual biases among neuropathologists, and also is a reflection of the percentages of needle biopsies at each institution with their inherent sampling problems. This poses a therapeutic challenge now that special chemotherapeutic agents are being used for mixed oligodendroglioma-astrocytoma.[50]

Regions of both neoplastic oligodendroglia and neoplastic astrocytic glia as described in previous sections must be conspicuous before this diagnosis can be issued. Oligoastrocytomas can progress to grade III neoplasms and to glioblastomas.

### Glioblastoma Multiforme (Glioblastoma)—Grade IV

Most glioblastomas are supratentorial; however, they also are found in brainstem, cerebellum, and spinal cord.[88] These tumors may occur at any age, and are most common between 45 and 60 years. Often a hemispheric glioblastoma extends across the midline via the corpus callosum to produce a "butterfly" lesion that simulates other conditions.[16,136] In various classifications, glioblastomas are considered either the most malignant glioma, or they are interpreted as undifferentiated neuroectodermal tumors. We prefer the former interpretation, and consider them the most malignant variant of an astrocytoma.

Glioblastomas are the most frequent type of glioma to occur after radiotherapy.[99] Anaplastic astrocytomas and oligodendrogliomas also develop following irradiation.[80,170] The latent period ranges between 5 and 25 years, and most of these tumors develop after patients receive treatment for a pituitary adenoma or a craniopharyngioma.

Nelson and co-workers[118] recognized the importance of *coagulation necrosis* in glioblastoma multiforme (Fig. 2-43). Presence of this type of necrosis predicted the median survival of patients with high-grade supratentorial astrocytoma to be 8 months, compared with 28 months for those lacking necrosis. The latest WHO classification suggests that prominent vascular cell proliferation without coagulation necrosis constitutes the point of distinction between anaplastic astrocytoma and glioblastoma (Fig. 2-44). Accordingly, a glioma with sufficient pleomorphism and cellular density for anaplastic astrocytoma is considered a glioblastoma if the neoplasm also has prominent vascular cell proliferation. Either this feature or coagulation necrosis defines glioblastoma according to these criteria.[81] The impact of this reclassification is under study.[71]

The term "endothelial proliferation" is commonly used to describe vascular cell proliferation. The latter term is more accurate, because cells in the vessel wall other than endothelial cells, including smooth muscle cells, proliferate. The conventional term "endothelial proliferation" as well as the more accurate term "vascular cell" proliferation are both used in this chapter

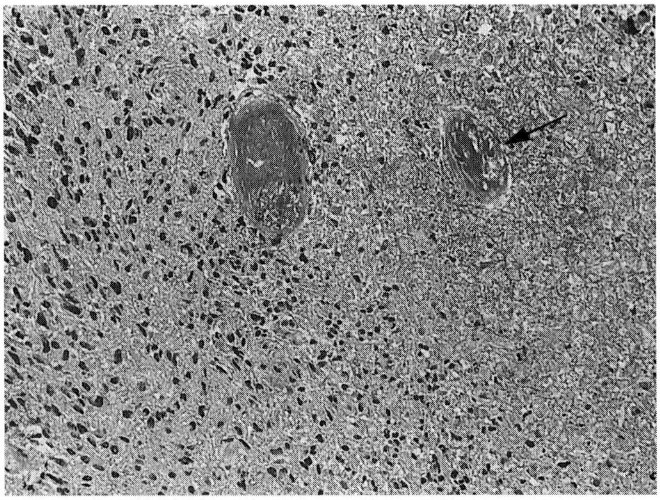

2-43

**Figs. 2-43, 2-44.** Glioblastoma. The 69-year-old patient had a right posterior temporal and parietal mass. **Fig. 2-43,** Zone of coagulation necrosis includes necrotic ghosts of vessels (*arrow*). (×200.) **Fig. 2-44,** Vascular cell proliferation. The vascular wall is thickened by cells with lightly stippled nuclear chromatin (*arrow*) in the neoplasm composed of highly pleomorphic fibrillar parenchymal cells. (×400.)

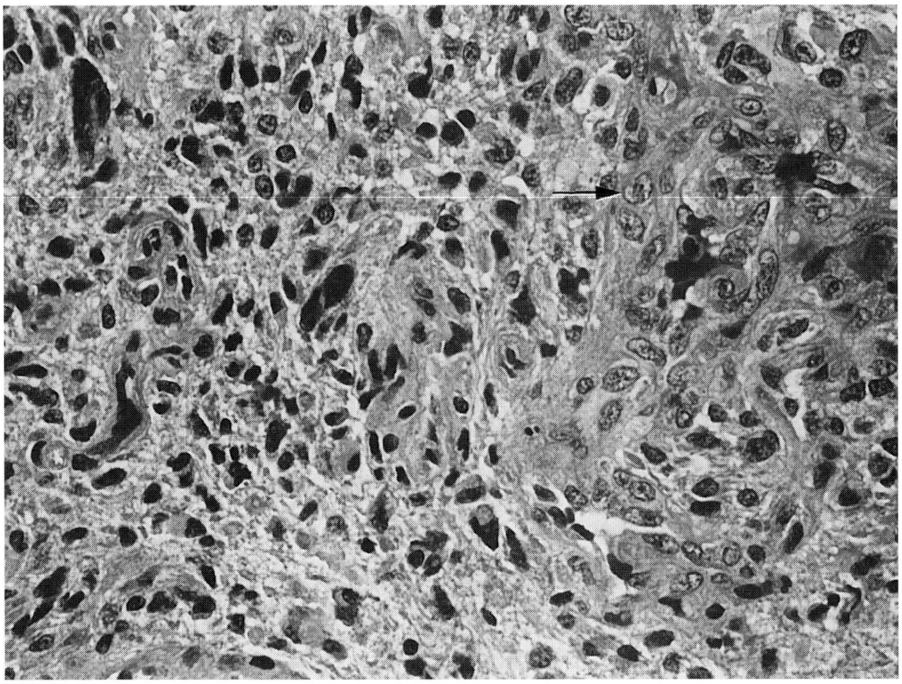

2-44

with the same meaning. We prefer "vascular cell" proliferation.

Other histopathologic features of glioblastoma are bizarre cells and nuclei and multinucleated tumor cells. The fibrillarity in these tumors varies, but some cellular processes can be found in most (Fig. 2-45). The frequency of these features varies among subtypes of glioblastoma, but they tend to be common in so-called giant cell glioblastoma.

Glioblastoma can mimic malignant meningioma and carcinoma. The biology of glioblastoma is such that glioblastoma is more often a solitary lesion when first encountered than is the metastatic carcinoma. Glioblastomas are fibrillar, not epithelioid like carcinoma or syncytial like meningioma. The microscopic margin around glioblastoma shows invasion by individual neoplastic glia; however, the presences of secondary structures of Scherer (see the section on gliosis versus glioma) are even more conclusive discriminators. Immunocytochemistry identifies each of these three malignancies (Chapter 4).

The median survival of glioblastoma among patients treated with radiotherapy is 1 year, but a few patients survive longer. Special techniques have been used to predict longer survival.[102,104]

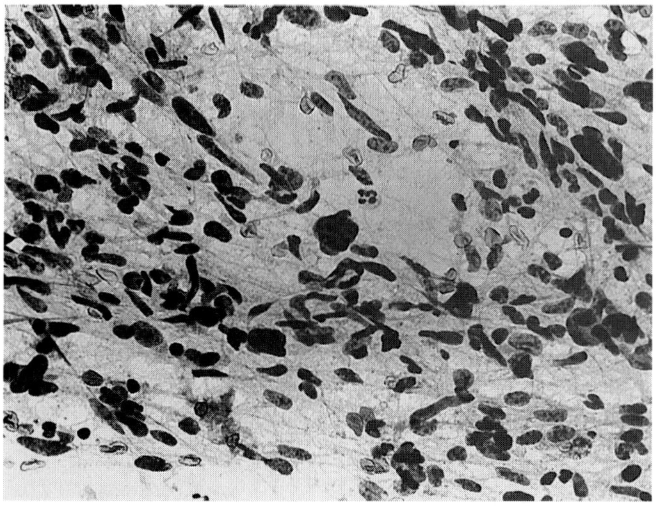

**Fig. 2-45.** Cytologic preparation of glioblastoma. This preparation of a fresh surgical specimen highlights the cellular and nuclear pleomorphism, some nuclei devoid of cytoplasm, and the fibrillar cellular processes of this glioblastoma. (×400.)

**Gliosarcoma—grade IV.** It is somewhat surprising that superficial gliosarcomas in situ often seem more circumscribed than the glioblastoma, and they closely resemble a meningioma. Gliosarcoma is considered to be a mixture of glioblastoma and sarcoma (Fig. 2-46). Regions of sarcoma cells that may originate from neoplastically transformed cells of the vascular tunica adventita bridge the glioblastoma in a marbled configuration. These regions with malignant nuclei and mitotic figures can be found on H&E or trichrome stains, but better confirmation is obtained by immunocytochemistry (Chapter 4). In situ hybridization identifies the sarcoma cells as being the source of collagen in these tumors.[106] Some neuropathologists distinguish another entity, "sarcoglioma," in which sarcoma predominates.

Gliosarcoma is said to be more likely to metastasize than glioblastoma; however, the evidence for this is inconclusive. Gliosarcomas can evolve into a pure sarcoma that lacks GFAP-positive cells.[103,105,160] The median survivals for both gliosarcoma and glioblastoma are similar.[107]

**Other malignant variants.** Kepes and co-workers,[75,77] Rubinstein and associates,[141] and Mörk and co-

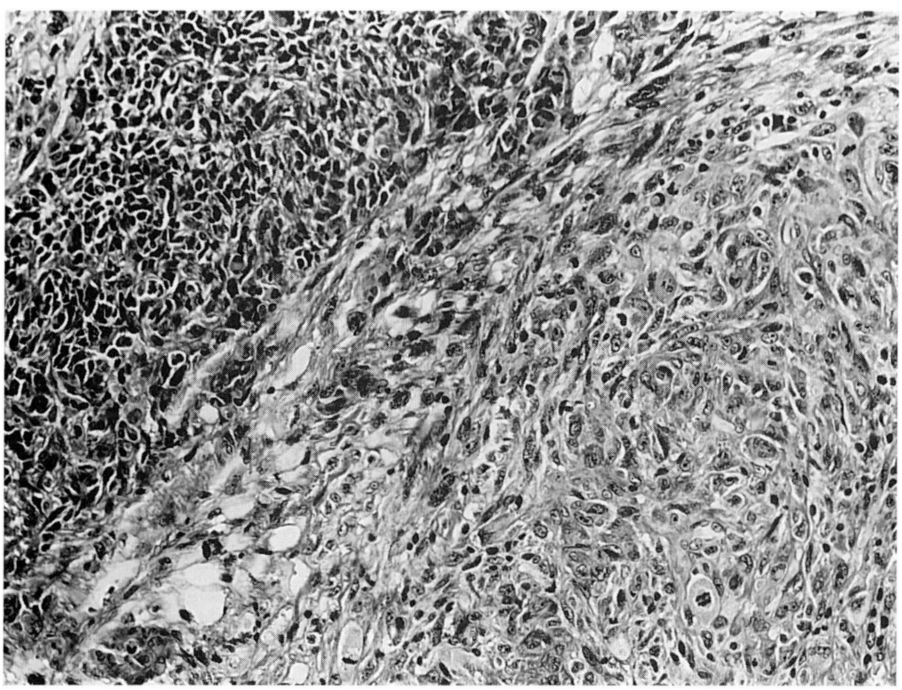

**Fig. 2-46.** Gliosarcoma. Masson's trichrome stains the collagen and the large bubbly nuclei of cells in the sarcomatous region in the lower portion of the illustration. Cells with very dark and pleomorphic nuclei in the upper left comprise the gliomatous portion. Both portions contain mitosing malignant cells. The 73-year-old woman had recent onset of dysphagia, and a left temporal lobe mass. (×200.) (Reprinted from McKeever PE, and Blaivas M: The brain, spinal cord, and meninges, In Sternberg SS, and others, editors: Diagnostic Surgical Pathology, ed 2, New York, 1994, Raven Press.)

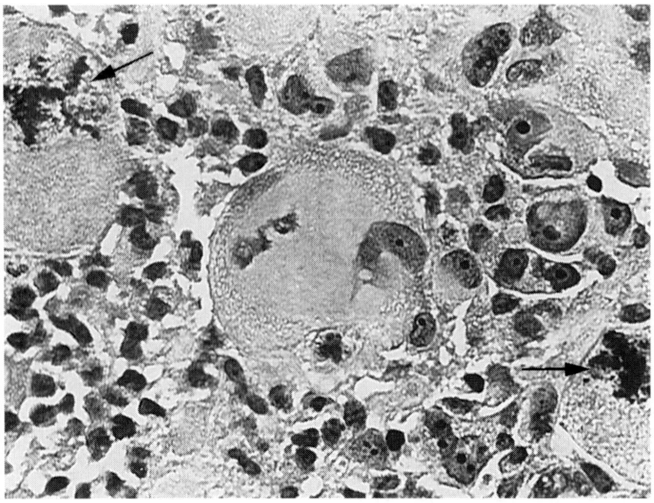

**Fig. 2-47.** Giant cell glioblastoma. Bizarre cellular and nuclear pleomorphism, conspicuous cellular gigantism, and abnormal mitotic spindles (*arrows*) are features of this glioblastoma. (×400.)

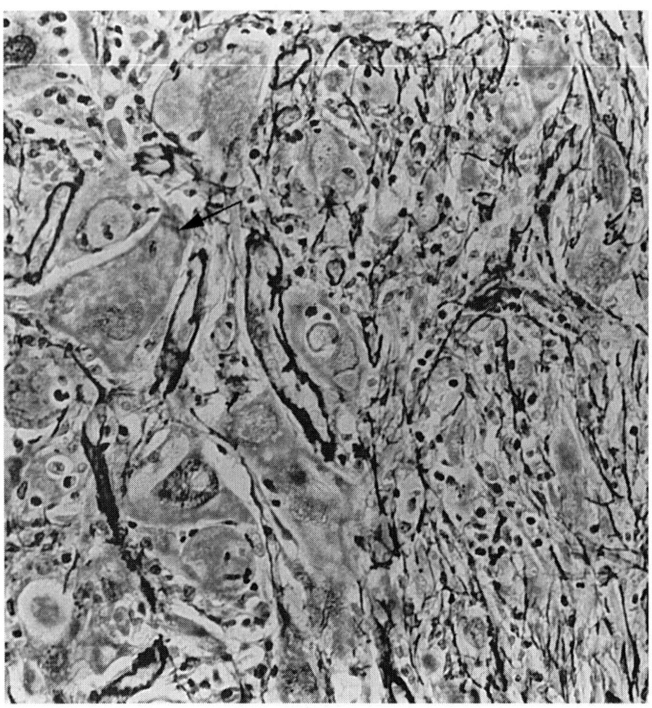

**Fig. 2-48.** Giant cell glioblastoma. Grotesque giant cells (*arrow*) intermix with smaller cells and black reticulin fibers. Snook's reticulin stain with nuclear fast red counterstain. (×200.)

workers[115] each described glioblastomas and gliosarcomas that produce adenoid or epithelial foci. These regions resemble metastatic carcinoma, and immunostain as a carcinoma (Chapter 4). Some glioblastoma cells contain lipid droplets.[140]

Previous classifications recognized a tumor with large, bizarre, slightly fibrillar cells as a monstrocellular sarcoma.[172] This term has been replaced by giant cell glioblastoma following recognition that these cells express GFAP (Figs. 2-47 and 2-48).[81]

## NEURONAL TUMORS

Most brain tumors containing abundant or prominent neurons visible on H&E are benign or low-grade. Their proper identification is important because they often have a better prognosis than the gliomas they resemble (Tables 2-4 and 2-5). Nonetheless, rare malignant forms of neuronal tumors such as anaplastic ganglioglioma, ganglioneuroblastoma, and CNS neuroblastoma do occur.

Modern identification of neurons and interpretation of whether they are part of the neoplasm depends on electron microscopy and immunocytochemistry (Chapters 3 and 4). The central neurocytoma was thought to be an oligodendroglioma for years. It was ultimately defined ultrastructurally.* This should alert pathologists who feel comfortable using a single H&E slide for all diagnoses to be more cautious. Although the presence of large and abnormal neurons in gangliogliomas and gangliocytomas aids in their recognition, ultrastructural or immunocytochemical confirmation of neuronal tumors is advised.

### Ganglioglioma—Grade I-II

This neoplasm most often occurs in the temporal lobe; other sites in the cerebrum, cerebellum, brainstem, and spinal cord are rarely affected.[72] The ganglioglioma is composed of both neoplastic glia (usually astrocytoma) and large neoplastic neurons (Figs. 2-49, 2-50). Visible on H&E stains, these neurons also may be distinguished from glia with axonal or Nissl stains.[98] Neuronal neoplasia is confirmed by hypercellularity and disarray of neurons, binucleated neurons (Fig. 2-51), and pleomorphism. Degenerative changes may be visible in such neurons (Fig. 2-50).[122] One subset of gangliogliomas contains heavy bands of fibrous tissue. Others have perivascular lymphocytes; some others are cavitary (Fig. 2-49).

**Anaplastic ganglioglioma—grade III.** The glial component of a ganglioglioma may evolve into one of these malignant tumors, but this progression is rare. The histologic criteria of anaplasia are the same ones applied for the diagnosis of anaplastic astrocytomas and oligodendrogliomas.

Another rare tumor, the ganglioneuroblastoma, reflects neuronal differentiation in a neuroblastoma (Fig. 2-52).

* Refs.: 8, 18, 38, 110, 120, 121, 126, 159, 163, 164, 169.

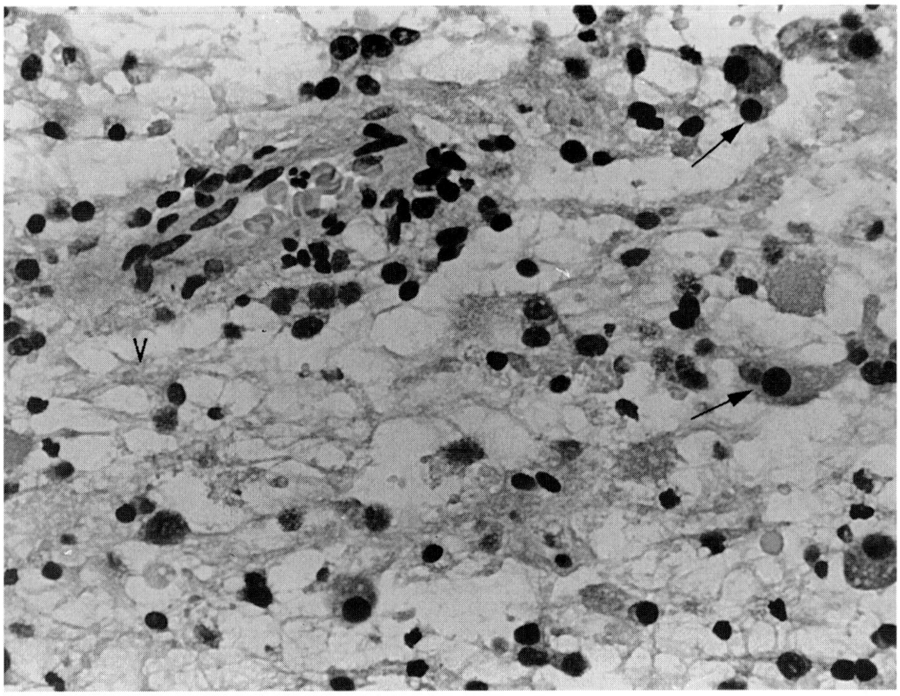

**Fig. 2-49.** Ganglioglioma. Juxtaposed and binucleated neurons (*arrows*) mix with neoplastic glia in a microcystic background. Protein droplet degeneration (*arrowhead*) resembles that in pilocytic astrocytoma. Small mononuclear cells surround a thick-walled vessel in the upper left portion of illustration. The 50-year-old woman with neurofibromatosis had a 4-cm cystic frontal mass. (×400.) (Courtesy of Dr. Patricia M. Novak, Jackson, MI.)

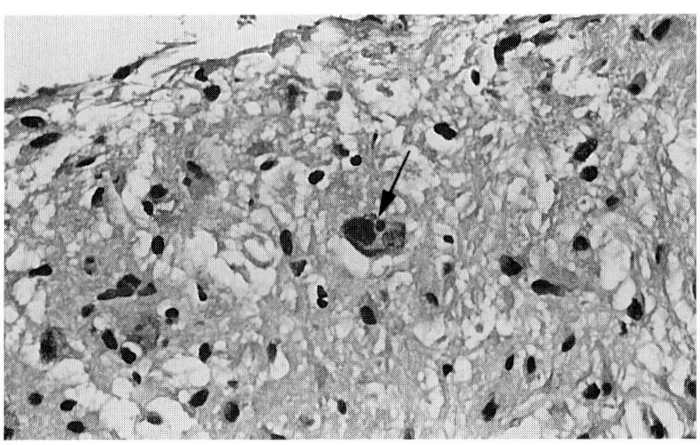

**Fig. 2-50.** Ganglioglioma. Misshapen large, multinucleated neuron with Nissl substance at the periphery of the cytoplasm (*arrow*) is surrounded by sparse neoplastic and reactive astrocytes. The 10-year-old girl had a long history of seizures and a nonenhancing lesion within her left temporal lobe. (×330.)

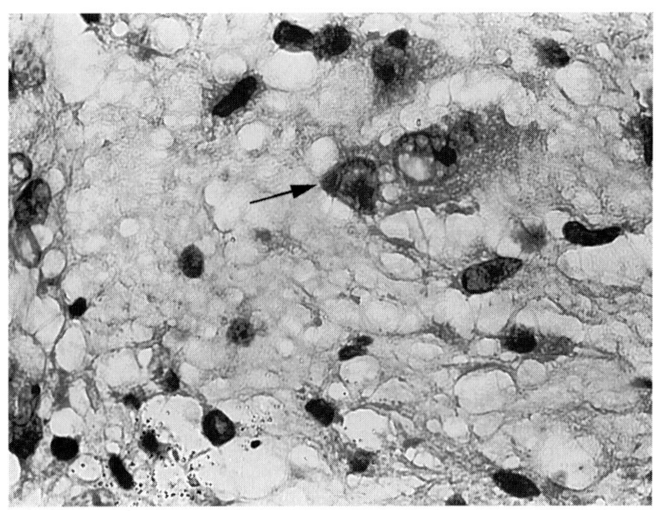

**Fig. 2-51.** Ganglioglioma. Binucleated neurons (*arrow*) aid identification of the ganglioglioma. The 19-year-old woman had nystagmus for years and an intrinsic brainstem mass beneath her fourth ventricle. (×1000.)

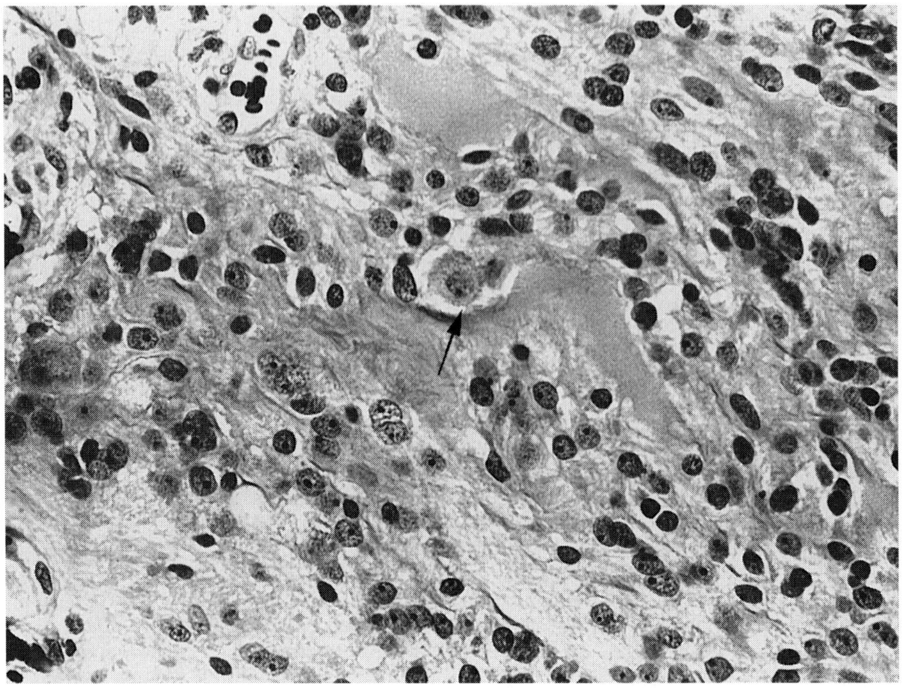

**Fig. 2-52.** Ganglioneuroblastoma. Most of the small, round neuronal nuclei lack cytoplasm or are surrounded by clear halos. Some neurons are larger and better differentiated (*arrow*). The background is fibrillar. The 38-year-old man had seizures and a focally slightly enhancing right temporal lesion. (×330.)

### Gangliocytoma—Grade I

Gangliocytomas occur principally in the pediatric age group in the temporal lobe or hypothalamic regions. Their ganglion cells can be recognized on H&E stains, and their features are similar to those of a ganglioglioma (Fig. 2-53). Unlike gangliogliomas, gangliocytomas do not contain neoplastic glia and are not known to progress to anaplasia.

### Dysembryoplastic Neuroepithelial Tumor—Grade I

This recently described tumor frequently is associated with a long-standing partial complex seizure disorder in children and young adults.[28] It is multinodular and occurs within the cerebral cortex, most often of the temporal lobe. It is composed of a hamartomatous mixture of neurons and glia mixed with acid mucopolysaccharide that stains with Alcian blue.[28] Its prominent cells resemble oligodendroglia,[29,132] and the tumor is histologically benign (Fig. 2-54). The low proliferation index, typical of these tumors, their gross features, and their association with cortical dysplasia all suggest a maldevelopmental origin.[133]

### Central Neurocytoma—Grade I

The grade I central neurocytoma is a recently recognized tumor that commonly grows from the septum pellucidum or from structures located near the foramen of Monro. Neurocytomas frequently extend into the lateral ventricle.[100,120,169] Central neurocytoma is the most common neoplasm to involve the septum pellucidum in young adults.[120] Magnetic resonance image characteristics include serpiginous flow voids and isointensity with cortex.[126]

The central neurocytoma closely resembles an oligodendroglioma by H&E stains (Fig. 2-55), and special stains for axons and Nissl substance are insufficient to differentiate these two tumors. Electron microscopy or immunoperoxidase stains are recommended to differentiate central neurocytoma from gliomas. A few neurocytomas show features suggestive of Homer Wright rosettes or ganglionic cells.[159,164]

Total surgical excision produces good results in most cases.[18,38] However, rare anaplastic variants have been reported.[163,169]

### Desmoplastic Infantile Ganglioglioma—Grade I

Desmoplastic infantile gangliogliomas (DIGs) occur in patients under 18 months of age, and frequently are cavitary. These tumors often involve the meninges, and attain considerable size.[160,161,171] DIG frequently resemble very fibrous gangliogliomas (Figs. 2-56 to 2-58). However, the ganglionic element is inconspicuous in some tumors.[171] Absence of ganglion cells in a tumor otherwise similar to a DIG prompts the classification of the lesion as a desmoplastic infantile astrocytoma (Figs. 2-59 to 2-61).

*Text continued on page 62.*

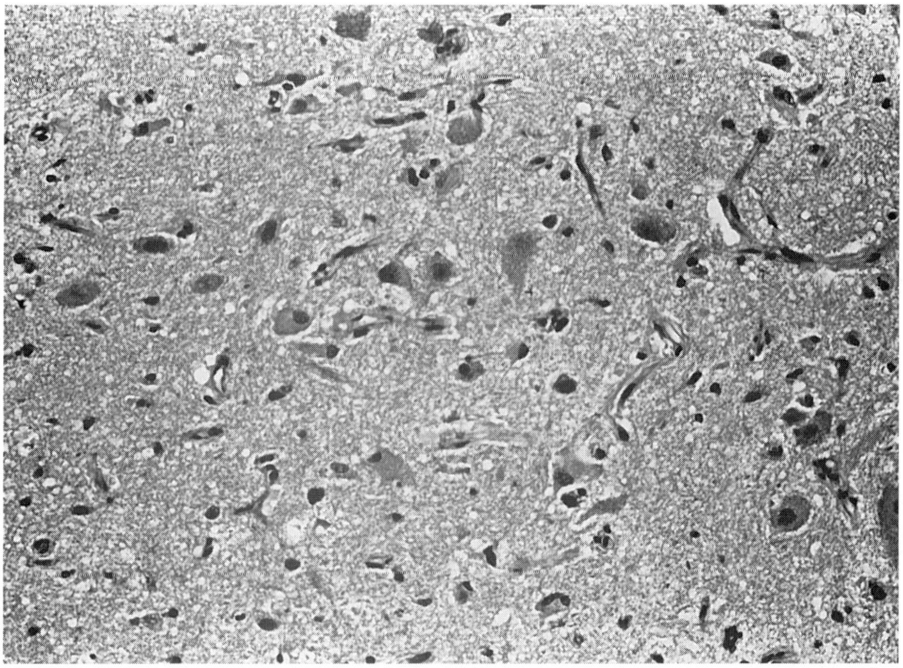

**Fig. 2-53.** Gangliocytoma. Varying in shape and orientation, large abnormal neurons are mixed with gliosis. The vessels are typically thin, branching, and arcuate. The 22-year-old man had an 8-year history of a nonenhancing right parietal lesion that was presumed to be a low-grade glioma. (×165.)

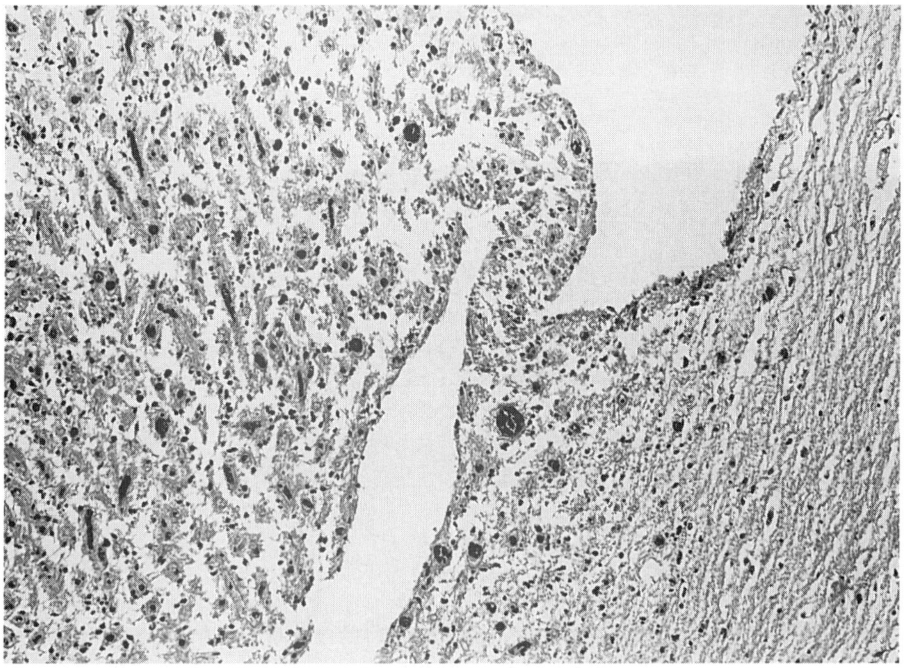

**Fig. 2-54.** Dysembryoplastic neuroepithelial tumor (DNT). This benign mixture of widely separated neurons and glia presents a pattern of fibrillar cords arranged around capillaries. The small, round nuclei of the majority of the cells resemble oligodendroglia. (×100.) (Courtesy of Dr. Jonathan D. Fratkin, Jackson, MS.)

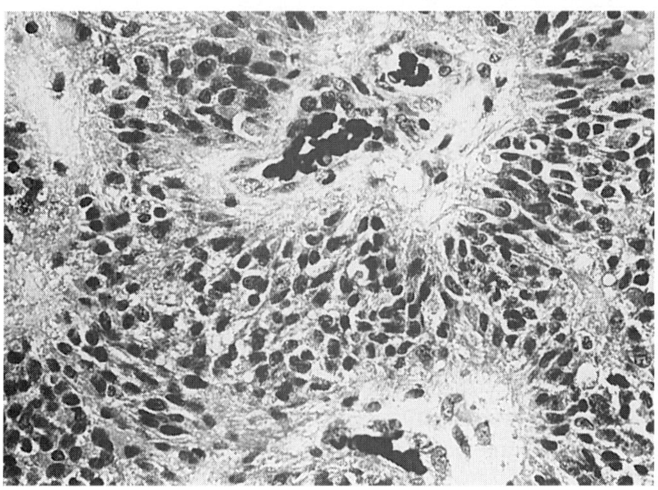

**Fig. 2-55.** Central neurocytoma. Cells with round and oval nuclei extend fibrillary cytoplasmic processes toward vessels as in ependymoma. Other cells with round nuclei and perinuclear halos resemble cells of an oligodendroglioma. These neurons require special procedures for their identification (Chapters 3, 4). (×400.)

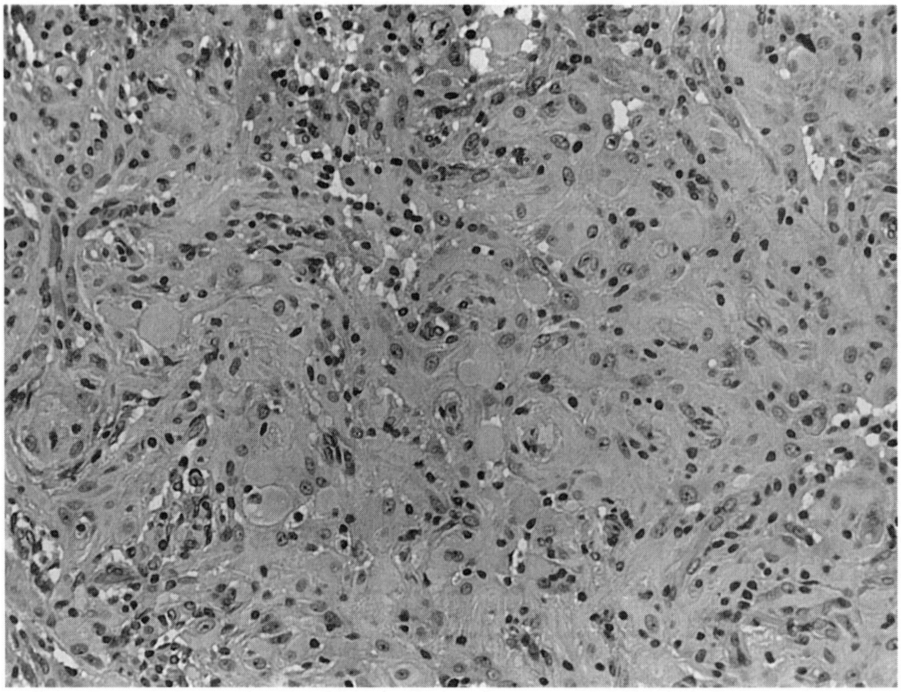

2-56

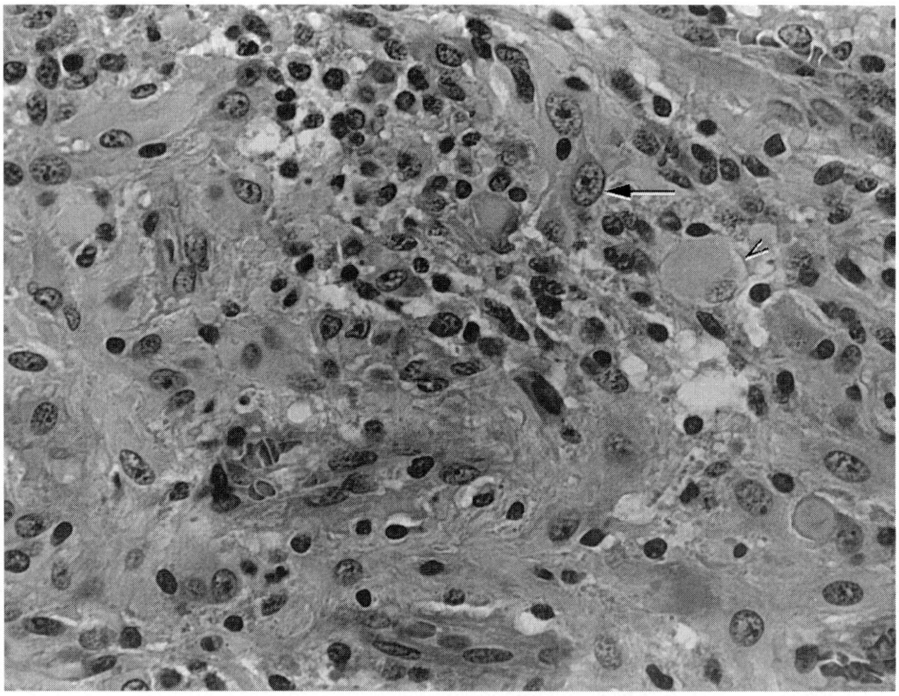

2-57

**Figs. 2-56 to 2-58.** Desmoplastic infantile ganglioglioma. This massive tumor occupied a third of the left cerebral hemisphere of a 9-month-old male infant. **Fig. 2-56,** The mixture of heterogeneous cells and fibrovascular septa produces a swirled and slightly lobulated pattern at low magnification. (×200.) **Fig. 2-57,** Neuronal (*arrow*), glial, and ambiguous elements are present in this tumor. The glia include gemistocytes (*arrowhead*). (×400.)

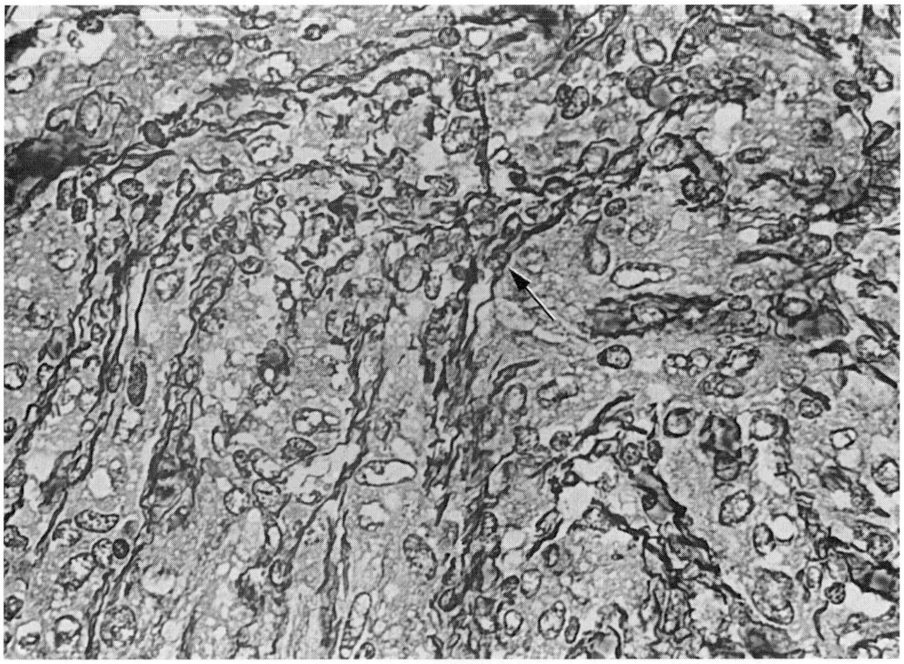

2-58

Fig. 2-58. Snook's silver stain for reticulin reveals the extensive fibrovascular component (*arrow*) of this tumor that made it firm to the touch. (×400.)

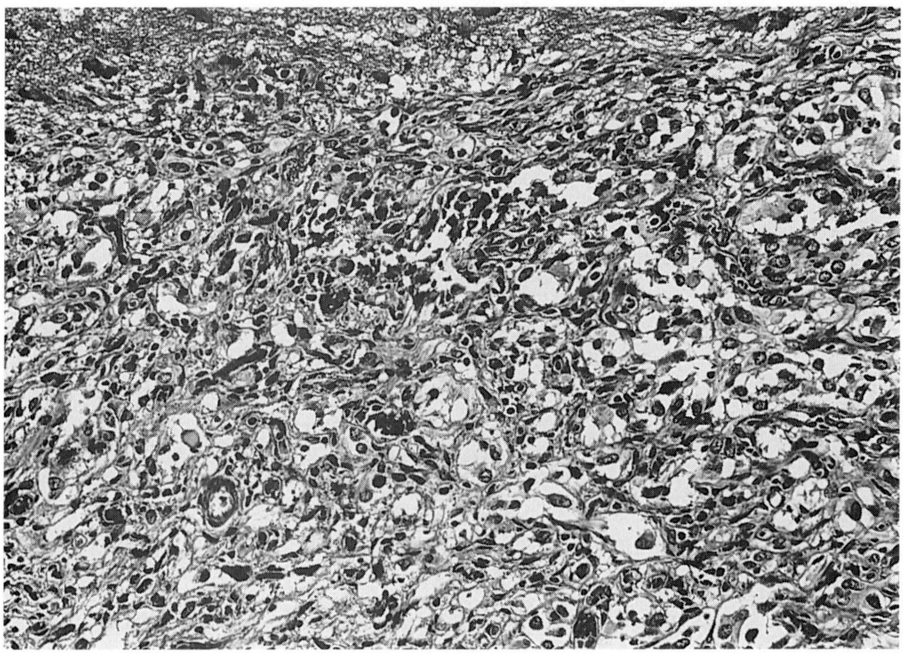

2-59

**Figs. 2-59 to 2-61.** Desmoplastic infantile astrocytoma. This large cystic and exophytic mass occupied a major portion of the left cerebral hemisphere of a 3-month-old boy. Its solid tissue was quite firm. **Fig. 2-59,** Mixed cellular elements form nests and swirled patterns. **Fig. 2-60,** Pleomorphic astrocytes mix with fibrovascular stroma. The collagenous tumor has a distinct margin with brain (*arrow*). Trichrome stain reveals nuclear features and collagenous regions. **Fig. 2-61,** Reticulin stain of a section near the two sections illustrated above highlights the fibrovascular stroma and the margin of the tumor (*arrow*). Immunohistochemistry is required to distinguish this tumor from a desmoplastic infantile ganglioglioma. (2-59 to 2-61, ×200; semiserial sections.)

2-60

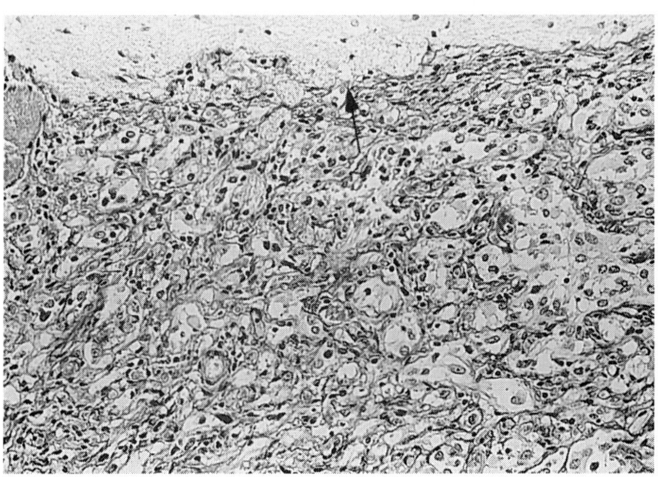

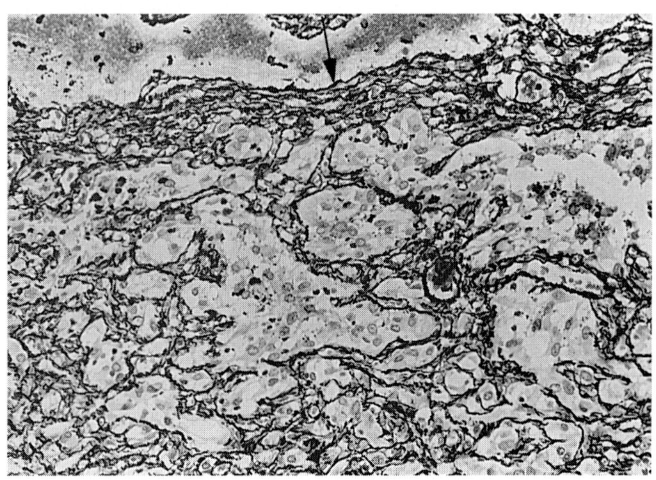

2-61

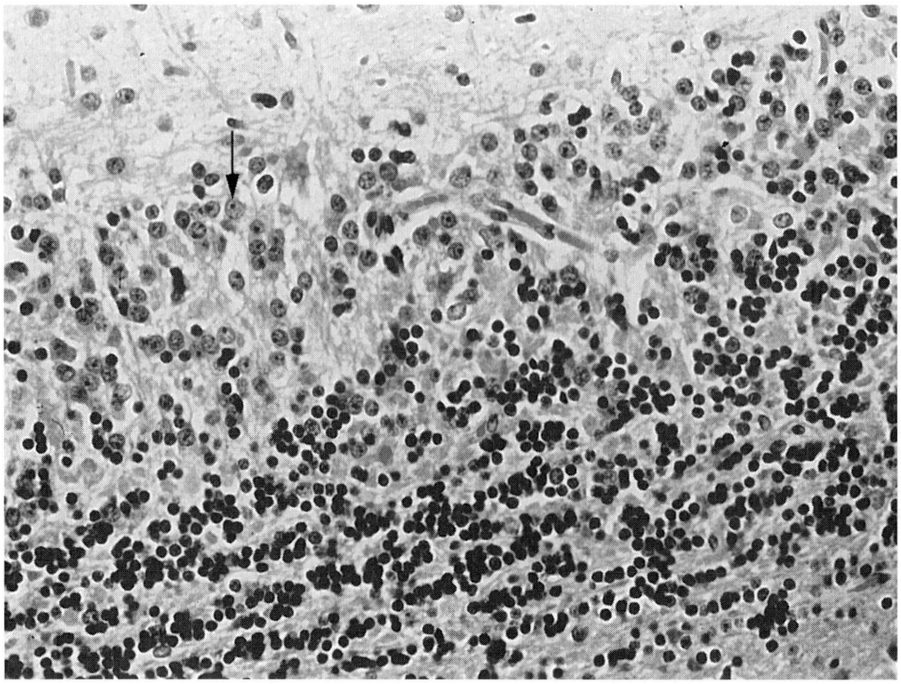

**Fig. 2-62.** Lhermitte-Duclos disease. Dysplastic granular cell neurons (*arrow*) lie in a band between the darker granular cell layer below and the molecular layer above. The 36-year-old man had headaches and visual disturbances, and a mass in his cerebellum. (×240.)

### Lhermitte-Duclos Disease

Lhermitte-Duclos Disease (LDD) or dysplastic gangliocytoma of the cerebellum is a rare enlargement of a portion of the cerebellar cortex by hyperplastic and disordered granule cell neurons (Fig. 2-62) that form a lesion resembling a hamartoma. The neoplastic nature of these cells is indicated by some cases in which the lesion recurred following surgical excision. Familial cases of LDD and an association with Cowden's syndrome, or multiple hamartoma-neoplasia syndrome, have been reported at least in one instance.[90]

### Pineocytoma—Grade II

Most pineocytomas become symptomatic among young adults.[27]

The normal pineal gland is composed of modified neurons, and this neoplasm is more cellular than, but otherwise similar to, the normal gland. Fibrillar cells with round nuclei form lobules between fibrovascular stroma or sheets of cells (Fig. 2-63). These cells sometimes orient their processes toward the vessels.[100] Silver impregnation for axons may demonstrate expansions at the tips of these processes that resemble clubs.

The diagnosis is simplified when enlarged fibrillary rosettes are found on H&E. These structures resemble Homer Wright rosettes and display massive accumulations of fibrils in the center. The diagnosis should be confirmed by electron microscopy and immunocytochemistry (Chapters 3 and 4).

Some pineocytomas contain neoplastic astrocytes.[145] In these cases the neoplasms may be distinguished from astrocytomas invading pineal gland by the macroscopic size and the microscopic nulear pleomorphism of the neuronal component of the tumor.

### Pineoblastoma—Grade IV

This tumor, which usually occurs in the first three decades of life, is found in the pineal region. The histologic features of pineoblastoma resemble those of medulloblastoma or primitive neuroectodermal tumor (PNET) (Fig. 2-64). Like these, pineoblastoma has been considered a multipotential neuroectodermal tumor. However, Flexner's rosettes, which are visible in some of these tumors, as well as their immunocytochemical and ultrastructural features all suggest a tendency toward retinal differentiation (Chapters 3 and 4). Fibrillary rosettes resemble those seen in medulloblastoma (see the section on medulloblastoma). Also, like medulloblastoma, these tumors of children spread through the CSF.

### Mixed Pineocytoma and Pineoblastoma

These recently recognized mixtures of both pineocytoma and pineoblastoma are relatively common among primary pineal tumors.[81] They also spread via the CSF.

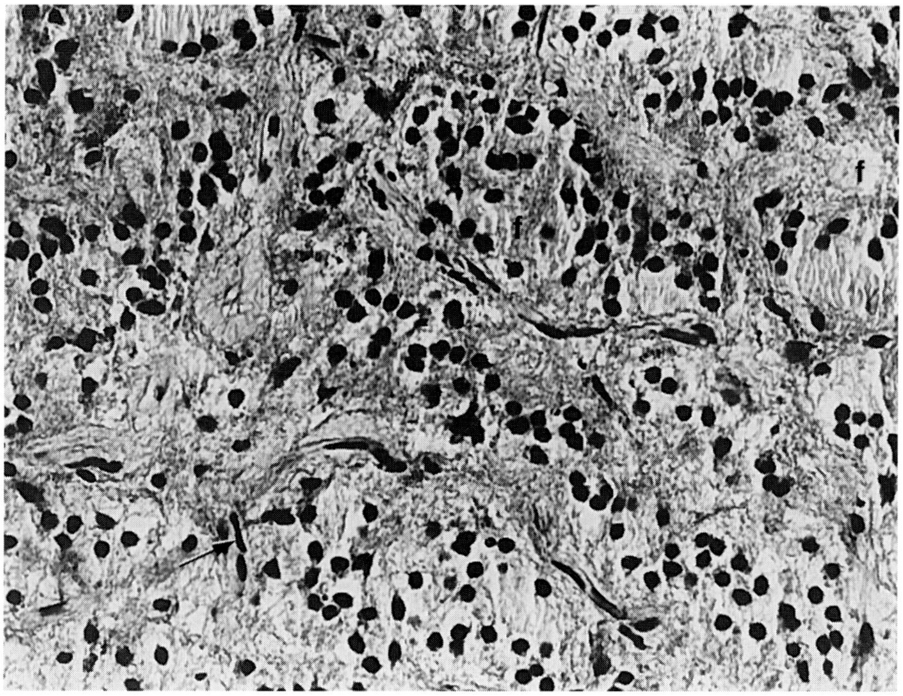


**Fig. 2-63.** Pineocytoma. Cells with small round nuclei and delicate fibrillary cytoplasmic processes mingle with small vessels. Some cellular fibrils touch vessels (*arrow*), others form large fibrillar rosettes (*f*). The 29-year-old man developed an unsteady gait. He had headaches for 3 months. (×400.) (Courtesy of Dr. Uma P. Kalyan-Raman, Peoria, IL.)

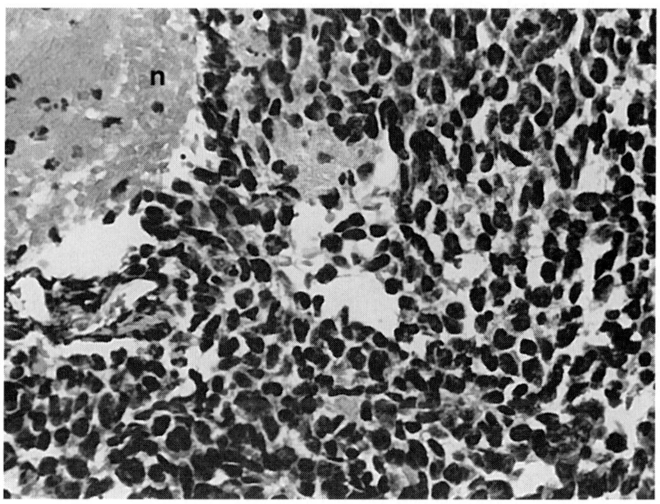


**Fig. 2-64.** Pineoblastoma. This pineal tumor is crowded with pleomorphic small cells that are mitotically active. They extend a few fibrillary cellular processes. The tumor contains small regions of necrosis (*n*). The 4-year-old girl had a tumor involving her pineal gland and posterior third ventricle. (×400.)

### Esthesioneuroblastoma (Olfactory Neuroblastoma)—Grade III

This neuroblastoma arises in the olfactory bulb and may invade the craniospinal vault. It is described in Chapter 5.

## MULTIPOTENTIAL NEUROECTODERMAL TUMORS

These neoplasms are malignant.[138] They tend to be crowded with cells of high nuclear-to-cytoplasmic ratio and contain abundant mitoses and apoptotic figures.[147] They commonly manifest differentiation of more than one cell lineage (i.e., neuronal, glial, epithelial, and others).

### Medulloblastoma—Grade IV

This multipotential neuroectodermal tumor arises in the cerebellum or in the roof of the fourth ventricle. Some neuropathologists prefer to call medulloblastomas primitive neuroectodermal tumors (PNET), and similar tumors that arise in cerebrum or spinal cord tend to be called PNETs.[42] Most medulloblastomas occur in the pediatric age group. They have been reported in the elderly, but are rare in patients over 35 years.[35,134,137]

The medulloblastoma is a malignant neoplasm composed of small cells (Table 2-7). On H&E stained slides and examined with the unaided eye it is a "blue tumor" owing to its nuclear crowding and high nuclear-to-cytoplasmic ratio (Fig. 2-65). The presence of cellular processes (fibrils) distinguishes a medulloblastoma from most other blue tumors except ependymoblastoma. These fibrils are difficult to see, and cytologic preparations make them more visible. However,

**Table 2-7.** Features of different brain tumors with small, crowded malignant cells

| Diagnosis* | Features | |
|---|---|---|
| | Structures | Locations† |
| Ependymoblastoma | Like PNET; ribbons/cords of cells; true ependymal rosettes | Cerebrum; cerebellum |
| Medulloblastoma/ pineoblastoma/ neuroblastoma/PNET | Slight fibrillarity; (Homer Wright rosettes); palisades; "carrot" nuclei; (neural or glial foci)‡ | Cerebellum; brainstem; pineal; CNS; (extraaxial) |
| Rhabdomyosarcoma/ medullomyoblastoma | Like PNET; muscle striations | Pineal; cerebellum; CNS |
| Hemangiopericytoma | Hypercellularity; thick pericellular matrix; mitoses | Falx, tentorium; meninges; (extracranial) |
| Lymphoma | Noncohesive round cells; vascular wall invasion | Deep cerebrum; CNS; meninges; may be multiple |
| Small cell carcinoma | Cohesive cells; (epithelioid); (desmosomes) | CNS; meninges; frequent multiple masses; systemic |

* Adapted from McKeever PE, and Blaivas M: The brain, spinal cord and meninges, In Sternberg S, and others, editors: Diagnostic Surgical Pathology, ed 2, New York, 1994, Raven Press.

† Most common or most specific craniospinal location is listed first.

‡ Parentheses around a differential feature indicate an uncommon feature very useful in differential diagnosis when found.

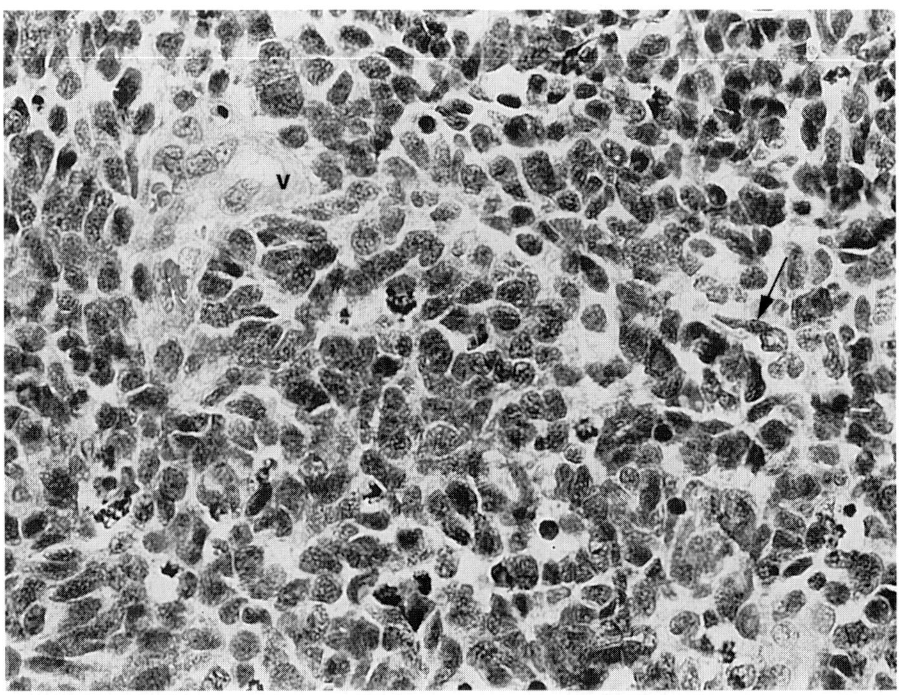


**Fig. 2-65.** Medulloblastoma. Round to carrot-shaped (*arrow*) nuclei crowd and indent one another in this medulloblastoma with abundant single cell necrosis. It lacks Homer Wright rosettes and shows only scant cellular fibrils. Cell bodies directly abut vessels (*v*). Many medulloblastomas require immunocytochemistry or electron microscopy for confirmation (Chapters 3, 4). The 11-year-old boy had a large mass in his fourth ventricle and hydrocephalus. (×400.)

they are best seen by electron microscopy (Chapter 3). Homer Wright rosettes, characteristic of medulloblastoma, are rosettes with cores that are filled with fibrils (Fig. 2-66). Unfortunately, biopsy samples often lack classic Homer Wright rosettes (Fig. 2-65). Some medulloblastomas have tumor cells arranged in rhythmic palisades alternating with fibrils. These palisades are more cellular than those seen in gliomas. Elongated nuclei shaped as carrots (Fig. 2-65) help distinguish medulloblastomas from carcinoma and lymphoma. Rare medulloblastomas contain melanin.[81]

Medulloblastomas spread along CSF pathways through the entire neuraxis. They commonly respond well to radiotherapy. About 5% of medulloblastomas metastasize to a systemic location, particularly to bone.[35]

**Desmoplastic medulloblastoma—grade IV.** These medulloblastomas contain excessive amounts of connective tissue (Table 2-5) and often are located superficially in the cerebellum (Fig. 2-67). Islands of medulloblastoma cells mingle with bands of fibrous

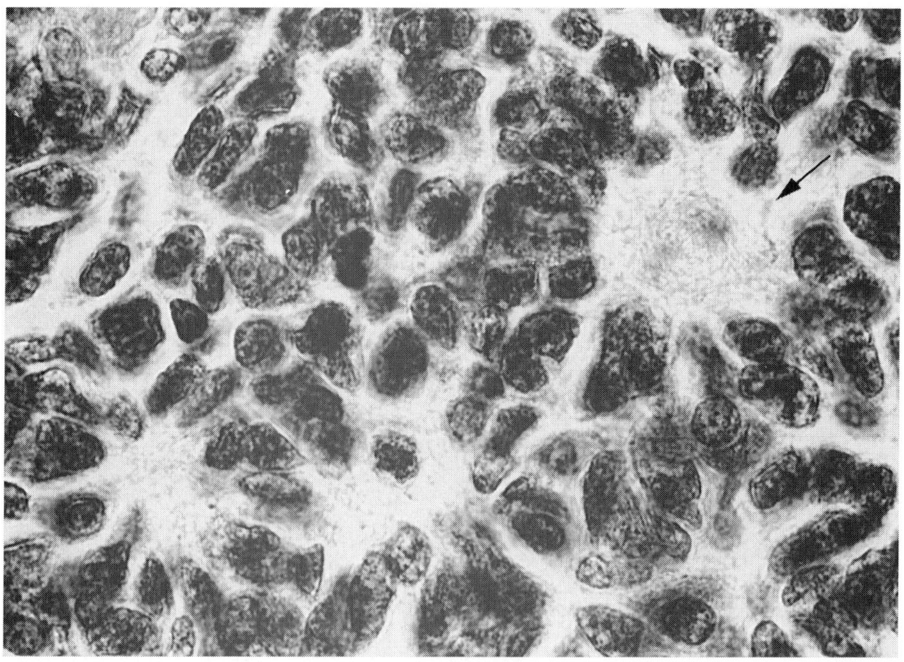

**Fig. 2-66.** Medulloblastoma. Homer Wright rosettes contain fibrillary cellular processes (*arrow*). These fibrils are the processes of nearby cells. (×1000.)

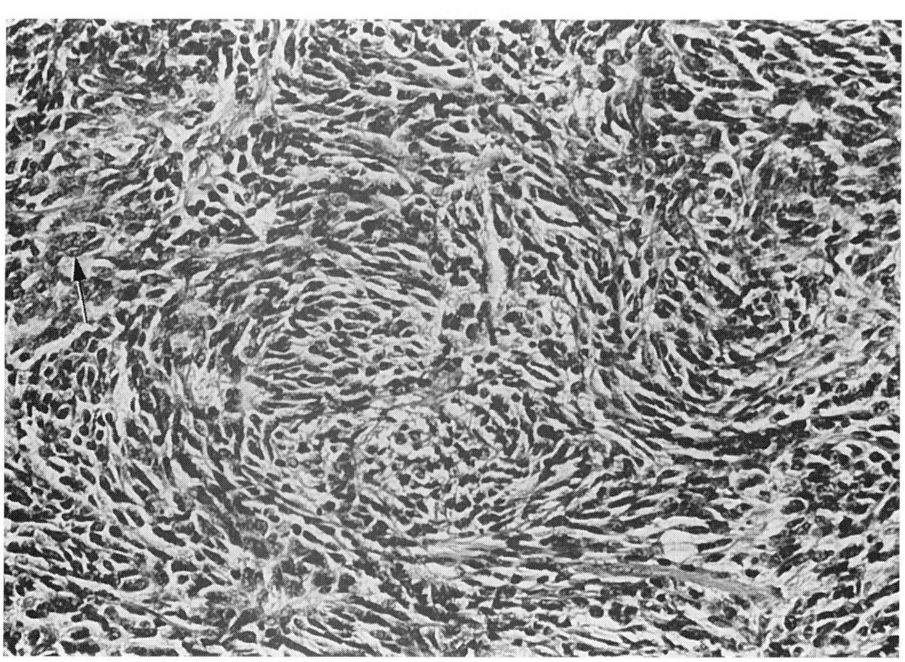

**Fig. 2-67.** Desmoplastic medulloblastoma. Clusters of neuroectodermal cells with sparse cytoplasmic processes are divided by desmoplastic regions of spindled cells with less hyperchromatic nuclei (*arrow*) and pink collagen, producing a swirled pattern of the two cell types. The 10-year-old boy had a tumor in his right cerebellum. (×200.) (Courtesy of Dr. John A. McGee, Jackson, MI.)

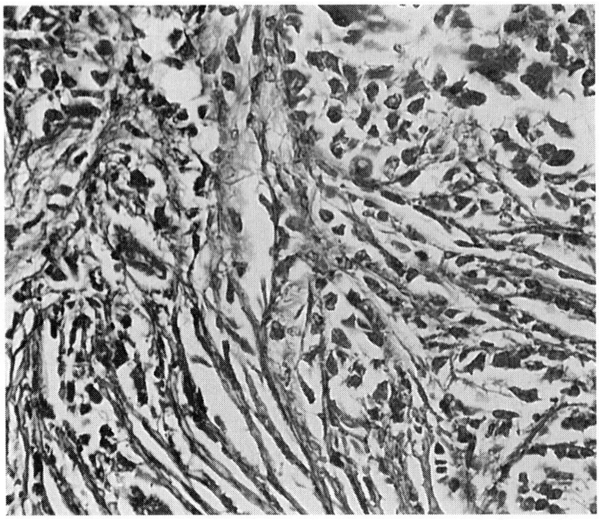

**Fig. 2-68.** Desmoplastic medulloblastoma. The trichrome stain distinguishes blue regions of desmoplasia from red regions of medulloblastoma cells. The 10-year-old boy had a tumor in his right cerebellum. (×400) (Courtesy of Dr. John McGee, Jackson, MI.) (See Plate 1C.)

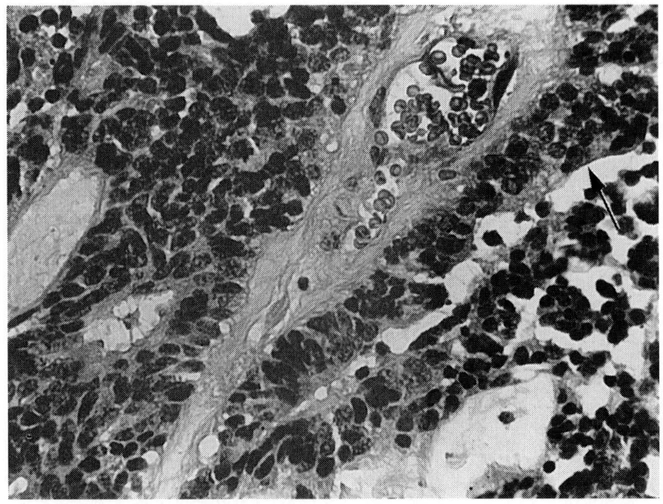

**Fig. 2-69.** Medulloepithelioma. Neoplastic cells resemble the medullary epithelium of the neural tube. They have both a basement membrane and thick material on their apical surface (*arrow*). Mitoses are abundant. (×300.)

tissue.[49,142] Stains for collagen distinguish these regions (Fig. 2-68, Plate 1C). Some pale groups of cells with perinuclear halos are made of neurons or neuroblasts.[73] Invasion of arachnoid membranes may explain the desmoplasia, but the potential for generating vascular proliferation also exists.[44]

**Lipomatous medulloblastoma.** This cerebellar neoplasm is a distinct pathologic entity that occurs in adults of mean age of 50 years.[154a] The tumor and its adipocytes are variably immunoreactive for neuronal and glial markers. The lipomatous variant resembles a medulloblastoma, but has low mitotic activity and a better prognosis.

**Medullomyoblastoma—grade IV.** This rare variant of medulloblastoma contains muscle fibers.[16,145] Immunocytochemistry is recommended to confirm this diagnosis (Chapter 4). Medulloblastoma can also contain mesenchymal cells other than muscle.[7,22]

### Polar Spongioblastoma

The primitive polar spongioblastoma is so rare that it is not graded. It had been cited as a tumor of children and adolescents. It contains rhythmic palisades of unipolar and bipolar cells with delicate cellular processes.[67] Patterns that resemble regions of spongioblastoma are more commonly seen in gliomas, neuroblastoma,[123] and medulloblastoma than the pure tumor itself.

### Medulloepithelioma—Grade IV

This rare tumor produces glandlike structures that resemble embryonic neural tube (Fig. 2-69) and has thick, eosinophilic material on both sides of the epithelium. This material is PAS-positive and resembles basal lamina.

Medulloepithelioma resembles carcinoma. Since it afflicts patients younger than 6 years, metastatic carcinoma is an unlikely differential diagnosis. However, choroid plexus carcinoma must be considered. To distinguish medulloepithelioma, its location away from the choroid plexus and the differentiation toward neuronal or glial features are helpful clues.

### Atypical Teratoid/Rhabdoid Tumor

This highly malignant neoplasm occurs in infants and young children; it usually grows in the posterior fossa or brainstem. Metastases via CSF may be present upon initial encounter. The histologic features resemble those of a medulloblastoma, but individual neoplastic cells have more pink cytoplasm and are more epithelial than are the cells of medulloblastoma. Moreover, these cells may have rhabdoid features and may be vacuolated. Abnormalities of chromosome 22 help to distinguish them from other primitive neuroectodermal tumors.[15,139]

## INTRINSIC CHOROID PLEXUS TUMORS

These papillary tumors are uncommon. Most appear in childhood. Location in the choroid plexus aids in their recognition (Table 2-6). They occur more fre-

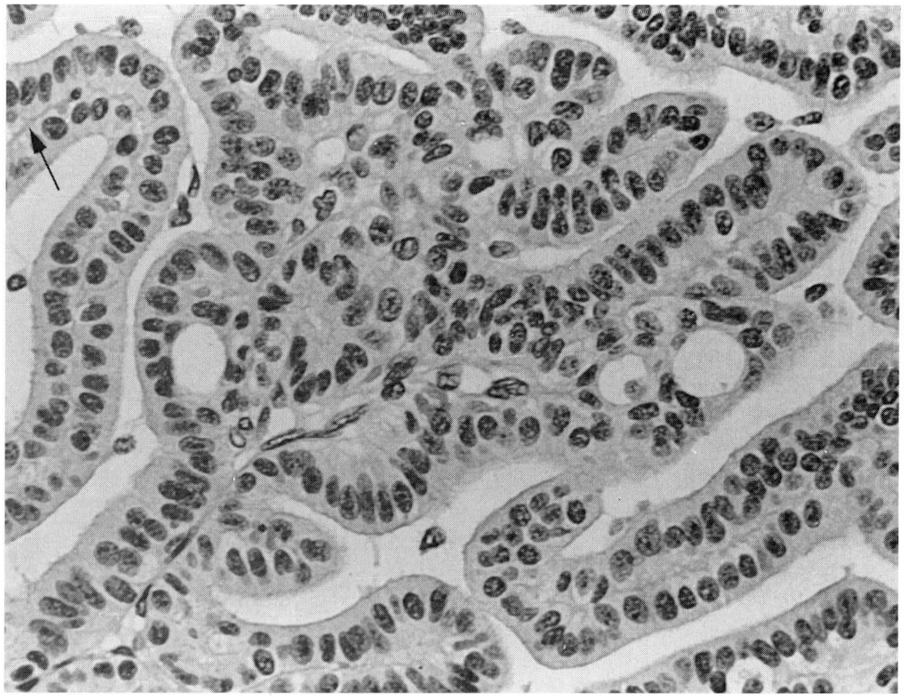

**Fig. 2-70.** Choroid plexus papilloma. Epithelial cells line up along thin fibrovascular septa (*arrow*). The 15-month-old patient had a history of lethargy, irritability, and vomiting and a large fourth ventricular mass. (×400.)

quently in the lateral ventricles of children or in the fourth ventricle of adults.[100]

### Choroid Plexus Papilloma—Grade I

This tumor may present clinically with signs of hydrocephalus. Since the microscopic features of choroid plexus papilloma are very similar to normal choroid plexus, the tumor should be larger than a normal choroid plexus to establish the diagnosis of choroid plexus papilloma. Thus, needle biopsy is not recommended because of the unavoidable sampling error.

The choroid plexus papilloma has a layer of well-differentiated columnar to cuboidal epithelial cells over a basement membrane and fibrovascular stroma (Fig. 2-70). The epithelial lining of some papillomas is pseudostratified, but one should not depend on this feature for diagnosis. Pigmented, oncocytic, osteogenic, and adenomatous variants of papillomas are rare.[6,165]

The choroid plexus papilloma resembles papillary ependymoma, and distinguishing these tumors is best done by immunocytochemistry (Chapter 4).[96] However, its reticulin staining pattern is also different from that seen in ependymoma. It has epithelium on a basement membrane forming papillae. In contrast, ependymomas have solid parenchyma without reticulin.

### Choroid Plexus Carcinoma—Grade III

The choroid plexus carcinoma (anaplastic choroid plexus papilloma) is a rare neoplasm. It resembles undifferentiated carcinoma or adenocarcinoma.[65] Epithelial cells are pleomorphic, hyperchromatic, and mitotically active (Fig. 2-71). Necrosis occurs spontaneously (Fig. 2-72).

Metastatic carcinoma must be carefully excluded before making this diagnosis.[145] If sufficient specimen is available, it may reveal a zone of gradual transition between papilloma and carcinoma of the choroid plexus, supporting the interpretation. Primary systemic carcinomas are sufficiently rare in children as to increase the likelihood of choroid plexus carcinoma when a malignant epithelial tumor is found in this age group.

## TUMORS OF MENINGES AND RELATED COVERINGS

### Meningiomas—Grade I

Meningeal location distinguishes the meningioma from primary glial and neuronal tumors. Most meningiomas occur in adults and are attached to the dura. Some grow locally into the dura, a fact that does not indicate malignancy. However, dural invasion can complicate total surgical removal, for example when the lesion involves dural sinuses.

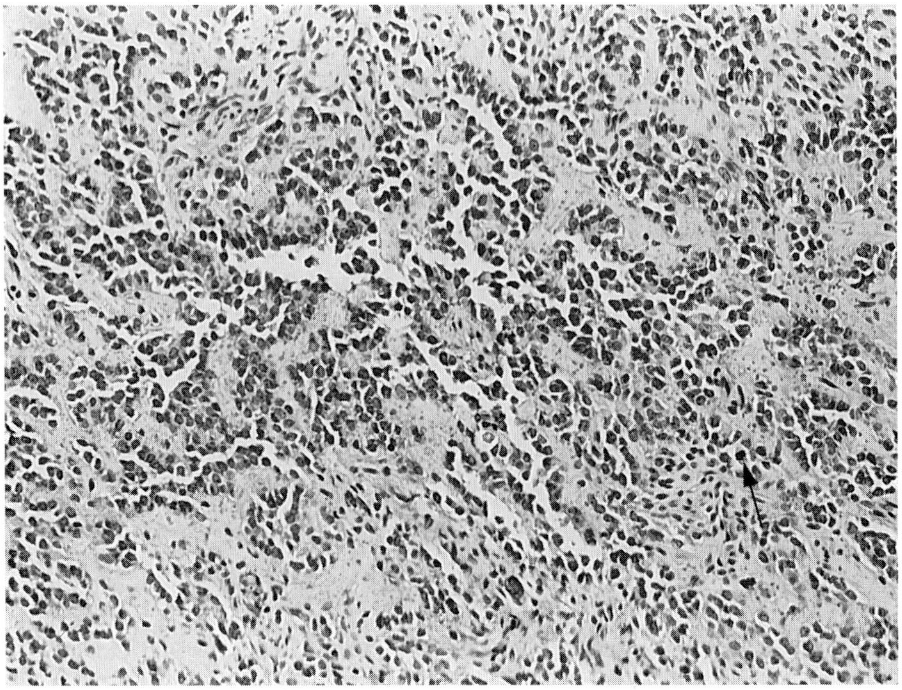

2-71

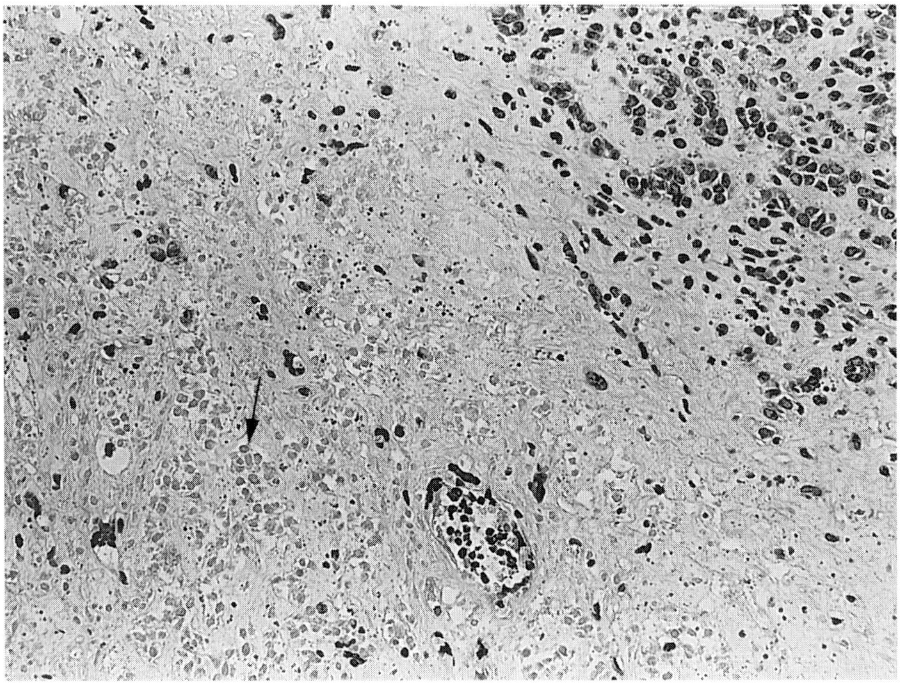

2-72

**Figs. 2-71, 2-72.** Choroid plexus carcinoma. The 5-year-old girl had a large tumor in her lateral ventricle. **Fig. 2-71,** Papillae are crowded with malignant epithelial cells with mitoses (*arrow*). (×200.) **Fig. 2-72,** Spontaneous coagulation necrosis shows ghostly remnants (*arrow*) of carcinoma cells. (×250.)

**Table 2-8.** Features of different brain tumors with "syncytial" cells

| Diagnosis* | Features: Structures | Features: Locations† |
|---|---|---|
| Meningiomas | Whorls; psammoma bodies; interdigitating cell processes and desmosomes; (thick collagen)‡ | Falx, tentorium; meninges; choroid plexus; (extracranial) |
| Anaplastic meningioma | Decrease in above features; mitoses; necrosis; CNS invasion | Above locations |
| Hemangiopericytoma | Hypercellularity; thick pericellular matrix; mitoses | Above locations |
| Choriocarcinoma | Syncytium usually mixed with cytotrophoblast | Pineal; suprasellar |

* Adapted from McKeever PE, and Blaivas M: The brain, spinal cord and meninges, In Sternberg S, and others, editors: Diagnostic Surgical Pathology, ed 2, New York, 1994, Raven Press.
† Most common or most specific craniospinal location is listed first.
‡ Parentheses around a differential feature indicate an uncommon feature very useful in differential diagnosis when found.

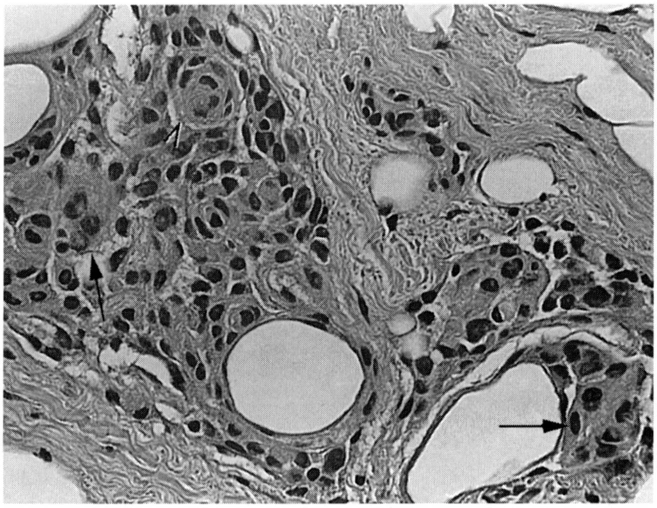

2-73

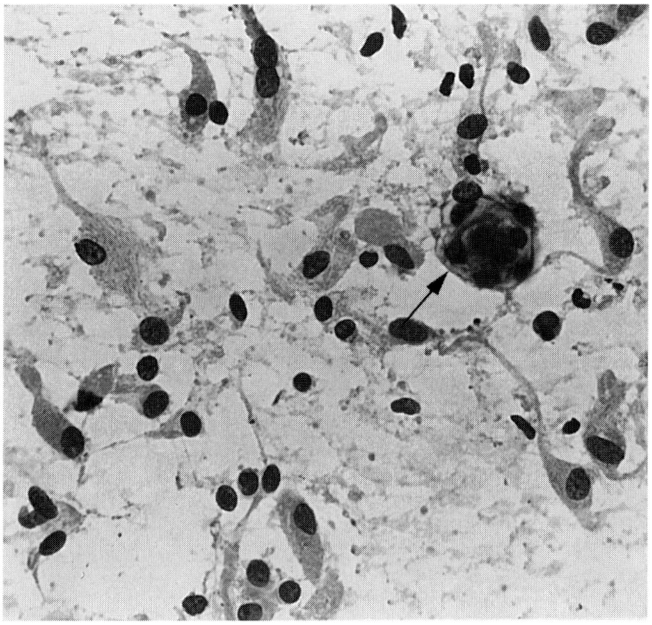

2-74

**Figs. 2-73, 2-74.** Meningioma. The 71-year-old woman had a recurrent meningioma in her sphenoid ridge 2 years after first surgery and decreased vision in her left eye. **Fig. 2-73,** Meningioma outside of skull. Meningothelial cells are growing in the fibroadipose tissue of the scalp. Both syncytial patterns (*arrows*) and whorls (*arrowhead*) are present. (×400.) **Fig. 2-74,** Individual meningothelial cells show round to oval nuclei and scant thick cellular processes. A whorl (*arrow*) is composed of similar cells. (Cytologic preparation; ×400.)

Meningiomas are much less common in the ventricles and are very rare within the brain tissue itself.[146] Multiple meningiomas occur in 1% to 6% of the cases. Some are associated with von Recklinghausen's neurofibromatosis.[78]

It is difficult to generalize about the histology of a tumor with so many variants. Nevertheless, certain features provide strong evidence of meningioma.[100] For example, a distinctive "syncytial" pattern (Fig. 2-73; Table 2-8), is ubiquitous in meningothelial meningiomas and occurs focally in other subtypes (Fig. 2-82). Such a pattern is best appreciated ultrastructurally (Chapter 3).

Cellular whorls and psammoma bodies are quite typical of a meningioma. Whorls are concentric clusters of flat cells that resemble cabbage leaves or onion bulbs (Figs. 2-73 to 2-75).[101] Psammoma bodies are concentrically laminated calcifications (Fig. 2-76).

Meningiomas that involve the sellar region are described in Chapter 5. Histologically benign meningiomas occasionally escape the craniospinal vault, particularly following surgery (Fig. 2-73).

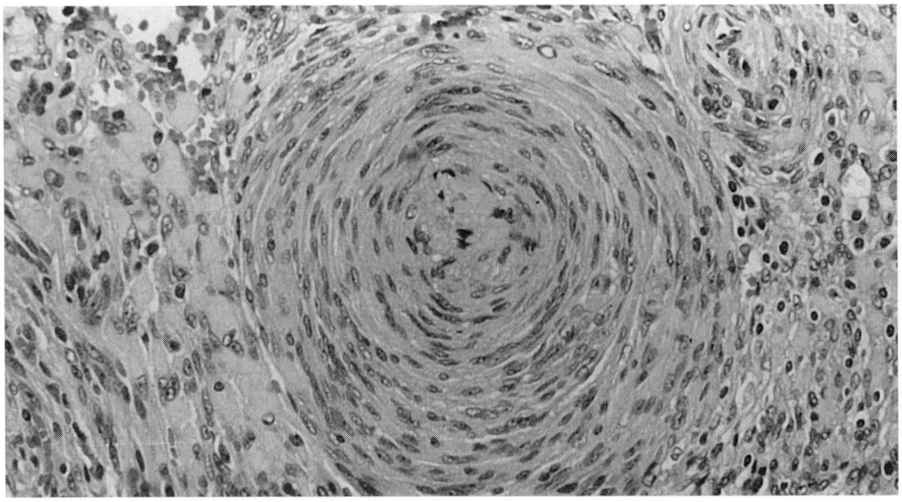

**Fig. 2-75.** Whorls. Occasional whorls are quite large, as in this meningioma. The 57-year-old man had headaches, balance impairment, and a large mass of his right cerebellar convexity. (×250.)

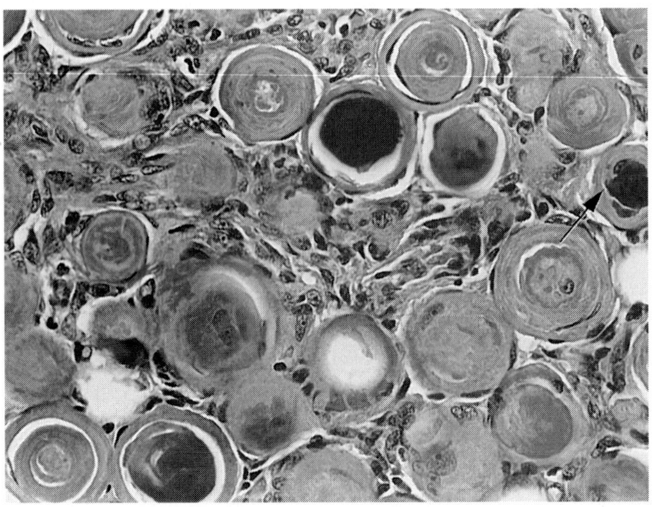

**Fig. 2-76.** Psammomatous meningioma. Round psammoma bodies with variable calcification (*arrow*) predominate in this meningioma. (×400.)

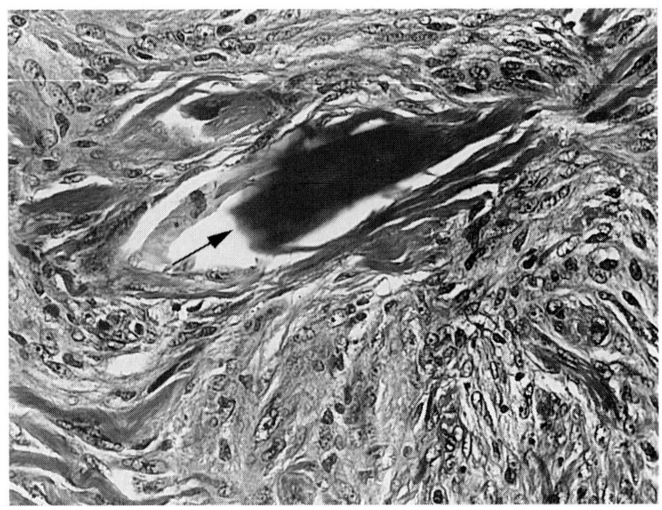

**Fig. 2-77.** Calcified fibrous meningioma. Thick bundles of collagen have calcified (*arrow*) in this tumor composed of spindle-shaped meningothelial cells. The 71-year-old patient had this asymptomatic but radiographically apparent suboccipital meningioma resected 2 years after its previous incomplete resection. (×400.)

**Fibrous meningioma (fibroblastic meningioma)—grade I.** Fibrous meningiomas are firm tumors. Some contain considerable glycosylated collagen that can be identified by reticulin stains.[98] They are composed of spindle cells (Fig. 2-77).

Fibrous meningiomas may mimic schwannomas and, occasionally, solitary fibrous tumors. Schwannoma can be a particular diagnostic challenge in tumors located in the cerebellopontine angle and around spinal nerve roots. Useful features to identify meningiomas include whorls, psammoma bodies, and very thick bundles of collagen. These bundles occasionally calcify (Fig. 2-77). Psammoma bodies scattered within the meningioma exclude schwannoma from the differential diagnosis,[53] but some schwannomas form whorls (see Figs. 2-95, 2-97). Electron microscopy and immunocytochemistry are recommended to distinguish refractory schwannomas and solitary fibrous tumors (Chapters 3 and 4).

**Meningotheliomatous meningioma (syncytial meningioma)—grade I.** This is the prototypic meningioma with "syncytial" features because the individual boundaries between the cells are indistinct on paraffin sections. Whorls and psammoma bodies often are sparse. Meningothelial meningioma occasionally resembles ependymoma.[74] For example, differentiation from myxopapillary ependymoma can be difficult in the region of cauda equina. Immunocytochemistry is recommended to distinguish these entities (Chapter 4).

Meningiomas can be confused with oligodendrogliomas, particularly if they lack meningeal attachment. The margin of the meningioma with brain tissue is more discrete than the margin of this glioma. In difficult cases the diagnosis is made by electron microscopy (Chapter 3).

**Transitional meningioma (mixed meningioma)—grade I.** Transitional meningiomas are the simplest to identify. They show both syncytial and fibroblastic features (Fig. 2-75). Most specimens contain an adequate sample of whorls, psammoma bodies, and clusters of "syncytial" cells to confirm the interpretation.

**Psammomatous meningioma—grade I.** Psammomatous meningiomas show a predominance of psammoma bodies (Fig. 2-76). They are often in the spinal canal. Syncytial cells fill spaces between the conspicuous, concentrically laminated psammoma bodies.

**Hemangioblastic, angioblastic, and angiomatous meningiomas—grade I.** A few meningiomas resemble hemangioblastoma (Fig. 2-78). Sometimes only topography, such as attachment to the dura and supratentorial location, can distinguish meningiomas from classic hemangioblastoma. Foamy cells and meningothelial cells concentrically wrapped around small blood vessels and capillaries are considered evidence of meningioma.[78]

The angiomatous meningioma lacks the vacuolated stromal cells of hemangioblastic meningioma. The angiomatous type has numerous small or large vascular channels (Fig. 2-79).[81]

**Other benign meningiomas.** When a distinctive region predominates in a meningioma, a new variant is proposed. The importance of recognizing these variants is to distinguish them from other tumors, including more ominous ones. In addition, meningiomas with chordoid and clear cell types may be more aggressive. Lipoblastic,[87] arachnoid trabecular,[66] cystic,[85] glycogen-rich,[150] clear cell, microcystic (Fig. 2-80), osteogenic,[79] chordoid (Fig. 2-81),[81] cartilaginous,[79] and secretory (Fig. 2-82)[21,92,167] variants have been described. Most of these variants contain foci of cells with meningothelial features that help in the diagnosis. Adequate sampling for regions that contain a syncytial pattern, whorls, or a pattern with cells encircling vessels is recommended. If the diagnosis is still doubtful, electron microscopy usually is definitive (Chapter 3).

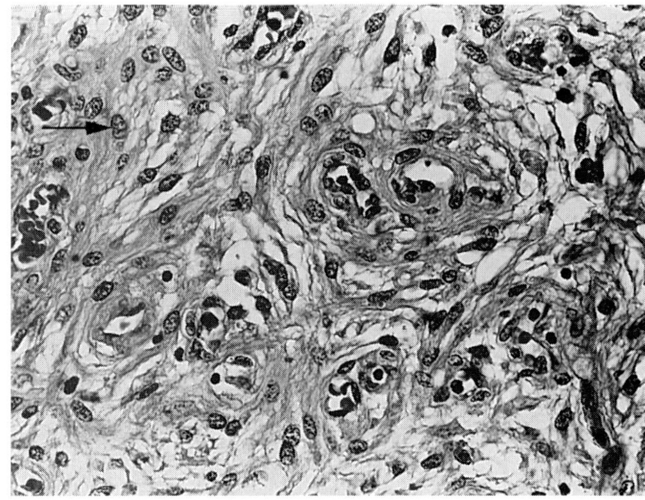

**Fig. 2-78.** Hemangioblastic meningioma. This highly vascular meningioma has numerous small vessels with vacuolated meningothelial cells (*arrow*) in between them. While it resembles a hemangioblastoma, its more elongated meningothelial cells wrap concentrically around vessels as if they were forming a whorl. The 72-year-old woman had syncope, headaches, and a left frontotemporal dural mass with an angiographic blush. (×400.)

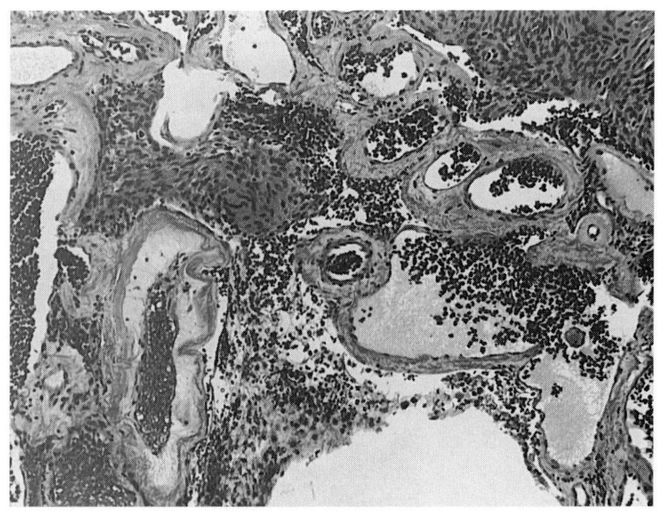

**Fig. 2-79.** Angiomatous meningioma. Vessels predominate around scattered clusters of meningothelial cells in this meningioma. (×125.)

A rare condition termed meningiomatosis or meningioangiomatosis[145] occurs as a dysplastic/malformative lesion in patients with central neurofibromatosis (Figs. 2-83, 2-84). It presents as "en plaque" meningioma, contains numerous psammoma bodies, and infiltrates the brain by way of parenchymal blood vessels.

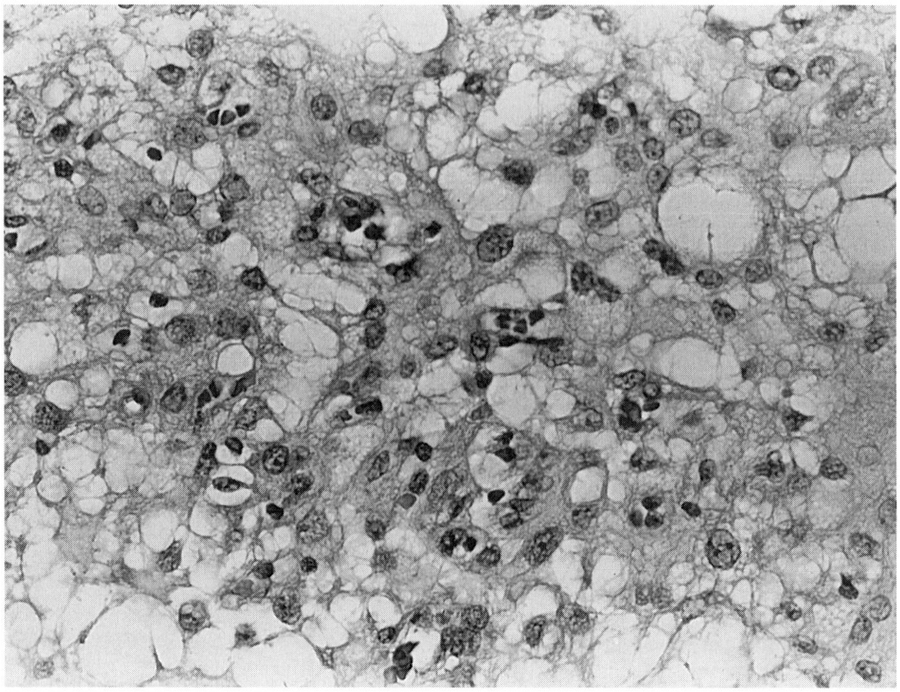

**Fig. 2-80.** Microcystic meningioma. Numerous large cysts, some containing wisps of eosinophilic material, characterized this dural-based neoplasm. (×400.)

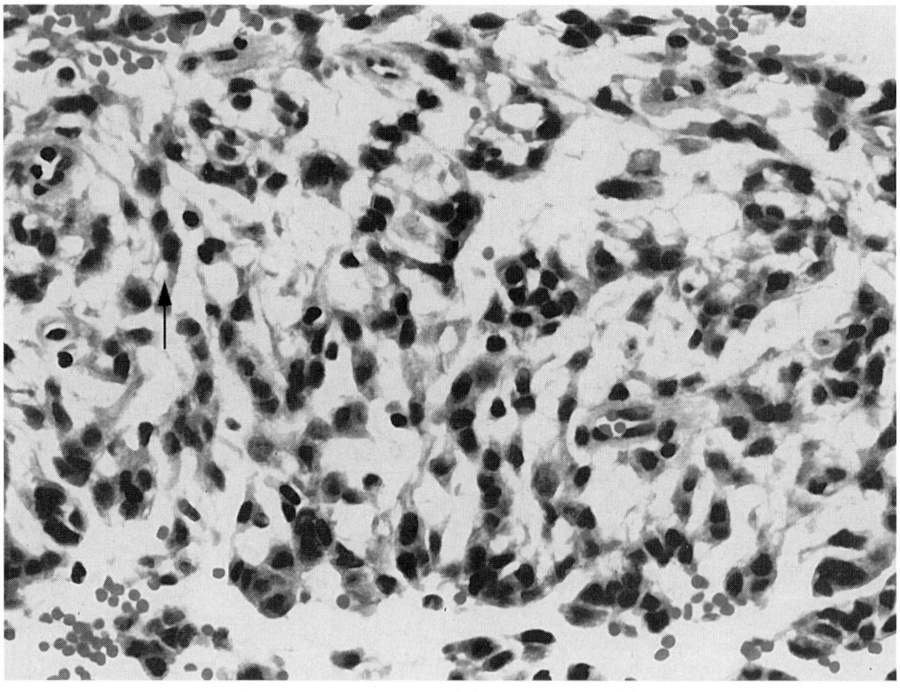

**Fig. 2-81.** Chordoid meningioma. Chains of eosinophilic cells contain a few cytoplasmic vacuoles (*arrow*). Focal meningothelial features were present elsewhere in this tumor. (×300.)

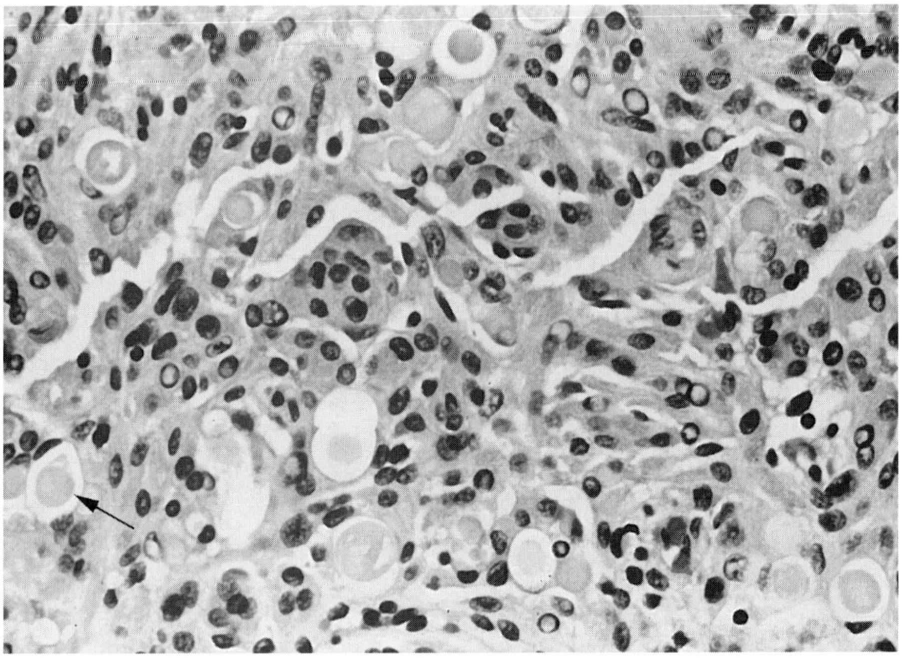

**Fig. 2-82.** Secretory meningioma. Meningothelial cells that look syncytial surround globules of pale eosinophilic material (*arrow*). The 75-year-old man had headaches and memory difficulties. A mass was removed from the subfrontal region. (×200.)

**Figs. 2-83, 2-84.** Meningioangiomatosis. **Fig. 2-83,** Densely cellular tissue is formed by a flattened wavy arrangement of meningothelial cells sharply demarcated from lighter brain parenchyma. (×80.) **Fig. 2-84,** Parenchymal island (*i*) is encased within this meningothelial tissue that contains whorls with and without psammoma bodies (*arrow*). (×330.) (Courtesy of Dr. Peter Smythe, Toledo, OH.)

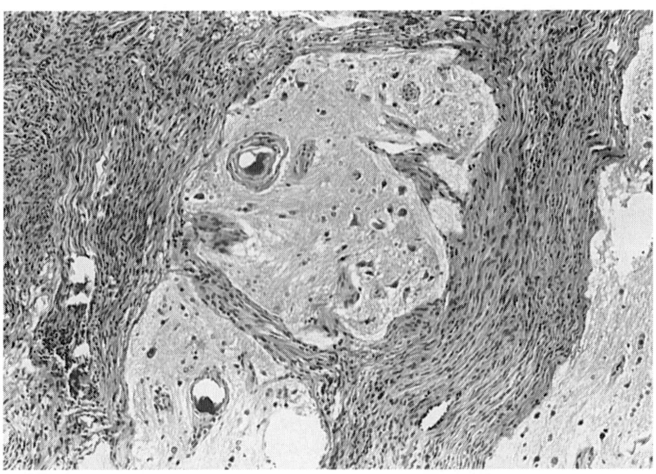

2-83

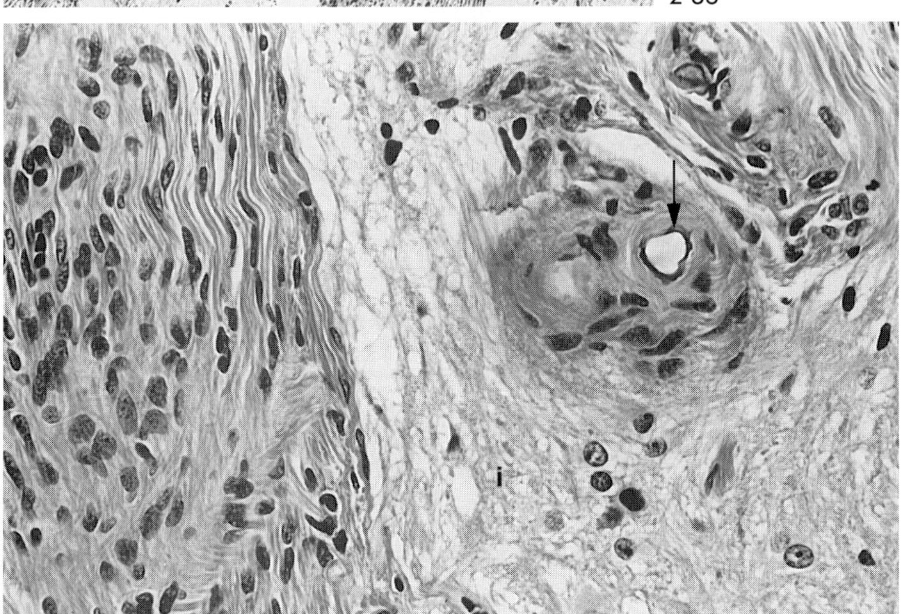



2-84

**Atypical meningioma—grade II.** Atypical meningiomas are more cellular and mitotically active than grade I meningiomas (Fig. 2-85). They may have patternless sheetlike growth (Fig. 2-86) and foci of necrosis.[81] (Fig. 2-85). While the diagnostic criteria for this meningioma are subjective, it is recognized as a distinct diagnostic entity with histopathologic features between benign and malignant meningioma. It is likely to recur locally. Chromosomal abnormalities in addition to standard loss of chromosome 22 may be early evidence of increased aggressiveness.[19]

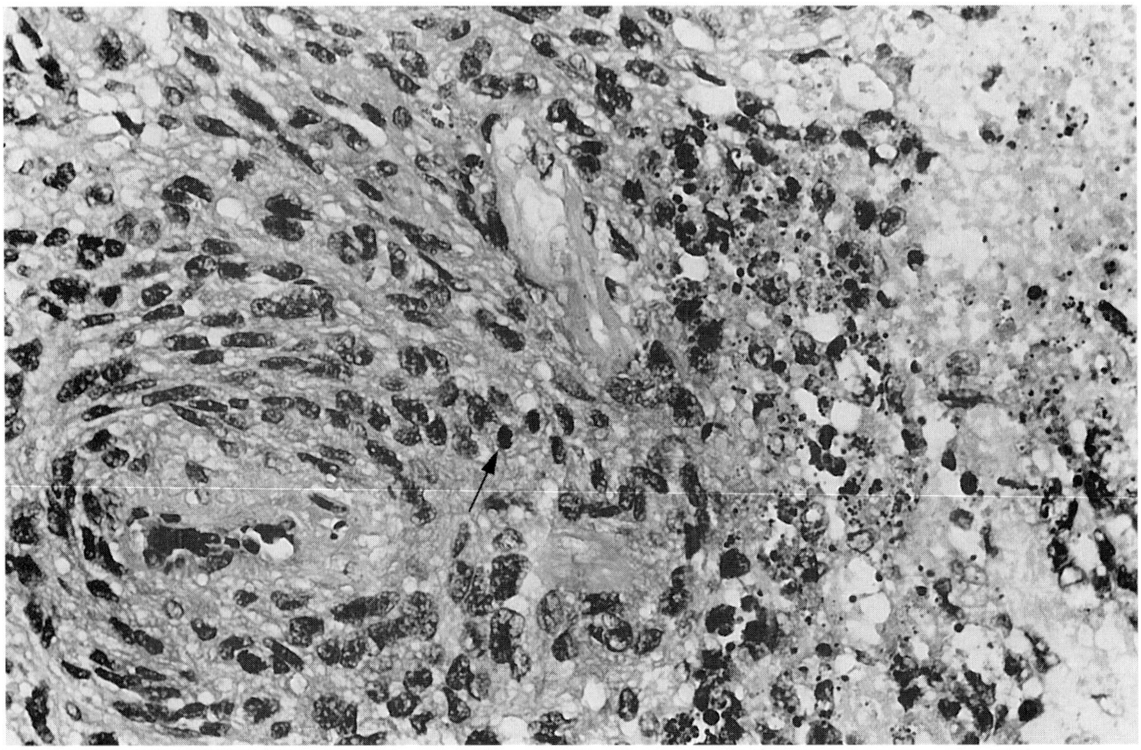

**Fig. 2-85.** Atypical meningioma. The tendency of its meningothelial cells to swirl around vessels and other objects on the left is still apparent. However, spontaneous necrosis shown on the right and mitotic activity (*arrow*) of crowded cells are features of a grade higher than grade I. The totality of features corresponds to grade II. (×400.)

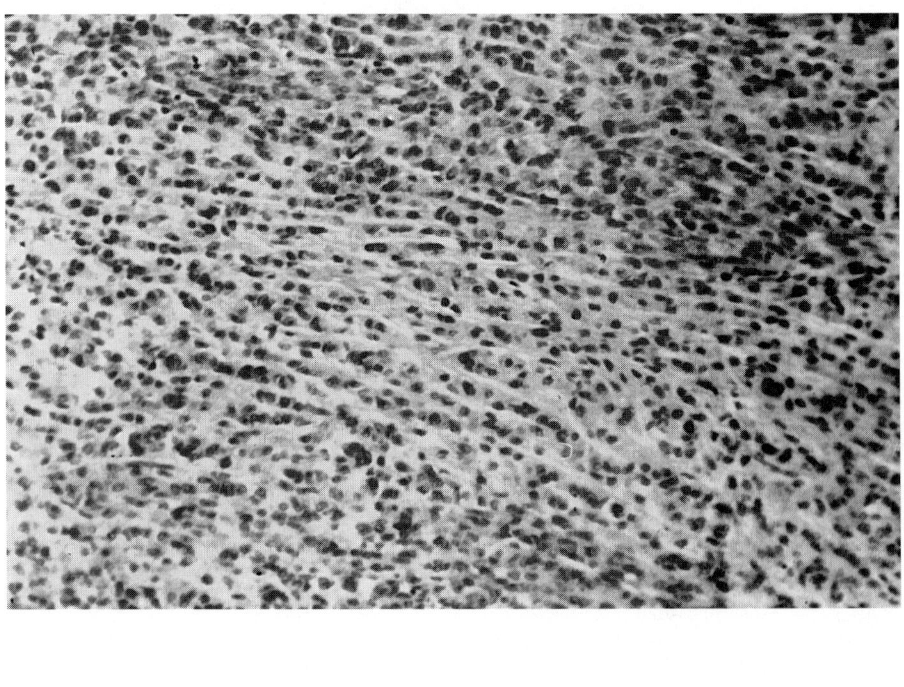

**Fig. 2-86.** Monotonous sheets of cells are a feature of atypical and malignant meningiomas. (×120.)

**Anaplastic meningioma (malignant meningioma)—grade III.** These tumors retain enough features to be recognized as meningiomas, but in addition have qualitatively more malignant cytology, conspicuous mitoses, spontaneous tumor necrosis, and—very importantly—brain invasion (Fig. 2-87). Kepes[78] recommends a close follow-up of patients with tumors in which any of these features are present. The action of meningioma cells breaking through pia into brain parenchyma is a particularly ominous sign.[15] When all of these features are evident, the meningioma is anaplastic. Clinical history is important to determine whether necrosis is spontaneous or simply a result of preoperative embolization.

Metastases indicate malignant biologic behavior, but histopathologic features do not correlate well with metastatic potentials of individual meningiomas. Most malignant meningiomas are aggressive only locally, but occasional tumors have metastasized through the CSF. Pulmonary, abdominal, or bone metastases are rare.[15,78]

Anaplastic meningiomas occasionally may be confused with glioblastomas and carcinomas. Immunocytochemistry is recommended to distinguish these entities (Chapter 4).

**Papillary meningioma—grade II to III.** Papillary configurations in meningiomas need to be recognized because they are associated with high rates of local recurrence and metastases. The papillae are formed by meningioma cells arranged around a vascular core (Fig. 2-88). Necrosis and loosening of the surrounding tumor cells may produce them.[78]

Papillary ependymomas, choroid plexus papillomas, and carcinomas may mimic this meningioma. However, the papillary meningioma usually shows foci with features characteristic of meningioma, such as syncytial appearance, whorls, or psammoma bodies. Immunocytochemistry helps to identify these tumors when these features are absent (Chapter 4).

### Hemangiopericytoma—Grade II

This highly cellular and mitotically active neoplasm occurs in the meninges and has the appearance of a "blue tumor" when viewed with the naked eye on an H&E stained histology slide. Its hypercellularity and high mitotic index are helpful features in the diagnosis; however, the most distinctive feature is the tendency of the neoplastic cells to bulge into vascular lumina (Fig. 2-89). Hemangiopericytomas have regions rich in reticulin where these fibers surround individual cells (Fig. 2-90). These features distinguish hemangiopericytomas from other malignant neoplasms like gliomas and metastatic carcinomas. Eighty percent of all hemangiopericytomas recur, and 23% of them eventually metastasize.[56,70]

### Chordoma

Approximately 40% of chordomas arise in the clivus and more than 45% in the sacral portions of the spinal canal. The remainder are distributed along the spinal cord. All are midline lesions. Chordomas are described in detail in Chapter 5 on tumors of the pituitary gland region.

### Chondroma and Chondrosarcoma

Chondroid neoplasms are uncommon brain tumors (Fig. 2-91). They form cartilage and sometimes need to be distinguished from chordoma by immunocytochemistry (Chapter 4).[10,23,86] They occur infrequently

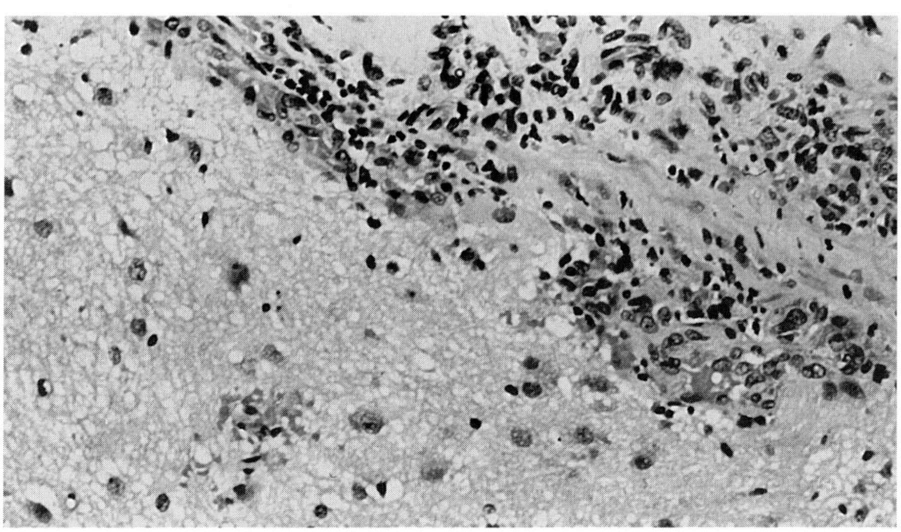

**Fig. 2-87.** Anaplastic meningioma margin. Meningioma cells in the hypercellular region of this picture both infiltrate brain parenchyma and cluster around nearby vessels. Surrounding brain has reactive astrocytosis. The 42-year-old woman had a large partially enhancing neoplasm involving her right posterior parasagittal falx. (×165.)

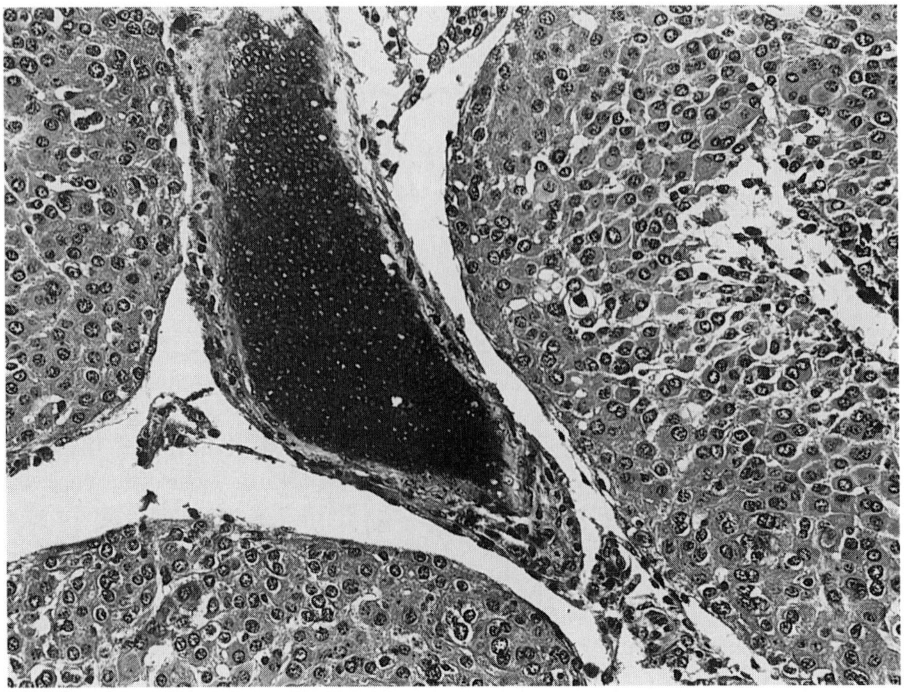

**Fig. 2-88.** Papillary meningioma. Papillae have vascular cores. (×200.)

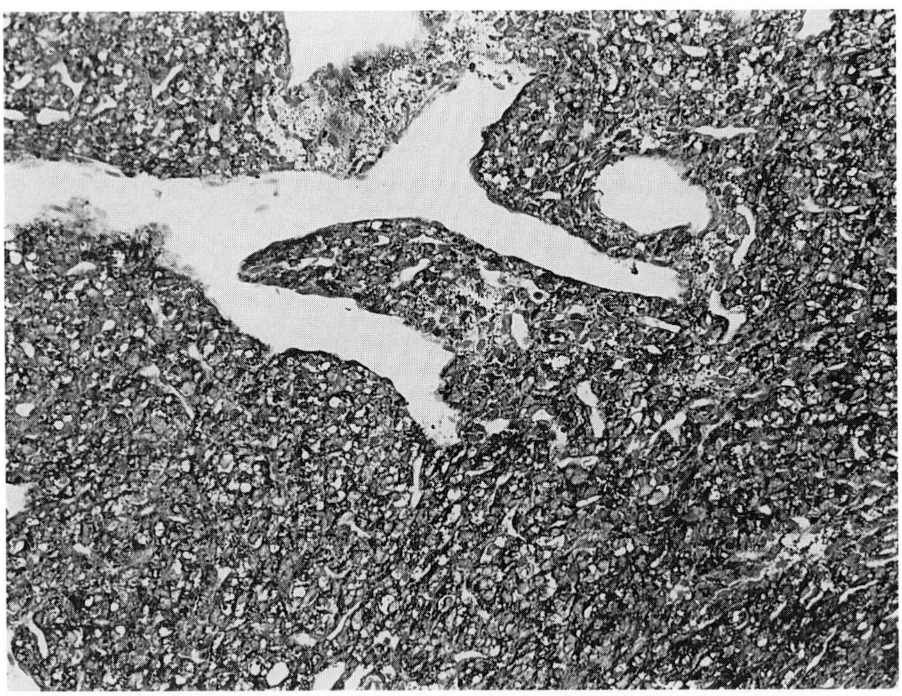

**Fig. 2-89.** Hemangiopericytoma. Crowds of cells with high nuclear-to-cytoplasmic ratio compress vascular lumina to form peculiar shapes like this "staghorn" vessel. PAS stain reveals pericellular basement membrane material. The 32-year-old woman had a mass in her temporal fossa causing bone erosion and cranial nerve pain. (×200.)

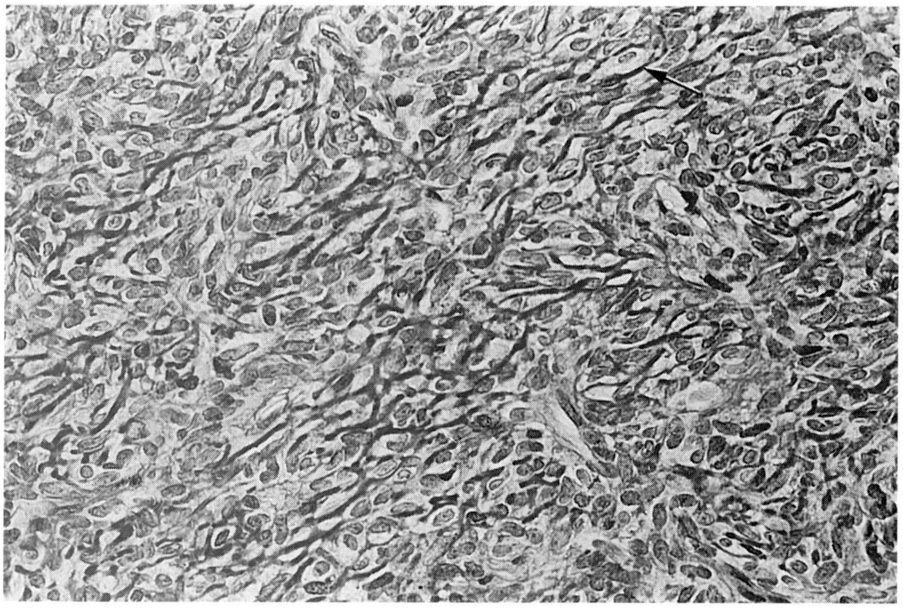

**Fig. 2-90.** Hemangiopericytoma. Reticulin stain highlights basement membrane material (*arrow*) encompassing many cells. The 40-year-old woman had a large right parietal tumor involving her dura and brain. (×400.)

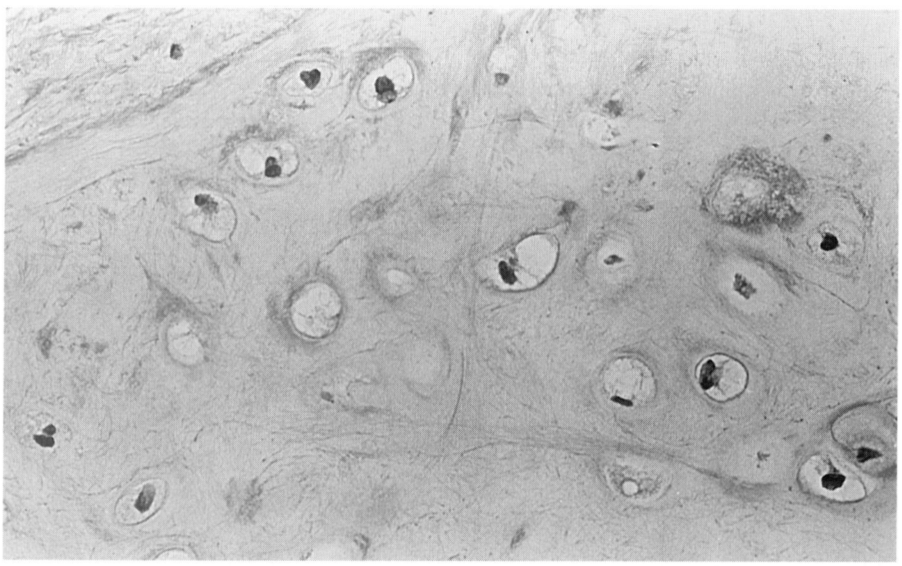

**Fig. 2-91.** Extensive cartilage formation distinguishes this neoplasm. The low cellularity and differentiated appearance of this chondroid tumor suggest chondroma; however, it has been locally invasive and impossible to eradicate surgically from the skull base despite numerous resections over more than a decade. (×400.)

in the skull or meninges, and rarely within the brain or choroid plexus.

Chondromas are well-differentiated chondroid tumors that produce extensive cartilage. When binucleated cells and nuclear pleomorphism are evident within this neoplasm, a diagnosis of low-grade chondrosarcoma needs to be considered.

The mesenchymal chondrosarcoma is a rare tumor of the meninges. It occurs in childhood and young adulthood.[144] Histologically, it resembles a hemangiopericytoma that contains islands of cartilage.[16]

Poorly differentiated chondrosarcomas are rare. They usually involve the meninges. Evidence of cartilage production often is sparse.

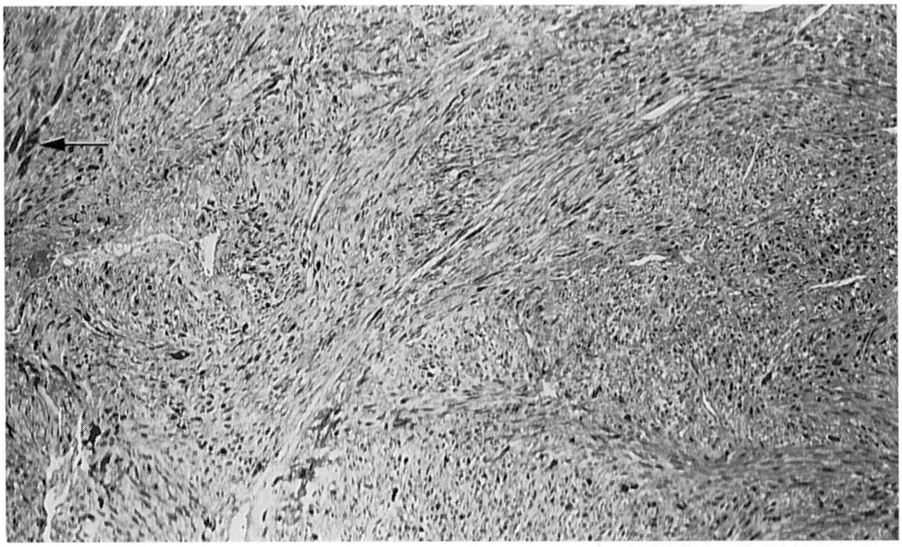

**Fig. 2-92.** Leiomyosarcoma. Large nuclei with very dark chromatin (*arrow*) and mitoses distinguish this invasive malignancy from more benign spindle-cell tumors. The 46-year-old woman had a uterine leiomyosarcoma metastatic to her T4 vertebral body and epidural region. (×100.)

### Sarcomas Other Than Chondrosarcoma—Grade IV

Sarcomas may arise as a primary meningeal tumor, as a brain parenchymal tumor, or as a metastasis from a systemic primary.[12,128] In each case they are rare tumors. Reported incidences of primary intracranial sarcomas vary from 0.08% to 4.3%.[128] Our own experience is closer to the lower percentage. Malignant fibrous histiocytoma (MFH), myogenic sarcoma, fibrosarcoma, liposarcoma, leiomyosarcoma (Fig. 2-92), and rhabdomyosarcoma have been described within the craniospinal vault.* More infiltrative growth and lack of meningothelial features distinguishes sarcomas from anaplastic meningioma.

Diffuse leptomeningeal sarcoma is a rare and fatal entity.[81] Immunocytochemistry is recommended to exclude leptomeningeal gliomatosis and other malignancies.

Intracranial sarcomas are associated with a history of radiation to the head (Chapter 5). They occur in the sellar region after radiotherapy for craniopharyngioma or adenoma.[3,99,130,156] Patients with sarcomas that follow sellar radiation succumb within months as a result of local tumor invasion.

## NERVE SHEATH TUMORS

Most benign nerve sheath tumors are either schwannoma or neurofibroma. Within the craniospinal vault, malignant nerve sheath tumors fortunately are rare outside of the context of neurofibromatosis.

* Refs. 12, 97, 111, 117, 125, 128, 153.

### Schwannoma (Neurilemoma, Neuroma, Neurinoma)—Grade I

Most schwannomas of the brain are attached to the eighth cranial nerve (Fig. 2-93). Their clinical appellation is "acoustic neuroma." Involvement of the fifth or seventh cranial nerves is uncommon, and involvement of the others is rare. Spinal schwannomas usually are attached to a nerve root (Fig. 2-94). Schwannomas that originate in central nervous parenchyma are very rare. Odd locations, multiple tumors, or mixtures with meningeal proliferations invite suspicion of neurofibromatosis of NF2 type (Fig. 2-95).[46]

Schwannomas usually are solid, but can contain cysts (Fig. 2-94). They are composed of spindle-shaped cells that are well-differentiated neoplastic Schwann cells. Antoni A patterns show these cells lined up in parallel arrays to produce fascicles (Fig. 2-96). Antoni B patterns suggest the mnemonic "**B**" for **B**ubbles. They are a looser arrangement of cells and vacuoles (Fig. 2-94). Verocay bodies are repeating palisades of parallel nuclei and fibrils found in Antoni A regions (Figs. 2-95 to 2-98). Verocay bodies are more characteristic of schwannomas than are the Antoni A and B patterns, but are not seen in all of them. They may resemble rhythmic palisades of gliomas and medulloblastomas, but have many more reticulin fibers.

The histologic appearance of schwannoma is similar to that of fibrous meningioma, tanycytic ependymoma, and subependymoma. Noninvasive attachment to a peripheral nerve suggests the correct diagnosis. Schwannoma can be distinguished from these gliomas

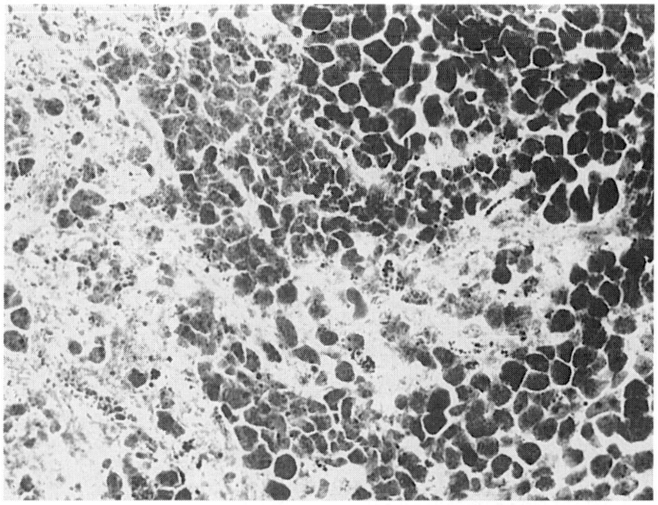

**Fig. 2-93.** Melanotic schwannoma. This tumor attached to the eighth cranial nerve contains cells filled with melanin. (×150.)

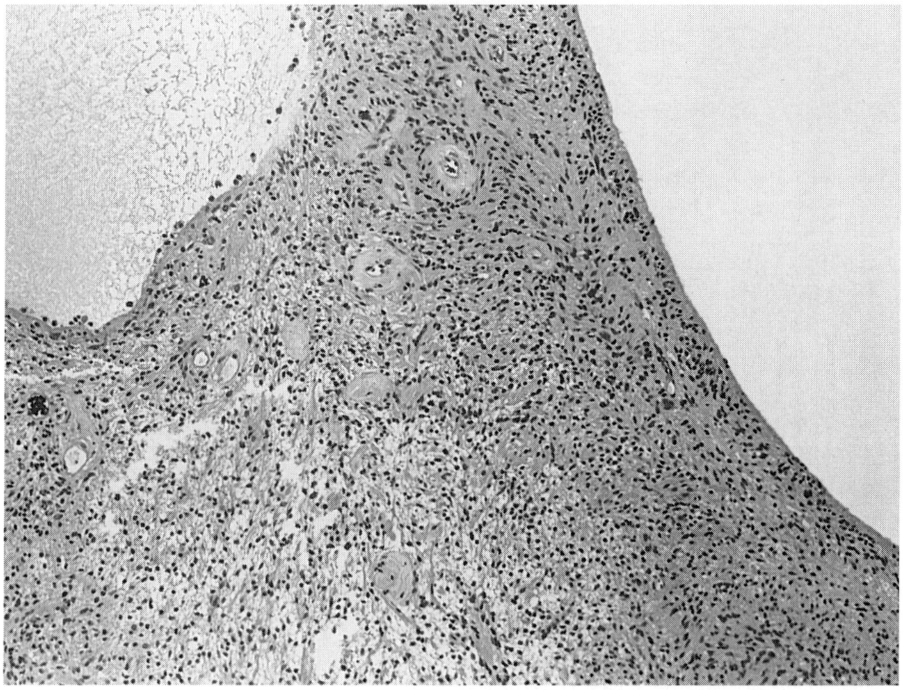

**Fig. 2-94.** Cystic schwannoma. Antoni A tissue lies closer to the cysts, and Antoni B tissue occupies the bottom center of the illustration. The 43-year-old woman had pains radiating to her arms and hands, and a 6×18 mm tumor attached to her spinal nerve root at T1. (×100.)

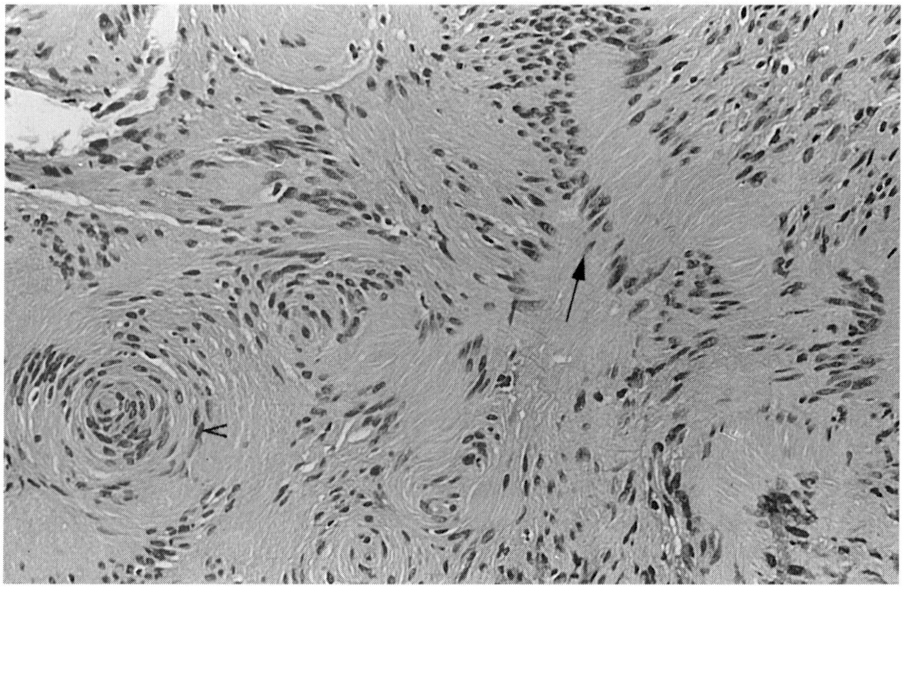

**Fig. 2-95.** Verocay bodies (*arrow*) and whorls (*arrowhead*) in a schwannoma. This large encapsulated tumor was attached to the side of a nerve root in the cauda equina of a man with type 2 neurofibromatosis, multiple schwannomas, and a meningioma. Electron microscopy will distinguish schwannoma from meningioma when light microscopy is not distinctive. (×200.)

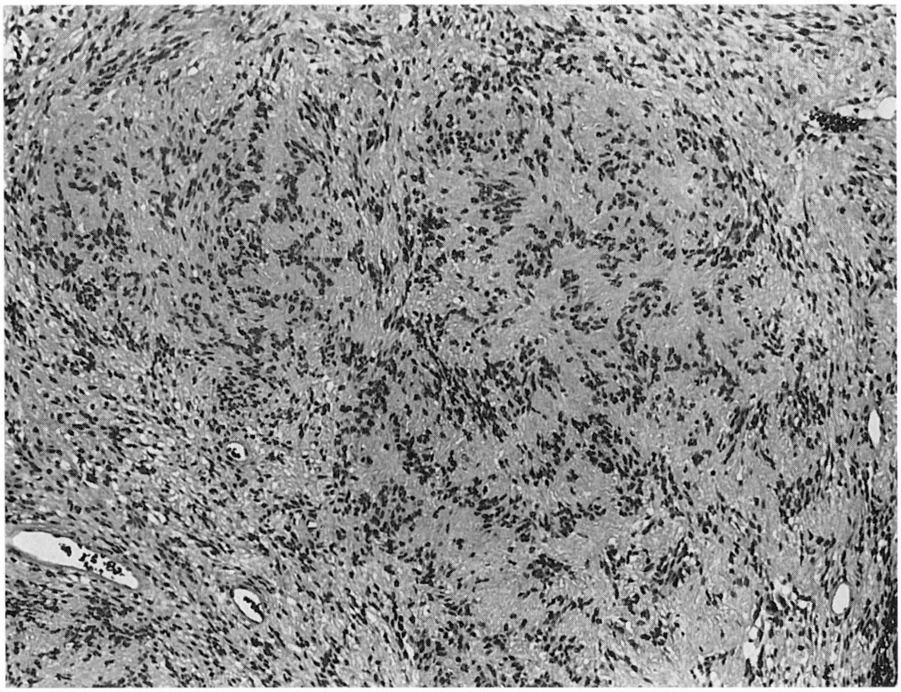

**Fig. 2-96.** Schwannoma. Rhythmic palisades of nuclei and fibrils produce Verocay bodies within Antoni A tissue of this schwannoma. The 53-year-old woman had a 3-year history of weak lower extremities and a tumor in her cauda equina. (×100.)

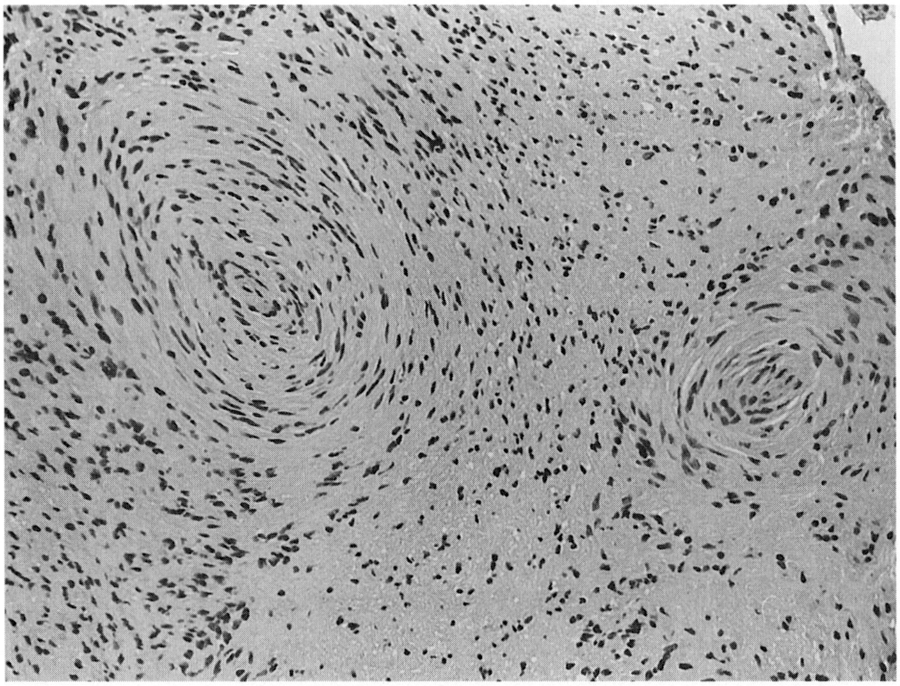

2-97

**Figs. 2-97, 2-98.** Schwannoma. **Fig. 2-97,** This schwannoma mimics a meningioma, forming large and small "whorls." (×165.) **Fig. 2-98,** Loosely arranged palisading nuclei of Verocay bodies and absence of psammoma bodies identify it as a schwannoma. (×80.)

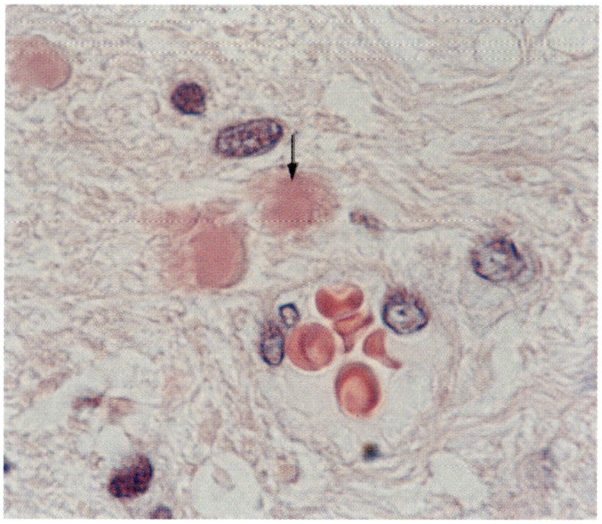

**Plate 1A.** Rosenthal fibers. The Rosenthal fibers (*arrow*) in this pilocytic astrocytoma are more pink and more heterogeneous in size and shape than the orange, biconcave erythrocytes in the vessel below them. (×1600.)

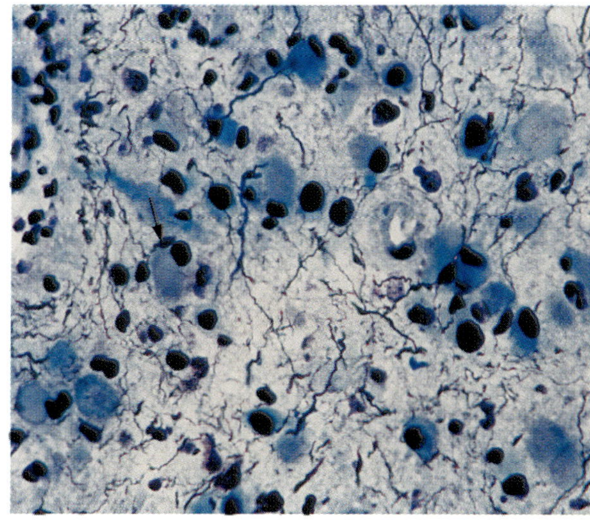

**Plate 1B.** Gemistocytic astrocytoma. Black axons of cerebral white matter are infiltrated and spread apart by neoplastic gemistocytes (*arrow*) of a gemistocytic astrocytoma. Axons do not originate in neoplastic cells. Similar infiltration is common among gliomas of grade II and higher, such as fibrillary astrocytomas. (LFB/Holmes stain; ×400.)

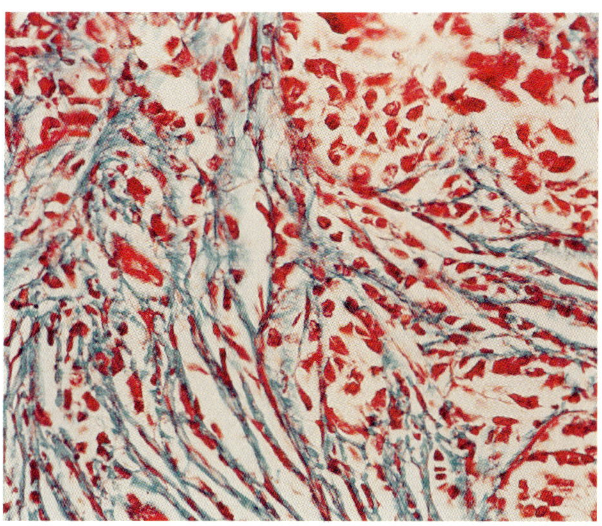

**Plate 1C.** Desmoplastic medulloblastoma. The trichrome stain distinguishes blue regions of desmoplasia from red regions of medulloblastoma cells. The 10-year-old boy had a tumor in his right cerebellum. (×400.) (Courtesy of Dr. John McGee, Jackson, MI.)

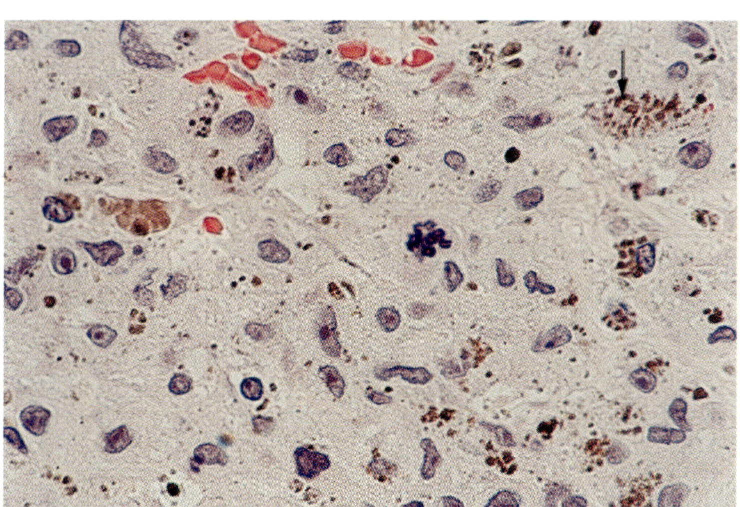

**Plate 1D.** Melanin and hemosiderin. Melanin granules (*arrow*) are smaller and darker than hemosiderin. This method of pigment identification on H&E is not entirely reliable, and special stains are recommended for critical cases. The 35-year-old patient had left trigeminal neuralgia for 1 year, and a primary melanocytic tumor in Meckel's cave. (×1000.) (Courtesy of Dr. George K. Tong, Saginaw, MI.)

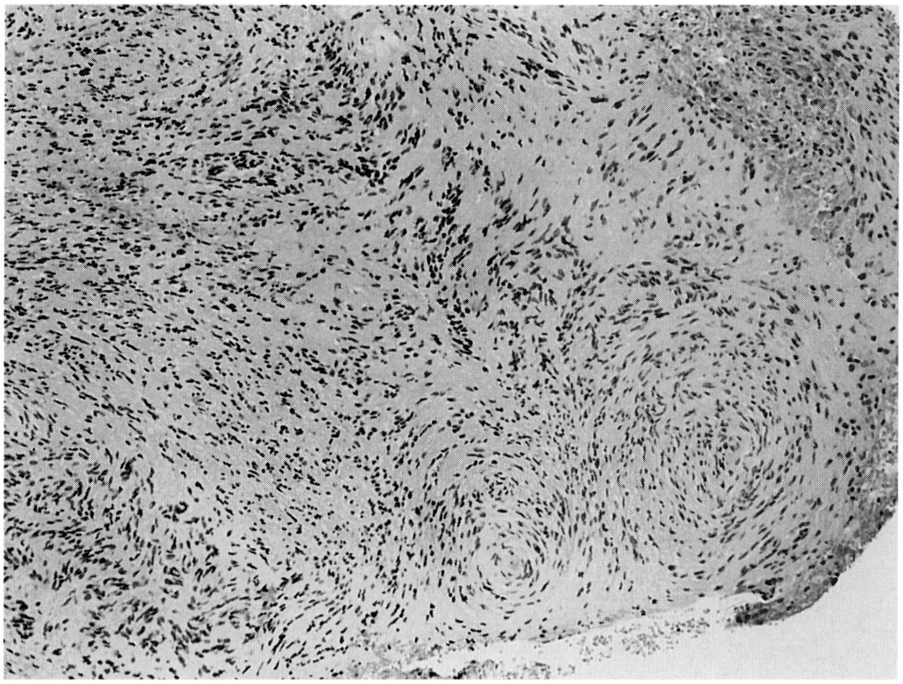

2-98

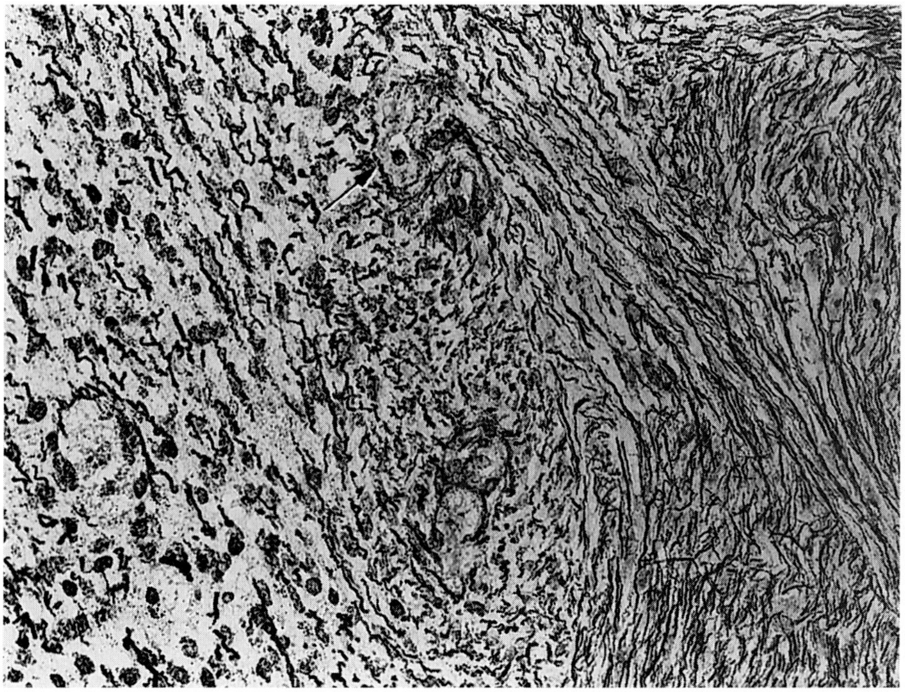

**Fig. 2-99.** Schwannoma. Snook's silver stain for reticulin stains most of the basement membrane material that surrounds each cell (*arrow*). The 36-year-old woman had an intradural tumor near her conus medullaris. (×400.)

by its abundant parenchymal reticulin (Fig. 2-99). Fibrous meningiomas without specific meningothelial features are difficult to distinguish from schwannomas, particularly since schwannomas occasionally show whorls (Figs. 2-95, 2-97). Electron microscopy is recommended in such cases (Chapter 3).

Variants of schwannoma rarely encountered within the craniospinal vault include cellular, plexiform, and melanotic schwannomas (Fig. 2-93).[81] The last of these may be hereditary and should prompt examination for Carney's triad.

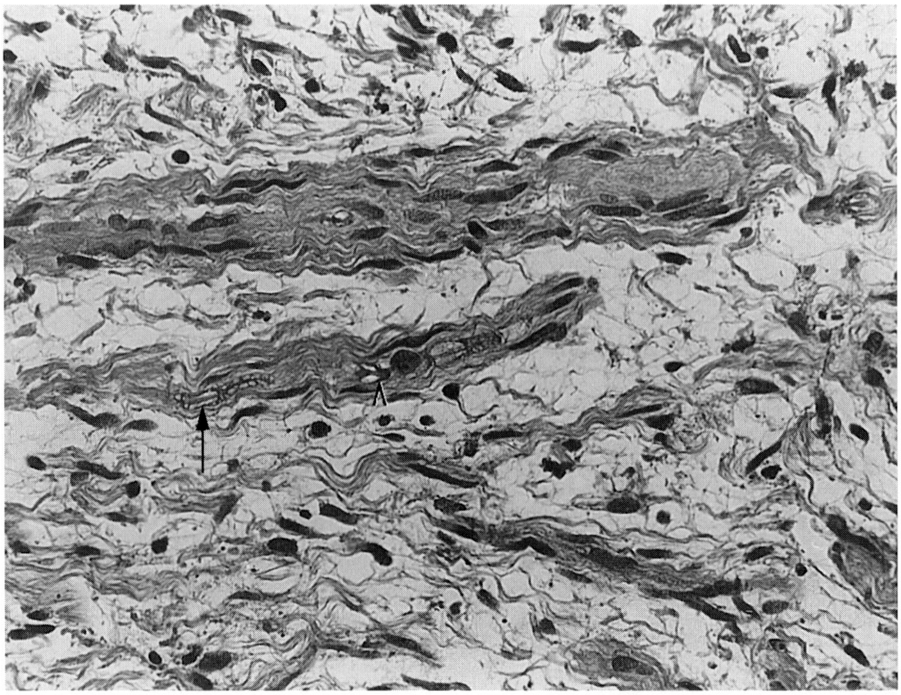

**Fig. 2-100.** Neurofibroma. Loose, myxoid cellular arrangement and scarce myelinated axons (*arrow* and *arrowhead*) within the tumor itself distinguish this neurofibroma from a schwannoma. Artifactual "herringbone" vacuolization of myelin around axons in paraffin sections help to identify them (*arrowhead*). (×400.)

### Neurofibroma—Grade I

The key to recognition of the few neurofibromas that occur inside the craniospinal vault near the brainstem and spinal cord is their primary involvement of the nerve root rather than brain or cord. The specimen usually comes with part of the spinal (or cranial) nerve in continuation with the tumor because the lesion infiltrates the nerve. This is also reflected microscopically: unlike schwannomas, neurofibromas contain stainable axons running through the tumor itself and divided by neoplastic cells. When myelinated, these axons are visible in H&E stained sections by artifactual disruption of the myelin, producing a pattern like a herringbone (Fig. 2-100) that is especially prominent in frozen material. They are easier to identify with a silver stain for axons[100] or by immunocytochemistry (Chapter 4). The neoplasm itself is a swelling of the nerve with a mixture of Schwann cells, fibroblasts, collagen, and a variable amount of mucoid material. A neurofibroma within the craniospinal vault raises suspicion about the possibility of von Recklinghausen's disease, NF1.

### Malignant Peripheral Nerve Sheath Tumor—Grade III–IV

Malignant peripheral nerve sheath tumors are very rare within the cranial cavity and raise suspicion of NF1. They are difficult to subclassify, but there is a consensus that most are malignant counterparts of neurofibroma. Doubtful cases require immunocytochemical confirmation (Chapter 4). Those that arise as malignant transformation within a neurofibroma are most easily recognized. They exhibit intense hypercellularity and increased nuclear pleomorphism, multiple mitoses per one microscopic field, abnormal mitoses, and invasion of surrounding tissue (Fig. 2-101).

## NEUROENDOCRINE TUMORS

The most common primary intracranial endocrine tumor is the pituitary adenoma (Chapter 5). Others are described below.

### Paraganglioma—Grade I

Paragangliomas arise within the spinal canal[152,154] or as a glomus jugulare tumor. They occasionally are reminiscent of ependymomas, but their cells "sit" right on the vessel walls, whereas ependymoma cells keep their distance by sending their processes toward the vessel walls. Paraganglioma cells nest between thin-walled vessels. These nests or balls of cells appropriately are referred to as "Zellballen" (Fig. 2-102). The paraganglioma cells contain granules barely visible at high magnification on H&E stain (Fig. 2-103). Grimelius stain highlights these granules, but immu-

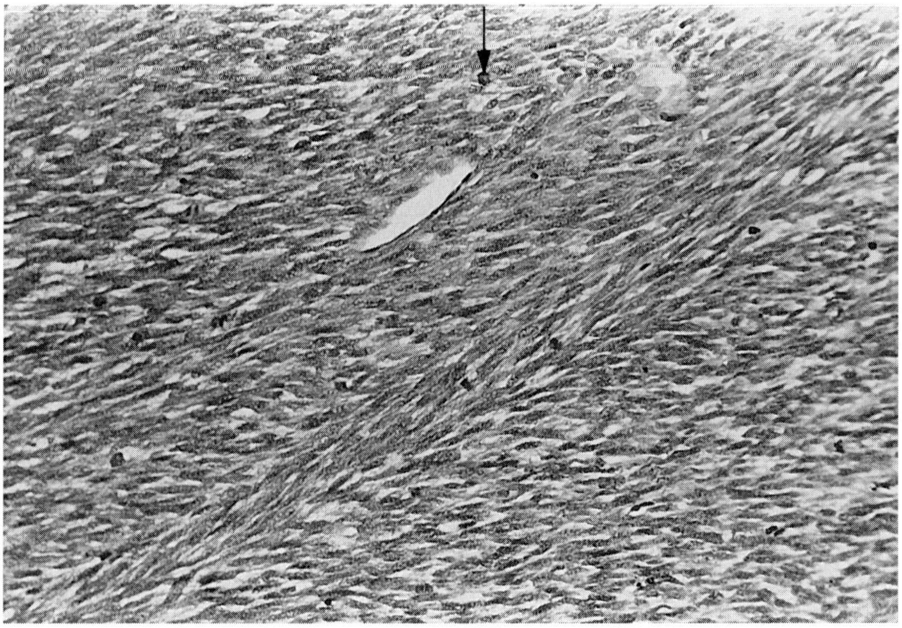

**Fig. 2-101.** Malignant peripheral nerve sheath tumor (MPNST). This densely cellular spindle-cell neoplasm has many mitoses (*arrow*). The 45-year-old woman had this large tumor invading her nerve roots in the cauda equina. (×200.)

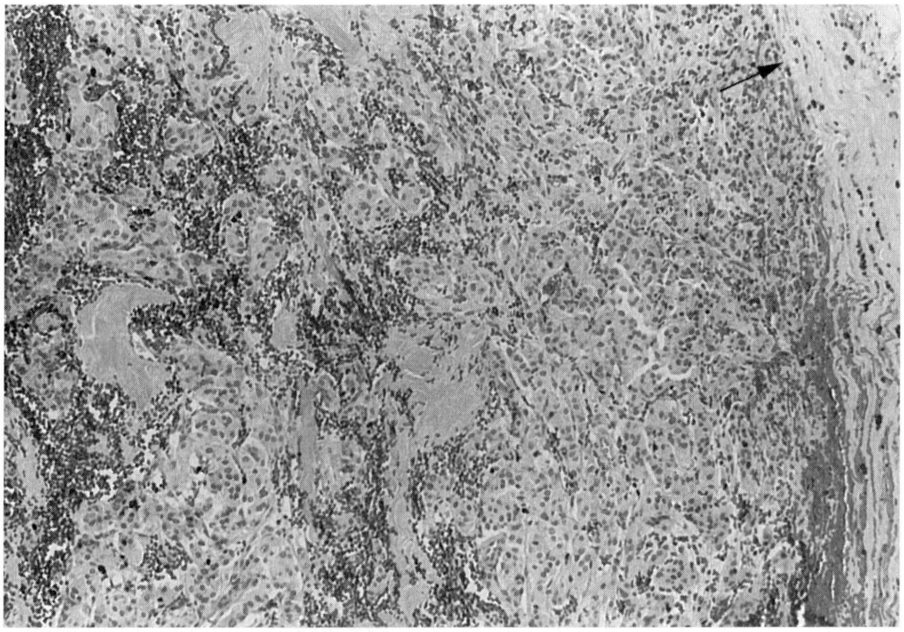

2-102

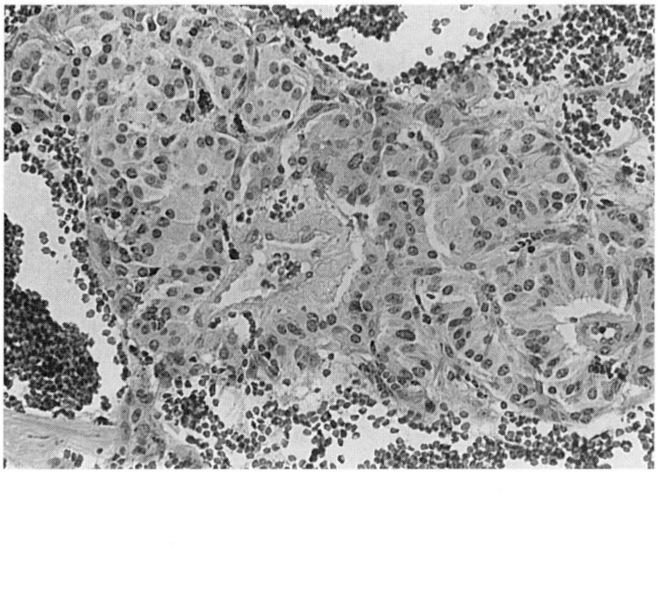

2-103

**Figs. 2-102, 2-103.** Paraganglioma. The 54-year-old patient had leg pain and numbness for over a year, and an intradural extramedullary spinal tumor in the cauda equina. **Fig. 2-102,** This highly vascular tumor is entirely encapsulated by fibrous tissue (*arrow*). The cells cluster into *Zellballen*. (×100.) **Fig. 2-103,** Clusters of cells with pink cytoplasmic granules and round nuclei with prominent nucleoli are divided by spindled cells and fibrovascular stroma congested with blood. (×250.)

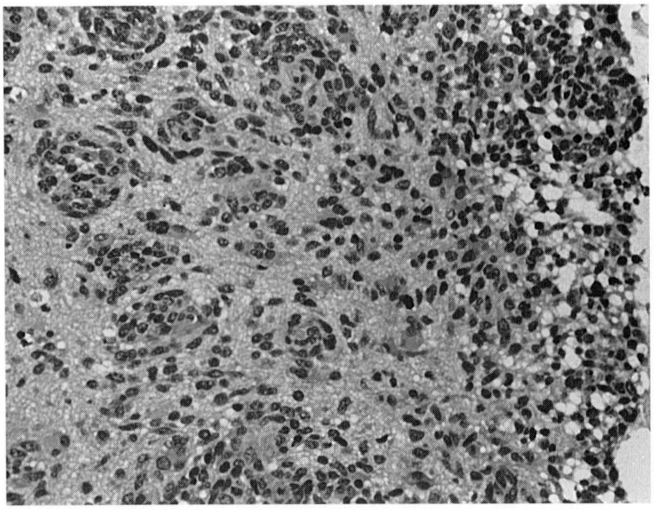

**Fig. 2-104.** Neuroendocrine small cell carcinoma. This carcinoma has small cells that invade brain like a medulloblastoma or glioma. Search for a pulmonary or other primary; identification with immunocytochemistry or electron microscopy is prudent. (×200.)

nocytochemical or ultrastructural confirmation is more definitive (Chapters 3 and 4).

### Neuroendocrine and Small Cell Carcinoma—Grade IV

Neuroendocrine carcinomas of brain originate from systemic primaries, like oat cell carcinoma of the lung. Local invasion from the paranasal region is also possible (Chapter 3). The cells are small with high nuclear-to-cytoplasmic ratios and numerous mitoses. Oat cell and related small cell carcinoma represent one of a triad of malignant "blue tumors" on H&E slides that can be difficult to identify, the other two being lymphoma and medulloblastoma. Cytologic preparations on fresh tissue are helpful. A rim of epithelial cytoplasm and cohesive nonfibrillar cells distinguish small cell carcinoma from lymphoma and medulloblastoma (PNET). Immunocytochemistry is recommended to confirm difficult cases (Fig. 2-104). Most helpful is a biopsy of the primary tumor.

## GERM CELL TUMORS

Germ cell tumors are described in Chapter 5.

## HEMATOPOIETIC AND LYMPHOID NEOPLASMS

### Lymphoma—Grade IV

Lymphomas from two sources are found in the craniospinal vault. The first and more common is the primary malignant lymphoma of the CNS that originates in brain.[4,9] Primary lymphomas can be subcategorized like systemic lymphomas.[81] Parasellar lymphomas are discussed in Chapter 5.

The second source is systemic lymphoma. These lesions mainly involve the meninges. Lymphomas that arise outside the brain do not often involve it secondarily. Nonetheless, they can cause clinical problems in regions where meningeal infiltration produces neurologic symptoms, particularly in the narrow spinal canal.

Diagnosis of primary CNS lymphomas (PCNSL) is facilitated by clinical awareness and by procuring adequate specimens. One must keep in mind that there is association between lymphoma and HIV, and also a linkage between lymphoma and lymphomatoid granulomatosis as well as systemic Hodgkin's disease.[5,31,33,108,135] The radiographic appearance, particularly of the multicentric variety,[2] helps with the diagnosis.

To procure adequate tissue, steroid treatment before biopsy should be minimized as much as clinically feasible, since this therapy lyses the neoplastic cells. Whenever a crowded accumulation of small to medium-sized malignant cells is seen in frozen section, the pathologist should take care to acquire tissue for possible immunostaining and electron microscopy. If the biopsy is of sufficient size to include the tumor margin, lymphomas usually demonstrate a characteristic vasocentric growth pattern that aids interpretation. Needle biopsy samples frequently miss this feature (Fig. 2-105).

A cytologic preparation of tissue immediately fixed in ethanol is helpful, provided there is no mutilation of cells.[48] Lymphomas show round noncohesive cells of small to medium size, high nuclear-to-cytoplasmic ratio, and prominent nucleoli (Fig. 2-106).

PCNSL invasion into vascular walls is best appreciated with a stain that both highlights the wall and demonstrates fine nuclear morphology, such as Masson's trichrome or PAS with hematoxylin, or an immunocytochemical stain. Immunocytochemistry is recommended to confirm and subclassify all lymphomas (Chapter 4). The vast majority of PCNSL are B-cell lymphomas.[100] Nonetheless, immunophenotyping is essential, since T-cell lymphomas run a more favorable course than B-cell lymphomas.[37]

Classification schemes for systemic lymphomas have been applied to PCNSL.[69,114] There is no consensus about the prognostic value of these attempts to subclassify PCNSL.[54,57,109,124] On the other hand, PCNSL that arise in immunocompromised patients carry a distinctly poorer prognosis than PCNSL in the immunocompetent.[39,41] Prognostic indicators in AIDS patients with PCNSL are the extent of immunosuppression, Karnovsky clinical score prior to therapy, and spread of tumor.[20,41]

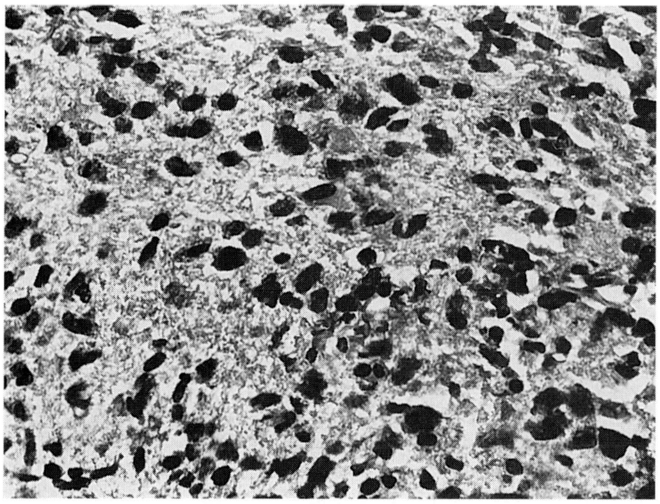

2-105

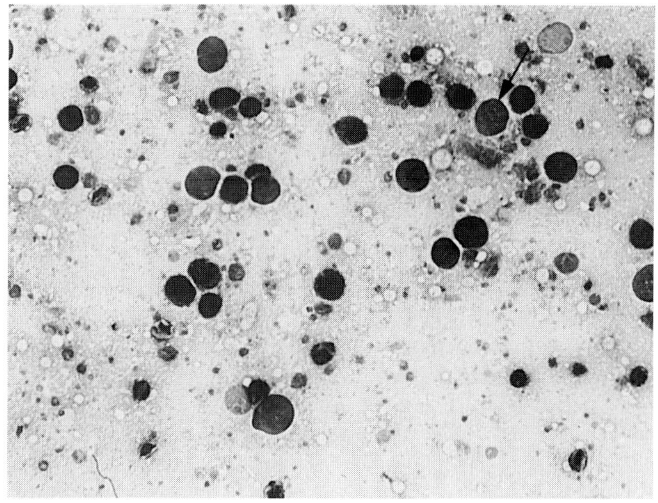

2-106

**Figs. 2-105, 2-106.** Primary CNS lymphoma. The 64-year-old patient had a right frontal lobe tumor. Subsequent immunophenotyping as described in Chapter 5 revealed a B-cell lymphoma. **Fig. 2-105,** Cells invade gliotic brain parenchyma in a manner resembling an infiltrating glioma. Their lack of cellular processes is obscured by the infiltrated brain tissue. (×500.) **Fig. 2-106,** Cytologic preparation reveals that the discohesive, round lymphoma cells (*arrow*) have high nuclear-to-cytoplasmic ratios and lack cellular processes. (×500.)

### Leukemia

Cerebrospinal fluid (CSF) cytology usually establishes the diagnosis of CNS leukemia.[4,9] Terminal brain hemorrhages reflect blast crises of more than 300,000 leukocytes per cubic millimeter and intravascular leukostasis. Cerebral vasculitis is rarely associated with leukemia.[93] Peripheral eosinophilia may suggest that the focal masses in brain parenchyma are leukemic cells.[60]

### Histiocytosis

Histiocytosis is a disease that usually affects children and young adults. Brain involvement is generally secondary to bony or systemic involvement, but rare cases appear first in brain. Various regions including the parasellar region are involved.[34,94,95,99] Collagen fibers mix with histiocytes and inflammatory cells (Fig. 2-107).[95,100] Electron microscopy is recommended for confirmation and differentiation of histiocytoses of Langerhans cell origin from others[52] (Chapters 3 and 4).

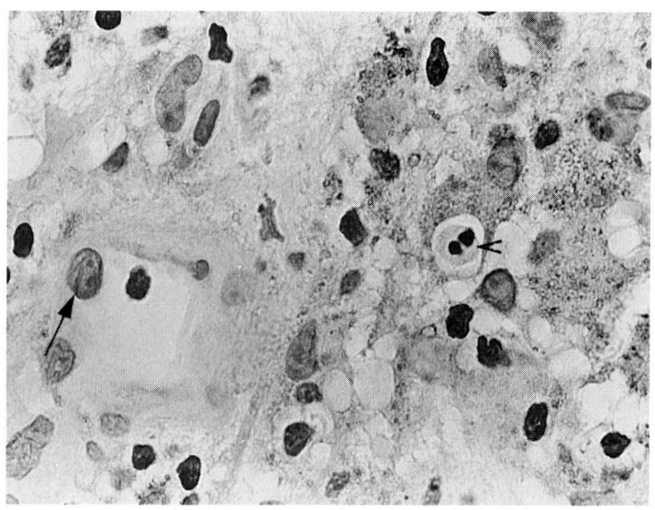

**Fig. 2-107.** Rosai-Dorfman disease. Large histiocytes with reniform and oval nuclei with nuclear clefts (*arrow*) have granules and occasional leukocytes (*arrowhead*) in their cytoplasm. Collagen is present between histiocytes. This is from an intrinsic brainstem mass in a 6-year-old girl who lacked clinical evidence of lymph node involvement. Extranodal sinus histiocytosis with massive lymphadenopathy mimics gliomas in the cranial vault. (×1000.)

## MISCELLANEOUS INTRACRANIAL OR SPINAL MASSES

### Lipoma—Grade I

Lipomas are found in midline locations, near the corpus callosum, quadrigeminal plate, hypothalamus, spinal canal, or cauda equina. They consist of mature adipose tissue, but also may contain Schwann cells, bone, cartilage, or blood vessels.[16]

### Amyloidoma—Grade I

Amyloidoma is a rare tumor. Intensely congophilic, multiple pink granules larger than surrounding cells contain amyloid.[55] The amyloid originates from immunoglobulin light chain protein.[149]

### Hemangioblastoma (Capillary Hemangioblastoma)—Grade I

The capillary hemangioblastoma resembles an endocrine neoplasm in its structural arrangement of close juxtaposition of capillary and stromal cells (Figs. 2-108 and 2-109).[36] A gland of origin, however, has not been found. The stromal cells are epithelioid and contain variable quantities of lipid and glycogen that can be stained in appropriate sections.[17]

On paraffin sections, the epithelioid nature of the hemangioblastoma is usually more apparent than on frozen sections. It resembles a well-differentiated renal cell carcinoma, which can be distinguished immunocytochemically (Chapter 4). Some hemangioblastomas are a manifestation of the von Hippel-Lindau complex.[68] This complex should be considered clinically, particularly with hemangioblastomas that are multiple or that occur in unusual locations.[143]

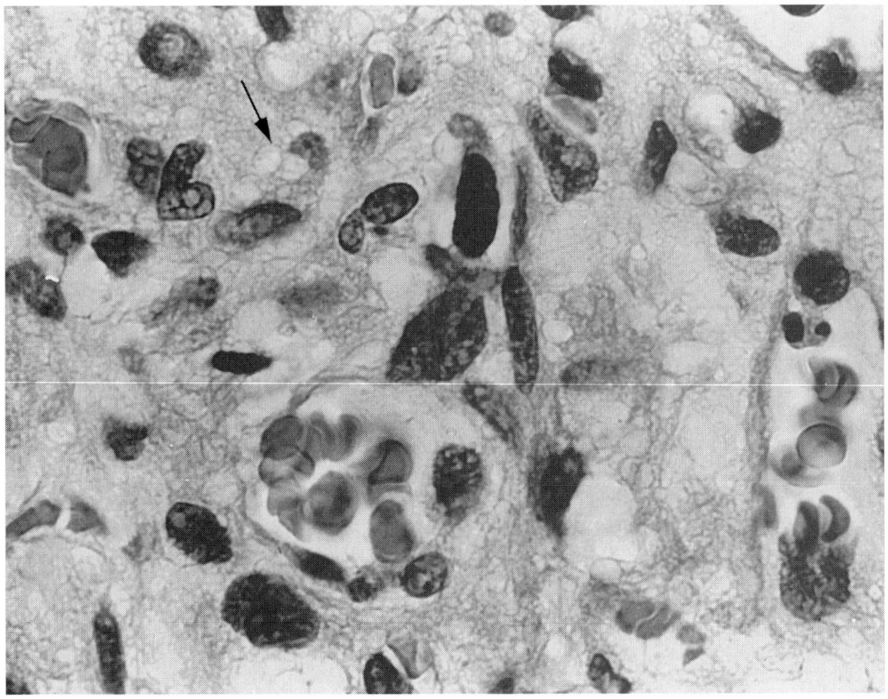

**Fig. 2-108.** Hemangioblastoma. Vacuolated stromal cells (*arrow*) mingle between capillaries. While occasional stromal cell nuclei are large, there is little clumping or margination of chromatin within them. The 28-year-old man had a vascular tumor in his cerebellum. (×1000.) (Courtesy of Dr. Patricia M. Novak, Jackson, MI.)

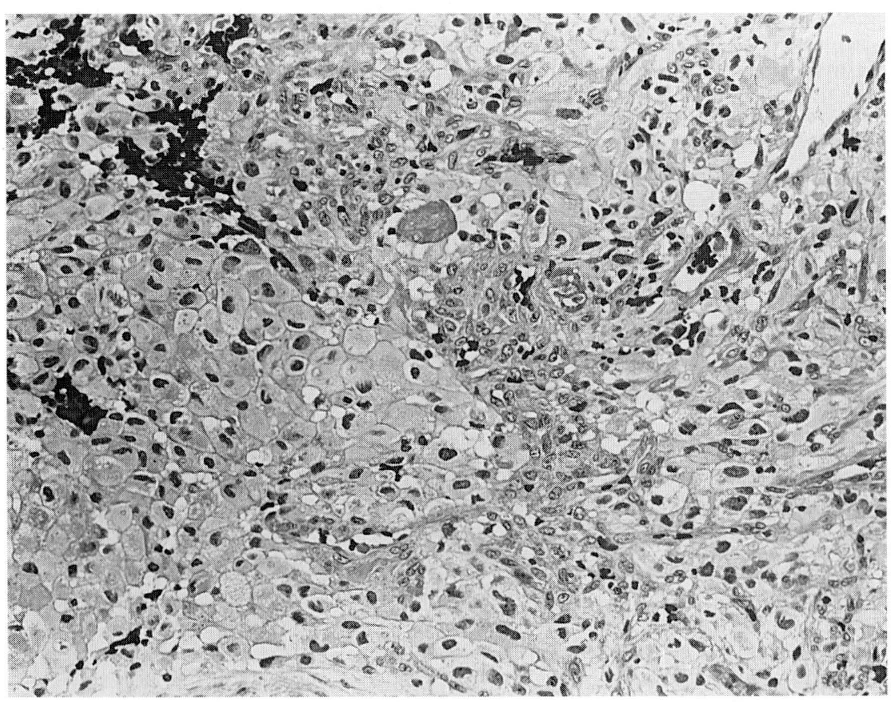

**Fig. 2-109.** Hemangioblastoma. Epithelioid stromal cells intermix with vessels in this cerebellar tumor from a patient with von Hippel-Lindau disease. Vacuoles in some of the stromal cells contained lipid prior to processing through paraffin. (×200.)

**Desmoplastic Small Round-Cell Tumor**

This aggressive neoplasm of children and young adults usually occurs in the abdomen. It is composed of well-defined nests of small, round, primitive cells separated by abundant desmoplastic stroma. It consistently shows a (t11;22)(p13;q12) chromosomal translocation. One case has been found in the cranial vault.[157]

## METASTATIC TUMORS

### Carcinoma—Grade IV

Carcinoma has a distinctively epithelial structure that differentiates it from many brain tumors (Fig. 2-110). Most carcinomas in the craniospinal vault are metastatic from a systemic primary. Less common are locally invasive head and neck carcinomas (Figs. 2-111 to 114).[99] Primary brain carcinomas are rare. They occur in the choroid plexus (Figs. 2-68, 2-69), or arise from germ cell tumors of the pineal and suprasellar regions (Chapter 5), or from cysts.[99,166,168]

Metastatic carcinomas are found almost anywhere in the brain and meninges. They metastasize to regions of the brain approximately in proportion to the volume of target brain tissue, hence their frequency in cerebrum. Typical features of metastatic carcinoma are an epithelial appearance of cohesive cells and a *distinct tumor margin* with brain tissue.

Within brain, few tumors other than glioblastoma, malignant astrocytoma, lymphoma, or malignant meningioma show the intensity of pleomorphism, profuse mitotic abnormalities, or tumor necrosis of metastatic carcinomas.[43,99] *Distinct borders* of malignant epithelial cells and lack of fibrillar cytoplasmic processes contrast with the pattern of these high-grade gliomas.[74] Lymphoma cells are discohesive. If malignant meningioma is in the differential, electron microscopy is advised (Chapter 3).

Carcinomatous meningitis is uncommon. Clinical features resemble inflammatory meningitis. Positive CSF cytology provides definitive diagnosis.[166]

Specific types of carcinoma with a propensity to metastasize to brain are described below. Some of these can be distinguished ultrastructurally or immunocytochemically (Chapters 3 and 4).

**Pulmonary and mammary carcinoma.** Carcinoma of the lung accounts for more than one third and the breast for one fifth of brain metastases.[16] Except for small cell carcinoma, discussed with neuroendocrine tumors, these usually are either adenocarcinomas, which form acini and produce mucin, or are undifferentiated carcinomas (Figs. 2-115, 2-116).

After location of the primary tumor, male gender is the most useful feature in choosing metastatic pulmonary over mammary cancer. Nonetheless, as a group, lung cancer cells tend to be more pleomorphic than breast cancer cells. Their abnormal mitotic spindles

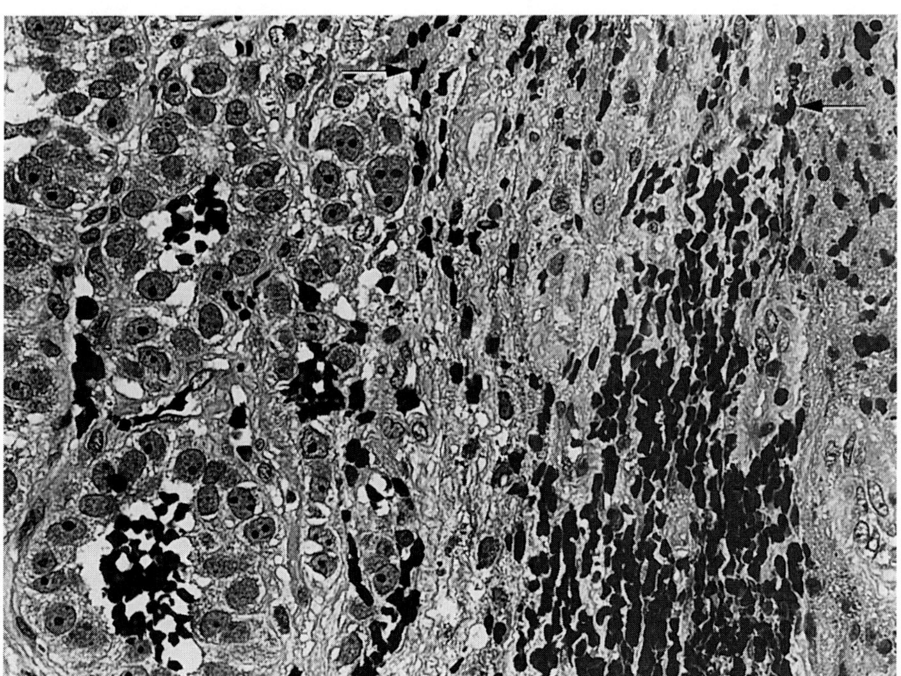

**Fig. 2-110.** Metastatic thyroid carcinoma. Epithelioid cells on left are more uniform than most lung cancers metastatic to the brain. Their large nuclei are round. There is a fibrovascular capsule (*arrows*) between the carcinoma and gliotic brain to the far right. The 63-year-old woman had this solitary cerebellar tumor 2 years after an invasive moderately differentiated follicular adenocarcinoma was excised from her right thyroid gland. (×400.)

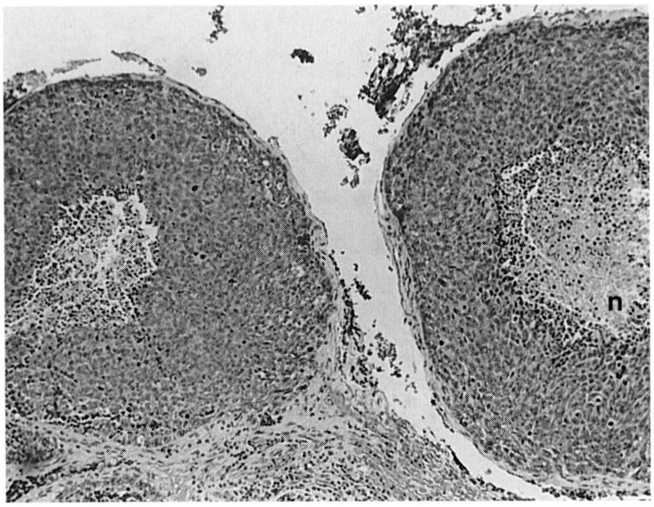

**Fig. 2-111.** Sinonasal undifferentiated carcinoma (SNUC). Malignant cells produce a lobulated pattern of growth within fibrous tissue and vessels. Central regions are necrotic (*n*). (×100.)

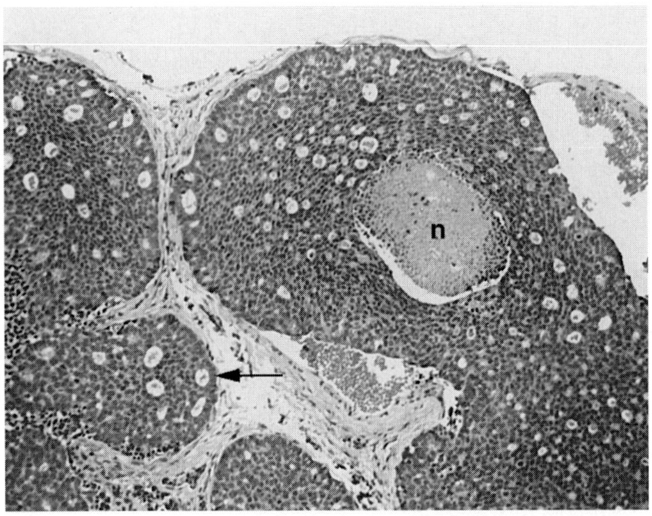

**Fig. 2-112.** Adenoid cystic carcinoma. This skull-base tumor was near the brainstem. The lobulated tumor produces numerous acini (*arrow*). Some lobules are centrally necrotic (*n*). The 60-year-old woman presented with visual blurring and left-sided facial numbness. A skull-based tumor involved cranial nerves and brainstem. Later, a left parotid primary was found. (×125.)

tend to be more bizarre and their nucleoli larger than their counterparts in breast cancer. Immunocytochemistry promises to be more definitive in the future, but there is still no substitute for proper clinical evaluation.

**Renal cell carcinoma (hypernephroma).** Metastatic renal cell carcinomas consist of variably pleomorphic cells with variable mitotic activity. They possess clear or vacuolated cytoplasm and distinct epithelial cell

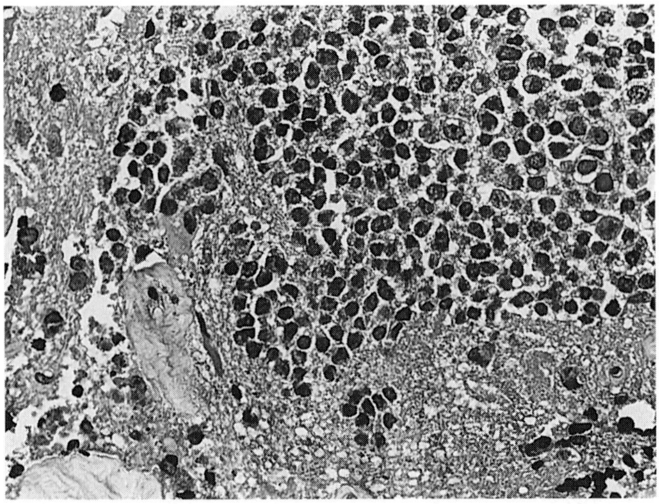

2-113

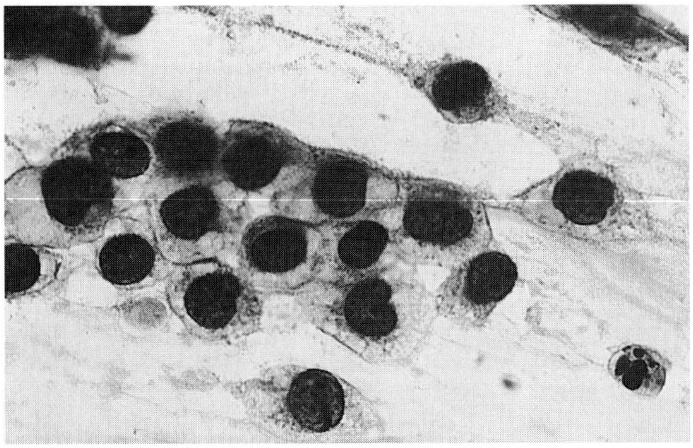

2-114

**Figs. 2-113, 2-114.** Carcinoma ex pleomorphic adenoma. This 52-year-old man had a skull-base tumor compressing his left temporal lobe. The invasive neoplasm had previously involved his left parotid gland and temporal bone. **Fig. 2-113,** Sheets of epithelial cells with round nuclei and high nuclear-to-cytoplasmic ratio invade brain tissue. (×400.) **Fig. 2-114,** Carcinoma ex pleomorphic adenoma, cytologic preparation. Cohesive epithelial cells have distinct borders typical of carcinoma. They have round nuclei. (×1000.)

borders (Fig. 2-117). Abundant glycogen (demonstrated by PAS stain with and without diastase) is often a feature. Renal cell carcinomas tend to bleed, and can present clinically as spontaneous intracranial hemorrhage.

Renal cell carcinomas resemble malignant oligodendroglioma and malignant meningioma. Immunocytochemistry aids the former and ultrastructure aids the latter differential (Chapters 3 and 4). Indolent renal cell carcinomas resemble hemangioblastomas. Immunocytochemistry is recommended for this differential.

**Small cell carcinoma.** This malignancy is described in the section on neuroendocrine tumors, this chapter.

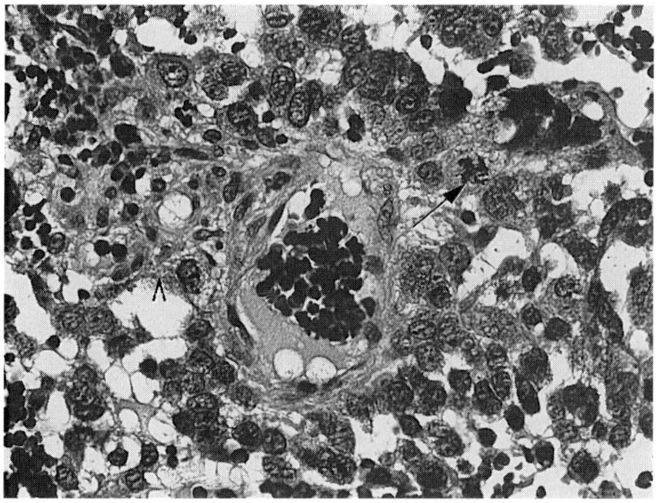

**Fig. 2-115.** Metastatic pulmonary carcinoma. Abnormal mitoses (*arrow*) occur among undifferentiated epithelial cells. Inflammatory cells cluster in a desmoplastic region (*arrowhead*). The 57-year-old woman had a carcinoma excised from her lung years previously. This is her solitary cerebellar metastasis. (×400.)

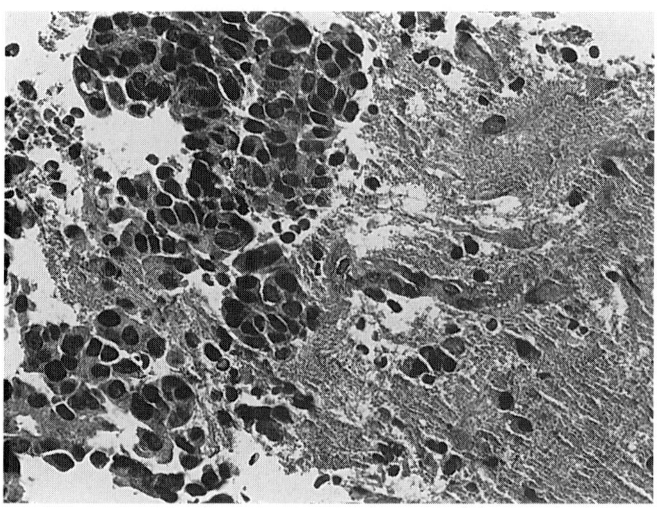

**Fig. 2-116.** Metastatic mammary carcinoma. Cohesive epithelial cells with hyperchromatic nuclei abut brain parenchyma on the right with little invasion of gliotic and edematous brain tissue. The 46-year-old woman had a poorly differentiated ductal carcinoma excised from her left breast, and this similar tumor in her right temporal lobe. (×400.) (Reprinted from McKeever PE, and Blaivas M: The brain, spinal cord, and meninges, In Sternberg SS, and others, editors: Diagnostic Surgical Pathology, ed 2, New York, 1994, Raven Press.)

**Choriocarcinoma and embryonal carcinoma.** Systemic choriocarcinoma has a high propensity to metastasize to the brain. It is fortunate that the primary tumor is rare and treatable, which has almost eliminated metastatic choriocarcinoma in developed countries. Metastatic choriocarcinoma and embryonal carcinoma occur outside of the pituitary-pineal axis (Chapter 5). In brain, choriocarcinoma is frequently hemorrhagic. Rare occult choriocarcinomas have produced spontaneous intracranial bleeding. Immunohistochemistry is recommended to distinguish choriocarcinoma from other carcinomas, other germ cell tumors, and glioblastomas (Chapters 4 and 5).

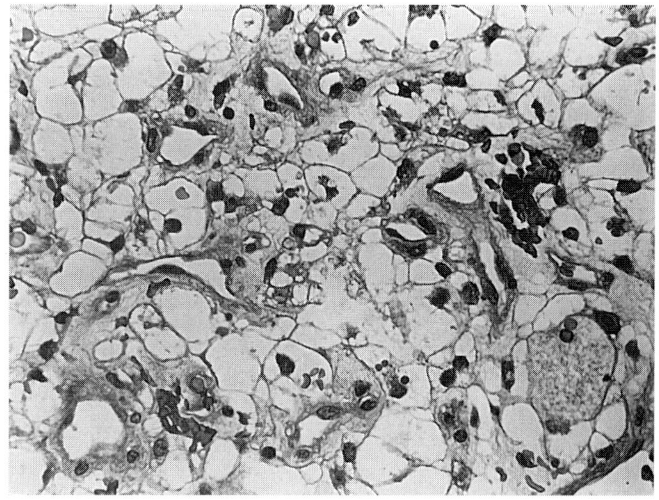

**Fig. 2-117.** Renal cell carcinoma. Cytoplasmic vacuoles and extensive vascularity resemble those of hemangioblastoma. However, the vacuoles are larger than the typical cytoplasmic vacuoles of hemangioblastoma. The 68-year-old patient had this carcinoma in her left parietal lobe. Subsequently, a primary renal cell carcinoma was found. (×300.)

**Gastrointestinal carcinoma.** Considered as a group, gastrointestinal carcinomas are a relatively common source of brain metastases, exceeded only by pulmonary and mammary carcinomas. Although some are undifferentiated, many retain specific epithelial or organotypic features (Figs. 2-118 to 2-120). Colonic and rectal carcinomas tend to produce mucin (Fig. 2-118). Hepatocellular carcinomas occasionally make bile or form cords (Fig. 2-120). Only rarely are features sufficiently specific to indicate the site of an occult primary carcinoma metastatic to brain. Care should be taken in the interpretation of brain lesions in patients with carcinomas of the gastrointestinal system, since both second primaries of the brain[158] and intracranial hemorrhages are associated with these cancers.

### Melanoma and Melanocytoma

Most melanomas in the craniospinal vault are metastatic and are considered malignant or grade IV (Fig. 2-121). Variable features of individual melanomas determine the difficulty of their diagnosis. Metastatic malignant melanomas with a known cutaneous primary and multiple brain masses, an epithelial histologic ap-

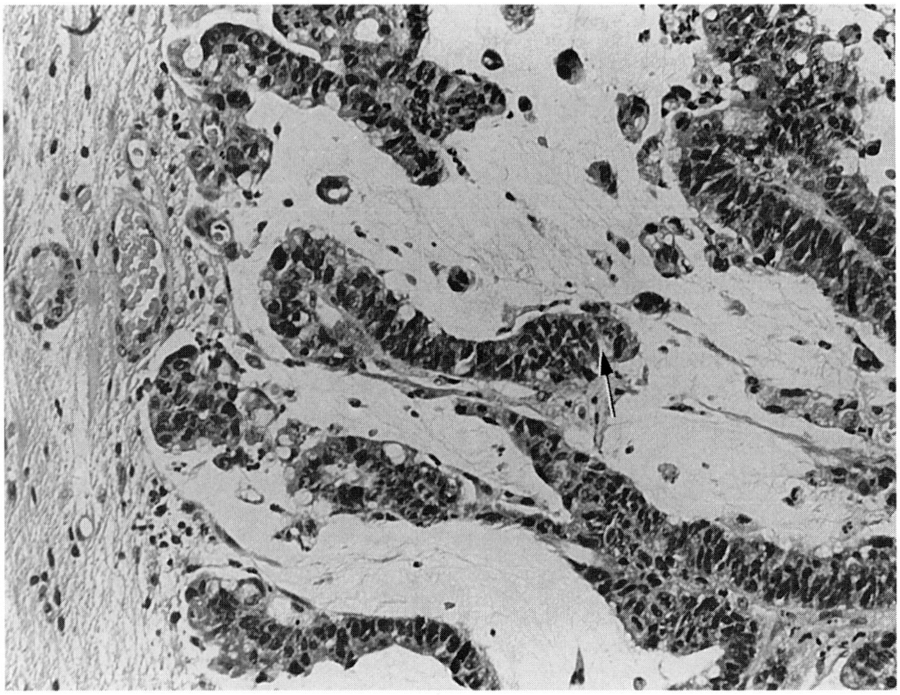

**Fig. 2-118.** Metastatic colorectal adenocarcinoma. Mucinous (*arrow*), stratified epithelium of malignant cells with elongated nuclei abut gliotic brain parenchyma at the left of the illustration. The 51-year-old man had an adenocarcinoma that invaded through his colonic wall, and this frontal lobe metastasis. (×200.)

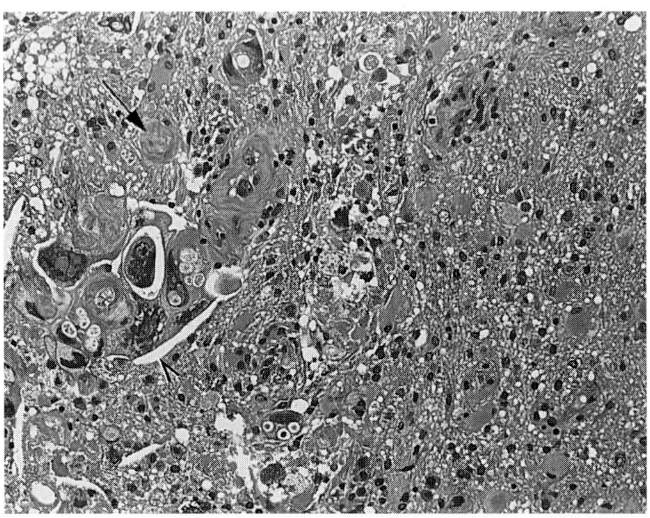

**Fig. 2-119.** Metastatic esophageal carcinoma. Keratin (*arrow*), cholesterol clefts (*arrowhead*), and bizarre epithelial cells characterize this squamous cell carcinoma metastatic from an esophageal primary. The right side of illustration shows gliotic brain. (×200.)

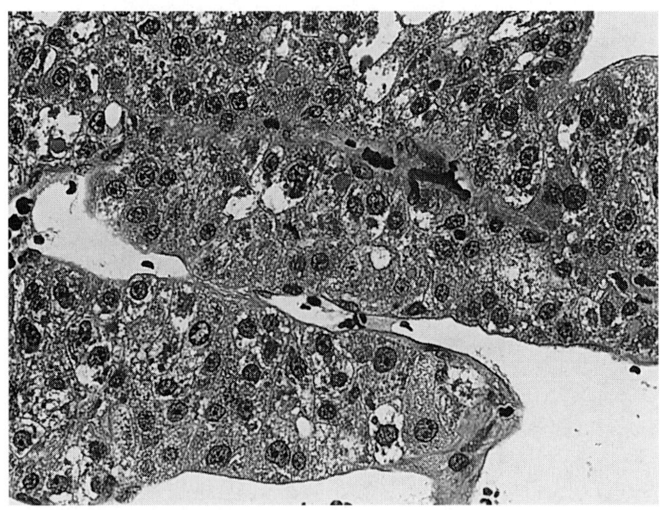

**Fig. 2-120.** Metastatic hepatocellular carcinoma. Neoplastic hepatocytes form cords of polygonal cells. The 50-year-old patient had this solitary 3-cm left frontal lobe mass excised 1 year after diagnosis of primary hepatocellular carcinoma. (×400.)

pearance, features of malignancy, and presence of melanin are easy to interpret. Solitary nonpigmented tumors with fibrillar or spindle cells and no known primary are at the other end of the spectrum of difficulty. In such cases, including melanoma in the differential diagnosis is critical.

Primary melanocytic tumors confined to the craniospinal vault are rare (Fig. 2-122; Fig. 2-123, Plate 1D). Most arise from meningeal melanocytes, with a propensity to involve the meninges. For example, the benign melanocytoma tends to involve Meckel's cave and the thoracic leptomeninges. Its cells often have promi-

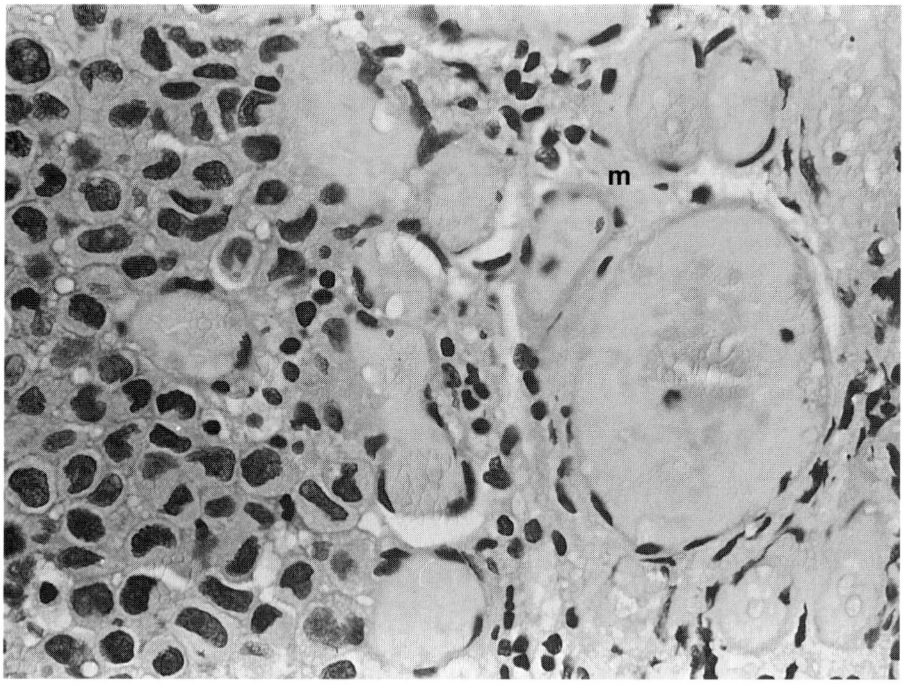


**Fig. 2-121.** Metastatic melanoma. Pleomorphic epithelioid cells on left are mitotically active, and have a highly vascular margin (*m*) with brain, but no visible melanin granules. The 32-year-old patient presented with a solitary intraparenchymal left temporal lobe tumor surrounded by edema. Immunocytochemistry was necessary to confirm the diagnosis. Extracranial melanoma was found subsequently. (×400.)

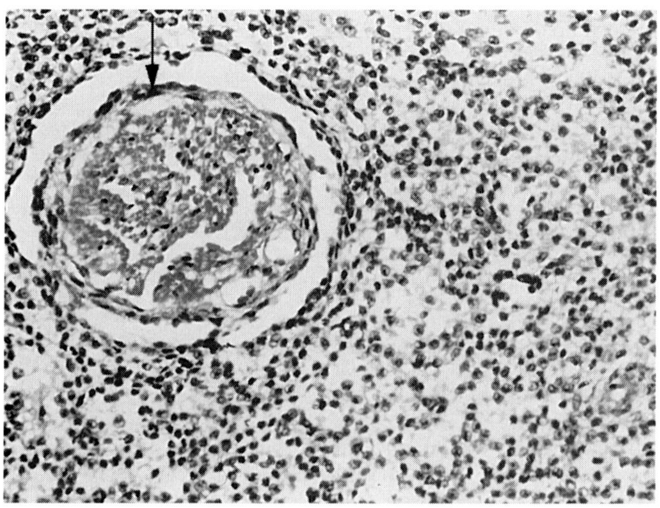

**Fig. 2-122.** Primary CNS melanoma. Malignant cells invade the subarachnoid space and surround a cranial nerve root (*arrow*). The 15-month-old infant had cranial enlargement and a subarachnoid tumor over her ventral brainstem and spinal cord. No other primary tumor was evident. (×200.)

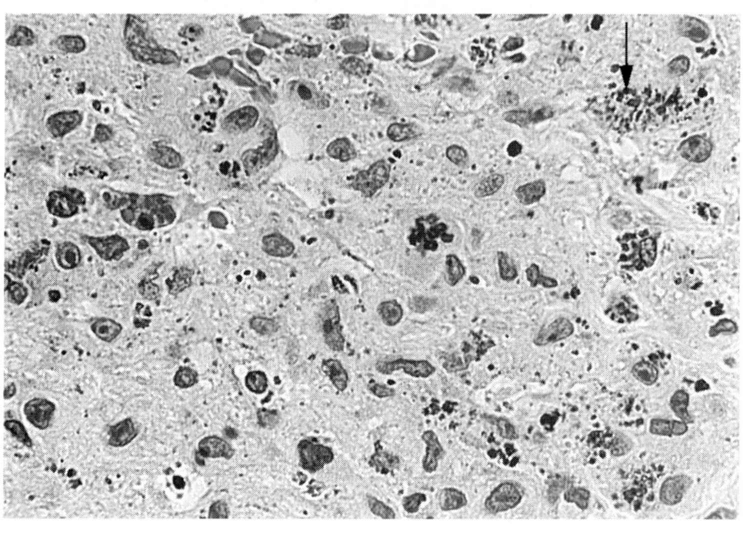

**Fig. 2-123.** Melanin and hemosiderin. Melanin granules (*arrow*) are smaller and darker than hemosiderin. This method of pigment identification on H&E is not entirely reliable, and special stains are recommended for critical cases. The 35-year-old patient had left trigeminal neuralgia for 1 year, and a primary melanocytic tumor in Meckel's cave. (Courtesy of Dr. George K. Tong, Saginaw, MI.) (×1000.) (See Plate 1D.)

nent nucleoli but inconspicuous mitoses. These hyperpigmented tumors may need to be bleached[98] to reveal these cytologic features. Special stains for melanin like Fontana-Masson's and for iron like Perl's Prussian blue will distinguish melanin from hemosiderin.[98]

Primary malignant melanoma can be leptomeningeal (Fig. 2-122) or parenchymal. Its pigmentation, pleomorphism, mitoses, and infiltration of surrounding structures are highly variable. Melanomas that involve the sella are described in Chapter 5. Meningeal melanomatosis is diffuse infiltration of the leptomeninges by melanocytes. About 25% of these two primary melanocytic malignancies are associated with neurocutaneous melanosis.[81]

Melanin is found in normal melanocytes of the arachnoid and can be seen on MRI.[45] These can be distinguished from melanocytic neoplasms by their sparse distribution and benign nuclear features. Constituent cells of meningioma, schwannoma (Fig. 2-93), ependymoma, neuroblastoma, medulloblastoma, and PNET rarely contain melanin.[15,145] Each of these cell types can be identified by their features described in previous pages of this chapter.

## ACKNOWLEDGMENTS

We thank Ms. Dianna Banka and Ms. Dawn Banka for skillfully preparing and editing the manuscript. Mr. Mark Deming and Mr. Randal Stegmeyer provided photographic prints of high quality.

### REFERENCES

1. Albright AL, Price RA, and Guthkelch AN: Diencephalic gliomas of children. A clinicopathologic study, Cancer 55:2789-2793, 1985.
2. Amendola BE, and others: Primary large-cell lymphoma of the central nervous system, Am J Clin Oncol 9:204-208, 1986.
3. Amine AR, and Sugar O: Suprasellar osteogenic sarcoma following radiation for pituitary adenoma, J Neurosurg 44:88-91, 1976.
4. An-Foraker SH: Cytodiagnosis of malignant lesions in cerebrospinal fluid. Review and cytohistologic correlation, Acta Cytol (Baltimore) 29:286-290, 1985.
5. Anders KH, and others: Lymphomatoid granulomatosis and malignant lymphoma of the central nervous system in the acquired immunodeficiency syndrome, Hum Pathol 20:326-334, 1989.
6. Andreini L, Doglioni C, and Giangaspero F: Tubular adenoma of choroid plexus: a case report, Clin Neuropathol 10:137-140, 1991.
7. Anwer UE, and others: Medulloblastoma with cartilaginous differentiation, Arch Pathol Lab Med 113:84-88, 1989.
8. Barbosa MD, and others: Intraventricular neurocytoma: a clinical and pathological study of three cases and review of the literature, Neurosurgery 26:1045-1054, 1990.
9. Bigner SH, and Johnston WW: The cytopathology of cerebrospinal fluid. I. Nonneoplastic conditions, lymphoma and leukemia, and II. Metastatic cancer, meningeal carcinomatosis and primary central nervous system neoplasms, Acta Cytol (Baltimore) 25:345-353; 461-479, 1981.
10. Brooks JJ, LiVolsi VA, and Trojanowski JQ: Does chondroid chordoma exist? Acta Neuropathol 72:229-235, 1987.
11. Bruner JM: Oligodendroglioma: diagnosis and prognosis, Semin Diagn Pathol 4:251-261, 1987.
12. Buff BL, Schick RM, and Norregaard T: Meningeal metastasis of leiomyosarcoma mimicking meningiomas: CT and MR findings, J Comput Assist Tomogr 15:166-167, 1991.
13. Burger PC: Use of cytologic preparations in the frozen section diagnosis of central nervous system neoplasia, Am J Surg Pathol 9:344-354, 1985.
14. Burger PC, and others: Clinicopathologic correlations in the oligodendroglioma, Cancer 59:1345-1352, 1987.
15. Burger PC, and Scheithauer BW: Atlas of tumor pathology. Tumors of the central nervous system. Washington, 1994, Armed Forces Institute of Pathology.
16. Burger PC, Scheithauer BW, and Vogel FS: Surgical pathology of the nervous system and its coverings, ed 3, New York, 1991, Churchill-Livingstone.
17. Burger PC, and Vogel FS: Frozen section interpretation in surgical neuropathology. I. Intracranial lesions. II. Intraspinal lesions, Am J Surg Pathol 1:323-347; 2:81-95, 1977-8.
18. Casadei GP, and others: Central neurocytoma. A clinicopathologic study of five cases, Tumori 77:323-327, 1991.
19. Cerdá-Nicolás M, and others: Histologic and cytogenetic patterns in benign, atypical, and malignant meningiomas. Does correlation with recurrence exist? Int J Surg Pathol 2:301-310, 1995.
20. Chamberlain M: Long survival in patients with acquired immune deficiency syndrome-related primary central system lymphoma, Cancer 73:1728-1730, 1994.
21. Chen WYK, and Kepes JJ: Extensive intracellular mucoid changes in meningiomas: a manifestation of polyvinylpyrrolidone (PVP) effect on tissues with mesenchymal characteristics, J Neuropathol Exp Neurol 44:360, 1985.
22. Chimelli L, Hahn MD, and Budka H: Lipomatous differentiation in a medulloblastoma, Acta Neuropathol (Berl) 81:471-473, 1991.
23. Chu TA: Chondroid chordoma of the sacrococcygeal region, Arch Pathol Lab Med 111:861-864, 1987.
24. Clark GB, Henry JM, and McKeever PE: Cerebral pilocytic astrocytoma, Cancer 56:1128-1133, 1985.
25. Coakley KJ, and others: Pilocytic astrocytomas: Well-demarcated magnetic resonance appearance despite frequent infiltration histologically, Mayo Clin Proc 70:747-751, 1995.
26. Cohen ME, and others: Prognostic factors in brainstem gliomas, Neurology 36:602-605, 1986.
27. D'Andrea AD, and others: Pineocytomas of childhood. A reappraisal of natural history and response to therapy, Cancer 59:1353-1357, 1987.
28. Daumas-Duport C: Dysembryoplastic neuroepithelial tumors, Brain Pathol 3:283-295, 1993.
29. Daumas-Duport C, and others: Dysembryoplastic neuroepithelial tumors of young patients with intractable partial seizures: report of 39 cases, Neurosurgery 23:545-556, 1988.
30. Daumas-Duport C, Scheithauer BW, and Kelly PJ: A histologic and cytologic method for the spatial definition of gliomas, Mayo Clin Proc 62:435-449, 1987.
31. Davenport RD, and others: Non-Hodgkin's lymphoma of the brain following Hodgkin's disease: an immunohistochemical study, Cancer 67:440-443, 1991.
32. De Recondo J, and Haguenau M: Neuropathologic survey of the phakomatoses and allied disorders. In Vinken PJ, Bruyn GW, editors: Handbook of clinical neurology, New York, 19–91, 1972, American Elsevier.
33. Deangelis LM, and others: Primary CNS lymphoma: managing patients with spontaneous and AIDS-related disease, Oncology 1:52-62, 1987.
34. Eriksen B, and others: Primary histiocytosis X of the parieto-occipital lobe, Hum Pathol 19:611-614, 1988.

35. Farwell JR, Dohrmann GJ, and Flannery JT: Medulloblastoma in childhood: an epidemiological study, J Neurosurg 61:657-664, 1984.
36. Feldenzer JA, and McKeever PE: Selective localization of gamma-enolase in stromal cells of cerebellar hemangioblastomas, Acta Neuropathol (Berl) 72:281-285, 1987.
37. Ferracini R, and others: Primary T-cell lymphoma of the central nervous system, Clin Neuropathol 14:125-129, 1995.
38. Figarella-Branger D, and others: Central neurocytomas. Critical evaluation of a small-cell neuronal tumor, Am J Surg Pathol 16:97-109, 1992.
39. Fine H, and Mayer R: Primary central nervous system lymphoma, Ann Intern Med 119:1093-1104, 1993.
40. Forsyth PA, and others: 51 cases of supratentorial pilocytic astrocytomas: a clinicopathologic, prognostic, and flow cytometric study, Cancer 72:1335-1342, 1993.
41. Forsyth P, Yahalom J, and DeAngelis L: Combined-modality therapy in the treatment of primary central nervous system lymphoma in AIDS, Neurology 44:1473-1479, 1994.
42. Freyer DR, Hutchinson RJ, and McKeever PE: Primary primitive neuroectodermal tumor of the spinal cord associated with neural tube defect, Pediatr Neurosci 15:181-187, 1989.
43. Galloway PG, and Roessmann U: Anaplastic astrocytoma mimicking metastatic carcinoma, Am J Surg Pathol 10:728-732, 1986.
44. Gaudin PB, and Rosai J: Florid vascular proliferation associated with neural and neuroendocrine neoplasms. A diagnostic clue and potential pitfall, Am J Surg Pathol 19:642-652, 1995.
45. Gebarski SS, and Blaivas MA: Imaging of normal leptomeningeal melanin, Am J Neuroradiol 17:55-60, 1996.
46. Geddes JF, Sutcliffe JC, and King TT: Mixed cranial nerve tumors in neurofibromatosis type 2, Clin Neuropathol 14:310-313, 1995.
47. Geddes JF, and others: Granular cell change in astrocytic tumors, Am J Surg Pathol 20:55-63, 1996.
48. Ghandur-Mnaymneh L: Tissue imprints in surgical pathology, with a modified fixation procedure, Hum Pathol 14:11-13, 1983.
49. Giangaspero F, and others: "Desmoplastic" versus "classic" medulloblastoma: comparison of DNA content, histopathology and differentiation, Virchows Arch A Pathol Anat Histopathol 418:207-214, 1991.
50. Glass J, and others: The treatment of oligodendrogliomas and mixed oligodendroglioma-astrocytomas with PCV chemotherapy. J Neurosurg 76:741-745, 1992.
51. Grant JW, and Gallagher PJ: Pleomorphic xanthoastrocytoma. Immunohistochemical methods for differentiation from fibrous histiocytomas with similar morphology, Am J Surg Pathol 10: 336-341, 1986.
52. Hammond RR, and MacKenzie IRA: Xanthoma disseminatum with massive intracranial involvement, Clin Neuropathol 14: 314-321, 1995.
53. Hardman JM, and Hong-Yi Y: The central nervous system, In Silverberg SG, editor: Principles and practice of surgical pathology, New York, 1983, John Wiley.
54. Hardwidge C, and others: Primary cerebral lymphoma—a clinico-pathological study, Clin Neuropathol 9:217-223, 1990.
55. Harris JH, and Rayport M: Primary "cerebral amyloidoma," J Neuropathol Exp Neurol 38:318, 1979.
56. Hart LL, and Weinberg JB: Metastatic hemangiopericytoma with prolonged survival, Cancer 60:916-920, 1987.
57. Hayakawa T, and others: Primary central nervous system lymphoma in Japan: A retrospective, co-operative study by CNS-Lymphoma Study Group in Japan, J Neurol Oncol 19:197-215, 1994.
58. Hayostek C, and others: Astrocytomas of the cerebellum. A comparative clinicopathologic study of pilocytic and diffuse astrocytomas. Cancer 72:856-869, 1993.
59. Healey EA and others: The prognostic significance of postoperative residual tumor in ependymoma, Neurosurgery 28:666-671, 1991.
60. Henson JW, and Wiley RG: CNS chloromas in patients presenting with eosinophilia, Neurology 39:1386-1388, 1989.
61. Herpers MJ, and Budka H: Glial fibrillary acidic protein (GFAP) in oligodendroglial tumors: gliofibrillary oligodendroglioma and transitional oligoastrocytoma as subtypes of oligodendroglioma, Acta Neuropathol (Berl) 64:265-272, 1984.
62. Hoag G, Sima AA, and Rozdilsky B: Astroblastoma revisited: a report of three cases. Acta Neuropathol (Berl) 70:10-16, 1986.
63. Hood TW, and others: Stereotaxic biopsy of intrinsic lesions of the brain stem, J Neurosurg 65:172-176, 1986.
64. Hood TW, Venes JL, and McKeever PE: Stereotactic biopsy of pediatric brain stem tumors, J Pediatr Neurosci 2:79-88, 1986.
65. Imaya H and Kudo M: Malignant choroid plexus papilloma of the IV ventricle, Childs Nerv Syst 7:109-111, 1991.
66. Ito H, and others: Meningiomas differentiating to arachnoid trabecular cells: a proposal for histological subtype "arachnoid trabecular cell meningioma," Acta Neuropathol (Berl) 82:327-330, 1991.
67. Jansen GH, Troost D, and Dingemans KP: Polar spongioblastoma: an immunohistochemical and electron microscopical study, Acta Neuropathol (Berl) 81:228-232, 1990.
68. Jeffreys R: Pathological and haematological aspects of posterior fossa haemangioblastomata, J Neurol Neurosurg Psychiatry 38: 112-119, 1975.
69. Jellinger K, and Paulus W: Primary central nervous system lymphomas: an update, J Cancer Res Clin Oncol 119:7-27, 1992.
70. Jellinger K, and Slowik F: Histological subtypes and prognostic problems in meningiomas, J Neurol 208:279-298, 1975.
71. Junck L, and others: Prognostic value of PET-FDG scans in untreated gliomas, Neurology 45(Suppl 4):A387, 1995.
72. Karamitopoulou E, and others: Ganglioglioma of the brain stem: neurological dysfunction of 16-year duration, Clin Neuropathol 14:162-168, 1995.
73. Katsetos CD, and others: Cerebellar desmoplastic medulloblastomas. A further immunohistochemical characterization of the reticulin-free pale islands, Arch Pathol Lab Med 113:1019-1029, 1989.
74. Kepes JJ: Differential diagnostic problems in brain tumors, In Minckler J, editor: Pathology of the nervous system, New York, 1971, McGraw-Hill, Blakiston.
75. Kepes JJ, Fulling KH, and Garcia JH: The clinical significance of "adenoid" formations of neoplastic astrocytes, imitating metastatic carcinoma, in gliosarcomas. A review of five cases, Clin Neuropathol, 1:139-150, 1982.
76. Kepes JJ, Rubinstein LJ, and Eng LF: Pleomorphic xanthoastrocytoma: a distinctive meningocerebral glioma of young subjects with relatively favorable prognosis: a study of 12 cases, Cancer 44:1839-1852, 1979.
77. Kepes JJ, Sher J, and Oliver MG: Light and electron microscopic study of "adenoid" components in gliomas. Fibroblastic activity of neoplastic astrocytes, J Neuropathol Exp Neurol 44:359, 1985.
78. Kepes JJ: Meningiomas: biology, pathology, and differential diagnosis, Chicago, 1982, Year Book.
79. Kepes JJ: Presidential address: The histopathology of meningiomas. A reflection of origins and expected behavior, J Neuropathol Exp Neurol 45:95-107, 1986.
80. Kitanaka C, and others: Postradiation astrocytoma: report of two cases, J Neurosurg 70:469-474, 1989.
81. Kleihues P, Burger PC, and Scheithauer BW: Histological typing of tumours of the central nervous system, ed 2. International Histological Classification of Tumours, vol 21, Berlin, 1993, Springer-Verlag.
82. Kros JM, de Jong AA, and van der Kwast TH: Ultrastructural characterization of transitional cells in oligodendrogliomas, J Neuropathol Exp Neurol 51:186-193, 1992.

83. Kros JM, Vecht CJ, and Stefanko SZ: The pleomorphic xanthoastrocytoma and its differential diagnosis: a study of five cases, Hum Pathol 22:1128-1135, 1991.
84. Krouwer HGJ, and others: Gemistocytic astrocytomas: a reappraisal, J Neurosurg 74:399-406, 1991.
85. Kulah A, Ilcayto R, and Fiskeci C: Cystic meningiomas, Acta Neurochir (Wien) 111:108-113, 1991.
86. Lam R: The nature of cytoplasmic vacuoles in chordoma cells. A correlative enzyme and electron microscopic histochemical study, Pathol Res Pract 186:642-650, 1990.
87. Lattes R, and Bigotti G: Lipoblastic meningioma: "vacuolated meningioma," Hum Pathol 22:164-171, 1991.
88. Levine SA, McKeever PE, and Greenberg HS: Primary cerebellar glioblastoma multiforme, J Neurooncol 5:231-236, 1987.
89. Levy RA, Allen R, and McKeever P: Pleomorphic xanthoastrocytoma presenting with massive intracranial hemorrhage, AJNR 17:154-156, 1996.
90. Lindboe CF, Helseth E, and Myhr G: Lhermitte-Duclos disease and giant meningioma as manifestations of Cowden's disease, Clin Neuropathol 14:327-330, 1995.
91. Lombardi D, and others: "Angioglioma" and the arteriovenous malformation-glioma association, J Neurosurg 75:589-599, 1991.
92. Louis DN, and others: Pseudopsammomatous meningioma with elevated serum carcinoembryonic antigen: a true secretory meningioma. Case report, J Neurosurg 74:129-132, 1991.
93. Lowe J, and Russel NH: Cerebral vasculitis associated with hairy cell leukemia, Cancer 60:3025-3028, 1987.
94. Lulenski GC, Singleton EF, and Oberman HA: Histiocytosis X. An unusual cause of salivary gland enlargement, Arch Otolaryngol 100:319-321, 1974.
95. MacCumber MW, and others: Opthalmic involvement in aggressive histiocytosis X, Opthalmology 72:22-27, 1990.
96. Mannoji H, and Becker LE: Ependymal and choroid plexus tumors: cytokeratin and GFAP expression, Cancer 61:1377-1385, 1988.
97. Matsukado Y, Yokota A, and Marubayashi T: Rhabdomyosarcoma of the brain, J Neurosurg 43:215-221, 1975.
98. McKeever PE, and Balentine JD: Histochemistry of the nervous system, In Spicer SS editor: Histochemistry in pathologic diagnosis, New York, 1987, Marcel Dekker.
99. McKeever PE, Blaivas M, and Sima AAF: Neoplasms of the sellar region, In Lloyd RV editor: Surgical pathology of the pituitary gland, Philadelphia, 1992, WB Saunders.
100. McKeever PE, and Blaivas M: The brain, spinal cord, and meninges, In Sternberg SS and others, editors: Diagnostic surgical pathology, ed 2, New York, 1994, Raven Press.
101. McKeever PE, and Brissie NT: Scanning electron microscopy of neoplasms removed at surgery: surface topography and comparison of meningioma, colloid cyst, ependymoma, pituitary adenoma, schwannoma and astrocytoma, J Neuropathol Exp Neurol 36:875-896, 1977.
102. McKeever PE, Burger PC, and Nelson JS: Introduction to neurooncology, In Nelson JS, Parisi JF, and Schochet SS Jr, editors: Principles and practice of neuropathology. St Louis, 1993, CV Mosby.
103. McKeever PE, Davenport RD, and Shakui P: Patterns of antigenic expression in cultured glioma cells, In Nelson JS, editor: Critical reviews in neurobiology, Boca Raton, FL, 1991, CRC Press.
104. McKeever PE, and others: Nuclear parameters as prognostic indicators in glioblastoma patients, J Neuropathol Exp Neurol 49:71-78, 1990.
105. McKeever PE, and others: Sarcoma arising from a gliosarcoma, South Med J 77:1027-1032, 1984.
106. McKeever PE, and others: Type IV collagen messenger RNA localizes within cells of abnormal vascular proliferations of glioblastoma and sarcomatous regions of gliosarcoma, J Histochem Cytochem 41:1124, 1993.
107. Meis JM, Martz KL, and Nelson JS: Mixed glioblastoma multiforme and sarcoma: a clinicopathologic study of 26 radiation therapy oncology group cases, Cancer 67:2342-2349, 1991.
108. Michaud J, Banerjee D, and Kaufmann JCE: Lymphomatoid granulomatosis involving the central nervous system: complication of a renal transplant with terminal monoclonal B-cell proliferation, Acta Neuropathol (Berl) 61:141-147, 1983.
109. Miller D, and others: Pathology with clinical correlations of primary central nervous system non-Hodgkin's lymphoma, Cancer 74:1383-1397, 1994.
110. Miller DC, and others: Synaptophysin: a sensitive and specific marker for ganglion cells in central nervous system neoplasms, Hum Pathol 21:271-276, 1990.
111. Min KW, Gyorkey F, and Halpert B: Primary rhabdomyosarcoma of the cerebrum, Cancer 35:1405-1411, 1975.
112. Molloy PT, and others: Brainstem tumors in patients with neurofibromatosis type 1, Neurology 45:1897-1902, 1995.
113. Montine TJ, and others: Prognostic significance of Ki-67 proliferation index in supratentorial fibrillary astrocytic neoplasms, Neurosurgery 34:674-678, 1994.
114. Morgello S: Pathogenesis and classification of primary central nervous system lymphoma: an update, Brain Pathol 5:383-393, 1995.
115. Mörk SJ, and others: Patterns of epithelial metaplasia in malignant gliomas: II. Squamous differentiation of epithelial like formations in gliosarcomas and glioblastomas, J Neuropathol Exp Neurol 47:101-118, 1988.
116. Mörk SJ, and Rubinstein LJ: Ependymoblastoma: a reappraisal of a rare embryonal tumor, Cancer 55:1536-1542, 1985.
117. Nanda A, Hirsh LF, and Antoiniades K: Malignant fibrous histiocytoma in a recurrent thoracic chordoma: case report and literature review, Neurosurgery 28:588-592, 1991.
118. Nelson JS, and others: Necrosis as a prognostic criterion in malignant supratentorial, astrocytic gliomas, Cancer 52:550-554, 1983.
119. Newton HB, Rosenblum MK, and Malkin MG: Turcot's syndrome. Flow cytometric analysis, Cancer 68:1633-1639, 1991.
120. Nishio S, and others: Tumors of the lateral ventricular wall, especially the septum pellucidum: clinical presentation and variations in pathological features, Neurosurgery 27:224-230, 1990.
121. Nishio S, and others: Intraventricular neurocytoma: clinicopathological features of six cases, J Neurosurg 68:665-670, 1988.
122. Oberc-Greenwood MA, and others: A human ganglioglioma containing paired helical filaments, Hum Pathol 15:834-838, 1984.
123. Ojeda VJ, Spagnolo DV, and Vaughan RJ: Palisades in primary cerebral neuroblastoma simulating so-called polar spongioblastoma. A light and electron microscopical study of an adult case, Am J Surg Pathol 11:316-322, 1987.
124. O'Neill B, and Illig J: Primary central nervous system lymphoma, Mayo Clin Proc 64:1005-1020, 1989.
125. Pasquier B, and others: Primary rhabdomyosarcoma of the central nervous system, Acta Neuropathol (Berl) 1975;33:333-342, 1975.
126. Patil AA, and others: Intraventricular neurocytoma: a report of two cases, Neurosurgery 26:140-144, 1990.
127. Paulus W, and Peiffer J: Intratumoral histologic heterogeneity of gliomas. A quantitive study, Cancer 64:442-447, 1989.
128. Paulus W, Slowik F, and Jellinger K: Primary intracranial sarcomas: histopathological features of 19 cases, Histopathology 18:395-402, 1991.
129. Pell MF, Revesz T, and Thomas DG: Multicentric malignant glioma, Br J Neurosurg 5:631-634, 1991.

130. Powell HC, Marshall LF, and Igneizi RJ: Post-irradiation pituitary sarcoma, Acta Neuropathol (Berl) 39:165-167, 1977.
131. Powell SZ, and others: Divergent differentiation in pleomorphic xanthoastrocytoma. Evidence for a neuronal element and possible relationship to ganglion cell tumors, Am J Surg Pathol 20: 80-85, 1996.
132. Prayson RA, and Estes ML: Dysembryoplastic neuroepithelial tumor, Am J Clin Pathol 97:398-401, 1992.
133. Prayson RA, and others: Dysembryoplastic neuroepithelial tumor: a clinicopathologic and immunohistochemical study of 11 tumors including MIB1 immunoreactivity, Clin Neuropathol 15:47-53, 1996.
134. Ramsay DA, and others: Medulloblastomas in late middle age and the elderly: report of 2 cases, Clin Neuropathol 14:337-342, 1995.
135. Reddick RL, and others: Immunoblastic sarcoma of the central nervous system in a patient with lymphomatoid granulomatosis, Cancer 42:652-659, 1978.
136. Rieth KG, and others: Primary demyelinating disease simulating glioma of the corpus callosum: report of three cases, J Neurosurg 55:620-624, 1981.
137. Roberts RO, and others: Medulloblastoma: a population-based study of 532 cases, J Neuropathol Exp Neurol 50:134-144, 1991.
138. Rorke LB, and others: Revision of the World Health Organization classification of brain tumors for childhood brain tumors, Cancer 56:1869-1886, 1985.
139. Rorke LB, Packer R, and Biegel J: Central nervous system atypical teratoid/rhabdoid tumors of infancy and childhood, J Neurooncol 24:21-28, 1995.
140. Rosenblum MK, Erlandson RA, and Budzilovich GN: The lipid-rich epithelioid glioblastoma, Am J Surg Pathol 15:925-934, 1991.
141. Rubinstein LJ, and others: Squamous differentiation of epithelial-like formations in glioblastoma and gliosarcoma, J Neuropathol Exp Neurol 45:327, 1986.
142. Rubinstein LJ, and Northfield DWC: The medulloblastoma and the so-called "arachnoidal cerebellar sarcoma." A critical re-examination of a nosological problem, Brain 87:379-412, 1964.
143. Rubio A, and others: Hemangioblastoma of the optic nerve, Hum Pathol 25:1249-1251, 1994.
144. Rushing EJ, Mena H, and Smirniotopoulos JG: Mesenchymal chondrosarcoma of the cauda equina, Clin Neuropathol 14:150-153, 1995.
145. Russell DS, and Rubinstein LJ: Pathology of tumours of the nervous system, Baltimore, 1989, Williams & Wilkins.
146. Salvati M, and others: Intramedullary meningioma: case report and review of the literature, Surg Neurol 37:42-45, 1992.
147. Schiffer D, and others: Apoptosis and cell proliferation in human neuroepithelial tumors, Neuroscience Lett 195:81-84, 1995.
148. Schiffer D, and others: Histologic prognostic factors in ependymoma, Child Nerv Syst 7:177-182, 1991.
149. Schroder R, and others: Intracerebral Aλ amyloidoma diagnosed by stereotactic biopsy, Clin Neuropathol 14:347-350, 1995.
150. Shiraishi K: Glycogen-rich meningioma. Case report and short review, Neurosurg Rev 14:61-64, 1991.
151. Shyn PB, and others: Primary intracranial ependymoblastoma presenting as spinal cord compression due to metastasis, Child Nerv Syst 2:323-325, 1986.
152. Silverstein AM, Quint DJ, and McKeever PE: Intradural paraganglioma of the thoracic spine, Am J Neuroradiol 11:614-616, 1990.
153. Skullerud K, and others: Intracranial primary leiomyosarcoma arising in a teratoma of the pineal area, Clin Neuropathol 14: 245-248, 1995.
154. Sonneland PR, and others: Paraganglioma of the cauda equina region. Clinicopathologic study of 31 cases with special reference to immunocytology and ultrastructure, Cancer 58:1720-1735, 1986.
154a. Soylemezoglu F, and others: Lipomatous medulloblastoma in adults. A distinct clinicopathological entity, Am J Surg Pathol 20:413-418, 1996.
155. Taratuto AL, Sevlever G, and Piccardo P: Clues and pitfalls in stereotactic biopsy of the central nervous system, Arch Pathol Lab Med 115:596-602, 1991.
156. Terry RD, Hyams VJ, and Davidoff LM: Combined nonmetastasizing fibrosarcoma and chromophobe tumour of the pituitary, Cancer 12:791-798, 1959.
157. Tison V, and others: Intracranial desmoplastic small-cell tumor. Report of a case, Am J Surg Pathol 20:112-117, 1996.
158. Tiszlavicz L: Multiple primary intracranial tumors and association of intra- and extracranial tumors. An autopsy study, Clin Neuropathol 12:204-210, 1993.
159. Townsend JJ, and Seaman JP: Central neurocytoma—a rare benign intraventricular tumor, Acta Neuropathol (Berl) 71:167-170, 1986.
160. Vandenberg SR, Herman MM, and Rubinstein LJ: Embryonal central neuroepithelial tumors: current concepts and future challenges, Cancer Metastasis Rev 5:343-365, 1987.
161. VandenBerg SR, and others: Desmoplastic supratentorial neuroepithelial tumors of infancy with divergent differentiation potential ("desmoplastic infantile gangliogliomas"). Report on 11 cases of a distinctive embryonal tumor with favorable prognosis, J Neurosurg 66:58-71, 1987.
162. Vertosick FT Jr, Selker RG, and Arena VC: Survival of patients with well-differentiated astrocytomas diagnosed in the era of computed tomography, Neurosurgery 28:496-501, 1991.
163. von Deimling A, and others: Patterns of differentiation in central neurocytoma. An immunohistochemical study of eleven biopsies, Acta Neuropathol (Berl) 79:473-479, 1990.
164. von Deimling A, and others: Histogenesis and differentiation potential of central neurocytomas, Lab Invest 64:585-591, 1991.
165. Watanabe K, and others: Choroid plexus papilloma containing melanin pigment, Clin Neuropathol 14:159-161, 1995.
166. Weller M, and others: Tumor cell dissemination triggers an intrathecal immune response in neoplastic meningitis, Cancer 69: 1475-1480, 1992.
167. Winek RR, Scheithauer BW, and Wick MR: Meningioma, meningeal hemangiopericytoma (angioblastic meningioma), peripheral hemangiopericytoma, and acoustic schwannoma: a comparative immunohistochemical study, Am J Surg Pathol 13: 251-261, 1989.
168. Wong SW, Ducker TB, and Powers JM: Fulminating parapontine epidermoid carcinoma in a four-year-old boy, Cancer 37: 1525-1231, 1976.
169. Yasargil MG, and others: Central neurocytoma: histopathological variants and therapeutic approaches, J Neurosurg 76:32-37, 1992.
170. Zampieri P, and others: Radiation-associated cerebral gliomas. A report of two cases and review of the literature, J Neurosurg Sci 33:271-279, 1989.
171. Zuccaro G, Taratuto AL, and Monges J: Intracranial neoplasms during the first year of life, Surg Neurol 26:29-36, 1986.
172. Zülch KJ: Histologic typing of tumours of the central nervous system. International Histological Classification of Tumours, vol 21, Geneva, 1979, World Health Organization.

C • H • A • P • T • E • R

3

# Tumors: Applications of Ultrastructural Methods

**Robert E. Mrak***



* Dr. Mrak was a full-time Federal employee at the time of writing and thus the material in this chapter is in the public domain.

## INTRODUCTION

Thirty years have passed since the seminal investigations of Terry and Harkin,[368] Luse,[220] Van Breeman,[382] Webster and Spiro,[395a] and others* opened the field of ultrastructural neuropathology. Following the advances of the 1960s, the decade of the 1970s brought increasing recognition of the diagnostic usefulness of this new tool.† Today, even with the new addition of biochemical and immunohistochemical analyses, electron microscopy remains a valued tool in the evaluation of difficult or unusual cases. Most modern diagnostic applications of electron microscopy fall into one of four categories:

1. Identification of etiologic agents. The demonstration of polyoma virus particles in cases of progressive multifocal leukoencephalopathy is an example.
2. Demonstration of intracellular "storage" material in metabolic deficiencies. GM-2 ganglioside in Tay Sachs disease and galactocerebroside in Krabbe's (globoid cell) leukodystrophy are examples.
3. Demonstration of submicroscopic changes in certain hereditary or "degenerative" diseases. Examples include neuroaxonal dystrophy, various peripheral neuropathies, and unusual congenital myopathies.
4. Classification (or subclassification) of tumors for which light microscopy is inconclusive.

Most applications, in our experience, fall into the latter two categories. Viral antigens are now usually identified by means of immunohistochemistry, in situ hibridization, and polymerase chain reaction, and metabolic defects generally are identified either histologically or biochemically. The third category includes many peripheral nerve biopsies and some cases of congenital myopathies; and electron microscopy is an important tool in evaluating such cases. The usefulness of electron microscopy in the diagnosis of nervous system tumors, is the topic of this chapter.

### Ultrastructural Tumor Diagnosis

Within the field of tumor diagnosis, five general types of problems can be identified for which electron microscopy may be of use. These are:

1. Histologic look-alikes. This problem is an especially thorny one with tumors of the spinal canal. As discussed below, ependymomas of the spinal cord may be mistaken for astrocytomas, schwannomas, or even meningiomas. Generally these are readily distinguished by electron microscopy. Another example is peripheral spindle cell tumors. Tumors originating from Schwann cells, smooth muscle, and fibroblasts may appear similar by light microscopy, but are usually quite distinct ultrastructurally.
2. Poorly differentiated or undifferentiated tumors. These tumors, by definition, lose their identifying histopathologic features. Such identifying features may remain, however, at the ultrastructural level. Among large cell undifferentiated tumors, electron microscopy may assist in distinguishing carcinoma, lymphoma, amelanotic melanoma, and glioblastoma. Small cell undifferentiated tumors are another source of confusion. Electron microscopy may be useful in distinguishing neuroblastoma, medulloblastoma, and other primitive neuroectodermal tumors, Ewing's sarcoma, rhabdomyosarcoma, lymphoma, small cell carcinoma, and occasionally oligodendroglioma and astrocytoma.
3. Rare tumors or unusual presentations of common tumors. In such cases, electron microscopy may bolster confidence in a tentative diagnosis or may provide diagnostic information. Examples include ependymoblastoma and intraparenchymal schwannoma.
4. Identification of unique, submicroscopic structures. Examples of this rather classic use of electron microscopy include the demonstration of Birbeck granules in cases of histiocytosis X, premelanosomes in amelanotic melanoma, and Weibel-Palade bodies in tumors derived from endothelial cells.
5. Identification of primary site for metastatic adenocarcinoma of unknown origin. The application of ultrastructural analysis as a means to identify a primary site in these cases is underrecognized and underutilized. This method is noninvasive (i.e., requires no further procedures beyond the already-performed biopsy) and is relatively inexpensive (in comparison with a full clinical workup).

It is worth noting that an area in which electron microscopy is *not* useful is the determination of malignancy. The power of ultrastructural analysis lies in identification of tumor cell type (histogenesis), whereas assessment of malignant potential is better accomplished by light microscopy. An exception to this exists among cases in which the identification of cell type itself carries prognostic import. For example, a peripheral spindle cell tumor with occasional atypical cells and mitotic figures may be considered benign if composed of Schwann cells,[126] while a histologically similar tumor of smooth muscle derivation has greater potential for recurrence and invasion.[332] Similarly, a

* Refs. 82, 336, 367, 369, 395, 416, 418.

† Refs. 23, 95, 115, 148, 183, 226, 251.

malignant plexosarcoma may mimic a benign leiomyoma on histologic evaluation.[139]

Samples of tumors submitted for electron microscopy generally arrive with a short list of diagnostic possibilities based on clinical, histologic, and immunohistochemical results. The electron microscopist is then responsible for choosing among these possibilities. At times there may be only a single diagnostic possibility, but sufficient doubt remains to prompt ultrastructural confirmation. Usually the correct diagnosis is among those considered before ultrastructural examination, but occasionally electron microscopy suggests another diagnosis that was not in the differential. This, in fact, is one advantage of electron microscopy over immunohistochemistry—the ability to answer questions not asked. Immunohistochemical techniques, by their very nature, only provide yes-or-no answers to specific questions.

Diagnostic uncertainties and a consequent request for ultrastructural examination are more common with some tumor types than with others, and certain groups of tumors are more likely to be confused with one another. Consequently, this chapter is organized around such common diagnostic problems, and the descriptions and illustrations are chosen to illustrate points that are important in differential diagnosis. For more thorough descriptions of particular tumors, the reader is referred to the literature cited and to several pertinent monographs and reviews.[60,63,74,133]

### Specimen Preparation

The ideal specimen for electron microscopy is one that is received promptly from the surgeon, cut into small cubes or rectangular solids no more than 1–2 mm in thickness, and fixed in buffered glutaraldehyde. This is a relatively simple procedure, and a prudent approach would be to process all but the most obvious neoplasms this way upon receipt. Then, if electron microscopy is not required, the specimen may be discarded later.

Unfortunately, all too often this is not done, and ultrastructural consultation is only sought later, usually after an exhaustive histologic and immunohistochemical work-up has been completed. In such cases, samples that may approach the quality of glutaraldehyde-fixed specimens may be obtained from tissue originally fixed and stored in buffered formalin. Provided it is adequately buffered to a neutral pH, 10% to 20% formalin (4% to 8% formaldehyde) is an entirely adequate fixative for most diagnostic ultrastructural work. In addition to adequate buffering, promptness of fixation is important. Most poor-quality, uninterpretable results blamed on "formalin fixation" are in fact the result of delayed fixation or of inadequate buffering of the formalin, and are not attributable to inadequacies of formalin as a fixative. Because the tissue penetration of the fixative is relatively slow, one should select a superficial (and, hence, rapidly-fixed) portion of the specimen, cut this into small cubes as described above, and submit these still in formalin. Postfixing a specimen with glutaraldehyde that already has been thoroughly fixed in formalin confers no known benefit.

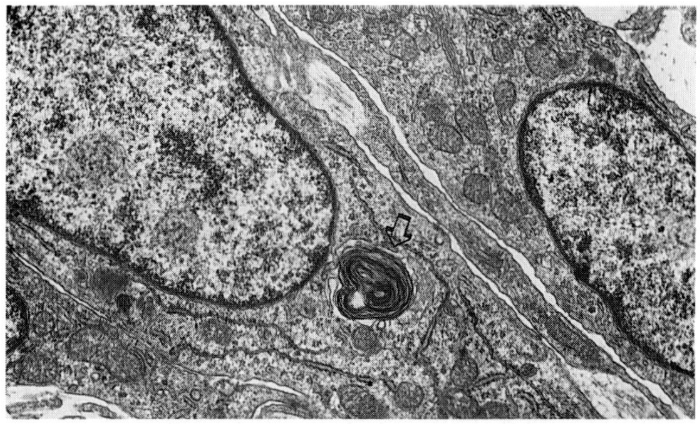

**Fig. 3-1.** Artifactual membranous whorl (*arrow*) in a gastric spindle cell tumor. Specimen held in glutaraldehyde for 7 days. (×9500.)

Length of fixation is of some concern. Prolonged fixation in formalin or glutaraldehyde extracts proteins and lipids from tissue, resulting in some loss of crispness of detail and in the appearance of some artifacts, especially myelin-like membranous whorls (Fig. 3-1). However, these problems, while detracting from the esthetic quality of the resulting electron micrographs, rarely interfere with diagnostic interpretation. Thus, while 2 to 4 hours is an ideal length of fixation, tissues fixed for days, weeks, or in some cases months or years, may still provide useful diagnostic information.[146] For example, Zu Rhein and Chou[418] first demonstrated viral particles in a case of progressive multifocal leukoencephalopathy using tissue that had been stored in 10% formalin for 2 years.

As a last resort, tissue for electron microscopy may be excised from a paraffin block (or even recovered from paraffin sections on glass slides).[108] We have had good results with this approach in occasional cases (see Fig. 3-78). Unfortunately, however, the more common result is a specimen of rather poor quality. The important parameters relate to the original fixation and embedding of the tissue. The technique is rather straightforward: The excised tissue (again, a small piece) is incubated in xylene (a minimum of 90 minutes, but often overnight) to extract the paraffin, and is then rehydrated by means of a series of ethanol/water mixtures (or acetone/water mixtures) until the specimen is returned to an aqueous buffered medium. The tissue is then postfixed with osmium and further processed as usual. Alternatively, the osmication step (and consequently the necessity for rehydration) may be omitted and the tissue transferred from xylene to ethanol to propylene oxide for embedding. This shortcut requires insertion of a toluidine blue staining step so that the tissue can be seen during processing.[400]

### Special Techniques for Immunocytochemistry

Routine specimens are postfixed in osmium tetroxide, dehydrated in a series of ethanol/water (or acetone/water) mixtures, and embedded in a hydrophobic resin such as Epon, Araldite, or Spurr. This technique gives excellent ultrastructural preservation. However, antigenic determinants of tissue components are frequently extracted, altered, or obscured, and this is of concern in light of growing interest in ultrastructural immunocytochemistry.[57,185] Numerous strategies have been devised to preserve tissue antigens. In general, the greater the preservation of antigens, the poorer the quality of ultrastructural appearance, and usually some compromise is settled upon depending on the individual stability of the particular antigen of interest. Excellent reviews of such techniques are now available,[132,137,388] and the following is only a brief and rather superficial survey of possible approaches.

1. The simplest procedure modification is to substitute a partially *hydrophilic* resin such as LR-white. This allows introduction of the resin to a specimen in 70% ethanol and avoids the final (and most damaging) dehydration steps. Disadvantages include loss of ultrastructural detail and loss of stability of the final tissue blocks (which must be stored desiccated).[137,268,269]
2. A somewhat less simple procedure, but one that involves minimal expense, is cryofixation and freeze-substitution. The fresh, unfixed tissue is swiftly clamped in a pair of liquid-nitrogen cooled cryopliers (available from Ted Pella, Redding, CA). The tissue is then introduced to cold, pure acetone (−80° C) containing a small amount of osmium and maintained there for several days. A surrounding acetone/dry ice mixture in an insulated container, placed in an ordinary freezer (or even refrigerator) and refilled with dry ice daily, is satisfactory, although more complicated protocols are available.[67] The specimen is then warmed to 4° C, transferred to fresh acetone, warmed to room temperature, and embedded directly in a hydrophobic resin. Alternatively, low-temperature resins can be used, allowing embedding and polymerization without warming the specimen.[67,161,338] This *freeze-substitution technique* avoids all but the mildest fixation and gives reasonably good ultrastructural preservation[171,338] (Figs. 3-2, 3-3). The disadvantages of this technique are the extremely small size of the specimen (even by EM standards) and the additional length of time required for such processing.
3. The technique described above can be improved upon with purchase of specialized equipment. Thus, automated quick-freeze devices are available (Gentleman Jim, Energy Beam Sciences, Agawam, MA; CF 100 Cryofixation System, LifeCell Corp, The Woodlands, TX) as well as automated freeze-substitution units (MDD-C Molecular Distillation Dryer, LifeCell Corp; CS Auto, Reichert Jung, Vienna, Austria).
4. The ultimate approach in preparing thin sections without antigenic damage is freeze-fixation followed by cryo-thin sectioning.[213,338] This is a technically demanding approach requiring some specialized equipment, but primarily specialized training, practice, patience, and persistence.
5. If all else fails, immunocytochemical reactions may be performed in fresh tissue prior to processing.[80] This technique is simple and guarantees antigen integrity. However, aggressive tissue treatments are required to provide antibody access to intracellular antigens, the reaction is limited to the superficial portions of the tissue, and ultrastructural preservation is unsatisfactory.

### Thick Sections

Following fixation, dehydration, and resin embedding of specimens, it is important to cut a 1.0 μm thick section (a semithin, or "thick" section) and stain this for examination by light microscopy (this is commonly done with toluidine blue or paraphenylenediamine). This allows histopathologic correlation with paraffin-embedded material, assessment of adequacy of tissue sampling, and a preliminary survey of the material prior to ultrastructural examination. Such semithin sections of resin-embedded material provide much greater light microscopic detail than do standard paraffin sections, and thus may themselves provide diagnostically useful information (see Figs. 3-4, 3-64, 3-83, and 3-96).

## CENTRAL SPINDLE CELL TUMORS

Ependymomas, schwannomas, meningiomas, and astrocytomas all occur in the spinal canal, where they collectively account for approximately three quarters of primary tumors.[309] Although "typical" examples show distinguishing histologic features, there is enough overlap in the histologic appearances of these tumors to generate diagnostic uncertainty in many cases. Thus, a fibroblastic meningioma may mimic a schwannoma, and a schwannoma with whorls may be mistaken for a meningioma. Intraspinal ependymomas are a frequent source of diagnostic uncertainty.[87] Examples occur in which perivascular palisading (pseudorosette formation) is not prominent and in which

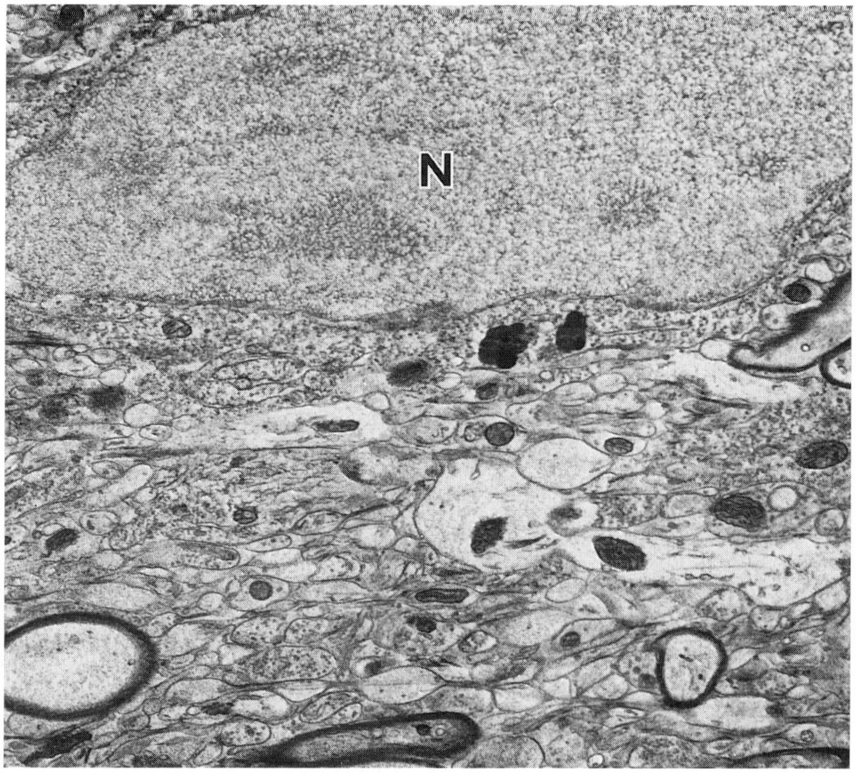


**Fig. 3-2.** Mouse cerebral cortex freeze-fixed using commercial cryopliers and freeze-substituted in a dry-ice-cooled acetone prior to embedding in epoxy resin. There is slight mechanical compression (top to bottom) and slight ice crystal artifact (bubbly appearance) of nuclear chromatin *(N)*. Preservation of neuronal cytoplasm and of neuropil elements is comparable to conventionally processed specimens. (×10,500.)

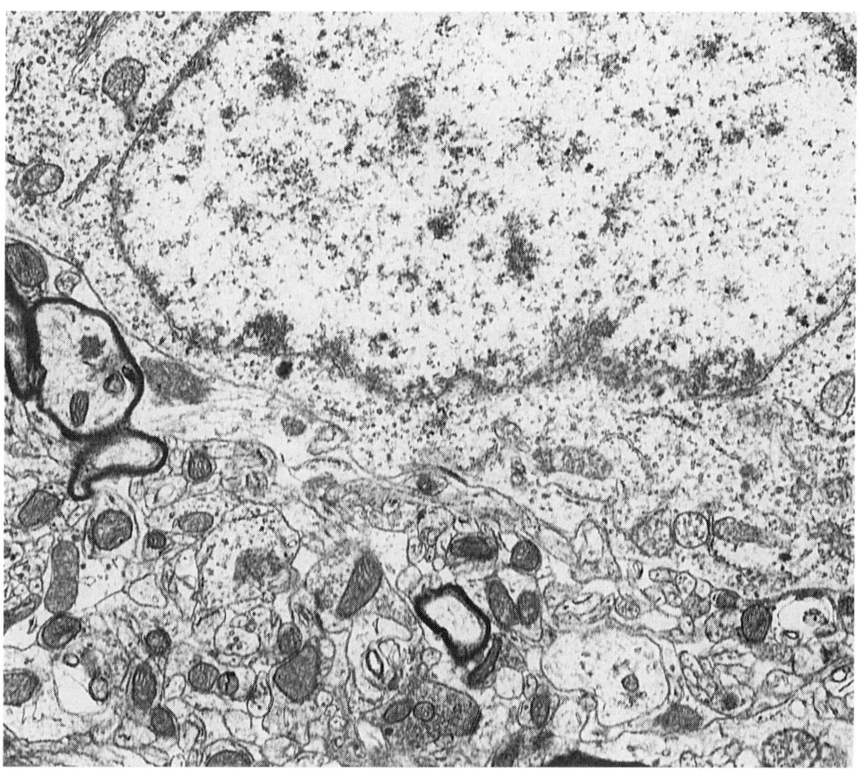

**Fig. 3-3.** Specimen from same animal as Fig. 3-2, processed conventionally. (×10,500.)

the component cells tend toward elongation. These intraspinal ependymomas may thus approach the histologic appearance of a fibroblastic meningioma, of Antoni A areas of schwannoma, or of a pilocytic astrocytoma. Ultrastructurally, however, these tumors are all quite distinct, and electron microscopy is thus often of practical use in the differential diagnosis of intraspinal tumors.

Within the cranium, fibroblastic meningiomas of the cerebellopontine angle occasionally may be confused with acoustic schwannomas, and here, too, electron microscopy can be of value in differential diagnosis. Meningiomas with pseudoglandular patterns have been described[194] that may be mistaken for metastatic adenocarcinoma by light microscopy. The distinction between intracranial ependymoma and schwannoma or meningioma is less likely to present a problem in differential diagnosis. However, some clear cell ependymomas may resemble the histological features of oligodendrogliomas or hemangioblastomas.[191,328] Occasionally, common tumors create diagnostic confusion because of their uncommon location. For instance, astrocytomas occasionally are encountered in an extraparenchymal location,* and both intraparenchymal schwannomas[103,104,237] and extraspinal ependymomas[255,372] have been reported. In these instances electron microscopy may bolster confidence in a histologic diagnosis that appears to be at odds with the diagnosis suggested by the clinical information. Primary intracerebral fibrosarcomas have also been described, and ultrastructural examination is useful in confirming this diagnosis.[239]

## Ependymoma

Ependymomas† generally are readily diagnosed by electron microscopy, even on casual inspection of random electron micrographs (Figs. 3-4 to 3-7). A much-sought but infrequently found histologic feature of ependymoma is the true ependymal rosette or glandlike space lined by ependymal cells. The histologic rarity of these structures results not from their absence but from their size. By electron microscopy most ependymomas show prominent and frequent evidence of such epithelial features. There are small intercellular or intracellular lumina lined by microvilli and, often, cilia and specialized junctional devices between cells. Indeed, cilia-containing intracellular lumina appear to be unique to ependymomas.[158a] Lest this description suggest a similarity to metastatic carcinoma, it should be pointed out that ependymoma cells also show ultrastructural evidence of their glial origin in the form of filament-rich processes similar to those seen in astrocytomas. Indeed, astrocyte-like cells are common in ependymomas and may even be the dominant cell type.[218] A diagnosis of astrocytoma, however, is ruled out in the presence of the characteristic epithelial features of ependymoma.

A common (and commonly misdiagnosed) variant of ependymoma, often found as a spinal intramedullary lesion, is the *tanycytic* variant described by Friede and Pollak.[87] These tumors are composed of slender, elongated, bipolar cells. Ultrastructurally, one pole of each cell shows a microvillus-bearing surface that may be crowded against an adjacent cell rather than lining an identifiable lumen. The opposite pole of the tumor cells abuts a basal lamina, usually adjacent to a blood vessel (see Fig. 3-37).

*Papillary ependymomas* are described below under papillary tumors.

## Schwannoma

Schwannomas* also have readily obvious features on ultrastructural examination, although occasional examples may require more serious study. The ultrastructural features of intracranial schwannomas[49,220,294] do not differ from those of spinal and peripheral examples. Characteristically there are long, often quite thin cytoplasmic processes that in Antoni A areas show extensive intertwining with similar processes from adjacent cells (Figs. 3-8 to 3-10). This may, on occasion, be so marked as to form lamellar whorls reminiscent of myelin formation.[174] The overall impression in a two-dimensional electron micrograph is one of widely separated "cells" (actually nucleated perikarya), with the "intercellular" (interperikaryal) space filled with numerous thin cytoplasmic sheets or processes of indeterminant origin. This feature alone, however, is not diagnostic, as meningiomas may show a somewhat similar feature—extensive interdigitation of adjacent cell processes. Another feature of schwannomas is the presence of basal lamina (basement membrane). This lamina usually encircles each tumor cell completely, and is often reduplicated in the space between the intertwining processes. In contrast, meningiomas do not display well-formed basal lamina, instead meningioma cells display scattered small deposits of electron-dense basal lamina-like material in interstices between the tumor cells. Finally, schwannomas quite commonly contain abnormal collagen fibers that are abnormally thick and show an unusually long periodicity to their banding structure. Such "fibrous long-spacing collagen" or "Luse bodies"[220] are frequently florid in schwannomas,[50] to the point that many electron microscopists will not be content with a diagnosis of schwannoma until they have found some of these Luse bodies. They are not, however, necessary for diagnosis and are not, unfortu-

* Refs. 12, 159, 164, 187, 196, 201, 332a, 358.

† Refs. 74, 87, 106, 124, 131, 157, 158a, 204, 220, 221, 294, 328, 355.

* Refs. 49, 74, 76, 85, 174, 210, 220, 294, 391.

*Text continues on page 107.*

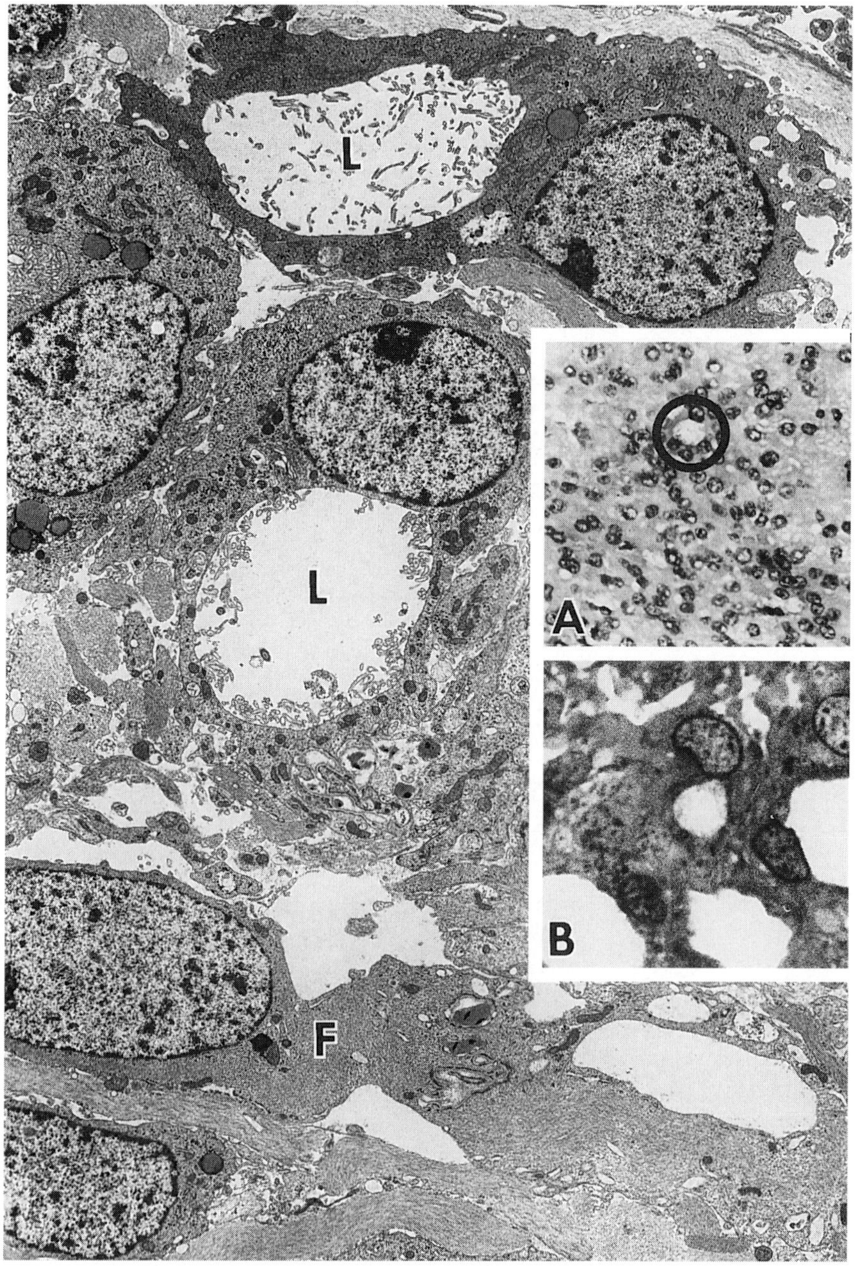


**Fig. 3-4.** Ependymoma of fourth ventricle in a 45-year-old man. Two tumor cells contain intracellular lumens *(L)* lined by microvilli. At the bottom there are tumor cell processes containing densely matted filaments *(F)* resembling those seen in astrocytomas. **Inset A,** Histologic appearance of tumor. A small "space" (*circle*) cannot be resolved as a lumen. **Inset B,** Semithin section of epoxy-embedded material. In such preparations microvilli sometimes can be discerned by light microscopy (*center*). (**Fig.**, ×4050; **Inset A,** ×195; **Inset B,** ×1050.)

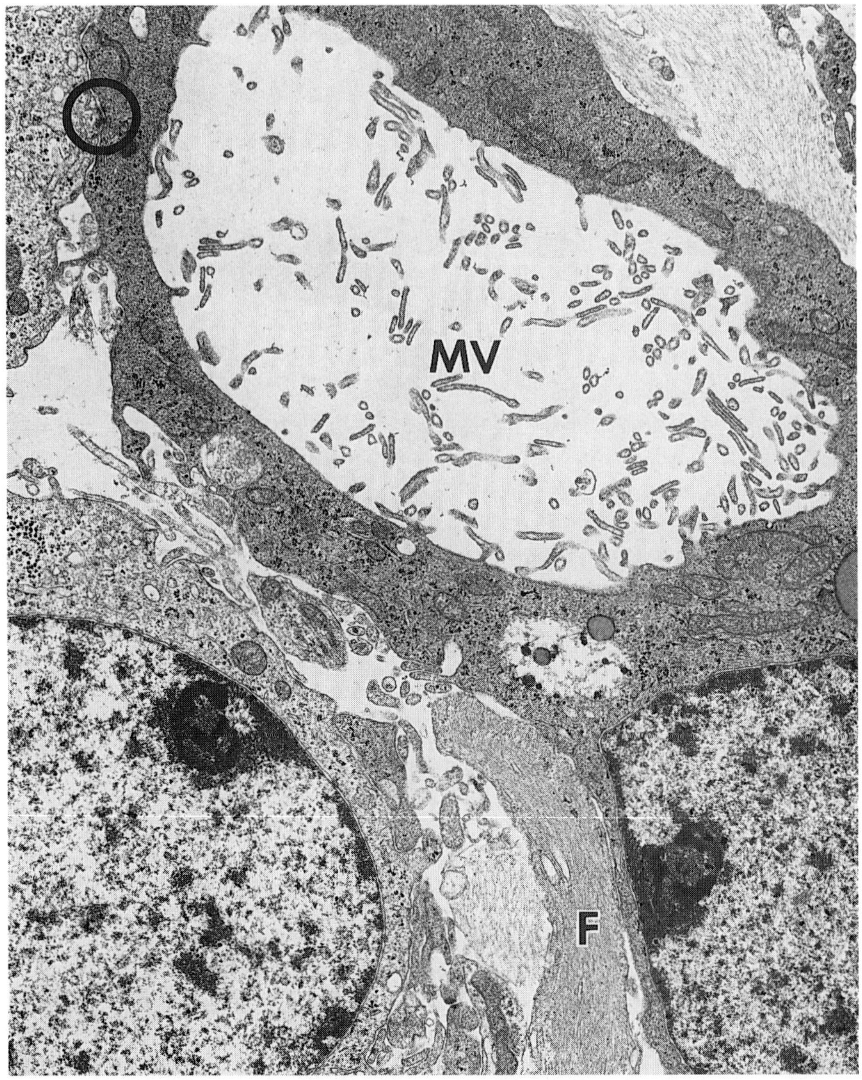


**Fig. 3-5.** Ependymoma; detail from Fig. 3-4. Luminal microvilli (*MV*), intercellular junctions (*circle*) and a filament-containing cell process *(F)* are evident. (×10,500.)

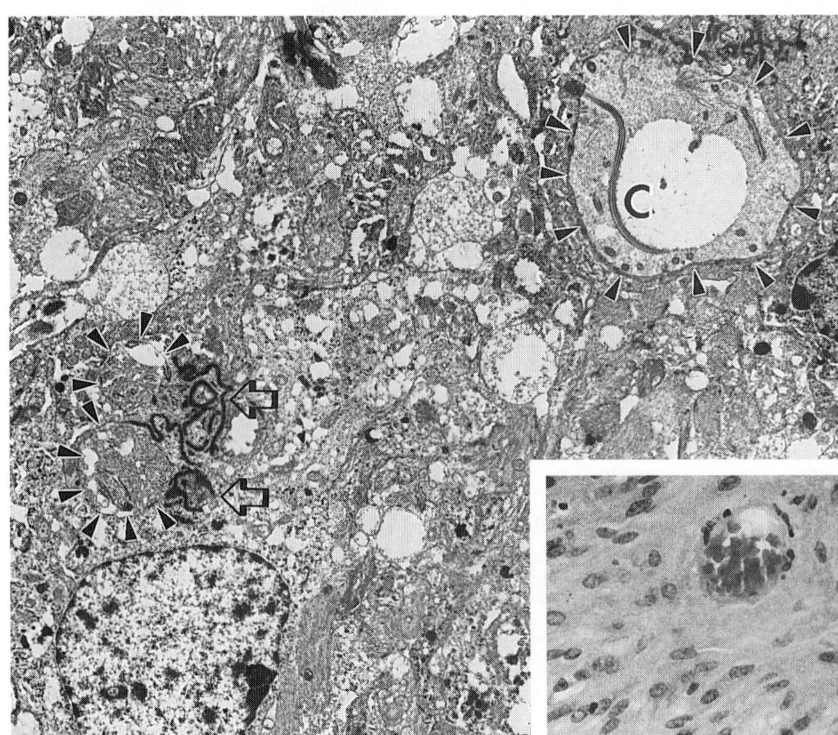


**Fig. 3-6.** Ependymoma of the spinal cord in a 14-year-old boy. Three microvillus-containing lumina are evident (*arrowheads*) as well as numerous filament-containing cell processes. Complex, elongated intercellular junctions (*arrows*) attract the eye to two of these lumina, and cilia *(C)* are evident in the other. **Inset**, Histologic appearance of tumor. (**Fig.**, ×4050; **Inset**, ×195.)

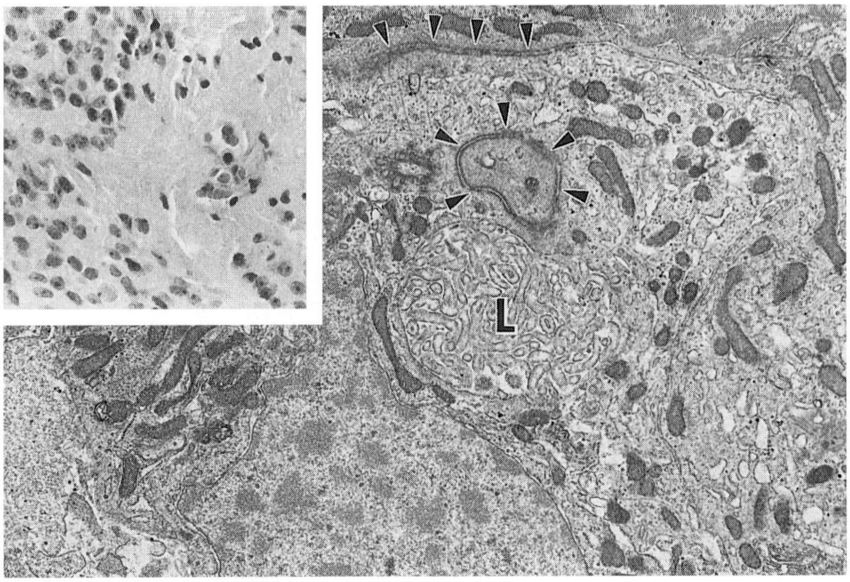


**Fig. 3-7.** Ependymoma of the spinal cord, recurrent in a 53-year-old man. A lumen *(L)* filled with microvilli is seen adjacent to elongated intercellular junctions (*arrowheads*). **Inset,** Histologic appearance of tumor. (**Fig.,** ×10,500; **Inset,** ×195.)

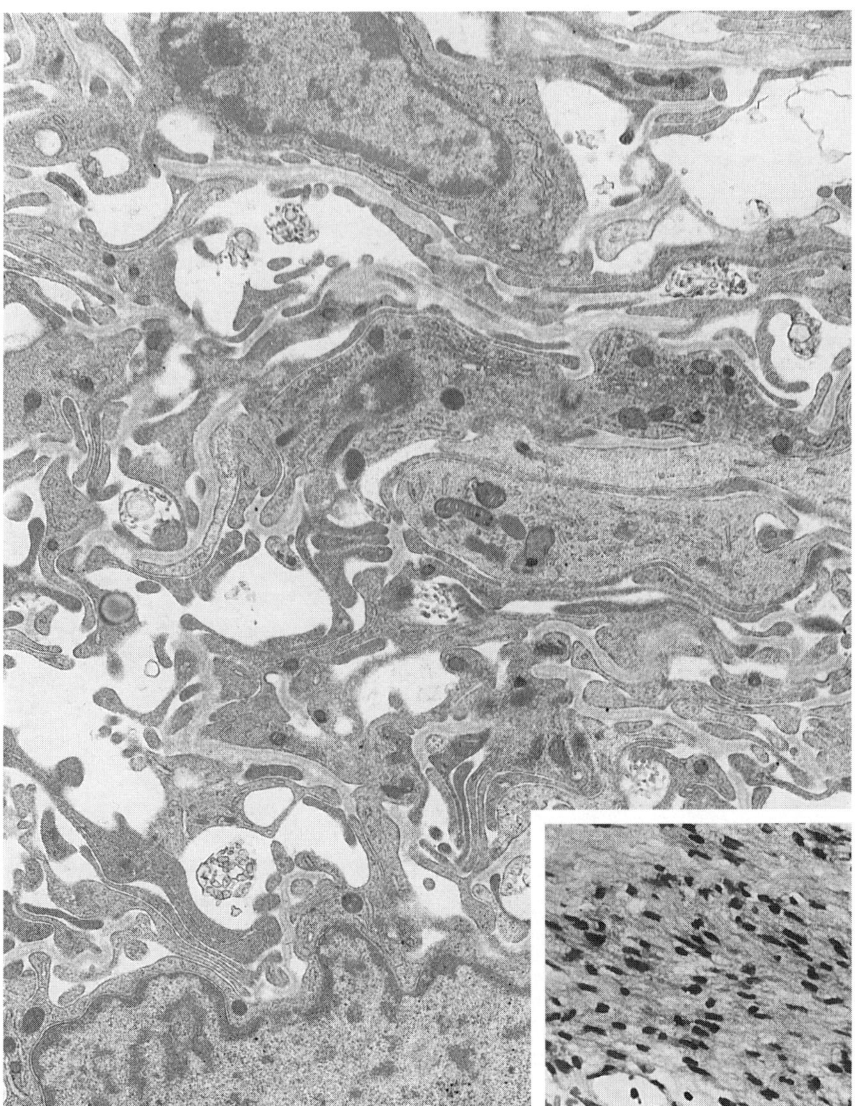

**Fig. 3-8.** Acoustic schwannoma in a 68-year-old woman. The area between tumor cell perikaryal areas is filled with numerous entangled cell processes, many of which are lined by a basal lamina. **Inset,** Histologic appearance of tumor. (**Fig.,** ×10,500; **Inset,** ×195.)

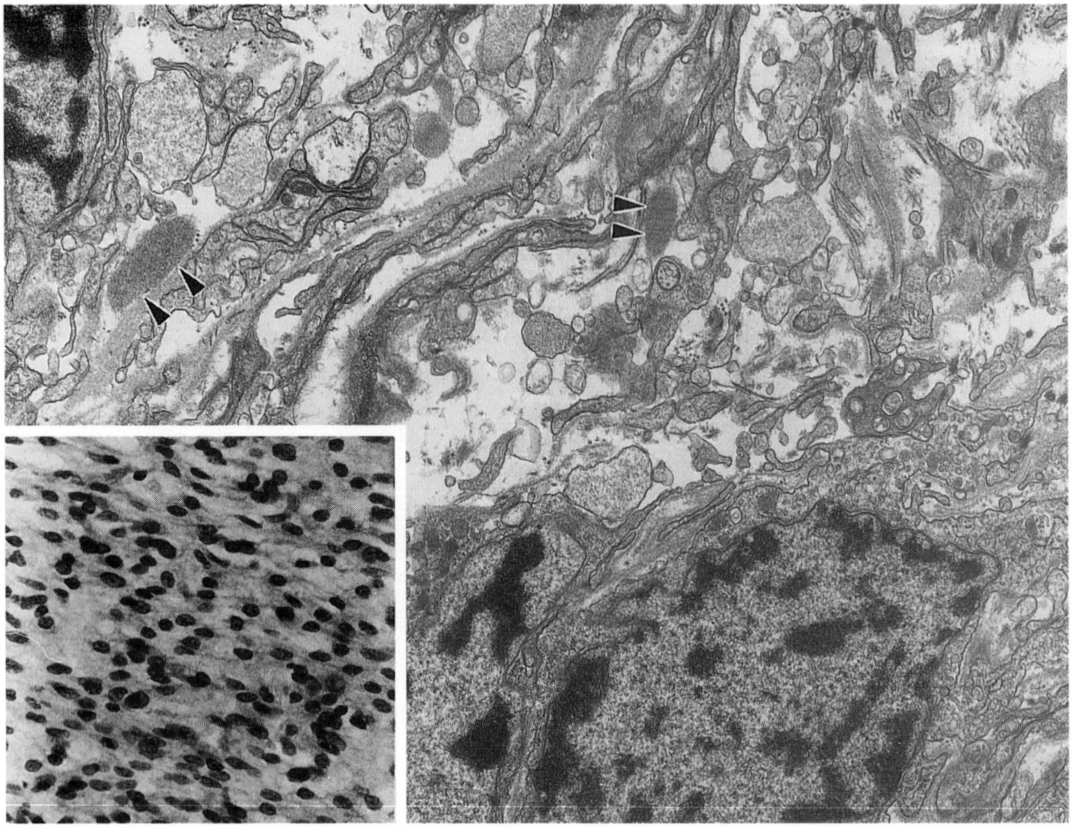

**Fig. 3-9.** Schwannoma of the cauda equina in a 14-year-old boy. Numerous intertwining, basal lamina-lined cell processes are evident, as well as at least two Luse bodies (*arrowheads*). **Inset**, Histologic appearance of tumor. (**Fig.**, ×9600; **Inset**, ×240.)

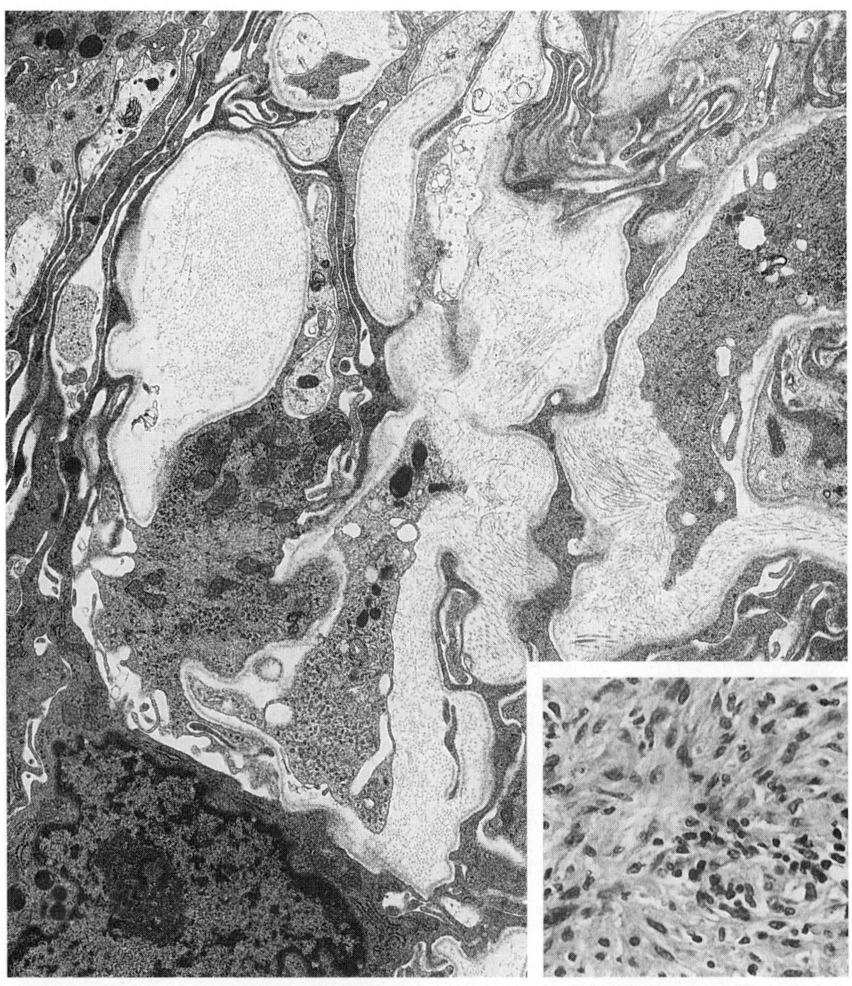

**Fig. 3-10.** Schwannoma of the spinal canal. The intercellular areas are larger in this tumor and contain fair numbers of collagen fibrils. Intertwining, basal lamina-lined processes, however, are still readily apparent. **Inset**, Histologic appearance of tumor. (**Fig.**, ×8750; **Inset**, ×195.)

nately, specific for schwannoma. Luse bodies have been reported in a wide variety of tissues and tumors,[100] including astrocytomas,[297] but rarely are Luse bodies as conspicuous and numerous as they are in schwannomas.

## Meningioma

Meningiomas* are readily distinguished from the other tumors discussed in this section, although additional care may be required in the examination of fine structures, particularly cell junctional devices and intracellular filaments. Meningiomas frequently show complex interdigitation of cell processes, in a manner reminiscent of schwannoma. Basal lamina, however, are lacking, except for the scattered, electron-dense "splotches" found in intercellular spaces (Figs. 3-11 to 3-14). In contrast to schwannomas, however, meningiomas frequently show well-formed desmosome junctions. Desmosomes may be found in schwannomas, but here they are infrequent. Meningiomas also show prominent cytoplasmic filaments. These filaments are vimentin type rather than glial, and react with antivimentin antibodies rather than with antiglial fibrillary acid protein antibodies. Ultrastructurally these filaments usually have a "loose," matted appearance, in contrast to the dense, homogeneous glial filaments of astrocytes. Glial filaments tend to fill cell processes completely and thus impart a homogeneous appearance to the cytoplasm at low magnification, an appearance generally not seen in meningiomas. The filaments of meningioma are further distinguished by their attachment to desmosomes (reminiscent of squamous carcinomas). Occasional fine filaments may be found within the cytoplasm of schwannomas, but they are not as prominent or dense as those in meningioma, and they do not attach to desmosomes. Fibroblastic meningiomas may not show striking interdigitation of cell processes and may be poor in filaments and desmosomes. They do, however, have extracellular "splotches" of basal lamina-like material that distinguish meningiomas from basal lamina-rich schwannomas on the one hand and basal lamina-free fibroblastic tumors on the other. The rare "secretory" variant of meningioma shows minute intracellular lumens lined

* Refs. 36, 47, 74, 172, 220, 263, 294, 410.

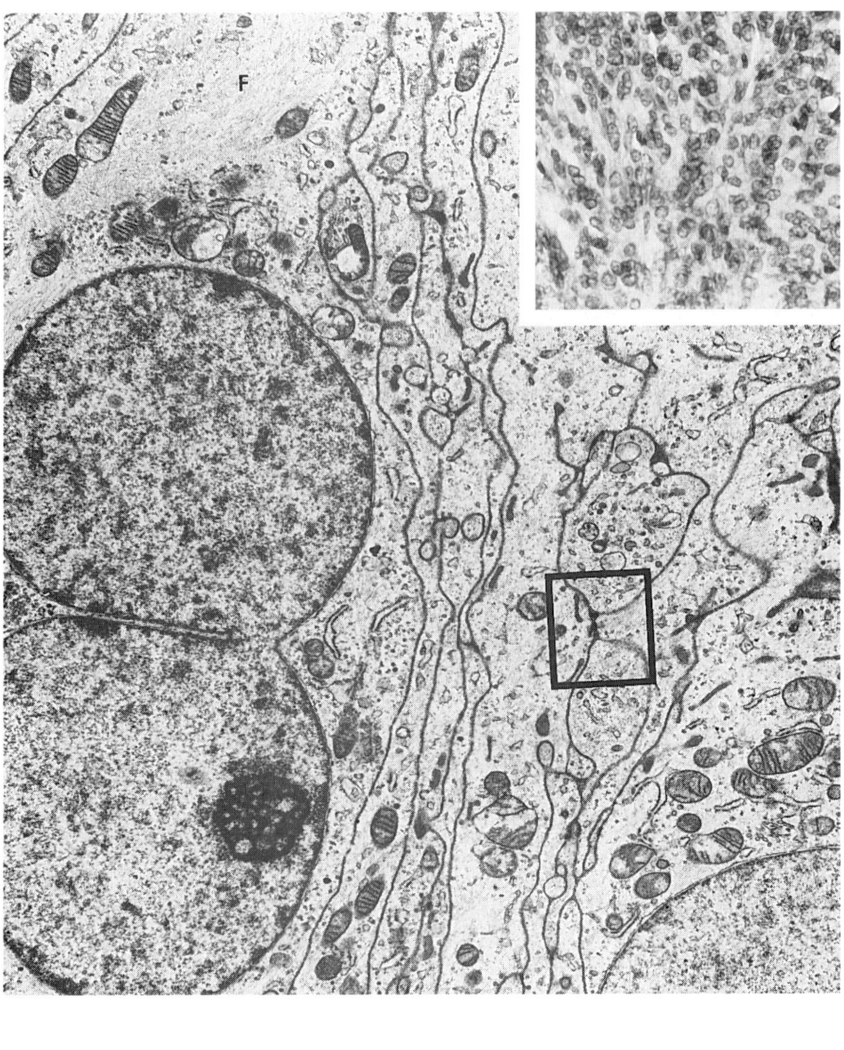


**Fig. 3-11.** Posterior fossa meningioma in a 16-year-old-boy with bilateral acoustic neurofibromatosis. Numerous entangled cell processes are present in the interperikaryal areas, but these processes lack basal lamina. Note cytoplasmic filaments *(F)*. The area in the box is shown in greater detail in Fig. 3-12. **Inset,** Histologic appearance of tumor. (**Fig.,** ×7780; **Inset,** ×195.)

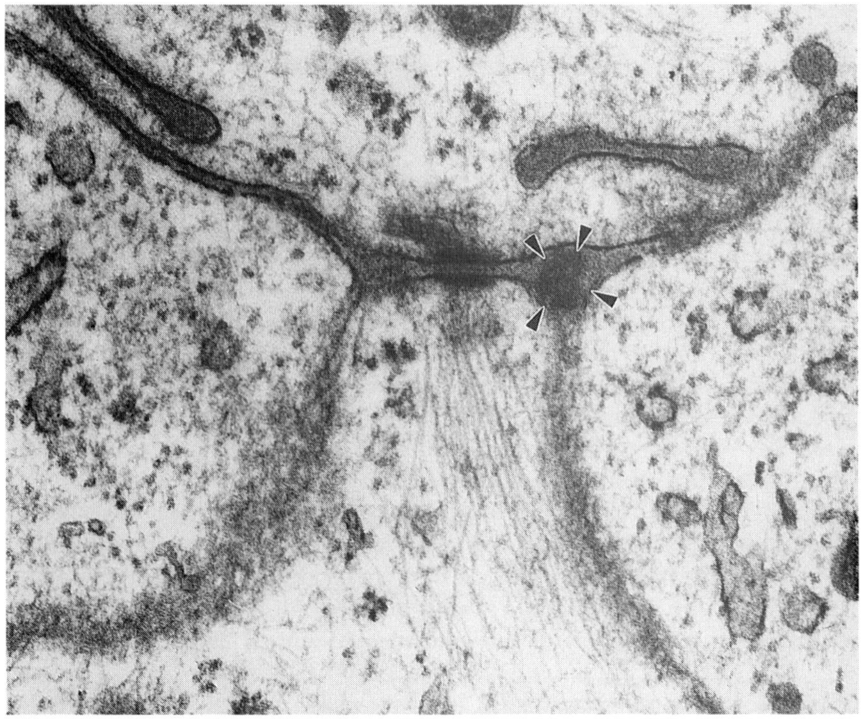

**Fig. 3-12.** Meningioma: detail from Fig. 3-11 shows a well-formed intercellular desmosome with attachment of cytoplasmic filaments. A small deposit of basal lamina-like material is present in the intercellular space (*arrowheads*), but there is no well-defined basal lamina. (×6250.)

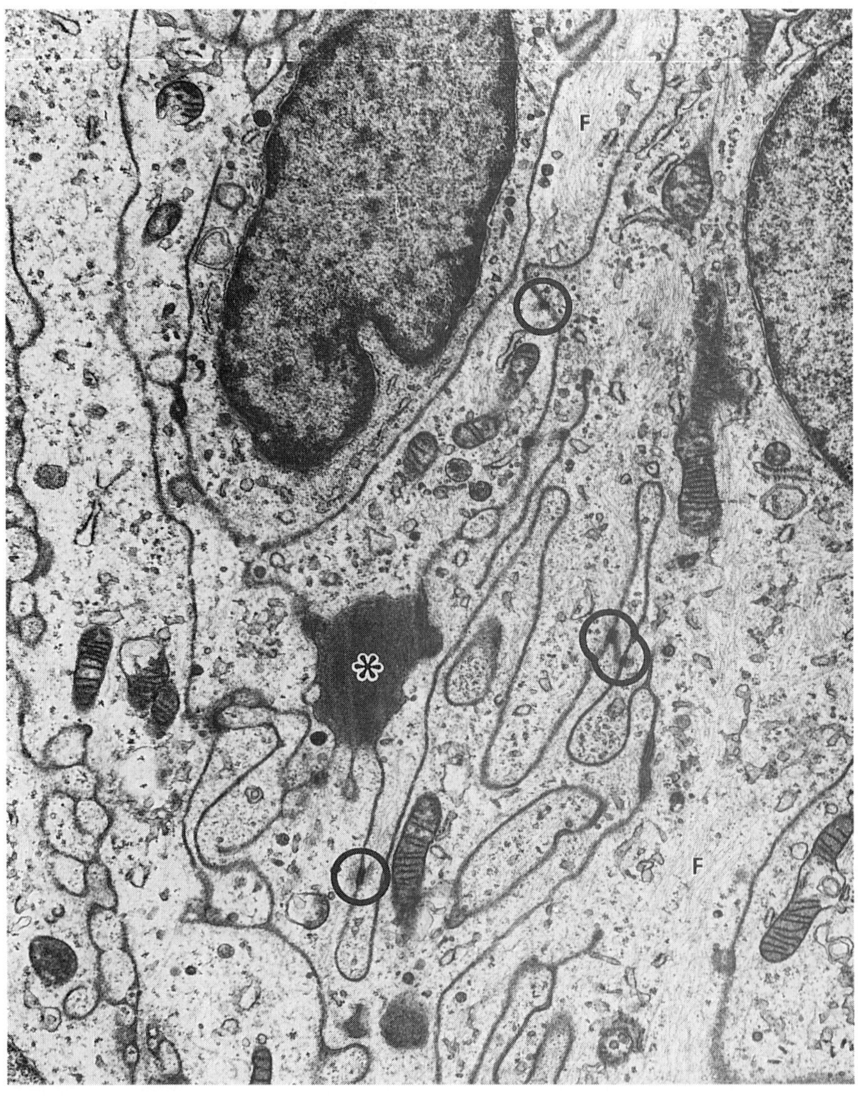


**Fig. 3-13.** Meningioma (same case as Fig. 3-11). A large "splotch" of basal lamina-like material is present between cytoplasmic processes (*asterisk*), but no true basal lamina is present. There are cytoplasmic filaments *(F)* and numerous intercellular junctions (*circles*). (×10,500.)

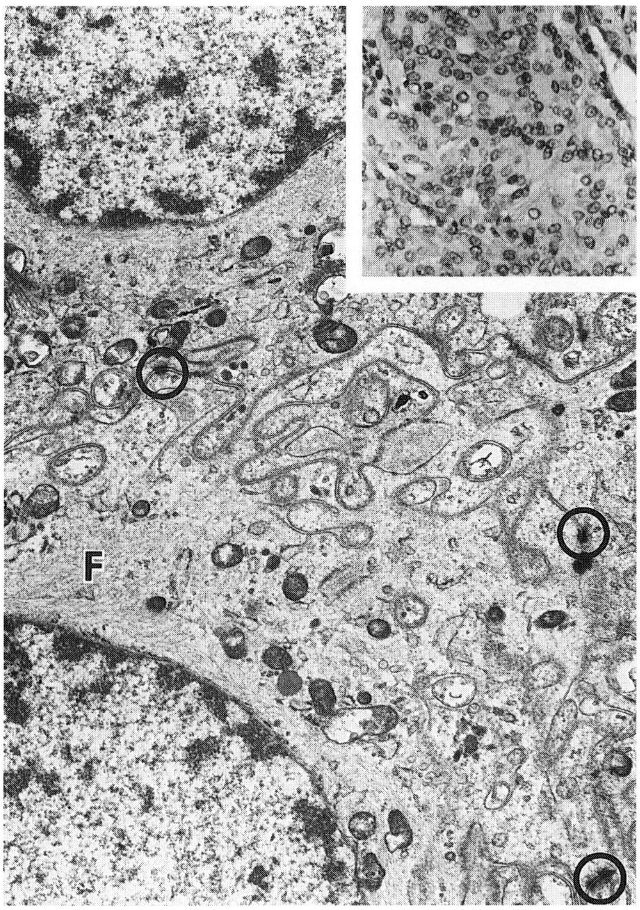


**Fig. 3-14.** Intraspinal, extradural meningioma in a 21-year-old man. Cytoplasmic filaments *(F)* are prominent in this case, as well as entangled cell processes and numerous intercellular junctions (*circles*). **Inset**, Histologic appearance of tumor. (**Fig.**, ×9500; **Inset**, ×175.)

by microvilli.[192] Cilia have been reported in meningiomas,[36] but they are rare.

### Astrocytoma

Astrocytomas* may be confused with ependymomas, especially in the spinal cord. Confusion with schwannoma or meningioma is less common but does occur[164,319] (see Fig. 3-8). Antibodies against glial fibrillary acidic protein are useful in identifying astrocytic tumors, but atypical astrocytomas may be submitted for ultrastructural examination with a tentative alternative diagnosis.

Ultrastructurally, the distinguishing feature of astrocytomas is the presence of numerous cytoplasmic processes filled with dense filaments (Figs. 3-15 to 3-17). In contrast to schwannoma and meningioma, these processes are usually separated by amorphous intercellular "matrix"; individual cells do not have desmosomes or basal lamina (extra-axial astrocytomas, however, are an exception to this rule; see the section on astroblastoma). The filaments typically fill these processes and render them homogeneous in appearance at low magnification. Individual constituent cells of ependymomas may also show long, filament-filled processes, but astrocytomas are readily distinguished from ependymomas by their lack of "epithelial" features, such as lumina, microvilli, and junctional complexes.

* Refs. 35, 64, 74, 124, 168, 220, 294, 321.

### Superficial (Extra-Axial) Astrocytoma

Superficial (extra-axial) astrocytomas differ from intraparenchymal examples in the presence of basal lamina and of a mesenchymal (fibroblastic) component.* Normal astrocytes abut upon a basement membrane at areas of mesenchymal contact such as the glia limitans, beneath the pia mater, and the basal lamina of intraparenchymal capillaries, and this feature appears to be reproduced in astrocytic tumors growing in extraparenchymal tissues. The basal lamina may surround groups of cells or individual cells, but it is found only around the astrocytic component of mixed astrocytic/fibroblastic tumors (Figs. 3-18 to 3-20). These features are also seen in parenchymal astrocytomas that secondarily invade the meninges.

### Astroblastoma

Astroblastomas are rare tumors of children and young adults, in which the component cells show a polarized structure and orientation to blood vessels reminiscent of the perivascular pseudorosettes of ependymoma. Astroblastomas are well circumscribed and often cavitary. Both low- and high-grade subtypes exist.[25]

Ultrastructural studies of five cases are available.[160,173,203,312] Intermediate filaments within tumor cell perikarya and within cell processes are described in all cases, although these filaments vary in prominence from case to case and area to area. In addition, Rubinstein and Herman[312] have described rudimentary ependymal features in the form of (1) apical microvilli arising from a narrow base ("purse-string" appearance); (2) occasional long intercellular junctional devices interrupted by "microrosettes" (intercellular spaces lined by microvilli); and (3) interdigitation of tumor cell cytoplasm along their lateral borders. Basally, along the capillary walls, there were cytoplasmic infoldings and a lining basal lamina. This duality of astrocytic and epithelial features recalls the tanycytic variant of ependymoma, although both the astrocytic and epithelial features are considerably more rudimentary in astroblastomas than those seen in ependymomas.

* Refs. 164, 196, 205, 321, 358, 398.

*Text continues on page 113.*

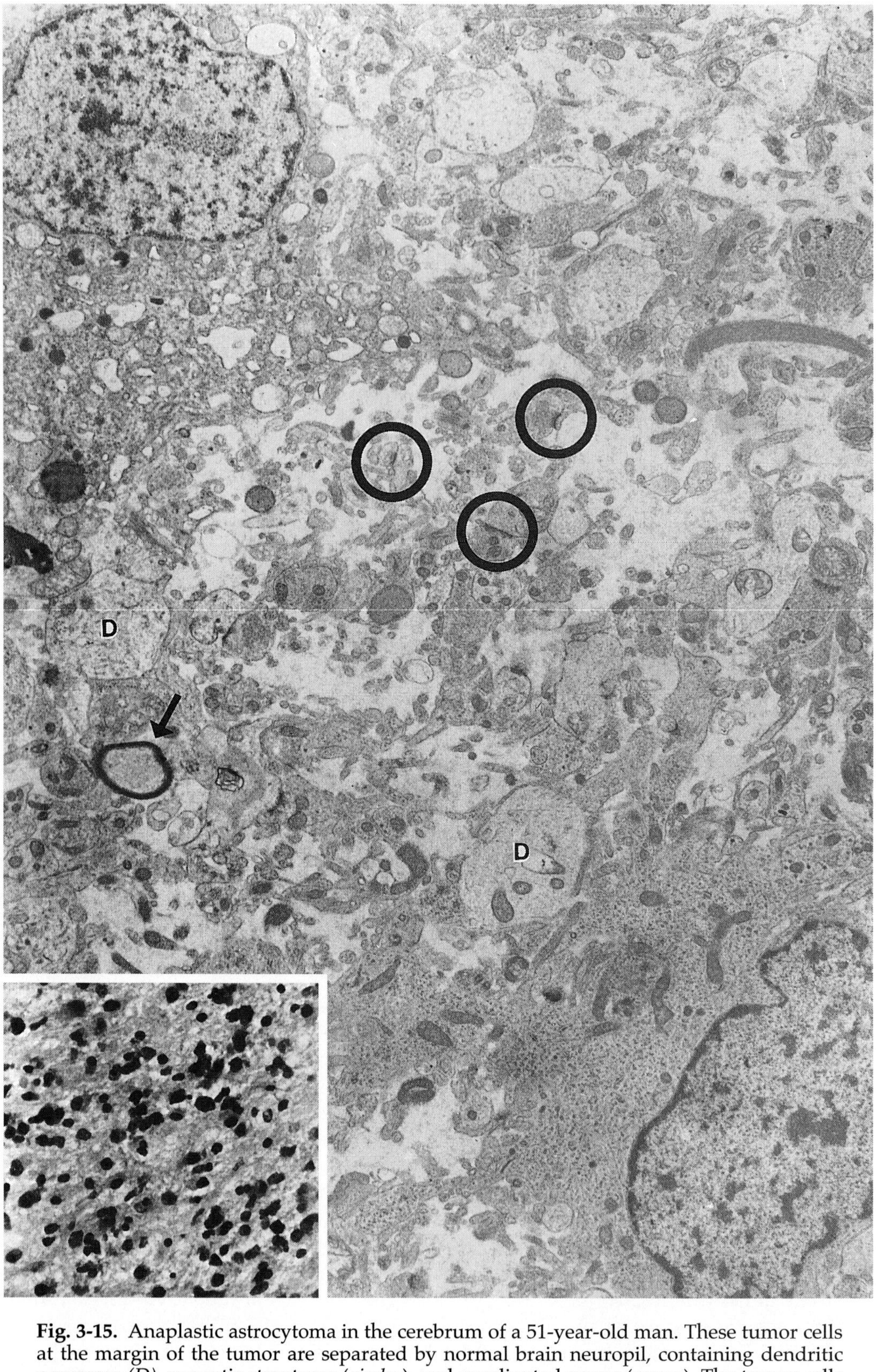


**Fig. 3-15.** Anaplastic astrocytoma in the cerebrum of a 51-year-old man. These tumor cells at the margin of the tumor are separated by normal brain neuropil, containing dendritic processes *(D)*, synaptic structures (*circles*), and myelinated axons (*arrow*). The tumor cells show numerous cytoplasmic processes and show some cytoplasmic filaments that are difficult to resolve at this magnification. **Inset**, Histologic appearance of tumor. (**Fig.**, ×6240; **Inset**, ×195.)

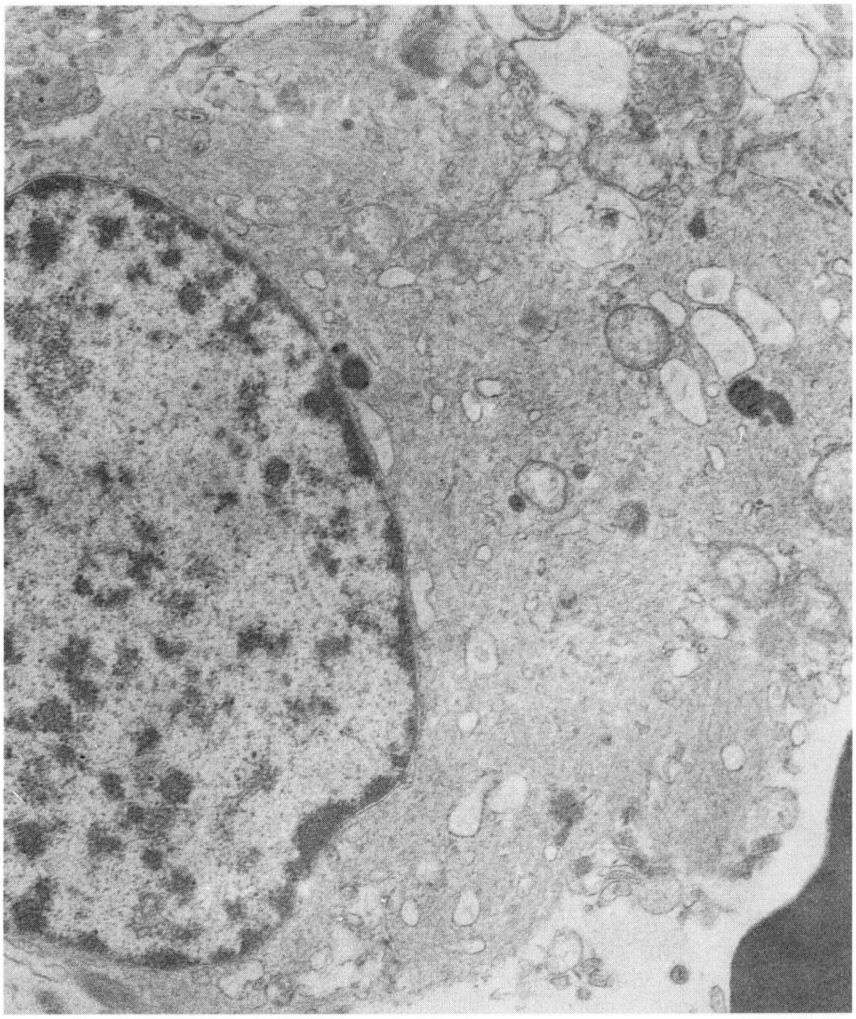

**Fig. 3-16.** Astrocytoma (same case as Fig. 3-15). Cytoplasmic filaments are prominent in this cell. They are matted and contain entangled organelles. (×15,400.)

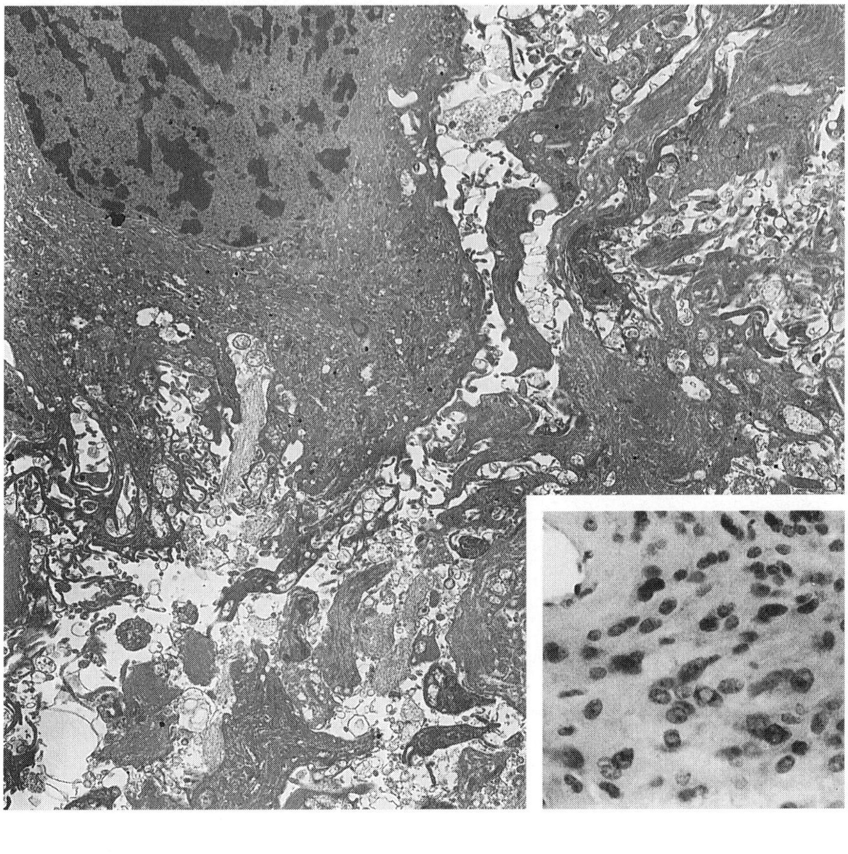

**Fig. 3-17.** Astrocytoma of the spinal cord in an 11-year-old boy. Filaments are prominent both in the tumor cell cytoplasm and in the numerous cytoplasmic processes. These processes are more widely separated than those of most meningiomas and schwannomas, and there are no junctions and no basal lamina or extracellular basal lamina-like material. **Inset**, Histologic appearance of tumor. (**Fig.**, ×4050; **Inset**, ×195.)

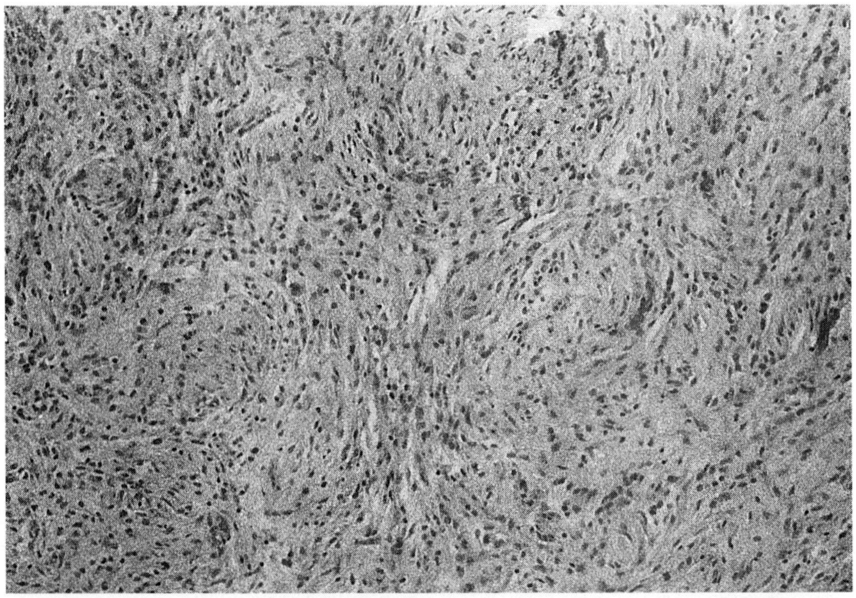

**Fig. 3-18.** Superficial astrocytoma. Four-month-old boy with suprasellar mass invading optic tracts, third ventricle, and brain stem. By light microscopy this tumor resembles a meningioma. (H&E; ×105.)

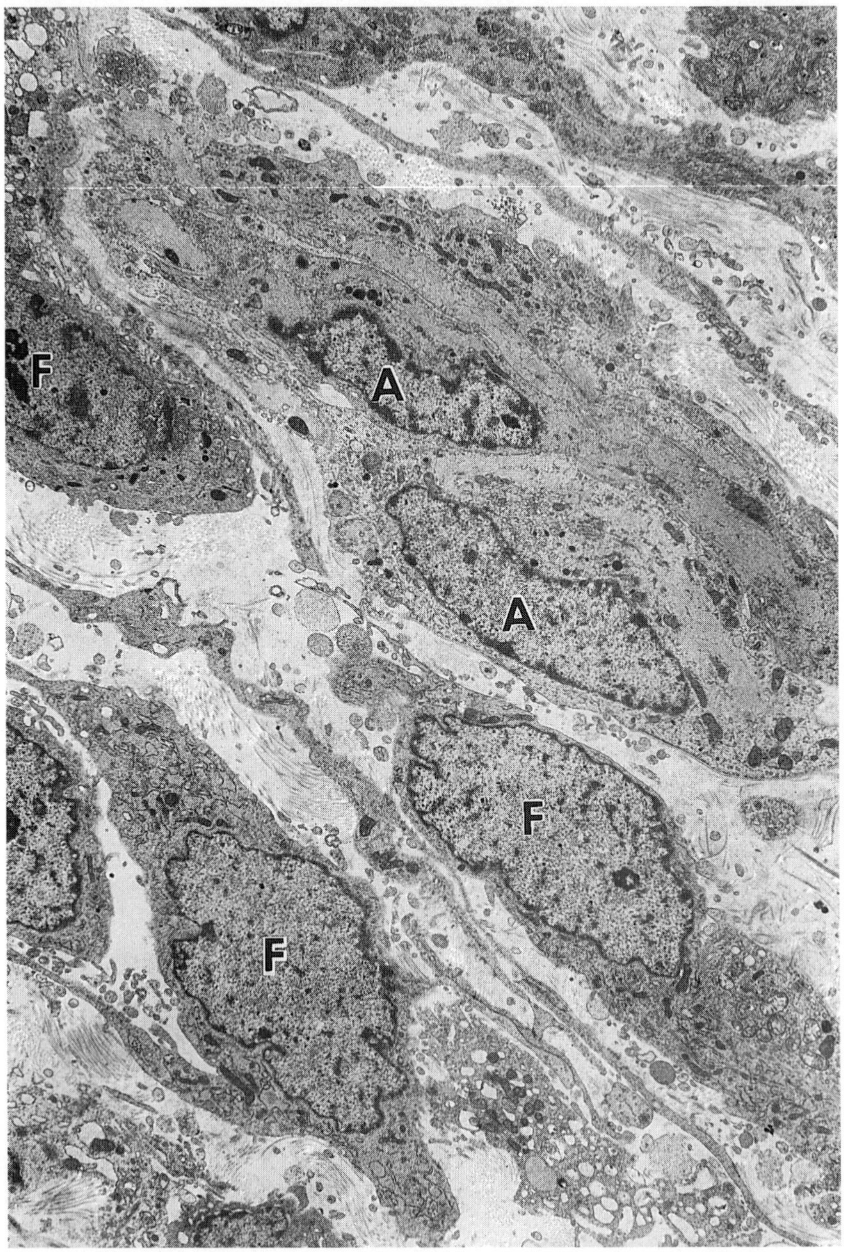


**Fig. 3-19.** Superficial astrocytoma (same case as Fig. 3-18). Ultrastructurally there are two component cell types, both of which are spindle shaped. Loosely cohesive fibroblast-like cells *(F)* show polar cytoplasmic regions with modest numbers of dilated rough endoplasmic reticulum cisterns, while closely apposed astrocytic cells *(A)* are rich in cytoplasmic filaments. (×4050.)

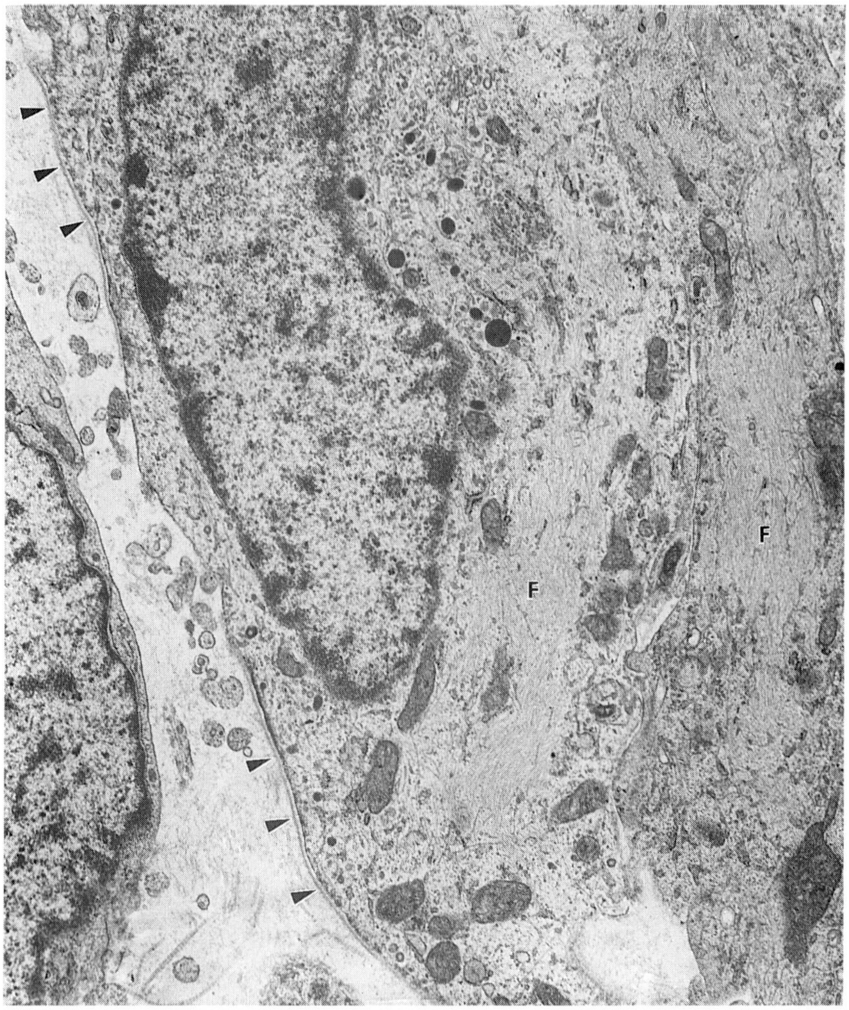


**Fig. 3-20.** Superficial astrocytoma; detail of Fig. 3-19. The astrocytic cells show cytoplasmic filaments *(F)* and a basal lamina (*arrowheads*). (×10,500.)

## PERIPHERAL SPINDLE CELL TUMORS

The distinction between peripheral nerve sheath tumors and other spindle cell tumors is a common histopathologic challenge,[81,125] and one for which electron microscopy has proved useful.[43,59,182,348,364] Benign and well-differentiated spindle cell tumors can be correctly classified by electron microscopy in virtually all cases,[59] while malignant spindle cell tumors can be so classified in most, if not all, cases.* Such histogenetic classification may actually assist in the assessment of malignancy. A moderately cellular spindle cell neoplasm with occasional mitotic figures may be considered benign if it is shown to be of Schwann cell origin,[126] while a histologically similar tumor may be considered a low-grade malignancy if shown to be of smooth muscle origin.[332] Similarly, the benign-appearing plexosarcoma, which may be mistaken for a leiomyoma on histologic examination, generally pursues an aggressive clinical course.[139]

Leiomyosarcomas and fibrosarcomas rarely metastasize to the central nervous system.[54,96,272,417] Dal Canto and Valsamis[54] have described one such patient who presented with neurologic symptoms. Primary intracerebral fibrosarcomas have also been described.[239] Ultrastructural examination can be helpful in such cases.

### Nerve Sheath Tumors

Schwannomas* are generally quite easily diagnosed by electron microscopy (Figs. 3-21, 3-22). Peripheral schwannomas are ultrastructurally similar to central schwannomas (discussed above), and only a few points of relevance to differentiation from other peripheral tumors will be mentioned here. The two cardinal features of schwannomas are long, intertwining cell processes and the presence of basal lamina that usually surround individual cells and often are redundant. Smooth muscle tumors (but not fibroblastic tumors)

* Refs. 27, 58, 76, 182, 254, 364.

* Refs. 59, 72, 74, 76, 85, 210, 220, 294, 300, 333, 391.

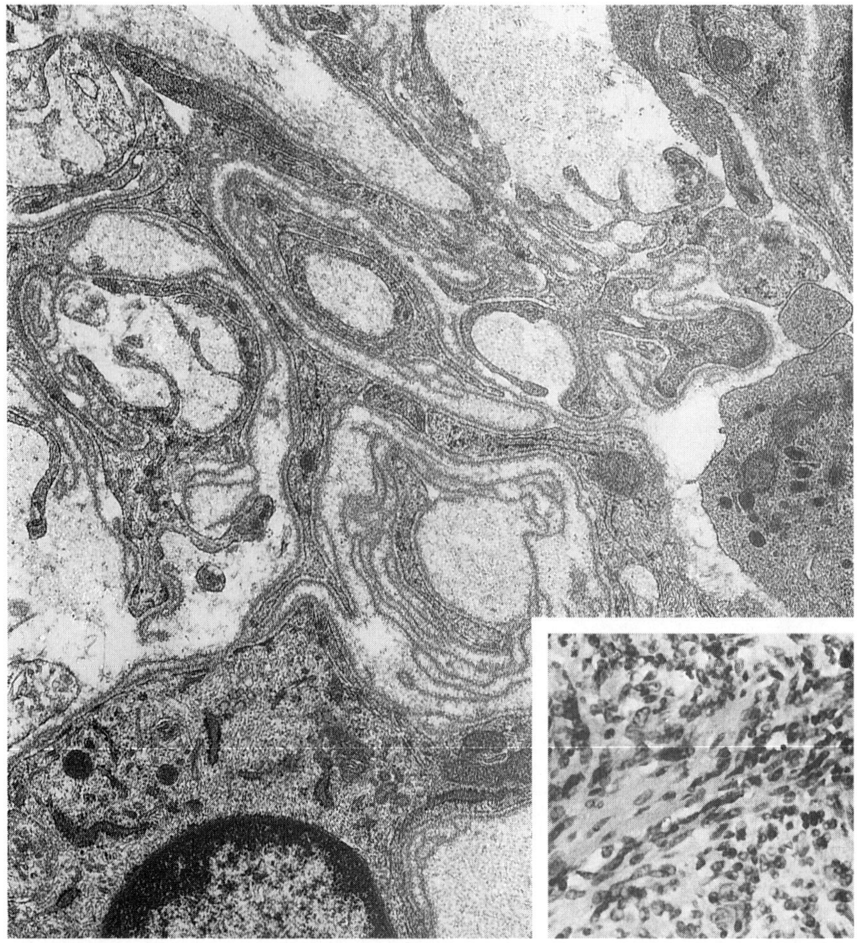

**Fig. 3-21.** Schwannoma of thigh in a man. There are intertwining cell processes and a prominent basal lamina that is focally redundant. **Inset**, Histologic appearance of tumor. (**Fig.**, ×17,800; **Inset**, ×195.)

may also have basal lamina, but the long intertwining cell processes are (in this context) unique to Schwann cell tumors. These processes may occasionally encircle portions of extracellular matrix to produce an appearance reminiscent of axonal ensheathment.[59,72,76,333] Additional features of note, but less important diagnostically, are the presence of fibrous long-spacing collagen ("Luse bodies"), infrequent dense-core granules (evidence of the neural crest origin of Schwann cells), and occasional cells containing prominent tertiary lysosomes (reflecting the phagocytic capabilities of Schwann cells). Several unusual variants of peripheral schwannoma merit mention: *Cellular schwannomas*[72,76] and *epithelioid schwannomas*[363] appear less well differentiated by light microscopy but are generally similar to "classic" schwannomas ultrastructurally. *Pigmented (melanotic) schwannomas* contain melanosomes and premelanosomes in addition to showing features of schwannoma.[59,72] This rare tumor, evidence of the common neural crest origin of Schwann cells and melanocytes, is readily distinguished from melanoma by the presence of characteristic schwannoma-type cell processes and basal lamina. *Granular cell schwannomas,* in contrast, show less well-developed schwannian features.[59] In particular, cell processes are not well-developed, and the basal lamina often encircles groups of cells rather than individual cells. The striking ultrastructural feature of these tumors, of course, is the myriad secondary lysosomes that fill the cytoplasm, a feature that these tumors share with other, nonschwannian, granular cell tumors.[259]

*Malignant peripheral nerve sheath tumors* (PNSTs)* show various degrees of anaplasia. Taxy and co-workers[364] found diagnostic ultrastructural features in 8 of 15 tumors classified as malignant PNSTs by gross (arising from a nerve) and histologic criteria, and Erlandson and Woodruff[76] found diagnostic ultrastructural features in 5 of 10 such tumors. The diagnostic ultrastructural features consist of long, overlapping, tightly packed cytoplasmic processes and occasional fragments of basal lamina. Neither of these features is as well developed as in benign schwannomas. The cell processes are broader and sparser than those of benign schwannoma, and basal lamina is present as occasional

* Refs. 5, 43, 58, 72, 74, 76, 151, 331, 348, 364.

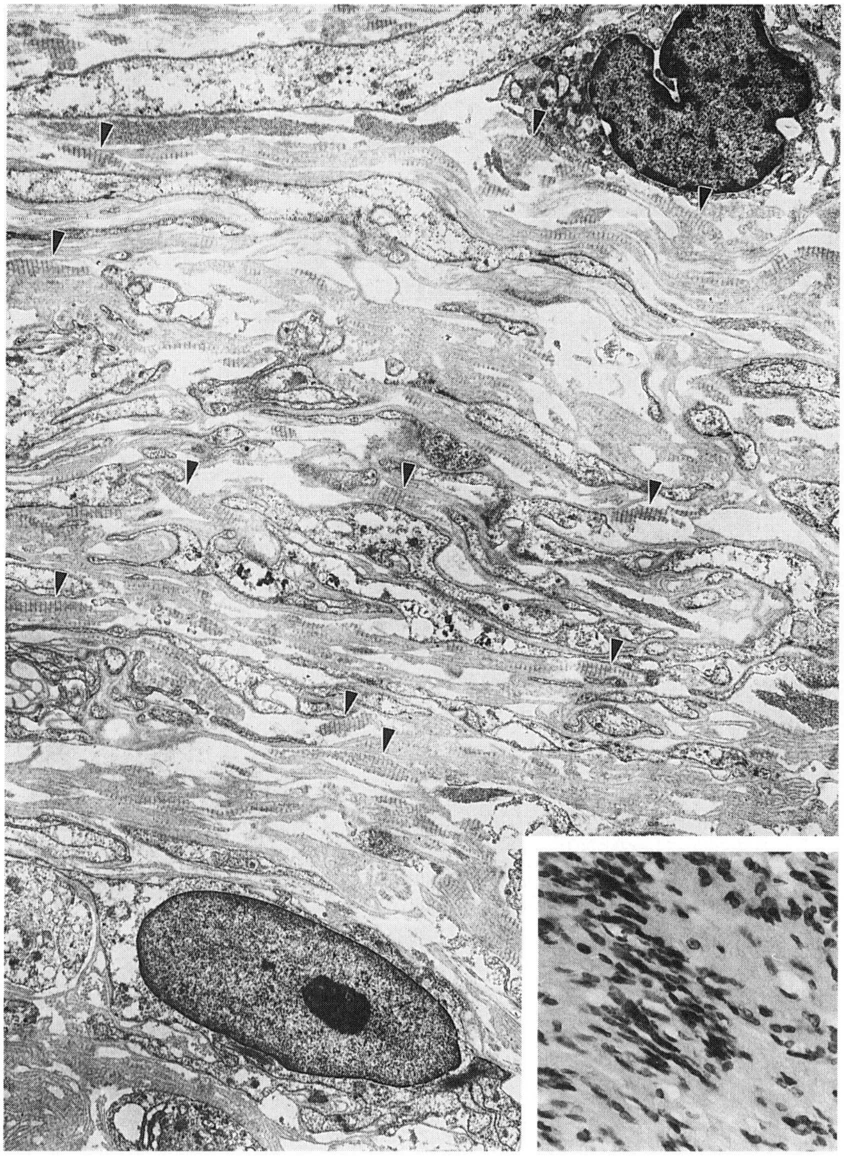

**Fig. 3-22.** Schwannoma of index finger in a 50-year-old man. Numerous Luse bodies are present (*arrowheads*). **Inset**, Histologic appearance of tumor. (**Fig.**, ×4050; **Inset**, ×195.)

pericellular fragments or extracellular scrolls or whorls. Luse bodies are found only rarely.[43,76,364] The occasional occurrence of ciliated cells[283] is an interesting, but not diagnostically useful feature.

## Smooth Muscle Tumors

Leiomyomas invariably show diagnostic ultrastructural features, with the notable exception of gastric "leiomyomas" (see below). The most important feature is the presence of actin-containing microfilaments, usually arranged longitudinally, with periodic small, oval, or spindle-shaped electron-dense patches (dense bodies) in contact with the filaments (Fig. 3-23). These dense bodies distinguish smooth muscle filaments from the ubiquitous and nonspecific intermediate filaments that can be found in almost any cell type. A variant of the (cytoplasmic) dense body is the attachment plaque, which differs only in its location adjacent to the plasma membrane. Two additional helpful, but less specific, features are a pericellular basal lamina (also seen in schwannomas, but a distinguishing feature from fibromas) and prominent pinocytotic activity along the plasma membrane.

The demonstration of microfilaments with dense bodies is generally considered conclusive proof of smooth muscle differentiation. However, smooth muscle differentiation is different from smooth muscle origin. Fibroblasts, too, may differentiate along smooth muscle lines to produce myofibroblasts as a component of fibroblastic and fibrous histiocytic tumors* (see below). In these cells, however, the filaments and dense bodies are usually restricted to a narrow subplasma-

* Refs. 3, 45, 58, 162, 349, 380.

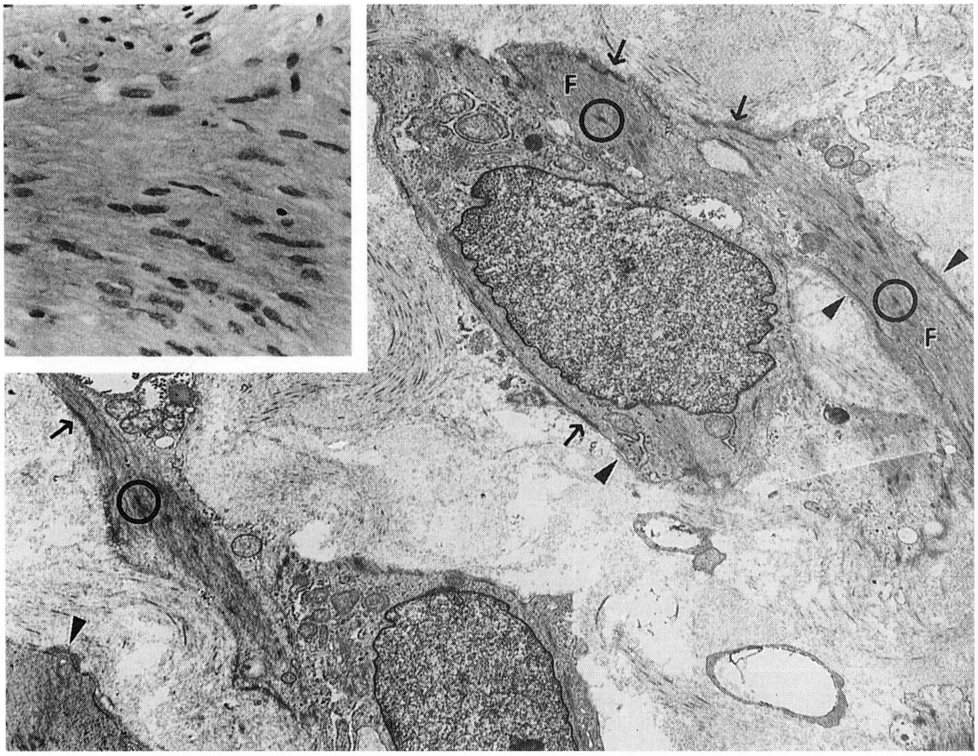


**Fig. 3-23.** Leiomyoma of kidney in a 63-year-old man. There are cytoplasmic filaments *(F)* with associated dense bodies (*circles*), plasmalemmal attachment plaques (*arrows*) and basal lamina (*arrowheads*). **Inset**, Histologic appearance of tumor. (**Fig.**, ×9800; **Inset**, ×220.)

lemmal zone in a cell that otherwise resembles a fibroblast (dilated rough endoplasmic reticulum, no basal lamina). Thus, a cytoplasm full of filaments and dense bodies and dense plaques, or the presence of these features in a cell that also has a basal lamina, indicates a cell of smooth muscle derivation. Pinocytotic vesicles are a nice additional finding, as these are rarely seen in fibroblastic tumors or schwannomas.[43] They are, however, seen in neurofibromas.[59,76,211]

An entity deserving of special note is the gastric "leiomyoma" (Figs. 3-24, 3-25). This benign spindle cell tumor has long been known for its paucity of ultrastructural smooth muscle features.[233,254,399] Mazur and Clark[233] found ultrastructural evidence of smooth muscle origin in only 2 of 12 gastric stromal tumors examined by electron microscopy. One showed well-developed schwannian features (interlacing cell processes and well-developed basal lamina), while the remaining nine showed somewhat more irregular, overlapping cell processes and focal patches of basal lamina. These findings suggest that most gastric tumors classified as "leiomyomas" by light microscopy are, in fact, benign peripheral nerve sheath tumors.

Leiomyosarcomas[79,254,267,332,348] like malignant peripheral nerve sheath tumors show a range of ultrastructural differentiation (Fig. 3-26). Morales and coworkers[254] found filaments with dense bodies in 7 of 14 sarcomas classified histologically as leiomyosarcomas. An additional four tumors showed other, less specific smooth muscle features, such as basal lamina, pinocytotic vesicles, or filaments without dense bodies. Even these features, however, may be of diagnostic significance in the correct context. Fibroblastic tumors do not have basal lamina, so the presence of convincing tumor cell-associated basal lamina or basal lamina fragments excludes fibrosarcoma. Similarly, pinocytotic vesicles are seen rarely, if ever, in malignant spindle cell tumors of nerve sheath origin (with the possible exception of malignant epithelioid schwannoma[5]),[43] and the finding of even modest numbers of pinocytotic vesicles thus excludes this diagnosis. Intracytoplasmic filaments alone, unfortunately, are not very helpful, as they may be found in schwannian or fibroblastic tumors as well as smooth muscle tumors. Finally, it should be noted that three of the "leiomyosarcomas" examined by Morales and associates[254] showed no ultrastructural features of smooth muscle at all. Such tumors may best be classified as fibrosarcomas or simply as undifferentiated sarcomas.

Spindle cell sarcomas originating in the stomach, like their benign counterparts (see above), frequently lack evidence of smooth muscle differentiation,[233,397]

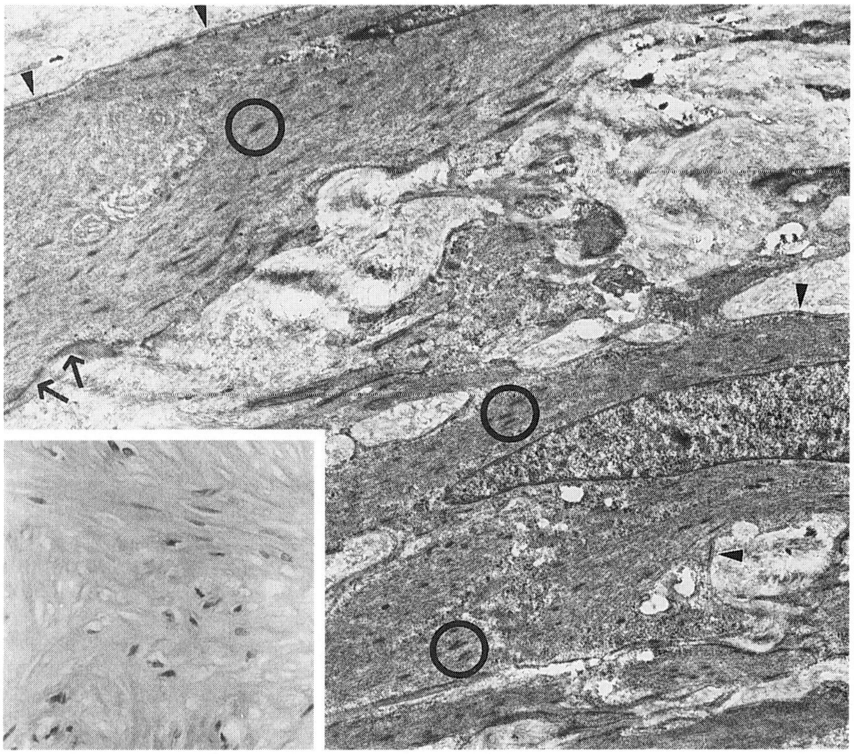

**Fig. 3-24.** True gastric leiomyoma in a 70-year-old man. Filaments, dense bodies (*circles*), attachment plaques (*arrows*) and basal lamina (*arrowheads*) are evident. **Inset**, Histologic appearance of tumor. (**Fig.**, ×6250; **Inset**, ×195.)

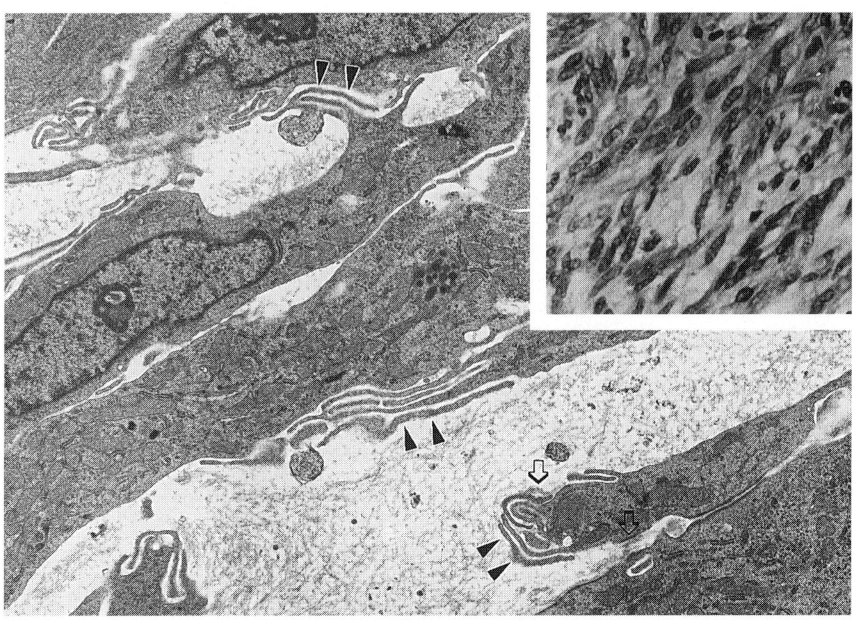

**Fig. 3-25.** Benign gastric stromal tumor, classified as leiomyoma by light microscopy. Ultrastructural examination showed cell processes (*arrowheads*) and focal basal lamina formation (*arrows*) reminiscent of peripheral nerve sheath tumors, and an absence of smooth muscle features. **Inset**, Histologic appearance of tumor. (**Fig.**, ×6250; **Inset**, ×195.)

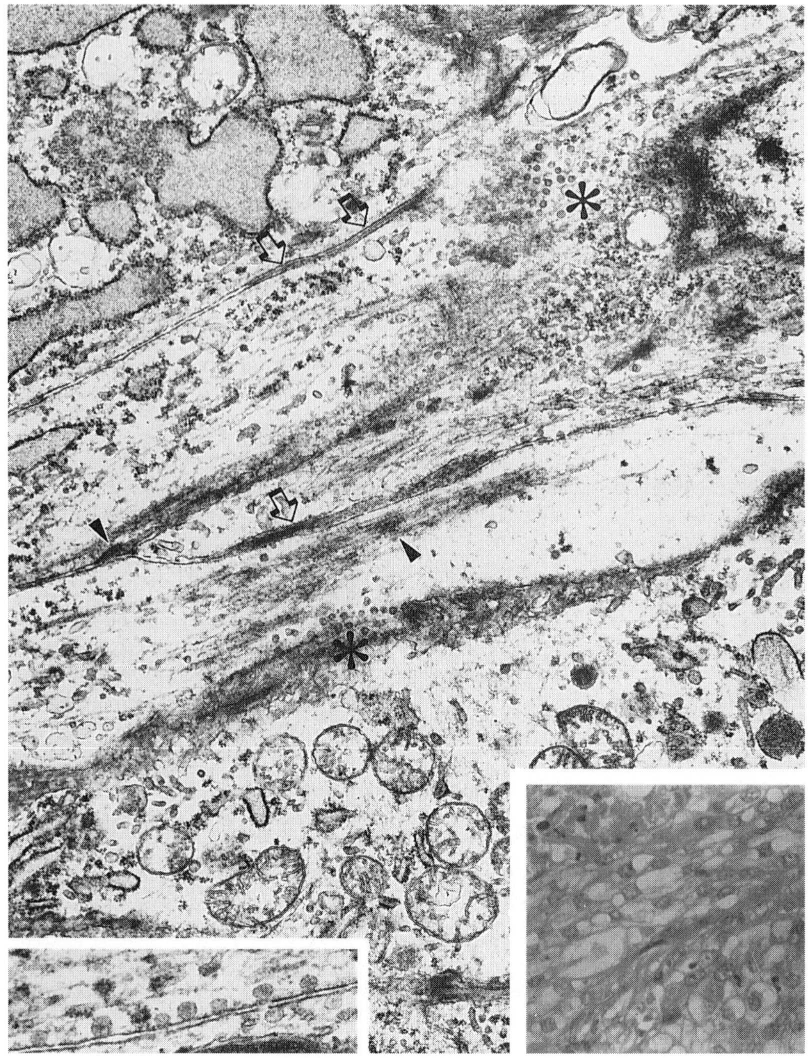

**Fig. 3-26.** Leiomyosarcoma metastatic to temporal lobe of a 62-year-old woman from primary in breast. There are intracellular filaments with rudimentary dense bodies and some suggestion of attachment plaques (*arrowheads*). Focal basal lamina is present (*arrows*) as well as small collections of pinocytotic vesicles (*asterisks*). **Left inset**, Detail showing pinocytotic vesicles oriented along the cell membrane. **Right inset**, Histologic appearance of tumor. (**Fig.**, ×16,150; **Left inset**, ×38,250; **Right inset**, ×205.)

and, like their benign counterparts, actually may be peripheral nerve sheath tumors.[233]

### Fibroblastic Tumors

*Fibromas* and *fibrosarcomas* are composed of fibroblasts, a cell type that is ultrastructurally rather undistinguished. Although the ultrastructural appearance of fibroblasts is characteristic (see below), no ultrastructural features can be said to be diagnostic, and the ultrastructural diagnosis of a fibroblastic lesion is, to a large extent, one of exclusion.

Fibroblasts are spindle shaped cells distinguished primarily by moderate cytoplasmic accumulations of rough endoplasmic reticulum cisterns and by a tendency of these cisterns to be dilated and to contain material of moderate electron density (Figs. 3-27, 3-28). This material appears amorphous at low or medium magnifications but may appear finely fibrillar at higher magnifications. A "close" association with extracellular collagen fibers is also frequently cited as a feature of fibroblasts. In the context of differential diagnosis of spindle cell tumors it is important to point out features that fibroblasts do *not* display. These include basal lamina (indeed, the finding of even fragments of basal lamina excludes a fibroblastic histogenesis), pinocytotic vesicles, and complex, intertwining cell processes. Cytoplasmic filaments, in contrast, may be found in purely fibroblastic cells. In fact, cytoplasmic filaments associated with dense bodies (indicative of smooth muscle differentiation) may be found as a component of myofibroblasts, a common component of fibroblastic tumors.* These cells generally have a thin "band" of such smooth muscle-type filaments along the plasma membrane on one edge of the cell (Fig. 3-29). Other features of smooth muscle differentiation (basal lamina, pinocytotic vesicles) are absent in such cells.

Published descriptions of fibromas[349] and fibrosarcomas† are sparse. More attention has been accorded

---

* Figs. 3, 45, 58, 162, 349, 380.

† Refs. 45, 81, 182, 239, 348, 349.

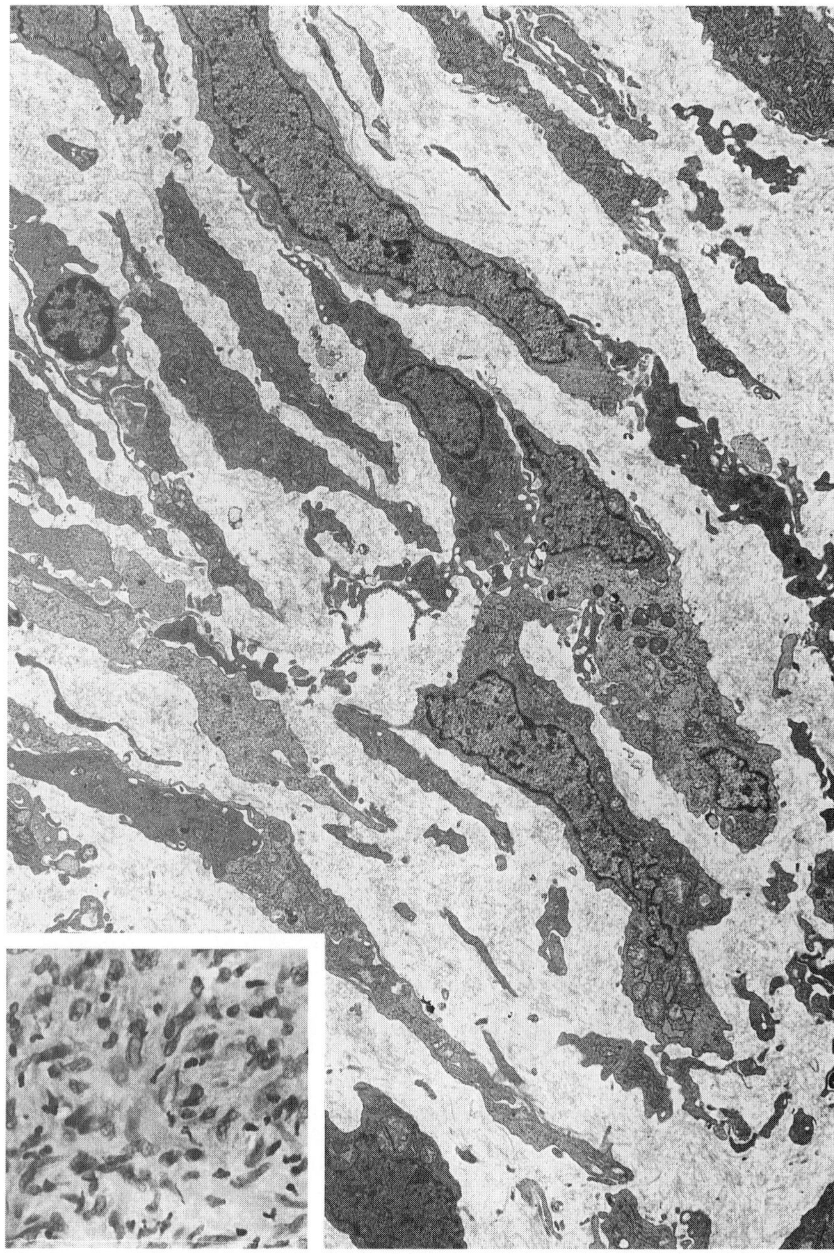

**Fig. 3-27.** Storiform malignant spindle cell neoplasm arising in the posterior mediastinum of a 75-year-old man, classified as a neurogenic sarcoma by light microscopy. Immunohistochemical studies were not helpful, and ultrastructural examination showed fibroblast-like cells devoid of Schwann cell features. The tumor was reclassified as a storiform fibrosarcoma (or malignant fibrous histiocytoma). **Inset**, Histologic appearance of tumor. (**Fig.**, ×4050; **Inset**, ×195.)

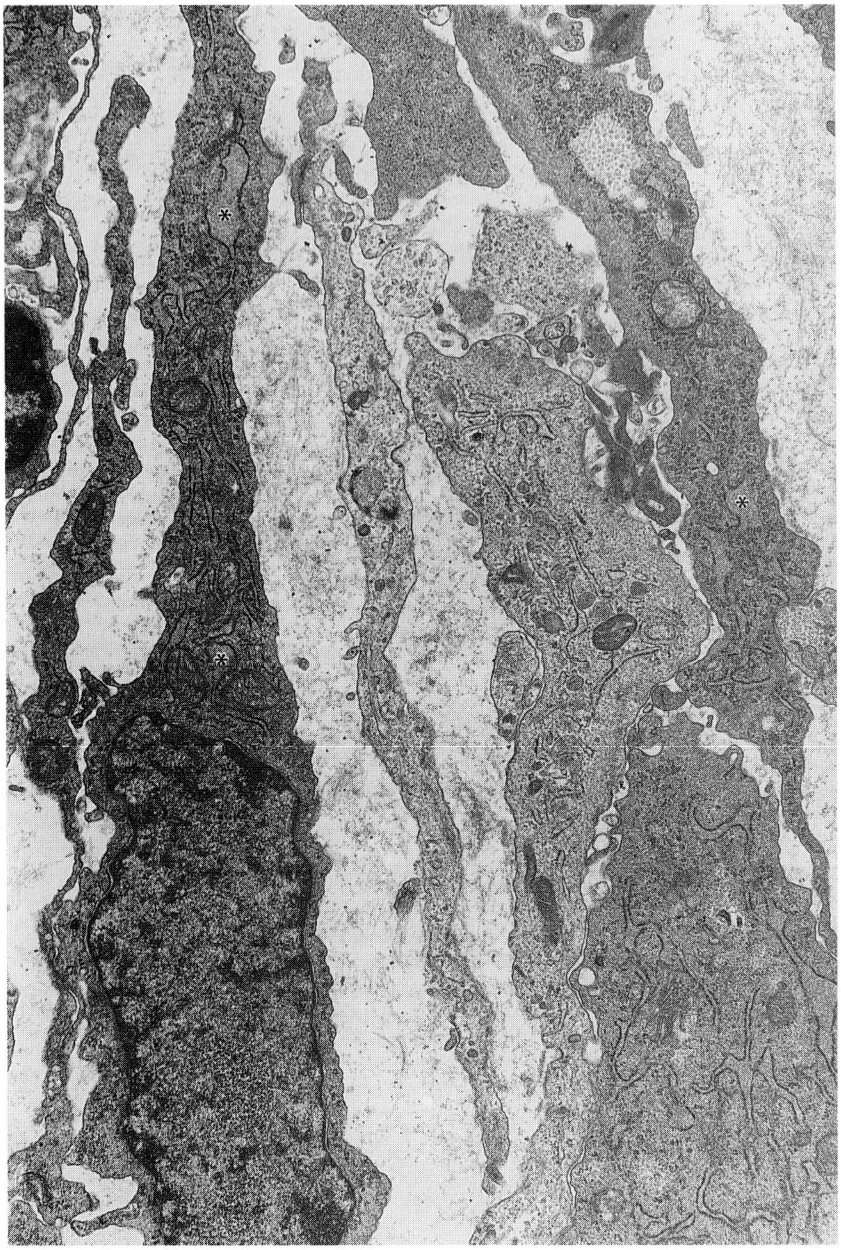

**Fig. 3-28.** Fibrosarcoma (same case as Fig. 3-27). Higher magnification shows dilated rough endoplasmic cisterns, containing finely granular amorphous material in the paranuclear areas (*asterisk*). There is no basal lamina, and the intercellular space contains collagen fibrils. (×10,500.)

the entity of malignant fibrous histiocytoma.* Although histiocytic cells have been reported in most of these tumors,[3,90,207,215,362,380] there is some controversy about their role in the neoplastic process. One study found convincing neoplastic histiocyte-like cells in only 3 of 11 malignant fibrous histiocytomas studied ultrastructurally and suggested that most of these tumors would be better classified as fibrosarcomas.[58,162]

* Refs. 3, 45, 58, 90, 91, 162, 207, 215, 362, 380.

### Plexosarcoma (Gastrointestinal Autonomic Nerve Tumors)

A recently recognized entity is a stromal tumor of the stomach[393] or small intestine[135,139,140] that appears to originate from neural elements of the enteric plexus. By light microscopy these "plexosarcomas" may appear as bland spindle cell tumors similar to leiomyomas, but this belies a clinical course characterized by widespread metastases and short survival. Ultrastructurally, the component cells of plexosarcomas have in-

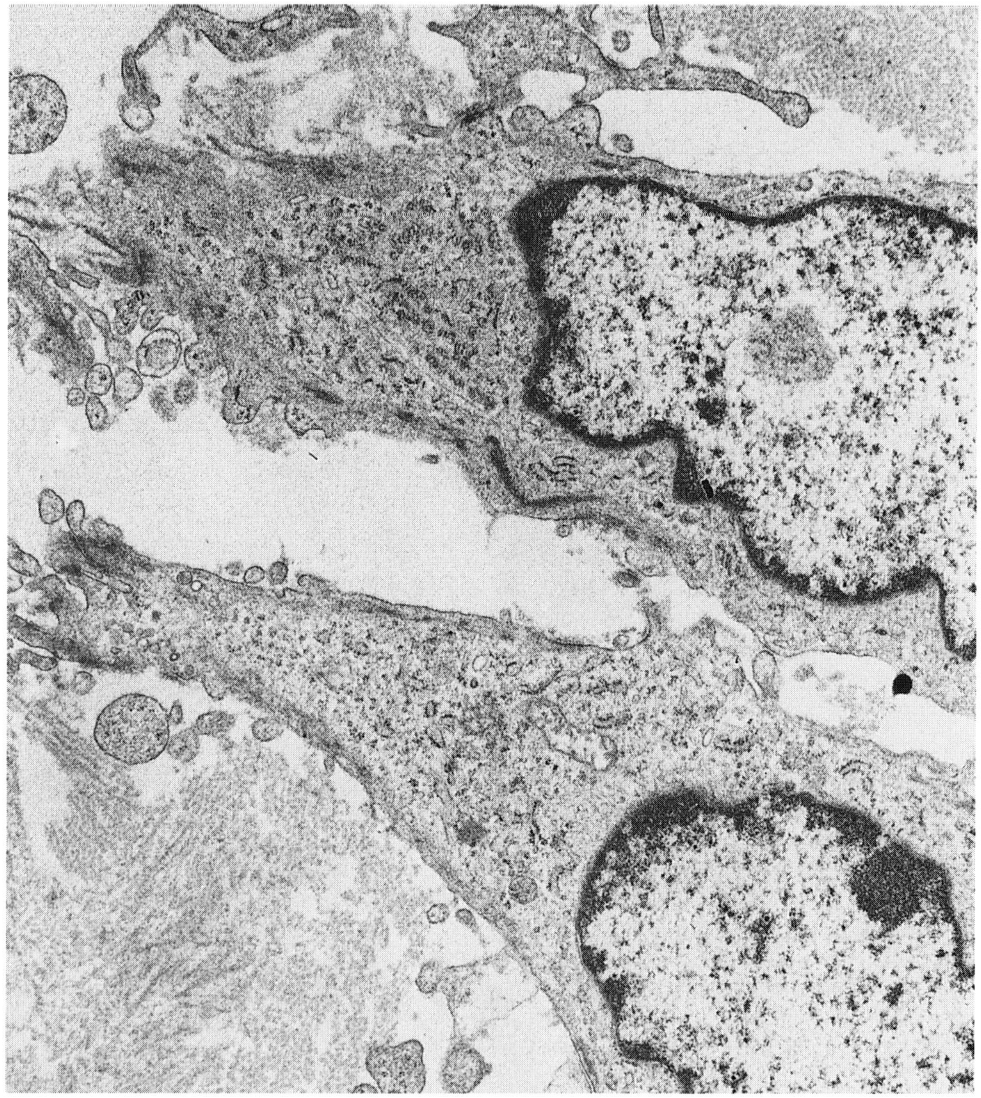

**Fig. 3-29.** Myofibroblasts. Nodular fasciitis of the parotid gland in a 21-year-old woman. The cells appear "fibroblastic" with spindled shape, paranuclear rough endoplasmic reticulum, and no basal lamina. Smooth muscle features are limited to a thin band of filaments with dense bodies immediately beneath the cell membrane. (×13,400.)

tertwined cell processes (neurites) containing both dense-core and empty synaptic-type vesicles, as well as filaments (Fig. 3-30). These cells do not have basal lamina, filaments with dense bodies, or attachment plaques.

## PAPILLARY TUMORS

Papillary tumors of the nervous system include choroid plexus tumors, papillary ependymomas, "papillary" (actually pseudopapillary) meningiomas, and metastatic carcinomas. The papillae of "papillary" meningioma (Fig. 3-31) are artifacts of tumor necrosis and of processing, and these tumors show ultrastructural features similar to those of nonpapillary meningiomas, described earlier. Metastatic carcinomas are discussed in a later section.

### Choroid Plexus Tumors

Both benign (papillomas) and malignant (adenocarcinomas) tumors arise in the choroid plexus. The former are unusual, and the latter are rare. The differential diagnosis of such lesions includes papillary ependymoma and metastatic adenocarcinoma. Of these possibilities, papillary ependymoma is readily distinguished from the rest by electron microscopy. Electron microscopy also may be useful in identifying metastatic adenocarcinoma in some cases, if identifying features of the primary site are retained in the tumor (see

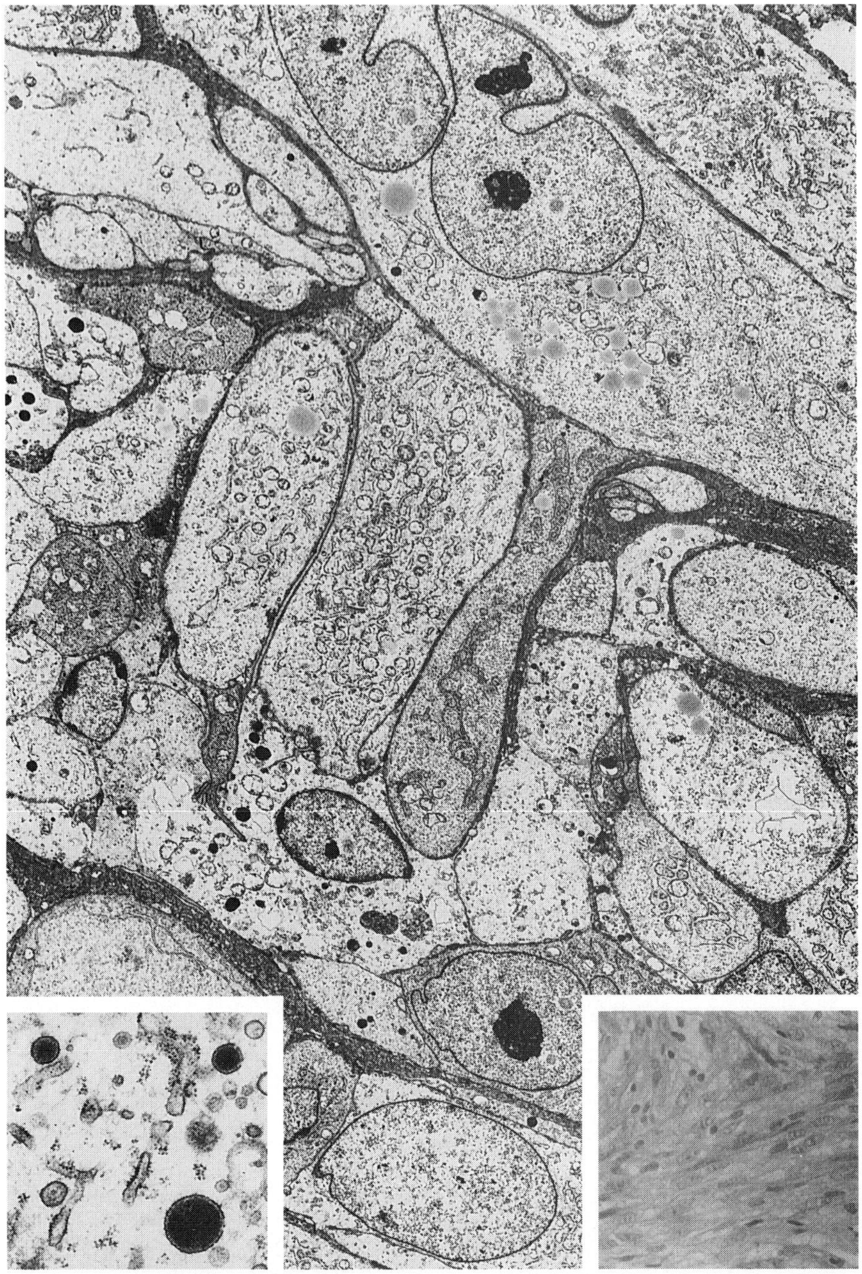

**Fig. 3-30.** Plexosarcoma originating from the small bowel of a 66-year-old woman. Note numerous cross- and longitudinally-sectioned cell processes between perikaryal areas. There are also a number of dense-core, neurosecretory-type granules present. **Left inset**, Detail showing neurosecretory granules. **Right inset**, Histologic appearance of tumor. (**Fig.**, ×3300; **Left inset**, ×20,250; **Right inset**, ×195.)

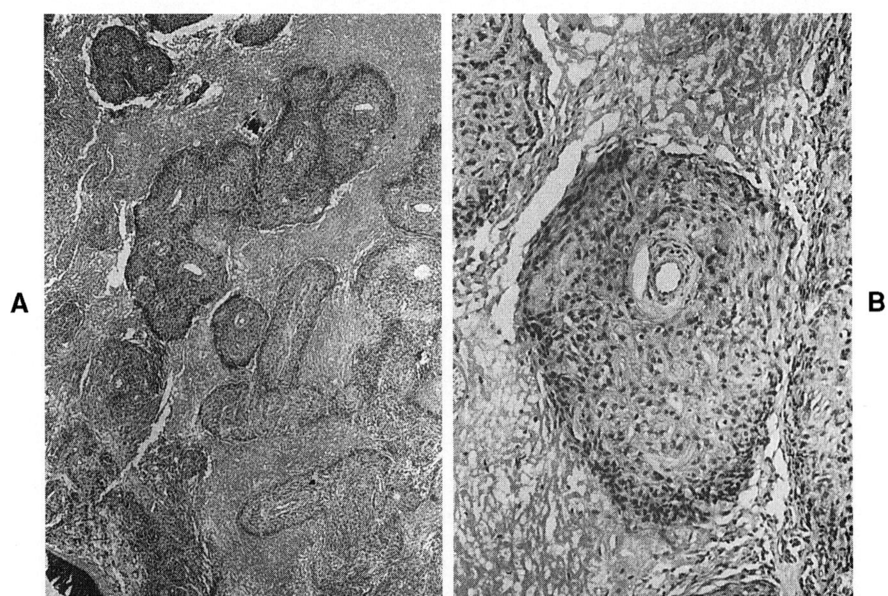


**Fig. 3-31.** "Papillary" meningioma. Frontoparietal tumor in a 58-year-old man. The perivascular "papillae" are surrounded by necrotic material and organizing thrombus. The ultrastructural appearance of this tumor was similar to that of "ordinary" meningiomas (not shown). (**A**, ×14; **B**, ×72.)

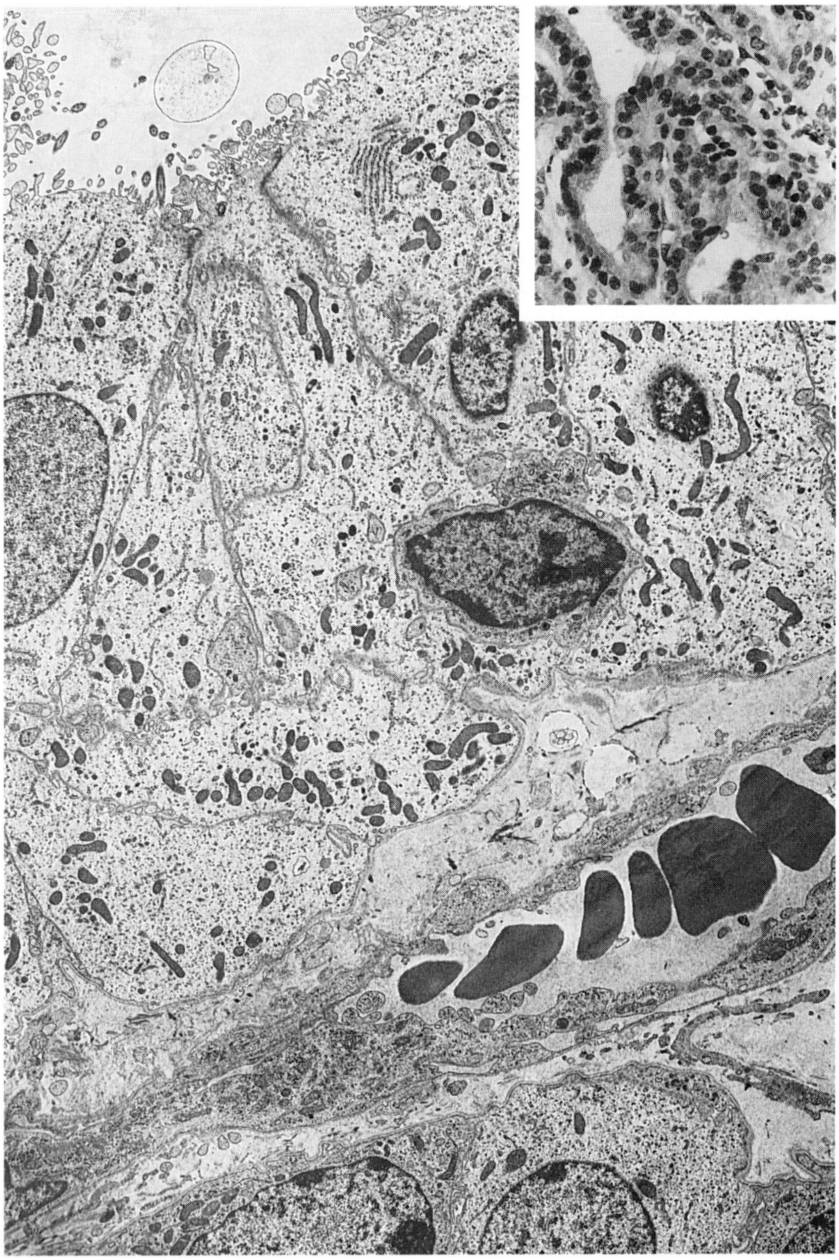

**Fig. 3-32.** Choroid plexus papilloma in a 1-year-old girl. Tall, columnar epithelial cells show apical microvilli and cilia (*upper left*). Basally, they rest on a papillary core containing a capillary (*bottom right*). **Inset**, Histologic appearance of tumor. (**Fig.**, ×4050; **Inset**, ×195.)

section on identification of primary site for metastatic adenocarcinoma of unknown origin). Electron microscopy cannot unequivocally establish a diagnosis of choroid plexus adenocarcinoma, but it may support such a diagnosis through the demonstration of features that recall normal choroid plexus. The distinction between choroid plexus papilloma and choroid plexus adenocarcinoma is best accomplished by light microscopy.

Ultrastructurally, both papillomas and adenocarcinomas of the choroid plexus show features recalling the fine structure of normal choroid plexus.* Important diagnostic points are the presence of a fibrovascular core containing collagen and vessels with fenestrated endothelium, and a basal lamina separating the tumor cells from this core (Figs. 3-32, 3-33). Within this core, a second basal lamina surrounds individual capillaries. These features distinguish choroid plexus tumors from papillary ependymomas (see the section on papillary ependymomas). Additional ultrastructural features of

* Refs. 32, 102, 124, 220, 232, 236, 257, 262, 264, 311.

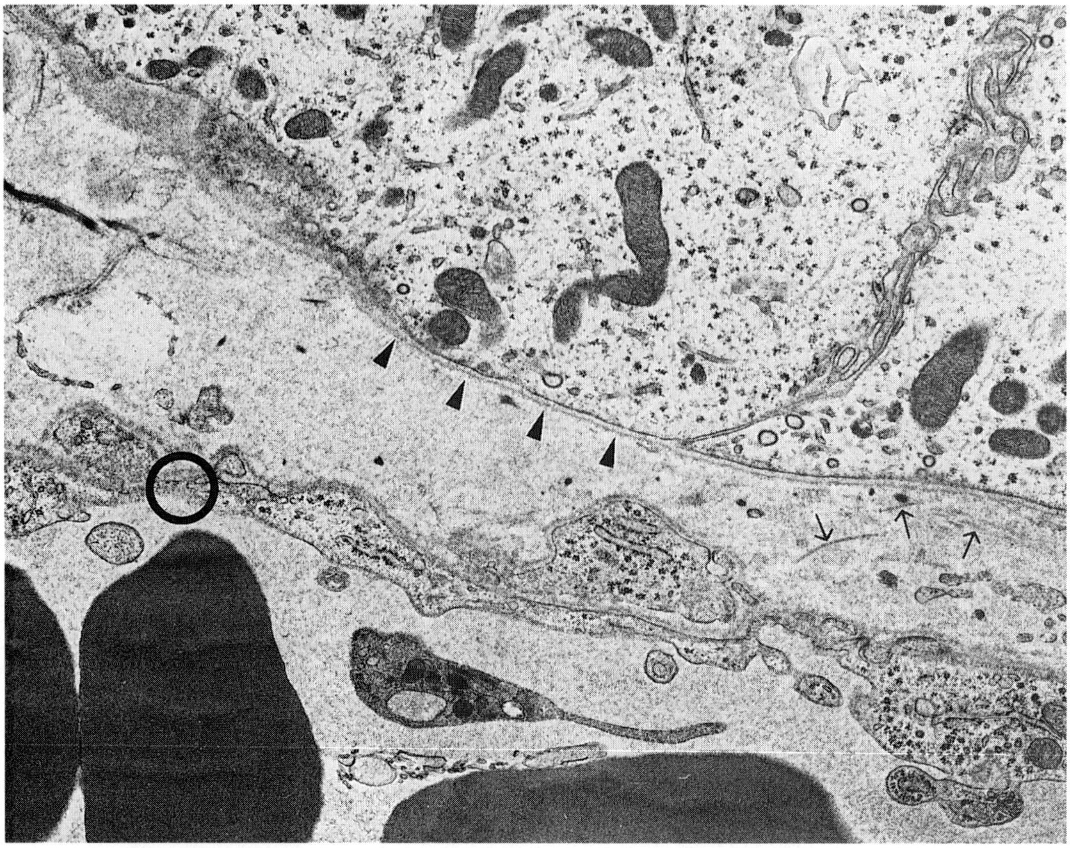

**Fig. 3-33.** Choroid plexus papilloma. Detail of Fig. 3-32 showing basal aspect of tumor cells with basal lamina (*arrowheads*), intercellular space containing collagen fibrils (*arrows*), and a capillary with its own basal lamina. The capillary endothelium is fenestrated (*circles*), but this is difficult to resolve at this magnification. (×13,000.)

choroid plexus tumors include the "epithelial" features of surface microvilli (and occasionally cilia) and apical junctional specializations between cells. Cytoplasmic microtubules have also been described.

### Papillary Ependymomas

The ultrastructural differentiation of papillary ependymomas from choroid plexus tumors rests on the nature of their papillary cores. Papillary ependymomas and choroid plexus tumors both have a perivascular eosinophilic zone by light microscopy. For choroid plexus tumors, as described above, this zone consists of a collagen-containing fibrovascular core, delineated from the tumor cells by a basal lamina. In contrast, ependymomas have a gliovascular core in which the perivascular eosinophilic zone is composed of filament-containing glial (ependymal) processes instead of extracellular collagen. There is, consequently, no basal lamina at the outer margin of the perivascular zone because the ependymal foot processes continue across this zone to abut directly upon the capillary basal laminas (Figs. 3-34, 3-35). These capillaries are of the "central nervous system type," without endothelial fenestrations, in contrast to the "systemic type" of capillaries with endothelial fenestrations seen in choroid plexus tumors. At the surface of the ependymoma papillae one may find "epithelial" features similar to those seen in choroid plexus tumors (microvilli, cilia, and junctional specializations), and these features are thus not helpful in distinguishing these tumors (see section on ependymomas, above).

A distinctive variant of ependymoma is the *myxopapillary ependymoma*. Ultrastructurally, these tumors show a continuous basal lamina along the basal aspects of the component cells, with an adjacent collagenous matrix[299,344] (Figs. 3-36, 3-37). In this regard, they resemble more closely a choroid plexus tumor than they do the papillary ependymomas described above. However, the almost exclusive localization of these tumors to the region of the cauda equina[314] precludes diagnostic confusion. Indeed, there is only a single case report of an intracranial example.[318] A more likely source of confusion is the rare occurrence of *paragangliomas* in the cauda equina region.[343a] These tumors, which may

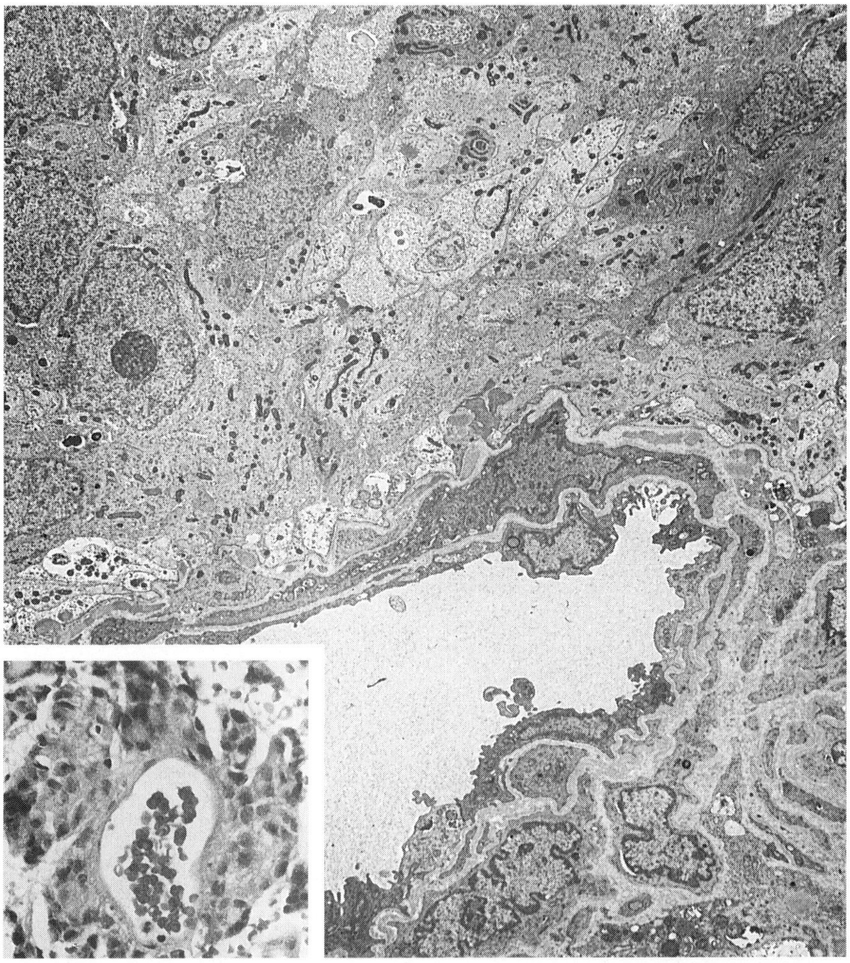

**Fig. 3-34.** Ependymoma showing perivascular area. Fourth ventricle tumor in a 54-year-old female. Tumor cell processes abut directly upon the capillary, without an intervening collagenous stroma. **Inset**, Histologic appearance of tumor. (**Fig.**, ×3000; **Inset**, ×195.)

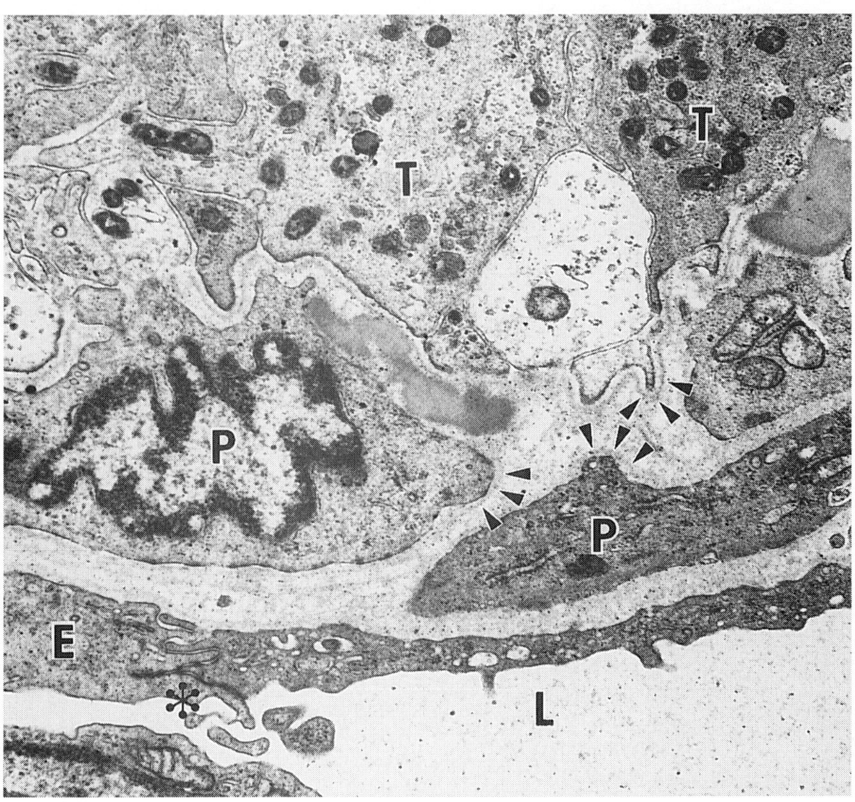


**Fig. 3-35.** Ependymoma showing perivascular area (same case as Fig. 3-34). Ependymoma tumor cell cytoplasm *(T)* is separated from capillary pericytes *(P)* and endothelial cells *(E)* by a double layer of basal lamina (*arrowheads*). Note endothelial tight junctions (*asterisk*) and absence of endothelial fenestrations. *L* = capillary lumen. (×15,400.)

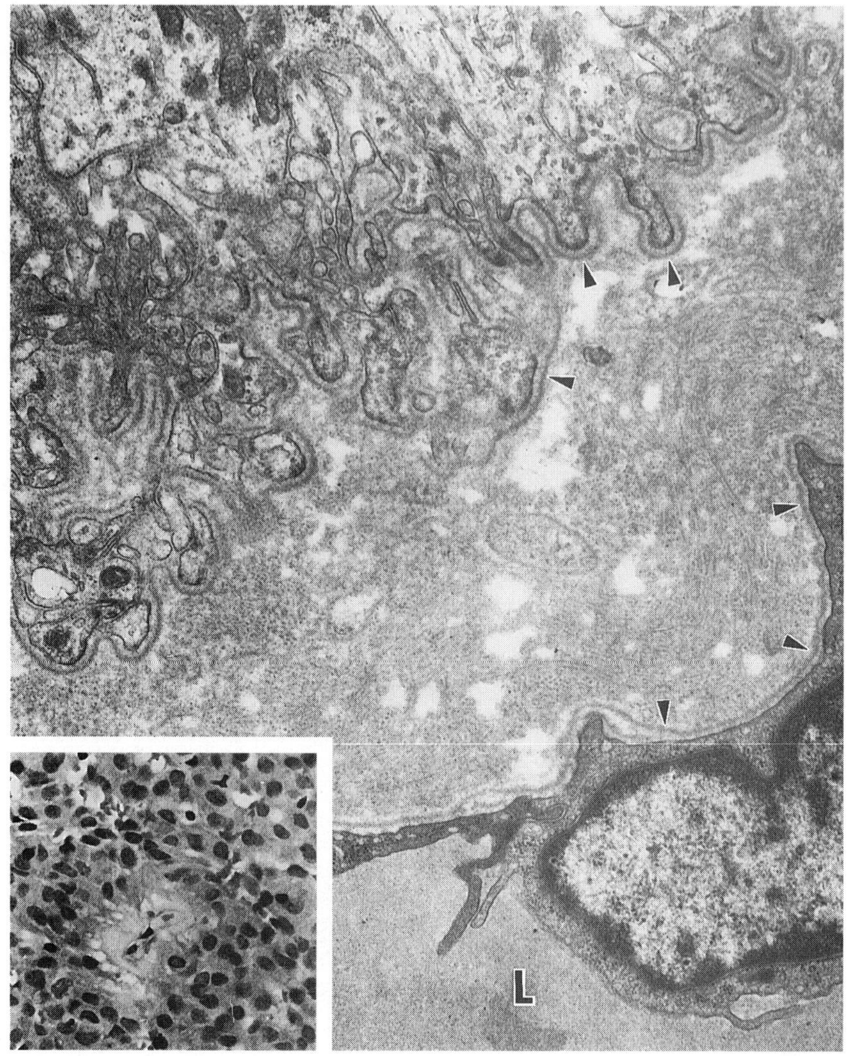


**Fig. 3-36.** Myxopapillary ependymoma of the filum terminale in a 17-year-old girl. The perivascular region shows separation of the tumor cells from a capillary by two basal laminae (*arrowheads*) and an intervening, collagen-containing space. This ultrastructural appearance is similar to that seen in choroid plexus papillomas. $L$ = capillary lumen. **Inset,** Histologic appearance of tumor. (**Fig.,** ×15,400; **Inset,** ×195.)

resemble myxopapillary ependymomas by light microscopy, are distinguished ultrastructurally by prominent cytoplasmic dense-core granules.

## ANGIOBLASTIC MENINGIOMA

Among tumors of the meninges, rare occurrences of vasoformative tumors have long been recognized. These were originally described as part of a group entitled "angioblastic meningiomas"[11] that also included highly vascular but nonvasoformative tumors of meningothelial cells. These "angioblastic meningiomas" were subclassified into three groups[52] that are recognized today under the following terminology:

(1) Hemangiopericytomas of the meninges (also called angioblastic meningioma, hemangiopericytic type).
(2) Highly vascular meningioma or angiomatous meningioma (not a vasoformative tumor).
(3) Hemangioblastoma (sometimes called hemangioendothelioma) with dural attachment.

This three-part division is universally accepted, although there remains some controversy over the nosologic interrelationship of these entities.[165,287] It is clear that this is a prognostically important classification. Tumors in the first group (hemangiopericytomas) have a propensity for local recurrence and for late (5 to 10 years) appearance of extraneural metastases.[114,178a,202a,235a] Such aggressive behavior is not typical of the other two groups (highly vascular meningiomas and hemangioblastomas with dural attachment).

In most cases, these three groups can be distinguished by light microscopy. Hemangiopericytomas of the meninges resemble hemangiopericytomas elsewhere; highly vascular meningiomas are identified by the presence of typical meningothelial cells between the blood vessels; and hemangioblastomas with dural attachment do not differ in appearance from those without dural attachment[165] (which occur most commonly in the cerebellum). There is some overlap in histologic appearance, however, and in such cases electron microscopy can be helpful.

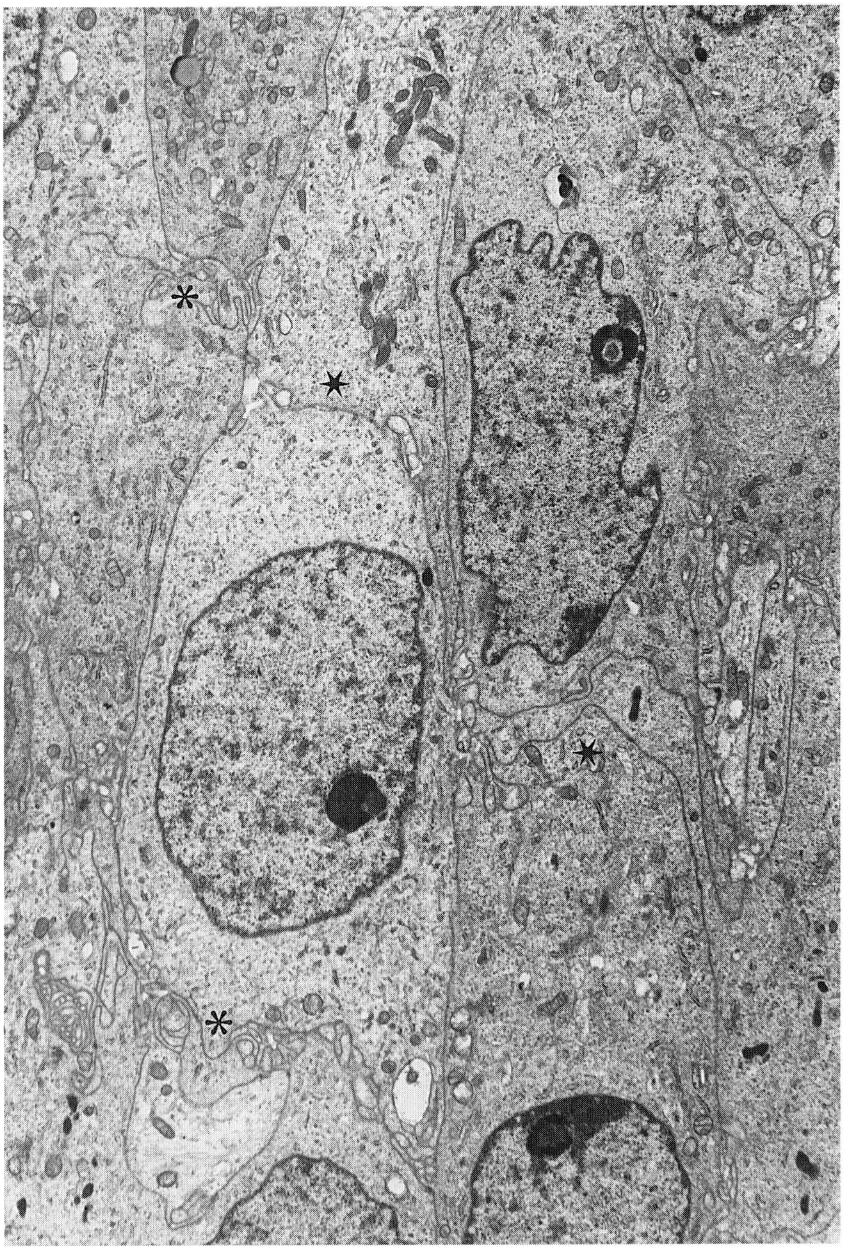

**Fig. 3-37.** Myxopapillary ependymoma (same case as Fig. 3-36). The tumor cells in this area show a "stacked" or "brick-wall" appearance. Complex processes at one end of some tumor cells (*asterisks*) suggest microvilli inspissated against adjacent cells. Such areas alternate with blunt tumor cell ends (*stars*). A similar appearance may be found in tanycytic variants of intramedullary spinal cord ependymomas. (×6250.)

## Hemangiopericytoma

Hemangiopericytomas of the meninges* are similar in ultrastructural appearance to extracranial hemangiopericytomas,[291] but do show some differences in the frequency of some of the ultrastructural features.[55] Two important ultrastructural features are: (1) the presence of normal-appearing capillary endothelial cells and (2) the relative paucity of interdigitating tumor cell processes and intercellular junctional devices (Figs. 3-38 to 3-43). The former feature distinguishes hemangiopericytoma from hemangioblastoma, whereas the latter feature distinguishes hemangiopericytoma from vascular meningiomas.

* Refs. 44, 55, 165, 261, 287, 291, 298.

At low magnification, the capillaries of hemangiopericytoma are lined with flattened normal-appearing endothelial cells having intercellular tight junctions and pinocytotic vesicles. There is a well-defined surrounding basal lamina separating the endothelial cells from the adjacent tumor cells. This basal lamina may extend outward to separate individual tumor cells, but more commonly one simply finds irregular intercellular deposits of basal lamina-like material scattered between tumor cells. In this respect, meningeal hemangiopericytomas differ somewhat from extracranial examples, which tend to have better development of basal lamina around individual tumor cells.[55]

The tumor cells of hemangiopericytoma have enlarged euchromatic ("active-appearing") nuclei that

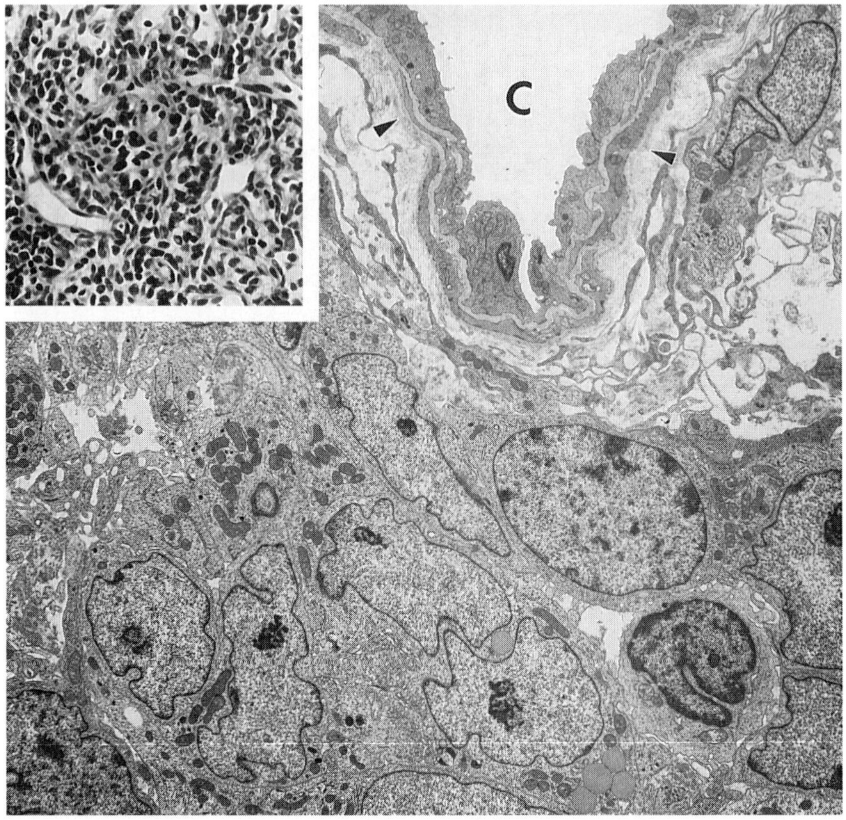


**Fig. 3-38.** Hemangiopericytoma arising in the orbit of a 56-year-old woman. A similar tumor had been excised 33 years previously. A capillary *(C)* is separated from the tumor cells by a basal lamina (*arrowheads*), but there is little or no basal lamina between tumor cells. **Inset**, Histologic appearance of tumor. (**Fig.**, ×3000; **Inset**, ×195.) (Reproduced with permission from Rice et al.[302])

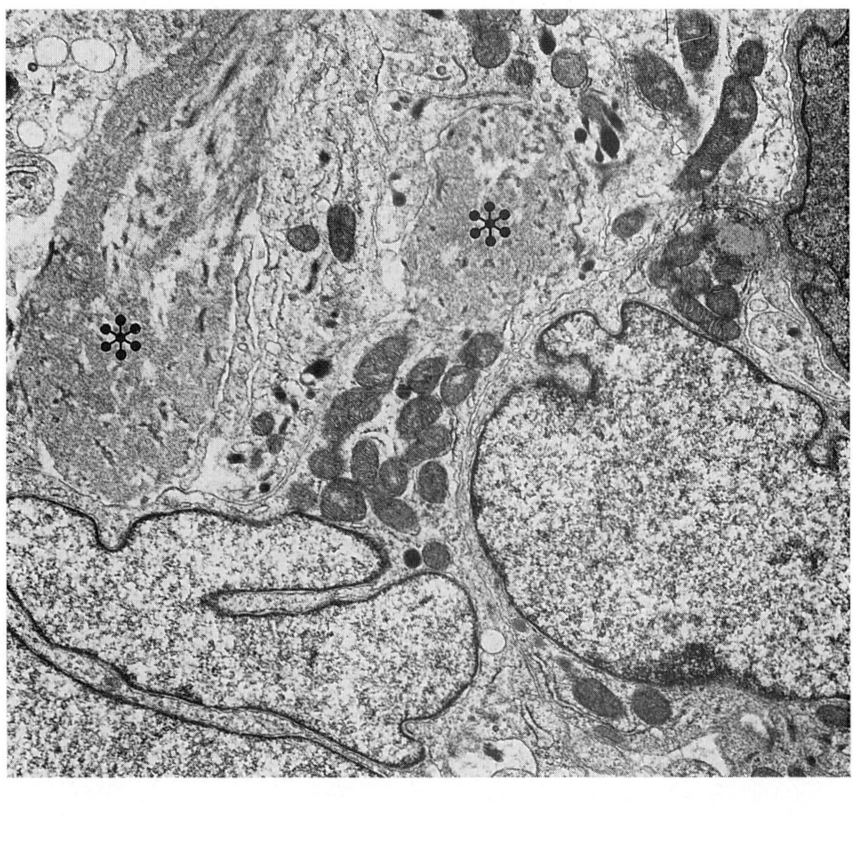

**Fig. 3-39.** Hemangiopericytoma (same case as Fig. 3-38). Intercellular deposits of basal lamina-like, electron-dense material (*asterisks*) are found between tumor cells, but well-defined basal lamina is sparse. (×10,500.) (Reproduced with permission from Rice et al.[302])

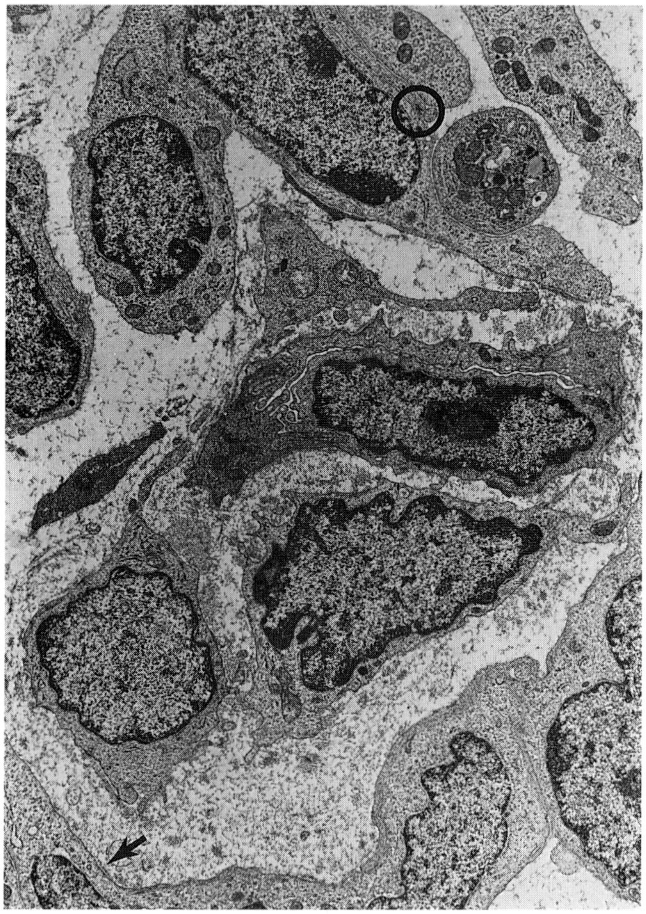

**Fig. 3-40.** Hemangiopericytoma. A small capillary with slit-like lumen is surrounded by layers of tumor cells. The intercellular spaces contain basal lamina material and collagen. *Arrow*: segmental basal lamina. *Circle*: intercellular junction. (×6280.) (Courtesy of Dr. Khang-Loon Ho, Department of Pathology, Henry Ford Hospital, Detroit, MI.)

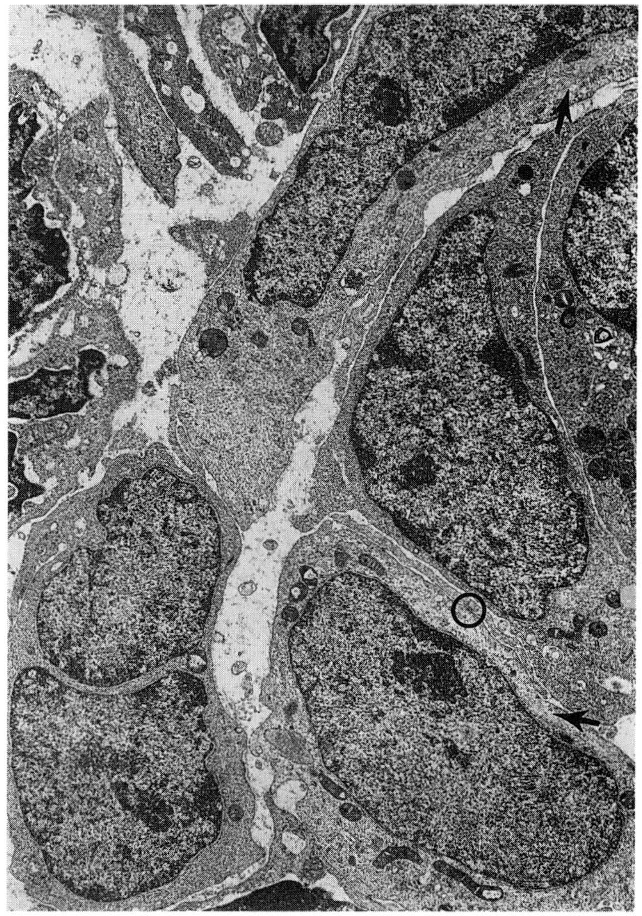

**Fig. 3-41.** Hemangiopericytoma. The tumor cells, closely arranged in sheets, are oval or fusiform with occasional intercellular attachments (*circle*). Elongated slender cytoplasmic processes are often interspersed among tumor cells. *Arrows*: intracytoplasmic bundles of microfilaments. (×6280.) (Courtesy of Dr. Khang-Loon Ho, Department of Pathology, Henry Ford Hospital, Detroit, MI.)

contrast sharply with the flattened, heterochromatic ("resting") nuclei of the endothelial cells. The tumor cells generally show few cytoplasmic processes, few interdigitations of cytoplasmic processes, and only sparse and rudimentary intercellular junctional devices. (The latter feature represents another departure from peripheral hemangiopericytomas, in which junctional devices are somewhat more prominent.[55]) Occasional cells contain cytoplasmic filaments and (rarely) dense bodies, suggestive of smooth muscle differentiation[261,287]; these dense bodies, however, are so rare as to be diagnostically useless.

## Vascular Meningioma

Highly vascular meningiomas[165,291] differ from typical meningothelial meningiomas only by their rich vascularity. The vessels are mature in appearance and are surrounded by a basal lamina, as they are in hemangiopericytoma. The tumor cells, however, show the same prominent interdigitation of cytoplasmic processes, intercellular filaments, and abundant, well-formed desmosome junctions that characterize less vascular meningiomas (see above), and these features distinguish these tumors from hemangiopericytomas. Both hemangiopericytomas and highly vascular meningiomas contain irregular interstitial deposits of basal lamina-like material. Vascular meningiomas react immunohistochemically with antibodies to epithelial membrane antigen,[270,325] whereas hemangiopericytomas do not.[404]

## Hemangioblastoma

Hemangioblastomas* show many ultrastructural similarities to hemangiopericytoma.[34,298] They are consequently readily distinguished from vascular meningioma by means of the same criteria described above.

* Refs. 29, 34, 40, 152–156, 158, 178, 188, 190, 298, 329.

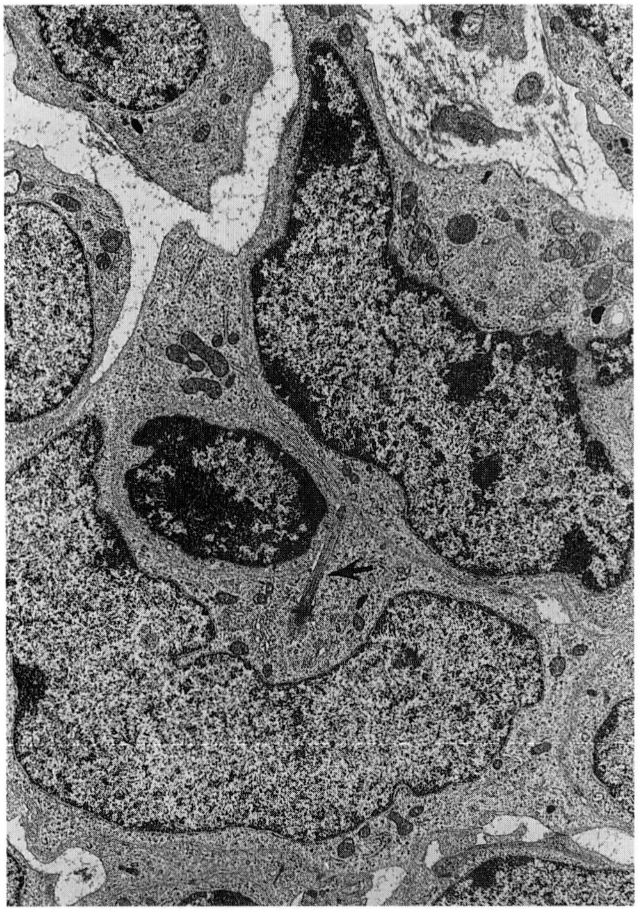

**Fig. 3-42.** Hemangiopericytoma. The nuclei of tumor cells are either oval or irregularly shaped and contain one or two distinct nucleoli. An intranuclear inclusion body is occasionally visible. The cytoplasm contains rough endoplasmic reticulum cisternae, mitochondria, bundles of microfilaments, and prominent Golgi apparatus. Intracytoplasmic cilia are also present (*arrow*). (×6280.) (Courtesy of Dr. Khang-Loon Ho, Department of Pathology, Henry Ford Hospital, Detroit, MI.)

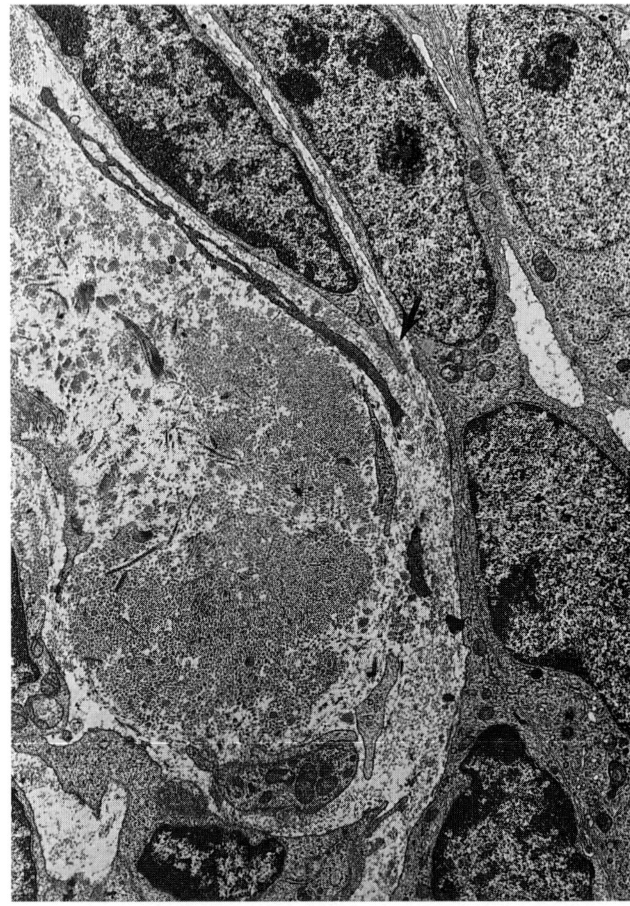

**Fig. 3-43.** Hemangiopericytoma. Intercellular spaces are often distended by mature collagen fibers, basal lamina material, and cellular processes. *Arrow*: sequential basal lamina. (×6000.) (Courtesy of Dr. Khang-Loon Ho, Department of Pathology, Henry Ford Hospital, Detroit, MI.)

The distinction between hemangiopericytoma and hemangioblastoma rests on the following criteria (Figs. 3-44 to 3-47):

(1) Appearance of the endothelial cells. These are more numerous than those seen in hemangiopericytoma or in normal capillaries, and they bulge into the vessel lumen instead of appearing flattened.[40,190,298] In addition, Weibel-Palade bodies are more common in these cells than in the endothelial cells of hemangiopericytoma or in normal cerebral capillaries[152,190] (Figs. 3-44, 3-46). Weibel-Palade bodies are cylindrical organelles with a characteristic tubular substructure.[396] They are morphologic markers for endothelial cells, and they are rich in von Willebrand protein.[392]

(2) Appearance of the stromal cells. These are somewhat more heterogeneous in appearance than those of hemangiopericytoma.[34,152,298] Indeed, this heterogeneity may suggest transitional forms between the endothelial cells and the stromal cells,[40,190] but interconvertability of the two cell types is not supported by tissue culture experiments.[345] The stromal cells often contain lipid (but not glycogen) and may contain unusual whorled arrangements of endoplasmic reticulum.[158] The absence of glycogen is an important feature in distinguishing hemangioblastomas from metastatic renal cell carcinomas,[178] with which they are occasionally confused at the light microscopic level. Hemangioblastomas are further distinguished from metastatic renal cell carcinomas by lack of epithelial features such as lumen formation, apical microvilli, and immunohistochemical reaction for epithelial membrane antigen.[86] A frequent and possibly helpful feature in the identification of hemangioblastomas is the presence of fair numbers of histiocytes[34,153,190] (Fig. 3-46).

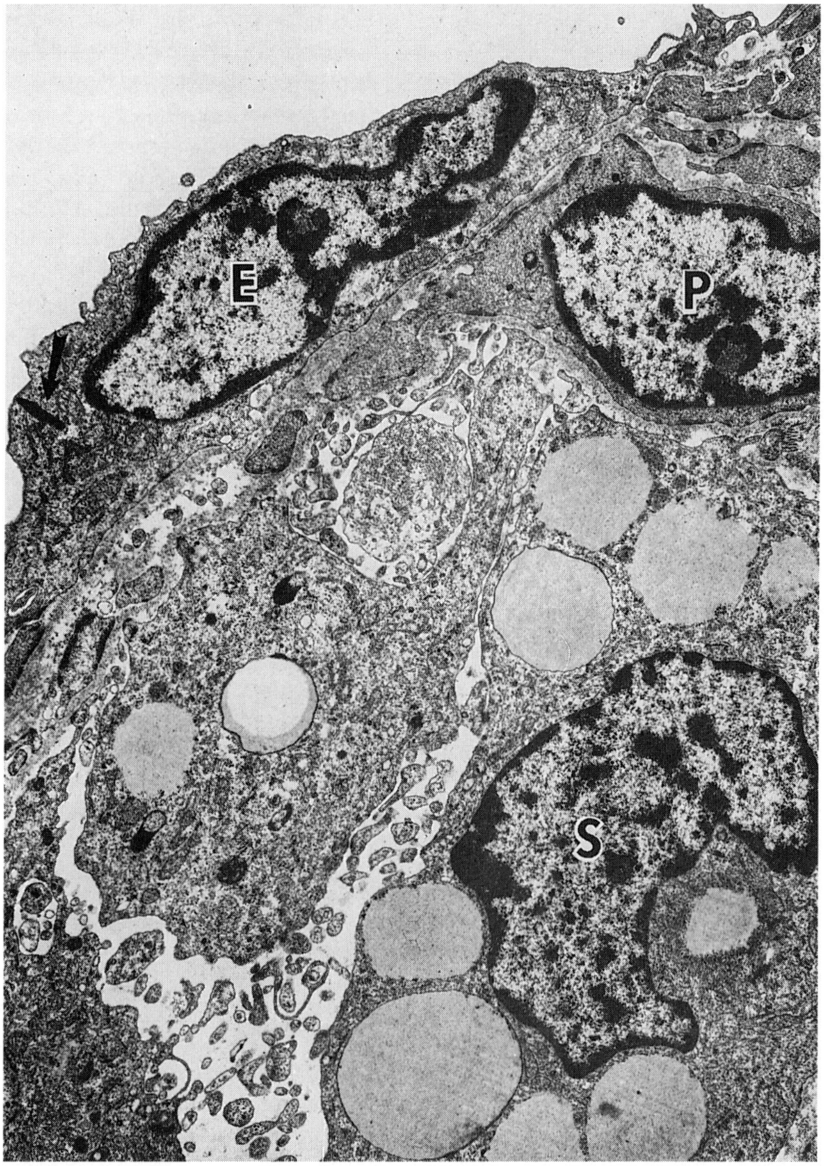


**Fig. 3-44.** Hemangioblastoma. Three main cell types are identified in hemangioblastoma. The endothelial cells *(E)* and their associated pericytes *(P)* form the capillary meshworks. Weibel-Palade bodies (*arrow*) are seen frequently within endothelial cells. The stromal cells *(S)* often contain lipid droplets. (×6630.) (Courtesy of Dr. Khang-Loon Ho, Department of Pathology, Henry Ford Hospital, Detroit, MI.)

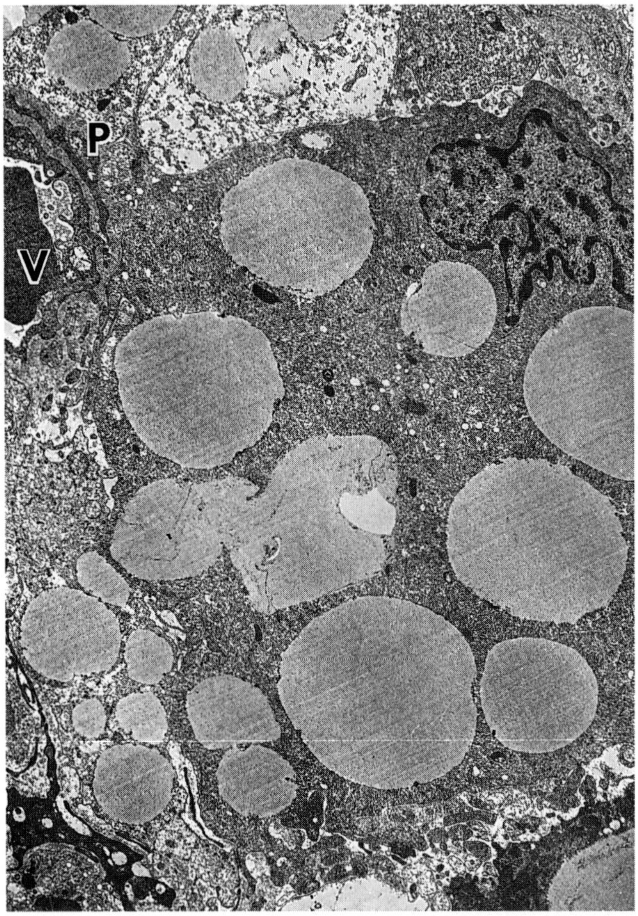


**Fig. 3-45.** Hemangioblastoma. A lipidized stromal cell contains lipid droplets that distend the cytoplasm and displace the nucleus. *V*: capillary, *P*: pericyte. (×5300.) (Courtesy of Dr. Khang-Loon Ho, Department of Pathology, Henry Ford Hospital, Detroit, MI.)

## LARGE CELL TUMORS

Poorly differentiated tumors tend to have a common histologic appearance. Metastatic carcinoma, amelanotic melanoma, and lymphoma may appear similar; glioblastoma or anaplastic astrocytoma may even mimic a poorly differentiated metastatic carcinoma.[93,193,309] Glioblastoma, on occasion, may also be confused with ganglioglioma, a rare tumor of childhood and early adulthood. Further examination of additional areas will often clarify histogenesis, but this is not always possible with small neurosurgical specimens. Such tumors, lacking distinguishing histologic features, may retain differentiating antigen structures (demonstrable by immunocytochemistry) or differentiating ultrastructural features.

### Glioblastoma

Glioblastomas[74,117,220,294,321] retain characteristic astrocytic features, particularly cytoplasmic filaments and surface processes, with a paucity of cell-to-cell contacts and few intercellular junctional devices (Fig. 3-48). The filaments are often loosely distributed throughout the tumor cell cytoplasm, around and between the other organelles, which consequently appear randomly scattered. These filaments generally are not densely matted, as are those of low-grade astrocytomas (see the section on astrocytomas), and on occasion may be overlooked on casual inspection of low-magnification electron micrographs. There is generally some space between adjacent glioblastoma cells. Junctional devices between these cells may be found, but these are sparse and rudimentary and generally found between cell processes rather than cell bodies.[293,321,354] An occasional glioblastoma displays prominent cytoplasmic lipofuscin pigment. This is discernible by light as well as electron microscopy.

### Ganglioglioma

Gangliogliomas are rare tumors of children and young adults that usually are well demarcated and slowly growing. Abnormal, neoplastic neurons are intermixed with neoplastic glial cells (usually astrocytes). By light microscopy these tumors may be confused with glioblastomas containing a mixture of small and large cells. Diagnosis of ganglioglioma is thus dependent on (1) the demonstration of both glial and neuronal elements in the tumor and (2) the demonstration of the neoplastic nature of both of these elements. The latter requirement is addressed by light microscopy, using criteria such as heterotopia, clustering, and abnormal cytology of the neuronal elements[314]; the former requirement can be met by ultrastructural examination. In the closely related tumor ganglioneuroma, electron microscopy can also assist in identifying the poorly differentiated cellular component of the tumor as composed of neuroblasts.

The ultrastructural confirmation of a neuronal tumor component rests on the demonstration of neuronal features in the large cells. These features include stacks of rough endoplasmic reticulum cisternae (Nissl substance), microtubule-containing neuritic processes, synaptic complexes between cell processes, and dense-core neurosecretory-type vesicles (similar features are seen in neuroblastic tumors: see Figs. 3-61 to 3-68, 3-72, 3-73). The latter feature (dense-core vesicles) has been emphasized in the two available ultrastructural reports.[310,353] The glioma component in these two cases showed ultrastructural features of astrocytes.

A single available ultrastructurally examined *ganglioneuroma*[305] demonstrated mature neuronal or

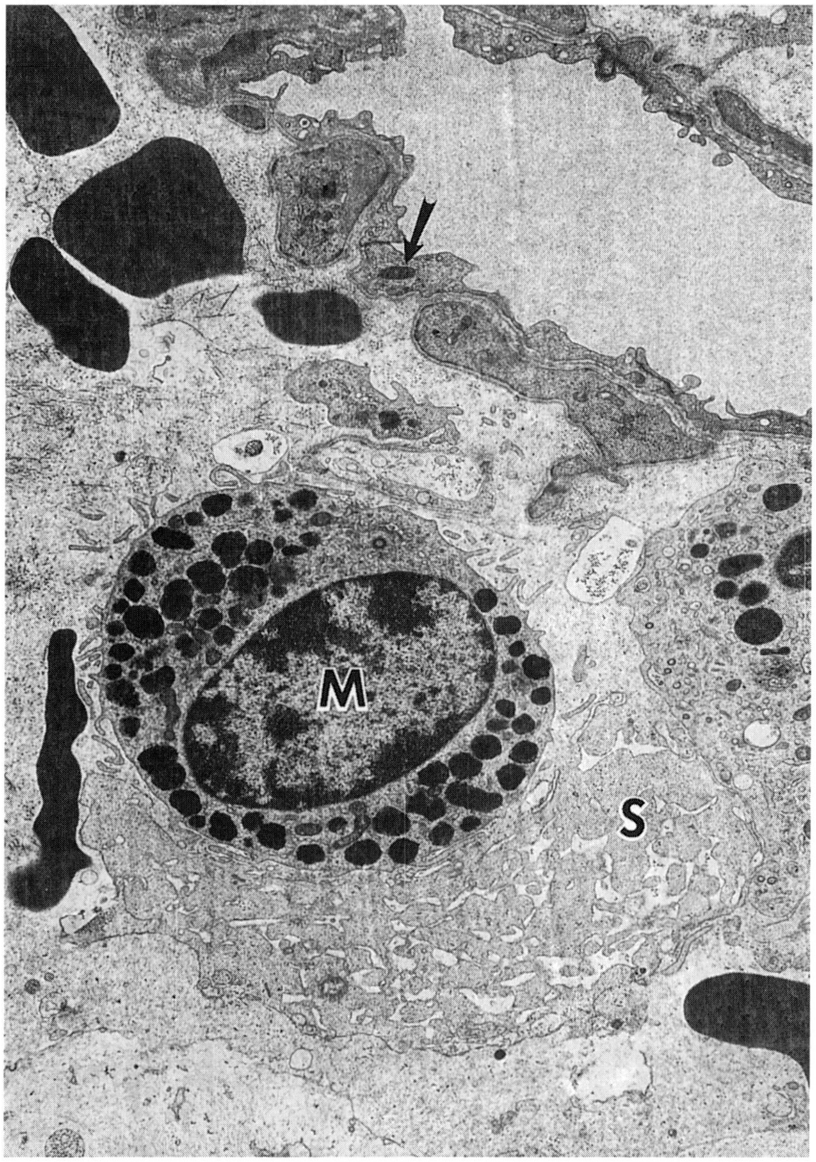


**Fig. 3-46.** Hemangioblastoma. A mast cell *(M)* containing numerous electron-dense granules is located in the intervascular space close to the capillary wall. *S*: stromal cell with dilated endoplasmic reticulum. *Arrow*: Weibel-Palade body in endothelial cell. (×6630.) (Courtesy of Dr. Khang-Loon Ho, Department of Pathology, Henry Ford Hospital, Detroit, MI.)

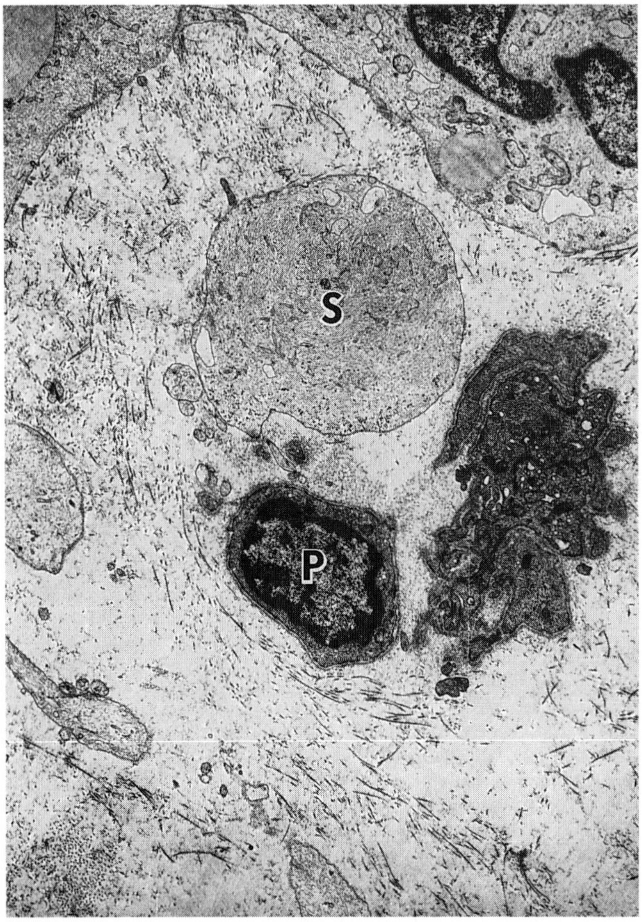


**Fig. 3-47.** Hemangioblastoma. A small collapsed capillary with a distended perivascular space containing an isolated pericyte *(P)*, processes of stromal cells, and mature collagen. Abundant intracytoplasmic microfilaments are common in nonlipidized stromal cells *(S)*. (×5300.) Courtesy of Dr. Khang-Loon Ho, Department of Pathology, Henry Ford Hospital, Detroit, MI.)

ganglion cells similar to those described above and, in addition, small neuroblasts characterized by cell processes containing small vesicles.

## Carcinoma

Metastatic carcinoma cells are generally polygonal. They may show surface microvilli or microvillus-like projections, but the longer, more irregular surface processes characteristic of glial tumor cells are not seen. The most important distinguishing feature of metastatic carcinoma is the presence of intercellular junctional devices—either well-formed desmosomes or the more common but less striking "desmosome-like" junctions (Fig. 3-49). These are usually found between tumor cell bodies and are present in fair numbers. There is also usually a greater degree of cell-to-cell contact than is seen with glioblastomas. Metastatic carcinomas may contain cytoplasmic filaments, generally in the form of small, dense perinuclear bundles of filaments rather than the widely distributed loose filaments of glioblastoma. These small perinuclear filament bundles are not limited to metastatic squamous carcinomas but may be seen in adenocarcinomas as well. In contrast, peripheral filament bundles showing attachment to intercellular desmosome junctions are an identifying feature of squamous cell carcinoma, and this feature is not seen in other undifferentiated large cell tumors.

## Melanoma

Amelanotic melanomas[23,31,234] are diagnostic problems wherever they are found. This "great imitator" of tumors serves as a yardstick of one's skill as a surgical pathologist. The usefulness of electron microscopy in such cases rests on the ability to identify melanocytic differentiation (i.e., the presence of cytoplasmic melanin granules or melanosomes) that is not detectable by the light microscope. The failure of histologic methods to find these structures may result from a paucity of melanosomes or from the presence of unduly small melanosomes (less than 250 nm).[97] As it is only such difficult and poorly differentiated cases that come to the attention of the electron microscopist, these tumors are a diagnostic challenge at the ultrastructural level as well (Figs. 3-50 to 3-55). It is usually necessary to spend a fair amount of time scanning these tumors at relatively high magnifications seeking the diagnostic granules. This is generally complicated by the presence of numerous cytoplasmic structures—lysosomes, mitochondria and others—that at first glance resemble melanosomes. Despite all of these qualifications, electron microscopy is often the best method to establish a diagnosis of melanoma in particularly troublesome cases.[97] The diagnostic feature—the melanosome—undergoes a maturation process that starts with an undistinguished (and nonspecific) empty-appearing membrane-bound organelle, evolves through several stages characterized by a filamentous (or perhaps membranous) internal structure with a characteristic (and diagnostic) transverse banding, and ends with another nonspecific structure, an opaque electron-dense organelle indistinguishable from a tertiary lysosome. It is thus the diagnostic intermediate stages of melanosome maturation that are sought (Figs. 3-52, 3-54). While "normal" melanosomes are round or oval with longitudinally oriented filaments, neoplastic melanocytes may contain pleomorphic melanosomes that have coils or spirals of filaments. For the purpose of

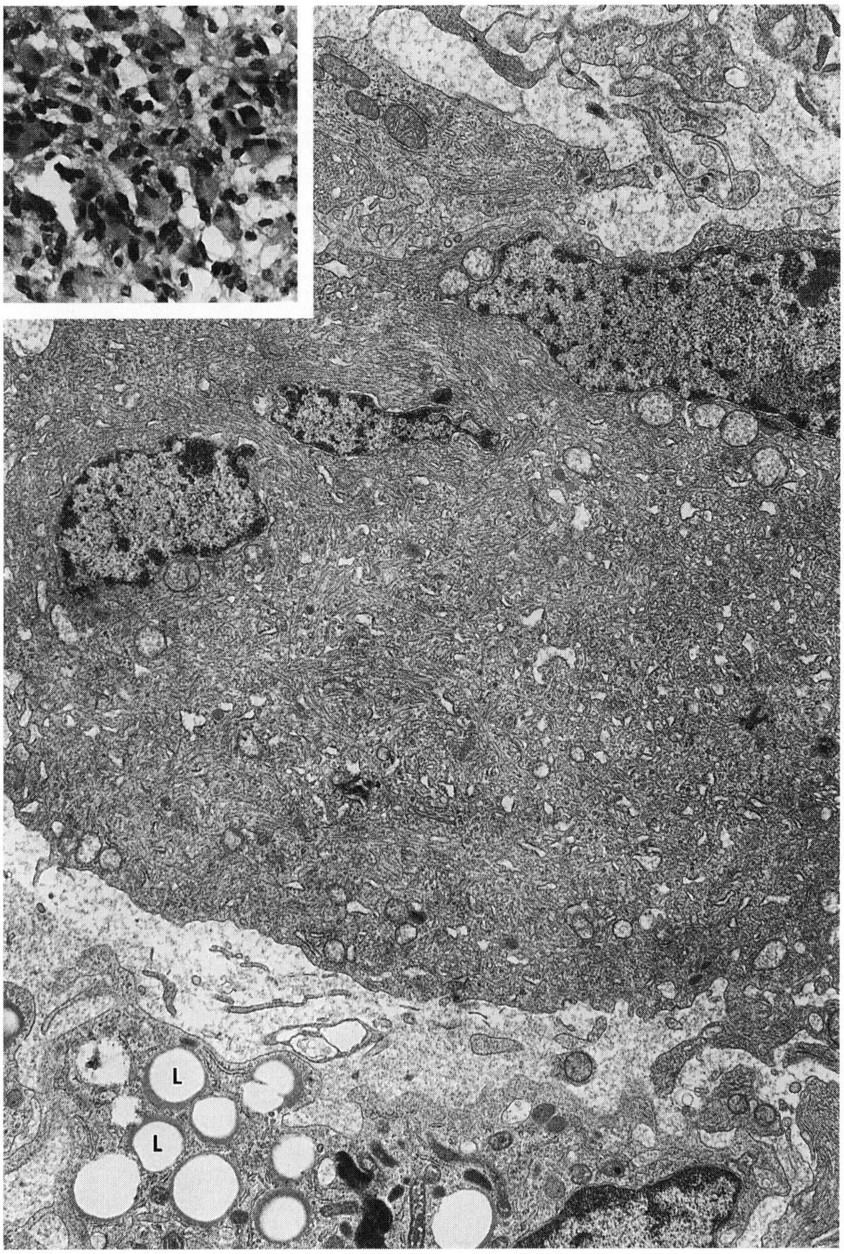


**Fig. 3-48.** Glioblastoma of the left occipital lobe in a 52-year-old man. This large tumor cell contains abundant fine filaments, loosely matted and interwoven with cytoplasmic organelles. An adjacent cell (*below*) contains lipid droplets (*L*). There are irregular cell processes in the space between the tumor cells, and some of these processes contain filaments. There is little cell-to-cell contact, and no junctions are evident in this area. **Inset,** Histologic appearance of tumor. (**Fig.,** ×7775; **Inset,** ×195.)

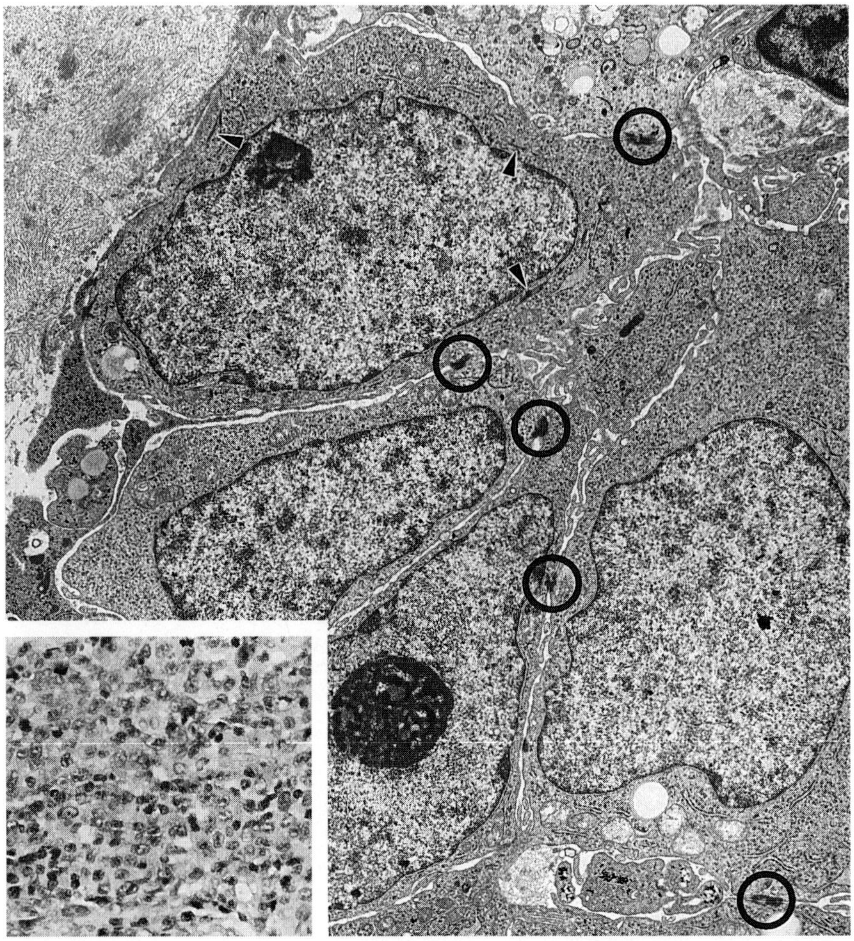

**Fig. 3-49.** Undifferentiated carcinoma; unknown primary, metastatic to cerebrum in a 67-year-old man. The tumor cells are more cohesive than those of glioblastoma, with frequent intercellular junctions (*circles*). Occasional cytoplasmic filaments are present (*arrowheads*) that are more densely packed than those of glioblastoma and do not entangle cytoplasmic organelles. Cell processes, when present, are more uniform than those of glioblastoma and do not contain filaments. **Inset**, Histologic appearance of tumor. (**Fig.**, ×8750; **Inset**, ×195.)

establishing a diagnosis of melanoma, it is mandatory that a suspected "melanosome" be shown within a tumor cell. The granules of both mast cells and basophils have been mistaken for melanosomes, as have the rod-shaped microtubulated bodies (Weibel-Palade bodies) of vascular endothelial cells[97] (see Figs. 3-44, 3-46). A high-magnification electron micrograph of a long-sought melanosome should be followed by a low-magnification electron micrograph of the same area to show the location of the structure.

In addition to the diagnostic melanosomes, a few other ultrastructural features of melanoma merit mention. First, junctional devices are rare in melanomas, if they occur at all. The finding of even modest numbers of junctional devices in a tumor submitted for a "melanosome hunt" should reassure the electron microscopist that the tumor is not a melanoma. Second, lest the absence of junctional devices tempt one to consider a diagnosis of lymphoma, melanoma cells generally have more pleomorphic nuclei, greater amounts of cytoplasm, and a richer organelle content than do lymphomas. Third, occasional melanomas contain microtubules within the lumina of cytoplasmic rough endoplasmic cisterns, and these filaments may condense into "crystalloid" arrangements (Fig. 3-55). Such structures, when present, may bolster interest in hunting for melanosomes.

Melanosomes may occur, rarely, in tumors other than melanoma. These include pigmented schwannomas[59,72] and melanotic neuroectodermal tumors of infancy.[320] Both subjects are discussed in the section on peripheral small cell tumors.

*Text continues on page 141.*

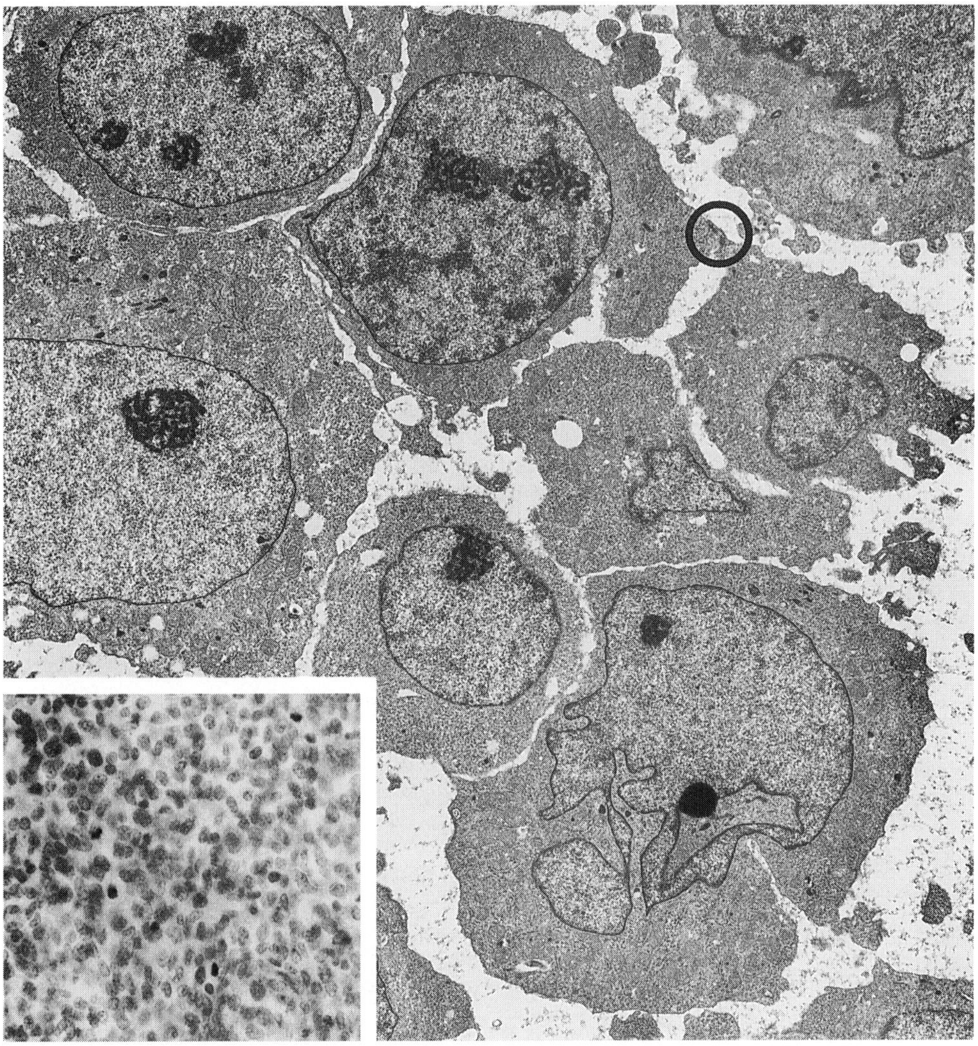

**Fig. 3-50.** Melanoma metastatic to left frontal lobe of a 45-year-old man. The tumor cells in this example are loosely cohesive, with sparse intercellular junctions (*circle*). Initially interpreted as a poorly differentiated carcinoma, this case was proved to be a melanoma on subsequent rebiopsy. **Inset**, Histologic appearance of tumor. (**Fig.**, ×4550; **Inset**, ×220.)

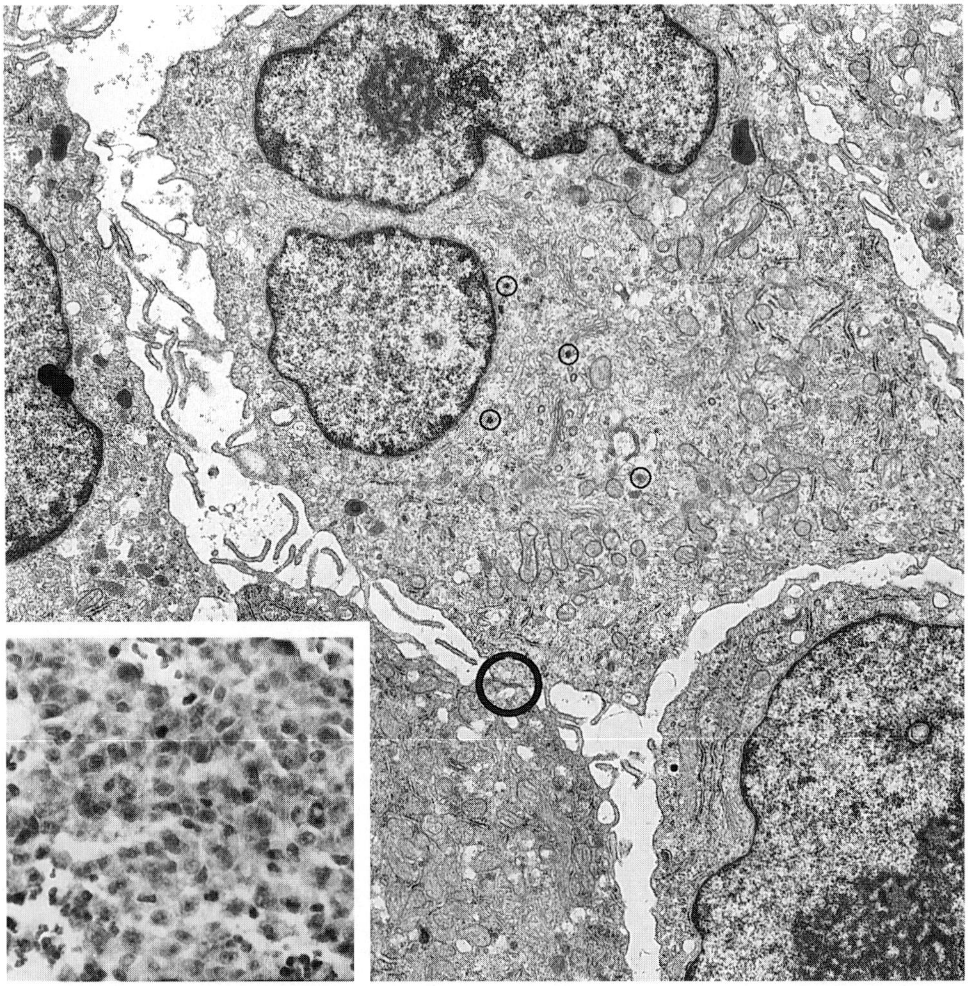

**Fig. 3-51.** Melanoma metastatic to right frontal lobe in a 57-year-old man. The tumor cells are again loosely cohesive, with sparse intercellular junctions (*large circle*). The cytoplasm is somewhat richer in organelles than that of lymphomas, and these organelles include scattered electron-dense bodies (*small circles*). **Inset**, Histologic appearance of tumor. (**Fig.**, ×8740; **Inset**, ×220.)

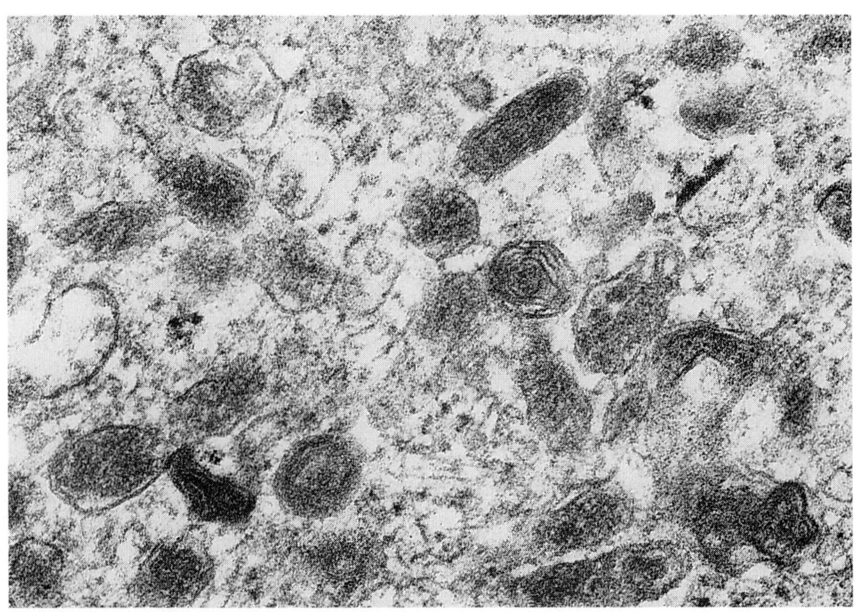

**Fig. 3-52.** Melanoma (same case as Fig. 3-51). Several diagnostic intermediate melanosomes are present, showing longitudinal or circular filamentous structures with a transverse periodicity and bounded by a unit membrane. (×62,400.)

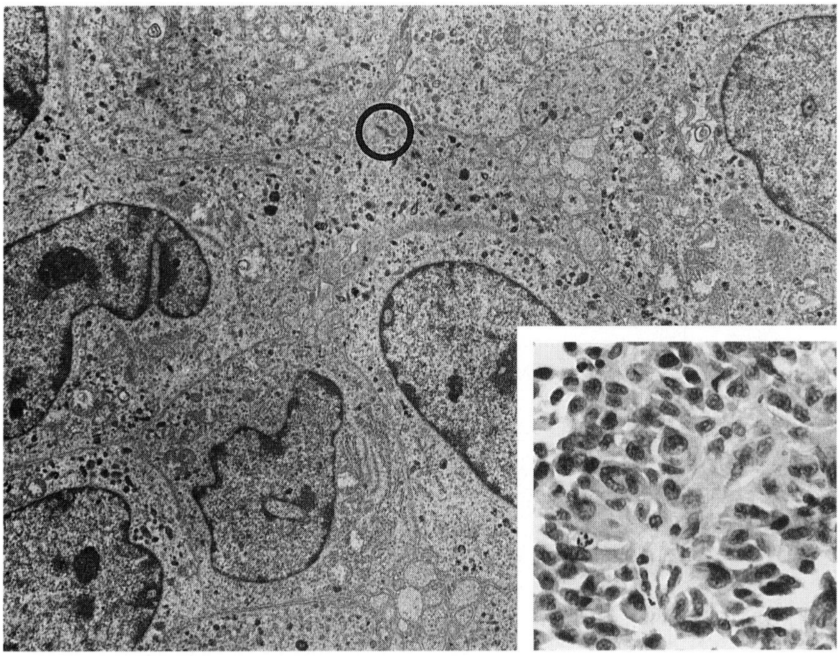

**Fig. 3-53.** Melanoma metastatic to parieto-occipital lobe in a 62-year-old man. The tumor cells here are closely apposed to one another, but intercellular junctions are again infrequent (*circles*). Numerous electron-dense cytoplasmic bodies suggest (but do not establish) a diagnosis of melanoma. **Inset**, Histologic appearance of tumor. (**Fig.**, ×4050; **Inset**, ×195.)

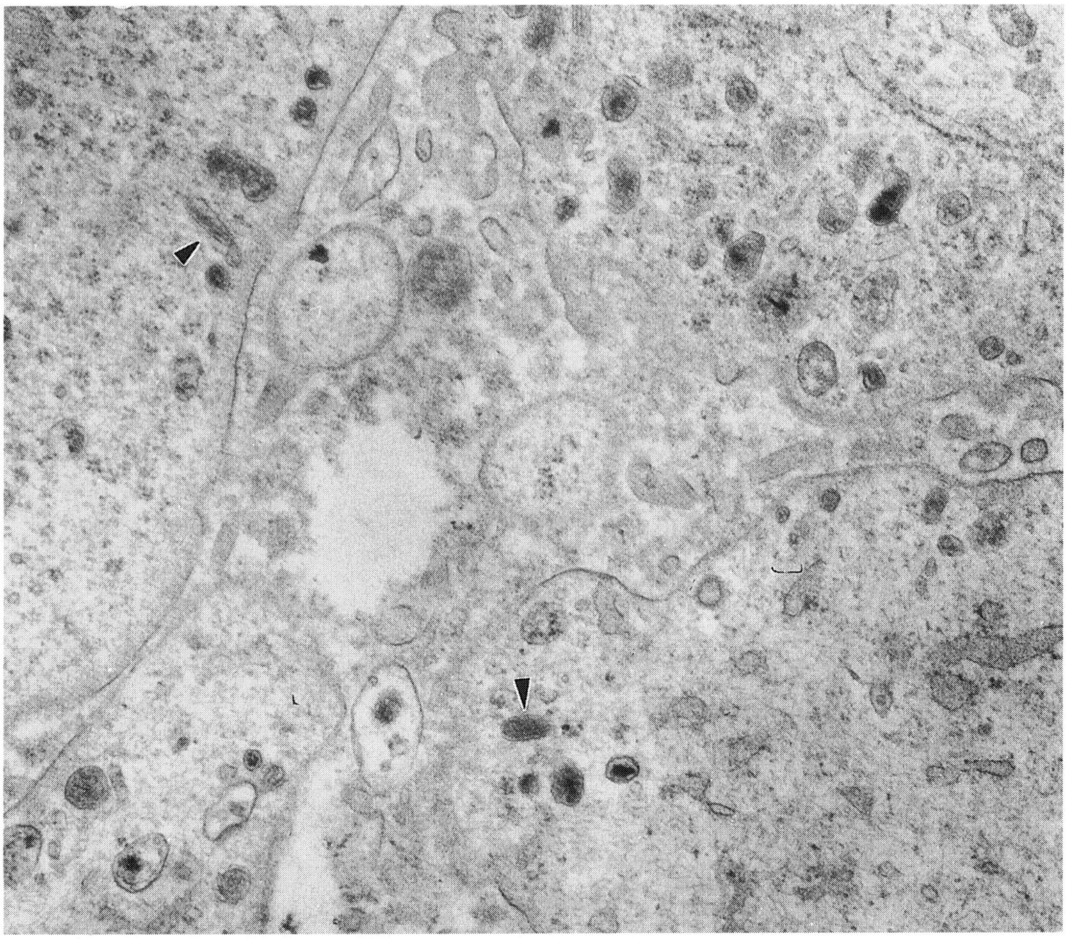

**Fig. 3-54.** Melanoma (same case as Fig. 3-54). Most of the small, dark structures shown here are probably melanosomes, but only a few show the diagnostic internal filaments with transverse periodicity (*arrowheads*). (×27,000.)

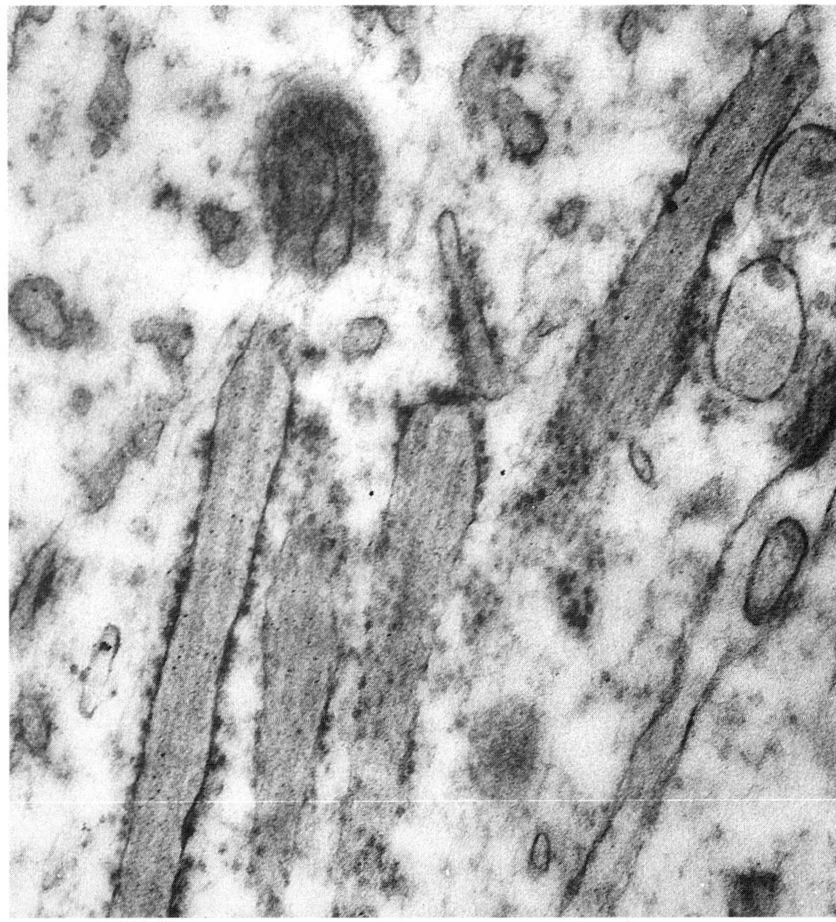

**Fig. 3-55.** Microtubules within the lumina of cytoplasmic rough endoplasmic cisterns ("crystalloids") in a malignant melanoma metastatic to the ovary of a 47-year-old woman. Note also presence of an atypical melanosome. (×63,400.)

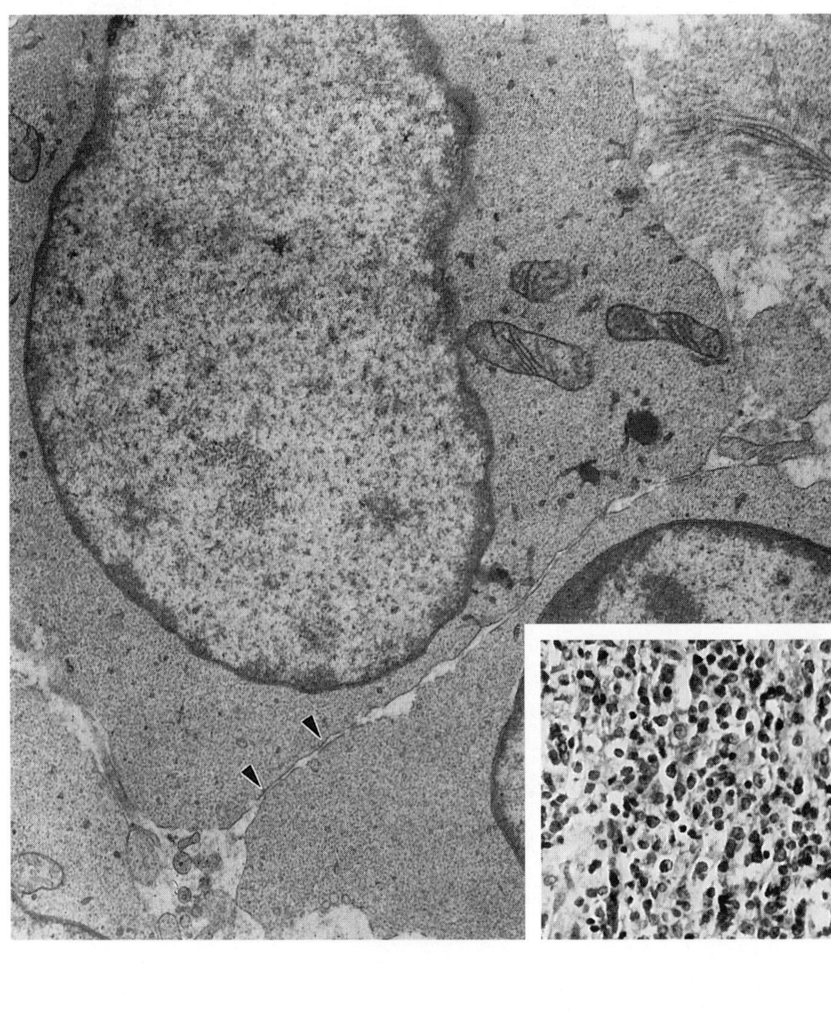

**Fig. 3-56.** Large cell lymphoma in the chest wall of a 58-year-old man. The homogeneous, organelle-poor, gray-appearing cytoplasm (reflecting innumerable polyribosomes) is characteristic. Focal slight "thickenings" of the plasma membranes (*arrowheads*) are artifacts and do not represent intercellular junctions. **Inset,** Histologic appearance of tumor. (**Fig.**, ×10,500; **Inset**, ×195.)

### Lymphoma

Lymphomas[134,315] are, ultrastructurally, a diagnosis of exclusion. Their constituent cells are distinguished more by what they do not show than by what they do. Thus, lymphomas never have junctional devices. The discovery of even one unequivocal junction involving one unequivocal tumor cell is sufficient to rule out lymphoma. Lymphoma cells do not have epithelial features (lumina, microvilli, cilia, etc.), although they do have irregular cytoplasmic projections along their surfaces that may be florid in rare "anenome cell" or "filiform" lymphomas.[8,18,75,334,361] Lymphoma cells do not have any distinctive cytoplasmic organelles. What they do have is a high nuclear-to-cytoplasmic ratio and an abundance of free polyribosomes, giving the cytoplasm a homogeneous medium- to dark-gray appear-

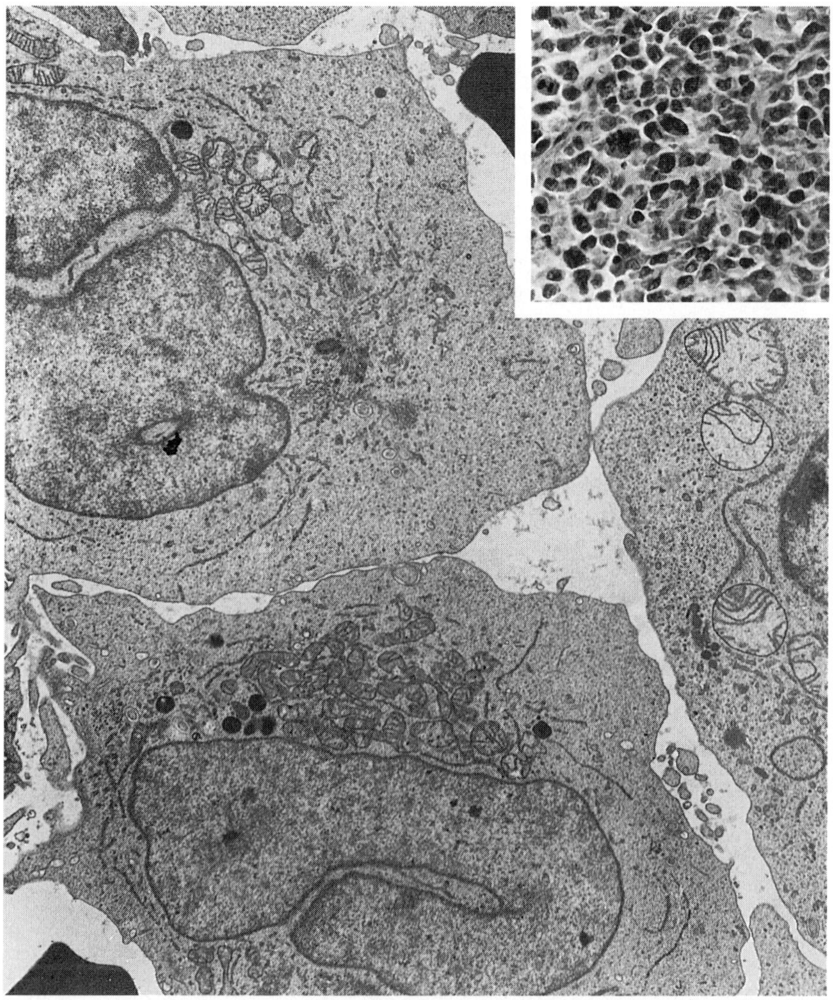

**Fig. 3-57.** Large cell lymphoma in an axillary lymph node of a 58-year-old man. This tumor is somewhat richer in cytoplasmic organelles than that shown in Fig. 3-56, but the homogeneous gray cytoplasm and lack of intercellular junctions are again seen. **Inset**, Histologic appearance of tumor. (**Fig.**, ×6250; **Inset**, ×195.)

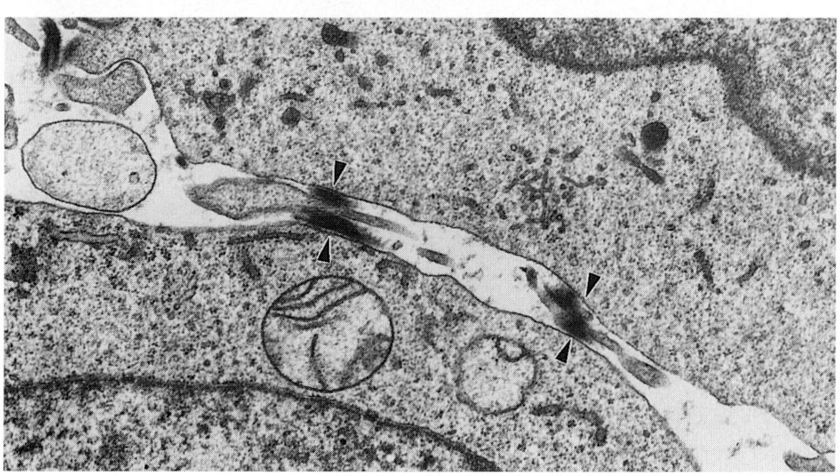

**Fig. 3-58.** Large cell lymphoma (same case as Fig. 3-57). Intercellular deposits of fibrin (*arrowheads*) should not be mistaken for junctions or for basal lamina material. (×15,400.)

ance at low magnification (Figs. 3-56 to 3-58). This appearance is characteristic and distinctive once one has seen it several times, but it is not diagnostic. Lymphoma cells also have a few scattered mitochondria; short, usually single cisterns of rough endoplasmic reticulum; and, occasionally, small, perinuclear collections of filaments of the type seen from time to time in epithelial and mesenchymal tumor cells. True *histiocytic lymphomas*, which are quite rare, may show well-developed Golgi apparatus with associated lysosomes.*

Primary cerebral lymphomas are ultrastructurally similar to extracerebral examples.[50,147,167,177]

* Refs. 75, 92, 247, 370, 383, 384.

## OLIGODENDROGLIOMA-LIKE TUMORS

Oligodendrogliomas are rather undistinguished tumors ultrastructurally, and the histogenesis and nosology of these tumors have recently been questioned.[269a] The features of oligodendrogliomas may be contrasted with histologically similar, primary intracerebral tumors of adults that show clear evidence of neuronal differentiation by electron microscopy.[56,128,273,374,403] These recently recognized tumors, presenting in adults as calcified intraventricular masses, appear to have relatively favorable prognosis and are now known as central neurocytomas.[128,273,374] A malignant counterpart to these tumors exists, distinguished from benign neurocytomas by its diffuse cerebral spread and histologic features of malignancy, and distinguished from childhood neuroblastomas by its larger cell size (with a histologic resemblance to malignant oligodendroglioma) and by its occurrence in adolescents and adults.[258a] In contrast to these oligodendroglioma-like tumors, the common, highly malignant small cell variant of glioblastoma may, in some cases, represent not a glial tumor at all, but instead a high-grade neuroblastoma of adults.[276,406] Finally a *clear cell variant of ependymoma* histologically resembles oligodendroglioma.[191,328] These tumors show under the EM, ependymal features as described in the section on central spindle cell tumors.

### Oligodendroglioma

Oligodendrogliomas* are composed of small round cells that may have a few, short, branching processes (Figs. 3-59, 3-60). The tumor cell cytoplasm generally contains only sparse organelles, although occasionally there are abundant mitochondria, microtubules, or ribosomes. Microfilaments and secretory vesicles are absent in these tumor cells. These tumors are thus rather undistinguished ultrastructurally, and this diagnosis is to some extent one of exclusion. Exceptionally, an oligodendroglioma may show concentric membrane laminations reminiscent of myelin formation.[168,306] Unfortunately, these laminations are not only rare, but nonspecific,[189] and consequently of limited diagnostic value.

* Refs. 74, 94, 168, 220, 221, 294, 316.

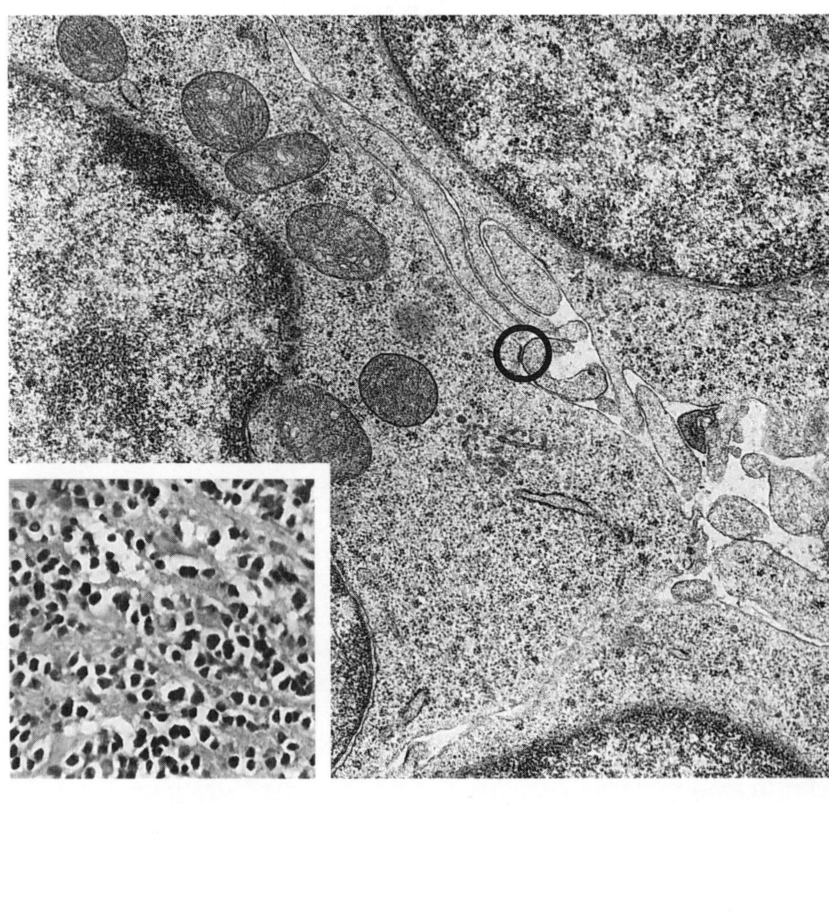

**Fig. 3-59.** Cerebral oligodendroglioma in a 60-year-old man. Ultrastructurally undistinguished cells containing polyribosomes and a few mitochondria. A few short, blunt cell processes are present, and occasional junctions can be found (*circle*). **Inset**, Histologic appearance of tumor. (**Fig.**, ×17,800; **Inset**, ×195.)

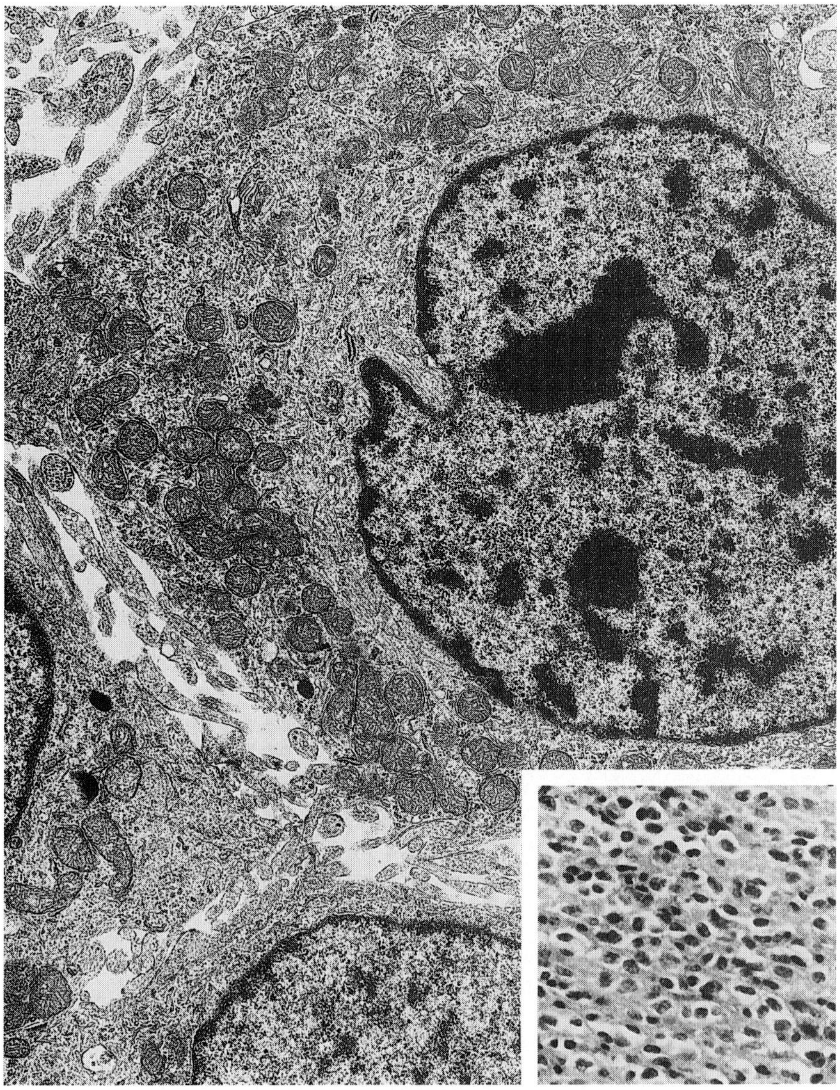

**Fig. 3-60.** Oligodendroglioma of the right frontal lobe in an adult man. This tumor contains more mitochondria than the one shown in Fig. 3-59. **Inset,** Histologic appearance of tumor. (**Fig.**, ×10,900; **Inset**, ×195.)

## Central Neurocytoma

Central neurocytoma is a recently-described benign tumor, often calcified and usually found in the lateral ventricles of young adults.[56,128,273,374,403] These tumors consist of cells with small, uniform nuclei and clear cytoplasm that are easily mistaken for oligodendrogliomas on histologic examination. Ultrastructurally, there is striking neurocytic differentiation, including microtubule-containing cell processes (neurites) and synapse- and synaptic boutonlike contacts between cells (Figs. 3-61 to 3-63). These ultrastructural features easily establish the correct diagnosis (for comparison, see the descriptions of central and peripheral neuroblastomas).

## Malignant Neurocytic Tumor

This recently described tumor[258b] shares the ultrastructural features of central neurocytoma, but differs in having an obviously malignant presentation (a diffuse cerebral tumor), a distinct and clearly malignant histologic appearance (with vague oligodendrocytic features but with obvious cytologic malignancy), and a rapidly lethal clinical course (death within months). Clinically and histologically these tumors are likely to be confused with glioblastoma or malignant oligodendroglioma rather than central neurocytoma. Ultrastructurally, both the resemblance to central neurocytoma and the distinction from either glioblastoma or malignant oligodendroglioma are readily apparent (Figs. 3-64 to 3-68).

*Text continues on page 149.*

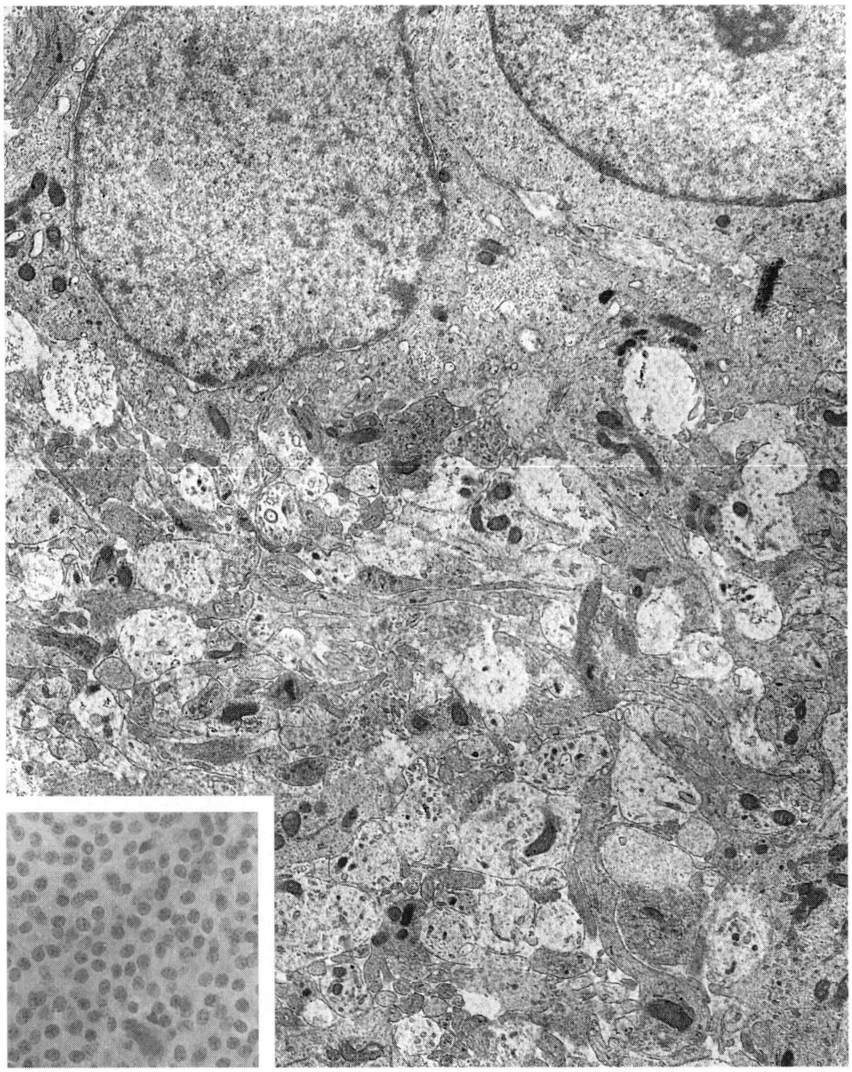

**Fig. 3-61.** Central neurocytoma presenting as a calcified mass in the lateral ventricle of a 32-year-old woman. Patient remained asymptomatic 3 years after partial resection of tumor with no postoperative radio- or chemotherapy. Note numerous cross- and longitudinally sectioned cell processes (neurites) filling the interperikaryal space (lower half of figure). **Inset**, Histologic appearance of tumor. (**Fig.**, ×8750; **Inset**, ×195.)

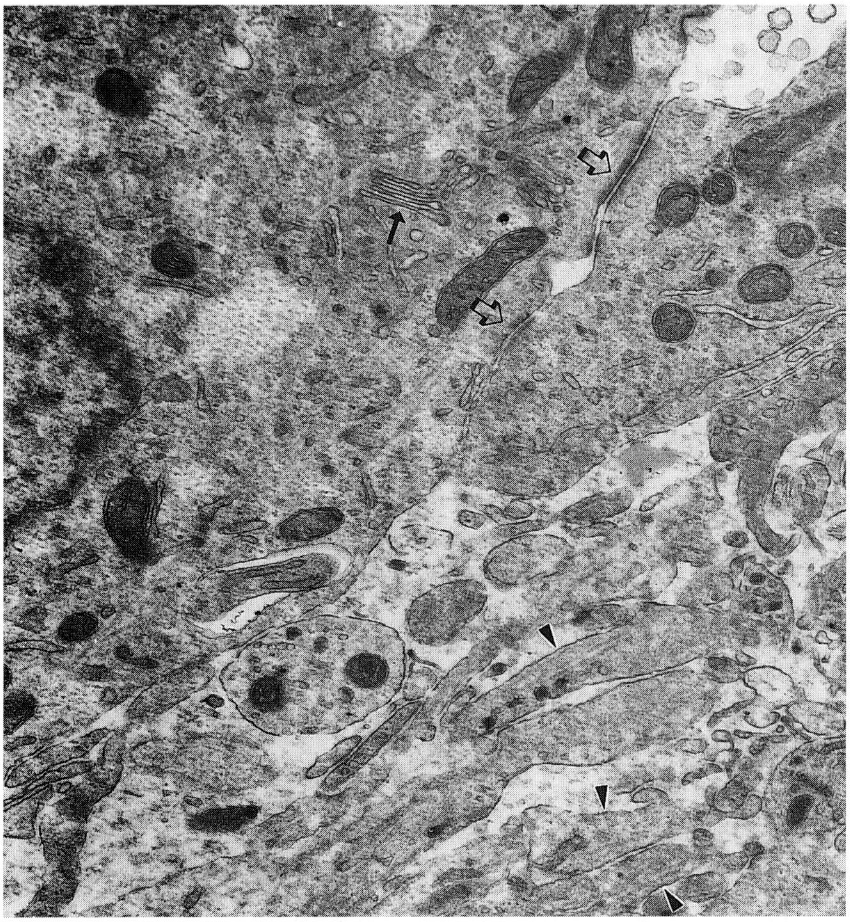

**Fig. 3-62.** Central neurocytoma (same case as Fig. 3-61). Neuronal features include synapselike intercellular junctional devices (*open arrows*), Nissl-like stacks of endoplasmic reticulum (*closed arrow*), and microtubules within neuritic cell processes (*arrowheads*). (×23,150.)

A

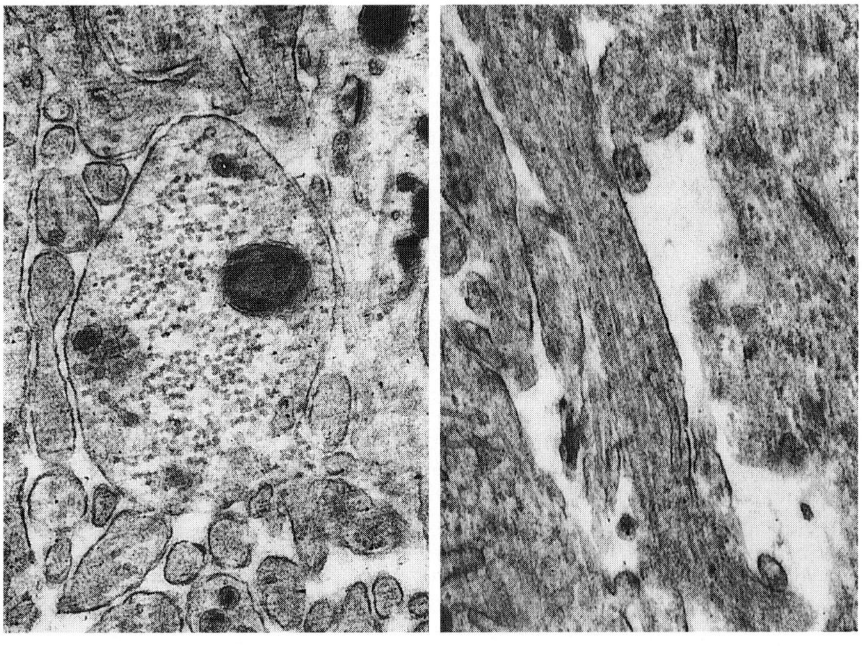

B

**Fig. 3-63.** Central neurocytoma (same case as Fig. 3-61). **A**, Synaptic boutonlike structure filled with small, uniform, empty-appearing synaptic-type vesicles (*center*) surrounded by microtubule-containing neuritic cell processes. **B**, Longitudinally sectioned cell process (neurite) containing oriented parallel microtubules. (**A**, ×43,500; **B**, ×43,500.)

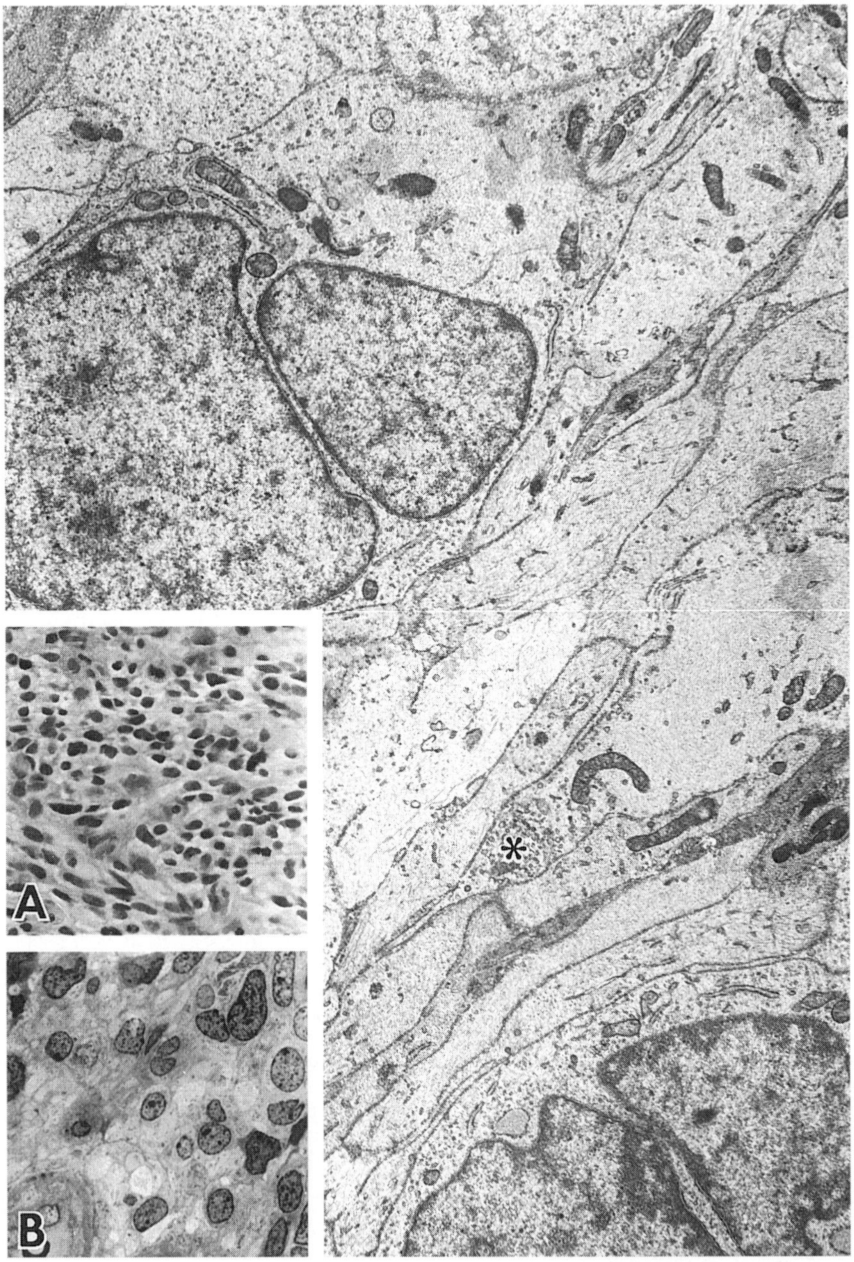


**Fig. 3-64.** Malignant neurocytic tumor. Striking neurocytic differentiation in a diffuse frontal lobe tumor in a 14-year-old girl. The tumor cells have irregular nuclei with a moderate amount of perikaryal cytoplasm. Numerous long, slender, microtubule-containing neurite-like processes are found in the interperikaryal areas. One of these (*asterisk*) contains clear synaptic type vesicles. The ultrastructural features of this tumor are similar to those of benign, intraventricular tumors of young adults that have been designated "neurocytomas." **Inset A**, Histologic appearance of tumor. **Inset B**, Semithin section of epoxy-embedded material. Some of the tumor cell processes can be resolved by light microscopy in such plastic sections. (**Fig.**, ×7775; **Inset A**, ×195; **Inset B**, ×485.)

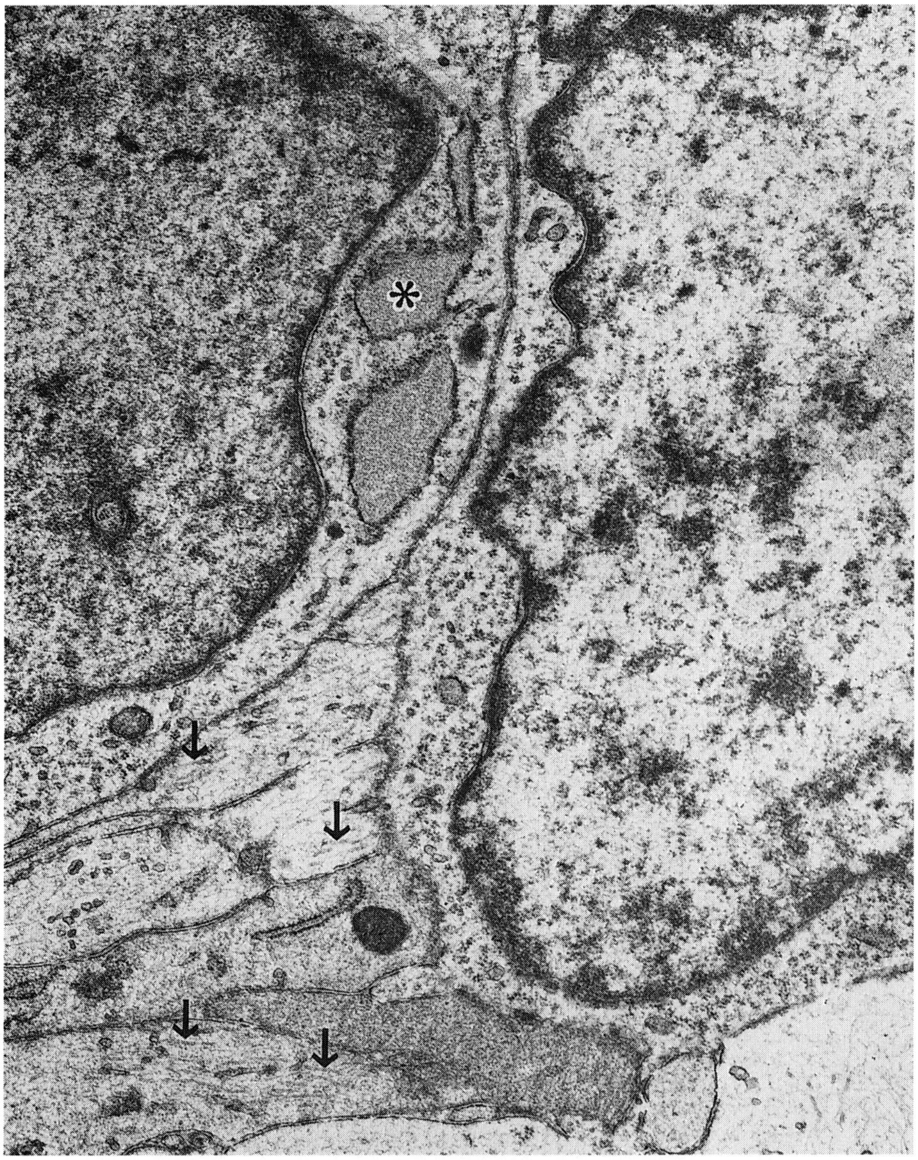

**Fig. 3-65.** Malignant neurocytic tumor (same case as Fig. 3-64). The microtubule-containing processes are well demonstrated at this magnification (*arrows*). The perikaryal areas contain occasional collections of rough endoplasmic reticulum cisterns (*asterisk*) reminiscent of Nissl substance. (×17,300.)

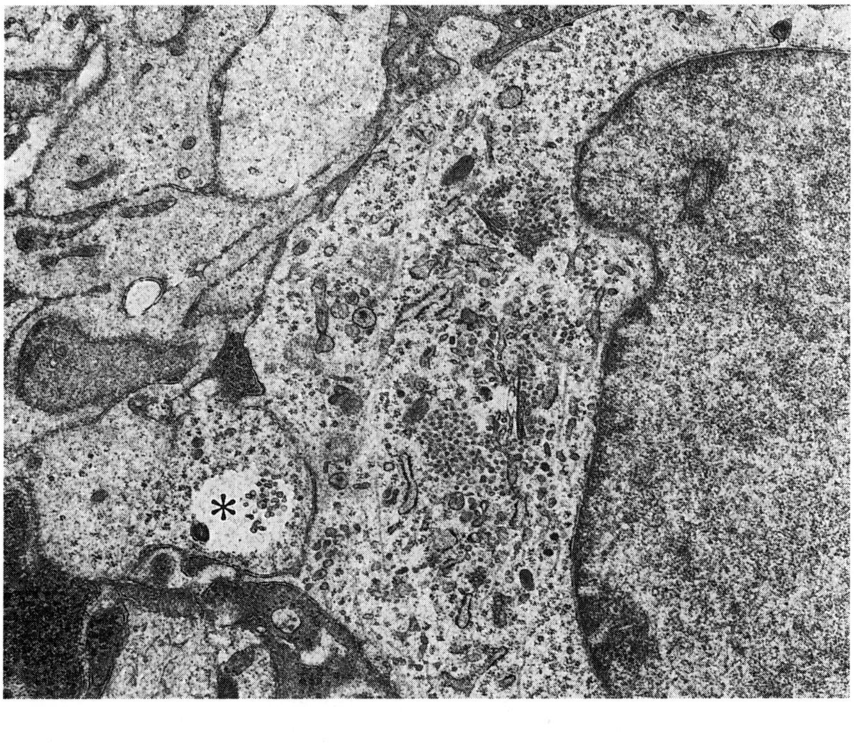

**Fig. 3-66.** Malignant neurocytic tumor (same case as Fig. 3-64). A cellular process (*asterisk*) containing clear synaptic-type vesicles abuts a tumor cell perikaryon. (×12,150.)

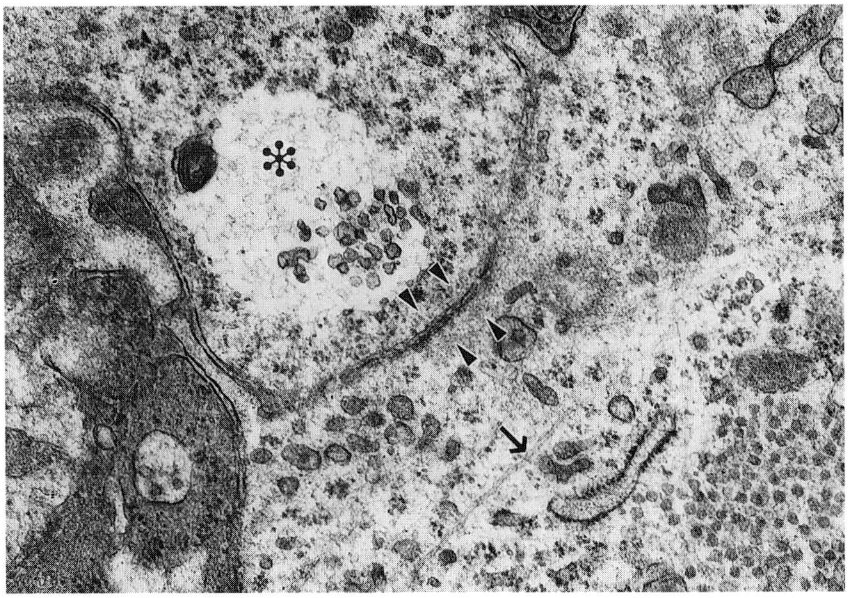

**Fig. 3-67.** Malignant neurocytic tumor. Detail of Fig. 3-66 showing synapselike structure. The vesicle-containing process (*asterisk*) and the adjacent tumor cell perikaryon show some membrane thickening where they meet (*arrowheads*), reminiscent of synaptic contact. Note microtubule (*arrow*) in tumor cell cytoplasm. (×30,000.)

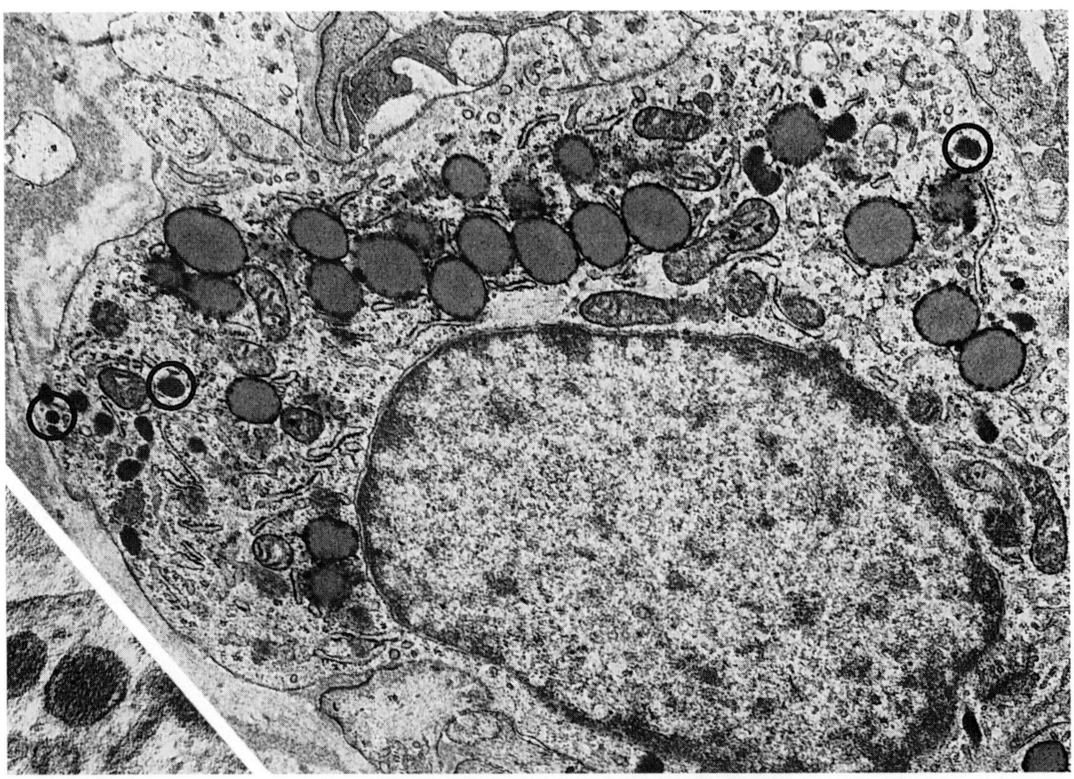

**Fig. 3-68.** Malignant neurocytic tumor (same case as Fig. 3-64). Dense-core neurosecretory-type granules are found within the perikaryon of a tumor cell (*circles*). **Inset**, Detail showing dense-core granules with limiting unit membranes. (×77,000.)

## CENTRAL SMALL CELL TUMORS OF CHILDHOOD

Few entities encountered in surgical neuropathology are the source of as much confusion and uncertainty as are those tumors composed of small, round, "blue" cells.[16] Indeed, it is common practice to classify these tumors as much on clinical (age of the patient) and anatomic (site) data as on histologic appearance. Thus, similar-appearing tumors in children may be called medulloblastomas when found in the cerebellar vermis, and may be called neuroblastomas or primitive neuroectodermal tumors when found in the cerebral hemispheres. In an elderly adult, a similar-appearing tumor will most likely be called a metastatic pulmonary carcinoma. This system is not an esthetically satisfying approach, and it is not infallible. Thus, truly primitive tumors similar to medulloblastomas are found in the cerebral hemispheres (where they are properly known as primitive neuroectodermal tumors), and true neuroblastomas are found in the cerebellum* as well as in the cerebrum. Some such tumors are neither "primitive" nor neuroblastic but, in fact, are ependymoblastomas.[148,149]

Peripheral small cell tumors (discussed below) may also appear in the central nervous system, either as metastases[385] (lymphoma, Ewing's sarcoma,[96,230,238] rhabdomyosarcoma[96,77]) or rarely as primary tumors (rhabdomyosarcoma).[407] Primary cerebral lymphomas are ultrastructurally similar to lymphomas originating extracerebrally.[50,147,167,177]

Electron microscopy is of great value in classifying (or in some cases even in defining) these small round cell tumors. In the central nervous system, ultrastructural analysis can define the following cell types as components of small cell tumors: undifferentiated cells (medulloblasts or "primitive neuroectodermal cells"), neuroblasts and specialized variants, and ependymoblasts.

* Refs. 37, 148, 150, 284, 330, 408, 409.

### Medulloblastoma and Primitive Neuroectodermal Tumors

Medulloblastomas of the cerebellum* and primitive neuroectodermal tumors of the cerebrum[16,21,124,228] are composed of rather unremarkable, undifferentiated cells with a paucity of distinguishing cytoplasmic features (Fig. 3-69 to 3-71). Intercellular junctional devices are a common feature of medulloblastomas but are apparently less frequent in cerebral primitive neuroectodermal tumors. These junctional devices are usually simple in type (desmosome-like puncta adherens, or larger zonula adherens), although one reported medulloblastoma contained classic desmosomes.[9] Some reports comment on the occurrence of focal differentiation within these tumors, where evidence of neuroblastic, astroglial, or even ependymal differentiation can be discerned[16,28,74,228,258] (see Fig. 3-75). Other reported cases, however, lack such features.[21,231] While focal or rudimentary neuroblastic differentiation is usual in primitive neuroectodermal tumors, well-developed and widespread neuroblastic differentiation should prompt reclassification of a tumor as a neuroblastoma. The ultrastructural identification of neuroblastic or ependymoblastic differentiation within me-

* Refs. 9, 16, 28, 74, 124, 130, 186, 221, 231, 258.

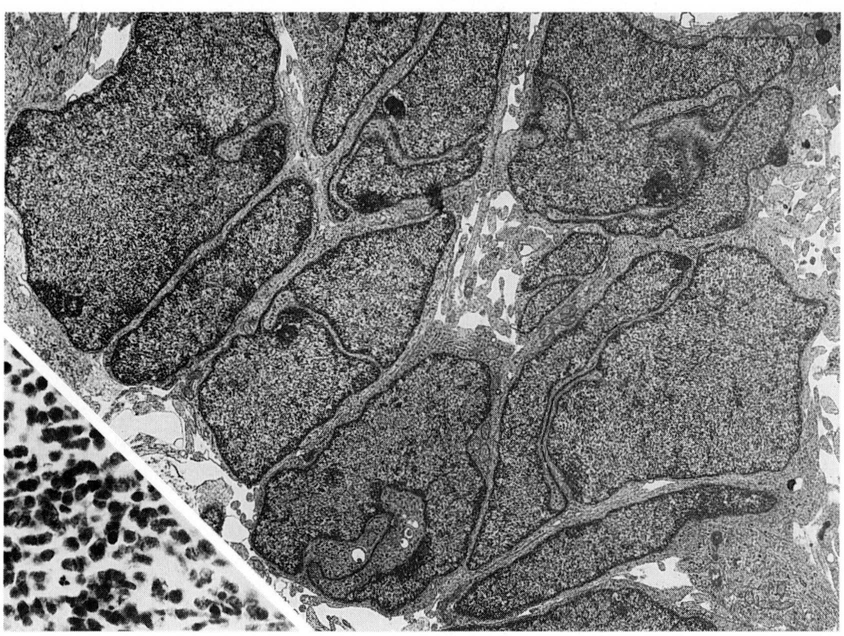

**Fig. 3-69.** Medulloblastoma. Primitive cells with a high nuclear-to-cytoplasmic ratio are closely apposed in some areas, while elsewhere there are tumor cell processes between perikaryal areas. **Inset**, Histologic appearance of tumor. (**Fig.**, ×8750; **Inset**, ×195.)

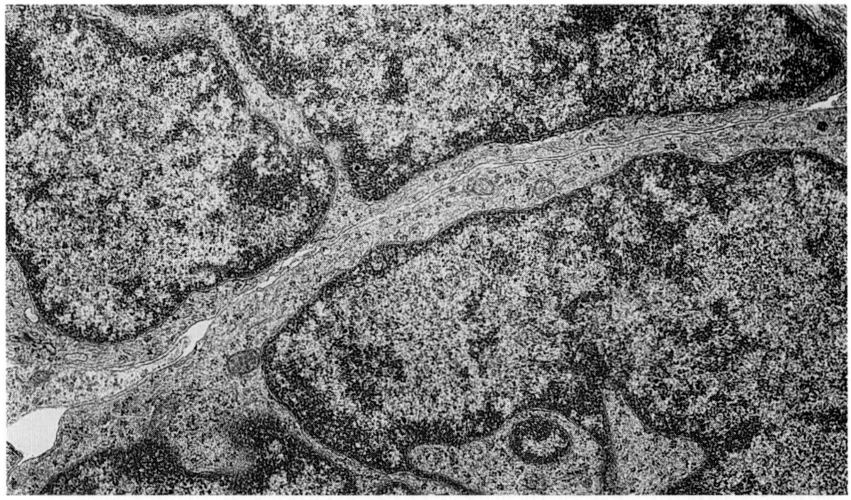

**Fig. 3-70.** Medulloblastoma (same case as Fig. 3-69). The sparse tumor cell cytoplasm contains few distinguishing features. Intercellular junctions are sparse in this example but may be more numerous in some tumors. (×17,800.)

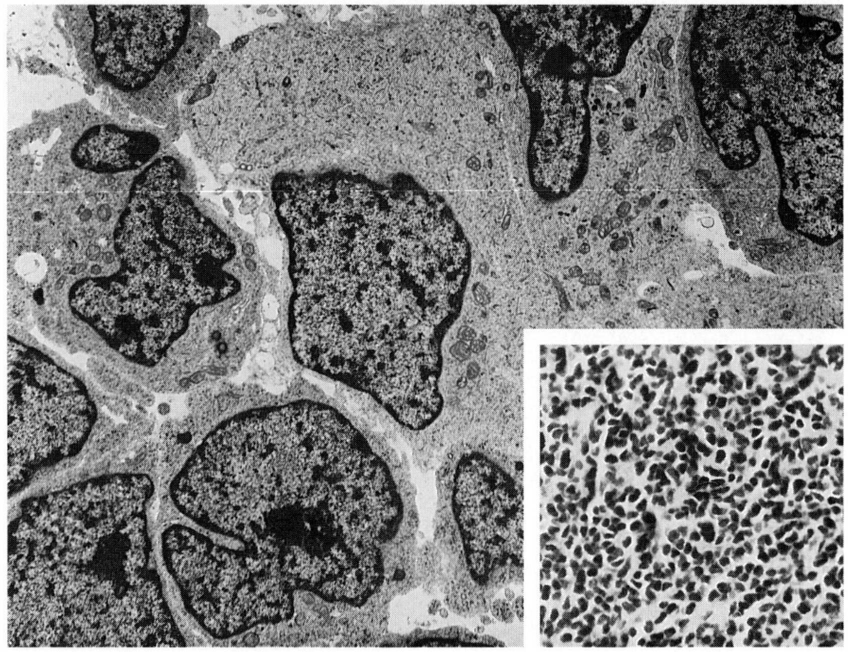

**Fig. 3-71.** Primitive neuroectodermal tumor of cerebrum. Primitive and featureless tumor cells resemble those of cerebellar medulloblastoma. Elsewhere this tumor showed focal neuroblastic differentiation. **Inset**, Histologic appearance of tumor. (**Fig.**, ×5250; **Inset**, ×195.)

dulloblastomas and primitive neuroectodermal tumors is fairly straightforward, according to criteria described below. As always, of course, sampling error is a problem in electron microscopy, and careful correlation of light microscopy (semithin, or one-micron thick sections) with ultrastructure is essential. It is advisable to obtain several samples from different portions of any small cell tumor. In contrast to the ease of identification of the cell types mentioned above, the identification of astroglial differentiation within these tumors is frequently subject to the criticism that the observed astrocytic elements may represent entrapped normal or reactive astrocytes rather than neoplastic components of the tumor.

### Neuroblastoma and Specialized Variants

The diagnosis of neuroblastoma, either in the cerebrum* or in the cerebellum† is frequently dependent on electron microscopy. Indeed, some reported cases were initially misdiagnosed histologically as astrocytoma[246] or polar spongioblastoma.[38] An ependymoma-like histologic appearance has also been reported in some primary brain neuroblastomas.[246] The salient ultrastructural feature of neuroblastoma is the presence of neuritic processes (Fig. 3-72). These are seen as slen-

* Refs. 10, 107, 124, 246, 301, 373.

† Refs. 38, 148, 150, 284, 330, 408, 409.

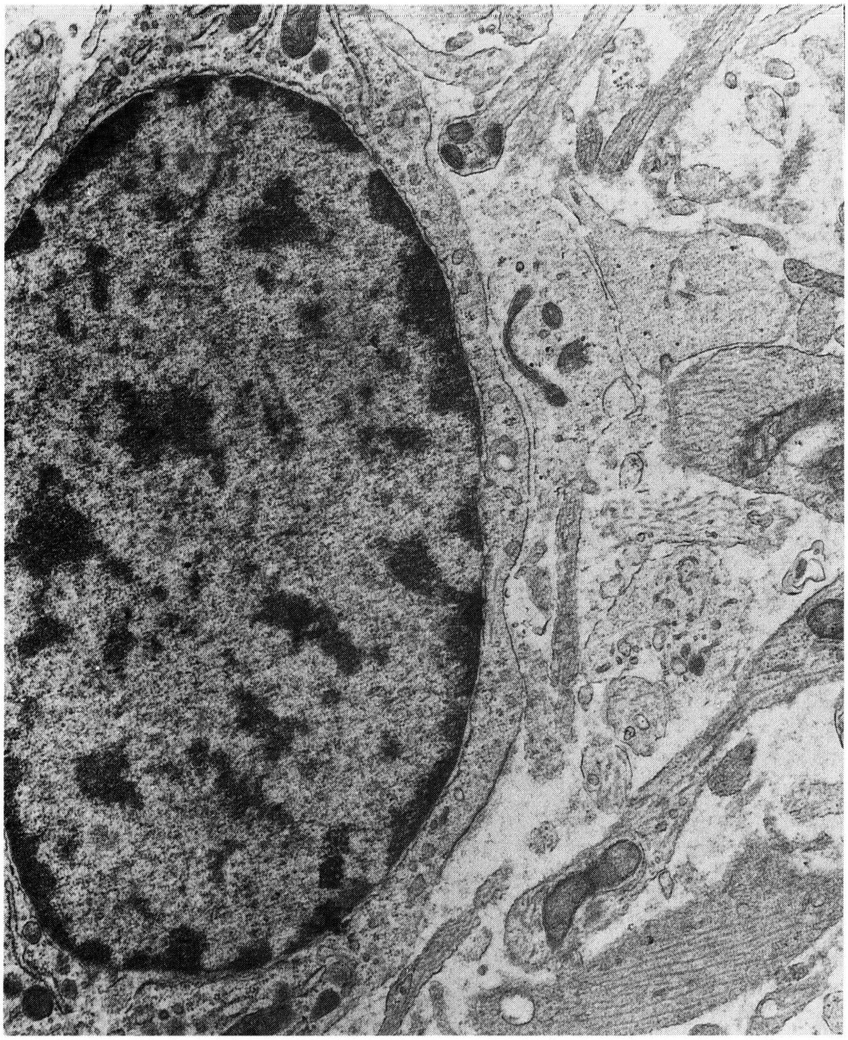

**Fig. 3-72.** Neuroblastoma in the frontal lobe of a 5-year-old boy. Microtubule-containing processes are evident adjacent to a tumor cell perikaryon. (×15,400.)

der cell processes, of more or less constant diameter, present in longitudinal or cross sections that fill the space between adjacent perikarya. Occasionally such masses of processes form an "intercellular" area large enough to be discerned histologically as a Homer Wright rosette. The processes usually contain longitudinally oriented microtubules and variable numbers of dense-core neurosecretory-type granules, although such granules are generally more frequent in the cell perikarya. Some tumors show synapselike contacts between processes or between processes and perikarya, sometimes complete with small, clear vesicles reminiscent of synaptic vesicles. The presence of characteristic neuritic processes in combination with any of the other distinguishing features is strong evidence of a neuroblastic histogenesis. Oligodendrogliomas may show both processes and microtubules, but the processes are short, tapering, and branching, and the microtubules are largely confined to the perikaryal area. Oligodendrogliomas do not contain secretory vesicles, clear vesicles, or synapselike structures. Occasional neuroblastomas show scattered "differentiating" cells with neuronal features (Fig. 3-73).

Specialized variants of neuroblastoma include retinoblastoma, olfactory neuroblastoma, and pineoblastoma. *Retinoblastomas*[62,289,290,377–379] show characteristic evidence of photoreceptor differentiation in the form of rosettes, within which there are: (1) elongated apical mitochondria-filled cytoplasmic extensions (presumably developing inner segment ellipsoids) protruding into the lumen; (2) apical junctional complexes that include tight junctions, reminiscent of epithelial-type terminal bars; and (3) apical cilia with a 9 + 0 microtubule doublet pattern typical of photosensory neurons. These specialized rosettes have been called "fleurettes." In contrast to such ultrastructural specialization in retinoblastomas, descriptions of *olfactory neuroblastomas* (esthesioneuroblastomas) are simi-

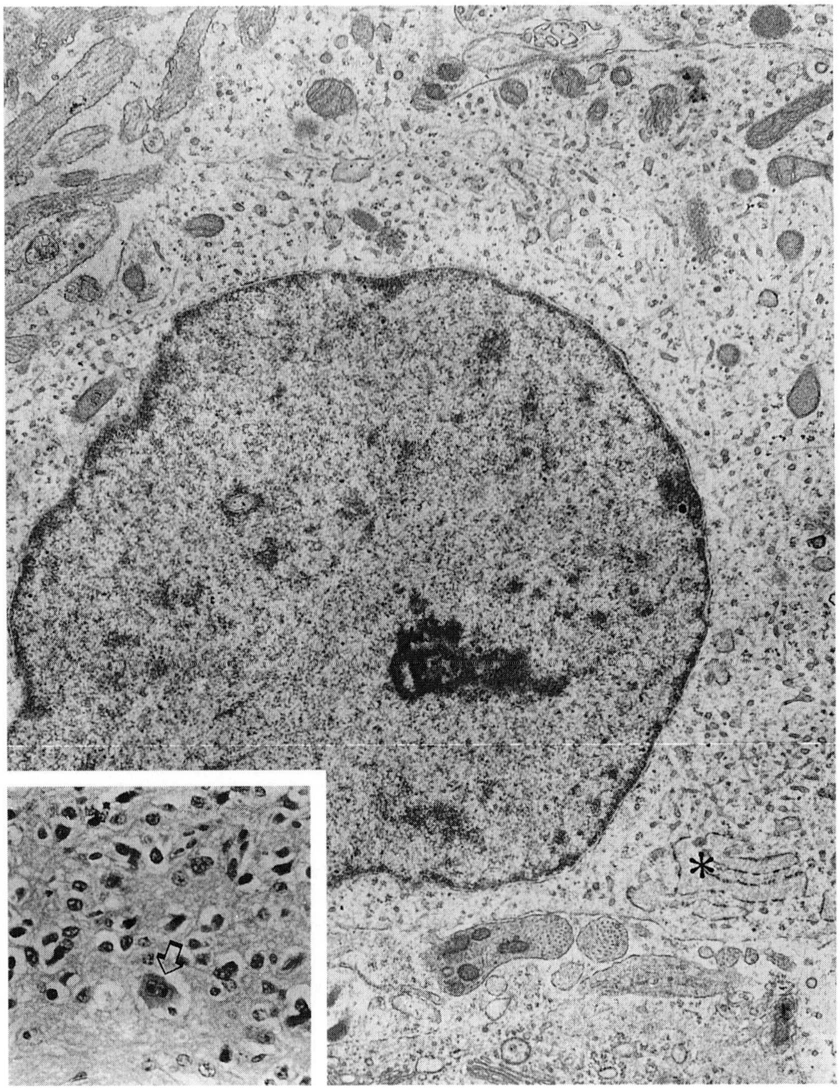

**Fig. 3-73.** Neuronal differentiation in a cerebral neuroblastoma (same case as Fig. 3-72). This tumor cell has an enlarged nucleus with a nucleolus and a moderate amount of cytoplasm, within which there is a Nissl substancelike stack of rough endoplasmic reticulum cisternae (*asterisk*). **Inset**, Histologic preparation shows dysplastic neuron (*arrow*) in an area of relatively low cell density. (**Fig.**, ×10,500; **Inset**, ×195.)

lar to those of nonolfactory neuroblastomas,[39,242,365,366] with the exception of the *neuroendocrine carcinoma* variant of olfactory neuroblastoma.[335a] These latter tumors are found in older patients (mean age 50 years) than the classic olfactory neuroblastomas (mean age 20 years) and resemble paragangliomas. They thus lack the neurites found in olfactory (and other) neuroblastomas, but do contain neurosecretory granules (Fig. 3-74). An *esthesioneuroepithelioma* showed a tubular arrangement with a basal lamina at the periphery of the tubule and microvilli and junctional complexes at the luminal apices. These epithelial features were combined with long tapering cell processes containing microtubules and clear vesicles but without dense-core neurosecretory-type vesicles.[127] *Pineoblastomas* may appear similar to medulloblastomas or primitive neuroectodermal tumors[229] or may show evidence of rudimentary photoreceptor differentiation.[202]

### Pineocytoma

Pineocytomas differ somewhat from the tumors described above. These pineal-derived neoplasms are less densely cellular, containing cells with more abundant cytoplasm. Orientation of tumor cells around

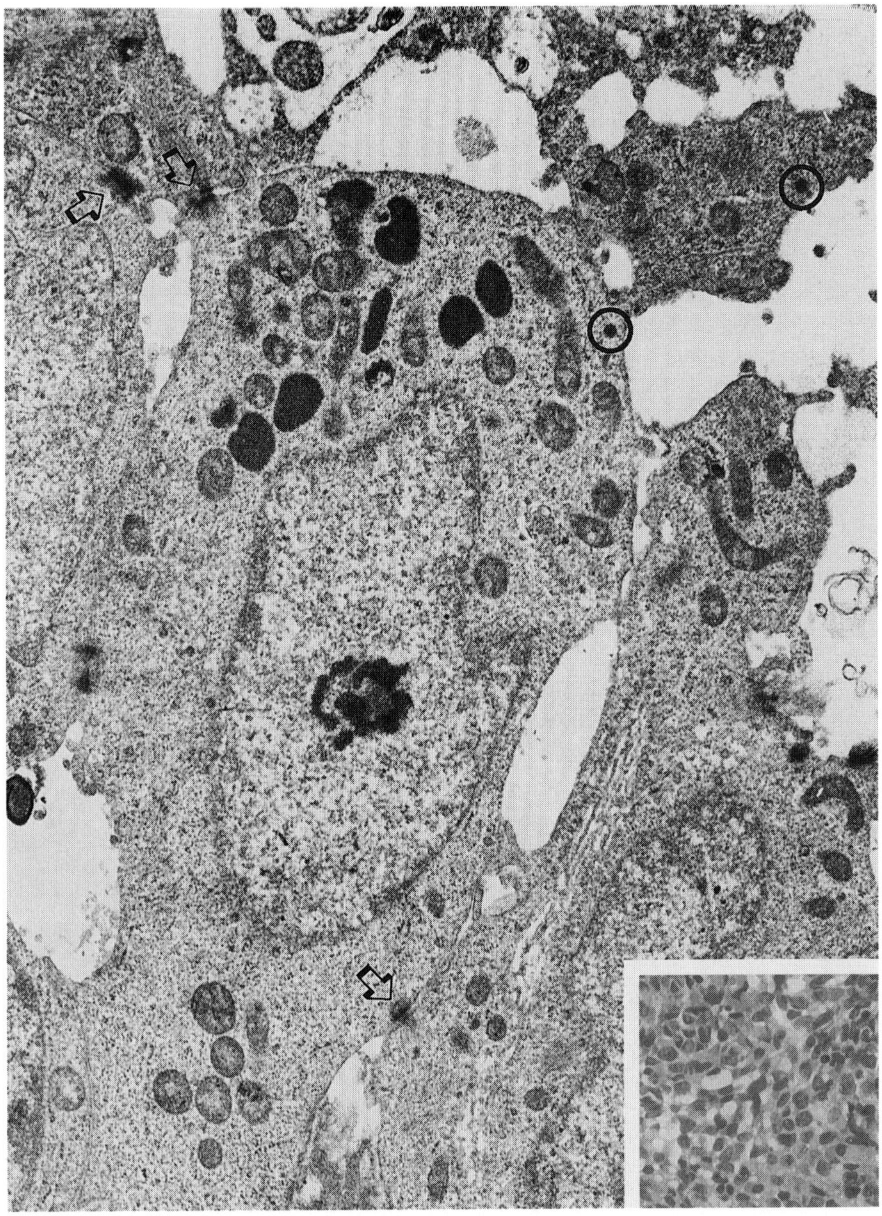

**Fig. 3-74.** Neuroendocrine variant of esthesioneuroblastoma arising in the nasal cavity of a 65-year-old man. Neuroblastic features are confined to sparse neurosecretory granules (*circles*). Intracellular junctional devices (*arrows*) are also present. **Inset**, Histologic appearance of tumor. (**Fig.**, ×12,900; **Inset**, ×230.)

blood vessels is common, producing perivascular pseudorosettes. Ultrastructurally,[129,143,229,271] these tumors show evidence of both astrocytic and neuronal differentiation, the former as cells with filament-rich processes and the latter as cells with microtubule-containing processes, dense-core and clear vesicles, and occasionally linear or arciform synapselike densities adjacent to plasma membranes. The histologic and ultrastructural features of these tumors forms a spectrum that merges with pineoblastoma at one end,[143,229] and with ganglioglioma at the other.[314]

### Ependymoblastoma

Ultrastructural descriptions of ependymoblastomas are sparse.[51,148,149,208] Such tumors may be poorly differentiated medulloblastoma-like tumors by light microscopy,[148,149] may show ependymoma-type perivascular pseudorosettes, or may even show true ependymal rosettes histologically.[51,208] Ultrastructurally, these tumors show minute intercellular lumina with apical basal bodies and adjacent, well-developed apical junctional specializations (Fig. 3-75). Microvilli and cilia are seen in the better-differentiated cases.[51,208]

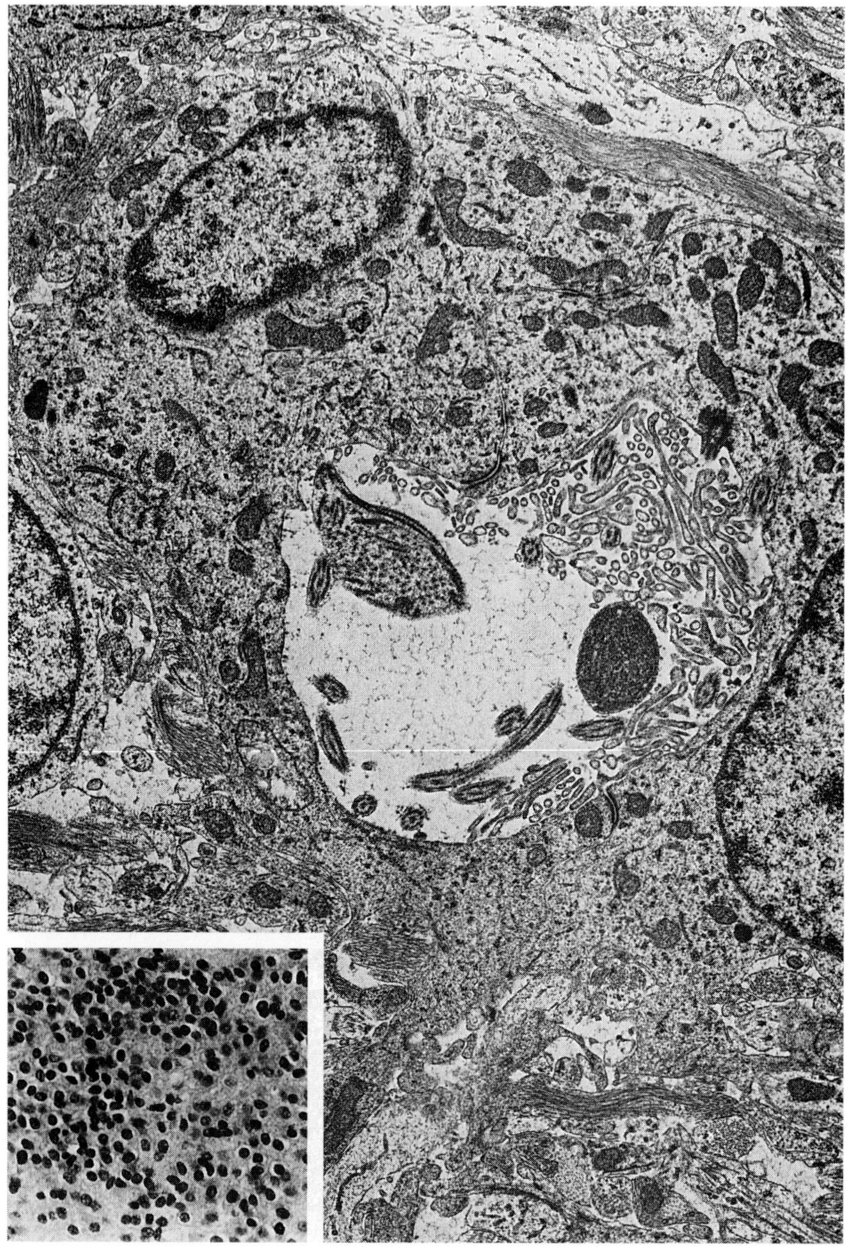

**Fig. 3-75.** Ependymoblastic differentiation in a primitive neuroectodermal tumor. Encapsulated midline cerebellar mass in a 21-month-old boy. Intercellular lumen formation by tumor cells with apical microvilli, cilia, and gap junctions. Adjacent to these cells are numerous fibrillated cell processes. **Inset**, Histologic appearance of tumor. (**Fig.**, ×10,500; **Inset**, ×195.)

## PERIPHERAL SMALL CELL TUMORS OF CHILDHOOD

The differentiation of peripheral small cell tumors is at least as great a problem as the differentiation of central small cell tumors.[376] The childhood tumors neuroblastoma, rhabdomyosarcoma, Ewing's sarcoma, and to a lesser extent lymphoma and nephroblastoma may be confused with one another. Neuroblastomas of bone have been reported both in children[181] and adults.[225,347] A recently described childhood malignant small cell tumor of the thoracopulmonary region ("Askin tumor") may represent a peripheral primitive neuroectodermal tumor.[7,109,216,323] Electron microscopy can be of assistance in distinguishing these tumors. In adults, peripheral small cell tumors are almost always carcinomas, although peripheral neuroblastomas do occur in adults, even into the eighth decade.[224] As is the case with intracranial neuroblastomas, peripheral neuroblastomas appear to follow a somewhat more favorable course in adults.

### Neuroblastoma

Peripheral neuroblastomas* resemble their central counterparts, with minor, mostly quantitative differ-

* Refs. 74, 89, 111, 116, 222–224, 248, 307, 356, 360, 376, 413.

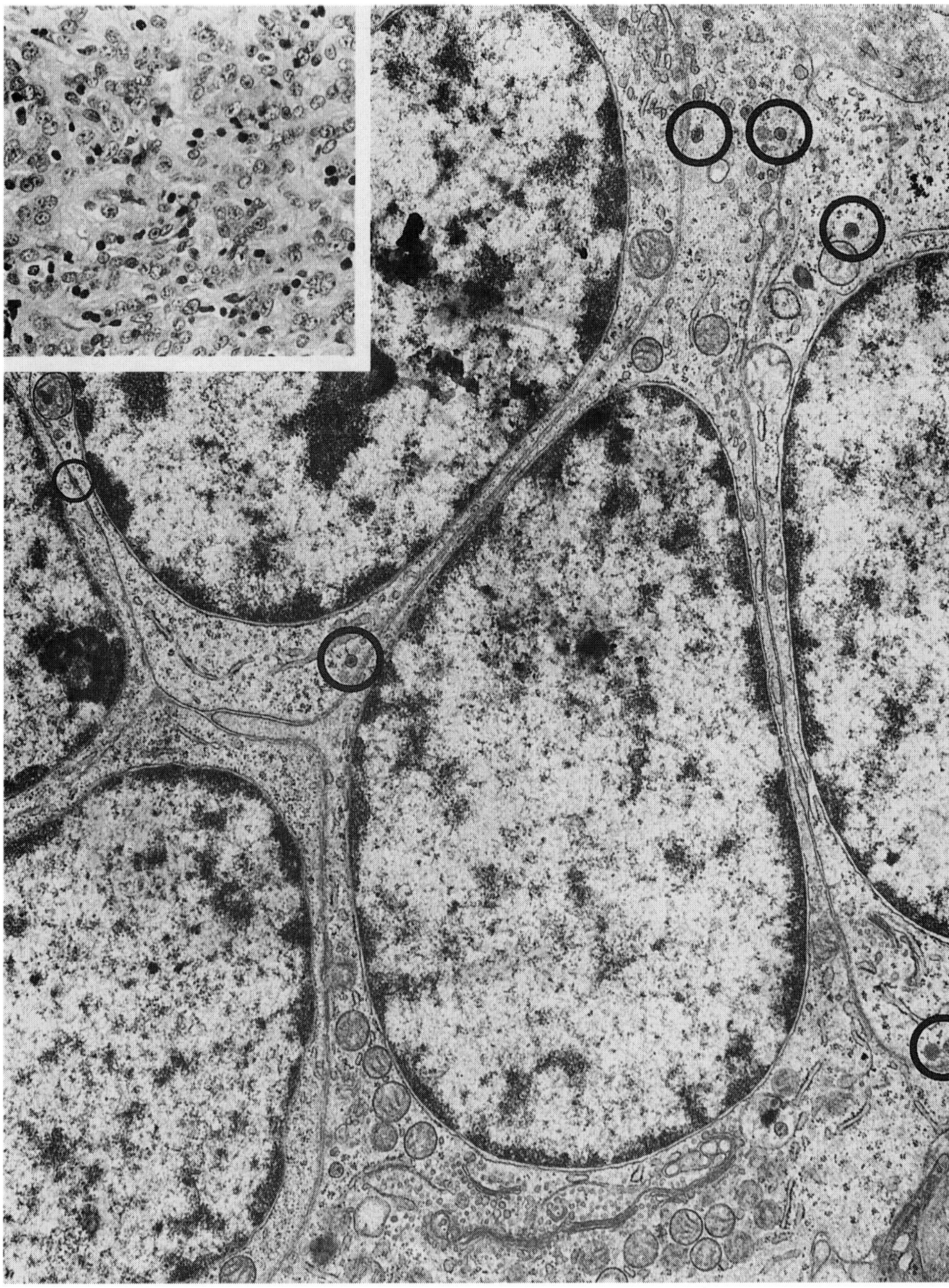

**Fig. 3-76.** Neuroblastoma in a cervical lymph node of a 7-month-old boy. Occasional junctions (*small circle*) and dense core vesicles (*large circles*) are present. There are few neuritic processes in this area. **Inset**, Histologic appearance of tumor. (**Fig.**, ×11,700; **Inset**, ×215.)

ences. In particular, dense-core granules are somewhat more frequent in peripheral neuroblastomas and usually are found clustered in (neuritic) cell processes. Synapselike structures, although described,[222] are quite rare.[246] The presence of cytoplasmic processes with dense-core, neurosecretory-type granules is a constant, well-developed, and diagnostic feature[224,360] (Figs. 3-76 to 3-78), and the prominence of granules in the cell processes (as opposed to the cell perikarya) distinguishes peripheral neuroblastomas from those found in the central nervous system. Small cell carcinomas of adults may also show processes and dense-core granules, but the former are rudimentary and the latter are sparse and scattered in the perinuclear cytoplasm. Processes and granules are not found in other small cell tumors. The number of neuritic processes in peripheral neuroblastomas (but not other ultrastructural features) may correlate with the degree of tumor differentiation.[224]

A rare and generally benign tumor, *melanotic neuroectodermal tumor* of infancy, may present as a small

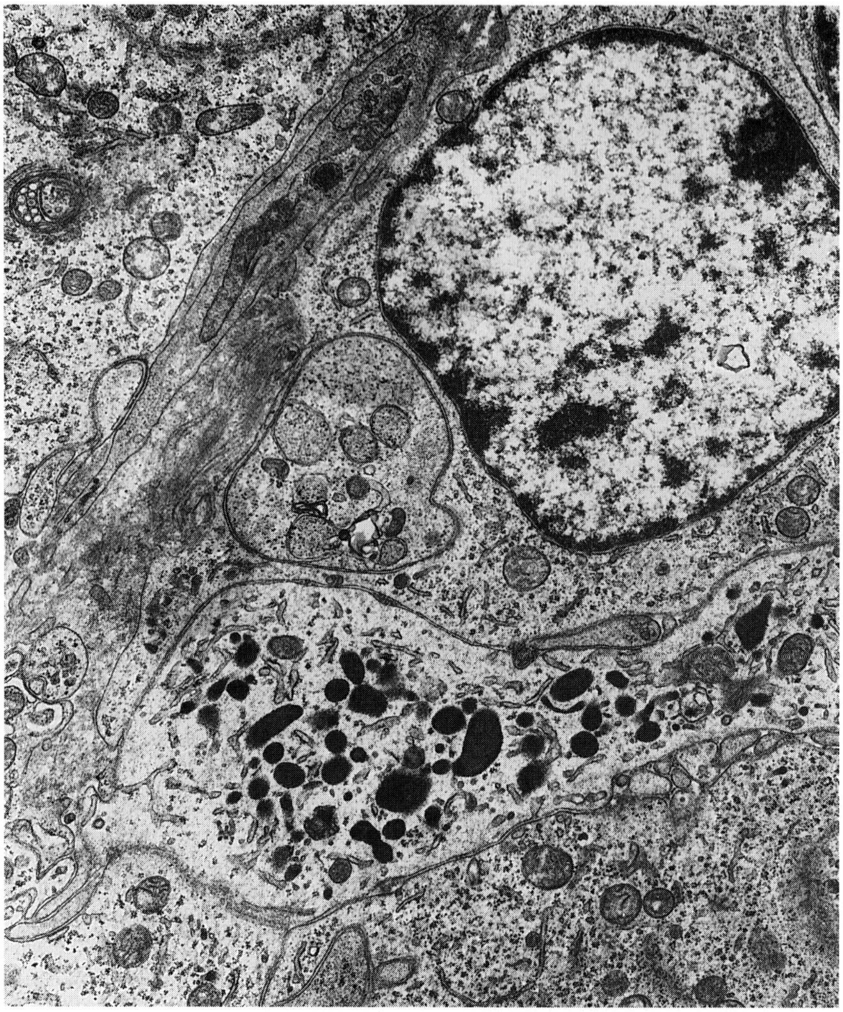

**Fig. 3-77.** Neuroblastoma (same case as Fig. 3-76). A process with dense-core vesicles courses between tumor cell perikarya. (×10,500.)

round cell tumor of bone or soft tissue. These tumors contain both dense-core granule-containing neuroblast-like cells and melanosome-containing cells.[320]

### Rhabdomyosarcoma

The fully developed ultrastructural picture of rhabdomyosarcoma is striking, diagnostic, and immediately recognizable.* The cells in these tumors contain both thick and thin filaments, in parallel array on longitudinal section and in hexagonal array in cross section. Irregular electron-dense masses reminiscent of Z-lines may be present, sometimes arrayed with organized filaments to recapitulate sarcomere formation (Fig. 3-79). There may also be an external lamina investing the tumor cells. Unfortunately, these features, or at least convincing thick and thin filaments, are found in only about one half of histologically diagnosed childhood rhabdomyosarcomas, and even here the diagnostic features may be present in as few as 1% of the tumor cells.[244] A typical case may thus require diligent search for such minimal evidence of skeletal muscle differentiation.

Poorly differentiated rhabdomyosarcomas are a diagnostic problem, one for which there is little agreement as to acceptable criteria. Many authorities[98,252,386] will accept nothing less than thick and thin filaments in a fibrillar array for a confident ultrastructural diagnosis of rhabdomyosarcoma. In contrast, Triche and Askin[376] find these criteria too restrictive and point out that even tangled feltworks of intermediate filaments (Fig. 3-80) weigh against other small cell tumors (neuroblastoma, Ewing's lymphoma). Similarly these au-

* Refs. 26, 46, 73, 162a, 166, 223, 244, 252, 386, 407.

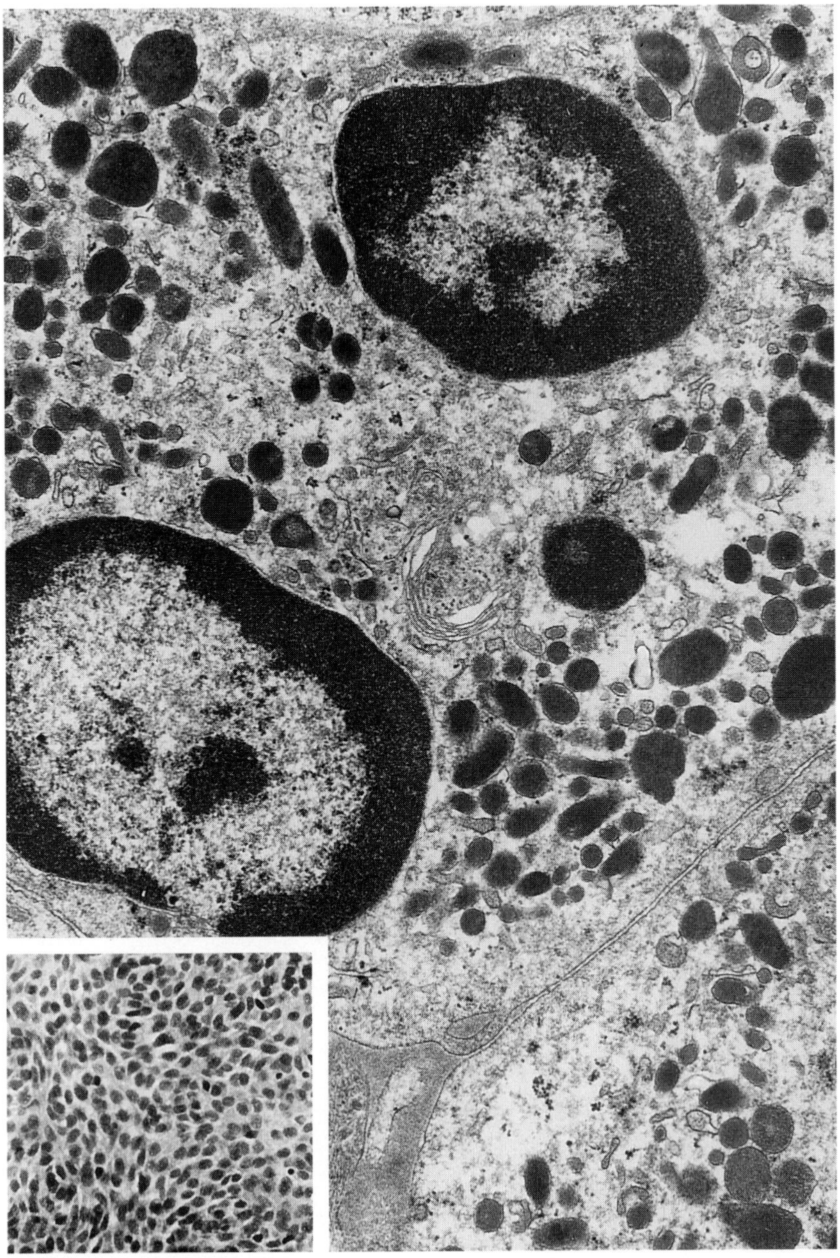

**Fig. 3-78.** Retroperitoneal neuroblastoma in a 14-year-old boy. Numerous dense-core neurosecretory-type vesicles are present in the perinuclear cytoplasm. This specimen was carved from a paraffin block, deparaffinized, and processed for electron microscopy. **Inset**, Histologic appearance of tumor. (**Fig.**, ×26,300; **Inset**, ×195.)

thors suggest that intracytoplasmic phagocytosed collagen, or evidence of an external lamina are diagnostic features of rhabdomyosarcoma within the context of the histologic differential diagnosis of a small, round, "blue cell" tumor.

Even within those rhabdomyosarcomas showing diagnostic thick and thin filaments there may be numerous tumor cells without such filaments. These latter cells resemble Ewing's sarcoma cells,[46] and distinguishing these two tumors can present a serious challenge in differential diagnosis. However, these two tumors do differ somewhat in the appearance of their nuclei. The nuclei of rhabdomyosarcomas generally show greater pleomorphism and more heterochromatin than the typical round, uniform, euchromatic nuclei of Ewing's sarcoma.[73,223]

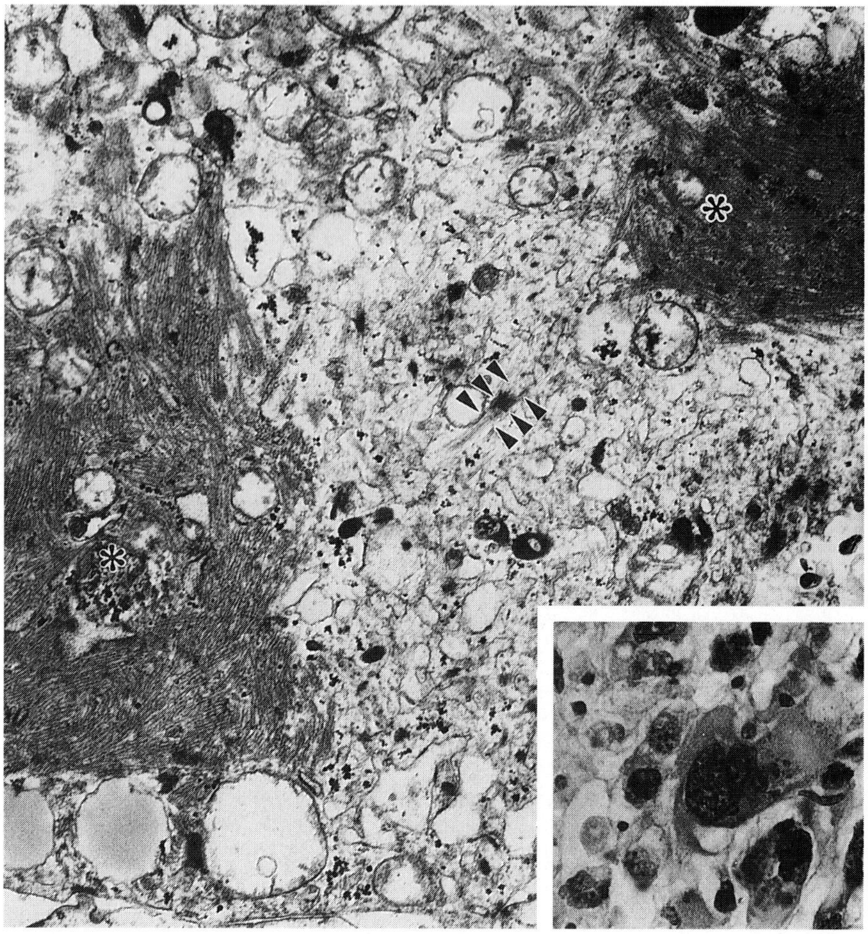

**Fig. 3-79.** Rhabdomyosarcoma metastatic to brain in a 68-year-old man. Autopsy specimen. There are tangled masses of filaments (*asterisks*), including easily identified thick filaments and less obvious thin filaments. Also present are bundles of thin filaments attached to Z-line-like densities (*arrowheads*). **Inset**, By light microscopy this rhabdomyosarcoma is an "adult" pleomorphic type. (**Fig.**, ×13,300; **Inset**, ×200.)

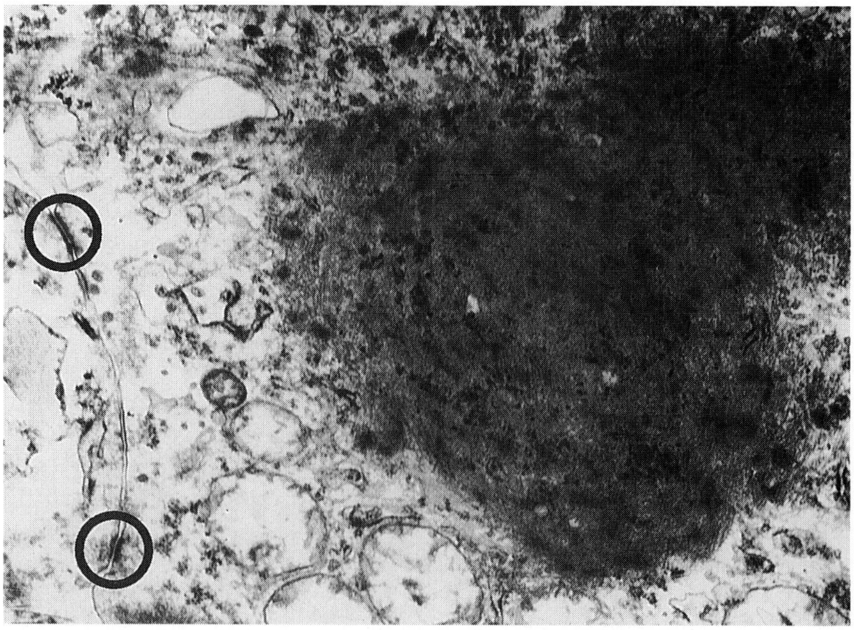

**Fig. 3-80.** Rhabdomyosarcoma (same case as Fig. 3-79). A tangled mass of filaments and irregular electron densities is present, without obvious evidence of sarcomere-like structures. Areas such as these support a diagnosis of rhabdomyosarcoma and should prompt a more thorough search for myofibrillar arrangements. Note intercellular junctions (*circles*). (×17,800.)

## Nephroblastoma (Wilms' Tumor)

Nephroblastomas[13,322,357,375,402] are generally not a diagnostic problem because their site of origin and their specialized histologic features are usually well defined. By electron microscopy these tumors contain undifferentiated (and nondiagnostic) small cells that occasionally arrange themselves into tubular or "pre-tubular" formations that may have diagnostic significance. These arrangements consist of a small group of cells with a surrounding basal lamina and a central lumen. Occasionally these structures may be so rudimentary as to be histologically unresolvable.[357] The lumen-lining cells may also show apical microvilli and lateral intercellular junctional devices. Additional features are the presence of epithelial cell masses reminiscent of glomerular epithelial cells and occasional evidence of mesenchymal (including rhabdomyoblastic) differentiation.[375]

## Ewing's Sarcoma

In contrast to the myriad interesting ultrastructural features of neuroblastoma, rhabdomyosarcoma, and nephroblastoma, Ewing's sarcomas* are rather nondescript. The cells are generally closely apposed to one another, without the cell processes typical of neuroblastic tumors. The cytoplasm is sparse and contains few organelles, the sole distinguishing feature being the presence of large pools of glycogen in most (but not all) cases (Fig. 3-81). Such glycogen granules are generally cited as being *the* distinguishing feature of Ewing's sarcoma, and on a statistical basis this is true. However, glycogen accumulations also can occur in neuroblastomas[415] and other tumors, and may be absent in as many as 14% of Ewing's cases;[227] therefore, neither the presence nor the absence of glycogen con-

* Refs. 58, 73, 88, 89, 105, 115, 169, 219, 223, 227, 292, 352, 401.

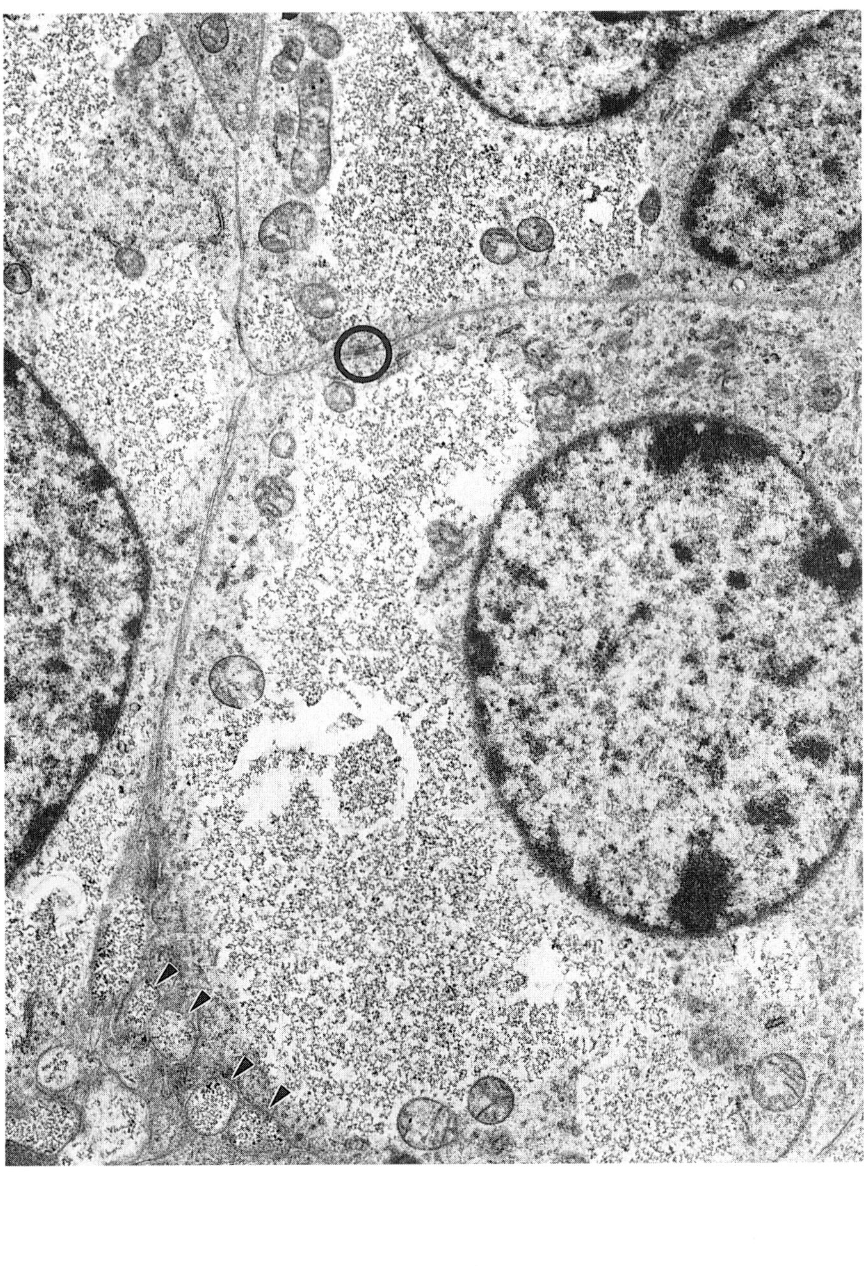

**Fig. 3-81.** Ewing's sarcoma metastatic to brain in a 24-year-old man. Primary tumor identified 5 years previously in a rib. Note uniform, round nuclei with finely dispersed chromatin. Note also abundant cytoplasmic glycogen, sparse cytoplasmic processes (*arrowheads*), and simple intercellular junctions (*circle*). (×13,050.) (Courtesy of Dr. Alan D. Glick, Department of Pathology, Vanderbilt University School of Medicine, Nashville, TN.)

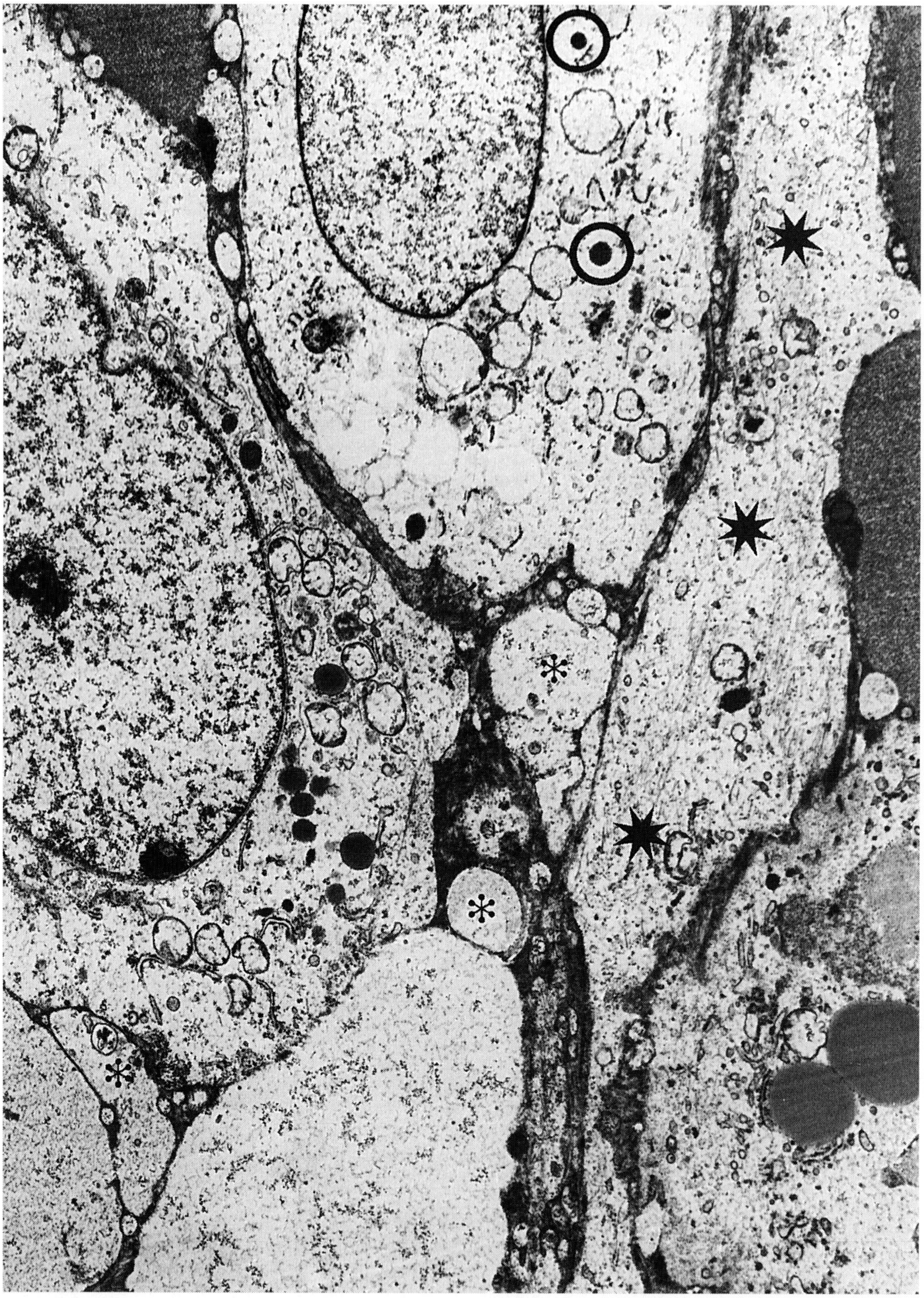

**Fig. 3-82.** Extraskeletal Ewing's sarcoma (peripheral primitive neuroectodermal tumor) in the popliteal soft tissue of a 35-year-old man. Blunt cytoplasmic processes are seen in cross section (*asterisks*) and in longitudinal section (*stars*). These and scattered neurosecretory-type dense-core granules (*circles*) suggest a neural origin. (×9600.)

A 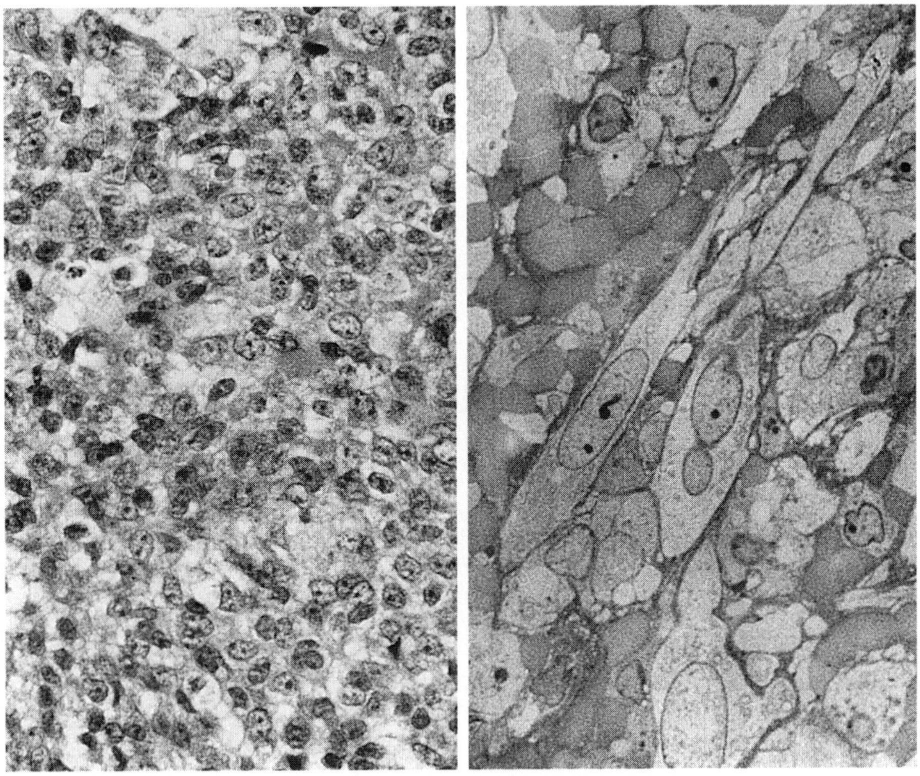 B

**Fig. 3-83.** Extraskeletal Ewing's sarcoma (peripheral primitive neuroectodermal tumor). Light microscopy of tumor shown in Fig. 3-82. **A,** Histologic appearance of tumor. **B,** Semithin section of epoxy-embedded material. Some of the cellular processes can be resolved by light microscopy in this plastic-embedded material. (**A,** ×340; **B,** ×865.)

fers diagnostic certainty in individual cases. Some Ewing's sarcomas have primitive intercellular junctional devices,[169,292,352] a point that may help distinguish them from lymphomas; however, the lack of junctional devices does not rule out Ewing's sarcoma. Most Ewing's sarcoma cells have fairly uniform round nuclei with finely dispersed chromatin, a feature that may be of some help in distinguishing these tumors from rhabdomyosarcomas.[73,223]

### Extraskeletal Ewing's Sarcoma (Peripheral Primitive Neuroectodermal Tumor)

Extraskeletal Ewing's sarcomas[105,352,401] share many ultrastructural features with skeletal examples of the same tumor.* However, they do have a tendency to display less glycogen, more numerous cytoplasmic processes, and occasional electron-dense granules, thus suggesting some affinity to neuroblastic tumors.[243] Askin and associates[7] separated a group of these tumors that presented as malignant childhood small cell tumors of the thoracopulmonary region, and have identified them as peripheral primitive neuroectodermal tumors. Ultrastructurally, these tumors display cytoplasmic cell processes, variable in size and number; dense-core, neurosecretory-type granules, often atypical in shape; and sometimes microtubules.* (Figs. 3-82, 3-83). Whether such tumors should be considered extraskeletal Ewing's sarcomas with evidence of neuroblastic differentiation or should be recognized as a distinct entity is a matter of controversy.†

### Lymphoma

The ultrastructure of small cell lymphomas[73,89,134, 315,376] is not markedly different from the ultrastructure of large cell lymphomas, described earlier in the section on large cell tumors. As stated, the constituent cells of lymphomas are largely devoid of distinguishing ultrastructural features, and the diagnosis of lymphoma by electron microscopy is one of exclusion. The cytoplasm of lymphoma cells has a distinctive, uniform gray color that reflects the presence of numerous polyribosomes (Figs. 3-84, 3-85). Occasional filaments and small collections of glycogen granules may be seen in lymphoma cells, but other distinguishing features, including junctional devices, secretory granules, and basal lamina, are lacking.[89,376] Nodular lymphomas contain dendritic cells in addition to lym-

* Refs. 88, 89, 169, 219, 227, 292.

* Refs. 7, 74, 109, 216, 279, 323.

† Refs. 71, 109, 110, 243, 279, 308, 323, 324, 414.

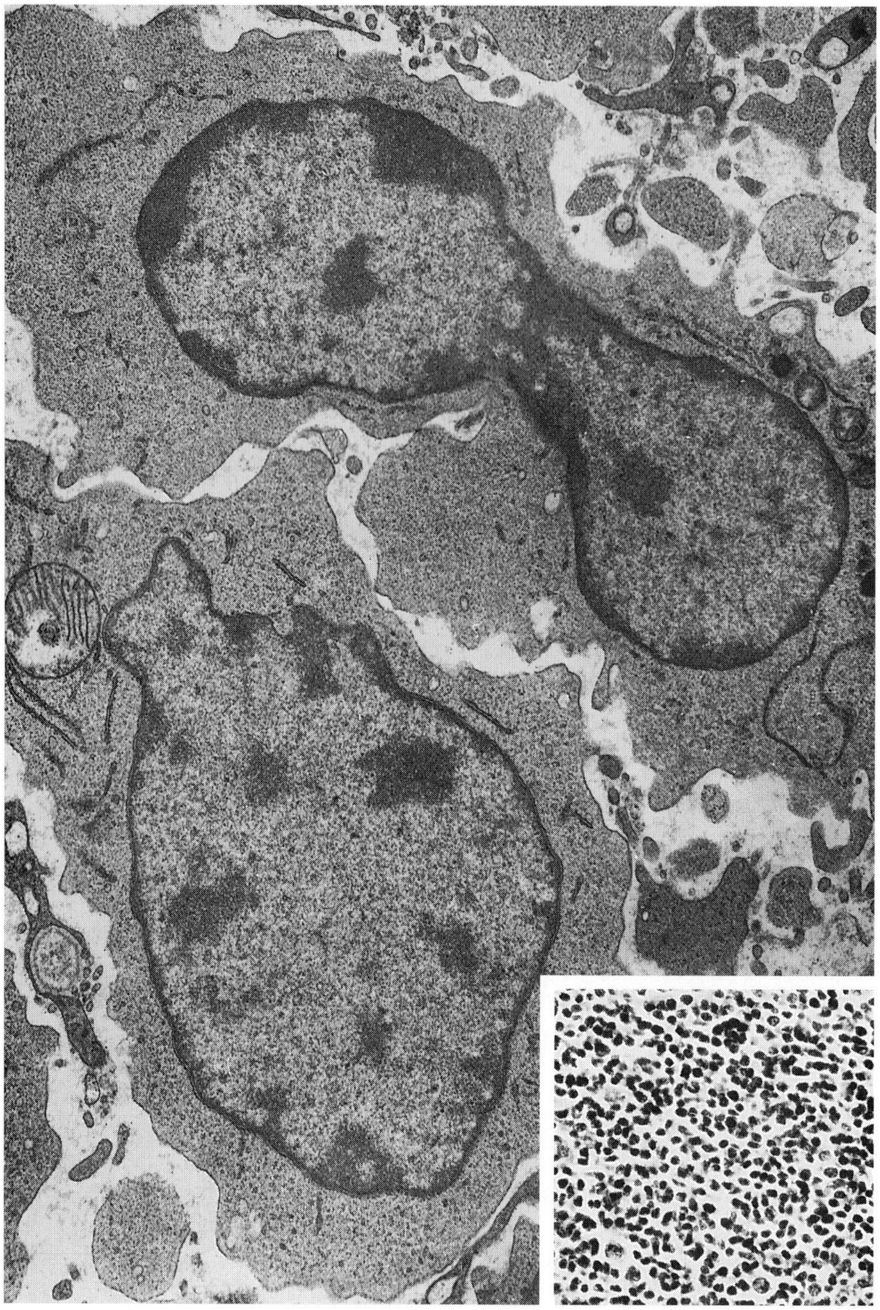

**Fig. 3-84.** Small cell lymphoma in a cervical lymph node of a 71-year-old man. Note nuclear irregularity, uniform, gray cytoplasm with sparse organelles, and loose arrangement of tumor cells without intercellular junctions. **Inset**, Histologic appearance of tumor. (**Fig.**, ×10,500; **Inset**, ×190.)

phoma cells, and these dendritic cells possess desmosomes.[315] However, such nodular lymphomas are less of a diagnostic problem than are the diffuse types. T-cell lymphomas may be distinguished from B-cell tumors by the presence of cells with extremely irregular or convoluted nuclei.[315]

## METASTATIC ADENOCARCINOMA OF UNKNOWN ORIGIN

Metastatic tumors account for about one third of lesions that present as a single supratentorial mass,[390] and adenocarcinomas make up about a third of these.[42] In a significant number of such patients (again, about

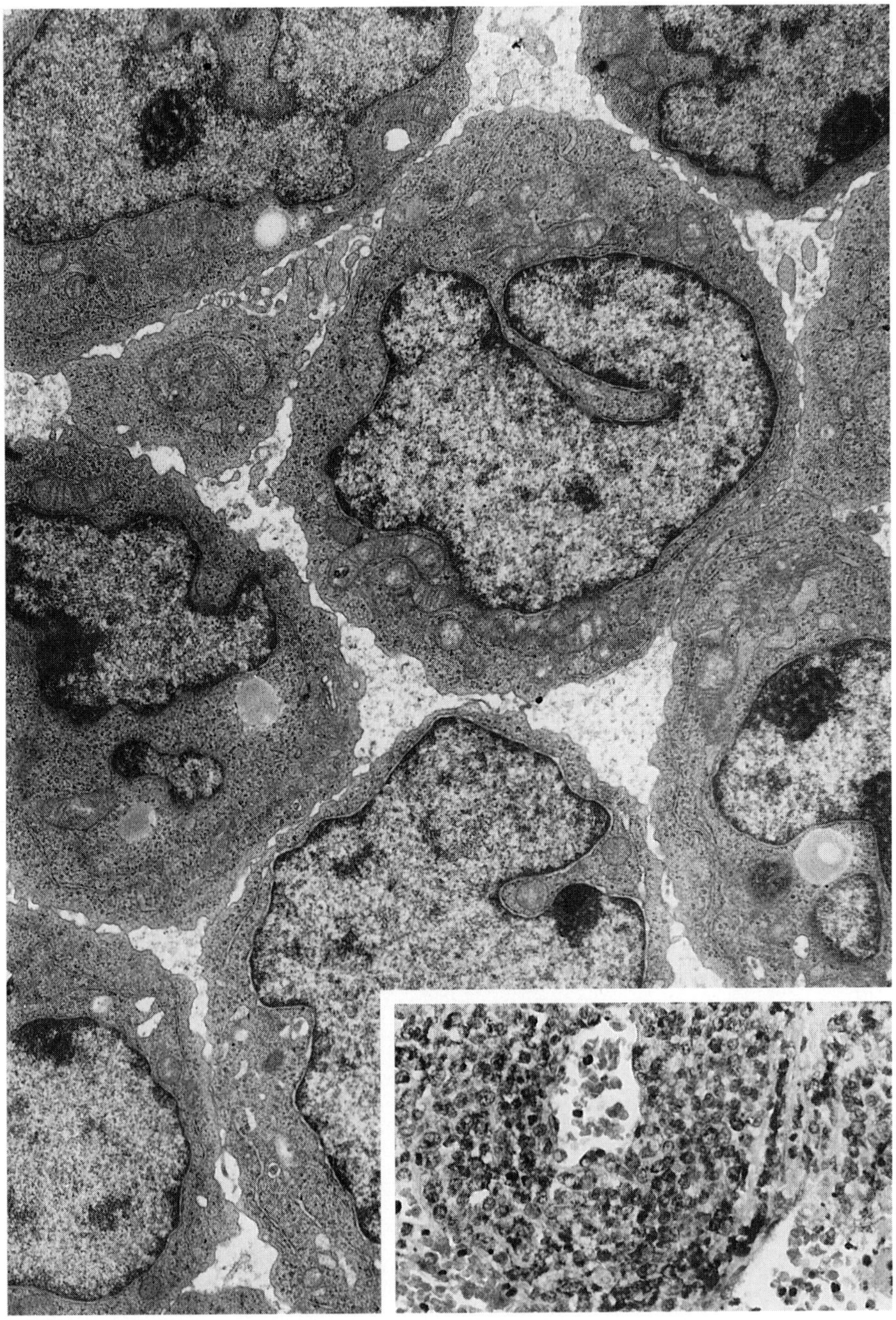

**Fig. 3-85.** Primary intracerebral small cell lymphoma in an adult man. Cytoplasmic polyribosomes are slightly more prominent in this case, imparting a "speckled" appearance to the tumor cell cytoplasm. The tumor cells are otherwise similar to those seen in Fig. 3-84. **Inset**, Histologic appearance of tumor. (**Fig.**, ×7775; **Inset**, ×195.)

a third,) the metastatic lesion is the first manifestation of a systemic cancer.[390] Among patients for whom the primary tumor is known or subsequently discovered, the common primary sites are lung, kidney, and colon.[390] Carcinoma of the breast commonly metastasizes to the brain,[6,389] but only rarely does so in the absence of an obvious primary lesion.[42,390] Prostatic adenocarcinomas rarely present as brain metastases[33] but may present as spinal or spinal cord metastases.[14] Other less common sources of metastatic adenocarcinoma include upper gastrointestinal tract, pancreas, and thyroid gland.[6,66,303]

Well-differentiated and moderately differentiated adenocarcinomas frequently (and poorly differentiated adenocarcinomas occasionally) retain ultrastructural features that allow identification of their site of origin,[65,121,141,258b] and as many as 80% to 90% of such metastatic tumors can be traced to a specific anatomic site of origin on the basis of their ultrastructural appearances.[141,258b] Electron microscopy, therefore, is a potentially useful tool in the evaluation of patients with metastatic adenocarcinomas of unknown origin.

### General Features

Adenocarcinoma cells are generally large and polygonal, with closely apposed plasma membranes that may or may not have complex interdigitations. Lumen formation is an important feature, with apical microvilli and junctional complexes that include tight junctions. Laterally, these usually are desmosomes, or simpler "desmosome-like" junctions, and basally there is frequently a basal lamina. The cytoplasm of adenocarcinoma cells generally has a good complement of organelles, including endoplasmic reticulum cisternae, Golgi apparatus, and secretory vesicles.

Important features in distinguishing the origin of metastatic adenocarcinomas include the fine structure of microvilli and adjacent glycocalyx (if present) and the nature of cytoplasmic granules. Other features that occasionally are helpful include the presence of more than one cell type (or direction of differentiation), intracellular lumen formation, and striking cytoplasmic content of glycogen, lipid, or rough or smooth endoplasmic reticulum.

It is important to survey a large number of cells and, if possible, several areas of the tumor. Many of the features cited below are not unique, but merely well developed in particular adenocarcinomas. As is the case in light microscopy, diagnoses based on single cells (or single organelles) should be avoided.

### Pulmonary Adenocarcinomas

Pulmonary adenocarcinomas, which make up the largest group of adenocarcinomas metastatic to the central nervous system,[258a] also show the greatest ultrastructural diversity. Ultrastructurally, pulmonary adenocarcinomas are composed of one or more of three basic cell types: mucus-secreting cells, Clara cells, and

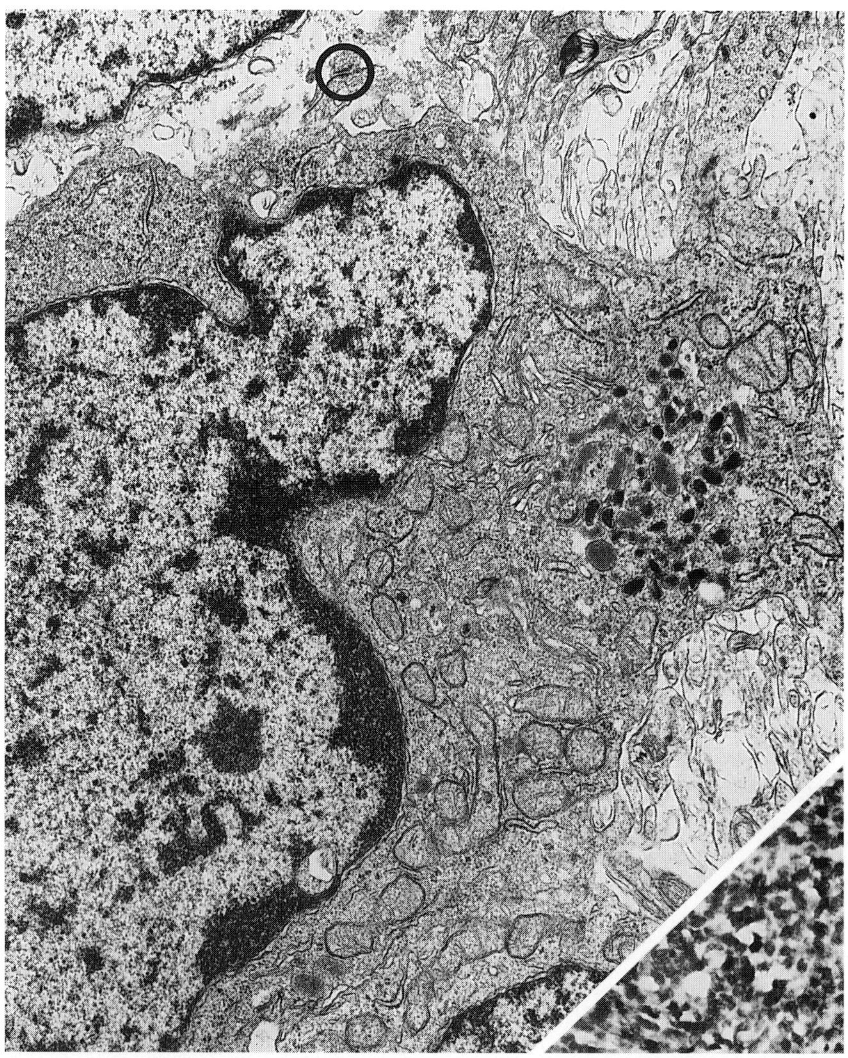

**Fig. 3-86.** Small cell ("oat cell") carcinoma of lung metastatic to brain in a 78-year-old man. There is a small collection of cytoplasmic dense-core granules. A junctional device is also evident (*circle*). **Inset**, Histologic appearance of tumor. (**Fig.**, ×15,400; **Inset**, ×195.)

alveolar (type II pneumocyte) cells.* These ultrastructural categories do not correspond with recognized histopathologic categories.[30,296] Pulmonary adenocarcinomas also may contain cells showing squamous or neuroendocrine (oat cell) differentiation (Figs. 3-86, 3-87), and evidence of such multidirectional differentiation is a useful feature in identifying adenocarcinomas of pulmonary origin.[141,258a]

*Mucus cell adenocarcinomas* of pulmonary origin are distinguished primarily by the presence of cytoplasmic mucin granules. This by itself is not a particularly helpful differentiating feature, and evidence of Clara or alveolar cell differentiation or of a squamous or oat cell component should be sought in such tumors. Mucus cell adenocarcinomas are composed of cells having short, nonbranching microvilli that are generally sparser than those of colonic adenocarcinomas.[138] They also usually lack the prominent core rootlets and adjacent glycocaliceal bodies of colonic adenocarcinomas (see below). However, careful search of these tumors will reveal foci of such colonlike microvilli and glycocaliceal bodies in many pulmonary mucus cell adenocarcinomas,* and the distinction of colonic from pulmonary mucus cell adenocarcinomas is generally based on the prominence and omnipresence of these features in colonic tumors rather than findings in occasional isolated tumor cells.[136,296] Rarely, primary pulmonary adenocarcinomas will show widespread "colonic" features on ultrastructural examination, and these tumors are thus difficult to identify as pulmonary tumors.[119,396a]

*Clara cell adenocarcinomas* are distinguished by a characteristic bell, or hobnail cell shape,[119,123] bushy, branching microvilli,[138,141,142] and the presence of Clara-type cytoplasmic granules† (Figs. 3-88 to 3-92). These granules are apically located, moderately large (50 to 150 nm), round or oval, and membrane-bound, and contain homogeneous electron-dense material. They must be distinguished from the somewhat more heterogeneous and ubiquitous tertiary lysosomes.

The shape of these Clara tumor cells, with an apical "dome" and deep extracellular "gullies" between the cells, combined with the bushy, branching microvilli,

* Refs. 22, 24, 30, 68, 123, 138, 142, 199, 250.

* Refs. 17, 69, 112, 119, 123, 142, 206, 296.

† Refs. 22, 30, 68, 119, 123, 138, 141, 142, 180, 199, 206, 250.

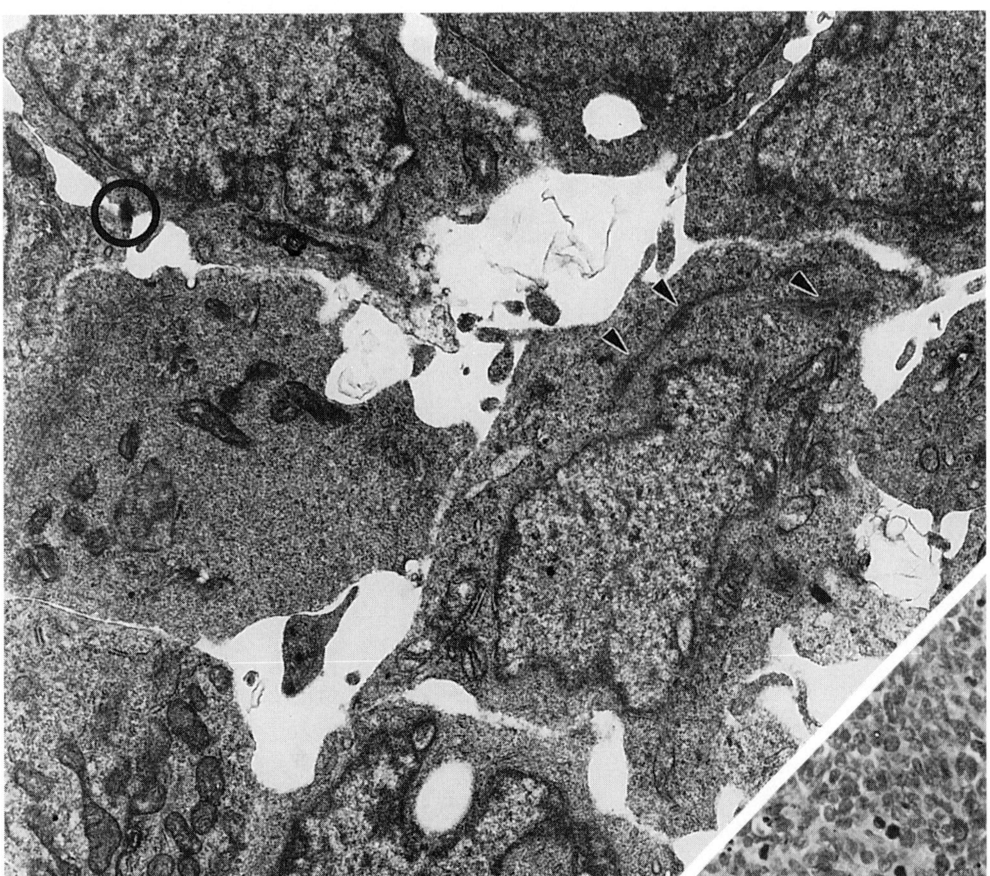

**Fig. 3-87.** Small cell squamous carcinoma of lung metastatic to brain in a 59-year-old man. Condensed bundles of tonofilaments (*arrowheads*) and intercellular junctions (*circles*) are present. **Inset**, Histologic appearance of tumor. (**Fig.**, ×11,800; **Inset**, ×220.)

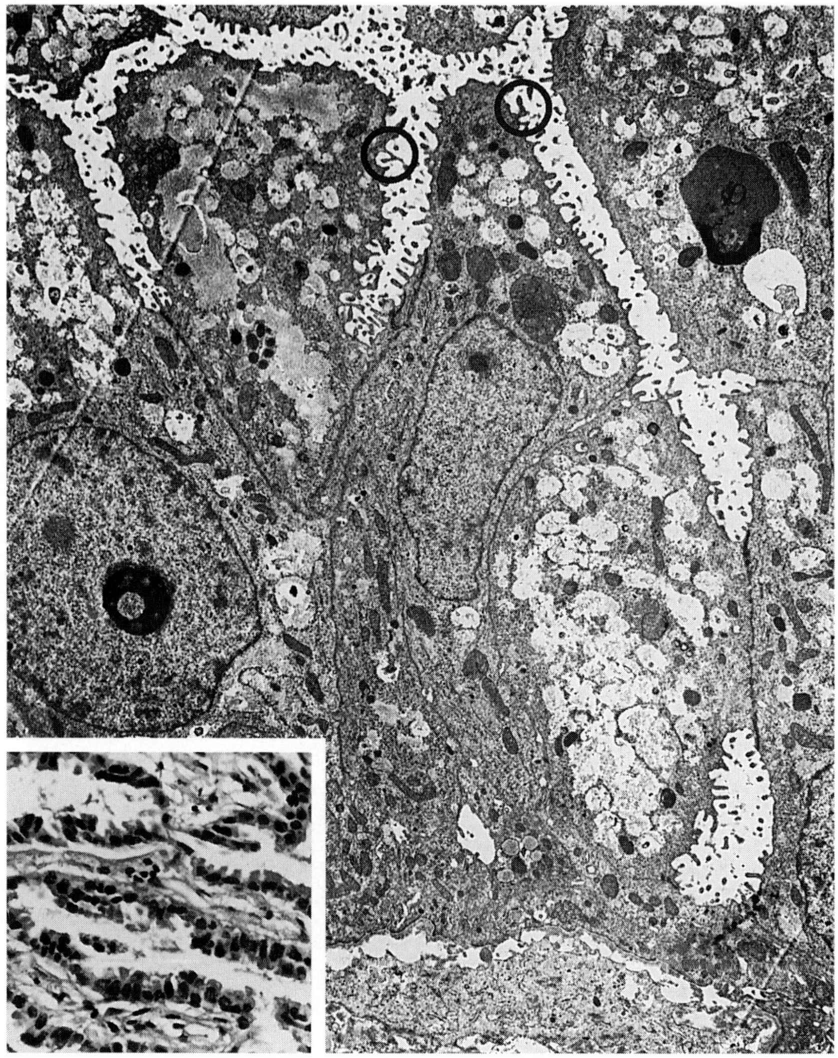

**Fig. 3-88.** Adenocarcinoma of lung in a 73-year-old man. Note deep "gullies" between tumor cells, with abundant, irregular, occasionally branching microvilli (*circles*). **Inset**, Histologic appearance of tumor. (**Fig.**, ×4050; **Inset**, ×195.)

often produces a characteristic appearance of circumferential microvilli on tangential sections of tumor cells,[250] an appearance that may be exaggerated in metastatic lesions. This appearance, which also may be seen in alveolar cell adenocarcinomas (see below), is cited by Herrera and Reimann[141] as an important feature in identifying metastatic adenocarcinomas as being of pulmonary origin.

*Alveolar cell adenocarcinomas* are distinguished by bushy, branching microvilli similar to those seen in Clara cell adenocarcinomas,[24,120,142] and by the presence of lamellar cytoplasmic bodies* (Figs. 3-93 to 3-95) that are an expression of surfactant production.[387] An additional feature is the presence, in occasional tumors, of prominent intranuclear inclusions consisting of packed masses of tubules.[30,53,120,337] The lamellar bodies are particularly helpful in identifying metastatic adenocarcinomas as pulmonary tumors[65,101,121,141] because they occur only rarely in other adenocarcinomas.[20,119,170] These lamellar bodies must, however, be distinguished from the ubiquitous "myelin figures" that appear in degenerated, autolyzed, poorly fixed, or overly fixed cells (see Figs. 3-1, 3-97, 3-106). As a general rule, the lamellar bodies should be cytoplasmic, unassociated with degenerating mitochondria or other organelles, and present within cells that appear well preserved, in tissue that has not been held for days or weeks on fixative.

In summary, important ultrastructural features in identifying pulmonary adenocarcinomas include the presence of divergent lines of cellular differentiation, circumferential branching microvilli without filamentous cores or glycocaliceal bodies, and surfactant-type lamellar cytoplasmic bodies.

*Text continues on page 171.*

* Refs. 1, 22, 24, 30, 65, 68, 119–121, 123, 138, 142, 180, 199, 212, 335.

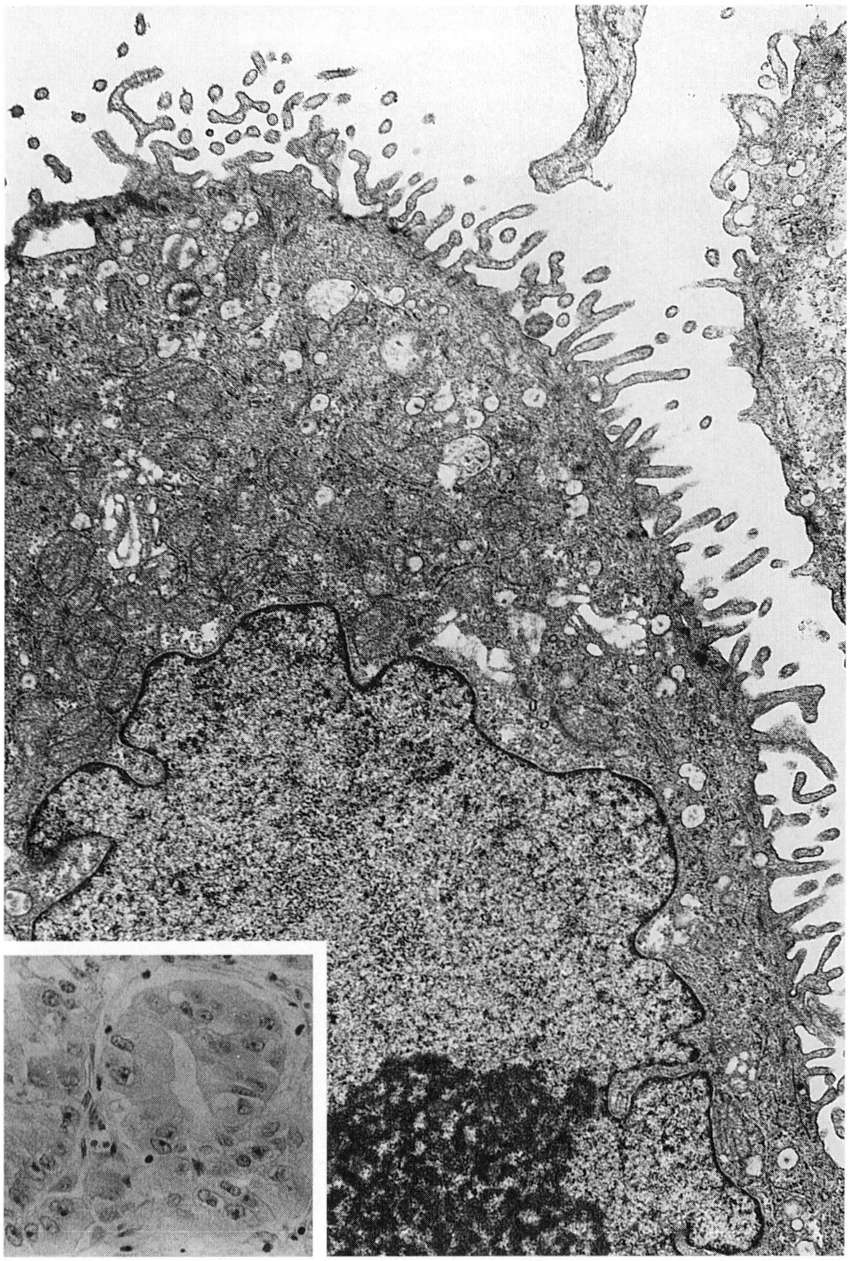

**Fig. 3-89.** Adenocarcinoma metastatic to left cerebellar hemisphere of a 61-year-old man. Primary unknown. There are abundant, irregular, occasionally branching microvilli around this tumor cell, suggesting a pulmonary primary. **Inset**, Histologic appearance of tumor. (**Fig.**, ×10,500; **Inset**, ×195.)

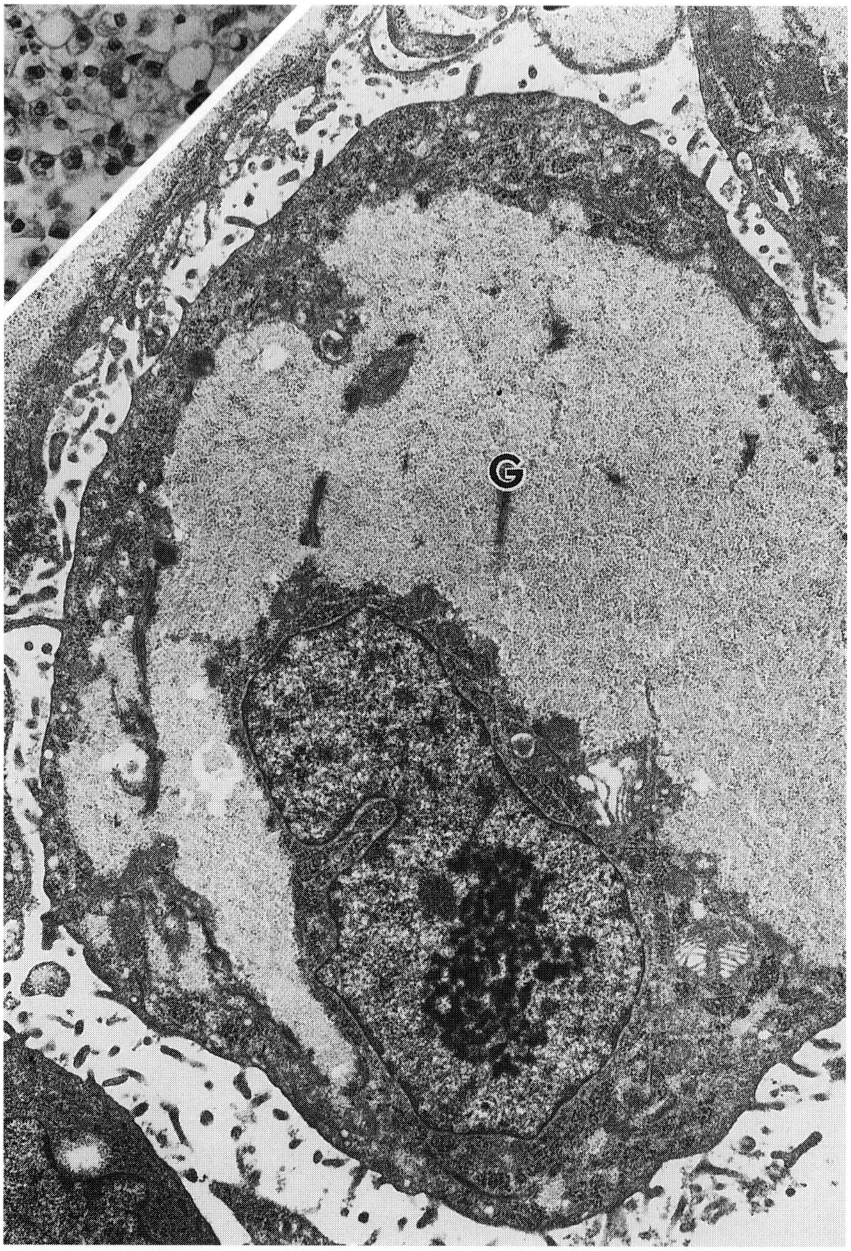


**Fig. 3-90.** Adenocarcinoma of lung, "clear cell" type, presenting as metastasis to brain in a 61-year-old woman. This tumor cell shows circumferential, irregular, occasionally branching microvilli, suggestive of a pulmonary primary. A large pool of glycogen particles *(G)* occupies most of the tumor cell cytoplasm, accounting for the clear appearance by light microscopy. Subsequent autopsy revealed a primary pulmonary adenocarcinoma. **Inset,** Histologic appearance of tumor. (**Fig.**, ×10,500; **Inset**, ×195.)

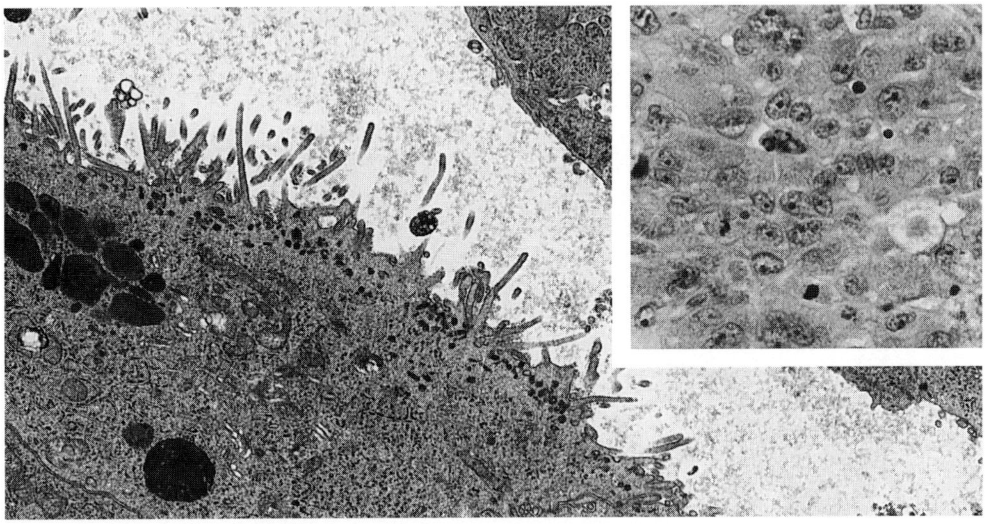

**Fig. 3-91.** Adenocarcinoma metastatic to cerebellum in a 58-year-old man. Primary unknown. Numerous small subapical irregular dense bodies reminiscent of Clara cell granules suggest a pulmonary primary. **Inset**, Histologic appearance of tumor. (**Fig.**, ×9800; **Inset**, ×220.)

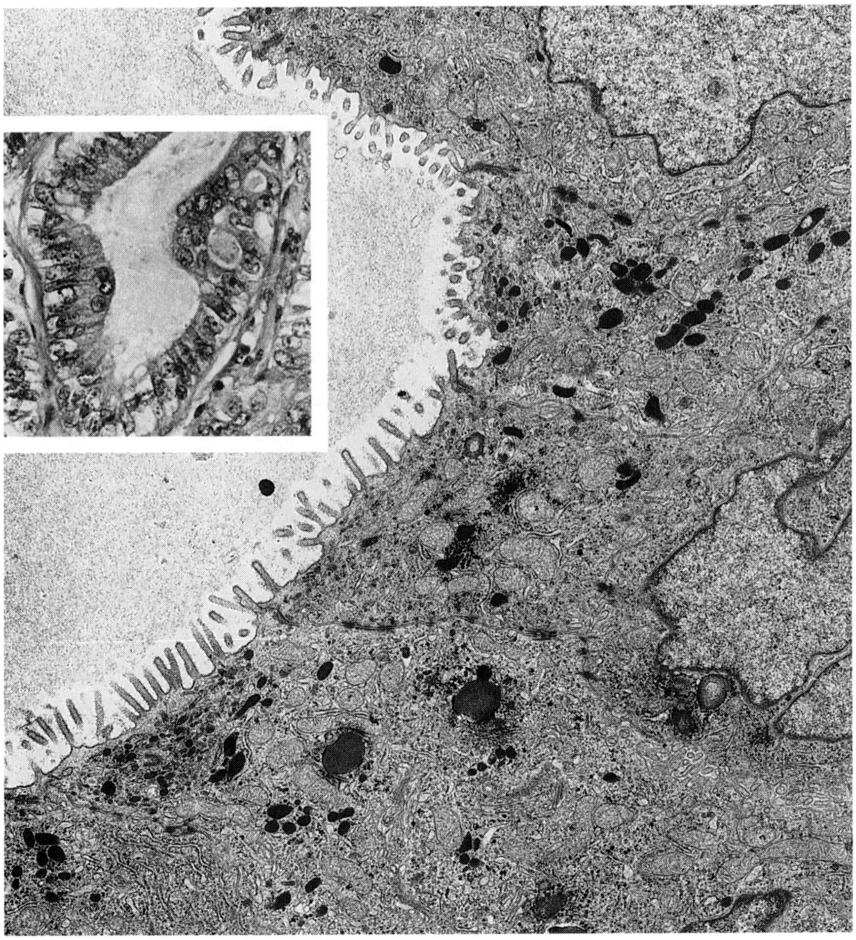

**Fig. 3-92.** Adenocarcinoma metastatic to left frontal lobe of a 62-year-old man. Primary unknown. Numerous subapical dense bodies again suggest a pulmonary origin. The microvilli are more regular than those seen in most pulmonary adenocarcinomas, and focally there was evidence of core rootlets and terminal web formation (not shown). Radiographic and endoscopic studies revealed no evidence of an intestinal lesion, and serial chest radiographs showed an enlarging perihilar mass. **Inset**, Histologic appearance of tumor. (**Fig.**, ×8750; **Inset**, ×195.)

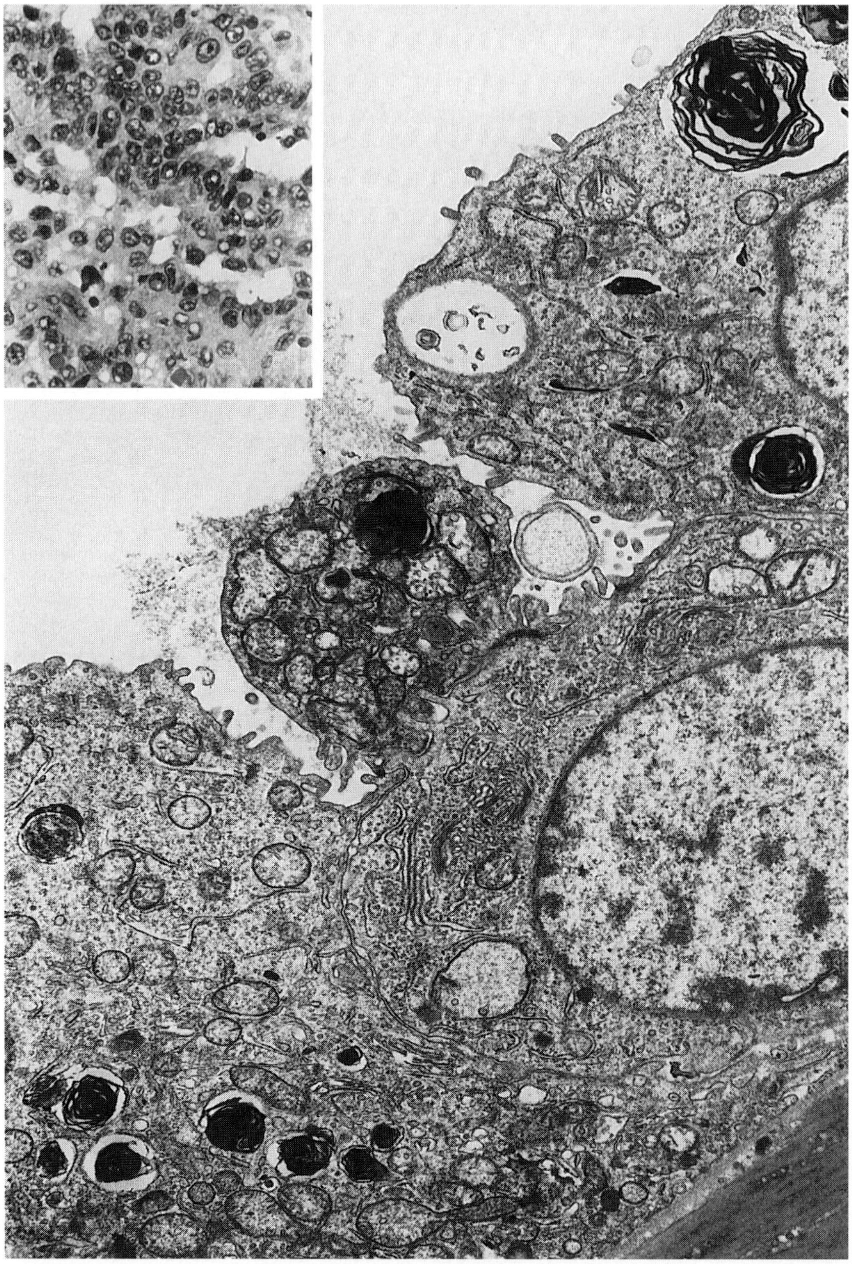

**Fig. 3-93.** Pulmonary adenocarcinoma, bronchiolo-alveolar type, in a 68-year-old man. Numerous cytoplasmic membranous whorls are present, reminiscent of surfactant production. **Inset**, Histologic appearance of tumor. (**Fig.**, ×10,500; **Inset**, ×195.)

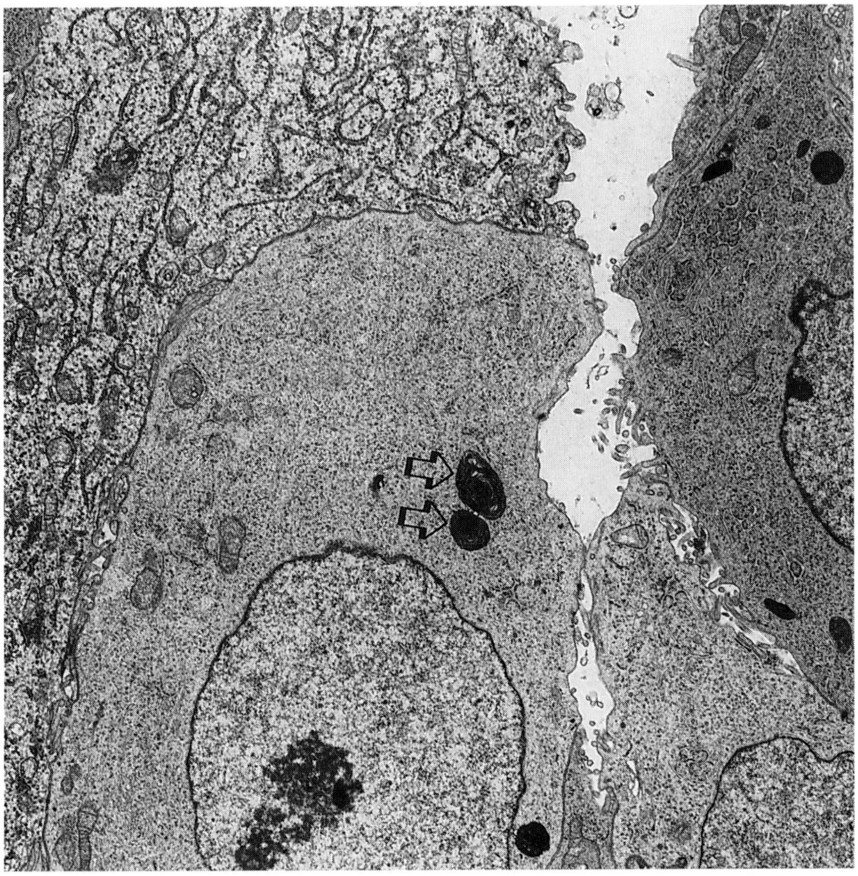

**Fig. 3-94.** Adenocarcinoma metastatic to cerebellum; primary unknown (same case as Fig. 3-91). Here microvilli are inauspicious and Clara-type granules are not seen. There are, however, cytoplasmic membranous whorls (*arrows*), suggesting alveolar cell differentiation in a pulmonary adenocarcinoma. (×8750.)

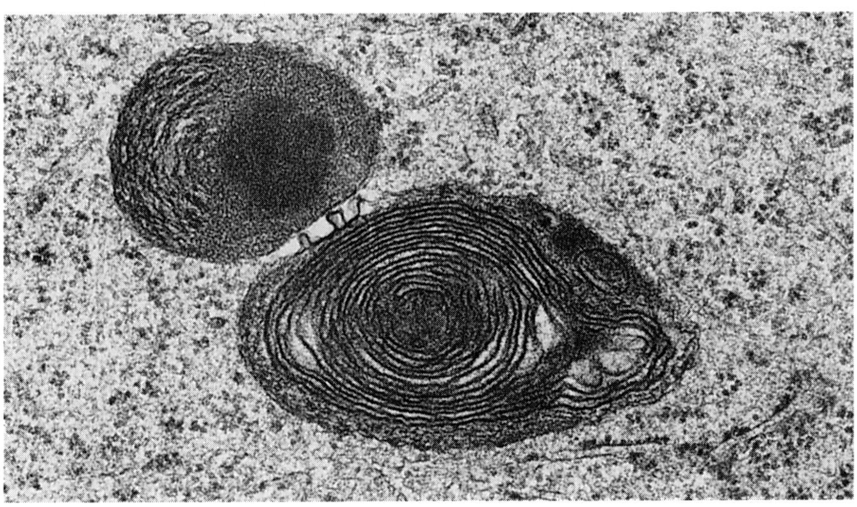

**Fig. 3-95.** Adenocarcinoma metastatic to cerebellum. Detail of Fig. 3-94 showing membranous whorls. (×43,900.)

## Renal Adenocarcinomas

Most metastatic renal cell carcinomas are clear cell carcinomas, and these are identified ultrastructurally by the presence of glycogen and lipid in copious amounts and by the absence of mucin* (Figs. 3-96, 3-97). The presence of cytoplasmic glycogen granules is an important distinguishing feature from capillary hemangioblastoma, which may resemble metastatic renal cell carcinoma histologically[178] (Fig. 3-96). Additional features helpful in distinguishing these two tumors are lumen formation, apical microvilli, and immunohistochemical reaction for epithelial membrane antigen. These features are seen in renal cell carcinomas but not in hemangioblastomas. In addition to clear

* Refs. 84, 121, 141, 275, 327, 350, 351, 357.

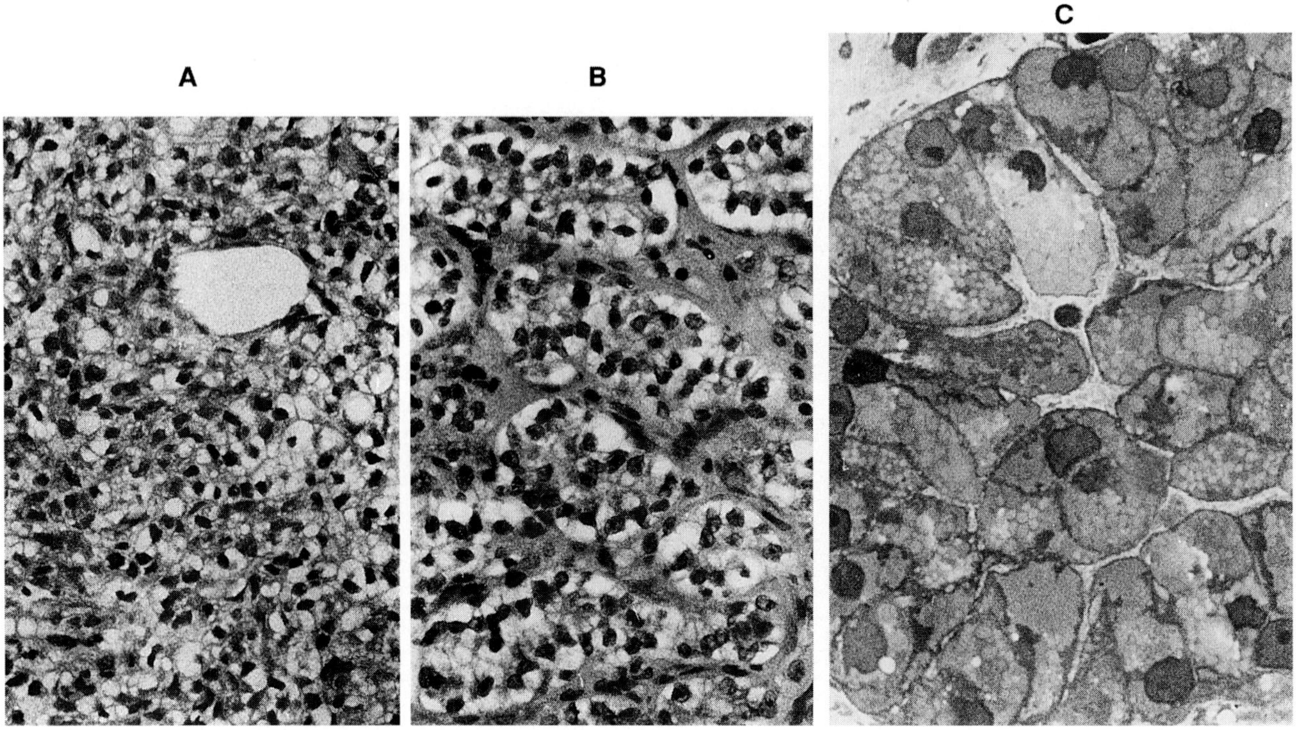


**Fig. 3-96.** Metastatic renal cell carcinoma in a 61-year-old man. Patient presented with a solitary cerebellar lesion and no known extracranial tumor. **A**, By light microscopy this tumor resembled a capillary hemangioblastoma. **B**, Some areas showed packeting of cells ("zellballen"), but intercellular lumina could not be discerned. **C**, Semithin sections of epoxy embedded material allowed resolution of fine intercellular luminal spaces lined by microvilli in the "zellballen" areas. These features suggested a metastatic renal cell carcinoma, and subsequent sonographic examination revealed an inferior renal mass. (**A**, ×290; **B**, ×290; **C**, ×820.)

cells, renal cell carcinomas also may have granular cells. These granular cells contain generous numbers of cytoplasmic mitochondria, but cytoplasmic lipid and glycogen are generally still evident.[350,357] Additional ultrastructural features that may be observed in better differentiated examples of renal cell carcinomas include apical pinocytotic vesicles, basilar mitochondria and basal lamina infoldings,[84,141,327,357] and intracytoplasmic tubulofilamentous structures.[121]

### Adenocarcinomas from the Colon and Rectum

Colon and rectal adenocarcinomas are generally readily identifiable ultrastructurally by their distinctive apical cell surfaces.[65,121,141,145,217] These are lined by well-organized, nonbranching microvilli with prominent filamentous cores that extend deeply into the underlying apical cell cytoplasm ("core rootlets") (Fig. 3-98). Overlying these microvilli there is a prominent glycocalyx containing minute, round ringlike structures ("glycocaliceal bodies") (Fig. 3-99). In addition to these features, mucin production usually is evident.

The specialized microvillous and glycocaliceal structure of colonic and rectal adenocarcinomas is a prominent and consistent ultrastructural feature, but it is not unique. Occasional mucous pulmonary adenocarcinomas may show scattered foci of (and rare pulmonary tumors may show widespread evidence of[119,396a]) similar-appearing microvilli. The distinction generally rests on the extent of such microvillous specialization, as well as on the presence or absence of distinguishing pulmonary features.

### Mammary Adenocarcinomas

Mammary adenocarcinomas, as mentioned above, only rarely metastasize to the central nervous system in the absence of a clinically obvious primary lesion, and thus only rarely present as an adenocarcinoma of unknown origin. A more common problem is exemplified by the patient with a previous history of mastectomy who returns at a later time with a brain metastasis. It may be necessary to distinguish a late metastasis from the breast from a new metastasis from an unrecognized second primary tumor.

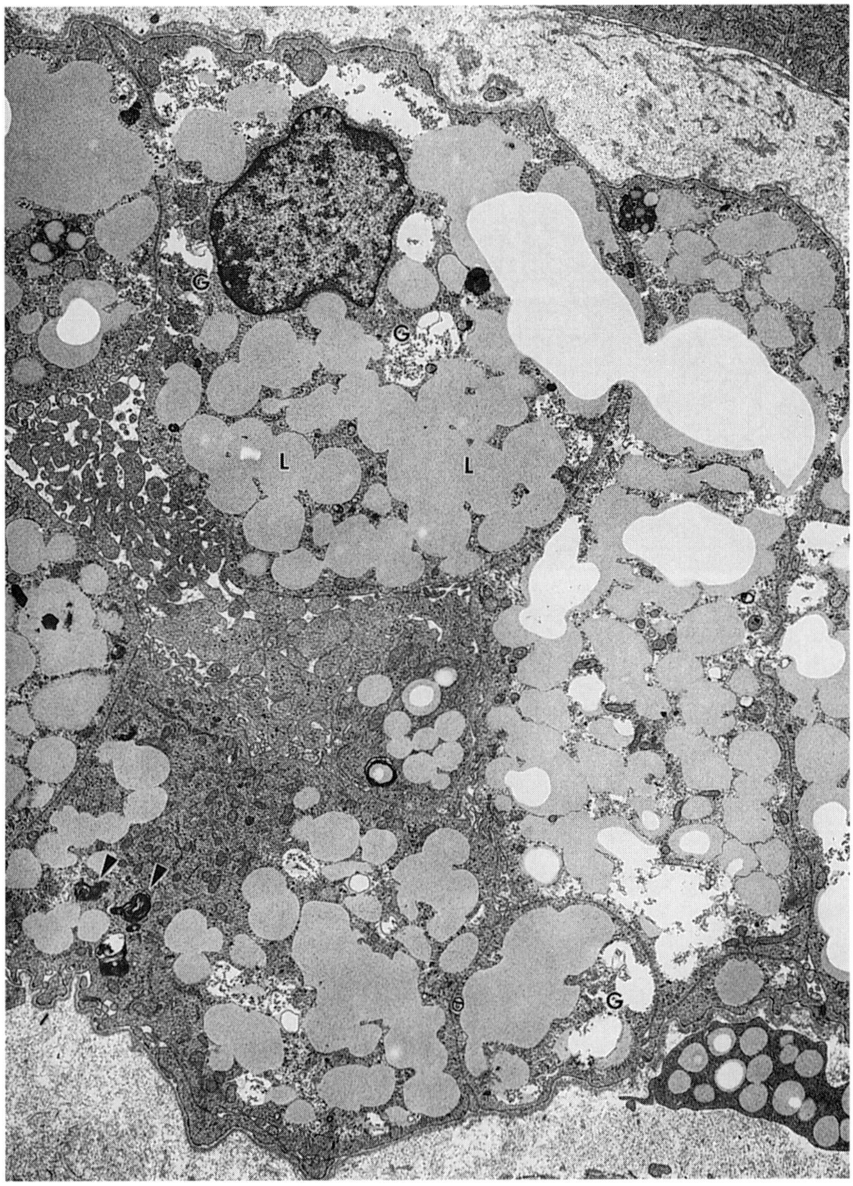


**Fig. 3-97.** Renal cell carcinoma. There is abundant cytoplasmic glycogen *(G)* and lipid *(L)*. Note membranous whorls in tumor cell cytoplasm (*arrowheads*). (×5250.)

An unusual and distinguishing feature of mammary adenocarcinomas is the presence of small, round intracellular spaces lined with slender, uniform, nonbranching microvilli[15,83,265,341] (Fig. 3-100). These "intracellular lumina" may appear empty or may contain granular material. There may be adjacent filaments, secretory vesicles, or "condensed cytoplasm." Like most ultrastructural findings, these are not unique to breast adenocarcinomas, as they have been found in adenocarcinomas from kidney, thyroid, stomach, lung, ovary and sweat glands, as well as in some tumors other than adenocarcinoma,[99,341] including meningiomas.[192] However, intracellular lumina are found most often and in greatest numbers in adenocarcinomas of the breast, and their presence in a metastatic adenocarcinoma is considered strongly suggestive of mammary origin.*

Additional helpful features in the recognition of mammary adenocarcinomas include a dual cell population of glandular and myoepithelial cells, cytoplasmic filaments in bundles, and "lakes" of cytoplasmic glycogen.[141]

---

* Refs. 15, 99, 121, 141, 265, 341.

A

B

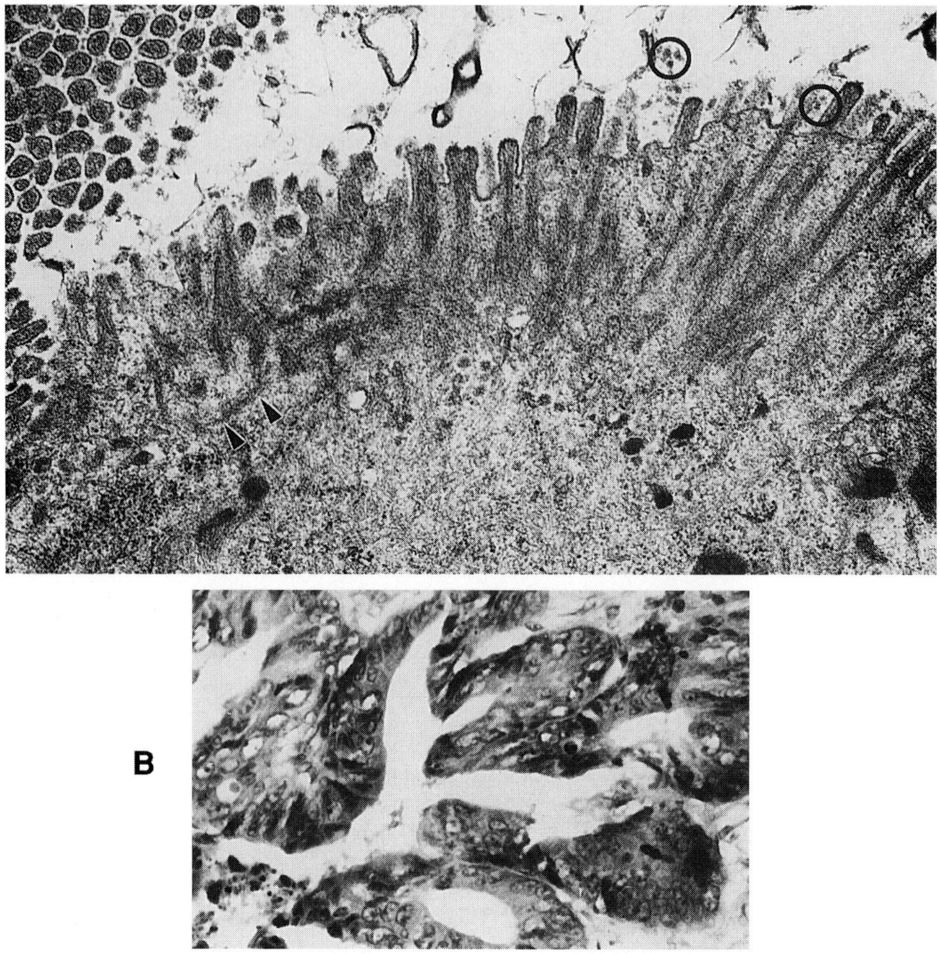

**Fig. 3-98.** Colonic adenocarcinoma metastatic to pelvis in a 72-year-old man. **A**, Detail of apical cytoplasm shows well-formed, uniform microvilli with filamentous cores extending down into the underlying cytoplasm (core rootlets). There is some suggestion as well of filaments running perpendicular to these rootlets (terminal web formation, *arrowheads*). Glycocalyx is not as apparent in this example as it is in many such tumors, but occasional small ringlike structures (glycocaliceal bodies) can be found "floating" above the tumor cell cytoplasm (*circles*). **B**, Histologic appearance of tumor. (**A**, ×43,700; **B**, ×220.)

## Prostatic Adenocarcinomas

Metastatic prostatic adenocarcinomas rarely come to ultrastructural examination for diagnosis. Metastases of suspected prostatic origin (a category that includes many spinal lesions) may be evaluated by immunohistochemistry, and intracranial metastases are distinctly unusual. The ultrastructure of prostatic adenocarcinomas is, however, distinctive (Figs. 3-101 to 3-103). The most important features are prominent cytoplasmic vacuolization and numerous pleomorphic lysosomal bodies.[70,115,141,179] The latter are membrane-bound bodies, often with eccentric, crescentic, electron-dense cores. Additional features are prominent, although somewhat disorganized-appearing, microvilli without colonic type filaments, and the absence of mucin. Neuroendocrine (oat cell) differentiation is found in 5% to 10% of prostatic adenocarcinomas.[381]

## Miscellaneous Adenocarcinomas

*Gastric adenocarcinomas*[217,266,411] may resemble colonic adenocarcinomas, often with abundant cytoplasmic mucin. However, both the microvillus core rootlets and the glycocaliceal bodies are generally much less prominent in gastric tumors than are those seen in colonic adenocarcinomas (Figs. 3-104, 3-105). *Pancreatic adenocarcinomas*[141,282,394] also may show microvilli with attenuated filamentous cores and a glycocalyx. These tumors usually contain cells with abun-

*Text continues on page 178.*

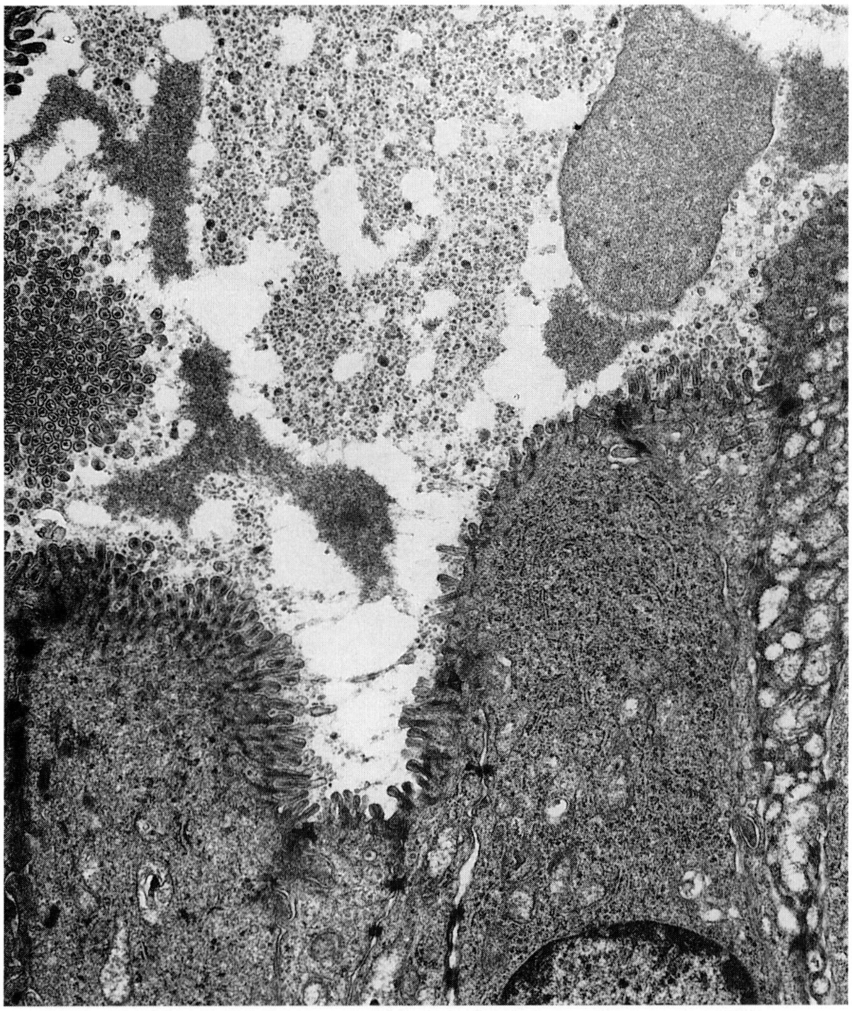

**Fig. 3-99.** Colonic adenocarcinoma. Glycocalyx and innumerable glycocaliceal bodies are well demonstrated in this example. (×10,500.)

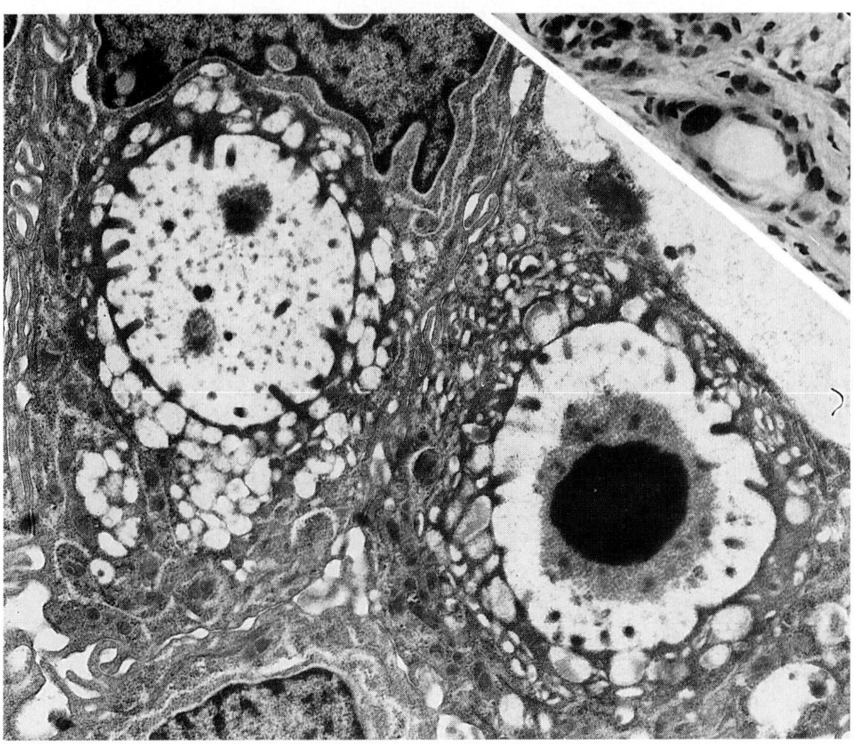

**Fig. 3-100.** Adenocarcinoma metastatic to liver in a 65-year-old woman. Primary unknown. Prominent and numerous intracytoplasmic lumina suggest a mammary origin. **Inset**, Histologic appearance of tumor. (**Fig.**, ×10,500; **Inset**, ×195.)

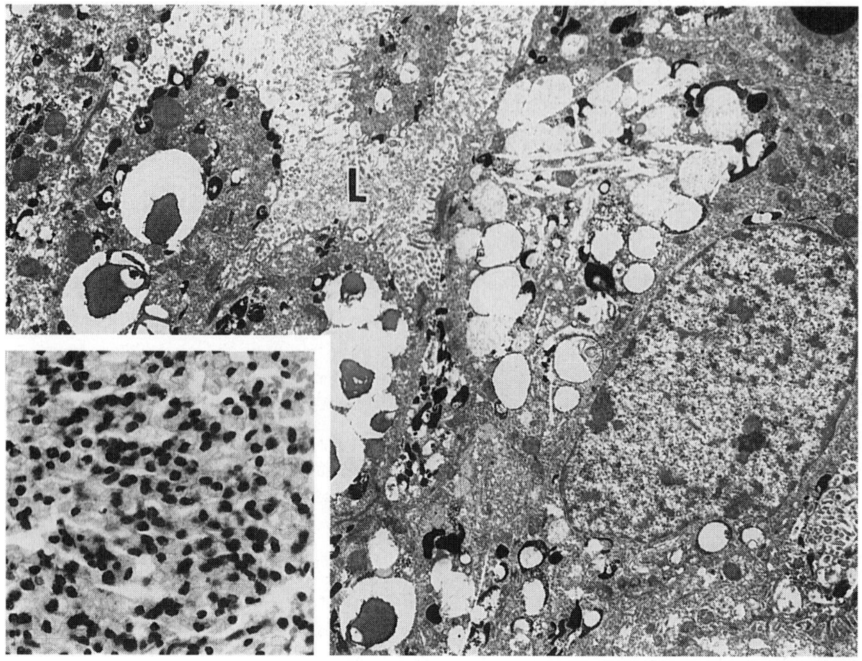


**Fig. 3-101.** Adenocarcinoma of prostate, metastatic to cavernous sinus in a 74-year-old man with known prostatic primary. Numerous pleomorphic lysosomes, vacuoles, and lipid droplets are apparent at low magnification, as well as lumen formation *(L)* and apical microvilli. **Inset**, Histologic appearance of tumor. (**Fig.**, ×4050; **Inset**, ×195.)

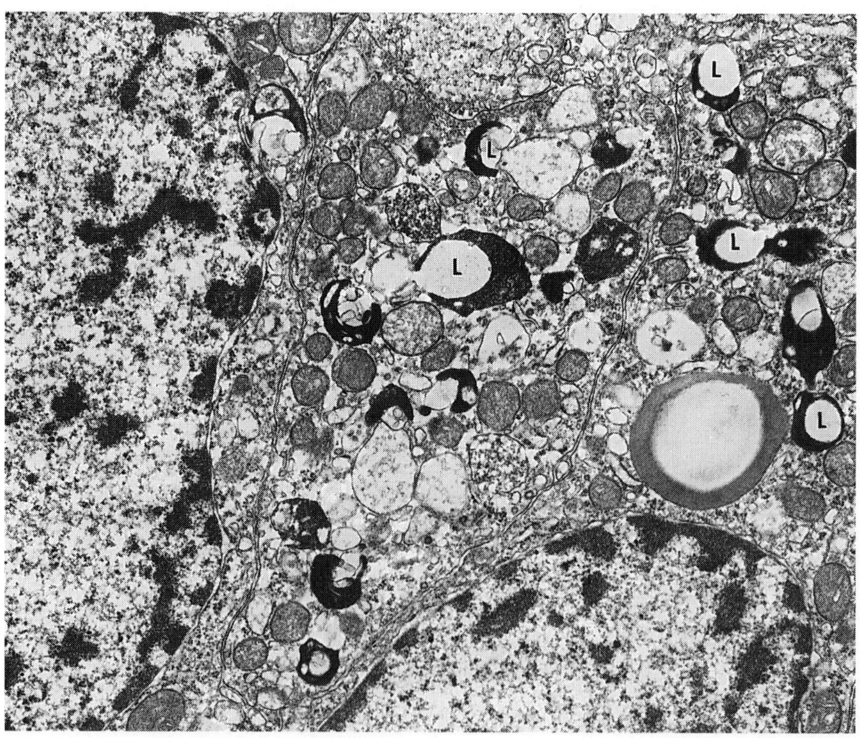


**Fig. 3-102.** Metastatic prostatic adenocarcinoma (same case as Fig. 3-101). Pleomorphic lysosomes *(L)* are seen, often with eccentric, crescentic, electron-dense cores. (×10,500.)

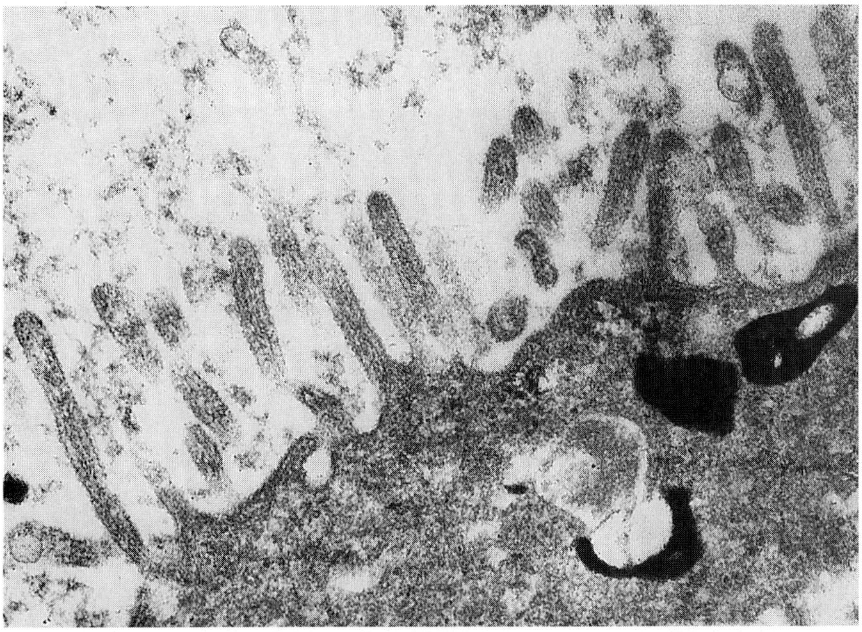

**Fig. 3-103.** Metastatic prostatic adenocarcinoma (same case as Fig. 3-101). Well-formed but short apical microvilli show fine filamentous cores but lack core rootlets. (×40,900.)

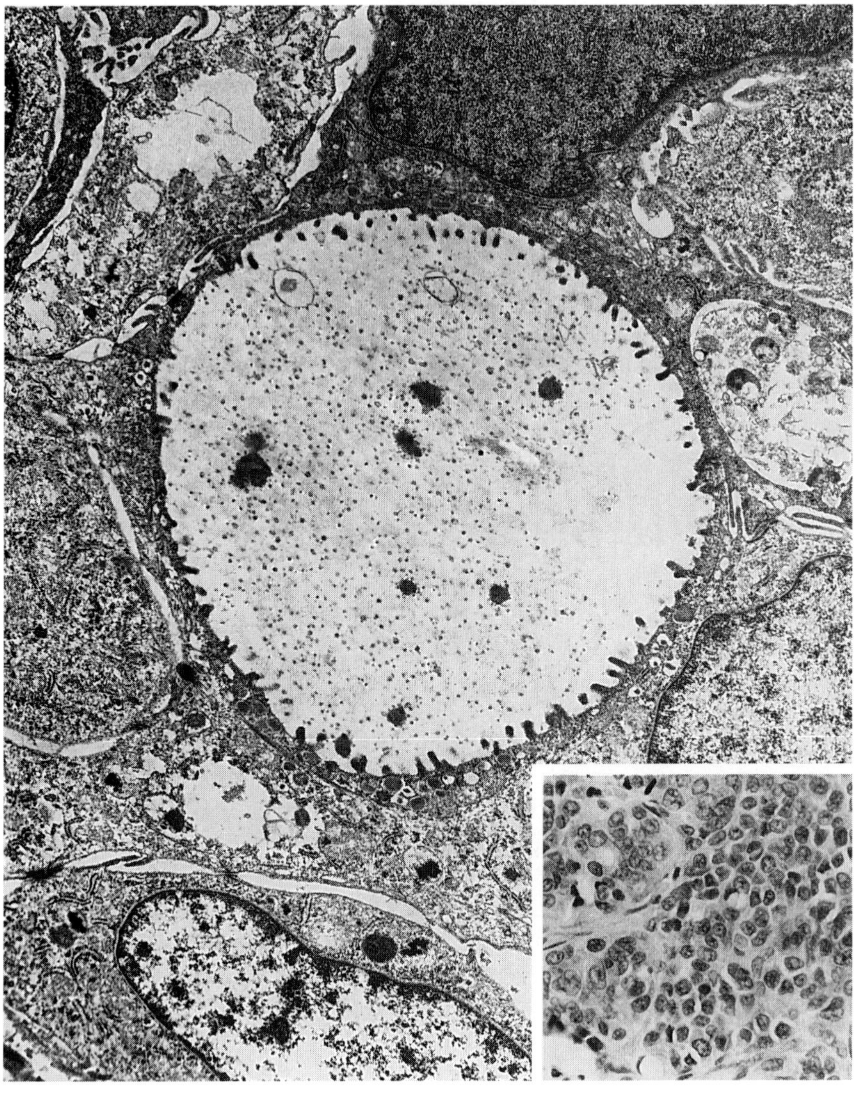

**Fig. 3-104.** Adenocarcinoma of stomach presenting as metastasis of unknown origin to skin in an adult man. Ultrastructural examination showed short, blunt microvilli and glycocalyx (fuzzy luminal contents). **Inset**, Histologic appearance of tumor. (**Fig.**, ×7700; **Inset**, ×195.)

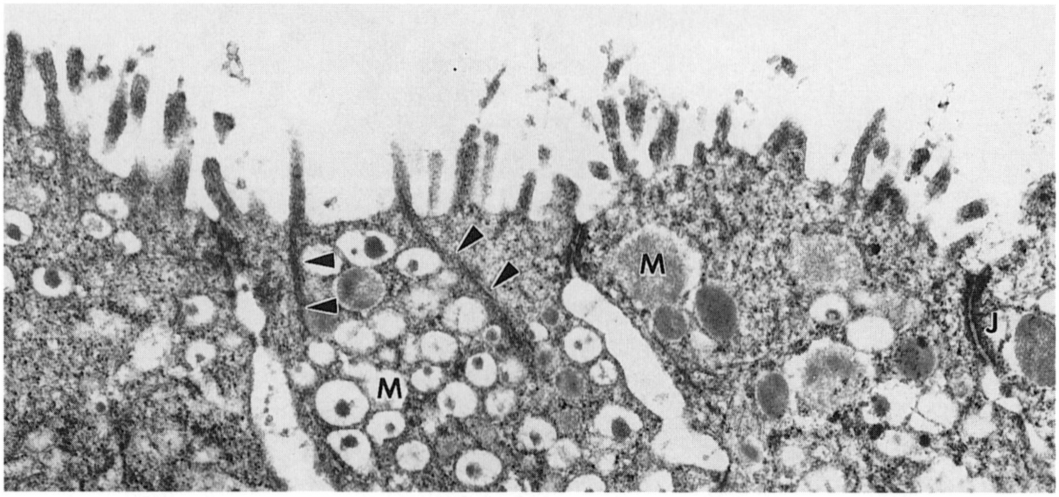


**Fig. 3-105.** Adenocarcinoma of stomach metastatic to skin (same case as Fig. 3-104). Higher magnification shows microvillous filamentous cores with occasional core rootlets (*arrowheads*), some overlying glycocalyx (not well shown) but no glycocaliceal bodies, and abundant cytoplasmic mucin vacuoles *(M)*. Note also apical junctional complex *(J)*. An upper gastrointestinal origin was suggested, and gastroscopic biopsy confirmed gastric adenocarcinoma. (×19,000.)

dant lamellae of rough endoplasmic reticulum and with zymogen granules. The latter are exceedingly large (250 to 1000 nm), round, membrane-bound granules containing homogeneous electron-dense material. *Thyroid adenocarcinomas** show colloid-filled lumina, tall apical microvilli without core rootlets, and small apical lysosomes (Fig. 3-106). Occasional oncocytic cells contain abundant, ultrastructurally abnormal mitochondria. *Ovarian adenocarcinomas* are noted for their bushy, branching microvilli that arise from small cytoplasmic "hillocks" ("staghorn microvilli").[121,141,240] Published descriptions are also available for other adenocarcinomas.†

## OTHER METASTATIC TUMORS

### Histiocytosis X

Histiocytosis X is thought to be a disorder of immune regulation that results in a tumorlike reactive proliferation of histiocytes, especially Langerhans cells. These are dendritic cells that normally are residents of skin and mucous membranes, lymph nodes, and perhaps lung.[78,304] The tumorlike lesions of histiocytosis X may be localized to bone, including spine or skull, or may be disseminated throughout visceral organs. In neurosurgical practice, this entity is encountered as a skull or spinal bone lesion, or, rarely, in the form of an intraparenchymal mass.‡

* Refs. 61, 121, 141, 184, 342, 343.

† Refs. 2, 4, 19, 41, 118, 163, 198, 200, 235, 241, 249, 260, 280, 281, 313, 405, 412.

‡ Refs. 122, 144, 176, 195, 197, 256, 317, 339, 340, 371.

Identification of the component cells as histiocytes is generally accomplished histopathologically, and the role of electron microscopy in such cases is the identification of Birbeck granules (Figs. 3-107, 3-108). These unique subcellular organelles identify the component cells as Langerhans cells and thus establish a (nonspecific) histiocytic lesion as a (specific) histiocytosis X lesion.

Birbeck granules (or Langerhans cell granules) are cytoplasmic rodlike structures of variable length but constant width that appear as two closely apposed membranes with a central, parallel line between them.* Birbeck granules are most numerous at the periphery of the cell, where they may appear continuous with the cell membrane and have a vesicular expansion at one end, imparting a "tennis racquet" appearance. These granules are generally quite easy to find in well fixed material, being present in 10 to 60% of sectioned cells.[78,245] Even in poorly fixed tissue or tissue retrieved from paraffin they may be demonstrable, albeit with somewhat more difficulty.[245] Birbeck granules must be distinguished from other, superficially similar structures, including intercellular "zipperlike" contacts and short segments of endoplasmic reticulum.

In addition to the diagnostic Birbeck granules, the component cells of histiocytosis X have the general ultrastructural features of histiocytes: irregular, indented nuclei; cytoplasmic lysosomes; phagosomes and Golgi bodies; and irregular cell boundaries without intercellular junctional devices.

* Refs. 78, 115, 245, 253, 326, 359.

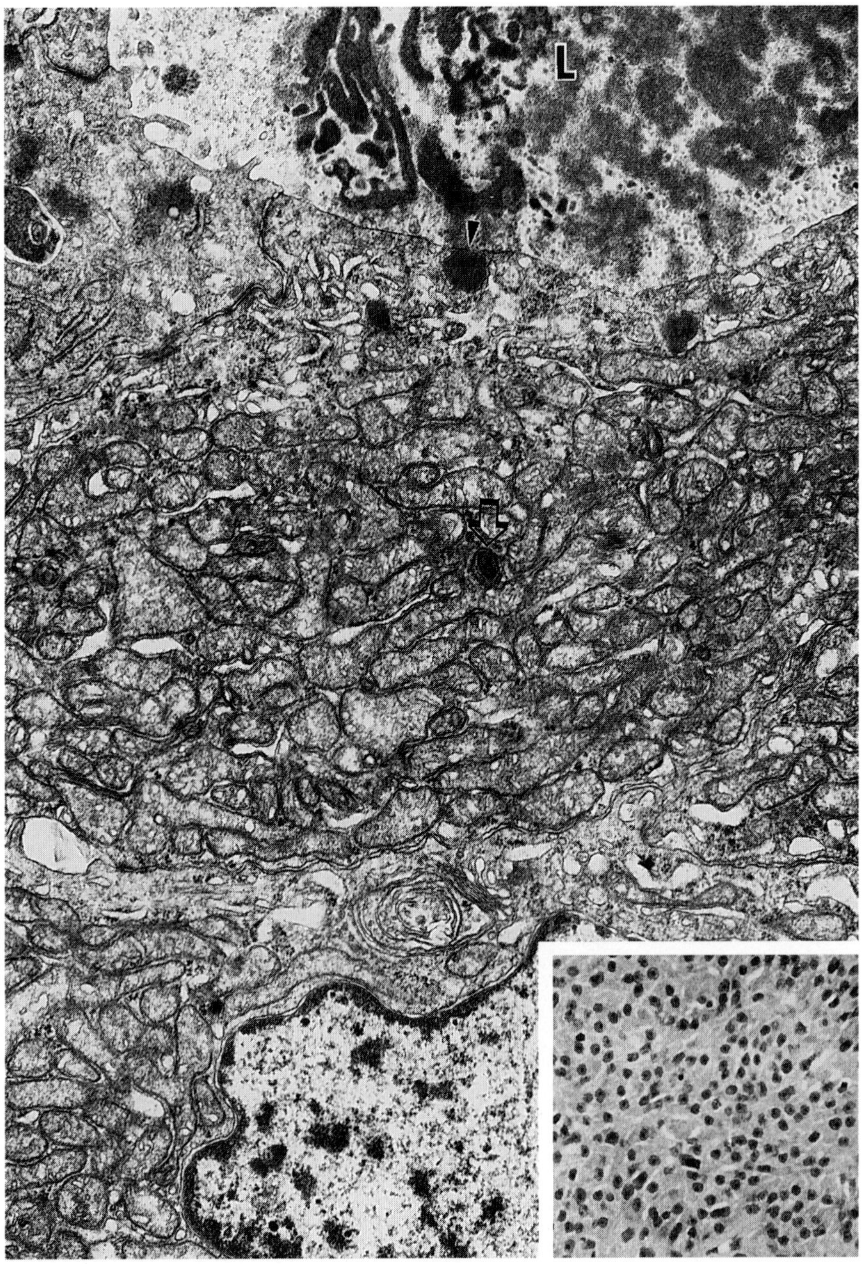


**Fig. 3-106.** Thyroid tumor in a 70-year-old man. Abundant cytoplasmic mitochondria, apical dense bodies (*arrowhead*), and short, irregular apical microvilli are characteristic. Note also colloid-containing lumen *(L)* and finely clumped nuclear chromatin. There is a cytoplasmic membranous whorl (*arrow*), probably artifactual. **Inset**, Histologic appearance of tumor. (**Fig.**, ×15,400; **Inset**, ×195.)

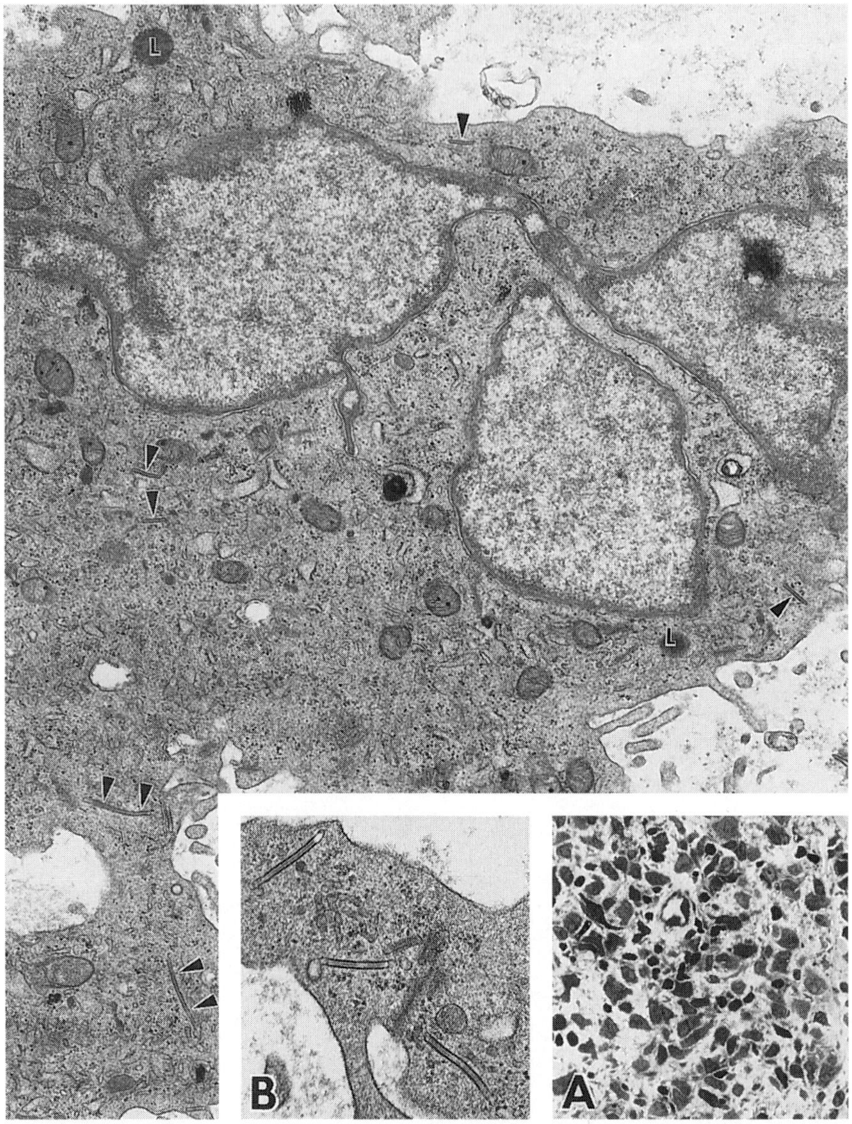

**Fig. 3-107.** Histiocytosis X. Dermal infiltrate in a 66-year-old woman. General histiocytic features include irregular, eccentrically located nucleus, tertiary lysosomes *(L)*, and irregular cell surface without intercellular junctions. Several Birbeck granules (*arrowheads*) are present. **Inset A**, Light microscopic appearance of infiltrate (semithin sections of epoxy-embedded material). **Inset B**, Higher magnification of Birbeck granules, including one with an empty-appearing, vacuolar "head." (**Fig.**, ×15,400; **Inset A**, ×195; **Inset B**, ×27,550.)

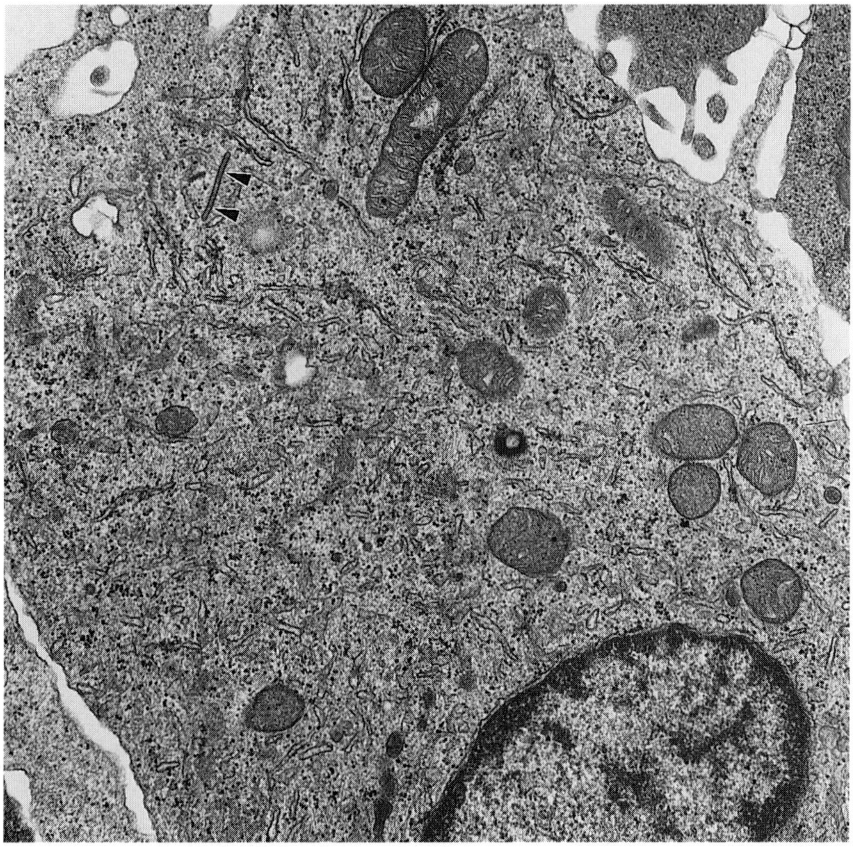

**Fig. 3-108.** Histiocytosis X. Cells prepared from spinal fluid. A Birbeck granule (*arrowheads*) lies within the cytoplasm of a histiocytic cell. (×17,800.)

### Alveolar Soft Part Sarcoma

Alveolar soft part sarcomas are unusual tumors. They do, however, metastasize to brain more commonly than do most sarcomas.[214A] They are distinguished ultrastructurally by unusual rhomboidal cytoplasmic paracrystalline inclusions (Fig. 3-109).[84a,329a]

### Small Cell Carcinoma

Among "ordinary" small cell carcinomas, electron microscopy has shown histogenetic diversity. Ultrastructural subclassification of these tumors carries prognostic importance and may have therapeutic relevance as well. The presence of scattered, small, dense-core neurosecretory granules in small cell carcinomas is well known (see Fig. 3-86). Frequently this feature, alone or in combination with some sparse, simple junctional devices, is the only distinguishing ultrastructural feature of small cell carcinomas. However, 30 to 50% of such tumors show evidence of epithelial differentiation when examined ultrastructurally.[48,175,214] These features may be squamous (tonofilaments, desmosomes) or glandular (intercellular or intracellular lumina; microvilli; junctional complexes; abundant rough endoplasmic reticulum; cilia; large, mucin-type secretory granules)[48,175,214,274] (Figs. 3-87, 3-110). Such features are more common among small cell carcinomas of intermediate cell type or small cell carcinomas with atypical features than they are among classic "oat cell" carcinoma.[274] Patients with such "small cell squamous carcinomas" or "small cell adenocarcinomas" apparently follow a somewhat more favorable clinical course than do those whose tumors possess neurosecretory granules alone or have no differentiating ultrastructural features.[175,214]

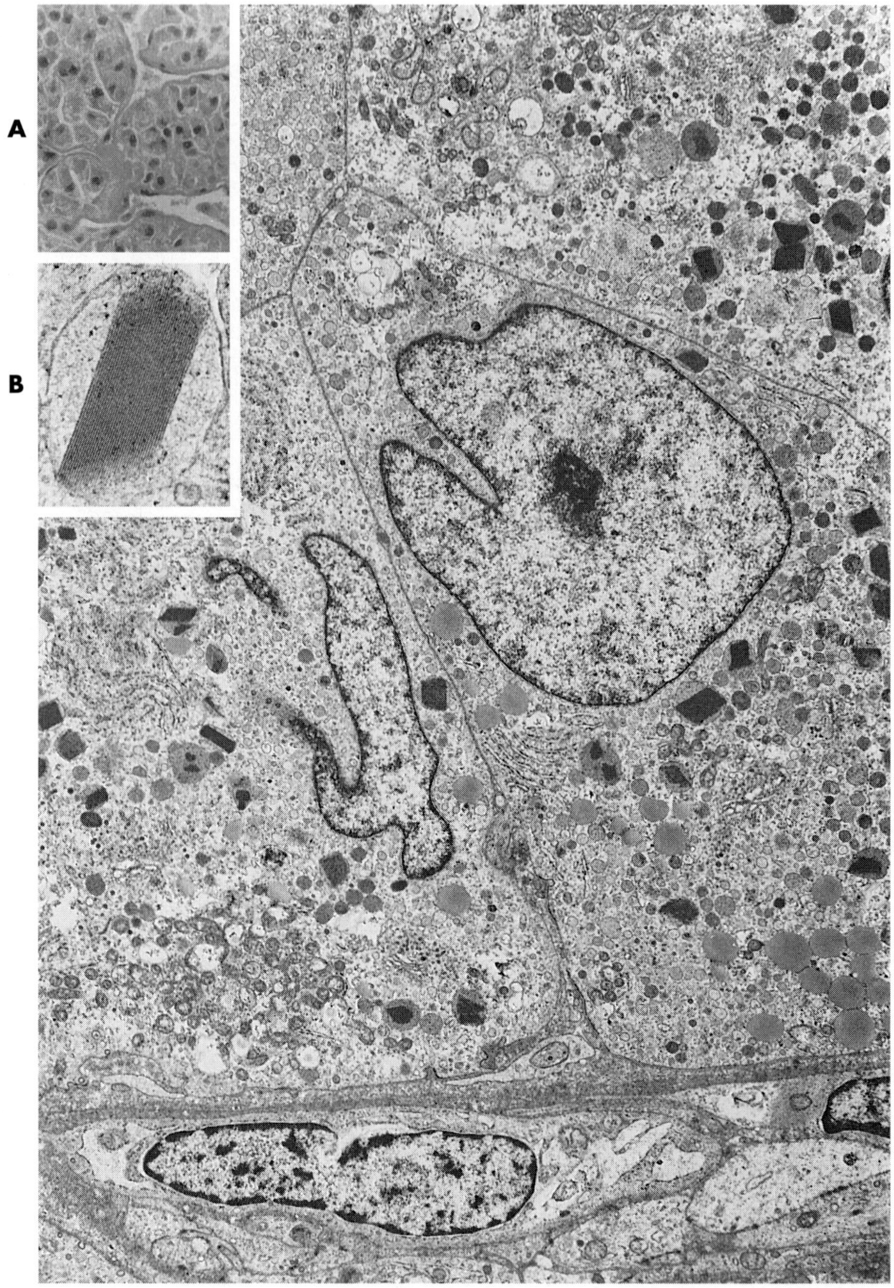

**Fig. 3-109.** Alveolar soft part sarcoma arising in the thigh of a 44-year-old female. Note polygonal tumor cells (top portion of photomicrograph) adjacent to spindle-shaped stromal cell (*bottom*). The tumor cells contain numerous membrane-bound granules containing rhomboid crystals. **Inset A**, Histologic appearance of tumor. **Inset B**, Detail showing rhomboid crystal with 10-nm periodicity of parallel, linear lamellae. (**Fig.**, ×6550; **Inset A**, ×195; **Inset B**, ×43,750.)

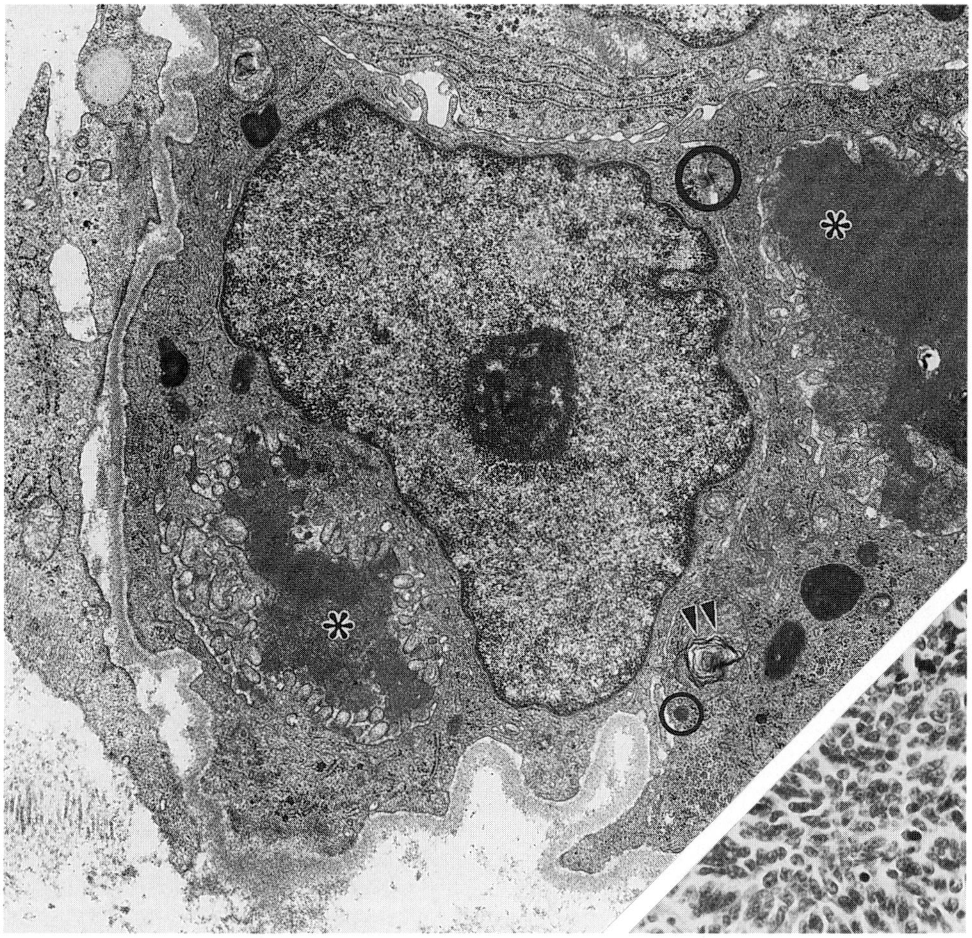

**Fig. 3-110.** Small cell adenocarcinoma of lung in a 74-year-old man. Intracellular lumina are present (*asterisks*). There are also basal lamina, cytoplasmic dense-core granules (*small circle*), intercellular junctions (*large circle*), and cytoplasmic membranous whorls (*arrowheads*). **Inset**, Histologic appearance of tumor. (**Fig.**, ×12,300; **Inset**, ×220.)

## REFERENCES


1. Adamson JS, Senior RM, and Merrill T: Alveolar cell carcinoma. An electron microscopic study, Am Rev Resp Dis 100: 550-557, 1969.
2. Aikawa M, and Ng ABP: Mixed (adenosquamous) carcinoma of the endometrium: electron microscopic observations, Cancer 31:385-397, 1973.
3. Alguacil-Garcia A, Unni KK, and Goellner JR: Malignant fibrous histiocytoma. An ultrastructural study of six cases, Am J Clin Pathol 69:121-129, 1978.
4. Alpert LI, and others: Cholangiocarcinoma. A clinicopathologic study of five cases with ultrastructural observations, Hum Pathol 5:709-728, 1974.
5. Alvira MM, Mandybur TI, and Menefee MG: Light microscopic and ultrastructural observations of a metastasizing malignant epthelioid schwannoma, Cancer 38:1977-1982, 1976.
6. Aronson SM, Garcia JH, and Aronson BE: Metastatic neoplasms of the brain: their frequency in relation to age, Cancer 17:558-563, 1964.
7. Askin FB, and others: Malignant small cell tumor of the thoracopulmonary region in childhood. A distinctive clinicopathologic entity of uncertain histogenesis, Cancer 43:2438-2451, 1979.
8. Azar HA, and others: "Undifferentiated" large cell malignancies: an ultrastructural and immunocytochemical study, Hum Pathol 13:323-333, 1982.
9. Azzarelli B, Muller J, and Mirkin LD: Medulloblastoma (?) with epithelioid features, Acta Neuropathol (Berl) 61:109-115, 1983.
10. Azzarelli B, and others: Central neuroblastoma. Electron microscopic observations and catecholamine determinations, J Neuropathol Exp Neurol 36:384-397, 1977.
11. Bailey P, Cushing H, and Eisenhardt I: Angioblastic meningioma, Arch Pathol 6:953-990, 1928.
12. Bailey P, and Robitaille Y: Primary diffuse leptomeningeal gliomatosis, Can J Neurol Sci 12:278-281, 1985.
13. Balsaver AM, Gibley CW Jr, and Tessmer CF: Ultrastructural studies in Wilms's tumor, Cancer 22:417-427, 1968.
14. Barron KD, and others: Experiences with metastatic neoplasms involving the spinal cord, Neurology 9:91-106, 1954.
15. Battifora H: Intracytoplasmic lumina in breast carcinoma. A helpful histopathologic feature, Arch Pathol 99:614-617, 1975.
16. Becker LE, and Hinton D: Primitive neuroectodermal tumors of the central nervous system, Hum Pathol 14:538-550, 1983.
17. Bedrossian CWM, and others: Ultrastructure of human bronchiolo-alveolar cell carcinoma, Cancer 36:1399-1413, 1975.
18. Bernier V, and Azar HA: Filiform large-cell lymphomas. An ultrastructural and immunohistochemical study, Am J Surg Pathol 11:387-396, 1987.
19. Bibro MC, LiVolsi VA, and Schwartz PE: Adenosarcoma of the uterus: ultrastructural observations, Am J Clin Pathol 71: 112-117, 1979.

20. Bignold LP, and others: Adenocarcinoma of rectosigmoid colon, Ultrastruct Pathol 12:569-575, 1988.
21. Boesel CP, Suhan JP, and Bradel EJ: Ultrastructure of primitive neuroectodermal neoplasms of the central nervous system, Cancer 42:194-201, 1978.
22. Bolen JW, and Thorning D: Histogenetic classification of pulmonary carcinomas. Peripheral adenocarcinomas studied by light microscopy, histochemistry, and electron microscopy, Pathol Annu 17(Part 1):77-100, 1982.
23. Bonikos DS, Bensch KG, and Kempson RL: The contribution of electron microscopy to the differential diagnosis of tumors, Beitr Path Bd 158:417-444, 1976.
24. Bonikos DS, Hendrickson M, and Bensch KG: Pulmonary alveolar cell carcinoma. Fine structural and in vitro study of a case and critical review of this entity, Am J Surg Pathol 1:93-108, 1977.
25. Bonnin JM, and Rubinstein LJ: Astroblastomas: A pathological study of 23 tumors, with a postoperative follow-up in 13 patients, Neurosurgery 25:6-13, 1989.
26. Bundtzen JL, and Norback DH: The ultrastructure of poorly differentiated rhabdomyosarcomas: a case report and literature review, Hum Pathol 13:301-313, 1982.
27. Bures JC, Barnes L, and Mercer D: A comparative study of smooth muscle tumors utilizing light and electron microscopy, immunocytochemical staining and enzymatic assay, Cancer 48:2420-2426, 1981.
28. Camins MB, and others: Medulloblastoma: an ultra structural study—evidence for astrocytic and neuronal differentiation, Neurosurgery 6:398-411, 1980.
29. Cancilla PA, and Zimmerman HM: The fine structure of a cerebellar hemangioblastoma, J Neuropathol Exp Neurol 24: 621-628, 1965.
30. Carlson C, and Sibley RK: Ultrastructural features of pulmonary neoplasms. In Russo J, and Sommers SC, editors: Tumor diagnosis by electron microscopy, vol 3, New York, 1990, Field & Wood.
31. Carstens PHB, and Kuhns JG: Ultrastructural confirmation of malignant melanoma, Ultrastruct Pathol 2:147-149, 1981.
32. Carter LP, Beggs J, and Waggener JD: Ultrastructure of three choroid plexus papillomas, Cancer 30:1130-1136, 1972.
33. Catane R, and others: Brain metastasis from prostatic carcinoma, Cancer 38:2583-2587, 1976.
34. Cervós-Navarro J: Elektronenmikroskopie der Hämangioblastome des ZNS und der angioblastischen Meningiome, Acta Neuropathol (Berl) 19:184-207, 1971.
35. Cervós-Navarro J, and others: The fine structure of gliomatosis cerebri, Virchows Arch A 411:93-98, 1987.
36. Cervós-Navarro J, and Vazquez JJ: An electron microscopic study of meningiomas, Acta Neuropathol (Berl) 13:301-323, 1969.
37. de Chadarévian J-P, Guyda HJ, and Hollenberg RD: Hypothalamic polar spongioblastoma associated with the diencephalic syndrome, Virchows Arch Pathol Anat 402:465-474, 1984.
38. de Chadarévian J-P, and others: Maturation of cerebellar neuroblastoma into ganglioneuroma with melanosis. A histologic, immunocytochemical, and ultrastructural study, Cancer 59: 69-76, 1987.
39. Chaudhry AP, and others: Olfactory neuroblastoma (esthesioneuroblastoma). A light and ultrastructural study of two cases, Cancer 44:564-579, 1979.
40. Chaudhry AP, Montes M, and Cohn GA: Ultrastructure of cerebellar hemangioblastoma, Cancer 42:1834-1850, 1978.
41. Chen SY, and others: Acinic cell adenocarcinoma of minor salivary glands, Cancer 42:678-685, 1978.
42. le Chevalier T, and others: Sites of primary malignancies in patients presenting with cerebral metastases. A review of 120 cases, Cancer 56:880-882, 1985.
43. Chitale AR, and Dickersin GR: Electron microscopy in the diagnosis of malignant schwannomas. A report of six cases, Cancer 51:1448-1461, 1983.
44. Choux R, and others: Hémangiopéricytome cérébral. Étude ultrastructurale d'un cas, J Neurol Sci 28:361-371, 1976.
45. Churg AM, and Kahn LB: Myofibroblasts and related cells in malignant fibrous and fibrohistiocytic tumors, Hum Pathol 8: 205-218, 1977.
46. Churg AM, Ringus J: Ultrastructural observations on the histogenesis of alveolar rhabdomyosarcoma, Cancer 41:1355-1361, 1978.
47. Copeland DD, Bell SW, and Shelburne JD: Hemidesmosome-like intercellular specializations in human meningiomas, Cancer 41:2242-2249, 1978.
48. Copple B, Wright SE, and Moatamed F: Electron microscopy in small cell lung carcinomas: clinical correlation, J Clin Oncol 2:910-915, 1984.
49. Cravioto H: The ultrastructure of acoustic nerve tumors, Acta Neuropathol (Berl) 12:116-140, 1969.
50. Cravioto H: Human and experimental reticulum cell sarcoma (microglioma) of the nervous system, Acta Neuropathol (Berl) Suppl VI:135-140, 1975.
51. Cruz-Sanchez FF, and others: Ependymoblastoma: a histological, immunohistological and ultrastructural study of five cases, Histopathology 12:17-27, 1988.
52. Cushing H, and Eisenhardt L: The Meningiomas, Springfield, IL, 1938, Charles C Thomas.
53. Dairaku M, and others: Immunohistological analysis of surfactant-apoprotein in the bronchiolo-alveolar carcinoma, Virchows Arch Pathol Anat 400:223-234, 1983.
54. Dal Canto M, and Valsamis MP: Fibrosarcoma metastatic to the brain. An unusual case, Arch Pathol 96:108-110, 1973.
55. Dardick I, Hammar SP, and Scheithauer BW: Ultrastructural spectrum of hemangiopericytoma: a comparative study of fetal, adult, and neoplastic pericytes, Ultrastruct Pathol 13:111-154, 1989.
56. Dehner LP, Abenoza P, and Sibley RK: Primary cerebral neuroectodermal tumors: neuroblastoma, differentiated neuroblastoma, and composite neuroectodermal tumor, Ultrastruct Pathol 12:479-494, 1988.
57. DeLellis RA: Ultrastructural immunocytochemistry: An overview of methodology in diagnostic pathology. In Russo J, Sommers SC, editors: Tumor diagnosis by electron microscopy, vol 2, Philadelphia, 1988, Field & Wood.
58. Dickersin GR: The contributions of electron microscopy in the diagnosis and histogenesis of controversial neoplasms, Clin Lab Med 4:123-164, 1984.
59. Dickersin GR: The electron microscopic spectrum of nerve sheath tumors, Ultrastruct Pathol 11:103-146, 1987.
60. Dickersin GR: Central nervous system neoplasms. Diagnostic electron microscopy: A text atlas, New York, 1988, Ikagu-Shoin.
61. Dickersin GR, Vickery AL Jr, and Smith SB: Papillary carcinoma of the thyroid, oxyphil cell type, "clear cell" variant. A light- and electron-microscopic study, Am J Surg Pathol 4:501-509, 1980.
62. Dickson DH, Ramsey MS, and Tonus JG: Synapse formation in retinoblastoma tumours, Br J Ophthalmol 60:371-375, 1976.
63. Dolman CL: Ultrastructure of brain tumors and biopsies, a diagnostic atlas (Methods in laboratory medicine, vol 3), New York, 1984, Praeger.
64. Duffell D, and others: Electron microscopic observations on astrocytomas, Am J Pathol 43:539-554, 1963.
65. Dvorak AM, and Monahan RA: Metastatic adenocarcinoma

of unknown primary site. Diagnostic electron microscopy to determine the site of tumor origin, Arch Pathol Lab Med 106: 21-24, 1982.

66. Earle KM: Metastatic and primary intracranial tumors of the adult male, J Neuropathol Exp Neurol 13:448-454, 1954.
67. Edelmann L: Freeze substitution and low temperature embedding, Inst Phys Conf Ser 98:763-768, 1990.
68. Eimoto T, and others: Ultrastructure of well-differentiated adenocarcinomas of the lung with special reference to bronchioloalveolar carcinoma, Ultrastruct Pathol 8:177-190, 1985.
69. Engstrand DA, England DM, and Oberley TD: Limitations of the usefulness of microvillous ultrastructure in distinguishing between carcinoma primary in and metastatic to the lung, Ultrastruct Pathol 11:53-58, 1987.
70. Erlandson RA: Diagnostic transmission electron microscopy of human tumors, New York, 1981, Masson.
71. Erlandson RA: Ewing's sarcoma with intermediate filaments, Ultrastruct Pathol 5:323-328, 1983.
72. Erlandson RA: Peripheral nerve sheath tumors, Ultrastruct Pathol 9:113-122, 1985.
73. Erlandson RA: The ultrastructural distinction between rhabdomyosarcoma and other undifferentiated "sarcomas," Ultrastruct Pathol 11:83-101, 1987.
74. Erlandson RA: Electron microscopy of tumors of the central and peripheral nervous system including meninges. In Russo J, Sommers SC, editors: Tumor diagnosis by electron microscopy, vol 2, Philadelphia, 1988, Field & Wood.
75. Erlandson RA, and Filippa DA: Unusual non-Hodgkin's lymphomas and true histiocytic lymphomas, Ultrastruct Pathol 13:249-273, 1989.
76. Erlandson RA, and Woodruff JM: Peripheral nerve sheath tumors: an electron microscopic study of 43 cases, Cancer 49: 273-287, 1982.
77. España P, Chang P, and Wiernik PH: Increased incidence of brain metastases in sarcoma patients, Cancer 45:377-380, 1980.
78. Favara BE, McCarthy RC, and Mierau GW: Histiocytosis X, Hum Pathol 14:663-676, 1983.
79. Ferenczy A, Richart RM, and Okagaki T: A comparative ultrastructural study of leiomyosarcoma, cellular leiomyoma, and leiomyoma of the uterus, Cancer 28:1004-1018, 1971.
80. Ferrari C, de Panfilis G, and Manara GC: Preembedding immunogold staining of cell surface-associated antigens performed on suspended cells and tissue sections. In Hayat AT, editor: Colloidal gold. Principles, methods and applications, vol 2 San Diego, 1989, Academic Press.
81. Fine G, and Horn RC: Soft tissue tumors. Aids in differential diagnosis, Pathol Annu, 211–229, 1969.
82. Finean JB, and Woolf AL: An electron microscope study of denenervative changes in human cutaneous nerve, J Neuropathol Exp Neurol 21:211–229, 1962.
83. Fisher ER: Ultrastructure of the human breast and its disorders, Am J Clin Pathol 66:291-375, 1976.
84. Fisher ER, and Horvat B: Comparative ultrastructural study of so-called renal adenoma and carcinoma, J Urol 108:382-386, 1972.

84a. Fisher ER, and Reidbord H: Electron microscopic evidence suggesting the myogenous derivation of the so-called alveolar soft part sarcoma, Cancer 27:150-159, 1971.

85. Fisher ER, and Vuzevski VD: Cytogenesis of schwannoma (neurilemoma), neurofibroma, dermatofibroma and dermatofibrosarcoma as revealed by electron microscopy, Am J Clin Pathol 49:141-154, 1968.
86. Frank TS and others: A detailed immunohistochemical analysis of cerebellar hemangioblastoma: an undifferentiated mesenchymal tumor, Mod Pathol 2:638-651, 1989.
87. Friede RL, and Pollak A: The cytogenetic basis for classifying ependymomas, J Neuropathol Exp Neurol 37:103-118, 1978.
88. Friedman B, and Gold H: Ultrastructure of Ewing's sarcoma of bone, Cancer 22:307-322, 1968.
89. Friedman B, and Hanaoka H: Round-cell sarcomas of bone. A light and electron microscopic study, J Bone Joint Surg 53A: 1118-1136, 1971.
90. Fu Y-S, and others: Malignant soft tissue tumors of probable histiocytic origin (malignant fibrous histiocytomas): general considerations and electron microscopic and tissue culture studies, Cancer 35:176-198, 1975.
91. Fukuda T, Tsuneyoshi M, and Enjoji M: Malignant fibrous histiocytoma of soft parts: an ultrastructural quantitative study, Ultrastruct Pathol 12:117-129, 1988.
92. Furukawa F, and others: True histiocytic lymphoma, Arch Dermatol 116:915-918, 1980.
93. Galloway PG, and Roessmann U: Anaplastic astrocytoma mimicking metastatic carcinoma, Am J Surg Pathol 10:728-732, 1986.
94. Garcia JH, and Lemmi H: Ultrastructure of oligodendroglioma of the spinal cord, Am J Clin Pathol 54:757-765, 1970.
95. Garcia JH, and Mena H: The diagnosis of central nervous system disorders by transmission electron microscopy. In Trump BF, Jones RT, editors: Diagnostic electron microscopy, vol 2, New York, 1979, John Wiley & Sons.
96. Gercovich FG, Luna MA, and Gottlieb JA: Increased incidence of cerebral metastases in sarcoma patients with prolonged survival from chemotherapy, Cancer 36:1843-1851, 1975.
97. Ghadially FN: Is it a melanoma? Diagnostic electron microscopy of tumours, ed 2, London, 1985, Butterworths.
98. Ghadially FN: Is it a myosarcoma? Diagnostic electron microscopy of tumours, ed 2, London, 1985, Butterworths.
99. Ghadially FN: Intracytoplasmic lumina. Diagnostic electron microscopy of tumours, ed 2, London, 1985, Butterworths.
100. Ghadially FN: Fibrous long-spacing collagen. Ultrastructural pathology of the cell and matrix, ed 3, London, 1988, Butterworths.
101. Ghadially FN, Harawi S, and Khan W: Diagnostic ultrastructural markers in alveolar cell carcinoma, J Submicrosc Cytol 17:269-278, 1985.
102. Ghatak NR, and McWhorter JM: Ultrastructural evidence for CSF production by a choroid plexus papilloma, J Neurosurg 45:409-415, 1976.
103. Ghatak NR, Norwood CW, and Davis CH: Intracerebral schwannoma, Surg Neurol 3:45-47, 1975.
104. Gibson AAM, Hendrick EB, and Conen PE: Intracerebral schwannoma. Report of a case, J Neurosurg 24:552-557, 1966.
105. Gillespie JJ, and others: Extraskeletal Ewing's sarcoma. Histologic and ultrastructural observations in three cases, Am J Surg Pathol 3:99-108, 1979.
106. Goebel HH, and Cravioto H: Ultrastructure of human and experimental ependymomas. A comparative study, J Neuropathol Exp Neurol 31:54-71, 1972.
107. Goldammer D, and Goebel HH: Dense core vesicles in the desmoplastic variant of cerebral neuroblastoma, Acta Neuropathol (Berl) 50:81-83, 1980.
108. Gonzales-Angulo A, de Chavez IR, and Casteneda M: A reliable method for electron microscopic examination of specific areas from paraffin-embedded tissue mounted on glass slides, Am J Clin Pathol 70:697-699, 1978.
109. Gonzalez-Crussi F, and others: Peripheral neuroectodermal tumors of the chest wall in childhood, Cancer 54:2519-2527, 1984.
110. Gould VE, and others: Immunohistochemical analysis of Ewing's tumors, Lab Invest 56:28A (Abstr 163), 1987.
111. Greenberg R, Rosenthal I, and Falk GS: Electron microscopy of human tumors secreting catecholamines: correlation with biochemical data, J Neuropathol Exp Neurol 28:475-500, 1969.
112. Greenberg SD, Smith MN, and Spjut HJ: Bronchiolo-alveolar carcinoma—cell of origin, Am J Clin Pathol 63:153-167, 1975.

113. Reference deleted in proofs.
114. Guthrie BL, and others: Meningeal hemangiopericytoma: histopathological features, treatment, and long-term follow-up of 44 cases, Neurosurgery 25:514-522, 1989.
115. Gyorkey F, and others: The usefulness of electron microscopy in the diagnosis of human tumors, Hum Pathol 6:421-441, 1975.
116. Hachitanda Y, Tsuneyoshi M, and Enjoji M: An ultrastructural and immunohistochemical evaluation of cytodifferentiation in neuroblastic tumors, Mod Pathol 2:13-19, 1989.
117. Hadfield MG, and Silverberg SG: Light and electron microscopy of giant-cell glioblastoma, Cancer 30:989-996, 1972.
118. Hameed K, and Morgan DA: Papillary adenocarcinoma of the endometrium with psammoma bodies. Histology and fine structure, Cancer 29:1326-1335, 1972.
119. Hammar SP: Adenocarcinoma and large cell undifferentiated carcinoma of the lung, Ultrastruct Pathol 11:263-291, 1987.
120. Hammar SP, Bockus D, and Remington F: Metastatic tumor of unknown origin, Ultrastruct Pathol 10:281-288, 1986.
121. Hammar SP, Bockus D, and Remington F: Metastatic tumors of unknown origin: an ultrastructural analysis of 265 cases, Ultrastruct Pathol 11:209-250, 1987.
122. Hammar SP, Weaver RA, and Keranen VJ: Left temporal lobe cortex mass in a 19-year-old male, Ultrastruct Pathol 10:583-591, 1986.
123. Hammar SP, and others: Ultrastructural and immunohistochemical features of common lung tumors: an overview, Ultrastruct Pathol 9:283-318, 1985.
124. Harb JM: The ultrastructural appearance of pediatric brain tumors, EMSA Bull 20(1):64-72, Spring, 1990.
125. Hare HG, and Cerny MJ: Soft tissue sarcoma. A review of 200 cases, Cancer 16:1332-1337, 1963.
126. Harkin JC, and Reed RJ: Tumors of the peripheral nervous system, Washington, DC, 1969, Armed Forces Institute of Pathology.
127. Hassoun J, and others: Esthesioneuroepithelioma, a true neurosensorial tumor. Light- and electron-microscopic study of a case with endocranial extension, Acta Neuropathol (Berl) 55: 77-80, 1981.
128. Hassoun J, and others: Central neurocytoma. An electron-microscopic study of two cases, Acta Neuropathol (Berl) 56:151-156, 1982.
129. Hassoun J, and others: Specific ultrastructural markers of human pinealomas. A study of four cases, Acta Neuropathol (Berl) 62:31-40, 1983.
130. Hassoun J, Hirano A, and Zimmerman HM: Fine structure of intercellular junctions and blood vessels in medulloblastomas, Acta Neuropathol (Berl) 33:67-78, 1975.
131. Haustein J, Cruz-Sanchez F, and Cervós-Navarro J: On the ultrastructure of ependymomas—a semiquantitative analysis of diagnostic criteria in 21 cases with special reference to glycogen as a marker, Neurosurg Rev 11:67-76, 1988.
132. Hayat AT: Colloidal gold. Principles, methods and applications, vol 2, San Diego, 1989, Academic Press.
133. Henderson DW, and Papadimitriou JM: Section three: Neural tumors. Ultrastructural appearances of tumours. A diagnostic atlas, Edinburgh, 1982, Churchill Livingstone.
134. Henry K: Electron microscopy in the non-Hodgkin's lymphomata, Br J Cancer 31 suppl II:73-93, 1975.
135. Herrera GA: Limitations of the usefulness of microvillous ultrastructure in distinguishing between carcinoma primary in and metastatic to the lung, Ultrastruct Pathol 12:151(letter), 1988.
136. Herrera GA: Small bowel neoplasm, Dig Dis Sci 30:698, 1985.
137. Herrera GA: Ultrastructural postembedding immunogold labeling: applications to diagnostic pathology, Ultrastruct Pathol 13:485-499, 1989.
138. Herrera GA, Alexander CB, and DeMoraes HP: Ultrastructural subtypes of pulmonary adenocarcinoma. A correlation with patient survival, Chest 84:581-586, 1983.
139. Herrera GA, and Reimann BEF: Electron microscopy in determining origin of metastatic adenocarcinomas, South Med J 77: 1557-1566, 1984.
140. Herrera GA, Turbat-Herrera EA, and Alexander CB: Ultrastructural heterogeneity of pulmonary scar adenocarcinomas: correlation with patients' survival, Ultrastruct Pathol 12:265-277, 1988.
141. Herrera GA, and others: Gastrointestinal autonomic nerve tumors: "plexosarcomas," Arch Pathol Lab Med 113:846-853, 1989.
142. Herrera GA, and others: Malignant small bowel neoplasm of enteric plexus derivation (plexosarcoma): light and electron microscopic study confirming the origin of the neoplasm, Dig Dis Sci 29:275-284, 1984.
143. Herrick MK, and Rubinstein LJ: The cytological differentiating potential of pineal parenchymal neoplasms (true pinealomas), Brain 102:289-320, 1979.
144. Hewlett RH, and Ganz JC: Histiocytosis X of the cauda equina, Neurology 26:472-476, 1976.
145. Hickey WF, and Seiler MW: Ultrastructural markers of colonic adenocarcinoma, Cancer 47:140-145, 1981.
146. Hirano A: Electron microscopy in neuropathology, Prog Neuropathol 1:1-61, 1971.
147. Hirano A: A comparison of the fine structure of malignant lymphoma and other neoplasms in the brain, Acta Neuropathol Suppl VI: 141-145, 1975.
148. Hirano A: Some contributions of electron microscopy to the diagnosis of brain tumors, Acta Neuropathol (Berl) 43:119-128, 1978.
149. Hirano A, Ghatak NR, and Zimmerman HM: Some new fine structure of ependymoblastoma, J Neuropathol Exp Neurol 32:144-152, 1973.
150. Hirano A, and Shin W-Y: Unattached presynaptic terminals in a cerebellar neuroblastoma in the human, Neuropathol Appl Neurobiol 5:63-70, 1979.
151. Hirose T, Sano T, and Hizawa K: Heterogeneity of malignant schwannomas, Ultrastruct Pathol 12:107-116, 1988.
152. Ho K-L: Ultrastructure of cerebellar capillary hemangioblastoma I. Weibel-Palade bodies and stromal cell histogenesis, J Neuropathol Exp Neurol 43:592-608, 1984.
153. Ho K-L: Ultrastructure of cerebellar capillary hemangioblastoma II. Mast cells and angiogenesis, Acta Neuropathol (Berl) 64:308-318, 1984.
154. Ho K-L: Ultrastructure of cerebellar capillary hemangioblastoma III. Crystalloid bodies in endothelial cells, Acta Neuropathol (Berl) 66:117-126, 1985.
155. Ho K-L: Ultrastructure of cerebellar capillary hemangioblastoma IV. Pericytes and their relationship to endothelial cells, Acta Neuropathol (Berl) 67:254-264, 1985.
156. Ho K-L: Ultrastructure of cerebellar capillary hemangioblastoma V. Large pinocytic vacuolar bodies (megalopinocytic vesicles) in endothelial cells, Acta Neuropathol (Berl) 70:117-126, 1986.
157. Ho K-L: Abnormal cilia in a fourth ventricular ependymoma. Acta Neuropathol (Berl) 70:30-37, 1986.
158. Ho K-L: Ultrastructure of cerebellar capillary hemangioblastoma VI. Concentric lamellar bodies of endoplasmic reticulum in stromal cells, Acta Neuropathol (Berl) 74:345-353, 1987.
158a. Ho K-L, Caccamo DV, and Garcia JH: Intracytoplasmic lumina in ependymomas: an ultrastructural study, Ultrastruct Pathol 18:371-380, 1994.

159. Ho K-L, Hoschner JA, and Wolfe DE: Primary leptomeningeal gliomatosis. Symptoms suggestive of meningitis, Arch Neurol 38:662-666, 1981.
160. Hoag G, Sima AAF, and Rozdilsky B: Astroblastoma revisited: a report of three cases, Acta Neuropathol (Berl) 70:10-16, 1986.
161. Hobot JA: Lowicryls and low-temperature embedding for colloidal gold methods. In Hayat AT, editor: Colloidal gold. Principles, methods and applications, vol 2, San Diego, 1989, Academic Press.
162. Hoffman MA, and Dickersin GR: Malignant fibrous histiocytoma: An ultrastructural study of eleven cases, Hum Pathol 14:913-922, 1983.
162a. Hogan MJT, and Wood I: Orbital rhabdomyosarcoma: an electron microscopic study, Trans Am Ophthalmol Soc 70:131-153, 1972.
163. Horie A, Kotoo Y, and Hayashi I: Ultrastructural comparison of hepatoblastoma and hepatocellular carcinoma, Cancer 44: 2184-2193, 1979.
164. Horoupian DS, Lax F, and Suzuki K: Extracerebral leptomeningeal astrocytoma mimicking a meningioma, Arch Pathol Lab Med 103:676-679, 1979.
165. Horten BC, and others: The angioblastic meningioma: a reappraisal of a nosological problem, J Neurol Sci 31:387-410, 1977.
166. Horvat BL, Caines M, and Fisher ER: The ultrastructure of rhabdomyosarcoma, Am J Clin Pathol 53:555-564, 1970.
167. Horvat BL, Pêna C, and Fisher ER: Primary reticulum cell sarcoma (microglioma) of brain. An electron microscopic study, Arch Pathol 87:609-616, 1969.
168. Hossmann K-A, and Wechsler W: Ultrastructural cytopathology of human cerebral gliomas, Oncology 25:455-480, 1971.
169. Hou-Jensen K, Priori E, and Dmochowski L: Studies on ultrastructure of Ewing's sarcoma of bone, Cancer 29:280-286, 1972.
170. Hull MT, and Eble JN: Myelinoid lamellated cytoplasmic inclusions in human renal adenocarcinomas: an ultrastructural study, Ultrastruct Pathol 12:41-48, 1988.
171. Humbel BM, and Schwarz H: Freeze-substitution for immunocytochemistry. In Verkleij AJ, Leunissen JLM, editors: Immunogold labeling in cell biology, Boca Raton, FL, 1989, CRC Press.
172. Humeau C, and others: The fine structure of meningiomas: an attempted classification, Virchows Arch A Path Anat Histol 382:201-216, 1979.
173. Husain AN, and Leestma JE: Cerebral astroblastoma: immunohistochemical and ultrastructural features, J Neurosurg 64: 657-661, 1986.
174. Hwang WS, and Benediktsson H: Lamellar bodies in benign and malignant schwannomas, Acta Pathol Microbiol Immunol Scand Sect 90:89-93, 1982.
175. Iglehart JD, and others: Electron microscopy in selection of patients with small cell carcinoma of the lung for medical versus surgical therapy, J Thorac Cardiovasc Surg 90:351-360, 1985.
176. Iraci G, and others: Histiocytosis X of the central nervous system: clinical and pathological report of a case with predominant cerebellar involvement, Childs Brain 5:116-130, 1979.
177. Ishida Y: Fine structure of primary reticulum cell sarcoma of the brain, Acta Neuropathol (Berl) Suppl VI: 147-153, 1975.
178. Ishwar S, Taniguchi RM, and Vogel FS: Multiple supratentorial hemangioblastomas. Case study and ultrastructural characteristics, J Neurosurg 35:396-405, 1971.
178a. Jääkeläinen J, and others: Intracranial hemangiopericytoma: radiology, surgery, radiotherapy and outcome in 21 patients, Surg Neurol 23:227-236, 1985.
179. Jablokew VR, and others: Testicular nodule incidentally found in elderly male, Ultrastruct Pathol 10:87-91, 1986.
180. Jacques J, and Currie W: Bronchiolo-alveolar carcinoma: a Clara cell tumor? Cancer 40:2171-2180, 1977.
181. Jaffe R, and others: The neuroectodermal tumor of bone, Am J Surg Pathol 8:885-894, 1984.
182. Jakobiec FA, and Tannenbaum M: The ultrastructure of orbital fibrosarcoma, Am J Ophthalmol 77:899-917, 1974.
183. Johannessen JV, editor: Nervous system, sensory organs, and respiratory tract, vol 6, Electron microscopy in medicine, New York, 1979, McGraw Hill.
184. Johannessen JV, and Sobrinho-Simões M: The fine structure of follicular thyroid adenomas, Am J Clin Pathol 78:299-310, 1982.
185. Johnson JE, and others: New perspectives of electron microscopy in medicine. In Russo J, Sommers SC, editors: Tumor diagnosis by electron microscopy, vol 2, Philadelphia, 1988 Field & Wood.
186. Kadin ME, Rubinstein LJ, and Nelson JS: Neonatal cerebellar medulloblastoma originating from the fetal external granular layer, J Neuropathol Exp Neurol 29:583-600, 1970.
187. Kalyan-Raman UP, Cancilla PA, and Case MJ: Solitary, primary malignant astrocytoma of the spinal meninges, J Neuropathol Exp Neurol 42:517-521, 1983.
188. Kamitani H, and others: Capillary hemangioblastoma: histogenesis of stromal cells, Acta Neuropathol (Berl) 73:370-378, 1987.
189. Kamitani H, and others: Ultrastructure of concentric laminations in primary human brain tumors, Acta Neuropathol (Berl) 71:83-87, 1986.
190. Kawamura J, Garcia JH, and Kamijyo Y: Cerebellar hemangioblastoma: histogenesis of stroma cells, Cancer 31:1528-1540, 1973.
191. Kawano N, Yada K, and Yagishita S: Clear cell ependymoma. A histological variant with diagnostic implications, Virchows Arch A Pathol Anat 415:467-472, 1989.
192. Kepes JJ: The fine structure of hyaline inclusions (pseudopsammoma bodies) in meningiomas, J Neuropathol Exp Neurol 34:282-289, 1975.
193. Kepes JJ, Fulling KH, and Garcia JH: The clinical significance of "adenoid" formations of neoplastic astrocytes, imitating metastatic carcinoma in gliosarcomas. A review of five cases, Clin Neuropathol 1:139-150, 1982.
194. Kepes JJ, Goldware S, and Leoni R: Meningioma with pseudoglandular pattern. A case report, J Neuropathol Exp Neurol 42:61-68, 1983.
195. Kepes JJ, and Kepes M: Predominantly cerebral forms of histiocytosis X: a reappraisal of "Gagels hypothalamic granuloma," "granuloma infiltrans of the hypothalamus," and "Ayala's disease" with a report of four cases, Acta Neuropathol (Berl) 14:77-98, 1969.
196. Kepes JJ, Rubinstein LJ, and Eng LF: Pleomorphic xanthoastrocytoma: a distinctive meningocerebral glioma of young subjects with relatively favorable prognosis, Cancer 44:1839-1852, 1979.
197. Khan A, and others: Focal histiocytosis X of the parietal lobe: case report, J Neurosurg 52:431-433, 1980.
198. Kihara I, and others: Cholangiocarcinoma with hypercalcemia: a case report studied by electron microscope and radioimmunoassay, Acta Pathol Jpn 23:791-804, 1973.
199. Kimula Y: A histochemical and ultrastructural study of adenocarcinoma of the lung, Am J Surg Pathol 2:253-264, 1978.
200. King GS, Yu X-R, and Fenoglio-Preiser CM: Electron microscopic and immunocytochemical features of the normal and abnormal endometrium. In Russo J, Sommers SC, editors: Tumor diagnosis by electron microscopy, vol 1, New York, 1986, Field & Wood.
201. Kitahara M, and others: Diffuse form of primary leptomeningeal gliomatosis, J Neurosurg 63:283-287, 1985.
202. Kline KT, and others: Pineoblastoma: An electron microscopic study, Cancer 44:1692-1699, 1979.

202a. Kochanek S, Schröder R, and Firsching R: Hemangiopericytoma of the meninges. I. Histopathological variability and differential diagnosis, Zentralbl Neurochir 47:183-190, 1986.
203. Kubota T, and others: The fine structure of astroblastoma, Cancer 55:745-750, 1985.
204. Kubota T, and others: Abnormal cilia in a malignant ependymoma, Acta Neuropathol (Berl) 71:100-105, 1986.
205. Kuhajda FP, and others: Pleomorphic xanthoastrocytoma: Report of a case with light and electron microscopy, Ultrastruct Pathol 2:25-32, 1981.
206. Kuhn C: Fine structure of bronchiolo-alveolar cell carcinoma, Cancer 30:1107-1118, 1972.
207. Lagáce R: The ultrastructural spectrum of malignant fibrous histiocytoma, Ultrastruct Pathol 11:153-159, 1987.
208. Langford LA: The ultrastructure of the ependymoblastoma, Acta Neuropathol (Berl) 71:136-141, 1986.
209. Reference deleted.
210. Lassmann H, and others: Different types of benign nerve sheath tumors. Light microscopy, electron microscopy and autoradiography, Virchows Arch A Pathol Anat Histol 375:197-210, 1977.
211. Lazarus SS, and Trombetta LD: Ultrastructural identification of a benign perineural cell tumor, Cancer 41:1823-1829, 1978.
212. Leong AS-Y: The relevance of ultrastructural examination in the classification of primary lung tumours, Pathology 14:37-46, 1982.
213. Leunissen JLM, and Verkleij AJ: Cryo-ultramicrotomy and immuno-gold labeling. In Verkleij AJ, Leunissen JLM, editors: Immuno-gold labeling in cell biology. Boca Raton, FL, 1989, CRC Press.
214. Li W, and others: Unpredictable course of small cell undifferentiated lung carcinoma, J Thorac Cardiovasc Surg 81:34-43, 1981.
214a. Lieberman PH, and others: Alveolar soft-part sarcoma, JAMA 198:1047-1051, 1966.
215. Limacher J, Delage C, and Lagáce R: Malignant fibrous histiocytoma. Clinicopathologic and ultrastructural study of 12 cases, Am J Surg Pathol 2:265-274, 1978.
216. Linnoila RI, and others: Evidence for neural origin and PAS-positive variants of the malignant small cell tumor of thoracopulmonary region ("Askin tumor"), Am J Surg Pathol 10:124-133, 1986.
217. Listrom MB, and Fenoglio-Preiser CM: The ultrastructure and immunocytochemistry of gastrointestinal tumors. In Russo J, Sommers SC, editors: Tumor diagnosis by electron microscopy, vol 3, New York, 1990, Field & Wood.
218. Liu HM, McLone DG, and Clark S: Ependymomas of childhood II. Electron-microscopic study, Childs Brain 3:281-296, 1977.
219. Llombart-Bosch A, Blache R, and Peydro-Olaya A: Ultrastructural study of 28 cases of Ewing's sarcoma: typical and atypical forms, Cancer 41:1362-1373, 1978.
220. Luse SA: Electron microscopic studies of brain tumors, Neurology 10:881-905, 1960.
221. Luse SA: Ultrastructural characteristics of normal and neoplastic cells, Prog Exp Tumor Res 2:1-35, 1961.
222. Luse SA: Synaptic structures occurring in a neuroblastoma, Arch Neurol 11:185-190, 1964.
223. Mackay B, Donner L, and Ordonez NG: Small round cell tumors. In Russo J, Sommers SC, eds: Tumor diagnosis by electron microscopy, vol 3, New York, 1990, Field & Wood.
224. Mackay B, Luna MA, and Butler JJ: Adult neuroblastoma: electron microscopic observations in nine cases, Cancer 37:1334-1351, 1976.
225. Mackay B, and Ordonez NG: Adult neuroblastoma of bone. A case report, Ultrastruct Pathol 11:455-464, 1987.
226. Mackay B, and Silva EG: Diagnostic electron microscopy in oncology, Pathol Annu 15 Part 2:241-270, 1980.
227. Mahoney JP, and Alexander RW: Ewing's sarcoma: A light- and electron-microscopic study of 21 cases, Am J Surg Pathol 2:283-298, 1978.
228. Markesbery WR, and Challa VR: Electron microscopic findings in primitive neuroectodermal tumors of the cerebrum, Cancer 44:141-147, 1979.
229. Markesbery WR, Haugh RM, and Young AB: Ultrastructure of pineal parenchymal neoplasms, Acta Neuropathol (Berl) 55: 143-149, 1981.
230. Marsa GW, and Johnson RE: Altered pattern of metastasis following treatment of Ewing's sarcoma with radiotherapy and adjuvant chemotherapy, Cancer 27:1051-1054, 1971.
231. Matakas F, Cervós-Navarro J, and Gullotta F: The ultrastructure of medulloblastoma, Acta Neuropathol (Berl) 16:271-284, 1970.
232. Matsushima T: Choroid plexus papillomas and human choroid plexus. A light and electron microscopic study, J Neurosurg 59:1054-1062, 1983.
233. Mazur MT, and Clark HB: Gastric stromal tumors. Reappraisal of histogenesis, Am J Surg Pathol 7:507-519, 1983.
234. Mazur MT, and Katzenstein A-LA: Metastatic melanoma: the spectrum of ultrastructural morphology, Ultrastruct Pathol 1: 337-356, 1980.
235. McCarty KS Jr, and others: Gonadal dysgenesis with adenocarcinoma of the endometrium: an electron microscopic and steroid receptor analysis with a review of the literature, Cancer 42:512-520, 1978.
236. McComb RD, and Burger PC: Choroid plexus carcinoma. Report of a case with immunohistochemical and ultrastructural observations, Cancer 51:470-475, 1983.
237. McCormick WF: Intramedullary spinal cord schwannoma. A unique case, Arch Pathol 77:378-382, 1964.
238. Mehta Y, and Hendrickson FR: CNS involvement in Ewing's sarcoma, Cancer 33:859-862, 1974.
239. Mena H, and García JH: Primary brain sarcomas. Light and electron microscopic features, Cancer 42:1298-1307, 1978.
240. Michael H, and Roth LM: The value of electron microscopy in the differential diagnosis of ovarian tumors. In Russo J, Sommers SC, editors: Tumor diagnosis by electron microscopy, vol 3, New York, 1990, Field & Wood.
241. Michael RG, and others: Ceruminous gland adenocarcinoma: a light and electron microscopic study, Cancer 41:545-553, 1978.
242. Michaeu C: A new histochemical and biochemical approach to olfactory esthesioneuroma. A nasal tumor of neural crest origin, Cancer 40:314-318, 1977.
243. Mierau GW: Extraskeletal Ewing's sarcoma (peripheral neuroepithelioma), Ultrastruct Pathol 9:91-98, 1985.
244. Mierau GW, and Favara BE: Rhabdomyosarcoma in children: ultrastructural study of 31 cases, Cancer 46:2035-2040, 1980.
245. Mierau GW, Favara BE, and Brenman JM: Electron microscopy in histiocytosis X, Ultrastruct Pathol 3:137-142, 1982.
246. Mierau GW, and others: Primary cerebral neuroblastoma, Ultrastruct Pathol 13:281-289, 1989.
247. Mirchandani I, and others: True histiocytic lymphoma. A report of four cases, Cancer 52:1911-1918, 1983.
248. Misugi K, Misugi N, and Newton WA Jr: Fine structural study of neuroblastoma, ganglioneuroblastoma, and pheochromocytoma, Arch Pathol 86:160-170, 1968.
249. Mohamed AH, and Cherrick HM: Glycogen-rich adenocarcinoma of minor salivary glands. A light and electron microscopic study, Cancer 36:1057-1066, 1975.
250. Montes M, and others: Clara cell adenocarcinoma. Light and electron microscope studies, Am J Surg Pathol 1:245-253, 1977.
251. Morales AR: Electron microscopy of human tumors, Prog Surg Pathol 1:51-70, 1980.
252. Morales AR, Fine G, and Horn RC Jr: Rhabdomyosarcoma: an ultrastructural appraisal, Pathol Annu 7:81-106, 1972.
253. Morales AR, and others: Langerhans cells in a localized lesion of the eosinophilic granuloma type, Lab Invest 20:412-423, 1969.

254. Morales AR, and others: The ultrastructure of smooth muscle tumors with a consideration of the possible relationship of glomangiomas, hemangiopericytomas, and cardiac myxomas, Pathol Annu 10:65-92, 1975.
255. Morantz RA, and others: Extraspinal ependymomas. Report of three cases, J Neurosurg 51:383-391, 1979.
256. Moscinski LC, and Kleinschmidt-DeMasters BK: Primary eosinophilic granuloma of the frontal lobe: diagnostic use of S-100 protein, Cancer 56:284-288, 1985.
257. Moss TH: Electron microscopic observations on malignant choroid plexus papilloma, Neuropathol Appl Neurobiol 9:225-235, 1983.
258. Moss TH: Evidence for differentiation in medulloblastomas appearing primitive on light microscopy: an ultrastructural study, Histopathology 7:919-930, 1983.
258a. Mrak RE: Origins of adenocarcinomas presenting as intracranial metastases: an ultrastructural study, Arch Pathol Lab Med 117:1165-1169, 1993.
258b. Mrak RE: Malignant neurocytic tumor, Hum Pathol 25:747-752, 1994.
259. Mrak RE, Baker GF: Granular cell basal cell carcinoma, J Cutan Pathol 14:37-42, 1987.
260. Mrak RE, Husain MM, and Schaefer RF: Ultrastructure of metastatic rete testis adenocarcinoma, Arch Pathol Lab Med 114: 84-88, 1990.
261. Nakamura M, and others: Analysis of hemangiopericytic meningiomas by immunohistochemistry, electron microscopy and cell culture, J Neuropathol Exp Neurol 46:57-71, 1987.
262. Nakashima N, and others: Choroid plexus papilloma, light and electron microscopic study, Virchows Arch Pathol Anat 400:201-211, 1983.
263. Napolitano L, Kyle R, and Fisher ER: Ultrastructure of meningiomas and the derivation and nature of their cellular components, Cancer 17:233-241, 1964.
264. Navas JJ, and Battifora H: Choroid plexus papilloma: Light and electron microscopic study of three cases, Acta Neuropathol (Berl) 44:235-239, 1978.
265. Nesland JM, and others: Diagnostic problems in breast pathology: The benefit of ultrastructural and immunocytochemical analysis, Ultrastruct Pathol 11:293-311, 1987.
266. Nevalainen TJ, and Järvi OH: Ultrastructure of intestinal and diffuse type gastric carcinoma, J Pathol 122:129-136, 1977.
267. Nevalainen TJ, and Linna MI: Ultrastructure of gastric leiomyosarcoma, Virchows Arch Pathol Anat Histol 379:25-33, 1978.
268. Newman GR: LR white embedding medium for colloidal gold methods. In Hayat, AT, editor: Colloidal gold. Principles, methods and applications, vol 2, San Diego, 1989, Academic Press.
269. Newman GR, and Hobot JA: Role of tissue processing in colloidal gold methods. In Hayat AT, editor: Colloidal gold. Principles, methods and applications, vol 2, San Diego, 1989, Academic Press.
269a. Ng H-K, and Ko CW: Immunohistochemical and ultrastructural studies of oligodendrogliomas reveal features of neuronal differentiation [Abstract], J Neuropathol Exp Neurol 52: 326, 1993.
270. Ng H-K, Tse CCH, and Lo STH: Meningiomas and arachnoid cells: an immunohistochemical study of epithelial markers, Pathology 19:253-257, 1987.
271. Nielsen SL, and Wilson CB: Ultrastructure of a "pineocytoma," J Neuropathol Exp Neurol 34:148-158, 1975.
272. Nirmel KN, and others: Leiomyosarcoma metastatic to the brain, Surg Neurol 10:147-151, 1978.
273. Nishio S, and others: Intraventricular neurocytoma: clinicopathological features of six cases, J Neurosurg 68:665-670, 1988.
274. Nomori H, and others: Subtypes of small cell carcinoma of the lung: morphometric, ultrastructural, and immunohistochemical analyses, Hum Pathol 17:604-613, 1986.
275. Oberling C, Rivière M, and Haguenau F: Ultrastructure of the clear cells in renal carcinomas and its importance for the demonstration of their renal origin, Nature 186:402-403, 1960.
276. Ojeda VJ, Spagnolo DV, and Kakulas BA: Cerebral gliomas with palisading necrosis: glioblastoma multiforme or high grade cerebral neuroblastoma? A light and electron microscopical study of three cases, Pathology 19:167-172, 1987.
277. Reference deleted in proofs.
278. Reference deleted in proofs.
279. Ordóñez NG, Huang W-L, and Mackay B: Peripheral neuroectodermal tumor of the chest wall in a 19-year-old female, Ultrastruct Pathol 13:301-306, 1989.
280. Ordóñez NG, and Mackay B: Ultrastructure of liver cell and bile duct carcinomas, Ultrastruct Pathol 5:201-241, 1983.
281. Osborn DA: Morphology and the natural history of cribiform adenocarcinoma—adenoid cystic carcinoma, J Clin Pathol 30: 195-205, 1977.
282. Osborne BM, and others: Acinar cell carcinoma of the pancreas in a 9-year-old child: case report with electron microscopic observations, South Med J 70:370-372, 1977.
283. Park P, Manabe S, and Ohno T: Incidence and ultrastructure of rudimentary cilia in benign and malignant peripheral nerve tumors, Ultrastruct Pathol 12:407-418, 1988.
284. Pearl GS, and Takei Y: Cerebellar "neuroblastoma": nosology as it relates to medulloblastoma, Cancer 47:772-779, 1981.
285. Reference deleted in proofs.
286. Reference deleted in proofs.
287. Peña CE: Intracranial hemangiopericytoma. Ultrastructural evidence of its leiomyoblastic differentiation, Acta Neuropathol (Berl) 33:279-284, 1975.
288. Pitkethly DT, and others: Angioblastic meningiomas. Clinicopathologic study of 81 cases, J Neurosurg 32:539-544, 1970.
289. Popoff NA, and Ellsworth RM: The fine structure of nuclear alterations in retinoblastoma and in the developing human retina: in vivo and in vitro observations, J Ultrastruct Res 29: 535-549, 1969.
290. Popoff NA, and Ellsworth RM: The fine structure of retinoblastoma. In vivo and in vitro observations, Lab Invest 25:389-402, 1971.
291. Popoff NA, Malinin TI, and Rosomoff HL: Fine structure of intracranial hemangiopericytoma and angiomatous meningioma, Cancer 34:1187-1197, 1974.
292. Povýšil C, and Matějovský Z: Ultrastructure of Ewing's tumour, Virchows Arch Pathol Anat Histol 374:303-316, 1977.
293. Quinonez G, and Simon GT: Cellular junctions in a spectrum of human malignant tumors, Ultrastruct Pathol 12:389-405, 1988.
294. Raimondi AJ, Mullan S, and Evans JP: Human brain tumors: an electron-microscopic study, J Neurosurg 19:731-753, 1962.
295. Raino P: Ultrastructure of neoplastic cells in different histologic subtypes of pulmonary adenocarcinoma, Pathol Res Pract 176:216-235, 1983.
296. Raino P, Sutinen S, and Sutinen SH: Histological subtypes or grading of pulmonary adenocarcinoma. A histochemical and electron microscopic study, Acta Pathol Microbiol Immunol Scand (Section A) 91:227-234, 1983.
297. Ramsey HJ: Fibrous long-spacing collagen in tumors of the nervous system, J Neuropathol Exp Neurol 24:40-48, 1965.
298. Ramsey HJ: Fine structure of hemangiopericytoma and hemangio-endothelioma, Cancer 19:2005-2018, 1966.
299. Rawlinson DG, Herman MM, and Rubinstein LJ: The fine structure of a myxopapillary ependymoma of the filum terminale, Acta Neuropathol (Berl) 25:1-13, 1973.
300. Razzuk MA, and others: Electron microscopical observations

on mediastinal neurolemmoma, neurofibroma, and ganglioneuroma, Ann Thorac Surg 15:73-83, 1973.
301. Rhodes RH, and others: Primary cerebral neuroblastoma: a light and electron microscopic study, Acta Neuropathol (Berl) 41:119-124, 1978.
302. Rice CD, Kersten RC, and Mrak RE: An orbital hemangiopericytoma recurrent after 33 years, Arch Ophthalmol 107:552-556, 1989.
303. Richards P, and McKissock W: Intracranial metastases, Br Med J 1:15-18, 1963.
304. Risdall RJ, and others: Histiocytosis X (Langerhans' cell histiocytosis). Prognostic role of histopathology, Arch Pathol Lab Med 107:59-63, 1983.
305. Robertson DM, Hendry WS, and Vogel FS: Central ganglioneuroma: a case study using electron microscopy, J Neuropathol Exp Neurol 23:692-705, 1964.
306. Robertson DM, and Vogel FS: Concentric laminations of glial processes in oligodendroglioma, J Cell Biol 15:313-334, 1962.
307. Romansky SG, Crocker DW, and Shaw KNF: Ultrastructural studies on neuroblastoma. Evaluation of cytodifferentiation and correlation of morphology and biochemical and survival data, Cancer 42:2392-2398, 1978.
308. Rosai J, Sibley RK, and Dehner LP: A case for the panel: anaplastic malignant round cell tumor of chest wall, Ultrastruct Pathol 3:387-392, 1982.
309. Rubinstein LJ: Tumors of the central nervous system, Washington, 1972, Armed Forces Institute of Pathology.
310. Rubinstein LJ, and Herman MM: A light- and electron-microscopic study of a temporal-lobe ganglioglioma, J Neurol Sci 16: 27-48, 1972.
311. Rubinstein LJ, and Herman MM: Recent advances in neuro-oncology, Recent Adv Neuropathol 1:179-223, 1979.
312. Rubinstein LJ, and Herman MM: The astroblastoma and its possible cytogenic relationship to the tanycyte. An electron microscopic, immunohistochemical, tissue- and organ-culture study, Acta Neuropathol 78:472-483, 1989.
313. Ruebner BH, Gonzalez-Licea A, and Slusser RJ: Electron microscopy of some human hepatomas, Gastroenterology 53:18-30, 1967.
314. Russell DS, and Rubinstein LJ: Pathology of tumours of the nervous system, ed 5, Baltimore, 1989, Williams & Wilkins.
315. Said JW, Hargreaves HK, and Pinkus GS: Non-Hodgkin's lymphomas. An ultrastructural study correlating morphology with immunologic cell type, Cancer 44:504-528, 1979.
316. Salcman M, Quest DO, and Mount LA: Histiocytosis of the spinal cord: case report, J Neurosurg 41:383-386, 1974.
317. Sarkar C, Roy S, and Tandon PN: Oligodendroglial tumors. An immunohistochemical and electron microscopic study, Cancer 61:1862-1866, 1988.
318. Sato H, and others: Myxopapillary ependymoma of the lateral ventricle. A study on the mechanism of its stromal myxoid change, Acta Pathol Jpn 33:1017-1025, 1983.
319. Sceats DJ Jr, and others: Primary leptomeningeal glioma mimicking an acoustic neuroma: case report with review of the literature, Neurosurgery 19:649-654, 1986.
320. Scheck O, and others: Melanotic neuroectodermal tumor of infancy occurring in the left thigh of a 6-month old infant, Ultrastruct Pathol 13:23-33, 1989.
321. Scheithauer BW, and Bruner JM: The ultrastructural spectrum of astrocytic neoplasms, Ultrastruct Pathol 11:535-581, 1987.
322. Schmidt D, and others: Wilm's tumor: review of ultrastructure and histogenesis, Pathol Annu 12:281-300, 1982.
323. Schmidt D, Harms D, and Burdach S: Malignant peripheral neuroectodermal tumours of childhood and adolescence, Virchows Arch Pathol Anat 406:351-365, 1985.
324. Schmidt D, Mackay B, and Ayala AG: Ewing's sarcoma with neuroblastoma-like features, Ultrastruct Pathol 3:143-151, 1982.
325. Schnitt SJ, and Vogel H: Meningiomas. Diagnostic value of immunoperoxidase staining for epithelial membrane antigen, Am J Surg Pathol 10:640-649, 1986.
325a. Schröder R, Firsching R, and Kochanek S: Hemangiopericytoma of the meninges. II. General and clinical data, Zentralbl Neurochir 47:191-199, 1986.
326. Schuler G, and others: Coated Langerhans cell granules in histiocytosis X cells, Ultrastruct Pathol 5:77-82, 1983.
327. Seljelid R, and Ericsson JLE: Electron microscopic observations on specializations of the cell surface in renal clear cell carcinoma, Lab Invest 14:435-447, 1965.
328. Severi B, and others: Ependymoma of the foramen of Monro: Ultrastructural characterization, Ultrastruct Pathol 13:35-42, 1989.
329. Shimura T, Hirano A, and Llena JF: Ultrastructure of cerebellar hemangioblastoma. Some new observations on the stromal cells, Acta Neuropathol (Berl) 67:6-12, 1985.
329a. Shipkey FH, and others: Ultrastructure of alveolar soft part sarcoma, Cancer 17:821-830, 1964.
330. Shin W-Y, and others: Fine structure of a cerebellar neuroblastoma, Acta Neuropathol (Berl) 42:11-13, 1978.
331. Shivshanker K, and Bennetts R: Neurogenic sarcoma of the gastrointestinal tract, Am J Gastroenterol 75:214-217, 1981.
332. Shmookler BM, and Lauer DH: Retroperitoneal leiomyosarcoma. A clinicopathologic analysis of 36 cases, Am J Surg Pathol 7:269-280, 1983.
332a. Shuangshoti S, and others: Solitary primary intracranial extracerebral glioma, J Neurosurg 61:777-781, 1984.
333. Sian CS, and Ryan SF: The ultrastructure of neurilemoma with emphasis on Antoni B tissue, Hum Pathol 12:145-160, 1981.
334. Sibley R, Rosai J, and Froehlich W: A case for the panel: Anenome cell tumor, Ultrastruct Pathol 1:449-453, 1980.
335. Sidhu GS: The ultrastructure of malignant epithelial neoplasms of the lung, Pathol Annu 17 (part 1):235-266, 1982.
335a. Silva EG, and others: Neuroblastomas and neuroendocrine carcinomas of the nasal cavity: a proposed new classification, Cancer 50:2388-2405, 1982.
336. Silverman L, and Rubinstein LJ: Electron microscopic observations on a case of progressive multifocal leukoencephalopathy, Acta Neuropathol (Berlin) 5:215-224, 1965.
337. Singh C, Katyal SL, and Torikata C: Carcinoma of type II pneumocytes. PAS staining as a screening test for nuclear inclusions of surfactant specific apoprotein, Cancer 50:946-948, 1982.
338. Sitte H, Neumann K, and Edelman L: Cryosectioning according to Tokayasu vs rapid-freezing, freeze-substitution and resin embedding. In Verkleij AJ, Leunissen JLM, editors: Immuno gold labeling in cell biology, Boca Raton, FL, 1989, CRC Press.
339. Sivalingam S, and others: Focal eosinophilic granuloma of the temporal lobe: case report, J Neurosurg 47:941-945, 1977.
340. Smolik EA, and others: Histiocytosis X of the optic chiasm of an adult with hypopituitarism: case report, J Neurosurg 29: 290-295, 1968.
341. Sobrinho-Simões MA, Johannessen JV, and Gould VE: The diagnostic significance of intracytoplasmic lumina in metastatic neoplasms, Ultrastruct Pathol 2:327-335, 1981.
342. Sobrinho-Simões MA, and others: Transmission electron microscopy and immunocytochemistry in the diagnosis of thyroid tumors, Ultrastruct Pathol 9:255-275, 1985.
343. Sobrinho-Simões MA, Nesland JM, and Johannessen JV: Ultrastructural features of neoplastic lesions of the thyroid gland. In Russo J, Sommers SC, editors: Tumor diagnosis by electron microscopy, vol 3, New York, 1990, Field & Wood.
343a. Sonneland PRL, and others: Paraganglioma of the cauda equina region, clinicopathologic study of 31 cases with special reference to immunocytology and ultrastructure, Cancer 58: 1720-1735, 1986.
344. Specht CS, and others: Myxopapillary ependymoma of the

filum terminale. A light and electron microscopic study, Cancer 58:310-317, 1986.

345. Spence AM, and Rubinstein LJ: Cerebellar capillary hemangioblastoma: its histogenesis studied by organ culture and electron microscopy, Cancer 35:326-341, 1975.
346. Srigley JR, and others: Selected ultrastructural aspects of urothelial and prostatic tumors, Ultrastruct Pathol 12:49-65, 1988.
347. Steiner GC, Graham S, and Lewis MM: Malignant round cell tumor of bone with neural differentiation (neuroectodermal tumor), Ultrastruct Pathol 12:505-512, 1988.
348. Stembridge VA, Luibel FJ, and Ashworth CT: Soft tissue sarcomas: electron microscopic approach to histogenetic classification, South Med J 57:772-779, 1964.
349. Stiller D, and Katenkamp D: Cellular features in desmoid fibromatosis and well-differentiated fibrosarcomas, Virchows Arch Pathol Anat Histol 369:155-164, 1975.
350. Sun CN, and others: Spectrum of ultrastructural patterns of renal cell adenocarcinoma, Urology 9:195-200, 1977.
351. Syrjänen K, and Hjelt L: Ultrastructural characteristics of human renal cell carcinoma in relation to the light microscopic grading, Scand J Urol Nephrol 12:57-65, 1978.
352. Szakacs JE, Carta M, and Szakacs MR: Ewing's sarcoma, extraskeletal and of bone. Case report with ultrastructural analysis, Ann Clin Lab Sci 4:306-322, 1974.
353. Takahashi H, and others: Ultrastructural alterations of neuronal cells in a brain stem ganglioglioma, Acta Neuropathol (Berl) 74:307-312, 1987.
354. Tani E, and Ametani T: Intercellular contacts of human gliomas, Prog Neuropathol 1:218-231, 1971.
355. Tani E, and Higashi N: Intercellular junctions in human ependymomas, Acta Neuropathol (Berl) 22:295-304, 1972.
356. Tannenbaum M: Ultrastructural pathology of adrenal medullary tumors, Pathol Annu 5:145-171, 1970.
357. Tannenbaum M: Ultrastructural pathology of human renal cell tumors, Pathol Annu 6:249-277, 1971.
358. Taratuto AL, and others: Superficial cerebral astrocytoma attached to dura. Report of six cases in infants, Cancer 54:2505-2512, 1984.
359. Tarnowski WM, and Hashimoto K: Langerhans' cell granules in histiocytosis X. The epidermal Langerhans' cell as a macrophage, Arch Dermatol 96:298-304, 1967.
360. Taxy JB: Electron microscopy in the diagnosis of neuroblastoma, Arch Pathol Lab Med 104:355-360, 1980.
361. Taxy JB, and Almanaseer IY: "Anenome" cell (villiform) tumors: Electron microscopy and immunohistochemistry of five cases, Ultrastruct Pathol 7:143-150, 1984.
362. Taxy JB, and Battifora H: Malignant fibrous histiocytoma. An electron microscopic study, Cancer 40:254-267, 1977.
363. Taxy JB, and Battifora H: Epithelioid schwannoma: Diagnosis by electron microscopy, Ultrastruct Pathol 2:19-24, 1981.
364. Taxy JB, and others: Electron microscopy in the diagnosis of malignant schwannoma, Cancer 48:1381-1391, 1981.
365. Taxy JB, and others: The spectrum of olfactory neural tumors. A light-microscopic immunohistochemical and ultrastructural analysis, Am J Surg Pathol 10:687-695, 1986.
366. Taxy JB, and Hidvegi DF: Olfactory neuroblastoma. An ultrastructural study, Cancer 39:131-138, 1977.
367. Tellez-Nagel I, and Harter DH: Subacute sclerosing leukoencephalitis: ultrastructure of intranuclear and intracytoplasmic inclusions, Science 154:899-901, 1965.
368. Terry RD, and Harkin JC: Regenerating peripheral nerve sheaths following Wallerian degeneration, Exp Cell Res 13:193-197, 1957.
369. Terry RD, and Weiss M: Studies in Tay-Sachs disease II. Ultrastructure of the cerebrum, J Neuropathol Exp Neurol 22:18-55, 1963.
370. Thomas P, and others: True histiocytic lymphoma: an immunohistochemical and ultrastructural study of two cases, Am J Clin Pathol 81:243-248, 1984.
371. Tibbs PA, Challa V, and Mortara RH: Isolated histiocytosis X of the hypothalamus: case report, J Neurosurg 49:929-934, 1978.
372. Timmerman W, and Bubrick MP: Presacral and postsacral extraspinal ependymoma. Report of a case and review of the literature, Dis Colon Rectum 27:114-119, 1984.
373. Torres LF, and others: Intracerebral neuroblastoma. Report of a case with neuronal maturation and long survival, Acta Neuropathol (Berl) 68:110-114, 1985.
374. Townsend JJ, and Seaman JP: Central neurocytoma—a rare benign intraventricular tumor, Acta Neuropathol (Berl) 71:167-170, 1986.
375. Tremblay M: Ultrastructure of a Wilms' tumour and myogenesis, J Pathol 105:269-277, 1971.
376. Triche TJ, and Askin FB: Neuroblastoma and the differential diagnosis of small-, round-, blue-cell tumors, Hum Pathol 14:569-595, 1983.
377. Ts'o MOM, Fine BS, and Zimmerman LE: The Flexner-Wintersteiner rosettes in retinoblastoma, Arch Pathol 88:664-671, 1969.
378. Ts'o MOM, Fine BS, and Zimmerman LE: The nature of retinoblastoma II. Photoreceptor differentiation: an electron microscopic study, Am J Ophthalmol 69:350-359, 1970.
379. Ts'o MOM, and others: Photoreceptor elements in retinoblastoma, Arch Ophthalmol 82:57-59, 1969.
380. Tsuneyoshi M, Enjoji M, and Shinohara N: Malignant fibrous histiocytoma. An electron microscopic study of 17 cases, Virch Arch Pathol Anat 392:135-145, 1981.
381. Turbat-Herrera EA, and others: Neuroendocrine differentiation in prostatic carcinomas. A retrospective autopsy study, Arch Pathol Lab Med 112:1100-1105, 1988.
382. Van Breeman VL: Ultrastructure of human muscle II. Observations on dystrophic striated muscle fibers, Am J Pathol 37:333-341, 1960.
383. van der Valk P, and others: Histiocytic sarcoma (true histiocytic lymphoma): a clinicopathological study of 20 cases, Histopathology 8:105-123, 1984.
384. van der Valk P, and others: Malignant lymphoma of true histiocytic origin: histiocytic sarcoma. A morphological, ultrastructural, immunological, cytochemical and clinical study of 10 cases, Virchows Arch Pathol Anat 391:249-265, 1981.
385. Vannucci RC, and Baten M: Cerebral metastatic disease in childhood, Neurology 24:981-985, 1974.
386. Vartio T, and others: Rhabdomyosarcoma of the oesophagus: light and electron microscopic study of a rare tumor, Virchows Arch Pathol Anat Histol 386:357-361, 1980.
387. Vasquez M, and Sidhu GS: Surfactant production by neoplastic type II pneumocytes. Ultrastruct Pathol 12:605-612, 1988.
388. Verkleij AJ, and Leunissen JLM, editors: Immuno gold labeling in cell biology, Boca Raton, FL, 1989, CRC Press.
389. Vieth RG, and Odom GL: Intracranial metastases and their neurosurgical treatment, J Neurosurg 23:375-383, 1965.
390. Voorhies RM, Sundaresan N, and Thaler HT: The single supratentorial lesion. An evaluation of preoperative diagnostic tests, J Neurosurg 53:364-368, 1980.
391. Waggener JD: Ultrastructure of benign peripheral nerve sheath tumors, Cancer 19:699-709, 1966.
392. Wagner DD, Olmsted JB, and Marder VJ: Immunolocalization of von Willebrand protein in Weibel-Palade bodies of human endothelial cells, J Cell Biol 95:355-360, 1982.
393. Walker P, and Dvorak AM: Gastrointestinal autonomic nerve (GAN) tumor: Ultrastructural evidence for a newly recognized entity, Arch Pathol Lab Med 110:309-316, 1986.
394. Webb JN: Acinar cell neoplasms of the exocrine pancreas, J Clin Pathol 30:103-112, 1977.

395. Webster HDeF: Schwann cell alterations in metachromatic leukodystrophy: preliminary phase and electron microscopic observations, J Neuropathol Exp Neurol 21:534-554, 1962.

395a. Webster HDeF, and Spiro D: Phase and electron microscopic studies of experimental demyelination. I. Variations in myelin sheath contour in normal guinea pig sciatic nerve, J Neuropathol Exp Neurol 19:42-69, 1960.

396. Weibel ER, and Palade GE: New cytoplasmic components in arterial endothelia, J Cell Biol 23:101-112, 1964.

396a. Weidner N: Pulmonary adenocarcinoma with intestinal-type differentiation, Ultrastruct Pathol 16:7-10, 1992.

397. Weiss RA, and Mackay B: Malignant smooth muscle tumors of the gastrointestinal tract: an ultrastructural study of 20 cases, Ultrastruct Pathol 2:231-240, 1981.

398. Weldon-Linne CM, and others: Pleomorphic xanthoastrocytoma. Ultrastructural and immunohistochemical study of a case with a rapidly fatal outcome following surgery, Cancer 52:2055-2063, 1983.

399. Welsh RA, and Meyer AT: Ultrastructure of gastric leiomyoma, Arch Pathol 87:71-81, 1969.

400. Widehn S, and Kindblom L-G: A rapid and simple method for electron microscopy of paraffin-embedded tissue, Ultrastruct Pathol 12:131-136, 1988.

401. Wigger HJ, Salazar GH, and Blane WA: Extraskeletal Ewing's sarcoma. An ultrastructural study, Arch Pathol Lab Med 101: 446-449, 1977.

402. Williams AO, and Ajayi O: Ultrastructure of Wilms' tumor (nephroblastoma), Exp Mol Pathol 24:35-47, 1976.

403. Wilson AJ, Leaffer DH, and Kohout ND: Differentiated cerebral neuroblastoma: a tumor in need of discovery, Hum Pathol 16:647-649, 1985.

404. Winek RR, Scheithauer BW, and Wick MR: Meningioma, meningeal hemangiopericytoma (angioblastic meningioma), peripheral hemangiopericytoma and acoustic schwannoma. A comparative immunohistochemical study, Am J Surg Pathol 13:251-261, 1989.

405. Wright JD, and Font RL: Mucinous sweat gland adenocarcinoma of eyelid. A clinicopathologic study of 21 cases with histochemical and electron microscopic observations, Cancer 44:1757-1768, 1979.

406. Wyche M, and others: High-grade cerebral neuroblastoma: a case study, Med J Austral 150:505-507, 1989.

407. Yagashita S, and others: Primary rhabdomyosarcoma of the cerebrum, Acta Neuropathol (Berl) 45:111-115, 1979.

408. Yagashita S, and others: Morphological investigations on cerebellar "neuroblastoma" group, Acta Neuropathol (Berl) 56:22-28, 1982.

409. Yagashita S, and others: Cerebellar neuroblastoma. A light and ultrastructural study, Acta Neuropathol (Berl) 50:139-142, 1980.

410. Yamashima T, Kida S, and Yamamoto S: Ultrastructural comparison of arachnoid villi and meningiomas in man, Mod Pathol 1:224-234, 1988.

411. Yamashiro K, Suzuki H, and Nagayo T: Electron microscopic study of signet-ring cells in diffuse carcinoma of the human stomach, Virchows Arch Pathol Anat Histol 374:275-284, 1977.

412. Yasutake S, Nakao K, and Matsunaga Y: Fine structure of human hepatoma, Kurume Med J 9:193-204, 1962.

413. Yokoyama M, and others: Ultrastructural and biochemical study of neuroblastoma and ganglioneuroblastoma, Invest Urol 9:156-163, 1971.

414. Yunis EJ: Ewing's sarcoma with neuroblastoma-like features (letter), Ultrastruct Pathol 5:323-328, 1983.

415. Yunis EJ, and others: Glycogen in neuroblastomas. A light- and electron-microscopic study of 40 cases, Am J Surg Pathol 3:313-323, 1979.

416. Zeman W, and Donahue S: Fine structure of the lipid bodies in juvenile amaurotic idiocy, Acta Neuropathol (Berl) 3:144-149, 1963.

417. Zucker DK, and others: Sarcomas metastatic to the brain: case report of a metastatic fibrosarcoma and review of the literature, Surg Neurol 9:177-180, 1978.

418. Zu Rhein GM, and Chou S: Particles resembling papova viruses in human cerebral demyelinating disease, Science 148: 1477-1479, 1965.

C • H • A • P • T • E • R

# 4

# *Tumors: Applications of Immunocytochemical Methods*

**Dario V. Cáccamo**
**Lucien J. Rubinstein***



Progress in immunohistochemistry in the past two decades has resulted in considerable advances in neurosurgical diagnosis. These advances have been paralleled by similar developments in other branches of surgical oncology. Its potential is so great that immunohistochemistry techniques have become almost routine in the histopathology laboratory. Diagnosis has been considerably refined, new entities have been uncovered, and known disorders better outlined. But a stage is reached in which it is apparent that too exclusive a reliance on immunochemistry can raise a num-

* The earliest version of this manuscript was completed shortly before the untimely death of Lucien J. Rubinstein in January, 1990.

ber of diagnostic problems and even, in some cases, result in misinterpretation. Immunohistochemical procedures must be carefully managed by positive and negative controls, and are delicate and sometimes unpredictable. The methods employed are subject to various artifacts and to cross-reactivities that diminish the specificity of immunohistochemistry. A critical evaluation of the appearances must be made in the light and context of other morphologic data. Although evidence provided by immunoreactive methods is often regarded as "hard," the problems raised by these procedures are of the same order of difficulty as those of other special staining techniques: they are often uneven, they are usually variable, and they do not absolve the observer from independent judgment, even if it means dismissing the immunohistochemical findings when they are obviously at variance with other morphologic evidence. This is especially true in the case of markers that have not been fully tested over a wide range of normal and abnormal cells. Thus, the results of electron microscopy and of special stains, especially silver impregnations for reticulin and Mallory's phosphotungstic acid-hematoxylin (PTAH), retain their value and continue to be contributory. Some of the technical pitfalls, the need for reliable positive and negative controls, and the superiority of long incubation periods at low temperature and with high dilutions of the primary antibodies, have been emphasized elsewhere.[168] It has also become apparent that too much weight has been given to immunohistochemical markers in their application as indicators of cyto- or histogenesis, whereas often these markers merely indicate differentiation.[184]

Many immunohistochemical applications are well known. The demonstration of cytoplasmic and cell surface antigens that play a role as glial, neuronal, or other markers of differentiation in neural tumors has been repeatedly reviewed in detail from this and from other laboratories.* Because of the increasing number of contributions published in the field, regular progress reports have become necessary, with frequent revision of the data and their interpretation. These reviews largely lay stress on the immunohistochemical markers most often relied on and on the more recent work performed to demonstrate them. In the present review, only the most important publications in this still rapidly expanding field need to be quoted, with emphasis on work published after those reviews were prepared.

The differentiation markers to be considered play an important role in nervous system structure and function, but their neural specificity is, with few exceptions, only relative. Some of these markers implicate cytoskeletal structures or other organelles; others are related to the cell membranes. Both types are generally known as structural proteins. Other markers function as enzymes, which may be either systemic or local endocrine carriers, or which may behave as neurotransmitters. These proteins are usually soluble. This chapter is mainly concerned with the utilization of these markers in the diagnostic interpretation of central nervous system (CNS) tumors, but it is likely that future applications will include the recognition of different cellular subpopulations in which single or multiple discriminating markers may be expressed. An important aspect of immunohistochemistry is currently being studied at several centers for the demonstration of the kinetic parameters of brain tumors, in particular by using monoclonal antibodies raised against bromodeoxyuridine (BrdU), a thymidine analog incorporated into DNA during the S phase, or Ki-67, a monoclonal antibody that recognizes a human antigen expressed on proliferating and dividing cells. Such an approach may be of significant value in predicting the postoperative behavior of cerebral tumors following exploratory or therapeutic surgery.

This chapter is divided in two main sections. In the first, the principal markers employed in diagnostic neuropathology are discussed. The markers are classified in the following main groups:

**Proteins Associated with the Central Nervous System**

Structural proteins of CNS cells:

- **Intermediate filament proteins:** Glial fibrillary acidic protein (GFA protein), neurofilament proteins
- **Microtubule-associated proteins:** Neuron-associated types of $\beta$-tubulin, microtubule-associated proteins, tau protein
- **Other structural proteins:** Synaptophysin

Non-structural proteins of CNS cells:

- **Nervous system-related enzymes:** Glutamine synthetase, aldolase, carbonic anhydrase, neuron-specific enolase, calcineurin
- **Other nervous system-related proteins:** S-100 protein, myelin-basic protein (MBP), myelin-associated glycoprotein (MAG), retinal S-antigen
- **Growth factor receptors and oncogenes:** p53 tumor suppressor gene, nerve growth factor, epidermal growth factor
- **Neuropeptides and neurotransmitters**
- **Shared lymphoid and neural markers:** CD57 (Leu 7)
- **Neuroectodermal oncofetal markers**

**Non-Neural-Associated Markers**

- **Epithelial markers:** cytokeratins, epithelial membrane antigen, transthyretin
- **Desmin**
- **Vimentin**
- **Markers for germ cell tumors**
- **Lymphoid markers**
- **Apolipoprotein A**

* Refs. 16, 17, 107, 168, 179, 184, 185, 187.

**Laminin, fibronectin, and other extracellular matrix glycoproteins**
**Tenascin**
**Glial hyaluronate-binding protein**
**Endothelial cell markers**
**Hystiocytic markers**
**Markers for microglial cells**

Kinetic markers
**Bromodeoxyuridine, Proliferating Cell Nuclear Antigen (PCNA), Ki-67, and MIB 1**

The second part of the chapter concerns the immunohistochemistry of selected CNS tumors in the following order:

Gliomas: astrocytic neoplasms, ependymomas, oligodendrogliomas
Choroid plexus papillomas and carcinomas
Medulloblastomas and other embryonic CNS tumors
Neuronal neoplasms, including pineal parenchymal tumors, central neurocytoma, and dysembryoplastic neuroepithelial tumors (DNT)
Meningiomas
Cerebellar hemangioblastoma
Schwannomas and neurofibromas
Rhabdoid tumors
CNS histiocytosis
Chordomas, including chondroid chordomas

## PROTEINS ASSOCIATED WITH THE CENTRAL NERVOUS SYSTEM

### Glial Fibrillary Acidic (GFA) Protein

This intermediate filament (IF) protein is widely regarded as the most useful immunocytochemical marker currently available to surgical neuropathologists. Originally described by Eng and co-workers in 1971,[48] it has become an almost indispensable tool for the study of astroglial cells in health and disease. GFA is a cytoskeletal acidic protein with a molecular weight of 55 kilodaltons (kD), which polymerizes in vitro to form smooth, curvilinear or rectilinear 10-nm intermediate filaments. There is very little cross-reactivity between GFA and other neural and non-neural antigens. Excellent monoclonal antibodies (Mabs) and polyclonal antisera are commercially available and work reliably well in routinely fixed and processed tissues. Antigenicity is adequately retained after formalin fixation and can be readily demonstrated in paraffin sections. It is not surprising, then, that GFA protein immunohistochemistry has largely replaced the demonstration of fibrous astrocytes by silver carbonate preparations, although Mallory's PTAH remains a valuable special stain. There appear to be several subtypes of GFA protein, which can be distinguished with specific sets of Mabs[59,201]; however, the distribution of subtypes in specific cellular subpopulations or in altered states of the astrocyte has hardly been studied.[201]

In the normal adult central nervous system (CNS), GFA protein immunostaining is restricted to the cytoplasm of normal and reactive astrocytes (Plate 2A) and some ependymal cells. In the maturing CNS, GFA can be demonstrated in developing astrocytes, oligodendrocytes, ependyma, and choroid plexus epithelium. Outside the CNS, GFA is detected, among others, in the Schwann cells of unmyelinated nerves, in enteric glia, and in the folliculo-stellate glands.[107,187] It is also found in fetal and neonatal cartilage as well as in adult laryngeal and bronchial cartilage.[103,222] Several explanations have been proposed to account for the presence of a glial filament in nonglial cells; these include the sharing of common antigenic determinants with other intermediate filaments (mainly vimentin) and the occasional expression of GFA protein by cells that usually produce other types of intermediate filament protein.[187]

GFA protein is an excellent marker of glial differentiation in CNS tumors. Practically all astrocytomas are GFA protein-positive, with the exception of some protoplasmic astrocytomas. Immunoreactive cells are found in virtually all other subtypes, such as the fibrillary, gemistocytic, and pilocytic variants, the astroblastoma (Plate 2B) the pleomorphic xanthoastrocytoma, the subependymal giant cell astrocytoma, the giant cell glioblastoma (Plate 2C), the superficial astrocytoma attached to the dura, the heavily lipidized glioblastoma, and the astrocytic component of the desmoplastic infantile ganglioglioma.* In glioblastomas (Plate 2D) GFA reactivity is generally focal and restricted to the better differentiated areas; the small anaplastic cells and areas of necrosis are usually negative. Neoplastic astrocytes forming perivascular, perineuronal, and subpial aggregates (the secondary structures of Scherer) are usually GFA-positive.

The astrocytic component of gliosarcomas is also strongly positive (Plate 2E) and contrasts with the negatively stained sarcomatous element.[187] In these circumstances, the protein is invaluable in the differential diagnosis of meningeal sarcoma. GFA reactivity also permits the distinction between pleomorphic xanthoastrocytoma[104] and fibrous xanthoma, and between an extensively lipidized glioma and a xanthosarcoma. In contrast, GFA reactivity does not by itself allow for differentiation of astrocytomas from oligodendrogliomas and ependymomas, since the last two may also contain GFA protein-positive cells (see below). Neoplasms outside the CNS that may show positivity include a variable proportion of schwannomas and neurofibromas, salivary gland epithelial tumors, some tumors of Müllerian origin, and, of course, teratomas

* Refs. 16, 17, 27, 107, 187, 219.

with glial differentiation.* Sustentacular cells in paragangliomas are also GFA- (and S-100) protein positive.[108]

### Neurofilament Proteins

Neurofilament proteins (NFP) are the major intermediate filament proteins of neurons. In contrast to other intermediate filament proteins, NFP are composed of three different subunits, or isoforms, of about 70, 170, and 200 kD in molecular weight. Because there are small variations in their molecular weights in different mammalian species, it is preferable to refer to them as low (L), middle (M), and high (H) molecular weight neurofilament subunits.[214,215] Early studies yielded contradictory results on whether the different subunits were simultaneously coexpressed in central and peripheral nervous system neurons. Subsequent studies using NFP subunit-specific Mabs have shown convincingly that at least some nerve cells (i.e., Purkinje cells) express all three NFP subunits.[217]

To a large extent, many of the biochemical, immunochemical, and immunohistochemical properties of the NFP subunits are affected by their state of phosphorylation. The phosphate content of NFP subunits increases with their molecular weight: NFP-L is the least and NFP-H the most phosphorylated of the subunits.[214] Recently synthesized NF subunits (i.e., NF proteins that have not yet undergone posttranslational modifications) are less phosphorylated than posttranslationally modified neurofilaments. Thus, both heavily and poorly phosphorylated forms of NF-H occur, and they appear to be selectively localized within nerve cells. Heavily phosphorylated NF-H predominates in axons, whereas less phosphorylated NF-H is more abundant in perikarya and dendrites.[214,215] Some of the commercially available anti-NF Mabs react selectively with phosphorylated determinants (e.g., clone SMI 31, Sternberger Immunocytochemicals, Jarretsville, MD) or with nonphosphorylated NF (e.g., SMI 32, Sternberger). Thus, immunostaining is found predominantly in the axonal neurites or in the perikarya, respectively.[205] During fetal development, NF-L is the first of the subunits to appear in the cells of the primitive neural tube, whereas NF-H, which is considered a major factor in determining the diameter of the axon, appears last.[82,194]

In CNS tumors, NF subunits are demonstrated immunohistochemically in differentiated neoplastic neurons and their processes, such as those found in ganglioцytoma, ganglioglioma, and desmoplastic infantile ganglioglioma.[168,215–217,219] In embryonal tumors, such as medulloblastomas, immunoreactivity is present in delicate neurites elaborated by the primitive neoplastic cells, especially in the pale islands of desmoplastic medulloblastomas.[98] In medulloepitheliomas, immunoreactivity for NF cannot be demonstrated in the primitive neuroepithelial elements, but can be found in areas of neuroblastic and ganglionic differentiation.[27] Outside the CNS, immunostaining is found in a variety of peripheral nervous system (PNS) tumors, such as neuroblastomas, paragangliomas, chemodectomas, pheochromocytomas, carcinoid tumors, and neuroendocrine carcinomas, including small cell tumors. NFP subunits are often coexpressed with keratins, and the demonstration of NFP immunoreactivity often requires the use of frozen sections.[127]

### Neuron-Associated Isotypes of β-tubulin

Cytoplasmic microtubules in neurons and in all other eukaryotic cells are predominantly composed of tubulin. This protein is a 100 kD heterodimer, composed of monomers of $\alpha$ and $\beta$-tubulin. There are several different isotypes of $\beta$-tubulin, each of them sharing with the others a constant region sequence but differing in the polypeptide sequence in the variable region, which is located near the carboxyl terminal group of the polypeptide chain.[207] Significant advances have been made in our knowledge and understanding of the structure and expression of $\beta$-tubulin isotypes. In mammals, six functional genes have been identified and sequenced; each of them codifies a different $\beta$-tubulin isotype, classified as I to VI. The class III isotype is expressed in neurons (Plate 2F), but not in glia or in non-neural cell types, except for the Sertoli cell of the testis.[53,207] In addition to its specificity, the class III tubulin appears to be one of the earliest markers indicative of nerve cell differentiation. For instance, in the chick embryo, this isotype can be detected in placodal precursors of the trigeminal ganglion, when the cells are still in the cuboidal epithelial stage.[132] Therefore, the demonstration of its immunoreactivity can be useful to determine neuroblastic or neuronal commitment in a CNS tumor. Employing a monoclonal antibody (TUJ1), we have detected class III tubulin in a number of animal and human neuroepithelial tumors (Plate 3A).

In animal tumors with neuroepithelial differentiation, we have found this isotype in primitive cells forming medulloepithelial rosettes at a very early stage of differentiation, i.e., when other proteins indicative of neuronal or glial differentiation cannot yet be demonstrated.[26,28] In a study of human cerebral medulloepithelioma, we have detected the class III tubulin in the primitive cells of solid areas of the tumor and in the medulloepithelial rosettes (Plate 3B), which morphologically resemble the primitive stages of neural tube formation.[27] Immunoreactivity for this isotype is also found in foci of neuroblastic and neuronal differentiation in these tumors, but not in areas of ependymoblastic, ependymal, or mesenchymal differentiation. The

* Refs. 99, 107, 125, 168, 187, 201.

presence of this tubulin isotype in the cells of the "pale islands" of human cerebellar desmoplastic medulloblastomas has been interpreted as evidence of neuroblastic differentiation.[98]

Current data thus suggest that the class III $\beta$-tubulin isotype is one of the earliest and most specific markers indicative of neuroblastic differentiation. Tubulin isotype-specific Mabs are not yet commercially available.

### Microtubule-Associated Proteins

The microtubule-associated proteins (MAPs) are a group of proteins that copurify with tubulin in brain extracts. MAPs constitute about 5% of purified microtubules and are thought to play an important role in the assembly and stabilization of these structures. The two best studied microtubule proteins are MAP1 and MAP2, but other types also exist, including "juvenile" types mostly detectable in the developing brain.[119,157] In nerve cells, MAP1 is found mainly in axons but is also present in non-neuronal cells. Its diagnostic value is limited. In contrast, MAP2 is a highly specific neuronal microtubular protein. During development, it is transiently expressed in axonal neurites, but in mature neurons MAP2 is mostly found in the perikarya and dendrites.[119] Monoclonal antibodies to MAP2 are very sensitive and specific in demonstrating nerve cells and their processes. MAP2 is easily detected in neuroblasts, but, in contrast to the neuron-associated $\beta$-tubulin isotype, is not detected in the primitive cells of medulloepitheliomatous rosettes of the mouse teratoma.[26] In human tumors, MAP2 is found in adrenal neuroblastomas (Plate 3C), in neuroblastic cells of cerebellar medulloblastomas and cerebral medulloepitheliomas, and in cultures of retinoblastoma cells.[6,27,76,98] MAP2 can be demonstrated in routinely fixed and embedded tissues and should therefore be regarded as a sensitive marker of neuroblastic differentiation in the CNS and PNS.

### Tau Protein

This protein, or group of proteins, is predominantly found in the axons of the adult CNS, where it seems to play an important role in facilitating the assembly and stabilization of microtubules.[14] Unfortunately, its potential as a marker of CNS neoplasms is largely hindered by its poor preservation in routinely fixed tissues. Trojanowski and associates[218] have investigated its immunoreactivity using a monoclonal antibody to a phosphate-independent form of tau. These authors detected tau in axons of neocortex, hippocampus, and cerebellum, with little immunoreactivity in the spinal cord and in the PNS, and none in glial cell lines. Its antigenicity was poorly preserved in formalin-fixed tissues, but Bouin's fixative yielded better results.

Several studies have examined the distribution of tau in Alzheimer's disease and related conditions,[161] but very little is known about the distribution of this protein on human CNS neoplasms. We found tau immunoreactivity in delicate neurites of neuroblastic cells in animal tumors with neuroepithelial differentiation when fixed in Bouin's solution.[26] If properly fixed tissues are available, tau demonstration could be a useful indication of neuroblastic differentiation in CNS neoplasms.

### Synaptophysin

This 38-kD glycoprotein was first isolated from rat and bovine brain in 1985. Synaptophysin is an integral calcium-binding membrane protein of presynaptic vesicles in neurons and neurosecretory granules in neuroendocrine cells.[62,227] The most widely employed Mab to synaptophysin, SY38 (Boehringer Mannheim, Mannheim, Germany), is commercially available and works well both in frozen sections and in routinely fixed and embedded tissues. In normal cerebral cortex, the pattern consists of a delicate punctate staining of the neuropil and around the cytoplasmic membranes of cortical neurons, with less intense staining of the perikarya. This pattern probably reflects the distribution of synapses and of synaptic vesicles. In contrast, in the neuroendocrine system, synaptophysin stains rather evenly throughout the cytoplasm of neuroendocrine cells.[62]

Synaptophysin is a reliable marker for differentiated neuronal tumors, such as ganglioneuromas or the mature elements of ganglioneuroblastomas[62,129] (Plate 3D). In neuroblastomas and cerebellar medulloblastomas, the pattern of reactivity is more delicate and needs to be carefully evaluated, but definite staining is evidence for the neuroblastic nature of a tumor.

### Nervous System-Related Enzymes

**Glutamine synthetase.** This is a cytoplasmic enzyme of astrocytes that plays a role in the detoxification of ammonia and the metabolism of glutamate.[156] It can be detected in astrocytomas and in areas of astrocytic differentiation in cerebellar medulloblastomas.[187]

**Aldolase.** Aldolase is a glycolytic enzyme that may be detected in normal and well-differentiated neoplastic astrocytes.[187]

**Carbonic anhydrase.** This enzyme is a metalloprotein involved in the hydration of carbon dioxide and plays an important role in the regulation of ionic and acid-base balance in various organs, including the CNS. The isoenzyme C is the form present in the CNS that has been found both in normal oligodendrocytes of the human and rodent brain, as well as in Müller cells of the retina.[146] Some oligodendrogliomas contain a small number of cells immunopositive for this isoenzyme, but other CNS and extra-CNS tumor cells are also frequently immunopositive, including normal and neoplastic astrocytes, many ependymomas, meningiomas, schwannomas, and neurofibromas.[146] Carbonic anhydrase has been proposed as a marker for choroid plexus neoplasms.[226] In our view, its reactivity is found in such a wide variety of tumors as to render its diagnostic value in neuropathology marginal.

**Neuron-specific enolase.** Neuron-specific enolase (NSE) remains a widely employed marker in diagnostic neuropathology, as well as in other areas of surgical pathology. First isolated by Moore and co-workers from brain tissue in 1965, NSE is an isoenzyme of the glycolytic enzyme enolase.[117,118,133] There are five different types of dimeric isoenzymes, each of them composed of two out of three immunologically distinct subunits ($\alpha$, $\beta$, and $\gamma$). Nervous tissue contains a mixture of three isoenzymes, two homodimers ($\alpha\alpha$ and $\gamma\gamma$) and one heterodimer ($\alpha\gamma$). The $\gamma$ subunit, as the $\gamma\gamma$) homodimer or the $\alpha\gamma$ heterodimer, constitutes about 2% of the total soluble brain protein.[118] Much lower levels of the $\gamma$ subunit are found in extraneural tissues, such as the liver and skeletal muscle. In the CNS, the $\gamma\gamma$ homodimer is largely confined to neurons, whereas the $\alpha\gamma$ heterodimer is found in glial, meningothelial, and Schwann cells. Neuroblasts appear to contain initially the $\alpha\gamma$ heterodimer, but they switch to produce the $\gamma\gamma$ homodimer when migration is completed and synaptogenesis is initiated.[117] Most commercially available anti-NSE antisera do not discriminate between the neuron-specific $\gamma\gamma$ isoenzyme and the $\alpha\gamma$ heterodimer.

Although NSE is a sensitive marker for cells of neuronal lineage in normal tissues, (Plate 3E) a positive immunostain in a CNS tumor should be interpreted with caution. Positivity can generally be regarded as characteristic, but not specific, of tumors of neuroblastic or neuronal lineage—including cerebellar medulloblastomas, neuroblastomas, ganglioneuroblastomas, and neurocytomas—and of parenchymal pineal tumors, as in pineocytomas and pineoblastomas. However, a large number of glioblastomas, astrocytomas, oligodendrogliomas, meningiomas, choroid plexus tumors, and schwannomas may also show variable NSE reactivity.[60,223] The stromal cells (but not the endothelial cells) of capillary hemangioblastomas may also be NSE-positive. In our experience, although the aforementioned non-neuronal tumors are immunopositive, their staining is often not as widespread or intense as in tumors of neuronal origin.

NSE is also widely used to demonstrate certain neuroendocrine cells and the tumors originated from them, including pancreatic islet cell tumors, medullary thyroid carcinomas, carcinoid tumors, and pulmonary small cell carcinomas, as well as neuron-containing tumors of the PNS such as paragangliomas and pheochromocytomas (Plate 3F). However, positive immunostaining has also been reported in many melanomas, schwannomas, chordomas, and a variety of non-neuroendocrine carcinomas. Possibly, increased glycolytic activity occurs in many proliferating cells so as to meet the needs of rapid cell division. The newer monoclonal antibodies have shown a higher degree of specificity for neuronal and neuroendocrine neoplasms than the commercially available polyclonal antisera.[193]

In summary, NSE remains a useful adjunct in the diagnosis of central and peripheral neuronal and neuroendocrine tumors, but other immunohistochemical or ultrastructural confirmatory evidence must also be available. NSE cannot be used as the only marker to establish the neuronal or neuroendocrine nature of a tumor. The role of NSE as a neuronal marker will probably be superseded by more specific markers, such as synaptophysin, chromogranin, and neuronal microtubular proteins.

**Calcineurin.** This calcium-dependent, calmodulin-stimulated phosphatase is very abundant in the brain, but its function is unknown. Calcineurin is detected in neuronal cells of CNS and PNS tumors, including retinoblastomas and medulloblastomas.[61]

### Other Nervous System-Related Proteins

**S-100 protein.** This thermolabile protein was first isolated by Moore in 1965 from bovine brain, together with NSE.[133] It is an acidic protein with a molecular weight of 20-25 kD, and was named S-100 because of its complete solubility in a solution of 100% ammonium sulfate at neutral pH.[45] S-100 protein consists of two polypeptide chains of 93 and 91 amino acids, which are designated as the $\alpha$ and $\beta$ subunits. The subunits may form homodimers ($\alpha\alpha$, $\beta\beta$) or a heterodimer ($\alpha\beta$). The physiologic role of these dimers is not known. Over 90% of the cerebral S-100 belong to the $\beta$ fraction.[45,94]

S-100 is a calcium-binding protein that may be found bound to the membranes of mitochondria, endoplasmic reticulum, and other organelles, or as a soluble cytoplasmic protein. It can also be found in the cell nucleus, where it may stimulate RNA polymerase I. Other putative roles of S-100 protein include the promotion of neurite outgrowth during development, microtubule disassembly, and the phosphorylation and dephosphorylation of proteins, but its exact function remains unclear.[45]

Although originally thought to be a protein specific for the nervous system, S-100 has been detected in a large number of other cell types. In the brain, although it is found in some neurons, it is fundamentally a protein of glial cells, including astrocytes, oligodendrocytes, and ependymal cells, and also of Schwann cells. Positive tumors include astrocytomas, oligodendrogliomas, ependymomas, glioblastomas, and schwannomas.[147] S-100 reactivity is positive in some nonglial intracranial neoplasms, such as chordomas and the adamantinomatous component of craniopharyngiomas, and in many neoplasms outside the CNS, such as pleomorphic adenomas of the salivary glands, chondrosarcomas, liposarcomas, medullary carcinomas of the breast, and others.[147] Practically all melanocytic neoplasms, including amelanotic melanomas, are strongly positive.[203] S-100 is also useful in the identification of Langerhans cells and in the diagnosis of histiocytosis.

Despite its widespread distribution, S-100 remains a useful marker in certain situations. In neuro oncology, its main application is in the study of tumors with spindle cell features, since it is consistently detected in schwannomas and neurofibromas. However, a significant fraction of malignant schwannomas are negative (see below). Together with other markers, S-100 also permits the distinction between Schwann cells and perineurial cells, which are the presumed cells of origin of perineuriomas, also known as hypertrophic neuropathy or localized neurofibrosis.[5,202,224] Perineurial cells are negative for S-100, but positive for the epithelial membrane antigen (see below).

**Myelin basic protein (MBP) and myelin-associated glycoprotein (MAG).** These two myelin-specific proteins are present in both the central and peripheral nervous systems. Both have been detected in the developing immature oligodendrocytes of the rat; MBP has also been found in oligodendrocytes of the developing human brain.[87,206] Following demyelination, during the period immediately prior to and during remyelination, both MBP and MAG can be demonstrated in oligodendrocytes.[234] Tissue culture studies have also suggested that MAG could represent a marker for immature oligodendrocytes, whereas the presence of MBP would be indicative of advanced maturation and differentiation.[183]

Despite initial hopes that MBP and MAG would be significant markers for oligodendrogliomas and Schwann cell tumors, neither is useful for the identification of these neoplasms. In our experience, the neoplastic cells of oligodendrogliomas are not positive for MBP, which can be detected only in remnants of myelin sheaths. In a personal study of 32 oligodendrogliomas, none was positive for MBP, and only two showed focal reactivity for MAG.[145] Somewhat better results were obtained by Tanaka and co-workers,[211] who detected MBP positivity in 14 of 28 oligodendrogliomas. However, some of the cells immunoreactive for MBP in their study could be astrocytes, since these cells also reacted for GFA protein. In peripheral nerve sheath tumors, immunoreactivity for MBP or MAG cannot, in our experience, be demonstrated in schwannomas, neurofibromas, or granular cell tumors. Johnson and co-workers[95] confirmed this failure to detect MBP immunoreactivity in benign nerve sheath tumors or in sarcomas; the only MBP-positive lesions were traumatic "neuromas."

**Retinal S-antigen.** Retinal S-antigen, also known as arrestin, is a 48-kD protein that can be detected immunohistochemically in retinal photoreceptors and in the pinealocytes of several vertebrates, including humans (Plate 4A). In retinal photoreceptors and in submammalian pineal photoreceptors, the protein is thought to be involved in the transduction of light; its function in mature pinealocytes is unclear.[164,169]

In our study of 18 retinoblastomas, S-antigen immunoreactivity was found in all differentiated, but in only 1 of 11 undifferentiated, tumors. The differentiated cells forming Flexner rosettes were also positive for NSE and for the 200 kD subunit of NF. Glial markers were found only in reactive neuroglia. The presence of these markers is interpreted as evidence for the neuronal potential of retinoblastoma cells, thus supporting the view that the tumor is of neuroblastic origin and may arise from precursors of photoreceptor cells.[164]

In tumors of the pineal parenchyma, S-antigen has been found in some well-differentiated pineocytomas and in pineoblastomas. Two examples of malignant pineocytoma were negative.[169] Korf and associates[109] conducted a study on S-antigen in the cerebrospinal fluid of 13 patients with tumors of the pineal region. Immunoreactivity was detected in one patient with a pineocytoma; other nonparenchymatous tumors of the pineal region were negative.

S-antigen also can be detected immunohistochemically in some of the cells of cerebellar medulloblastomas.[15,42] In our experience, S-antigen is not found in cerebral neuroblastomas, in central neurocytomas, or in other intracranial tumors such as meningiomas.[168]

### Growth Factor Receptors and Oncogenes

**p53 tumor suppressor gene.** Tumor suppressor genes such as p53 may play an important role in the pathogenesis of human gliomas. In fact, p53 mutations are the most common genetic alterations in human tumors. The p53 gene located in the short arm of chromosome 17 encodes for a nuclear phosphoprotein that controls key elements of the cell cycle. One of the earliest events of glioma progression entails loss of genetic information from the short arm of chromosome 17, where the p53 gene is located.[36,209] Since turnover of the normal p53 product is rapid, the very small amount of the protein present under normal conditions is not detectable immunohistochemically. Mutations of p53 in neoplastic cells lead to a slow turnover and accumulation of the p53 protein in both the nucleus and cytoplasm of the tumor cells that can be detected immunohistochemically by using polyclonal and monoclonal antibodies such as Pab 1801. In general, the immunohistochemical detection of p53 in gliomas correlates well with p53 mutations detected by molecular genetic techniques such as restriction fragment length polymorphism analysis, but not all p53 mutations can be detected immunohistochemically.[114] Several groups have detected accumulation of p53 protein in human gliomas in situ and in human glioma cell lines.[209] In general, high-grade gliomas, such as anaplastic astrocytomas and glioblastomas show greater accumulation of p53 than do better differentiated tumors.[47] In some cases, progression of a well-differentiated astrocytoma to an anaplastic tumor has coincided with accumulation of p53.[47] Pilocytic astrocytomas, non-neoplastic gliosis, and normal brain contain no or very little p53.[19] Some authors have suggested immunohistochemical detection of p53 as a potential means to distinguish between reactive and neoplastic astrocytes.[8] The practical value of p53 immunohistochemical detection in gliomas remains to be established, but p53 detection could play an important role in future studies of glioma progression.

**Nerve growth factor.** Nerve growth factor (NGF) is a polypeptide essential for the differentiation and survival of sympathetic and sensory neurons derived from the neural crest. In cultures of the PC12 rat pheochromocytoma line, NGF induces neuronal differentiation, promoting the outgrowth of neurites. A number of Mabs recognize NGF-binding proteins or receptors (NGFR). In addition to sympathetic and sensory neuroma, NGFR can be detected in non-neuronal cells, such as Schwann cells in culture or fetal Schwann cells in vivo. NGFR immunoreactivity has also been identified in neurofibromas of patients with von Recklinghausen's disease and in traumatic neuromas.[230]

A regulatory role has been proposed for NGFR in both neuronal and non-neuronal tissue and tumors. Using Mabs to NGF in either frozen or paraffin-embedded sections, Garin-Chesa and co-workers[54] detected immunoreactivity in peripheral nerves, ganglion cells, and Schwann cells, but not in CNS tumors. NGFR was also found in keratinocytes, breast epithelium, the basal layer of the esophageal epithelium, renal glomeruli, prostatic epithelium, lymphocytes, and perivascular mesenchymal tissues. In tumors, NGFR was detected in embryonal rhabdomyosarcomas, skin and breast carcinomas, lymphomas, ganglioneuromas, schwannomas, meningiomas, and melanomas, but NGFR was not present in neuroblastomas, astrocytomas, and nevi. In contrast, Perosio and Brooks,[171] using the avidin-biotin-complex (ABC) method in paraffin-embedded tissues, found NGFR positivity in epineurium and endoneurium, but not in ganglion cells or in axons. Immunoreactive tumors to NGFR include granular cell tumors, benign and malignant peripheral nerve sheath tumors, neuroblastomas, synovial sarcomas, and hemangiopericytomas. Infrequent positivity was found in fibrous and fibrohistiocytic tumors. Ewing's sarcomas were negative. Although additional studies are needed, NGFR may be a potentially useful marker in very restricted situations; in the distinction of undifferentiated small cell tumors, an NGFR-positive neuroblastoma could possibly be differentiated from an NGFR-negative Ewing's sarcoma.

**Epidermal growth factor.** The epidermal growth factor receptor (EGFR) is a polypeptidic cellular mitogen sharing a common plasma membrane receptor for signal transduction. Epidermal growth factor is encoded by the erb-B oncogene located on chromosome 7. In a study of meningiomas, strong immunoreactivity for EGFR was detected in the endothelial cells of 6 of 12 tumors; very weak reactivity was found in the neoplastic meningothelial cells.[198] Interestingly, normal leptomeningeal vessels do not display any immunoreactivity. No correlation was found between the immunoreactivity and the histologic type of meningioma. EGFR may help promote the growth of stromal vessels of meningiomas, but a diagnostic role for this marker remains to be established.

### Neuropeptides and Neurotransmitters

More than 200 substances have been demonstrated or suggested as neurotransmitters and regulatory neuropeptides in the mammalian brain.[83] Although the immunohistochemical demonstration of these compounds can be interpreted as evidence of the neuronal or neuroendocrine nature of a tumor, relatively few studies have looked for their presence in CNS neoplasms. This is probably because their demonstration calls for stringent requirements of tissue fixation and processing. Also, in contrast to neuroendocrine tumors—in which neuropeptides are relatively abundant—the amount of these substances in normal and neoplastic ganglion cells is probably small. The appropriate fixation of these small and soluble neuropeptides and neurotransmitters is especially challenging.[197,220] In a study of a rodent tumor with neuroepithelial differentiation, we found that formalin fixation is a poor preservative of antigenicity. In contrast, fixation in Bouin's solution or in Zamboni's fluid yields better results.[26] Also the positive immunohistochemical demonstration of a small neuropeptide or a neurotransmitter should be interpreted with caution. Most studies have used polyclonal antisera in which the neuropeptide, as a hapten, is coupled with a large carrier protein (e.g., albumin). The possibility that such antisera react with an antigenic determinant of the carrier protein rather than with the specific neuropeptide should be ruled out. It is therefore essential to confirm a positive staining by absorbing the antiserum with its corresponding neuropeptide; the preabsorbed antiserum should extinguish the reactivity detected with the untreated antiserum.[204]

Few studies have explored the presence of neuropeptides in tumors of the PNS. Opioid peptides (met- and leu-enkephalin, $\beta$-endorphin), somatostatin, vasoactive intestinal peptide (VIP), substance P, neuropeptide Y, and cholecystokinin are examples of the best known neuropeptides. In a study comparing benign and malignant paragangliomas, Linnoila and associates[112] showed that malignant tumors immunostain for fewer neuropeptides (average two) than do benign (average five). In another study of functional and nonfunctional extraadrenal paragangliomas, the immunohistochemical demonstration of neuropeptide Y, met-enkephalin, and the enzyme tyrosine hydroxylase correlated with the secretion of biologically active substances.[71]

There are even fewer studies as yet on the distribution of neuropeptides and neurotransmitters in CNS tumors. Immunopositivity for somatostatin, leu- and met-enkephalin, substance P, and serotonin exists in cerebral gangliocytomas and ganglioneuromas,[210] and the presence of VIP has been documented in a gangliocytoma of the cerebellum.[90] Although neuropeptides can be detected biochemically in glial tumors, Przedborski and associates[174] showed that these substances are contained in neuronal elements entrapped within the tumor, while neoplastic glial cells do not contain neuropeptides. We have shown an opioid peptide, serotonin, and GABA-like reactivity in the immature cells of rodent ovarian tumors with neuroepithelial differentiation.[26] There seems to be an interesting correlation with the normal embryonic development of peptidergic systems, since the above-named substances are the earliest neuropeptides to appear in the developing vertebrate brain. In summary, provided that adequately fixed and processed tissue is available and appropriate control procedures are employed, the demonstration of neuropeptide-like immunoreactivity could be used as evidence for the neuronal lineage of a CNS tumor.

### Shared Lymphoid and Neural Markers

**Leu 7 monoclonal antibody.** This commercially available mouse monoclonal antibody (Beckton Dickinson, Mountain View, CA) was originally raised against a human T-cell lymphoblastoid cell line.[1] Although initially regarded as a specific marker of cells with natural killer activity (HNK) and of antibody-dependent killer cells, Leu 7 antibody recognizes normal and neoplastic elements of the rodent and human CNS and PNS.[189] In the cluster designation (CD), Leu 7 is the CD57 antigen. The antibody apparently reacts with a carbohydrate epitope on MAG and also recognizes antigenic determinants in neuroendocrine cells and tumors, including small cell carcinomas of the lung and normal, hyperplastic, and malignant prostatic epithelium.[120] Generally, immunoreactivity to Leu 7 is seen on the cytoplasmic membranes of the cells and the myelin sheaths, but occasionally it is visible as a diffuse cytoplasmic staining.

In the PNS, one of the most useful applications resides in Leu 7's ability to recognize normal and neoplastic Schwann cells.[166] Thus, most benign schwannomas and neurofibromas are immunoreactive. In our experience, most malignant schwannomas and neurofibrosarcomas are also reactive,[166] as confirmed by others[208]; however, other authors have found no reactivity in nerve sheath sarcomas.[95] In contrast to Schwann cells, normal and neoplastic perineurial cells are Leu 7-negative. Other non-schwannian neoplasms, such as meningiomas, leiomyomas, leiomyosarcomas, and fibrohistiocytomas are Leu 7-negative. In conjunction with S-100 protein and EMA, this antibody therefore forms a triad of useful markers in peripheral nerve sheath tumors (see below).

In CNS tumors, Leu 7 reacts with more than 90% of oligodendrogliomas, but it also recognizes many other neoplastic cell types, including those of astrocytomas, glioblastomas, astroblastomas, and, to an extent, ependymomas.[138,145,167] Some of the cells in polar spongioblastomas, pineoblastomas, medulloblastomas, and esthesioneuroblastomas are also recognized.[167] Despite its reactivity with diverse tumor cells, Leu 7 remains a useful tool in the diagnosis of oligodendrogliomas; the number of positive cells in oligodendrogliomas is generally much greater than that seen in other CNS tumors. The antibody seems to especially recognize the cell membranes, particularly in well-differentiated tumors, whereas anaplastic variants tend to be immunonegative. Meningiomas are negative, thus Leu 7 may be helpful in distinguishing this tumor from an oligodendroglioma invading the arachnoid membrane.

Leu 7 is therefore of value in diagnostic neurooncology, as in the examples quoted above. The physiologic role of the cell membrane and myelin proteins that bind with this antibody needs further study.

### Neuroectodermal Oncofetal Markers

A number of polyclonal antisera and monoclonal antibodies have been produced that react with antigens shared by human fetal brain, human neuroepithelial tumors, and cell lines derived from glioma, neuroblastoma, and melanoma.[22,228] Their pattern of immunoreactivity is rather complex and related to the considerable antigenic heterogeneity of human gliomas and their cell lines. For instance, Mab UJ13A selectively reacts with tissues of neuroectodermal origin and their neoplasms.[3] This pan-neuroectodermal Mab has been applied to distinguish neuroectodermal tumors from metastatic neoplasms and lymphomas. However, the practical use in human neurooncology of this and other human brain-associated antigens is very limited, owing to the marked phenotypic variations of human neuroectodermal tumors and the inability of these antigens to define specific human histocompatibility complex (HLA) determinants. Moreover, most Mabs raised to glioma-associated antigens cross-react extensively with normal neuroepithelial cells and with extraneural tissues. The antigenic determinants are also very sensitive to routine fixation and are inactivated by formalin; special techniques are necessary to maintain adequate antigenicity.

## NON-NEURAL-ASSOCIATED MARKERS

### Cytokeratins

The cytokeratins are a group of proteins with a molecular weight ranging between 40 and 68 kD that constitute the intermediate filament proteins associated with epithelial cells.[143] At least 19 subtypes have been demonstrated in human epithelial cells, with an additional group of four to eight "hard" keratins also detected in hair-forming cells. Based on their molecular weight and isoelectric point, Moll and colleagues have classified the keratins in subgroups 1 to 19.[131] Subsequently, a cytokeratin has been designated cytokeratin 20 with a limited range of expression, primarily confined to gastric and intestinal epithelium, certain endocrine cells, and Merkel's cells in the epidermis. Keratins 1 to 8 constitute the neutral-basic keratins, and 9 to 19 the group of acidic keratins. Acidic and basic keratins occur as obligate pairs, forming heteropolymers in all epithelial cells. Cytokeratin filaments are, apparently, tetrameric units consisting of two acidic and two basic proteins. Thus, each epithelial cell type possesses its own subset of keratins, usually composed of two to ten classes.[175] Each subset consists of at least one pair, formed by one basic and one acidic keratin. Importantly, the subsets are heterogeneous and vary according to the specific epithelium under consideration, and also according to the stage of embryonic development and the degree of differentiation. For example, simple cuboidal or columnar epithelia usually contain keratins 7 or 8 (basic) and 18 or 19 (acidic). Stratified epithelium usually possesses one basic keratin of class 4, 5, or 6, and one acidic keratin belonging to class 13 or 14.[143] Of significance to the surgical pathologist is the fact that these patterns of keratin production are retained in the tumors originating from simple or stratified epithelia.

A meaningful comparison of the results of keratin immunochemistry requires that special attention be given to the methodology employed by different groups. In some instances, keratin positivity was identified in frozen sections or after pretreatment of tissue sections with proteases.[7] The subject of keratin immunohistochemistry in brain tumors is therefore complex, and contradictory results are not unusual. Nevertheless, keratins have some utility in a number of diagnostic neuropathologic situations. A first, almost obvious use is the identification of epithelial elements in a poorly differentiated carcinoma metastatic to the brain. Immunostains for keratin play a specially important role in the common situation of metastatic carcinoma to the brain in a patient with no known primary malignancy (Plate 4B). In this situation, demonstration of keratin immunoreactivity is of the greatest importance to confirm the diagnosis of metastatic carcinoma. Moreover, future availability of monoclonal antibodies with selective reactivity for specific keratins may be useful to lead the clinician to the most likely primary site. For instance, a monoclonal antibody against keratin 7 is more likely to react against adenocarcinomas from ovary, lung, or breast and less likely to react with carcinomas of the gastrointestinal tract. A metastatic carcinoma to the brain of unknown primary that reacts with cytokeratin 20 is more likely to originate from the gastrointestinal tract than from the breast or lung.

Cytokeratin immunoreactivity also can be useful in the detection of epithelial elements in intracranial and spinal teratomas, and in identifying the epithelial elements of craniopharyngiomas. However, keratin immunoreactivity has also been detected in primary neuroepithelial tumors, where its occurrence is apparently unexpected.

A potentially serious pitfall in the interpretation of keratin immunoreactivity in brain tumors is the well-established fact that some gliomas are keratin positive. For instance, Ng and Lo[151] identified keratin in about 60% of glioblastomas and anaplastic astrocytomas and in 40% of well-differentiated astrocytomas. These results were obtained with Mabs AEI/AE3, but not with other keratin antibodies (CAM 5.2 and PKK-1). The highly sensitive avidin biotin complex (ABC) method was employed in that study. Isolated neoplastic astrocytes and oligodendrocytes showing immunoreactivity to keratin were identified in 50% of oligodendrogliomas. Ependymomas showed no immunoreactivity. Similar results were obtained in another study, also employing Mabs AE1/AE3, and again using the ABC method; most (83%) anaplastic astrocytomas and glioblastomas showed positivity.[38] Many of the keratin-positive tumors were also reactive for vimentin, and all were reactive for GFA protein. In our practice, when we use keratin to confirm a diagnosis of metastatic carcinoma, we employ a "restricted cocktail" of anti-keratin monoclonal antibodies that include monoclonal antibody CAM 5.2 but not AE1/AE3. This limited cocktail decreases the potential reactivity of normal and neoplastic glial cells to keratin and produces a more specific stain for truly epithelial elements. Nevertheless, keratin immunoreactivity is an example of a circumstance in which immunohistochemistry must be interpreted in conjunction with routine stains and with the rest of the clinical and radiologic features of the patient.

Epithelial-like areas have been described in gliosarcomas,[102] and they contain cells that immunostain for keratin by the peroxidase-antiperoxidase (PAP) technique.[136] Both in gliosarcomas and glioblastomas, epithelial-like whorls identical to the keratin pearls of a squamous cell carcinoma rarely may be found. Such whorls are strongly immunopositive for keratin and the epithelial membrane antigen.[136,187] Here immunohistochemical and conventional light microscopy findings reinforce each other strongly. They suggest an extreme example of metaplasia (namely squamous) in a malignant glial tumor. But when such confirmatory evidence is lacking, the diagnostic significance of keratin immunoreactivity in poorly or well-differentiated primary gliomas is uncertain. Keratin positivity has also been reported in smooth muscle tumors, including leiomyosarcomas.[64]

Chordomas are also keratin-positive. These tumors, which may occasionally invade the brain parenchyma, have a complex immunohistochemical pattern. They also react for vimentin, S-100 protein, and the epithelial membrane antigen.

Intracranial germ cell tumors may display immunoreactivity for keratin. Tumor cells in 3 of 11 intracranial germinomas showed focal immunoreactivity while seemingly equivalent gonadal tumors, namely testicular seminomas and ovarian dysgerminomas, did not immunostain for keratin.[144] Other intracranial germ cell tumors, namely the epithelial elements of teratomas and large areas of endodermal sinus tumors and embryonal carcinomas, also immunoreact for keratin (Plate 4C).

### Epithelial Membrane Antigen

The epithelial membrane antigen (EMA) is a glycoprotein first demonstrated in human milk fat globules.[78] Studies using polyclonal antisera and monoclonal antibodies have shown that EMA is an excellent marker for normal and neoplastic epithelia. The immunoreactivity is resistant to various fixatives and well preserved in paraffinized sections. In contrast to keratin, which EMA complements or sometimes advantageously replaces in the study of epithelial neoplasms, frozen sections or protease pretreatment are not necessary.

EMA shows wide reactivity with the cells of epithelial neoplasms, with the exception of hepatocellular and adrenal carcinomas.[172] Mesotheliomas, synovial and epithelioid sarcomas, as well as chordomas are also EMA positive. Paradoxically, the most important use of EMA in neuro oncology is related to non epithelial tumors.

Most meningiomas are EMA positive. This percentage varies in different studies but is always high; in two large series it was 100% and 90%, respectively.[152,191] The positivity generally is confined to the cell membranes, but, occasionally, intracytoplasmic immunoreactivity is found. Normal arachnoid granulations also display EMA positivity,[152] which exists in all histologic types of meningioma, with the important exception of the angioblastic (hemangiopericytic) meningioma.[229]

The luminal lining surface of normal ependymal cells is positive for EMA. Occasional cells of the normal choroid plexus are also positive. Positivity also may be found in ependymomas. In a study by Cruz-Sanchez et al.,[40] 18 of 27 ependymomas showed EMA positivity in the luminal and the apical surfaces of cells lining ependymal rosettes; in contrast, anaplastic ependymomas showed no immunoreactivity. The nature of the immunoreactive material in ependymoma cells that cross-reacts with a glycoprotein of human milk fat globules is unknown.

Areas showing squamous differentiation in the epithelial-like areas of gliosarcomas and glioblastomas are strongly EMA positive.[168,187] Occasional positivity also may be found in some cells of malignant astrocytomas but oligodendrogliomas are consistently negative. EMA immunoreactivity may also be demonstrated in intracranial germ cell tumors, such as the epithelial components of teratomas, in cells of endodermal sinus tumors and embryonal carcinomas, and in a small number of cells in germinomas.[144]

Some studies[5,165,202] report that perineurial cells of normal nerves and the cells of perineuriomas are strongly EMA positive. Schwannomas, neurofibromas, granular cell tumors, and neurothekeomas show no positivity, except for the entrapped perineurial cells. Traumatic and Morton neuromas display bundles of nerve cell processes wrapped in layers of EMA-positive perineurial cells. Thus, EMA is a marker of perineurial cells and their neoplasms and should be used in conjunction with the standard Schwann cell marker S-100 protein in the study of peripheral nerve tumors. The concept that perineurial and arachnoidal cap cells may share a common embryologic origin is supported by the fact that both are EMA immunoreactive.[5]

### Transthyretin

Transthyretin (TTR), also known as prealbumin, is a thyroxine-binding protein that also intervenes in the transport of retinol. TTR is composed of four identical subunits, and its molecular weight is about 55 kD.[91,92]

The liver apparently is the major source of serum TTR, but the choroid plexus epithelium also has been identified as another site of TTR synthesis. Other putative sites of synthesis are the A (glucagon) cells of the pancreas. Transthyretin immunoreactivity also has been shown in glucagonomas and malignant insulinomas of the pancreas.[91,92]

Because the epithelium of the normal choroid plexus is strongly immunoreactive for TTR, this protein could be a useful marker for choroid plexus papilloma and, especially, choroid plexus carcinoma, a tumor that may present significant diagnostic problems. The immunoreactivity has also been investigated in colloid cysts of the third ventricle, a lesion with a histogenetic origin that is a matter of controversy. In a preliminary study, we did not detect TTR immunoreactivity in colloid cysts. Some metastatic carcinomas are also immunoreactive for TTR; however, since choroid plexus carcinomas occur predominantly in infants and newborns, detecting TTR immunoreactivity in a poorly differentiated intraventricular neoplasm supports the diagnosis of choroid plexus carcinoma.

### Desmin

Desmin is the intermediate filament protein of all muscle cells. Its immunohistochemical demonstration can be useful in rare CNS tumors with rhabdomyoblastic differentiation, as in medullomyoblastoma or rhabdomyosarcoma. However, most polyclonal antisera or monoclonal antibodies commercially available show rather low sensitivity when used in formalin-fixed tissue and give good results only in alcohol or Carnoy-fixed tissue, or on cryostat-cut sections. We have noted nonspecific immunoreactivity of this antigenic determinant with some malignant glioma cells; the reasons for this reactivity are still unclear. Commercial Mabs to muscle-specific actin (such as the clone HHF 35) have been developed; this Mab works well in routinely fixed and embedded tissues and thus is more useful than desmin or myoglobin in the study of tumors with suspected muscle differentiation.[9]

### Vimentin

This 57-kD intermediate filament protein exists in most normal and neoplastic mesenchymal cells, including endothelial cells, fibroblasts, macrophages, lymphocytes, chondrocytes, and vascular smooth muscle cells. Vimentin was believed to be a useful marker for the distinction of nonepithelial from epithelial-derived neoplasms,[160] but recent reports indicate that epithelial cells can switch to synthesize vimentin when they are grown in tissue culture or when they are detached in vivo and suspended in effusion fluid.[176] Moreover, a number of solid epithelial neoplasms may coexpress keratin and vimentin, including among others, renal, lung, gastric, and ovarian carcinomas.[7] Thus, the specificity of vimentin as a mesenchymal marker and therefore its diagnostic value are severely limited. Vimentin reactivity is best preserved in alcohol-fixed tissues,[7] but good reactivity is usually obtained in formalin-fixed tissues. Treating histologic sections with proteolytic enzymes does not improve vimentin reactivity.

During CNS development, vimentin is the first intermediate filament protein to appear in the primitive cells of the neural tube. Neuronal precursors rapidly switch to synthesize NF proteins, and glial precursors start to produce GFA protein soon.[11] In mature and neoplastic astroglia, vimentin and GFA protein coexist. Whether the presence of vimentin in glioma cells is indicative of tumor dedifferentiation and, thus, of a poor prognosis, is a matter of controversy. Some studies have indicated that vimentin reactivity is quite common in astrocytic and ependymal gliomas, regardless of the differentiation of the tumor, even though the more anaplastic tumors show increased frequency of vimentin positivity; virtually all malignant astrocytomas and ependymomas and all glioblastomas are positive.[38,40,89] Other vimentin-positive CNS neoplasms include a large proportion of meningiomas, schwannomas and hemangioblastomas, chordomas, and rare CNS sarcomas.[16,107,168,187] With the possible exception of meningiomas (see below), in none of these tumors does vimentin immunoreactivity play a significant role in the differential diagnosis, and markers for each of them better than vimentin are readily available.

### Markers for Germ Cell Tumors

Intracranial germ cell tumors generally display immunohistochemical markers similar to those found in their gonadal equivalents. Thus, the demonstration of $\beta$-human chorionic gonadotrophin ($\beta$-hCG) in syncytiotrophoblasts, of $\alpha$-fetoprotein in cells of endodermal sinus tumors, and of placental alkaline phosphatase (PLAP) in germinoma cells is useful in the diagnosis of intracranial germ cell tumors.[2,144] Angiotensin-converting-enzyme (ACE) has been detected in intracranial and gonadal germinomas. In one patient with a suprasellar germinoma, elevated plasma levels of ACE dramatically decreased after surgery, suggesting that monitoring plasma ACE could be useful in the follow-up of selected patients.[188] There may be immunohistochemical differences between intracranial germinomas and their gonadal equivalents; some of the cells in intracranial germinomas display immunoreactivity for keratin, EMA, and vimentin, while all gonadal seminomas and dysgerminomas were immunonegative for these determinants.[144]

### Lymphoid Markers

Primary lymphomas of the CNS are relatively rare tumors, representing in most series less than 2% of primary brain neoplasms. However, their incidence is increasing, and they are conspicuous in immunocompromised patients, including organ transplant recipients and those with the acquired immune deficiency syndrome (AIDS).[81] The histologic subtypes of CNS lymphomas are the same as those of nodal or extranodal origin. A marked predominance of diffuse, large cell lymphomas exists, while nodular lymphoma and Hodgkin's disease of the CNS are very rare. It would be preferable to study CNS lymphomas with the same thoroughness as their nodal counterparts, but most immunohistochemical studies of CNS lymphoma are performed on formalin-fixed, paraffin-embedded tissues.

The first diagnostic problem is often the differential diagnosis with other primary or metastatic brain tumors, including gliomas and poorly differentiated anaplastic carcinomas. For this purpose, the most useful antigen is the leukocyte common antigen (LCA) (CD45RB), a cell surface antigen detectable in virtually all hematolymphoid proliferations (Plates 4D and 4E).[111] The commercially available monoclonal antibodies recognizing this antigen are reliable, and some of these antisera work well on paraffin sections. Immunohistochemical detection of LCA strongly indicates a lymphoid proliferation. Confirmatory evidence such as negative staining for GFA protein and epithelial markers (keratin or EMA) also should be sought. Of note, some lymphomas such as anaplastic large cell lymphomas may be negative for LCA and positive for some epithelial markers such as EMA. In these instances, overinterpretation of immunostains without taking into account the morphology of the tumor cells may lead to an erroneous diagnosis of metastatic poorly differentiated carcinoma. In such cases, CD30 (BerH2) may be useful to demonstrate the lymphoid nature of the tumor cells. Plasma cells and Reed-Sternberg cells are also frequently negative for LCA.

Most primary brain lymphomas are B-cell neoplasms.[81,187] Each of 20 cases, reported by Garson and co-workers, were of B-cell origin, as determined by a monoclonal antibody specific for B lymphocytes.[55] This and other pan-B-cell markers such as L26 (CD20) (Dako Corporation, Santa Barbara, CA), can be demonstrated in paraffin sections.[30] In most CNS lymphomas, an infiltrate of reactive small T lymphocytes is also present. These lymphocytes may be identified by their reactivity for T-cell markers, such as polyclonal CD3 or UCHL1 (CD45RO). Because nearly one half of the brain lymphomas express cytoplasmic immunoglobulins, a monoclonal staining pattern for heavy and light chains is further evidence of a neoplastic B cell proliferation.

### Apolipoprotein A

Apolipoprotein A (Apo A) is a 34-kD lipophilic protein that circulates in plasma as a constituent of chylomicrons and of very low-density and high-density lipoproteins.[140] Apo A is synthesized principally in the liver, but the adrenal, kidney, and brain are additional sources. The protein can be demonstrated immunohistochemically in astrocytes and to a lesser extent in Bergmann glia, but not in neurons, oligodendrocytes, or choroid plexus cells. In tumors, Apo A has been found in astrocytomas and glioblastomas and in the astrocytic component of mixed oligodendrocytomas-astrocytomas.[140] In cell cultures, cells derived from well-differentiated astrocytomas secrete Apo A into the medium, thus suggesting that immunoreactive Apo A in glial tumors is not merely absorbed to neoplastic glial cells. Nevertheless, the demonstration of Apo A does not offer any significant advantage over GFA protein immunostaining, a procedure that reacts much more intensely in glioma cells.

### Laminin, Fibronectin, and Other Extracellular Matrix Glycoproteins

Basement membranes are complex structures composed of several different macromolecules, especially laminin, type IV collagen, heparin and chondroitin sulfate proteoglycans, entactin, and nidogen. In addition, fibronectin and type V collagen are localized at the interface of the basement membrane and the underlying stroma. These and other complex macromolecules of the extracellular matrix are putatively involved in the biology of malignant neoplasms, such as tumor invasion, metastases, and host immune responses.[123]

Some immunohistochemical studies have explored the usefulness of detecting these substances in diagnostic neuropathology. McComb and associates[122] investigated the distribution of collagen type VI, fibronectin, and glioma-mesenchymal extracellular matrix (GMEM) glycoprotein in normal brain and gliomas. In normal brain, type VI collagen was found in the blood vessels and the leptomeninges, whereas in neoplasms both type VI collagen and fibronectin were codistributed in the vasculature and connective stromal tissues. In contrast, GMEM glycoprotein was localized not only in blood vessels and connective tissue, but also within the tumor parenchyma. The glycoprotein was found in some astrocytomas but was practically absent from pilocytic astrocytomas and medulloblastomas. Both GMEM glycoprotein and proteoglycans are the only extracellular matrix components associated with glioma cells in vivo.

The expression of extracellular proteins may change with the progression of gliomas in vitro.[124] Malignant tumors may become rich in fibronectin, while GFA protein decreases; no differences in laminin and in collagen type IV production were detected between GFA protein-positive and GFA-negative glioma cells. This progression may be the result of an early switch from GFA protein to fibronectin production by glioma cells in the artificial milieu of culture, or it could be an overgrowth of these cultures by mesenchymal cells present in the original tumor. The issue is unsettled. High-grade gliomas contain urokinase-like plasminogen activator (uPA), an enzyme that may enhance the invasiveness and dissemination of these aggressive tumors.[29]

Schwann cells produce both type IV collagen and laminin. Thus, both schwannomas and neurofibromas display linear immunostaining for these substances.[56,178] There is also a differential distribution of collagen subtypes in nerve sheath tumors.[158] Antoni A areas in schwannomas, which are composed of tightly packed spindle cells, are almost exclusively immunoreactive for collagen type IV, indicating an abundance of basement membranes; in the less cellular Antoni B areas, types I, III, IV, and VI collagen can be demonstrated. These findings suggest that neoplastic Schwann cells may produce diverse types of collagen according to the regional organization of the tumor.

### Tenascin

This extracellular matrix glycoprotein is found in human glioma cell lines, in glioma xenografts of athymic mice, and in human gliomas in vivo, but not in normal adult and fetal brain.[70,232] Tenascin is also found in many other tumor types, including fibrosarcoma, carcinoma of the breast, and Wilms' tumors, as well as in normal liver and spleen sinusoids. A radioiodinated antitenascin Mab (81C6) exhibits therapeutic potential against subcutaneous and intracranial human glioma xenografts in athymic mice and rats. The selective localization of tumors using Mab 81C6 in patients with gliomas and other intracranial malignancies also has been reported.[232]

### Glial Hyaluronate-Binding Protein

Hyaluronectin is a hyaluronic acid-binding protein localized in the nodes of Ranvier of central and peripheral nerve fibers, as well as in connective tissue and in the stroma of some tumors. Bignami and Dahl[13] isolated a glial hyaluronate-binding protein (GHAP), which is related to but different from hyaluronectin. GHAP, which shows structural similarities with cartilage proteoglycans, is found mainly in brain and in the white matter astrocytes of the spinal cord, where it colocalizes with GFA protein, but is not found outside the CNS.[170] In a study with anti-GHAP Mabs, no reactivity existed in 13 primary brain tumors, except for areas of polar spongioblastoma in one astrocytoma;[12] neoplastic and reactive GFA protein-positive astrocytes showed no GHAP positivity. Polar spongioblastoma, it has been suggested, may derive from GHAP-positive, GFA protein-negative glial precursor cells.

### Endothelial Cell Markers

The endothelium of blood vessels, but not that of lymphatic vessels, is immunoreactive for both laminin and type IV collagen. However, the two most widely used markers of endothelial cell differentiation are factor VIII-related antigen and Ulex Europaeus lectin. The factor VIII-related antigen is one of the three functional components of the antihemophilic factor; factor VIII-related antigen is synthesized in vascular endothelial cells, but it can also be identified in megakaryocytes, platelets, and mast cells.[67,139] It is a reliable marker for normal endothelial cells and benign angiogenic tumors, but many malignant tumors of vascular origin, especially poorly differentiated angiosarcomas, are often negative.[4]

Ulex Europaeus I is a fucose-binding lectin that reacts with a surface glycoprotein of human endothelial cells and erythrocytes. The bound lectin can be detected with an anti-Ulex polyclonal antiserum in a modified immunoperoxidase reaction. Ulex Europaeus-binding activity is a good marker of endothelial cells and is more sensitive than the factor VIII-related antigen.[159] However, the lectin may also react with carcinomas and some sarcomas because of the expression of blood group isoantigen H by epithelial cells.

Immunodetection of CD34-related antigen has become a new and useful marker to identify endothelial-derived tumors. CD34 is a 100-kD protein expressed in hematopoietic cells and in endothelial cells. In non hematopoietic tissue, CD34 reactivity is largely confined to endothelial cells.[51] The role of CD34 antigen related protein in endothelial cells is not known, but it may be involved in cell adhesions and interactions. In routinely-fixed and embedded sections, CD34 is superior to factor VIII in identifying normal and neoplastic endothelial cells in CNS and non-CNS tissues. Vascular tumors positive for CD34 include most angiosarcomas and the spindle cells of Kaposi's sarcoma, among several other tumors.[177] Spindle cells of certain cutaneous tumors, such as dermatofibrosarcoma protuberans are also positive. The use of endothelial cell markers in the study of CNS hemangioblastomas is discussed below.

### Histiocytic Markers

Alpha-1-antichymotrypsin (AACT), alpha-1-antitrypsin, and lysozyme are often used in the study of histiocytic tumors, especially in the recognition of malignant fibrous histiocytoma (MFH), a tumor that rarely occurs in the CNS and needs to be distinguished from the more common pleomorphic xanthoastrocytoma (PXA).[46,65,104] However, the results of applying those markers to the study of CNS and extra-CNS lesions should be interpreted with considerable caution. Immunoreactivity for AACT is very widespread and can be detected in 80% of carcinomas, sarcomas, melanomas, and lymphomas.[200] In CNS tumors, 77% of all gliomas stained for both AACT and alpha-1-antitrypsin, metastatic carcinomas, melanomas, and sarcomas were also positive for both markers.[150] Pleomorphic xanthoastrocytomas and the lipidized cells of some gliomas are also AACT immunoreactive. The lack of specificity of these histiocytic markers precludes their use in distinguishing MFH or related atypical fibroxanthomas from PXA, lipidized gliomas, or non-neuroepithelial tumors. The tumor cells of PXA, including those infiltrating the leptomeninges, are positive for GFA protein, thus indicating their astrocytic nature.[104]

### Markers Reactive for Microglial Cells

Activated microglial cells can be recognized with HAM 56,[25,86] an IgM antibody that reacts with an epitope of the CD68 cluster region antigen. Other monoclonal antibodies that react with CD68 and that may be useful to detect activated microglial cells are KP1 and EBM11. HAM56 also reacts with the multinucleated giant cells of HIV-infected brains. Activated microglial cells also may be detected with biotinylated lectin *Ricinus communis* agglutinin (RCA-1).

## KINETIC MARKERS

Modern advances in immunohistochemistry have made possible the in situ investigation of cell kinetics in human brain tumors and other neoplasms.[24] These methods tend to replace older more laborious methods such as those employing autoradiography with tritiated thymidine. The newer procedures allow the in situ evaluation of proliferation potential in human brain tumors in a short period of time and do not require the use of radioactive or myelotoxic substances.

Five basic modern methods allow the study of proliferation rate in a brain tumor: bromodeoxyuridine, proliferating cell nuclear antigen (PCNA), Ki 67, nucleolar organizer regions, and flow cytometry. Of these, the last two methods are not immunohistochemical techniques, and their discussion is beyond the scope of this chapter.

Bromodeoxyuridine (BrdU) is a thymidine analogue that is incorporated into the nuclear DNA during the S-phase of DNA replication.[134,231] Nuclei that incorporated BrdU can be detected by anti-BrdU Mabs after procedures that denature their DNA. The fraction or proportion of cells in S-phase can be calculated by determining the percentage of nuclei so labeled. Because BrdU appears to have no toxic effects, it can be administered to patients with brain tumors, and an estimate of the proliferation potential of the neoplasm can be determined 1 or 2 days after the tumor biopsy has been obtained or the entire tumor is resected. BrdU labeling methods in tissue sections and flow cytometry of brain tumors yield comparable results.[41] The labeling pattern can be heterogeneous; therefore, different areas of the tumor must be evaluated. Initially, studies of BrdU labeling had to be performed on frozen sections or on alcohol-fixed, paraffin-embedded sections. However, good results can be obtained in tissues routinely prepared using enzymatic pretreatment with trypsin, pepsin and, especially, protease.[75]

Kinetic studies with BrdU have been performed mostly in rapidly growing tumors, such as anaplastic astrocytomas, glioblastomas, medulloblastomas, and malignant meningiomas. Hoshino and co-workers analyzed the results obtained in 143 patients with gliomas of astrocytic origin[85]: the glioblastomas had median labeling indices (LI) of 7.5%, and three quarters of these tumors had an LI greater than 5%. The anaplastic astrocytomas showed an LI varying from less than 1% to over 5%; these results suggest that tumors with similar phenotypic features have different proliferating potentials and that kinetic growth information may be important to predict postoperative prognosis and for devising tumor-specific regimens of treatment.

BrdU also can be applied to more slowly growing neoplasms, as in pilocytic astrocytomas. Here labeling of the stromal endothelial cells may be more conspicuous than that of the tumor cells themselves. In one study of spinal and intracranial ependymomas, the authors found that most tumors have an LI of less than 1%; those with an LI between 3% and 5% recurred within 2 years.[141]

Proliferating cell nuclear antigen (PCNA) or cyclin is a 36-kD DNA polymerase-$\delta$ auxiliary protein that accumulates in the nucleus during the S-phase.[113] Several monoclonal antibodies such as PC10 recognize PCNA in formalin-fixed, paraffin-embedded sections and give an estimate of the cells engaged in replicating DNA. Kiel-67 or Ki 67 is a monoclonal antibody that reacts with a nuclear antigen detectable in all proliferating and dividing cells. The antigen is present in the nuclei of cells in the $G_1$, $G_2$, S, and M phases, but not in $G_0$ cells.[57,58] In contrast to BrdU, which must be administered to patients before tumor biopsy, patient preparation is not necessary for the detection of PCNA or Ki 67. One initial major disadvantage of Ki 67 was that the method works only on frozen sections and brain smears; for this reason, studies based on paraffin embedded tissues were not possible. More recently, several monoclonal antibodies such as MIB 1 and MIB 3 have become available; these are equivalent to Ki 67 and can be demonstrated in routinely fixed and embedded tissues, needing only simple antigen-retrieval tecniques such as microwave oven processing.[31] Most proliferation cell studies of brain tumors have used PCNA in paraffin sections or Ki 67 in frozen sections. The LI obtained in these studies reflects the grade of malignancy of the tumor; the proportion of positive cells may be as high as 40% to 60% in metastatic carcinomas, or 10% to 40% in glioblastomas and anaplastic astrocytomas and medulloblastomas.[24,44,196] In contrast, LI may be as low as 0.6% in pilocytic astrocytomas or 0.2% in benign schwannomas (Plates 4F and 5A). The LI values obtained in gliomas with Ki 67 increase with the histologic grade of the tumor and may have prognostic implications. For instance, in the series of Zuber and associates,[233] five patients with malignant gliomas showing LI lower than 2.5% survived over 40 months. Some researchers claim that glioblastomas can be divided into two different prognostic groups based on the estimates of the proliferation indices.[213] Haapasalo and co-workers have reported 1-year survival of 56 (or 17%) in a group of patients with glioblastoma that had a low LI with PCNA.[68] In addition, some authors have attempted to estimate the extent of the tumor resection in gliomas by estimating the labeling of tumor cells at the margins.[105]

Several studies show a good correlation between the results obtained with bromodeoxyuridine, PCNA, Ki 67, MIB 1, and with nonimmunohistochemical techniques that estimate the proliferative activity of brain tumors.[72,135,142,173] All of these studies require a quantitative assessment of the number of positive cells, expressed as the percentage of the number of neoplastic cells per unit surface ($mm^2$) of neoplastic tissue. For this the observer can count the percentage of labeled tumor nuclei per 500 or 1000 tumor cells. In our experience, the best results are obtained with monoclonal antibody MIB 1 used in paraffin sections. This method provides an easy distinction between stained and nonstained neoplastic cells, and also between neoplastic cells and stromal or non-neoplastic cells, something difficult to accomplish in frozen sections.[96] Regardless of the method used, results with these still novel techniques must be cautiously interpreted. Proliferation indices between tumors should be compared only with results obtained using the same method and technique (for instance, an LI of 5% obtained with PCNA may not be equivalent to an LI of 5% obtained with Ki 67 or MIB1). Moreover, the marked heterogeneity and different rates of growth in different areas of the same tumor are other reasons to be cautious in interpreting these indices; this is especially true in the evaluation of small specimens.[37]

## IMMUNOHISTOCHEMISTRY OF SELECTED NEURAL TUMORS

### Astrocytic Neoplasms

Undoubtedly, GFA protein remains the most valuable marker for normal and neoplastic astrocytes. In astrocytic tumors, immunostaining decreases with progressive dedifferentiation, but some cells retain immunopositivity even in the most anaplastic astrocytomas and glioblastomas.[187,22] With the exception of some protoplasmic astrocytomas, tumors entirely devoid of GFA protein immunoreactivity are not astrocytomas. In general, the staining is predominantly cytoplasmic in gemistocytic and anaplastic astrocytomas; staining of cell processes predominates in the fibrillary and pilocytic variants. Reactivity of Rosenthal fibers in pilocytic tumors is variable, but usually there is a rim of positive staining.[199] The eosinophilic globules of fibrillary astrocytomas are strongly GFA protein positive.[199]

S-100 protein immunoreactivity in astrocytomas parallels that of GFA protein.[106] Better differentiated astrocytomas are usually strongly immunoreactive, with less staining in anaplastic astrocytomas and glioblastomas. Since schwannomas, neurofibromas, and metastatic melanomas are also S-100 positive, this protein offers no real advantage over GFA protein in the diagnostic work-up of astrocytic neoplasms. S-100 protein immunoreactivity occasionally can be detected in the nuclei of neoplastic astrocytes as well as in their cytoplasm.

The subependymal giant cell astrocytoma is a distinctive type of tumor, characteristically associated with tuberous sclerosis, but also found in patients without that condition. A variable number of GFA protein-positive neoplastic cells can be found in most, if not all, subependymal astrocytomas unassociated with the disease. In tumors associated with tuberous sclerosis, GFA protein immunoreactivity is often not detectable: in these cases, the cells may be positive for S-100, NSE, and even, occasionally, NF protein.[187] The tumor probably originates from a dysplastic cell in which the potential for astrocytic and, to a lesser extent, neuronal differentiation, is incompletely expressed.

Vimentin is also often detectable in astrocytic neoplasms as well as in reactive astrocytes. Vimentin is expressed during early astrogliogenesis, and is codistributed with GFA protein in the same intermediate filament system of malignant glioma cells in vivo.[163] Whether vimentin immunoreactivity is more predominant in poorly differentiated astrocytomas is controversial. Several studies have found no evidence for such an association.[39,190]

### Ependymomas

The only confirmatory evidence of the ependymal nature of a cell or a neoplasm is electron microscopic. There are no specific immunohistochemical markers for ependymal cells. Positivity for GFA protein is frequent, but not constant, and GFA protein is detected in different variants of ependymoma, such as the epithelial, papillary, and myxopapillary types, and in subependymomas.[89,115,128] In general, positivity in ependymomas is mostly found in the delicate glial processes of perivascular rosettes, but this is not constant. S-100 protein-positive cells also can be detected, paralleling the demonstration of GFA protein, and Leu 7 positivity is occasionally found in ependymoma cells. Immunoreactivity for EMA can be detected on the luminal surface of cells lining ependymal rosettes (Plate 5B), and vimentin can be demonstrated in ependymal and ependymoblastic rosettes.[27,40] In most ependymomas, cytokeratins cannot be demonstrated, but myxopapillary and papillary ependymomas, and ependymoblastomas have shown focal luminal positivity.[115,154] However, ependymomas do not show the diffuse intracytoplasmic positivity seen in metastatic carcinomas or choroid plexus tumors.

### Oligodendrogliomas

An entirely satisfactory or specific marker for oligodendrogliomas is not available. Immunoreactivity with a Mab recognizing Leu 7 represents the best available option. Although not specific, the number of Leu 7-reactive cells in oligodendrogliomas surpasses the number of positive cells found in other gliomas, schwannomas, or neuroblastomas.[145] GFA protein-positive cells may also be found in oligodendrogliomas. These can be entrapped reactive astrocytes, neoplastic astrocytes in mixed oligoastrocytomas, or truly GFA protein-positive neoplastic oligodendrocytes.[145] The synthesis of GFA protein by neoplastic oligodendrocytes probably is related to the transient expression of the protein by oligodendrocytes in the early phase of myelinogenesis.[32] The combination of numerous cells with surface Leu 7 immunoreactivity, with occasional GFA protein-positive neoplastic cells, is useful in confirming the diagnosis of oligodendroglioma. As mentioned earlier, myelin-associated proteins are not useful or specific markers in oligodendrogliomas.

### Choroid Plexus Papillomas and Carcinomas

Choroid plexus papillomas, especially the anaplastic or malignant variants, may present diagnostic difficulties and must be differentiated from other papillary intraventricular tumors, such as papillary ependymoma and metastatic carcinoma. Embryonal CNS tumors with a papillary pattern such as the medulloepithelioma and the papillary form of immature teratoma must be considered in the differential diagnosis, especially since these tumors typically occur in the same age group, i.e., young children.

Glial markers such as GFA and S-100 proteins often can be demonstrated focally in choroid plexus papillomas. Cells positive for these markers do not differ in their morphology from neighboring protein-negative epithelial cells. This feature, which has been interpreted as focal divergent glial, presumably ependymal, differentiation,[186] may be helpful in the distinction from a metastatic carcinoma. Adult choroid plexus epithelium is negative for GFA protein, but focal immunoreactivity can be detected in the choroid plexus of the newborn.[97]

Other intermediate filament proteins such as vimentin and keratin can also be demonstrated in choroid plexus papillomas and also exist in the normal adult choroid plexus epithelium.[110,115] In contrast to most ependymomas, both benign and malignant epithelial choroid plexus tumors are keratin-positive. In malignant examples, keratin positivity is found in the papillary rather than in the solid areas. The desmosomal plaque proteins desmoplakin I and II, and the carcinoembryonic antigen (CEA) can also be detected in choroid plexus neoplasms; CEA is especially common in anaplastic choroid plexus tumors.[34] Other markers such as EMA, S-100 protein, and Leu 7 have also been present. However, none of these antigens distinguish choroid plexus papillomas from ependymoma, a tumor that may also display EMA, keratin, and vimentin reactivity. Immunoreactivity for transthyretin may support the diagnosis of choroid plexus tumor, but its specificity is not absolute, and poorly differentiated choroid plexus tumors may be negative for this protein.

### Medulloblastomas and Other Embryonic CNS Tumors

The potential of medulloblastomas has been investigated with a number of immunohistochemical markers for glial and neuronal differentiation. Immunoreactivity for GFA protein exists in a variable number of cells in both the classic and desmoplastic variants of medulloblastomas.[41,116] Despite some opinions to the contrary,[33] most authors agree that some of the GFA protein-positive cells are truly neoplastic,[23,41,116,187] although clearly reactive, entrapped astrocytes can also be found within medulloblastomas. Furthermore, GFA protein-positive medulloblastoma cells may, rarely, infiltrate the subarachnoid space or metastasize outside the CNS.[187]

The frequency of GFA protein-positive neoplastic cells in medulloblastoma ranges from rare[33] to as frequent as 40[41] and 50%[180] of the tumors. S-100 immunoreactivity in neoplastic cells has also been demonstrated.[41,106]

Neuronal markers identified in medulloblastomas include synaptophysin,[98,107,192] NSE,[23] PGP9.5,[41] and proteins of the neuronal cytoskeleton such as the NF subunits, MAP2, and class III neuronal-associated $\beta$-tubulin isotype.[98] Immunoreactivity for the last group of markers is well demonstrated in the pale islands of the desmoplastic medulloblastomas, but immunoreactivity for GFA protein is also found in these structures, indicating their potential for dual divergent differentiation.[98] S-antigen and rhodopsin, markers of retinal and pineal differentiation, have been also found in a significant proportion of medulloblastomas.[15,42]

In the primitive areas of cerebral medulloepitheliomas—the prototype of embryonic CNS neoplasms—focal immunoreactivity for vimentin, GFA protein, and the class III neuronal-associated $\beta$-tubulin isotype in foci has been detected.[27] These foci indicate, in the case of the last two markers, an early commitment to glial and neuronal differentiation, respectively. The tumor often displays areas of frank neuroblastic, ganglionic, astrocytic, and ependymal differentiation, and those areas will then demonstrate the relevant immunohistochemical markers.

### Neuronal Neoplasms, Including Pineal Parenchymal Tumors

Tumors composed partially or entirely of well-differentiated ganglionic cells, such as gangliocytomas, gangliogliomas, ganglioneuromas, ganglioneuroblastomas, and desmoplastic infantile gangliogliomas, are usually easily recognizable with conventional stains supplemented with Bielschowsky's silver impregnations for neurites. The ganglionic cells immunoreact with most neuronal markers, including neurofilament subunits, MAP2, class III $\beta$-tubulin, NSE, synaptophysin, and neurotransmitters. Less well differentiated neuroblastic neoplasms are more difficult to recognize. However, neuronal markers can be helpful in identifying neuronal components in neoplastic cells. Synaptophysin, MAP2, and the class III $\beta$-tubulin are probably the most useful ones[6,129]; all three are demonstrable in routinely fixed and embedded tissues. Immunoreactivity for chromogranin also may be detected, especially in tumors composed of differentiated neuroblasts.[69] NSE positivity cannot be used as the only marker to establish the neuroblastic nature of a tumor. In the central neurocytoma,[73,155] a tumor presenting as an intraventricular calcified neoplasm in young adults, the microscopic appearances are almost indistinguishable from those of an oligodendroglioma. Moreover, the cells are immunoreactive with Leu 7, further complicating its differential diagnosis.[167] Presence of synaptophysin, MAP2, and the class III $\beta$-tubulin suggest the neuroblastic nature of this tumor, but the need to obtain confirmatory electron microscopy cannot be overemphasized in this type of case. This important aspect is well discussed in a contribution by Mierau and associates.[126] Synaptophysin is extremely useful to distinguish central neurocytoma from oligodendroglioma, its main differential diagnosis. The cells and, especially, the fibrillary areas of central neurocytoma are positive for synaptophysin and NSE, but generally negative for chromogranin. Central neurocytomas are also positive for class III $\beta$-tubulin and neurofilament proteins.[74,77] Scattered reactive astrocytes may be positive for GFAP.

In pineal parenchymal tumors (pineoblastomas and pineocytomas), markers of neuronal differentiation such as synaptophysin and neurofilament proteins may be detected.[35] Retinal S-antigen, a more specific indicator of the pineal parenchymatous nature of the tumor, may be demonstrable in some, but not all, examples of pineoblastoma and pineocytoma.[169]

Dysembryoplastic neuroepithelial tumor (DNT) is a rare tumor associated with a long history of partial complex seizures. DNTs tend to occur in the cortex of the temporal lobes and present as multiple intracortical nodules composed of neurons and oligodendrocyte-like cells that are often separated by abundant extracellular substance rich in acid mucopolysaccharides.[43] Immunostains such as synaptophysin, NSE, or neurofilament proteins may be useful to confirm the presence of neurons, and GFAP may highlight a small astrocytic component. Oligodendrocyte-like cells in some DNT are strongly positive for S-100 protein and, to a lesser extent, for GFAP and class III $\beta$-tubulin; this suggests that DNT may consist of a heterogeneous population of cells with glial and early neuronal differentiation.[79] However, more important than a given immunostain pattern, the diagnosis of DNT is mainly based in the low-power identification of distinct cortical multinodularity with the characteristic cell components.

### Meningiomas

In most meningiomas, the histologic pattern is so characteristic as to make immunohistochemistry unnecessary. However, immunohistochemical stains can help in certain situations, especially when an anaplastic malignant meningioma must be distinguished from other primary or metastatic tumors, such as a glioma infiltrating the meninges, a malignant schwannoma, or a secondary carcinoma.

The immunohistochemical pattern of meningiomas, as well as that of arachnoidal cap cells, is complex, as these cells share markers of both mesenchymal and epithelial tissues.[101] Most histologic subtypes, with the exception of the controversial hemangiopericytic variant, have common immunohistologic characteristics. Vimentin is present in virtually all meningiomas. Epithelial membrane antigen is also very commonly detected in meningiomas; the more characteristic pattern is of immunoreactivity restricted to the plasma membrane of the neoplastic cells, whereas weak and diffuse cytoplasmic positivity for EMA is of less diagnostic value. The combination of cytoplasmic vimentin and surface EMA positivity is highly characteristic of meningiomas (Plates 5C and 5D). In many meningiomas, immunoreactivity for desmoplakins I and II, the major proteins of desmosomal plaques,[130] is readily demonstrable.[80] Cytokeratin can be detected focally in some cases, especially in areas of psammoma bodies and in the secretory variant.[152,229] In the secretory variant of meningioma, the luminal contents of this tumor display positivity for carcinoembryonic antigen as well. Double-labeling studies have shown cytokeratin and vimentin to be localized in different cells of meningiomas.[212] Extracellular matrix glycoproteins such as laminin, fibronectin, and type V collagen also have been identified, especially in association with whorl formation and psammoma bodies.[121] In an exceptional case of malignant hemangiopericytic and papillary meningioma, the triple detection of vimentin, keratin, and GFA protein has been documented,[21] but this example is, as far as we are aware, unique. Results for S-100 protein in meningiomas have been highly variable,[187] showing generally weak results as compared with the strong positivity of schwannomas and neurofibromas.

Hemangiopericytoma of the meninges, previously classified as hemangiopericytic meningiomas (HGP) have been the object of considerable controversy.[187] Regardless of their precise histogenesis, their identification is important because they are frequently associated with aggressive behavior. Mixed papillary and hemangiopericytic patterns are frequently present. Unlike hemangiopericytomas originating in soft tissues and unlike normal pericytes, the meningeal tumors are vimentin-positive.[84] Evidence of EMA activity has been contradictory; most authors report immunonegativity,[88,137,153,229] but immunopositivity for EMA has also been reported in an angioblastic papillary meningioma.[212] Immunopositivity for factor XIIIa in CNS and extra-CNS hemangiopericytomas may be useful to distinguish this tumor from other vascular tumors.[149]

### Cerebellar Hemangioblastoma

The presence of three cell types in this tumor is characteristic—namely, endothelial cells, pericytes, and stromal cells. Stromal cells are unique to this tumor and have no counterpart in the normal or developing brain. Numerous immunohistochemical studies have attempted to define their origin. Possible histogenesis of stromal cells have included vascular cells (either endothelial cells, pericytes, or primitive angiogenic mesenchymal cells), histiocytes, microglia, astrocytes, leptomeningeal pial cells, and even peptidergic neurons. Another point of great practical importance is the sometimes difficult distinction from a metastatic tumor, especially renal cell carcinoma.

Immunohistochemical studies have not helped clarify the histogenesis of these tumors and the origin of stromal cells. However, it seems clear that stromal cells are not antigenically related to endothelial cells; factor VIII-related antigen and Ulex europaeus I lectin in most studies are consistently negative.[49,66] Stromal cells are also negative for CD 34 antigen, a more recently introduced and sensitive marker of endothelial differentiation[100] (Plate 5E). In contrast, these cells stain with a variety of markers that include vimentin, S-100 protein, NSE, keratin, Leu M1,[195] Leu 7, and GFA protein. Immunoreactivity for erythropoietin and for renin has been demonstrated in some of the cells of capillary hemangioblastomas, a finding probably responsible for the secondary polycythemia often associated with hemangioblastomas.

The interpretation of such complex immunohistochemical patterns has led to many controversies. The detection of focal GFA and S-100 protein staining in some of the stromal cells has been interpreted as representing the uptake, by micropinocytotic stromal cells, of proteins liberated from reactive astrocytes.[187] A similar explanation has been suggested for the occasional presence of GFA protein-positive neoplastic cells in metastatic carcinomas. Despite this rare feature, difficulties in the differential diagnosis from cerebellar astrocytomas usually do not arise since the latter are uniformly and intensely GFA protein-positive. NSE immunoreactivity in stromal cells is more common and more diffuse than it is the staining for GFA and S-100 proteins. But the presence of NSE, together with the finding of neuropeptide-like immunoreactivity, suggests a possible origin from primitive neurons or neuroendocrine cells. Becker and associates[10] found immunoreactivity for NSE, synaptophysin, and neuropeptides (substance P and neuropeptide Y), while Frank and co-workers[52] found none for chromogranin, and Grant and co-workers[66] none for synaptophysin, chromogranin, or any of eight polypeptide hormones. More recently, the stromal cells of CNS hemangioblastomas are reported immunoreactive for factor XIIIa. The reaction is found mostly in the cytoplasm of small stromal cells with few vacuoles, whereas larger multivacuolated cells are less immunoreactive[100,148] (Plate 5F). We have not detected factor XIIIa immunoreactivity in normal cerebellar tissue; thus factor XIIIa may be a useful marker for the diagnosis of CNS hemangioblastoma, especially in small biopsies where the characteristic pattern of the tumor may not be readily identifiable. Metastatic renal cell carcinoma may be difficult to differentiate from hemangioblastomas of the cerebellum. In this situation, in addition to factor XIIIa, EMA is also a helpful marker, since it is positive in the clear cells of metastatic renal carcinoma and negative in the stromal cells of capillary hemangioblastoma.[52]

### Schwannomas and Neurofibromas

S-100 protein (especially its $\beta$-subunit) is the standard marker for normal Schwann cells, and practically all benign schwannomas and neurofibromas are S-100 positive. The staining is more intense in Antoni A than in Antoni B and hyalinized areas.[225] In neurofibromas, both S-100-positive and S-100-negative cells are found, reflecting the heterogeneous composition of these tumors. A significant proportion (about 50%) of the malignant peripheral nerve sheath tumors also show S-100 positivity[225]; the number of positive cells is highly variable and, in some tumors, only a few cells are immunoreactive. The differential diagnosis from a meningioma is facilitated by the detection of Leu 7 immunoreactivity, as most schwannomas and a significant number of neurofibromas react with this antibody, whereas meningiomas are negative.[168] Staining for neurofilament proteins may disclose the presence of axons in both schwannomas and neurofibromas, especially in the latter. As discussed earlier, EMA is a valuable marker for the distinction of the proliferating cells in perineuriomas (localized hypertrophic neuropathy) and traumatic neuromas.[5,165,201] Finally, both schwannomas and neurofibromas show, in a variable proportion of cases, positive immunoreactivity for GFA protein with both polyvalent antisera and monoclonal antibodies.[63,125,201]

### Rhabdoid Tumors

CNS rhabdoid tumors are rare neoplasms composed of cells similar to those found in malignant rhabdoid tumors of the kidney. In the CNS, they are more common in the cerebellum and may contain, in addition to rhabdoid cells, areas resembling medulloblastomas or other embryonal CNS tumors. Some tumors also contain malignant mesenchyma or squamous or glandular elements (thus the designation of atypical teratoid/rhabdoid tumor proposed by some authors). The prognosis of these tumors is in general worse than that of medulloblastoma. Rhabdoid cells may express EMA, vimentin, or smooth muscle antigens (such as HHF35 or muscle-specific antigen), GFAP, keratin, or neurofilament protein,[162,182] but the diagnosis depends more on identification of the characteristic rhabdoid cells than on a specific immunohistochemical profile.

### CNS Histiocytosis

Histiocytosis X (Langerhans cell histiocytosis) may involve the brain by extension from a nearby area of bone involvement, such as the spine or the base of the skull. More rarely, unifocal or multifocal involvement of the CNS parenchyma may occur, especially in the hypothalamic/third ventricle region. The histiocytic infiltrate may induce a brisk astrocytic reaction that, when the characteristic Langerhans cells are not identified, may be confused with a fibrillary or pilocytic astrocytoma. Langerhans cells have well-known light and electron microscopic features, but immunohistochemistry may be useful to confirm the diagnosis. Langerhans cells are positive for CD1 (OKT6), a marker that can be demonstrated only in frozen tissue. More practical is S-100 protein, which works well in formalin-fixed, paraffin-embedded tissue and produces a strong reaction in the cytoplasm of Langerhans cells.[25] These cells, in contrast to tissue histiocytes, lack lisozyme and CD68 (an antigen detected with Mab KP-1) and do not react with MAC 387, an antibody that reacts with a human antigen expressed in granulocytes and histiocytes.[50] Langerhans cells are also negative for GFAP.

### Chordomas, Including Chondroid Chordomas

Immunohistochemistry may be useful to support a distinction between chordomas and low-grade chondromas of the base of the skull or sacrum. Chordomas display positivity for cytokeratin, epithelial membrane antigen, vimentin, S-100 protein, and carcinoembryonic antigen. Chondrosarcomas are S-100 and vimentin positive but negative for epithelial markers. Chondroid chordomas are histologically biphasic neoplasms that display both chordoid and chondroid differentiation. These tumors occur almost exclusively in the base of the skull of younger patients and are said to have a better progonosis than classic chordomas. The precise morphologic and immunohistochemical criteria necessary for the identification of chondroid chordomas are very controversial.

Very few of the tumors show biphasic differentiation by immunohistochemistry, i.e., positive for reactivity epithelial markers in chordoid areas but negative in the chondroid areas. Some authors who found that both the chordoid and chondroid areas are negative for epithelial markers conclude that chondroid chordomas are better classified as low-grade chondrosarcomas.[18] In other authors' experiences, both components were positive for epithelial antigens, indicating that chondroid chordoma may merely represent a variant of chordomas.[93,181]

## ACKNOWLEDGMENTS

The studies described in this review were partly supported by Research Grant CA 31271 from the National Cancer Institute, US Department of Health and Human Services. We thank Dr. Paul McKeever, Department of Pathology, University of Michigan, for his helpful comments and criticism.

## REFERENCES

1. Abo T, and Balch TA: Differentiation antigen of human NK and K cells identified by a monoclonal antibody (HNK-1), J Immunol 127:1024-1029, 1981.
2. Aguzzi A, and others: Intracranial mixed germ cell tumor with syncytiotrophoblastic giant cells and precocious puberty, Acta Neuropathol 75:427-431, 1988.
3. Allan PM, and others: Biological characterization and clinical applications of a monoclonal antibody recognizing an antigen restricted to neuroectodermal tissues, Int J Cancer 31:591-598, 1983.
4. Alles JU, and Bosslet K: Immunocytochemistry of angiosarcomas. A study of 19 cases with special emphasis on the applica-

bility of endothelial cell specific markers to routinely prepared tissues, Am J Clin Pathol 89:463-471, 1988.

5. Ariza A, Bilbao JM, and Rosai J: Immunohistochemical detection of epithelial membrane antigen in normal perineurial cells and perineurioma, Am J Surg Pathol 12:679-683, 1988.
6. Artlieb U, Krepler R, and Wiche C: Expression of microtubule-associated proteins, Map-1 and Map-2, in human neuroblastomas and differential diagnosis of immature neuroblasts, Lab Invest 53:684-691, 1985.
7. Azumi N, and Battifora H: The distribution of vimentin and keratin in epithelial and non-epithelial neoplasms. A comprehensive immunohistochemical study on formalin- and alcohol-fixed tumors, Am J Clin Pathol 88:286-296, 1987.
8. Barbareschi M, and others: p53 protein expression in central nervous system neoplasms, J Clin Pathol 45:583-586, 1992.
9. Battifora H: Clinical applications of the immunohisto-chemistry of filamentous proteins, Am J Surg Pathol (Suppl 1)12:24-42, 1988.
10. Becker I, Paulus W, and Roggendorf W: Histogenesis of stromal cells in cerebellar hemangioblastomas. An immunohistochemical study, Am J Pathol 134:271-275, 1989.
11. Bennett GS: Changes in intermediate filament composition during neuronogenesis, Curr Top Dev Biol 21:151-183, 1987.
12. Bignami A, and others: Glial hyaluronate-binding protein in polar spongioblastoma, J Neuropathol Exp Neurol 48:187-196, 1989.
13. Bignami A, and Dahl D: Brain-specific hyaluronate-binding protein: an immunohistological study with monoclonal antibodies of human and bovine central nervous system, Proc Natl Acad Sci USA 83:3518-3522, 1986.
14. Binder LI, Frankfurter A, and Rebhun LI: The distribution of tau in the mammalian central nervous system, J Cell Biol 101: 1371-1378, 1985.
15. Bonnin JM, and Perentes E: Retinal S-antigen immunoreactivity in medulloblastomas, Acta Neuropathol 76:204-207, 1988.
16. Bonnin JM, and Rubinstein LJ: Immunohistochemistry of central nervous system tumors. Its contribution to neurosurgical diagnosis, J Neurosurg 60:1121-1133, 1984.
17. Bouldin TW: Immunohistology of intracranial tumors. In Jennette JC, editor: Immunohistology in diagnostic pathology, Boca Raton, 1989, CRC Press.
18. Brooks JJ, LiVolsi V, and Trojanowski JQ: Does chondroid chordoma exist? Acta Neuropathol 72:229-235, 1987.
19. Bruner JM, Saya M, and Moser RP: Immunocytochemical detection of p53 in human gliomas, Mod Pathol 4:671-674, 1991.
20. Bruner JM, Langdorf L, and Fuller G: Neuropathology, cell biology and newer diagnostic methods, Curr Op Oncol 5:441-449, 1993.
21. Budka H: Non-glial specificities of immunocytochemistry for the glial fibrillary acidic protein (GFAP), Acta Neuropathol 72: 43-54, 1986.
22. Bullard DE, and Bigner DD: Applications of monoclonal antibodies in the diagnosis and treatment of primary brain tumors, J Neurosurg 63:2-16, 1985.
23. Burger PC, and others: Differentiation in the medulloblastoma. A histological and immunohistological study, Acta Neuropathol 73:115-123, 1987.
24. Burger PC, Shibata T, and Kleihues P: The use of the monoclonal antibody Ki-67 in the identification of proliferating cells: application to surgical neuropathology, Am J Surg Pathol 10:611-617, 1986.
25. Burger PC, and Scheithauer BW: Tumors of the Central Nervous System. In Atlas of Tumor Pathology, third series, Washington, DC, 1993, Armed Forces Institute of Pathology.
26. Caccamo DV, and others: An immunohisto-chemical study of neuropeptides and neuronal cytoskeletal proteins in the neuroepithelial component of a spontaneous ovarian teratoma. Primitive neuroepithelium displays immunoreactivity for neuropeptides and neuron-associated $\beta$-tubulin isotype, Am J Pathol 135: 801-813, 1989.
27. Caccamo DV, Herman MM, Rubinstein LJ: An immunohistochemical study of the primitive and maturing elements of human cerebral medulloepitheliomas, Acta Neuropathol 79: 248-254, 1989.
28. Caccamo DV, and others: Immunohisto-chemistry of a spontaneous murine ovarian teratoma with neuroepithelial differentiation. Neuron-associated $\beta$-tubulin as a marker for primitive neuroepithelium, Lab Invest 60:390-398, 1989.
29. Caccamo DV, Keohane ME, and McKeever P: Tissue plasminogen activators and inhibitors in human gliomas. An immunohistochemical study. Mod Pathol 7:99-104, 1994.
30. Cartun RW, Coles FB, and Pastuszak WT: Utilization of monoclonal antibody L26 in the identification and confirmation of B-cell lymphomas. A sensitive and specific marker applicable to formalin and B5-fixed, paraffin-embedded tissues, Am J Pathol 129:415-421, 1987.
31. Cattoreti G, and others: Monoclonal antibodies against recombinant parts of the Ki-67 antigen (MIB1 and MIB3) detect proliferating cells in microwave-processed formalin-fixed paraffin sections, J Pathol 168:357-363, 1992.
32. Choi BH, and Kim RC: Expression of glial fibrillary acidic protein in immature oligodendroglia, Science 223:407-409, 1984.
33. Coffin CM, Mukai K, and Dehner LP: Glial differentiation in medulloblastomas. Histogenic insight, glial reaction, or invasion of brain, Am J Surg Pathol 7:555-565, 1983.
34. Coffin CM, and others: Choroid plexus neoplasms. Clinicopathologic and immunohistochemical studies, Am J Surg Pathol 10: 394-404, 1986.
35. Collins VP: Pineocytoma with neuronal differentiation demonstrated immunocytochemically, Acta Pathol Microbiol Immunol Scan Sect 95:113-117, 1987.
36. Collins VP, and James CD: Gene and chromosomal alterations associated with the development of human gliomas, FASEB J 7:926-930, 1993.
37. Coons S, and Johnson P: Regional heterogeneity in the proliferative index of human gliomas as measured by the Ki-67 labelling index, J Neuropathol Exp Neurol 52:609-618, 1993.
38. Cosgrove M, and others: Intermediate filament expression in astrocytic neoplasms, Am J Surg Pathol 13:141-145, 1989.
39. Cruz-Sanchez FF, and others: Epithelial membrane antigen expression in ependymomas, Neuropathol Appl Neurobiol 14: 197-205, 1988.
40. Cruz-Sanchez FF, and others: An immunohistological study of 66 ependymomas, Histopathology 12:443-454, 1988.
41. Cruz-Sanchez FF, and others: Medulloblastoma. An immunohistological study of 50 cases, Acta Neuropathol 79:205-210, 1989.
42. Czerwionka M, and others: Differentiation in medulloblastomas: correlation between the immunocytochemical demonstration of photoreceptor markers (S-antigen, rhodopsin) and the survival rate in 66 patients, Acta Neuropathol 78:629-636, 1989.
43. Daumas-Duport C: Dysembryoplastic neuroepithelial tumor, Brain Pathol 3:285-295, 1993.
44. Deckert M, Reifenberger G, and Wechsler W: Determination of the proliferative potential of human brain tumors using the monoclonal antibody Ki-67, J Cancer Res Clin Oncol 115:179-188, 1989.
45. Donato R: S-100 proteins, Cell Calcium 7:123-145, 1986.
46. Elema JD, and Atmosoerokjo-Briggs JE: Langerhans cells and macrophages in eosinophilic granuloma: an enzyme histochemical, enzyme cytochemical and ultrastructural study, Cancer 54:2174-2179, 1984.
47. Ellison DW, and others: Expression of the p53 protein in a spectrum of astrocytic tumors, J Pathol 168:383-386, 1992.

48. Eng LF, and others: An acidic protein isolated from fibrous astrocytes, Brain Res 28:351-374, 1971.
49. Epstein JI, White CL III, and Mendelsohn G: Factor VIII related antigen and glial fibrillary acidic protein immunoreactivity in the differential diagnosis of central nervous system hemangioblastomas, Am J Clin Pathol 8:285-292, 1984.
50. Fartasch M, and others: Immunohistochemical and ultrastructural study of histiocytosis X and non-X histiocytosis, Am J Acad Dermatol 23:885-892, 1990.
51. Fima L, and others: Expression of the CD34 antigen in vascular endothelial cells, Blood 75:2417-2426, 1990.
52. Frank TS, and others: A detailed immunohistochemical analysis of cerebellar hemangioblastoma: an undifferentiated mesenchymal tumor, Mod Pathol 2:638-651, 1989.
53. Frankfurter A, Binder LI, and Rebhun LI: Limited tissue distribution of a novel beta-tubulin isoform, J Cell Biol 103. 273(abstract), 1986.
54. Garin-Chesa P, and others: Immunohistochemical analysis of nerve growth factor receptor expression in normal and malignant human tissues, J Histochem Cytochem 36:383-389, 1988.
55. Garson JA, and others: Immunohistological diagnosis of primary brain lymphoma using monoclonal antibodies: confirmation of B-cell origin, Neuropathol Appl Neurobiol 14:19-37, 1988.
56. Gay RE, Gay S, and Jones RE Jr: Histological and immunohistological identification of collagens in basement membranes of Schwann cells of neurofibromas, Am J Dermatopathol 5:317-325, 1983.
57. Gerdes J: An immunohistological method for estimating cell growth fractions in rapid histopathological diagnosis during surgery, Int J Cancer 35:169-171, 1985.
58. Gerdes J, and others: Production of a mouse monoclonal antibody reactive with a human nuclear antigen associated with cell proliferation, Int J Cancer 31:13-20, 1983.
59. Gheuens J, and others: Identification of several forms of the glial acidic fibrillary protein, or alpha-albumin, by a specific monoclonal antibody, J Neurochem 43:964-970, 1984.
60. Ghobrial M, and Ross ER: Immunocytochemistry of neuron-specific enolase: a re-evaluation. In: Zimmerman HM, editor: Progress in neuropathology, vol 6, New York, 1986, Raven Press.
61. Goto S, and others: An immunocytochemical demonstration of calcineurin in human nerve cell tumors. A comparison with neuron-specific enolase and glial fibrillary acidic protein, Cancer 60:2948-2957, 1987.
62. Gould VE, and others: Synaptophysin: a novel marker for neurons, certain neuroendocrine cells, and their neoplasms, Hum Pathol 17:979-983, 1986.
63. Gould VE, and others: The intermediate filament complement of the spectrum of nerve sheath neoplasms, Lab Invest 55:463-474, 1986.
64. Gown AM, and others: Smooth muscle cells can express cytokeratins of "simple" epithelium, Am J Pathol 132:223-232, 1988.
65. Grant JW, and Gallagher PJ: Pleomorphic xanthoastrocytoma. Immunohistochemical methods for differentiation from fibrous histiocytomas with similar morphology, Am J Surg Pathol 10: 336-341, 1986.
66. Grant JW, Gallagher PJ, and Hedinger C: Hemangioblastoma. An immunohistochemical study of ten cases, Acta Neuropathol 76:82-86, 1988.
67. Guarda LA, and others: Immunoperoxidase localization of factor VIII in angiosarcomas, Arch Pathol Lab Med 106:515-516, 1982.
68. Haapasalo H, and others: Comparison of the quantitation methods for PCNA immunostaining: applicability and relation to survival in 83 astrocytic tumors, J Pathol 171:207-214, 1993.
69. Hachitanda Y, Tsuneyoshi M, and Enjoji M: Expression of panneuroendocrine proteins in 53 neuroblastic tumors, Arch Pathol Lab Med 113:381-384, 1989.
70. Halfter W, Chiquet-Ehridsmann R, and Tucker RP: The effect of tenascin and embryonic basal lamina on the behavior and morphology of neural crest cells in vitro, Dev Biol 132:14-25, 1989.
71. Hamid Q, and others: Extra-adrenal paragangliomas. An immunocytochemical and ultrastructural report, Cancer 60:1776-1781, 1987.
72. Hara A, and others Correlation between nucleolar organizer region staining and Ki-67 immunostaining in human gliomas, Surg Neurol 33:320-324, 1990.
73. Hassoun J, and others: Central neurocytoma. An electron microscopy study of two cases, Acta Neuropathol 56:151-156, 1982.
74. Hassoun J, and others: Central neurocytoma: a synopsis of clinical and histological patterns, Brain Pathol 3:297-306, 1993.
75. Hayashi Y, and others: Effects of fixation time and enzymatic digestion on immunohistochemical demonstration of bromodeoxyuridine in formalin-fixed paraffin-embedded tissue, J Histochem Cytochem 36:511-514, 1988.
76. Herman MM, and others: Neuroblastic differentiation potential of the human retinoblastoma cell lines Y-79 and WERI-Rb1 maintained in an organ culture system. An immunohistochemical, electron microscopic and biochemical study, Am J Pathol 134:115-132, 1989.
77. Hessler R, and others: Cytoskeletal immunohistochemistry of central neurocytomas, Am J Surg Pathol 16:1031-1038, 1992.
78. Heyderman E, Steele K, and Ormerod MG: A new antigen on the epithelial membrane: its immunoperoxidase localization in normal and neoplastic tissue, J Clin Pathol 32:35-39, 1979.
79. Hirose T, and others: Dysembryoplastic neuroepithelial tumors (DNT). An immunohistochemical and ultrastructural study, J Neuropathol Exp Neurol 53:184-195, 1994.
80. Hitchcock K, and Morris CS: Immunocytochemistry of intracranial meningiomas, J Neurooncol 5:357-368, 1987.
81. Hochberg FH, and Miller DC: Primary central nervous system lymphoma, J Neurosurg 68:835-853, 1988.
82. Hoffman PN, Griffin JW, and Price DL: Control of axonal caliber by neurofilament transport, J Cell Biol 99:705-714, 1984.
83. Hökfelt T, Johansson O, and Goldstein M: Chemical anatomy of the brain, Science 225:1326-1334, 1984.
84. Holden J, Dolman CL, and Churg A: Immunohistochemistry of meningiomas including the angioblastic type, J Neuropathol Exp Neurol 46:50-56, 1987.
85. Hoshino T, and others: Variability in the proliferative potential of human gliomas, J Neurooncol 7:137-143, 1989.
86. Hulette CM, Downey BT, and Burger PC: Macrophage markers in diagnostic neuropathology, Am J Surg Pathol 16:493-499, 1992.
87. Itoyama T, and others: Immunocytochemical method to identify myelin basic protein in oligodendroglia and myelin sheaths of the human nervous system, Ann Neurol 7:157-166, 1980.
88. Iwaki T, and others: Hemangiopericytoma of the meninges: a clinicopathological and immunohistochemical study, Clin Neuropathol 7:93-99, 1988.
89. Izukawa D, and Lach B: Immunocytochemical analysis of intermediate filaments in human ependymal tumors, Can J Neurol Sci 15:114-118, 1988.
90. Izukawa D, Lach B, and Benoit B: Gangliocytoma of the cerebellum: ultrastructure and immunohistochemistry, Neurosurgery 22:576-581, 1988.
91. Jacobsson B, and others: Transthyretin in endocrine pancreatic tumors, Am J Pathol 134:465-471, 1989.
92. Jacobsson B, and others: Transthyretin immunoreactivity in

human and porcine liver, choroid plexus, and pancreatic islets, J Histochem Cytochem 37:31-37, 1989.

93. Jeffrey P, Biava C, and Davis R: Chondroid chordomas. A hyalinized chordoma without cartilaginous component, Am J Clin Pathol 103:271-279, 1995.
94. Jensen A, and others: Characterization of human brain S-100 fraction: amino acid sequence of S-100 beta, J Neurochem 45: 700-705, 1985.
95. Johnson MD, Glick AD, and Davis BW: Immunohistochemical evaluation of Leu-7, myelin basic protein, glial fibrillary acidic protein, and LN3 immunoreactivity in nerve sheath tumors and sarcomas, Arch Pathol Lab Med 112:155-160, 1988.
96. Karamitopoulou E, and others: Ki-67 immunoreactivity in human central nervous system tumors: a study with MIB 1 monoclonal antibody on archival material, Acta Neuropathol 87:47-54, 1994.
97. Kasper M, Stosiek P, and Karsten U: Age-related changes in the expression of cytokeratin and vimentin immunoreactivity in human choroid plexus, J Hirnforsch 30:1-4, 1989.
98. Katsetos CD, and others: Cerebellar desmoplastic medulloblastomas. A further immunohistochemical characterization of the reticulin-free pale islands, Arch Pathol Lab Med 113:1019-1029, 1989.
99. Kawahara WE, and others: Expression of glial fibrillary acidic protein (GFAP) in peripheral nerve sheath tumors, Am J Surg Pathol 12:115-120, 1988.
100. Keohane ME, Caccamo DV, and Ho K-L: Factor XIIIa and the CD34 antigen in hemangioblastomas of the CNS, Am J Clin Pathol 98:349, 1992 (abstract).
101. Kepes JJ: The histopathology of meningiomas. A reflection of origins and expected behavior? J Neuropathol Exp Neurol 45: 95-107, 1986.
102. Kepes JJ, Fulling KH, and Garcia JH: The clinical significance of "adenoid" formations of neoplastic astrocytes, imitating metastatic carcinoma, in gliosarcoma, Clin Neuropathol 1:139-150, 1982.
103. Kepes JJ, and Perentes E: Glial fibrillary acidic protein in chondrocytes of elastic cartilage in the human epiglottis: an immunohistochemical study with polyvalent and monoclonal antibodies, Anat Rec 220:296-299, 1988.
104. Kepes JJ, Rubinstein LJ, and Eng LF: Pleomorphic xanthoastrocytoma: a distinctive meningocerebral glioma of young subjects with relatively favorable prognosis. A study of 12 cases, Cancer 44:1389-1852, 1979.
105. Kim D, and others: Detection of proliferating cell nuclear antigen in gliomas and adjacent resection margins, Neurosurgery 33:619-625, 1993.
106. Kimura T, Budka H, and Soler-Federsppiel S: An immunocytochemical comparison of the glial-associated proteins glial fibrillary acidic protein (GFAP) and S-100 protein in human brain tumors, Clin Neuropathol 5:21-27, 1986.
107. Kleihues P, Kiessling M, and Janzer RC: Morphologic markers in neuro-oncology, Cur Top Pathol 77:307-338, 1987.
108. Kliewer KE, and others: Paragangliomas: Assessment of prognosis by histologic, immunohistochemical and ultrastructural techniques, Hum Pathol 20:29-39, 1989.
109. Korf HW, and others: Immunoreactive S-antigen in cerebrospinal fluid: a marker of pineal parenchymal tumors? J Neurosurg 70:682-687, 1989.
110. Kouno M, and others: An immunohistochemical study of cytokeratin and glial fibrillary acidic protein in choroid plexus papilloma, Acta Neuropathol 75:317-320, 1988.
111. Kurtin PJ, and Pinkus GS: Leukocyte common antigen—a diagnostic discriminant between hematopoietic and nonhematopoietic neoplasms in paraffin sections using monoclonal antibodies, Hum Pathol 16:353-365, 1985.
112. Linnoila RI, and others: Decreased expression of neuropeptides in malignant paragangliomas. An immunohistochemical study, Hum Pathol 19:41-50, 1988.
113. Louis DN, and others: Proliferating cell nuclear antigen and Ki-67 immunohistochemistry in brain tumors: a comparative study, Acta Neuropathol 81:675-679, 1991.
114. Louis DN, and others: Molecular genetics of pediatric brain stem gliomas. Application of PCR techniques to small and archival brain tumor specimens, J Neuropathol 52:507-515, 1993.
115. Mannoji H, and Becker LE: Ependymal and choroid plexus tumors. Cytokeratin and GFAP expression, Cancer 61:1377-1385, 1988.
116. Mannoji H, and others: Glial fibrillary acidic protein in medulloblastoma, Acta Neuropathol 55:63-69, 1981.
117. Marangos PJ: Neuron-specific enolase: a neural and neuroendocrine protein. In Marangos PJ, Campbell IC, Cohen RM, editors: Neuronal and glial proteins. Structure, function and clinical application, New York, 1988, Academic Press.
118. Marangos PJ, and others: Measurement of neuron-specific (NSE) and non-neuron (NNE) isoenzymes of enolase in rat, monkey and human nervous tissue, J Neurochem 33:319-329, 1979.
119. Matus A: Microtubule-associated proteins: their potential role in determining neuronal morphology, Ann Rev Neurosci 11: 29-44, 1988.
120. May EE, and Perentes E: Anti-Leu 7 immunoreactivity with 83 tumors: its value in the diagnosis of prostatic adenocarcinoma, Histopathology 11:295-304, 1987.
121. McComb RD, and Bigner DD: Immunolocalization of laminin in neoplasms of the central and peripheral nervous systems, J Neuropathol Exp Neurol 44:242-253, 1985.
122. McComb RD, Moul JM, and Bigner DD: Distribution of type VI collagen in human gliomas: comparison with fibronectin and glioma-mesenchymal matrix glycoproteins, J Neuropathol Exp Neurol 46:623-633, 1987.
123. McDonald JA: Extracellular matrix assembly, Ann Rev Cell Biol 4:183-207, 1988.
124. McKeever PE, and others: Products of cells cultured from gliomas. VII. Extracellular matrix proteins of gliomas which contain glial fibrillary acidic protein, Lab Invest 60:286-295, 1989.
125. Memoli VA, Brown EF, and Gould VE: Glial fibrillary acidic protein (GFAP) immunoreactivity in peripheral sheath tumors, Ultrastruct Pathol 7:269-275, 1984.
126. Mierau GW, and others: Primary cerebral neuroblastoma, Ultrastruct Pathol 13:281-289, 1989.
127. Miettinen M: Synaptophysin and neurofilament proteins as markers for neuroendocrine tumors, Arch Pathol Lab Med 11: 813-818, 1987.
128. Miettinen M, Clark R, and Virtanen I: Intermediate filament proteins in choroid plexus and ependyma and their tumors, Am J Pathol 123:231-240, 1986.
129. Miettinen M, and Rapola J: Synaptophysin: an immunohistochemical marker for childhood neuroblastoma, Acta Pathol Microbiol Immunol Scand (sect A) 95:167-170, 1987.
130. Moll R, and others: Desmosomal proteins: new markers for identification and classification of tumors, Lab Invest 54:4-25, 1986.
131. Moll R, and others: The catalog of human cytokeratins: patterns of expression in normal epithelia, tumors and cultured cells, Cell 31:11-24, 1982.
132. Moody SA, Quigg MS, and Frankfurter A: Development of the peripheral trigeminal system in the chick revealed by an isotype-specific anti-beta tubulin monoclonal antibody, J Comp Neurol 279:567-580, 1989.
133. Moore BW: Brain-specific proteins: S-100 protein, 14.3.2 protein, and glial fibrillary acidic protein, Adv Neurochem 1:137-155, 1975.

134. Morimura T, Kitz K, and Budka H: In situ analysis of cell kinetics in human brain tumors, Acta Neuropathol 77:276-282, 1989.
135. Morimura T, and others: Determination of proliferation activities in human brain tumor specimens: a comparison of three methods, J Neurooncol 10:1-11, 1991.
136. Mörk SJ, and others: Patterns of epithelial metaplasia in malignant gliomas: II. Squamous differentiation of epithelial-like formations in gliosarcomas and glioblastomas, J Neuropathol Exp Neurol 47:101-118, 1988.
137. Moss THE: Immunohistochemical characteristics of hemangiopericytic meningiomas: comparison with typical meningiomas, hemangioblastomas and hemangiopericytomas from extracranial sites, Neuropathol Appl Neurobiol 13:467-480, 1987.
138. Motoi M, and others: Immunohistochemical studies on human brain tumors using anti-Leu 7 monoclonal antibody in paraffin-embedded specimens, Acta Neuropathol 66:75-77, 1985.
139. Mukai K, Rosai J, and Burgdorf WHC: Localization of factor VIII-related antigen in vascular endothelial cells using an immunoperoxidase method, Am J Surg Pathol 4:273-276, 1980.
140. Murakami M, and others: Immunohistochemical localization of apolipoprotein E in human glial neoplasms, J Clin Invest 82: 177-188, 1988.
141. Nagashima T, and others: The proliferative potential of human ependymomas measured by in situ bromodeoxyuridine labeling, Cancer 61:2433-2438, 1988.
142. Nagashima T, and others: Comparison of bromodeoxyuridine labeling indices obtained from tissue sections and flow cytometry of brain tumors, J Neurosurg 68:388-392, 1988.
143. Nagle RB: Intermediate filaments: efficacy in surgical pathology diagnosis, Am J Clin Pathol 91(suppl):S14-18, 1989.
144. Nakagawa Y, and others: Immunohistochemical differences between intracranial germinomas and their gonadal equivalents. An immunoperoxidase study of germ cell tumours with epithelial membrane antigen, cytokeratin, and vimentin, J Pathol 156: 67-72, 1988.
145. Nakagawa Y, Perentes E, and Rubinstein LJ: Immunohistochemical characterization of oligodendrogliomas. An analysis of multiple markers, Acta Neuropathol 72:15-22, 1986.
146. Nakagawa Y, Perentes E, and Rubinstein LJ: Non-specificity of anti-carbonic anhydrase as a marker in human neurooncology, J Neuropathol Exp Neurol 46:451-460, 1987.
147. Nakajima T, and others: An immunoperoxidase study of S-100 protein distribution in normal and neoplastic tissues, Am J Surg Pathol 6:715-727, 1982.
148. Nemes Z: Fibrohistiocytic differentiation in capillary hemangioblastoma, Hum Pathol 23:805-810, 1992.
149. Nemes Z: Differentiation markers in hemangiopericytomas, Cancer 61:133-142, 1992.
150. Ng HK, and Lo STH: Immunostaining for $\alpha$-1-antichymotrypsin and $\alpha$-1-antitrypsin in gliomas, Histopathology 13:79-87, 1988.
151. Ng HK, and Lo STH: Cytokeratin immunoreactivity in gliomas, Histopathology 14:359-368, 1989.
152. Ng HK, Tse CCH, and Lo STH: Meningiomas and arachnoid cells: an immunohistochemical study of epithelial markers, Pathology 19:253-257, 1987.
153. Ng HK, Tse CCH, and Lo STH: Hemangiopericytic meningiomas are epithelial membrane antigen-negative, Pathology 20: 90, 1988.
154. Ng HK, Tse CCH, and Lo STH: Ependymomas: an immunohistochemical study of 14 cases, Histopathology 13:462-465, 1988.
155. Nishio S, and others: Intraventricular neurocytoma: clinicopathological features of six cases, J Neurosurg 68:665-670, 1988.
156. Norenberg MD: The distribution of glutamine synthetase in the rat central nervous system. J Histochem Cytochem 27:756-762, 1979.
157. Nuñez J: Differential expression of microtubule components during brain development, Dev Neurosci 8:125-141, 1986.
158. Oda Y, and others: Immunohistochemical studies on the tissue localization of collagen types I, III, IV, VI and VI in schwannomas, Virchows Archiv B Cell Pathol 50:153-163, 1988.
159. Ordoñez NG, and Batsakis JG: Comparison of Ulex europaeus I lectin and factor VIII-related antigen in vascular lesions, Arch Pathol Lab Med 108:129-132, 1984.
160. Osborn M, and Weber K: Intermediate filaments: cell-type specific markers in differentiation and pathology, Cell 31:303-306, 1982.
161. Papasozomenos SC: Tau protein immunoreactivity in dementia of the Alzheimer type. I. Morphology, evolution distribution and pathogenetic implications, Lab Invest 60:123-137, 1989.
162. Parham D, Weeks D, and Beckwith J: The clinicopathological spectrum of putative extrarenal rhabdoid tumors. An analysis of 42 cases with immunohistochemistry and electron microscopy, Am J Surg Pathol 18:1010-1029, 1994.
163. Paulus W, and Roggendorf W: Vimentin and glial fibrillary acidic protein are codistributed in the same intermediate filament system of malignant gliomas cells in vivo, Virchows Archiv B Cell Pathol 56:67-70, 1988.
164. Perentes E, and others: Immunohisto-chemical characterization of human retinoblastomas in situ with multiple markers, Am J Ophthalmol 103:647-658, 1987.
165. Perentes E, and others: Expression of epithelial membrane antigen in perineurial cells and their derivates. An immunohistochemical study with multiple markers, Acta Neuropathol 75: 160-165, 1987.
166. Perentes E, and Rubinstein LJ: Immunohistochemical recognition of human nerve sheath tumors by anti-Leu 7 (HNK-1) monoclonal antibody, Acta Neuropathol 68:319-324, 1985.
167. Perentes E, and Rubinstein LJ: Immunohistochemical recognition of human neuroepithelial tumors by anti-Leu 7 (HNK-1) monoclonal antibody, Acta Neuropathol 69:227-233, 1986.
168. Perentes E, and Rubinstein LJ: Recent applications of immunoperoxidase histochemistry in human neuro-oncology. An update, Arch Pathol Lab Med 111:796-812, 1987.
169. Perentes E, and others: S-antigen immunoreactivity in human pineal glands and pineal parenchymal tumors. A monoclonal antibody study, Acta Neuropathol 71:224-227, 1986.
170. Perides G, and others: Isolation and partial characterization of a glial hyaluronate-binding protein, J Biol Chem 264:5981-5987, 1989.
171. Perosio PM, and Brooks JJ: Expression of nerve growth factor receptor in paraffin-embedded soft tissue tumors, Am J Pathol 132:152-160, 1988.
172. Pinkus GS, and Kurtin PJ: Epithelial membrane antigen: a diagnostic discriminant in surgical pathology: immunohisto-chemical profile in epithelial, mesenchymal and hematopoietic neoplasms using paraffin sections and monoclonal antibodies, Hum Pathol 16:929-940, 1985.
173. Plate K, and others: Proliferative potential of human brain tumors as assessed by nucleolar organizer regions (AgNORs) and Ki-67 immunoreactivity, Acta Neurochir 104:103-109, 1990.
174. Przedborski S, and others: Neuropeptide Y, somatostatin, and cholecystokinin neurone preservation in anaplastic astrocytomas, Acta Neuropathol 76:507-510, 1988.
175. Quinlan RA, and others: Patterns of expression and organization of cytokeratin intermediate filaments, Ann NY Acad Sci 455:282-306, 1985.
176. Ramaekers FCS, and others: Coexpression of keratin- and vimentin-type intermediate filaments in human metastatic carcinoma cells, Proc Natl Acad Sci USA 80:2618-2622, 1983.
177. Ramani P, Bradley N, and Fletcher C: QEBND/10, a new monoclonal antibody to endothelium: assessment of its diagnostic utility in paraffin sections, Histopathology 17:237-242, 1990.

178. Reibel J, Wever U, and Albrechtsen R: The pattern of distribution of laminin in neurogenic tumors, granular cell tumors, and nevi of the oral mucosa, Acta Pathol Microbiol Immunol Scand Sect 93:41-47, 1985.
179. Reifenberger G, Szymas J, and Wechsler W: Differential expression of glial- and neuronal-associated antigens in human tumors of the central and peripheral nervous system, Acta Neuropathol 74:105-123, 1987.
180. Roessmann U, and others: Neuronal and astrocytic differentiation in human neuroepithelial neoplasm. An immunohistochemical study, J Neuropathol Exp Neurol 42:113-121, 1983.
181. Rosenberg A, and others: Chondroid chordoma: a variant of chordoma, Am J Clin Pathol 101:36-41, 1994.
182. Rourke L, Packer R, and Biegel J: CNS atypical teratoid/rhabdoid tumors of infancy and childhood, J Neuroncol 24:21-28, 1995.
183. Roussel G, and others: An immuno-histochemical study of two myelin-specific proteins in enriched oligodendroglial cell cultures combined with an autoradiographic investigation using $^{3}$H-thymidine, Dev Brain Res 8:193-204, 1983.
184. Rubinstein LJ: Immunohistochemical signposts—not markers—in neural tumor differentiation, Neuropathol Appl Neurobiol 12:525-537, 1986.
185. Rubinstein LJ: Diagnostic markers in human neuro-oncology. A progress report, Ann NY Acad Sci 540:78-90, 1988.
186. Rubinstein LJ, and Brucher JM: Focal ependymal differentiation in choroid plexus papillomas. An immunoperoxidase study, Acta Neuropathol 53:29-33, 1981.
187. Russell DS, and Rubinstein LJ: Pathology of tumours of the nervous system, ed 5, London, 1989, Edward Arnold.
188. Saint-André JP, and others: Angiotensin-I-converting enzyme in germinomas, Hum Pathol 19:208-213, 1988.
189. Sato S, and others: Antigenic determinant shared between myelin-associated glycoprotein from human brain and natural killer cells, Biomed Res 4:489-494, 1983.
190. Schiffer D, and others: Immunohistochemical demonstration of vimentin in human cerebral tumors, Acta Neuropathol 70:209-219, 1986.
191. Schnitt SJ, and Vogel H: Meningiomas. Diagnostic value of immuno-peroxidase staining for epithelial membrane antigen, Am J Surg Pathol 10:640-649, 1986.
192. Schwechheimer K, Wiedenmann B, and Franke WW: Synaptophysin: a reliable marker for medulloblastomas, Virchows Archiv A Pathol Anat Histol 411:53-59, 1987.
193. Seshi B, and others: Immunohistochemical characterization of a set of monoclonal antibodies to human neuron-specific enolase, Am J Pathol 131:258-269, 1988.
194. Shaw G, and Weber K: Differential expression of neurofilament triplet proteins in brain development, Nature 298:277-279, 1982.
195. Sheibani K, and others: Leu M1 antigen in human neoplasms: an immunohistologic study of 300 cases, Am J Surg Pathol 10: 227-236, 1986.
196. Shibata T, and Burger PC: The use of the monoclonal antibody Ki-67 in determination of the growth fraction in pediatric brain tumors, Child Nerv System 3:364-367, 1987.
197. Shiosaka S, and Tohyama M: Immunohistochemical techniques, Prog Brain Res 66:3-32, 1986.
198. Shiurba RA, and others: Epidermal growth factor receptor in meningiomas is expressed predominantly on endothelial cells, Cancer 62:2139-2144, 1988.
199. Smith DA, and Lantos PL: Immunocytochemistry of cerebellar astrocytomas: with a specific note on Rosenthal fibers, Acta Neuropathol 66:155-159, 1985.
200. Soini Y, and Miettinen M: Widespread immunoreactivity for alpha-1-antichymotrypsin in different types of tumors, Am J Clin Pathol 89:131-136, 1988.
201. Stanton C, and others: GFA protein reactivity in nerve sheath tumors: a polyvalent and monoclonal antibody study, J Neuropathol Exp Neurol 46:634-643, 1987.
202. Stanton C, and others: The immunohisto-chemical demonstration of early perineurial change in the development of localized hypertrophic neuropathy, Hum Pathol 19:1455-1457, 1988.
203. Stefansson K, and others: S-100 protein in soft tissue tumors derived from Schwann cells and melanocytes, Am J Pathol 106: 261-268, 1982.
204. Sternberger LA: Immunocytochemistry, 3 ed, New York, 1986, John Wiley & Sons.
205. Sternberger LA, and Sternberger NH: Monoclonal antibodies distinguish phosphorylated and nonphosphorylated forms of neurofilaments in situ, Proc Natl Acad Sci USA 80:6126-6130, 1983.
206. Sternberger NH, and others: Myelin-associated glycoprotein demonstrated immunocytochemically in myelin-forming cells of developing rat, Proc Natl Acad Sci USA 76:1510-1514, 1979.
207. Sullivan KF: Structure and utilization of tubulin isotypes, Ann Rev Cell Biol 4:687-716, 1988.
208. Swanson PE, Manivel JC, and Wick MR: Immunoreactivity for Leu-7 in neurofibrosarcoma and other spindle cell sarcomas of soft tissue, Am J Pathol 126:546-560, 1987.
209. Tabuchi K, and others: Altered structure and expression of the p53 gene in human neuroepithelial tumors, Neurologia Medicochirurgica 32:725-732, 1992.
210. Takahashi H, and others: Neuroendocrine markers in central nervous system neuronal tumors (gangliocytoma and ganglioglioma), Acta Neuropathol 77:237-243, 1989.
211. Tanaka J, Hokama Y, and Nakamura H: Myelin basic protein as a possible marker for oligodendroglioma, Acta Pathol Jpn 38:1297-1303, 1988.
212. Theaker JM, and others: Epithelial membrane antigen and cytokeratin expression by meningiomas: an immunohistological study, J Clin Pathol 39:435-439, 1986.
213. Torp SH, and others: Relationship between Ki-67 labelling index, amplification of the epidermal growth factor receptor gene, and prognosis in human glioblastomas, Acta Neurochir 117:182-186, 1992.
214. Trojanowski JQ: Cytoskeletal proteins and neuronal tumors. In Colvin RB, Bhan AK, McCluskey RT, editors: Diagnostic immunopathology, New York, 1988, Raven Press.
215. Trojanowski JQ: Immunohistochemistry of neurofilament proteins and their diagnostic applications. In De Lellis R, editor: Advances in Immunohistochemistry, New York, 1988, Raven Press.
216. Trojanowski JQ, Lee VMY, and Schlaepfer WW: An immunohistochemical study of human central and peripheral nervous system tumors, using monoclonal antibodies against neurofilaments and glial filaments, Hum Pathol 15:248-257, 1984.
217. Trojanowski JQ, Obrocka MA, and Lee VMY: Distribution of neurofilament subunits in neurons and neuronal processes. Immunohistochemical studies of bovine cerebellum with subunit-specific monoclonal antibodies, J Histochem Cytochem 33:557-563, 1985.
218. Trojanowski JQ, and others: Distribution of tau proteins in the normal human central and peripheral nervous system, J Histochem Cytochem 37:209-215, 1989.
219. VandenBerg SR, and others: Desmoplastic supratentorial neuroepithelial tumors of infancy with divergent differentiation potential ("desmoplastic infantile gangliogliomas"). Report of 11 cases of a distinctive embryonal tumor with favorable prognosis, J Neurosurg 66:58-71, 1987.
220. Van Noorden S, and Varndell IA: Regulatory peptide immunocyto-chemistry at light and electron microscopical levels, Experientia 43:724-735, 1987.

221. Velasco ME, and others: Immunohistochemical localization of glial fibrillary acidic protein in human glial neoplasms, Cancer 45:484-494, 1980.
222. Viale G, and others: Glial fibrillary acidic protein immunoreactivity in human respiratory tract cartilage and pulmonary chondromatous hamartomas, Am J Pathol 133:363-373, 1988.
223. Vinores S, and others: Immunohisto-chemical demonstration of neuron-specific enolase in neoplasms of the CNS and other tissues, Arch Pathol Lab Med 108:536-540, 1984.
224. Weidenheim KM, and Campbell WG Jr: Perineurial cell tumor. Immunocytochemical and ultrastructural characterization. Relationship to other peripheral nerve tumors with review of the literature, Virchows Archiv A Pathol Anat Histol 408:375-383, 1986.
225. Weiss SW, Langloss JM, and Enzinger FM: Value of S-100 protein in the diagnosis of soft tissue tumors with particular reference to benign and malignant Schwann cell tumors, Lab Invest 49:299-308, 1983.
226. Weller RO, Stewart PV, and Moore IE: Carbonic anhydrase C as a marker antigen in the diagnosis of choroid plexus tumors: an immunoperoxidase study. In Walker MD, Thomas DGT, editor: Biology of brain tumors, Boston, 1986, Nijhoff.
227. Wiedenmann B, and Franke WW: Identification and localization of synaptophysin, an integral membrane glycoprotein of MW 38,000 characteristic of presynaptic vesicles, Cell 41:1017-1028, 1985.
228. Wikstrand CJ, and others: Human fetal brain antigen expression common to tumors of neuroectodermal origin: gliomas, neuroblastomas, and melanomas, J Neuroimmunol 3:43-62, 1982.
229. Winek RR, Scheithauer BW, and Wick MR: Meningioma, meningeal hemangiopericytoma (angioblastic meningioma), peripheral hemangiopericytoma and acoustic schwannoma. A comparative immunohistochemical study, Am J Surg Pathol 13: 251-261, 1989.
230. Yasuda T, and others: Nerve growth factor receptor immunoreactivity in human benign peripheral nerve sheath tumor, Acta Neuropathol 77:591-598, 1989.
231. Yoshii Y, and others: Estimation of growth fraction with bromodeoxyuridine in human central nervous system tumors, J Neurosurg 65:659-663, 1986.
232. Zalutsky MR, and others: Pharmacokinetics and tumor localization of $^{131}$I-labeled anti-tenascin monoclonal antibody 81C6 in patients with gliomas and other intracranial malignancies, Cancer Res 49:2807-2813, 1989.
233. Zuber P, Hanou MF, and de Tribolet N: Identification of proliferating cells in human gliomas using the monoclonal antibody Ki-67, Neurosurgery 22:364-368, 1988.
234. Zurbriggen A, and others: Myelin-associated glycoprotein is produced before myelin basic protein in cultured oligodendrocytes, J Neuroimmunol 6:41-49, 1984.

C • H • A • P • T • E • R

# 5

# *Tumors of the Pituitary Region*

Paul E. McKeever
Ricardo V. Lloyd



## ADENOMAS

### Introduction

Most pituitary neoplasms are benign. The *etiology* of pituitary neoplasms in humans is unknown, although in animal models hormonal induction of pituitary tumors is fairly common. For example, chronic estrogen treatment can lead to prolactin cell hyperplasia and prolactin-producing neoplasms in rats and mice.[97] Although estrogens may stimulate the growth of preexisting prolactinomas in humans,[392] there is no strong evidence, except for anecdotal cases, that estrogens can induce pituitary neoplasms in humans.[108] End organ failure, as in chronic hypothyroidism and Addison's disease, may be associated with hyperplasia of specific pituitary cell types and pituitary tumor development.

Small pituitary tumors are commonly found at autopsy, and in various series this incidence has ranged from 3.2 to 27% of examined pituitaries.[50,54,62] The contributions of geographic and environmental factors versus examination techniques to this eightfold variation in incidence are uncertain. In most large series examined by immunohistochemical staining, prolactinomas and nonfunctioning or null cell adenomas are the most common incidental neoplasms.[182,224,284]

Pituitary adenomas can be divided into microadenomas (tumors less than 10 mm in diameter) and macroadenomas (tumors 10 mm or greater in diameter). A more complete classification by *level of invasiveness* has been described by Hardy[118] and includes the following: Grade 1 tumors are usually confined to the sella turcica and are less than 10 mm in size. Grade 2 tumors are larger than 10 mm but remain intrasellar. There is usually sellar enlargement, but no destruction of bony structure. Grade 3 tumors usually cause localized erosion of the sella, while grade 4 tumors represent invasive adenomas with extensive destruction of bony structures. Invasive tumors have been discussed by Scheithauer and associates.[330] Most adenomas are in the lower grade numbers and do not infiltrate their surroundings.[85]

In general, *magnetic resonance imaging* (MRI) exceeds computed tomography (CT) in defining pituitary adenomas, particularly microadenomas. Nevertheless, CT complements MRI in some cases.[390] Specific imaging procedures for receptors and secretory proteins are being developed.[217]

Pituitary tumors have been classified in recent years by immunohistochemical and ultrastructural studies. These methods are necessary for precise classification of pituitary neoplasms. They also provide prognostic information on subtotally resected and invasive adenomas.[183,330] Their specificity for pituitary hormones and secretory granules also provides decisive means to distinguish adenomas from other sellar neoplasms of similar histology. For example, immunoreactivity for growth hormone (GH) distinguishes GH adenoma from chordoma, which would be nonreactive. This level of specificity improves upon the specificity of S-100 protein, a common marker of chordoma, because a few adenomas contain S-100 protein.[126,138,397] Recently, subtypes of hormone-secreting adenomas have been characterized on cytologic touch preparations by immunocytochemistry.[168]

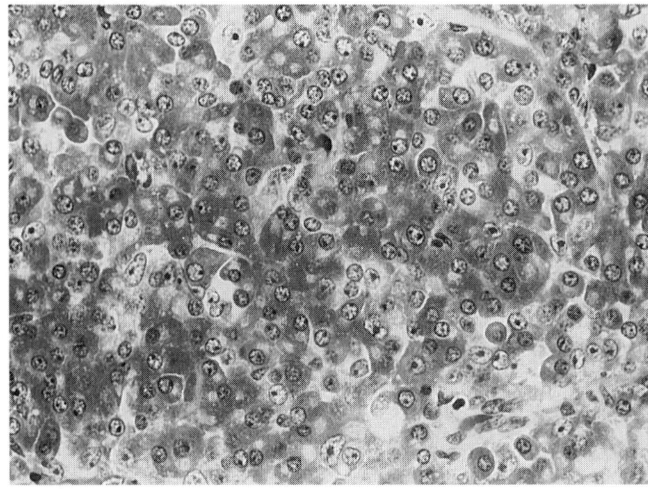

**Fig. 5-1.** GH adenoma with prominent acidophilic cells. (×350.)

Radioimmunoassays have greatly aided the recognition of small pituitary adenomas in the last few decades. Molecular biologic techniques such as in situ hybridization, the polymerase chain reaction, and examination of clonality of pituitary neoplasms have contributed to our understanding and to the classification of these neoplasms within the last few years.*

*General histologic features* shared by most pituitary adenomas include sheets of epithelioid cells of nearly uniform size and round to polygonal shape.[228,232] Fibrovascular stroma intersect these epithelioid sheets, but rarely encloses them completely, distinguishing them from acini of adenohypophysis (see the section on the anterior pituitary gland). Single round nuclei predominate in adenoma cells. Cytoplasmic granules are barely visible with hematoxylin and eosin stains (Fig. 5-1). Specific features that classify types of pituitary adenomas are described next.

### Growth Hormone Adenomas

Growth hormone adenomas made up about 14% of neoplasms in a large series of surgically resected adenomas (see Table 5-2). These neoplasms are usually acidophilic on hematoxylin and eosin staining (Fig. 5-1). A variable degree of nuclear pleomorphism may be seen in these tumors. Growth hormone adenomas show diffuse positive immunoreactivity after staining with growth hormone antibodies, and many adenomas may also show focal positive immunoreactivity for prolactin and for the alpha-subunit of the glycoprotein hormones[172] (Figs. 5-2, 5-3). Growth hormone adeno-

* Refs. 5, 123, 145, 206, 209, 356.

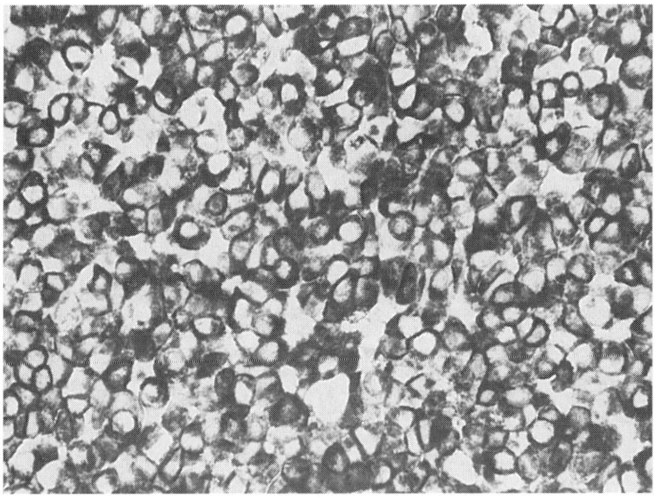

**Fig. 5-2.** Adenoma with intense cytoplasmic immunoreactivity with GH antiserum. (×350.)

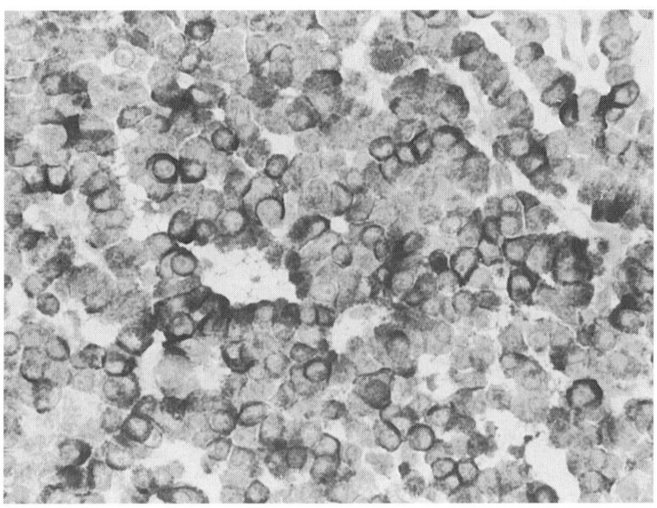

**Fig. 5-3.** The same GH adenoma in Fig. 5-2 also contained many immunoreactive PRL cells. (×350.)

mas have been divided into *two subtypes* based on ultrastructural features.* These include densely granulated and sparsely granulated growth hormone adenomas.

The *densely granulated* adenomas usually have a strong positive immunoreactivity after staining with growth hormone antibodies. Ultrastructural features show polyhedral or elongated cells with spherical or slightly irregular nuclei (Fig. 5-4). Nucleoli are often prominent. The tumor cells have a globular Golgi complex that may contain immature secretory granules. The secretory granules range from 150 to 600 nm in diameter.

*Sparsely granulated* growth hormone adenomas may be chromophobic on hematoxylin and eosin staining. These tumors are slightly more common than the acidophilic variant and may be more aggressive and have a more rapid growth rate. Immunoreactive growth hormone is usually present predominantly in the Golgi region, and the message for growth hormone is less than in the other subtype.[399] Ultrastructural features of sparsely granulated growth hormone adenomas include eccentric crescent-shaped or pleomorphic nuclei and variable amounts of rough endoplasmic reticulum. *Fibrous bodies* are commonly associated with sparsely granulated growth hormone adenomas. These fibrous bodies are spherically arranged aggregates of type 2 microfilaments, which are usually present in the Golgi region. The secretory granules range from 100 to 200 nm in diameter. Endocrine amyloid may be seen in both sparsely and densely granulated growth hormone adenomas.[191,248,322]

Among patients who have been treated with long-acting *somatostatin analogs*, adenomas often have morphologic changes at the time of surgery. There may be a variable reduction in tumor size. Perivascular fibrosis and variable increases in the number of secretory granules have also been observed[24,192] (Figs. 5-5, 5-6).

Patients with acromegaly may have a mixed picture of growth hormone-producing tumors.[172] These may include: (1) A *mixed* growth hormone cell and prolactin cell adenoma in which separate cells produce each hormone. These tumors generally respond better to dopamine agonist therapy than do pure GH adenomas.[270] (2) An *acidophilic stem cell adenoma* is often an invasive neoplasm in which the tumor cells produce prolactin and growth hormone. Hyperprolactinemia is often present with this neoplasm. Excess growth hormone production with acromegaly is uncommon. This menacing tumor has a poorer prognosis than the others and may even metastasize.[146] It is characterized ultrastructurally by giant mitochondria[172] that should be sought to confirm the diagnosis. (3) *Mammosomatotroph* cell adenoma, in which the same cell produces both prolactin and growth hormone. (4) *Plurihormonal* adenomas, in which growth hormone production is associated with acromegaly and with at least one other cell type. Rare cases of mixed growth hormone and TSH production by the same neoplasm have been reported. These patients usually have acromegaly and hyperthyroidism.[174,175] In a recently described silent growth hormone adenoma the tumor cells contained immunoreactive growth hormone and there was ultrastructural evidence of growth hormone secretory granules in the tumor cells, but the patients did not show evidence of acromegaly.[181] In situ hybridization analyses of this tumor have shown that the messenger RNA for growth

* Refs. 173, 237, 320, 332, 378.

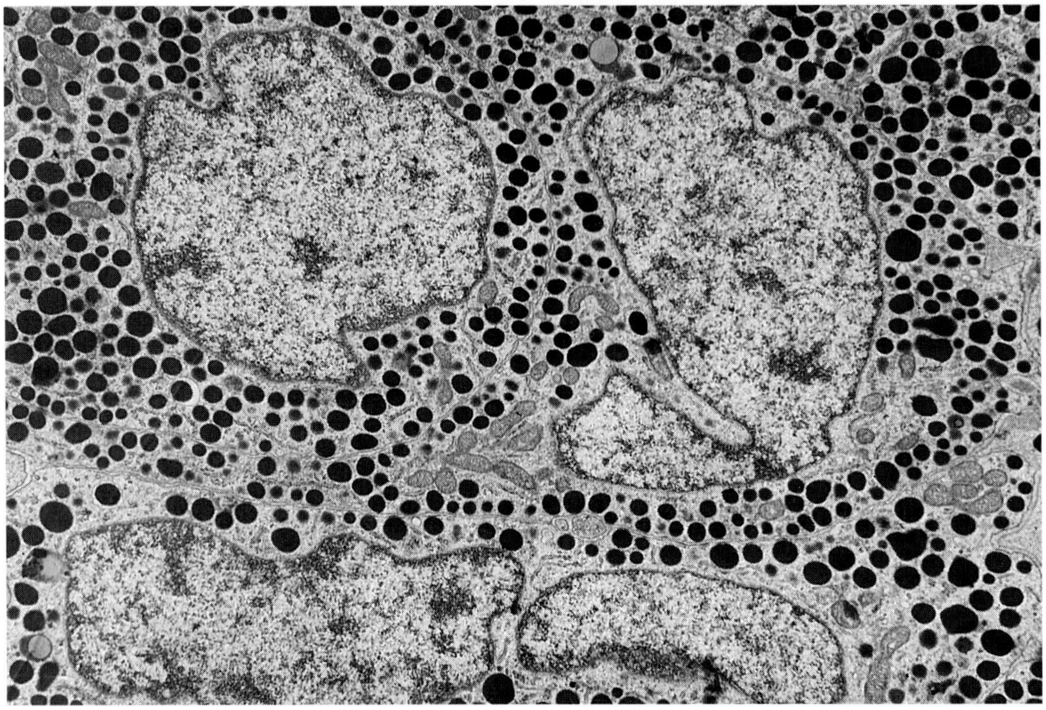

**Fig. 5-4.** Ultrastructural features of a densely granulated GH adenoma with abundant large secretory granules of 150–600 nm. (×8800.)

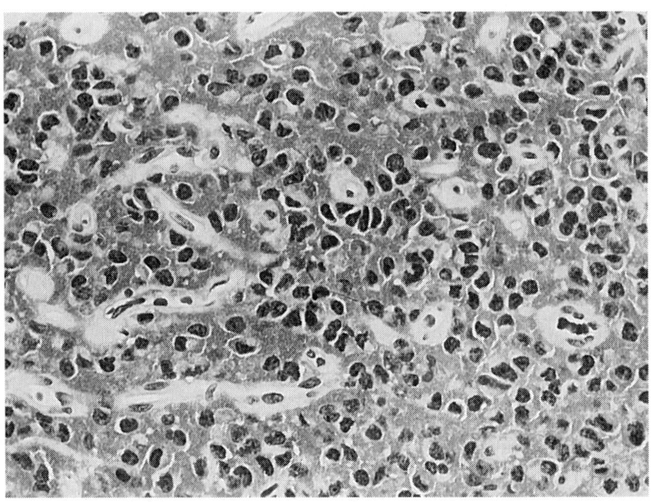

**Fig. 5-5.** GH adenoma after 1 month of treatment with the somatostatin analog SMS 201–995. Perivascular fibrosis is prominent. (×350.)

hormone was present in the tumor cells. Analysis of a series of growth hormone tumors by immunohistochemistry and in situ hybridization has shown that most growth hormone-secreting tumors are mixed neoplasms and that they contain the messenger RNAs for both growth hormone and prolactin.[206,296]

### Prolactin-Producing Adenomas

Prolactin-producing adenomas are the *most common* surgically resected adenohypophyseal neoplasm. These tumors constituted approximately 30% of adenomas in a large series (see Table 5-2). In autopsy series, prolactinomas may represent up to 50% of pituitary adenohypophyseal neoplasms. Easy to recognize symptoms (amenorrhea and galactorrhea) in women facilitate their early detection. In men, these adenomas may be confused with other tumors.[61]

Prolactinomas may range from acidophilic to chromophobic tumors on hematoxylin and eosin staining (Fig. 5-7). Calcification is seen in many of these neoplasms, and cystic changes may also be present. Amyloid production is present in a small percentage of prolactinomas.[35] Immunohistochemical staining often reveals prolactin immunoreactivity in most tumor cells (Fig. 5-8). Most prolactinomas are *sparsely granulated,* and densely granulated prolactinomas have been observed rarely. The sparsely granulated prolactinomas are chromophobic or slightly acidophilic by hematoxylin and eosin staining. Ultrastructural features of untreated sparsely granulated prolactinomas include highly-organized rough endoplasmic reticulum with nebenkern formation. The Golgi complex is usually oval or crescent-shaped and very prominent. Immature granules in the Golgi's sacculi are often pleomorphic, while most of the storage granules are spherical.

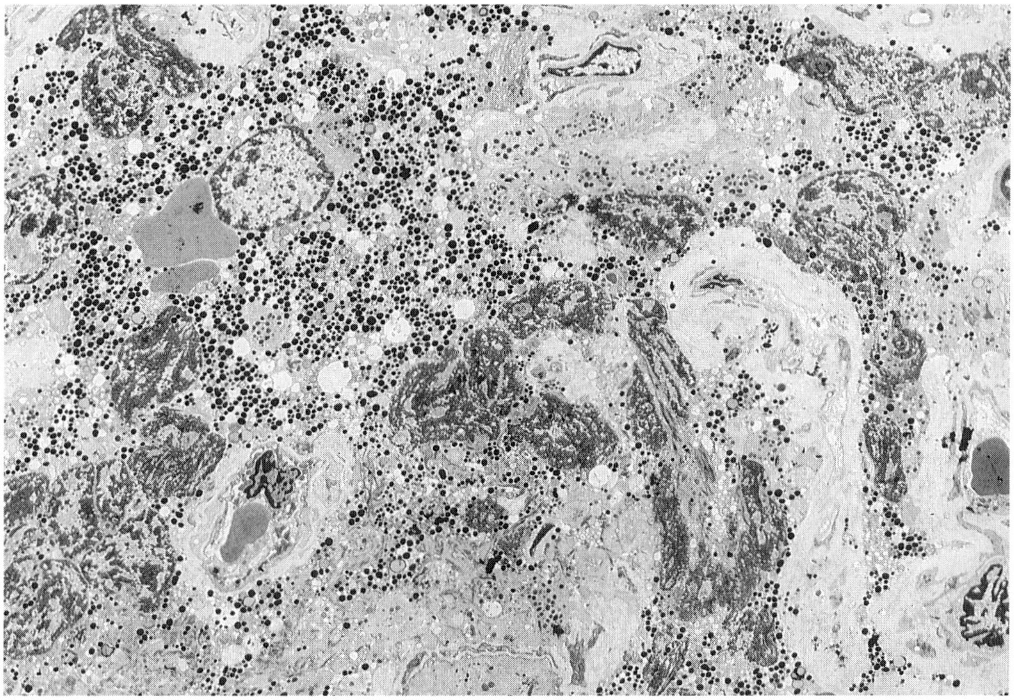

**Fig. 5-6.** GH adenoma after SMS 201–995 treatment shows densely granulated cells and prominent perivascular fibrosis. (×3800.)

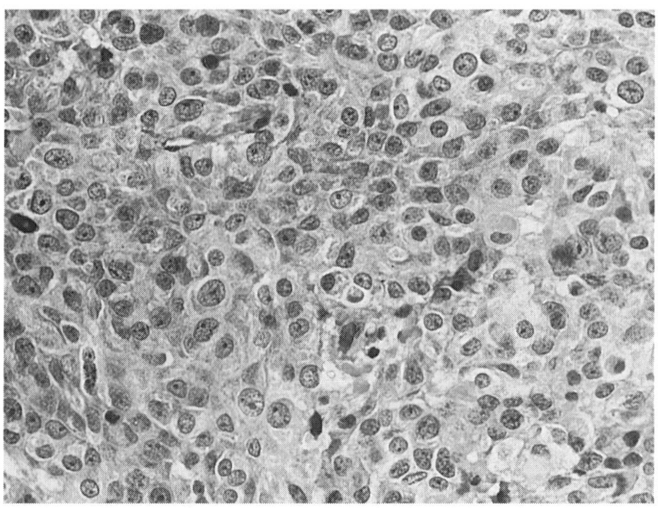

**Fig. 5-7.** PRL adenoma with sheets of uniform cells. (×350.)

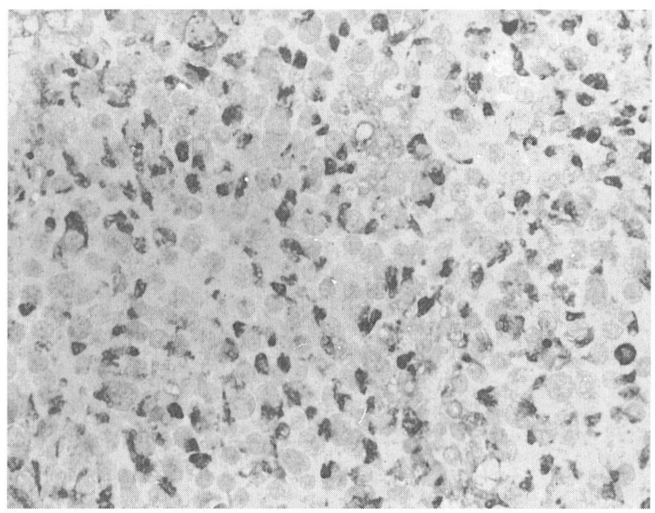

**Fig. 5-8.** Immunostaining of a PRL adenoma showing prominent juxtanuclear staining in most tumor cells. (×350.)

The storage granules range in diameter from 150 to 300 nm (Fig. 5-9). Reverse exocytosis or extrusion of secretory granules into the extracellular space is a characteristic feature of prolactin-producing adenomas in the human pituitary and is the most important diagnostic feature of prolactinomas[172] (Fig. 5-10).

Densely-granulating prolactin adenomas are extremely rare. They are deeply acidophilic on hematoxylin and eosin staining and strongly immunoreactive for prolactin. Ultrastructural studies show a well-developed Golgi complex and secretory granules that range in size from 300 to 700 nm in diameter. Granule extrusion is also common in these neoplasms. Many cases of densely-granulated prolactin cell adenomas

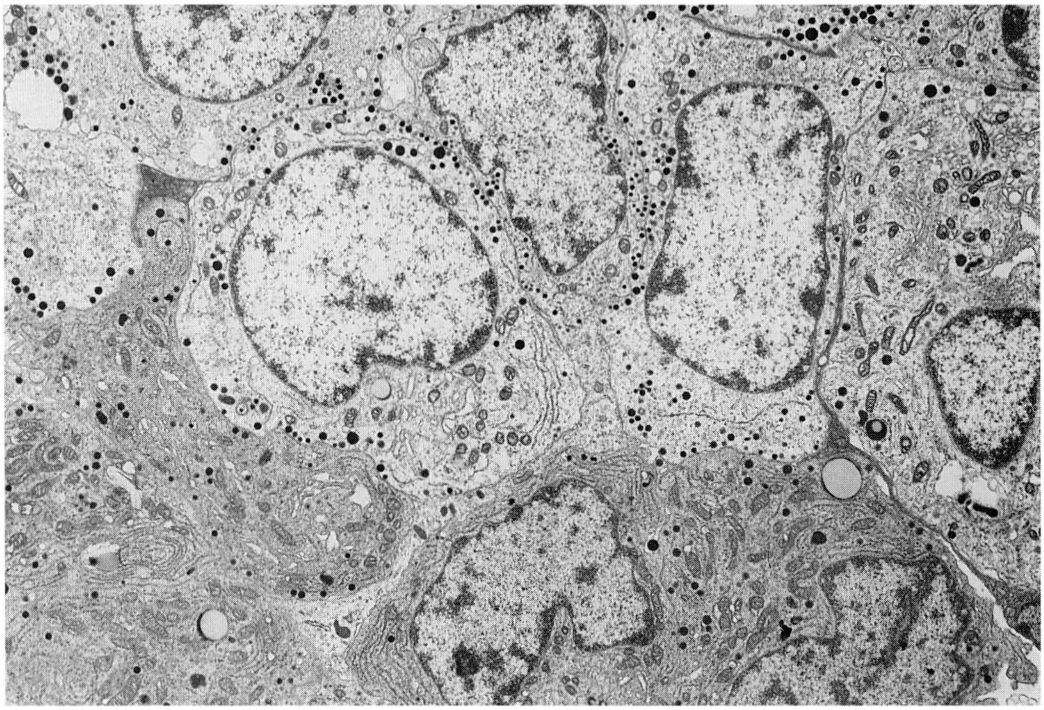

**Fig. 5-9.** Ultrastructure of a sparsely granulated PRL adenoma with prominent rough endoplasmic reticulum. (×6000.)

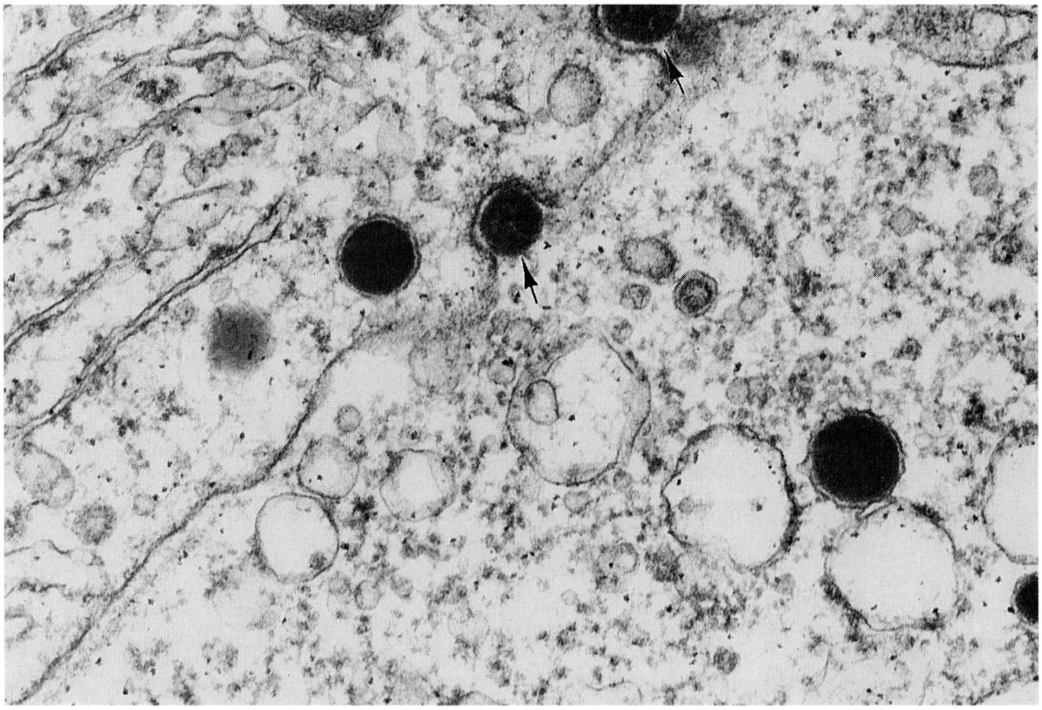

**Fig. 5-10.** Prolactinomas showing reverse exocytosis (*arrows*). (×50,000.)

have been associated with medical treatment of the patient for their neoplasm before surgery. Such treatment has included *bromocriptine* and related ergot alkaloid drugs, and usually leads to marked shrinkage of the tumor with reduction in nuclear and cytoplasmic volumes.* Ultrastructural studies of prolactin-producing tumors after ergot alkaloid treatment show small cytoplasm with scanty rough endoplasmic reticulum and involuted Golgi complexes. The size and volume density of secretory granules usually do not show significant changes, and granular extrusion may still be seen. After termination of treatment there is a rapid reestablishment of the original morphologic features of the neoplasm, with an increase in serum prolactin levels.

Prolonged treatment of prolactin-producing adenomas with ergot alkaloids leads to an increase in the amount of fibrosis and retrogressive changes in the neoplasm.[82,193] The responsiveness of prolactin-producing adenomas to these ergot alkaloids places a premium on the immunocytochemical detection of prolactin, even in adenomas that secrete other hormones.[270]

Rare prolactinomas present as aggressive skull base tumors.[11] These cellular tumors with epithelial-lined microcysts require immunocytochemical or ultrastructural confirmation.

### Corticotroph Cell Adenomas

Adrenocorticotrophin hormone (ACTH)-producing adenomas may be functional or clinically silent. Neoplasms producing *Cushing's* or *Nelson's syndrome* usually are small basophilic microadenomas with a characteristic sinusoidal pattern (Fig. 5-11). These tumors are strongly PAS positive. Some ACTH-producing tumors may be only 1 to 2 mm in diameter. These small tumors may be easily lost during surgery or tissue processing, and this may explain why a small percentage of patients with Cushing's disease are cured by surgery even though a tumor was not seen by the pathologist. In some cases, multiple sections of the same paraffin block may be needed to demonstrate a small adenoma.

Hormone from small ACTH-producing adenomas that are laterally displaced in the gland can be detected prior to surgery by simultaneous bilateral sampling of the right and left inferior *petrosal sinuses*.[56,274] Since approximately four out of five of these tumors are laterally displaced,† petrosal sinus sampling can guide the surgical removal of the appropriate side of the gland when the adenoma cannot be identified. Petrosal sampling is superior to radiographic methods for detcting small microadenomas.

* Refs. 101, 210, 246, 376.

† Refs. 34, 56, 187, 216.

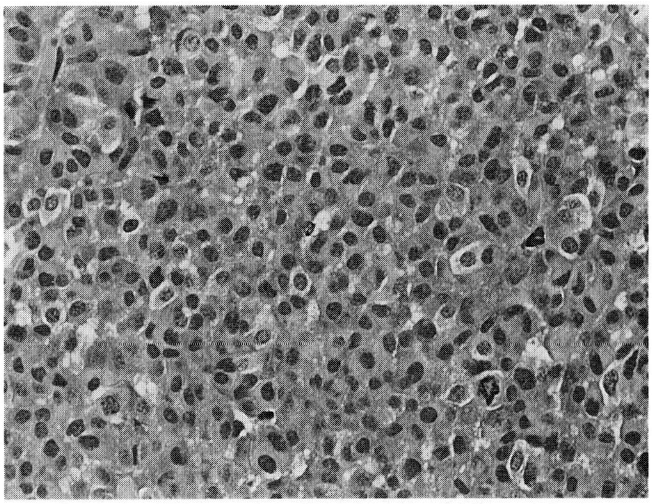

**Fig. 5-11.** ACTH adenoma with slightly basophilic tumor cells. (×350.)

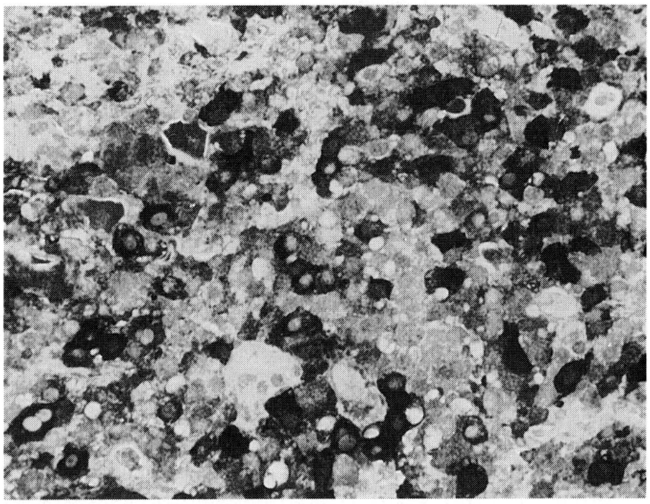

**Fig. 5-12.** Immunostaining of the adenoma in Fig. 5-11 shows a heterogeneous pattern of positivity for ACTH. (×350.)

Immunohistochemical stains usually show ACTH immunoreactivity (Fig. 5-12) as well as positive immunostaining for pro opiomelanocortin (POMC) cleavage products, including beta endorphin and melanocyte-stimulating hormone.[172,233] The POMC immunoreactivities are often restricted to the peripheral part of the cytoplasm, indicating subplasmalemmal accumulation of secretory granules. The prohormone convertase enzymes that process secretory hormones are present in different ratios in corticotroph adenomas than in other adenomas.[212]

Ultrastructural studies of functional corticotroph adenomas often reveal round cells with ovoid nuclei. The rough endoplasmic reticulum is randomly distributed and tends to be slightly dilated. The secretory

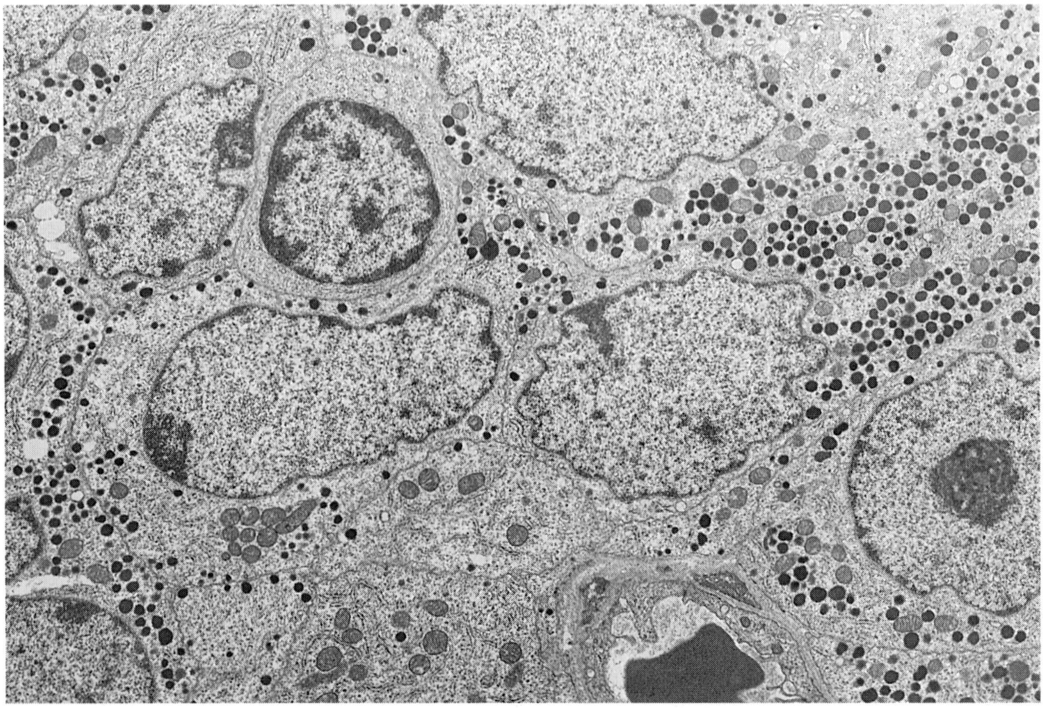

**Fig. 5-13.** Ultrastructure of an ACTH adenoma showing tumor cells with oval nuclei and secretory granules of 150–450 nm. (×5500.)

granules range from 150 to 450 nm in diameter (Fig. 5-13). The Golgi complex is usually spherical and often contains maturing granules within the dilated sacculi. Corticotroph adenomas have characteristic type 1 microfilaments, which form bundles around the nucleus.[86,133,308]

Although *Crooke's hyaline change* is usually seen in the non-neoplastic ACTH cells associated with Cushing's disease, some corticotroph adenomas show Crooke's hyaline changes. Ultrastructural features of these cells are similar to those of Crooke's cells. Clinically silent corticotroph adenomas have been divided into various subtypes according to the ultrastructural features[134] (subtype 1 adenomas are similar to the densely-granulated ACTH tumors). These neoplasms have microfilaments and increased lysosomal activity. Subtype 2 silent adenomas have secretory granules measuring 150 to 400 nm in diameter but no cytoplasmic microfilaments. Subtype 3 microadenomas may represent a heterogeneous group. They contain small secretory granules up to 200 nm and many lysosomes. The subtype 3 tumor has been described as a new class of pituitary adenoma.[136]

### Gonadotroph Cell Adenomas

Gonadotroph tumors are associated with elevated serum levels of follicle-stimulating hormone (FSH) and/or luteinizing hormone (LH). The alpha-subunit of glycoprotein hormones may also be increased in the

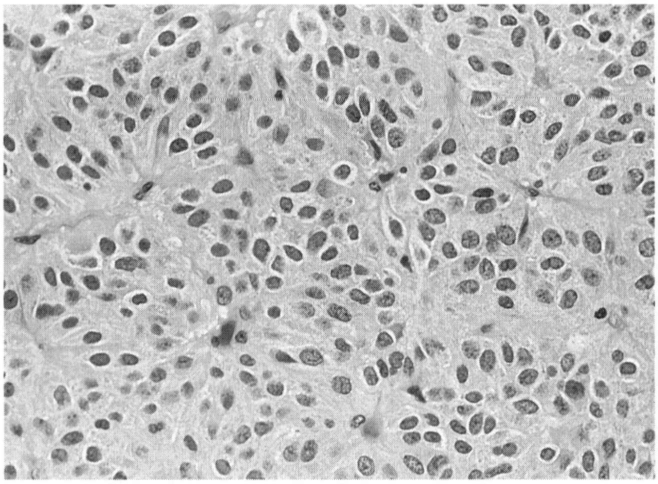

**Fig. 5-14.** Gonadotroph adenoma with oval to spindle cells. (×350.)

serum. (Gonadotroph expression in clinically nonfunctional adenomas is described in the section on null cell adenomas.) Gonadotroph adenomas are usually chromophobic on H&E staining (Fig. 5-14). PAS staining is variably positive. Immunohistochemical staining is positive for FSH and/or LH in the cytoplasm (Fig. 5-15, *A* to *C*), although LH is less commonly elevated in the serum.*

* Refs. 66, 131, 176, 179, 379.

A

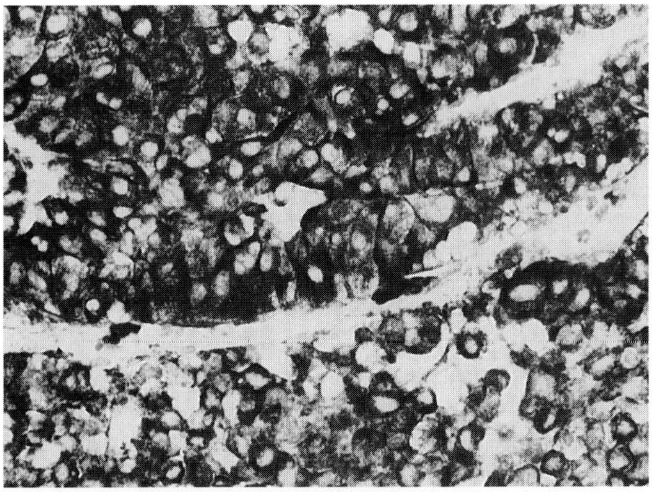

B

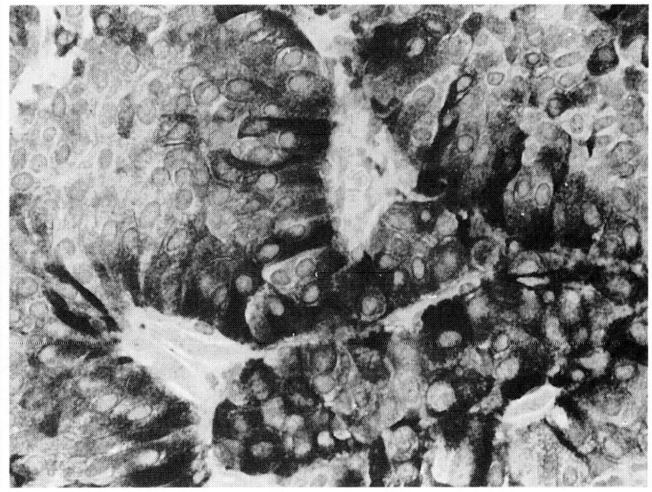

C

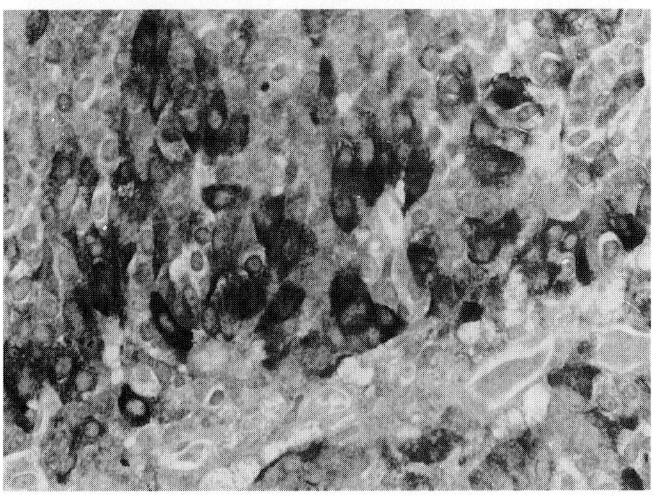

**Fig. 5-15.** The tumor cells of the gonadotroph adenoma are strongly positive for **A**, chromogranin A, **B**, FSH, and **C**, LH. (**A** to **C**, ×400.)

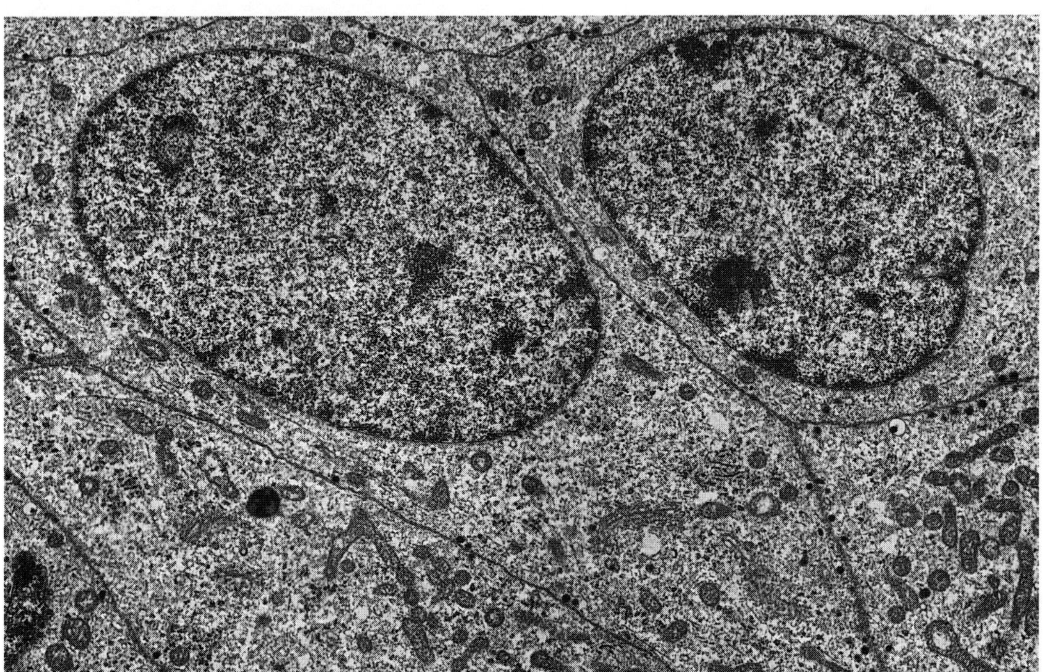

**Fig. 5-16.** Ultrastructural features of a male pattern of gonadotroph adenoma with small secretory granules up to 150 nm and an inconspicuous Golgi region. (×8800.)

The ultrastructural features of gonadotroph adenomas show a striking *sexual dimorphism*. The well-differentiated (female type) tumors consist of stacks of rough endoplasmic reticulum, rod-shaped mitochondria, and Golgi complexes with a honeycomb appearance. The cells are fairly uniform, and the secretory granules are usually less than 150 nm in diameter. The ultrastructural features of the male pattern of differentiation are variable (Fig. 5-16). The secretory granules measure up to 250 nm in diameter and are unevenly distributed in the tumor cells. Secretory granules are more prominent within cell processes. The characteristic Golgi complex pattern in women with gonadotroph adenoma is a very helpful diagnostic feature.[172] Because of the usual elevation of FSH and LH levels in the serum of women after menopause, often it has been difficult to clinically diagnose gonadotroph adenomas in postmenopausal women. However, studies[66] have shown that these neoplasms are also as common in older women as they are in older men.

### Thyrotroph Cell Adenomas

Thyrotroph cell adenomas are uncommon neoplasms in surgical series.* These tumors may be associated with chronic hypothyroidism or they may develop spontaneously and be associated with hyperthyroidism. Thyrotroph cell adenomas may be basophilic or chromophobic. The tumor cells show variable immunoreactivity after staining with TSH antibodies. Ultrastructural studies show a great variation in tumor cells. Many tumors consist of elongated cells with abundant rough endoplasmic reticulum and a prominent Golgi complex. Secretory granules vary in number and tend to be present in cytoplasmic processes. Granules range from 150 to 200 nm in diameter.

* Refs. 2, 105, 172, 319.

### Null Cell or Undifferentiated Adenomas

These tumors were defined by Kovacs and coworkers as clinically nonfunctioning pituitary tumors without histologic, immunocytochemical, or ultrastructural features to reveal their cellular derivation.[177] Numerous studies have characterized null cell adenomas in recent years. Many of these neoplasms stain positively for alpha-subunit of gonadotroph hormones and many also express the messenger RNA for gonadotrophic hormones or alpha-subunit.[14,144,218] The tumor cells are often chromophobic and vary from spindled to round (Fig. 5-17). Immunohistochemistry reveals staining for chromogranin A,[312] and cells may be positive for gonadotrophic hormone and for alpha-subunit[327] (Fig. 5-18, *A* and *B*). Based on immunocytochemical and molecular biological data, null cell and gonadotroph cell adenomas seem closely related.[211] Ultrastructural

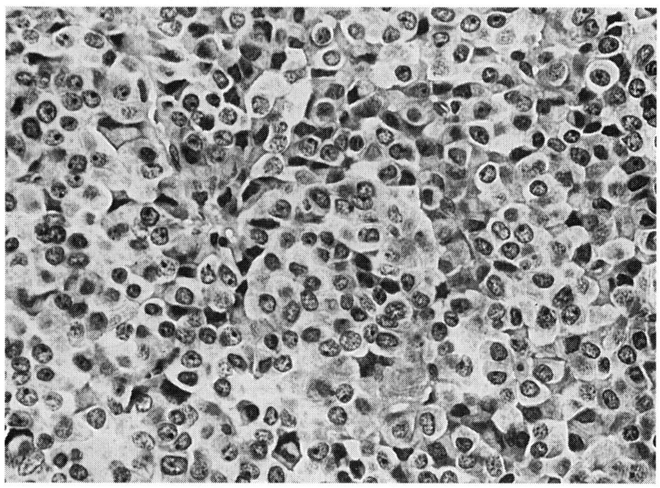

**Fig. 5-17.** Null cell adenoma with round to oval tumor cells. (×350.)

A

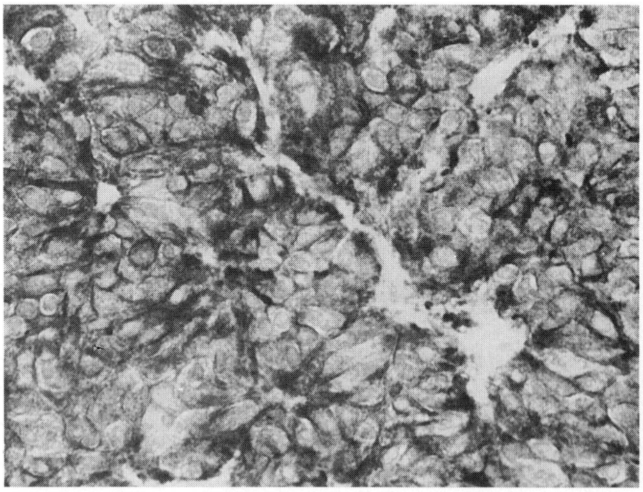

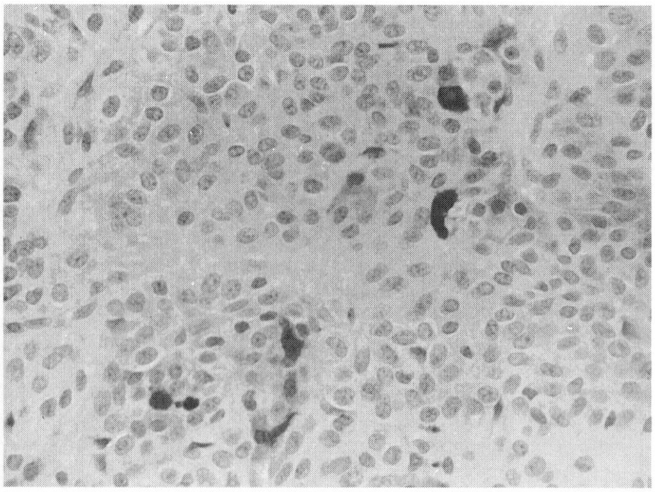

B

**Fig. 5-18.** Null cell adenoma staining positively and diffusely for **A,** chromogranin A and **B,** focally for alpha-subunit of human chorionic gonadotropin. (×350.)

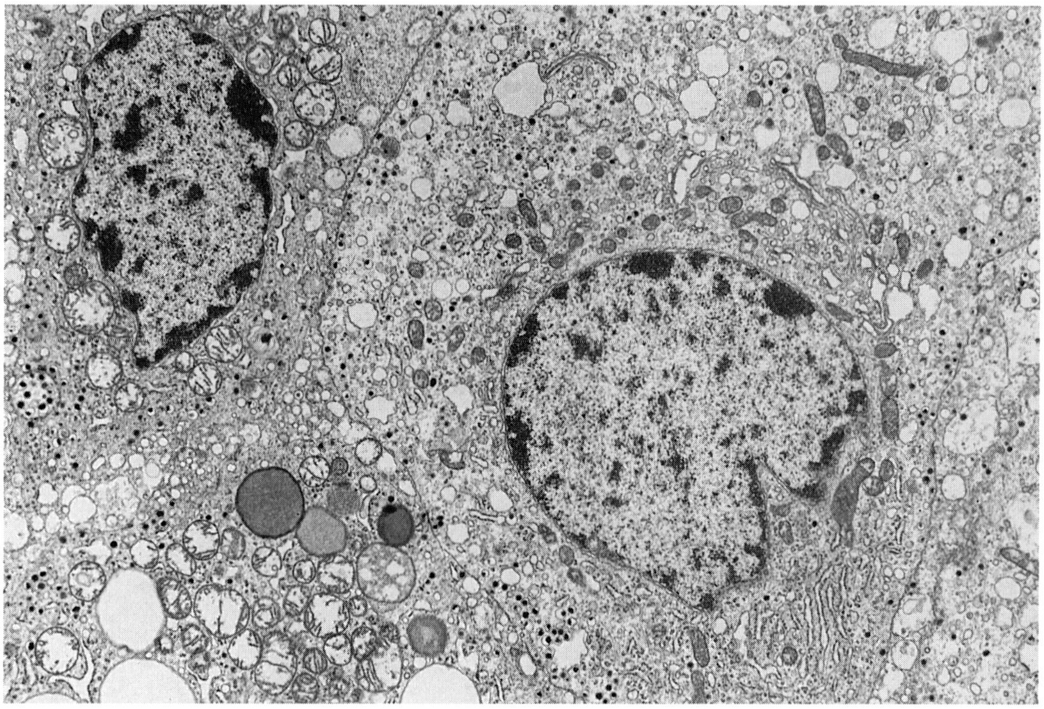

**Fig. 5-19.** Null cell adenoma with sparse numbers of small secretory granules 50–250 nm in diameter and poorly developed rough endoplasmic reticulum. (×8800.)

studies of null cell adenomas show small polyhedral cells with scanty amounts of poorly developed rough endoplasmic reticulum and Golgi complexes. Small secretory granules measuring 50 to 250 nm are often present (Fig. 5-19).

### Oncocytomas

Oncocytomas may be considered a variant of null cell adenomas.[174,194] These cells are acidophilic but may also be chromophobic. Immunohistochemical staining shows features similar to null cell adenomas. The striking ultrastructural feature is the large number of *mitochondria* within the cytoplasm of these cells. Mitochondria may occupy up to 50% of the cytoplasmic area of these neoplasms. Immunoreactivity for chromogranin A and focal immunoreactivity for LH and alpha-subunit may be present within these tumors.

### Plurihormonal Adenomas

A small percentage of pituitary neoplasms have unusual combinations of pituitary hormones by immunohistochemical staining and ultrastructural studies.* Based on morphologic studies, these tumors may be monomorphous, with a uniform cell population, or plurimorphous, consisting of two or more morphologic cell types. Some adenomas may produce hormones of one cell line such as growth hormone or prolactin. Other adenomas may contain hormones of two cell lines, such as eosinophilic and basophilic cells producing growth hormone and TSH; prolactin and TSH; growth hormone, prolactin, and TSH; or growth hormone, ACTH, and related peptides. Other adenomas may produce hormones from three cell lines such as growth hormone, ACTH, and alpha-subunit; or prolactin, TSH, alpha-subunit, and pro-opiomelanocortin cleavage products. However, even these rare adenomas do not show the full spectrum of hormone-producing cells evident in normal adenohypophysis. The cellular derivation of these plurihormonal adenomas remains unknown. The plurihormonal adenomas may be similar to pancreatic endocrine tumors in which immunohistochemical analysis may show a variety of hormones, even though the patient usually has clinical signs and symptoms from excessive production of only one or two hormones.

* Refs. 73, 135, 175, 278, 345.

### Double Adenomas

Double adenomas are two structurally or immunocytochemically distinct tumors occurring in one patient. The adenomas may be regionally or temporally distinct. They are rare. In one study, they represented one third of 1% of surgically removed adenomas.[169] They usually cannot be identified in routine sections of surgical material without immunocytochemical or ultrastructural studies.

### Ectopic Pituitary Adenomas

Pituitary tissue is found outside the sphenoid sinus in over 90% of patients in some autopsy series.[36,236] Adenomas may arise from these ectopic foci.[208] Functional or nonfunctional pituitary adenomas may be found in the sphenoid bone, clivus, nasal pharynx, or buccal region. Most ectopic adenomas coexist with normal intrasellar pituitary tissue, but they may associate with hyperplastic or with neoplastic intrasellar pituitary tissue.* These adenomas are most likely derived from the pharyngeal pituitary or from other ectopic foci of pituitary cells. The sphenoid sinus has been the most common site of ectopic pituitary adenomas.[36]

Immunohistochemical stains to characterize these tumors show that prolactin and growth hormone-producing tumors are the common adenomas. This is similar to the general incidence of these adenomas among surgically resected tumors. Another subtype of ectopic pituitary adenomas include the suprasellar tumors, which may arise from the anterior lobe cells attached to the suprasellar portion of the pituitary stalk. Although most ectopic pituitary adenomas are solitary, one report found two separate ectopic adenomas that originated in the sphenoid and suprasellar areas.[36] Patients with ectopic adenomas commonly present with evidence of an expanding mass and compression of adjacent structures. Most of these neoplasms are low-grade, and routine immunohistochemistry can prevent inappropriately aggressive therapy.[382] The use of CT scans may be helpful in the diagnosis of ectopic adenomas.

## LESIONS ASSOCIATED WITH PITUITARY ADENOMA: HEMORRHAGE AND INFARCTION

Adenomas have been associated with extensive hemorrhagic infarction (*pituitary apoplexy*).[307,315] Pituitary apoplexy has been found in cases with growth hormone-producing tumors, in which dramatic improvement of the patient's symptoms may occur after infarction of the adenoma. Pituitary apoplexy is also commonly associated with other large adenomas, including the frequently occurring null cell and other clinically nonfunctioning adenomas. Lack of clinical endocrinologic signs allows these tumors to grow large enough to infarct prior to detection. Pituitary infarction can be associated with vascular occlusion or simply hypoperfusion leading to necrosis and cell death.

Infarcts also occur in non-neoplastic pituitary glands. Small pituitary infarcts may be present in up to 8% of cases at the time of autopsy. Hypopituitarism usually develops only after extensive loss of anterior pituitary tissues. More than 75% of the anterior pituitary tissue must be lost before moderate symptoms of hypopituitarism develop, while severe hypophyseal insufficiency becomes apparent when there is loss of more than 90% of the hormone-producing cells.[130] *Sheehan's syndrome* is a form of pituitary necrosis occurring in the postpartum period in which there is massive infarction of the adenohypophysis. This can lead to permanent anterior pituitary insufficiency.[341] Vasospasm may be the initiating trigger of ischemia leading to infarction. Necrosis may be focal or very extensive in the adenohypophysis. The posterior pituitary with its rich arterial blood supply, which is independent of the portal vasculature, is usually not severely affected.[342]

Hemorrhage in the pituitary may occur with traumatic head injury or secondary to bleeding into the subarachnoid space. Hemorrhage may extend into the subarachnoid space of the pituitary.

## ANTERIOR LOBE ABNORMALITIES CONFUSED WITH ADENOMA

Two abnormalities that have been confused with adenoma are discussed here. Neither abnormality is neoplastic.

### Pituitary Hyperplasia

Hyperplasia of the anterior pituitary is an uncommon condition. The diagnosis is very difficult to make on small biopsy specimens, because hyperplasia shares features with both adenoma and normal pituitary. Hyperplasia can be divided into primary or idiopathic hyperplasia and secondary hyperplasia resulting from non-neoplastic production of hypothalamic releasing hormone, hypothalamic hamartomas, hypothalamic releasing hormone-producing tumors, or organ failure.* Difficulties in establishing the diagnosis of pituitary hyperplasia stem from the variable distribution of various cell types in the anterior lobe. For example, corticotroph cells are more numerous in the mucoid wedge; therefore, small biopsies from this area may lead to an erroneous diagnosis of ACTH cell hyperplasia. Hyperplasia may be diffuse or nodular. The *nodular form* of hyperplasia may be easier to recognize in histologic sections (Fig. 5-20). Special stains such as the reticulin and immunohistochemical staining are helpful in establishing the diagnosis. Reticulin stains may show expansion of the normal acinar structure. Immunohistochemical stains may show enlarged cells of a specific lineage admixed with other cell types. End organ failure may lead to pituitary hyperplasia. Anencephaly is associated with decreased ACTH cells in the pituitary.†

Patients with untreated Addison's disease may show diffuse and/or nodular hyperplasia of ACTH cells.[331] ACTH hyperplasia is seen in patients who died

* Refs. 36, 61a, 208, 396.

* Refs. 17, 18, 132, 150, 180, 207, 230, 251, 331, 333, 374.

† Refs. 27, 121, 247, 323.

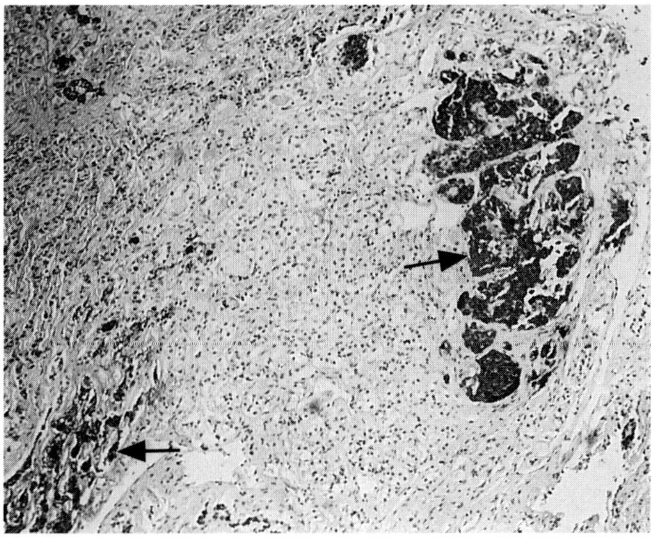

**Fig. 5-20.** Two separate dark nodules of ACTH hyperplasia (*arrows*) are from a patient who had Cushing's disease that did not respond to partial excision. Immunostained for ACTH. (×65.) (Reprinted from McKeever PE, and others: Refractory Cushing's disease caused by multinodular ACTH hyperplasia, J Neuropathol Exper Neurol 41:490-499, 1982.)

of fully developed AIDS.[249] Patients with untreated hypothyroidism have been reported to have hyperplasia of TSH and prolactin cells.[295] Well-documented cases of nodular hyperplasia of ACTH cells corroborated by postmortem examination of the entire pituitary[230] have shown its bilateral multifocal distribution. The stimulus for primary hyperplasia may not be readily identified in many patients.

### Inflammatory Lesions of the Pituitary

Autoimmune hypophysitis or *lymphocytic hypophysitis* may appear like a pituitary neoplasm clinically. It has been described by several authors.* This lesion usually affects young women and often causes enlargement of the pituitary gland. Most patients are pregnant or in the postpartum period. Postmenopausal cases are rare.[142] Antipituitary antibodies have been identified in some cases, supporting an autoimmune etiology. Autoimmune hypophysitis has also been described in association with inflammatory disorders of the thyroid, adrenals, and other endocrine tissues. Histologic examination usually reveals cellular infiltrates of lymphocytes and some plasma cells. Follicle and germinal center formation may be seen. Immunofluorescence studies have failed to show immune complex deposition.

Acute inflammatory lesions of the pituitary are uncommon and rarely confused with adenoma. Patients with sepsis may develop purulent hypophysitis with *abscess* formation. Cysts of the pituitary gland may be a predisposing factor for abscess formation.[271] The anatomic structures adjacent to the pituitary, such as the sphenoid bone, may be involved with purulent inflammation such as sphenoid sinusitis, bacterial meningitis, and purulent otitis media, which can cause suppurative inflammation of the pituitary.[72,202]

The pituitary gland may be involved with various *granulomatous* inflammatory lesions, including sarcoidosis, fungal infection, and tuberculosis.[306,385] The histologic changes seen in the pituitary with these infections are similar to those seen in the lung and other tissues. Culture, microbiologic and/or immunohistochemical, and other special stains can be used to characterize the infectious agents. Sarcoidosis affecting the pituitary gland is a diagnosis of exclusion. Sarcoidosis occurs more commonly in the posterior pituitary. It can also involve the hypothalamus, leading to pituitary insufficiency and destruction of the neurons that produce various regulatory peptides. Sarcoidosis has been associated with hyperprolactinemia in some of these cases.[130]

* Refs. 12, 148, 223, 234, 298, 353.

## ANTERIOR, INTERMEDIATE, AND POSTERIOR PITUITARY GLAND

The pituitary is the tissue most frequently confused with adenoma. An understanding of its anatomy and histology is critical to distinguishing it. As elaborated below, features of particular importance are the small size of the gland, its venous drainage, its acinar configuration, and the different mixtures of secretory cells in different portions of the gland.

### Development and Anatomy

The pituitary gland is composed of the adenohypophysis and the neurohypophysis. The pars distalis, pars intermedia, and pars tuberalis form the adenohypophysis; the posterior lobe, neural stalk, and infundibulum make up the neurohypophysis. During embryonic development, the invagination of the stomodeal ectoderm and Rathke's pouch develop into the adenohypophysis. The neurohypophysis is derived from the floor of the diencephalon. The neurohypophysis has a connection with the brain via the infundibular stalk.

The *fetal* pituitary gland can be recognized by the third month of gestation.[72] Acidophil and basophil cells can be readily identified, and various cell types can be characterized by immunohistochemical stains in the adenohypophysis.[107] All of the various cell types of the adult adenohypophysis can be identified immunohistochemically in the pituitary by 3 months of gestation.* The early studies of Baker and Jaffe[23] characterized the various cell types in the adenohypophysis of

* Refs. 27, 32, 276, 277.

the human fetus by immunohistochemistry. Other studies have shown that ACTH and beta endorphin can be detected immunohistochemically by the eighth week of gestation. Growth hormone cells can also be detected at this time, while the $\alpha$-subunit of the glycoprotein hormones and the $\beta$-subunit of TSH, FSH, and LH are identified immunohistochemically by 12 weeks of development.[16,276] Prolactin cells are identified by the twelfth week of gestation, and there is a marked increase of prolactin cells by term.[16]

The pituitary gland is located in the sella turcica, a midline cavity of the sphenoid bone. It is bilaterally symmetric and weighs approximately 100 mg at birth. The adult gland weighs between 400 and 900 mg, and the anterior lobe constitutes about 80% of the total pituitary. The small size of the anterior pituitary distinguishes it from macroadenomas of the pituitary. Macroadenomas are larger than 10 mm in diameter (discussed in the introduction to the section on pituitary adenoma).

The anterior pituitary increases in size during *pregnancy* secondary to prolactin cell hyperplasia. The gland may weigh over 1000 mg during late pregnancy. As a consequence of the increase in the numbers of prolactin cells, the pituitary gland of multiparous women usually weighs more than that of nulliparous women.[18]

The pituitary is covered by the dura mater, which is a dense layer of connective tissue covering the brain. The roof of the sella turcica is covered by the diaphragm sella, which is part of the dura mater. The hypophyseal stalk is connected to the rest of the pituitary through a small hole about 5 mm wide in the diaphragm sella. When the diaphragm sella is incomplete or absent, a condition known as the *empty sella syndrome* develops. In this condition, the diaphragm sella is more widely open, and increased cerebrospinal fluid pressure leads to enlargement of the sella and compression of the pituitary. The pituitary may be very flattened and may appear like a thin layer of tissue at the bottom of the sella. This flattened pituitary can be mistaken radiographically for a neoplasm.[156] Considerable compression atrophy and loss of pituitary tissue ordinarily produce few clinical signs of hypopituitarism. This "pituitary reserve" calls for generous sampling to find occult adenomas in other patients. The relatively common empty sella syndrome should not be confused with the rare congenital absence of anterior pituitary gland.[41,303] Congenital absence is commonly associated with multiple endocrine abnormalities.[32,360]

Connective tissue penetrates the gland along fibrovascular septae that surround individual acini. The number of cells per acinus averages 30 or fewer in standard histologic sections, with a considerable range between individual acini. The pattern of *fibrovascular stroma* encircling individual acini resembles chicken-wire (Fig. 5-21). This normal pattern is distinctly different from that of most adenomas, which have stroma that do not completely encircle parenchymal cells.[231] In adenomas, the reticulin pattern resembles chicken-wire cut open and broken apart (Fig. 5-22).

The pituitary gland receives its *blood supply* from the branches of the internal carotid arteries, which include

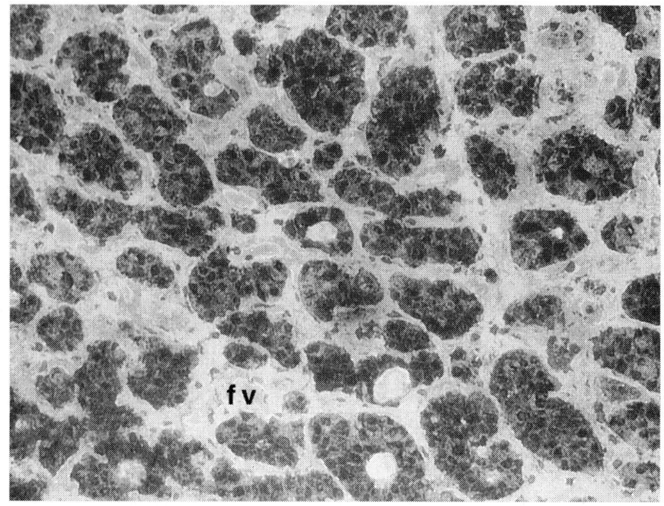


**Fig. 5-21.** Frozen section of a biopsy specimen of adenohypophysis stained with the fluorescein labeled lectin *Ricinus communis* agglutinin. The fibrovascular (fv) stroma that surrounds acini stains brightly in a pattern that resembles "chicken-wire." (×250.) (Reprinted from McKeever PE, and others: Stromal and nuclear markers for rapid identification of pituitary adenomas at biopsy, Arch Pathol Lab Med 109:509-514, 1985.)

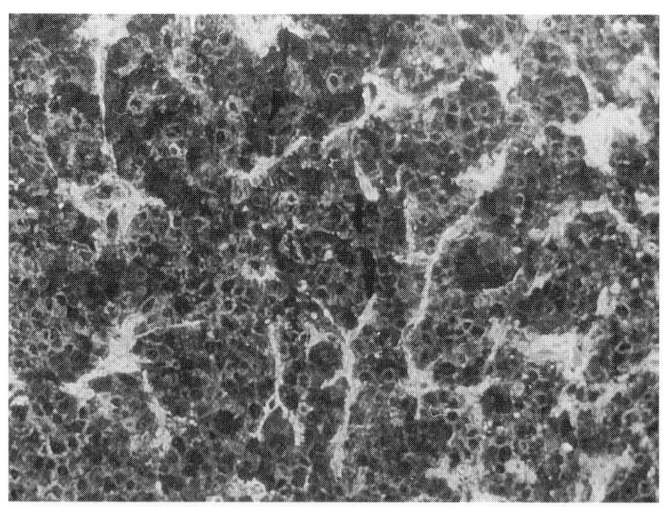

**Fig. 5-22.** Frozen section of biopsy specimen of pituitary adenoma stained with fluorescein labeled lectin *Ricinus communis* agglutinin. The bright bands of fibrovascular stroma do not interconnect around acini. Instead they are individual linear and branching strips of fluorescent light. (×250.) (Reprinted from McKeever PE, and others: Stromal and nuclear markers for rapid identification of pituitary adenomas at biopsy, Arch Pathol Lab Med 109:509-514, 1985.)

the superior hypophyseal arteries. The long portal vessels and the short vessels carry about 70 to 90% of the blood to the adenohypophysis. These vessels also contain hypothalamic releasing hormones, which regulate secretion of anterior pituitary hormones. The middle and inferior hypophyseal arteries are connected to the neurohypophysis; thus, the neurohypophysis has a more direct arterial blood supply, which explains why metastatic neoplasms to the pituitary gland are more common in the neurohypophysis.

Venous drainage is lateralized into the left and right inferior petrosal sinuses. These can be individually sampled.[274] Laterally displaced secretory adenomas produce a gradient of increased hormone in the sinus ipsilateral to the adenoma. This is particularly valuable for the detection of ACTH microadenomas, as elaborated in the section on corticotroph cell adenomas.

The *posterior pituitary* has direct contact with the hypothalamus. The posterior pituitary is composed of nerve fibers, pituicytes, and axon terminals that contain neurosecretory granules, including vasopressin, oxytocin, and the carrier protein neurophysin. The adenohypophysis has minimal innervation, with only a few sympathetic neural fibers that penetrate the anterior lobe adjacent to capillaries. The neural connections to the neurohypophysis are very important. For example, atrophy of the neurohypophysis occurs after interruption of hypothalamic innervation.[67] The pituitary capillaries are lined with fenestrated epithelium.[172]

*Ectopic* or pharyngeal pituitary tissue is a common finding at autopsy.[36,38,236] This extrasellar adenohypophyseal tissue is usually found along the path of fetal development of the pars distalis.[78] Ectopic pituitary tissue may occasionally give rise to pituitary adenomas.

### Normal Pituitary Gland

The *anterior pituitary gland* is composed of many cell types with various functions (Table 5-1). After staining with H&E, the cells of the anterior pituitary appear acidophilic, basophilic, and chromophobic. These traditional histochemical stains do not reliably indicate the specific hormone being produced by specific cell types or neoplasms. These classic stains have largely been replaced by immunohistochemical staining methods and ultrastructural studies for the analysis of normal pituitary cells and pituitary adenomas.[232]

As explained below, all regions of normal anterior pituitary gland contain a variety of secretory cells that contain different pituitary hormones.[232] The resulting mosaic of immunoreactive cells is more polymorphous than immunoreactivity of pituitary adenomas, even the adenomas that are plurihormonal. This feature is critical in differentiating normal adenohypophysis from adenoma.

The most abundant cell type in the adenohypophysis is the *GH cell.* These cells make up approximately 40 to 50% of the total adenohypophyseal cell population. The cells are medium size and often stain intensely with growth hormone antibodies. Ultrastructural studies show that the cells have secretory granules ranging in size from 250 to 700 nm in diameter. The GH cells are present predominantly in the lateral wings of the anterior lobe (Fig. 5-23) but can be found in most areas of the adenohypophysis. The conspicuous abundance of GH cells in the lateral wings can cause confusion with growth hormone adenomas (see Figs. 5-2, 5-23). Look for cell types that are virtually nonexistent in GH adenomas, particularly gonadotrophs. A complete battery of immunostains will show a broader range of cell types in lateral wings than in GH, or even plurihormonal, adenomas.

*Prolactin (PRL) cells* are the second most common cell type in the adenohypophysis. PRL cells constitute between 15 and 25% of the anterior pituitary cells and are present throughout the pars distalis. PRL cells may be acidophilic or chromophobic with H&E stains. PRL cells are abundant in the term fetus and neonate, possibly due to maternal estrogens. The number of PRL cells decreases after birth and remains low during childhood, and there is prolactin cell hyperplasia during pregnancy and lactation. Two types of PRL cells can be recognized in the human pituitary gland with immunohistochemical staining and ultrastructural studies.[172] One PRL cell type stains strongly and diffusely for PRL hormone, while the second cell type stains strongly only in a juxtanuclear pattern. The first cell type has secretory granules measuring 500 to 700 nm in diameter, while the second cell type has secretory granules measuring 200 to 350 nm in diameter. Several studies have identified cells that contain both PRL and GH in the normal pituitary gland in both humans and other vertebrates.[205,267]

The ACTH-producing cells are the third most abundant in the anterior pituitary gland and constitute

**Table 5-1.** Principal anterior pituitary cells

| Cell type | Percent of cells | Secretory granule diameter (nm) |
|---|---|---|
| Growth hormone (GH) | 50 | 250–600 |
| Prolactin | 15–25 | 500–700 |
| Adrenocorticotropin | 15–20 | 200–350 |
| Follicle-stimulating hormone (FSH) | 10* | 200–300 |
| Luteinizing hormone (LH) | 10* | 300–500 |
| Thyroid-stimulating (TSH) hormone | 5 | 100–300 |
| Folliculo-stellate cells | <1 | None |

* Most gonadotropic cells contain both FSH and LH.

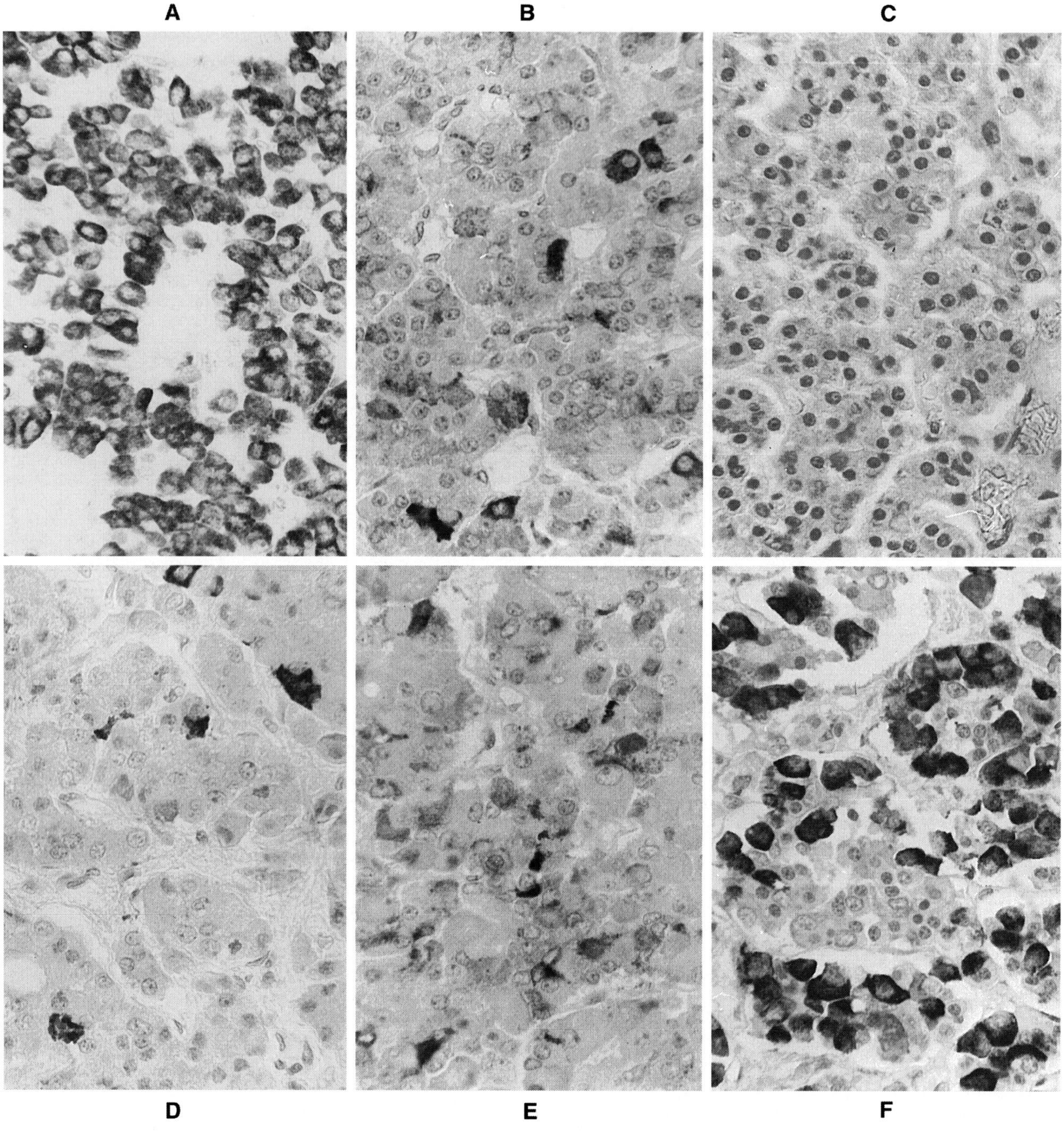


**Fig. 5-23.** Topographic variation in the normal abundance of adenohypophyseal cells. Top three panels are sections of lateral wing, and bottom three panels are from the mucoid wedge. Left panels are GH cells, middle panels are PRL cells, and right panels are ACTH cells.

about 15% of the total secretory cells. These cells stain positively with periodic acid-Schiff (PAS). ACTH cells are located in the central mucoid wedge of the pars distalis (Fig. 5-23). Immunohistochemical studies show strong staining for ACTH, beta lipotropin, endorphin, and alpha and beta melanocyte-stimulating hormone. Ultrastructural studies show secretory granules ranging from 250 to 700 nm in diameter. Type 1 microfilaments are often seen in the cytoplasm adjacent to the nucleus. When endogenous or exogenous glucocorticoid excess is present, the ACTH cells undergo a distinct morphologic change and acquire a glassy homogeneous material in the cytoplasm that pushes the ACTH immunoreactive granules to the periphery of the cells. This condition is known as Crooke's hyaline change.[63] The hyaline material stains positively for cytokeratin intermediate filament and is composed of type 1 microfilaments.[178,263]

Most *gonadotroph cells* produce FSH and LH by immunohistochemical staining. A small percentage of gonadotrophic cells produce only FSH or LH.[287] Gonadotroph cells constitute about 10% of the anterior pituitary cells. Ultrastructural studies show two granule populations of 200 to 300 nm and 300 to 500 nm in diameter. With chronic gonadectomy, the gonadotroph cells assume a "signet-ring" appearance and have been designated as "castration cells." They are composed of widely dilated rough endoplasmic reticulum and decreased numbers of secretory granules.

*Thyroid-secreting hormone* (*TSH*) *cells* comprise about 5% of anterior pituitary cells. These PAS-positive cells are often angular and stain intensely with TSH antibodies. Ultrastructural studies reveal secretory granules ranging in size from 100 to 300 nm in diameter. The secretory granules are usually adjacent to the cytoplasmic membranes. With chronic hypothyroidism, the anterior pituitary gland develops "thyroidectomy cells," which consist of enlarged thyrotrophs with prominent Golgi complexes, dilated rough endoplasmic reticulum, and decreased numbers of secretory granules.

Other cell types in the pars distalis include the *follicular cells* or folliculo-stellate cells. These nonsecretory cells are angular and contain prominent junctional complexes. Groups of these cells may form a central lumen. Folliculo-stellate cells are strongly positive for S-100 acidic protein.[254] In experimental animals, these cells contain fibroblast growth factor and interleukins, as well as a novel heparin-binding growth factor specific for vascular endothelial cells.[22,87,88] The folliculo-stellate cells may have various functions, including a phagocytic function, and they also have a paracrine function and can regulate secretion of adjacent anterior pituitary hormone cells.[22,95,363]

The pars tuberalis forms part of the adenohypophysis. Several anterior pituitary hormone cells are present in this area, and these may give rise to neoplasms. Immunohistochemical stains often show FSH and LH cells with occasional ACTH and TSH cells.[15]

The *pars intermedia* is not as well developed in humans as it is in lower animals, but is considered part of the adenohypophysis in humans. The pars intermedia consists of cavities of varying sizes lined by single layers of cuboidal epithelium, which may be partially ciliated. The lumina of these cavities are often filled with colloid material, which may show ACTH immunoreactivity.[172]

ACTH-positive basophilic cells often extend into the pars nervosa and deeply into the neural lobe of the pituitary.[232] These ACTH cells increase in number with age and are often referred to as "*basophil invasion*" of the posterior pituitary. If not recognized as a normal anatomic feature, these clusters can be mistaken for infiltrating adenoma. Recognition of their small size, linear growth pattern, and lack of compression of surrounding tissue help to avoid this misinterpretation.

The *posterior lobe* of the pituitary is considered part of the nervous system. It consists of storage secretory granules containing oxytocin, vasopressin, and neurophysin carrier proteins. The hormones oxytocin and vasopressin are produced in the supraoptic and paraventricular nuclei of the hypothalamus and are then transported to the posterior lobe for storage and subsequent release. The secretory granules containing oxytocin and vasopressin range in size from 100 to 200 nm in diameter when examined ultrastructurally. These hormones are bound to neurophysins, which are sulfur-rich proteins of about 10 kilodaltons. The principal cell in the posterior pituitary is the pituicyte, which is the glial cell of the posterior lobe. These cells have supportive and phagocytic functions. The posterior lobe is highly vascularized, and the capillaries are lined by fenestrated epithelium.

*Hypothalamic hormones* regulate the synthesis and secretion of anterior pituitary hormones. The hypothalamic hormones include releasing hormones as well as a few inhibiting hormones, such as somatostatin and dopamine, which inhibit release of GH and PRL, respectively. The releasing hormones include corticotropin-releasing hormone (CRH), which stimulates ACTH release; gonadotropin-releasing hormone (GnRH), which stimulates LH and FSH release; thyrotropin-releasing hormone (TRH), which stimulates TSH and PRL release; growth hormone-releasing hormone (GHRH), which stimulates GH release; and vasoactive intestinal polypeptide (VIP), which stimulates PRL release.

The posterior lobe sometimes confounds the interpretation of pituitary biopsy specimens by its gross appearance in situ. The surgeon searching through adenohypophysis for a sign of a microadenoma may seize upon the discrete white posterior pituitary, thinking it to be the encapsulated adenoma. The pathologist must be prepared to interpret the true nature of the tissue. Stained with H&E, posterior pituitary is quite fibrillary and resembles brain tissue more closely than adenoma (or anterior pituitary). Unlike a collagenous "capsule" of dura or compressed atrophic acini, posterior pituitary does not polarize white-yellow and does not stain blue or green with Masson's trichrome for collagen (except for its discontinuous fibrovascular stroma). Axons are much more abundant in posterior pituitary than adenoma or its "capsule." These can be stained with immunoperoxidase anti-neurofilament or conventional silver stains for axons.[189,232]

## CARCINOMAS

Carcinoma is a problem in the diagnosis of pituitary adenomas from two points of view. First, the epithelioid cells of well-differentiated carcinomas resemble adenoma cells (Fig. 5-24). Second, sellar cysts and tumors easily distinguished from adenoma in their benign form can degenerate to structures that may be confused with adenoma.

There are four *sources of carcinoma* in the pituitary. Fortunately, these are not common. Primary pituitary carcinomas are malignant counterparts of pituitary adenomas composed of malignant endocrine cells. Rare intrasellar and suprasellar carcinomas arise from other tumors and cysts. Still others like nasopharyngeal carcinomas arrive by local invasion of surrounding structures. Metastases to pituitary from distant primary carcinomas also occur.

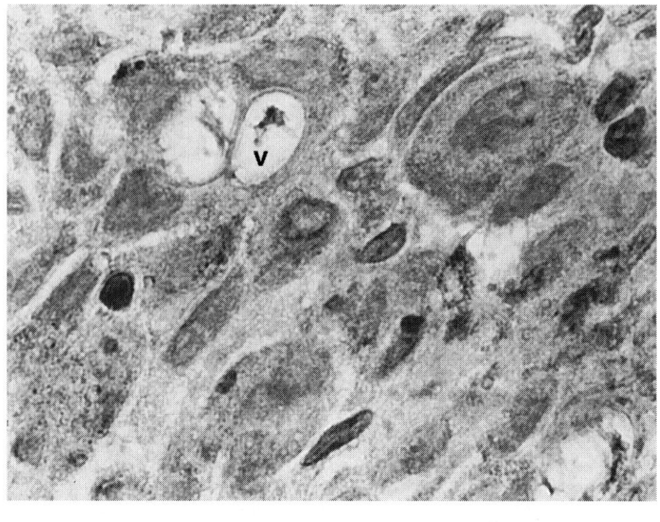


**Fig. 5-24.** Nuclear pleomorphism and cytoplasmic vacuoles (*v*) are the conspicuous features that distinguish the epithelial cells of this metastatic adenocarcinoma from adenoma. Note resemblance to chordoma (Fig. 5-25). (×1200.)

### Pituitary Carcinomas

Malignant neoplasms composed of pituitary cells are extremely uncommon. Invasion of adjacent tissues, such as with grade 4 adenomas, is usually not regarded as evidence of malignancy.[118,172,330] Some investigators emphasize that a diagnosis of pituitary carcinoma should be made only when *distant metastases* are present.[172] In some reported series, metastatic pituitary carcinoma to lymph nodes, liver, heart, lung, and bones has been reported.[55] Pituitary carcinomas can be acidophilic, basophilic, or chromophobic. Mitotic figures are usually more common than in adenomas.[127,343] However, the tumors are usually well differentiated. Immunohistochemical stains may reveal prolactin, growth hormone, ACTH, or other hormones. In some cases, the carcinomas may be clinically silent.

### Carcinomas Arising from Other Sellar Abnormalities

Carcinoma arises in craniopharyngioma[259] and epidermoid cyst.[200,325] Such malignant transformation is rare. Features of these malignant regions include nuclear pleomorphism, hyperchromaticity, and indentation of adjacent nuclei. There is significant mitotic activity. Invasion of brain and small veins can occur. Features of individual cells include dyskaryosis and dyskeratosis.

These carcinomas show focal *squamous differentiation.* This helps distinguish them from endocrine adenomas. Their mitoses are more numerous and their nuclear features more pleomorphic than well-differentiated adenomas. While necrosis may be present, this does not necessarily distinguish them from adenomas. Important features that distinguish these carcinomas from adenomas and metastatic carcinomas are vestiges of the benign neoplasm in which they occurred.[259,325] Their immunohistochemical profile is not well described. However, they are likely to differ from primary pituitary carcinoma and adenoma in regard to peptide hormones.

### Local Carcinomas That Invade the Sellar Region

The nasopharyngeal carcinomas are a heterogeneous group of neoplasms. Some are squamous cell carcinomas, others are nonkeratinizing carcinomas, and still others are undifferentiated carcinomas.[137,242,340] Sinusoidal adenocarcinomas resemble intestinal carcinoma.[92] Undifferentiated carcinomas include lymphoepithelioma, oat cell carcinoma, and sinonasal undifferentiated carcinoma (SNUC).[242] Some of these are not relevant to primary pituitary neoplasia because of their distinctly different morphology, and others do not invade near the sella. Two carcinomas potentially confused with primary pituitary neoplasia are mentioned next.

Nasopharyngeal *oat cell carcinomas* resemble their counterparts in the lung. Their cells are small, and their degree of epithelial differentiation is variable. Their dark, pleomorphic nuclei produce a high ratio of nuclear to cytoplasmic area. Spontaneous tumor necrosis is common.

*Sinonasal undifferentiated carcinomas* contain larger cells than oat cell carcinomas. These epithelial cells produce a number of histologic patterns, including clusters divided by stroma and sheets. Their round and oval nuclei are often less pleomorphic than might be expected in such a malignant tumor. They often kill in less than a year.[95] Mitoses are regionally variable and can be numerous. Extensive vascular invasion and central necrosis of cell nests are frequent.[242] These are of significant value in recognizing SNUC.

Anatomic relationships, anaplasia, and antigens

(AAA) are primary considerations in distinguishing nasopharyngeal carcinomas from primary pituitary neoplasms. Most pituitary adenomas are solitary neoplasms confined within the sella. *Anatomically,* nasopharyngeal carcinomas are not a serious concern in these cases. In contrast, 2% of pituitary adenomas grow into the nasal cavity by local invasion through the sella.[157] A tumor discovered in both locations presents a diagnostic challenge. While one fifth of malignant nasopharyngeal tumors have already invaded the skull base at diagnosis, the sella is not a preferential site of invasion.[336,339] Sphenoid sinus, clivus, or petrous regions are more commonly involved. Thus, radiographic confirmation is useful.

An additional consideration in a nasopharyngeal mass without sellar invasion is an ectopic pituitary adenoma. These are rare compared to neoplastic sellar invasion.[219,313]

Nasopharyngeal carcinoma cells are generally more *anaplastic* than cells of pituitary adenomas, even invasive adenomas. However, the spectrum of these features in each group varies. This causes partial overlap between relatively well-differentiated nasopharyngeal carcinomas and pleomorphic or mitotically active pituitary adenomas.

If anatomic relationships and anaplasia fail to confirm the nature of a neoplasm, the third "A" in the AAA triad should be considered: *Antigens.* Staining for pituitary peptide antigens is recommended. Shared epithelial and neuroendocrine features of nasopharyngeal and primary pituitary tumors limit the utility of cytokeratin and chromogranin staining in distinguishing them. Pituitary peptide antigens, in contrast, are sufficiently unique and stable to routine processing that even their absence (negative staining) may be diagnostically important as evidence of a nasopharyngeal carcinoma. Many other antigenic tumor markers are not as reliable as the pituitary peptides.

### Metastatic Carcinomas

Carcinomas metastatic to the pituitary gland have been reported in many series.* Carcinoma of the *breast* in women and carcinoma in the *lung* in men are the most common primary sites. In addition, tumors from the prostate, colon, stomach, pancreas, kidney, thyroid, and gonads are known to metastasize to the pituitary. Ultrastructure and immunocytochemistry (Chapters 3, 4) may help determine a site of origin when clinical approaches fail. Most metastatic carcinomas have anaplastic nuclear features that distinguish them from adenomas (Fig. 5-24). Rarely, these metastases may present a confusing clinical picture by stimulating pituitary hormone production.[102]

Metastasis to the posterior lobe of the pituitary is more common than to the anterior lobe. This is most likely related to the direct systemic arterial blood supply to this region. Some metastatic foci in the anterior lobe probably result from direct extension from the posterior lobe or via the portal vessels. Most pituitary glands with metastatic disease may be grossly normal in appearance. Only about one quarter of affected glands with metastatic diseases are enlarged. The mean survival of patients with pituitary metastases is less than 1 year after diagnosis. This is most likely a reflection of the extent of metastatic disease to other organs at the time of diagnosis.

* Refs. 39, 115, 129, 171, 261, 299, 371.

## CAVERNOUS ANGIOMA

Cavernous angiomas rarely involve the sellar region.[361] They can produce pituitary dysfunction. Their magnetic resonance images are valuable aids to their diagnosis. Some of these vascular malformations include islets of adipose tissue.[188]

## CHORDOMA

Chordomas are common parasellar neoplasms. Two of 41 neoplasms in the region of the sella were chordomas in one series.[190] Chordomas of this region represent at least one third of all chordomas.[48,386] They arise near the *clivus,* where the most cranial portion of the fetal notochord and notochordal remnants may exist.[21] Most other chordomas arise in the spinal canal.[386]

In theory, chordomas should not be difficult to distinguish from pituitary adenomas for two major reasons. First, their clival origin is anatomically distinct from the confines of the sella, where most adenomas originate. Second, classic chordomas contain cords of cells in linear array with huge cytoplasmic vacuoles that are not features of adenomas. The vacuolated cells are called physaliphorous (or bubbly). They resemble bubbles or a line of beads on a string. The vacuoles are highly variable in size. They range up to a whole cell diameter (Fig. 5-25). The largest are larger than macrophage vacuoles. Unlike watery perinuclear oligodendroglial vacuoles that surround nuclei, they contain "*mucin*" and lie *beside* cellular nuclei. These features must be sought and considered. They often help to establish the diagnosis. However, individual cases escape the predicted pattern and confound identification by simple anatomic and histologic criteria.

Chordomas commonly *destroy bone* of the clivus and sella.[21,290] After a chordoma has grown and invaded the sella, its intrasellar versus clival origin is obscured. A few adenomas exit the sella by invasion, so that a tumor spanning both locations can be confusing. Erosion of the tip of the clivus and sclerotic bone reactions are common in chordomas. These can be detected by radiography.[93,159,386] Their presence is a significant feature to consider in the pathologic diagnosis. These

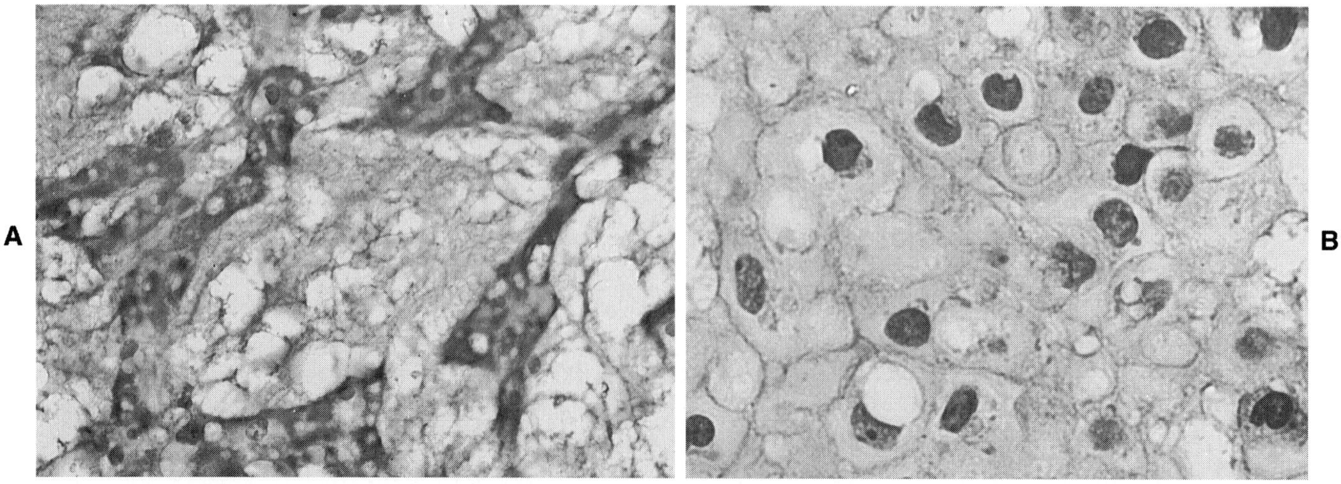

**Fig. 5-25.** Large cytoplasmic vacuoles are accentuated by the highly S-100-positive cytoplasm of these chordoma cells. **A,** Chordoma matrix is in center of field. **B,** shows another chordoma that has a less typical appearance more likely to be confused with other neoplasms. (**A,** ×400; **B,** H&E; ×1000.)

changes, especially when detected early, decrease the likelihood of adenoma.

Chordomas may remain confined within the sella.[28,222] Their anatomic location increases the likelihood of confusion with adenoma. Fortunately, totally intrasellar chordomas are rare.

Portions of a chordoma may not show the typical physaliphorous appearance. Portions may be very epithelioid with the cells containing few vacuoles and thus resembling a pituitary adenoma, meningioma, or low-grade carcinoma.[21,386] The pathologist requires the entire tissue specimen to optimize evaluation.

Although less specific than physaliphorous cells, other features of chordoma tissue include their multilobular, gelatinous, and myxoid macroscopic appearance. Chordomas are often firmer than untreated pituitary adenomas. Some chordoma cells lie within a substantial *myxoid extracellular matrix* that stains with Alcian blue. While its staining characteristics are like mucin, this material is probably a highly glycosylated, acidic ground substance.

Immunocytochemistry and electron microscopy improve the interpretation of questionable cases.[90,170] A panel of antibodies is recommended. Chordomas typically stain strongly for two intermediate filaments (cytokeratin and vimentin) and S-100 protein (Fig. 5-25).* Lack of these proteins suggests a neoplasm other than chordoma. Pituitary adenomas have less vimentin reactivity and are usually S-100 negative (discussed in the folliculo-stellate cells part in the section on Gliomas). Chromogranin or pituitary peptide hormone positive adenomas are distinctively different from chordomas. Immunohistochemical panels for distinguishing chordomas from tumors other than adenomas have been recently published.[226,227]

The distinction between chordoma and low-grade chondrosarcoma is difficult to make. Immunohistochemistry is recommended for making this distinction, and for excluding carcinoma and paraganglioma (Chapter 4).

The large vacuoles of *physaliphorous cells* ultrastructurally contain sparse, short microvilli protruding into their lumina.[158] These large vacuoles contain matrix material like the extracellular matrix of chordomas. Smaller cytoplasmic vacuoles appear to be dilated rough endoplasmic reticulum (RER) in continuity with mitochondria.[158,283] Still other vacuoles contain glycogen.[81,125] When present, these vacuoles distinguish chordomas from adenomas and most other parasellar tumors. Pituitary *adenomas* and *plasmacytomas* have abundant RER but lack the large cytoplasmic vacuoles lined with microvilli of chordoma. Vacuoles of *macrophages* are phagocytic vacuoles that differ from RER.

*Mitochondrial-RER complexes* typify chordomas.[81] These are alternating layers of RER and elongated mitochondria. The mitochondria have bulbous ends protruding from these complexes in a dumbbell configuration.[80] The entire complex suggests coalescence to juxtapose energy close to the protein production facilities of these cells.

Chordomas of the clivus invade surrounding structures, compromise critical neuroanatomic structures, and eventually kill. They occasionally compress the internal carotid artery[195] and rarely cause hemorrhage.[163] Despite this invasion, many chordomas have a low proliferative rate and very slow growth. The incidence of metastases varies between studies from rare

* Refs. 37, 60, 235, 240, 253, 256, 273, 318, 324, 334, 391.

to up to 43%.[227,386] Average survival of patients with intracranial chordoma is 4 years. Studies of proliferative capacity may eventually be of prognostic value in chordomas.[227]

## CRANIOPHARYNGIOMA

One fifth of these tumors occur in the sella, and over nine tenths occur above the sella turcica. The overlap in these portions reflects tumors with both intrasellar and suprasellar components. The epithelial appearance of craniopharyngioma is so distinctive that it virtually assures diagnosis on H&E stained sections. Multiple layers of epithelium in a mass or nodule are the histologic hallmark. Craniopharyngiomas may be solid or cystic, but even cystic craniopharyngiomas have a nodule of tissue that distinguishes them from a simple epidermoid cyst. This nodule needs to be provided as part of the surgical specimen to assure a correct diagnosis.

*Adamantinomatous* craniopharyngiomas show loose arrangements of squamous epithelium (stellate reticulum) with a prominent and more compact basal epithelial layer. Keratinizing cells and their nuclei become huge and orange-pink as they die to produce ghost cells. Cholesterol accumulates in "motor oil" dark brown fluid, where its crystals are visible by polarized light. In paraffin sections there are clefts of dissolved cholesterol and calcifications.

*Papillary* craniopharyngiomas contain well-differentiated squamous epithelium in sheets that separate to resemble papillae. They generally lack cholesterol and dark brown fluid.[47]

Sampling only the intensely gliotic margin around a craniopharyngioma can suggest a pilocytic astrocytoma. Both tumors are associated with juvenile predominance, location near the third ventricle, and presence of Rosenthal fibers. Rare presentation of craniopharyngioma in the optic chiasm can be particularly confusing. Communication with the neurosurgeon or the neuroradiologist usually can clarify the differential diagnosis. Microscopically, the reactive gliosis surrounding a craniopharyngioma differs from pilocytic astrocytoma by its lower cellularity and lack of microcysts. Cholesterol deposits suggest craniopharyngioma.

Immunocytochemistry usually is not necessary to diagnose properly sampled craniopharyngiomas. They are keratin- and cytokeratin-positive, and they may express human chorionic gonadotropin and P-glycoprotein.[128,185,367]

The prognostic import of squamous papillary versus adamantinomatous variants is controversial.[1,64,241] Numerous attempts have been made to identify prognostically meaningful subgroups.* Different morphologic criteria for these subgroups have hindered a consensus. Nonetheless, it is possible that papillary features, squamous epithelial subtype, lack of calcification, and tumors under 3 cm predict a better prognosis when compared with that of tumors lacking the above features.

* Refs. 1, 151, 152, 292, 366.

## GANGLIOCYTOMA

These tumors are composed of mature neurons. They are uncommon in the sella and generally are found in children and young adults. Some are associated with endocrine symptoms and pituitary adenomas.*

Irregularly oriented and unevenly spaced neurons characterize gangliocytomas. Binucleated neurons aid in their identification. They may be mixed with, juxtaposed to, or unassociated with adenoma tissue. In some cases, the neurons contain releasing factor for the hormone secreted by the adenoma.

Gangliocytomas are benign. Surgical removal effects a cure.

## GERM CELL TUMORS

Almost all primary germ cell tumors of the brain are found along the midline in the pineal and suprasellar regions.[147] About one tenth of these tumors involve both regions, and one fourth originate in the suprasellar cistern.[141,147] Metastases of germ cell tumors to other areas of the brain from the suprasellar-pineal axis and from systemic primaries are uncommon.[100,279,388]

### Germinoma

This tumor is the most common germ cell neoplasm of brain, and it is the predominant germ cell tumor found near the sella. Most germinomas become symptomatic in adolescence and puberty.[147] Most originate above the sella in the hypothalamus, but one fifth involve the sella.[103,280]

Although germinoma is part of the differential diagnosis of adenomas, careful attention to clinical and structural differences can avoid confusion. Two thirds of patients with germinoma are diagnosed in *adolescence*.[141,147] This suggests that pubertal changes activate growth of these tumors. In contrast, most adenomas are diagnosed in older patients. Nearly all patients with suprasellar germinoma have *diabetes insipidus*.[43,197] Signs of hypopituitarism (hypogonadism, hypocortisolism, hypothyroidism, growth delay, and pubertal delay) are almost as common. These endocrinologic deficiencies contrast with selective hormonal overactivity produced by pituitary adenomas that are endocrinologically active.

In contrast to adenomas, most germinomas displace

* Refs. 17, 19, 29, 46, 91, 153, 302.

the third ventricle. Germinomas tend not to displace the optic chiasm or carotid artery.[154,305] Radiographically, suprasellar germinomas neither calcify nor erode the dorsum sellae.[154,197] On neuroimaging studies germinomas appear as a soft tissue density or hyperdense mass. The mass enhances with contrast dye on CT.[197] Germinomas tend to show isodensity on T1-weighted magnetic resonance images and hyperintensity on T2-weighted images.[154,197] However, in the normally hyperintense posterior pituitary, less intensity of the T1-weighted image is an important differential feature.[96]

Intrasellar germinomas are less common and have radiologic images different from those of suprasellar germinomas. They are capable of expanding the sella.[25] Intrasellar germinomas may have the clinical and radiographic features of a prolactinoma.[344]

While clinical manifestations help to distinguish germinomas from adenomas, confirmation by structural features is needed. Fortunately, histologic features are distinctive when an adequate sample of tissue is obtained. Like testicular seminoma and ovarian dysgerminoma, germinomas feature *two distinct cell populations.* Large, neoplastic, epithelioid cells contain glycogen. They have large, round vesicular nuclei with irregular and pleomorphic nucleoli (Fig. 5-26). The second cell population is composed of polyclonal small lymphocytes, occasionally mixed with granulomatous inflammation.[184,281] This pattern is diagnostic if the specimen is adequate. Problems arise from small biopsies and from mechanical problems in removal of the firm and fibrous tumors that distort their architecture. The lymphocytes crush and smear easily, leaving streaks of hematoxylin as the only clues of their prior existence.

All biopsies of suspected germinomas should be monitored with frozen sections and cytologic preparations.[265] For cytology, we prefer touch preparations because lymphocytes streak less, but squash preparations reveal more cells from collagenous germinomas. Careful sampling and handling are needed to preserve the described features. Small samples may show only the lymphocytes. This may be mistaken for inflammation, lymphoma, or adenoma.

If there is a complication of incomplete sampling or atypical histology, immunostaining may provide welcome evidence of the diagnosis. *Placental alkaline phosphatase* (PLAP) is expressed in up to 93% of germinomas.* It predominates on the surface of the large cells (Fig. 5-26). Unfortunately, a few metastatic carcinomas also express PLAP,[394] compromising its specificity for germinoma. Angiotensin-I-converting enzyme (ACE) is a new marker of germinomas discussed further elsewhere.[227] Distinctive ultrastructural features of germinomas are intranuclear membranous profiles and fenestrated nucleoli.[120,165]

The small cells in germinomas are a mixture of T lymphocytes, B lymphocytes, and natural killer (NK) cells.† The T and B lymphocytes can be immunostained (Chapter 4).

The histiologic pattern and the extent of disease influence survival of germinoma patients.[147] Tumor in the third ventricle or spinal cord significantly de-

* Refs. 141, 164, 275, 400.

† Refs. 281, 321, 329, 383.

A

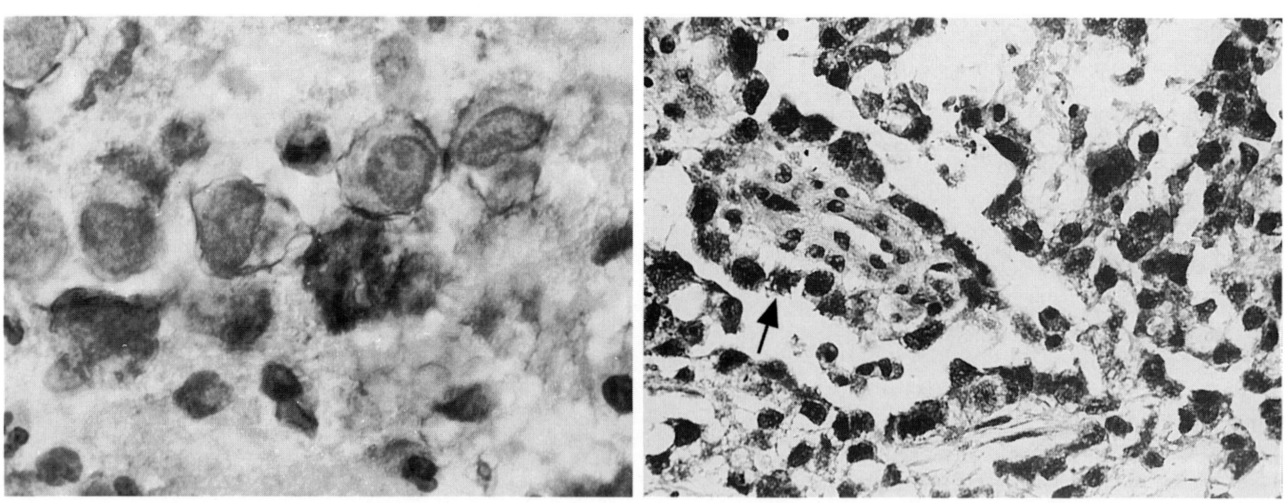

B

**Fig. 5-26. A,** Huge cells with large nuclei and nucleoli have placental alkaline phosphatase concentrated in their plasma membranes. Small cells at periphery of field are lymphocytes. **B,** an endodermal sinus tumor in the sellar region of an adolescent boy. It resembled an adenoma except for the following: Nucleoli are large and pleomorphic. It has a Schiller-Duval body (*arrow*). Other regions of the neoplasm were typical germinoma. (**A,** ×1000; **B,** ×400.)

creases survival. Presence of substantial choriocarcinoma, embryonal carcinoma, or endodermal sinus tumors mixed with germinoma predicts poorer survival than does pure germinoma.[227] These tumors without coexisting germinoma in other locations are rare in the sella (Fig. 5-26). Rare germinomas are associated with dysgenetic syndromes.[167,350,365]

### Teratoma

Teratomas are a mixture of a variety of tissues derived from all three germinal layers. *Mature teratomas* have well-differentiated representatives of all three layers, including neuroectodermal.[227] Regions of epithelium are mixed with glandular or tubular structures. Mesenchymal proliferation and glial and neuronal tissue are common. Cartilage is occasionally present. The diagnosis can be made on an adequate sample of tissue stained with H&E. However, sampling problems occur with needle biopsies as described above.

*Immature teratomas* are less differentiated than teratomas. Their embryonic elements originate from all or any of the three germinal layers. Prognostically important elements include embryonal neuroepithelial structures that resemble medulloepithelioma, neuroblastoma, retinoblastoma, or ependymoblastoma.[317] The 1-year survival of patients with intracranial immature teratomas is 50%.[147] Teratomas can be mixed with elements of another, less benign, germ cell tumor.[31,269] The most malignant germ cell element found in any significant amount determines the prognosis of teratomas.[227]

### Other Germ Cell Tumors

*Choriocarcinoma* is composed of huge syncytial and smaller trophoblastic cells usually recognizable on H&E stains. *Embryonal carcinoma* is composed of primitive epithelial cells with many mitoses and necrosis. The cells of *endodermal sinus tumors* contain Schiller-Duvall bodies (Fig. 5-26).[227] These are papillae and channels lined by cuboidal epithelium. Compared with germinoma, lymphocytes are relatively sparse in pure choriocarcinoma, embryonal carcinoma, or endodermal sinus tumors.

These other germ cell tumors are found mixed with germinoma. Patient survival does not equal that of germinoma, making their correct classification especially important. The identification of each element and evaluation of whether a significant amount is present should be done with the aid of immunocytochemistry (Chapter 4).

## GLIOMAS

The term *glioma* describes the group of glial neoplasms, including astrocytoma, ependymoma, oligodendroglioma, and their anaplastic counterparts; mixed gliomas like oligoastrocytoma; and glioblastoma (Chapter 2).[402]

Astrocytomas of various grades of malignancy represent the most common intracranial gliomas. The pilocytic variant of astrocytoma is found in the sella,[338] but it is more common in the hypothalamus and infundibulum. It is also known as infundibuloma, and bears a close resemblance to the pituicytoma.[203] All of these gliomas are easily distinguished from pituitary adenoma by their fibrillar cellular processes. Although GFAP-positive, these processes are usually recognizable on H&E stains. Since pilocytic astrocytomas are so easily distinguished from adenomas, only their distinctive features will be mentioned briefly here. "Pilocytic" means "*hair-cell,*" one of the major distinguishing features of this astrocytoma. Parallel bundles of elongated, fibrillar, cytoplasmic processes resemble mats of hair. These hairlike fibrillar cellular processes contain large amounts of glial filaments that stain well with either PTAH or immunoperoxidase for GFAP.[289] *Rosenthal fibers* are highly eosinophilic hyaline structures. They are round, oval, or beaded with slightly irregular margins.[59] Their beaded appearance results from their formation within glial processes. They must be distinguished from erythrocytes by their pink rather than orange color and their greater variation in size and shape. *Eosinophilic droplets* of protein are sometimes found in association with Rosenthal fiber formation. These protein droplets are usually intracellular but occasionally extracellular and up to 40 $\mu$ in diameter.[226]

The following categories of gliomas have an association with pituitary adenomas. Oligodendrogliomas and ependymomas bear a close morphologic resemblance to adenomas. Gliomas of high-grade malignancy exemplified by glioblastomas have occurred after radiotherapy for pituitary adenomas.

### Gliomas That Resemble Pituitary Adenoma

Nonastrocytic gliomas are less fibrillar than astrocytomas, and their cells are epithelioid (Fig. 5-27). Pituitary adenomas are also epithelioid. Their features resemble nonastrocytic gliomas, particularly oligodendrogliomas and ependymomas.

*Perinuclear halos* are an important feature of biopsy specimens of oligodendroglioma (Figs. 5-27, 5-28). As strikingly illustrated by Burger, Scheithauer, and Vogel, the perinuclear halo is an effect of delayed fixation.[48] Thus, the absence of perinuclear halos does not rule out oligodendroglioma and may merely reflect prompt fixation. Their absence on frozen sections is common. Well-differentiated oligodendrogliomas usually have remarkably round and regular nuclei centrally placed within the cell, resembling fried eggs. Their vessels are usually numerous fine capillaries that sometimes segregate the parenchyma into small lob-

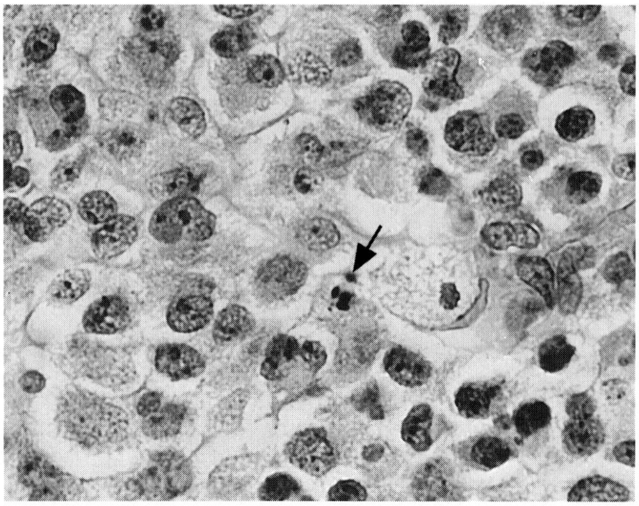

**Fig. 5-27.** Epithelioid cells, only a portion of which have perinuclear halos, resemble adenoma cells. This anaplastic oligodendroglioma has an apoptotic nucleus in fragments (*arrow*) and pleomorphic nuclei. Elsewhere it had mitoses. (×1000.)

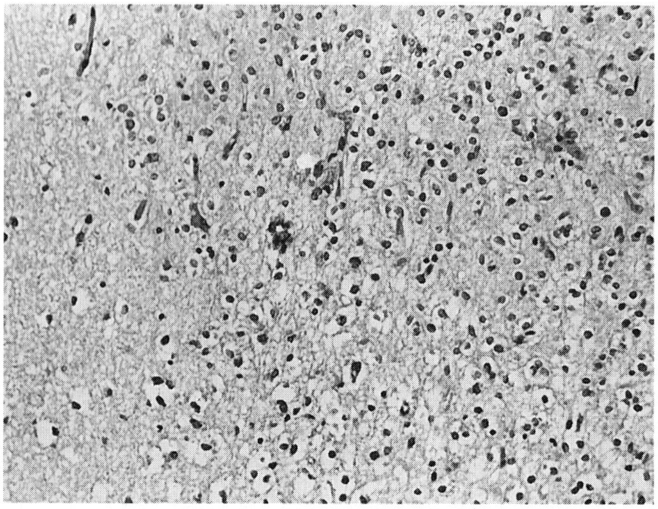

**Fig. 5-28.** This tumor resembled an adenoma. However, extrasellar invasion of brain shows a diffuse, infiltrative margin typical of a glioma. The epithelioid cells have perinuclear halos of oligodendroglioma cells. (×200.) (Reprinted from McKeever PE, and Blaivas M: The brain, spinal cord, and meninges. In Sternberg SS, and others, editors: Diagnostic surgical pathology, ed 2, New York, 1994, Raven Press.)

ules.[42] These features may be duplicated by adenomas.

Precise *anatomic location* is critical, because oligodendrogliomas do not originate from the adenohypophysis and rarely invade the sella. Because oligodendrogliomas originate in brain parenchyma dorsal to the sella, and pituitary adenomas originate within the sella, only tumors that span both locations generate this differential. Fortunately, such tumors represent minor fractions of adenomas and oligodendrogliomas.

Rare tumors grow in both sella and brain, and thereby abut CNS parenchyma. If the margin of the neoplasm is sampled in addition to the central region, even macroscopically discrete oligodendrogliomas will show a more *diffuse margin* with CNS parenchyma than adenomas. Individual neoplastic oligodendroglia infiltrate the parenchyma and are not excluded or restricted to vessels like nonglial neoplasms (Fig. 5-28). Secondary structures of Scherer where neoplastic glia surround brain tissue structures are frequent, especially perineuronal gliomatosis.

In distinguishing an oligodendroglioma from a pituitary adenoma, immunocytochemical markers of oligodendrogliomas may help (Chapter 4).[288] One note of caution should be considered. Cells with strong GFAP and/or S-100 reactivity are found in less than 5% of adenomas and probably represent folliculo-stellate cells.[126,397] Most important, immunoreactivity for chromogranin or a pituitary hormone clearly indicates adenoma.[210,225]

Ependymomas are like oligodendrogliomas with respect to their extrasellar origins. Thus, only tumors in both sellar and suprasellar locations require serious consideration of both adenoma and ependymoma in a diagnostic differential.

The cellular conformations of ependymomas vary between *fibrillar* and *epithelial*. Epithelial cells have distinct cellular borders that in aggregate resemble cobblestones in a street. These produce special problems of differentiation from pituitary adenomas. This differentiation is facilitated by recalling that even epithelioid ependymomas frequently stain with *anti-GFAP* (Chapter 4), have distinctive ultrastructure (Chapter 3), and will contain at least a few cells with fibrillar processes. A good place to look for these few fibrillar processes is around vessels.[226]

Look for rosettes to confirm suspicion of an ependymoma. The *true ependymal rosette* or luminal rosette is the most characteristic and may be found in individual cases of any of the ependymoma variants, but some specimens do not show these rosettes.[47] The ependymal rosette consists of ependymal cells evenly spaced around a lumen, having a superficial resemblance to cells lining a duct (Fig. 5-29). The resemblance ends at the outer portion of the rosettes, which blends into parenchyma without a basement membrane. Cilia protruding into the lumen from the ependymal lining are sometimes evident. Some cases show expanded ependymal rosettes; others show long ependymal linings that do not close into rosettes.

The *perivascular rosette* or pseudorosette is the most frequently encountered rosette of ependymoma. It consists of slender cellular fibrils perpendicularly oriented toward a blood vessel, like spokes on a wheel. Perivascular rosettes of ependymomas should have a fibrillar zone (spokes of the wheels) that is at least two nuclear or three erythrocyte diameters (measured from vascular adventitia) out to the beginning of the zone of parenchymal nuclei. Perivascular rosettes are common in many ependymomas, producing distinctive patterns of halos around vessels at low magnification. The processes should taper to become very thin as they radiate from the cells to the vascular adventitia. With the majority of tumor vessels involved, a characteristic pattern resembling atolls with light sandy beaches is evident on H&E stains at low magnification.[226]

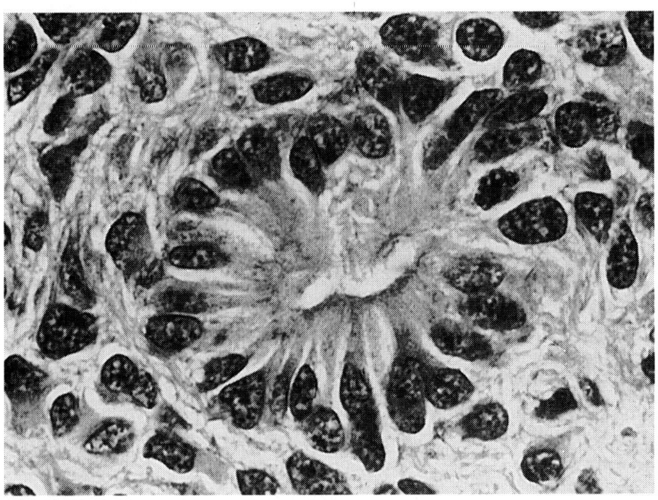

**Fig. 5-29.** True rosettes with lumina formed by neoplastic cells help to distinguish ependymoma. Neoplastic glia are epithelioid and fibrillar. (×1200.) (Reprinted from McKeever PE, and Blaivas M: The brain, spinal cord, and meninges. In Sternberg SS, and others, editors: Diagnostic surgical pathology, ed 2, New York, 1994, Raven Press.)

Light microscopic features described above will distinguish the majority of ependymomas from the pituitary adenomas and other parasellar neoplasms. Electron microscopy is recommended for the few remaining cases (Fig. 5-30).

### Gliomas That Follow Sellar Radiotherapy

Glioblastomas and anaplastic astrocytomas are the most common gliomas in patients following sellar radiation.[227] Of a total of 14 published cases, six patients had glioblastomas and six had anaplastic astrocytomas, together accounting for 85% of all postradiation gliomas.* The hallmark of the 12 astrocytic high-grade gliomas was their fibrillarity. This and their malignancy clearly distinguished them from adenomas. Another patient had an anaplastic oligodendroglioma.[138] One half of these patients had previous radiation for pituitary adenomas, and the other half had been radiated for craniopharyngiomas. Their total radiation dose ranged between 45 and 66 Gy.

The designation "anaplastic" emphasizes the grade of malignancy: grade III (Chapter 2). Features of anaplasia that are common to gliomas of high grades (III and IV) of malignancy are increased *cellular density*, increased *cellular* and *nuclear pleomorphism*, and increased *nuclear hyperchromaticity*.

* Refs. 113, 138, 139, 162, 166, 204, 215, 220, 293, 354, 364, 381, 401.

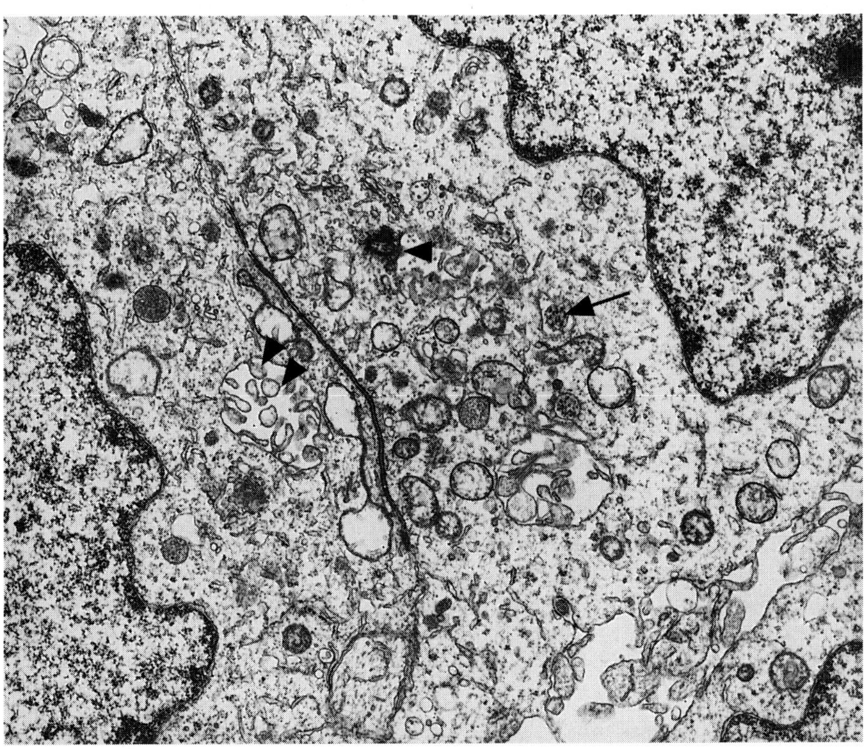

**Fig. 5-30.** Cytoplasmic cilia (*arrow*), basal body (*arrowhead*), and microvilli (*double arrowhead*) and an extensively elongated intercellular junction characterize these ependymoma cells. (×10,000.) (Reprinted from McKeever PE, and Blaivas M: The brain, spinal cord, and meninges. In Sternberg SS, and others, editors: Diagnostic surgical pathology, ed 2, New York, 1994, Raven Press.)

*Vascular proliferation* (increased density of cells in vascular walls) is an important characteristic. Recent classifications consider significant vascular proliferation to be a criterion of glioblastoma. Vascular proliferation is relatively easy to recognize in either of its two forms. One form is simply an increase in the nuclei within the vascular wall, and the other form is multiple lumina within the vascular structure that resembles a renal glomerulus. The lack of vascular proliferation and lack of foci of coagulation necrosis distinguish anaplastic astrocytomas from glioblastoma,[47] but individual cells with pyknotic nuclei may be interspersed within anaplastic astrocytomas.

The diagnosis of glioblastoma multiforme is established if there is coagulation *necrosis* in a glioma composed of malignant astrocytes.[260] While spontaneous coagulation necrosis and vascular proliferation are key to diagnosis of glioblastoma, other malignant features of glioblastomas are similar to those of anaplastic astrocytoma, but they are present to a greater degree. These include hypercellularity, bizarre nuclei, multinucleated cells, and mitoses.[226]

The *latency period* between parasellar radiation and diagnosis of malignant glioma varies between *4 and 24 years,** with an average latency of 10 years. Since the total survival of treated anaplastic astrocytoma was less than 3 years and glioblastoma less than 1 year during the time of these studies, these gliomas probably were not present at the time of radiation. These data combined with the conspicuous difference between adenomas and malignant gliomas indicate that these gliomas occurring in the previous field of radiation meet Cahan's criteria for correlation with radiation (discussed in the section on Meningioma).

High-grade gliomas that occur within fields of parasellar radiation delivered a decade before are not always confined to the sella. Some involve the temporal or ventral frontal lobes, the diencephalon, or the optic chiasm.* As more focused radiotherapy beams are now employed and will be in the future, study of the anatomic distributions of subsequent gliomas should prove interesting.

The histologic features of high-grade gliomas occurring after sellar radiation duplicate those in patients who never received therapeutic radiation.[226] In contrast to the effects of radiation upon preexisting neoplasm,[221] no "radiation-specific" histologic feature has been found.

Since these gliomas occur in the sellar region years after radiotherapy, clinical circumstances and tumor histology establish the differential diagnosis. Pituitary adenomas are epithelioid tumors that lack the fibrillary cytoplasmic processes of astrocytic gliomas and are negative for glial fibrillary acidic protein (GFAP). Parasellar sarcomas and meningiomas also occur subsequent to radiation. These are more difficult to distinguish from high-grade gliomas because spindled cells of glioblastomas resemble those of sarcoma and fibroblastic meningioma. GFAP is usually sufficient to identify the glioma (Chapter 4).[229]

* Refs. 113, 138, 139, 162, 166, 204, 215, 220, 293, 354, 364, 381, 401.

## GRANULAR CELL TUMOR (CHORISTOMA, GRANULAR MYOBLASTOMA)

Granular cell tumors are very common incidental tumors that predominate in the *posterior pituitary* and stalk.[214] Most are smaller than 0.5 cm and asymptomatic. While they grow slowly, some become symptomatic by middle age.[384] Their location and structural features are sufficiently similar to adenomas to cause problems in recognition. While their radiographic features overlap, location in the posterior lobe and high vascularity are particularly associated with granular cell tumors.[26]

Although structural features vary among individual cases, *granular cytoplasm* in a circumscribed nodule of medium to large cells suggests granular cell tumor.[214,227] The cytoplasmic granules are a mixture of vacuoles, dense bodies, multivesicular bodies, and membrane-bound organelles.[71,98] They are stained with periodic acid Schiff (PAS) stain after diastase treatment.[225,227] These granular cells are difficult to distinguish from adenoma cells without ultrastructural or immunohistochemical examination. Their larger cytoplasm with granules larger than those found in most adenomas can help to make this distinction (Fig. 5-31).

An appropriate panel of immunohistochemical stains would include pituitary hormones, chromogranin, and S-100 protein. Negative reactivity for all markers except S-100 protein suggests granular cell tumor. S-100-positive folliculo-stellate cells in a few adenomas caution against sole reliance upon S-100 reactivity to confirm suspicion of a granular cell tumor.[126,397] Doubtful cases may require electron microscopy, which distinguishes the endocytic structures of granular cell tumors from pituitary secretory granules.[71,98]

Granular cell tumors of the sella are benign. In this regard, their biologic behavior differs from systemic granular cell tumors, which can be malignant, albeit rarely.[272,375]

## LYMPHOMA (RETICULUM CELL SARCOMA—MICROGLIOMA)

Two general categories of lymphoma occur in the sellar region: metastatic and primary. Both can usually be distinguished from adenomas with critical attention to their precise anatomic site or sites of origin and to pertinent histologic features.

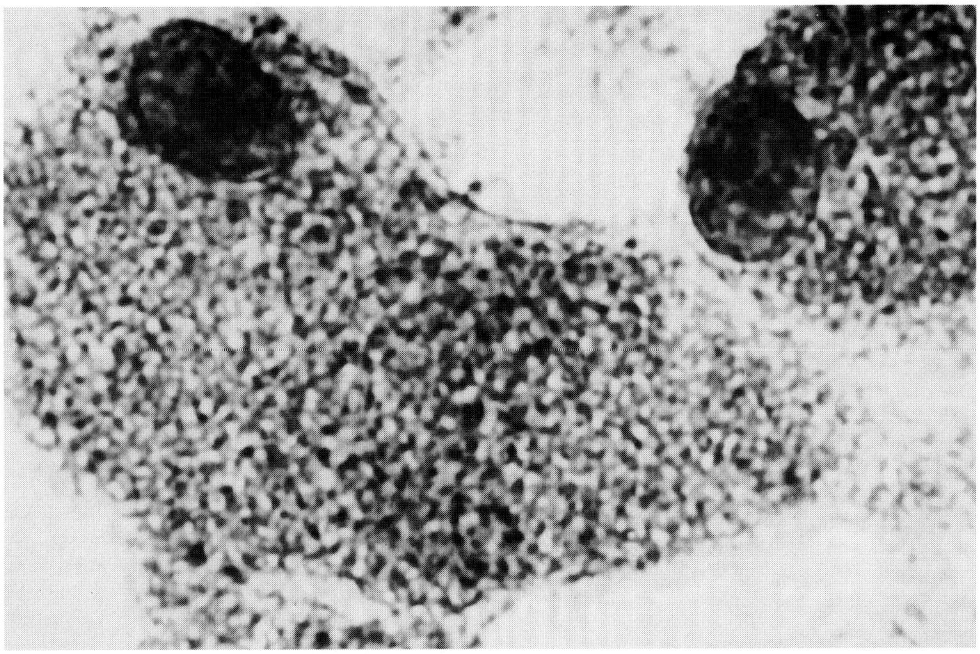

**Fig. 5-31.** Touch preparation reveals extreme cytoplasmic granularity of cells in this granular cell tumor. The nuclear to cytoplasmic ratio is lower than in most pituitary adenomas. (×3000.)

*Primary lymphomas* involve the hypothalamus in preference to the adenohypophysis. Although these structures are close to each other, they can be distinguished radiographically. This can show the distinct difference in location of lymphoma from that of adenoma. Presenting symptoms reflect hypothalamic dysfunctions. *Diabetes insipidus,* hypoglycemia, or weight loss may signal hypothalamic invasion by lymphomas.* On T1-weighted magnetic resonance images, suprasellar lymphomas are nearly isointense, but hyperintense on spin density and T2-weighted images.[154]

A significant percentage of primary CNS lymphomas are *multicentric.*[7] Multiple tumors plus hypothalamic signs suggest CNS lymphomas with hypothalamic involvement. Most *primary CNS lymphomas* are composed of B cells.[99,226,257] Their immunoglobulin marker expression historically identified them as lymphomas.[99] They range from small cell and plasmacytoid to large cell and immunoblastic. While the number is small, histiocytic lymphoma is represented among hypothalamic lymphomas.[252,257,310]

*Sinonasal lymphoma* can invade the parasellar region, with destruction of bone. Unlike adenomas, sinonasal lymphomas preferentially involve multiple regions of the nasal cavity. Sinonasal lymphomas usually are composed of B cells.[242]

*Systemic lymphomas* metastasize to the pituitary late in the course of the disease. As with leukemia, the incidence of metastasis may be high, particularly if micrometastases are considered.[44,262] Confusion with adenoma or other neoplasm can often be minimized by good clinical-pathologic correlation, since a primary tumor is likely to have been known or at least suspected prior to pituitary involvement.

Among 49 autopsied patients with acquired immunodeficiency syndrome (AIDS), no lymphomas invaded the pituitary despite the occurrence of 12 CNS lymphomas.[326]

Histologic features suggestive of lymphoma are a crowded accumulation of small to medium-sized *malignant cells* that are nonfibrillar and noncohesive. Neoplastic cells often grow around vessels and within vascular walls (Fig. 5-32). Although adenoma cells are variably cohesive, they avoid growing within vascular walls. Stains that differentiate vascular walls and parenchyma while simultaneously demonstrating benign versus neoplastic features of nuclei highlight vascular invasion. Masson trichrome is recommended for the sellar region.[225,226,277]

Cytologic features of some lymphomas, particularly the large cell immunoblastic lymphomas common in the CNS, are clearly more malignant than adenomas (Fig. 5-33). Problems arise with the more indolent lymphoproliferative disorders with low-grade features. These may resemble adenoma or inflammation. If these occur at biopsy, portions can be fixed in glutaraldehyde for electron microscopy (Chapter 3) and a portion frozen for analysis of DNA.[194,352] Unfortu-

* Refs. 20, 114, 124, 286, 291, 357.

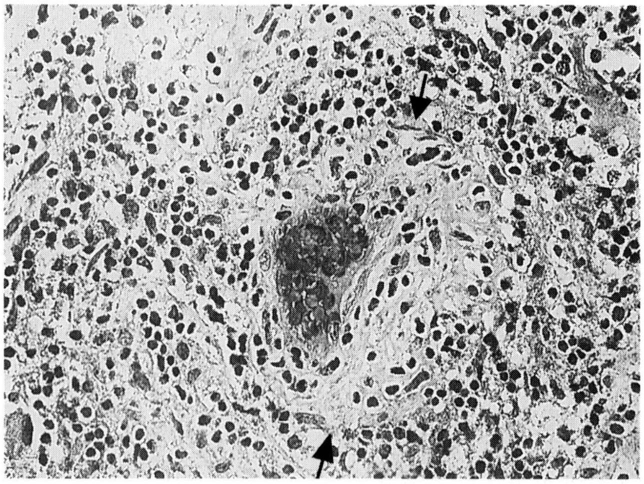

**Fig. 5-32.** Vascular wall invasion provides evidence that these small neoplastic cells are lymphoma cells. Masson's trichrome stain allows critical evaluation of pleomorphic nuclei and tinctorial delineation of vascular wall (*arrows*) from surrounding lymphoma. (×400.)

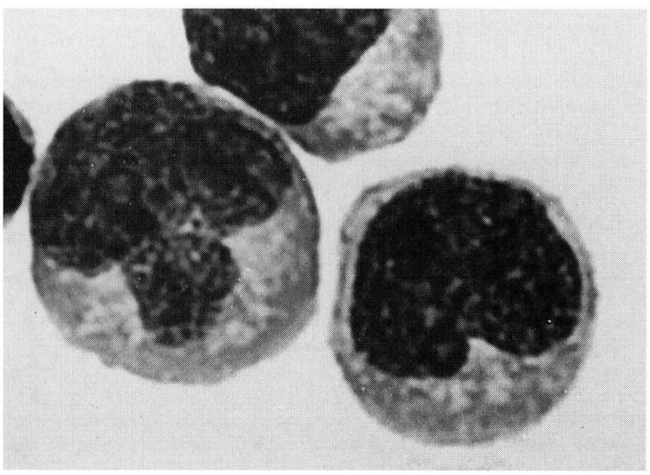

**Fig. 5-33.** High nuclear-to-cytoplasmic ratio and pleomorphic nuclei distinguish this lymphoma from a pituitary adenoma. The cells are obviously discohesive. This is a feature shared by many adenomas that have weak intercellular junctions. (Whole cells, Wright's stain; ×2000.)

nately, the critical functions of the hypothalamic-pituitary axis may hinder access to the desired amount of tissue. The advent of reliable immunohistochemical and in situ hybridization markers for paraffin sections facilitates diagnosis of lymphomas from such cases.[68,255] Future combinations of polymerase chain reactions with Southern blots may facilitate analyses of tiny fragments of difficult cases.[117]

For confirmation of lymphoma and immunophenotyping, the *immunostaining panel* should include leukocyte common antigen (LCA, CLA) (CD45 antigen), L26 (CD20 antigen) marker of B cells, and A6 antibody or

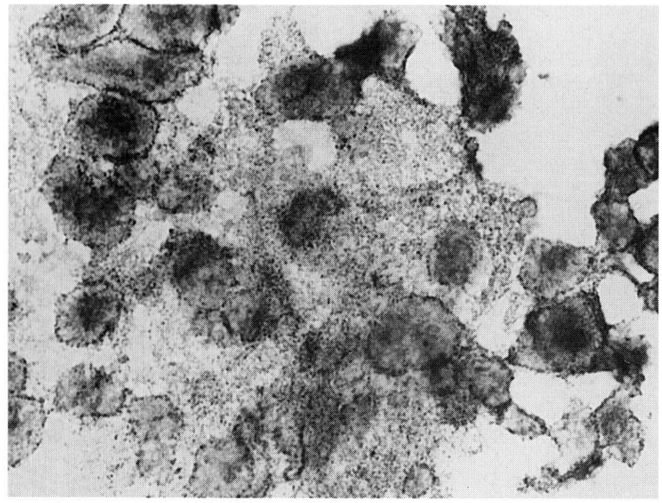

**Fig. 5-34.** Monoclonal surface antigen expression of kappa immunoglobulin light chains confirms this lymphoma on frozen sections. The lymphoma was lambda negative. Cytoplasmic background staining is common in such preparations. (×1200.)

UCHL-1 antibody (CD45RO antigen) marker of T cells.* These markers survive paraffin embedding. A frequent result shows all lymphoid cells positive with CLA, lymphoma cells additionally positive with L26, and smaller focal reactive lymphocytes—some L26-positive but most of which are UCHL-1-positive. Additional markers for refractory cases include MB2, MT2, and KP1 (CD68).[68,252] Monoclonal antibodies LN-1, LN-2, and LN-3 are also useful in B-cell lymphomas. Immunostaining for monoclonal expression of kappa or lambda immunoglobulin light chains is best reserved for frozen sections due to the small amount of surface antigen (Fig. 5-34). Lymphomas lack immunostaining markers related to pituitary peptide hormone secretion, chromogranin, and cytokeratin.[226,227]

## MELANOMA

Primary melanomas occur within the pituitary, where they might be confused with adenoma.[258,311,337] Fortunately, the rarity and the pigmentation of primary sellar melanomas minimize their chance of being mistaken for adenoma. Other melanomas metastasize to the pituitary, some with little pigment. Careful attention to malignant cytologic features and dermatologic history should be applied to such cases.

Melanomas expand the pituitary fossa and erode the dorsum sellae.† Melanomas invade meninges.[58,104,250,393] In the sella, their growth may resemble pituitary carcinoma or invasive adenoma.

* Refs. 10, 76, 186, 268, 347, 384, 389.

† Refs. 155, 250, 337, 348, 393.

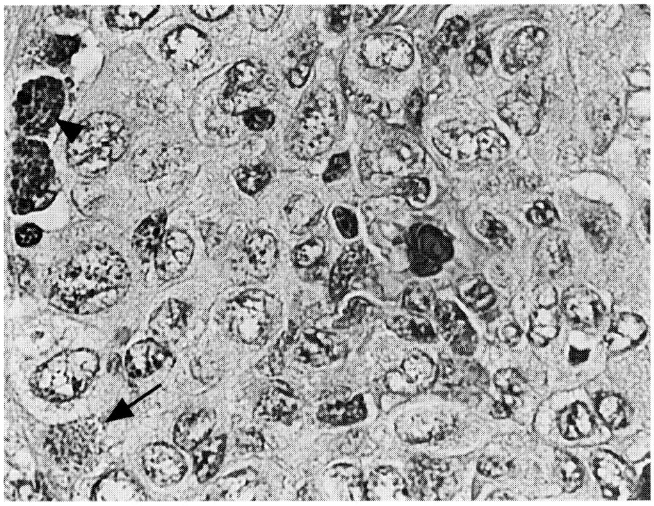

**Fig. 5-35.** Two sizes of granules are evident in these epithelioid cells. The smaller granules are typical dark brown and black melanin granules (*arrows*). However, the large granules at the edge of the image of this melanoma are also melanin (*arrowhead*). They represent cytoplasmic coalescence of granules, which, except for their chemical composition, could be mistaken for hemosiderin. Both granules were positive with Fontana stain and negative with Perls' stain. (×800.)

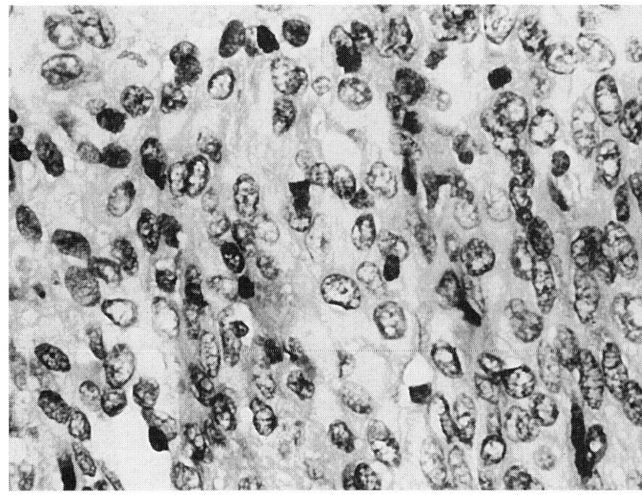

**Fig. 5-36.** Epithelioid cells of this tumor are not quite as well demarcated as pituitary adenoma cells. This and the slightly more elongated nuclei suggest the correct diagnosis of meningioma. (×600.)

The origin of intrasellar melanomas is not known. Possible sources include pigmented cells in the pars nervosa, Rathke's pouch remnants, and meninges.[258,337]

Most primary sellar and parasellar melanomas are *pigmented.* They are gray to black, with soft regions of necrosis.* Their malignant epithelioid to spindled cells contain melanin (Fig. 5-35). These tiny cytoplasmic granules are darker than hemosiderin. Melanoma nuclei and nucleoli are pleomorphic. Nucleoli are large in individual tumors. Regional and individual cell necrosis is common. However, pleomorphism and heterogeneity characterize melanomas, so that individual sellar melanomas have papillae and few mitoses.[337]

Fine granules of dark brown pigment reactive with the Fontana stain suggest melanoma.[225] Melanin granules will bleach when exposed to oxidants. This property helps to confirm them as melanin.

Melanomas express S-100 protein.[226,349,393] This marker is often negative in adenomas (discussed in the section on ectopic pituitary adenoma). The combination of strong S-100 and vimentin and lack of cytokeratin immunoreactivity distinguishes melanoma from adenoma, carcinoma, and chordoma.[102]

The *HBM-45* monoclonal antibody detects melanocytic cells, including cells of melanoma. The specificity of HMB-45 is more restricted than S-100. It may be useful when pigment is not evident on standard H&E or Fontana stains.[74] However, many HMB-45 antibodies are not strongly reactive with their epitopes so that minimal positivity may be overlooked. Avidin-biotin or immunoglobulin bridge enhancement is recommended.[225] While HMB-45 has theoretical value in confirming melanomas in the sella, the spectrum of reactivity of sellar tumors for HMB-45 remains to be comprehensively evaluated. Electron microscopy is the best method to establish the diagnosis of melanoma (Chapter 3).

* Refs. 155, 258, 311, 337, 348.

## MENINGIOMAS

### Resemblance to Adenoma

Meningiomas are common in the region of the sella.[227] Approximately 40% of these are meningothelial meningiomas.* This and the similarity of meningothelial meningioma to pituitary adenoma create considerable risk of confusion.

*Meningothelial meningiomas* contain sheets of cells with round and oval nuclei (Fig. 5-36). Their uniform appearance is interrupted by variable amounts of fibrovascular stroma and parenchymal reticulin. Most parasellar meningothelial meningiomas are benign with uncommon to inconspicuous mitoses like those in adenomas.[160,227,232]

Anatomic site is not as helpful in identifying sellar meningiomas as it is in identifying meningiomas in the cerebral fossae, partly because of the small distances between structures. Some meningiomas are associated with the sphenoid ridge, anterior clinoid process, or diaphragma sellae.† This may suggest their diagnosis.

* Refs. 77, 111, 119, 161, 301, 398.

† Refs. 50, 70, 111, 112, 119, 201, 282, 398.

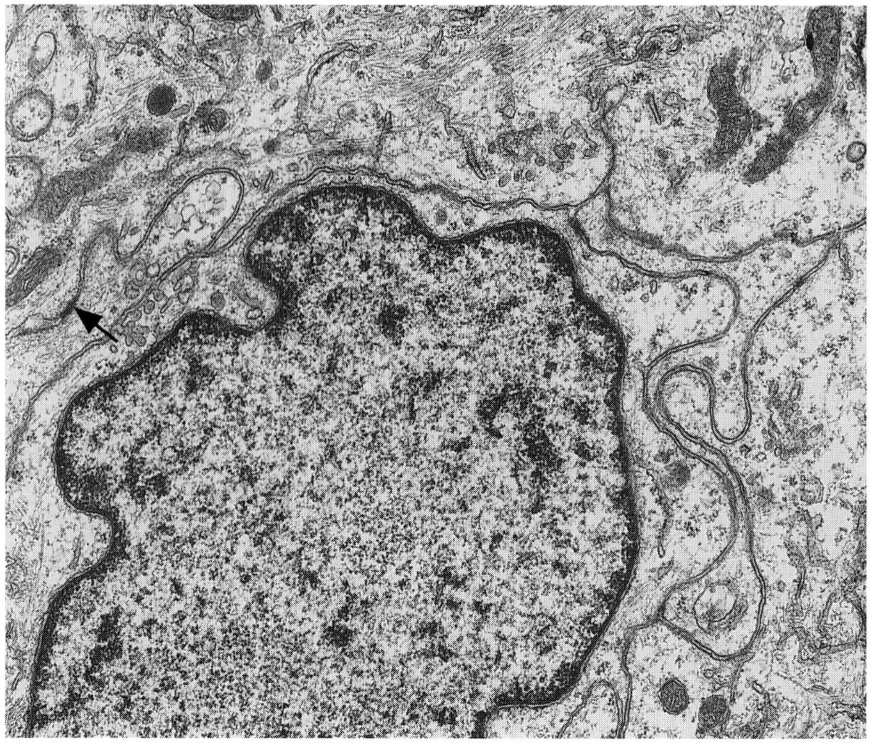

**Fig. 5-37.** Extensively interdigitating cellular processes focally connected with desmosomes (*arrow*) characterize this meningothelial meningioma. (×16,000.) (Reprinted from McKeever PE, and Blaivas M: The brain, spinal cord, and meninges. In Sternberg SS, and others, editors: Diagnostic surgical pathology, ed 2, New York, 1994, Raven Press.)

Certain features should be sought in any sellar tumor suspected of being meningioma. A *syncytial* appearance is a distinctive feature of meningiomas and is particularly prominent in meningothelial meningioma (Fig. 5-36). The structural bases of this syncytial appearance are plasma membranes and numerous tightly interdigitating cellular processes riveted by desmosomes (Fig. 5-37). These characteristic structures hold meningioma cells tightly together during routine tissue processing, in contrast to pituitary adenomas. The presence of these structures, coupled with few uniquely positive histochemical and immunochemical markers of meningioma cells, maintains electron microscopy as an important procedure for the diagnosis of difficult cases (Chapter 3). On the other hand, immunochemical pituitary hormone stains will distinguish adenomas.

Some meningiomas contain epithelial cells rather than syncytial cells,[160,226] requiring further discriminating features. Meningothelial *whorls* are characteristic of meningiomas. Whorls should be sought around calcifications to distinguish the calcifications from those that are prominent in some prolactinomas. Lack of cytoplasmic granularity on H&E stain is a feature of meningioma of only modest value in this differential, remembering that rare meningiomas resemble granular cell tumors.[94]

Meningiomas other than the meningothelial variant occur in the sellar region. These are mentioned only briefly, since they do not look like pituitary adenomas. Fibroblastic meningiomas are composed of long, slender, spindle cells often enmeshed in collagen.[77,160,226] Transitional meningiomas combine the meningothelial and fibroblastic features described previously.[77,355] Psammomatous meningiomas are crowded with conspicuous, concentrically laminated psammoma bodies among syncytial cells.[226]

### Meningiomas Associated with Adenoma

Meningiomas occur in association with pituitary adenomas. In some cases the meningioma has been in the cerebral fossa,[140,213] and in others, the sellar region.[40,116,398] These anecdotal associations have been dismissed as coincidental.[398] However, there is an unexpectedly common association between the chromophobe adenoma and meningothelial meningioma found in its immediate vicinity. From studies that report the type of meningioma, four such cases have been described.* This represents 50% of a total of eight associations of any type between these two tumors. Random association of chromophobe adenomas (Table 5-2) with parasellar meningothelial meningiomas[77] would permit maximally a 43% × 61% = 26% occurrence. While the number of actual cases is too small to be conclusive, the percentages suggest a *nonrandom association* between chromophobe adenomas and parasellar meningothelial meningiomas. These figures emphasize the importance of accurately distinguishing these two tumors, which closely resemble one another.

* Refs. 40, 45, 116, 140, 161, 227, 301, 398.

**Table 5-2.** Frequency of surgically resected pituitary adenomas

| Tumor type | Percent of cases* |
|---|---|
| Densely granulated GH adenoma | 6.7 |
| Sparsely granuated GH adenoma | 7.3 |
| Densely granulated PRL adenoma | 0.6 |
| Sparsely granulated PRL adenoma | 26.6 |
| Mixed GH-PRL adenoma | 4.8 |
| Acidophil stem cell adenoma | 2.2 |
| Mammosomatotroph cell adenoma | 1.4 |
| Functioning corticotroph cell adenoma | 8.0 |
| Silent corticotroph cell adenoma | 6.0 |
| Thyrotroph cell adenoma | 1.0 |
| Gonadotroph cell adenoma | 6.4 |
| Null cell adenoma | 16.3 |
| Oncocytoma | 8.9 |
| Plurihormonal adenoma | 3.7 |

* From 1043 biopsies in unselected surgical material. The percentage of cases is based on data from Horvath E, and Kovacs K: Pituitary gland, Pathol Res Pract 183:129–142, 1988.

### Meningioma Following Radiotherapy for Adenoma

Most authorities attribute these *criteria* for consideration of a correlation between radiation exposure and a second tumor to Cahan and associates[52,358]: (1) the second tumor is located within the irradiated region; (2) the first and second tumors are histologically confirmed to be different types; and (3) asymptomatic latency interval was sufficiently long to indicate that the second tumor was not present at the time of irradiation. Their criteria have been modified by many, including us. Unlike some others, we do not automatically exclude cases that arise in the context of a phakomatosis if the above criteria are met.

Seven instances of meningiomas have been reported after radiotherapy for pituitary adenoma.* Most of these fulfill the above criteria of correlation between radiation exposure and a second tumor. However, in two cases of acromegaly the initial adenoma was not verified histologically.[33,196] One patient died of other causes, resulting in a short latency interval of 1 year.[285] This patient had a very small incidental meningioma at autopsy. The radiation doses ranged from 35 to 70 Gy, and the average *latency interval* was 13 years.

Neglected in most reports are epidemiologic and statistical evaluations of appropriate populations at risk to determine the likelihood of correlation between parasellar radiation and subsequent meningioma. One study by Spallone provides data from one institution of two postradiation meningiomas among 192 patients at risk following radiation for their pituitary adenomas.[358] This suggests an incidence of 1% of the irradiated patient population at risk. Although the incidence of meningioma in an appropriate control population was not compared, it is certainly less than 1%. Historical control populations of different groups of patients suggest an incidence of meningiomas of 0.01% in nonirradiated subjects.[245] Thus, an association between previous radiation and these meningiomas is suggested.

* Refs. 33, 196, 239, 285, 358, 362.

## OLFACTORY NEUROBLASTOMA (ESTHESIONEUROBLASTOMA)

Olfactory neuroblastomas arise from the superior portion of the *nasal cavity* among the olfactory sensory cells.[244,304] While they occur in patients of all ages, their peak incidences are during the second and sixth decades.[79] They may present with epistaxis and nasal obstruction.[4,336]

Olfactory neuroblastomas are rare around the sella because they arise rostral and inferior to this structure.[75] Intracranial involvement is usually secondary to local extension from its origin near the cribriform plate, or occasionally by metastasis into the cranial vault.[309] Thus, despite histologic similarities to adenoma, precise radiographic and surgical *anatomic information* should suggest the correct diagnosis in most instances. Computerized tomography reveals tumors of mixed density that are often large before discovery.* Erosion of cribriform plate, sinus walls, and other bones of the skull base frequently occurs.[199,266] The bone lesions are more apparent on CT images than on magnetic resonance images (MRI). MRI is more informative than CT when the tumor is within the cranial fossa.[199]

Unfortunately, rare olfactory neuroblastomas present in the sellar and parasellar regions.[49,328] Their precise site of origin is unknown, but ganglionic origins have been suggested.[143,328] Olfactory neuroblastomas in this location must be distinguished from the more common pituitary adenoma. Rare adenomas arise in ectopic locations, including the nasopharynx (discussed in the section on ectopic pituitary adenomas). These also must be distinguished from olfactory neuroblastomas.

The neoplastic parenchyma of olfactory neuroblastoma is moderately to highly cellular. Moderately cellular examples overlap the cellular density commonly encountered in adenomas. However, unlike adenomas, olfactory neuroblastoma cells extend *fibrillary cellular processes*. This fibrillarity is critical to their differentiation and is evident in more than 80% of cases stained with H&E[243] (Fig. 5-38). Silver stains for neurites or immunostains for neurofilaments (Chapter 4) often stain these filaments, but not always. Equivocal cases should be examined ultrastructurally (Chapter 3). Homer Wright rosettes with fibrillary cores, olfac-

* Refs. 49, 266, 313, 368.

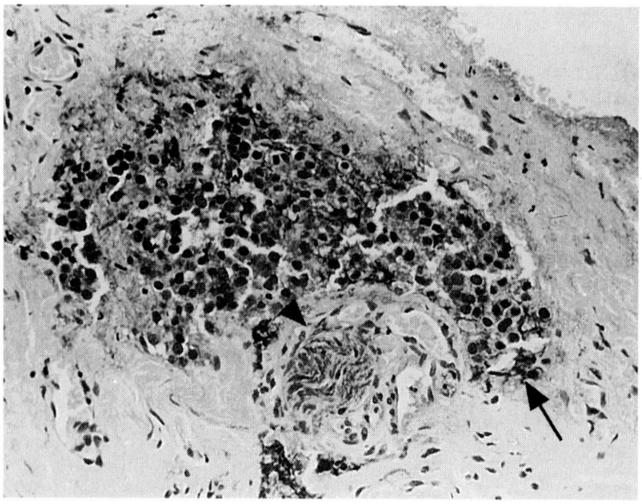

**Fig. 5-38.** Small cells with round nuclei and prominent nucleoli first appear epithelioid but upon close inspection are slightly fibrillar in this invasive margin of an olfactory neuroblastoma. Dark S-100 positive neoplastic cells (*arrow*) partially surround an S-100 positive neurovascular bundle (*arrowhead*). (×200.)

tory rosettes with ciliated lumina and mucin, or Flexner rosettes with central lumina rimmed by distinct pink borders are valuable diagnostic features.[266] However, these rosettes are not always evident.

While olfactory neuroblastomas vary morphologically between cases, perinuclear cytoplasm is usually minimal.[336] Nuclei are small and round with minimal to moderate pleomorphism. Mitoses vary substantially between cases. The amount of fibrovascular stroma varies and in some tumors it is very thick, resembling the desmoplasia of carcinoma.[266] In other cases, the stroma is minimal.[242]

*Neuronal markers* like synaptophysin, neurofilament, beta-tubulin, and microtubule-associated protein-2 can help identify olfactory neuroblastoma (Chapter 4). However, immunostaining does not detect these markers on all neuroblastomas.* The intermingling of neuronal elements with adenomas requires careful morphologic interpretation of tumors, even when the more specific neuronal markers are applied to distinguish adenomas from olfactory neuroblastomas.† Pituitary peptide hormones, noted in the section on adenomas, help to distinguish pituitary adenomas from neuroblastoma.

Neoplasms other than adenoma that might be confused with olfactory neuroblastoma include *lymphoma* and *melanoma*.[4,84] Both of these lack the true neuronal markers described above. Absence of cellular processes and of cohesion, as well as the presence of lymphocytic markers should distinguish lymphomas.

* Refs. 94a, 242, 370, 377.

† Refs. 13, 109, 189, 333, 351.

Melanomas can be more difficult to distinguish because melanoma and neuroblastoma both have S-100 reactivity and can produce melanin.[65,370] However, most melanomas have larger cells, nuclei, and nucleoli than olfactory neuroblastomas. Electron microscopy or immunoperoxidase of neurosecretory granules or neuronal markers distinguish the olfactory neuroblastoma (Chapters 3, 4).[57,369]

The neoplasm most frequently confused with olfactory neuroblastoma is the *sinonasal undifferentiated carcinoma* (SNUC).[242,266] Distinguishing the olfactory neuroblastoma from SNUC is clinically important because neuroblastomas have a better prognosis.[243] Olfactory neuroblastomas do not invade vessels like SNUC.[227] The fibrillar cells of the olfactory neuroblastoma differ from the clusters and ribbons of small epithelioid cells in the SNUC.[89,198] Homer Wright, olfactory, or Flexner *rosettes* identify neuroblastoma, if evident. Immunocytochemistry for *neuronal markers* can distinguish olfactory neuroblastoma from SNUC. Some neuroblastomas stain for neurofilaments or neurotubules, which SNUCs lack.[314,370] *Synaptophysin* and S-100 protein are specific markers for olfactory neuroblastoma in this context and should be employed in difficult cases.[314]

## PLASMACYTOMA (MYELOMA)

The sellar plasmacytoma fortunately is a rare entity,* since a solitary plasmacytoma or the first presentation of multiple myeloma in the sella displays extraordinary similarity to a pituitary adenoma (Fig. 5-39). This simulation of endocrine by hematopoietic neoplasia is even more extraordinary owing to their major differences in cellular lineages. However, both neoplasms synthesize and secrete large amounts of product. This produces similarities in appearance.

The term plasmacytoma is used here for the solitary neoplasm composed of plasma cells. If subsequent studies of the patient reveal multiple lesions of systemic involvement, the neoplasm is then called *multiple myeloma*.

Most extramedullary plasma cell neoplasms occur in the head and neck.[242] Since at least 75% of these involve the sinonasal region, direct extension around the sella is a concern. Careful review of the previous studies of such cases is indicated and may confirm the diagnosis.

*Primary intrasellar plasmacytomas* may be more common than recognized. Two cases were initially diagnosed as pituitary adenomas. The subsequent systemic course of the illness did not occur until 3 to 5 months later, stimulating a reevaluation of the initial diagnosis.[30,297] A solitary plasmacytoma that did not progress to multiple myeloma might elude correct diagnosis in

* Refs. 30, 53, 83, 297, 380.

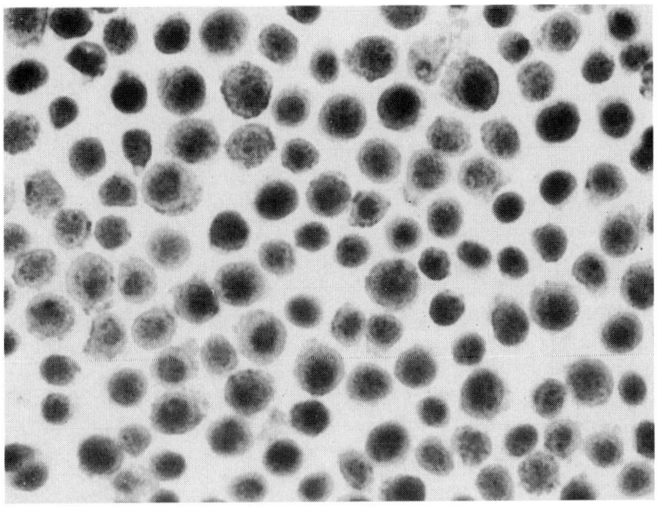

**Fig. 5-39.** Monotonous collection of discohesive cells have purple cytoplasm. Features of this particular myeloma that distinguish it from adenoma include high nuclear to cytoplasmic ratio, extreme paucity of fibrovascular stroma, and a separate neoplasm with these features outside of the sella. (×800.)

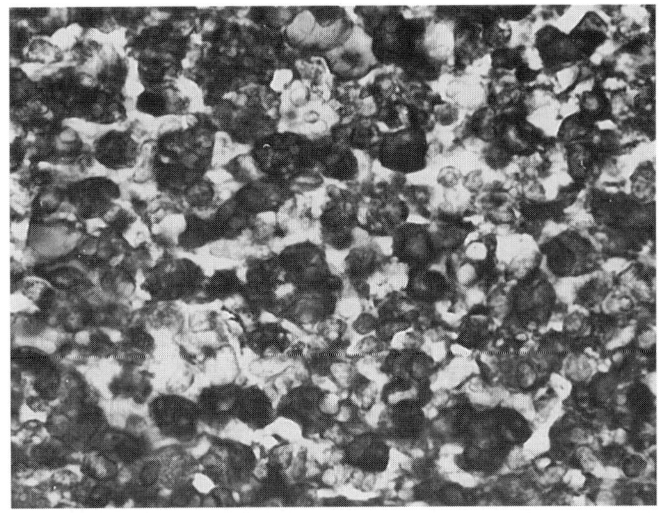

**Fig. 5-40.** Monoclonal expression of IgG distinguishes this solitary parasellar plasmacytoma from an adenoma. (×800.)

the sella because its light microscopic features resemble pituitary adenoma.

The light microscopic features of intrasellar plasmacytomas consist of sheets of round to oval cells separated by fibrovascular septae.[297,380] Tumor cells are uniform, with round and oval nuclei and with few binucleated cells. Mitoses are sparse. Peripheral nuclear chromatin suggests cartwheels. Some nuclei are eccentric.

Different clinical manifestations provide keys to distinguishing plasmacytomas from pituitary adenomas. The sellar lesion can be *lytic,* with a sharp margin in bone. Radiologic evidence of other "punched-out" lesions in the skull or other bones may suggest multiple myeloma.[30,297] Laboratory data are of paramount importance to the pathologist who encounters such a plasmacytoma. Serum or urinary protein abnormalities may indicate a *monoclonal gammopathy.*[30] Patients with multiple myeloma presenting in the sella often have systemic manifestations.[297] A second tumor, lytic lesion, or protein abnormality should immediately raise suspicion of a myeloma.

Most solitary plasmacytomas have been recognized with electron microscopy, a procedure eminently suited to distinguish plasmacytoma from adenoma. Myeloma cells lack hormone storage granules, intercellular junctions, and basement membranes. These are present in pituitary adenomas.[380]

If electron microscopy cannot be obtained, immunocytochemistry is recommended. *Monoclonal* expression of an *immunoglobulin* (Ig) heavy chain subtype and a kappa or lambda light chain distinguish myeloma from pituitary adenoma (Fig. 5-40).[380] As with other differentials involving pituitary adenomas, positive chromogranin and pituitary peptide hormone staining can be critical in identifying an adenoma.

## RATHKE'S CLEFT CYSTS

These are fluid-filled cysts rather than tumors and are described in detail elsewhere.[227] They are mentioned here because they may clinically or radiographically resemble adenomas.[372]

The histopathologic features of Rathke's cysts are characteristic. The cysts contain mucin. A thin cuboidal to columnar epithelium rests directly upon fibrovascular connective tissue. When squamous epithelial change occurs, it does not fill the cyst with keratin. Pseudostratification of this simple epithelial layer may occur. Goblet cells are often mixed with ciliated cells.

## SARCOMA

Sellar sarcomas are rare tumors. They are related to pituitary adenomas by virtue of *radiotherapy* of these adenomas. Nearly all sellar sarcomas occur 2 to 22 years after radiation to the region of origin.* About half of these received 30–50 Gy, and half more than 50 Gy. With the exception of "collision tumors" discussed below, their features differ unmistakably from adenomas. Thus, all of Cahan and associates' criteria for consideration of correlation with radiotherapy are met by most sellar sarcomas.[52] In contrast to the long interval between radiation and diagnosis, the interval between diagnosis and death averages only 4.3 months.[346]

The relationship between sellar sarcomas and prior radiation is critical to their *early recognition.* Repeated

---

* Refs. 8, 106, 110, 238, 264, 294, 300, 316, 346, 359, 373, 387.

specimens have yielded mesenchymal tissues ranging from not clearly neoplastic, through benign neoplasm, to frank sarcoma.[346,373] These may reflect tumor heterogeneity or tumor progression over time. They place a premium upon the realization of the clinical setting in which sarcomas are likely to occur.

Frank sarcomas contain pleomorphic spindled and stellate cells with many mitoses, including bizarre mitoses.[264,373] Most resemble *fibrosarcomas,* although the question whether they include malignant fibrous histiocytomas has not been critically addressed. Their cellular density is high. Early samples of tissue may not demonstrate the features described.[373] These tumors may resemble benign neoplastic spindled cells of lower cellular density and some may even resemble dense connective tissue.

Mixed mesenchymal and epithelial neoplasms often occur in this group of tumors.* Individual cases have been interpreted as "collision tumors" between the adenoma and the subsequent sarcoma.[346] In such a situation, the sarcoma would have presumably originated in parasellar mesenchyme and invaded the adenoma. *Local invasion* is typical of parasellar sarcomas, often compromising critical neuroanatomic regions, including pituitary, hypothalamus, brainstem, and cranial nerves.

The configurations of *mixed tumors* are variable and sometimes confusing. Adenoma may predominate, intersected by fibrous and cellular bands that may be interpreted as stromal reaction or neoplasm. Sarcoma may predominate, dividing adenoma cells into small residual islands.[346,373] In other cases, an exuberant growth of pleomorphic mesenchymal and epithelial cells may suggest mixed sarcoma and carcinoma.

While most sellar sarcomas resemble fibrosarcomas, about 20% of them are *osteosarcomas.*† A typical osteosarcoma in this region has extremely pleomorphic spindled and polyhedral cells with multinucleated tumor cells and monstrous forms. Nucleoli are prominent. Select regions of tumor contain abundant eosinophilic stroma or osteoid.[8,238]

*Spontaneous sellar sarcomas* are rarer than sarcomas following radiation.[9,227,395] Spontaneous sarcomas metastasize more frequently than postradiation sarcomas.[395] Fibrosarcoma and leiomyosarcoma are represented.

## ACKNOWLEDGMENTS

We thank Ms. Peggy Otto, Dianna Banka, and Dawn Banka for their skillful typing and editorial assistance. Drs. Mila Blaivas and Anders Sima provided citations and comments. Mr. Craig Biddle, Mark Deming, and Randal Stegmeyer provided high-quality illustrations.

* Refs. 69, 264, 346, 373.

† Refs. 3, 6, 8, 69, 106, 110, 238, 264, 294, 300, 316, 346, 359, 373, 387.

## REFERENCES

1. Adamson TE, and others: Correlation of clinical and pathological features in surgically treated craniopharyngiomas, J Neurosurg 73:12-17, 1990.
2. Afrasiabi A, Valenta L, and Gwinup GA: A TSH-secreting pituitary tumour causing hyperthyroidism: presentation of a case and review of the literature, Acta Endocrinol (Copenh) 92:448-454, 1979.
3. Ahmad K, and Fayos JV: Pituitary fibrosarcoma secondary to radiation therapy, Cancer 42:107-110, 1978.
4. Albert RW: Esthesioneuroblastoma, Ear Nose Throat J 60:522-526, 1981.
5. Alexander JM, and others: Clinically nonfunctioning pituitary tumors are monoclonal in origin, J Clin Invest 86:336-340, 1990.
6. Amendola BE, and others: Radiation associated sarcoma: a review of 23 patients with postradiation sarcoma over a 50-year period, Am J Clin Oncol 12:411-415, 1989.
7. Amendola BE, and others: Primary large-cell lymphoma of the central nervous system, Am J Clin Oncol 9:204-208, 1986.
8. Amine ARC, and Sugar O: Suprasellar osteogenic sarcoma following radiation for pituitary adenoma, J Neurosurg 44:88-91, 1976.
9. Anderson WR, Cameron JD, and Tsai SH: Primary intracranial leiomyosarcoma. Case report with ultrastructural study, J Neurosurg 53:401-405, 1980.
10. Aozasa K, and others: Malignant lymphoma of the central nervous system in Japan: histologic and immunohistologic studies, Int J Cancer 45:632-636, 1990.
11. Arnesen M, and Scheithauer BW: Aggressive small cell tumor of the skull base, Ultrastruct Pathol 18:191-197, 1994.
12. Asa SL, and others: Lymphocytic hypophysitis of pregnancy resulting in hypopituitarism: a distinct clinicopathologic entity, Ann Intern Med 95:166-171, 1981.
13. Asa SL, and others: Hypothalamic neuronal hamartoma associated with pituitary growth hormone cell adenoma and acromegaly, Acta Neuropathol 52:231-234, 1980.
14. Asa SL, and others: Gonadotropin secretion in vitro by human pituitary null cell adenomas and oncocytomas, J Clin Endocrinol Metab 62:1011-1019, 1986.
15. Asa SL, Kovacs K, and Bilbao JM: The pars tuberalis of human pituitary. A histologic, immunohistochemical, ultrastructural and immunoelectron microscopic analysis, Virchows Arch 399: 49-59, 1983.
16. Asa SL, and others: Human fetal adenohypophysis. Histologic and immunocytochemical analysis, Neuroendocrinology 43: 308-316, 1986.
17. Asa SL, and others: Cushing's disease associated with an intrasellar gangliocytoma producing corticotrophin-releasing factor, Ann Intern Med 101:789-793, 1984.
18. Asa SL, and others: Prolactin cells in the human pituitary. A quantitative immunocytochemical analysis, Arch Pathol Lab Med 106:360-363, 1982.
19. Asa SL, and others: A case of hypothalamic acromegaly: a clinicopathological study of six patients with hypothalamic gangliocytomas producing growth hormone-releasing factor, J Clin Endocrinol Metab 58:796-803, 1984.
20. Ashworth B: Cerebral histiocytic lymphoma presenting with loss of weight, Neurology 32:894-896, 1982.
21. Austin MB, and Mills SE: Neoplasms and neoplasm-like lesions involving the skull base, Ear Nose Throat J 65:25-52, 1986.
22. Baes M, Allaerts W, and Denef C: Evidence for functional communication between folliculo-stellate cells and hormone-secreting cells in perfused anterior pituitary cell aggregates, Endocrinology 120:685-691, 1987.
23. Baker BL, and Jaffe RB: The genesis of cell types in the adenohypophysis of the human fetus as observed with immunocytochemistry, Am J Anat 143:137-161, 1975.

24. Barkan AL, and others: Preoperative treatment of acromegaly with somatostatin analog SMS 201-995: shrinkage of invasive pituitary macroadenoma and improved surgical remission, J Clin Endocrinol Metab 67:1040-1048, 1988.
25. Baskin DS, and Wilson CB: Transsphenoidal surgery of intrasellar germinomas. Report of two cases, J Neurosurg 59:1063-1066, 1983.
26. Becker DH, and Wilson CB: Symptomatic parasellar granular cell tumor, Neurosurgery 8:173-180, 1981.
27. Begeot M, Dubois MP, and Dubois PM: Growth hormone and ACTH in the pituitary of normal and anencephalic human fetuses: immunocytochemical evidence for hypothalamic influences during development, Neuroendocrinology 24:208-220, 1977.
28. Belza J: Double midline intracranial tumors of vestigial origin: contiguous intrasellar chordoma and suprasellar craniopharyngioma: Case report, J Neurosurg 25:199, 1966.
29. Bevan JS, and others: Intrasellar gangliocytoma containing gastrin and growth hormone-releasing hormone associated with a growth hormone-secreting pituitary adenoma, Clin Endocrinol 30:213-224, 1989.
30. Bitterman P, and others: Multiple myeloma mimicking pituitary adenoma, Computerized Radiol 10:201-205, 1986.
31. Bjornsson J, and others: Intracranial germ cell tumors: pathobiological and immunohistochemical aspects of 70 cases, J Neuropathol Exp Neurol 44:32-46, 1985.
32. Blizzard RM, Alberts M: Hypopituitarism, hypoadrenalism and hypogonadism in the newborn infant, J Pediatr 48:782-792, 1956.
33. Bogdanowicz WM, and Sachs E Jr: The possible role of radiation in oncogenesis of meningioma, Surg Neurol 2:379-383, 1974.
34. Boggan JE, Tyrrell JB, and Wilson CB: Transsphenoidal microsurgical management of Cushing's disease. Report of 100 cases, J Neurosurg 59:195-200, 1983.
35. Bononi PL, and others: Amyloid deposits in a prolactin-producing pituitary adenoma, J Endocrinol Invest 16:339-343, 1993.
36. Borit A, and Blanshard TP: Sphenoidal pituitary adenoma, Hum Pathol 10:93-96, 1979.
37. Bouropoulou V, and others: Immunohistochemical investigation of chordomas: histogenetic and differential diagnostic aspects, Current Top Pathol 80:183-203, 1989.
38. Boyd JD: Observations on the human pharyngeal hypophysis, J Endocrinol 14:66-77, 1956.
39. Branch CL Jr, and Laws ER Jr: Metastatic tumors of the sella turcica masquerading as primary pituitary tumors, J Clin Endocrinol Metab 65:469-474, 1987.
40. Brennan TG Jr, and others: Case report: tandem lesions. Chromophobe adenoma and meningioma, J Comput Assist Tomogr 1:517-520, 1977.
41. Brewer D: Congenital absence of the pituitary gland and its consequences, J Pathol Bacteriol 73:59-67, 1957.
42. Bruner JM: Oligodendroglioma: diagnosis and prognosis, Semin Diagn Pathol 4:251-261, 1987.
43. Buchfelder M, and others: Endocrine disturbances in suprasellar germinomas, Acta Endocrinol (Copenh) 120:337-342, 1989.
44. Buchmann E, and Schweisinger G: Hypophyse und Hamoblastosen, Zentralbl Neurochir 40:35, 1979.
45. Bunick EM, Mills LC, and Rose LI: Association of acromegaly and meningiomas, JAMA 240:1267-1268, 1978.
46. Burchield KJ, Shaw COM, and Kelly WA: A mixed functional microadenoma and ganglioneuroma of the pituitary fossa. Case Report, J Neurosurg 58:416-420, 1983.
47. Burger PC, and Scheithauer BW: Tumors of the central nervous system. In Rosai J, and Sobin LH, editors. Atlas of tumor pathology, Washington, DC, Third Series Fascicle 10, 1994, Armed Forces Institute of Pathology.
48. Burger PC, Scheithauer BW, and Vogel FS: Surgical Pathology of the Nervous System and its Coverings, ed 3, New York, 1991, Churchill Livingstone.
49. Burke DP, and others: Radiology of olfactory neuroblastoma, Radiology 137:367-372, 1980.
50. Burrow GN, and others: Microadenomas of the pituitary and abnormal sellar tomograms in an unselected autopsy series, N Engl J Med 304:156-158, 1981.
51. Busch E, and Mahneke A: A case of meningioma from the diaphragm of the sella turcica, Zentralbl Neurochir 14:25-28, 1954.
52. Cahan WG, and others: Sarcoma arising in irradiated bone. Report of eleven cases, Cancer 1:3-29, 1948.
53. Calvo A, and others: Tumors of the sellar region and the cavernous sinus. Evaluation of diagnostic procedures and therapeutic orientation, Acta Neurol Latinoam 26:111-122, 1980.
54. Camaris C, Balleine R, and Little D: Microadenomas of the human pituitary, Pathology 27:8-11, 1995.
55. Cartwright DM, Miller TR, and Nasr AJ: Fine-needle aspiration biopsy of pituitary carcinoma with cervical lymph node metastases: a report of two cases and review of the literature, Diagn Cytopathol 11:68-73, 1994.
56. Chandler WF, and others: Surgical treatment of Cushing's disease, J Neurosurg 66:204-212, 1987.
57. Chaudhru AP, and others: Olfactory neuroblastoma (esthesioneuroblastoma): a light and ultrastructural study of two cases, Cancer 44:554-579, 1979.
58. Christensen E: Two cases of primary intracranial melanomata, Acta Chir Scand 85:90-98, 1941.
59. Clark GB, Henry JM, and McKeever PE: Cerebral pilocytic astrocytoma, Cancer 56:1128-1133, 1985.
60. Coindre JM, and others: Immunohistological study in chordomas, J Pathol 150:61-63, 1986.
61. Cook RJ, and others: Prolactinomas in men masquerading as invasive skull base tumor, Br J Neurosurg 8:51-55, 1994.
61a. Corenblum B, LeBlanc FE, and Watanabe M: Acromegaly with an adenomatous pharyngeal pituitary, JAMA 243:1456-1457, 1980.
62. Costello RT: Subclinical adenoma of the pituitary gland, Am J Pathol 12:205-216, 1936.
63. Crooke AC: A change in the basophil cells of the pituitary gland common to conditions which exhibit the syndrome attributed to basophil adenoma, J Pathol Bacteriol 41:339-349, 1935.
64. Crotty T, and others: Papillary craniopharyngiomas: a morphological and clinical study of 46 cases, Endocr Pathol 3 Suppl 1: S6, 1992.
65. Curtis JL, and Rubinstein LJ: Pigmented olfactory neuroblastoma. A new example of melanotic neuroepithelial neoplasm, Cancer 49:2136-2143, 1982.
66. Daneshdoost L, and others: Recognition of gonadotroph adenomas in women, N Engl J Med 324:589-594, 1991.
67. Daniel PM, and Prichard MML: Studies of the hypothalamus and the pituitary gland, Acta Endocrinol *Kbh* 86:S1-S216, 1975.
68. Davey FR, Elghetany MT, and Kurec AS: Immunophenotyping of hematologic neoplasms in paraffin-embedded tissue sections, Am J Clin Pathol 93:S17-S26, 1990.
69. del Regato JA: Eosinophilic adenoma of the pituitary with sarcomatous changes, Cancer Semin 3:77-80, 1962.
70. Demailly PW, and Guiat G: Meningomes du diaphragme sellaire, Bull Soc D'Ophthalm 2:191-193, 1970.
71. Dickson DW, and others: Cerebral granular cell tumor: immunohistochemical and electron microscopic study, J Neuropathol Exp Neurol 45:304-314, 1986.
72. Domingue JN, and Wilson CB: Pituitary abscesses. Report of seven cases and review of the literature, J Neurosurg 46:601-608, 1977.
73. Duello TM, and Halmi NS: Pituitary adenoma producing thyrotropin and prolactin. An immunohistochemical and electron microscopic study, Virchows Arch 376:255-265, 1977.

74. Duray PH, Ernstoff MS, and Titus-Ernstoff L: Immunohistochemical phenotyping of malignant melanoma: A procedure whose time has come in pathologic practice, Pathol Annu 25(2): 351-377, 1990.
75. Durham JC: Olfactory neuroblastoma, Ear Nose Throat J 68: 185-186, 1989.
76. Egerter DA, and Beckstead JH: Malignant lymphomas in the acquired immunodeficiency syndrome. Additional evidence for a B-cell origin, Arch Pathol Lab Med 112:602-606, 1988.
77. Ehlers N, and Malmros R: The suprasellar meningioma. A review of the literature and presentation of a series of 31 cases, Acta Ophthalmol Scand Suppl 121:1-73, 1973.
78. Ehrlich RM: Ectopic and hypoplastic pituitary with adrenal hypoplasia; case report, J Pediatr 51:377-384, 1957.
79. Elkon D, and others: Esthesioneuroblastoma, Cancer 44:1087-1094, 1979.
80. Erlandson RA: Diagnostic Transmission Electron Microscopy of Human Tumors: The Interpretation of Submicroscopic Structures in Human Neoplastic Cells, New York, 1983, Masson.
81. Erlandson RA, and others: Ultrastructure of human chordoma, Cancer Res 28:2115-2125, 1968.
82. Esiri MM, and others: Effect of bromocriptine treatment on the fibrous tissue content of prolactin-secreting and nonfunctioning macroadenomas of the pituitary gland, J Clin Endocrinol Metab 63:383-388, 1986.
83. Estopinan V, and others: Intrasellar plasmacytoma simulating a pituitary adenoma (letter), Med Clin (Barc) 89:128, 1987.
84. Fagan MF, and Rone R: Esthesioneuroblastoma: cytologic features with differential diagnostic considerations, Diagn Cytopathol 1:322-326, 1985.
85. Farnoud MR, and others: Interactions between normal and tumoral tissues at the boundary of human anterior pituitary adenomas. An immunohistochemical study, Virchows Arch 424: 75-82, 1994.
86. Felix IA, Horvath E, and Kovacs K: Massive Crooke's hyalinization in corticotroph cell adenomas of the human pituitary. A histological, immunocytological, and electron microscopic study of three cases, Acta Neurochir (Wien) 58:235-243, 1981.
87. Ferrara N, and Henzel WJ: Pituitary follicular cells secrete a novel heparin-binding growth factor specific for vascular endothelial cells, Biochem Biophys Res Commun 161:851-858, 1989.
88. Ferrara N, and others: Pituitary follicular cells produce basic fibroblast growth factor, Proc Natl Acad Sci (*USA*) 84:5773-5777, 1987.
89. Ferris CA, and others: Olfactory neuroblastoma. Cytodiagnostic features in a case with ultrastructural and immunohistochemical correlation, Acta Cytol 32:381-385, 1988.
90. Finley JL, and others: Chordoma: Diagnosis by fine-needle aspiration biopsy with histologic, immunocytochemical, and ultrastructural confirmation, Diagn Cytopathol 2:330-337, 1986.
91. Fischer EG, Morris JH, and Kettyle WM: Intrasellar gangliocytoma and syndromes of pituitary hypersecretion, J Neurosurg 59:1071-1082, 1983.
92. Franquemont DW, Fechner RE, and Mills SE: Histologic classification of sinonasal intestinal-type adenocarcinoma, Am J Surg Pathol 15:368-375, 1991.
93. Franquemont DW, Katsetos CD, and Ross GW: Fatal acute pontocerebellar hemorrhage due to an unsuspected spheno-occipital chordoma, Arch Pathol Lab Med 113:1075-1078, 1989.
94. Friede RL, and Yasargil MG: Suprasellar neoplasm with a granular cell component, J Neuropath Exp Neurol 36:769-782, 1977.
94a. Frierson HF Jr, and others: Olfactory neuroblastoma: additional immunohistochemical characterization, Am J Clin Pathol 94: 553-574, 1990.
95. Frierson HF Jr, and others: Sinonasal undifferentiated carcinoma. An aggressive neoplasm derived from Schneiderian epithelium and distinct from olfactory neuroblastoma, Am J Surg Pathol 10:771-779, 1986.
96. Fujisawa I, and others: Magnetic resonance imaging of neurohypophyseal germinomas, Cancer 68:1009-1014, 1991.
97. Furth J, Meda G, and Clifton KH: The pathophysiology of pituitaries and their tumors. Methodological advances, Methods Cancer Res 10:210-277, 1973.
98. Gambini C, and others: Intracerebral granular cell tumor. Case report, Pathologica 82:83-88, 1990.
99. Garvin AJ, Spicer SS, and McKeever PE: The cytochemical demonstration of intracellular immunoglobulin. II. In neoplasms of lymphoreticular tissue, Am J Pathol 82:457-478, 1976.
100. Gay JC, Janco RL, and Lukens JN: Systemic metastases in primary intracranial germinoma. Case report and literature review, Cancer 55:2688-2690, 1985.
101. Gen M, and others: Necrotic changes in prolactinomas after long term administration of bromocriptine, J Clin Endocrinol Metab 59:463-470, 1984.
102. Genka S, and others: Acromegaly, diabetes insipidus, and visual loss caused by metastatic growth hormone-releasing hormone-producing malignant pancreatic endocrine tumor in the pituitary gland. Case Report, J Neurosurg 83:719-723, 1995.
103. Ghatak NR, Hirano A, and Zimmerman HM: Intrasellar germinomas: a form of ectopic pinealoma, J Neurosurg 31:670, 1969.
104. Gibson JB, Burrows D, and Weir WP: Primary melanoma of the meninges, J Pathol Bacteriol 74:419-438, 1957.
105. Girod C, Trouillas J, and Claustrat B: The human thyrotropic adenoma: pathologic diagnosis in five cases and critical review of the literature. Semin Diagn Pathol 3:58-68, 1986.
106. Goldberg MB, Sheline GE, and Malamud N: Malignant intracranial neoplasms following radiation therapy for acromegaly, Radiology 80:465-470, 1963.
107. Goodyer CG, Guydan HJ, and Giroud CJP: Development of the hypothalamic-pituitary axis in the human fetus. In Tolis G, and others, editors: Clinical Neuroendocrinology: a pathophysiological Approach, New York, 1979, Raven Press.
108. Gooren LJG, and others: Estrogen-induced prolactinoma in a man, J Clin Endocrinol Metab 66:444-446, 1988.
109. Graber H, and Kersting G: Pubertas praecox bei Hamartie des mediobasalen Hypothalamus mit heterotoper Retinaanlage, Deut Z Nervenheilk 173:1-11, 1955.
110. Greenhouse AH: Pituitary sarcoma. A possible consequence of radiation, JAMA 190:269-273, 1964.
111. Grisoli F, and others: Intrasellar meningioma, Surg Neurol 20: 36-41, 1983.
112. Guiat G, and others: Meningiomes suprasellaries retrochiasmatiques, Neurochirurgie 16:273-285, 1970.
113. Gutjahr P, and Dieterich E: Risikozweiter manligne Neoplasien nach erfolgreicher Tumor behandlung im Kindersalter, Dtsch Med Wochenschr 104:969-972, 1979.
114. Hadfield MG, Vennart GP, and Rosenblum WI: Hypoglycemia: Invasion of the hypothalamus by lymphosarcoma. Metastasis to blood glucose regulating centers, Arch Pathol 94:317-321, 1972.
115. Hagerstrand I, and Schonebeck J: Metastases to the pituitary gland, Acta Pathol Microbiol Scand 75:64-70, 1969.
116. Hainer V, and others: Meningioma in contact with eosinophilic adenoma in a patient with acromegaly, Cas Lek Cesk 117:829-831, 1978.
117. Handt S, and Hofstadter F: What's new in the application of Southern blot analysis of malignant lymphomas? Path Res Pract 184:455-463, 1989.
118. Hardy J: Transphenoidal surgery of hypersecretory pituitary tumors. In Kohler PO, and Ross GT, editors: Diagnosis and treatment of pituitary tumors. International Congress Series No 1. 303, Amsterdam, 1973, Excerpta Medica.
119. Hardy J, and Robert F: Un meningiome de la sella turcique variete sous diaphragmatique (exerse par voie transphenoidale), Neurochirurgie 15:535-544, 1969.

120. Hassoun J, and others: Germinomas of the brain. Light and electron microscopic study. A report of seven cases, Acta Neuropathol Suppl (Berl) 7:105-108, 1981.
121. Hatakeyama S: Electron microscopic study of the anencephalic adenohypophysis with reference to the adrenocorticotrophs and their correlation with the functional differentiation of the hypothalamus during the fetal life, Endocrinol Jpn 16:187-203, 1969.
122. Heitz PU: Neuroendocrine tumor markers, Curr Pathol 77:279-306, 1987.
123. Herman V, and others: Clonal origin of pituitary adenomas, J Clin Endocrinol Metab 71:1427-1433, 1990.
124. Hirata K, and others: A case of primary hypothalamic malignant lymphoma with diabetes insipidus, No Shinkei Geka 17: 461-466, 1989.
125. Ho KL: Ecchordosis physaliphora and chordoma: a comparative ultrastructural study, Clin Neuropathol 4:77-86, 1985.
126. Hofler H, Walter GF, and Denk H: Immunohistochemistry of folliculo-stellate cells in normal human adenohypophyses and in pituitary adenomas, Acta Neuropathol (Berl) 65:35-40, 1984.
127. Hoi Sang U, and Johnson C: Metastatic prolactin-secreting pituitary adenoma, Hum Pathol 15:94-96, 1984.
128. Honegger J, and others: Human chorionic gonadotrophin immunoactivity in cystic intracranial tumours, Clin Endocrinol (Oxf) 42:235-241, 1995.
129. Horikoshi T, and others: Renal cell carcinoma metastatic to the hypophysis—case report, Neurol Med Chir (Tokyo) 28:78-82, 1988.
130. Horvath E, and Kovacs K: Pathology of the pituitary gland. In Ezrin C, and others, editors: Pituitary Diseases, Boca Raton, Florida, 1980, CRC Press.
131. Horvath E, and Kovacs K: Gonadotroph adenomas of the human pituitary: sex-related fine structural dichotomy. A histologic, immunocytochemical and electron microscopic study of 30 tumors, Am J Pathol 117:429-440, 1984.
132. Horvath E, and Kovacs K: The adenohypophysis. In Kovacs K, and Asa SL, editors: Functional Endocrine Pathology, Boston, 1991, Blackwell Scientific Publications.
133. Horvath E, Kovacs K, and Josse R: Pituitary corticotroph cell adenoma with marked abundance of microfilaments, Ultrastruct Pathol 5:249-255, 1983.
134. Horvath E, and others: Silent corticotropic adenomas of the human pituitary gland. A histologic, immunocytologic and ultrastructural study, Am J Pathol 98:617-638, 1980.
135. Horvath E, and others: Pituitary adenomas producing growth hormone, prolactin and one or more glycoprotein hormones, Ultrastruct Pathol 5:171-183, 1983.
136. Horvath E, and others: A novel type of pituitary adenoma: morphological features and clinical correlations, J Clin Endocrinol Metab 66:1111-1118, 1988.
137. Hsu YC, and others: Pathology of nasopharyngeal carcinoma. Proposal of a new histologic classification correlated with prognosis, Cancer 59:945-951, 1987.
138. Huang CI, Chiou WH, and Ho DM: Oligodendroglioma occurring after radiation therapy for pituitary adenoma, J Neurol Neurosurg Psychiatry 50:1619-1624, 1987.
139. Hufnagel TJ, and others: Malignant glioma of the optic chiasm eight years after radiotherapy for prolactinoma, Arch Ophthalmol 106:1701-1705, 1988.
140. Hyoda A, and others: Pituitary adenoma and meningioma in the same patient, Neurochirurgia (Stuttg) 25:66-67, 1982.
141. Inoue HK, Haganuma H, and Ono N: Pathobiology of intracranial germ-cell tumors: Immunochemical, immunohistochemical, and electron microscopic investigations, J Neurooncol 5: 105-115, 1987.
142. Ito K, and others: Lymphocytic adenohypophysitis with sudden onset of diabetes insipidus in menopausal female—case report, Neurol Med Chir (Tokyo) 32:346-350, 1992.
143. Jakumeit HD: Neuroblastoma of the olfactory nerve, Acta Neurochir 25:99-108, 1971.
144. Jameson JL, and others: Glycoprotein hormone genes are expressed in clinically nonfunctioning pituitary adenomas, J Clin Invest 80:1472-1478, 1987.
145. Jameson JL, Lindell CM, and Habener JF: Gonadotropin and thyrotropin $\alpha$ and $\beta$-subunit gene expression in normal and neoplastic tissues characterized using specific messenger ribonucleic acid hybridization probes, J Clin Endocrinol Metab 64: 319-327, 1987.
146. Jamjoom A, and others: Cervical lymph node metastases from a pituitary carcinoma, Br J Neurosurg 8:87-92, 1994.
147. Jennings MT, Gelman R, and Hochberg F: Intracranial germ-cell tumors: natural history and pathogenesis, J Neurosurg 63: 155-167, 1985.
148. Jensen MD, and others: Lymphocytic hypophysitis with isolated corticotropin deficiency, Ann Intern Med 105:200-203, 1986.
149. Johnson PC: Ultrastructural study of two central nervous system lymphomas, Acta Neuropathol Suppl (Berl) 6:155-160, 1975.
150. Judge DM, and others: Hypothalamic hamartoma: a source of luteinizing hormone-releasing factor in precocious puberty, N Engl J Med 296:7-10, 1977.
151. Kahn EA, and others: Forty-five years experience with the craniopharyngiomas, Surg Neurol 1:5-12, 1973.
152. Kahn LB: Esthesioneuroblastoma: a light and electron microscopic study, Hum Pathol 5:364-371, 1974.
153. Kamel OW, Horoupian DS, and Silverberg GD: Mixed gangliocytoma-adenoma. A distinct neuroendocrine tumor of the pituitary fossa, Hum Pathol 20:1198-1203, 1983.
154. Karnaze MG, and others: Suprasellar lesions: evaluation with MR imaging, Radiology 161:77-82, 1986.
155. Kasumova S, and Inauri GA: Melanotic tumor of the hypophysis, Vopr Onkol 26:64-66, 1980.
156. Kaufman B, and Chamberlin WB Jr: The ubiquitous "empty" sella turcica, Acta Radiol 13:413-425, 1972.
157. Kay S, Lees JK, and Stout AP: Pituitary chromophobe tumors of the nasal cavity, Cancer 3:695-704, 1950.
158. Kay S, and Schatzki PF: Ultrastructural observations of a chordoma arising in the clivus, Hum Pathol 3:403-413, 1972.
159. Kendall BE: Cranial chordomas, Br J Radiol 50:687-698, 1977.
160. Kepes JJ: Meningiomas: biology, pathology and differential diagnosis, Chicago, 1982, Mosby.
161. Kitamura K, and others: Primary brain tumors, Brain Nerve 17: 109-117, 1965.
162. Kitanaka C, and others: Postradiation astrocytoma: report of two cases, J Neurosurg 70:469-474, 1989.
163. Koga N, and others: A case of clivus chordoma showing hemorrhage in the posterior fossa, No Shinkei Geka 16:1417-1421, 1988.
164. Koide O, Iwai S, and Matsumura H: Intranuclear membranous profiles in germinoma cells—a variant of nuclear pockets and intranuclear annulate lamellae, Acta Pathol Jpn 35:605-619, 1985.
165. Koide O, and others: Isoenzymes of alkaline phosphatase in germinoma cells, Am J Clin Pathol 89:611-616, 1988.
166. Komaki S, and others: Radiation and drug induced intracranial neoplasm with angiographic demonstration, Neurol Med Chir (Tokyo) 17:55-62, 1977.
167. Konig R, Schonberger W, and Grimm W: Mediastinal teratocarcinoma and hypophyseal stalk germinoma in a patient with Klinefelter syndrome, Klin Padiatr 202:53-56, 1990.
168. Kontogeorgos G, and others: Diagnosis of pituitary adenomas on touch preparations assisted by immunocytochemistry, Acta Cytol 39:141-52, 1995.

169. Kontogeorgos G, and others: Double adenomas of the pituitary: a clinicopathological study of 11 tumors, Neurosurgery 31:840-849, 1992.
170. Kontozoglou T, and others: Chordoma: cytologic and immunocytochemical study of four cases, Diagn Cytopathol 2:55-61, 1986.
171. Kovacs K: Metastatic cancer of the pituitary gland, Oncology 27:533-542, 1973.
172. Kovacs K, and Horvath E: Pathology of growth hormone-producing tumors of the human pituitary, Semin Diagn Pathol 3: 18-33, 1986.
173. Kovacs K, and Horvath E: Pituitary "chromophobe" adenoma composed of oncocytes. A light and electron microscopic study, Arch Pathol 95:235-239, 1973.
174. Kovacs K, and Horvath E: Tumors of the pituitary gland. Atlas of tumor pathology, Second Series, Fascicle 21, Washington, DC, 1986, Armed Forces Institute of Pathology.
175. Kovacs K, and others: Adenoma of the human pituitary producing growth hormone and thyrotropin: A histologic, immunocytologic and fine-structural study, Virchows Arch [A] 395:59-68, 1982.
176. Kovacs K, Horvath E, Rewcastle NB, and others: Gonadotroph cell adenoma of the pituitary in a woman with long-standing hypogonadism, Arch Gynecol 229:57-65, 1980.
177. Kovacs K, and others: Null cell adenoma of the human pituitary, Virchows Arch 387:165-174, 1980.
178. Kovacs K, and others: Cytoplasmic microfilaments in the anterior lobe of the human pituitary gland, Acta Anat (Basel) 87: 414-426, 1974.
179. Kovacs K, and others: Pituitary adenomas associated with elevated blood follicle-stimulating hormone levels. A histologic, immunocytologic and electron microscopic study of two cases, Fertil Steril 29:622-628, 1978.
180. Kovacs K, and others: Pituitary prolactin cell hyperplasia, Horm Res 12:87-95, 1980.
181. Kovacs K, and others: Silent somatotroph adenomas of the human pituitary. A morphologic study of three cases including immunocytochemistry, electron microscopy, in vitro examination and in situ hybridization, Am J Pathol 134:345-353, 1989.
182. Kovacs K, and others: Pituitary adenomas in old age, J Gerontol 35:16-22, 1980.
183. Kovalic JJ, and others: Immunohistochemistry as a predictor of clinical outcome in patients given postoperative radiation for subtotally resected pituitary adenomas, J Neurooncol 16:227-232, 1993.
184. Kraichoke S, Cosgrove M, and Chandrasoma PT: Granulomatous inflammation in pineal germinoma. A cause of diagnostic failure of stereotaxic brain biopsy, Am J Surg Pathol 12:655-660, 1988.
185. Kubo O, and others: Immunohistochemical study of craniopharyngiomas, Noshuyo Byori Brain Tumor Pathol, 10:131-134, 1993.
186. Kurtin PJ, and Pinkus GS: Leukocyte common antigen—a diagnostic discriminant between hematopoietic and nonhematopoietic neoplasms in paraffin sections using monoclonal antibodies: Correlation with immunologic studies and ultrastructural localization, Hum Pathol 16:353-365, 1985.
187. Kuwayama A, and Kageyama N: Current management of Cushing's disease. Part II, Contemp Neurosurg 7:1-6, 1985.
188. Lach B, and Lesiuk H: Intracranial suprasellar angiolipoma: ultrastructural and immunohistochemical features, Neurosurgery 34:163-167, 1994.
189. Lamberts SW, de Lange SA, and Stefanko SZ: Adrenocorticotropin-secreting pituitary adenomas originate from the anterior or the intermediate lobe in Cushing's disease: differences in the regulation of hormone secretion, J Clin Endocrinol Metab 54: 286, 1982.
190. Lana-Peixoto MA, Pittella JE, and Arouca EM: Primary intracranial tumors: Analysis of a series of consecutive autopsies and biopsies, Arq Neuropsiquiatr 39:13-24, 1981.
191. Landolt AM, Kleihues P, and Heitz PU: Amyloid deposits in pituitary adenomas, Arch Pathol Lab Med 111:453-458, 1987.
192. Landolt AM, Osterwalder V, and Stuckman G: Pre-operative treatment of acromegaly with SMS 201-995: surgical and pathological observations. In Tolis G, Ludeke DK, editors: Growth hormone, New York, 1988, Raven Press.
193. Landolt AM, and Osterwalder V: Perivascular fibrosis in prolactinomas: is it increased by bromocriptine? J Clin Endocrinol Metab 58:1179-1183, 1984.
194. Landolt AM, and Oswald UW: Histology and ultrastructure of an oncocytic adenoma of the human pituitary, Cancer 31:1099-1105, 1973.
195. Launay M, and others: Narrowing and occlusion of arteries by intracranial tumors: review of the literature and report of 25 cases, Neuroradiology 14:117-126, 1977.
196. Lawrence JH, and others: Successful treatment of acromegaly: metabolic and clinical studies in 145 patients, J Clin Endocrinol Metab 31:180-198, 1970.
197. Legido A, and others: Suprasellar germinomas in childhood, Cancer 63:340-344, 1989.
198. Levine PA, and others: Sinonasal undifferentiated carcinoma: a distinctive and highly aggressive neoplasm, Laryngoscope 97:905-908, 1987.
199. Levine PA, and others: MRI vs high resolution CT scanning: evaluation of the anterior skull base, Otolaryngol Head Neck Surg 96:260-267, 1987.
200. Lewis AJ, and others: Squamous cell carcinoma arising in suprasellar epidermoid cysts, J Neurosurg 59:538-541, 1983.
201. Ley A, and Gabas E: Meningiomas of the tuberculum sellae, Acta Neurochir Suppl (Wien) 28:402-404, 1979.
202. Lindholm J, Rasmussen P, and Korsgaard O: Intrasellar or pituitary abscess, J Neurosurg 38:616-619, 1973.
203. Liss L, Kahn EA: Pituicytoma: tumor of the sella turcica. A clinicopathologic study, J Neurosurg 15:481-488, 1958.
204. Liwnicz BH, and others: Radiation-associated gliomas: a report of four cases and analysis of postradiation tumors of the central nervous system, Neurosurgery 17:436-445, 1985.
205. Lloyd RV, and others: Analysis of mammosomatotropic cells in normal and neoplastic human pituitary tissues by the reverse hemolytic plaque assay and immunocytochemistry, J Clin Endocrinol Metab 66:1103-1110, 1988.
206. Lloyd RV, and others: Human growth hormone and prolactin secreting pituitary adenomas analyzed by in situ hybridization, Am J Pathol 134:605-613, 1989.
207. Lloyd RV, and others: The spectrum of ACTH-producing pituitary lesions, Am J Surg Pathol 10:618-626, 1986.
208. Lloyd RV, and others: Ectopic pituitary adenomas with normal anterior pituitary gland, Am J Surg Pathol 10:546-552, 1986.
209. Lloyd RV, and others: Analysis of endocrine active and clinically silent corticotropic adenomas by in situ hybridization, Am J Pathol 137:479-488, 1990.
210. Lloyd RV, Gikas PW, and Chandler WF: Prolactin and growth hormone producing pituitary adenomas. An immunohistochemical and ultrastructural study, Am J Surg Pathol 7:251-260, 1983.
211. Lloyd RV, and others: Analysis of pituitary hormones and chromogranin A mRNAs in null cell adenomas, oncocytomas, and gonadotroph adenomas by situ hybridization, Am J Pathol 139: 553-564, 1991.
212. Lloyd RV, and others: Analysis of the chromogranin A post-translational cleavage product pancreastatin and the prohormone convertases PC2 and PC3 in normal and neoplastic human pituitaries, Am J Pathol 146:1188-1198, 1995.

213. Love JG, and Blackburn CM: Association of intracranial meningioma with pituitary adenoma, Minnesota Med 37:335-336, 1955.
214. Luse SA, and Kernohan JW: Granular cell tumors of the stalk and posterior lobe of the pituitary gland, Cancer 8:616-622, 1955.
215. Maat-Schiemann MLC, and others: Malignant astrocytoma following radiotherapy for craniopharyngioma, Br J Radiol 48: 480-482, 1985.
216. Magiakou MA, and others: Cushing's syndrome in children and adolescents. Presentation, diagnosis, and therapy, N Engl J Med 331:629-636, 1994.
217. Magnani P, and others: Combined use of 111 in-labeled pentetreotide and three-step immunoscintigraphy with antichromogranin A monoclonal antibody in the diagnosis of pituitary adenomas, Cell Biophys 24-25:307-313, 1994.
218. Martinez AJ: The pathology of nonfunctional pituitary adenomas, Semin Diagn Pathol 3:83-94, 1986.
219. Martins AN, Hayes GJ, and Kempe LG: Invasive pituitary adenomas, J Neurosurg 22:268-276, 1965.
220. Marus G, Levin VC, and Rutherfoord GS: Malignant glioma following radiotherapy for unrelated primary tumors, Cancer 58:886-894, 1986.
221. Masunaga S-I, Ono K, and Abe M: A method for the selective measurement of the radiosensitivity of quiescent cells in solid tumors—combination of immunofluorescence staining of BrdU and micronucleus assay, Radiation Res 125:243-247, 1991.
222. Mathews W, and Wilson CB: Ectopic intrasellar chordoma: Case report, J Neurosurg 40:260, 1974.
223. Mayfield RK, and others: Lymphoid adenohypophysitis presenting as a pituitary tumor, Am J Med 69:619-623, 1980.
224. McComb DJ, and others: Subclinical adenomas of the human pituitary. New light on an old problem, Arch Pathol Lab Med 107:488, 1983.
225. McKeever PE, and Balentine JD: Nervous system. In Spicer SS, editor: Histochemistry in pathologic diagnosis, vol 22, Schwartz MK, editor: Clinical and biochemical analysis, New York, 1987, Marcel Dekker.
226. McKeever PE, and Blaivas M: Surgical pathology of the brain, spinal cord, and meninges. In Sternberg SS, and others, editors: Diagnostic surgical pathology, New York, 1994, Raven Press.
227. McKeever PE, Blaivas M, and Sima AAF: Neoplasms of the sellar region. In Lloyd RV, editor: Surgical pathology of the pituitary gland. Philadelphia, 1993, WB Saunders.
228. McKeever PE, and Brissie NT: Scanning electron microscopy of neoplasms removed at surgery: surface topography and comparison of meningioma, colloid cyst, ependymoma, pituitary adenoma, schwannoma and astrocytoma, J Neuropathol Exp Neurol 36:875-896, 1977.
229. McKeever PE, Davenport RD, and Shakui P: Patterns of antigenic expression of human glioma cells, Crit Rev Neurobiol 6: 119-147, 1991.
230. McKeever PE, and others: Refractory Cushing's disease caused by multinodular ACTH-cell hyperplasia, J Neuropathol Exp Neurol 41:490-499, 1982.
231. McKeever PE, and others: Stromal and nuclear markers for rapid identification of pituitary adenomas at biopsy, Arch Pathol Lab Med 109:509-514, 1985.
232. McKeever PE, and Spicer SS: The pituitary: contributions of cytochemistry to pathological diagnosis. In Spicer SS, editor: Histochemistry in pathologic diagnosis, New York, 1987, Marcel Dekker.
233. McNicoll AM: Patterns of corticotropic cells in the adult human pituitary in Cushing's disease, Diagn Histopathol 4:335-341, 1981.
234. Meichner RH, and others: Lymphocytic adenohypophysitis causing pituitary mass, Neurology 37:158-161, 1987.
235. Meis JM, and Giraldo AA: Chordoma: an immunohistochemical study of 20 cases, Arch Pathol Lab Med 112:553-556, 1988.
236. Melchionna RH, Moore RA: The pharyngeal pituitary gland, Am J Pathol 14:763-771, 1938.
237. Melmed S, and others: Pathophysiology of acromegaly, Endocrinol Rev 4:271-290, 1983.
238. Meredith JM, Mandeville FB, and Kay S: Osteogenic sarcoma of the skull following roentgen ray therapy for benign pituitary tumor, J Neurosurg 17:792-799, 1960.
239. Meyrignac C, and others: Meningiome post radique. Complication tardive de l'irradiation de la selle turcique, Nouv Presse Med 10:3246-3247, 1981.
240. Miettinen M, and others: Differential diagnosis of chordoma, chondroid, and ependymal tumors as aided by anti-intermediate filament antibodies, Am J Pathol 112:160-169, 1983.
241. Miller DC: Pathology of craniopharyngiomas: clinical import of pathological findings, Pediatr Neurosurg 21 Suppl 1:11-17, 1994.
242. Mills SE, and Fechner RE: Undifferentiated neoplasms of the sinonasal region: differential diagnosis based on clinical, light microscopic, immunohistochemical, and ultrastructural features, Semin Diagn Pathol 6:316-328, 1989.
243. Mills SE, and Frierson HF Jr: Olfactory neuroblastoma. A clinicopathologic study of 21 cases, Am J Surg Pathol 9:317-327, 1985.
244. Miyaguchi M, and others: Clinical and histopathological studies of olfactory neuroblastoma, Auris Nasus Larynx 16:157-163, 1989.
245. Modan B, and others: Radiation induced head and neck tumor, Lancet 1:277-279, 1974.
246. Molitch ME, and others: Bromocriptine as primary therapy for prolactin-secreting macroadenoma: results of a prospective multicenter study, J Clin Endocrinol Metab 60:698-705, 1985.
247. Moncrieff MW, and others: Congenital absence of pituitary gland and adrenal hypoplasia, Arch Dis Child 47:136-137, 1972.
248. Mori H, and others: Growth hormone-producing pituitary adenoma with crystal-like amyloid immunohistochemically positive for growth hormone, Cancer 55:96-102, 1985.
249. Mosca L, and others: Hypophyseal pathology in AIDS, Histol Histopathol 7:291-300, 1992.
250. Moseley RP, and others: Neoplastic meningitis in malignant melanoma: diagnosis with monoclonal antibodies, J Neurol Neurosurg Psychiatry 52:881-886, 1989.
251. Mosier HD: Hypoplasia of the pituitary and adrenal cortex, J Pediatr 48:633-639, 1956.
252. Murphy JK, O'Brien CJ, and Ironside JW: Morphologic and immunophenotypic characterization of primary brain lymphomas using paraffin-embedded tissue, Histopathology 15:449-460, 1989.
253. Nakajima T, and others: An immunoperoxidase study of S-100 protein distribution in normal and neoplastic tissues, Am J Surg Pathol 6:715-727, 1982.
254. Nakajima T, Yamaguchi H, and Takahashi K: S-100 protein in folliculostellate cells of the rat pituitary anterior lobe, Brain Res 191:523-531, 1980.
255. Nakamine H, and others: Non-Hodgkin's lymphoma involving the brain. Diagnostic usefulness of stereotactic needle biopsy in combination with paraffin-section immunohistochemistry, Acta Neuropathol (Berl) 78:462-471, 1989.
256. Nakamura Y, Becker LE, and Marks A: S-100 protein in human chordoma and human and rabbit notochord, Arch Pathol Lab Med 107:118-120, 1983.

257. Nakhleh RE, and others: Central nervous system lymphomas: immunohistochemical and clinicopathologic study of 26 autopsy cases, Arch Pathol Lab Med 113:1050-1056, 1989.
258. Neilson J McE, Moffat AD: Hypopituitarism caused by a melanoma of the pituitary gland, J Clin Pathol 16:144-149, 1963.
259. Nelson GA, and others: Malignant transformation in craniopharyngioma, Neurosurgery 22:427-429, 1988.
260. Nelson JS, and others: Necrosis as a prognostic criterion in malignant supratentorial, astrocytic gliomas, Cancer 52:550-554, 1983.
261. Nelson PB, Robinson AG, and Martinez AJ: Metastatic tumor of the pituitary gland, Neurosurgery 21:941-944, 1987.
262. Nemoto K, Ohnishi Y, and Tsukada T: Chronic lymphocytic leukemia showing pituitary tumor with massive leukemic cell infiltration, and special reference to clinicopathological findings of CLL, Acta Pathol Jpn 28:797, 1978.
263. Neumann PE, and others: Cytoplasmic filaments of Crooke's hyaline change belong to the cytokeratin class: an immunocytochemical and ultrastructural study, Am J Pathol 116:214-222, 1984.
264. Newton TH, Borhenne HJ, and Palubinskas AJ: Primary carcinoma of the pituitary, AJR 87:110-120, 1962.
265. Ng HK: Cytologic diagnosis of intracranial germinomas in smear preparations, Acta Cytol 39:693-697, 1995.
266. Ng HK, and others: Intracranial olfactory neuroblastoma mimicking carcinoma: report of two cases, Histopathology 12:393-403, 1988.
267. Nikitovitch-Winer MB, Atkin J, and Maley BE: Colocalization of prolactin and growth hormone within specific adenohypophyseal cells in male, female and lactating female rats, Endocrinology 121:625-631, 1987.
268. Nishiyama A, and others: An immunohistochemical analysis of T cells in primary B cell malignant lymphoma of the brain, Acta Neuropathol (Berl) 79:27-29, 1989.
269. Norgaard-Pedersen B, and others: Alpha-fetoprotein and human chorionic gonadotropin in a patient with a primary intracranial germ cell tumor, Cancer 41:2315-2320, 1978.
270. Nyquist P, Laws ER Jr, and Elliott E: Novel features of tumors that secrete both growth hormone and prolactin in acromegaly, Neurosurgery 35:179-183, 1994.
271. Obenchain TG, and Becker DP: Abscess formation in a Rathke's cleft cyst. Case Report, J Neurosurg 36:359-362, 1972.
272. O'Donovan DG, and Kell P: Malignant granular cell tumor with intraperitoneal dissemination, Histopathology 14:417-428, 1989.
273. Okajima K, Honda I, and Kitagawa T: Immunohistochemical distribution of S-100 protein in tumors and tumor-like lesions of bone and cartilage, Cancer 61:792-799, 1988.
274. Oldfield EH, and others: Preoperative lateralization of ACTH-secreting pituitary microadenomas by bilateral and simultaneous inferior petrosal venous sinus sampling, N Engl J Med 312: 100-103, 1985.
275. Ono N, and others: Diagnosis of germinal neoplasm in the thalamus and basal ganglia, Surg Neurol 26:24-28, 1986.
276. Osamura RY: Functional prenatal development of anencephalic and normal anterior pituitary glands in human and experimental animals studied by peroxidase-labeled antibody method, Acta Pathol Jpn 27:495-509, 1977.
277. Osamura RY, and Watanabe K: Histogenesis of the cells of the anterior and intermediate lobes of human pituitary glands: Immunohistochemical studies, Int Rev Cytol 95:103-129, 1985.
278. Osamura RY, and Watanabe K: Immunohistochemical colocalization of growth hormone (GH) and alpha-subunit in human GH secreting pituitary adenomas, Virchows Arch 411:323-330, 1987.
279. Packer RJ, and others: Intracranial embryonal cell carcinoma, Cancer 54:520-524, 1984.
280. Page RB, and others: Intrasellar mixed germ-cell tumor: Case report, J Neurosurg 58:766, 1983.
281. Paine JT, and others: Suprasellar germinoma with shunt metastasis: Report of a case with an immunohistochemical characterization of the lymphocyte subpopulations, Surg Neurol 25:55-61, 1986.
282. Papo I, and others: Angioblastic parasellar extradural tumours, Acta Neurochir, Suppl 28:438-444, 1979.
283. Pardo-Mindan FJ, and others: A comparative ultrastructural study of chondrosarcoma, chordoid sarcoma, and chordoma, Cancer 47:2611-2619, 1981.
284. Parent AD, Brown B, and Smith EE: Incidental pituitary adenomas: a retrospective study, Surgery 92:880-883, 1982.
285. Pask SG, and Uzmanova RR: On primary multiple brain tumours, Zdravookhr Kazakhstana 8:42-43, 1965.
286. Patrick AW, and others: Primary cerebral lymphoma presenting with cranial diabetes insipidus, Postgrad Med J 65:771-772, 1989.
287. Pelletier G, Robert F, and Hardy J: Identification of human anterior pituitary cells by immunoelectron microscopy, J Clin Endocrinol Metab 46:534-542, 1978.
288. Perentes E, and Rubinstein LJ: Immunohistochemical recognition of human neuroepithelial tumors by anti-Leu 7 (HNK-1) monoclonal antibody, Acta Neuropathol (Berl) 69:227-233, 1986.
289. Perentes E, and Rubinstein LJ: Recent applications of immunoperoxidase histochemistry in human neuro-oncology. An update, Arch Pathol Lab Med 111:796-812, 1987.
290. Perzin KH, and Pushparaj N: Nonepithelial tumors of the nasal cavity, paranasal sinuses, and nasopharynx, Cancer 57:784-796, 1986.
291. Peters FT, Keuning JJ, and deRooy HA: Primary cerebral malignant lymphoma with endocrine defect. Case report and review of the literature, Neth J Med 29:406-410, 1986.
292. Petito CK, DeGirolami U, and Earle KM: Craniopharyngiomas, Cancer 37:1944-1952, 1976.
293. Piatt JH Jr, and others: Glioblastoma multiforme after radiotherapy for acromegaly, Neurosurgery 13:85-89, 1983.
294. Pieterse S, Dinning TAR, and Blumbergs PC: Postirradiation sarcomatous transformation of a pituitary adenoma; a combined pituitary tumor, J Neurosurg 56:283-286, 1982.
295. Pioro EP, and others: Combined thyrotroph and lactotroph cell hyperplasia simulating prolactin-secreting pituitary adenoma in long-standing primary hypothyroidism, Surg Neurol 29:218-226, 1988.
296. Pixley S, Weiss M, and Melmed S: Identification of human growth hormone messenger ribonucleic acid in pituitary adenoma cells by in situ hybridization, J Clin Endocrinol Metab 65:575-580, 1987.
297. Poon M-C, and others: Multiple myeloma masquerading as chromophobe adenoma, Cancer 43:1513-1516, 1979.
298. Portocarrero CJ, and others: Lymphoid hypophysitis: an unusual cause of hyperprolactinemia and enlarged sella turcica, JAMA 246:1811-1812, 1981.
299. Post KD, and others: Metastatic carcinoma to pituitary adenoma. Report of two cases, Surg Neurol 30:286-292, 1988.
300. Powell HC, Marshall LF, and Ignelzi RJ: Post-irradiation pituitary sarcoma, Acta Neuropathol (Berl) 39:165-167, 1977.
301. Probst VA: Kombination eines Cushing-Syndromes, Hypophysenadenoms und suprasellaren Meningeoms, Fallbericht Abl Neurochir 32:75-82, 1971.
302. Puchner MJ, and others: Cushing's disease in a child caused by a corticotropin-releasing hormone-secreting intrasellar gangliocytoma associated with an adrenocorticotropic hormone-secreting pituitary adenoma, Neurosurgery 33:920-924, 1993.
303. Reid JD: Congenital absence of the pituitary gland, J Pediatr 56:658-664, 1960.
304. Reznik M, and others: Neuroendocrine tumor of the nasal cav-

ity (esthesioneuroblastoma). Apropos of a case with paraneoplastic Cushing's syndrome, Ann Pathol 7:137-142, 1987.
305. Richmond I, and Wilson CB: Parasellar tumors in children. I. Clinical presentation, preoperative assessment, and differential diagnosis, Child's Brain 7:73-84, 1980.
306. Rickards AG, and Harvey PW: "Giant cell granuloma" and the other pituitary granulomata, QJM 47:425-440, 1954.
307. Rigolosi RS, Schwartz E, and Glick SM: Occurrence of growth-hormone deficiency in acromegaly as a result of pituitary apoplexy, N Engl J Med 279:362-364, 1968.
308. Robert F, and Hardy J: Human corticotroph cell adenomas, Semin Diagn Pathol 3:34-41, 1986.
309. Rodas RA, Erkman-Balis B, and Cahill DW: Late intracranial metastasis from esthesioneuroblastoma: case report and review of the literature, Neurosurgery 19:622-627, 1986.
310. Roggli VL, and others: Pituitary microadenoma and primary lymphoma of brain associated with hypothalamic invasion, Am J Clin Pathol 71:724-727.
311. Roos B: Isolated melanoma of the pituitary, Fortschr Hals Nasen Ohrenheilkd 12:193-198, 1965.
312. Rosa P, and others: Widespread occurrence of chromogranins/secretogranins in the matrix of secondary granules of endocrinologically silent pituitary adenomas, J Histochem Cytochem 40:523-533, 1992.
313. Rosengren JE, and others: Radiographic features of olfactory neuroblastoma, Am J Roentgenol 132:945-948, 1979.
314. Reference deleted in proofs.
315. Rovit RL, and Fein JM: Pituitary apoplexy: a review and reappraisal, J Neurosurg 37:280-288, 1972.
316. Rubinstein LJ: Tumors of the central nervous system. In Atlas of tumor pathology, 2nd series, fascicle 6, Washington, DC, 1972, Armed Forces Institute of Pathology.
317. Russell DS, and Rubinstein LJ: Pathology of tumours of the nervous system, London, 1988, Williams & Wilkins.
318. Rutherford GS, and Davies AG: Chordomas—ultrastructure and immunohistochemistry: a report based on the examination of six cases, Histopathology 11:775-787, 1987.
319. Saeger W, and Ludecke DK: Pituitary adenomas with hyperfunction of TSH. Frequency, histological classification, immunocytochemistry and ultrastructure, Virchows Arch [A] 394: 255-267, 1982.
320. Saeger W, and others: Electron microscopical morphometry of GH-producing pituitary adenomas in comparison with normal GH cells, Virchows Arch [A] 411:467-472, 1987.
321. Saito T, and others: Tumor-infiltrating lymphocytes and histocompatibility antigens in primary intracranial germinomas, J Neurosurg 70:81-85, 1989.
322. Saitoh Y, and others: Accumulation of amyloid in pituitary adenomas, Acta Neuropathol (Berl) 68:87-92, 1985.
323. Salazar H, and others: The human hypophysis in anencephaly. I. Ultrastructure of the pars distalis, Arch Pathol 87:201-211, 1969.
324. Salisbury JR, and Isaacson PG: Demonstration of cytokeratins and an epithelial membrane antigen in chordomas and human fetal blood, Am J Surg Pathol 9:791-797, 1985.
325. Salyer D, and Carter D: Squamous carcinoma arising in the pituitary gland, Cancer 31:713-718, 1973.
326. Sano T, and others: Pituitary pathology in acquired immunodeficiency syndrome, Arch Pathol Lab Med 113:1066-1070, 1989.
327. Sano T, and Yamada S: Histologic and immunohistochemical study of clinically nonfunctioning pituitary adenomas: special reference to gonadotropin-positive adenomas, Pathol Int 44: 697-703, 1994.
328. Sarwar M: Primary sellar-parasellar esthesioneuroblastoma, AJR 133:140-141, 1979.
329. Sawamura Y, and others: Immunohistochemical and in vitro functional analysis of pineal-germinoma infiltrating lymphocytes: report of a case, Neurosurgery 25:454-457, 1989.
330. Scheithauer BW, and others: Pathology of invasive pituitary tumors with special reference to functional classification, J Neurosurg 65:733-744, 1986.
331. Scheithauer BW, Kovacs K, and Randall RV: The pituitary gland in untreated Addison's disease. A histologic and immunocytologic study of 18 adenohypophyses, Arch Pathol Lab Med 107: 484-487, 1983.
332. Scheithauer BW, and others: Pathology of excessive production of growth hormone, Clin Endocrinol Metab 15:655-681, 1986.
333. Scheithauer BW, and others: Hypothalamic neuronal hamartoma and adenohypophyseal neuronal choristoma: Their association with growth hormone adenoma of the pituitary gland, J Neuropathol Exp Neurol 42:633-663, 1983.
334. Schmitt FC, and Bacchi CE: S-100 protein: Is it useful as a tumor marker in diagnostic immunocytochemistry? Histopathology 15:281-288, 1989.
335. Schmitt HP: Rapid anaplastic transformation in gliomas of adulthood. "Selection" in neuro-oncogenesis, Pathol Res Pract 176:313-318, 1983.
336. Schochet SS Jr and others: Intracranial esthesioneuroblastoma. A light and electron microscopic study, Acta Neuropathol (Berl) 31:181-189, 1975.
337. Scholtz CL, and Siu K: Melanoma of pituitary. Case report, J Neurosurg 45:101-103, 1976.
338. Scothorne CM: Glioma of the posterior lobe of the pituitary gland, J Pathol 69:109-112, 1955.
339. Sham JST, and others: Cranial nerve involvement and base of the skull erosion in nasopharyngeal carcinoma, Cancer 68:422-426, 1991.
340. Shanmugaratham K, and others: Histopathology of nasopharyngeal carcinoma. Correlations with epidemiology, survival rates and other biological characteristics, Cancer 44:1029-1044, 1979.
341. Sheehan HL, and Stanfield JP: The pathogenesis of post-partum necrosis of the anterior lobe of the pituitary gland, Acta Endocrinol (Copenh) 37:479-510, 1961.
342. Sheehan HL, and Whitehead R: The neurohypophysis in post-partum hypopituitarism, J Pathol 85:145-169, 1963.
343. Sheldon WH, Golden A, and Bondy PK: Cushing's syndrome produced by a pituitary basophil carcinoma with hepatic metastasis, Am J Med 17:134-142, 1954.
344. Shen DY, and others: Primary intrasellar germinoma in a woman presenting with secondary amenorrhea and hyperprolactinemia, Neurosurgery 15:417-420, 1984.
345. Sherry SH, and others: Concurrent production of adrenocorticotropin and prolactin from two distinct cell lines in a single pituitary adenoma: A detailed immunohistochemical analysis, J Clin Endocrinol Metab 55:947-955, 1982.
346. Shi T, Farrell MA, and Kaufman JCE: Fibrosarcoma complicating irradiated pituitary adenoma, Surg Neurol 22:277-283, 1984.
347. Shibata S: Sites of origin of primary intracerebral malignant lymphoma, Neurosurgery 25:14-19, 1989.
348. Shinbor T, and others: An autopsy case of malignant melanoma possibly originating in the sphenoid sinus, Rinsho Shinkeigaku 28:636-642, 1988.
349. Shoup SA, and others: A panel of antibodies useful in the cytologic diagnosis of metastatic melanoma, Acta Cytol 34:385-392, 1990.
350. Shuangshoti S: Combined occurrence of third ventricular germinoma and hypothalamic mixed glioma, J Surg Oncol 31:148-152, 1986.
351. Slowik F, and others: Intrasellar hamartoma associated with pituitary adenoma, Acta Neuropathol 80:328-333, 1990.
352. Slowik F, and Jellinger K: Membranous changes in primary malignant CNS lymphomas, Acta Neuropathol 79:86-93, 1989.

353. Sobrinho-Simoes M, and others: Lymphoid hypophysitis in a patient with lymphoid thyroiditis, lymphoid adrenalitis and idiopathic retroperitoneal fibrosis, Arch Pathol Lab Med 109: 230-233, 1985.
354. Sogg RL, Donaldson SS, and Yorke CH: Malignant astrocytoma following radiotherapy of a craniopharyngioma, J Neurosurg 48:622-627, 1978.
355. Solero CL, Giombini S, and Morello G: Suprasellar and olfactory meningiomas. Report on a series of 153 personal cases, Acta Neurochir 67:181-194, 1983.
356. Spada A, and others: Clinical, biochemical and morphological correlates in patients bearing growth hormone-secreting pituitary tumors with or without constitutively active adenylyl cyclase, J Clin Endocrinol Metab 71:1421-1426, 1990.
357. Spalke G, Mennel HD, and Martin G: Histogenesis of olfactory neuroblastoma. I. Electron microscopy of typical human case, Pathol Res Pract 180:516-520, 1985.
358. Spallone A: Meningioma as a sequel of radiotherapy for pituitary adenoma, Neurochirurgia 25:68-72, 1982.
359. Sparagana M, and others: Osteogenic sarcoma of the skull: a rare sequela of pituitary irradiation, Cancer 29:3176-1379, 1972.
360. Steiner MM, and Boggs JD: Absence of pituitary gland, hypothyroidism, hypoadrenalism and hypogonadism in a 17-year-old dwarf, J Clin Endocrinol Metab 25:1591-1598, 1965.
361. Stephenson G, and Afshar F: Suprasellar cavernous angioma causing pituitary and hypothalamic dysfunction, Br J Neurosurg 8:225-227, 1994.
362. Stock JM, Ghatak NR, and Oppenheimer JH: Unsuspected meningioma in a patient with pituitary gigantism. Case report with autopsy findings, Metabolism 24:767-775, 1975.
363. Storkreef JC, Reifel CS, and Shin SH: A possible phagocytic role for folliculostellate cells of anterior pituitary following estrogen withdrawal from primed male rats, Cell Tissue Res 243:255-261, 1986.
364. Suda Y, and others: Malignant astrocytoma following radiotherapy in pituitary adenoma: Case report, No Shinkei Geka 17:783-788, 1989.
365. Sugita K, and others: Cornelia de Lange syndrome associated with a suprasellar germinoma, Brain Dev 8:541-546, 1986.
366. Szeifert GT, and others: Pathological characteristics of surgically removed craniopharyngiomas: analysis of 131 cases, Acta Neurochir (Wien) 124:139-143, 1993.
367. Tachibana O, and others: Immunohistochemical expression of human chorionic gonadotropin and P-glycoprotein in human pituitary glands and craniopharyngiomas, J Neurosurg 80:79-84, 1994.
368. Takahashi H, and others: Esthesioneuroepithelioma: a tumor of true olfactory epithelium origin. An ultrastructural and immunohistochemical study, Acta Neuropathol (Berl) 75:147-155, 1987.
369. Takahashi H, and others: Esthesioneuroblastoma: a nasal catecholamine-producing tumor of neural crest origin. Demonstration of tyrosine hydroxylase-immunoreactive tumor cells, Acta Neuropathol (Berl) 76:522-527, 1988.
370. Taxy JB, and others: The spectrum of olfactory neural tumors. A light-microscopic immunohistochemical and ultrastructural analysis, Am J Surg Pathol 10:687-695, 1986.
371. Teears RJ, and Silverman EM: Clinicopathologic review of 88 cases of carcinoma metastatic to the pituitary gland, Cancer 36: 216-220, 1975.
372. Teramoto A, and others: Incidental pituitary lesions in 1,000 unselected autopsy specimens, Radiology 193:161-164, 1994.
373. Terry RD, Hyams VJ, and Davidoff LM: Combined nonmetastasizing fibrosarcoma and chromophobe tumour of the pituitary, Cancer 12:791-798, 1959.
374. Thorner MO, and others: Somatotroph hyperplasia: successful treatment of acromegaly by removal of the pancreatic islet tumor secreting a growth hormone-releasing factor, J Clin Invest 70:965-977, 1982.
375. Thunold S, Von Eyben FE, and Maehle B: Malignant granular cell tumor of the neck: immunohistochemical and ultrastructural studies of a case, Histopathology 14:655-662, 1989.
376. Tindall GT, and others: Human prolactin-producing adenomas and bromocriptine: a histological, immunocytochemical, ultrastructural and morphometric study, J Clin Endocrinol Metab 55:1178-1183, 1982.
377. Trojanowsky JQ, and others: Neuronal origin of human esthesioneuroblastoma demonstrated with antineurofilament monoclonal antibodies, N Engl J Med 307:159-161, 1982.
378. Trouillas J, and others: Morphological and biochemical relationships in 31 human pituitary adenomas with acromegaly, Virchows Arch 389:127-142, 1980.
379. Trouillas J, and others: Human pituitary gonadotropic adenoma: histological, immunocytochemical, ultrastructural and hormonal studies in 8 cases, J Pathol 135:315-336, 1981.
380. Urbanski SF, and others: Intrasellar solitary plasmacytoma terminating in multiple myeloma: a report of a case including electron microscopical study, Surg Neurol 14:233-236, 1980.
381. Ushio Y, and others: Glioblastoma after radiotherapy for craniopharyngioma: Case report, Neurosurgery 21:33-38, 1987.
382. van der Lely AJ, and others: Nasopharyngeal presentation of pituitary tumors. Differential diagnosis and treatment, J Clin Endocrinol Metab 74:811-813, 1992.
383. Vaquero J, and others: Immunohistochemical study of natural killer cells in tumor-infiltrating lymphocytes of primary intracranial germinomas, J Neurosurg 72:616-618, 1990.
384. Vaquero J, and others: Granular pituicytomas of the pituitary stalk, Acta Neurochir 59:209-215, 1981.
385. Vesely DL, Maldonodo A, and Levey GS: Partial hypopituitarism and possible hypothalamic involvement in sarcoidosis. Report of a case and review of the literature, Am J Med 62:425-431, 1977.
386. Volpe R, and Mazabraud A: A clinicopathologic review of 25 cases of chordoma, Am J Surg Pathol 7:161-170, 1983.
387. Waltz TA, and Brownell B: Sarcoma: A possible late result of effective radiation therapy for pituitary adenoma. Report on two cases, J Neurosurg 24:901-907, 1966.
388. Wara WM, and others: Tumors of the pineal and suprasellar region: Childrens Cancer Study Group treatment results 1960-1975, Cancer 43:698-701, 1979.
389. Warnke RA, and others: Diagnosis of human lymphoma with monoclonal antileukocyte antibodies, N Engl J Med 309:1275-1281, 1983.
390. Webb SM, and others: Computerized tomography versus magnetic resonance imaging: a comparative study in hypothalamic-pituitary and parasellar pathology, Clin Endocrinol (Oxf) 36: 459-465, 1992.
391. Weiss SW, Langloss JM, and Enzinger FM: Value of S-100 protein in the diagnosis of soft tissue tumors with particular reference to benign and malignant Schwann cell tumors, Lab Invest 3:299-308, 1983.
392. White MC, and others: Heterogeneity of prolactin responses to estradiol benzoate in women with prolactinoma, Lancet I:1394-1396, 1981.
393. Wick MR, Stanley SJ, and Swanson PE: Immunohistochemical diagnosis of sinonasal melanoma, carcinoma, and neuroblastoma with monoclonal antibodies HMB-45 and anti-synaptophysin, Arch Pathol Lab Med 112:616-620, 1988.
394. Wick MR, Swanson PE, and Manivel JC: Placental-like alkaline phosphatase reactivity in human tumors: an immunohistochemical study of 520 cases, Hum Pathol 18:946-954, 1987.

395. Willis RA: Pathological study of tumors of the pituitary region, Med J Aust 1:281-291, 1938.

396. Wong K, and others: Pituitary adenoma as an unsuspected clival tumor, Am J Surg Pathol 19:900-903, 1995.

397. Yagishita S, and others: Follico-stellate cell adenoma of the pituitary: a light- and electron-microscopic study, Acta Neuropathol (Berl) 62:340-344, 1984.

398. Yamada K, and others: Coincidental pituitary adenoma and parasellar meningioma. Case report, Neurosurgery 19:267-270, 1986.

399. Yamada S, and others: Growth hormone and prolactin gene expression in human densely and sparsely granulated somatotroph adenomas by in situ hybridization with digoxigenin-labeled probes, Diagn Mol Pathol 3:46-52, 1994.

400. Yamagami T, and others: An immunohistochemical study of intracranial germ cell tumours, Acta Neurochir 86:33-41, 1987.

401. Zampieri P, and others: Radiation-associated cerebral gliomas. A report of two cases and review of the literature, J Neurosurg Sci 33:271-279, 1989.

402. Zülch KJ: Histological typing of tumors of the central nervous system. International Histological Classification of Tumours, Geneva, Switzerland, 1979, World Health Organization.

C • H • A • P • T • E • R

# 6

# Vascular Diseases

**Julio H. Garcia**
**Hernando Mena**



The rubric *vascular diseases of the CNS* covers a large group of disorders that lead to the development of one of these abnormalities in the brain: ischemia, edema, and hemorrhage. In a significant number of instances, the etiology of these abnormalities can be traced to diseases of the blood vessels, in particular those in the arterial tree. However, other factors such as hematologic abnormalities and hemodynamic alterations also can induce ischemic and hemorrhagic injuries to the CNS. For didactic purposes the description of diagnosis of diseases covered in this chapter is separated into: (1) ischemic disorders, (2) hemorrhages (intracerebral and subarachnoid), (3) edema associated with ischemic and hemorrhagic injuries to the brain, and (4) selected angiopathies of the CNS.

Increased interest in stroke has followed the report of the successful therapeutic intervention with a thrombolytic agent (tissue plasminogen activator) in a discrete group of stroke patients.[305] The term *stroke* is used in the medical literature with two different connotations. Applied to an individual patient, stroke describes the development of a focal neurologic deficit that on account of its suddenness is thought to be the result of a vascular event, i.e., occlusion or rupture of a brain vessel. In the epidemiologic literature, stroke is used as a generic designation for several groups of diseases. These are: ischemic strokes, intracerebral hemorrhage, subarachnoid hemorrhage, and miscellaneous disorders. The latter category includes a relatively small group of patients who eventually are diagnosed as having CNS neoplasms, demyelinating diseases, and migrainous attacks. Stroke, as defined

**Table 6-1.** Ischemic Disorders

| |
|---|
| Secondary to Hemodynamic Crises (Global) |
| Subcortical Arteriosclerotic Leukoencephalopathy |
| Secondary to Arterial Occlusions (Focal) |
| Brain Infarcts: Anemic, Hemorrhagic |
| Venous Infarcts |
| Incomplete Brain Infarcts |
| Ischemic Lesions of the Spinal Cord |
| Lacunes |

above, is the third most important cause of death and the outstanding cause of disability in the US and other industrialized countries.[257] Ischemic events secondary to arterial occlusions are the leading cause of strokes; among these, the lacunae or lacunar lesions are the most common.[196]

## ISCHEMIC DISORDERS (Table 6-1)

Ischemia, or inadequate blood supply, can be categorized according to its severity. Moderate ischemia refers to a 40% to 50% decrease in the normal average cerebral blood flow (55 ml/100 gm/min). A decrease in the cerebral blood flow (CBF) of 75% or greater is considered severe ischemia. The tolerable period of time after which reversibility of the functional loss can be achieved is directly proportional to the degree to which CBF decreases.[127] Depending on the etiology, two kinds of ischemic conditions can affect the CNS: (1) those secondary to hemodynamic crises, such as exist during hypotensive episodes and transient cardiac arrest, and (2) ischemic events caused by the occlusion of one or more cerebral arteries.

### Ischemic Injuries of Hemodynamic Origin

The autoregulatory capacity of the brain, which keeps constant an average CBF of 55 ml/100 g/min, is lost in normotensive individuals when the mean arterial blood pressure drops below 60 mm Hg.[164] Cardiac arrest, severe hypotension, cardiac dysrhythmias, and cardiac valve disease can all result in insufficient blood flow to the CNS. Because under these circumstances the ischemic conditions apply to the entire CNS, this type of ischemic injury is called *global* to differentiate it from the focal injury induced by an arterial occlusion. Either of the two events, if severe enough, can induce brain *infarctions*. These are defined as areas of coagulation necrosis caused by an ischemic event, usually secondary to an arterial occlusion.[70] However, there are significant differences in the patterns of brain injury that result from these two types of ischemia, global and focal.

The global nature of the injury produced by a transient cardiac arrest does not result in a uniform or predictable pattern of brain lesions. The reasons for this are twofold: (1) the architecture of the arterial tree supplying the CNS, and (2) the differential vulnerability of selected neuronal groups.[269,287]

**Angioarchitectonic factors.** The pattern of arterial supply to the brain and spinal cord determines that certain areas of the CNS parenchyma will be marginally irrigated by blood during a hypotensive crisis. These regions are called *arterial border zones* ("watershed areas") or *boundary zones*. In the cerebral hemispheres, the region situated between the end of the MCA and the ACA territories is an area where ischemic lesions are likely to be more pronounced, probably because during a hypotensive crisis the regional CBF drops at these sites to lower levels than noted in the rest of the brain. Comparable areas of increased vulnerability to the effects of global ischemia exist in the cerebellum and in the spinal cord. The midthoracic segments of the cord are supplied by the terminal branches of the anterior spinal artery (from above) and the terminal branches of the large radicular artery of Adamkiewicz (from below). Therefore, during a hypotensive crisis this segment of the cord is more likely to be more severely injured than is the rest of the cord. Different patterns of blood supply exist in the cortex, basal ganglia, and cerebral white matter. The penetrating branches that irrigate the cortex have abundant anastomotic connections, whereas the long penetrating arterioles that supply the cerebral white matter are considered terminal vessels because they do not anastomose with one another. The lenticulostriate arteries that irrigate the basal ganglia are also terminal vessels devoid of anastomotic connections. For this reason, it is likely that during hypotensive crises the cerebral white matter and the basal ganglia are more vulnerable to the effects of global ischemia than is the rest of the brain.

**Selective vulnerability.** The designation *selective vulnerability* applies to the selective injury of isolated neuronal groups in response to systemic conditions such as global ischemia and hypoglycemia that presumably affect all cells equally. Vogt and Vogt[319] introduced the concept of selective vulnerability to the hippocampus as well as groups of neurons such as the cerebellar Purkinje cells, neurons in layers 3 to 5 of the cerebral neocortex, and neurons of the globus pallidum, among many others. The reason for this selective destruction of cells that do not share a common arterial supply prompted Spatz[287] and Scholz[269] to suggest that there may be intrinsic (or topistic) characteristics in these neuronal groups that make them uniquely vulnerable to an ischemic injury that does not affect other neurons located in the same region.

Experimentally, forebrain ischemia secondary to bilateral carotid artery clamping of 5-minutes' duration induces *delayed neuronal injury* in the hippocampus of gerbils and rats.[154] The number of necrotic neurons in the CA-1 sector of the hippocampus increases in these experiments in proportion to the duration of the postischemic period. Brains from experiments terminated on day 4 have more abundant necrotic neurons than do those from experiments terminated on day 1.[154] Comparable effects may exist in human brains of survivors of cardiac arrest. In autopsy specimens of these patients, the extent of the hippocampal injury was greater in those who survived a longer time after the transient episode of global ischemia.[232] A possible explanation for the selective vulnerability of the hippocampal neurons is offered by the observation that forebrain ischemia in gerbils raises by several fold the interstitial concentration of glutamate.[25] The neurons of the CA-1 sector of the hippocampus are glutamatergic; therefore, it is assumed that these cells are particularly susceptible to the effects of ischemia because glutamate facilitates the intracellular uptake of $Ca^{++}$, which in excessive concentrations is lethal to the mitochondria.[278]

### Global Ischemia: Effects on the Central Nervous System

Several clinical conditions can result in global injury to the brain through a combination of hypoxic-ischemic disturbances. These include transient cardiac arrest, severe hypotension, increased intracranial pressure (of the type commonly observed in victims of head trauma), open-heart surgery, subarachnoid hemorrhage, hanging, strangulation, and near drowning.[99] The neurologic syndromes observed in patients who develop brain injuries localized to the watershed areas, or arterial boundary zones, vary according to the topographic distribution of the lesions. The most frequently observed syndrome is attributed to the involvement by the ischemic injury of brain regions located in the border zone stradling the territories of the anterior and middle cerebral arteries. Bilateral cerebral lesions at these sites are responsible for a syndrome of bilateral brachial paralysis with maximum involvement of the proximal limb muscles. The neurologic deficits thus induced have been described under the designation of "man-in-a-barrel" syndrome. Several other syndromes are described in association with injuries in other cerebral locations.[178] The pathogenesis of the arterial border zone infarct in human brains includes three different categories: (1) global ischemia; (2) multiple small emboli into the territory of the internal carotid artery; and (3) idiopathic causes.[308] The time limits of reversibility after a severe global ischemic crisis generally are said to be 4 to 6 minutes. However, this applies only to adult normothermic persons. Under hypothermic conditions, complete recovery of neurologic function has been documented in at least two instances of cardiac arrest that lasted 35 minutes.[274] In a group of 8 patients who were resuscitated after suffering out-of-the-hospital cardiac arrest, neuroimaging studies performed 2 to 6 days later showed bilateral symmetrical, partly hemorrhagic brain lesions (infarctions ?) involving basal ganglia, thalamic nuclei, and substantia nigra.[92a] The clinical sequelae of global ischemia include transient or persistent amnestic syndromes, miscellaneous motor deficits, cortical blindness, cerebellar ataxia, dystonias, involuntary movements, and several others. Each of these syndromes develops secondary to the involvement by the ischemic injury of specific brain regions. For example, ataxia predominates among patients who suffer primary injury to the cerebellum. Systemic hypoxic-ischemic conditions also develop in premature newborns through a combination of the inability of the immature lung to appropriately oxygenate blood and the accompanying hypotensive crises that characterize this condition. In children who suffer hypoxic-ischemic injuries to the brain during the perinatal period, the resulting clinical syndrome frequently is designated cerebral palsy.[320]

The morphologic changes induced in the brain by global ischemia are influenced primarily by the time elapsed after the injury. In the immediate postischemic period the brain is markedly swollen, and the large blood vessels are dilated and hyperemic (Figs. 6-1, 6-2). This results in an increase in brain weight accompanied by narrowing of the sulci and of the ventricular caliber. The abundant erythrocytes filling the lumen of distended small blood vessels impart a dark grayish discoloration to the cortical ribbon. This is particularly pronounced at the bottom of the cerebral gyri and in multiple scattered sites of the cerebellar cortex[97] (Fig. 6-1). Among persons who survive days or weeks after the ischemic event, the structural abnormalities affecting the brain include patterns of tissue injury known as laminar necrosis, hippocampal sclerosis, granular atrophy, and subcortical leukoencephalopathy. In neonates and young children, the brain lesions of presumed hypoxic-ischemic origin include germinal matrix hemorrhages, pontosubicular necrosis, periventricular leukomalacia, multicystic encephalomalacia, ulegyria, and status marmoratus.[107a]

*Laminar or pseudolaminar necrosis* describes a pattern of brain injury in which layers 3 to 5 of the cerebral cortex are preferentially or more severely injured after a global hypoxic-ischemic event. The pattern of laminar necrosis may be more pronounced in the arterial boundary zones, but frequently the lesions are randomly distributed (Fig. 6-3). At the site of the injury there is necrosis of variable numbers of neurons (selective neuronal injury) and astroglia with or without macrophage infiltration. In many instances the most superficial layer of the cerebral cortex (i.e., the molecu-

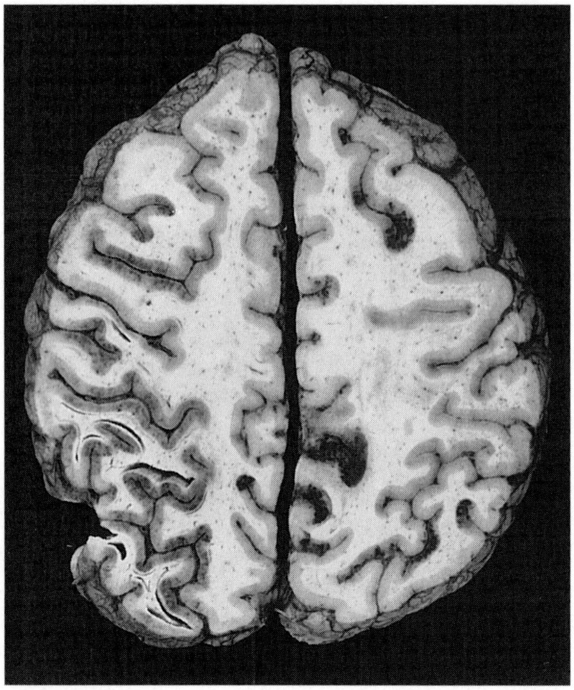

**Fig. 6-1.** Axial view of the cerebral hemispheres. Demonstration of the diffuse pattern of cortical injury. Global ischemia (transient cardiac arrest) occurred 3 days before death. Hyperemic vessels and petechial hemorrhages are visible throughout.

lar layer) survives the ischemic injury. The layered pattern of necrosis of the cerebral cortex spreading over several adjacent gyri accounts for the designation of laminar necrosis. In addition to the injury to the neocortex, global ischemic crises also can affect the cerebellum, the basal ganglia, the brainstem, and the spinal cord. Frequently, regardless of the location, the lesions of global ischemia are bilateral and relatively symmetric in distribution. In an individual case it is extremely difficult to predict in the acute postictal state the extent or the distribution of the lesions. Probably this is because in addition to the duration of the ischemic event, many factors, including the age of the patient, the condition of the vascular tree, body temperature, and levels of serum glucose at the time of injury, can all influence the consequences of a global ischemic episode.[258] Furthermore, after re-establishing circulation, many areas remain hypoperfused for reasons that are not fully defined. The duration of this "postischemic hypoperfusion" (also known as "no-reflow" phenomenon) is another factor that influences the outcome of a global ischemic crisis.

***Hippocampal sclerosis.*** Selective injury to the neurons of the CA-1 sector and the end folium of the hippocampus accompanied by gliosis was originally observed at autopsy in the brains of persons who had a longstanding history of chronic epilepsy.[285] The presumed causes of this injury in these patients are the repeated apneic episodes that accompany severe epileptic events. This is the assumption made from the observation that global ischemia and hypoglycemia also can selectively injure the neurons in the Sommer sector or CA-1 sector.[210] The proliferation of astrocytes at the site of neuronal necrosis forms a scar that explains the designation of hippocampal sclerosis, which is the most frequent pathologic finding in patients with temporal lobe epilepsy. This type of injury has been presumed to be the result of perinatal hypoxemic events, and for over a century it has been debated widely whether hippocampal sclerosis can be the cause, but not the result, of temporal lobe seizures. A recent study of a large number of temporal lobe specimens, surgically resected from patients with temporal lobe seizures, revealed findings that the authors interpreted as supporting the hypothesis that hippocampal sclerosis and granule cell dispersion are not the consequence of repetitive seizures beginning at an early developmental age but that the changes are the most likely cause of epilepsy in these patients.[181]

*Periventricular leukomalacia (PVL)* describes areas of coagulation necrosis involving the periventricular white matter of the cerebral hemispheres and the centrum semiovale. PVL affects premature newborns and frequently coexists with subependymal germinal matrix hemorrhages. The etiology of PVL is incompletely defined, but most authors opine that PVL is the result of an undefined metabolic disorder associated with ischemic conditions that affect watershed areas in the cerebral white matter. Neonatal hypoxemia and hypotension are the main risk factors for PVL.[321] The issue is fully discussed in Chapter 13 of this book.

*Pontosubicular necrosis (PSN)* originally was described as neuronal necrosis involving the subiculum and isolated nuclei in the pons. More recent studies have shown that the cerebellar cortex and several thalamic nuclei are also involved in most instances of PSN. These lesions were the most common brain injuries in a group of 96 preterm infants evaluated at autopsy.[281] The frequent coexistence of PSN, PVL, and germinal matrix hemorrhages in the same specimen suggests that all three lesions may be produced by a common etiologic mechanism.[281] Multicystic encephalomalacia and ulegyria are descriptive terms for destructive lesions of the brain that are associated with perinatal asphyxia, severe cyanosis, and delayed parturition.[91] Each one of these entities is fully described and illustrated in Chapter 13 of this book.[262]

### Ischemic Brain Lesions of Arterial Occlusive Origin

Ischemic strokes are significantly heterogeneous lesions in terms of their etiology, natural progression,

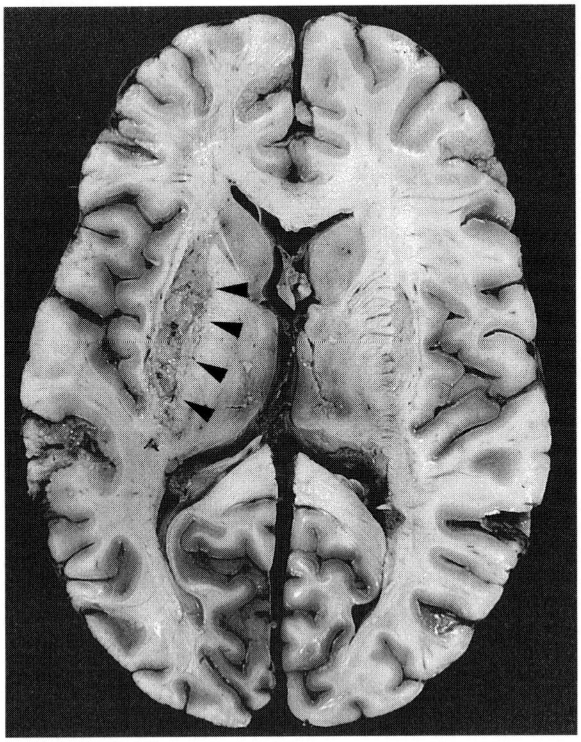

**Fig. 6-2.** The effects of global ischemia, which preceded death by 4 days, are visible in the occipital cortex (i.e., hyperemia) as well as in the putamen (*arrowheads*).

and mortality. The diagnosis of ischemic stroke, secondary to large-artery occlusion (e.g., branch of the MCA), versus one produced by the occlusion of a small penetrating artery (e.g., lenticulostriate) is based, during the initial few hours, purely on the clinical evaluation of the patient. This is because conventional CT and MRI do not detect definitive abnormalities in most ischemic strokes until about 12 to 18 hours after the stroke.[203] Most neuroimaging studies of patients with ischemic strokes are based on the analysis of brain lesions secondary to the occlusion of one MCA. This is probably explained by the fact that this artery supplies the largest territory in the brain and that the MCA is the artery most commonly involved in ischemic strokes of the large-artery etiology.[196] Conventional CT or MRI do not reveal an infarct during the first 24 hours after the stroke.[203] There are two reasons for this: (1) the initial changes induced by the arterial occlusion are microscopic (and in some instances reversible); and (2) the CT attenuation is linearly proportional to the water content of the brain. For each 1% change in water content, there is a 2.6-fold change in Hounsfield units (HU). The CT abnormality becomes obvious when the hypodensity corresponds to 20 to 30 HU.[241] Repeated CT evaluations of 100 patients with ischemic strokes in the MCA territory revealed early (about 6 to 8 hours after the beginning of symptoms) tissue density abnormalities that involved only small regions of the arterial territory such as the caudoputamen, the insular cortex, or isolated cortical gyri. In most of these patients a second CT, within 10 days of the first one, showed extension of the hypodensity to an area much larger than that revealed by the initial evaluation.[203] The difficulty that exists in defining the microscopic abnormalities induced by early ischemia in human brains has been overcome by studies on experimental models of ischemic stroke. In one study, Wistar rats with MCA occlusion of variable duration (30 minutes to 7 days) developed brain lesions that evolved at a rate of progression comparable to that observed in human lesions evaluated by CT. In these animals, the correlation between neuroimaging studies (diffusion-weighted MR) and ultrastructural analysis revealed that among the earliest changes induced by the arterial occlusion is swelling of dendrites, astrocytes, and endothelial cells of microvessels.[169] In a separate study, utilizing the same experimental model, the progression of ischemic (reversible) changes to infarction evolved over a period of 3 to 4 days after the arterial occlusion.[110]

### Brain Infarcts

Infarcts are areas of coagulation necrosis that develop at sites of severe ischemia, usually secondary to an arterial occlusion. Coagulation necrosis is a tissue abnormality characterized by the loss of affinity for hematoxylin, which normally binds to the cell nucleic acids. Areas of coagulation necrosis (in hematoxylin and eosin preparations) appear as sites where the cell boundaries are still recognizable, but the necrotic cells completely lose their hematoxylinophilia.

The occlusion of an intracranial artery creates ischemic conditions that are significantly patchy and heterogeneous; some portions of the arterial territory will be severely ischemic within a matter of minutes, whereas in others the blood supply will be either normal (via the collateral anastomosis) or only moderately decreased. The conditions initiated by an arterial occlusion are governed by as yet undefined dynamic processes that make the multiple scattered lesions evolve into a homogeneous area of coagulation necrosis. Thus, in experimental animals as well as in humans, there is an interval of several hours between the clinical event (ischemic stroke) and the appearance of the brain infarct. The possible causes for the progression of the brain lesion are discussed in several review articles under the heading of Pathophysiology of Brain Ischemia.[94,95,96,223,278]

Brain infarcts may be created either as a result of vascular occlusions or as a consequence of hemodynamic failures. Localized zones of coagulation necrosis that develop after a severe hypotensive episode or after transient cardiac arrest sometimes are designated as areas of encephalomalacia, or brain softening; their his-

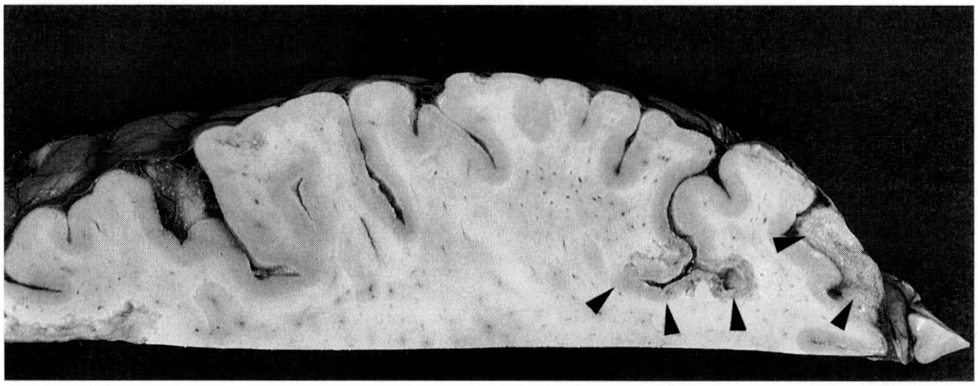

**Fig. 6-3.** Laminar necrosis (*arrowheads*) involves the bottom of two adjacent gyri.

tologic features and their etiology are comparable to those of a lesion produced by an arterial occlusion. Brain lesions secondary to venous occlusions are also called infarcts, but their histologic characteristics are somewhat different from those of arterial and hemodynamic infarcts. Moreover, the clinical syndromes produced by intracranial venous occlusions do not fulfill the criteria of ischemic stroke. Patients with intracranial venous thrombosis do not develop sudden, localized neurologic deficits; instead, over 80% of these patients complain of persistent, dull, unrelenting headache, which frequently is accompanied by papilledema.[76]

**Arterial infarcts (white or anemic).** Brain lesions secondary to the occlusion of an artery traditionally are classified into bland or white (when the lesion is devoid of any hemorrhagic component) and red or hemorrhagic when the area of evolving infarct develops multiple petechiae that usually are restricted to the gray matter. A sharp distinction between these two types is somewhat artificial; repeated computed tomography shows that many arterial infarcts begin as white lesions that spontaneously become red 2 to 3 days after the stroke. Because there are significant differences in the management and prognosis of these two types of lesions, it is customary to separate brain ischemic injuries into two large categories: those associated with large-artery occlusions (i.e., infarctions) and those presumed to be caused by disease of small blood vessels (i.e., lacunae).[196,197]

Clinically, the most significant ischemic stroke, and possibly the most common one in this category, is represented by occlusion of the middle cerebral artery. The typical case history may involve a 65-year-old slightly hypertensive man who upon awakening notices speech disorder (dysphasia) accompanied by weakness of the right hand. Computed tomography obtained 4 to 5 hours later is normal in most cases despite angiographic evidence of an arterial occlusion involving the stem of the left middle cerebral artery. A second CT scan several hours later will show blurring of the corticomedullary junction in the left insular cortex and surrounding gyri, and this will be followed by the appearance of hypodensity in a region that more or less corresponds to the territory supplied by the occluded artery.[323] On day 3 or 4 after the stroke, neuroimaging abnormalities may include deformity of the ipsilateral ventricular cavities and compression of the sulci secondary to the edematous expansion of the ischemic parenchyma. In severe cases there may be displacement of brain tissues across the midline (cingulate herniation) or transtentorially (uncinate herniation). Conventional MRI does not offer additional sensitivity in recognizing changes in tissue density, and neither of the two methods (CT or MRI) discriminates between areas of severe ischemia with probable irreversible injury and areas of moderate ischemia where the process of necrosis may be delayed by several hours or days.

Analyzing the sequential changes that develop in the brain from the moment the artery is occluded until an infarct becomes evident cannot be done in human specimens. Few patients die within minutes of an ischemic stroke, and conducting a detailed histologic study of the entire human brain injured by an arterial occlusion would be extremely onerous. For these reasons, it has become necessary to define in appropriate experimental animals the sequence of cellular events leading to an infarct. One of the most useful and readily available models is based on the intravascular occlusion of the middle cerebral artery in the adult Wistar rat. The procedure to occlude the artery is minimally invasive and does not alter the intracranial pressure; furthermore, the known variability in the biologic responses that follow an arterial occlusion can be compensated for by averaging the results of multiple experiments repeated at frequent intervals. The brain lesion induced by this method is restricted to the terri-

A 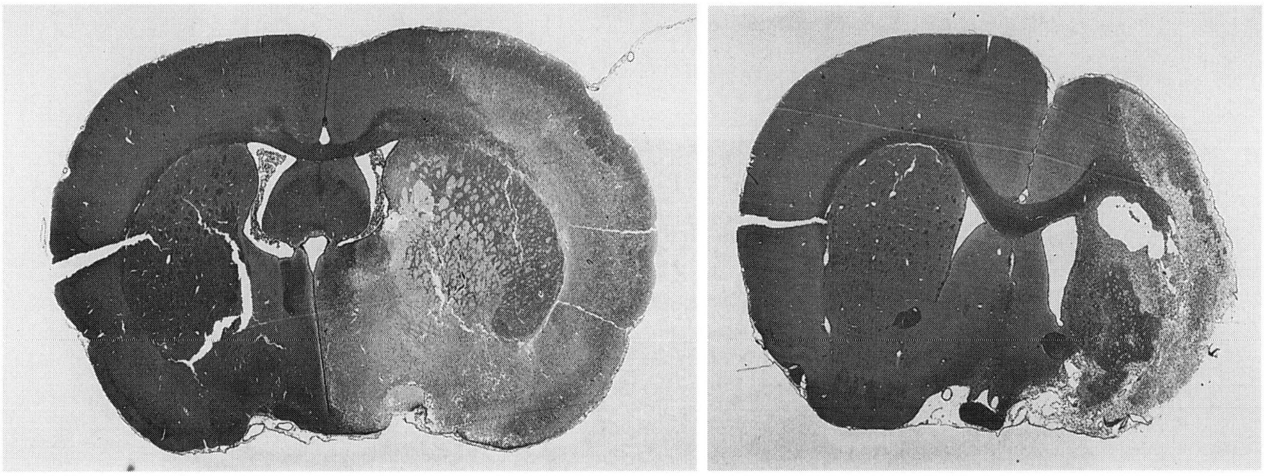 B

**Fig. 6-4.** Arterial brain infarct in a Wistar rat. **A**, Area of hypodensity limited to the territory of the MCA occluded 72 hours before death; ipsilateral edema resulted in a shift of the midline structures. **B**, Cavitation and tissue shrinkage are apparent 2 weeks after the arterial occlusion. (H&E; ×2.5.)

tory of the occluded artery, has the same histologic features of a mature human brain infarct, and is compatible with long-term survival[110] (Fig. 6-4, *A* and *B*).

In human autopsy specimens arterial brain infarcts are not detectable to the naked eye inspection until 3 to 4 days after the stroke.[200,231] One study addressed the description of the microscopic features of human arterial infarcts at earlier times, but the data are incomplete because the results were based on the evaluation of only one or two histologic samples from each brain, and the earliest time interval recorded was 16 hours after the ischemic stroke.[50] Our observations on several hundred experiments of MCA occlusion suggest that the morphologic features of the ischemic lesion can be modified significantly by reopening the artery at various times between 10 minutes to 1 hour.[109] Since the length of time of the arterial occlusion cannot be determined in most human ischemic strokes, this makes the accurate interpretation of the microscopic findings in human brains extremely difficult.

The following is a summary of the microscopic events characteristic of brain lesions induced in experimental animals by MCA occlusion. As is true of human lesions, the infarct (or area of pannecrosis) becomes visible only 72 to 96 hours after the arterial occlusion (Fig. 6-4, *A*). The earliest event recorded is based on evaluating changes in the translational movement of hydrogen ions by diffusion-weighted magnetic resonance imaging (DW-MRI).[169] This technique is extremely sensitive to alterations in the Brownian movement of hydrogen ions, which are reflected in changes in the apparent diffusion coefficient (ADC) of water. Five minutes after occluding one MCA in rats or rabbits ADC values change in isolated regions of the territory supplied by the occluded artery. This abnormality corresponds to structural changes that include marked swelling of astrocytes and endothelial cells of the microvessels accompanied by narrowing of the vascular lumina and intravascular retention of leukocytes and erythrocytes[169] (Fig. 6-5). Neuronal necrosis does not become evident until 6 hours after the arterial occlusion, and at this time only a limited number of neurons in the territory of the occluded artery exhibit the features of necrosis, as defined by Farber and others.[78]

The astroglial and microvascular changes are associated with concomitant abnormalities in the neuronal perikaryon (Fig. 6-6). These include swelling and shrinkage that involve a large number of neurons as early as 2 hours after the arterial occlusion (Figs. 6-7, 6-8). The features of neuronal necrosis (i.e., eosinophilia) involve a limited number of neurons 4 to 6 hours after MCA occlusion, but 24 hours later a limited number (40%) of cortical neurons still show signs of reversible injury; at the same time, almost the entire neuronal population of the caudoputamen exhibits signs of necrosis[106] (Fig. 6-9). A number of publications, based on observations made in various experimental models of brain ischemia, report that in addition to *necrosis* (causally associated with injury to plasma membranes), ischemic injury may be mediated in the brain by *apoptosis* (caused by activation of endonucleases and DNA scission).[151] However, the issue remains unsettled because the morphologic features of both conditions include nuclear fragmentation (or karyorrhexis) and also because the phenotype of cells expressing either necrosis or apoptosis is difficult to verify once lethal injury has occurred. Perhaps the most important issue concerning neuronal death in ischemia is that

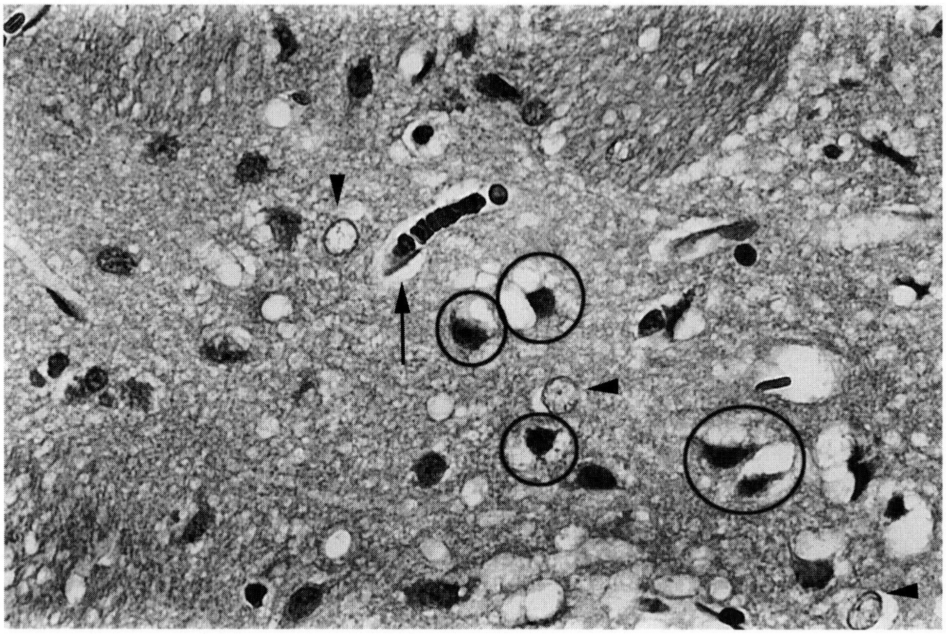

**Fig. 6-5.** Wistar rat, one hour after MCA occlusion; prominent changes at this site include: vacuolation of neuropil and white matter, swelling of astrocytes nuclei (*arrowheads*), shrinkage of neuronal perikarya with formation of perineuronal haloes (*circles*), and intravascular retention of erythrocytes (*arrow*). (H&E; ×160.)

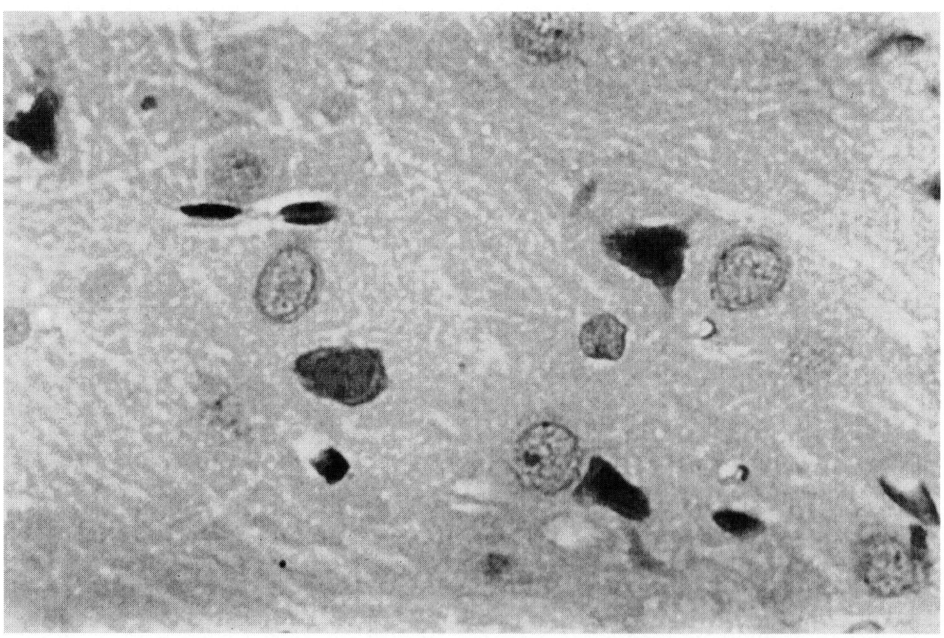

**Fig. 6-6.** Wistar rat. Dark neurons are visible in the hemisphere opposite the side of the arterial occlusion as well as in sham operated animals. These neuronal changes are not accompanied by visible alterations in neuropil, glia, or microvessels. (H&E; ×240.)

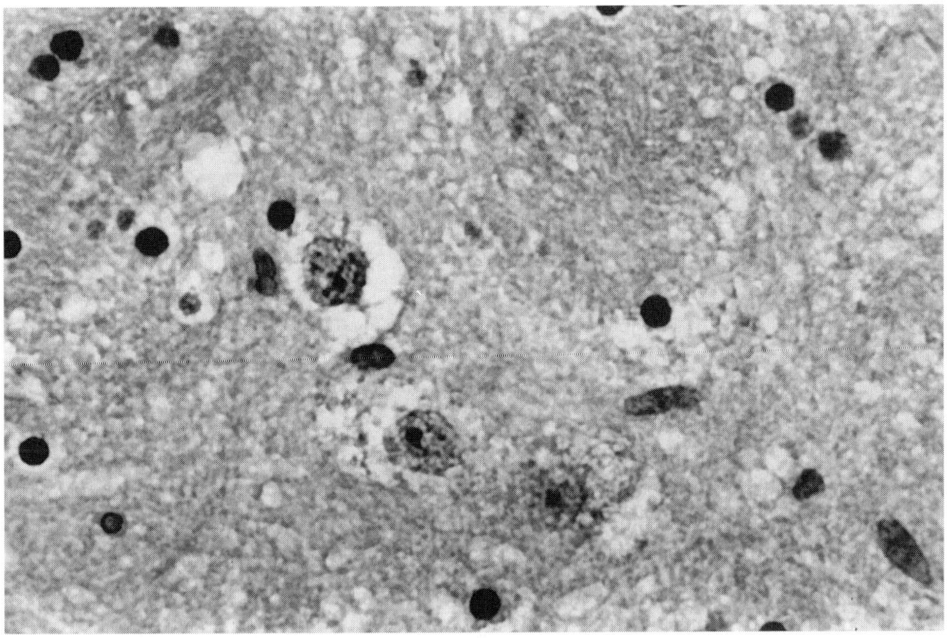

**Fig. 6-7.** Wistar rat. Swollen neurons, vacuolated neuropil, and pyknotic glial cells are abundant at this site 4 hours after MCA occlusion. (H&E; ×240.)

signs of irreversible injury do not involve all neurons simultaneously, and that significant numbers of eosinophilic neurons are identifiable, for the first time, 6 hours after a persistent arterial occlusion.[110]

The microvascular abnormalities that appear in isolated regions of the arterial territory include the influx of polymorphonuclear (PMN) leukocytes that begins within the first hour after the arterial occlusion and peaks 12 to 24 hours later (Fig. 6-10). Subsequently, PMN leukocytes migrate into the ischemic parenchyma through the endothelial lining of venules, and their numbers begin to decrease, although as late as 7 days after the MCA occlusion few PMN leukocytes are recognizable in the lesion[106] (Figs. 6-11, 6-12). It is important to emphasize that the previously described sequence of leukocyte influx applies to experiments of permanent MCA occlusion. The previously outlined cellular response undergoes significant modifications by reopening the artery at variable periods of time. The role of neutrophils in an evolving arterial infarct remains incompletely defined.

Coagulation necrosis in experimental models of permanent arterial occlusion can be demonstrated only 3 to 4 days later; at earlier times only a portion of the involved territory shows pannecrosis, while necrosis in the surrounding tissues affects mostly isolated, scattered neurons and this is accompanied by survival of many of the glial and vascular components. In experiments in which the artery is reopened within 30 to 60 min, the resulting lesion exhibits morphologic features significantly different from those of an infarct. These lesions, for which the designation *incomplete brain infarct* has been suggested,[164] are characterized by a marked decrease in the number of identifiable neurons, or neuronal "loss," accompanied by proliferation of microglia (that do not evolve into macrophages) and an increased number of reactive astrocytes[109] (Fig. 6-13).

Tissues injured by coagulation necrosis in organs such as the heart, kidney, and liver eventually are replaced by a fibroblastic scar. In the brain, necrotic tissues are removed by macrophages that leave behind a fluid-filled cavity (Figs. 6-14, 6-15). This has prompted some authors to describe the evolution of a brain infarct as a process in which coagulation necrosis is followed by liquefaction necrosis. This is probably incorrect, because the term liquefaction necrosis more appropriately applies to the formation of pus at sites made necrotic by the biologic action of microorganisms. Cavitation at a site of coagulation necrosis in the brain can be easily recognized by modern neuroimaging methods, as a sharply circumscribed area of low attenuation (in CT) or low density (in MR).[203] The beginning of cavitation can be seen as early as 7 days after permanent experimental MCA occlusion. In experiments of *transient* MCA occlusion, coagulation necrosis seldom develops, and cavitation is almost never observed. Thus, the tissue responses are influenced by the duration of the arterial occlusion, and this is something that in most human cases is extremely difficult to determine. Therefore, estimating the age of a human brain infarct on the basis of its histologic features can be inaccurate, especially when several weeks have elapsed between the clinical event (stroke) and the his-

*Text continues on page 275.*

A

B

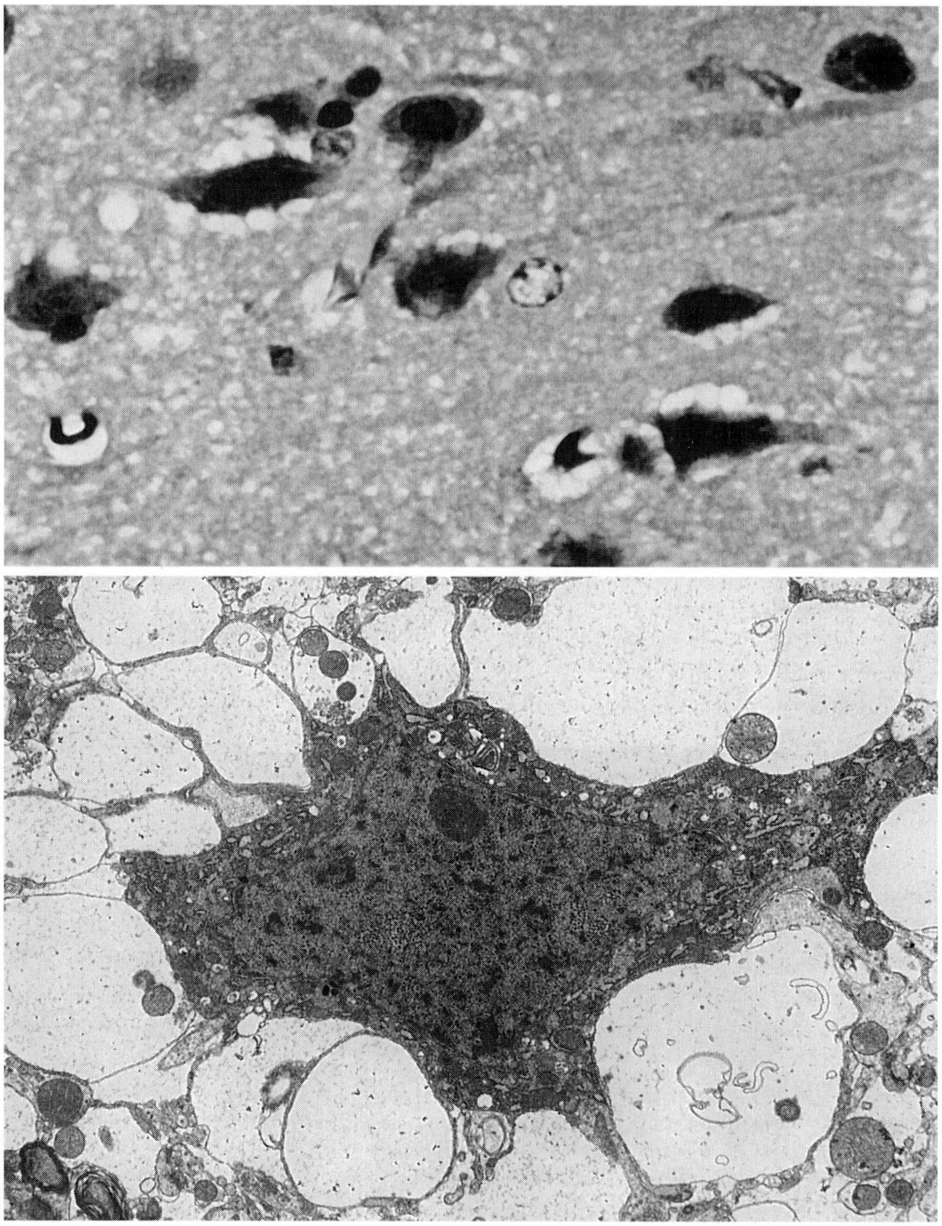

**Fig. 6-8.** **A**, The scalloped appearance of these neuronal perikarya corresponds to the swelling of astroglial cell processes **B**, Detail of one of the neurons shown in **A** from a Wistar rat with MCA occlusion of a few hours' duration. (**A**, H&E; ×240; **B**, ×8100.)

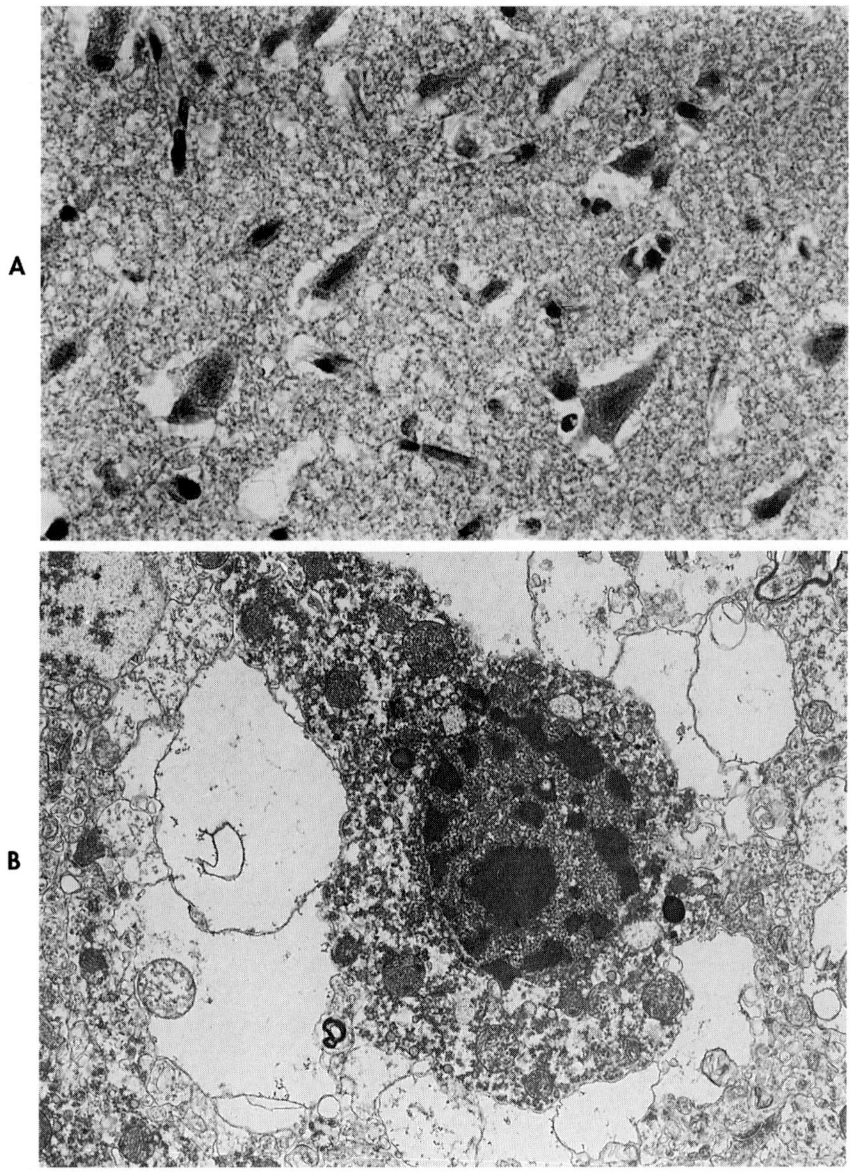


**Fig. 6-9.** **A**, Eosinophilic (red) neurons in the cerebral cortex of a Wistar rat. MCA had been occluded 72 hours before death. **B**, Detail of one of the neuronal perikarya shown in **A**. (**A**, H&E; ×160; **B**, ×9800.)

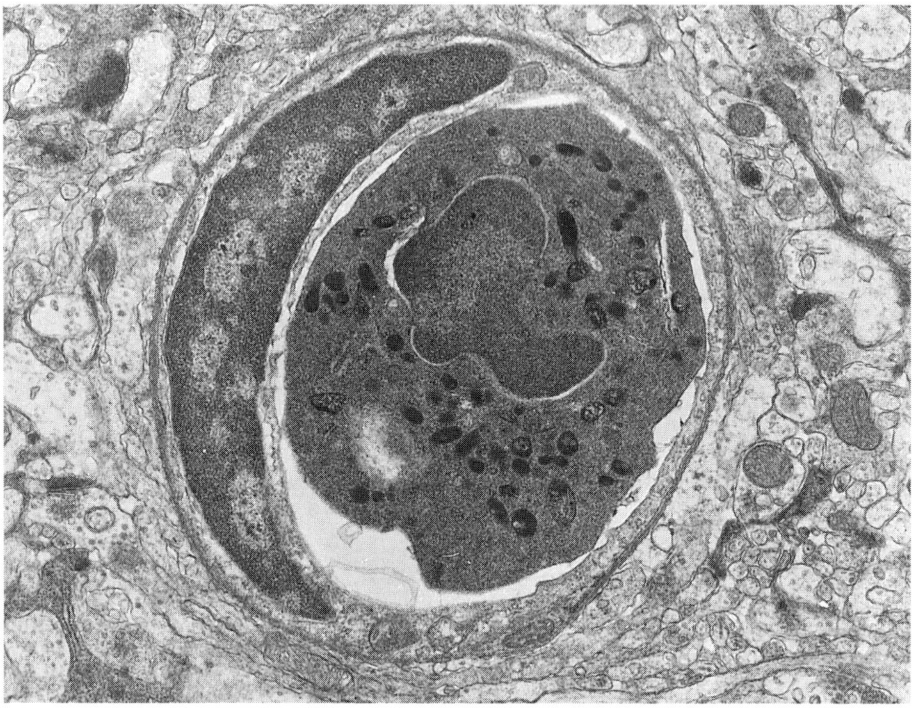

**Fig. 6-10.** Polymorphonuclear leukocytes are found, in increasing numbers, in the lumen of microvessels within the territory of the occluded MCA. This preparation is from a Wistar rat; the artery was occluded 1 hour before death. (×8550.) (Reproduced with permission from American Journal of Pathology 144:188-199, 1994.)

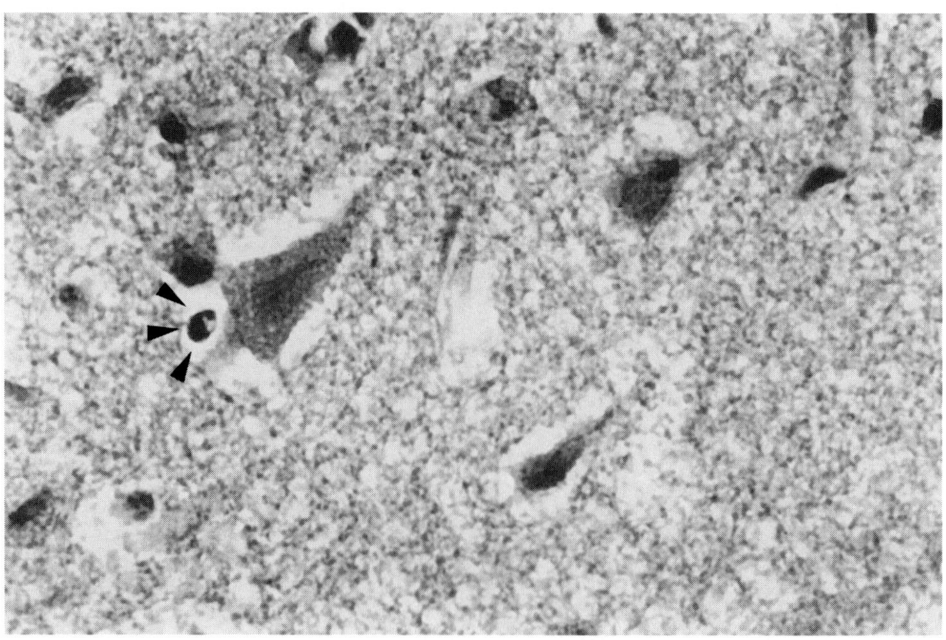

**Fig. 6-11.** Polymorphonuclear leukocyte *(arrowheads)* next to an eosinophilic neuron in the cerebral cortex of a Wistar rat, 72 hours after MCA occlusion. (H&E; ×240.)

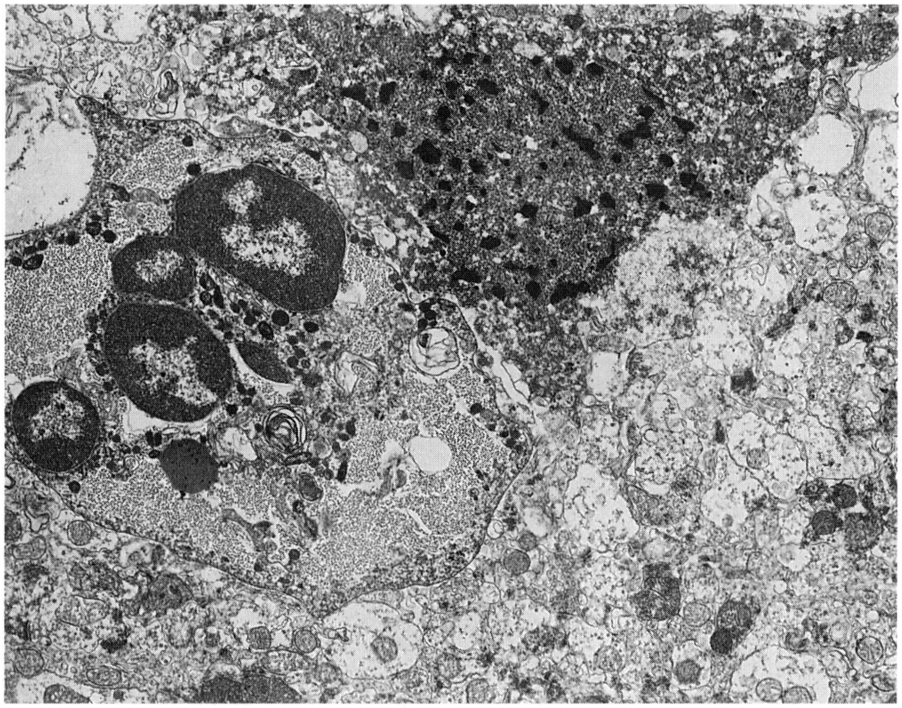

**Fig. 6-12.** PMN leukocyte next to a necrotic cell (neuron); basal ganglia of a Wistar rat. MCA was occluded 24 hours before death. (×6750.)

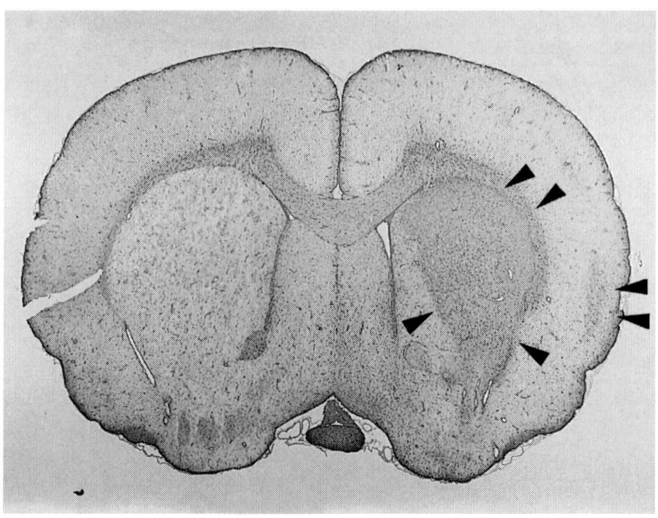

**Fig. 6-13.** Wistar rat with MCA occlusion of 25 minutes' duration, followed by 2 weeks' reperfusion. At the sites of partial neuronal necrosis (incomplete infarction) there is increased gliosis (*arrowheads*). (GFAP; ×2.5.)

tologic evaluation of the brain tissues. The fact that an arterial occlusion creates regions where ischemia has variable degrees of severity suggests that the histologic responses at each of these regions should be significantly different. Regions where ischemia is severe will develop coagulation necrosis (i.e., infarction) within a few hours, with abundant influx of neutrophils, activation of monocyte/macrophages, and eventual cavitation. These regions are called in some publications the *core* of the lesion. Regions injured by ischemia of moderate severity, sometimes referred to as the *penumbra,* evolve into areas where *selective neuronal injury* predominates (i.e., incomplete infarction). At these sites, necrosis of a limited number of neurons is accompanied by activation of microglia that do not evolve into macrophages and by hypertrophy of astrocytes. Influx of PMN leukocytes is not as prominent a feature of this type of brain lesion as it is in experiments of permanent MCA occlusion.[105,109]

Among ischemic stroke patients who do not improve spontaneously one of the most significant clinical events is determined by the formation of edema within the ischemic brain. The retention of fluid by the brain increases the intracranial pressure, and this decreases the perfusion pressure, thus worsening the ischemia. The conditions responsible for the postischemic edema are not clearly known, but in both humans and animals postischemic brain edema peaks 3 to 4 days after the arterial occlusion (Fig. 6-16). At such time brain edema and its deleterious effects on the integrity of the brainstem may be a significant contributor to the mortality of these patients; however, it is also known that postischemic brain swelling disappears spontaneously at the same rate at which it develops. Brain edema secondary to a hemispheric arterial infarct

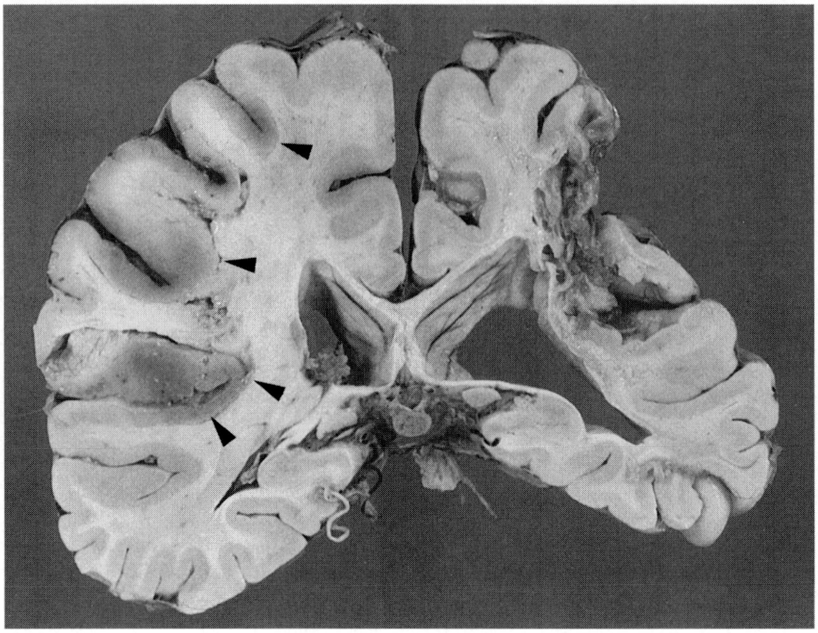

**Fig. 6-14.** The appearance of a cavitary infarction on the right hemisphere contrasts with the tissue abnormalities visible on the left hemisphere (*arrowheads*). Mitral valve disease accompanied by vegetations has led to two embolic episodes to the brain. The earliest occurred 18 months before death (*right*) and the more recent, 10 days before death (*left*).

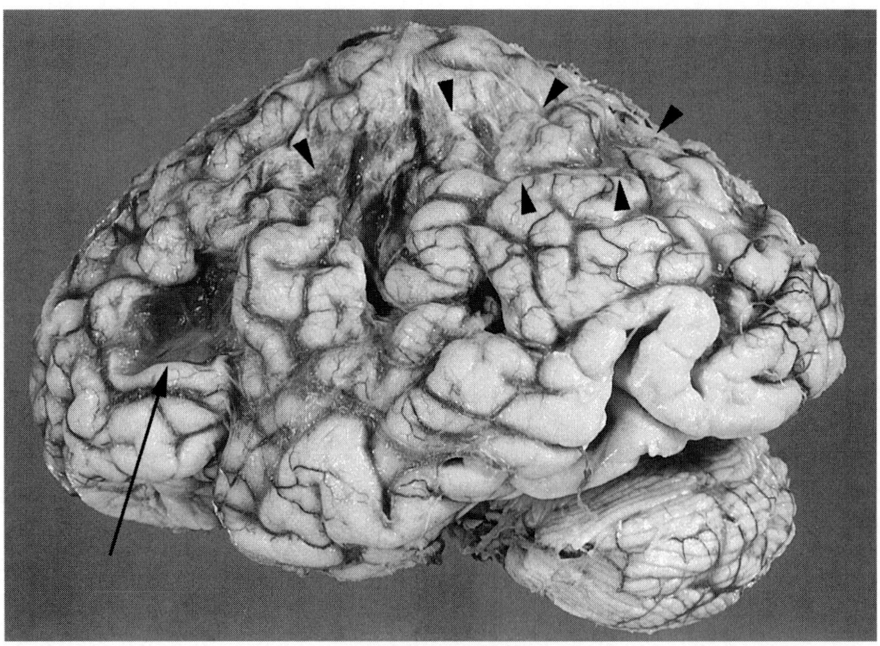

**Fig. 6-15.** Cavitary infarct in the left frontal lobe (*arrow*) is accompanied by arterial-border-zone infarction (*arrowheads*) in a patient with severe ipsilateral internal carotid artery atherosclerosis.

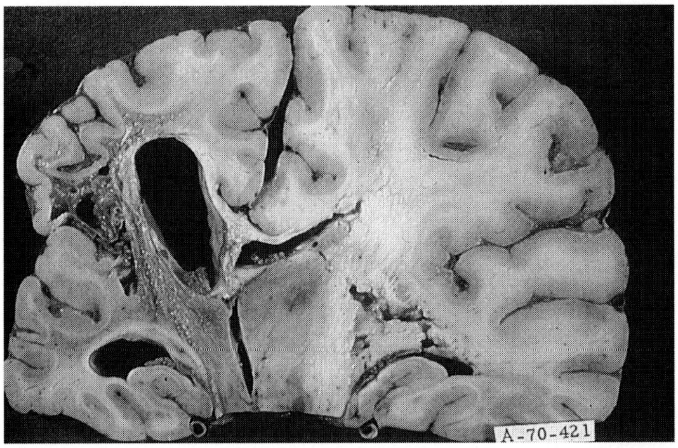


**Fig. 6-16.** Post-ischemic edema in the right hemisphere peaked 4 days after the occlusion of the ipsilateral internal carotid artery (right). An ischemic occlusive event had led to necrosis and cavitation in the opposite hemisphere several months earlier (left).

causes displacement or herniation of brain tissues that can further aggravate the conditions created by the arterial occlusion. Cingulate gyrus herniation results in stretching and compression of the anterior cerebral arteries, and this may result in secondary infarcts in the territory supplied by those vessels. Herniation of the uncinate gyrus results in extrinsic compression of the posterior cerebral artery, which may be complicated by infarction of the occipital lobe; uncinate herniation also interferes with the blood supply to the upper midbrain with consequent injury to the reticular activating substance and related structures. Changes in the blood-brain barrier permeability to macromolecules are described under the heading of Brain Edema.

In summary, the structural abnormalities induced in the brain by an arterial occlusion can be divided into those responsible for injury to the neurons (which cannot be visualized by neuroimaging methods) and those responsible for changes in the tissue density (which are primarily a reflection of abnormalities in the ionic pumps leading to the retention of water in the ischemic territories). Diffusion-weighted MR imaging has demonstrated exquisite sensitivity to early ischemic brain changes. In the future, characterization of brain perfusion by hemodynamic imaging and changes in the distribution of relevant molecules by MR spectroscopy together with the observations made on the appropriate experimental models should considerably increase our understanding of the acute events in human ischemic strokes.[158]

**Hemorrhagic infarcts (red).** Ischemic brain lesions that appear hemorrhagic to naked eye inspection are known as hemorrhagic or red infarcts (Fig. 6-17). Repeated CT evaluation of patients with ischemic strokes

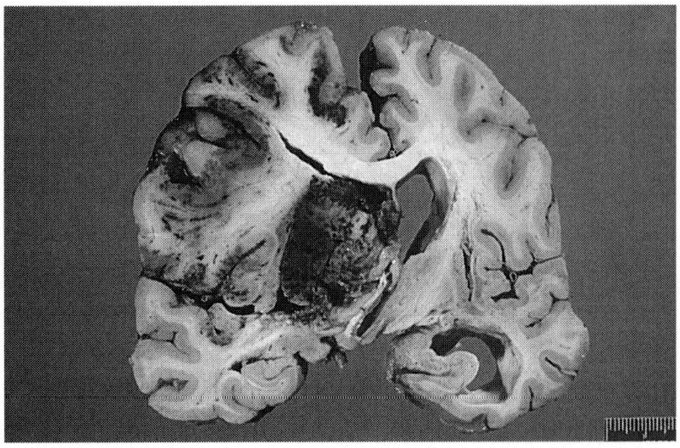

**Fig. 6-17.** Hemorrhagic infarction in the territory of the left MCA. A stroke occurred about 5 and one half days earlier.

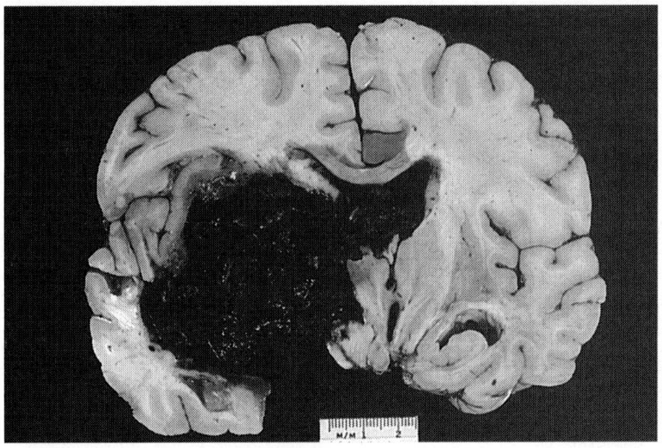

**Fig. 6-18.** In the first 24 hours after the stroke, CT had shown an area of hypodensity in the basal ganglia. Subsequent deterioration and death 3 days later were attributed to the development of a large hemorrhage that obliterated the original site of hypodensity.

has revealed that the hemorrhagic transformation of initially anemic or white infarcts is a relatively frequent event. Two types of hemorrhagic transformation are recognized: (1) The appearance of a few petechiae in the gray matter of a previously pale infarct is an event that is not accompanied by clinical deterioration or overt change in the condition of most patients. This type of transformation is the most common of the two and seemingly takes place a few days after the initial stroke (Fig. 6-17). (2) A second type of hemorrhagic transformation is accompanied by clinical deterioration and involves the appearance of a relatively large hematoma at the site of the original ischemic stroke (Fig. 6-18). This occurrence sometimes is lethal and is more frequent among patients receiving thrombolytic therapy for the treatment of either coronary or intracranial artery occlusions. Among patients with ischemic stroke who received tPA within the first 6 hours of the beginning of symptoms, an increased mortality rate (30%) on days 2 and 3 was directly related to the appearance of a large hemorrhage at the site of the evolving ischemic lesion.

The mechanisms responsible for the hemorrhagic transformation of a brain infarct are not known. Analysis of human autopsy material led two authors to suggest that the hemorrhagic transformation could follow the reperfusion of an ischemic territory after the spontaneous reopening of the occluded artery.[102,103] Spontaneous lysis of an arterial thromboembolus is relatively common within 12 hours after the initial arterial occlusion. This was the interpretation given to a study of nearly 100 patients with ischemic stroke in whom angiography showed an occluded artery in over 90%, if the procedure was completed within less than 12 hours after the stroke. In contrast, angiograms performed in the same group of patients after 96 hours showed occluded arteries in only 64%.[284] However, the rate of hemorrhagic transformation is less frequent than the rate of arterial recanalization. This suggests that the arterial reopening is not the only factor involved in the hemorrhagic transformation of ischemic lesions (Figs. 6-19, 6-20). Sudden changes in perfusion

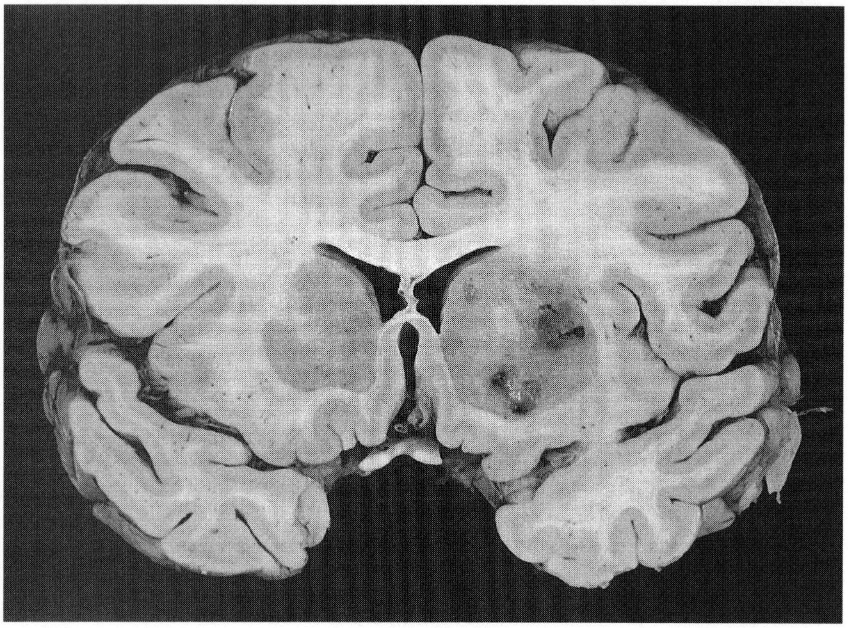

**Fig. 6-19.** Hemorrhagic components as seen in these basal ganglia infarcts are more common among lesions of cardiac embolic origin. These infarcts were accompanied by non-bacterial vegetations in the mitral valve.

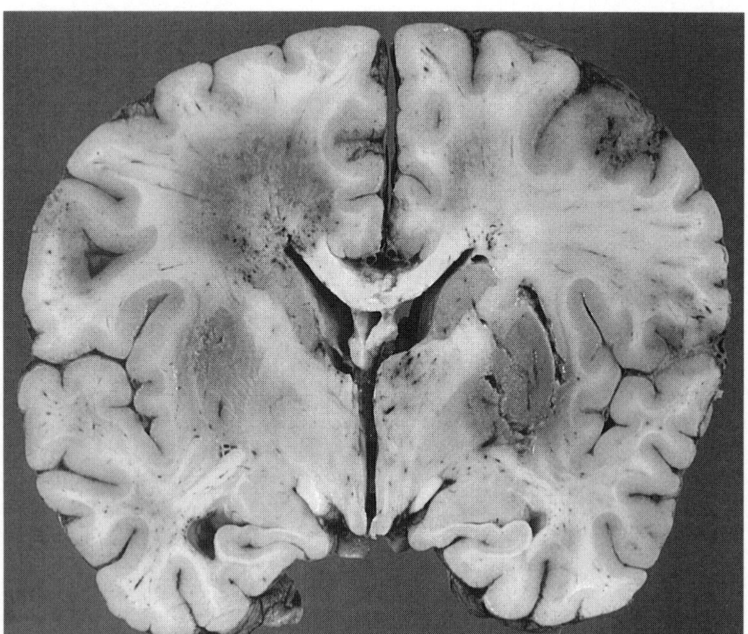

**Fig. 6-20.** Multiple, bilateral infarcts with hemorrhagic components in a case of disseminated aspergillosis complicated by multiple thromboses of cerebral arteries.

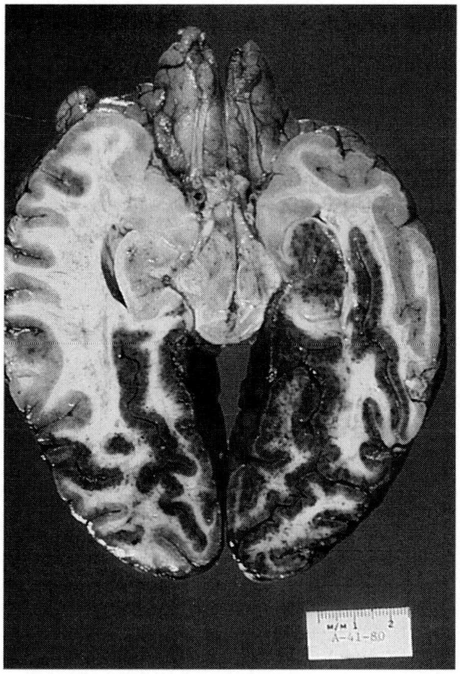

**Fig. 6-21.** Hemorrhagic infarction of the occipital lobes in a case of basilar-artery thrombosis; the supply of blood through the posterior communicating arteries probably accounts for the abundant hemorrhages.

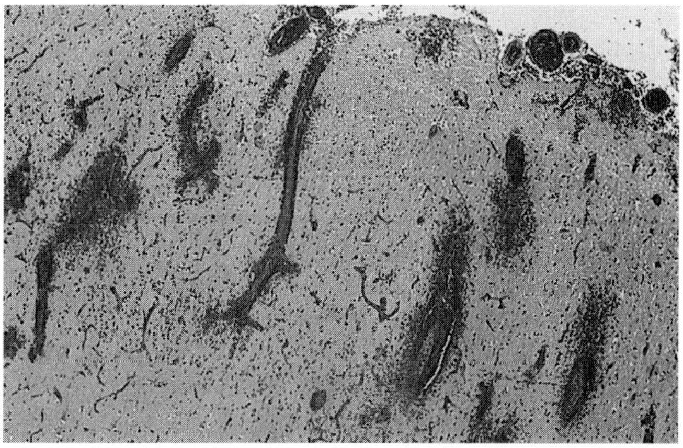

**Fig. 6-22.** Cerebral cortex showing coagulation necrosis accompanied by multiple petechiae in a hemorrhagic infarction with occlusion of the MCA. (H&E; ×25.)

pressure, as may occur during bouts of hypertension, may be important causes of bleeding into a nascent infarct. This hypothesis is supported by observations of hemorrhagic transformation among patients who had angiographically proven arterial occlusion at the time bleeding appeared in the infarct. Also, reopening the occluded artery is not indispensable; hemorrhagic features have been shown in brain infarcts examined in autopsy specimens in which the arteries remained occluded by thromboemboli.[211a] Hemorrhagic infarcts are also common in cases of incomplete arterial occlusion; for example, extrinsic compression of the posterior cerebral artery by a herniated uncinate gyrus frequently results in an infarction of the occipital lobe (Fig. 6-21). These lesions often contain numerous petechiae. The reason for the hemorrhagic component in these lesions may be explained by the fact that the artery, though severely narrowed, is not totally occluded. A similar circumstance may prevail in infarcts associated with arterial dissections; the brain lesions that accompany arterial dissections almost always have hemorrhagic components.[266] Additional factors responsible for the hemorrhagic transformation of ischemic brain lesions have been uncovered in experimental animal models in which bleeding into the brain parenchyma has been induced via intracerebral injection of collagenase. This enzyme selectively targets the basal lamina of microvessels.[249] Activation of collagenases and similar proteases as the consequence of an arterial occlusion is a subject of current investigation. The clinical diagnosis of hemorrhagic infarct can be made in most cases by CT: this technique is sufficiently sensitive to demonstrate the presence of confluent petechiae.[72]

The histologic features of hemorrhagic infarcts are not significantly different from those of white or anemic infarcts, except for the presence of extravasated red blood cells (Fig. 6-22). At the microscopic level the difference between white and red infarcts is more a matter of degree, as extravasated erythrocytes are seldom absent in white infarcts.

**Venous infarcts.** Intracranial sinus-venous thrombosis (SVT) has become an increasingly important entity on account of its demonstrated frequent occurrence. Before the era of neuroimaging, SVT was considered a rare condition; however, active screening of persons with chronic headaches and papilledema has uncovered among these a significant number of patients with SVT.[76] Our understanding of SVT has also been modified as we learn that spontaneous recovery is relatively common among many of these patients. More significant, the effectiveness of treating SVT with heparin seems to be well demonstrated.[76]

The three most common signs and symptoms of SVT in a large group of patients who had angiographic demonstration of venous/sinus occlusion, were longstanding and persistent headache, papilledema, and seizures.[36]

The brain parenchymal lesions are sometimes minimal and include massive brain edema (evidenced by narrowing of the sulci), occasional subcortical hemorrhages, and (in the case of thrombosis of the superior sagittal sinus [SSS]) marked dilatation of the ventricular system with a massive increase in the intracranial pressure (Fig. 6-23). This picture has been observed following sickle-cell crises accompanied by thrombosis

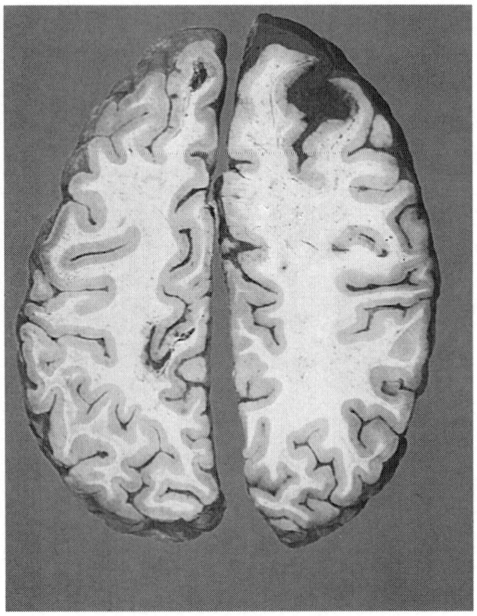

**Fig. 6-23.** Marked, diffuse bilateral hemispheric brain edema accompanied by a few subcortical hemorrhages. These brain injuries followed the occlusion of the superior sagittal sinus in a patient with sickle-cell disease.

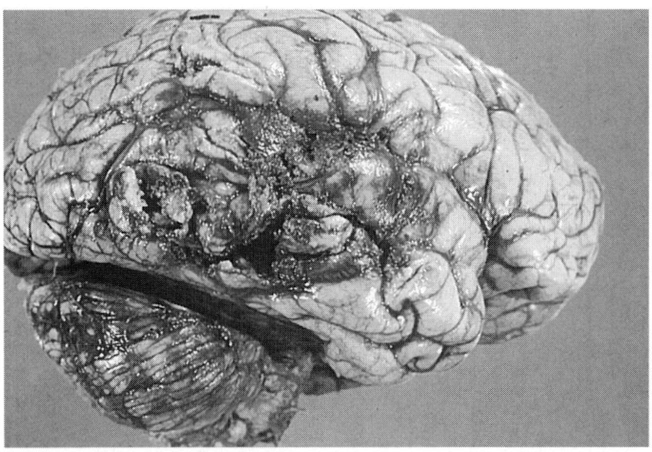

**Fig. 6-24.** Cortical vein thrombosis accompanied by subarachnoid hemorrhage localized to the lateral surface of the temporal lobe.

of the SSS.[98] Cortical venous thrombosis produces localized lesions accompanied by hemorrhage into the brain parenchyma and the subarachnoid space (Fig. 6-24). The distribution of the lesion does not conform to the territory of an arterial branch, and in contrast to the gray matter petechiae of arterial infarcts here the hemorrhage spreads widely into the white matter. Each of these features can be readily appreciated on neuroimaging studies. The microscopic features that make venous lesions different from those secondary to arterial occlusion include marked sponginess (edema) of the brain and profuse, diffuse infiltration by PMN leukocytes.[98]

**Incomplete brain infarcts.** The clinical deficit produced by an arterial occlusion evolves along a course that is difficult to predict at the time of the stroke. In several series of prospectively evaluated patients with ischemic stroke, 26% to 43% experienced worsening of their neurologic deficit; these figures were unchanged whether the evaluation was conducted 6 to 8 hours or 1 to 2 days after the onset of symptoms.[84] In contrast, a significant percentage of patients spontaneously begin recovering as early as 2 hours after an ischemic stroke.[21] Several mechanisms have been proposed to explain recovery, including reorganization of cortical maps and amelioration of remote functional depression, but these remain conjectural. One mechanism of early recovery, through reperfusion or recovery of nearly normal blood flow via collateral anastomoses, involves the survival of an initially functionless tissue at risk for infarction.[93] According to this theory, patients whose symptoms disappear within 24 hours are said to have had a transient ischemic attack (TIA) or a condition characterized by the temporary occlusion of the artery. Interestingly, despite the recovery of neurologic integrity, 17% to 40% of TIA patients have changes, demonstrable by either CT or MR, that correspond (in terms of their topographic location) to the symptoms present at the time of the stroke.[79] The neuropathologic features of these "silent ischemic lesions" have not been defined in human specimens. Experiments on Wistar rats based on the transient (5 to 25 minutes) occlusion of one MCA followed by reperfusion periods of 1 to 28 days' duration disclose brain lesions with structural features significantly different from those of an infarction (see Fig. 6-13). Coagulation necrosis did not develop in any of the 120 experimental animals. Among the 63% that developed brain lesions, necrosis (or eosinophilia) of isolated, scattered neurons in the caudoputamen and the cortex was accompanied by marked hypertrophy of astrocytes and activation of the perivascular microglia. In addition to the absence of coagulation necrosis, two other features differentiate this brain lesion from an infarct: (1) paucity of PMN leukocytes influx, and (2) lack of cavitation, which is attributed to the facts that microglia do not evolve into macrophages and circulating monocytes seemingly do not enter the areas of injured brain.[109] Tissue responses induced by moderate ischemia ought to be markedly different from those developing at sites of severe ischemia. Moderate ischemia, we presume, exists whenever the arterial occlusion is of short duration, i.e., less than 30 minutes. Moderate ischemia also prevails at sites where the collateral anastomoses are sufficiently robust to compensate for the conditions created by the arterial occlusion (Figs. 6-25, 6-26). Because this moderate type of ischemia does not induce either coagulation necrosis or cavitation (the essential components of infarction), we propose to designate these as *incomplete*

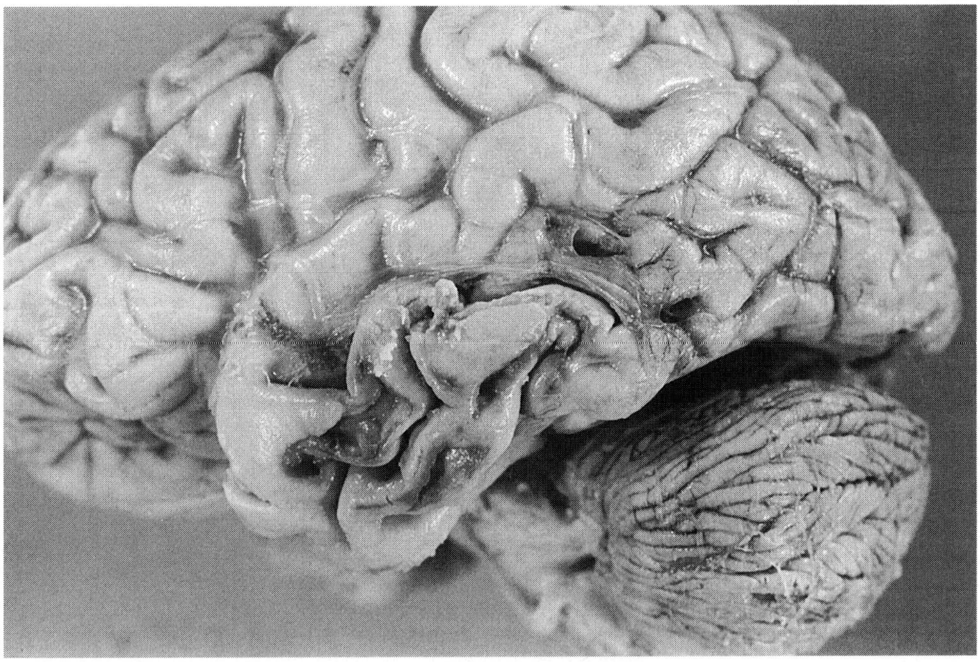

**Fig. 6-25.** Scarring rather than cavitation developed at this site of occlusive ischemic injury. The stroke occurred over two years before death. The incomplete infarction of this tissue may have been the result of early spontaneous reperfusion.

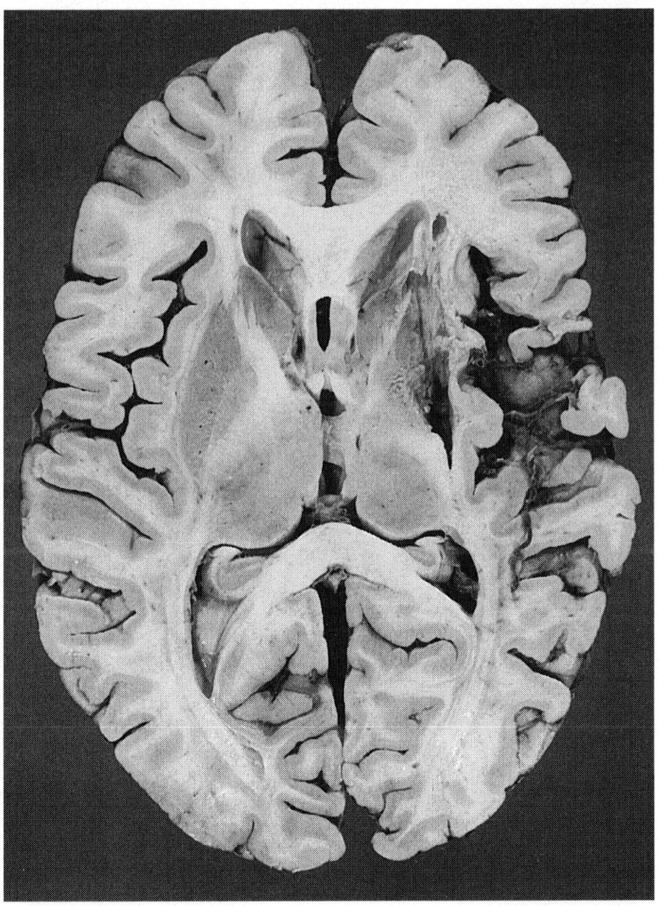

**Fig. 6-26.** Two different responses are visible in the territory of the right MCA. The occlusion of this artery was angiographically proven 14 months before death. Cavitation involves mostly putamen and subcortical white matter. Good collateral circulation may have partially preserved the integrity of the cerebral cortex.

*infarcts* or lesions where only a limited number of cells, primarily neurons, succumb to the conditions created by the arterial occlusion.[101] Imaging areas of incomplete infarction has been attempted following the injection of specific radiotracers in combination with single-photon emission CT. In appropriately selected patients with ischemic strokes this method has revealed decreased (but not absent) uptake of the radiotracer in areas where the CT was normal.[205]

### Ischemic Lesions of the Spinal Cord

These are much less common than the equivalent lesions in the brain. The sharp distinction that exists, in terms of their topographic distribution, between brain ischemic lesions of occlusive origin and brain lesions of hemodynamic etiology is less apparent in the cord. The morphologic features, according to the etiology of ischemia, are more difficult to separate in the spinal cord. Several medical and surgical procedures may be complicated by ischemic injury to the spinal cord. These include thoracolumbar sympathectomy, surgical repair of the abdominal aorta, pneumonectomy, aortography, and spinal angiography.[261] Ischemic events of occlusive origin have been associated with embolism originating from the cardiac chambers or from aortic atheromatous plaques. Surprisingly, fragments of cartilaginous material have been demonstrated in the lumina of branches of the radicular spinal arteries in patients who had ischemic spinal cord lesions and neurologic symptoms appropriate for the location of the lesion.[147] The presumed source of this intravascular material is the nucleus pulposus of the intervertebral disc, but the mechanism by which fibrocartilage fragments enter the arterial branch is unclear.

Following episodes of global ischemia (secondary to cardiac arrest, ruptured aorta, or severe hypotensive crises) the spinal segment most commonly involved is T9.[51] The occlusion of the anterior spinal artery results in a characteristic syndrome that reflects infarction of the anterior or ventral two thirds of the cord. Spinal cord hemisection, which is clinically expressed in the Brown-Séquard syndrome, is the result of the occlusion of the sulcocommissural artery.[51] Practically all the etiologic causes of occlusion affecting the intracranial arteries can apply to the vessels in the spinal cord; however, in contrast to the cerebral arteries, aortic disease, in particular atherosclerosis, is one of the most common sources of embolism with consequent ischemic injury to the cord. The risk of spinal cord infarction from atheromatous material increases with the surgical manipulation of the abdominal aorta. The hypothesis that there is a midthoracic zone of ischemic vulnerability in the spinal cord is not supported by clinical observations or autopsy studies, including more than 50 cases of ischemic injury to the spinal cord. In these series, the area of vulnerability was centered in the T9 to T10 segments[6,51]

### Lacunae (Lacunar Infarcts)

At the beginning of the 20th century, Pierre Marie described a neurologic syndrome in patients of geriatric age characterized by changes in mentation, and *marche à petit pas*, or a gait abnormality characterized by short steps.[177] The pathologic evaluation of these patients' brains showed small holes or *lacunae* in the basal ganglia and in the centrum semiovale (Fig. 6-27). These holes or lacunae in the brain are usually multiple, but an individual lacunae usually does not exceed a diameter of 1.5 cm. Marie described two types of grossly visible abnormalities: *état lacunaire (or lacunar state)* and *état crible* (or cribriform state); the former describes a conglomerate of destructive or cavitary lesions recognizable under the microscope by their contents (lipid-laden macrophages) and by the presence of reactive astrocytes at the edges of the cavity. The cribriform state, in contrast, represents a conglomerate of enlarged spaces each containing a blood vessel surrounded by a dilated Virchow-Robin space (Figs. 6-27, 6-28).

In the 1950s, Fisher revived the entities originally described by Marie and delineated a large number of clinical syndromes associated with lacunar states.[83] The most common syndromes are the pure hemimotor syndrome (associated with involvement of the knee of the internal capsule by a lacuna), the pure hemisensory syndrome (associated with involvement of the posterior limb of the internal capsule by a lacuna), and the sensory motor syndrome.[11] Fisher[83] ascribed the origin of lacunae to disease of the penetrating small arteries and arterioles; however, his observations were based

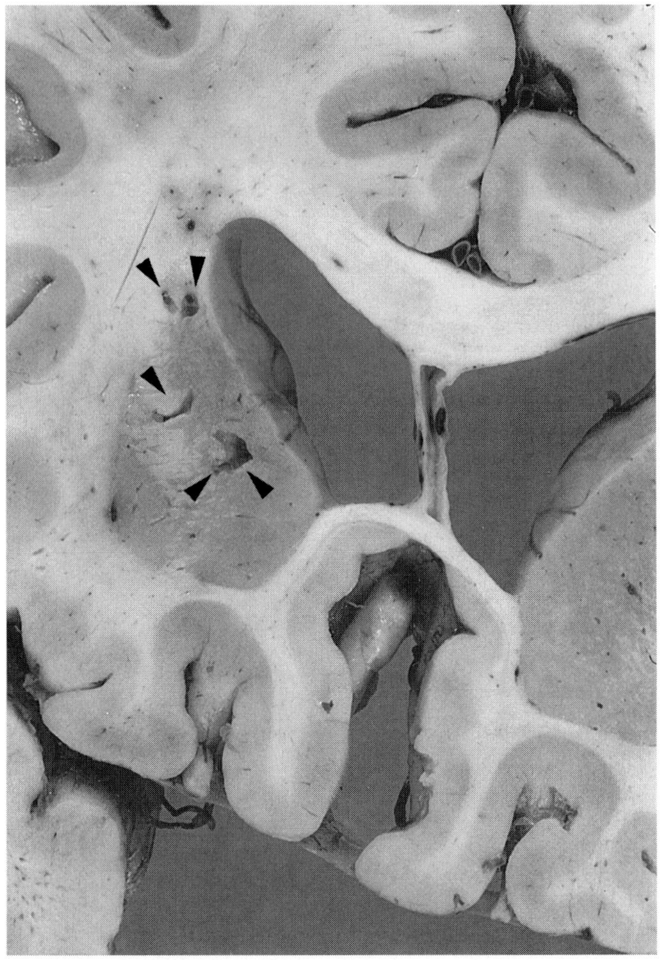

**Fig. 6-27.** Multiple lacunes are visible in the caudoputamen (*arrowheads*). Other, smaller holes (especially well seen in the subcortical white matter) represent dilated perivascular spaces.

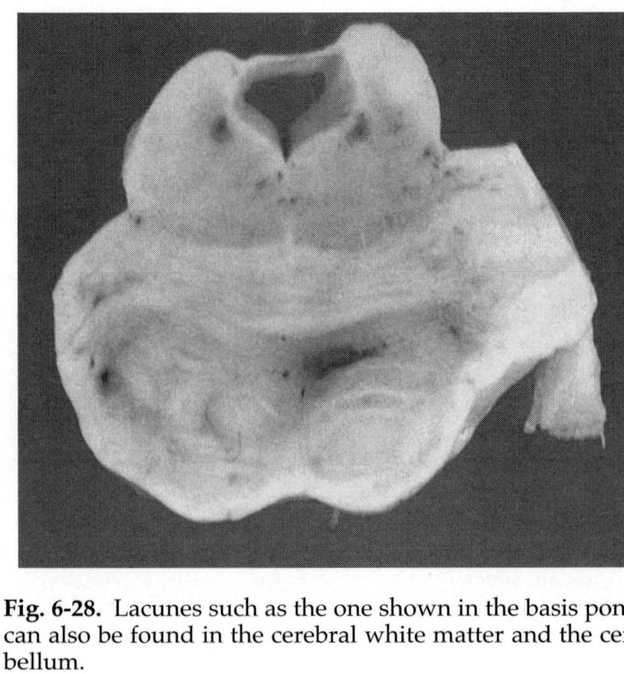

**Fig. 6-28.** Lacunes such as the one shown in the basis pontis can also be found in the cerebral white matter and the cerebellum.

on detailed histologic examination of only a few brain specimens. This prompted some authors to question the validity of assigning all lacunae an etiology based on small blood vessel disease. These authors suggest that some lacunae may result from embolism into the small blood vessels of material detached from the origin of the internal carotid in the neck.[190] The significance of this observation resides on the fact that patients with lacunar lesions should not be automatically assigned to the category of small blood-vessels disease; some lacunes may be the result of embolism from the carotid artery.

Most lacunar states evaluated at autopsy exist in specimens that have, in addition, extensive changes in the white matter (vacuolation and astrogliosis) as well as structural abnormalities such as arteriolarsclerosis involving the penetrating arteries that supply the subcortical white matter. Some of these abnormalities were recorded by Fisher under the descriptive name of lipohyalinosis. This structural change seemingly represents a combination of atheromatous disease (i.e., lipid deposits in the tunica intima) and arteriolosclerosis (or a condition characterized by replacement of the tunica media by collagen fibers) (see the section on arteriolosclerosis).

**Subcortical arteriosclerotic leukoencephalopathy.** Multiple lacunae located in the white matter of the frontal lobes coexist with a condition known in persons of geriatric age as subcortical leukoencephalopathy, or diffuse white matter rarefaction. Seemingly, this is one of the anatomic substrates of some dementing syndromes commonly known as vascular dementias.[100,221] This designation emphasizes the general concept that unspecified diseases of the cerebral blood vessels and the consequent changes in the blood supply to the brain may be responsible for some of dementias of old age. The suggestion that some dementing syndromes originate with injury to the cerebral white matter was first proposed by Binswanger[30] and subsequently was endorsed by Alzheimer,[7] who also hypothesized that the changes in the white matter could be the result of structural abnormalities in the blood vessels that supply the subcortical cerebral white matter. Such hypothesis remains plausible but still unconfirmed.

In 1894, Binswanger described three types of mental deterioration that, in his opinion, could have a vascular origin: (1) encephalitis subcorticalis chronica progressiva (ESCP); (2) cerebral arteriosclerotic degeneration; and (3) dementia postapoplexiam. Binswanger reported the clinical history of only one patient with ESCP. Eight years later, Alzheimer discussed the relationship between cerebrovascular diseases and cognitive impairment and suggested that there might be two types of dementing syndromes associated with vascular diseases, one affecting mainly the cortex (through alterations of the large arteries), and the other affecting the white matter (through involvement of small penetrating blood vessels). Thus, Alzheimer seems to have been the first to suggest a possible causal relationship between dementing syndromes and diseases of the small cerebral blood vessels. At present, three types of diseases affecting the penetrating blood vessels of the brain have been associated with structural abnormalities primarily confined to the white matter. These are: (1) arteriolosclerosis, (2) cerebral amyloid angiopathy, (3) and cerebral autosomal dominant arteriopathy with subcortical infarcts and leukoencephalopathy (CADASIL). Only the last of these three angiopathies has been clearly associated with a dementing syndrome and with changes in the white matter presumed to be secondary to the angiopathy.[309]

Changes in the cerebral hemispheric white matter, detectable with increasing frequency by modern neuroimaging methods, are associated with aging and may contribute to the development of specific cognitive deficits. In some series, as many as 20% of asymptomatic persons over the age of 65 may have white matter rarefactions identifiable by CT or MRI.[222] Some authors favor the use of the term *Binswanger's disease* (BD) to designate changes in the cerebral white matter that may or may not be associated with cognitive deficits. This practice is discouraged because the definition of BD is extremely vague. The original author reported only one case, and each of the subsequent writers who described cases of presumptive BD seems to describe a different type of disease.[221] Two descriptive designations are recommended: *leukoaraiosis* for the abnormalities visible on neuroimaging studies, and *subcortical leukoencephalopathy* for the structural abnormalities visible under the microscope that consist of decreased numbers of myelinated fibers, decreased numbers of oligodendrocytes, and increased numbers of hyperplastic astrocytes[225a] (Figs. 6-29, 6-30). Two patterns of leukoraraiosis have been identified in MRI studies: (1) smooth periventricular rims or thin caps located near the ependymal lining; and (2) extensive periventricular rims as well as both patchy or confluent hyperintensities. The former have been tentatively ascribed to breakdowns in the ependymal lining with accompanying disturbances in the flow of the CSF. The extensive white matter hyperintensities are thought to be the result of either ischemia or edema.[152,153]

Age and hypertension are univariate predictors of leukoaraiosis, and the condition is more prevalent in patients with Alzheimer disease than in matched controls.[152,153] Cerebral amlyloid angiopathy, a disease of small blood vessels, may be involved in the mechanisms responsible for leukoaraiosis in patients with Alzheimer disease. In one autopsy series close to 60% of Alzheimer disease cases had cerebral white matter changes that the authors interpreted as being indepen-

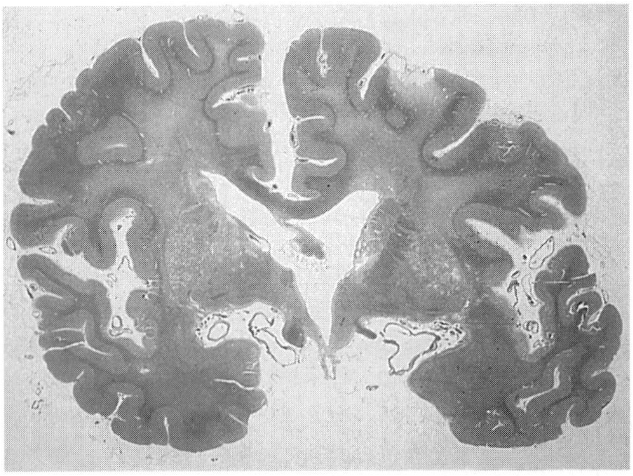

**Fig. 6-29.** Diffuse subcortical leukoencephalopathy accompanied by arteriolosclerosis in a demented patient whose brain had no changes of Alzheimer disease. (H&E; ×1.5.)

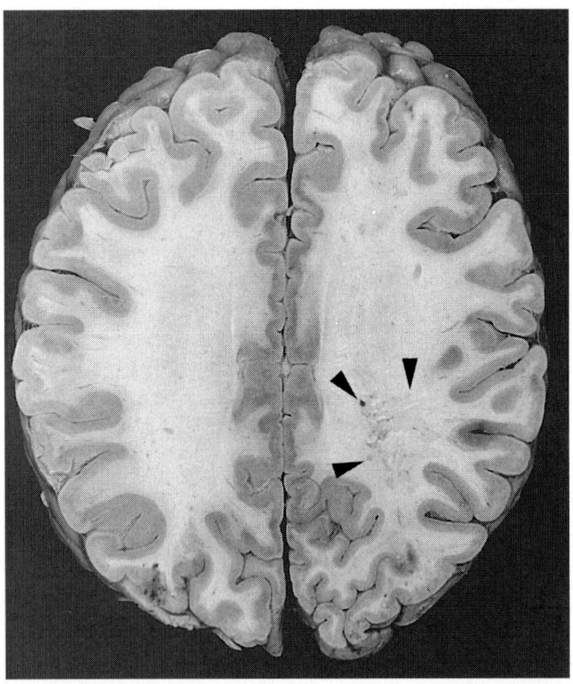

**Fig. 6-30.** Focal subcortical leukoencephalopathy (*arrowheads*) that occurred 10 days before death in a survivor of transient cardiac arrest.

dent of the structural abnormalities affecting the cortex.[39]

The authors of a review of over 100 publications dealing with the anatomy and physiology of the arterial circulation to the cerebral white matter and with the pathogenesis of leukoaraiosis suggest that some types of this condition may be the result of ischemic injury to the brain. Both structural changes affecting the small blood vessels of the brain, which in most instances are the result of chronic hypertension and aging, and the conditions created by the unique pattern of blood supply to the hemispheric white matter seem to contribute to the development of leukoraraiosis. Based on the information available in this review, the authors suggest that the conditions responsible for these white matter changes may involve transient repeated events characterized by moderate drops in regional cerebral blood flow.[223,224] This hypothesis is based on the observation that in animal models of regional ischemia significant structural alterations are observed in oligodendrocytes and axons as early as 3 hours after the occlusion of an intracranial artery (Fig. 6-31). At this time pyknosis in oligodendrocytes and segmental axonal swelling become prominent in the subcortical white matter of Wistar rats with MCA occlusion. Contemporaneous neuronal injury in adjacent gray matter is minimal or nonexistent, suggesting that this type of leukoencephalopathy develops independently of damage to the neuronal perikaryon.[225a]

## HEMORRHAGES

### Intracerebral Hemorrhage

Spontaneous bleeding into the brain parenchyma (intracerebral hemorrhage or ICH) and the subarachnoid space (subarachnoid hemorrhage or SAH) are collectively known in the epidemiologic literature as *hemorrhagic strokes*. These conditions account for about 20% of all strokes with ICH occurring twice as often as SAH. Hemorrhagic strokes have different etiologies and associated risk factors, but ICH are more common in hypertensive than in normotensive individuals.[43] In contrast, over 50% of instances of SAH among persons older than 50 years of age are associated with the rupture of a saccular aneurysm. Arterial hypertension, diabetes mellitus, anticoagulant treatment, and alcohol intake are more commonly associated with ICH than with SAH, which is, however, associated more frequently with cigarette smoking.[142] In addition to the volume and location of the hematoma, age and amount of alcohol ingested within 1 week of the ictus are independent determinants of the long-term outcome of ICH.[142] In contrast, during the acute postictal state, volume of ICH and presence of blood in the ventricular cavities are the two main determinants of the outcome.[142]

Several unexplained issues in the epidemiology of ICH include variation in hemorrhage rates among different racial groups. The incidence of ICH is highest in Asians, intermediate in blacks, and lowest in Caucasians. The disease has often been called "hypertensive" and there is little doubt that increased blood pressure promotes ICH. However, other factors influence the occurrence of ICH, including low serum cholesterol, heavy alcohol consumption, cigarette smoking, dietary patterns, and use of oral contraceptives. Intake of illicit

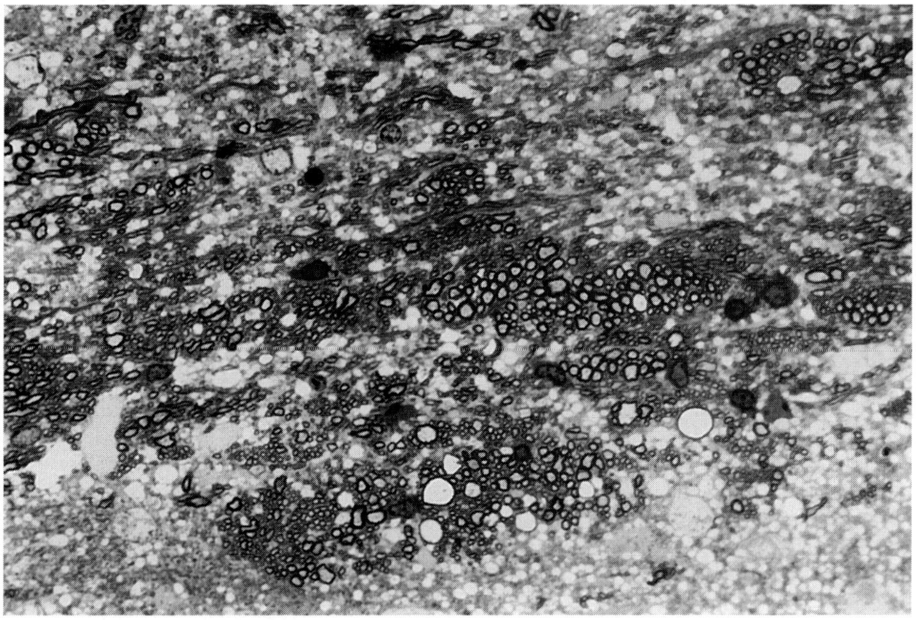

**Fig. 6-31.** Cerebral white matter from a Wistar rat with MCA occlusion of four hours' duration. The vacuolation and pallor of the injured white matter contrasts with the appearance of the preserved white mater bundles. (Toluidine blue; ×240.)

drugs, including cocaine and amphetamines, by oral, nasal, or intravenous routes also has been associated with an increased incidence of ICH.[331]

The earliest symptoms of ICH are focal in nature and vary according to the region of the brain where the hemorrhage begins.[44] The brain parenchyma does not contain pain-sensitive nerve endings; therefore, blood within the brain should not cause pain or headache unless pain-sensitive fibers in the meningeal blood vessels are stimulated by blood. The neurologic symptoms begin, evolve, and progress gradually, usually during a period of minutes. Several studies have documented progressive bleeding in patients with intracerebral hemorrhage, but the factors that lead to progressive bleeding have not been clarified. Most data from large series and registries have shown that most hemorrhages occur during activities of daily living; only 10% occurred during physical activity or emotional duress. Vomiting, loss of consciousness, and headache are common with ICH in the infratentorial compartment. Some patients with ICH may have arrhythmias and electrocardiographic changes consistent with ischemic myocardial injury.[45] Based on a study of consecutive evaluations of ICH by CT, the authors concluded that most patients with ICH that enlarge the hematoma did so during the first 6 hours after the ictus. In about 17% of the patients, enlargement of the hematoma occurred up to 24 hours later. Beyond this time, rebleeding at the site of an ICH is extremely rare.[150]

The causes of ICH are multiple and include systemic illnesses, especially hypertension, bleeding disorders,[65] vascular abnormalities such as amyloid angiopathy, vascular malformations, angiitis, and exogenous factors such as drug abuse and head trauma. In most large series, hypertension is the cause of ICH in about 37% to 66% of the cases.[146]

Cerebral angiography has demonstrated that ICH usually originates from a single artery or an arterialized vein. By neuroimaging methods secondary bleeding sites at the periphery of ICH have been identified as late as 20 days after the clinical onset. In this sense, intracerebral hematomas are heterogeneous lesions that slowly expand. Dul and Drayer[72] have summarized the stages of ICH as seen on CT as follows: In the acute stage, erythrocyte release of oxygen creates a relative concentration of deoxyhemoglobin. In the subacute phase, the oxidative denaturation of hemoglobin converts it into methemoglobin. Formation of methemoglobin begins at the periphery of the hematoma and progresses centrally concurrent with the ingrowth of macrophages and neovascularity at the periphery of the hematoma.[72] The diagnosis of acute ICH is relatively straightforward on CT, but the subacute and chronic stages have a less specific appearance. This is because the attenuation coefficient of the hematoma approximates that of the brain as the red blood cells are reabsorbed. In the hyperacute stage, blood is extravasated but not yet clotted. A direct linear relationship has been shown between the CT attenuation value and the hemoglobin concentration of the blood. Whole blood has an attenuation value of 56 HU, whereas the same value for cerebral hematoma is in the range of 85 HU.[72] In the acute stage, a cerebral hematoma becomes progressively dense as a result of thrombus formation and serum extrusion. The peripheral rim hypodensity reaches a maximum at approximately 5 to 7 days. During the subacute stage, the surrounding white matter edema begins to recede. The density of the ICH decreases first at the periphery and subsequently in the center. The presence of a hyperdense ring surrounding the hematoma has been tentatively explained on the basis of: (1) hypervascularity of granulation tissue, (2) loss of autoregulation with luxury perfusion, and (3) extravasation of contrast material associated with localized breakdown of the blood-brain barrier.[72]

In the chronic stage, ICH progresses from isodense to hypodense relative to the brain parenchyma. The displacement of nearby structures disappears and focal atrophy becomes apparent. On MR, the hyperacute ICH appears virtually identical to many brain lesions with high proton density. A few hours later, the surrounding edema and the serum from clot retraction give the high intensity perimeter on the T2-weighted images.[72] Subacute hematomas are characterized by their high signal intensity on T1-weighted images. The chronic stage of ICH evolution, as studied on MRI, begins as methemoglobin is phagocytized by macrophages and glial cells and is converted to hemosiderin. In summary, the clinical diagnosis of brain hemorrhage can be readily confirmed or excluded with the use of CT and MRI. Additionally, different causes of bleeding can show important variations from the temporal patterns characteristic of primary ICH.[72]

The morphologic description of the sequential changes in ICH is based on the evolution of basal ganglionic hemorrhages that occur in association with hypertension. Neumann recognized two pigmented layers within the hemorrhage: an inner layer called hematoidin and an outer layer containing abundant hemosiderin.[102] According to Spatz, three stages are typical in the evolution of ICH. The first one, lasting approximately 4 days, includes deformation, edema, and necrosis of the surrounding tissues. The second stage involves absorption of the hematoma and typically lasts 5 to 15 days. In the final stage, there is conversion of the hematoma into either a fibrous scar or a fluid-filled cavity.[102,103] In the acute stages, ICH consists of a liquid or semiliquid mass of blood displacing the surrounding brain tissue. Edema develops at the periphery of the hemorrhage after a few days and is particularly prominent in ICH located in the white matter, where it is common to see at this time multiple marginal hemorrhages. After a few days, the hematoma increases in consistency and adopts a brown color while edema at the periphery begins to recede. After several months or years, depending on the volume, the hematoma is replaced by a cavity lined by cells, mostly astroglial, containing brown or rusty pigment. Differences of opinion abound concerning the rate of evolution of ICH. Some authors contend that an ICH becomes a solid clot a few hours after the original bleeding; partial liquefaction develops only 12 to 15 hours later. Others report that clotting in ICH occurs only after the first day. Most authors believe that an ICH becomes at least partially liquefied by the end of the first week, but solid clots may persist for several weeks also. Large ICH become encapsulated by a fibroglial membrane that has been compared to the capsule of chronic subdural hematomas. This membrane, according to some authors, becomes established 5 to 6 weeks after the original bleeding.[102] After several hours or days, depending on the size and site of the hemorrhage, extracellular brain edema becomes evident in the parenchyma adjacent to the ICH. After approximately 4 to 10 days, the red blood cells begin to lyse, at which time cellular infiltrates, especially PMN leukocytes and activated microglia appear. Some of these microscopic events have been reproduced in experimental models in which small aliquots of the animal's own blood were injected into the brain; other models of ICH induced hemorrhagic lesions via the intracerebral injection of collagenases that have specificity for the basal lamina of microvessels.[249] In approximate order of frequency, ICH may start at one of the following sites: putamen, globus pallidus, thalamic nuclei, cerebral white matter (usually called lobar hemorrhages), cerebral ventricles, cerebellum, pons, and medulla[18,99] (Figs. 6-32 to 6-37). There are numerous etiologic factors for ICH; among the main categories are arterial hypertension, hematologic disorders (either primary or drug-induced), aneurysms and vascular malformations, cerebral amyloid angiopathy, drugs, head trauma, intracranial neoplasms, angiitis, and miscellaneous angiopathies.[146]

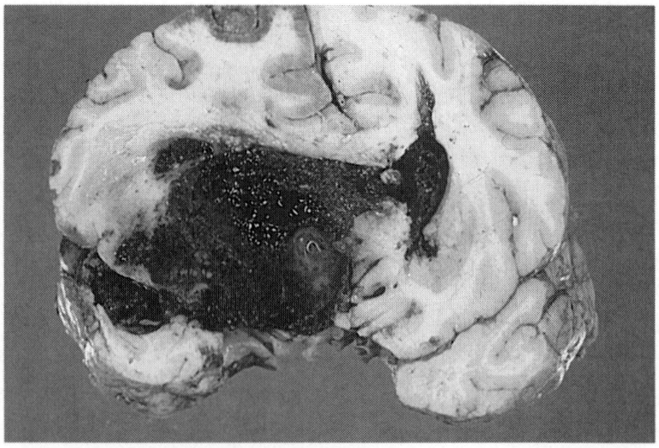

**Fig. 6-32.** Large, recent intracerebral hemorrhage at the basal ganglia. The location suggests a hypertensive etiology; however, a ruptured aneurysm of the anterior communicating artery was found in this specimen.

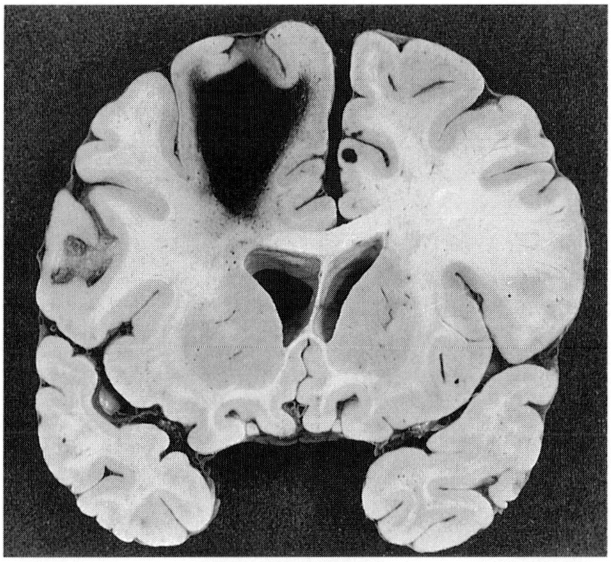

Fig. 6-33. Lobar hemorrhages associated with extensive cerebral amyloid angiopathy.

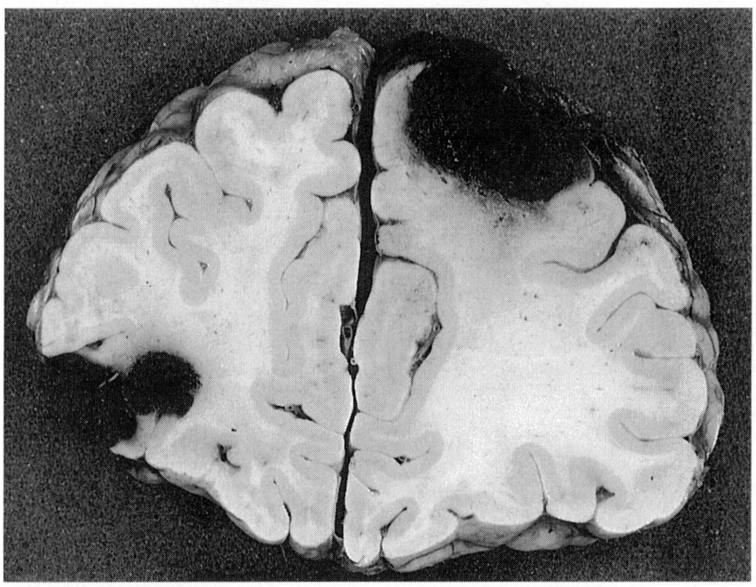

Fig. 6-34. Cerebral hemorrhages at the sites of metastatic choriocarcinoma. Extension of the parenchymal hemorrhage into the subarachnoid space (as shown here) is rare in ICH of hypertensive origin.

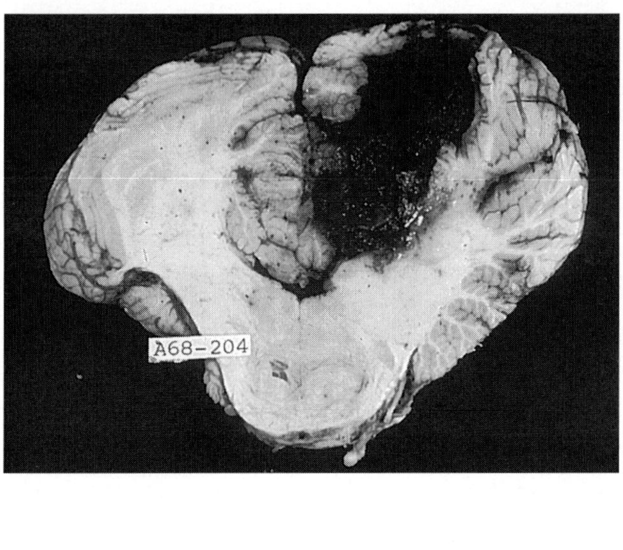


Fig. 6-35. Primary ICH of the left cerebellar hemisphere and a lacune in the basis pontis in a patient with a long-standing history of hypertension.

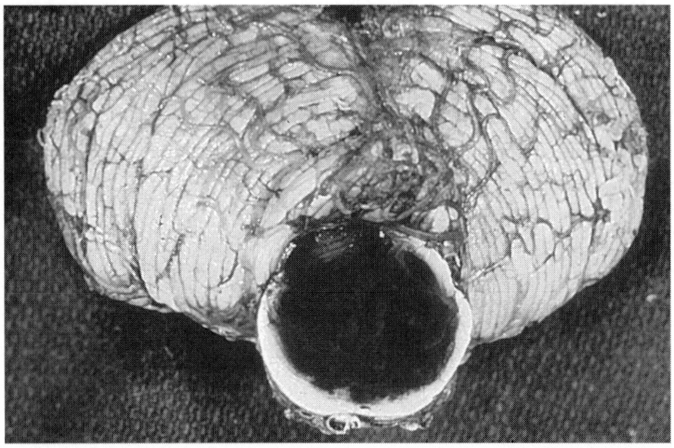

**Fig. 6-36.** Primary ICH of the pons in a specimen with marked arteriolosclerosis.

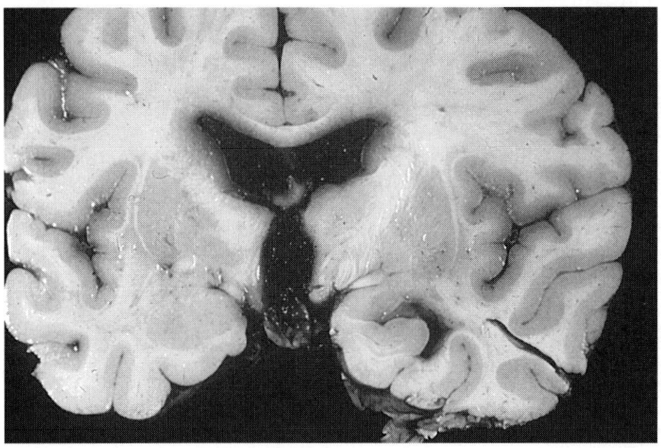

**Fig. 6-37.** Primary intraventricular hemorrhage associated with a cavernous hemangioma of the choroid plexus.

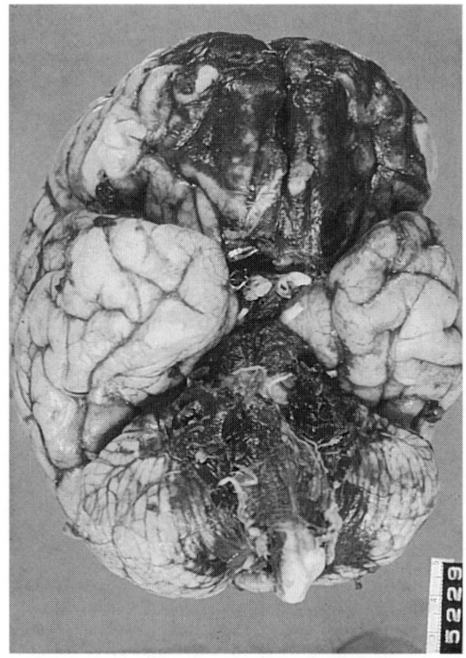

**Fig. 6-38.** Primary subarachnoid hemorrhage associated with rupture of a saccular aneurysm located at the junction of the ICA, MCA, and posterior communicating artery.

### Primary Subarachnoid Hemorrhage

Spontaneous bleeding in the subarachnoid space is responsible for slightly less than 10% of all strokes (Fig. 6-38). In contrast with the focal neurologic deficits that herald ischemic strokes and ICH, bleeding into the subarachnoid space is manifested by headache, usually of an excruciating nature.[180] The diagnosis of SAH is established by CT, which frequently can be analyzed to suggest the likely etiology of the hemorrhage. SAH of aneurysmal origin is more common among persons 55 to 58 years of age. In contrast, SAH in a younger population is more commonly associated with rupture of an arteriovenous malformation. Heros and Kistler[130] suggest that the following risk factors increase the likelihood of finding saccular aneurysms among patients admitted with the diagnosis of primary SAH: history of ruptured aneurysm in a member of the family, fibromuscular dysplasia, polycystic kidney, coarctation or hypoplasia of the aorta, Ehlers-Danlos syndrome, Marfan syndrome, and pseudoxanthoma elasticum. Almost all these conditions share abnormalities in the metabolism of stromal proteins. These defects are presumed to be reflected in the structural abnormalities of the arterial walls that make them susceptible to aneurysm formation and spontaneous rupture.

Approximately 12% of patients with SAH die before reaching the hospital. The main variable between this group and those who received medical attention was the frequency of posterior fossa aneurysms (38%) compared with 14% among those who received medical attention.[265] Angiography is necessary for the diagnosis of aneurysms and, in a few cases, leakage of contrast medium has been recorded during angiography.[87] The presence of blood in the subarachnoid space is a significant cause of severe headache. This is attributed to the fact that the large vessels at the base of the brain are abundantly innervated by fibers rich in substance P, which is the main tachykinin involved in the transmission of nociceptive information. These fibers originate from the trigeminal and the upper dorsal root ganglia.[173] This trigeminovascular system is thought to be intimately involved in the mechanisms of head pain and migrainous headaches. Loss of consciousness affects about 50% of patients who reach the hospital, and some complain of headache just before passing out. Approximately 40% of patients with SAH lack localizing neurologic signs.[316]

CT is the preferred method of diagnosing SAH. This is because CT is very sensitive in detecting blood in the CSF space and on selected occasions the location of the aneurysm can be deduced from the location of the hemorrhage (Fig. 6-39). Thus, a unilateral hematoma confined to the sylvian sulcus is likely to be the result of the rupture of a saccular aneurysm located at

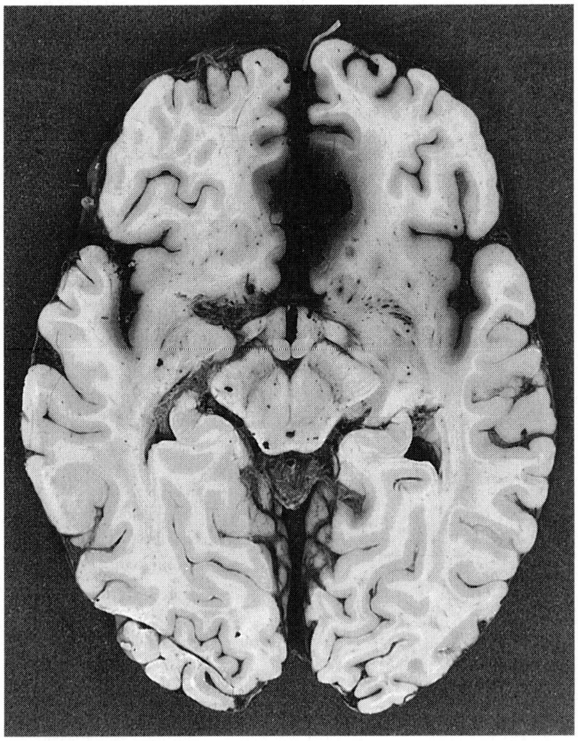

**Fig. 6-39.** Primary subarachnoid hemorrhage associated with rupture of a saccular aneurysm located at the anterior communicating artery.

the bifurcation of the MCA. The detection of blood in the subarachnoid space must be followed, in appropriately triaged cases, by angiographic evaluation of the intracranial vasculature.

In the last decade, a new entity called perimesencephalic nonaneurysmal subarachnoid hemorrhage (PNSH) has been described among patients who have subarachnoid hemorrhage confined to the basal cisterns surrounding the brainstem; the angiographic evaluation fails to disclose aneurysms or other sources of bleeding. The etiology of PNSH remains unclarified, although most authors suggest a venous origin. The original observation made by van Gijn and others[313] and its practical significance is that in contrast to aneurysmal SAH, PNSH has a benign course and these patients do not require extensive work up or detailed follow-up.[271] Compared with patients with SAH traceable to a ruptured aneurysm, the group of about 170 patients with PNSH tended to be younger, less hypertensive, and included a larger group of men.[271] The fatal consequences of aneurysmal subarachnoid hemorrhage in the acute state seem related to bleeding into the cerebral ventricles, development of acute pulmonary edema, and intraparenchymal hemorrhage.[265] After the initial stage, diffuse brain swelling, and ventricular dilatation (secondary to impaired drainage of spinal fluid) contribute to increase the intracranial pressure and, therefore, to decrease the brain perfusion pressure. This condition may be aggravated by spasm of the intracranial arteries, especially those branches located near the site of the bleeding. Although angiographically visible vasospasm of SAH is not always accompanied by neurologic symptoms, in some patients spasm is severe enough to cause brain infarction or to become the main cause of death.[316] Several blood components including serotonin, prostaglandins, and leukotrienes have been associated with the development of symptomatic intracranial vasospasm. The oral administration of nimodipine seems to be the only effective way of counteracting the ischemic effects attributed to vasospasm.[316]

## BRAIN EDEMA AND VASCULAR DISEASES

Both ischemic and hemorrhagic events in the brain are associated with increased parenchymal volume. This is an undesirable feature of the ischemic injury because increased tissue volume results in decreased perfusion pressure and therefore in further reduction in cerebral blood flow. The chronology of fluid retention in the brain has been mapped primarily on the basis of evaluations of ischemic strokes involving the cerebral hemispheres. After the occlusion of a large artery, such as the MCA, some patients undergo progressive swelling of the ischemic tissues that peaks 3 to 4 days after the stroke (Fig. 6-40) The consequences of this swelling are one of the potential causes of death among these patients.[94] The spontaneous disappearance of the swelling in survivors is almost as precipitous as the pattern observed during its induction. A comparable pattern of hemispheric swelling has been recorded in Wistar rats with experimental MCA occlusion (see Fig. 6-43). The timing of appearance and disappearance of edema is, in these animals, similar to that observed in humans.[110] Tissue edema during the first 90 minutes after the arterial occlusion has been traced to retention of protein-free fluid (i.e., water) primarily in the astrocyte compartment but also involving dendrites and endothelial cells of the microvessels.[169]

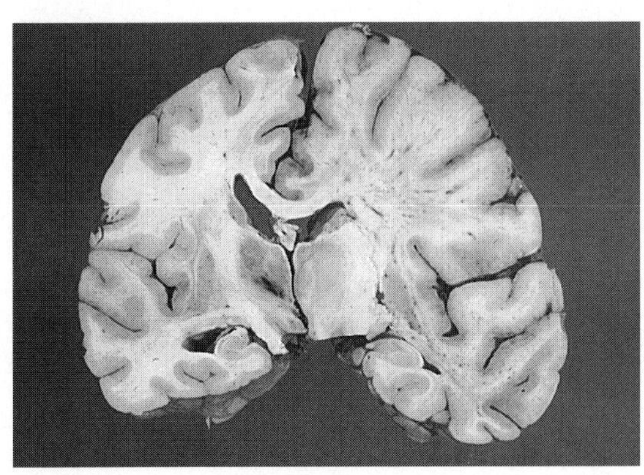

**Fig. 6-40.** Stroke associated with the occlusion of the MCA occurred 5 days before death. The specimen shows massive hemispheric swelling with secondary compression of the lateral ventricle and herniation of the cingulate and uncinate gyri.

The initial cell swelling is attributed to the deficit of energy-supplying metabolites, in particular ATP, which causes intracellular entry of $Na^+$ and cell extrusion of $K^+$.[278] Possible causes of the continuous deterioration of the microcirculation include the early arrival of PMN leukocytes and their adhesion to the endothelial surface of microvessels, the swelling of astrocytes/endothelial cells, and the consequent decrease in the patency of the microvascular channels through which erythrocytes must circulate.[106a] At some undetermined time after the arterial occlusion, the cerebral endothelium becomes permeable to circulating macromolecules in the area injured by the arterial occlusion. The timing of the BBB breakdown in ischemic strokes is incompletely defined largely because in most humans it is difficult to establish the length of time during which the artery remains occluded. Leakage of contrast medium (usually gadolinium) is observed 10 to 14 days after the stroke. The leakage observed at this time is presumptively attributed to the leaky condition of the newly formed microvessels at the periphery of the infarct. In experimental animals with MCA occlusion, leakage of horseradish peroxidase has been documented as early as 3 hours after the arterial occlusion. However, this leakage was transient; by 12 hours none was visible.[110]

The gross deformities produced by brain parenchymal expansions are known as herniations; the displacement of tissues can involve the cingulate gyrus, the uncus or uncinate gyrus (Fig. 6-40), the anterior hypothalamic structures (so-called central herniation), the superior cerebellar vermis, and the cerebellar tonsils. In most cases herniations impinge on the circulation of the compressed tissues and aggravate brain edema. Uncinate herniation can induce extrinsic compression on the posterior cerebral artery; this usually results in hemorrhagic infarction of the corresponding territory. In addition, uncinate herniation can impair the blood supply of the upper midbrain and pons. The consequence of this is the appearance, at these sites, of infarctions and hemorrhages (i.e., "Duret hemorrhages") that frequently remain confined to the tegmentum of the brainstem and are usually more numerous near the midline[94] (Fig. 6-41). The microscopic expression of postischemic brain edema is visible as vacuoles widely distributed throughout the neuropil and the white matter. During the acute postischemic stage, cellular swelling can be appreciated as neuronal haloes and as enlarged hypochromatic astrocyte nuclei.[110] In the white matter, acute ischemic edema is mainly axonal and periaxonal.[225a]

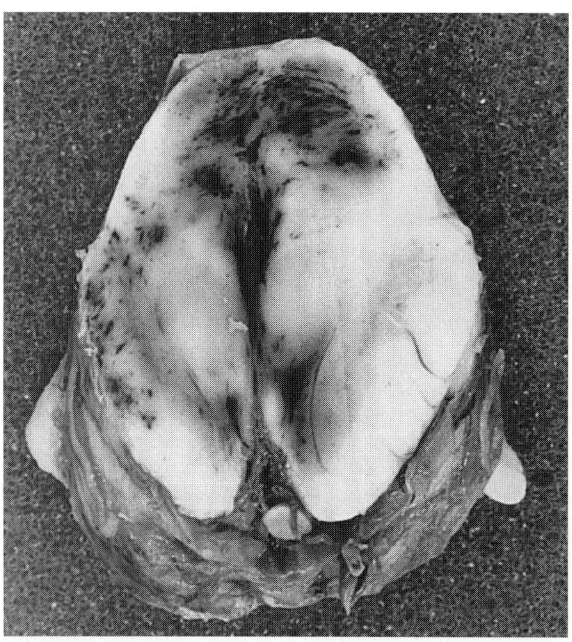

Fig. 6-41. Cross-section of upper midbrain showing the effects of uncinate herniation: narrowing of the interpeduncular fossa, as well as multiple petechiae in the tectum, tegmentum, and one of the cerebral peduncles.

## CENTRAL NERVOUS SYSTEM ANGIOPATHIES (Table 6-2)

### Anatomic Variations

The development of the vasculature of the CNS occurs as a concomitant event with the formation and evolution of the brain and spinal cord. At 3 weeks' gestation, angioblasts derived from the embryonic mesodermal layer start to form capillary plexuses at several sites of the developing CNS.[40] By a process of combination and reabsorption of the capillary plexuses the adult pattern of the arterial system takes place. Between 29 and 38 days' gestation the major intracranial arteries are identified, and by 42 to 44 days the circle of Willis is complete.[219] Additional changes occur, mainly in the size of the arteries, after 6 weeks' gestation. At birth the configuration of the circle of Willis is essentially that of an adult.[219]

The symmetric pattern of the circle of Willis with

**Table 6-2.** CNS Angiopathies

| |
|---|
| Anatomic variations |
| Malformations |
| Aneurysms |
| Atherosclerosis |
| Arteriolosclerosis |
| Cerebral embolism |
| Thrombosis: systemic, venous |
| Angiitis |
| Systemic angiopathies |
| Genetic angiopathies |
| Neoplastic angiopathies |
| Miscellaneous |

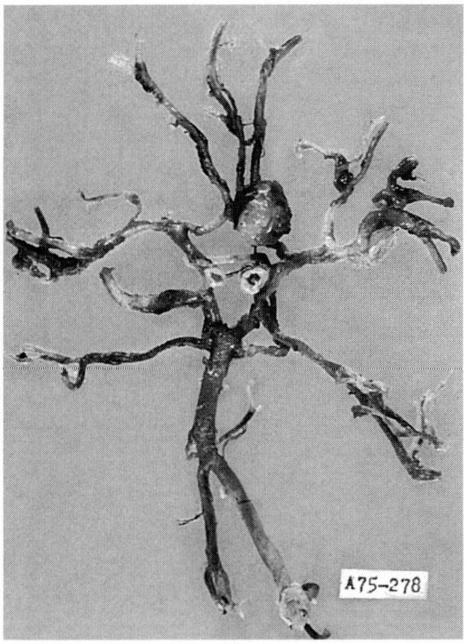


**Fig. 6-42.** Anatomic variations of the circle of Willis include hypoplasia of the left vertebral artery and persistence of three pericallosal arteries. An unruptured saccular aneurysm is visible at the junction of the anterior cerebral and anterior communicating arteries.

uniform communicating arteries connecting the internal carotid and vertebrobasilar systems is found in about 40% of the human population.[5a] In approximately 25% of individuals, one or both posterior communicating arteries retain their large fetal caliber and supply the ipsilateral posterior cerebral artery.[246] This variation may be associated with infarction in the territory supplied by the posterior cerebral artery in cases of occlusion of the common and internal carotid arteries. Other anomalies of the intracranial arteries that may be important in the development or absence of collateral circulation include agenesis, hypoplasia, duplication, and fenestration[40] (Fig. 6-42). Persistence of embryonic arteries is seldom encountered as an incidental finding either by angiography or at autopsy.[145] These carotid-basilar anastomoses are classified in three groups, including primitive trigeminal artery, primitive otic (acoustic) artery, and primitive hypoglossal artery.

**Primitive trigeminal artery.** During early embryonic life, the trigeminal artery connects the internal carotid artery with the paired longitudinal neural arteries that later fuse to form the basilar artery.[219] By the time the embryo is 14 mm in length, the trigeminal artery involutes. A persistent trigeminal artery may be found in adults, and it is the commonest anomaly of the above three types. The incidence of this abnormality is unknown, and until 1972 170 cases had been reported.[291] A persistent trigeminal artery may be the site of an occasional saccular aneurysm or an arteriovenous malformation.[291]

**Primitive otic (acoustic) artery.** The primitive otic artery that connects the internal carotid artery with the midportion of the basilar artery is usually the first of the primitive arteries to disappear when the embryo is 5 mm long.[291]

**Primitive hypoglossal artery.** The primitive hypoglossal artery joins the internal carotid artery with the basilar artery distal to the vertebral arteries.[99] Approximately 20 cases of a persistent hypoglossal artery are reported.[273]

In addition to conventional angiography, human intracranial vessels can be studied in vivo with Doppler ultrasonography. Moreover, magnetic resonance has been adapted to image arteries. Time-of-flight techniques have become the mainstay of noninvasive MRI angiography.[108]

### Malformations

The classification of vascular malformations proposed by McCormick stands as the most useful one.[184] Following are malformations included in the classification.

**Arteriovenous malformation (AVM).** This vascular lesion is characterized by a conglomerate of abnormal arteries and veins without an intervening capillary bed.[184] In most instances AVM are congenital abnormalities whose origin may take place very early in embryonic life within the capillary plexus.[219] The lesion tends to grow with the maturation of the nervous system. Most frequently AVM become symptomatic during the second and third decades of life. Another peak for the beginning of symptoms occurs during the fifth decade. Most common clinical manifestations involve intraparenchymal, subarachnoid, or intraventricular hemorrhages.[128] Other symptoms include seizures, headaches, or cerebral "steal syndromes."[174,230,310] Some malformations that are invisible on angiogram, referred to as "cryptic," may be the source of intracerebral hemorrhage in young persons.[183] AVMs are present throughout the brain and spinal cord.[185] Their location is grossly correlated with the mass volume of the area involved, the frontal lobe being the most common site. The lesion usually is single; multiple AVMs are described in about 19% of patients.[330] The size ranges from microscopic lesions to large AVMs that occupy one or more lobes of the brain. In the cerebral hemispheres AVM are pyramid-shaped lesions with the apex directed toward the center of the brain and the base in the meninges. Based on the number of feeding arteries and draining veins, several angiographic patterns are recognized: (1) the most common corresponds to the multiple-unit AVM in which several arteries feed a lesion drained by several veins; (2) single-

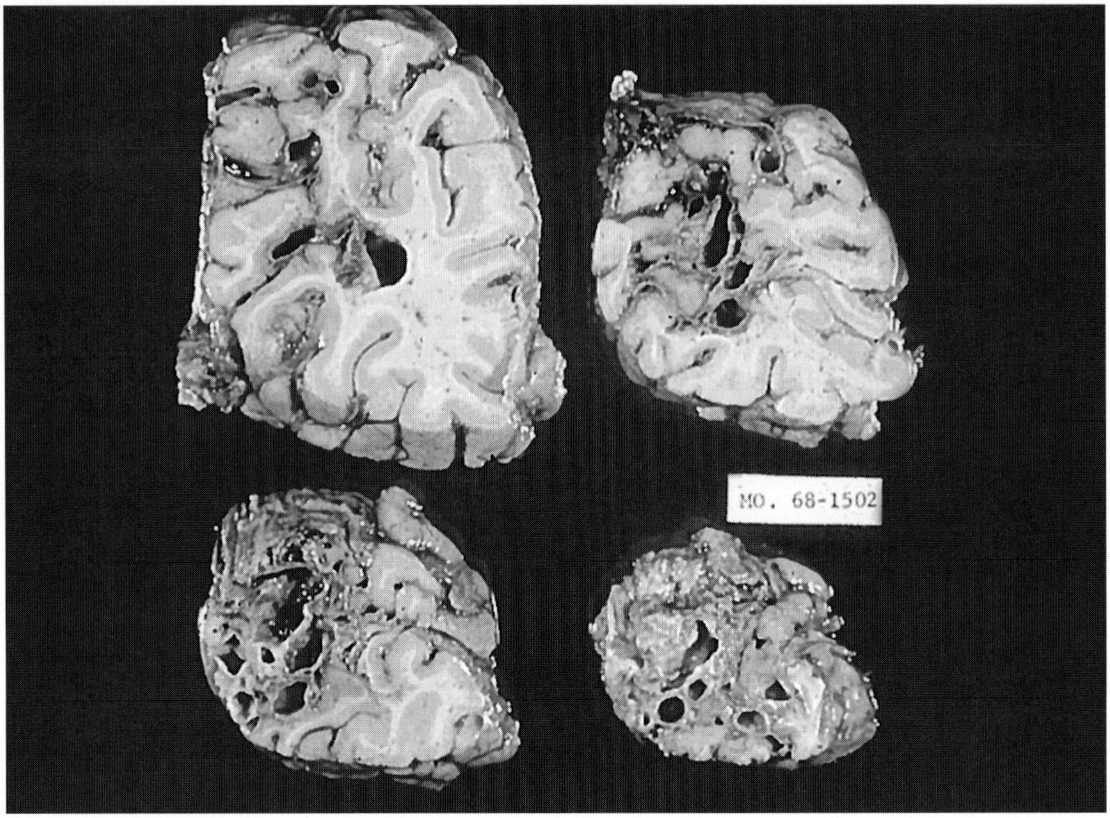


**Fig. 6-43.** Arteriovenous malformation that extends from the posterior parietal region into the occipital pole and is associated with parenchymal scarring. (Lindenberg collection, National Museum of Health and Medicine, Armed Forces Institute of Pathology.)

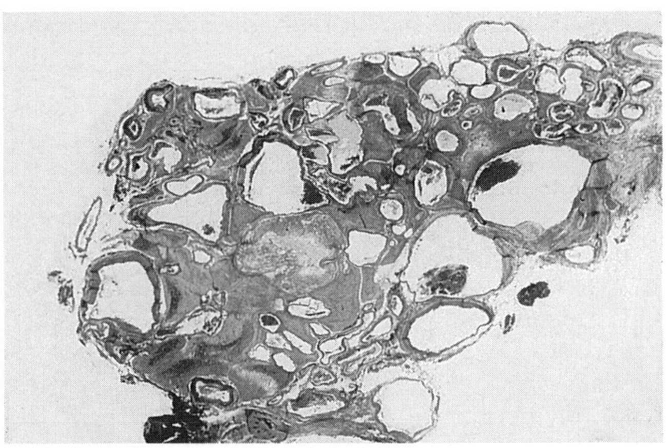

**Fig. 6-44.** Arteriovenous malformation composed of multiple vascular channels of variable caliber; some have fibrotic walls. (Trichrome stain; ×6.5.)

unit AVM is characterized by one feeding artery and one draining vein; (3) AVM with blood supply from intracranial and extracranial arteries; and (4) venous sinus wall type in which the feeding artery that usually is extracranial drains directly into the wall of one of the dural sinuses.[209,227,230] The gross inspection of surgically resected AVM discloses a tangle of vascular channels of variable caliber associated with firm, sometimes gritty neural tissue and areas of yellowish discoloration (Fig. 6-43). Some of the vessels are identified as arteries having elastic lamina or veins and arterialized veins, but many vascular channels exhibit irregular fibrous walls with abundant collagen deposition (Fig. 6-44). Other changes include recent and recanalized thrombi, calcium deposits, and in some cases bone formation.[254] The neural tissue shows increased numbers of reactive astrocytes and abundant astrocytic processes. Hemosiderin-laden macrophages are visible in some cases. Less common findings include aggregates of inflammatory mononuclear cells and deposits of amyloid. The selection of the mode of therapy is influenced by the size of the AVM, the pattern of venous drainage, and the eloquence of the brain parenchyma adjacent to the malformation.[288] Total surgical excision provides cure in most cases.[156,294]

**Varix of the vein of Galen.** The most dramatic example of this malformation is the varix or aneurysmal dilatation of the vein of Galen, which is an arteriovenous malformation in the region of the third ventricle or midbrain. In one type the feeding arteries are normal branches of the three main cerebral arteries, whereas in another type the vascular malformation empties into

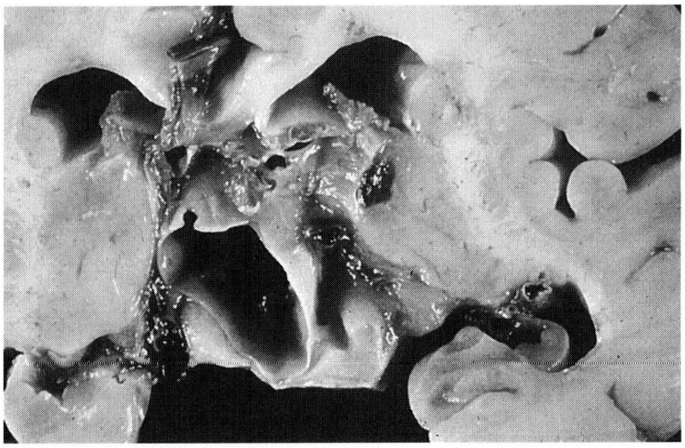

**Fig. 6-45.** Varix of vein of Galen with compression of the adjacent structures.

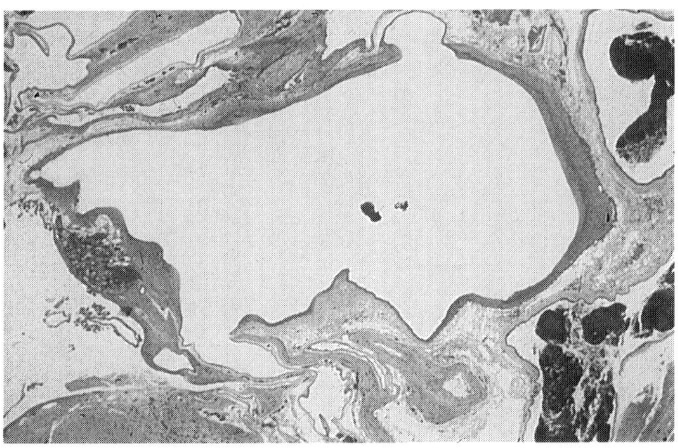

**Fig. 6-46.** Varix of vein of Galen. The vein of Galen exhibits focal fibrosis and an irregular, dilated lumen. (H&E; ×10.)

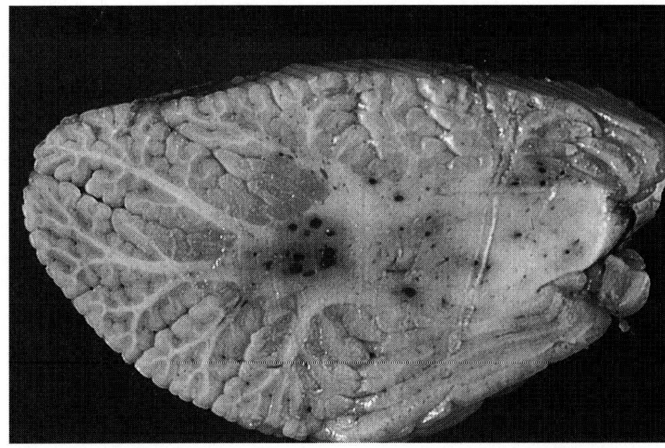

**Fig. 6-47.** Capillary telangiectasis of the cerebellar white matter showing multiple dilated vascular channels.

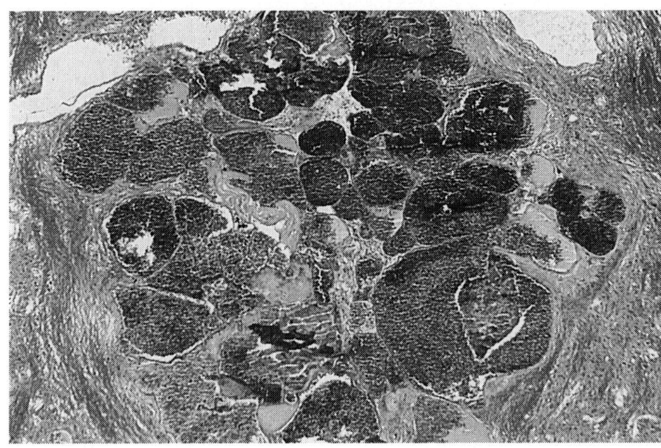

**Fig. 6-48.** Capillary telangiectasis composed of capillary-type vascular channels with delicate walls; intervening neural tissue has normal appearance. (Myelin stain; ×6.5.)

the vein of Galen.[48] The malformation becomes symptomatic most commonly in the neonatal period and early adolescence. The clinical presentation in neonates is associated with congestive heart failure and in infants with hydrocephalus.[8] Older children may present with hemorrhages or seizures. Pathologically, the vein of Galen is dilated and exhibits a wall of variable thickness (Figs. 6-45, 6-46). Dilatation of other adjacent vessels is also identified.

**Capillary telangiectasis.** This vascular malformation is characterized by dilated capillaries and absence of reactive changes within the intervening brain parenchyma. Most lesions are identified incidentally at postmortem examination as a small area of dark spots or petechial hemorrhages (Fig. 6-47). Each component blood vessel exhibits a single layer of endothelial cells supported by a scant number of reticulin fibers (Fig. 6-48). Smooth muscle cells are not present. Although the most common location is the basis pontis, other regions of the brain and spinal cord may be affected.[99] Capillary telangiectasis may be the occasional source of intraparenchymal bleeding or focal neurologic deficits.[81]

**Venous angiomas.** These are congenital abnormalities of the venous system of the CNS. They are the most common vascular malformation, not only in autopsy studies but also in series using the most modern imaging techniques.[52,112] Angiography reveals a characteristic pattern consisting of a single dilated vein fed by several tributary veins.[195] The most common site is the thoracic spinal cord, where the lesion may involve the parenchyma or leptomeninges.[332] Other regions are also involved (Fig. 6-49). The malformation is composed of a variable number of dilated veins lined by a single layer of endothelial cells associated with an irregular wall that contains smooth muscle cells, fibroblastic elements, and collagen fibers (Fig. 6-50). Arter-

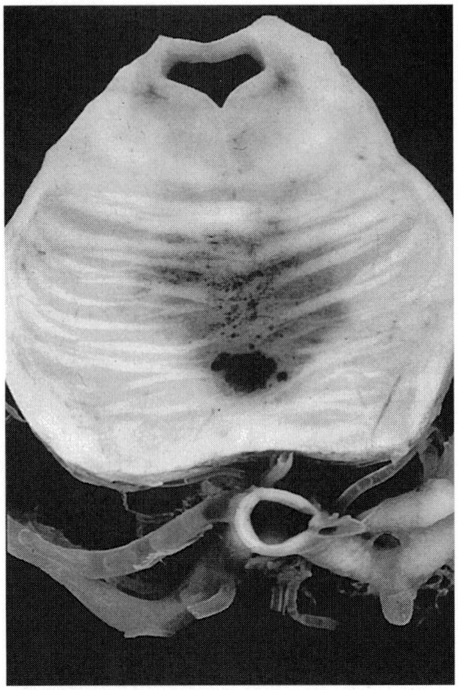

**Fig. 6-49.** Venous angioma with focal reddish discoloration in the adjacent pontine tissues.

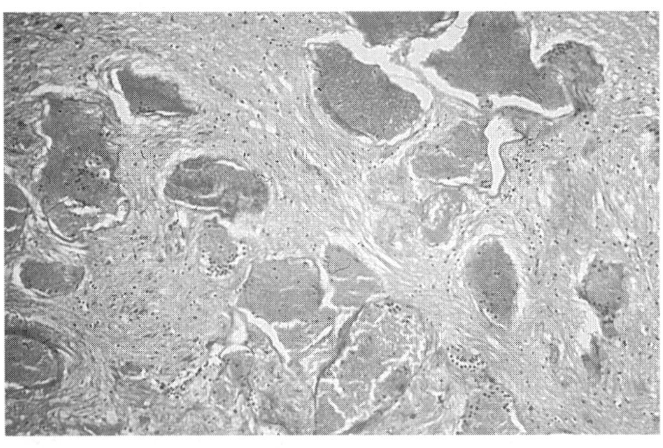

**Fig. 6-50.** Venous angioma composed of dilated veins with thin walls; focal hemosiderin deposition is also visible. (H&E; ×10.)

ies are not present and the intervening brain parenchyma is unremarkable. The alkaline phosphatase reaction of the vascular components is negative.[48] Symptomatic venous angiomas may be associated with other vascular malformations. Seizures, headaches, and hemorrhages are attributed to the presence of these malformations.[246]

**Cavernous angiomas.** These vascular malformations are found throughout the entire CNS, and symptoms are related to their specific location.[272,340] Most

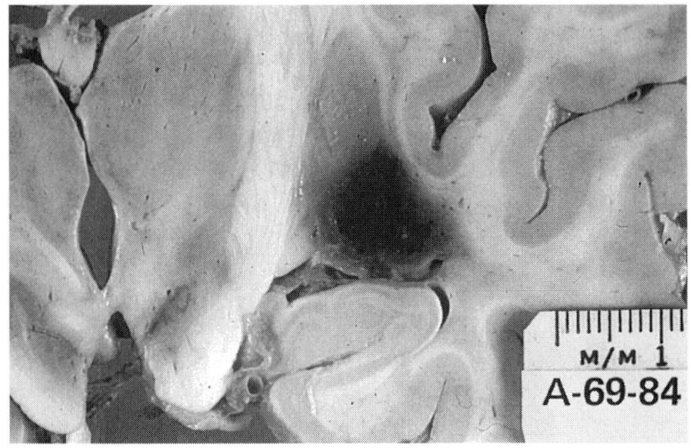


**Fig. 6-51.** Cavernous angioma with associated recent hemorrhage.

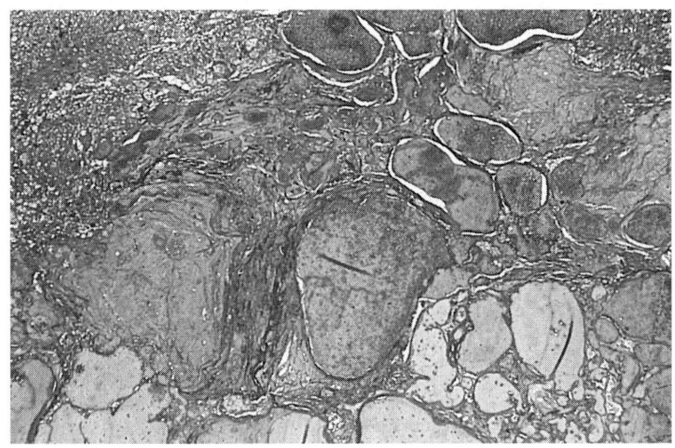

**Fig. 6-52.** Cavernous angioma exhibiting vascular channels with fibrous walls and luminal thrombosis. Neural tissue is not visible among the dilated blood vessels. (Trichrome stain; ×10.)

angiomas are seen in the cerebral white matter.[48] The malformation does not communicate with the arterial system and is invisible on angiography.[279] Angiomas are more frequently identified by CT and MRI of the brain.[238,239] Cavernous angiomas may be inherited as an autosomal dominant trait with multiple lesions that include retinal angiomas.[69] This familial occurrence is more frequent among persons of Hispanic descent.[243] The lesion is characterized by a conglomerate of vascular channels with fibrous walls without intervening brain or spinal cord parenchyma (Figs. 6-51, 6-52). Usually, there is evidence of old hemorrhage, gliosis at the periphery, and sometimes calcification of the vascular walls. A definitive classification of a lesion must be based on the knowledge that some angiomas coexist at the same site with other vascular anomalies.[242]

**Vascular malformations associated with genetic diseases.** Some vascular malformations may be a component of a hereditary disorder. This group of entities includes the following syndromes:

1. *Hereditary Hemorrhagic Telangiectasia (Osler-Weber-Rendu Disease)* is an autosomal dominant disorder characterized by telangiectasias involving skin, mucous membranes, lungs, and gastrointestinal and genitourinary systems.[111,121] A pulmonary arteriovenous fistula may be the source of paradoxic embolism to the brain with subsequent occlusive disease or, in cases of septic emboli, with abscess formation or meningitis.[280] Central nervous system vasculopathies are mainly arteriovenous malformations and telangiectases as well as intracranial aneurysms.[247]
2. *Wyburn-Mason Syndrome* is characterized by an arteriovenous malformation of the visual system that extends from the retina, following the optic nerves and chiasm into the midbrain and sometimes the occipital lobes.[189] The clinical manifestation, which occurs during childhood, is associated with progressive visual loss.[137] Less common symptoms include sudden loss of vision, epilepsy, and ataxia.
3. *Encephalofacial Angiomatosis (Sturge-Weber Syndrome)* is characterized by a facial cutaneous angioma (port-wine nevus) and ipsilateral angioma in the cerebral leptomeninges. The facial nevus usually involves the forehead and upper eyelid following the distribution of the trigeminal nerve.[5] In some patients the cutaneous angioma may involve other areas of the face or extend into the trunk and extremities.[312] The leptomeningeal angioma is typically unilateral, but bilateral lesions exist in about 15% of the patients.[34] The brain lesion consists of a proliferation of thin-walled veins and capillaries most commonly located in the parietal and occipital lobes. The adjacent cortex exhibits calcification in a gyriform pattern and atrophy with neuronal loss and gliosis (Fig. 6-53).

Cutaneous angiomas frequently herald the existence of complex vascular abnormalities affecting intracranial and extracranial arteries, the cerebellum, and less frequently the cerebral hemispheres. This association constitutes a relatively frequent neurocutaneous disorder for which the designation "cutaneous hemangioma-vascular complex syndrome" has been suggested.[228]

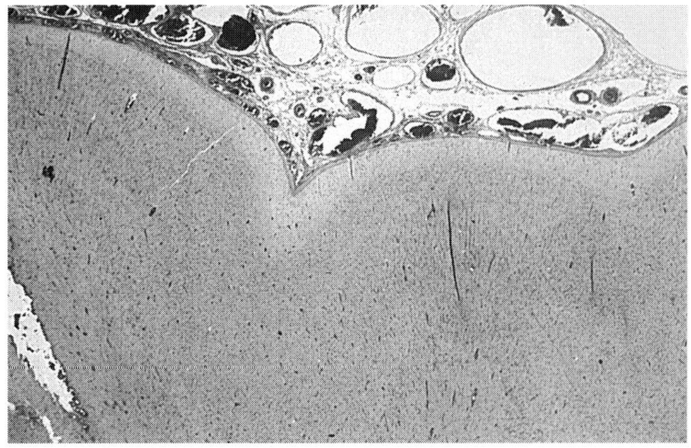

**Fig. 6-53.** Sturge-Weber syndrome with proliferation of thin-walled vascular channels in the leptomeninges and calcium-containing deposits in the cerebral cortex. (H&E; ×20.)

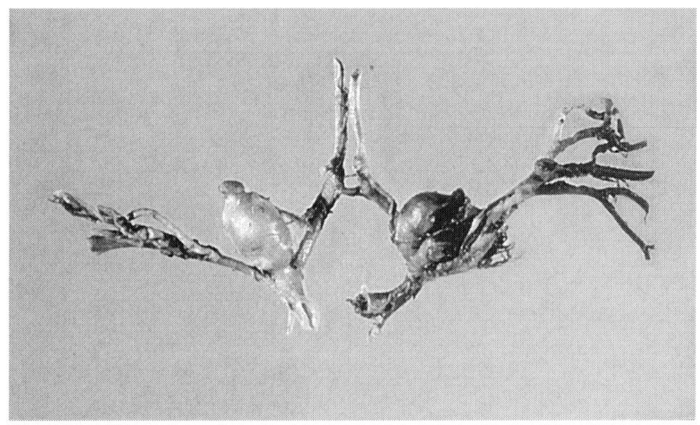

**Fig. 6-54.** Saccular aneurysms of the internal carotid arteries. Rupture is visible in the left internal carotid aneurysm. (Lindenberg collection, National Museum of Health and Medicine, Armed Forces Institute of Pathology.)

### Aneurysms

Intracranial aneurysms are classified as saccular, mycotic, and neoplastic.[199]

**Saccular aneurysms.** These aneurysmatic dilatations also are known as berry or congenital aneurysms.[252] Most are asymptomatic incidental autopsy findings. Approximately 5% of the population harbor saccular aneurysms.[138,311] The clinical presentation is most commonly associated with rupture and hemorrhage, either subarachnoid or intraparenchymal. Bleeding usually occurs between the ages of 55 and 60 years.[259] Saccular aneurysms also are present in children, in whom symptoms reflect intracranial hemorrhage that usually occurs before the age of 2 years or after 10 years.[217] About 90% of saccular aneurysms involve the internal carotid artery system with an equal distribution between the junction of the anterior cerebral and anterior communicating arteries, the junction of the internal carotid and posterior communicating arteries, and the bifurcation or trifurcation of the middle cerebral artery.[183] The bifurcation of the basilar artery into the posterior cerebral arteries is the most common site for saccular aneurysms of the vertebrobasilar system.[74] Multiple aneurysms exist in about 20% of cases (Fig. 6-54). The size of a saccular aneurysm is

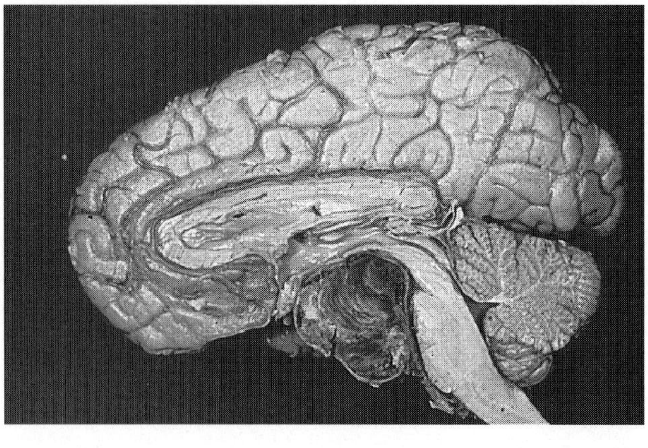

**Fig. 6-55.** Giant aneurysm at the dome of the basilar artery with thrombosis and compression of the pons and midbrain.

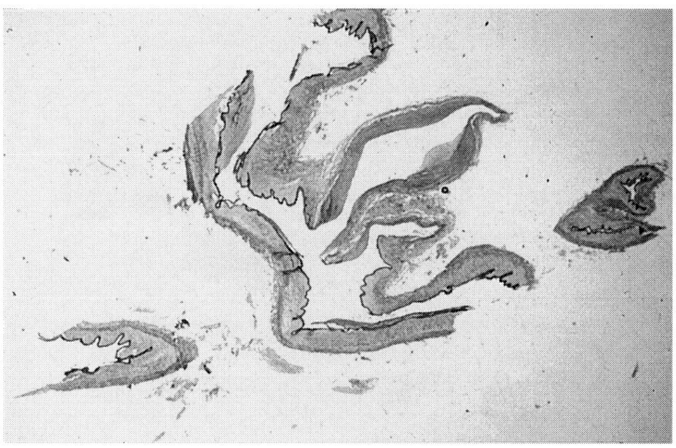

**Fig. 6-56.** Longitudinal section of a small unruptured saccular aneurysm and its parent artery. The aneurysmatic sac lacks internal elastic lamina. (Elastic stain; ×25.)

variable and ranges from a few millimeters to several centimeters. Rupture usually occurs in sacs larger than 5 mm. Saccular aneurysms greater than 2.5 cm in diameter are called *gigantic*. The clinical manifestations of these are similar to those of a tumor at the same location, or may be secondary to embolism of material originating within the aneurysmal sac[202] (Fig. 6-55). Complications that may occur either 2 or 3 days or 11 days after the initial bleeding episode include vasospasm of the arteries near the aneurysm, rebleeding, and hydrocephalus secondary to the adhesions between the leptomeninges.[199] Aneurysmal sacs have two components: the area proximal to the parent artery or neck, and the dome or apex. Most aneurysms rupture at the dome.[49] The aneurysmal wall is formed by a single layer of endothelial cells resting on fibrous stroma devoid of smooth muscle cells or elastic lamina. The muscle layer and the internal elastic lamina from the parent artery discontinue at the neck of the aneurysm (Fig. 6-56). The cause of saccular aneurysms is unknown.

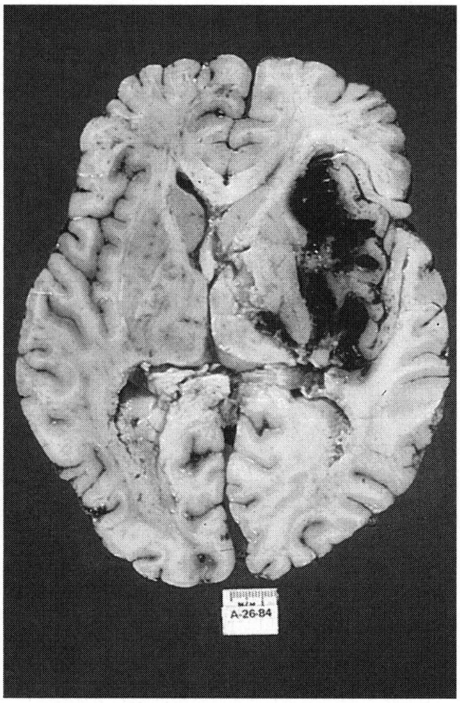



**Fig. 6-57.** Intraparenchymal hemorrhage associated with rupture of mycotic aneurysm of the middle cerebral artery.

Current theories include the following three categories: (1) *Congenital medial defects:* saccular aneurysms may originate at branching sites of the major cerebral arteries where the muscular layer is discontinuous.[85,259] (2) *Acquired defects:* degenerative changes may affect the muscular layer and elastic lamina as a result of hemodynamic factors.[292,293] (3) *Hereditary factors:* Saccular aneurysms are more common among persons with hereditary disorders of connective tissues, such as fibromuscular dysplasia, coarctation of the aorta, and polycystic kidney disease.[199]

**Mycotic aneurysms.** Mycotic aneurysms are localized sites of arteritis that develop secondary to septic embolism into the arterial wall. Most emboli originate from cardiac vegetations in cases of bacterial endocarditis.[21,301] Other sources of embolism include pulmonary infections and sepsis. The causal organisms usually are bacteria, but fungi also may be implicated.[3] Septic emboli may be systemic and involve arteries in several organs including spleen and kidney. In the brain, septic emboli with aneurysmal formation tend to involve peripheral branches of the main arteries, most commonly those of the middle cerebral artery[185] (Fig. 6-57). Once a septic embolus is wedged into the lumen of a blood vessel, microorganisms spread and colonize the wall, with subsequent dilatation, necrosis, and eventual rupture of the wall. A mycotic aneurysm is identified as a localized necrotizing panarteritis with acute inflammation (Fig. 6-58).

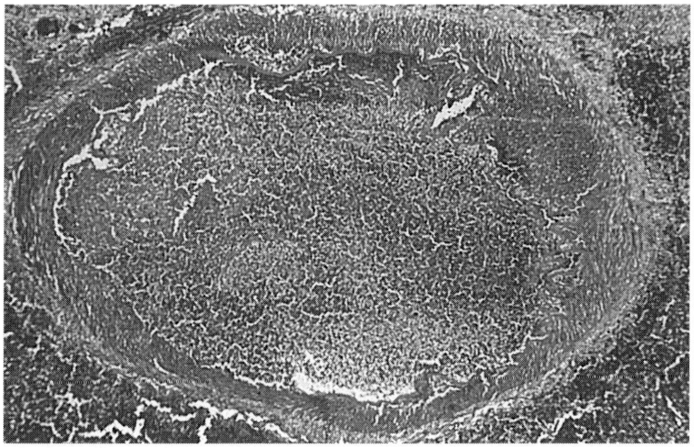

**Fig. 6-58.** Section of the middle cerebral artery showing occlusion by septic embolus and focal arteritis. Same case as in Fig. 6-57. (H&E; ×25.)

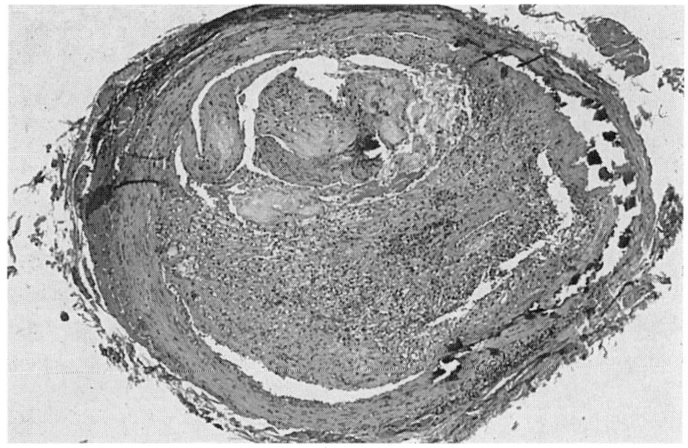

**Fig. 6-59.** Intracranial atherosclerosis complicated by thrombosis and luminal occlusion (H&E; ×25.)

**Neoplastic aneurysms** are associated with emboli from neoplasms located outside the nervous system. Cardiac myxomas of the left atrium are a recognized source of embolism to multiple organs, including the brain.[41] Choriocarcinoma is also associated with formation of neoplastic aneurysms.[133]

### Atherosclerosis

Atherosclerotic lesions are classified as fatty streaks, fibrous plaques, and complicated plaques. The fatty streak appears in the aorta and its major branches during late childhood and adolescence.[290] This lesion is characterized by subendothelial deposits of lipid-laden macrophages, free lipid, connective tissue elements, and T-lymphocytes.[101] Most macrophages originate from circulating monocytes, and few are smooth muscle cells that migrate from the tunica media through fenestrations in the internal elastic lamina into the subendothelial layer.[251] Fibrous plaques form at branching arterial sites and usually appear during adulthood. The lesion is characterized by a fibrous cap covered by endothelial cells. The fibrous cap contains macrophages, monocytes, free cholesterol and cholesterol esters, connective tissue elements including elastic fibers, calcium salts, and a necrotic core.[80] Complicated plaques are similar in composition to fibrous plaques; in addition, these lesions may be ulcerated, exhibit thrombus formation, calcification, and hemorrhage[82,155,187] (Fig. 6-59). Atherosclerosis in the cerebral circulation is more common at the origin of the internal carotid artery, vertebral arteries, basilar artery, posterior cerebral arteries, middle cerebral arteries, and the bifurcation of internal carotids (Figs. 6-60, 6-61). Some symptomatic plaques are associated with more than 70% narrowing of the lumen at the origin of the internal carotid and the basilar arteries. Risk factors implicated in symptomatic atherosclerosis include diabetes mellitus, hypertension, increased low density lipoprotein (LDL) cholesterol levels, cigarette smoking, and low estrogen levels.[33]

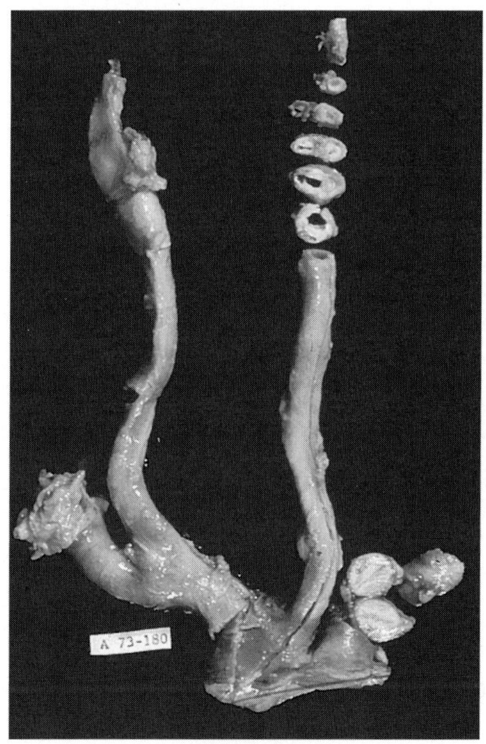


**Fig. 6-60.** Complicated atherosclerosis involving common, internal, and external carotid arteries.

### Arteriolosclerosis

These arteriolar changes are commonly associated with systemic hypertension, diabetes mellitus, and aging. The changes involve small intraparenchymal arteries and arterioles with a diameter of less than 500 μm.[82,234] The changes of arteriolosclerosis include mi-

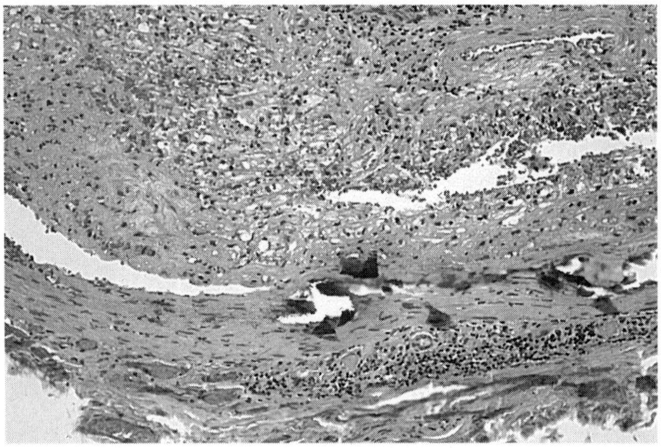

**Fig. 6-61.** Complicated atherosclerosis exhibiting calcification, macrophages, and inflammation. Same case as in Fig. 6-60. (H&E; ×16).

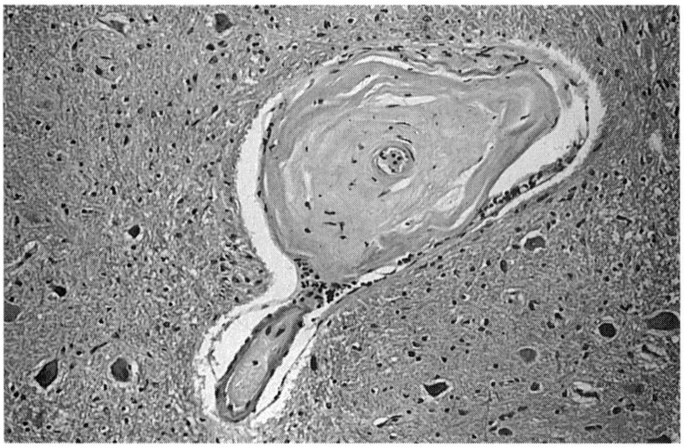

**Fig. 6-63.** Lipohyalinosis of small cerebral artery. The tunica media is replaced by homogeneous acellular material. The lumen is patent. (H&E; ×40.)

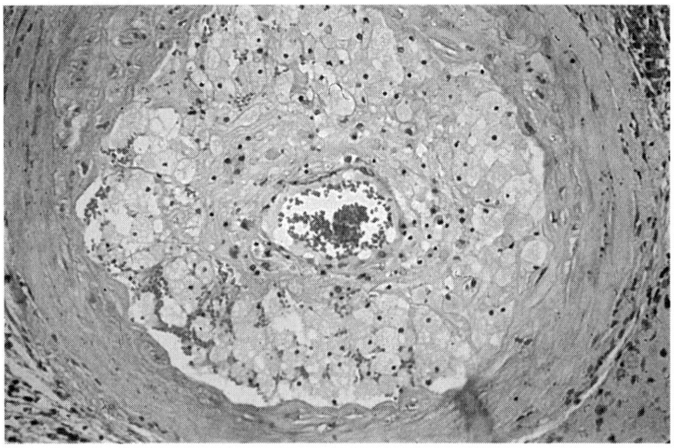

**Fig. 6-62.** Atheroma with prominent macrophages and narrowed lumen. (H&E; ×16)

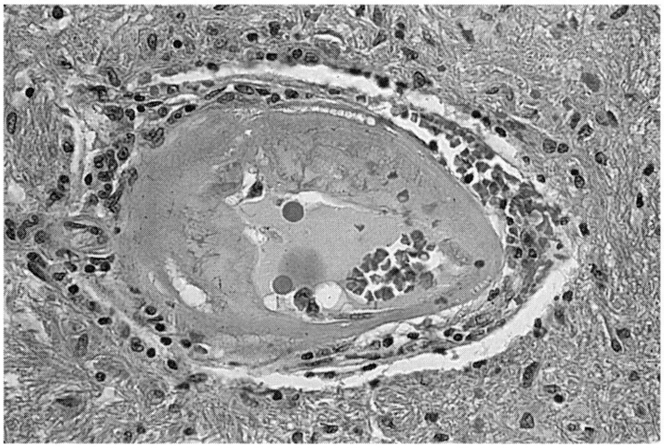

**Fig. 6-64.** "Fibrinoid" necrosis characterized by replacement of the smooth muscle cells by eosinophilic material. (H&E; ×40.)

croatheroma, lipohyalinosis, fibrinoid necrosis, and microaneurysms. Microatheroma is characterized by accumulation of lipid-laden macrophages in the subendothelial layer of a penetrating artery (Fig. 6-62). Lipohyalinosis describes a combination of hyaline change and aggregates of lipid-laden microphages in the vessel wall (Fig. 6-63). Fibrinoid necrosis designates bright eosinophilic material in the vascular wall that represents necrosis of smooth muscle cells and deposits of plasma proteins[289] (Fig. 6-64). Most microaneurysms of the penetrating vessels, or miliary aneurysms, represent ectasias and tortuosities of the arteriolar wall[47] (Fig. 6-65). Parenchymal brain lesions associated with hypertensive arteriolosclerosis are variable. Occlusion of a penetrating blood vessel may be associated with lacunar infarcts, and rupture of the vessel wall may lead to intracerebral hemorrhage.[82,83] Cerebral arteriolosclerosis is frequently associated with cerebral white matter rarefaction (or leukoaraiosis), especially among persons older than 60 years.[32,224]

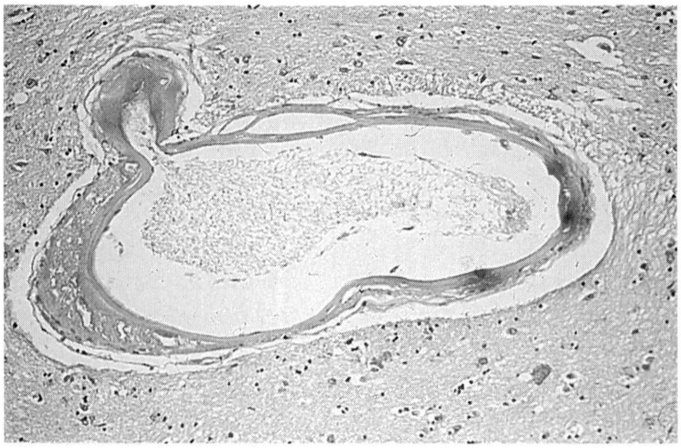

**Fig. 6-65.** Cerebral artery with aneurysmal dilatation. Other changes of arteriolosclerosis are also evident. (H&E; ×40.)

## Cerebral Embolism

Mural thrombi and vegetations in the cardiac chambers, as well as atherosclerosis of the ascending aorta and of the carotid arteries are common sources of brain embolism. Other sources include pulmonary disorders, trauma, coagulopathies and neoplasms associated with hypercoagulable states.[212,234] Cerebral embolism from cardiac lesions is the leading cause of strokes in children.[27,263] These lesions include congenital abnormalities, valvular lesions associated with bacterial or non-bacterial (marantic) vegetations and primary cardiac neoplasms. Conditions associated with brain embolism in adults include cardiac dysrhythmias (atrial fibrillation), myocardial infarction, and atherosclerosis of the aortic arch, and carotid arteries.[46] Pulmonary disorders associated with cerebral embolism include arteriovenous fistulae usually in cases of hemorrhagic hereditary telangiectasia, thrombosis of pulmonary vein and pulmonary and mediastinal tumors.[162,280] Trauma may allow the introduction of air or foreign substances into the systemic circulation.[6] Talc or cornstarch may embolize to the brain in drug abusers.[14] Air could be introduced into the circulation during cardiopulmonary bypass, cerebral angiography, cardiac surgery, cardiac catheterization, balloon angioplasty or as a consequence of mechanical ventilation.[24,325] Trauma is sometimes associated with embolism of intervertebral disc fragments.[307] Decompression sickness (Caisson disease) may be accompanied by the formation of nitrogen bubbles that frequently interfere with the spinal cord circulation.[125] Fat embolism usually occurs after fractures of long bones. Fat globules from the bone marrow enter the circulation and reach the lungs where their presence may be associated with respiratory distress. After reaching the brain through the arterial circulation, fat emboli cause neurological dysfunction through secondary injury to the endothelial lining of microvessels.[144] Most embolic brain lesions from a single source tend to involve the middle cerebral artery territory. Emboli usually lodge at branching sites of a major artery. Fragmentation of an embolus may be followed by occlusion of distal branches and reperfusion of the ischemic brain tissue. In instances of systemic embolism, the involved blood vessels are cerebral arterioles, capillaries, and venules and the parenchymal lesions are disseminated and hemorrhagic; these are described, on gross examination, as *brain purpura.* The embolic material can be identified as cholesterol clefts (Fig. 6-66) or as neoplastic cells. Special stains (e.g., Sudan black) are necessary to demonstrate neutral lipids in cases of fat embolism (Fig. 6-67). Phosphotungstic acid hematoxylin (PTAH) is a useful stain in the identification of fibrin thrombi (Fig. 6-68). Special stains for bacteria or fungi are recommended in cases of bacterial endocarditis and fun-

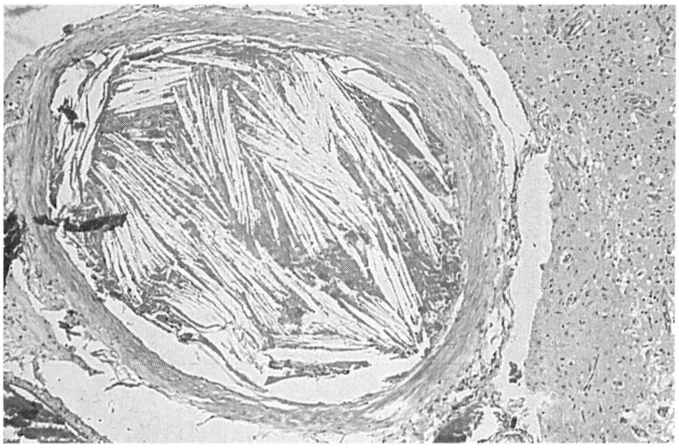

**Fig. 6-66.** Embolic material from atherosclerotic plaque that contains cholesterol crystal clefts. (H&E; ×40.)

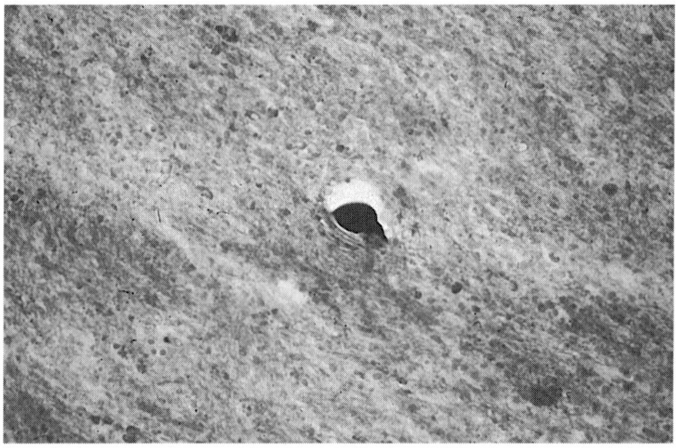

**Fig. 6-67.** Fat embolus occluding a small blood vessel in the cerebral white matter. (Oil-red-O stain; ×40.)

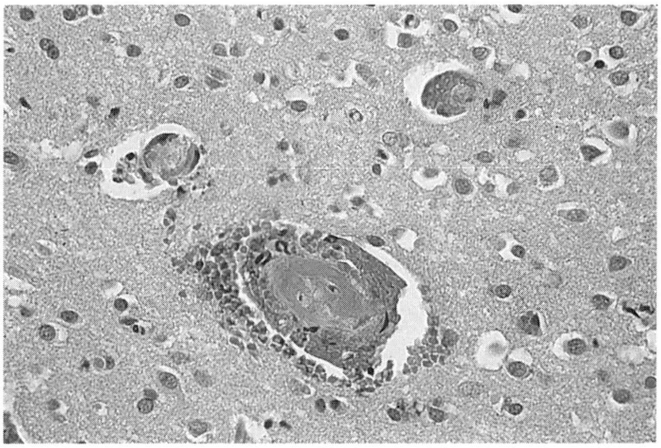

**Fig. 6-68.** Fibrin embolus from a case of non-bacterial endocarditis. (H&E; ×40.)

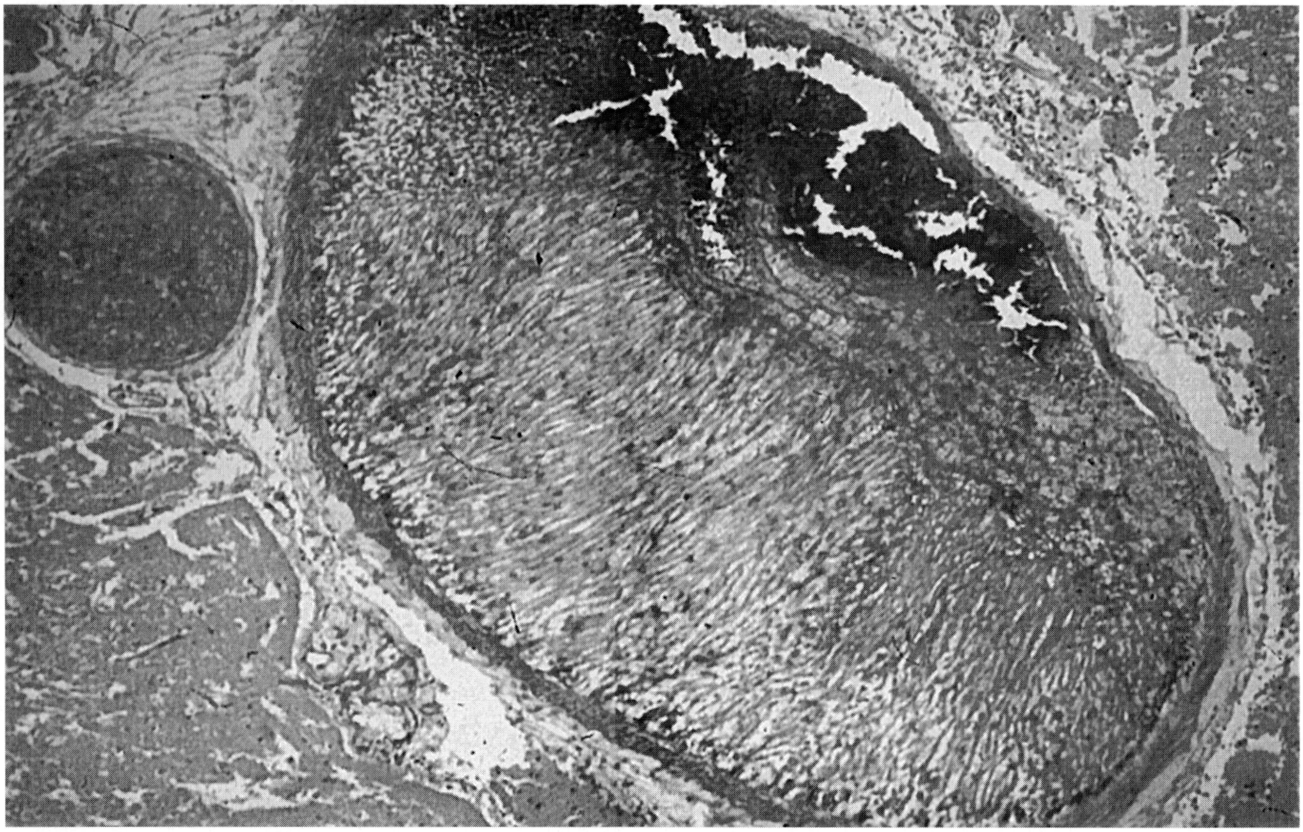

**Fig. 6-69.** Septic embolus with hyphae of Aspergillus. (H&E; ×40.)

gal infections[114] (Fig. 6-69). Air embolism is extremely difficult to demonstrate because it induces few specific structural changes in the brain.[104]

### Thrombotic Disorders

Intraparenchymal, subarachnoid, and subdural hemorrhages are the most common lesions of the CNS associated with a variety of congenital and acquired hematologic disorders. Some of these entities are also accompanied by occlusion of large and small blood vessels including arteries, arterioles, capillaries, venules, veins, and sinuses. The causes of thrombosis may be multifactorial and include activation of the coagulation cascade, increased concentration of coagulation factors, deficiency of an anticoagulant protein, limited activity of the fibrinolytic system, high concentrations of erythrocytes and platelets, platelet cell activation, increased adhesiveness of blood cells, and endothelial cell injury.[264] Tatlisumak and Fisher[303] have reviewed the medical literature dealing with hematologic disorders associated with ischemic strokes. These authors suggest the following classification of these disorders: (1) altered natural anticoagulants (heparin cofactor, antithrombin, protein C, protein S, activated protein C, and warfarin-induced ischemic necrosis); (2) antiphospholipid antibodies (in particular, lupus anticoagulant and anticardiolipin antibodies); (3) defects in fibrinolytic system; (4) erythrocyte disorders (polycythemia vera, paroxysmal nocturnal hemoglobinuria, and sickle-cell disease); (5) platelet disorders (essential thrombocytopenia, thrombotic thrombocytopenic purpura and heparin-associated thrombocytopenia); and (6) unusual hematological disorders associated with disseminated intravascular coagulation (DIC), and with malignant neoplasms.[303]

*Protein C deficiency* is a vitamin K-dependent plasma protein anticoagulant synthesized by the liver. Protein C deficiency can either be inherited or acquired. Inherited protein C deficiency is transmitted as an autosomal dominant trait. Acquired protein C deficiency may be secondary to liver disease, bone marrow transplantation, disseminated intravascular coagulation, sepsis, and L-asparaginase therapy.[179] Venous thrombosis is the most common complication of protein C deficiency; however, arterial thrombosis has may also been described.[73]

*Protein S deficiency* is another vitamin K-dependent anticoagulant plasma protein which functions as a cofactor for protein C. Deficiency can be either inherited or acquired. Acquired protein S deficiency is frequently associated with hepatic and renal failure, consumptive coagulopathy and inflammatory bowel dis-

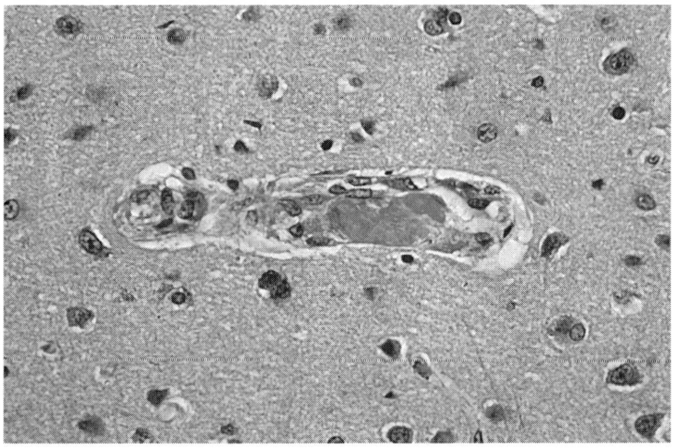

**Fig. 6-70.** Thrombotic thrombocytopenic purpura associated with hypertrophy of endothelial cells and occlusion of lumen by fibrin thrombus. (H&E; ×60.)

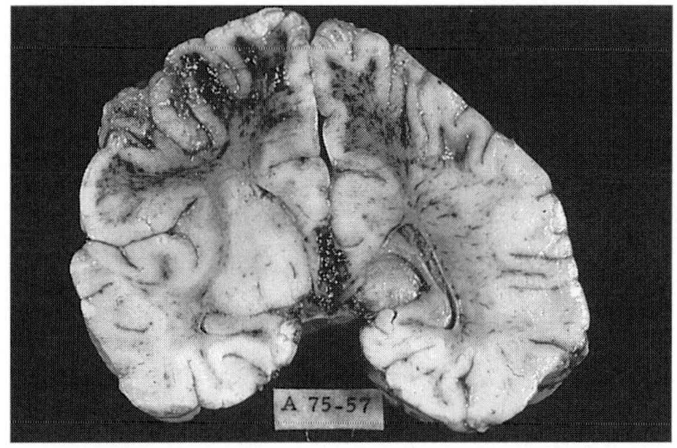



**Fig. 6-71.** Disseminated intravascular coagulation; petechiae and confluent hemorrhages are visible in the white matter.

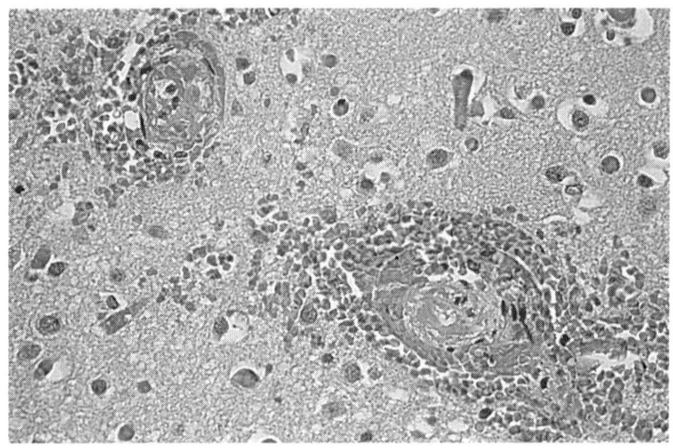

**Fig. 6-72.** Disseminated intravascular coagulation characterized by intravascular fibrin thrombi in cortical arterioles, and perivascular hemorrhages. (H&E; ×25.)

ease.[302] Protein S deficiency is a common cause of idiopathic stroke in children and young adults in whom the vascular lesions correspond to venous and, in fewer cases, to arterial thrombosis.[18]

*Antithrombin III Deficiency* is a plasma protein heparin cofactor which inactivates thrombin. Deficiency of this protein can be inherited as an autosomal dominant trait or acquired in association with nephrotic syndrome, protein-losing enteropathy, or L-asparaginase treatment. Deficiency of antithrombin III is most commonly associated with deep venous thrombosis and pulmonary embolism. Thrombosis of cerebral veins and arteries has been described in children and young adults.[322]

***Clotting factor excess.*** High concentration of some coagulation factors may be associated with ischemic strokes. Oral contraceptives and pregnancy may be complicated by intracranial venous or arterial thrombosis; this is probably related to altered coagulation factors including abnormal protein C and protein S activity.[248] Increased thrombin-antithrombin complexes are present during pregnancy, especially in hypertensive patients.[328] High concentrations of factors V and VIII may increase the risk for stroke in patients with AIDS and inflammatory bowel disease.

*Thrombotic thrombocytopenic purpura (TTP)* is characterized by thrombocytopenia, hemolytic anemia, fever, renal manifestations, and neurologic abnormalities.[59] TTP is most common in young healthy women. The brain lesions are usually hemorrhagic. Microscopically there is widespread occlusion of arterioles, capillaries, and venules by fibrin-platelet thrombi, accompanied by endothelial hypertrophy and hyperplasia (Fig. 6-70).

*Disseminated intravascular coagulation (DIC)* usually is a manifestation of a systemic disorder including infection, malignancy, trauma, shock, surgery, or obstetric complications.[115] The laboratory diagnosis includes thrombocytopenia, elevated prothrombin time (PT), activated partial thromboplastin time (aPTT), low fibrinogen, and elevated fibrin degeneration products (FDP). Brain lesions are characterized by multiple petechiae and occlusion of small vessels (arterioles, capillaries, and venules) by fibrin thrombi (Figs. 6-71, 6-72). A large intracranial hemorrhage may be the cause of death in some patients with DIC. This event has been described in association with bacterial endocarditis, sickle-cell disease, aortic aneurysm, leukemia, head trauma, and glioblastoma multiforme.[149]

*Hyperviscosity syndromes* are associated with plasma cell dyscrasias, hemoglobinopathies, and disorders of erythrocytes. Some of the hyperviscosity syndromes are associated with stroke. In plasma cell dyscrasias and disorders associated with polycythemia, the erythrocytes tend to form rouleaux that block terminal arterioles and capillaries. In hemoglobinopathies, such as sickle-cell disease, the erythrocytes may not flow freely

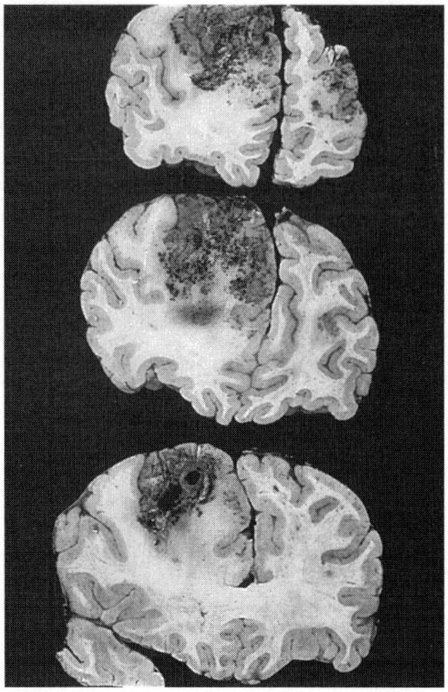

**Fig. 6-73.** Hemorrhagic infarction in the frontal lobe associated with superior sagittal sinus thrombosis.

because the increased rigidity of their membranes may lead to thrombosis and perfusion failure.[236]

### Venous and Sinus Thrombosis

Many disorders are associated with sinus and venous thrombosis. Some are risk factors, whereas others may be only coincidentally associated with the vascular event. Primary thrombosis usually is associated with a systemic disease. Secondary thrombosis is associated with systemic and local infections, including sinusitis, mastoiditis, otitis media, and meningitis. In children, the most common risk factors are dehydration and congestive heart failure.[58,334] Other common predisposing conditions include hematologic disorders such as polycythemia, hemoglobinopathies, coagulopathies, and leukemias. In adults, oral contraceptives, pregnancy, puerperium, inflammatory bowel disease, and systemic lupus erythematosus are on a long list of predisposing conditions. In a significant percentage of cases, the cause remains unknown.[36] The clinical presentation depends on the location of the thrombus and the presence of associated parenchymal lesions. Thrombosis of the anterior portion of the superior sagittal sinus may be asymptomatic.[99] Occlusion of the midportion or posterior superior sagittal sinus may be accompanied by thrombosis of superficial cerebral veins and cause increased intracranial pressure and focal neurologic deficits (Figs. 6-73, 6-74).[113] Unilateral thrombosis of a transverse sinus may have a clinical presentation similar to that of thrombosis of the superior sagittal sinus if the opposite transverse

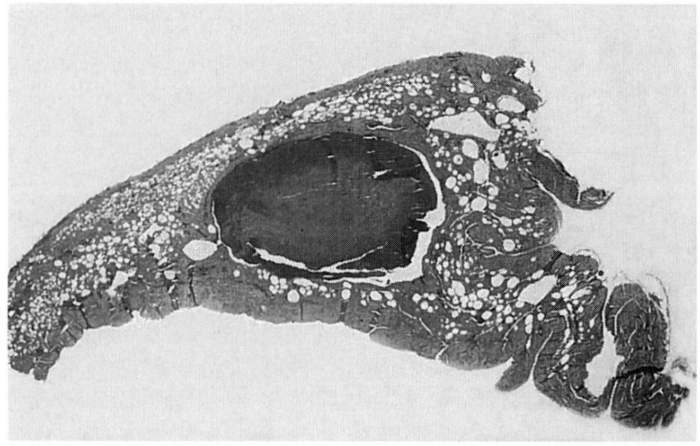

**Fig. 6-74.** Occlusion of superior sagittal sinus by organizing thrombus. Same case as in Fig. 6-73. (H&E; ×25.)

sinus is absent or poorly developed.[246] Cavernous sinus thrombosis usually is related to localized infections of the face or paranasal sinuses.[68] Parenchymal lesions caused by sinus/venous thrombosis tend to be hemorrhagic and localized to the territory drained by the thrombosed vessel. Thrombosis of the internal cerebral veins and the vein of Galen produces large, bilateral cerebral lesions involving thalamus, diencephalon, and the upper brainstem.[98]

### Infectious Angiitis

Bacterial, fungal, parasitic, viral, and rickettsial infections may be associated with CNS angiitis. Pyogenic bacterial infections with meningitis or abscess formation may involve leptomeningeal arteries and veins by an inflammatory process with abundant polymorphonuclear leukocytes.[119,132,292,300] Bacterial endocarditis or septicemia may result in embolization to the brain with development of a localized arteritis. Bacterial infections with granuloma formation, such as tuberculosis and syphilis, may mimic a panarteritis, of which Huebner's arteritis is a classic example[62,136] (Fig. 6-75). Parasitic infections associated with brain hemorrhage in children include cysticercosis and amebic meningitis.[4,119] The incidence of fungal infections of the CNS has increased among patients with immunodeficiencies. Fungi may be associated with meningitis, intraparenchymal abscesses, or angiitis; the latter group is most commonly found with infections caused by *Aspergillus fumigatus* species, phycomycetes, and *Candida albicans*.[176,326] Other agents associated with brain hemorrhages include *Petriellidium boydii, Pseudallescheria boydii* and *Coccidioides immitis*.[283] Viral infections of the CNS frequently are associated with meningitis and encephalitis. Vascular inflammation is frequent in infections with herpes zoster ophthalmicus and HIV.[131,161] The angiitis may become symptomatic in the form of a stroke or a sudden, focal neurologic deficit. Cerebro-

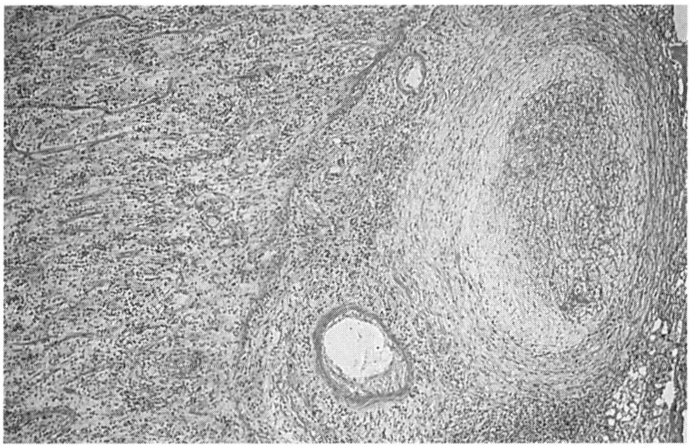

**Fig. 6-75.** Meningovascular syphilis with panarteritis obliterans. (H&E; ×25.)

vascular lesions secondary to the involvement of the intracranial arteries by HIV are rare. Rocky Mountain spotted fever may be associated with neurologic symptoms during the acute phase of the illness. This is related to the effects of the infection on the endothelial and smooth muscle cells of the small intraparenchymal blood vessels and the secondary thrombosis.[22] (Fig. 6-76).

## Noninfectious Angiitis

***Primary angiitis of the central nervous system.*** Primary angiitis of the central nervous system (PACNS), also known as *isolated angiitis of the CNS* and *granulomatous angiitis of the CNS,* is characterized by an inflammatory process similar to that of GCA. However, the process remains limited to arterioles and venules in the leptomeninges. The inflammatory infiltrate includes lymphocytes, plasma cells, occasional neutrophils, and eosinophils (Fig. 6-77). Multinucleated giant cells and noncaseating granuloma may be present.[61] This infiltrate extends through all layers of the vascular wall and may be associated with necrosis and mural rupture. The symptomatic inflammatory process is limited to cranial and spinal leptomeningeal blood vessels. However, autopsy studies of PACNS mention angiitis in other organs including lungs, kidneys, myocardium, and prostate.[13,88] Biopsy of leptomeninges and cerebral cortex is required to confirm the diagnosis of PACNS. Intracranial hemorrhage, either subarachnoid or intraparenchymal, is the most common complication of this disease. Hemorrhages can be small or large, single or multiple. Other complications include brain infarcts, spinal myelopathy, and thrombosis of large intracranial arteries. The disease may become

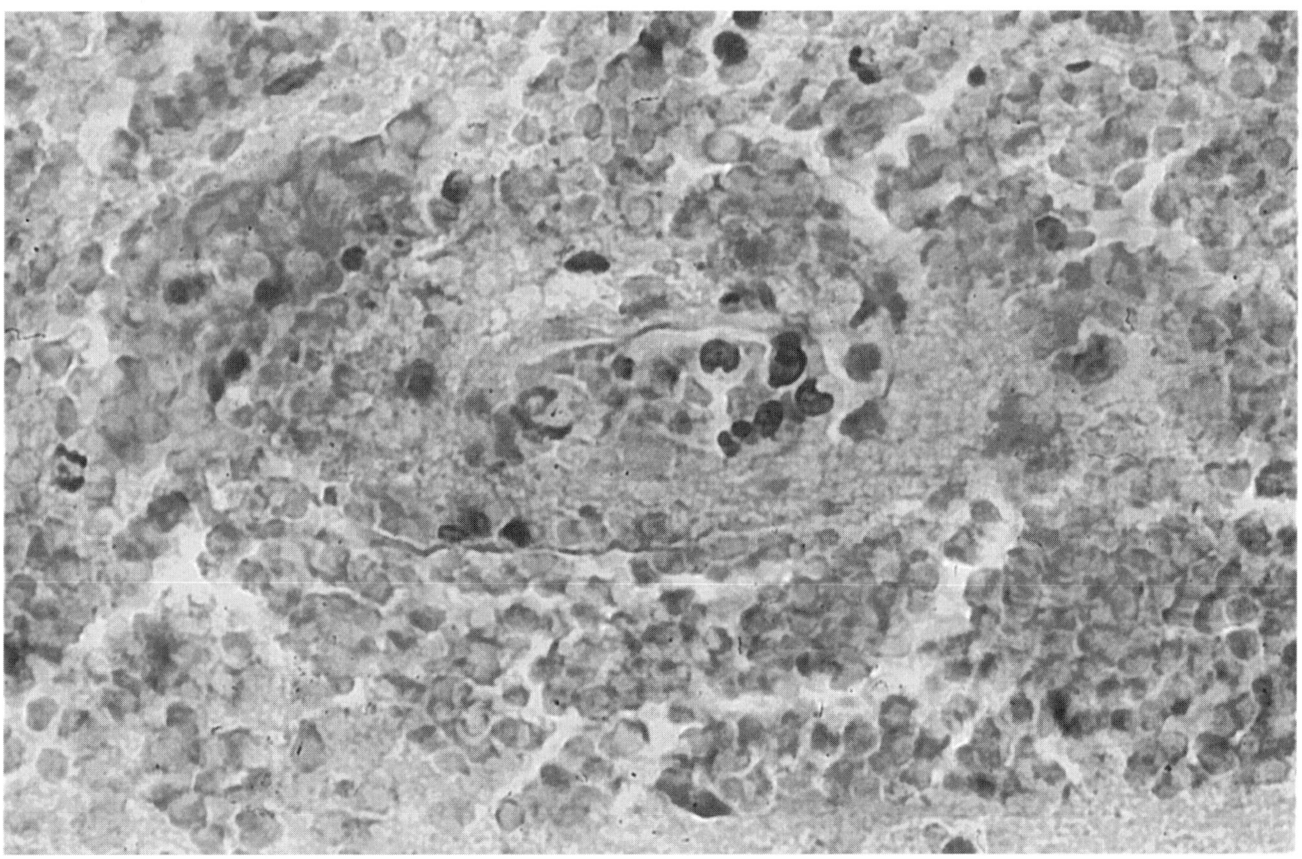

**Fig. 6-76.** Rocky mountain spotted fever associated with fibrinoid necrosis of the vascular wall and perivascular hemorrhage. Canine brain. (H&E; ×40.)

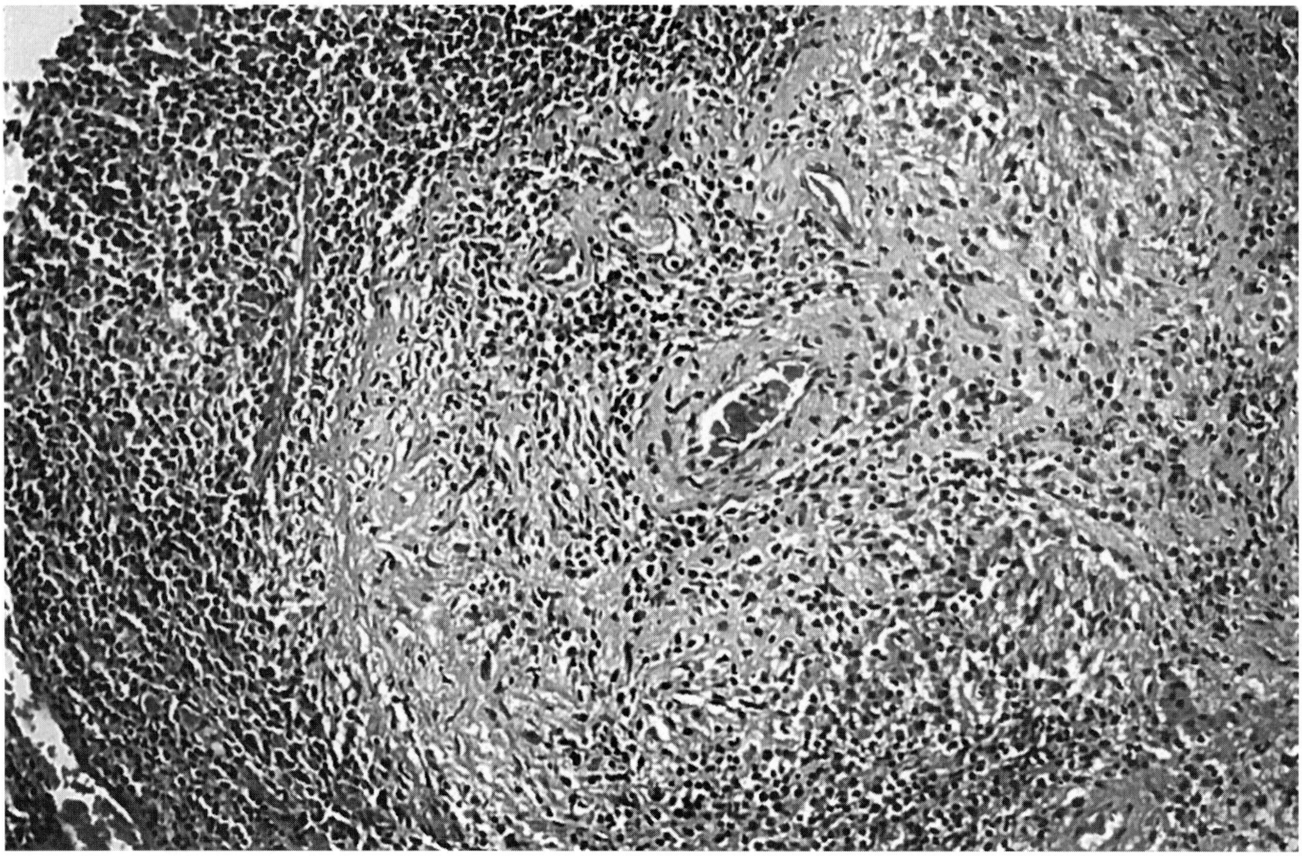

**Fig. 6-77.** Primary angiitis of the central nervous system. Biopsy of leptomeninges showing inflammatory infiltrate of mononuclear cells that involves blood vessel walls. (H&E; ×40.)

symptomatic at any age. The etiology is unknown and could be related to immunologic factors or infectious agents including varicella-zoster virus, HIV, and mycoplasma.[13,244,250,335] MRI reveals extensive white matter and subcortical changes that improve with appropriate steroid therapy. In a few instances, granulomatous angiitis has been found confined to the spinal cord in patients whose symptoms were limited to myelopathy.[42]

*Polyarteritis nodosa* is a systemic disease that affects medium and small arteries. All organs except the lungs and spleen may be involved. Peripheral neuropathy is the most common neurologic complication. Involvement of the CNS may become manifest as ischemic or hemorrhagic strokes.[86] The lesions usually are present in the main arteries of the circle of Willis and leptomeninges.[226] The necrotizing panarteritis may be associated with thrombosis. One half of the patients with polyarteritis nodosa have circulating immune complexes and one third have a hepatitis B antigenemia.[275]

*Wegener's granulomatosis (WG)* is a disease of the respiratory tract, kidneys, and vasculature characterized by angiitis with necrotizing granuloma.[134] The clinical diagnosis is based on the combined involvement of upper and lower respiratory tracts and the kidney. Some patients may present with lesions in a single organ or site. The lesions in the nervous system frequently involve the peripheral and cranial nerves.[71] Histopathologic diagnosis requires the demonstration of extravascular necrotizing granulomas and angiitis. The granulomas often have a central area of necrosis surrounded by macrophages with nuclei arranged in palisades; the inflammatory reaction frequently includes multinucleated giant cells, lymphocytes, plasma cells, neutrophils, and eosinophils. The vascular lesions, which are of different types, include necrotizing arteritis, cutaneous leukocytoclastic angiitis, pulmonary capillaritis, and granulomatous angiitis; the latter is considered diagnostic of the disease.[206,208] Tests for circulating antineutrophil cytoplasmic antibodies (C-ANCA) may facilitate the diagnosis. C-ANCA is found in 93% of patients with active generalized disease and may be a marker for disease activity.[315]

*Giant cell (temporal) arteritis (GCA)*, also known as *temporal arteritis*, is a generalized disorder affecting the aorta and its major branches. Involvement of arteries of the head and neck including vertebral, superior temporal, ophthalmic, posterior ciliary, and carotid accounts for the visual and neurologic symptoms.[233] The

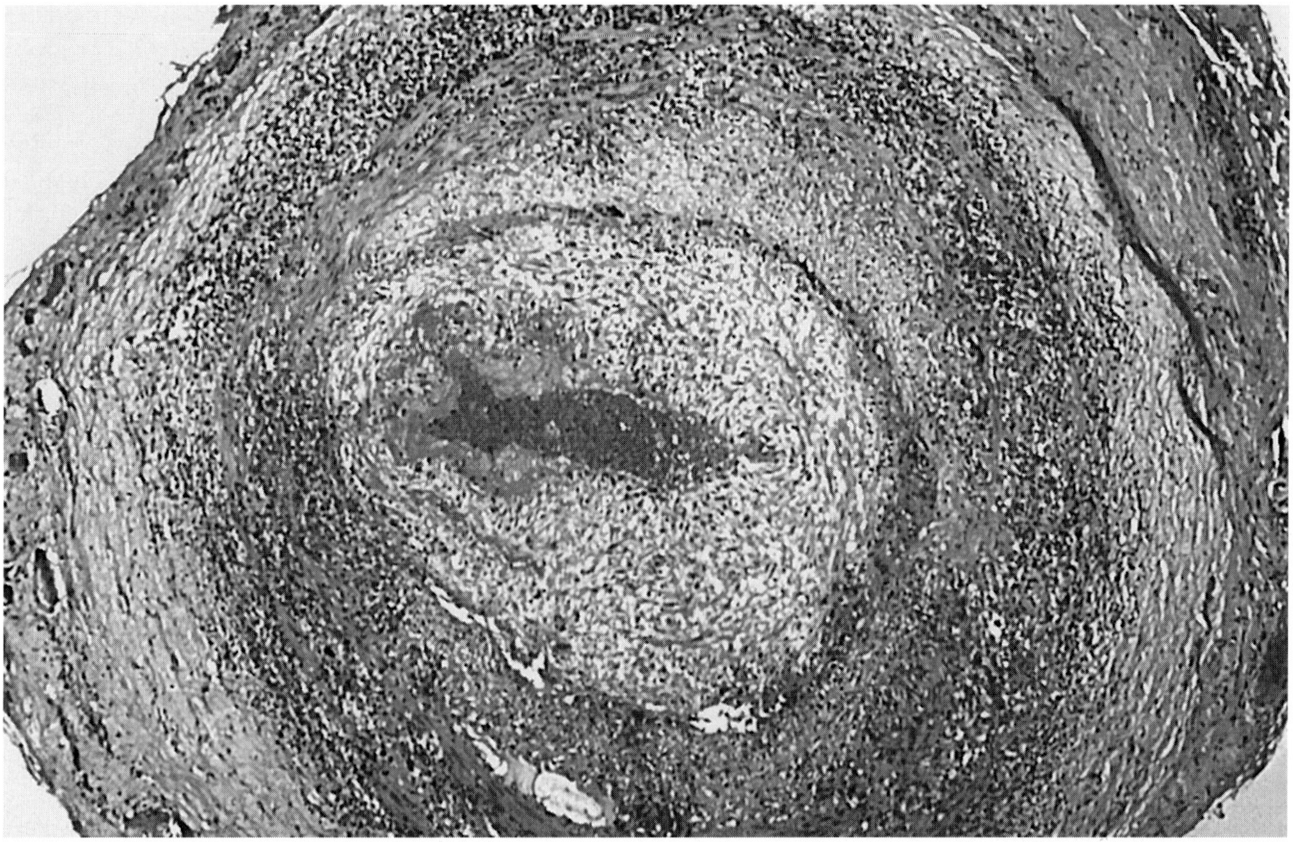

**Fig. 6-78.** Giant cell arteritis with narrowing of the lumen by fibrosis and prominent inflammation in the muscular layer. (H&E; ×25.)

disease is seldom symptomatic in persons younger than 50 years of age and is more common among women than men, and among Caucasians. The clinical presentation includes headaches, polymyalgia rheumatica, visual loss, and stroke. The erythrocyte sedimentation rate (ESR) usually is elevated.[26] The diagnosis is confirmed by biopsy, commonly of the temporal artery. The microscopic changes involve short segments of the artery, and for this reason multiple transverse sections should be examined. Pathologic features are noted in three main categories: (1) granulomas with multinucleated giant cells and other inflammatory cells are usually more prominent in the tunica media adjacent to the internal elastic lamina; (2) transmural cellular inflammation by lymphocytes, plasma cells, neutrophils, and eosinophils; and (3) intimal fibrosis (Figs. 6-78, 6-79). These changes may be accompanied by thrombosis or narrowing of the lumen and necrosis of the vascular wall.[168] The cause of the disease remains undetermined. Genetic predisposition may be related to an increased frequency of HLA-B8 and HLA-DR4 among patients with familial giant cell arteritis.[12] An immunologic reaction is supported by the presence of circulating immune complexes in the sera of some patients and by the demonstration of immunoglobu-

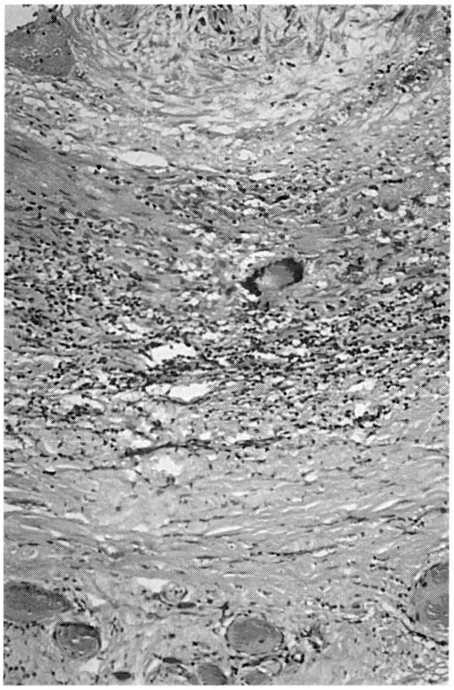

**Fig. 6-79.** Giant cell arteritis with granulomatous inflammation and multinucleated giant cells. Same case as in Fig. 6-78. (H&E.)

lins in biopsy specimens.[167,175] Elastin in the arterial wall could be the target for the immune reaction. The disease usually responds to steroid therapy.[277] Stroke, myocardial infarction, and ruptured aorta are some of the complications of GCA.[263]

*Takayasu's arteritis* affects the aorta and its major branches. The aortic arch is involved in about one third of the cases. The disease prevails among women between 11 and 30 years of age.[172] Most cases are reported from Asia. The clinical presentation is variable and correlates with the phase of the disease, the extent of the lesions, and the number of blood vessels involved. During the initial stages, the pathologic changes are confined to the adventitia and the outer muscle layer and consist of mononuclear cellular infiltrates that also involve the vasa vasorum. At a later stage, the inflammatory infiltrate may be more prominent in the tunica media and may include multinucleated giant cells. These changes are similar to those found in GCA.[122] In the late stages, the inflammatory reaction is less prominent, and fibrosis of the wall with narrowing of the lumen are the cardinal features. Thrombosis and aneurysmatic dilatations may develop at any stage. Narrowing or occlusion of the subclavian arteries is related to diminished or absent radial and brachial artery pulses, known as "pulseless disease." The disease may involve the carotid arteries in one half of the patients, and the vertebral arteries in one fifth.[172a] Neurologic manifestations include transient ischemic attacks and strokes.

***Churg-Strauss syndrome.*** This disorder is characterized by peripheral eosinophilia, systemic angiitis involving small to medium-sized vessels, and granulomatous lesions of the respiratory tract.[53] Other manifestations include peripheral neuropathy, glomerulonephritis, and myocardial ischemia. The vascular lesions may be indistinguishable from those of PAN and WG. The presence of ANCA suggests that Churg-Strauss syndrome may be a variant of WG.[329]

***Microscopic polyangiitis, microscopic polyarteritis, hypersensitivity angiitis, and leukocytoclastic angiitis.*** These names apply to a heterogeneous group of disorders associated with changes in small blood vessels including arterioles, capillaries, and venules. All lesions in each of the involved vessels are of the same age and are characterized by transmural infiltration of the vascular wall by neutrophils that exhibit karyorrhexis ("nuclear dust").[57] Fibrinoid necrosis may be present. The clinical manifestations are protean, and the lesions generally involve skin, mucous membranes, gastrointestinal tract, lungs, heart, kidneys, brain, and skeletal muscle. In some cases a precipitating factor (drug, infectious agent, protein) may be detected. Other cases may be associated with specific syndromes including Henoch-Schönlein purpura, essential mixed cryoglobulinemia, angiitis associated with mixed connective tissue disorders, and angiitis associated with malignant neoplasia.[103] P-ANCA are demonstrable in 70% of these patients.

***Angiopathies associated with opiates, amphetamines, and cocaine.*** Heroin is the most commonly abused substance of this group. Parenteral administration of heroin may be associated with bacterial endocarditis that could be complicated by stroke secondary to cerebral embolism, rupture of a mycotic aneurysm, or bacterial or fungal meningitis.[9] Intracerebral hemorrhage may be the result of a coagulopathy associated with hepatitis or hypertension due to heroin nephropathy. Other possible mechanisms of brain injury include widespread angiitis, hypotension, embolization of foreign material, and immune-mediated disorders. Ischemic and hemorrhagic strokes in adults and children may follow intravenous, oral, or intranasal intake of amphetamine. The brain lesions may be the result of angiitis, acute hypertension, or a combination of both. The cerebrovascular changes are visible on angiography and include segmental narrowing of large and medium-sized arteries and occlusion of small arteries.[256] The condition is regarded as a type of hypersensitivity angiitis.[338] Neurologic symptoms associated with cocaine use may be secondary to bacterial endocarditis, hepatitis, and HIV infection. Some ischemic strokes among cocaine users are attributed to angiitis, although vasospasm also could be an important contributor to the brain lesions.[160] Despite the angiographic evidence of "angiitis" reported in some cocaine abusers,[89] a postmortem evaluation of twelve hemorrhagic strokes associated with toxicologically proved presence of cocaine in serum and urine failed to detect angiitis or other abnormalities demonstrable by light microscopy.[2]

***Essential mixed cryoglobulinemia.*** This systemic disease is characterized by IgG-IgM deposits of cryoglobulins associated with cutaneous angiitis, synovitis, and glomerulonephritis. Some symptoms are secondary to hepatitis C infection.[37] Neurologic symptoms have been described in patients with angiographic abnormalities involving the arteries of the circle of Willis and thrombosis of the small vessels.[1]

***Anaphylactoid purpura (Henoch-Schönlein purpura).*** This syndrome, characterized by purpuric cutaneous lesions, gastrointestinal manifestations, arthralgia, and glomerulonephritis, is most frequent in children. The vascular lesions correspond to a systemic necrotizing angiitis with deposits of IgA in small arteries of the dermis.[268] Subdural, subarachnoid, and intraparenchymal brain hemorrhages have been reported in some of these patients.[23]

*Mucocutaneous lymph node syndrome (Kawasaki disease)* is a systemic angiitis of undetermined etiology most commonly affecting infants and children.[201] The disease manifestations include fever, mucocutaneous lesions, and enlargement of cervical lymph nodes. The vascular manifestations usually are restricted to the coronary arteries.[148] The arterial lesions are similar to those of polyarteritis nodosa. Complications such as encephalopathy, ataxia, and strokes are related to arterial occlusions.[304]

*Malignant atrophic papulosis (Köhlmier-Degos disease)* is a generalized disorder of blood vessels affecting skin and brain. Cerebral lesions correspond to multiple infarcts associated with an angiopathy characterized by intimal fibrous and thrombotic occlusion of large, medium, and small arteries.[186]

***Inflammatory bowel disease.*** Brain infarction or hemorrhage may affect patients with regional enteritis or ulcerative colitis.[170] The cause could be multifactorial, including coagulopathies and angiitis. Radiologic reports describe angiographic findings of cerebral angiitis, which has not been corroborated pathologically.[267]

### Systemic Angiopathies (Table 6-3)

*Sneddon's syndrome* is characterized by strokes, *livedo reticularis,* and hypertension.[282] Livedo reticularis may be associated with rheumatoid arthritis, polyarteritis nodosa, dermatomyositis, cryoglobulinemia, and systemic lupus erythematosus.[235] The most common neurologic manifestations are recurrent strokes. Many patients have antiphospholipid antibodies, including anticardiolipin and lupus anticoagulant or both. The vascular lesions include angiographic evidence of occlusion of medium-sized arteries and their branches. Angiopathic changes in the skin have a distinctive sequential pattern: initially, there is loosening and detachment of endothelial cells, accompanied by surface adhesion of inflammatory cells and fibrin deposition.[339]

**Table 6-3.** Systemic Angiopathies

| |
|---|
| Sneddon's Syndrome |
| Systemic Lupus Erythematosus |
| Rheumatoid Arthritis |
| Scleroderma |
| Mixed Connective Tissue Disease |
| Sjögren's Syndrome |
| Behçet's Disease |

*Systemic lupus erythematosus (SLE)* characteristically involves many organs. The etiology is unknown, but genetic, environmental, and immunologic factors all play important roles. Activation of helper T-cells and B-cells is associated with secretion of many different antibodies against several cell constituents including the nucleus and several cytoplasmic organelles.[57] The clinical manifestations are protean and correspond to the organs involved and the lesions present. Most patients are young women who develop hematologic abnormalities and involvement of the skin, joints, serous membranes, and kidney. Skeletal muscles, peripheral nerves and the CNS may be involved in 14% to 33% of patients. The arterial lesions include deposits of immunoglobulins, DNA, and C-3 protein. Clinical manifestations of CNS involvement in SLE are variable and in many cases non-specific; they include psychiatric disorders, encephalopathy, myelopathy, seizures, focal neurologic deficits, stroke, and extrapyramidal signs and symptoms.[140] Lack of correlation between the clinical symptoms and the microscopic abnormalities is noted in many cases. In a recently published series from the Armed Forces Institute of Pathology (AFIP), 5 of 11 cases of SLE had intraparenchymal and/or subarachnoid hemorrhages and five large or microscopic ischemic infarcts. There was no evidence of a necrotizing angiitis associated with the brain lesions.[129] That angiitis is rare as the source of CNS hemorrhagic or ischemic lesions has been mentioned by others.[77] Other important factors associated with occlusive intracranial disease include nonbacterial (marantic) endocarditis with embolism,[67] thrombotic thrombocytopenic purpura, antiphospholipid (lupus anticoagulant, anticardiolipin) antibodies and complications from infections and treatment.[143,165] The role of antineuronal antibodies remains to be determined.[31]

***Rheumatoid arthritis (RA).*** Neurologic complications occasionally may affect adults with chronic active rheumatoid arthritis. Some patients develop cranial neuropathies secondary to the formation of rheumatoid nodules in the meninges.[295] Cervical spinal cord compression is the most common neurologic manifestation of RA, usually as a result of subluxation of C1-C2 vertebrae. This condition occasionally may be complicated with infarcts in the vertebrobasilar territory.[327] CNS angiitis has been reported in a few cases of RA.[237]

*Scleroderma (systemic progressive sclerosis)* is seldom associated with neurologic manifestations. In some cases, CNS symptoms are a consequence of systemic hypertension, which in turn is the result of renal disease.[116]

***Mixed connective tissue disease.*** Some patients with mixed connective tissue disease, as well as with dermatomyositis, may develop neurologic complications attributed to angiitis.[117]

*Sjögren's syndrome* is characterized by *keratoconjunctivitis sicca* and xerostomia as the result of an immune reaction that destroys the lacrimal and salivary glands. Primary Sjögren's syndrome is not associated with autoimmune disease. The secondary form is related to autoimmune disorders such as RA, SLE, mixed connective tissue disease, polymyositis, vasculitis, scleroderma, and thyroiditis.[57] Neurologic complications of secondary Sjögren's syndrome usually are related to the primary collagen vascular disease. The reason for the CNS changes such as microinfarcts and meningitis that affect some patients with primary Sjögren's syndrome is uncertain.[29]

*Behçet's disease* is an immune-mediated angiitis clinically manifested by the triad of uveitis, oral or genital aphthous ulcers, and arthritis. Additional manifestations include cutaneous angiitis, thrombophlebitis, colitis, and CNS symptoms.[159] Angiitis has not been well documented as the cause of neurologic manifestations. The lesions described in the CNS include leptomeningeal thickening, parenchymal softening, gliosis, perivascular inflammation, hemorrhages, and demyelination.[253] HLA-B51 antigen recently was described as a potential marker for Behçet's disease among children with idiopathic strokes.[192]

### Genetic Angiopathies (Table 6-4)

Patients with heterogeneous hereditary disorders are at risk of developing strokes. This group includes hematologic disorders, metabolic diseases, coagulation disorders, vascular abnormalities, connective tissue diseases, and others. Strokes in children frequently are associated with genetic defects that result in structural or functional disorders of the cerebral blood vessels. Love has published an excellent review of these rare conditions.[171] Only a few of the metabolic diseases are described here.

*Homocystinuria* is an autosomal recessive disorder of methionine metabolism caused by a deficiency of cystathionine-$\beta$ synthase.[270] Affected persons excrete homocysteine or a mixed disulfide in the urine and have excessive amounts of homocysteine in plasma and tissues. Clinical manifestations include skeletal and cutaneous abnormalities, lens dislocation, mental retardation, and vascular lesions. The vascular abnormalities involve arteries and veins in many organs and may be accompanied by such complications as pulmonary thromboembolism, myocardial infarction, renovascular hypertension, and stroke.[204] Involvement of the intracranial vasculature may result in sinus/venous thrombosis or in arterial lesions indistinguishable from arteriosclerotic plaques with thrombotic occlusion.[123] The accumulation of homocysteine in the arterial wall may lead to endothelial cell injury thought to promote atherosclerosis.[64]

**Table 6-4.** Genetic Disorders

| |
|---|
| Homocystinuria |
| Mitochondrial Disorders |
| CADASIL |
| Select Cerebral Amyloid Angiopathies |

***Mitochondrial disorders.*** Some disorders of presumed mitochondrial origin may be associated with cerebrovascular complications. MELAS syndrome (myopathy, encephalopathy, lactic acidosis, and stroke) is the best characterized mitochondriopathy associated with brain infarcts.[229] The neurologic manifestations, which usually start during childhood or adolescence, include seizures, migraine, stroke, exercise intolerance, recurrent vomiting, and anorexia. The cerebral infarcts could be single or multiple and usually are not distributed in a specific arterial territory.[333] The most significant structural abnormality is an increased number of mitochondria in the smooth muscle cells of the small leptomeningeal and parenchymal penetrating arteries. Occlusive disease and inflammation usually are absent.[194] A mitochondrial dysfunction has been suggested as the cause of the ischemic cerebral lesions.

***Cerebral autosomal dominant arteriopathy with subcortical infarcts.*** Cerebral autosomal dominant arteriopathy with subcortical infarcts and leukoencephalopathy (CADASIL) is an entity originally described by Sourander[286] and recently recognized as a genetically transmitted angiopathy.[309] CADASIL is associated with an arteriopathy of undetermined etiology that involves several organs including central and peripheral nervous systems, skeletal muscle, and skin[255] (Fig. 6-80). The remarkable significance of CADASIL is underscored by the fact that this entity represents the first genetically determined disease in which several conditions (previously thought to be only tenuously or dubiously linked) appear to be clearly connected: angiopathy, strokes, leukoencephalopathy, and dementing syndromes. In the brain, the small leptomeningeal arteries and penetrating arteries of the subcortical white matter and basal ganglia are affected by deposits of granular osmiophilic material in the tunica media; sometimes these deposits are associated with duplication and fragmentation of the elastic lamina.[20] These vascular changes are associated with a subcortical leukoencephalopathy that spares the U-fibers and with lacunae in the cerebrum and pons. A locus for the disease has been mapped to chromosome 19q12.[309] Mutations, in CADASIL patients that cause serious disruption of the human *Notch 3* gene suggest that *Notch 3* could be the site of the defective protein in CADASIL

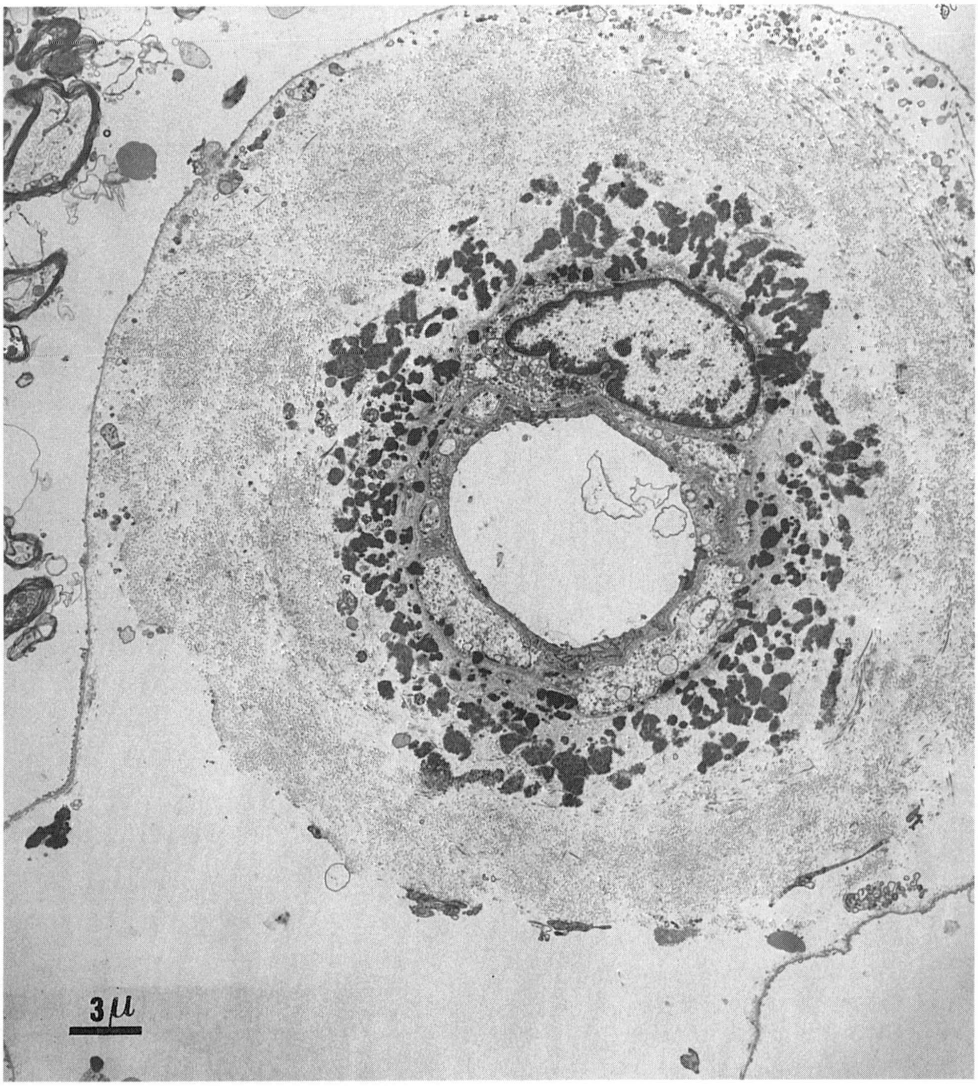


**Fig. 6-80.** CADASIL. Arteriole of the optic nerve showing characteristic granular osmiophilic deposits in the tunica media. (×18,900.) (Courtesy of Dr. M.M. Ruchoux; Lille, France.)

patients.[141] Amyloid angiopathies are described in the group of miscellaneous angiopathies.

## Neoplastic Angiopathies

*Intravascular lymphomatosis* is a proliferative lymphocytic neoplasia of B-cell or T-cell phenotype confined to the lumina of arteries, arterioles, capillaries and venules of several organs, most commonly the brain and the skin.[276,296] This malignancy usually becomes symptomatic in adults. Neurologic manifestations include dementia, stroke, and myelopathy. In most instances the clinical course is progressive and does not respond to treatment.[66] The diagnosis usually is made at postmortem examination, but a few cases are confirmed by brain biopsy. The lumina of leptomeningeal and parenchymal blood vessels contain mitotically active, atypical neoplastic cells that express B-cell or T-cell antigens (Fig. 6-81). In some cases, the

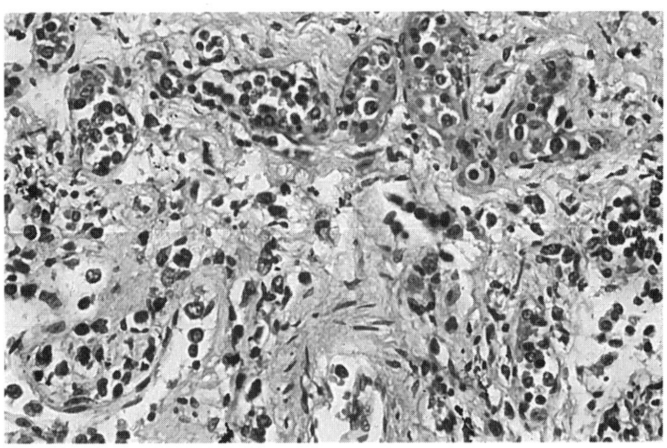

**Fig. 6-81.** Intravascular lymphomatosis: neoplastic cells are confined to the lumen of the cerebral blood vessels. (H&E; ×40.)

neoplastic cells may infiltrate the subintimal layer. This infiltration may be associated with endothelial cell proliferation and luminal narrowing. Most parenchymal brain lesions are ischemic or hemorrhagic infarcts.[55] Intravascular lymphomatosis usually affects the nervous system and skin, but generalized involvement also has been observed. The reasons for the selective involvement of the intravascular compartment are unknown, but expression of adhesion molecules that bind B-lymphocytes to endothelium could be involved in this rare syndrome.

*Lymphomatoid granulomatosis (LG)* is characterized by nodular, angiocentric infiltrates of atypical plasma cells, immunoblasts, and lymphoid cells. Pulmonary lesions are most frequent. Extrapulmonary involvement is present in 80% of cases, including the central and peripheral nervous systems.[260] In the CNS the lesions may be solid tumors, necrotic nodules, or infiltrates of the meninges and brain.[135] The vascular lesions may be associated with infarcts or parenchymal hemorrhages. LG is a lymphoproliferative disease that evolves into a malignant lymphoma in about 50% of the cases.[188] Association with Epstein-Barr Virus (EBV) has been documented in a few cases.[193] LG is more common among organ transplant recipients, patients with Sjögren's syndrome, and those infected with HIV.

### Miscellaneous Angiopathies (Table 6-5)

***Moyamoya disease.*** Initially described in Japan in 1955, moyamoya disease is now recognized as having a worldwide distribution.[207] The disease is identified by a bilateral occlusion of the intracranial segment of the internal carotid arteries, initial segments of the middle and anterior cerebral arteries, development of collateral circulation in the basal ganglia, and transdural anastomoses. Proliferation of a network of vascular channels among the involved arteries of the deep gray matter structures gives the characteristic angiographic appearance of a "puff of cigarette smoke," that in Japanese is "moyamoya"[298] (Fig. 6-82). The cause is unknown, and most authors would prefer the designation of spontaneous occlusions of the circle of Willis vessels. Vascular abnormalities mimicking moyamoya may be present in a diverse group of disorders including infections, hematologic disorders, metabolic diseases, genetic disorders, congenital abnormalities, neoplasms, drug abuse, and others.[337] The clinical presentation varies according to the age of the patient. Moyamoya is most commonly associated with cerebral infarction in children under the age of 10 years. In adults, intracranial hemorrhage (intraparenchymal, intraventricular, or subarachnoid) is more common than ischemic lesions, especially during the fourth decade (Fig. 6-83).

**Table 6-5.** Miscellaneous Angiopathies

| |
|---|
| Moyamoya Disease |
| Fibromuscular Dysplasia |
| Arterial dissection |
| Cerebral Amyloid Angiopathies |
| Radiation effects |

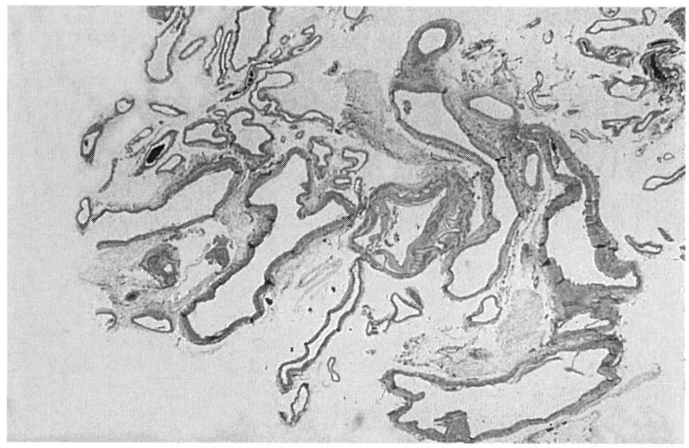

**Fig. 6-82.** Moyamoya disease. Sample from area adjacent to internal carotid artery showing small vascular channels, some with intimal fibrosis. Same case as in Fig. 6-83. (H&E.)

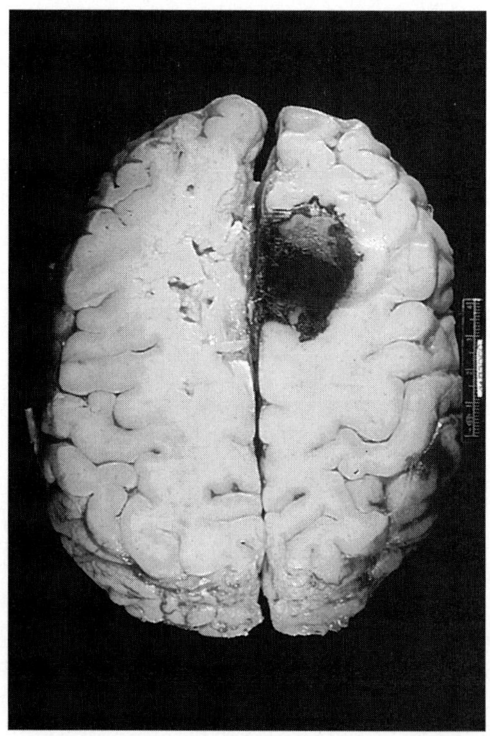

**Fig. 6-83.** Moyamoya disease: right frontal lobe hematoma and left frontal lobe cortical ischemic infarct. Prominent vascular markings are present in the white matter.

These parenchymal lesions are thought to be related to changes in the blood vessels. The main arteries of the internal carotid system exhibit intimal fibrosis, various degrees of stenosis or thrombotic occlusion of the lumen, atrophy of the tunica media, and reduplication of the internal elastic lamina (Fig. 6-84). These changes may be found in other intracranial arteries as well as in other organs, including the heart and the kidney. At present, moyamoya disease is regarded as a systemic vasculopathy. Cerebral intraparenchymal hemorrhages among moyamoya patients are most commonly located in the basal ganglia, thalamus, and white matter.[213] The source of these is attributed to arteriolosclerosis and rupture of microaneurysms present in the small collateral vascular channels.[182] Rupture of basilar artery aneurysms has been documented in some patients with moyamoya.

*Fibromuscular dysplasia (FMD)* is a systemic nonatherosclerotic vasculopathy of unknown cause that mainly affects medium-sized arteries, including renal, cephalic, visceral, and peripheral arteries. FMD is asymptomatic in most individuals. Clinical manifestations are frequent in women during the fourth and fifth decades of life. Renal artery stenosis is associated with systemic hypertension. Involvement of the cerebral vasculature is usually restricted to the extracranial portion of the internal carotid artery, where the lesion may be localized to a segment measuring up to 7 cm in length.[126] The vertebral artery in the cervical region is also occasionally involved. Confirmation of diagnosis requires imaging studies. An angiographic pattern showing alternating constriction and dilatation of the affected artery, described as "string of beads" appearance, is characteristic.[218] The microscopic changes may be particularly pronounced in any of the three layers of the arterial wall.[124] The most common form is *medial* fibromuscular dysplasia characterized by hyperplasia of the smooth muscle cells and fibrosis; the process causes, thickening of the tunica media and is associated with changes in the internal and external elastic laminae.[297] This medial thickening may be continuous or may alternate with areas of medial thinning and arterial dilatation. The other two patterns of FMD correspond to intimal and adventitial fibroplasia. Intimal fibroplasia describes fibrosis in the subintimal region with changes of the internal elastic laminae. In adventitial fibroplasia, fibrosis is localized to the adventitia and periarterial region. FMD may be associated with other lesions at the site of the arterial involvement, including luminal narrowing and occlusion, dissections, and aneurysmatic dilatations.[10,191] Neurologic complications of FMD include ischemic and hemorrhagic strokes.

***Arterial dissection.*** Cervicocephalic arterial dissection is a rare cause of stroke. Most dissections involve the cervical carotid artery in an area located between 1.5 cm and 3 cm from its common carotid artery origin. The extent of the dissection varies from a few millimeters to several centimeters. Additional sites of dissection include the intracranial segment of the internal carotid artery and proximal middle cerebral artery, cervical vertebral artery, and basilar artery (Fig. 6-85). Arterial dissections are characterized by intramural accumulations of blood that may remain localized either in the subintimal region (between the endothelial and muscular layers) or between the tunica muscularis and the adventitia.[92,211,336] Subendothelial hemorrhage may be associated with luminal stenosis or occlusion by thrombus formation (Fig. 6-85). The pathogenesis of arterial dissections is unclear. In many cases, the microscopic examination of the arterial segment involved fails to reveal any pathologic processes other than a dissection.[172] In a few cases, the dissection is associated with atherosclerosis, fibromuscular dyspla-

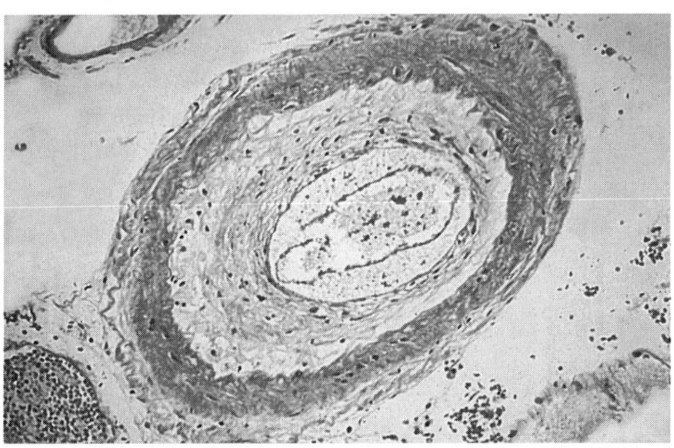

**Fig. 6-84.** Moyamoya disease. Section of internal carotid artery exhibiting subintimal fibrosis and thinned tunica media. Same case as in Figs. 6-82 and 6-83. (H&E; ×25.)

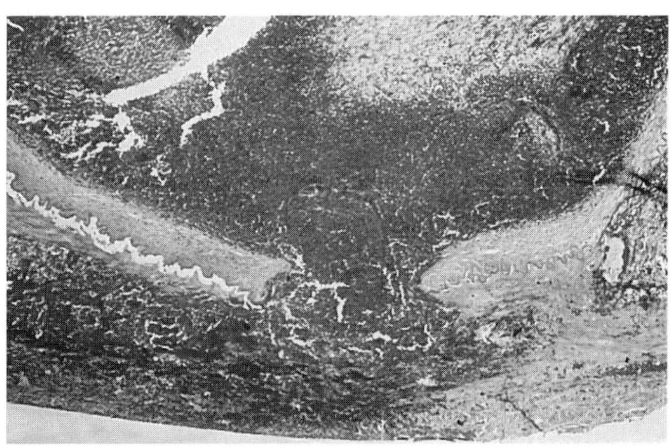

**Fig. 6-85.** Dissecting "aneurysm" of the basilar artery with hemorrhage within the tunicae media and adventitia, and organizing thrombus in the lumen. (H&E; ×10.)

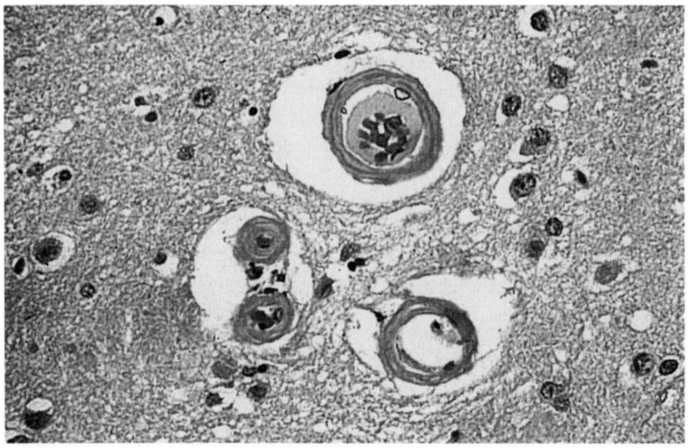

**Fig. 6-86.** Amyloid angiopathy with deposits of acellular material in small cerebral arteries and arterioles. (H&E; ×25.)

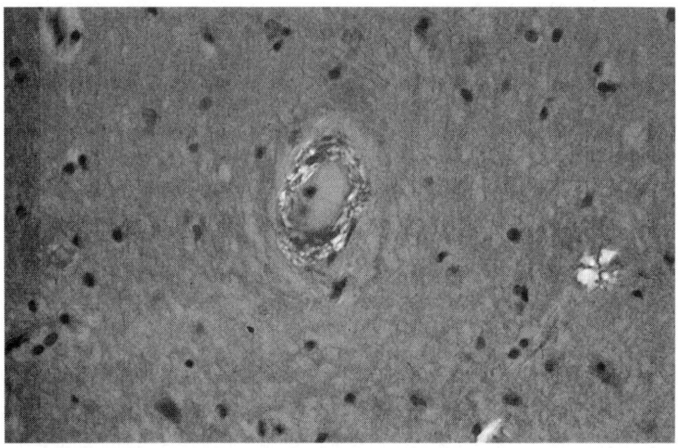

**Fig. 6-87.** Amyloid angiopathy. Small cerebral artery showing apple green birefringence under polarizing light. (Congo red stain; ×25.)

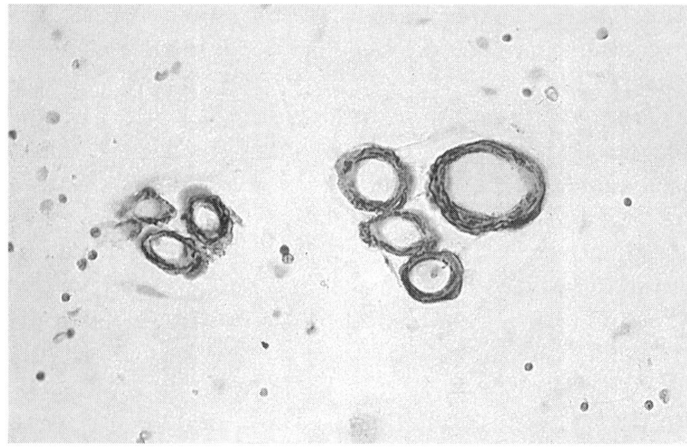

**Fig. 6-88.** Amyloid angiopathy. Cerebral blood vessels exhibit immunoreactivity for β-amyloid. (Avidin-biotin complex method.)

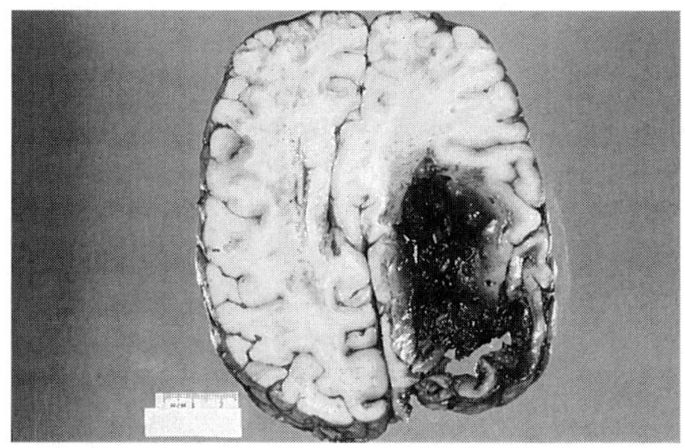

**Fig. 6-89.** Amyloid angiopathy associated with lobar hematoma in the right parietal occipital region.

sia, cystic medial necrosis, arteritis, or congenital defects of the arterial wall.[63] Marfan's syndrome, hypertension, and history of migraine are considered risk factors for arterial dissection.[15] Cervicocephalic arterial dissection has been associated with minor head trauma, a variety of physical activities, and with stress; in most patients the dissection is spontaneous.[266]

*Cerebral amyloid angiopathy (CAA) is* characterized by deposits of amyloid in small arteries and veins of the leptomeninges and cerebral cortex in the absence of systemic amyloidosis.[60] Amyloid can be identified by light microscopy (polarized light) with Congo red stain, by fluorescence microscopy with thioflavin S and T, by immunohistochemistry, and by electron microscopy through the identification of nonbranching filaments 9 nm in width (Figs. 6-86 to 6-88). CAA is rare before the age of 50 years. An increased incidence of intracerebral hemorrhage related to amyloid angiopathy is observed after 60 years of age.[317] Bleeding is most common in the cerebral subcortical white matter, and many of these hematomas involve the frontal lobe (Fig. 6-89).[318] Hemorrhages in the basal ganglia, thalamus, midbrain, and cerebellum are rare in CAA. Repeated intracerebral bleeding episodes are common in CAA but are not as common among CAA patients without hypertension.[38] The mechanism of bleeding is undetermined. Changes associated with hypertension including fibrinoid necrosis and microaneurysms are present in some patients with CAA and may contribute to the intracerebral hemorrhages.[214,324] Additional factors contributing to the hemorrhages in patients with CAA include angiitis, radiation effects, vascular malformations, head trauma, and neurosurgical procedures.[118,306]

Two familial forms of CAA have been described. The first familial syndrome is called hereditary cerebral hemorrhage with amyloidosis-Icelandic type (HCHWA-I).[216] This syndrome is inherited as a dominant trait and sometimes is associated with fatal intracerebral hemorrhage during the third decade of life. Amyloid is widely distributed and present not only in the cerebral blood vessels but also in extracranial organs, including lymph nodes and skin. The amyloid protein deposited in the vessel walls is cystatin-C or $\gamma$-trace. Hereditary cystatin-C amyloidosis can be detected preclinically by immunohistochemical demonstration of cystatin-C in skin biopsies and through the detection of the disease-causing mutation by molecular analysis.[299] The first clinical symptoms typically appear between 20 and 30 years of age. Small and large ICH and brain infarcts result in progressive mental deterioration; death supervenes within 10 years of the onset of symptoms.[120] The genetic defect is a point mutation in the cystatin-C gene on chromosome 20, with a substitution of glutamine for leucine at position 68 on the cystatin-C polypeptide chain.[220]

The other form of familial amyloidosis is known as hereditary cerebral hemorrhage with amyloidosis-Dutch type (HCHWA-D) and is also inherited as a dominant trait.[35] Intracerebral hemorrhage occurs in individuals with a mean age of 55 years of age. Dementia may also affect these patients. In this syndrome, as in sporadic CAA, the amyloid deposits are restricted to the cerebral cortical and leptomeningeal blood vessels and the protein is $\beta$ (or A4) amyloid. The genetic defect is in the $\beta$ protein precursor gene located in chromosome 21.[314] The single point mutation is the substitution of glutamine for glutamic acid at position 22 of the amyloid protein.[166] $\beta$-amyloid CAA may be hereditary or sporadic and share many features with Alzheimer disease. Both types of CAA derive from precursor proteins synthesized in situ by either astrocytes (cystatin C) or smooth muscle cells ($\beta$-amyloid). Both induce progressive degeneration of the vessel wall with eventual luminal closure or vascular rupture.[56] In a few cases, large collections of amyloid in the brain parenchyma (amyloidoma) have been clinically mistaken for a neoplastic growth.[54]

***Radiation.*** Neurologic complications of radiation therapy for neoplasms of the head and neck may develop several months or years after radiation. These include parenchymal necrosis, amyloid angiopathy, cerebral hemorrhage, accelerated atherosclerosis, and aneurysmatic dilatations of the intracranial arteries. After cranial radiation some children with midline tumors such as optic nerve glioma, craniopharyngioma, and hypothalamic gliomas may develop vascular changes similar to those of moyamoya disease.[215] Patients with head and neck tumors may develop accelerated atherosclerosis attributed to the effects of radiation.[139] Several radiation-induced intracranial aneurysms were described in a child with a suprasellar tumor.[17]

## REFERENCES


1. Abramsky O, and Slavin S: Neurological manifestations in patients with mixed cryoglobulinemia, Neurology (NY) 24:245-249, 1974.
2. Aggarwal SK, and others: Cocaine-associated intracranial hemorrhage: absence of vasculitis in 14 cases, Neurology 46: 1741-1743, 1996.
3. Ahuja GK, and others: Cerebral mycotic aneurysm of fungal origin, J Neurosurg 49:107-110, 1978.
4. Alarcón F, and others: Cerebral cysticercosis and stroke, Stroke 23:224-228, 1992.
5. Alexander GL, and Norman RM: Sturge-Weber Syndrome, Bristol, John Wright & Sons Ltd, 1960.

5a. Alpers BJ, and others: Circle of Willis in cerebrovascular disorders: The anatomic structure, Arch Neurol 8:398-405, 1963.

6. Alsofrom DJ, and others: Shotgun pellet embolization from the chest to the middle cerebral arteries, J Trauma 22:155-157, 1982.
7. Alzheimer A: Die Seelenstörungen auf arteriosclerotischer Grundlage (Allg Z Psychiatr Psych Gerichtl Med 59:695-711, 1902) translated by Förstl H, Howard R, Levy R: Mental disturbances of arteriosclerotic origin, Neuropsychiatr Neuropsychol Behav Neurol 5:106, 1992.
8. Amacher AL, and Shillito J: The syndromes and surgical treatment of aneurysms of the great vein of Galen, J Neurosurg 39:89-98, 1973.
9. Amine AR: Neurosurgical complications of heroin addiction: brain abscess and mycotic aneurysm, Surg Neurol 7:385-386, 1977.
10. Andersen CA, and others: Internal carotid artery occlusion associated with fibromuscular dysplasia, Vasc Surg 13:349, 1979.
11. Arboix A, Marti-Vilalta JL, and Garcia JH: Clinical study of 227 patients with lacunar infarcts, Stroke 21:842-847, 1990.
12. Armstrong RD, and others: Histocompatibility antigens in polymyalgia rheumatica and giant cell arteritis, J Rheumatol 10:659-661, 1983.
13. Arthur G, and Margolis G: Mycoplasma-like structures in granulomatous angiitis of the central nervous system: case report with light and electron microscopic studies, Arch Pathol Lab Med 101:382-387, 1977.
14. Atlee WE Jr: Talc and cornstarch emboli in eyes of drug abusers, JAMA 219:49-51, 1972.
15. Austin MG, and Schaefer RF: Marfan's syndrome with unusual blood vessel manifestations, Arch Pathol 64:205, 1957.
16. Azzarelli B, and Roessmann U: Diffuse anoxic myelopathy, Neurology 27:1049-1052, 1977.
17. Azzarelli B, and others: Multiple fusiform aneurysms following curative radiation therapy for suprasellar germinoma, J Neurosurg 61:1141-1145, 1984.
18. Barinagarrementeria F, and others: Progressive intracranial occlusive disease associated with deficiency of protein S. Report of two cases, Stroke 24:1752-1756, 1993.
19. Barinagarrementeria F, and Cantú C: Primary medullary hemorrhage. Report of four cases and review of the literature, Stroke 25:1684-1687, 1994.
20. Baudrimont M, and others: Autosomal dominant leukoencephalopathy and subcortical ischemic stroke: a clinicopathological study, Stroke 24:122-125, 1993.
21. Bell WE, and Butler C: Cerebral mycotic aneurysms in children, Neurology 18:81-86, 1968.
22. Bell WE, and Lascari AD: Rocky mountain spotted fever, Neurology 20:841-847, 1970.
23. Belman AL, and others: Neurologic manifestations of Schönlein-Henoch purpura: report of three cases and review of the literature, Pediatrics 75:687-692, 1985.

24. Benagale RC: Massive intracranial air embolism: a complication of mechanical ventilation, Am J Dis Child 134:799, 1960
25. Beneveniste H, and others: Ischemic damage in hippocampal CAI is dependent on glutamate release and intact innervation from CA3, J Cereb Blood Flow Metab 9:629-639, 1989.
26. Berlit P: Clinical and laboratory findings with giant cell arteritis, J Neurol Sci 111:1-12, 1992.
27. Biller J, and others: Non-bacterial thrombotic endocarditis, Arch Neurol 39:95-98, 1982.
28. Biller J, and others: Spontaneous improvement after acute ischemic stroke. A pilot study, Stroke 21:1008-1012, 1990.
29. Binder A, Snaith ML, and Isenberg D: Sjögren's syndrome: a study of its neurological complications, Br J Rheumatol 27: 275-280, 1988.
30. Binswanger O: Die Abgrenzung der allgemeinen progressive Paralyse, Berl Klin Wochenschr 31:1102-1105, 1137-1139, 1180-1186, 1894.
31. Bluestein HG, and Zvaifler NT: Antibodies reactive with central nervous system antigens, Hum Pathol 14:424-428, 1983.
32. Bogousslavsky J: Binswanger's disease. In Barnett HJM, and others, editors: Stroke, pathophysiology, diagnosis and management, ed 2, New York, 1992, Churchill-Livingstone.
33. Bogousslavsky J, Regli F, and Van Melle G: Risk factors and concomitants of internal carotid artery occlusion or stenosis: a controlled study of 159 cases, Arch Neurol 42:864-867, 1985.
34. Boltshauser E, Wilson J, and Hoare RD: Sturge-Weber syndrome with bilateral intracranial calcification, J Neurol Neurosurg Psychiatry 39:429-435, 1976.
35. Bornebroek M, and others: Hereditary cerebral hemorrhage with amyloidosis-Dutch type (HCHWA-D): I. A review of clinical, radiologic and genetic aspects, Brain Pathol 6:111, 1996.
36. Bousser MG, and Barnett HJM: Cerebral venous thrombosis. In Barnett HJM, and others, editors: Stroke, pathophysiology, diagnosis, and management, ed 2, New York, 1992, Churchill-Livingstone.
37. Brouet JC, and others: Biological and clinical significance of cryoglobulins. A report of 86 cases, Am J Med 57:775-788, 1974.
38. Brown RT, Coates RK, and Gilbert JJ: Radiographic-pathologic correlation in cerebral amyloid angiopathy, J Can Assoc Radiol 36:308-311, 1985.
39. Brun A, and Englund E: A white matter disorder in dementia of the Alzheimer type: a pathoanatomical study, Ann Neurol 19:253-262, 1986.
40. Burger PC, and Vogel FS: Cerebrovascular disease, Am J Pathol 92:253-313, 1978.
41. Burton E, and Johnson J: Multiple cerebral aneurysms and cardiac mysoma, N Engl J Med 181:35, 1970.
42. Caccamo DY, Garcia JH, and Ho KL: Isolated granulomatous angiitis of the spinal cord, Ann Neurol 32:580-582, 1992.
43. Calandre L, and others: Risk factors for spontaneous cerebral hematomas. Case-control study, Stroke 17:1126-1128, 1986.
44. Caplan LR: Intracerebral hemorrhage revisited, Neurology 38: 624, 1988.
45. Caplan LR: General symptoms and signs. In Kase CS and Caplan LR, editors: Intracerebral hemorrhage, Boston, 1994 Butterworth Heinemann.
46. Cerebral Embolism Task Force: Cardiogenic brain embolism, Arch Neurol 43:71, 1986.
47. Challa VK, Moody DM, and Bell MA: The Charcot-Bouchard aneurysm controversy: impact of a new histologic technique, abstracted, J Neuropathol Exp Neurol 51:264-271, 1992.
48. Challa VR, Moody DM, and Brown WR: Vascular malformations of the central nervous system, J Neuropathol Exp Neurol 54:609-621, 1995.
49. Chason JL, and Hindman WM: Berry aneurysms of the circle of Willis, Neurology 8:41, 1958.
50. Chauqui R, and Tapia J: Histologic assessment of the age of recent brain infarcts in man, J Neuropathol Exp Neurol 52: 481-489, 1993.
51. Cheshire WP, and others: Spinal cord infarction: etiology and outcome, Neurology 47:321-330, 1996.
52. Choeng WY, and Tan KP: Cerebral venous angioma—A misnomer? Ann Acad Med Singapore 22:736, 1993.
53. Chumbley LC, and others: Allergic granulomatosis and angiitis (Churg-Strauss syndrome). Report and analysis of 30 cases, Mayo Clin Proc 52:477-484, 1977.
54. Cohen M, and others: Amyloidoma of the CNS. I. Clinical and pathologic study, Neurology 42:2019-2023, 1992.
55. Colegial C, and others: Neuropathology of intravascular lymphomatosis, J Neuropathol Exp Neurol 55:625, 1996 (abstract).
56. Coria F, and Rubio I: Cerebral amyloid angiopathies, Neuropath Appl Neurobiol 22:216-227, 1996.
57. Cotran RS, Kumar V, and Robbins SL: Robbins pathologic basis of disease, ed 5, Philadelphia, 1994, WB Saunders.
58. Cottrill CM, and Kaplan S: Cerebral vascular accidents in cyanotic congenital heart disease, Am J Dis Child 125:484-487, 1973.
59. Coull BM, and Goodnight SH: Hematological abnormalities in stroke. In Adams HP, editor: Handbook of cerebrovascular diseases, New York, 1993, Marcel Dekker.
60. Crooks DA: Cerebral amyloid angiopathy, J Neurol Neurosurg Psychiatry 57:1457, 1994.
61. Cupps TR, Moore PM, and Fauci AS: Isolated angiitis of the central nervous system, Am J Med 74:97-105, 1983.
62. Dastur DK, and Lalitha VS: The many facets of neurotuberculosis: an epitome of neuropathology. In Zimmerman HM, editor: Progress in neuropathology, vol 2, New York, 1973, Grune & Stratton.
63. DeBaets P, and others: Atherosclerotic dissection of the cervical internal carotid artery—a case report, Angiology 41:161, 1990.
64. DeGroot RG, and others: Endothelial cell dysfunction in homocystinuria, Eur J Clin Invest 13:405, 1983.
65. del Zoppo GJ, and Mori E: Hematologic causes of intracerebral hemorrhage and their treatment, Neurosurg Clin N Am 3:637-658, 1992.
66. Demirer T, Dail DH, and Aboulafia DM: Four varied cases of intravascular lymphomatosis and a literature review, Cancer 73:1738-1745, 1994.
67. Devinsky O, Petito CK, and Alonso DR: Clinical and neuropathological findings in systemic lupus erythematosus. The role of vasculitis, heart emboli, and thromboti thromboytopenic purpura, Ann Neurol 23:380-384, 1988.
68. DiNubile MJ: Septic thrombosis of the cavernous sinuses, Arch Neurol 45:567-572, 1988.
69. Dobyns WB, and others: Familial cavernous malformations of the central nervous system and retina, Ann Neurol 21:578-583, 1987.
70. Dorland's Illustrated Medical Dictionary, ed 28, Philadelphia, 1994, WB Saunders.
71. Drachman DA: Neurological complications of Wegener's granulomatosis, Arch Neurol 8:145, 1963.
72. Dul K, and Drayer BP: CT and MR imaging of intracerebral hemorrhage. In Kase CS, Caplan LR, editors: Intracerebral hemorrhage, Boston, 1994, Butterworth Heinemann.
73. Dusser A, Boyer-Neumann C, and Wolf M: Temporary protein C deficiency associated with cerebral arterial thrombosis in childhood, J Pediatr 113:849-851, 1988.
74. Duvoisin RC, and Yahr MD: Posterior fossa aneurysms, Neurology 15:231, 1965.
75. Ehsan T, and others: Serial magnetic resonance imaging in isolated angiitis of the central nervous system, Neurology 45: 1462-1465, 1995.
76. Einhäupl KM, and Bousser MG: Cerebral venous and sinus

thrombosis. In Neurological disorders: course and treatment, New York, 1996, Academic Press.

77. Ellis SG, and Verity MA: Central nervous system involvement in systemic lupus erythematosus: a review of neuropathologic findings in 57 cases, 1955-1977, Semin Arthritis Rheum 8:212-221, 1979.
78. Farber JL: Biology of disease: membrane injury and calcium homeostasis in the pathogenesis of coagulation necrosis, Lab Invest 47:114-123, 1982.
79. Fazekas F, and others: Magnetic resonance imaging correlates of transient cerebral ischemic attacks, Stroke 27:607-611, 1996.
80. Feeley TM, and others: Histologic characteristics of carotid artery plaque, J Vasc Surg 13:719-724, 1991.
81. Farrell DF, and Forno LS: Symptomatic capillary telangiectasis of the brainstem without hemorrhage, Neurology 20:341-346, 1970.
82. Fisher CM, and others: Carotid artery plaques in the NASCET and ACAS projects, Neurol 42:(suppl 3) 204, 1992.
83. Fisher CM: Cerebral miliary aneurysms in hypertension, Am J Pathol 66:313, 1972.
84. Fisher M, and Garcia JH: Evolving stroke and the ischemic penumbra, Neurology 47:884-888, 1996.
85. Forbus WD: On the origin of miliary aneurysms of the superficial cerebral arteries, Bull Johns Hopkins Hosp 47:239, 1930.
86. Ford RG, and Siekert RG: Central nervous system manifestations of periarteritis nodosa, Neurology 15:114, 1965.
87. Franke CL, and Engelshove H: Subarachnoid haemorrhage, J Neurol Neurosurg Psychiatry 60:140, 1996.
88. Frayne JH, Gilligan BS, and Essex WB: Granulomatous angiitis of the central nervous system, Med J Aust 145:410-412, 1986.
89. Fredericks RK, and others: Cerebral vasculitis associated with cocaine abuse, Stroke 22:1437-1439, 1991.
90. Friede RL: Hemorrhages in asphyxiated premature infants. In Developmental neuropathology, ed 2, New York, 1989, Springer-Verlag.
91. Friede RL: Developmental neuropathology (ed 2, rev). Berlin, 1989, Springer-Verlag.
92. Friedman WA, and others: Cervical carotid dissecting aneurysms, Neurosurgery 7:207-214, 1980.
92a. Fujioka M, and others: Specific changes in the human brain following reperfusion after cardiac arrest, Stroke 25:2091-2095, 1994.
93. Furlan M, and others: Spontaneous neurological recovery after stroke and the fate of the ischemic penumbra, Ann Neurol 40: 216-226, 1996.
94. Garcia, JH: Evolution of the brain lesion induced by experimental focal ischemia. In Welch, and others, editors: Primer on cerebrovascular diseases, New York, 1997, Academic Press.
95. Garcia JH: Mechanisms of cell death in ischemia. In Caplan LR, editor: Brain ischemia: basic concepts and clinical relevance. London, 1995, Springer-Verlag.
96. Garcia JH: Pathophysiology of ischemic injury to the brain. In Nelson JS, and others, editors: Principles and practice of neuropathology, Philadelphia, 1993, Mosby–Year Book.
97. Garcia JH: Morphology of global cerebral ischemia: a review, Crit Care Med 16:979-987, 1988.
98. Garcia JH: Thrombosis of cranial veins and sinuses: the brain parenchymal effects. In Baethmann A, Kempski O, and Einhäupl K, editors: Experimental and clinical aspects of cerebral sinus thrombosis, New York, 1991, Plenum Press.
99. Garcia JH, and Anderson ML: Circulatory disorders and their effects on the brain. In Davis RL, and Robertson DM, editors: Textbook of neuropathology, ed 3, Baltimore, 1997, Williams & Wilkins.
100. Garcia JH, and Brown GG: Vascular dementia. Neuropathologic and metabolic brain changes, J Neurol Sci 109:121-131, 1992.
101. Garcia JH, and Geer JC: Atherosclerosis. In Wilkins RH, and Rengachary, S, editors: Neurosurgery, ed 2, New York, 1996, McGraw-Hill.
102. Garcia JH, Ho KL, and Caccamo DV: Intracerebral hemorrhage: pathology of selected topics. In Kase CS, and Caplan LR, editors: Intracerebral hemorrhage, Boston, 1994, Butterworth Heinemann.
103. Garcia JH, Ho KL, and Caccamo DV: Pathology of stroke. In Barnett HJM, and others, editors: Stroke, pathophysiology, diagnosis and management, ed 2, New York, 1992, Churchill-Livingstone.
104. Garcia JH, and others: Arterial air embolism: structural effects on the gerbil brain, Stroke 12:414-421, 1981.
105. Garcia JH, and others: Ischemic stroke and incomplete infarction, Stroke 27:161-165, 1996.
106. Garcia JH, Liu KF, and Ho KL: Neuronal necrosis after middle cerebral artery occlusion in Wistar rats progresses at different time intervals in the caudoputamen and the cortex, Stroke 26: 636-643, 1995.
106a. Garcia JH, and others: Influx of leukocytes and platelets in an evolving brain infarct (Wistar rat), Am J Pathol 144:188-199, 1994.
107. Garcia JH, and others: Neuronal ischemic injury: light microscopy, ultrastructure and biochemistry, Acta Neuropathol 43: 85-95, 1978.
107a. Garcia JH, and Pantoni L: Strokes in childhood, Semin Pediatr Neurol 2:180-191, 1995.
108. Garcia JH, Patel S, and Wagner S: The vasculature of the human brain. In Conn PM, editor: Neurosciences in medicine, Philadelphia, 1995, JB Lippincott.
109. Garcia JH, and others: Neurological deficit and extent of neuronal necrosis attributable to middle cerebral artery occlusion in rats, Stroke 26:627-635, 1995.
110. Garcia JH, and others: Progression from ischemic injury to infarct following middle-cerebral-artery occlusion in the rat, Am J Pathol 142:623-635, 1993.
111. Garland HG, and Anning ST: Hereditary hemorrhagic telangiectasia: a genetic and bibliographical study, Br J Dermatol Syph 62:289, 1950.
112. Garner TB, and others: The natural history of intracranial venous angiomas, J Neurosurg 75:715-722, 1991.
113. Gettelfinger DM, and Kokmen E: Superior sagittal sinus thrombosis, Arch Neurol 34:2-6, 1977.
114. Ghatak NR: Pathology of cerebral embolization caused by nonthrombotic agents, Hum Pathol 6:599-610, 1975.
115. Goodnight SH Jr: Bleeding and intravascular clotting in malignancy: a review, Ann NY Acad Sci 230:271-288, 1974.
116. Gordon RM, and Silverstein A: Neurologic manifestations in progressive systemic sclerosis, Arch Neurol 22:126-134, 1970.
117. Graf WD, Milstein JM, and Sherry DD: Stroke and mixed connective tissue disease, J Child Neurol 8:256-259, 1993.
118. Green GM and others: Surgical experience with cerebral amyloid angiopathy, Stroke 21:1545, 1990.
119. Griesemer DA, and others: Amebic meningoencephalitis caused by *Balamuthia madrillaris*, Pediatr Neurol 10:249-254, 1994.
120. Gudmundsson G, and others: Hereditary cerebral haemorrhage with amyloidosis, Brain 95:387-404, 1972.
121. Guillen B, and others: Hereditary hemorrhagic telangiectasia: report of 15 affected cases in a Mexican family, Clin Genet 32: 214, 1991.
122. Hall S, and others: Takayasu arteritis: a study of 32 North American patients, Medicine (Baltimore) 64:89-99, 1985.
123. Harker LA, and others: Homocystine-induced atherosclerosis, J Clin Invest 58:731-741, 1976.

124. Harrison EG Jr, and McCormack LJ: Pathologic classification of renal arterial disease in renovascular hypertension, Mayo Clin Proc 16:161-167, 1971.
125. Haymaker W, and Johnston AD: Pathology of decompression sickness. A comparison of the lesions in airmen with those in caisson workers and divers, Mil Med 117:285, 1955.
126. Healton EB: Cerebrovascular fibromuscular dysplasia, In Barnett HJM, and others, editors: Stroke, pathophysiology, diagnosis, and management, ed 2, New York, 1992, Churchill-Livingstone.
127. Heiss WD, and Rosner G: Functional recovery of cortical neurons as related to degree and duration of ischemia, Ann Neurol 14:294-301, 1983.
128. Henderson WR, and Gomez R: Natural history of cerebral angiomas, Br Med J 4:571-574, 1967.
129. Henry JM: Central nervous system manifestations of systemic lupus erythematosus, In Antonovych TT, editor: Pathology of systemic lupus erythematosus, Washington, 1995, Armed Forces Institute of Pathology.
130. Heros RC, and Kistler JP: Intracranial artery aneurysm—an update, Stroke 14:628-631, 1983.
131. Hilt DC, and others: Herpes zoster ophthalmicus and delayed contralateral hemiparesis caused by cerebral angiitis: diagnosis and management approaches, Ann Neurol 14:543, 1983.
132. Ho KL: Acute subdural hematoma and intra-cerebral hemorrhage: rare complications of rhinocerebral mucormycosis, Arch Otolaryngol 105:279-281, 1979.
133. Ho KL: Neoplastic aneurysm and intracranial hemorrhage, Cancer 50:2935-2940, 1982.
134. Hoffman GS, and others: Wegener granulomatosis: an analysis of 158 patients, Ann Intern Med 116:488-498, 1992.
135. Hogan PJ, Greenberg MK, and McCarthy GE: Neurologic complications of lymphoid granulomatosis, Neurology 31:619-620, 1981.
136. Hook EW III, and Marra CM: Acquired syphilis in adults, N Engl J Med 326:1060-1069, 1992.
137. Hopen G, and others: The Wyburn-Mason syndrome—concomitant chiasmal and fundus vascular malformations, J Clin Neuro-Ophthalmol 5:95, 1985.
138. Housepian EM, and Pool JL: A systematic analysis of intracranial aneurysms from the autopsy file of the Presbyterian Hospital, 1914 to 1956, J Neuropathol Exp Neurol 17:409, 1958.
139. Huvos AG, Leaming RH, and Moore OS: Clinicopathologic study of the resected carotid artery, Am J Surg 126:570, 1973.
140. Johnson RG, and Richardson EP: The neurological manifestations of systemic lupus erythematosus, Medicine 47:337, 1968.
141. Joutel A, and others: Notch 3 mutations in CADASIL, a hereditary adult-onset condition causing stroke and dementia, Nature 383:707-710, 1996.
142. Juvela S: Prevalence of risk factors in spontaneous intracerebral hemorrhage and aneurysmal subarachnoid hemorrhage, Arch Neurol 53:734-740, 1996.
143. Kaell AT, and others: The diversity of neurologic event in systemic lupus erythematosus—prospective clinical and computed tomographic classification of 82 events in 71 patients, Arch Neurol 43:273, 1986.
144. Kamenar E, and Burger PC: Cerebral fat embolism: study of a microembolic state, Stroke 11:477, 1980.
145. Kaplan HA: Collateral circulation of the brain, Neurology 11: 9, 1959.
146. Kase CS: Intracerebral hemorrhage: non-hypertensive causes, Stroke 17:590-595, 1986.
147. Kase CS, and others: Medial medullary infarction from fibrocartilaginous embolism to the anterior spinal artery, Stroke 14: 413-418, 1983.
148. Kato H, Koike S, and Yokoyama T: Kawasaki disease: effects of treatment on coronary artery involvement, Pediatrics 63: 175, 1979.
149. Kawakami Y, and others: Intracranial hemorrhage associated with nontraumatic disseminated intravascular coagulation: report of four cases, Neurol Med Chir 30:610, 1990.
150. Kazui S, and others: Enlargement of spontaneous intracerebral hemorrhage, Stroke 27:1783-1787, 1996.
151. Kerr JFR, and Harmon BV: Definition and incidence of apoptosis: an historical perspective. In Tomei LD, Cope FO, editors: Current communications in cell and molecular biology: apoptosis: the molecular basis of cell death. Cold Spring Harbor, NY, 1991, Cold Spring Harbor Laboratory Press.
152. Kidwell CS, and Saver JL: Causes and consequences of white matter hyperintensities. A meta-analysis, Facts and Research in Gerontology (suppl Stroke):137-150, 1996.
153. Kidwell CS, and Saver JL: Causes and consequences of leukoraraiosis: a review, facts and research in gerontology (suppl Stroke):115-135, 1996.
154. Kirino T, Tamura A, and Sano K: Delayed neuronal death in rat hippocampus following transient forebrain ischemia, Acta Neuropathol 64:139-147, 1984.
155. Klassbrun M, and Edelman ER: Biological and biochemical properties of fibroblast growth factors. Implications for the pathogenesis of atherosclerosis, Arteriosclerosis 9:269, 1989.
156. Kondziolka D, and others: Arteriovenous malformations of the brain in children: a forty year experience, Can J Neurol Scien 19:40, 1992.
157. Konzen JP, Levine SR, and Garcia JH: Vasospasm as a possible mechanism of stroke related to alkaloidal cocaine, Stroke 26: 1114-1118, 1995.
158. Koroshetz WJ: Imaging stroke in progress, Ann Neurol 39: 283-284, 1996.
159. Kozin F, Haughton V, and Bernhard GC: Neuro-Behcet disease: two cases and neuroradiologic findings, Neurology 27: 1148, 1977.
160. Krendel DA, and others: Biopsy-proven cerebral vasculitis associated with cocaine abuse, Neurology 40:1092, 1990.
161. Kure K, and others: Immunohistochemical localization of an HIV epitope in cerebral aneurysmal arteriopathy in pediatric acquired immunodeficiency syndrome (AIDS), Pediatr Pathol 9:655, 1989.
162. Kwee WS, and others: Neuroblastoma with a fulminant clinical course caused by tumor embolism, Eur J Pediatr 132:61, 1979.
163. Lassen NA, Ingvar DH, and Skinhoj E: Brain functions and blood flow, Sci Am 239:62, 1978.
164. Lassen NA: Incomplete cerebral infarction—focal incomplete ischemic necrosis not leading to emollision, Stroke 13:522, 1982.
165. Levine SR, and others: Cerebrovascular and neurologic disease associated with antiphospholipid antibodies: 48 cases, Neurology 40:1181, 1990.
166. Levy E, and others: Mutation of the Alzheimer disease amyloid gene in hereditary cerebral hemorrhage, Dutch type, Science 248:1124, 1990.
167. Liang GC, Simkin PA, and Mannik M: Immunoglobulins in temporal arteritis, Ann Intern Med 81:19, 1974.
168. Lie JT: The classification and diagnosis of vasculitis in large and medium-sized blood vessels. In Rosen PR, and Fechner RE, editors: Pathology Annual, Part I, Norwalk, Connecticut, 1987, Appleton-Century-Crofts.
169. Liu K-F, and others: Focal brain ischemia: endothelial-astrocyte swelling precedes neuronal necrosis, J Neuropathol Exp Neurol 55:621, 1996 (Abstract).
170. Lloyd-Still JD, and Tomasi L: Neurovascular and thromboembolic complications of inflammatory bowel disease in children, J Pediatr Gastroenterol Nutr 9:461, 1989.

171. Love BB: Rare genetic disorders predisposing to stroke. In Biller J, Matthews KD, and Love BB, editors: Stroke in young children and adults, Boston, 1994, Butterworth-Heinemann.
172. Luken MG, and others: Spontaneous dissecting aneurysms of the extracranial internal carotid artery, Clin Neurosurg 26:353, 1979.
172a. Lupi-Herrera E, and others: Takayasu arteritis. Clinical study of 107 cases, Am J Heart 93:94, 1977.
173. Macfarlane R, and Moskowitz MA: The innervation of pial blood vessels and their role in cerebral vascular regulation. In Caplan IR, editor: The scientific basis of stroke. New York, 1995, Springer-Verlag.
174. Mackenzie I: The clinical presentation of cerebral angioma: a review of 50 cases, Brain 76:184, 1953.
175. Malmvall BE, and others: Serum levels of immunoglobulin and complement in giant cell arteritis, JAMA 236:1876, 1976.
176. Marchevsky AM, and others: The changing spectrum of disease, etiology and diagnosis of mucormycosis, Hum Pathol 11:457, 1980.
177. Marie P: Des foyers lacunaires de desintegration et de differents autres états cavitaires du cerveau, Rev Med 21:281-298, 1901.
178. Marti-Vilalta JL, Arboix A, and Garcia JH: Brain infarcts in the arterial border zones: clinical-pathologic correlations, J Stroke Cerebrovasc Dis 4:114-120, 1994.
179. Martinez HR, Rangel-Guerra RA, and Marfil LJ: Ischemic stroke due to coagulation inhibitors. Report of 10 young adults, Stroke 24:19, 1993.
180. Masson RJ, and Day AL: Aneurysmal intracerebral hemorrhage, Neurosurg Clin N Am 3:539-550, 1992.
181. Mathern GW, and others: Human fascia dentata anatomy and hippocampal neuron densities differ depending on the epileptic syndrome and age at first seizure, Neuropathol Exp Neurol 56(2):199-212, 1997.
182. Mauro AI, and others: Lipohyalinosis and miliary aneurysms causing hemorrhage in a patient with moyamoya disease: a clinicopathological study, Stroke 11:405, 1980.
183. McCormick F: Vascular diseases. In Rosenberg RN, and others, editors: The clinical neurosciences, vol 3, New York, 1983, Churchill-Livingstone.
184. McCormick WF: The pathology of vascular ("arteriovenous") malformations, J Neurosurg 24:807, 1966.
185. McCormick WF, and Rosenfield DB: Massive brain hemorrhage. A review of 144 cases and an examination of their causes, Stroke 4:946, 1973.
186. McFarland HR, and others: Papulosis atrophicans maligna (Köhlmier-Degos disease): a disseminated occlusive vasculopathy, Ann Neurol 3:338, 1978.
187. McGill HC: The pathogenesis of atherosclerosis, Clin Chem 34:833, 1988.
188. Medeiros LJ, and others: Angiocentric immunoproliferative lesions. A molecular analysis of eight cases, Hum Pathol 22: 1150, 1991.
189. Mello LR, and Detoni XA: Bonnet-Dechaume-Blanc syndrome: report of a case with arteriovenous malformations, Acta Radiol 347:187, 1975.
190. Millikan C, and Futtrell N: The fallacy of the lacune hypothesis, Stroke 21:1251-1257, 1990.
191. Mettinger KL: Fibromuscular dysplasia and the brain. II. Current concept of the disease, Stroke 13:53, 1982.
192. Mintz M, Epstein LG, and Koenigsberger MR: Idiopathic childhood stroke is associated with human leucocyte antigen (HLA)-B51, Ann Neurol 31:675, 1992.
193. Mittal K, and others: Lymphomatoid granulomatosis in the acquired immunodeficiency syndrome. Evidence of Epstein-Barr virus infection and B-cell clonal selection without MYC rearrangement, Cancer 65:1150, 1990.
194. Mizukami K, and others: Central nervous system changes in mitochondrial encephalopathy: light and electron microscopic study, Acta Neuropathol 83:449, 1992.
195. Mohr JP, Hilal SK, and Stein BM: Arteriovenous malformations and other vascular anomalies, In Barnett HJM, and others, editors: Stroke, pathophysiology, diagnosis, and management, ed 2, New York, 1992, Churchill-Livingstone.
196. Mohr JP, and others: The Harvard cooperative stroke registry: a prospective registry, Neurology 28:754-762, 1978.
197. Mohr JP: Lacunes, Neurol Clin North Am 1:201-221, 1983.
198. Reference deleted.
199. Mohr JP, Kistler JP, and Fink ME: Intracranial aneurysms. In Barnett HJM and others, editors: Stroke, pathophysiology, diagnosis and management, ed 2, New York, 1992, Churchill-Livingstone.
200. Moossy J: Pathology of ischemic cerebrovascular disease. In: Wilkins RA, and Regachary SS, editors: Neurosurgery, New York, 1985, McGraw-Hill.
201. Morens DM, Anderson LJ, and Hurtwitz ES: National surveillance of Kawasaki disease, Pediatrics 65:21, 1980.
202. Morley TP, and Barr HWK: Giant intracranial aneurysms: diagnosis, course and management, Clin Neurosurg 16:73, 1968.
203. Moulin T, and others: Early CT signs in acute middle cerebral artery infarction: predictive value for subsequent infarct locations and outcome, Neurology 47:366-375, 1996.
204. Mudd SH, and others: The natural history of homocystinuria due to cystathione B-synthase deficiency, Am J Hum Genet 37:1, 1985.
205. Nakagawara J, and others: Incomplete brain infarction of early reperfused cortex may be quantified with iomazenil, Stroke 28:124–132, 1997.
206. Niles JL, and McCluskey RT: Vasculitis. In Colvin RB, and others, editors: Diagnostic immunopathology, ed 2, New York, 1995, Raven Press.
207. Nishimoto A, and Takeuchi S: Abnormal cerebral vascular network related to the internal carotid arteries, J Neurosurg 29: 255, 1968.
208. Nishino H, and others: Neurological involvement in Wegener's granulomatosis: an analysis of 324 consecutive patients at the Mayo Clinic, Ann Neurol 33:4, 1993.
209. Nishino A, and others: Superior petrosal sinus dural arteriovenous malformation with varix indenting brain stem. Report of a case and review of the literature, No To Shinkei 43:62, 1991.
210. Norenberg MD, and Bruce-Gregorios J: Nervous system manifestations of systemic disease. In Davis RL, and Robertson D, editors: Textbook of neuropathology, ed 3, Baltimore, 1997, Williams & Wilkins.
211. O'Connell BK, and others: Dissecting aneurysms of the head and neck, Neurology 35:993, 1985.
211a. Ogata J, and others: Hemorrhagic infarct of the brain without reopening the arteries in cardio-embolic stroke, Stroke 20:876-883, 1989.
212. O'Neill BP, Dinapoli RP, and Okazaki H: Cerebral infarction as a result of tumor emboli, Cancer 60:90, 1987.
213. Oka K: Cerebral hemorrhage in moyamoya disease at autopsy, Virchows Arch 392:247, 1981.
214. Okazaki H, Reagan TJ, and Campbell RJ: Clinicopathologic studies of primary cerebral amyloid angiopathy, Mayo Clin Proc 54:22, 1979.
215. Okuno T, Prensky AL, and Gado M: The moyamoya syndrome associated with irradiation of an optic glioma in children: report of two cases and review of the literature, Pediatr Neurol 1:311, 1985.
216. Olafsson E, Thorsteinsson L, and Jensson O: The molecular pathology of hereditary cystatin C amyloid angiopathy causing brain hemorrhage, Brain Pathol 6:121, 1996.

217. Orozco M, and others: Intracranial aneurysms in early childhood, Surg Neurol 9:247, 1978.
218. Osborne AG, and Anderson RE: Angiographic spectrum of cervical and intracranial fibromuscular dysplasia, Stroke 8: 617, 1977.
219. Padget DH: The development of the cranial arteries in the human embryo, Contrib Embryol Carnegie Inst 32:205, 1948.
220. Palsdottir A, and others: Mutation in cystatin C gene causes hereditary brain hemorrhage, Lancet 2:603-604, 1988.
221. Pantoni L, and Garcia JH: Cerebral ischemia and cognitive impairment in the elderly, Facts Res Gerontol, 1996; (supplement: Stroke):171-182, 1996.
222. Pantoni L, and Garcia JH: Binswanger's disease: Does it exist? Cerebrovasc Dis 6:255-263, 1996.
223. Pantoni L, and Garcia JH: Pathogenesis of leukoaraiosis: a review, Stroke 28:652–659, 1997.
224. Pantoni L, and Garcia JH: The significance of cerebral white matter abnormalities 100 years after Binswanger's report: a review, Stroke 26:1293-1301, 1995.
225. Pantoni L, Garcia JH, and Brown GG: Vascular pathology in three cases of progressive cognitive deterioration, J. Neurol Sci 135:131-139, 1996.
225a. Pantoni L, Garcia JH, and Gutierrez JA: Cerebral white matter is highly vulnerable to ischemia, Stroke 27:1641-1647, 1996.
226. Parker HL, and Kernohan JW: The central nervous system in periarteritis nodosa, Mayo Clin Proc 24:43, 1949.
227. Parkinson D, and Bachers G: Arteriovenous malformations: summary of 100 consecutive supratentorial cases, J Neurosurg 53:285, 1980.
228. Pascual-Castroviejo I, and others: Hemangiomas of the head, neck, and chest with associated vascular and brain anomalies: a complex neurocutaneous syndrome, AJNR 17:461-471, 1996.
229. Pavlakis SG, and others: Mitochondrial myopathy, encephalopathy, lactic acidosis, and stroke-like episodes: a distinctive clinical syndrome, Ann Neurol 16:481, 1984.
230. Peterson JH, and McKissock W: A clinical survey of intracranial angiomas with special reference to their mode of progression and surgical treatment: a report of 110 cases, Brain 79: 233, 1956.
231. Petito CK: Cerebrovascular diseases. In Nelson JS, Parisi JE, and Schochett SS, editors: Principles and practice of neuropathology, St. Louis, 1993, Mosby–Year Book.
232. Petito CK, and others: Delayed hippocampal damage in humans following cardiorespiratory arrest, Neurology (NY) 37: 1281, 1987.
233. Petty GW, and Mohr JP: Stroke in the setting of collagen vascular disease. In Barnett HJM and others, editors: Stroke, pathophysiology, diagnosis and management, ed 2, New York, 1992, Churchill-Livingstone.
234. Pullicino PM: The course and territories of cerebral small arteries. In Pullicino PM, Caplan LT, and Hommel M, editors: Advances in neurology: cerebral small artery disease, vol 62, New York, 1993, Raven Press.
235. Quimby SR, and Perry HO: Livedo reticularis and cerebrovascular accidents, J Am Acad Dermatol 3:377, 1980.
236. Ramadan NM, and Mitsias P: Nonatherosclerotic stroke. In Gorelic PB, editor: Atlas of cerebrovascular disease, Philadelphia, 1996, Current Medicine.
237. Ramos M, and Mandybur TI: Cerebral vasculitis in rheumatoid arthritis, Arch Neurol 32:271, 1975.
238. Rapacki TF, and others: Heterogeneity of cerebral cavernous hemangiomas diagnosed by MR imaging, J Comput Assist Tomogr 14:18, 1990.
239. Requena I, and others: Cavernomas of the central nervous system: clinical and neuroimaging manifestations in 47 patients, J Neurol Neurosurg Psychiatry 54:590, 1991.
240. Rhodes RH, and others: Primary angiitis and angiography of the central nervous system and their relationship to systemic giant cell arteritis, Arch Pathol Lab Med 19:334-349, 1995.
241. Reith KG, and others: Serial measurements of CT attentuation and specific gravity in experimental cerebral edema, Radiology 135:343-348, 1980.
242. Rigamonti D, and Spetzler RF: The association of venous and cavernous malformations. Report of four cases and discussion of the pathophysiological, diagnostic, and therapeutic implications, Acta Neurochir 92:100, 1988.
243. Rigamonti D, and others: Cerebral cavernous malformations—incidence and familial occurrence, N Engl J Med 319: 343, 1988.
244. Rhodes RH, and others: Primary angiitis and angiopathy of the CNS and their relationship to systemic giant cell arteritis, Arch Pathol Lab Med 119:334-349, 1995.
245. Roach MR, and Drake CG: Ruptured cerebral aneurysms caused by microorganisms, N Engl J Med 273:240, 1965.
246. Roach ES, and Riela AR: Pediatric cerebrovascular disorders, ed 2, Armonik, NY, 1995, Futura.
247. Roman G, and others: Neurological manifestations of hereditary hemorrhagic telangiectasia (Rendu-Osler-Weber disease): report of 2 cases and review of the literature, Ann Neurol 4: 130, 1978.
248. Roos KL, and others: Postpartum intracranial venous thrombosis associated with dysfunctional protein C and deficiency of protein S, Obstet Gynecol 76:492, 1990.
249. Rosenberg GA, and others: Bacterial collagenase disrupts extracellular matrix and open blood-brain barrier in rats, Neurosci Lett 160:117-119, 1993.
250. Rosenblum WI, and Hadfield MG: Granulomatous angiitis of the nervous system in cases of herpes zoster and lymphosarcoma, Neurology 22:348, 1972.
251. Ross R: The pathogenesis of atherosclerosis—update, N Engl J Med 314:488, 1986.
252. Ross-Russell RW: Observations on intracerebral aneurysms, Brain 86:425, 1963.
253. Rubinstein LJ, and Urich H: Meningo-encephalitis of Behcet disease: case report with pathological findings, Brain 86:151, 1963.
254. Rubinstein LJ: Tumors of the central nervous system, In Atlas of tumor pathology, second series, fascicle 6, Washington, 1972, Armed Forces Institute of Pathology.
255. Ruchoux MM, and others: Systemic vascular smooth muscle cell impairment in cerebral autosomal dominant arteriopathy with subcortical infarcts and leukoencephalopathy, Acta Neuropathol 89:500-512, 1995.
256. Rumbaugh CL, and others: Cerebral angiographic changes in the drug abuse patient, Radiology 101:335, 1971.
257. Sacco RL, and others: Infarcts of undetermined cause: the NINCDS stroke data bank, Ann Neurol 25:382-390, 1989.
258. Safar P: Cerebral resuscitation after cardiac arrest: a review, Circulation 74(Suppl IV):IV-138, 1986.
259. Sahs AL: Observations on the pathology of saccular aneurysms, J Neurosurg 24:792, 1966.
260. Saldana MJ, and others: Pulmonary angiitis and granulomatosis. The relationship between histological features, organ involvement, and response to treatment, Hum Pathol 8:391, 1977.
261. Sandson TA, and Friedman JH: Spinal cord infarction: report of 8 cases and review of the literature, Medicine (Baltimore) 68:282-292, 1989.
262. Sarnat HB: Perinatal hypoxic/ischemic encephalopathy: neuropathologic features. In Garcia JH, and others, editors: Neuropathology: The diagnostic approach, Philadelphia, 1997 Mosby–Year Book.

263. Säve-Söderbergh J and others: Giant cell arteritis as a cause of death: report of nine cases, JAMA 255:493, 1986.
264. Schaffer AI and Kroll MH: Nonatheromatous arterial thrombosis, Ann Rev Med 44:155, 1993.
265. Schievink WI, and others: Sudden death from aneurysmal subarachnoid hemorrhage, Neurology 45:871-874, 1995.
266. Schievink WI, Mokri B, and Piepgras DG: Spontaneous dissections of the cervicocephalic arteries in childhood and adolescence, Neurology 44:1607, 1994.
267. Schneiderman JH, Sharpe JA, and Sutton DMC: Cerebral and retinal vascular complications of inflammatory bowel disease, Ann Neurol 5:331, 1979.
268. Schoen FJ: Blood vessels, In Cotran RS, Kumar V, and Robbins SL, editors: Robbins pathologic basis of disease, Philadelphia, 1994, WB Saunders.
269. Scholz W: Die nicht zur Erweichung fuhrenden unvollständigen Gewebsnecrosen (Elektive Parenchymnekrose). In Lubarsch O, Rössle R, and Henke F, editor: Handbuch der speziellen pathologischen Anatomie und Histologie, XIII: Band Nervensystem, 1:Teil, Bandteil B. Berlin, 1957, Springer-Verlag.
270. Schuh S, and others: Homocystinuria and megaloblastic anemia responsive to vitamin B-12 therapy, N Engl J Med 310: 686, 1984.
271. Schwartz TH and Solomon RA: Perimesencephalic nonaneurysmal subarachnoid hemorrhage: review of the literature, Neurosurgery 39:433-440, 1996.
272. Scott RM, and others: Cavernous angiomas of the central nervous system in children, J Neurosurg 76:38, 1992.
273. Scott HS: Carotid basilar anastomosis—persistent hypoglossal artery, Br J Radiol 36:847, 1963.
274. Sekar TS, and others: Survival after prolonged submersion in cold water without neurologic sequelae: report of two cases, Arch Intern Med 140:775, 1980.
275. Sergent JS, and others: Vasculitis with hepatitis B antigenemia: long term observations in nine patients, Medicine (Baltimore) 55:1, 1976.
276. Sheibani K, and others: Further evidence that malignant angioendotheliomatosis is an angiotropic large cell lymphoma, N Engl J Med 314:943, 1986.
277. Shiiki H, Shimokama T, and Watanabe T: Temporal arteritis: cell composition and the possible pathogenetic role of cell-mediated immunity, Hum Pathol 20:1057, 1989.
278. Siesjö BK: Pathophysiology and treatment of focal cerebral ischemia. Part I: pathophysiology, J Neurosurg 77:169-184, 1992.
279. Simard JM, and others: Cavernous angioma: a review of 126 collected and 12 new clinical cases, Neurosurgery 18:162-172, 1986.
280. Sisel RJ, Parker BM, and Bahl OP: Cerebral symptoms in pulmonary arteriovenous fistula: a result of paradoxical emboli? Circulation 41:123, 1970.
281. Skullerud K, and Skjaeraasen J: Clinicopathological study of germinal matrix hemorrhage, pontosubicular necrosis, and periventricular leukomalacia in stillborn, Childs Nerv Syst 4: 88-91, 1988.
282. Sneddon JB: Cerebral vascular lesions in livedo reticularis, Br J Dermatol 77:180, 1965.
283. Sobel RA, and others: Central nervous system coccidioidomycosis: a clinicopathologic study of treatment with and without amphotericin B, Hum Pathol 15:980, 1984.
284. Solis OJ, and others: Cerebral angiography in acute cerebral infarction. Revista Interam Radiol 2:19-25, 1977.
285. Sommer W: Erkrankung des ammonshorns als aetiologisches Moment der Epilepsie, Arch Psychiatr Nervenkr 10:631-675, 1880.
286. Sourander P, and Walinder J: Hereditary multi-infarct dementia, Acta Neuropathol 39:247-254, 1977.
287. Spatz H: Pathologische Anatomie der Kreislaufstörungen, Z Neurol 167:301-324, 1939.
288. Spetzler RF, and Martin NA: A proposed grading systems for arteriovenous malformations, J Neurosurg 65:476, 1986.
289. Spiro D, Lattes RG, and Wiener J: The cellular pathology of experimental hypertension. I. Hypertension arteriolarsclerosis, Am J Pathol 47:19, 1965.
290. Stary HC: Evolution and progression of atherosclerosis in the coronary arteries of children and adults. In Bates GR, Gangloff EC, editors: Atherogenesis and aging, New York, 1987, Springer-Verlag.
291. Stehbens WE: Pathology of the cerebral blood vessels, St. Louis, 1972, CV Mosby.
292. Stehbens WE: Histopathology of cerebral aneurysms, Arch Neurol 8:272, 1963.
293. Stehbens WE: Ultrastructure of aneurysms, Arch Neurol 32: 798, 1975.
294. Stein BM: Surgical decisions in vascular malformations of the brain. In Barnett HJM, and others, editors: Stroke, pathophysiology, diagnosis and management, ed 2, New York, 1992, Churchill-Livingstone.
295. Steiner JW, and Gelboom AJ: Intracranial manifestations in two cases of systemic rheumatoid disease, Arthritis Rheum 2: 537, 1959.
296. Stroup RM, and others: Angiotropic (intravascular) large cell lymphoma: a clinicopathologic study of seven cases with unique clinical presentations, Cancer 66:1781, 1990.
297. Sukoff MH, and others: Intimal fibroplasia of the internal carotid arteries, Stroke 2:483, 1971.
298. Suzuki J, and Takaku A: Cerebrovascular myamoya disease, Arch Neurol 20:288, 1969.
299. Sveinbjörnsdótir S, and others: Progressive dementa and leukoencephalopahy as the initial presentation of late onset hereditary cystatin-C amyloidosis. Clinicopathological presentation of two cases, J Neurol Sci 140:101-108, 1996.
300. Taft TA, Chusid MJ, and Sty JR: Cerebral infarction in hemophilus influenza type B meningitis. Clin Pediatr 25:177, 1986.
301. Takeshita M, and others: Clinicopathological study of bacterial intracranial aneurysms, Neurol Med Chir (Tokyo) 31:508, 1991.
302. Talbot RW, and others: Vascular complications of inflammatory bowel disease, Mayo Clin Proc 61:140, 1986.
303. Tatlisumak T, and Fisher M: Hematologic disorders associated with ischemic stroke, J Neurol Sci 140:1-11, 1996.
304. Terasawa K, and others: Neurological complications in Kawasaki disease, Pediatr Neurol 8:235, 1992.
305. The National Institute of Neurological Disorders and Stroke and Stroke rt-PA Stroke Study Group: Tissue plasminogen activator for acute ischemic stroke, N Engl J Med. 333:1581-1587, 1995.
306. Torack RM: Congophilic angiopathy complicated by surgery and massive hemorrhage: a light and electron microscopic study, Am J Pathol 81:349, 1975.
307. Toro-Gonzalez G, and others: Acute ischemic stroke from fibrocartilaginous embolism to the middle cerebral artery, Stroke 24:738, 1993.
308. Torvik A: The pathogenesis of watershed infarcts in the brain, Stroke 15:221-223, 1984.
309. Tournier-Lasserne E, and others: Cerebral autosomal arteriopathy with subcortical infarcts and leukoencephalopathy maps on chromosome 19q12, Nat Genet 3:256, 1993.
310. Trussart V, and others: Epileptogenic cerebral vascular malformations and MRI, J Neuroradiol 16:273, 1989.
311. Turnbull HM: Intracranial aneurysms, Brain 41:50, 1918.

312. Uram M, and Zubillaga C: The cutaneous manifestations of Sturge-Weber syndrome, J Clin Neuro-Ophthalmol 2:245, 1982.
313. van Gijn J, and others: Perimesencephalic hemorrhage: a nonaneurysmal and benign form of subarachnoid hemorrhage, Neurology 35:493-497, 1985.
314. Van Broeckhoven C, and others: Amyloid B-protein precursor gene and hereditary cerebral hemorrhage with amyloidosis (Dutch), Science 248:1120, 1990.
315. Van Der Woude FJ, and others: Autoantibodies against neutrophils and monocytes: tool for diagnosis and marker of disease activity in Wegener's granulomatosis, Lancet 1:425, 1985.
316. Vermeulen M: Subarachnoid haemorrhage: diagnosis and treatment, J Neurol 243:496-501, 1996.
317. Vinters HV, and Gilbert JJ: Cerebral amyloid angiopathy: incidence and complications in the aging brain. II. The distribution of amyloid vascular changes, Stroke 14:924-928, 1983.
318. Vinters HV: Cerebral amyloid angiopathy: a critical review, Stroke 18:311, 1987.
319. Vogt C, and Vogt O: Erkrankungen der Grosshirnrinde im Lichte der Topistik, Pathoklise und Pathoarchitektonik, J Psychol Neurol 28:1, 1922.
320. Volpe JJ: Current concepts of brain injury in the premature infant, Am J Roentgenol 153:243-251, 1989.
321. Volpe JJ: Intraventricular hemorrhage and brain injury in the premature infant, Clin Perinatol 16:361, 1989.
322. Vomberg PP, and others: Cerebral thromboembolism due to antithrombin III deficiency in two children, Neuropediatrics 18:42, 1987.
323. von Kummer R, and others: Sensitivity and prognostic value of early CT in occlusion of the middle cerebral artery trunk, AJNR 15:9-15, 1994.
324. Vonsattel JP, and others: Cerebral amyloid angiopathy without and with cerebral hemorrhages: a comparative histological study, Ann Neurol 30:637, 1991.
325. Voorhies RM, and Fraser RAR: Cerebral air embolism occurring at angiography and diagnosed by computerized tomography, J Neurosurg 60:177, 1984.
326. Walsh TJ, Hier DB, and Caplan LR: Aspergillosis of the central nervous system: clinicopathological analysis of 17 patients, Ann Neurol 18:574, 1985.
327. Webb FWS, Hickman JA, and Brew DSJ: Death from vertebral artery thrombosis in rheumatoid arthritis, Br Med J 2:537, 1968.
328. Weibers DO: Ischemic cerebrovascular complications of pregnancy, Arch Neurol 42:1106, 1985.
329. Weinblatt ME, and Fienberg R: Case records of the Massachusetts General Hospital (Case 18-1987), N Engl J Med 316:1139, 1987.
330. Willinsky RA, and others: Multiple cerebral arteriovenous malformations (AVMs): review of our experience from 203 patients with cerebral vascular lesions, Neuroradiology 32: 207, 1990.
331. Wolf PA: Epidemiology of intracerebral hemorrhage. In Kas CS, and Caplan LR, editor: Intracerebral hemorrhage. Boston, 1994, Butterworth-Heinemann.
332. Wyburn-Mason R: The vascular abnormalities and tumors of the spinal cord and its membranes, London, 1943, Kimpton.
333. Yamamoto T, Beppu H, and Tsubaki T: Mitochondrial encephalomyopathy: fluctuating symptoms on CT, Neurology 34: 1456, 1984.
334. Yang DC, Sohn D, and Anand HK: Thrombosis of the superior longitudinal sinus during infancy, J Pediatr 74:570, 1969.
335. Yankner BA, and others: Cerebral granulomatous angiitis associated with isolation of human T-lymphotropic virus type III from the central nervous system, Ann Neurol 20:362, 1986.
336. Yonas H, and others: Dissecting intracranial aneurysms, Surg Neurol 8:407, 1977.
337. Yonekawa Y, Goto Y, and Ogata N: Moyamoya disease: diagnosis, treatment, and recent achievement. In: Barnett HJM, and others, editors: Stroke, pathophysiology, diagnosis, and management, ed 2, New York, 1992, Churchill-Livingstone.
338. Yu YJ, and others: Cerebral angiitis and intracerebral hemorrhage associated with amphetamine abuse, J Neurosurg 58: 108, 1983.
339. Zegler B, and others: Life history of cutaneous vascular lesions in Sneddon's syndrome, Hum Pathol 23:668-675, 1992.
340. Zimmerman RS, and others: Cavernous malformations of the brain stem, J Neurosurg 75:32, 1991.

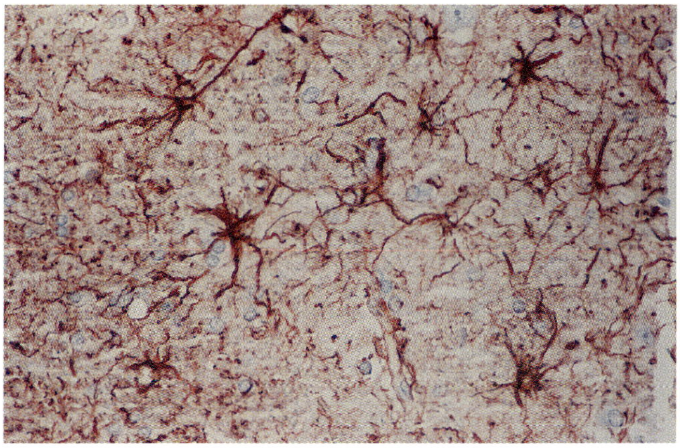

**Plate 2A.** Reactive astrocytes in a multiple sclerosis plaque are immunoreactive for GFA protein.

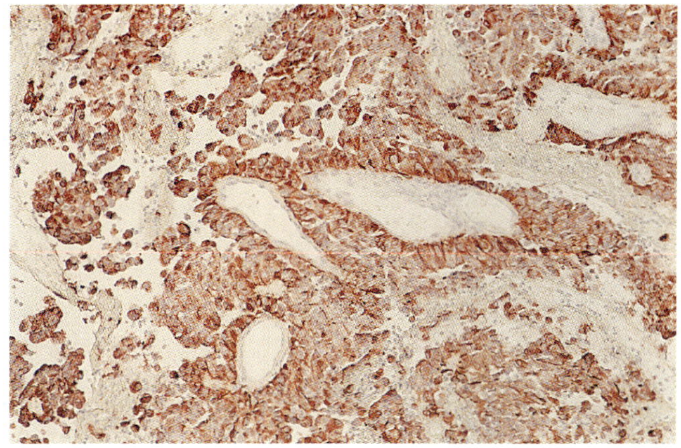

**Plate 2D.** Many GFA-positive cells are present in this glioblastoma.

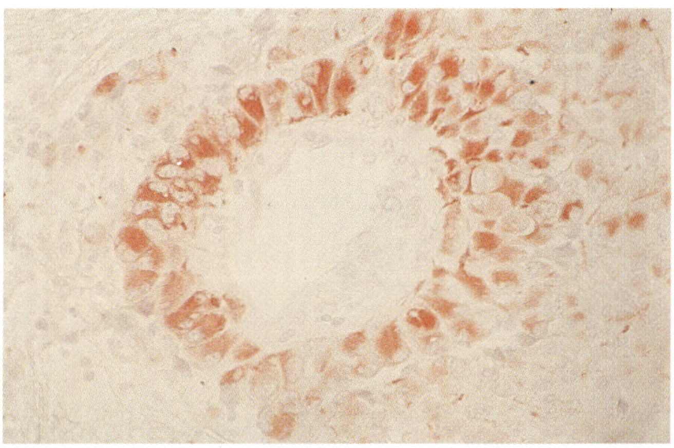

**Plate 2B.** Astroblastoma rosettes immunoreactive for GFA protein.

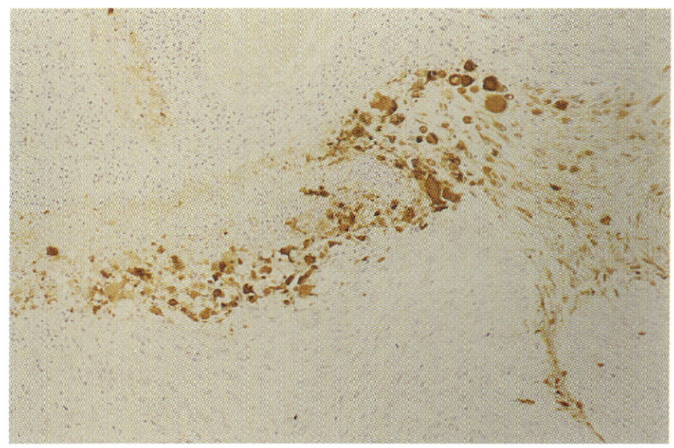

**Plate 2E.** GFA-positive neoplastic astrocytes contrast with negative stain fibrosarcoma elements in this gliosarcoma.

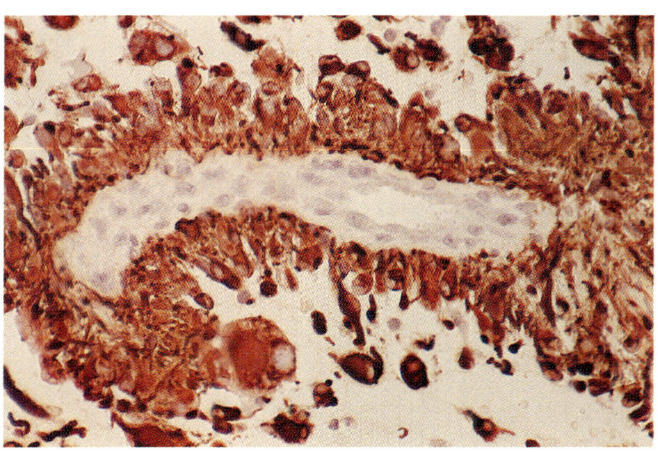

**Plate 2C.** Giant cell glioblastoma cells immunopositive for GFA protein.

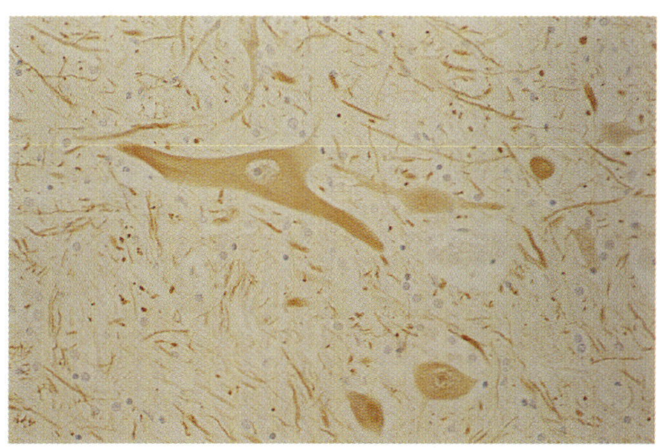

**Plate 2F.** Normal neurons and cell processes of the spinal cord show immunoreactivity for class III $\beta$-tubulin.

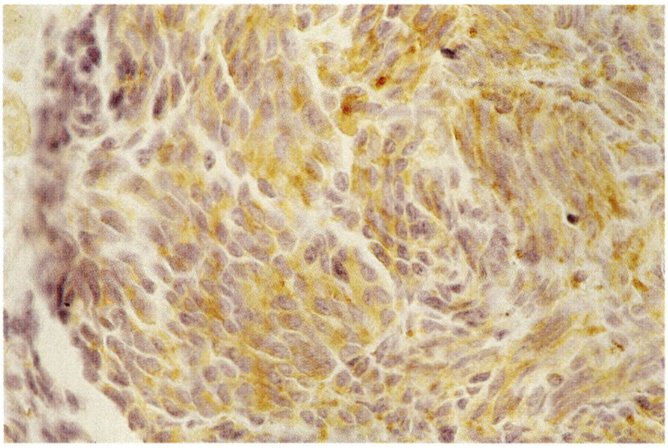

**Plate 3A.** Staining for class III beta-tubulin in delicate cell processes of a pineocytoma.

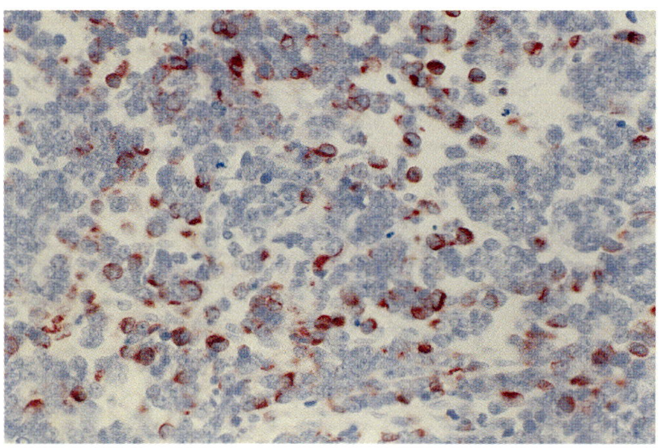

**Plate 3B.** Some of the primitive neoplastic cells in medulloepithelioma are positive for class III $\beta$-tubulin.

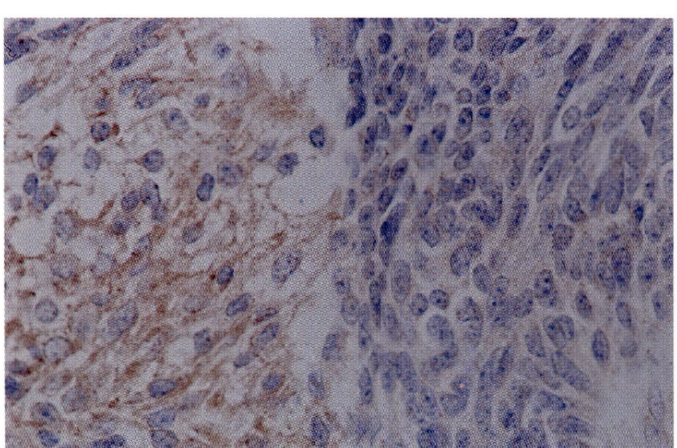

**Plate 3C.** MAP-2 positive cells and processes in neuroblastoma.

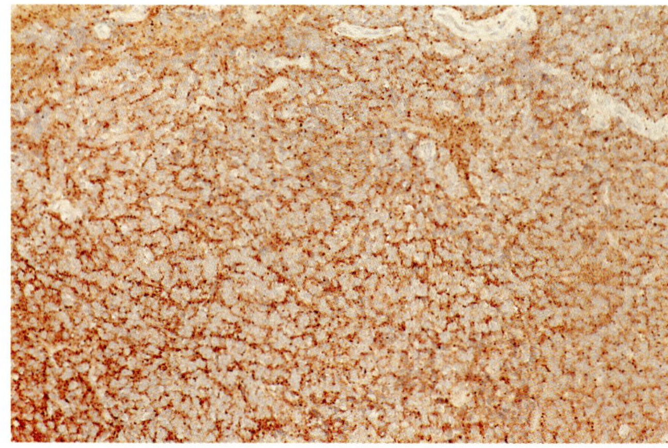

**Plate 3D.** Strong positivity for synaptophysin in central neurocytoma.

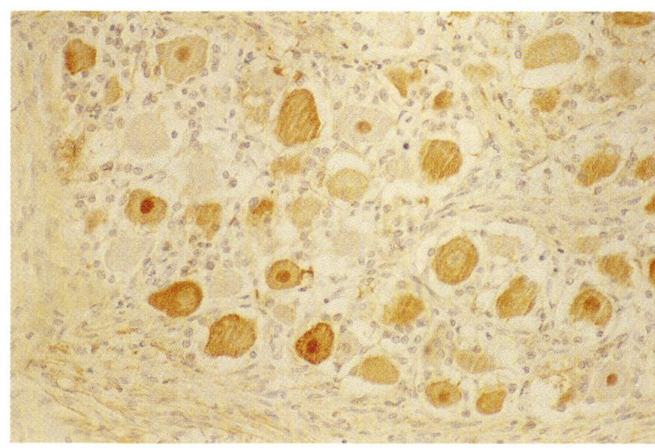

**Plate 3E.** Normal neurons from a dorsal root ganglion are positive for neuron-specific enolase.

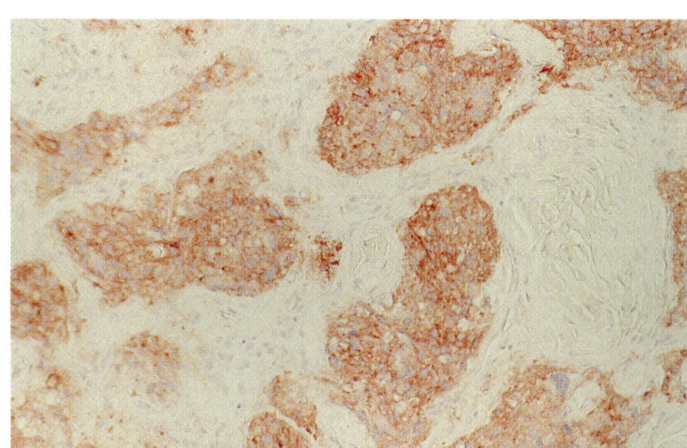

**Plate 3F.** Positive staining for neuron-specific enolase in tympanic paraganglioma.

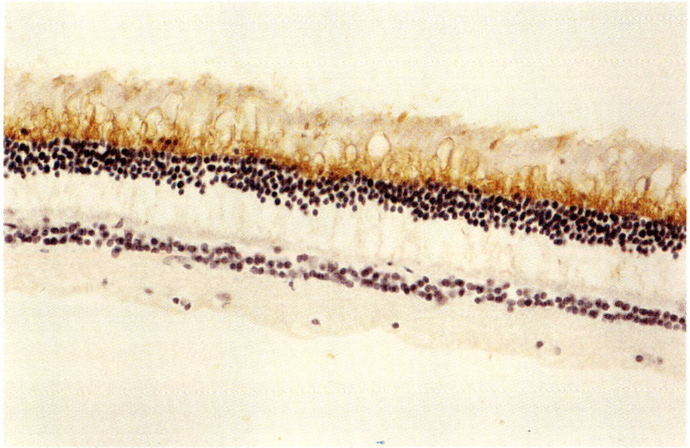

**Plate 4A.** S-retinal antigen staining of normal retina.

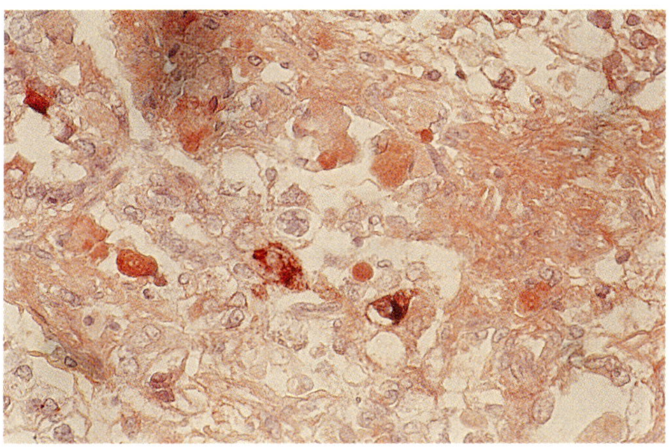

**Plate 4B.** Cytokeratin-positive cells in metastatic bronchogenic adenocarcinoma.

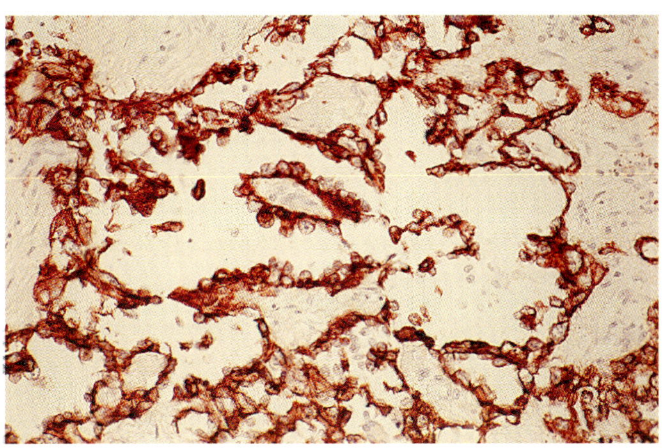

**Plate 4C.** The cells of primary embryonal cell carcinoma of the CNS show strong immunoreactivity for cytokeratins.

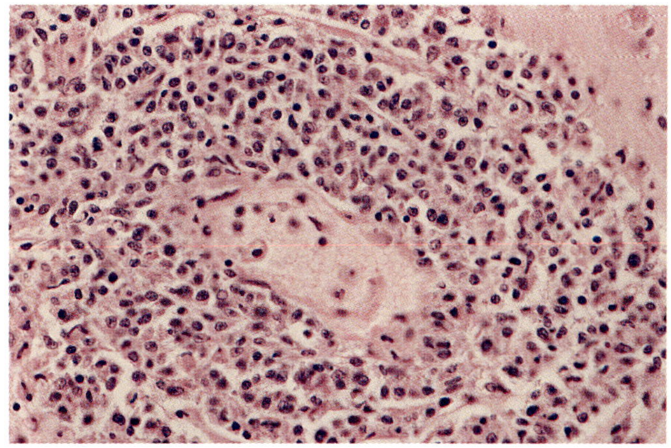

**Plate 4D.** Characteristic infiltration of blood vessel walls by neoplastic lymphocytes in primary CNS lymphoma. (H & E.)

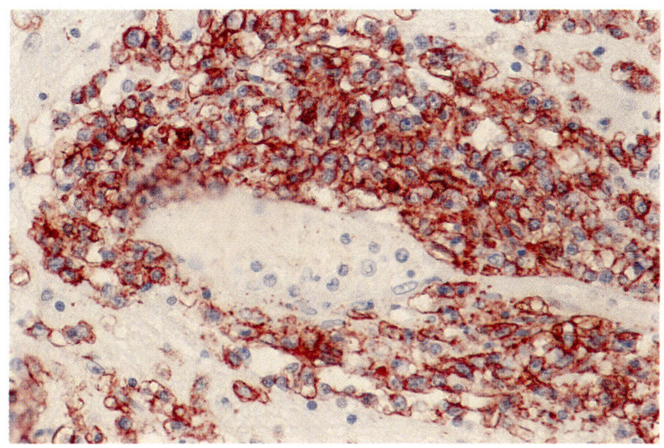

**Plate 4E.** Neoplastic lymphocytes immunoreactive for leukocyte common antigen in primary CNS lymphoma.

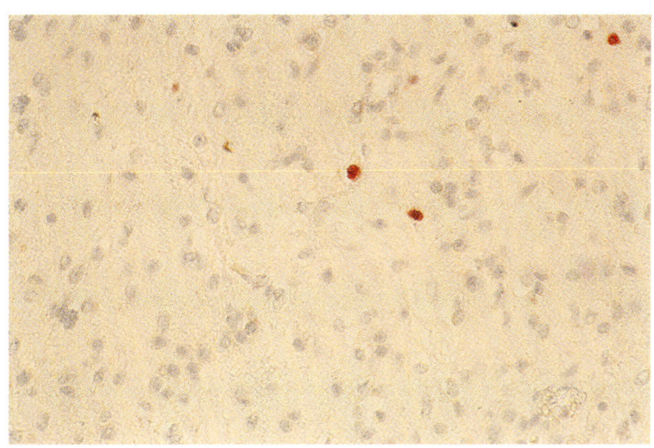

**Plate 4F.** Few cells of this well-differentiated astrocytoma show nuclear positivity for Ki-67 antigen (MIB-1 monoclonal antibody in paraffin sections).

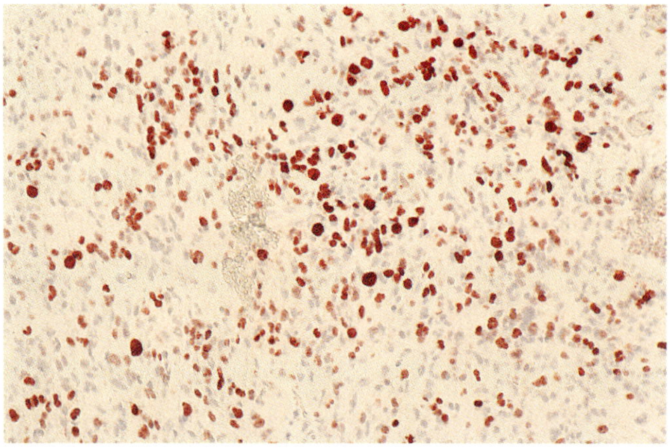

**Plate 5A.** Many glioblastoma cells show nuclear staining for Ki-67 (monoclonal antibody MIB 1 in paraffin sections).

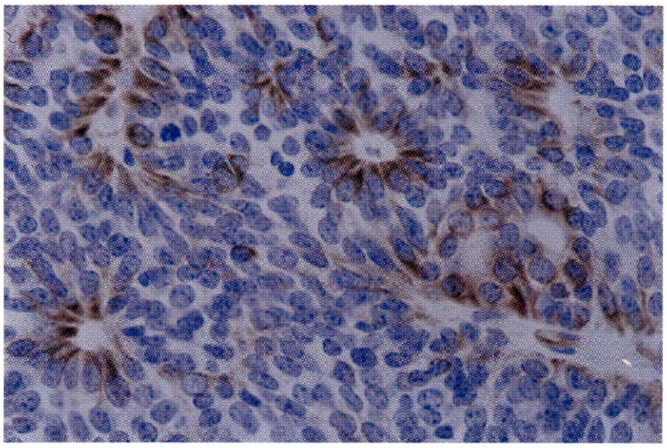

**Plate 5B.** Epithelial membrane antigen positivity is seen near the luminal surface of the rosettes of an ependymoma.

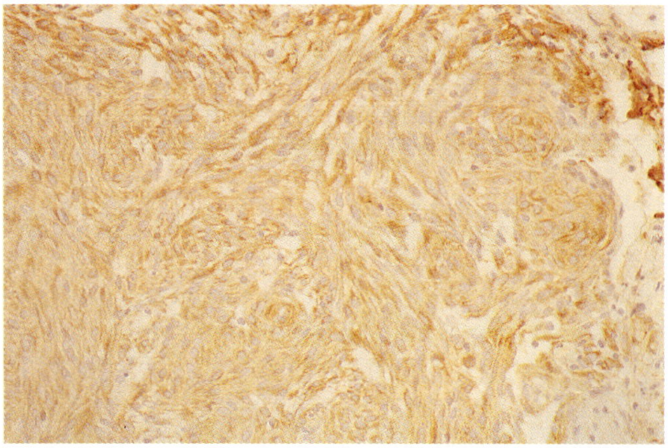

**Plate 5C.** Meningioma cells display immunopositivity for vimentin.

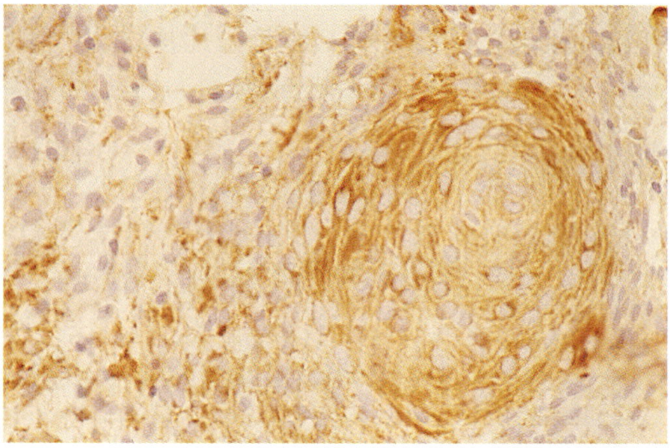

**Plate 5D.** Same case of meningioma as Plate 5C stained for epithelial membrane antigen. Positivity for vimentin and EMA is characteristic of many meningiomas.

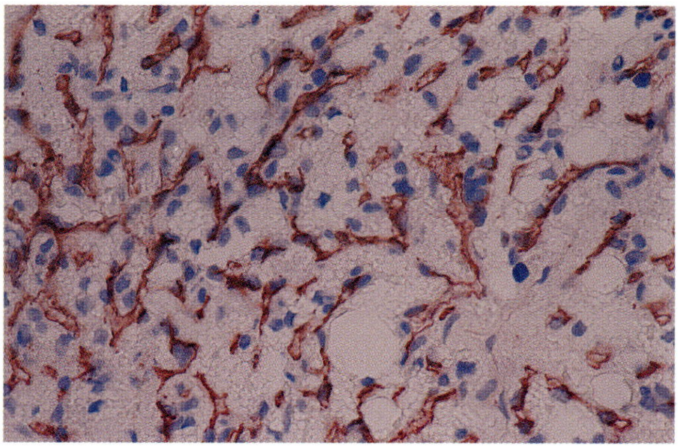

**Plate 5E.** CD34 antigen immunostain in cerebellar hemangioblastoma is positive in endothelial cells, but stromal cells are negative.

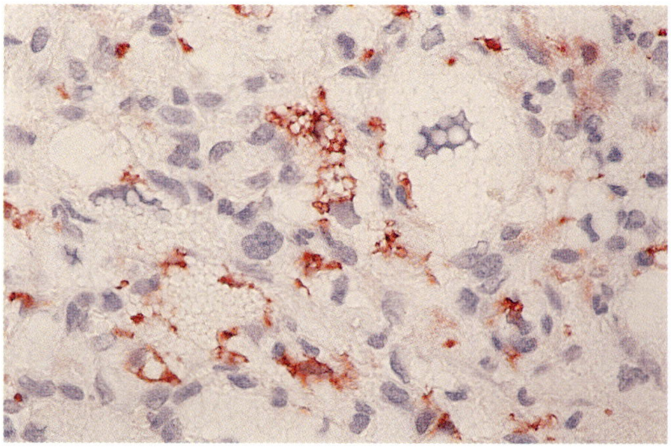

**Plate 5F.** Small stromal cells immunopositive for factor XIIIa in cerebellar hemangioblastoma.

C • H • A • P • T • E • R

# 7

# *Bacterial, Fungal, Protozoal, and Parasitic Infections*

**Ana Lia Taratuto**



Infectious diseases of the central nervous system (CNS) have long been recognized by neuropathologists, and the etiologic agents of these diseases have been identified on morphologic grounds by both light and electron microscopy, as well as by immunocytochemical means within the context of their histopathologic features. Microbiologic, parasitologic, or virologic studies, together with serologic assays, are commonly expected to aid in the diagnosis, especially when unfixed tissues are available. However, the diagnosis of these infections has become more challenging since the adoption of immunosuppressive therapy for organ transplantation and malignant neoplasms, as well as the increasing prevalence of the acquired immunodeficiency syndrome (AIDS).[135] Immunosuppression may modify host responses to infectious agents, rendering serology and morphology inadequate for diagnosis. Furthermore, the incidence of diseases classically related to poverty, malnutrition, or social backwardness has increased, even in industrialized countries, as a result of migrations, contaminated blood transfusions, and intravenous drug abuse. Brain biopsy by stereotaxic methods makes it necessary to deal efficiently with small tissue samples in order to reach a prompt diagnosis. Final diagnosis of infections of the brain is seldom obtained from cultures or other bacteriologic, parasitologic, or virologic routine techniques alone; therefore, adequate samples should be obtained during surgery for morphologic and complementary studies such as immunohistochemistry, in situ hybridization, and polymerase chain reaction (PCR). In the immunocompromised host, infection may manifest as a tumor with focal neurologic deficits accompanied at neuroimaging by a clearly localized lesion. Thus, certain mycotic and protozoan diseases may be diagnosed during surgery, particularly in smears, and such diagnosis on occasion may provide indirect evidence of immunosuppression.

Immunohistochemistry has greatly contributed to the routine diagnosis of infectious diseases, largely because most immunochemical methods can be applied to formaldehyde-fixed, paraffin-embedded samples and even to smears. Many commercially available polyclonal or monoclonal antibodies, within a given neuropathologic context and with adequate controls, may help confirm a diagnosis.

Both monoclonal (Mab) or polyclonal antibodies (Pab) can be used in formalin-fixed paraffin-embedded tissue. A recent review[26] listed many antibodies used in the diagnosis of infectious agents including some of those mentioned in this chapter, that is, *Listeria monocytogenes*, Mycobacteria spp, *Borrelia burgdorferi, Treponema pallidum,* Aspergillus spp, Candida spp, *Coccidioides immitis, Cryptococcus neoformans,* and *Entamoeba histolytica*. Other antibodies not commercially available also have been used with excellent results to confirm the diagnosis of infections by Amebae spp[165,166] and *Trypanosoma cruzi*.[124,155]

Moreover, molecular techniques including the PCR, in situ hybridization, sequence analysis, and immunoblotting have shortened the time required for identification of such infectious agents as *Mycobacterium tuberculosis* and *Toxoplasma gondii* from several weeks to 2 days.[126] PCR in situ has shown great promise in the diagnosis of infectious diseases.[109]

Bacterial pathogens detected by nucleic acid amplification include *Mycobacterium tuberculosis, M. leprae, M. avium intracellulare, Borrelia burgdorferi, Treponema pallidum, Escherichia coli, Rickettsia* spp. *Staphylococcus aureus,* Whipple's disease-associated bacterium, *Listeria monocytogenes, Neisseria meningitides* and *Haemophilus influenzae,* among others.[122] Recently, in an extensive review, J Weiss[172] listed parasitic infections detectable by DNA probes and PCR. These parasitic infections include *Plasmodium falciparum, P. vivax, Leishmania* spp., *Trypanosoma cruzi, T. brucei rhodesiense* and *gambiense, Toxoplasma gondii, Entamoeba histolytica, Naegleria fowleri, Schistosoma* spp., *Trichinella spiralis,* and *Echinococcus.* All of these parasitic infections are mentioned in this chapter.

An exhaustive review of diseases produced by each of the known infectious agents is beyond the scope of this chapter, and pertinent data may be readily found in bacteriology, parasitology, mycology, and neuropathology textbooks. Here I focus on the more prevalent entities, particularly those arising in immunosuppressed patients, in whom marked changes in the natural course of disease are common.

## BACTERIAL INFECTIONS

The main route of bacterial entry to the CNS is by hematogenous dissemination, either arterial or venous. On occasion microorganisms reach the brain by retrograde flow from the scalp and face or, alternatively, by direct entry through bone defects, open wounds, or surgical interventions. Shunting for hydrocephalus likewise may provide a portal of entry. Direct extension from neighboring infections such as facial sinusitis is not infrequent. Dural venous sinuses, the choroid plexus, and the cribriform plate are all sites from which microorganisms may reach the brain. The most frequent worldwide bacterial infections of the CNS among immunocompetent hosts are due to *Neisseria meningitides, Haemophilus influenzae* type B, *Streptococcus pneumoniae,* and, to a lesser extent, *Staphylococcus aureus,* Staphylococcus spp, *Pseudomonas aeruginosa,* and Enterobacteriaceae. *Listeria monocytogenes, Streptococcus agalactiae,* and *Escherichia coli* are bacteria that commonly infect the CNS of immunocompromised hosts. Gram-negative bacilli as well as Chlamydia spp and Rickettsiaceae, among others, may also infect the CNS, although these diseases are much less frequent than those mentioned above.

### Meningitis

Meningeal inflammations secondary to bacterial infections may involve separately either the dura mater or leptomeninges. The dura mater offers considerable resistance to bacterial penetration; thus, most infections remain localized to either surface of the dura. Epidural infections are spinal and focal; intracranial epidural infection is uncommon except in cases of penetrating wounds to the head. *Staphylococcus aureus* is the most frequent cause of epidural infection; often this event follows the infection of a vertebral body or a paranasal sinus. *Mycobacterium tuberculosis,* although uncommon, also may be the etiologic agent of spinal epidural infections.[74] Intracranial subdural empyemas are complications of penetrating injuries, the extension of purulent meningitis, or the result of neurosurgical procedures. *Staphylococcus aureus* and Streptococcus spp are the most frequent causes of these infections.

Leptomeningitis is an infection localized to the subarachnoid space that may extend to the brain paren-

A 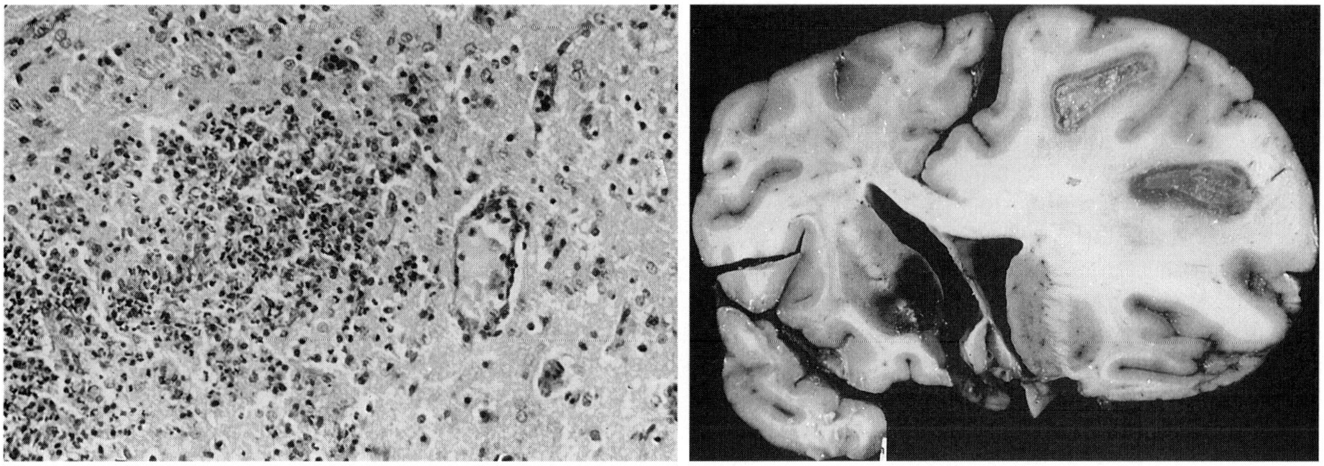 B

**Fig. 7-1.** **A**, Focal parenchymal infiltration by neutrophils in acute leptomeningitis caused by *Streptococcus pneumoniae*. **B**, Coronal section of cerebrum showing two well-demarcated abscesses, both of which are filled with pus. Swelling and cingulate herniation are visible. Recent ischemic infarction is visible on the opposite hemisphere. (**A**, H&E.) (Courtesy of Dr. L. Rorke.)

chyma (Fig. 7-1, *A*). Common manifestations include fever, malaise, headache, neck stiffness, photophobia, and impaired consciousness. CSF may be purulent, with increased protein level and decreased glucose content; bacteria may be visible on smears. Changes in CSF profile are influenced by the stage of the disease and by the nature of the treatment. The acute purulent stage is reflected in diffuse exudate accumulation in the sulci and basal cisterns; this is commonly associated with ventriculitis and choroid plexitis. The chronic or partially treated stages are reflected in mostly basal exudates. Cranial and spinal nerves may be involved in the infection. In the acute stage, polymorphonuclear leukocytes are visible in the subarachnoid and perivascular Virchow-Robin spaces. Blood vessels traversing exudate show cellular inflammation that may be complicated by thrombosis and parenchymal infarcts. Brain edema, neuronal injury, and microglial hyperplasia are constant features of leptomeningitis; slight hyperplasia of subpial astrocytes also may occur. After several days or weeks, in addition to neutrophils, mononuclear cells, lymphocytes, and plasmacytes appear in the infiltrates; further chronicity is characterized by formation of granulation tissue and fibroblastic proliferation. Meningeal fibrosis leads to obliteration of the subarachnoid space and consequent hydrocephalus. Vascular inflammation and thrombosis leading to ischemic brain lesions are typical complications of chronic leptomeningitis.

The inflammatory response by the host and the spread of the infectious process are influenced by several factors. Encapsulated bacteria, including those more frequently infecting CNS, resist opsonization as well as complement lysis, explaining the greater prevalence of meningitis in childhood, when opsonophagocytosis is decreased compared with the adult. Although the CSF is poorly endowed with defense factors, a wide spectrum of substances that modulate inflammatory response are released following bacterial invasion. Bacterial peptides and lipopolysaccharides stimulate chemotaxis of polymorphonuclear neutrophils (PMN) and enhance their activation as well as their adhesion to endothelium.[9,141] Tumor necrosis factor (TNF) secreted by macrophages among other substances[49,54] promotes endothelial adhesion of PMN; leukocyte adhesion glycoproteins also play a major role in leukocyte activation.[9] Macrophages derived from microglia and from blood monocytes may be activated by $\gamma$ interferon produced by natural killer T cells.[107] In turn, interleukin 1 (IL-1) produced by activated macrophages acts as a T cell mitogen, initiating and maintaining local and systemic inflammatory reaction, while TNF released by macrophages may exacerbate the clinical symptoms and accelerate the course of the disease.[82,167]

*Haemophilus influenzae* is the most common infectious agent in all ages, whereas *Streptococcus pneumoniae* predominates among infections in adults.[133] Mortality rate is high for neonatal meningitis, a disease commonly due to infections with group B streptococci and *Escherichia coli*. Strains having K1 capsular antigen, a polysaccharide that contributes to its invasiveness,[149] frequently affect neonates, premature infants, and children with meningomyelocele. *Listeria monocytogenes* also causes leptomeningitis in newborns, and the infection frequently is transmitted through the maternal genital tract, resulting in acute meningitis. Transplacental infections lead to widespread dissemination of the organism. Myocarditis and hepatosplenomegaly are seen as well as meningoencephalitis with microabscess formation. Microorganisms can be demonstrated in tissues by staining with the Gram method or by Warthin-Starry silver impregnations. *Haemophilus influenzae* type B, *Neisseria meningitides*, and *Streptococcus pneumoniae* cause leptomeningitis in infancy and early childhood when there is a transition from passive immunity from maternal antibodies to active immunity; this occurs from 4 months to 3 years of age. *N. meningitides* also affects young adults, and *S. pneumoniae* causes meningitis in the elderly or when predisposing risk factors affect the host. Obstructive hydrocephalus secondary to ventriculitis and obliteration of the subarachnoid space as well as encephalomalacia are sequelae of these infections in almost half of survivors.[15,45,81,121]

### Abscesses

Bacterial brain abscesses are infections that may spread from neighboring infected foci; brain parenchymal infections also can reflect hematogenous spread secondary to thromboembolism (infected endocarditis), or the infection may be the consequence of penetrating wounds. The paravertebral venous plexus lacks valves and allows bidirectional flow that may contribute to the entry into the CNS of microorganisms lodged at distant sites. Brain abscesses may be located in frontal, parietal, or temporal white matter; more frequently they occur at the gray-white junction (Fig. 7-1, *B*). Such posterior fossa contents as the cerebellum are less frequent sites of abscess formation.[39]

Clinical findings in brain abscesses can resemble those secondary to any other mass; neuroimaging is useful to diagnose and evaluate the abscess development. An abscess consists of a necrotic core where acute cerebritis with neutrophilic infiltration develops initially; within a few days the necrosis becomes liquefactive and purulent. Lymphocytes, plasmacytes, and macrophages invade the lesion in the ensuing days. At the end of the first week, microvessels proliferate at the periphery of the purulent site; this is accompanied by fibroblast proliferation and increased reactivity of astrocytes. A capsule then surrounds the abscess, and brain edema becomes apparent near the capsule. Both aerobic and anaerobic bacteria can cause brain abscesses; streptococci and staphylococci are the most frequent causes of brain abscesses, and in patients with open wounds staphylococcal infections are common. In addition to suppurative meningitis, *Listeria monocytogenes* may cause cerebritis and brain abscesses, as is well documented in patients with chronic leukemia, in recipients of renal transplants or immunosuppressive chemotherapy, and in patients with such chronic diseases as diabetes mellitus, cirrhosis, and ulcerative colitis. More recently Listeria infections have occurred among victims of AIDS.[66,82] Commercially available polyclonal antibodies that react with the antigen on histologically processed tissue are available for the diagnosis of *L. monocytogenes*.[26]

### Mycobacterial Infections

**Tuberculosis.** *M. tuberculosis*, an acid fast bacillus with worldwide distribution, still poses a major health hazard as a cause of childhood meningitis, especially in developing countries, where the disease is associated with poverty and malnutrition. In developed countries, the frequency of tuberculous infections has increased as a result of migrations and increasing AIDS prevalence. Signs and symptoms of tuberculous infections in AIDS patients may not be recognized easily. Infection with *M. tuberculosis* is acquired by droplet inhalation.

Primary tuberculosis occurs in individuals with no previous contact with tubercle bacilli. Bacilli proteins are responsible for tissue hypersensitivity, and this is responsible for a positive tuberculin skin test; almost one half of the patients with tuberculous meningitis have positive skin tests. Two to four weeks after the initial infection, delayed hypersensitivity to the tubercle bacillus develops. At this time, intradermal injection of purified protein derivative of *M. tuberculosis* (Mantoux reaction) to sensitized individuals will result in local induration greater than 5 mm, which indicates sensitivity but not active disease. After sensitization, the inflammatory response becomes granulomatous. The lesion contains epithelioid and giant Langhans' cells surrounded by lymphocytes and exhibits central caseous necrosis. At the same time an increase in resistance develops. The specific granulomatous lesion in the lung parenchyma subjacent to pleura frequently involves the lower part of one of the upper lobes; this lesion and the accompanying regional enlarged lymph nodes make up the primary Ghon complex. At this stage the infection is usually asymptomatic. It may either resolve spontaneously and become a calcified residual nodule, or the lesion may enlarge, become cavitated, and erode the bronchial wall and vessels. The infection may then disseminate through the bloodstream, causing a systemic and frequently fatal miliary tuberculosis that affects all organs.

This disseminated form may also result from secondary tuberculosis, which generally affects the apices of the lungs. "Secondary" is the name given to an active infection in a previously sensitized individual; it reflects either reactivation of dormant lesions or exogenous reinfection. The manifestations of secondary tuberculosis include night sweats, insidious fever, malaise, hemoptysis, and weight loss.

Miliary cortical or leptomeningeal lesions may remain dormant for years and then rupture into the subarachnoid space or the ventricles, infecting the spinal fluid and giving rise to tuberculous meningitis. The infection also may involve the choroid plexus, and the symptoms are similar to those caused by meningitis of other etiologies; these include headache, fever, vomiting, photophobia, and neck stiffness. On occasion immunosuppressed patients, in particular, may have a negative intradermal Mantoux reaction, and neuroimaging may not contribute to the diagnosis in the early stages of the neurologic infection. The characteristic changes in spinal fluid include increased pressure, increased protein concentration, and low glucose content, up to 1.6 mmol/L or even lower. These changes are accompanied by lymphocytic pleocytosis, although in the early stages of the disease neutrophils may predominate and glucose content may be normal. Tubercle bacilli may be difficult to demonstrate in either the spinal fluid or the tissues, and repeated sampling of CSF may be necessary. Guinea pig inoculation of CSF or laboratory cultures can be used to confirm the diagnosis, but either process may require up to 8 weeks for completion. Application of PCR shortens the considerable time required for detection of *M. tuberculosis* in spinal fluid samples.[52,115]

At autopsy, gross examination of the brain shows that the basal leptomeninges covering optochiasmatic and basilar cisterns are thickened, opaque, gelatinous, and greenish (Fig. 7-2, *A*); on the convexity, miliary tubercles may be visible. Obstruction of the CSF circulation commonly causes hydrocephalus, whereas involvement of the vessels by arteritis or endarteritis leads to vascular occlusions, ischemia, and infarcts. These lesions are more frequent in the basal ganglia as a result of the involvement of the perforating vessels by the infection. Histologically there is lymphocytic infiltration in the subarachnoid space that extends to the Virchow-Robin spaces (Fig. 7-2, *B*); typical tubercles feature a granuloma with caseous necrosis surrounded by epithelioid and giant multinucleated Langhans' cells, lymphocytes, and a few plasmacytes. Acid-fast bacilli measuring 1 to 3 $\mu$m may be readily disclosed in the giant cells, in histiocytes, or outside the cells in the necrotic debris by the Ziehl Neelsen staining method although on occasion it may prove troublesome to detect. Meningeal blood vessels may be involved by inflammation or by a secondary obliterative endarteritis. Early diagnosis and prompt treatment with specific antibiotic and chemotherapy may avoid the sequelae.[15,82,128] Tuberculomas are well-circumscribed single or multiple granulomas with a central necrotic area. Tuberculomas resemble neoplasms in their clinical symptoms and at neuroimaging. They may be located in the cerebrum, brainstem, or cerebellum. Tuberculomas are found more frequently in the cerebellum of children than in adults. However, the spinal cord of children are involved rarely. CNS tuberculomas are not uncommon in areas where tuberculosis is prevalent, such as South America and India. Brain tuberculomas and cysticercosis are frequent histological findings associated with epilepsy in India.[146]

**Mycobacterium avium-intracellulare.** *Mycobacterium avium-intracellulare* (MAI) is present in soil, water, dust, and animals; the organism infects humans through the respiratory or gastrointestinal tract.

In AIDS patients MAI is the most frequent opportunistic bacterial infection that can cause disseminated disease and CNS lesions, characterized by meningitis and encephalitis. The incidence of neurologic involvement is low (1.5% to 2%). In the brain the lesions may be confluent, appearing as a granuloma or an abscess visible on CT as a ring enhancing lesion. Disseminated disease is frequent among patients in whom CD4+ T lymphocyte count is below 100 per mm$^3$; in contrast,

A

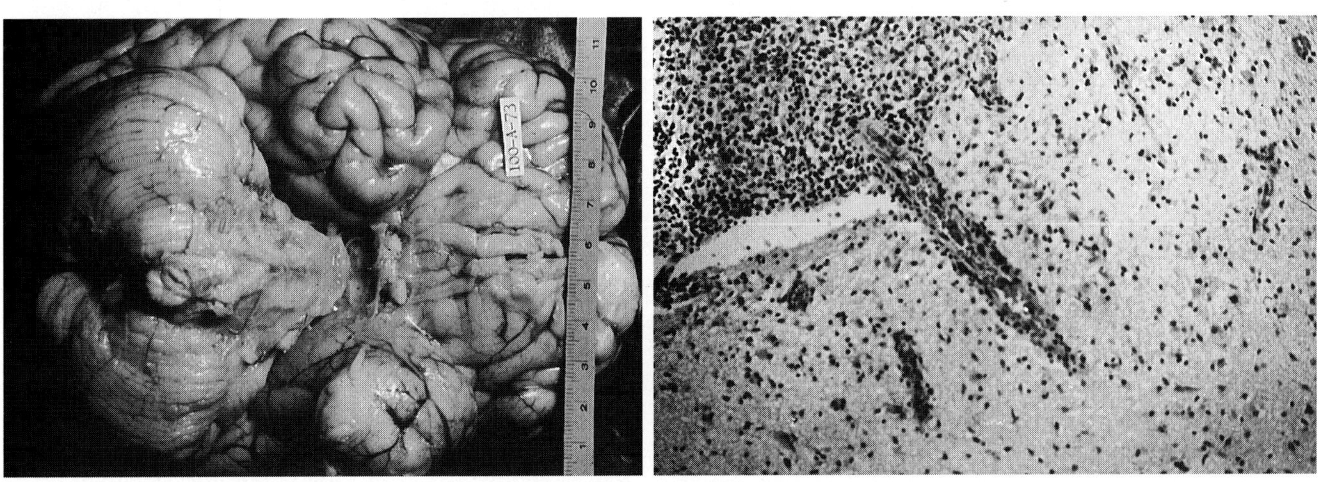

B

**Fig. 7-2. A,** Thickened, whitish, gelatinous exudate is visible in the basilar leptomeninges in a case of tuberculous leptomeningitis. **B,** Lymphocytic infiltration in the subarachnoid and Virchow-Robin spaces. Tuberculous leptomeningitis. (H&E.)

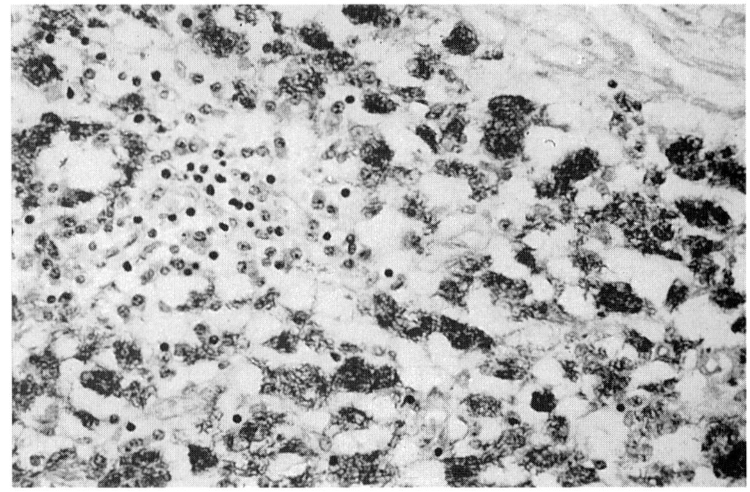

**Fig. 7-3.** *Mycobacterium avium intracellulare* are visible inside macrophages; brain biopsy from an AIDS patient. (Ziehl-Neelsen.)

focal infection is associated with zidovudine treatment (AZT) and higher CD4+ T counts.

At biopsy or autopsy, the leptomeningeal and brain perivascular infiltration of large pale histiocytes laden with acid-fast bacilli can be enhanced by Ziehl-Neelsen, Fite-Faracco, or Kinyoun stains (Fig. 7-3). These lesions are present mainly in areas where the blood-brain barrier is disrupted. Epithelioid or Langhans' cells are not frequent components of the lesion; localized fibrosis also is infrequent.*

**Leprosy.** Leprosy is a chronic infectious disease caused by an obligate intracellular parasite, *Mycobacterium leprae*. Although most leprosy patients live in the tropics, endemic foci exist all over the world, and nearly 11 million people are infected by this bacillus. Infection spreads by direct mucous or cutaneous contact. Patients with the lepromatous form of the disease shed abundant bacilli from the lesions, but patients with the other variants are contagious only during the reactive stage. There is a natural resistance to infection with *M. leprae*, and incubation periods range from 3 to 5 years. Following immunosuppression by thymectomy or total body irradiation, experimental infections have led to disseminated disease.[20]

The main clinical forms are *lepromatous*, characterized by minimal cell resistance to bacilli and extensive multiplication within macrophages, and *tuberculoid*, representing the opposite extreme. In the latter variety there is pronounced cellular immunity and tuberculoid reaction with abundant epithelioid cells and few bacilli. There is an *intermediate* or borderline, dimorphous form; an *indeterminate* form is the term reserved for early cases not yet susceptible to classification.

Lepromatous leprosy is characterized by erythematous or hypopigmented macular or infiltrated skin lesions that appear predominantly on the cooler parts of the body; the skin lesion is accompanied by extensive involvement of lymph nodes and many organs. Early lesions of tuberculoid leprosy are sharply defined, and during the healing process show a tendency to repigmentate in central areas. The Mitsuda lepromin test, a very useful prognostic tool, consists of an intradermal injection of heat-killed bacilli. The test is negative in the lepromatous form and positive in patients with the tuberculoid form, even within 24 to 48 hours when positive patients show an erythematous reaction similar to the tuberculin test (called the Fernandez Mitsuda test).

At this time neural involvement is restricted to the peripheral nerves. In fact peripheral nerve enlargement, especially ulnar, is observed in almost all forms of leprosy. In a biopsy of peripheral nerve, bacilli may be visible with Ziehl-Neelsen or Fite-Faracco stain within macrophages and Schwann cells (Fig. 7-4), preferentially in unmyelinated fibers. The perineurium invariably is involved by leprosy bacilli. Cellular inflammation may be profuse and eventually may lead to complete axonal loss and nerve destruction, with severe sensory disturbance as well as mutilation. In tuberculoid leprosy granulomas with epithelioid, Langhans' giant cells and occasionally caseous abscesses may destroy the nerve in spite of the scarcity of bacilli. *Mycobacterium leprae*, although present within circulating mononuclear cells, does not invade the CNS.

### Whipple Disease

Whipple disease is a rare infectious disease caused by *Tropheryma whippelii*, a rodshaped, Gram-positive, argyrophilic bacilliform bacterium that is intensely PAS positive and diastase resistant; the bacillus measures 1.5 $\mu$m in length and can be observed within macrophages in the lamina propia of the small bowel. Ultrastructurally, degenerating bacilli as well as fibrillar material may be visible within phagosomes.[4,143]

Patient age ranges from 40 to 70 years, and men

* Refs. 18, 48, 57, 58, 59, 101, 137, 164.

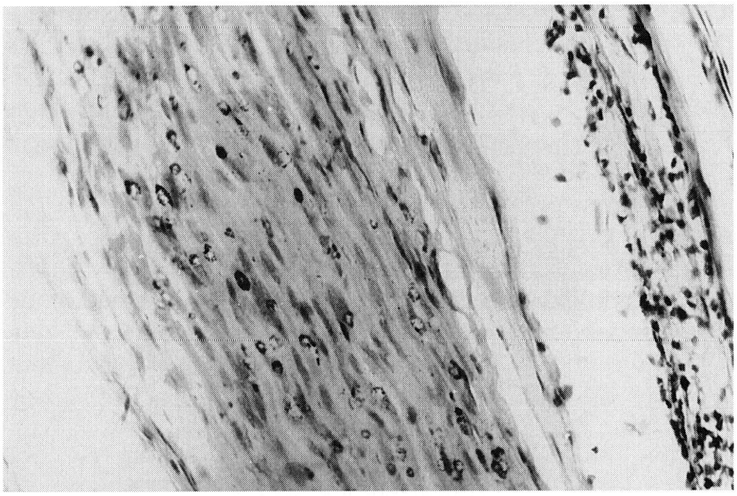

**Fig. 7-4.** *Mycobacterium leprae* are visible in macrophages and Schwann cells; there is inflammatory infiltration of the epineurium. Nerve biopsy. (Ziehl-Neelsen.)

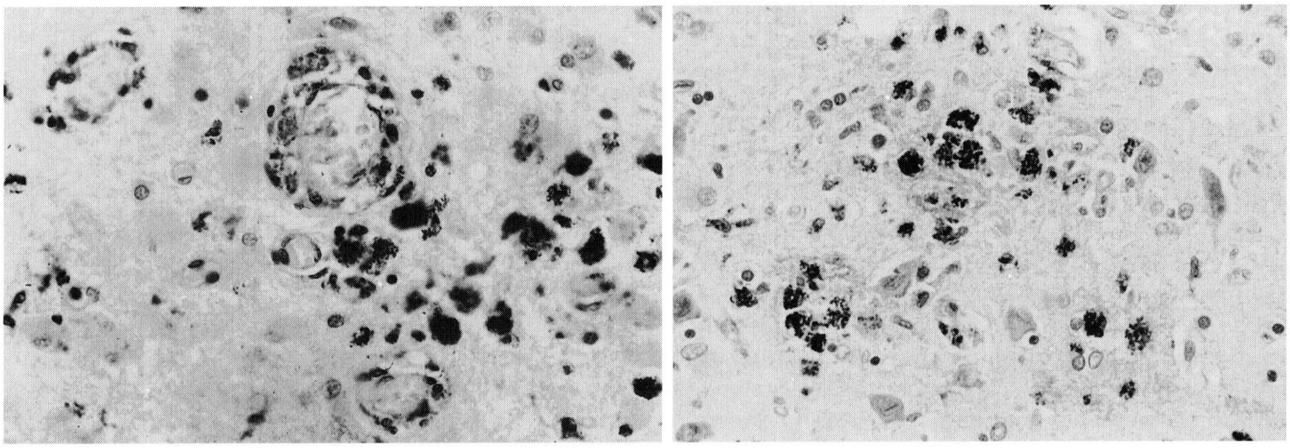


**Fig. 7-5. A, B,** Macrophages contain characteristic organisms in a brain biopsy from a patient with Whipple disease. (PAS.)

outnumber women. This infection affects mainly the small bowel, featuring cellular inflammation and foamy macrophages in the intestinal mucosa. This is accompanied by steatorrhea, malabsorption, and systemic compromise, including lymphadenopathy, endocarditis, polyserositis, and polyarthralgia. CNS involvement occurs in less than 10% of the cases, but may develop in the absence of intestinal disease.* The mechanism of dissemination of bacilli is still unclear, although intracellular forms may be seen within circulating neutrophils. Disseminated Whipple disease has been described in AIDS patients.[12]

Dementia, ophthalmoplegia, and myoclonus are the most characteristic clinical features of Whipple disease of the brain. The symptoms are attributed to involvement of cortical gray matter as well as the brainstem; in a few cases predominant neuroophthalmic manifestations have been reported.[46] Hypothalamic involvement may be responsible for polydipsia, hyponatremia, and thermodysregulation[24]; ataxia is attributable to cerebellar involvement. Extrapyramidal signs may be present in some patients, necessitating differential diagnosis with other dementias such as Creutzfeldt-Jakob disease. CSF cytology occasionally may be diagnostic, but CSF analysis may be normal in spite of granular ependymitis.

Magnetic resonance imaging (MRI) evaluations report abnormal high-signal intensity in the area about the hypothalamus, uncus, and medial temporal lobes; these changes together with appropriate clinical signs may suggest the diagnosis of Whipple disease.[4] The main lesion is a granulomatous polioencephalitis with cerebral gray matter involvement and predominating in the temporal lobes, hippocampi, and amygdaloid nuclei, hypothalamus, basal ganglia, brainstem, and cerebellum.

Microglial nodules and macrophages laden with intensely PAS-positive and silver methenamine-positive

* Refs. 4, 61, 83, 87, 132, 136.

bacilliform bacteria (Fig. 7-5, *A* and *B*) in a perivascular distribution, together with lymphocytes, occasional multinucleated giant cells, and reactive astrocytes with leptomeningeal involvement, are present in most of the lesions. Intraneuronal and free organisms also may be observed. Granular ependymitis may lead to the development of hydrocephalus, and granulomatous inflammation of arterioles may be accompanied by small infarcts.[77,125] A relatively good response occurs after treatment with appropriate antibiotics and a bactericidal combination of trimethoprim plus sulfamethoxazole. These drugs penetrate the blood-brain barrier; consequently, prompt diagnosis by brain biopsy is indicated in all cases.[4]

### Rickettsiae

Rickettsial diseases are transmitted by such arthropods as ticks and similar species that are responsible for the so-called spotted fevers such as the Rocky Mountain spotted fever (caused by *Rickettsiae rickettsii*), scrub typhus, which occurs in South East Asia, and epidemic typhus (caused by *Rickettsia prowazekii*). These obligate intracellular bacteria multiply in endothelial cells and cause widespread necrotizing vasculitis. Rocky Mountain spotted fever is no longer limited to the mountain area of the United States. The disease has spread to the U.S. East and Gulf coasts, and the reservoir has changed from mountain deer to dogs and other mammals. Young children and elderly adults are the most frequent victims. An acute disease may develop a few days after a tick bite. At this time blood cultures may prove negative,[180] and the Weil-Felix agglutination technique is not entirely specific. The clinical course depends on the accuracy of the diagnosis and prompt initiation of antibiotic treatment. Brain edema and abundant white matter petechiae are common in fatal cases. Light microscopy of brain samples discloses vessels surrounded by lymphocytes, in which microorganisms may be detected in endothelial cells by immunofluorescence.[168] These changes are accompanied by edema and gliosis in white matter. Abnormal higher intellectual functions are some of the sequelae noted in treated survivors.[56,82]

### Spirochetal Infections

**Neurosyphilis.** This disease is acquired through venereal transmission of *Treponema pallidum*. Asymptomatic meningeal involvement may be detected in a few cases during the secondary stage of syphilis, which follows a short while after the initial infection. Symptomatic acute meningitis may develop in a smaller number of patients with untreated secondary syphilis.[80]

CNS neurosyphilis includes: (1) meningovascular inflammation of large and medium-sized vessels (Heubner's endarteritis); (2) tabes dorsalis; (3) progressive general paresis; and (4) rarer than the first three, gumma. This tertiary syphilis occurs in a low percentage of untreated patients. Meningovascular involvement includes perivascular and adventitial infiltration by lymphocytes and plasma cells, intimal thickening with preservation of the elastic lamina, and secondary luminal occlusion and associated ischemic infarcts in cortical areas as well as in brainstem and spinal cord. Spirochetes are readily detectable with appropriate techniques, such as Steiner's silver impregnation, as spiral organisms measuring 5 to 12 $\mu$m in length. There is an increase in leukocyte count and globulin content in the CSF and positive VDRL and electrophoresis tests. Progressive arachnoiditis may lead to the development of cranial nerve palsies, pachymeningitis, and leptomeningeal fibrosis.

Tabes dorsalis is a slowly progressive degeneration of dorsal root ganglia, dorsal spinal roots, and posterior columns of the spinal cord. Involvement in most cases is pronounced mainly in lumbosacral and lower thoracic segments, as evidenced by myelin stains. These changes are accompanied by meningeal fibrosis and some mononuclear infiltration with dorsal ganglia involvement, but spirochetes have not been demonstrated in the spinal lesions; therefore, the spinal lesions of tabes dorsalis have been ascribed to the inflammation and fibrosis of the dorsal nerve roots.

Pupillary abnormalities described in neurosyphilis under the name of the Argyll Robertson sign are mostly but not exclusively associated with tabes dorsalis, and are a reflection of lesions involving intercalated neurons in the dorsal midbrain that receive and transmit light-generated impulses to the oculomotor nucleus.[94]

Progressive general paresis mainly affects males; symptoms appear many years after the primary infection, and the disease is characterized by parenchymal brain involvement with proliferation of typical elongated microglial cells or "rod" cells that contain iron and are readily stained blue with the Prussian blue method of Perls. Slight astroglial hyperplasia and neuronal depletion, perivascular plasma cell infiltrates, and abundant spirochetes are components of the disease that lead to rapid cortical frontal and striatal atrophy, with subsequent ventricular dilatation and granular ependymitis. All of these findings may not be present at autopsy of long-standing treated cases.[128]

Gummas, considered a hyperimmune tissue reaction, are infrequent lesions of coagulative necrosis that involve circumscribed sites of the brain parenchyma where spirochetes rarely can be demonstrated. Fibrosis and inflammatory infiltration by lymphocytes, plasma cells, epithelioid cells, and multinucleated giant cells can be observed at the periphery of the gumma.

Placental transmission can occur early in pregnancy; the symptoms of such infection may be manifest 2 to

5 years after the original infection. Congenital infection is seen in the form of the classic Hutchinson syndrome, with notched teeth, interstitial keratitis, and deafness secondary to eighth nerve involvement. Alternatively, perceptive deafness or meningovascular symptoms may be the only manifestations of congenital syphilis.

An increase in the incidence of syphilis has been reported in the United States, especially among persons at high risk for the acquired immunodeficiency syndrome. Neurosyphilis occurring in association with HIV-1 infection is prone to flare up and to progress very rapidly,[76] because of the decrease in cell-mediated immunity. This is evidenced by the young age at which CNS infections occur in these patients, with a latency period from the time of primary infection rarely exceeding 5 years. Failure of penicillin therapy to prevent subsequent neurosyphilis after positive serology has been reported in HIV-infected patients.[80]

Cerebral gumma seldom has been reported among HIV patients. High doses of intravenous, aqueous penicillin have led to both resolution of the lesion and nonreactive serologic tests in two out of three reported cases.[19,72] The gummatous lesion may be mistaken on neuroimaging for a neoplastic process or for opportunistic infections of different etiology. CT scanning discloses contrast enhancement lesions that may be accompanied by peripheral edema; MRI shows low intensity on T1-weighted and high intensity on T2-weighted images.[6,19] Neither previous penicillin treatment in doses insufficient to prevent neurosyphilis nor a negative CSF VDRL are reliable to rule out a diagnosis of neurosyphilis.[19] *T. pallidum* was identified in a cerebral syphilitic gumma by morphologic demonstration of the spirochete with a modified Steiner staining and by direct immunofluorescence for *Treponema pallidum;* DNA detection of the antigen was accomplished by PCR[176] and hybridization. Thus, biopsy is necessary to establish the etiologic diagnosis and identify the optimal treatment.[72,176]

Morgello and Laufer[106] suggest the concept of quaternary syphilis, featuring a process of brain tissue necrosis with numerous spirochetes. This condition was observed in an HIV-positive 22-year-old man, and it differs from the classic gumma of tertiary syphilis because in immunocompetent patients the immune response is prominent and spirochetes are either absent or difficult to detect.

**Lyme Borreliosis.** The *Borrelia burgdorferi* (Bb) spirochete causes lyme borreliosis (LB), a tickborne disease transmitted by tick bites that is widespread in North America and Europe. This is a multisystem infection, with neurologic symptoms in up to 15% of infected individuals[15,60]; asymptomatic infection is common. The clinical manifestations of LB have been classified on the basis of its resemblance to syphilis[120] into three main stages. The first is often self-limited and manifested by erythema migrans; later stages progress into severe and disseminated lesions unless appropriate treatment is instituted.

The early disseminated stage of the disease includes lymphocytic meningomyeloradiculoneuritis, sometimes accompanied by cranial neuropathy mainly of the seventh nerve. This may be associated with arthritis, myalgia, myocarditis, and lymphadenosis benigna cutis. The manifestations of peripheral nerve involvement may be protean and can include carpal tunnel syndrome, radiculitis, and mononeuritis multiplex. Spontaneous resolution of symptoms may occur after several months.

Evaluation of the CSF discloses pleocytosis with plasmacytes and lymphocytes. Atypical cytologic features in some of these cells may be misinterpreted as suggestive of a meningeal lymphoma.[50] After several weeks, analysis of sequentially obtained CSF specimens reveals intrathecal synthesis of specific antibodies, elevated total IgM and IgG, and the presence of oligoclonal bands.

Both indirect serologic assays including Western blot and enzyme-linked immunosorbent assay (ELISA) and direct methods of antigen detection such as PCR coupled with hybridization (PCR/H) for the detection of Borrelia DNA in the spinal fluid[101] are useful in the etiologic diagnosis. Samples of CSF are ideal to demonstrate the antigen[105] because Bb is hardly detectable in tissue samples or in other body fluids. Positive CSF cultures have been obtained from patients whose disease had evolved for less than 1 month.[50] For purposes of evaluating the response to therapy, titration of Bb-specific antibodies in serum is used in most instances,[63] although one must be aware of occasional false-positive serologic results.

In the late disseminated disease, in addition to skin and joint involvement, a chronic progressive meningoencephalomyelitis may develop several months or years after the onset of symptoms. Worsening of symptoms is the characteristic course of the disease, although some improvement may be achieved after instituting appropriate antibiotic treatment. White matter changes featuring a leukoencephalopathy or abnormalities mimicking those of multiple sclerosis may be disclosed by MRI; optic neuritis also has been documented in some cases of LB.[151]

Meningovascular involvement resembles the symptoms of tertiary syphilis.[50,86] Peripheral neuropathy, mainly involving sensory nerves, follows the topographic distribution of the skin disease and develops in most untreated patients. However, limbs free of cutaneous lesions also may display signs and symptoms of peripheral nerve axonopathy. Lymphocytic meningitis, mild encephalopathy, and cranial neuropathy are common manifestations of LB in children, whereas radicular involvement and peripheral neuropathy seldom occur in these patients. A pseudotumor-like syndrome has been observed in several pediatric patients.[50]

Neuropathologic studies on a few biopsy or autopsy specimens have shown microglial nodules and lymphoplasmacytic basal meningitis, but the microorganism rarely has been found in these specimens.[120] Meningovascular involvement is characterized by an obliterative inflammatory vasculopathy, similar to the syphilitic arteritis of Heubner, with secondary ischemic infarcts. Scattered spirochetes localized to the leptomeninges and surrounding subependymal vessels of the fourth ventricle were disclosed with the Warthin Starry silver method in one case.[86] Peripheral nerve involvement characterized by perivascular mononuclear cell infiltrates as well as axonal degeneration, probably caused by ischemia, has been documented in a few cases.[34,86]

Experimental Lyme neuroborreliosis (LNB) in rats inoculated intravenously with radiolabeled organisms provides a useful model to study the kinetics of Bb CNS invasion, both by examination of CSF and by autoradiography of whole brain sections.[50] In a separate study carried out on monkeys, CSF pleocytosis and MRI abnormalities closely correlated with the detection by PCR of Bb DNA in the cerebral white matter, supporting the concept that direct spirochetal invasion of the CNS is the main pathogenesis of LNB.[119,120] Complex immunologic damage, indirect injury associated with local production of cytokines, and direct vascular injury caused by Bb also should be considered in the pathogenesis of the lesions.[86]

Intravenous penicillin administered for a period of 2 to 4 weeks, ceftriaxone, and other antibiotics have been used successfully in the treatment of LB. The role of corticosteroids is not yet clearly established, but some patients given a combination of antibiotics and corticosteroids are said to recover faster than those receiving antibiotics alone.[50]

## MYCOTIC INFECTIONS

Most mycotic infections of the CNS are the result of hematogenous dissemination from such sites as lung and digestive tract. The disease also can be a direct extension from local infections in the skull or spine and paranasal sinuses; fungal infections also may be acquired after open head injury. Increased incidence of these infections is the result of the widespread treatment of malignancies with immunosuppressants, organ transplantation, and the worldwide rise in AIDS incidence. Some mycotic lesions in the brain that mimic neoplasms clinically and on neuroimaging grounds, pose a diagnostic challenge. This is especially true of intraoperative biopsies in which diagnosis is based on the quick evaluation of unprocessed tissues.[57,59,138]

### Candidiasis

Several species of this genus are a component of the flora normally found in the skin, cervix and vagina, oral cavity, and digestive tract. On occasion Candida may produce localized infections in patients with chronic debilitating diseases or may become invasive and disseminate through the blood stream. Conditions associated with disseminated and CNS Candida infections have been extensively reviewed; most are associated with spontaneous immunosuppression, as occurs in patients with leukemia or lymphoma. Additional risk factors include treatment for cancer, organ transplantation followed by immunosuppressive therapy, AIDS, long-term therapy with antibiotics or corticosteroids, intravenous drug abuse, indwelling central venous catheters, and instrumentation or surgery involving mucosal surfaces normally colonized by Candida.[71]

DNA sequences that are unique to *C. albicans* suitable for detection in blood by PCR have been identified in most of the conditions described above.[70] *C. albicans* is the species most frequently found in invasive CNS infections. Multiple small intracerebral microabscesses or large solitary ones frequently harbor PAS-positive and silver methenamine-positive pseudohyphae and yeast forms. The inflammatory reaction usually is slight and is a reflection of the immune status of the host. Granulomas, vasculitis, meningitis, and cerebral mycotic aneurysms due to *C. albicans* have been described.[93] In severely ill patients, prompt treatment with amphotericin B should be considered, even in the absence of a firm diagnosis.[71]

### Aspergillosis

*Aspergillus fumigatus* and allied species (*A. flavus, A. niger*, and others) causing human disease are ubiquitous fungi present in water, soil, and organic debris that form sporangia in contact with air. From a focal primary lung infection through hematogenous dissemination, these fungi may reach the CNS. Should the host's natural defenses be impaired, Aspergillus initiates progressive infection. Otherwise, macrophages and polymorphonuclear leukocytes provide adequate protection against the mycelial form.[67,139] Severe granulocytopenia and long-term exposure to high doses of corticosteroid compounds by recipients of organ transplants have been associated with disseminated aspergillosis. Among these latter patients CNS aspergillosis frequently is preceded by organ rejection requiring the administration of high-dose immunosuppressants and retransplantation.[160] Head trauma also has been implicated as a possible portal of entry of Aspergillus into the CNS.

Lesions of aspergillosis may be single or multiple, depending on the route of entry (local penetration or

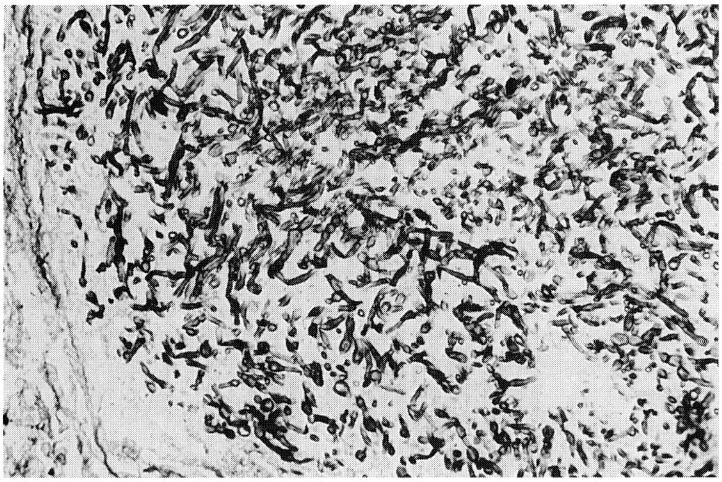

**Fig. 7-6.** *Aspergillus fumigatus*. Dichotomous branching septate hyphae are visible in a cerebellar lesion. (Grocott methenamine silver.)

hematogenous dissemination) and the immunologic status of the host. Focal granulomas or hemorrhagic necrotic foci may occur in either case. Dichotomous, branching, septate hyphae 6 to 8 μm thick, strongly positive with PAS stain and silver methenamine impregnation (Fig. 7-6), are present in most tissue samples. Aspergillus tends to invade vessel walls, causing secondary thrombosis and consequent ischemic necrosis of the brain; cerebral mycotic aneurysms with massive subarachnoid hemorrhage also have been reported among patients with aspergillosis.[73] A cerebellar granuloma with lymphocytes, plasma cells, epithelioid cells, and a few multinucleated giant cells containing hyphae having features consistent with those of Aspergillus can mimic an astrocytoma clinically and radiologically, as seen in a 9-year-old immunocompetent boy. The abscess developed following open head trauma and several craniotomies that included shunting (personal unpublished observation). A good response followed surgical excision of the aspergilloma and combined chemotherapy that included amphotericin B, as suggested by others.[177]

### Blastomycosis

North American blastomycosis, caused by *Blastomyces dermatitides*, appears mainly among farm workers or hunters in the central and southeastern United States. There are three main clinicopathologic forms. The mycosis may take the form of a benign localized cutaneous infection caused by inoculation of spores present in soil and rotting logs; a second expression includes a mild pneumonitis; less commonly, blastomycosis may become a generalized infection reaching the CNS through the bloodstream. On occasion, blastomycosis develops as an opportunistic infection among AIDS patients.[65]

Microorganisms may be found in tissues as budding yeasts 15 μm in diameter with a thick refractile cell wall and a single thick neck bud. These are found in association with single or multiple granulomas or abscesses where they are often found within multinucleated giant cells. PAS staining, silver methenamine impregnation, and specific immunofluorescence are useful tools for the identification of the organism in tissue sections. Diffuse or predominantly basal leptomeningitis with occlusion of subarachnoid space may lead to hydrocephalus. Prompt diagnosis followed by treatment with amphotericin B has been reported as successful in a few cases; however, widespread blastomycosis frequently is fatal.[90]

### Coccidioidomycosis

The etiologic agent, *Coccidioides immitis*, can be acquired by domestic animals and humans by inhalation of dust infected with arthrospores. The disease is endemic in South America, Mexico, and the southwestern United States.[82] It is particularly prevalent in hot, dry, semiarid areas where brief heavy rains carry the fungus into the subsoil. During dry, dusty, windy spells infective arthroconidia evolve, and these are capable of causing infection. The primary site of infection, the lung, often is asymptomatic, and the antigen is detectable only by skin reaction. More rarely, fungus affects skin, bones, pericardium, or CNS, where a basilar meningitis or a meningoencephalitis with secondary hydrocephalus may develop. Diagnosis is generally delayed, although microorganisms can be recognized easily in the CSF. The complement fixation test may be helpful. Severe and widespread disease has been documented in immunocompromised hosts.[92,179] Necrotizing granulomas may feature caseation necrosis, neutrophil infiltration, lymphocytes, plasmacytes, histiocytes, and multinucleated giant cells that harbor organisms, each measuring 25 to 35 μm in diameter and having a thick refractile capsule full of endospores.

### Paracoccidioidomycosis

South American paracoccidioidomycosis is caused by *Paracoccidioides brasiliensis*. The disease is endemic in Central and South America, with Brazil, Venezuela, Colombia, and Argentina reporting the highest incidence, most often in men aged 25 to 50 years who work in agriculture-related activities. Skin, mucous membranes, and lymph nodes may be involved by infection, although the disease is acquired through the respiratory tract with a well-established primary lung complex. Both asymptomatic infections and prolonged latency periods have been documented. Useful specific techniques for serodiagnosis are complement fixation, agar gel diffusion studies, and immunoenzymatic techniques. Advances in immunologic, cytochemical, antigenic, and ultrastructural studies as well as studies of host-parasite interactions have been fully documented in a review by Toro-Gonzalez.[158]

CNS involvement is not infrequent in endemic areas. We have seen two cases, one in the autopsy of an immunocompetent child who developed severe meningoencephalitis, and a second in a 40-year-old man who developed a tumor-like lesion (5.0 cm in diameter) resembling a falx meningioma. The latter patient remained asymptomatic after complete surgical resection of the mycotic mass and specific antifungal treatment. In the former case, the lymphocytic and plasmacytic infiltration involved the leptomeninges and the perivascular spaces of the brain. In the brain parenchyma, confluent inflammatory infiltrates included macrophages and multinucleated giant cells that harbored spherical yeasts 20 $\mu m$ in diameter. The presence of buds created a characteristic rudder-wheel appearance. In the patient with the pseudotumor, the dural lesion consisted of a tuberculoid granulomatous reaction with lymphocytes, histiocytes, and abundant giant cells laden with yeasts (unpublished observation).

Intrathecal administration of amphotericin B has been proposed as an effective treatment of paracoccidioidomycosis; in vitro and in vivo ketoconazole exerts both a fungistatic and a fungicidal effect.[112]

### Cryptococcosis

*Cryptococcus neoformans*, formerly known as *Torula histolytica*, is the cause of a disease that affects humans and domestic and wild animals. Infection with Cryptococcus is the most frequent cause of human mycotic basal meningitis; it has a worldwide distribution, and is associated in 30% to 50% of cases with immunosuppression caused by lymphoma or leukemia chemotherapy, by organ transplantation, and by long-term treatment with corticosteroids. This disease also can develop in immunocompetent individuals.[5,11,55] CD4+ T cells play a major defensive mechanism against Cryptococcus; therefore, cryptococcosis is a very common brain infection among AIDS patients.[79,85] Most humans acquire the infection through inhalation of bird excreta or dust contaminated with the fungi; the primary pulmonary infection then disseminates throughout the body.

*C. neoformans* is the only encapsulated fungus that invades the human CNS. The capsular polysaccharide confers serotype specificity; a positive latex test in the CSF is indicative of capsular antigens. Noncapsulated strains also may invade CNS and induce chronic infection with signs and symptoms of meningitis, meningoencephalitis, or a tumor. Parenchymal lesions or cryptococcomas may occur as multiple mucoid pseudocysts without any visible inflammatory host response. The lesions become encapsulated and manifest themselves as multiple contrast-enhanced lesions or as hyperdense or ring-type lesions on CT. Cryptococcomas of the choroid plexuses are characteristic of this infection and may be visible by MRI.[11]

The CSF in cryptococcosis may be clear or turbid and may have increased cellularity and protein content. Small floating particles may be mistaken for mononuclear cells, but India ink preparations may prove diagnostic in more than one half of the cases. In histology preparations, the organisms appear as budding yeasts, 15 to 20 $\mu m$ in diameter, that are both PAS-positive (Fig. 7-7, *A*) and impregnable with silver methenamine (Fig. 7-7, *B*) surrounded by a thick characteristic capsule that stains with mucicarmine and Alcian Blue. Commonly, the cryptococci elicit minimal cellular inflammation. Combined chemotherapy, including amphotericin B, must be instituted promptly, although the prognosis is poor in advanced cases. Shunting procedures to bypass sites of spinal fluid obstruction as well as surgical excision of cryptococcomas are indicated in some instances.[170]

### Histoplasmosis

*Histoplasma capsulatum* is a dimorphic fungus with a worldwide distribution. Infection is demonstrable by positive histoplasmin skin test in a variable percentage of the general population and in over half of adults in endemic areas. It is acquired in most cases by inhalation of dust containing spores from the mycelial form of the organism, which is frequently encountered in the soil. After entering the human body *H. capsulatum* adopts a yeast phase within the lungs and may disseminate to other organs via the bloodstream; most immunocompetent hosts are able to inhibit dissemination beyond the lung.[173] The primary lesions remain asymptomatic in the form of calcified nodules involving mediastinal lymph nodes, lungs, and occasionally kidney, liver, and adrenal glands. Active pulmonary and/or laryngeal infections in endemic areas have been widely recognized in healthy adults, predominantly

A 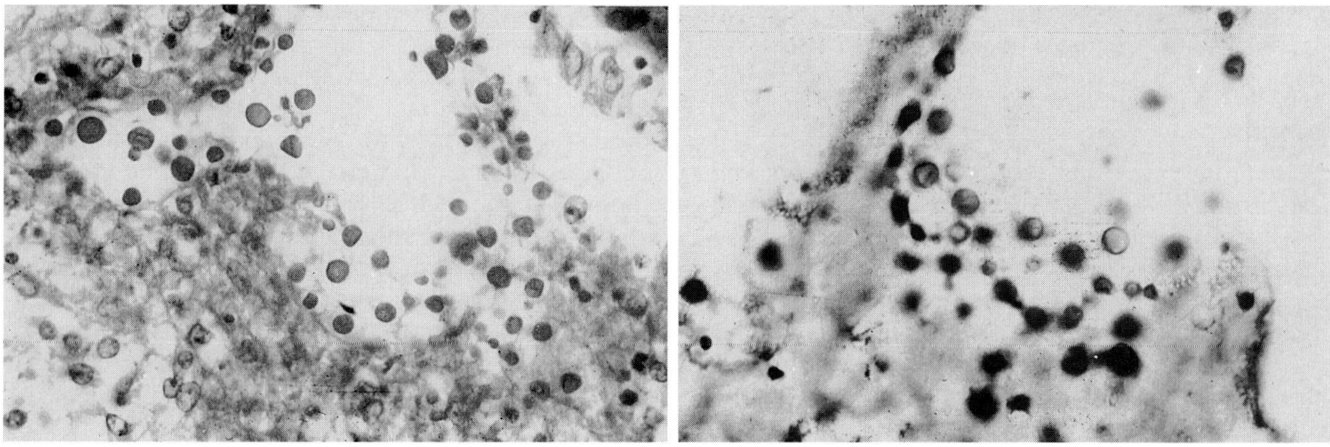 B

**Fig. 7-7.** *Cryptococcus neoformans*. Single budding yeasts are shown in the subarachnoid space in brain leptomeninges. (**A**, PAS; **B**, Grocott methenamine silver.)

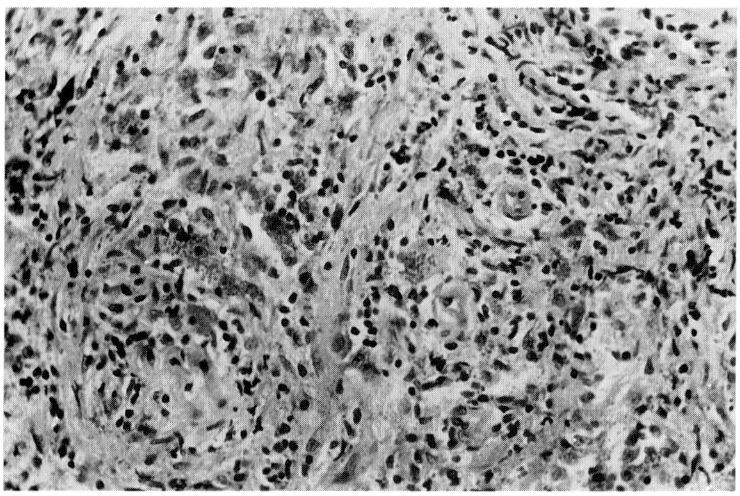

**Fig. 7-8.** Macrophages laden with *Histoplasma capsulatum* are shown in a spinal cord lesion from an immunosuppressed kidney transplant recipient. (PAS.)

males, but a more diffuse compromise of the reticuloendothelial system that involves lymph nodes, liver, and spleen also may occur, particularly during infancy and childhood. Although in the chronic stages of disseminated histoplasmosis immunodiffusion and complement fixation serologic tests often are negative, more sensitive radioimmunoassays in both serum and urine specimens may prove positive.[174] While infrequent, CNS involvement may occur in 20% to 50% of patients with disseminated histoplasmosis secondary to lung infection.[153,173] A diagnosis of histoplasmosis should be carefully considered in AIDS patients who have evidence of meningitis or intracranial mass effect lesions; this association between HIV and Histoplasma infections has been noted in a few cases in the recent past.[171] At neuroimaging histoplasmosis may present as isolated CT contrast-enhancing brain lesions.[8,163] A cervical spinal cord pseudoneoplastic lesion caused by histoplasmosis in a renal transplant recipient had neuroimaging features similar to those mentioned above (personal unpublished data). A fatal progressive myelopathy was the clinical expression of a chronic histoplasmosis reactivated by steroid treatment and diabetes mellitus.[153]

At autopsy, either diffuse or mostly basilar leptomeningitis is observed in chronic cases; vasculitis and granulomatous inflammation involving brain or spinal cord are common. The exudate consists of lymphocytes, plasmacytes, and organism-laden macrophages; most granulomas are well circumscribed by a fibrous capsule that surrounds a central area where caseous necrosis, epithelioid cells, and multinucleated giant cells may be visible. Almost invariably these lesions contain macrophages laden with intracytoplasmic ovoid budding yeasts, each measuring 2 to 5 $\mu$m in diameter. A typical clear halo in Histoplasma allows differential diagnosis from Toxoplasma and *Trypanosoma cruzi* amastigotes. *H. capsulatum* are intensely stained with PAS (Fig. 7-8) and easily impregnable with silver methenamine; the detection of antihistoplasma antibodies in serum and urine provides an easy means to diagnose disseminated histoplasmosis.[174]

### Nocardiosis

*Nocardia asteroides* and *brasiliensis* are both present in the soil and have a worldwide distribution, although *N. brasiliens* is found mainly in South America. Nocardia are filamentous, branching, aerobic organisms belonging to the family Actinomycetaceae that are pathogens in man. Following lung infection through the inhalation of spores, the nocardial brain lesion develops as single multiloculated or multiple partly encapsulated abscesses containing a dense purulent exudate, more commonly in the supratentorial compartment. Alternatively, nocardiosis may induce meningitis without abscesses. CT images resemble those of other brain abscesses with ring enhancement, but the additional findings of subependymal nodules and meningitis may suggest a diagnosis of nocardiosis, particularly when the brain lesions are associated with pulmonary infiltrates.[89] Data derived from experimental infections indicate that brain invasive nocardiae exhibit both an adhesin for attachment to endothelial cell membrane and an invasive factor that fosters microorganism penetration.[16]

At light microscopy, abscesses display a central necrotic area containing neutrophils, surrounded by both mononuclear and scavenger cells, reactive astrocytes, and fibrous tissue; multinucleated giant cells are present in some lesions. A dense cellular inflammatory infiltrate may be observed lining the ventricles as well as small subependymal abscesses. Nocardia organisms do not stain with H&E; PAS and Gridley stains also are not useful in the diagnosis of nocardiosis, but the microorganism may be stained with the Ziehl-Neelsen technique as long as a weak acid is used in the process of decolorization.[20] Gram stain and methenamine silver impregnation reveal Nocardia in tissues as delicate branching filaments 1 μm thick.

Nocardiosis is most commonly associated with chronic disease of the respiratory or of the immune system; meningoencephalitis and brain abscess also occur in both immunocompetent and immunosuppressed patients; systemic disease with widespread abscesses develops in intravenous drug abusers.[62,148] Although CNS nocardiosis is often fatal, good response has been achieved by combining medical therapy with complete surgical excision of the brain lesion.[2]

### Mucormycosis (Phycomycosis, Zygomycosis)

Three genera belong to the order Mucoraceae, namely, Mucor, Rhizopus, and Absidia, which may be found in the soil as saprophytes, are responsible for this severe, frequently fatal human disease. Infection may be acquired through inhalation of airborne spores and by accidental or surgical trauma. Mucoraceae also spread from the paranasal sinuses through veins that drain the orbital and adjacent parts of the brain. Hematogenous dissemination to the CNS from a primary pulmonary focus also is possible; the bowel mucosa and the skin are additional portals of entry for these fungi. Diabetic acidosis and immunosuppression therapies are both predisposing factors,[127] especially in the classic rhinocerebral type of mucormycosis, in which there is severe orbital edema and ocular globe protrusion. A rhinocerebral case of mucormycosis was seen in one patient following prolonged corticosteroid treatment of systemic lupus erythematosus (personal unpublished observation). AIDS also has been associated with CNS mucormycosis.[32,92] In the brain lesions, the fungi invade the blood vessel walls, leading to arterial occlusion and infarction. The agent of mucormycosis appears in tissue sections as broad nonseptate hyphae branching at right angles and measuring up to 50 μm in width. Silver methenamine (Fig. 7-9, *A*) and PAS are both useful to demonstrate hyphae (Fig. 7-9, *B*). An improved outcome has been reported following prompt surgical excision combined with amphotericin B treatment.[162]

## PARASITIC DISEASES

The description of these diseases here is limited to those that commonly involve the CNS.

### Nematodes

**Trichinosis.** Trichinosis is a worldwide zoonosis sparing only Australia and certain Pacific Islands. Sporadic outbreaks have been reported in North and South America, Europe, and Asia.[25,108]

Trichinosis is closely related to cultural and dietary habits. This disease occurs in lower animals and humans following the intake of under-cooked meat infected by the larvae of the nematode *Trichinella spiralis*. All of the members of *Trichinella* spp. complete their life cycle in a single host. Transmission occurs in both domestic or wild animals. Domestic transmission can involve pigs, rats, dogs, cats, and even herbivores such as horses. Wild transmission has been observed in foxes, boars, small rodents, wild canids, felids, and other sylvatic mammals.

Ingested larvae, after reaching the intestine, lose their capsules and invade the mucosa. After copulation, the adult male dies and the female lodges in the intestinal wall and multiplies. Newborn larvae ultimately enter the bloodstream, migrate to skeletal muscle and become encysted. The diaphragm, intercostal muscles, biceps, gastrocnemius, and extraocular muscles are infested to widely variable degrees.[53]

Clinical symptoms appear some two weeks after the ingestion of contaminated food and include vomiting and diarrhea, followed by periorbital and facial edema,

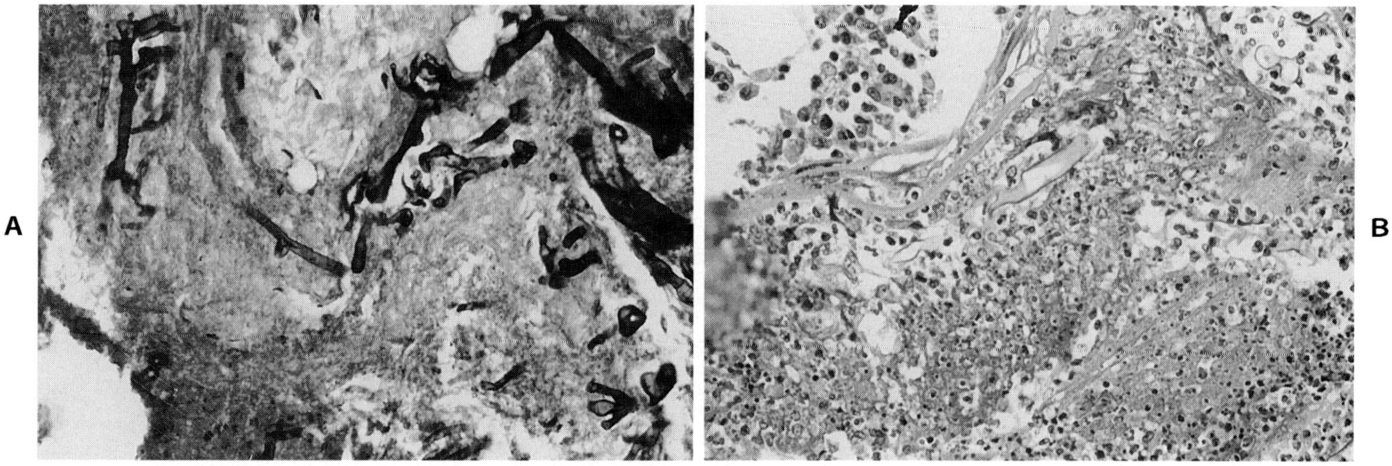


**Fig. 7-9. A**, *Mucor phycomycosis*. Broad nonseptate hyphae are visible in necrotic debris from the orbit. (Grocott methenamine silver.) **B**, *Mucor phycomycosis*. Broad nonseptate hyphae surrounded by necrotic tissue and inflammatory infiltrate in the wall of an intracranial artery in an AIDS patient. (PAS.)

fever, muscle weakness, and pain. Several organs may be involved via immune-mediated inflammatory infiltration or by migration and/or presence of parasites in tissues.

CNS involvement, originally estimated to be above 10%, appears to be declining in prevalence and may manifest as delirium, behavioral changes, higher function impairment, meningoencephalitic signs, and, on occasion, focal paresis. Anal and urinary sphincter dysfunction, vertigo, seizures, and cranial nerve palsies may also occur.[108]

Computed tomography discloses multiple small hypodense foci in cerebral white matter with ring enhancement[85] and, on occasion, small cortical infarcts. MRI shows bilateral high-signal intensity lesions in the white matter.[42] Such findings are usually associated with acute myocardial injury and/or infarction, marked eosinophilia, and increased levels of serum antibodies against *T. spiralis*.[23]

IgG, IgM, and IgE antibodies increase. IgE levels increase by up to tenfold at the peak of infection, subsiding thereafter. Diagnosis can be confirmed by positive serological tests, ELISA, and indirect immunofluorescence detection of antigen. Muscle biopsy from nodular tissue is also valuable in confirming the diagnosis (Fig. 7-10, *A*). Domestic *Trichinella* species can be differentiated from sylvatic species by recently developed DNA probes and PCR technology. This technology may soon be applied to meat screening.[172]

Inflammatory infiltration with eosinophils as well as granulomas may be visible where larvae are encysted within a modified host muscle fiber (a host nurse cell), surrounded by a host-derived connective tissue capsule rich in mucopolysaccharides. This connective tissue protects the host nurse cell–larva complex from immunological attack. The host cell differs from normal host muscle fibers in appearance and histochemical make-up (Fig. 7-10, *B* to *D*).[156] The presence of basophilic sarcoplasm, enlarged nuclei with prominent nucleoli, and increased acid and alkaline phosphatase activity in the host nurse cell suggest fiber regeneration. Such unique skeletal muscle fiber changes are the subject of active research.[36,75] These skeletal muscle fiber changes seem to be regulated at gene transcription level, together with a cell cycle repositioning, the muscle cell reentering the cell cycle, replicating its DNA, and becoming suspended in $G_2$ phase. The modified phenotype of the host nurse cell muscle fiber may be due to host regulatory pathways governed by cell cycle phase, which in turn may contribute to larval growth and development.[75]

CNS lesions can involve gray and white matter, cerebellum, pons, and the spinal cord. Inflammatory meningeal and parenchymal infiltration as well as *T. spiralis*-laden granulomas are usually evident mainly in white matter.[82] Small vascular thromboses and ischemic lesions may occur even in the absence of larvae. Besides direct larval effect, brain and myocardial lesions may occur because of the effects of toxemic and allergic factors, and by production of tumor necrosis factor $\alpha$ (TNF $\alpha$), which induces endothelial damage through eosinophil toxicity.[47] Thrombophlebitis of the brain and frequent ischemic lesions secondary to systemic embolism lend support to the hypothesis of endothelial injury.[41,51]

Treatment is partly symptomatic. Specific chemotherapy (e.g., levamisole, pyrantel, thiabendazole, albendazole, and/or mebendazole) works against the adult parasite and migrating larvae, but the effect on encysted larvae is questionable.

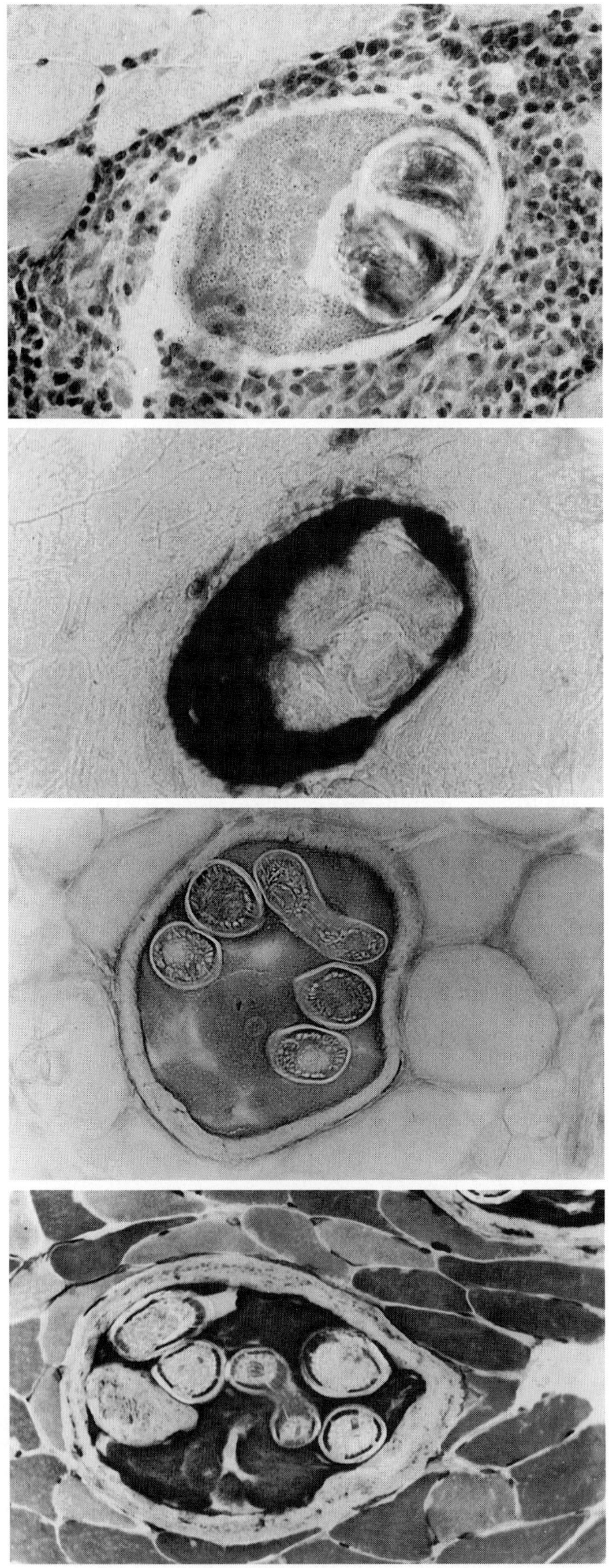


**Fig. 7-10.** **A**, Trichinosis larvae surrounded by inflammatory infiltrates in muscle biopsy. **B**, Host nurse cell, strong alkaline phosphatase activity; muscle biopsy, alkaline phosphatase. **C**, Host nurse cell, strong acid phosphatase activity; mouse experimental infection involving *T. spiralis*; acid phosphatase. **D**, Host nurse cell, strong ATPase activity; larval internal muscle is also reactive; mouse experiment involving *T. spiralis* infection; ATPase pH 4.6. (**A**, H&E.)

**Strongyloidiasis.** Strongyloidiasis is seen worldwide. The nematode, *Strongyloides stercoralis,* has a free-living phase in damp soil where eggs are deposited. The adult female is filariform and infects the intestinal mucosa of humans, dogs, and cats. After oviposition, eggs release rhabdoid larvae which, when evacuated with the feces, follow either of two cycles depending on environmental and/or genetic factors: direct (homogenic) or indirect (heterogenic). In the direct cycle, larvae become filariform and infective, whereas in the indirect cycle, rhabdoid larvae become adult males and females capable of independent life. Fertilized females deposit eggs in the soil and release rhabdoid larvae that become filariform. In both cases, filariform larvae become infective, penetrate the circulatory system through cutaneous abrasions, and migrate to the lungs. The larvae then travel through the trachea and esophagus, mature, and inhabit the duodenum and jejunum as adults. The female then produces larvae that either reenter the circulation or are excreted to reinfect a human host.

CNS complications include acute suppurative meningitis, abscesses, and localized granulomata that involve either leptomeninges or brain parenchyma. Disseminated strongyloidiasis with vascular invasion, subsequent thrombosis, and infarcts has been reported after long-term corticosteroid intake and in patients with lymphoma or AIDS.[24,106,111,131,181]

Serodiagnosis with an enzyme immunoassay is available from the Centers for Disease Control.[178] Thiabendazole, ivermectin, and albendazole are effective against *S. stercoralis.*

### Cestodes

**Cysticercosis.** Neurocysticercosis is a widespread CNS infection caused by *Cysticercus cellulosae,* the encysted larvae of the pig tapeworm, *Taenia solium;* this infection is endemic in Latin America, India, and China, and sporadically occurs in the rest of the world, especially among migrants.[35] Increased incidence of this infection in the United States, particularly in southern California, probably is related to the growing population of immigrants from Latin America.[102,140] Cases diagnosed in Argentina have involved patients originating from Bolivia, Colombia, and Ecuador (personal observation).

Man may be a definitive host after acquiring the infection through intake of undercooked pork meat containing encysted larvae; these become tapeworms in the small bowel and are eliminated in stools as proglottids, each containing thousands of ova. In turn, ova-contaminated food may be eaten by the pig, whose gastric juices dissolve the cyst and release immature larvae or oncospheres; the latter penetrate the stomach wall and reach the bloodstream to develop mainly in muscle tissue into a mature larval cyst (Fig. 7-11, *A*). Man becomes an intermediate host by ingesting food containing ova. Immature larvae or oncospheres tend to lodge in skeletal and heart muscle, but show a preference for the microvessels of the brain, penetrate these vessels, and reach the brain parenchyma and ventricles. Although the spinal cord is commonly spared, vertebrae may be involved and the lesion may cause secondary spinal cord compression. In one instance an intrarachidial encysted larva of *Cysticercus* mimicked an arachnoid cyst in the absence of brain lesions demonstrable by MRI (personal unreported observation) (Fig. 7-11, *B*). On occasion, a racemose form of the parasite develops within the ventricles, or in the subarachnoid space, affecting the basal meninges, obstructing the spinal fluid flow, and leading to intracranial hypertension. Clinical signs and symptoms of cysticercosis in most patients include seizures and hydrocephalus; signs of meningitis or intra-

A

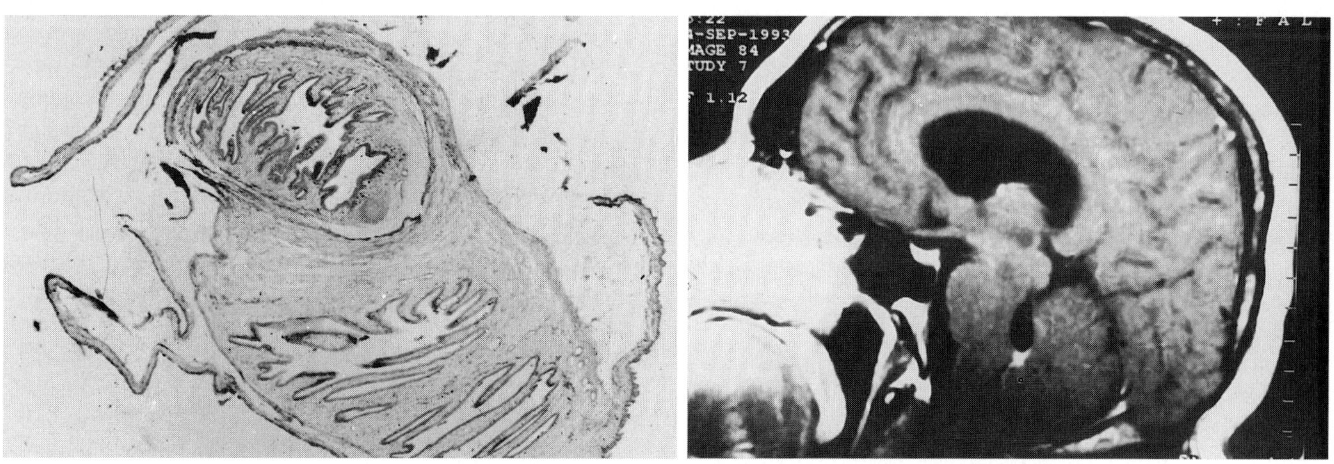

B

**Fig. 7-11. A,** Encysted larva of *Cysticercus cellulosae* in a brain biopsy. (H&E.) **B,** Hydrocephalus in a patient with *Cysticercus cellulosae* in the IV ventricle. Hyperintense lesion is visible by MRI T1-weighted image.

cranial tumors may pose differential diagnoses with neoplasms and granulomas of other etiologies. Ocular cysts may lead to blindness, especially in children. Brain neuroimaging may be diagnostic in cases in which multiple calcified cysts are visible.[102]

In the acute stage of the disease there is increased CSF cellularity that includes many lymphocytes and plasmacytes; a colloidal gold curve of the meningitic type also may be detectable. Complement fixation and ELISA tests may readily detect the antigen in the CSF; both tests have high sensitivity, but a recently developed immunoblot test identifies specific IgM and IgG with 100% specificity.[35,161] Serum indirect hemagglutinin titers may prove diagnostic in a high percentage of cases.

Autopsied cases have disclosed variable numbers of cysts in diverse locations, either intraparenchymal, intraventricular, or in the subarachnoid space. Cerebellar and spinal cysts are rare. Basal meninges are generally opalescent and thickened, and secondary hydrocephalus is frequent.

The cyst of *C. cellulosae* (Fig. 7-11, *A*) possesses a thin translucent wall filled with clear fluid and a four-sucker scolex with a double row of birefringent hooklets arising from the parenchymatous area. The external folded cuticular layer is 3 $\mu$m thick and is covered with microvilli; the middle layer displays a pseudoepithelial structure separated from the cuticle by mesenchymal fibers. The internal reticular layer consists of a fibrous network and a few calcareous bodies. Inflammatory reaction around the cyst occurs in most cases after parasite degeneration, and it is attributed to cyst fluid permeation. Cellular inflammation includes lymphocytes, plasmacytes, and eosinophils. Cysts located deep in the parenchyma may elicit considerable granulation tissue reaction, including foreign body giant cells, at times surrounded by a fibrous capsule, and vessels surrounded by inflammatory infiltrates.[35] Muscle biopsy disclosing encysted larvae may prove diagnostic, particularly in cases in which the disease has reached a chronic stage.

Therapeutic intervention has proved successful with pyrazino isaquinoline compounds. In some cases the drug is given with corticoids to avoid the risk of releasing Cysticercus antigens at the start of treatment. Surgical treatment and shunting procedures are indicated when the cysts reach a large size or become the cause of obstructive hydrocephalus (Fig. 7-11, *B*).

**Echinococcosis (hydatid disease).** A worldwide zoonosis,[40] echinococcosis is caused by the larval stage of *Echinococcus granulosus*, the dog tapeworm, although wild canides and other carnivores may act as definite hosts. The sheep, other domestic animals, and wild animals may act as intermediate hosts. Thus, the disease is more frequent in such sheep-raising areas as North Africa, Argentina, Australia, and New Zealand.[38] Humans become accidental intermediate hosts by ingesting food contaminated with canine feces containing ova; children are more frequently affected than adults because of their close contact with dogs. Ova hatch in the gastrointestinal tract, releasing a hexacanth invasive embryo that reaches the bloodstream and then the liver and lungs, where the primary sterile and fluid-filled hydatid cyst develops. Hydatid cysts are found in the liver in over 60% of cases and in the lungs in 10% to 40% of cases. Other sites, including the brain, periorbital tissue, pericardium, and kidneys, are involved in 5% of cases. DNA probes and PCR may be applied to diagnose *Echinococcus* spp.[172] Clinical symptoms are mostly related to the size and location of the cyst and include seizures and signs of spinal cord compression. Neuroimaging discloses cystic lesions, which allows presumptive diagnosis of hydatid disease in endemic areas (Fig. 7-12, *A*). Serology may be essential for diagnosis; immunoelectrophoresis or immunofiltration may demonstrate the presence of "arc 5," a finding highly specific for hydatid disease. ELISA determination of IgG and total and specific IgE levels is useful in detecting early progression of the disease and response to treatment.[38]

Brain cysts may be readily recognized at the time of surgery by their superficial location, bluish color, ovoid shape, and large size, an average of 4 to 10 cm in diameter in our experience in a pediatric series of 18 cases.[157] Each cyst contains a translucent fluid and daughter cysts, with an appearance similar to that of small, whitish grapes.

At light microscopy, hydatid cysts have an external or cuticular layer made of thick, multilamellated, nonnucleated, and eosinophilic material, and an inner germinal layer with many scolices (Fig. 7-12, *B*) that may be also recognizable in the multiple internal grapelike cysts. Although brain tissue reaction is minimal, focal infiltrates of lymphocytes, plasma cells, eosinophils, foreign giant cells, fibroblasts, and reactive astrocytes may surround the cyst; in organs other than the CNS, a thick fibrous adventitia develops around the cyst. The treatment of choice is complete surgical excision, avoiding cyst rupture to prevent further dissemination, and anaphylactic reaction.

Multilocular brain cysts with an alveolar-like pattern, difficult to eradicate surgically, are caused by *Echinococcus multilocularis*, which initially produce invasive pseudomalignant lesions within the liver, but is liable to metastasize to the lung or brain in 5% of cases.[79] This infection is transmitted by foxes, the definitive hosts; small rodents are intermediate hosts, and in cold climates can be the source of the infection. Alveolar echinococcosis requires surgery and chemotherapy.[14,15,17]

A

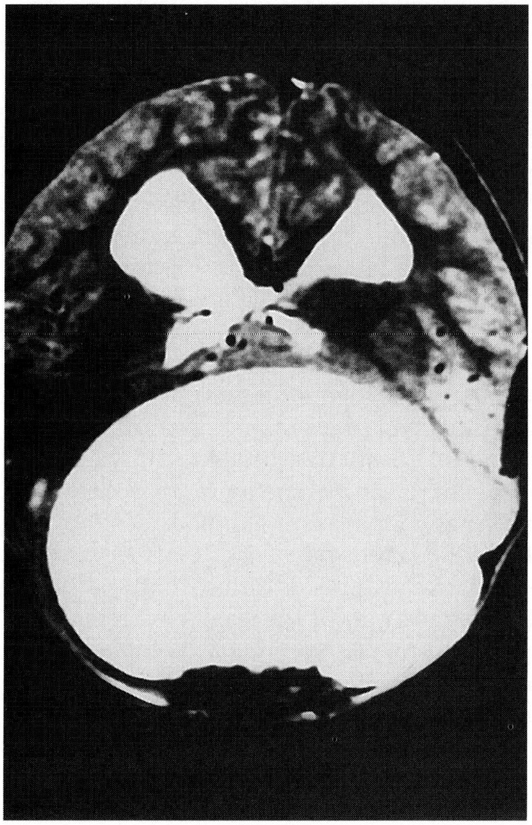

B

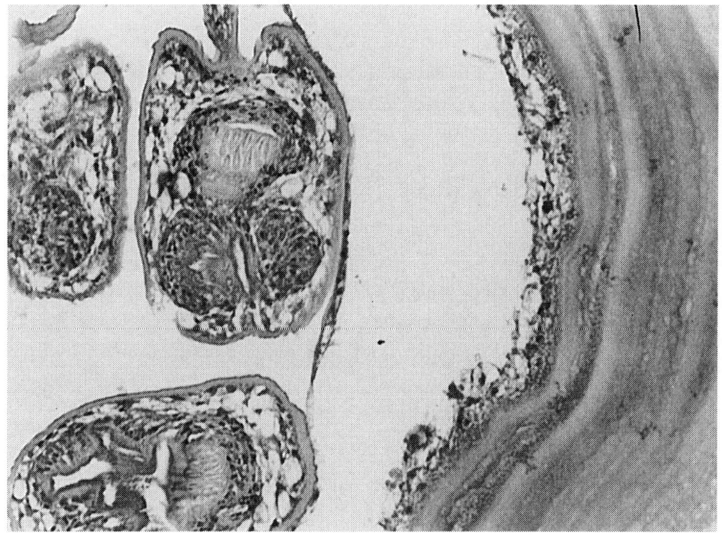

**Fig. 7-12. A**, Posterior fossa hydatid cyst; MRI T2-weighted image. **B**, Scolices with hooklets, germinative and laminated cuticle layer. Hydatid cyst, Brain biopsy, PAS.

### Trematodes

**Schistosomiasis.** Snails act as intermediate hosts for trematodes, such as *Schistosoma japonicum, S. mansoni,* and *S. hematobium,* the cause of this parasitic disease in Africa, South and Central America, and the Far East.[31] Frequent and large migrations have contributed to the geographic spread of the disease.

Once they enter the human body *S. japonicum* and *S. mansoni* predominantly inhabit superior and inferior mesenteric veins, whereas *S. hematobium* is found mainly in the veins around the urinary bladder. Eggs eliminated into water through feces or urine give rise to a miracidium that penetrates snails, where it reproduces asexually. Waterborne cercariae eliminated by snails gain entry through skin abrasions; after they become bloodborne, larvae reach first the lung through the veins and then the portal system, from which female worms travel to the peripheral veins. CNS involvement is an infrequent but severe complication. The spinal cord is more commonly involved by *S. haematobium* and *S. mansoni,* whereas brain is invaded by *S. japonicum*. Sphincter dysfunction and paraparesis are typical symptoms of conus medullaris involvement; lesions in this region produce a characteristic trident-shaped image at myelography.[38] Acute encephalitis may occur within months after the initial infection; chronic forms of schistosomiasis produce

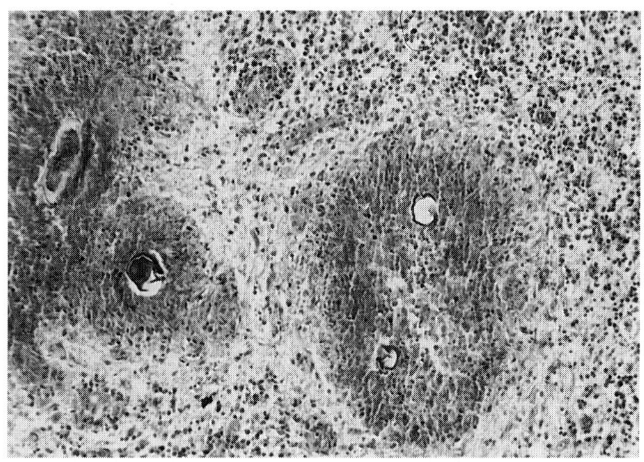

**Fig. 7-13.** *Schistosoma mansoni* ova surrounded by necrosis and inflammatory infiltrates in the brain. (H&E.)

either focal epileptic seizures or acute, subacute, or chronic myelitis. The immunologic diagnosis of this disease may be made either in the serum or the CSF. Granulomas in the form of tumors of variable size frequently develop in conus medullaris, and in the parietal and occipital lobes. At the site of brain involvement, the cortical vessels show yellowish granulations that contain calcified eggs surrounded by caseous necrotic tissue (Fig. 7-13); granulomatous inflammation with eosinophils, some multinucleated giant cells, and fibroblasts are also visible in the vessel wall. Surgical excision, in particular of lesions in the conus medullaris, may provide substantial improvement of symptoms.

## PROTOZOAL DISEASES

### Toxoplasmosis

This infection, caused by *Toxoplasma gondii*, may be acquired transplacentally, through intake of uncooked infected meat, and by inhaling or ingesting oocysts. Domestic cats acquire the disease from field mice and are the main reservoir and the main source of infection for humans.

Acquired toxoplasmosis often evolves with minimal symptoms; the early acute stage of infection is frequently followed by a chronic or late one. Most infected individuals remain almost asymptomatic, although on occasion, especially in immunosuppressed patients, cysts may rupture, leading to a particularly severe form of disease that includes CNS involvement. The dysfunction of cell-mediated immunity is paramount in determining the course of the infection. Moreover, evidence from experimental observations strongly suggests that steroids, cyclophosphamide, and total body irradiation may exacerbate chronic toxoplasmosis.[28]

A tropism of Toxoplasma for lymph nodes, muscle, myocardium, liver, and especially the CNS has been well recognized. Uveitis may occasionally present in adults, but lymphadenopathy accompanied by muscle aches, fever, and a transient skin manifestation are some of the acute expressions of infection.

The high percentage of positive serologic dye tests in the adult asymptomatic population (30% to 50%) reflects the profuse worldwide distribution of the acquired infection.[68] In addition to a dye test, hemagglutination and complement fixation tests are useful in the serologic diagnosis of toxoplasmosis. Serial serologic tests sometimes allow the differentiation between a recent infection and a chronic one, although only a small percentage of patients show increasing antibody titers.[110] In patients with encephalitis, detectable IgM antibody titers are suggestive of Toxoplasma infection, particularly when a fourfold increase in IgG antibody is demonstrable, but the diagnosis cannot be ruled out in patients whose antibody titers are low or undetectable. Susceptible patients and transplant recipients should be closely monitored with serial serum samples. Brain biopsy can be the only reliable procedure to diagnose toxoplasmic encephalitis.[28]

Primary maternal infection during pregnancy presents a high risk of placental transmission, especially after the end of the first trimester when the placenta is fully formed. The risk of fetal infection by Toxoplasma peaks at 6 to 7 months' gestation, although the extent of the CNS damage is milder than when transmission occurs early in gestation. Transplacental transmission may induce repeated abortion of infected fetuses or a congenital encephalopathy characterized, in its most severe form, by chorioretinitis, internal hydrocephalus, and extensive brain destruction. When brain destruction is less severe patients may develop seizures at a later date as the only clinical manifestation of congenital toxoplasmosis. Neuroimaging discloses dotted or curvilinear intracranial calcifications in periventricular locations. Indirect fluorescent antibody and IgM fluorescent antibody techniques may be useful for the diagnosis of congenital toxoplasmosis. In cases of severe congenital infection, the brain shows multiple foci of necrosis and calcification associated with the protozoal invasion of the brain parenchyma. In both gray and white matter and leptomeninges there is inflammatory infiltration of lymphocytes and plasmacytes; pseudocysts and free trophozoites also may be detected. Extensive necrosis may be the result of vascular inflammation and thrombosis secondary to contact between the Toxoplasma antigen and circulating passively transferred antibodies in the vessel walls.[138] Hydranencephaly is secondary to the destruction of the parenchyma as well as periependymal inflammation and aqueductal occlusion, with secondary thinning of the brain cortex (Fig. 7-14, *A*). The cerebellum, spinal cord, and nerve roots also may be involved in the inflammatory process.

Toxoplasmosis is the most frequent CNS opportunistic infection in patients with AIDS.[113] Immunosuppression promotes exacerbation of previous acquired infection that had remained latent in the form of pseudocysts; consequently, toxoplasmosis is a complication of organ transplantation and is often the initial expression of AIDS or HIV infection in otherwise asymptomatic patients.

On CT scan, Toxoplasma abscesses appear as isodense or hypodense single or multiple lesions in the cerebral parenchyma. Ring enhancement is particularly common in immunocompetent hosts; however, nonenhancing images also are compatible with a diagnosis of CNS toxoplasmosis.[147] In a clinical and neuropathologic study on cerebral toxoplasmosis complicating AIDS, CT scanning underestimated the number of lesions found at necropsy, whereas MRI had better sensitivity.[110] Imaging studies are hardly helpful in differentiating toxoplasmosis from lymphoma, although isolated brain lesions tend to be more common in lymphoma. Biopsy is essential to establish the diagnosis in patients presenting with single lesions at MRI.[27,29,31,44] Lack of improvement 2 weeks after starting specific treatment for toxoplasmosis or the appearance of a new lesion during therapy make a brain biopsy mandatory.[22]

Single or multifocal granulomatous lesions of toxo-

A B C D E

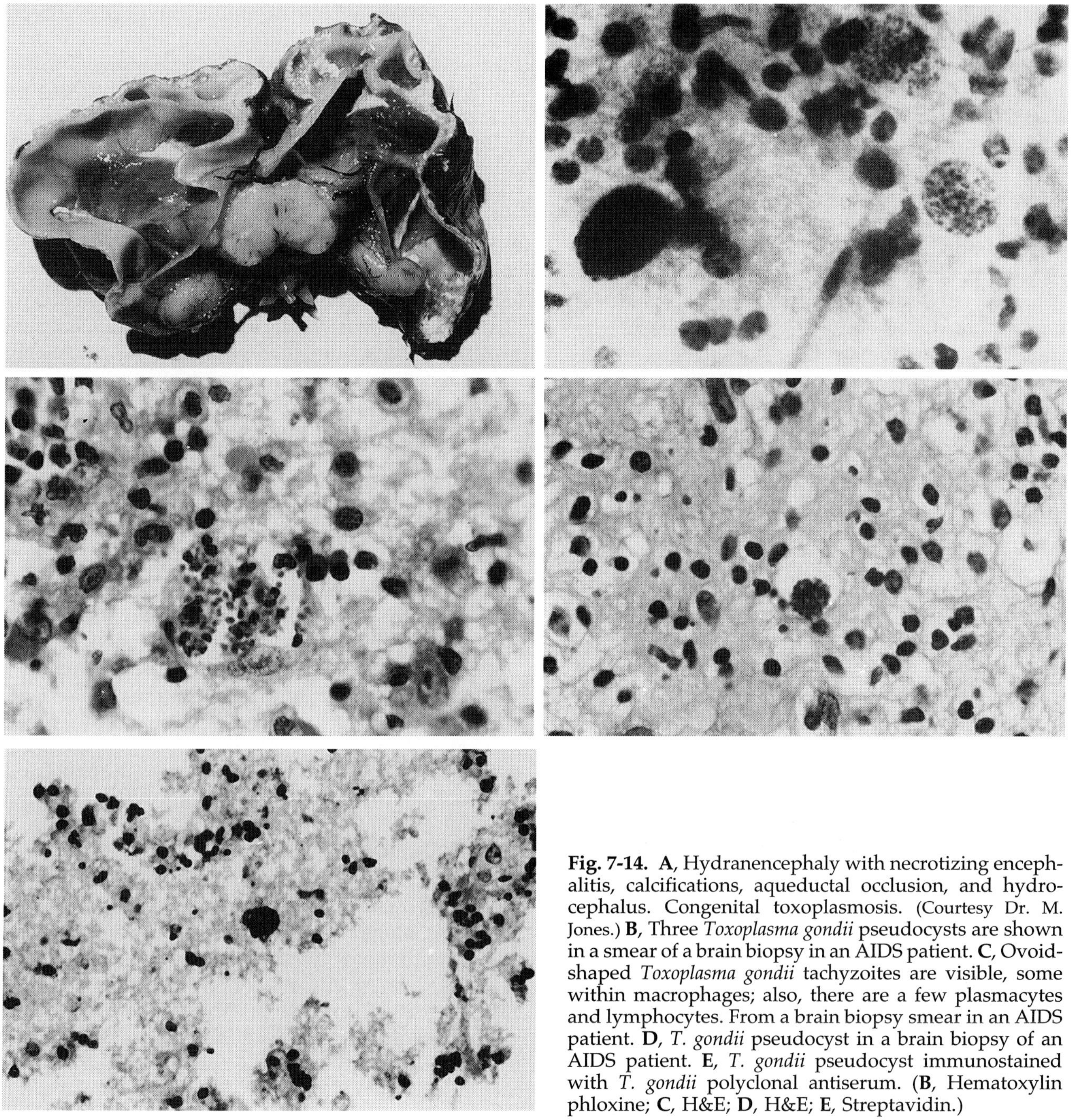

**Fig. 7-14. A**, Hydranencephaly with necrotizing encephalitis, calcifications, aqueductal occlusion, and hydrocephalus. Congenital toxoplasmosis. (Courtesy Dr. M. Jones.) **B**, Three *Toxoplasma gondii* pseudocysts are shown in a smear of a brain biopsy in an AIDS patient. **C**, Ovoid-shaped *Toxoplasma gondii* tachyzoites are visible, some within macrophages; also, there are a few plasmacytes and lymphocytes. From a brain biopsy smear in an AIDS patient. **D**, *T. gondii* pseudocyst in a brain biopsy of an AIDS patient. **E**, *T. gondii* pseudocyst immunostained with *T. gondii* polyclonal antiserum. (**B**, Hematoxylin phloxine; **C**, H&E; **D**, H&E; **E**, Streptavidin.)

plasmosis are located mainly in basal ganglia, thalamus, cerebellum, deep layers of the cortex, and white matter. At biopsy, most abscesses have a necrotic core where few tachyzoites are difficult to discern; often this area is surrounded by a vascular zone with macrophages full of trophozoites. Pseudocysts (or macrophages filled with organisms), inflammatory cells, isolated polymorphonuclear leukocytes, and an outer zone with reactive astrocytes make up the periphery of the lesion. Fibrinoid necrosis and thrombosis of blood vessels may occur when the necrotizing encephalitis is severe. As Toxoplasma are obligate intracellular parasites, they may be recognized at light microscopy in infected tissues as oval or crescent-shaped trophozoites measuring 3 to 6 $\mu$m in length inside macrophages or other cells, especially muscle fibers. Toxoplasma are also seen as rounded, 3-$\mu$m-diameter bradyzoites within a pseudocyst, where they may remain in a latent state. Staining with H&E or Giemsa allows recognition of pseudocysts or Toxoplasma-laden phagocytes; immunohistochemistry is useful to confirm the etiologic diagnosis by readily reacting with free trophozoites

(Fig. 7-14, *B* to *E*). Differential diagnosis with other intracellular organisms such as *Histoplasma capsulatum* is easy because of the characteristically strong staining of Histoplasma with PAS and Grocott's method. The main difference between tachyzoites and amastigotes is readily disclosed by the presence of a kinetoplast in the amastigote; the kinetoplast is evident at both light and electron microscopy.

A comparison between the cerebral lesions of toxoplasmosis among patients with early-onset and late-onset AIDS reported inflammatory cellular infiltration and fibrous capsule formation in the early diagnosis patients. Encapsulated bacterial abscesses superficially resemble those of toxoplasmosis. But Toxoplasma abscesses involve cerebral and cerebellar cortices as well as the overlying subarachnoid space, whereas bacterial abscesses usually remain confined to the white matter. Fibrous capsules are absent and neutrophils are abundant in Toxoplasma abscesses in AIDS patients whose untreated toxoplasmosis was a terminal complication of AIDS.[43,110]

Obtaining appropriate samples for diagnosis may be difficult because of the extensive coagulative necrosis and the alterations induced by the specific therapy. Toxoplasmosis, together with lymphoma and progressive multifocal leukoencephalopathy, have been the most frequent diagnoses of focal CNS lesions among AIDS patients.[29,31,46,147] JB Weiss has reviewed the detection of *T. gondii* DNA in human samples with DNA probes and PCR assays, including cases of immunocompromised HIV patients, congenital toxoplasmosis, and toxoplasmosis in immunocompetent subjects.[172] Treatments recommended for subclinical congenital toxoplasmosis include pyrimethamine and sulfadiazine, with folinic acid supplement. Spiramycin is alternated together with the above two drugs for subclinical and overt congenital infection.[95] In AIDS patients, induction therapy must be followed by maintenance anti-Toxoplasma therapy due to cyst resistance. Pyrimethamine plus sulfadiazine together with folinic acid is the regimen of choice, while steroids may be beneficial in severe cases.[96]

### Trypanosomiasis

**South American Trypanosomiasis (Chagas disease).** Chagas disease is endemic in Latin America. The etiologic agent, *Trypanosoma cruzi*, is a protozoan flagellate transmitted to humans by various species of hematophagous triatomine insects or reduviid bugs abundant in ramshackle dwellings. These insects nest in nooks and crannies and leave their shelters to feed at night. *T. cruzi* parasites in triatome feces gain entry through abrasions in the skin or mucous membranes. In tissues, the parasite adopts the amastigote form; after reproducing inside cells and provoking cell rupture, it invades the bloodstream as the trypomastigote form.[150] Acute disease in immunocompetent hosts is rare; this is because T lymphocytes play a major role in host defense against *T. cruzi*. Transmission of infection also may occur through blood transfusion[142] or transplacentally.

Most infected immunocompetent hosts remain asymptomatic for over 10 years, at which time they may develop megaesophagus, megacolon, and/or cardiomyopathy, lesions that are characteristic of chronic chagasic infection in endemic areas. Megaviscera are due to ganglion cell loss in the myenteric plexus secondary either to direct infection or antigenic responses. Cerebral neuronal "loss" in chronic disease has been attributed to the same pathogenesis. From a recent histopathologic and immunohistochemical study of the brain and heart in 50 patients with the chronic cardiac form, the authors concluded that there is no histopathologic basis to support the existence of the chronic CNS Chagas disease.[124] Acute cerebral involvement has been documented in children, generally 4 to 8 weeks after the infection. In endemic areas Machado-Guerreiro complement fixation test is routinely used in blood banks for the detection of the antigen. *T. cruzi* flagellates may be readily observed in the CSF and blood during acute infection.

Impaired cell-mediated immune systems among patients with neoplasia, in those receiving chemotherapy for chronic leukemia and lymphoma, and in organ transplant recipients make these patients susceptible to developing CNS trypanosomiasis secondary to reactivation of a previous infection, or to acquiring a new one through blood transfusion.

CT scanning may show one or multiple nodular brain lesions that enhance homogeneously with contrast; these lesions are frequently surrounded by a mild edematous region. Nonenhancing images also may be found in patients with cerebral trypanosomiasis[147] (Fig. 7-15, *A*). At MRI the lesions are hypointense and enhance with gadolinium-DTPA; more extensive areas of abnormality appear on T2-weighted images, and the mass effect is similar to the pattern of the lesions of toxoplasmosis.

The tissue responses of CNS trypanosomiasis may be those of a diffuse meningoencephalitis, or there may be single or multiple nodular lesions, soft in consistency and grayish with hemorrhagic areas. Brain cortex, cerebellum, and brainstem may all be involved by the process. Pseudotumoral nodular lesions (Fig. 7-15, *B*) similar to those of toxoplasmosis have been described in both HIV-infected patients and in immunosuppressed patients without HIV. Amastigotes measuring 2 to 5 $\mu$m, displaying a prominent nucleus, kinetoplast, and plasma membrane, can be readily seen even in intrasurgical smears either within macrophages (Fig. 7-15, *C*) or as individual organisms due to rupture of amastigote-laden macrophages. The ki-

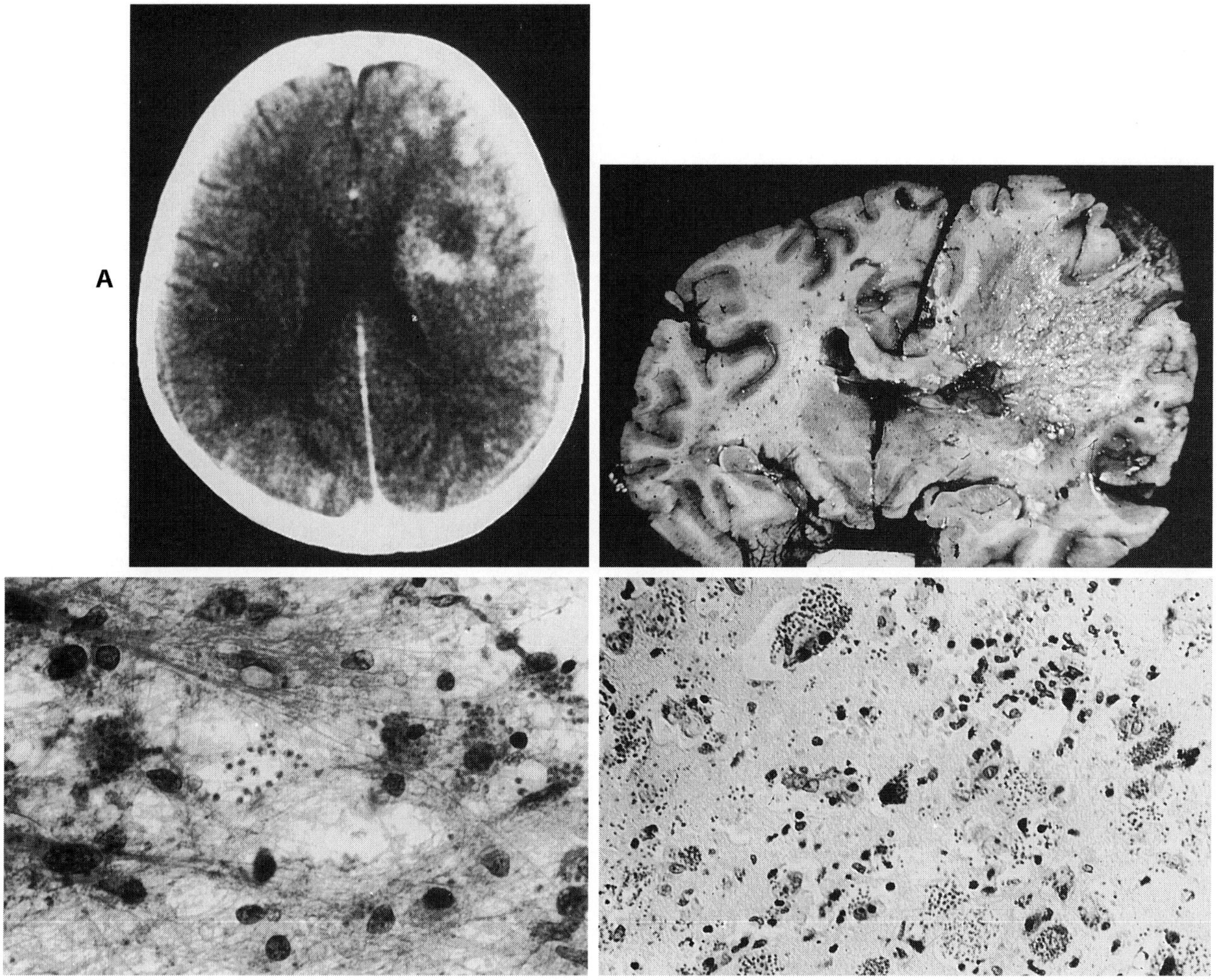


**Fig. 7-15.** **A**, Several cerebral lesions, the larger hypodense ones with ring enhancement are seen in Chagas infection in an immunosuppressed host. CT brain scan. **B**, Extensive pseudoneoplastic granulomatous chagasic lesion in the parietal lobe and centrum semiovale. Immunosuppression in the host was due to chemotherapy for leukemia. **C**, Macrophages laden with *T. cruzi* amastigote and a few free organisms are visible; nuclei and kinetoplast are evident. Smear of a brain biopsy in an AIDS patient. **D**, *T. cruzi* amastigotes in neurons and macrophages in brain autopsy samples of an immunosuppressed host receiving chemotherapy for Hodgkin's disease. **E**, *T. cruzi* immunostaining in amastigote-laden macrophages (*T. cruzi* polyclonal antiserum-streptavidin). **F**, *T. cruzi* amastigotes, nuclei, and kinetoplast are evident in brain samples from autopsy; fixation with formaldehyde. **G**, Acute chagasic myocarditis. Amastigotes within a myofiber. **H**, Trypomastigote of *T. cruzi* showing flagellum, nucleus, and terminal kinetoplast. Blood smear. (**C**, Hematoxylin phloxine; **D**, H&E; **F**, Electron microscopy; **G**, H&E; **H**, Giemsa.)

*Continued.*

netoplast is the main feature that differentiates Trypanosoma from Toxoplasma. Immunostaining with *T. cruzi* antiserum aids in the differentiation from other Trypanosoma and Leishmania. *T. gambiense* and *T. rhodesiense* are found in different endemic areas and fail to develop amastigotes within tissues; *T. rhodesiense* preferentially affects the skin and mucosa.

Coagulation necrosis, pyknotic debris, and a few inflammatory cells may be observed in most lesions of *T. cruzi*. Macrophages filled with amastigotes are the main component of the lesions; amastigotes also may be found in glial cells and neurons (Fig. 7-15, *C* to *F*) as well as in the myofibers (Fig. 7-15, *G*) of the heart and smooth muscle fibers of organs such as the bladder.

In HIV-positive hosts, a reactivation of a previous *T. cruzi* infection[134] or an increased susceptibility to infections through contaminated blood transfusions or cryoprecipitates may be the mechanisms of infection.[116] The possibility of iatrogenic infection is reinforced by the observation that immunosuppressed

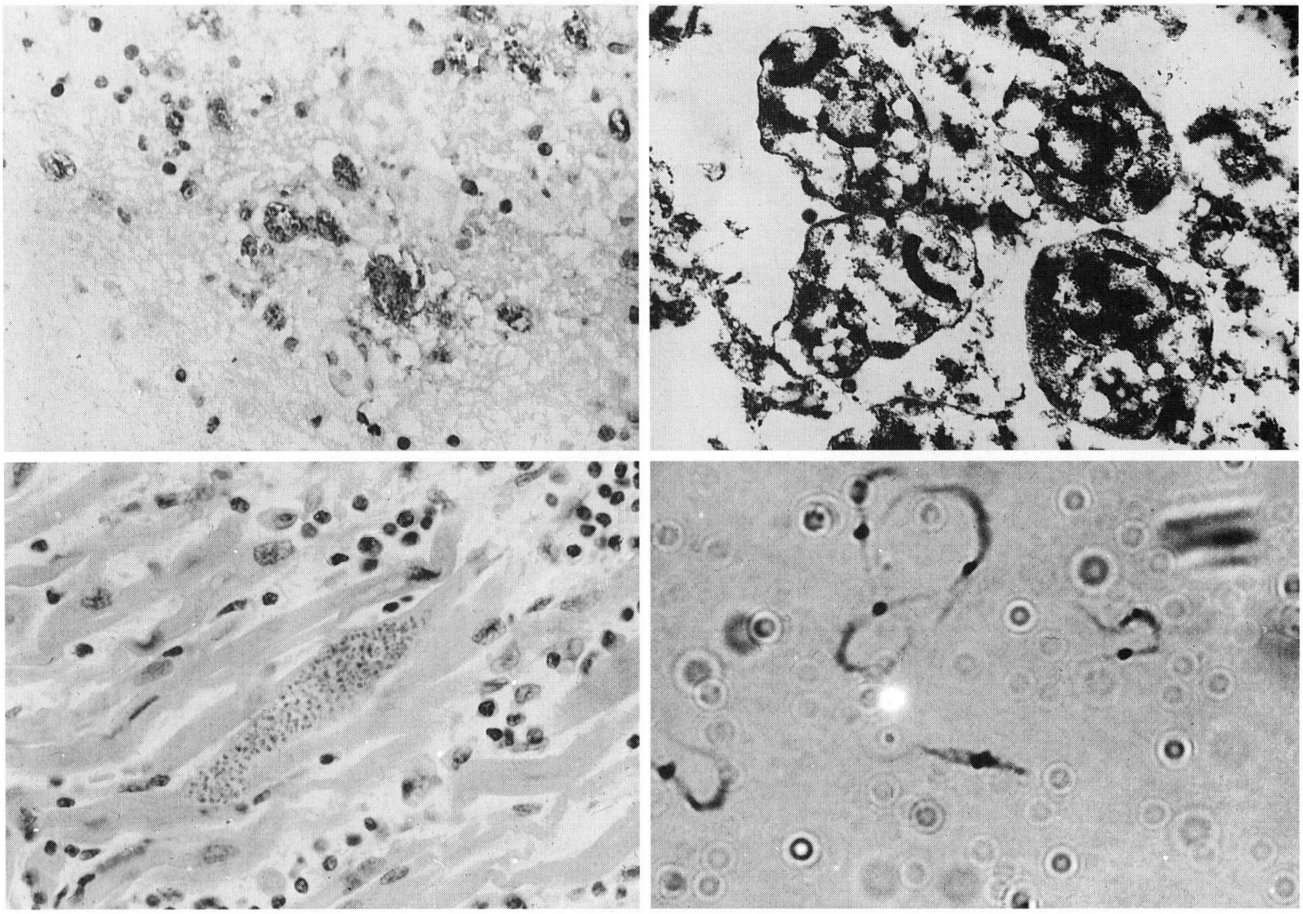


**Fig. 7-15, cont'd.** For legend see page 343.

children living in nonendemic areas may develop acute chagasic CNS lesions (personal unpublished observation).

We have studied four stereotaxic brain biopsies from HIV-positive adults with acute chagasic encephalitis, one of whom had received cryoprecipitates for hemophilia treatment.[147,155] Three open surgery brain biopsies were obtained from children, two of whom had received chemotherapy for chronic leukemia, and one of whom had hypogammaglobulinemia.[91] In addition, three CNS autopsies were from adult cases, one each with chronic leukemia, Hodgkin's disease, and kidney transplantation.[78,104] In all but one autopsy, chagasic CNS lesions displayed pseudotumoral features on clinical and neuroimaging grounds. In stereotaxic biopsied cases, the diagnosis of chagasic CNS provided the initial clue leading to the discovery of immunosuppression and HIV positivity.

Differential diagnosis from CNS toxoplasmosis or other opportunistic infections is impracticable on clinical and neuroimaging grounds alone without a brain biopsy, but in at least four of our cases *T. cruzi* flagellates were found in blood smears (Fig. 7-15, *H*) and in the bone marrow, both of which were examined after the brain biopsy was completed (unpublished personal observation). Direct examination of blood smears should precede invasive procedures in appropriately selected cases. In a recent review of the features of Chagas disease in AIDS and non-AIDS patients with fatal infections, only the immunosuppressed patients had chagasic lesions with tumorlike features.[129]

Prompt etiologic diagnosis of such pseudotumors is essential in order to start specific treatment with nitrofurans, even though complete recovery from the acute infection is seldom achieved.[78,104] Chagas disease should be considered in the differential diagnosis of acute CNS infections in immunosuppressed patients; the current migratory trends, particularly in individuals receiving repeated blood transfusions, make this diagnosis possible even in areas where trypanosomiasis is not endemic.[91] Since current serologic techniques present low specificity, a highly sensitive assay is required for diagnosis of *T. cruzi* infection. Several PCR assays have been developed to detect *T. cruzi* DNA directed to different gene targets and particularly useful for blood bank screening.[172]

**African trypanosomiasis.** *Trypanosoma gambiense* exists mainly in West Africa and *T. rhodesiense* in East

Africa; both are extracellular flagellate protozoa measuring up to 30 μm that may be found in body fluids and are the etiologic agents of African trypanosomiasis, a disease transmitted by the tsetse fly (genus Glossina). Humans and wild animals, respectively, are reservoirs for *T. gambiense* and *T. rhodesiense*. Over 50 million individuals are liable to contract the disease. Clinically a severe meningoencephalitis, known as sleeping sickness, may lead to death within a few months, especially in the more severe *T. rhodesiense* infections. A more protracted course of the disease may last for months or even years. Trypanosoma invades the bloodstream and promptly reaches the CNS, where it may remain latent and reenter the bloodstream. Clinical manifestations of the disease include cutaneous lesions at the portal of entry, followed 2 or 3 weeks later by fever and asthenia. Lymphadenopathy is characteristic in the *T. gambiense* infection, whereas hepatosplenomegaly and cardiac arrhythmias are more frequent with *T. rhodesiense*. Seizures and pyramidal and extrapyramidal signs may develop, together with impaired higher cortical functions; somnolence and nighttime restlessness are attributable to involvement by the infection of the ascending reticular activating system in the rostral mesencephalon.[23]

At autopsy, there is extensive leptomeningeal and perivascular infiltration by lymphocytes and plasmacytes full of Russell bodies that adopt a morular appearance. The brain parenchyma may show microglial nodules as well as profuse inflammatory infiltration in perivascular spaces. The cerebral cortex is primarily involved; secondary and severe autoimmune demyelination with subsequent gliosis involving cerebrum and cerebellum as well as generalized vasculitis (probably associated with autoimmune complexes) have been described. Intracellular leishmanoid or amastigote forms of *T. gambiense* and *T. rhodesiense* are not visible in many of the CNS lesions, although such intracellular forms latent in the choroid plexus have occasionally been described. The diagnosis of these infections may be achieved by detection of the Trypanosoma in the CSF, by inoculation of experimental animals, or by serum and CSF protein electrophoresis, showing a significant increase in IgG. Treatment with arsenical drugs that reach the CNS may prove toxic and lead to secondary hemorrhagic leukoencephalopathy.[3,38,82]

### Cerebral Malaria

Malaria, a widely distributed protozoan infection of humans, is produced by *Plasmodium vivax, falciparum, ovale,* and *malariae*. Each of these is transmitted to humans by the *Anopheles* mosquito that is abundant in tropical and subtropical regions; malaria also can be transmitted through blood transfusion. Almost one half million individuals are infected with plasmodia, and of those, around 50% are infected with *Plasmodium falciparum*, which produces a more severe type of disease,[152] including cerebral malaria in 1% of cases. Visitors entering endemic areas, infants and children, or immunosuppressed hosts lacking previous contact are more susceptible to clinical malaria.

The organism initially reaches the liver, where it develops and is later released as a merozoite that invades erythrocytes and completes its asexual cycle with extensive destruction of red blood cells, followed by further invasion of erythrocytes.

Symptoms at onset include lassitude and cephalea, accompanied by recurrent fever presenting intermittent peaks, on occasion associated with seizures that tend to be more severe in children and that may lead to status epilepticus, delirium, coma, and death from acute infection with *P. falciparum*.[169] Vomiting, diarrhea, and abdominal pain are common; impairment of high cortical functions suggests CNS tropism.

Several mechanisms have been proposed to explain the pathogenesis of cerebral malaria. The parasitized erythrocyte rapidly depletes blood glucose, and this causes hypoglycemia and lactic acidosis.[175] Parasitized red blood cells preferentially obstruct small vessels in the brain and adhere to the endothelial lining, a process enhanced by tumor necrosis factor (TNF) and other cytokines.[38,145]

Extensive brain capillary blockage by *P. falciparum*-laden erythrocytes best explains the severity of the lesions. Adherence to endothelial cells increases in the presence of electron-dense irregularities in the parasitized red blood cells; these form focal attachments to endothelial cells that are enhanced by development of endothelial pseudopodia.[103,117] Immune mechanisms also may be involved, as suggested by the demonstration of parasite-associated IgG and IgM in the capillary walls.[7,138]

Main findings at autopsy include opaque leptomeninges, diffuse brain edema, and abundant petechiae in the centrum ovale, internal capsule, and cerebellar white matter. Grayish discoloration of the cortex is the result of formation of a malarial pigment, hemozoin. By light microscopy merozoite-laden erythrocytes may be visible within obstructed capillaries (Fig. 7-16); this usually is accompanied by perivascular hemorrhages and focal brain necrosis, with some macrophages and reactive astrocytes visible in the white matter. Progressive gliosis of such lesions leads to the development of the so-called "Durk's granulomata."[159]

Searching for *Plasmodium* in blood smears usually is more fruitful than attempting diagnosis by serologic means alone.[38] Specific treatment with antimalarial drugs together with corticosteroids proves effective only when diagnosis is achieved early in the course of the infection.[33]

AIDS seemingly has not changed the course of cere-

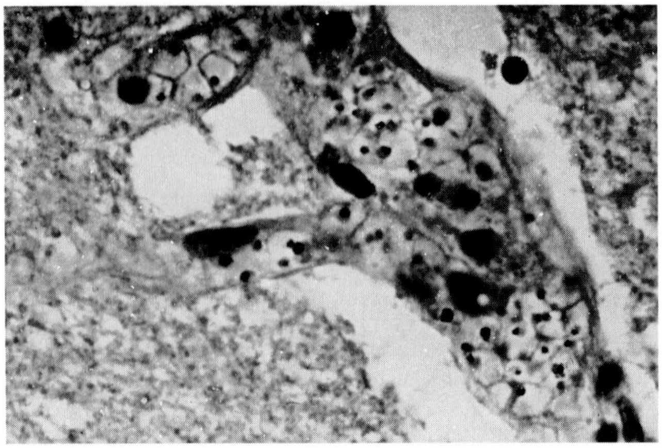

**Fig. 7-16.** Cerebral malaria. Cerebral venule packed with parasitized erythrocytes. Cerebral malaria. (Courtesy of Dr. L. Rorke.)

bral malaria.[88] Molecular biology techniques have been in use for *Plasmodium* DNA detection in whole blood samples by PCR.[172]

### Amebic Infection of the Central Nervous System

**Free-living amebic infection of the CNS.** Protozoa belonging to the genera *Naegleria, Acanthamoeba* and *Leptomyxidae* can infect both humans and animals.[97]

**Primary amebic meningoencephalitis.** Primary amebic meningoencephalitis (PAM) is a rapidly fatal meningoencephalitis induced by amebae of the genera *Naegleria,* which develop through trophozoite, cyst, or flagellate forms. The infection is acquired by immunocompetent hosts, mainly young adults, by swimming in stagnant water in swimming pools, or in artificial lakes. Entry is gained through the olfactory neuroepithelium. The amebae spread to the CNS along neural pathways; the incubation period is approximately 7 days, depending on the virulence and size of the inoculum. The clinical onset is abrupt, with progressive deterioration and fatal outcome in less than 2 weeks. CSF smears stained with Giemsa allow identification of characteristic trophozoites. A purulent leptomeningitis affects mainly the basilar cisternae and is accompanied by severe brain edema and small foci of hemorrhage. Necrosis, hemorrhage, mononuclear and polymorphonuclear infiltrates, vasculitis, and amebic trophozoites are all features of the disease. Trophozoites measure 10 to 20 $\mu$m in diameter; their cytoplasm frequently contains vacuoles and red blood cells; the nuclei have dense spherical nucleoli that contain a single large karyosome surrounded by a clear halo (Fig. 7-17, *A*). Processes called lobopodia emerging from the surface may be discerned in smears of the CSF. Cysts, measuring 10 $\mu$m in diameter, are spherical and refractile, but neither tissues nor body fluids disclose evidence of flagellates or cysts. Although trophozoites may readily be mistaken for macrophages in H&E stained histology sections, the amphophilic features of amebic nuclei and cytoplasm sharply contrast with the basophilic nuclei of macrophages.[114] Staining sections with Giemsa and iron hematoxylin is a useful means to identify amebae in tissues. The value of early diagnosis is highlighted by the survival of a few patients who received prompt treatment with amphotericin B.[144]

**Granulomatous amebic encephalitis.** Granulomatous amebic encephalitis (GAE) may be caused by different species of Acanthamoeba and by an agent of amebic meningoencephalomyelitis, order Leptomyxida,[10,165] classified as a new genus *Balamuthia* and described as *Balamuthia mandrillaris* (leptomyxid ameba; CDC VO39).[166] Both orders of amebae can be normal flora in healthy individuals; they have been found among others in samples of mineral water, in longstanding distilled water used for contact lenses, and in materials derived from dialysis machines. However, in immunodeficient hosts, including AIDS patients and organ transplant recipients, these opportunistic amebae are prone to induce disease. Amebic proliferation also occurs in weakened subjects with depressed cell-mediated immunity who may develop sudden infection of the CNS and other organs. Throughout the world over 100 cases of GAE have been attributed to infections with such free-living amebae. There were 65 cases in the United States, of which 30 involved HIV-positive subjects; 46 cases were secondary to infection with Acanthamoeba spp (29 with AIDS) and 21 with *Balamuthia mandrillaris* (2 with AIDS).[99] Latin American cases of GAE associated with Leptomyxida infections have been reported from Mexico,[130] Argentina,[154] Brazil,[30] and Venezuela,[98] thus highlighting the worldwide distribution of these organisms. Infection is acquired by hematogenous CNS invasion through a primary lung infection or skin abrasion; corneal ulcerations from a contact lens or infection of the olfactory mucous neuroepithelium also are possible routes of entry. The incubation period is roughly 10 days and the clinical course lasts several weeks. Multifocal lesions, showing contrast enhancement and tumor features on either CT brain scans or MRI T2-weighted images, may be observed (Fig. 7-17, *C*). Although hardly detectable on some lesions, the inflammatory infiltrate may feature lymphocytes and plasmacytes, with only a few polymorphonuclear leukocytes and multinucleated giant cells. Perivascular location and vasculitis are common. Individual trophozoites measuring 25 to 35 $\mu$m have a finely granular cytoplasm with vacuoles, a single nucleus with a central nucleolus (Fig. 7-17, *B* to *D*), and spinelike processes called acanthopodia evi-

A B C D

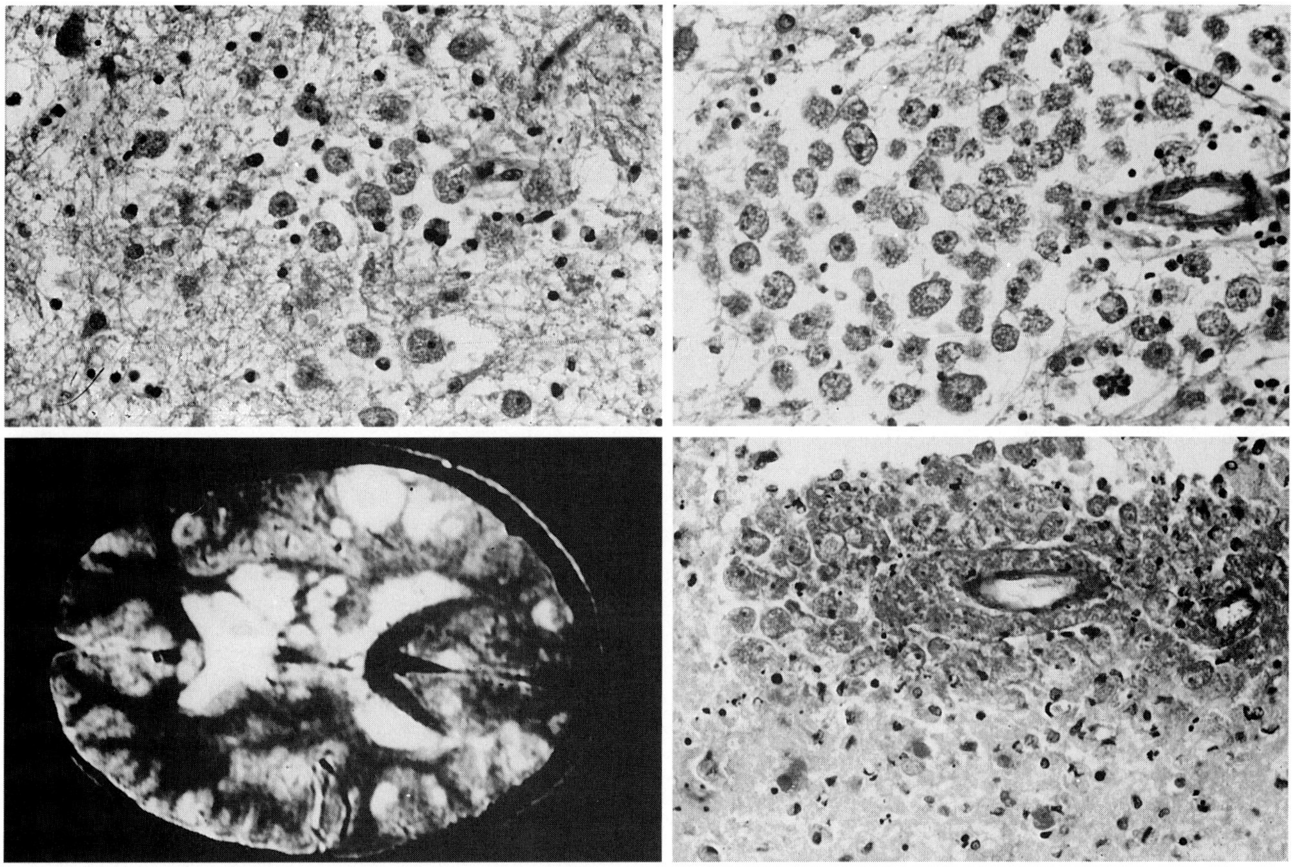

**Fig. 7-17.** **A**, *Naegleria* in brain autopsy from primary amebic meningoencephalitis. **B**, Perivascular acanthamoeba from brain autopsy of granulomatous amebic encephalitis. **C**, Multiple hyperintense round lesions in granulomatous amebic encephalitis in an immunosuppressed child. Brain MRI T2-weighted image. **D**, Perivascular leptomyxid from brain biopsy in a granulomatous amebic encephalitis in an immunosuppressed child. (**A**, H&E; **B**, H&E; **D**, Giemsa.)

dent at electron microscopy. Double-walled polygonal or spherical cysts, best discerned with PAS staining or methenamine silver impregnation, measure about 15 μm in diameter. Brain histology sections stained with H&E or Giemsa are useful in the diagnosis of amebic meningoencephalitis; differentiation of Naegleria from Acanthamoeba or Leptomyxid infections sometimes can be made on the basis of trophozoite size and the absence of cysts in Naegleria; however, precise characterization is based on immunofluorescence and immunoperoxidase assays with highly specific antisera. Rapid diagnosis allows early treatment, although Acanthamoeba is drug-resistant and response usually is poor.[82]

**Cerebral amebic abscess.** *Entamoeba histolytica*, the common etiologic agent of enteric infections, may lead to an amebic abscess in the brain through hematogenous dissemination. The organism may exist as a trophozoite or a cyst, although cysts do not appear in tissues. Brain abscesses coexist with similar lesions in the liver, may be single or multiple, and usually are rich in neutrophils and granulomatous tissue with lymphocytes and plasmacytes. Trophozoites, located at the edge of the lesions, are each 20 to 40 μm in diameter, have a round nucleus and nucleolus, and often harbor red blood cells in their cytoplasm.

## REFERENCES

1. Acha PN, and Szyfres B: Triquinelosis, in *Zoonosis y enfermedades transmisibles comunes al hombre y a los animales*. 503:865-879, 1986, Organización Panamericana de la Salud.
2. Adair JC, and others: Nocardial cerebral abscess in the acquired immunodeficiency syndrome, Arch Neurol 44:548-550, 1987.
3. Adams JH, and others: Human African trypanosomiasis (T.B. gambiense). A study of 16 fatal cases of sleeping sickness with some observations on acute reactive arsenical encephalopathy, Neuropathol Appl Neurobiol 12:81, 1986.
4. Adams M, and others: Whipple's disease confined to the central nervous system, Ann Neurol 21:104-108, 1987.
5. Agrawal, and others: Latex agglutination test negative cryptococcal meningitis in an immunocompetent individual: a case report, Clin Neurol Neurosurg 96:250-253, 1994.

6. Agrons GA, and others: MR imaging of cerebral gumma, Am J Neuroradiol 12:80-81, 1991.
7. Aikawa M: Human cerebral malaria, Am J Trop Med Hyg 39: 3-10, 1988.
8. Allo MDA, and others: Enlarging histoplasmosis following treatment of meningitis due to *Histoplasma capsulatum*, J Neurosurg 51:242-244, 1979.
9. Anderson DC, and Springer TA: Leukocyte adhesion deficiency: an inherited defect in the Mac-1, LFA-1 and p 150, 95 glycoproteins, Ann Rev Med 38:1975, 1987.
10. Anderson M: Leptomyxid ameba, a new agent of amebic meningoencephalitis in humans and animals, J Clin Microbiol 28: 2750-2756, 1990.
11. Andreula CF, Burdi N, and Carella A: CNS cryptococcosis in AIDS: spectrum of MRI findings. J Comput Assist Tomogr 17 (3):438-441, 1993.
12. Autran B, and others: AIDS in a Haitian woman with cardiac Kaposi's sarcoma and Whipple's disease (letter), Lancet 1:767-768, 1983.
13. Aydin Y, and others: Alveolar hydatid disease of the brain, J Neurosurg 65:115-119, 1986.
14. Ballard NB, and Vande Vusse FJ: *Echinococcus multilocularis* in Illinois and Nebraska, J Parasitol 69:790-791, 1983.
15. Bauserman SC, and Schochet SS Jr: Bacterial, fungal, and parasitic diseases of the central nervous system. In Nelson J, Parisi JE, and Schochet SS, editors: Principles and Practice of Neuropathology, St Louis, 1993, CV Mosby.
16. Beaman BL, and Ogata SA: Ultrastructural analysis of attachment to and penetration of capillaries in the murine pons, midbrain, thalamus and hypothalamus by Nocardia asteroides, Infect Immunol 61:955-965, 1993.
17. Bensaid AH, and others: Intracranial alveolar echinococcosis: CT and MRI Neuroradiology 36:289-291, 1994.
18. Benson CA: Disease due to Mycobacterium avium complex in patients with AIDS: epidemiology and clinical syndrome, Clin Infect Dis 18(Suppl 3):S218-222, 1994.
19. Berger JR, and others: Syphilitic cerebral gumma with HIV infection, Neurology 42:1282-1287, 1992.
20. Binford CH, and Meyers WM: Leprosy. In Binford CH, and Connor DH, editors: Pathology of Tropical and Extraordinary Diseases, Washington, 1976, Armed Forces Institute of Pathology.
21. Binford CH, and Dooley JR: Disease caused by fungi and Actinomycetes. In Binford CH, and Connor DH, editors: Pathology of Tropical and Extraordinary Diseases, Washington, 1976, Armed Forces Institute of Pathology.
22. Bise K, and others: The stereotactic biopsy diagnosis of focal intracerebral lesions in AIDS patients. Acta Neurol Scand 87: 228-233, 1993.
23. Brown J, and Voge M: Neuropathology of Parasitic Infections. New York, Oxford University Press, 1982.
24. Bruyn GW: Whipple disease. In Harris AA, editor: Handbook of Clinical Neurology, Amsterdam, 1988, Elsevier.
25. Campbell WC, and others: Clinical Aspects of Human Trichinellosis. In Veterinary Public Health Reports. Guidelines on Surveillance, Prevention and Control of Trichinellosis. Edit WHO and Inst. Sup di Sanitá, 1981.
26. Cartun RW: Immunohistologic diagnosis of infectious diseases: use of commercial reagents and methods, potential pitfalls and interpretation, United States and Canadian Academy of Pathology Meeting, Toronto 1995, booklet.
27. Ciricillo SF, and Rosenblum M: Use of CT and MR imaging to distinguish intracranial lesions and to define the need for biopsy in AIDS patients, J Neurosurg 73:720-724, 1990.
28. Couvrer J, and Desmonts G: Acquired and congenital toxoplasmosis. In Harris AA, editor: Handbook of Clinical Neurology. Amsterdam, 1988, Elsevier.
29. Chapell ET, Guthrie BL, and Orenstein J: The role of stereotactic biopsy in the management of HIV-related focal brain lesions, Neurosurgery 30:825-829, 1992.
30. Chimelli L, and others: Granulomatous amoebic encephalitis due to leptomyxid amoebae: report of the first Brazilian case, Trans R Soc Trop Med Hyg 86:635, 1992.
31. Chin LS, and others: Experience with image-directed stereotactic biopsy of CNS lesions in AIDS, J Neurosurg 72:355, 1990.
32. Cuadrado LM, and others: Cerebral mucormycosis in two cases of acquired immunodeficiency syndrome, Arch Neurol 45:109-111, 1988.
33. Daroff RB, and others: Cerebral malaria, JAMA 202:679-682, 1967.
34. Davis JP, and others: Recently recognized CNS infections: legionellosis, toxic shock syndrome, Lyme disease and Kawasaki disease. In Vinken PJ, and Bruyn GW, editors: Handbook of Clinical Neurology, Amsterdam, 1988, Elsevier.
35. Davis LE, and Kornfeld M: Neurocysticercosis: neurologic, pathogenic, diagnostic and therapeutic aspects, Eur Neurol 31: 229-240, 1991.
36. Despommier D, Symmans WF, Dell R: Changes in nurse cell nuclei during synchronus infection with *Trichinella Spiralis*, J Parasitol 77:290-295, 1991.
37. Di Lorenzo GA, Pagano MA, and Taratuto AL: Chagasic Granulomatous Encephalitis in Immunosuppressed Patients: computed tomography and magnetic resonance imaging findings, J Neuroimag 6:94-97, 1996.
38. Dumas M, Akani F, and Preux PM: Parasitology. In Duckett S, editor: Pediatric Neuropathology. Malvern PA, 1995, Williams & Wilkins.
39. Dyste GN, and others: Stereotaxis surgery in the treatment of multiple brain abscesses, J Neurosurg 69:188-194, 1988.
40. Eckert J, and others: Medical Aspects of Echinococcosis, Parasitology Today 11:273-276, 1995.
41. El Koussa S, and others: Trichinose e Occlusions sino-veineuses cerebrales, Rev Neurol 150:6-7, 446-447, 1994.
42. Ellrodt A, and others: Multifocal central nervous system lesions on three patients with trichinosis, Arch Neurol 44:432-434, 1987.
43. Falangola MF, Reichler BS and Petito CK: Histopathology of cerebral toxoplasmosis in human immunodeficiency virus infection: a comparison between patients with early-onset and late-onset acquired immunodeficiency syndrome, Hum Pathol 25:1091-1097, 1994.
44. Feiden W, and others: The stereotactic biopsy diagnosis of focal intracerebral lesions in AIDS patients, Acta Neurol Scand 87: 228-233, 1993.
45. Feigin RD, McCracken GH, and Klein JO: Diagnosis and management of meningitis, Pediatr Infect Dis J 11:785-814, 1992.
46. Finelli PF, and others: Whipple's disease with predominantly neuroophthalmic manifestations, Ann Neurol 1:247-252, 1977.
47. Fourestie V, and others: Neurotrichinosis: A cerebrovascular disease associated with myocardial injury and hypereosinophilia, Brain 116:603-616, 1993.
48. French MAH, Mallal SA, and Dawkins RL: Zidovudine induced restoration of cell mediated immunity to mycobacteria in immunodeficient HIV-infected patients, AIDS 6:1293-1297, 1992.
49. Gamble JR, and others: Stimulation of the adherence of neutrophils to umbilical vein endothelium by recombinant tumor necrosis factor, Proc Natl Acad Sci USA 82:8667, 1985.
50. Garcia-Monco JC, and Benach JL: Lyme neuroborreliosis. Ann Neurol 37:691-702, 1995.
51. Gay T, and others: Fatal CNS trichinosis, JAMA 247:1024-1025, 1982.
52. Gerda T, and others: Sensitivity and specificity of PCR for detection of *Mycobacterium tuberculosis*: a blind comparison study among seven laboratories, J Clin Microbiol 32:277-284, 1994.

53. Gherardi R, and others: Pathology of muscle in trichinosis: a series of 18 cases, J Neuropathol Exp Neurol 48:373, 1989.
54. Gimbrone MA Jr, Broch AF, and Schafer AI: Leukotriene B4 stimulates polymorphonuclear leukocyte adhesion to cultured vascular endothelial cells, J Clin Invest 74:1552-1557, 1984.
55. Giraldi C, and others: Cryptococcal meningoencephalitis in a non-immunocompromised patient: case report with necropsy, J Neurol Sci 14:79-81, 1993.
56. Gorman KJ, Saxon S, and Snead OC: Neurological sequelae of Rocky Mountain spotted fever, Pediatrics 67:354-361, 1981.
57. Gray F, Gherardi R, and Scaravilli F: The neuropathology of the acquired immune deficiency syndrome (AIDS): a review, Brain 111:245-266, 1988.
58. Gray F, and others: Pathology of the cerebral nervous system in 40 cases of acquired immunodeficiency syndrome (AIDS), Neuropathol Appl Neurobiol 14:365, 1988.
59. Gray F, and others: Neuropathologic study of 135 adult cases of acquired immunodeficiency syndrome (AIDS), Ann Pathol 4:236-247, 1991.
60. Halperin J, and Golightly M: Long Island Neuroborreliosis collaborative study group: Lyme borreliosis in Bell's palsy, Neurology 42:1268-1270, 1992.
61. Halperin J, Landis DMD, and Kleinman GM: Whipple's disease of the nervous system, Neurology 32:612-617, 1982.
62. Hanneman J, and others: Generalisierte nokardiose mit Meningoenzephalitis bei einer nicht immunosupprimier patientin, Dtsch Med Wochenschr 118:1281-1286, 1993.
63. Hansen K: Lyme neuroborreliosis: improvements of the laboratory diagnosis and a survey of epidemiological and clinical features in Denmark 1985-1990, Acta Neurol Scand 89(Suppl 151): 5-33, 1994.
64. Harcourt, and others: *Strongyloides stercoralis* hyperinfection in an HIV-positive patient, J Clin Pathol 44:346-348, 1991.
65. Harding CV: Blastomycosis and other opportunistic infections in patients with acquired immunodeficiency syndrome. Arch Pathol Lab Med 115:1133-1136, 1991.
66. Harris JO, and others: Listeria brain abscess in the acquired immunodeficiency syndrome, Arch Neurol 46:250, 1989.
67. Hartstein AI, and Winn RE: Aspergillosis. In Harris AA, editor: Handbook of Clinical Neurology. Amsterdam, 1988, Elsevier.
68. Hay J, and Hutchinson WM: *Toxoplasma gondii*: an environmental contaminant, Ecol Dis 2:33-43, 1983.
69. Hill JO, and Aguirre KM: CD4 T cell dependent acquired state of immunity that protects the brain against *Cryptococcus neoformans*, J Immunol 152:2344-2350, 1994.
70. Holmes AR, and others: Detection of *Candida albicans* and other yeasts in blood by PCR, J Clin Microbiol 32:1,228-231, 1994.
71. Hooper DC: Candidiasis. In Harris AA, editor: Handbook of clinical neurology. Amsterdam, 1988, Elsevier.
72. Horowitz H and others: Brief report: cerebral syphilitic gumma confirmed by the polymerase chain reaction in a man with human immunodeficiency virus infection, N Engl J Med 331: 1488-1491, 1994.
73. Horten BC, Abbot GF, and Porro RS: Fungal aneurysms of intracranial vessels, Arch Neurol 33:577-579, 1976.
74. Jamjoon ZAB and others: Intracranial epidural tuberculoma presenting as a scalp swelling. Surg Neurol 42:322-325, 1994.
75. Jasmer DP: *Trichinella spiralis*: subversion of differentiated mammalian skeletal muscle cells, Parasitology Today 11:185-188, 1995.
76. Johns DR, Tierney M, and Felsenstein D: Alteration in the natural history of neurosyphilis by concurrent infection with the human immunodeficiency virus. N Engl J Med 316:1569-1572, 1987.
77. Johnson L and Diamond Y: Cerebral Whipple's disease. Diagnosis by brain biopsy, Am J Clin Pathol 74:486-490, 1980.
78. Jost L, Turin M, and Taratuto AL: Meningoencefalitis chagasica en paciente con tratamiento immunosupresor por trasplante renal, Rev Neurol Arg 3:425-428, 1977.
79. Kammerer WS: Echinococcosis affecting the central nervous system, Semin Neurol 13(2):144-147, 1993.
80. Katz DA and Berger JR: Neurosyphilis in acquired immunodeficiency syndrome, Arch Neurol 46:895-898, 1989.
81. Kass PE, and Klein JO: Therapy of bacterial sepsis, meningitis and otitis media in infants and children: 1992 poll of directors of programs in pediatric infectious diseases. Pediatr Infect Dis J 11:702-705, 1992.
82. Kirkpatrick JB: Neurologic Infections due to bacteria, fungi and parasites. In Davis RL, and Robertson DM, editors: Textbook of Neuropathology, ed 2. Baltimore, 1991, Williams & Wilkins.
83. Kitamura T: Brain involvement in Whipple's disease: a case report, Acta Neuropathol 33:275-278, 1975.
84. Kovacs and others: Cryptococcosis in the acquired immunodeficiency syndrome. Ann Intern Med 102:533-538, 1985.
85. Kreel L, Poon WS, and Nainby-Luxmoore JC: Trichinosis diagnosed by computed tomography, Postgrad Med J 64:626-630, 1988.
86. Kuntzer T, and others: Borrelia rhombencephalomyelopathy, Arch Neurol 48:832-836, 1991.
87. Lahl R, and others: Zur diagnostischen Bedeutung des CT bei zerebraler Manifestation durch Morbus Whipple, Zentralbl Neurochir 47:301-310, 1986.
88. Leaver RJ, Haile Z and Watters DA: HIV and cerebral malaria. Trans R Soc Trop Med Hyg 84:201, 1990.
89. Le Blang SD, and others: CNS nocardia in AIDS patients: CT and MRI with pathologic correlation, J Comput Assist Tomogr 19:15-22, 1995.
90. Leers WD: North American blastomycosis. In Harris AA, editor: Handbook of Clinical Neurology. Amsterdam, 1988, Elsevier.
91. Leiguarda R, Roncoroni A, and Taratuto AL: Acute CNS infection by *Trypanosoma cruzi* (Chagas' disease) in immunosuppressed patients, Neurology 40:850-851, 1990.
92. Levy RM, Bredesen DE, and Rosenblum ML: Opportunistic central nervous system pathology in patients with AIDS, Ann Neurol 23, Suppl. 57, 7-12, 1988.
93. Lipton SA, and others: Candida infection in the central nervous system, Am J Med 76:101-108, 1984.
94. Lowenfeld IE: The Argyll Robertson pupil 1869-1969: A critical survey of the literature, Surv Ophthalmol 14:199-299, 1969.
95. Lowichik A, and Siegel JD: Parasitic infections of the central nervous system in children. I. Congenital infections and meningoencephalitis, J Child Neurol 10:4-17, 1995.
96. Lowichik A, and Siegel JD: Parasitic infections of the central nervous system in Children. II. Disseminated infections, J Child Neurol 10:77-87, 1995.
97. Martinez AJ: Free-living amebas: infection of the central nervous system, Mt Sinai J Med 60(4):271-278, 1993.
98. Martinez AJ, and others: Granulomatous amebic encephalitis: a review and report of a spontaneous case from Venezuela, Acta Neuropathol 87:430-434, 1994.
99. Martinez AJ and Visvesvara GS: Encephalitis by free-living amebas in the immunocompromised host, Brain Pathol 4:479, 1994.
100. Mawhorter SD, Kazura JM: Trichinosis of the central nervous system, Semin Neurol 13:148-152, 1993.
101. Michaud J: Neuropathology—Specialty Conference Handout, pages 4-5. United States and Canadian Academy of Pathology, Toronto, 1995.
102. McCormick GF, Zee Ch, and Heiden J: Cysticercosis cerebri. Review of 127 cases, Arch Neurol 39:534-539, 1982.
103. McPherson GG, and others: Human cerebral malaria. A quantitative ultrastructural analysis of parasitized erythrocyte sequestration, Am J Pathol 119:385-401, 1985.

104. Monteverde DA, Taratuto AL, and Lucatelli N: Meningoencefalitis chagasica aguda en pacientes immunosuprimidos, Rev Neurol Arg 2:260-266, 1976.
105. Morgello S, and Laufer H: Quaternary neurosyphilis in a Haitian man with human immunodeficiency virus infection, Hum Pathol 20:808-811, 1989.
106. Morgello S, and others: Central nervous system *Strongyloides stercoralis* in acquired immunodeficiency syndrome: a report of two cases and review of the literature, Acta Neuropathol 86: 285-288, 1993.
107. Munakata T, and others: Induction of interferon gamma production by human natural killer cells stimulated by hydrogen peroxide, J Immunol 134:2449-2455, 1985.
108. Murrel KD, and Bruschi F: Clinical Trichinellosis, Prog Clin Parasitol 4:117-148, 1994.
109. Naber SP: Molecular pathology—diagnosis of infectious disease, N Engl J Med 331:1212-1215, 1994.
110. Navia BA, and others: Cerebral toxoplasmosis complicating the acquired immune deficiency syndrome: clinical and neuropathological findings in 27 patients, Ann Neurol 19:224-238, 1986.
111. Neefe L, and others: Disseminated strongyloidiasis with cerebral involvement: a complication of corticosteroid therapy, Am J Med 55:832-838, 1973.
112. Negroni R: Estado actual del empleo de Ketoconazole en paracoccidioidomicosis (Ketoconazole 6 años después), Proceedings, International Conference on Paracoccidioidomycosis. Rionegro (Antioquia), Colombia. Corporación para Investigaciones Biológicas (CIB) 47, 1986.
113. Neuen JE, and others: Neuropathological studies in the brains of AIDS patients with opportunistic diseases, Int J Legal Med 105:339-350, 1993.
114. Niu MT, and Duma RJ: Amebic infections of the nervous system. In Harris AA, editor: Handbook of Clinical Neurology, 1988, Amsterdam, Elsevier.
115. Noordhoek GT, and others: Sensitivity of PCR for detection of *Mycobacterium tuberculosis*: a blind comparison study among seven laboratories: J Microbiol 32:2, 277-284, 1994.
116. Oddo D, and others: Acute Chagas' disease (*Trypanosomiasis americana*) in acquired immunodeficiency syndrome: report of two cases, Hum Pathol 23:41-44, 1992.
117. Oo MM, and others: Human cerebral malaria: pathological study, J Neuropathol Exp Neurol 46:223-231, 1987.
118. Pachner AR, and Delaney E: The polymerase chain reaction in the diagnosis of Lyme neuroborreliosis, Ann Neurol 34:544-550, 1993.
119. Pachner AR, and others: Inoculation of non-human primates with the N40 strain of *Borrelia burgdorferi* leads to a model of Lyme neuroborreliosis faithful to the human disease, Neurology 45:165-172, 1995.
120. Pachner AR, Duray P, and Steere AC: Central nervous system manifestations of Lyme disease, Arch Neurol 46:790-795, 1989.
121. Papasian CJ, and Parker JC: Bacterial and fungal infections. In Duckett S, editor: Pediatric Neuropathology. Malvern PA, 1995, Williams & Wilkins.
122. Persing DH, and others: Diagnostic Molecular Microbiology: Principles and Applications: American Society for Microbiology, Washington DC, Mayo Foundation, Rochester, 1993.
123. Pfister H, and others: Latent Lyme neuroborreliosis. Presence of *Borrelia burgdorferi* in the cerebrospinal fluid without concurrent inflammatory signs, Neurology 39:1118-1120, 1989.
124. Pittela JE, Meneguette C, and Barbosa AJ: Histopathological and immunohistochemical study of the brain and heart in the chronic cardiac form of Chagas' disease, Arch Neuropsiquiatr (Brasil) 51:8-15, 1993.
125. Powers JM, and Rawe SE: A neuropathologic study of Whipple's disease, Acta Neuropathol 48:223-226, 1979.
126. Powers J: Infectious diseases of the CNS, American Academy of Pathology Meeting, 1995, booklet.
127. Rangel Guerra R, Martinez HR, and Saenz C: Mucormycosis: a report of 11 cases, Arch Neurol 42:578-581, 1985.
128. Reid H, and Fallon RJ: Bacterial Infections. In Adams HJ and Duchen LW, editors: Greenfield's Neuropathology. London, 1992, Edward Arnold.
129. Rocha A, and others: Pathology of patients with Chagas' disease and acquired immunodeficiency syndrome, Am J Trop Med Hyg 50:261-268, 1994.
130. Rodriguez Jaramillo Y, and others: Encefalitis por una nueva ameba de vida libre, probablemente leptomyxid, Patologia (Mexico) 27:137-141, 1989.
131. Rogers W, and Nelson B: Strongyloidiasis and malignant lymphoma: "opportunistic infection" by a nematode, JAMA 195: 686-687, 1966.
132. Romanul FC, Radvany J, and Rosales RK: Whipple's disease confined to the brain: a case studied clinically and pathologically, J Neurol Neurosurg Psychiatry 40:901-909, 1977.
133. Roos KL, Tinkel AR, and Scheld WM: Acute bacterial meningitis in children and adults. In Scheld, Whitely RJ, Durack DT, editors: Infections of the Central Nervous System. Raven Press New York, 1991, Raven Press.
134. Rosenberg S, and others: Fatal meningoencephalitis caused by reactivation of *Trypanosoma cruzi* infection in a patient with AIDS, Neurology 42:640-642, 1992.
135. Rotterdam H: The acquired immunodeficiency syndrome and the evolution of new micro-organisms: a pathologist's view, Hum Pathol 24:935-936, 1993.
136. Ryser RJ, and others: Reversible dementia associated with Whipple's disease by trimethoprim-sulfomethoxazole, drugs that penetrate the blood-brain barrier, Gastroenterology 86:745-751, 1984.
137. Scaravilli F, and Gray F: Opportunistic infections. In Gray F, editor: Atlas of the Neuropathology of HIV infection. Oxford, 1993, Oxford University Press.
138. Scaravilli F: Parasitic and fungal infections. In Adams HJ, and Duchen LW, editors: Greenfield's Neuropathology. London, 1992, Edward Arnold.
139. Schaffner A, Douglas H, and Braude A: Selective protection against conidia by mononuclear and against mycelia by polymorphonuclear phagocytes in resistance to Aspergillus, J Clin Invest 69:617-631, 1982.
140. Scharf D: Neurocysticercosis. Two hundred thirty eight cases from a California hospital, Arch Neurol 45:777-780, 1988.
141. Schiffman E, and others: N-Formyl methionyl peptides as chemoattractants to leukocytes, Proc Natl Acad Sci USA 72: 1059, 1975.
142. Schmunis GA: Chagas' disease and blood transfusion. In Dodd RY, and Barker LF, editors: Infection, Immunity and Blood Transfusion. New York, 1984, Alan Liss.
143. Schochet SS, and Lampert PW: Granulomatous encephalitis in Whipple's disease. Electron microscopic observations, Acta Neuropathol 13:1-11, 1969.
144. Seidel JS, and others: Successful treatment of primary amebic meningoencephalitis. N Engl J Med 306:346-348, 1982.
145. Senaldi G, and others: Role of polymorphonuclear neutrophil leukocytes and their integrin CD11a (LF1) in the pathogenesis of severe murine malaria, Infect Immunol 62:1144-1149, 1994.
146. Sethi PP, and others: Ring or disc enhancing lesions in epilepsy in India, J Trop Med Hyg 97:347-353, 1994.
147. Sevlever G, and Taratuto AL: Stereotactic biopsy in HIV-related CNS lesions, Brain Pathol 4:486, 1994.
148. Sharer LR, and Kapila R: Neuropathologic observations in the acquired immunodeficiency syndrome, Acta Neuropathol 66: 188-198, 1985.

149. Smith AL, and Haas J: Neonatal bacterial meningitis. In Scheld WM, Whitley RJ, and Durack DT, editors: Infections of the Central Nervous System. New York, 1991, Raven Press.
150. Spina-Franca A, and Mattosinho-Franca LC: South American trypanosomiasis (Chagas disease). In Harris AA, editor: Handbook of Clinical Neurology. Amsterdam, 1988, Elsevier.
151. Steere AC, and others: Unilateral blindness caused by infection with Lyme disease spirochete, *Borrelia burgdorferi,* Ann Intern Med 103:382-384, 1985.
152. Sturchler D: How much malaria is there worldwide? Parasitol Today 5:39-40, 1989.
153. Tan V, and others: Histoplasmosis of the central nervous system, J Neurol Neurosurg Psychiatry 55:619-622, 1992.
154. Taratuto AL, and others: Leptomyxid *amoeba encephalitis*: report of the first case in Argentina, Trans R Soc Trop Med Hyg 85: 77, 1991.
155. Taratuto AL, Sevlever G, and Piccardo P: Clues and pitfalls in stereotactic biopsy of the central nervous system, Arch Pathol Lab Med 115:596-602, 1991.
156. Taratuto AL, and Venturiello SM: Trichinosis in Tropical Neuropathology, ed F. Scaravilli, Brain Pathol 7:663–672, 1997.
157. Taratuto AL, and Venturiello SM: Echinococcosis in Tropical Neuropathology, ed F. Scaravilli, Brain Pathol 7:673–680, 1997.
158. Toro-Gonzalez G: Paracoccidioidomycosis. In Harris AA, editor: Handbook of Clinical Neurology. Amsterdam, 1988, Elsevier.
159. Toro G, and Roman G: Cerebral malaria. A disseminated vasculomyelopathy, Arch Neurol 35:271-265, 1978.
160. Torre-Cisneros J, and others: CNS aspergillosis in organ transplantation: a clinicopathological study, J Neurol Neurosurg Psychiatry 56:188-193, 1993.
161. Tsang VCW, Brand JA, and Boyer AE: An enzyme-linked immunoelectrotransfer blot assay and glycoprotein antigens for diagnosing human cysticercosis (*Taenia solium*). J Infect Dis 159: 50-59, 1989.
162. Venezio FR, and Tucker PC: Zygomycosis (mucormycosis). In Harris AA, editor: Handbook of Clinical Neurology, Amsterdam, 1988, Elsevier.
163. Venger BH, Langdon G, and Rose JE: Solitary histoplasmoma of the thalamus: case report and literature review, Neurosurgery 20:784-787, 1987.
164. Vinters HV, and Anders KH: Neuropathology of AIDS. Boca Raton, Florida, 1990, CRC Press.
165. Visvesvara GS, and others: Leptomyxid ameba, a new agent of amebic meningoencephalitis in humans and animals, J Clin Microbiol 28:2750-2756, 1990.
166. Visvesvara GS, Schuster FL, and Martinez J: *Balamuthia madrillaris,* N. G., N. Sp., Agent of amebic meningoencephalitis in humans and other animals, J Euk Microbiol 40:504-514, 1993.
167. Waage A, and others: Association between tumour necrosis factor in serum and fatal outcome in patients with meningococcal disease, Lancet 1:355-356, 1987.
168. Walker DH, and Cain, BG: A method for specific diagnosis of Rocky Mountain spotted fever on fixed paraffin embedded tissue by immunofluorescence, J Infect Dis 137:206, 1978.
169. Warrell DA: Pathophysiology of severe falciparum malaria in man, Parasitology 94:853-876, 1987.
170. Weenink HR, and Bruyn GW: Cryptococcosis. In Harris AA, editor: Handbook of Clinical Neurology, Amsterdam, 1988, Elsevier.
171. Weidenheim KM, and others: Unusual patterns of *Histoplasma capsulatum* meningitis and progressive multifocal leukoencephalopathy in a patient with the acquired immunodeficiency virus. Hum Pathol 23:581-586, 1992.
172. Weiss JB: DNA Probes and PCR for Diagnosis of Parasitic Infections, Clin Microbiol Rev 8(1):113-130, 1995.
173. Wheat LJ, and Batteiger BE: Histoplasmosis. In Harris AA, editor: Handbook of Clinical Neurology. Amsterdam, 1988, Elsevier.
174. Wheat IJ, Kohler RB, and Tweari RP: Diagnosis of disseminated histoplasmosis by detection of *Histoplasma capsulatum* antigen in serum and urine specimens, N Engl J Med 314:83-88, 1986.
175. White NJ, and Looareesuwan S: Cerebral malaria. In Kennedy PGE, Johnson RT, editors: Infections of the nervous system, London, 1987, Butterworths.
176. Wicher K: Brief report: cerebral syphilitic gumma confirmed by the polymerase chain reaction in a man with human immunodeficiency virus infection, N Engl J Med 331:1488-1491, 1994.
177. Wiles CM, and others: Aspergillus granuloma of the trigeminal ganglion. J Neurol, Neurosurg Psychiatry 44:451-455, 1981.
178. Wilson M, and Schantz P: Nonmorphological diagnosis of parasitic infections in Balows A, and others, editors: Manual of Clinical Microbiology, ed 5, Washington DC, American Society for Microbiology, 1991.
179. Winn RE and Hartstein AI: Coccidioidomycosis, In Harris AA, editor: Handbook of Clinical Neurology. Amsterdam, 1988, Elsevier.
180. Woo ML, Leung JWC, and French GL: Rickettsial infection presenting as culture negative meningitis. Postgrad Med J 64:614, 1988.
181. Yim Y, and others: Fatal strongyloidiasis in Hodgkin's disease after immunosuppressive therapy, J Trop Med Hyg 73:245-249, 1970.

C • H • A • P • T • E • R

# 8

# *Viral Infections*

**Herbert Budka**



Neurovirology is one of the most fascinating fields in research on diseases of the nervous system. Interactions between the most sophisticated organ known and a group of highly versatile pathogens lead to an amazingly broad spectrum of disease manifestations that range from pathologic malformations to neoplastic lesions, necrotizing damage, inflammation and immunopathology, and primarily neurodegenerative processes. For decades a viral etiology has been sought for many neuropsychiatric diseases, such as multiple sclerosis and schizophrenia; when these early efforts met with disappointing results, much interest was lost. Recently, however, there has been renewed interest in this field, e.g., the relationship between Borna virus and neuropsychiatric illness.[107] When Richard T. Johnson published his classic textbook on viral diseases of the nervous system,[89] most chapters dealt with relatively rare, almost exotic conditions and our knowledge of their pathogenesis and therapy was very limited. Now, only 15 years later, the situation has changed dramatically. Our pathogenetic understanding, still incomplete, has improved, but these diseases are no longer truly rare. Enormous progress has been made in developing diagnostic tools and therapy. Thus neurovirology has come back to the center stage of both basic and clinical neurosciences.

Much of the recent increased interest in neurovirology has been caused by the acquired immunodeficiency syndrome (AIDS) pandemic. Viral infections of the nervous system are frequent complications of AIDS, with high morbidity and mortality. In addition to the still enigmatic effects on the brain of the human immunodeficiency virus (HIV) itself, the nervous system in AIDS is affected by two main groups of viruses: the herpesviruses [primarily cytomegalovirus (CMV), less frequently varicella zoster virus (VZV), and rarely herpes simplex virus (HSV)], and the papovaviruses. The herpesviruses cause variable neuropathologic manifestations, while the JC papovavirus produces a single, well-defined disease: progressive multifocal leukoencephalopathy (PML).

## CLINICAL AND VIROLOGIC DIAGNOSTIC ASPECTS OF VIRAL INFECTIONS OF THE NERVOUS SYSTEM AND THE NEUROPATHOLOGIST

Increasingly, neuropathologists must deal with diagnostic aspects of viral diseases, e.g., in stereotaxic brain biopsies or autopsies of HIV-infected patients. However, they are only part of the team responsible for the completion of optimal diagnostic procedures, which must also consider clinical and virologic investigations.

Clinical information is of paramount importance. It must include the results of neuroimaging studies, which serve as a guideline for adequate tissue sampling. Whenever possible, material should be preserved for virologic examination, especially for serology, culture assays, and the polymerase chain reaction (PCR). Many viral infections of the nervous system also involve the respiratory or gastrointestinal systems, and it is prudent to sample these organs as well whenever possible. When very little CNS tissue is available, e.g., in stereotaxic brain biopsies, it may be difficult to satisfy all tissue needs for additional diagnostic techniques. In such situations it is a matter of personal judgment to set priorities. While no general recommendations can be made and every case is individual and must be handled accordingly, neuropathologists must never forget that they are the first and most important line of diagnosis whenever tissue is sampled from the nervous system. Given that a suspected virus-induced lesion might turn out to be a tumor, an infarction, or some other pathologic condition, histologic examination still has top priority in working up a surgical specimen.

## NEUROPATHOLOGIC DIAGNOSIS OF VIRAL INFECTIONS OF THE NERVOUS SYSTEM

Fortunately, many viral infections run a favorable course, e.g., aseptic meningitis or mild meningoencephalitis, and only exceptionally represent a diagnostic task for the neuropathologist. More fulminant conditions may require neurosurgical biopsies or will be seen only at autopsy. Even if adequate material is available for further diagnostic tests, it is the histologic evaluation that decides primarily whether tissue pathology is suspicious for viral disease of the nervous system and whether (and which) other techniques may be useful. Although a wide variety of neuropathologic changes, as detailed later, may be found for specific viruses, it is mainly inflammation—at least in the immunocompetent host—in a given pattern that suggests viral disease. By plain histology, the essential features are the classic triad of the encephalitic (and/or myelitic) syndrome:

- parenchymal damage (e.g., neuronophagia or demyelination)
- reactive astrocytosis and microgliosis
- inflammatory cellular infiltration

Spatz[162] is credited for having emphasized the importance in etiologic considerations of determining the distribution and spread of these inflammatory changes. Of his six types of encephalitis, the patterns of continuous polioencephalitis (e.g., in subacute sclerosing panencephalitis [SSPE]) and of patchy-nodular polioencephalitis (e.g., in poliomyelitis, acute encephalitis by flaviviruses, togaviruses, and enteroviruses) are seen in viral infections. Only later was the predominant involvement of the white matter noted in PML, HIV encephalitis or leukoencephalopathy, and some cases of SSPE and VZV infection. In addition to the inflammatory quality and characteristic distribution of the tissue lesions, such cytologic features as inclusion bodies or cytomegalic cell change can give important diagnostic clues on routine stains, especially when the involved cell type is considered. Every viral infection of the nervous system usually features a fingerprint signature of selective vulnerability in the nervous system. Table 8-1 summarizes the characteristic cellular

**Table 8-1.** Cellular and regional tropism, as seen by productive tissue infection (ICC and/or ISH), in selected viral infections of the nervous system

| Disease | Cellular specificity | Regional selectivity |
|---|---|---|
| HSV encephalitis | Absent (all cell types affected) | High (limbic system) |
| VZV disease | Absent (all cell types affected) | Zoster: very high (ganglia, central projection nuclei)<br>VZV encephalomyelitis: variable |
| CMV disease | Absent (all cell types affected) | Moderate (preference of periventricular and superficial brain; cauda and roots) |
| Tick-borne encephalitis | High (neurons, ev. ependyma) | Moderate (preference of brainstem, cerebellum, spinal cord) |
| Poliomyelitis | High (neurons) | High (motoneurons) |
| SSPE | High (large neurons, oligodendroglia) | Low (usually cerebellum and spinal cord spared) |
| PML | High (oligodendroglia, astroglia) | Absent |
| Rabies | Very high (neurons) | Moderate (preference of hippocampus, cerebellum) to absent (progressed stage) |
| HIV encephalitis/ leukoencephalopathy | High (microglia/macrophages) | Moderate (preference of white matter, basal ganglia) to absent |

and regional tropism and Table 8-2 shows the distribution of inclusion bodies to specific neural cell populations in viral infections of the nervous system. Although inclusion bodies traditionally are held to be characteristic for viral infections, they are by no means specific, and their *absence* does not rule out a viral etiology. Unfortunately, immunosuppression and the effects of potent therapies notoriously modify, blur, or even wipe out the classic features of specific viral lesions. Again, only adequate clinical information can help one avoid diagnostic pitfalls. Nevertheless, most viral infections of the nervous system feature characteristic neuropathologic diagnostic hallmarks, and these are listed in this chapter for each major entity.

Neuropathologists can give an etiologic diagnosis only if they can visualize the virus or its products in diseased tissue. Thus it is productive virus infection of the nervous system that is the topic of this chapter.

**Table 8-2.** Distribution of inclusion bodies among neural cell populations in selected viral infections of the nervous system

| | Site of inclusion body | | Cell tropism of inclusion body | | |
|---|---|---|---|---|---|
| Virus/disorder | Intra-nuclear | Intra-cytoplasmic | Neurons | Glia | Other (vessels, meninges etc.) |
| Acute HSV encephalitis | + | | + | + | + − |
| CMV encephalitis | + | + | + | +* | + |
| VZV ganglionitis/encephalitis/ myelitis | + | | + | +* | + − |
| Rabies | | + | + | | |
| SSPE, measles inclusion body encephalopathy | + | + | + | +** | |
| PML | + | | | +*** | |

* May include ependyma, satellite and Schwann cells
** Usually oligodendroglia much more involved than astroglia
*** Almost exclusively in oligodendroglia

A B C

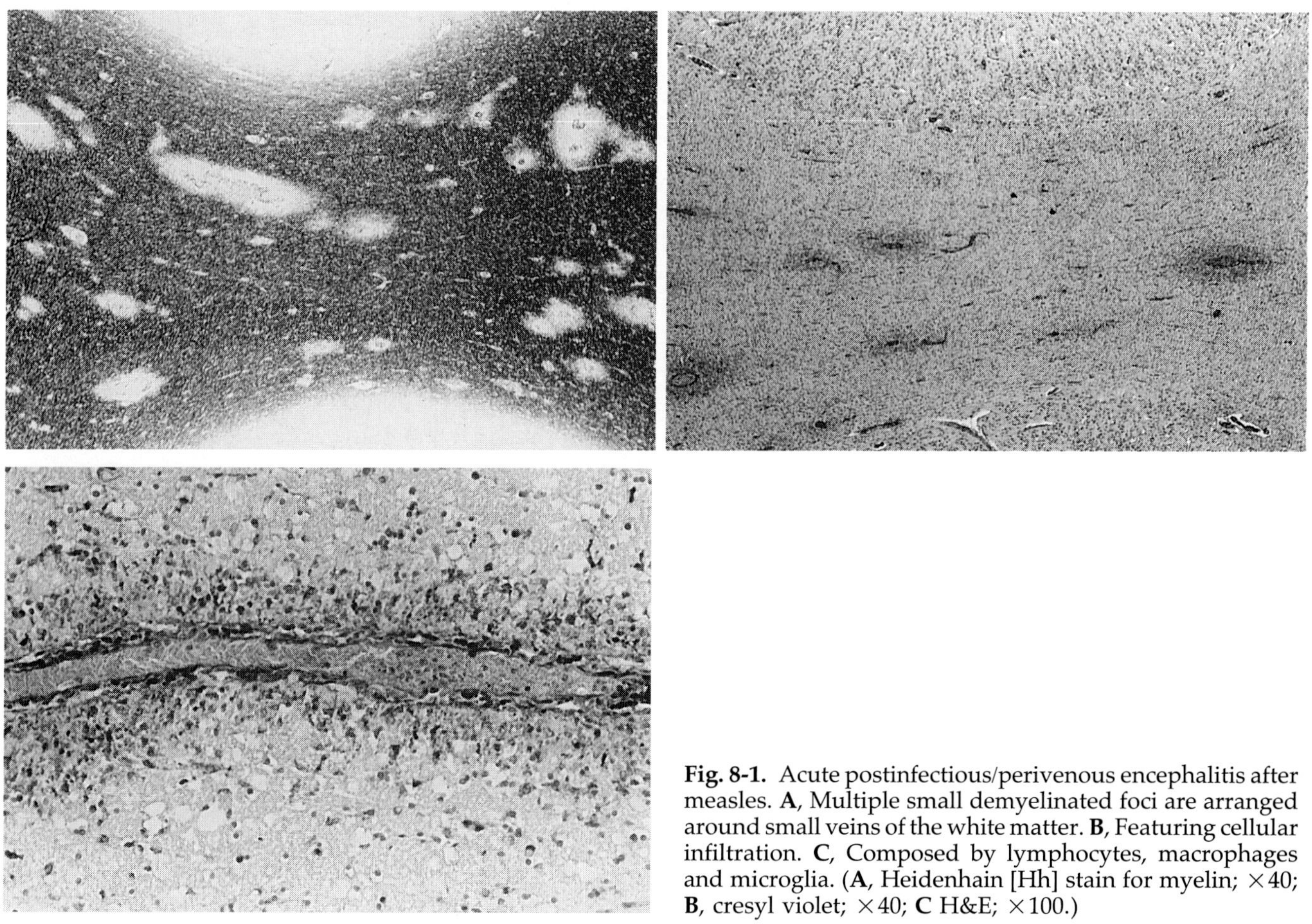

**Fig. 8-1.** Acute postinfectious/perivenous encephalitis after measles. **A**, Multiple small demyelinated foci are arranged around small veins of the white matter. **B**, Featuring cellular infiltration. **C**, Composed by lymphocytes, macrophages and microglia. (**A**, Heidenhain [Hh] stain for myelin; ×40; **B**, cresyl violet; ×40; **C** H&E; ×100.)

However, it must be remembered that viruses may damage the nervous system by indirect means as well. The best example of this damage is the postinfectious/perivenous encephalitis that occurs as immune-mediated sequel to exanthematous viral disease of childhood, e.g., measles, varicella, rubella or mumps, or influenza. This topic is not covered here, but is very important in making a differential diagnosis from productive viral encephalomyelitis: multiple small demyelinated foci are arranged around small veins of the white matter (Fig. 8-1, *A*), featuring cellular infiltration (Fig. 8-1, *B*) composed of lymphocytes, macrophages, and microglia (Fig. 8-1, *C*). Since this chapter aims at practical diagnostic work, it covers only selected infections that may be fatal and that exhibit more or less characteristic neuropathologic changes. Many systemic viral diseases common in the tropics also may involve the nervous system in one way or another, but these are not covered here.

Viruses have been considered as "neurotropic" as long as they demonstrate the classic triad: neuroinvasiveness (the ability to enter the nervous system), neurovirulence (the ability to cause disease in the nervous system), and the ability to replicate in nervous system elements proper.[89] With increased knowledge, this classic concept has to be reevaluated: the ability of HIV, for example, is still controversial in replicating in truly neuroectodermal elements, although both of the other criteria certainly apply.

Until the advent of special techniques, discussed in the next section, electron microscopy had a decisive role in neuropathologic diagnosis of viral infections. While interesting research information still can be obtained from ultrastructural studies, e.g., on the maturation process of viral particles in specific cell types, electron microscopy has lost much of its importance as a diagnostic tool for studying neuropathologic specimens and is now applied only in special situations.

### The Role of Special Techniques: Immunocytochemistry, In Situ Hybridization, Polymerase Chain Reaction

Perhaps the field of viral infections is where the techniques of immunocytochemistry (ICC), in situ hybridization (ISH), and polymerase chain reaction (PCR) have had the most profound impact on diagnosis in neuropathology. When done appropriately with adequate controls and adequate tissue selection, these techniques provide an etiologic diagnosis of high sensitivity and specificity. Nevertheless, there are caveats for situations in which they may not be diagnostic:

- Virus production may have burnt out or viral products may have become masked, resulting in negative ICC or ISH.
- Tissue preservation might be unsuitable for these techniques, e.g., ICC or ISH may be falsely negative in overfixed tissue, or nucleic acid amplification from paraffin-embedded tissue by PCR may be blocked by yet unidentified factors.
- Since PCR, and, to a much lesser degree, ISH, are extremely sensitive techniques, they might give positive results just by reflecting the mere presence of viral genomic information. This could result from dormant or latent infection and does not necessarily mean productive infection; thus, a "positive" result might have no pathogenetic relationship to tissue pathology.

Prerequisites for the use of ICC, ISH, or PCR for neuropathologic diagnosis of viral infections include:

- Simultaneous use of known positive and negative control tissues that were processed in the identical manner as the material to be examined.
- Availability of reagents (antibodies, probes, primers) with defined specificities.
- Adequate testing of reagents on control tissues for highest sensitivity (optimal signal-to-noise ratio) in the respective laboratory. To control sensitivity, it is wise to use material with a possible minimum of viral load rather than to use control sections loaded with virus.
- In many situations, experience with immunocytochemical antigen retrieval techniques such as enzyme digestion, microwave treatment, or autoclaving.

It is necessary for each laboratory to do its own testing. Never rely only on information given in product data sheets (or textbook articles such as this!). Both polyclonal and monoclonal antibodies may be suitable for diagnosis. For fixed tissues, polyclonal antibodies have the advantage of being able to bind to several antigenic sites, thus yielding some signal, even when some sites may be damaged by fixation. Monoclonal antibodies (McAb) sometimes work beautifully, e.g., on Western blots, but, for some poorly understood reasons, there is no guarantee that they will work similarly in ICC, and vice versa. If McAbs work, they have the advantage that batches do not differ in reactivity, and this may not be true for polyclonals. For many years, I have successfully used antibodies and DNA probes for neuropathologic diagnosis of selected viral infections on routinely processed (i.e., formaldehyde-fixed and paraffin-embedded sections) as listed in Table 8-3, which is presented as a guideline for source, tissue pretreatment, and optimal dilution range. For polyclonal antibodies, I use the peroxidase-antiperoxidase (PaP) detection system with diaminobenzidine (DAB) as chromogen; for monoclonals, the labeled biotin-avidin-proxidase complex (ABC) technique with

**Table 8-3.** Antibodies and DNA probes used for neuropathologic diagnosis of selected viral infections on routinely processed*

| Virus/viral product | Type | Clone | Tissue pretreatment | Optimal dilution in our lab | Source | Comment | Reference |
|---|---|---|---|---|---|---|---|
| CMV | mc | CCH2 | Protease | 1:20 | Dako | | 156 |
| HIV-1 p24 | mc | Kal-1.(1) | Protease | 1:5 | Dako | | 24,111,153 |
| HIV-1 gp41 | mc | | Boil in citrate buffer for 10 min. | 1:10 | DuPont | | 24,111,153 |
| SV40 T-antigen | mc | Pab 416 | Protease | 1:100 | Oncogene Science | Little sensitivity on paraffin sections | 155 |
| VZV gp | mc | 8 TDA 1986 | Protease | 1:2.000 | Dr. T. Kurata, Tokyo | Store at −20° C | 154 |
| VZV np | mc | 170.1 | Protease | 1:1.000 | Dr. T. Kurata, Tokyo | Store at −20° C | 154 |
| CEE/TBE (KV Hochosterwitz) | pc | | Protease | 1:20 | Dr. F. X. Heinz Vienna | Store at −20° C | 133 |
| HSV type 1 | pc | | | 1:100 | Dako | | 35 |
| HSV type 1 | pc | | Protease | 1:500 | Biomeda | Useful for typing | 151,152 |
| HSV type 2 | pc | | Protease | 1:200 | Dako | | 151,152 |
| HSV type 2 | pc | | | 1:50 | Biomeda | Useful for typing | 151,152 |
| Measles | pc | | | 1:100 | Dr. P. Halonen Turku | Store at −20° C | 29,33,38 |
| Papovavirus (81-298) | pc | | Protease | 1:200 | Dr. K. V. Shah, Baltimore | Genus-specific general antiserum; store at −20° C | 26,37,155 |
| JCV (80–140) | pc | | Protease | 1:20 | Dr. K. V. Shah, Baltimore | JCV-specific but little sensitivity on paraffin sections; store at −20° C | 37,155 |
| Rabies | pc (hamster) | | | 1:5.000 | Bundesanstalt f. Tierseuchenbekämpfung, Mödling | Store at −20° C | 26,35,36,112 |
| HSV types 1 & 2 | Bio-probe® | | Proteinase K | 1:5 in hybridization mix | ENZO | | 151,152 |
| CMV | Bio-probe® | | Proteinase K | 1:5 in hybridization mix | ENZO | | 156 |
| JCV | Bio-probe® | | Proteinase K | 1:5 in hybridization mix | ENZO | | 155 |
| SV40 virus | Bio-probe® | | Proteinase K | 1:5 in hybridization mix | ENZO | | 155 |
| VZV/H-N3 | DNA probe | | Proteinase K | 1:5 in hybridization mix, carrier DNA to be added | Dr. T. Kurata, Tokyo | | 154 |

* Formol-fixed and paraffin-embedded sections, listed for source, tissue pretreatment, and optimal dilutions in our laboratory. (Ms. H. Flicker, Head Technician). pc = polyclonal (rabbit if not otherwise specified); mc = monoclonal (mouse); protease pretreatment = protease type XXIV bacterial (Sigma) 0.03% at 37° C for 10 minutes (autopsies) or 5 minutes (biopsies); proteinase K pretreatment = proteinase K (Sigma) 0.04% at 37° C for 20 minutes.

Table 8-4. Acronyms

| Acronym | Definition |
|---|---|
| AIDS | Acquired immunodeficiency syndrome |
| BKV | BK virus |
| CEE | Central European encephalitis |
| CMV | Cytomegalovirus |
| EBV | Epstein-Barr virus |
| EEE | Eastern equine encephalitis |
| HAM | HTLV-I-associated myelopathy |
| HIV | Human immunodeficiency virus |
| HSV | Herpes simplex virus |
| ICC | Immunocytochemistry |
| ISH | in situ hybridization |
| JCV | JC virus |
| JE | Japanese encephalitis |
| LCM | Lymphocytic choriomeningitis |
| MIBE | Measles inclusion body encephalopathy |
| PCR | Polymerase chain reaction |
| PML | Progressive multifocal leukoencephalopathy |
| PRPE | Progressive rubella panencephalitis |
| SSPE | Subacute sclerosing panencephalitis |
| TBE | Tickborne encephalitis |
| TSP | Tropical spastic paraparesis |
| VEE | Venezuelan equine encephalitis |
| VZV | Varicella-zoster virus |
| WEE | Western equine encephalitis |

DAB; and for ISH, visualization of the biotinylated probe with the avidin-peroxidase complex and DAB.

### Neuropathologic Characteristics of Selected Viral Infections of the Nervous System

**Herpesviruses.** Human herpesviruses are notorious for acute reactivation after latency in peripheral nerve or other tissues, usually leading to encephalitis or myelitis in the limbic portions of the brain or in the brainstem (HSV), sensory projection areas (VZV), or diffuse or periventricular distribution (CMV). As a common feature, there is no specific cell tropism: all cell types of the CNS succumb to productive infection (Tables 8-1, 8-2).

***Herpes simplex virus.*** Herpes simplex virus type 1 is the most frequent causative agent of sporadic acute encephalitis in temperate parts of the world, with an untreated mortality rate of 51% to 76%.[62] The natural prevalence of HSV-1 infection increases gradually, beginning in childhood, and reaches 70% to 80% in later adult years.[48] HSV remains in a latent state in the trigeminal, superior cervical, and vagal ganglia.[52,176] The virus is transported intraaxonally to neurons of second and third order.[6] Mechanisms leading to reactivation from the latent stage have remained obscure.[62] Brain biopsy as an aggressive diagnostic procedure in suspected HSV encephalitis has become rare since the advent of the relatively nontoxic acyclovir treatment. A rapid, noninvasive in vivo method for the routine laboratory diagnosis of CNS infection due to HSV is PCR of the CSF.[8]

Herpes simplex virus type 2 (the "genital" type) is known to cause severe brain damage, usually multicystic encephalopathy, in septic infections in the newborn.[41,129] In the adult, HSV-2 caused encephalitis in two homosexual men with persistent lymphadenopathy[57] and thoracic myelitis in one AIDS patient.[19] HSV type 1 encephalitis is surprisingly rare in AIDS patients. In our autopsy series we identified only one case with nodular encephalitis and HSV DNA within the nodules.[152] HSV encephalitis does not seem to occur much more frequently in people with AIDS than in individuals who are immunocompetent; its clinical and pathologic features seem to be identical to those well known in immunocompetent patients.

*Acute herpes simplex virus encephalitis* — There are two major forms of HSV type 1 encephalitis. The form of paramount importance is the acute necrotizing type. The pathway of HSV to the brain in acute encephalitis has been a matter of controversy. In a significant portion of cases the virus appears to follow a transaxonal-olfactory route after intranasal infection, but hematogenous and transtrigeminal pathways, including spread via small meningeal nerves of the cranial base, also have been proposed.[62] In contrast to VZV infection of the CNS, spread via specific sensory projection areas is unlikely in the development of acute HSV encephalitis; trigeminal sensory nuclei are not usually affected or are involved only secondarily.[151]

**Diagnostic Hallmark: *Acute HSV Encephalitis***

- Necrotizing lesions of limbic areas
- Intranuclear inclusion bodies

Acute HSV encephalitis involves mainly the limbic brain with large, partly hemorrhagic necroses.[36] Temporal lobes, insular cortex, and orbital brain can be symmetrically or, more frequently, asymmetrically involved (Fig. 8-2, *A*). Additional macroscopic changes in the cingulate gyrus (Fig. 8-2, *B*) make the diagnosis almost certain at the time of gross inspection of the brain. There is prominent brain swelling and general congestion (Fig. 8-2, *A*); a frequent complication of the mass effect is transtentorial herniation. More advanced stages feature cortical necroses that sometimes have a cavitary component (Fig. 8-2, *C*). A meningeal infiltrate accompanies the extended necroses with frequent bleeding (Fig. 8-3, *A*); more advanced stages feature large fields of foamy macrophages intermixed with inflammatory infiltration of varying intensity (Fig. 8-3, *B*). For histologic diagnosis, it is useful to examine the border zone of necrotic areas, where eosinophilic intranuclear inclusion bodies of Cowdry type A are more

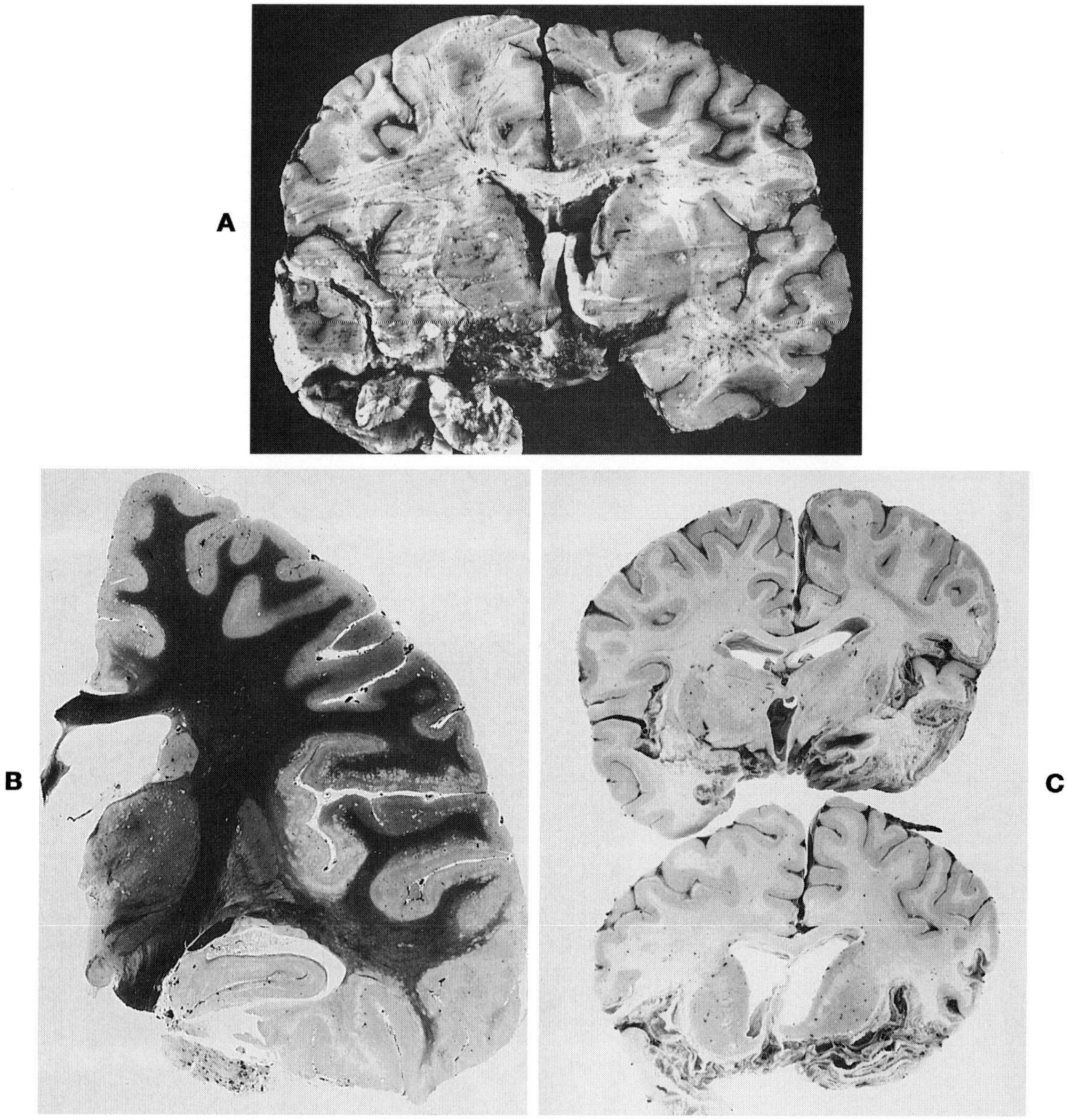


**Fig. 8-2.** Herpes simplex virus (HSV) encephalitis, macroscopical aspect. **A**, Mostly unilateral temporal necrosis, prominent brain swelling and general congestion. **B**, Large temporal cortico-subcortical necroses extend to the insular and cingulate cortex. **C**, Advanced stage with asymmetrical bitemporal and insular cystic necroses. (**B**, Hh stain.)

evident (Fig. 8-3, *C*) than within the necroses. However, inclusion bodies may be equivocal or even undetectable in a small fraction of cases confirmed by ICC.[36] Intranuclear inclusions may be found in various types of cells (Table 8-2). Inflammatory infiltrates may be relatively inconspicuous. Immunolabeled imprint preparations from the temporal lobe at autopsy or biopsy are a quick diagnostic tool, usually featuring many cells labeled for HSV antigen (Fig. 8-4, *A*). Most prominent viral involvement is seen in large (pyramidal) neurons in which the Nissl substance of the cytoplasm is converted into a factory of HSV proteins (Fig. 8-4, *B*); in contrast nuclear involvement is variable.[151] Electron microscopy may demonstrate herpesvirus particles in the nucleus even in less than ideally preserved autopsy tissue.[62] However, both ICC for HSV proteins and ISH for viral DNA have become easy and reliable tools for tissue diagnosis.[151] In our hands, they have, combined, a specificity of 84% in acute necrotizing encephalitis,[151] so that some cases remain with unproved etiology. Viral antigens usually are detectable only in cases with an acute course (4 weeks or less).[36] ISH is superior to ICC in demonstrating the virus in brain after a subacute course (longer than 1 month); however, only a

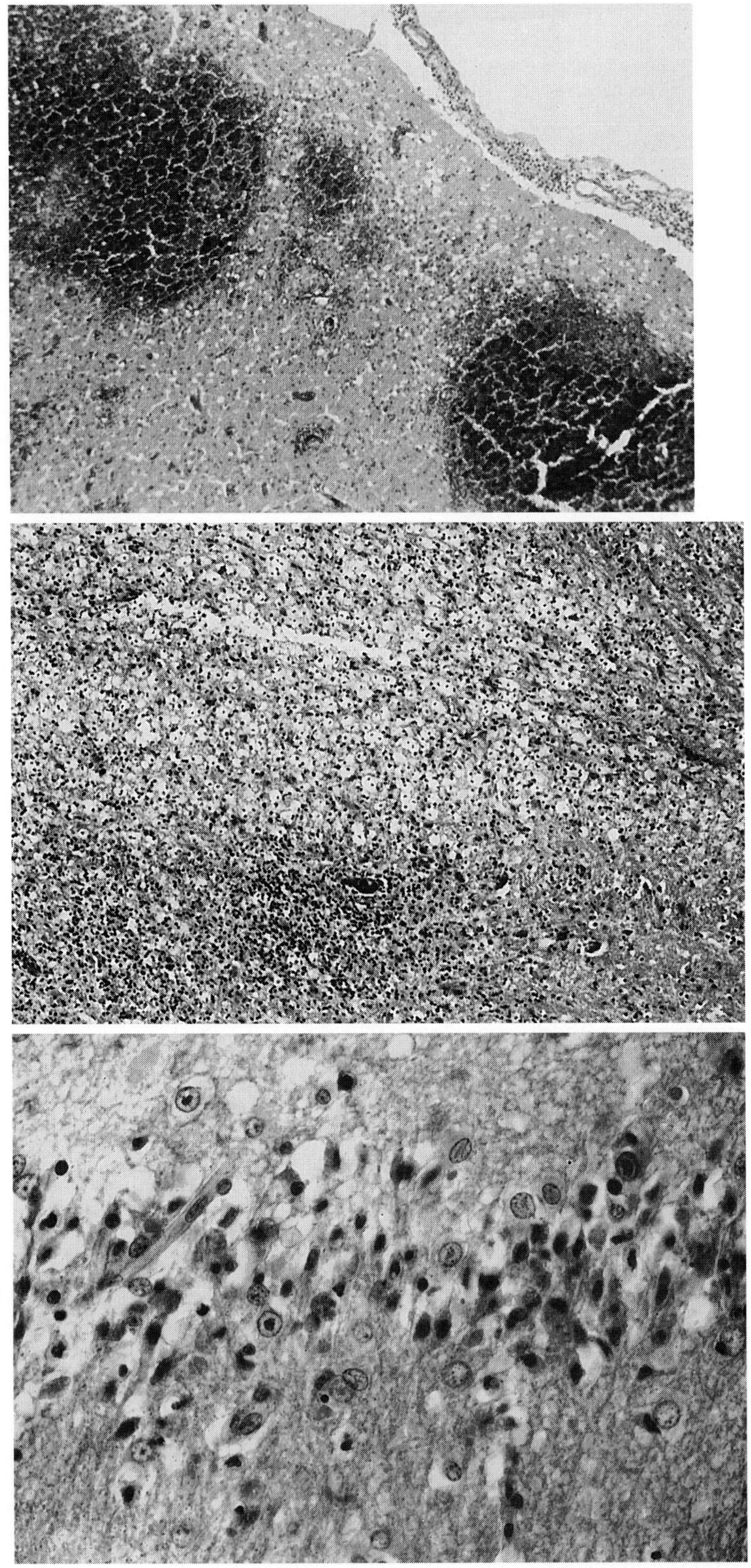


**Fig. 8-3.** Histology of HSV encephalitis. **A**, A meningeal infiltrate accompanies the extended necroses with hemorrhages. **B**, More advanced stages feature large fields of foamy macrophages intermixed with inflammatory infiltration. **C**, Numerous eosinophilic intranuclear inclusion bodies of type Cowdry A are evident in the Fascia dentata. (**A**, H&E; ×20; **B**, H&E; ×32; **C**, H&E; ×325.)

A

B

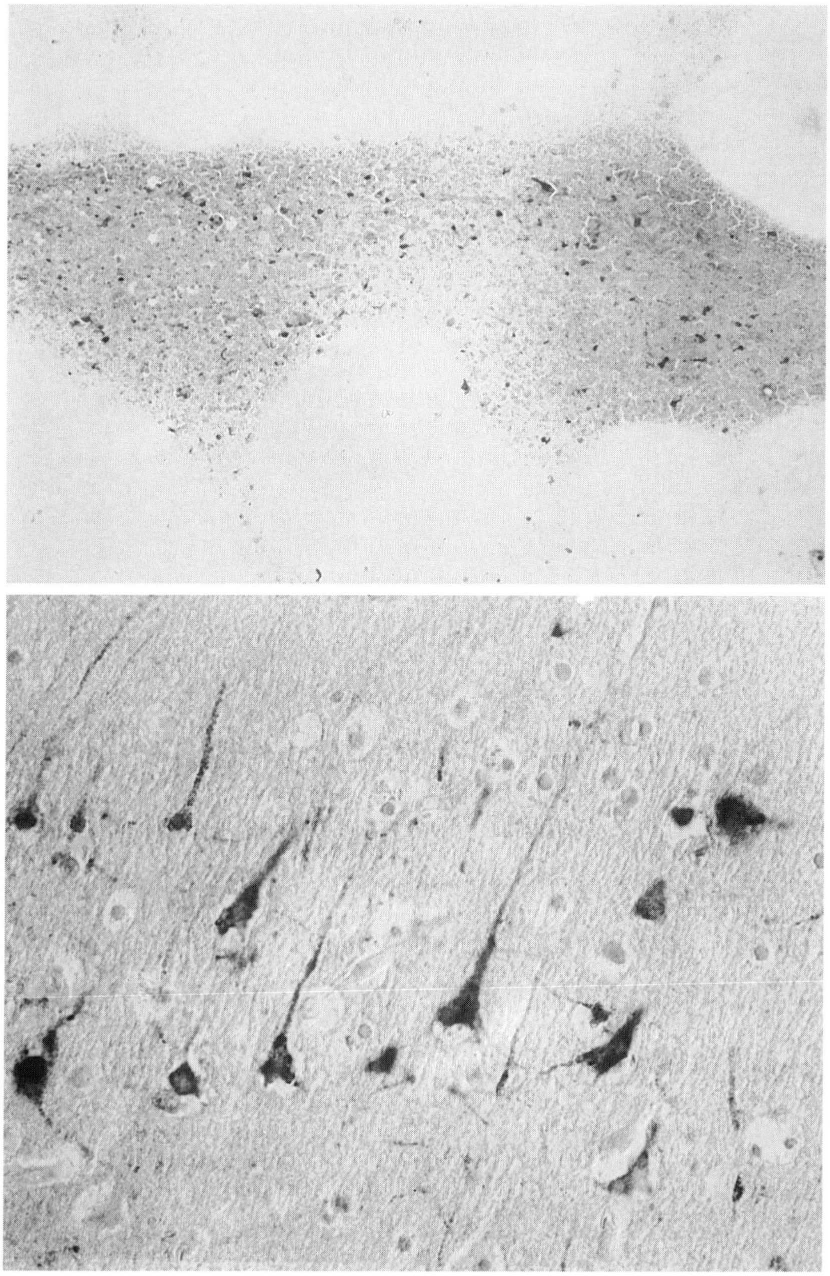

**Fig. 8-4.** Immunocytochemistry (ICC) of HSV encephalitis. **A**, Imprint preparation from temporal lobe reveals many labeled cells. **B**, Strong immunoreactivity in cytoplasm and processes of many pyramidal neurons. (**A**, ICC with anti-SV type 1 antiserum; ×63; **B**, ICC with anti-HSV type 1 antiserum; ×400.)

fraction of cases with prolonged course yield detectable HSV products.[151] Thus, long-standing temporal necroses usually are burnt-out and cannot be diagnosed by ICC and ISH; they can only be suspected as post-HSV encephalitic.

***Nodular herpes simplex virus encephalitis*** — This is the much less dramatic manifestation, featuring multiple microglial nodules with scant concomitant perivascular cuffing. Nodular encephalitis with minimal cellular inflammation frequently is seen at autopsy as a chance finding in the brainstem, especially in trigeminal projection sites, among patients with either severe or aggressively treated diseases. Inclusion bodies are not a feature. In almost half of the brains with micronodular brainstem encephalitis, HSV DNA was detected by ISH, whereas ICC was negative,[52] possibly reflecting early or restricted virus production. ISH-positive cells usually are seen near focal inflammatory infiltrates (Fig. 8-5).

***Cytomegalovirus (CMV).*** CMV infection is common, but CMV disease only exceptionally occurs in immunologically uncompromised adults as meningoencephalitis.[47] The most severe and pathologically varied manifestations of CMV infection of the nervous system are found in AIDS patients, whereas other immunosuppressive states, such as may exist among recipients of organ transplants, usually have milder man-

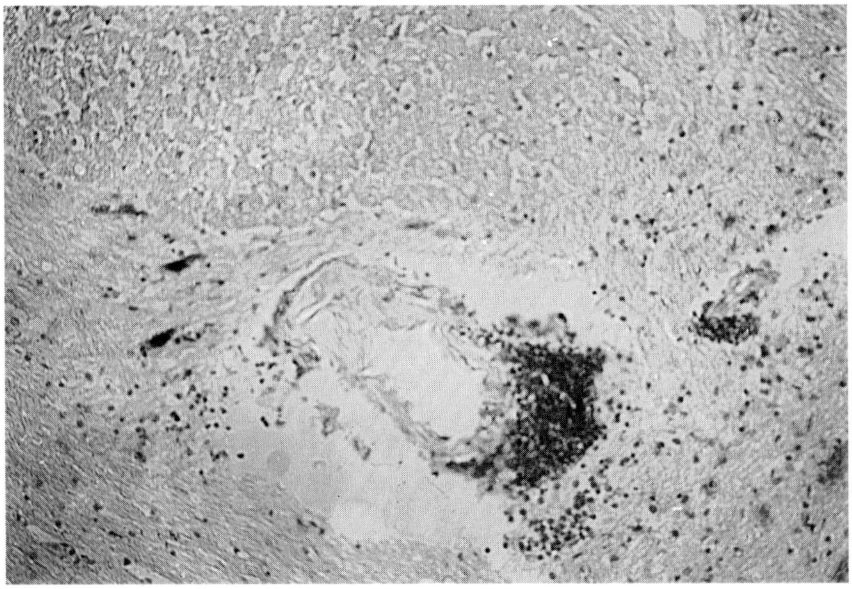

**Fig. 8-5.** Nodular HSV encephalitis in brainstem. Two large neurons adjacent to an inflammatory lesion contain HSV DNA. In situ hybridization with DNA probe for HSV-1. (Hematoxylin counterstain; ×160.)

ifestations, mostly as nodular encephalitis. CMV disease of the CNS generally develops in association with disseminated systemic CMV infection.[31,100,174] CMV disease may be due to reactivation of latent virus or to infection with exogenous virus that may be transmitted by contact with individuals who are shedding virus. CMV infection of the CNS rarely occurs in infants with congenital AIDS.[16]

Both productive CMV and HIV infections may develop within the same brain.[183] However, CMV usually is restricted to necrotizing lesions or microglial nodules, whereas HIV products are confined to lesions of HIV encephalitis.[24,156] Coinfection of multinucleated giant cells by HIV and CMV has been demonstrated in exceptional instances using immunocytochemical double-labeling techniques.[15] In our laboratory, double-labeling applied to several coinfected brains did not reveal cellular colocalization.

CMV probably enters the brain from the blood and then disseminates via the CSF before there is invasion into the brain parenchyma.[124] CMV replicates in several cell types of the nervous system, including astrocytes, ependymal cells, choroid plexus epithelium, vascular endothelium, meningeal cells, and neurons. In the peripheral nervous system, Schwann cells may be infected.[15] The histologic hallmark of CMV infection is the cytomegalic change ("owl's eye" cells) with large, round, or frequently sausage-shaped or even convoluted inclusion bodies in swollen distorted nuclei with an otherwise clear or "empty" nucleoplasm. Multiple smaller granular inclusions may be seen in the huge cytoplasm. In astrocytes, cytomegalic change is accompanied by a peculiar globular arrangement of glial filaments in the central perikaryon.[156] Cell infection does not always result in cytomegaly. Antigen-negative and structurally normal neurons and glial cells may contain CMV DNA fragments, indicating restricted intracellular replication of CMV.[184] Except for meningomyeloradiculitis, clinical presentation of CMV infection of the CNS is uncharacteristic. In some cases, CMV infection of the CNS was diagnosed by immunocytochemical demonstration of infected cells in the CSF.[163] Amplification of CMV DNA by PCR in the CSF has proved to be a rapid and reliable diagnostic method to detect CMV infection of the CNS.[46,69]

***Connatal cytomegalovirus encephalopathy***—Connatal cytomegalovirus encephalopathy develops in fetuses and neonates following in utero exposure. It may produce micrencephaly, congenital malformations, especially of the polymicrogyric type, and progressive neurologic disease after birth.[13] The spectrum of brain pathology ranges from relatively minor damage with few cytomegalic cells to panencephalic cystic necroses and prominent hydrocephalus with extensive periventricular calcification (Fig. 8-6, *A*). Cytomegalic cells may be found everywhere, especially in the malformed cortex (Fig. 8-6, *B*); they may even be found in the meninges.

***Necrotizing cytomegalovirus encephalitis/ventriculitis***—Necrotizing cytomegalovirus encephalitis/ventriculitis is the most severe manifestation, usually seen in AIDS patients. Macroscopically, CMV-infected brains may show no changes, focal parenchymal necrosis, or partly hemorrhagic necroses lining the ventricles (Fig. 8-7, *A*) and cerebral surfaces (Fig. 8-7, *B*). Focal parenchymal necrosis and necrotizing ventriculoencephalitis are characterized by a variable degree of inflammation accompanied by cytomegaly

A

B

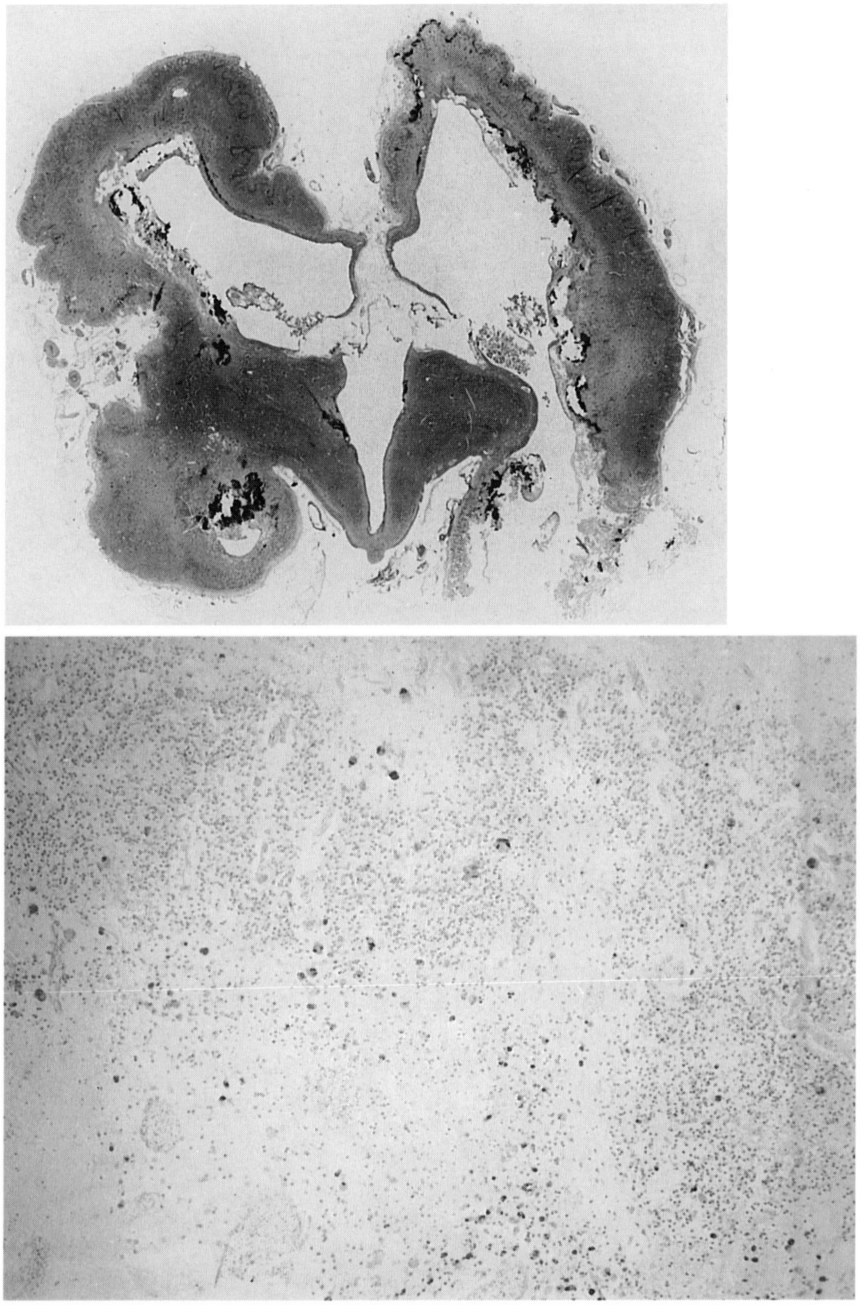

**Fig. 8-6.** Connatal CMV encephalopathy. **A**, Prominent hydrocephalus, periventricular calcifications, and severely malformed cortex. **B**, Micropolygyric cortex with numerous cells containing CMV DNA. ISH with probe for CMV. (**A**, H&E; ×2.5; **B**, H counterstain; ×63.)

with intranuclear and intracytoplasmic CMV inclusions in glial, ependymal, and endothelial cells and neurons (Table 8-2). Frequently, necrotizing lesions are associated with CMV nodular encephalitis in the same brain. Rarely, inclusion-bearing cells occur in an otherwise normal parenchyma. CMV inclusions can be readily identified by their characteristic size and shape with conventional light microscopy and by ICC and ISH (Fig. 8-8, *A* and *B*).[156] The latter techniques show that normal-appearing cells at the edges of the lesions also may contain virus. Focal parenchymal necrosis, ventriculoencephalitis, and isolated inclusion-bearing cells seem to be specific features of CMV brain disease in AIDS.[74] Ventriculoencephalitis may give rise to necrotizing radiculomyelitis by seeding via the CSF.[15,124]

**Diagnostic Hallmark:** ***CMV Encephalitis/Myelitis/Radiculitis***

- Cytomegalic cells ("owl's eye" cells)
- Necrotic lesions, frequently around ventricles, or in the conus medullaris/cauda equina region
- Microglial nodules

***Nodular cytomegalovirus encephalitis***—Historically, CMV was the first pathogen to be linked to the microglial nodules commonly observed in brains from

A
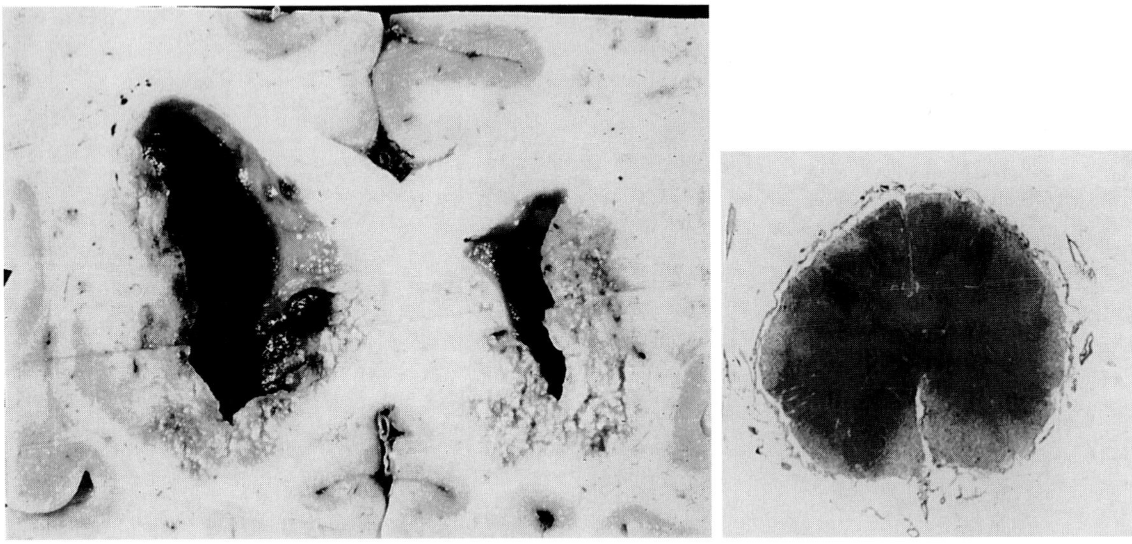
B

**Fig. 8-7.** Necrotizing CMV ventriculitis and encephalitis in AIDS. **A**, Partly hemorrhagic necroses line the ventricular walls. **B**, Almost circular necrotic zone outlines the surface of the lower medulla oblongata. (**B**, Luxol fast blue stain for myelin, counterstained with nuclear fast red; ×4.)

AIDS patients.[130] Histology shows relatively compact encephalitic nodules composed of lymphocytes, microglia, and monocytes/macrophages, and scattered diffusely in gray more than white matter, with, or often without, detectable CMV inclusion-bearing cells in many nodules (Fig. 8-8, *C*). Sometimes many nodules must be examined until diagnostic cytomegaly is found. Further descriptions of nodular encephalitis in AIDS are discussed in Chapter 9.

***Cytomegalovirus meningomyeloradiculitis*** — A few AIDS cases present with polyradiculomyelitis or spinal ganglionitis, causing a cauda equina syndrome. The clinical setting usually is a rapidly ascending polyradiculoneuropathy similar to Guillain-Barré syndrome,[119,174] but with a significant granulocytic CSF pleocytosis.

***Varicella-zoster virus.*** Varicella-zoster virus infects nearly 100% of the population in temperate parts of the world.[180,181] Among patients with the clinical syndrome of chickenpox, VZV apparently spreads into sensory ganglia via contiguous exteroceptive nerves. Although there is a strong association between immunosuppression and herpes zoster, with and without dissemination, only a few AIDS patients have been reported with neurologic complications associated with VZV. Presentations of VZV disease in AIDS are: multifocal leukoencephalitis with and without a noninflammatory vasculopathy;[72,123] encephalomyelitis, mainly involving the gray matter, possibly secondary to transsynaptic spread to the brain or spinal cord from VZV ophthalmical[48] trigeminal,[147] dermatomal,[116] or myotomal[154] infection; ependymitis/ventriculitis mimicking CMV infection with[44] and without[66] secondary meningomyeloradiculitis; and fulminant ascending myeloradiculopathy.[173] PCR of CSF for detection of VZV DNA has been proposed as a useful tool for the early diagnosis of VZV-associated neurologic disease.[143]

***Zosteric ganglionitis*** — The clinical syndrome of herpes zoster infection is assumed to be due to reactivation of a latent infection of the sensory ganglia[64] after decline of immunity.[62] Affected ganglia show partly hemorrhagic necroses, abundant viral products (Fig. 8-9, *A*) and Cowdry type A intranuclear inclusion bodies in ganglion and satellite cells (Fig. 8-9, *B*) as well as herpesvirus particles; there may be spread of inflammation, and even of necroses, into spinal nerves or roots.[154]

**Fig. 8-8.** ICC and ISH in necrotizing CMV ventriculitis (**A**) and encephalitis (**B**), and in nodular CMV encephalitis (**C**) in AIDS. **A**, Numerous strongly labeled, partly multinucleated cytomegalic cells in the ependymal and subependymal layer. **B**, Numerous strongly labeled cytomegalic cells in the cerebellar cortex. **C**, An encephalitic nodule contains a cytomegalic cell. (**A**, ISH, H counterstain; ×200; **B**, ICC with anti-CMV-antibody, Nomarski interference contrast optics; ×250; **C**, H&E; ×400.)

A

B

C

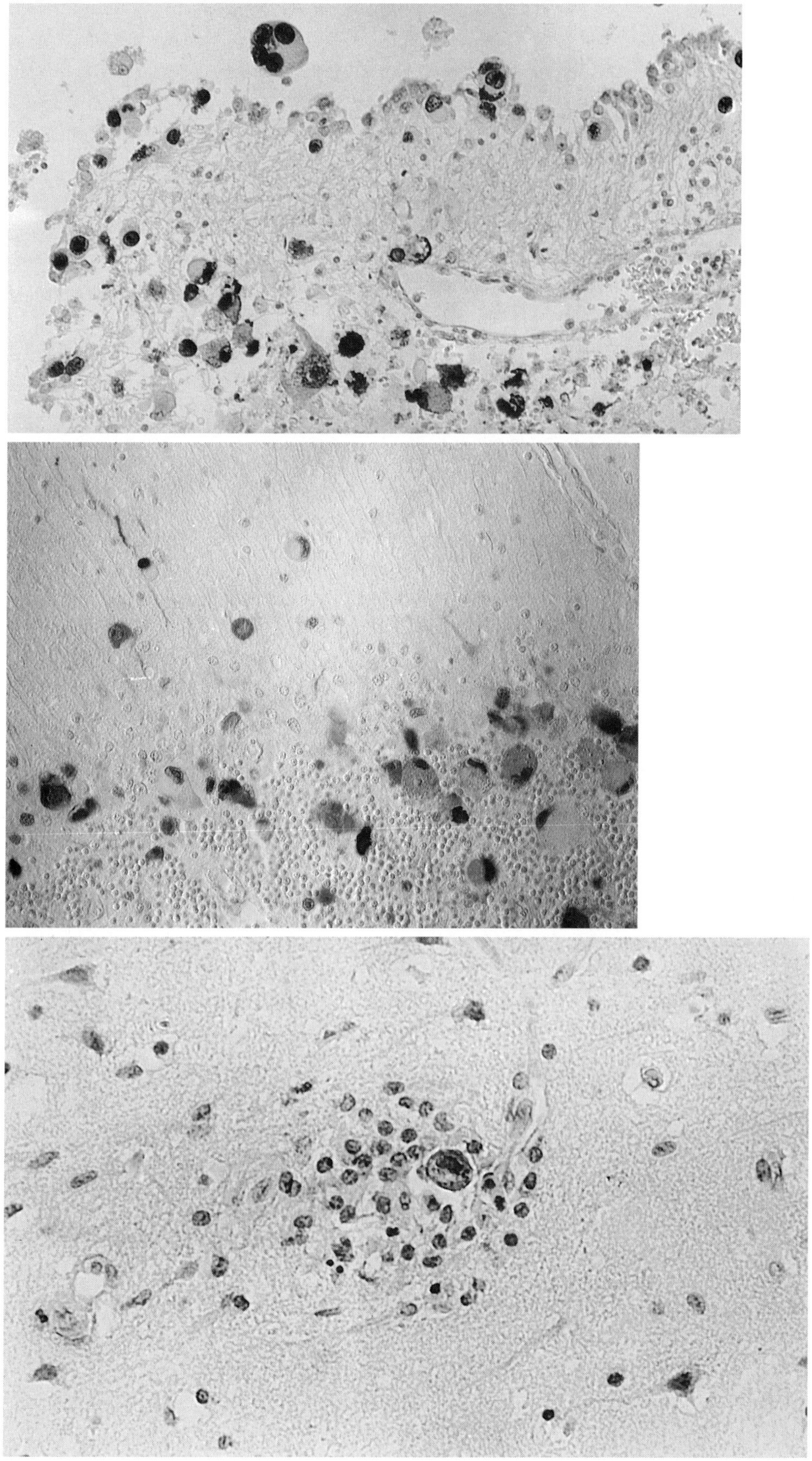

Fig. 8-8. For legend see opposite page.

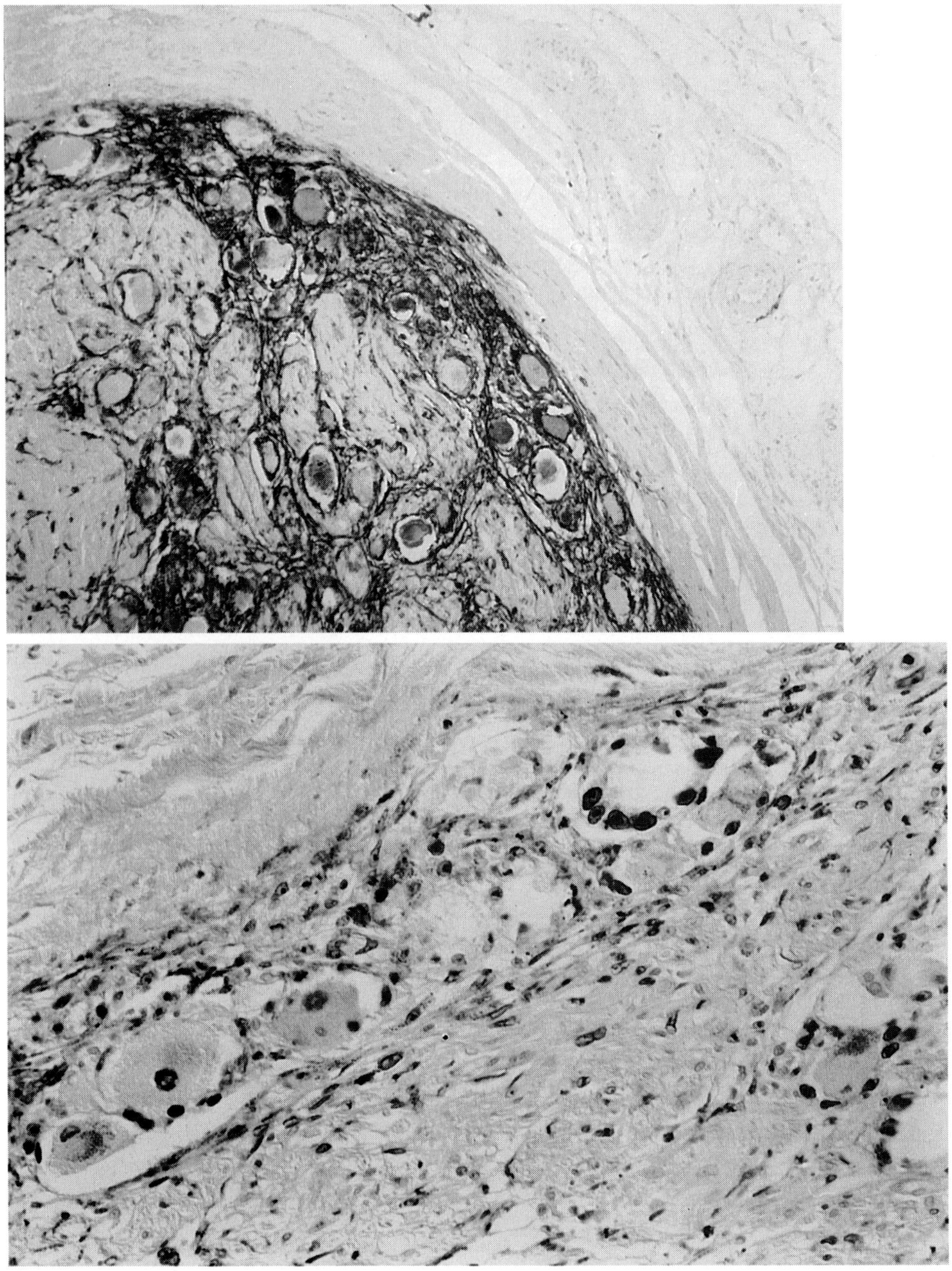

A

B

**Fig. 8-9.** Zosteric ganglionitis. **A,** Large amounts of varicella-zoster virus (VZV) in some ganglion cells and numerous satellite and interstitial cells. **B,** Nuclei and intranuclear inclusion bodies of many satellite and ganglion cells exhibit VZV antigen. (**A,** ICC with anti-VZV glycoprotein antibody; ×100; **B,** ICC with anti-VZV nucleoprotein antibody, H counterstain; ×250.)

***Varicella-zoster virus encephalomyelitis*** — There is frequent involvement of the CNS in herpes zoster, presenting as encephalitis and encephalomyelitis.[142,154] Nodular brainstem encephalitis due to VZV exceptionally may occur in a previously healthy individual[154] (Fig. 8-10, *A*). A detailed study on the development of productive VZV infection within nervous tissues[154] suggested several modes of virus spread to the CNS, including the classic transtrigeminal spread to specific projection nuclei. Eosinophilic intranuclear inclusions of Cowdry type A may be found in oligodendrocytes, astrocytes, occasional neurons, ependymal cells, endothelial cells, and Schwann cells (Table 8-2). VZV infection is verified by immunocytochemical and ISH techniques[154] (Fig. 8-10, *B*). The occurrence of a cutaneous herpes zoster eruption before or concomitant with the onset of neurologic signs is a useful although unreliable diagnostic clue.[72] In trigeminal infections by zoster,

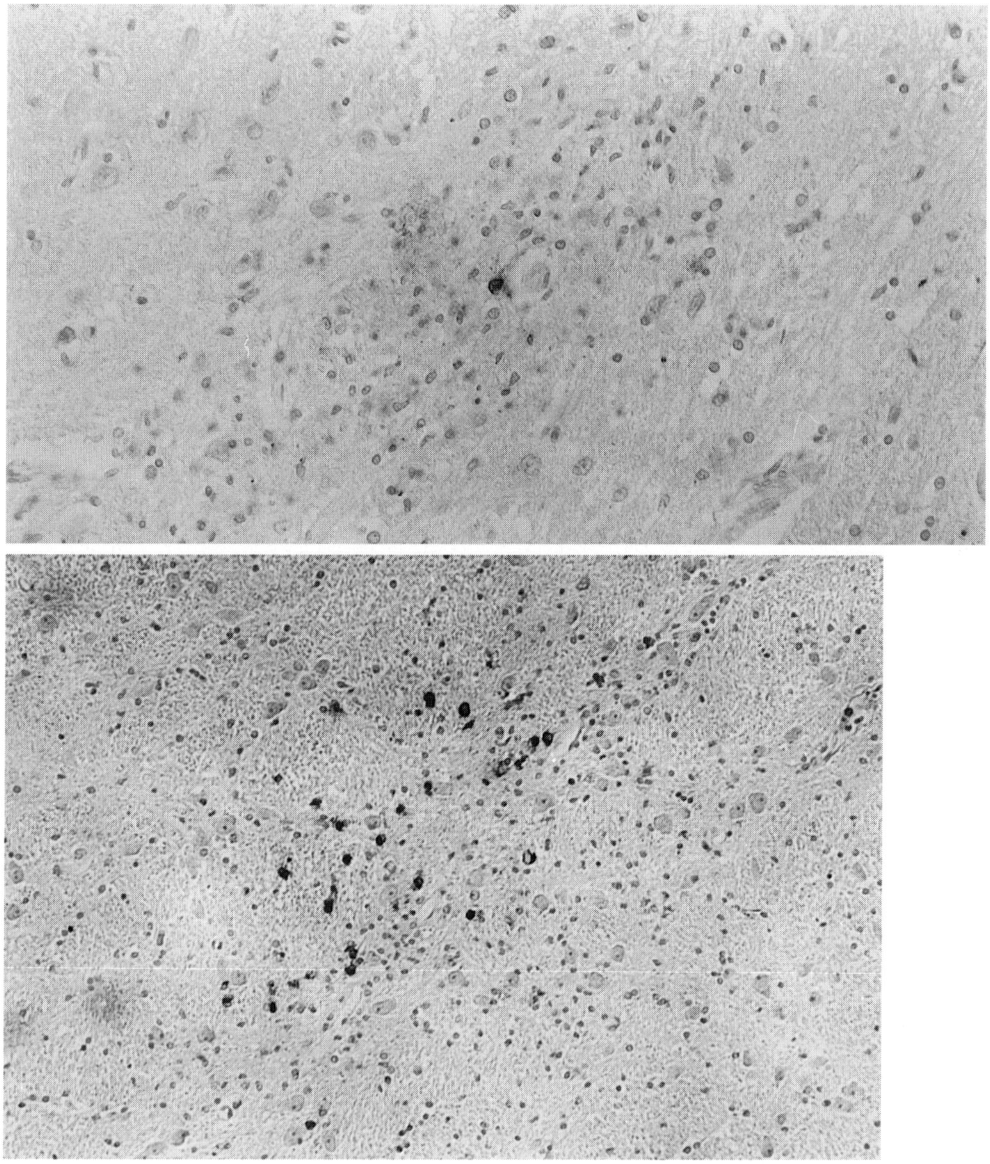

**Fig. 8-10.** **A**, VZV nodular brainstem encephalitis in a previously healthy young adult. Central cell labeled for VZV in an indistinct inflammatory infiltration. **B**, VZV encephalitis in herpes zoster. Numerous glial nuclei in the pons contain virus. (**A**, anti-VZV glycoprotein antibody; ×400; **B**, ICC with anti-VZV nucleoprotein antibody, H counterstain; ×200.)

a predominantly demyelinating lesion may be restricted to the ipsilateral spinal trigeminal tract and nucleus.[147] In spinal zoster, pathologic involvement is most severe in the dorsal root entry zone and posterior horn of the spinal cord segment corresponding to the involved dermatome.[54] In a rare case of congenital VZV infection, the neuropathologic examination revealed destructive and inflammatory lesions of cerebral cortex and white matter, thalamus, brainstem, and spinal cord; in addition there were cerebellar heterotopias and bilateral polymicrogyric malformations of the insular cortex.[77] One study group proposed that the mechanism of neurologic damage in VZV-associated syndromes is immune-mediated, there being increased expression of class II MHC antigens associated with persistent inflammation.[93]

**Diagnostic Hallmark:** ***VZV Encephalitis/Leukoencephalopathy/Myelitis/Vasculopathy***

- Intranuclear inclusion bodies
- Necrotic lesions, demyelinating areas, thrombotic vasculopathy

***Varicella-zoster virus leukoencephalopathy***—VZV leukoencephalopathy is the presentation most frequently seen in immunosuppression. Perivenous encephalomalacia[117] and leukoencephalopathy with and without brainstem involvement[117,149] have been reported. Neuropathologic examination reveals multifocal necrotic changes with numerous intranuclear Cowdry type A inclusion bodies in glial cells, endothelial cells, macrophages, and neurons, both within and around the lesions.[72] There also may be demyelinating lesions resembling those of PML; numerous cells with Cowdry type A intranuclear inclusions surround the lesions.[123] The demyelinating lesions, however, were reported as smaller and less coalescent than those seen in PML.[4]

*Cerebral varicella-zoster virus vasculopathy*—Cerebral VZV vasculopathy features a variety of clinicopathologic presentations. It was interpreted as the basic mechanism operating in most CNS manifestations of VZV infection.[4] However, we found vasculitis in only 2 of 19 zoster brains or spinal cords.[154] Vasculitis or noninflammatory vasculopathy with inclusion bodies or VZV products may involve medium-sized leptomeningeal vessels and lead to corticosubcortical or brainstem infarction.[61,72,154]

***Epstein-Barr virus.*** Various neurologic manifestations have been associated with Epstein-Barr virus (EBV), which may remain latent in circulating B lymphocytes.[62] However, convincing data are lacking, except for strong evidence that EBV is implicated in the pathogenesis of CNS lymphoma, both in the presence and absence of AIDS.* ICC against EBV products such as latent membrane protein,[14,40,110] EBNA-2 and viral capsid antigen,[14] dot blotting using a $^{32}$P-labeled fragment of EBV,[139] ISH with various probes,[75,40,110] and PCR for the EBNA-1 region and the first internal repeat segment of the EBV genome[51,122] were positive in a high percentage of cases. Immunoblast-rich lesions are more commonly associated with EBV than Burkitt-type tumors.[75] CNS-NHL in AIDS frequently are associated with macrophages and multinucleated giant cells that contain HIV.[49] However, PCR for the gag region of HIV failed to detect virus in any case of a series of 12 AIDS-associated CNS-NHL.[122] It was shown that PCR on CSF for EBV DNA is highly sensitive and specific for AIDS-associated CNS-NHL, and it may be useful as a diagnostic tumor marker.[45]

**Adenoviruses.** Adenoviral infections are very rarely associated with neurologic complications. Children with severe respiratory disease may be affected. At autopsy of a neonate, neuropathologic examination revealed diffuse edema, perivascular cuffing, and gliosis in the white matter; adenovirus type 11 was isolated from lung, hilar lymph node, and brain tissue.[134]

* Refs. 14, 40, 51, 75, 110, 122, 139.

**Papovaviruses**

***JC virus.*** Papovaviruses include three different subtypes: BK virus, JC virus (JCV), and SV40 virus.[158] PML has been linked to the latter two viruses, but all or almost all cases are caused by JCV, whereas the etiologic role of SV40 virus has remained controversial.[155,158] The name JCV derives from the initials of the index patient—there is no relation whatsoever with "Jakob-Creutzfeld virus"!

Antibodies against JCV are found in 70% of normal adults.[135] It is still unclear how the primary infection takes place, where the virus rests in seropositive, asymptomatic persons, and how it reaches the CNS.[10] However, JCV was found in extraneural sites, including kidney, spleen, and bone marrow.[58,84] During the primary infection, JCV may reach the CNS via the blood and from infected vascular endothelial cells, or, during immunosuppression, latent JCV dormant in the kidney and bone marrow may be reactivated and invade the brain.[10] Within the CNS, oligodendrocytes are fully permissive to infection, whereas astrocytes show a restricted infection.[37,73,115,158] Cell type specificity is regulated by the enhancer element[108] and transcription factors.[84] In vitro studies suggest that CMV might serve as helper virus for JCV replication in otherwise nonpermissive cells.[82]

*Progressive multifocal leukoencephalopathy*—Progressive multifocal leukoencephalopathy is exclusively a disease of the human CNS and was first described in 1958 in patients with chronic lymphocytic leukemia and Hodgkin's disease.[9] The ultrastructural studies of Zu Rhein and Chou[186] first demonstrated papovavirus within oligodendroglial nuclei, and JCV was isolated from infected brain tissue in 1971.[136] A promising new method for identification of JCV in neurologic disease is PCR of CSF.[121,177]

PML is found in a broad spectrum of different forms of immunosuppression, including AIDS, transplant recipients, treated malignancies, and collagen vascular diseases. In the pre-AIDS era[11] 11% of PML cases occurred in persons without obvious compromising conditions.[37] The autopsy incidence of PML among AIDS patients ranges between 2% and 11%;[74] most researchers believe that the incidence of PML is likely to increase in the future. In HIV-seropositive patients, PML has been noted even in the absence of other clinical manifestations of immunodeficiency.[88] JCV has been detected in brains of AIDS patients without clinically evident PML.[144] PML is one rare neurologic complication of HIV-infected children.[17] Neurologic symptoms are unspecific and include focal neurologic deficits or dementia.[175] Patients usually have a relentless downhill course. CT scans show low-density nonenhancing white matter lesions, and MRI demonstrates high-intensity signals on T2-weighted spin-echo images.

**Diagnostic Hallmark: *PML***

- PML cells
- Multiple, frequently coalescing demyelinating small foci and larger areas

Macroscopically, the white matter features multiple, bilateral, irregular, and ill-defined patches of discoloration and granular destruction, frequently in subcortical areas (Fig. 8-11). Lesions range in size from a few millimeters to extensive involvement of cerebral and cerebellar hemispheres. Parietooccipital regions are most frequently involved. Histologic sections stained for myelin demonstrate the characteristic small multifocal lesions of motheaten appearance, frequently at the border of large demyelinated areas (Fig. 8-12, *A*). In extremely severe cases, most of the cerebral myelin may disappear (Fig. 8-12, *B*).

Histologically, there are confluent foci of demyelination with many lipid-laden macrophages and reactive gliosis with occasional bizarre, giant astrocytic nuclei (Fig. 8-13, *A* and *B*). Mainly at the edge of the lesion (Fig. 8-13, *C*), greatly enlarged oligodendroglial nuclei are pathognomonic ("PML cells");[37] their chromatin is replaced by glassy amphophilic viral inclusion material (Fig. 8-13, *D*). Abundant JCV products are demonstrable by ICC[37] and ISH[155] in these cells; mitosis, although morphologically abnormal, may be visible in virus-packed cells (Fig. 8-13, *D*). Astroglial involvement is different. More in the center of PML lesions, huge and bizarre tumor-like astrocytes with giant nu-

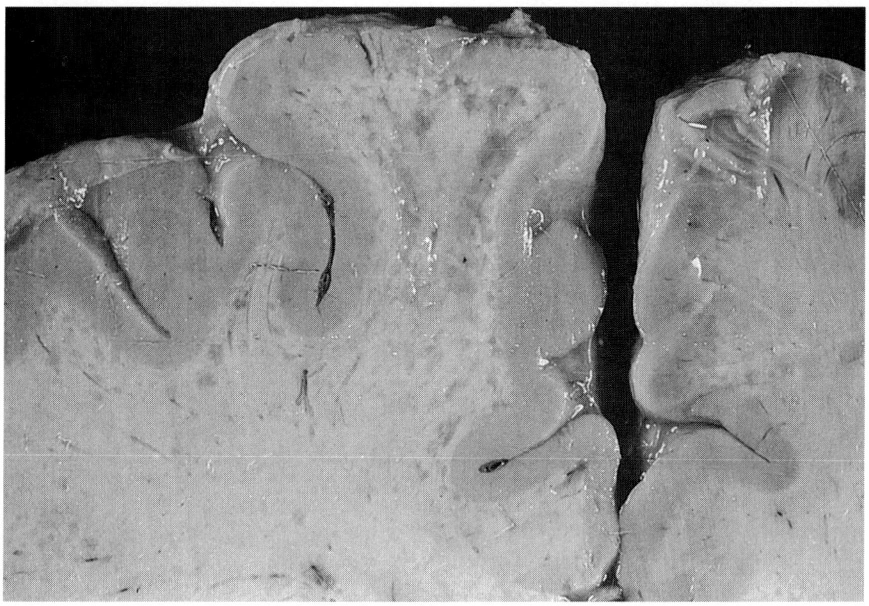

**Fig. 8-11.** Progressive multifocal leukoencephalopathy (PML), macroscopic aspect. The subcortical white matter contains numerous small dark gray foci.

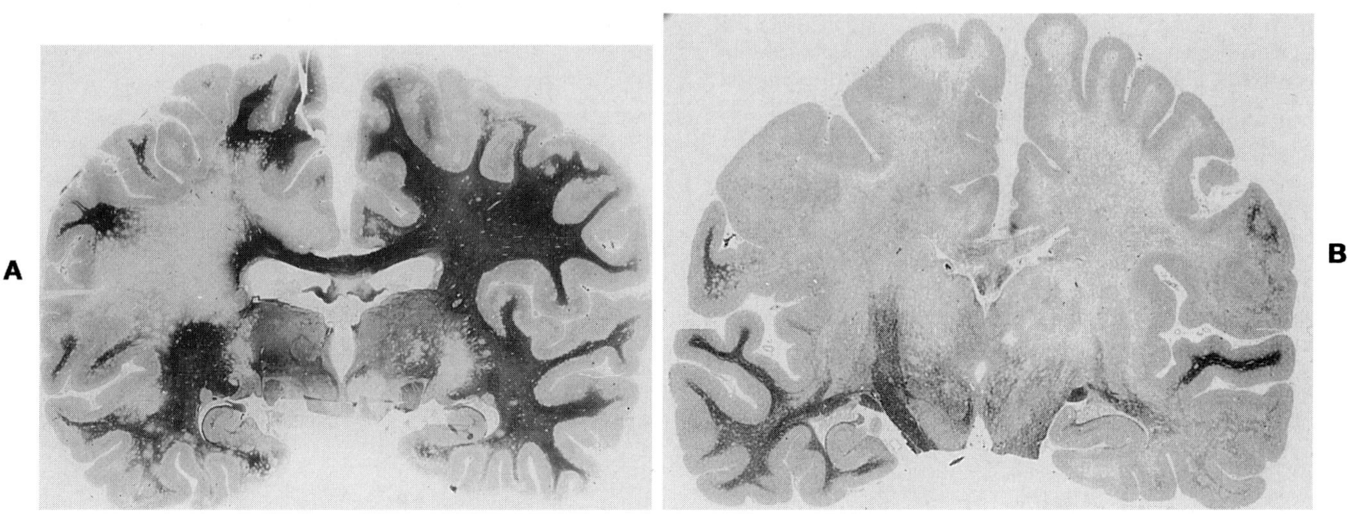

**Fig. 8-12.** Distribution of PML lesions. Large demyelinated areas may invest mainly one cerebral hemisphere (**A**, AIDS) or almost the whole white matter of a brain section (**B**, systemic lupus erythematosus). In addition, there are countless small lesions of moth-eaten appearance. (LFB-NFR stain.)

A B C D

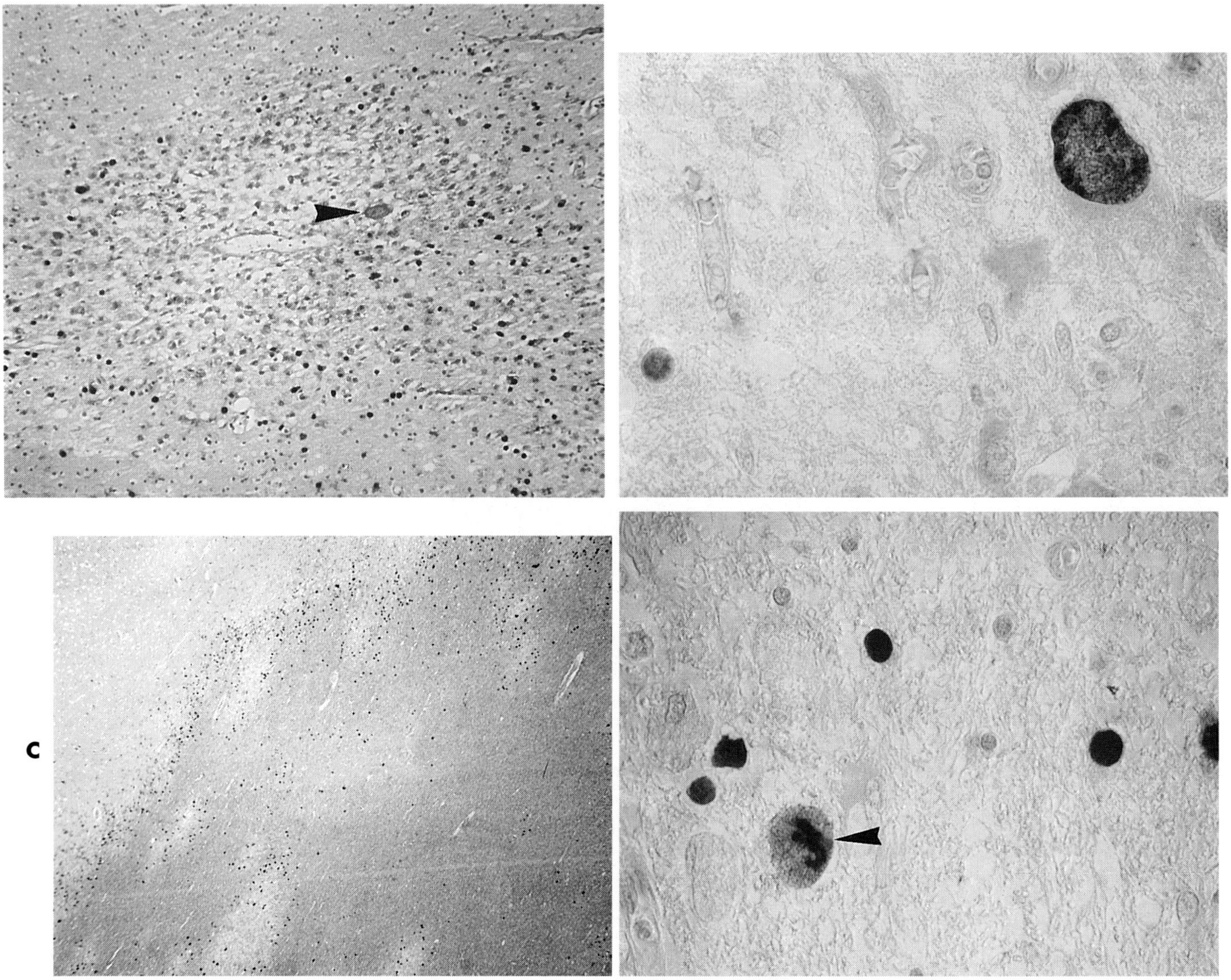

E

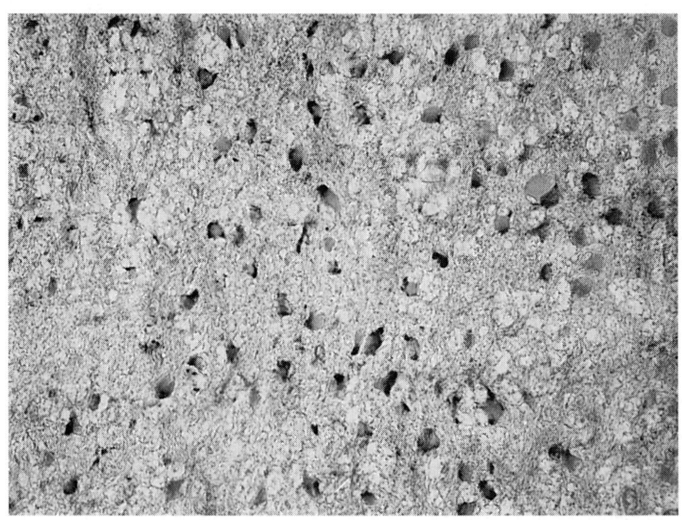

**Fig. 8-13.** Histology and viral products in PML. **A**, An actively demyelinating lesion features numerous macrophages, a giant astrocyte in the center (*arrowhead*), and numerous virus-laden PML signs at the lesion margin. **B**, In addition to an oligodendroglial nucleus, a giant astroglial nucleus contains much viral antigen. **C**, Virus-laden PML cells characteristically decorate the margin of demyelinated lesions. **D**, PML cells with swollen, homogeneously labeled nuclei and a labeled abnormal mitotic figure (*arrowhead*). **E**, Gemistogytic astroglia in a lesion with advanced demyelination contains virus antigen in the cytoplasmic periphery. **F**, Electron micrograph of papovavirus nucleocapsids with an approximate diameter of 55 nm in the nucleus of a PML cell. (**A**, ICC with antipapovavirus antiserum, H counterstain; ×100; **B**, ICC with antipapovavirus antiserum, slight H counterstain; ×630; **C**, ICC with antipapovavirus antiserum, slight H counterstain; ×63; **D**, ICC with antipapovavirus antiserum, NICO; ×630; **E**, ICC with antipapovavirus antiserum, slight H counterstain; ×250; **F**, ×315.000.) Courtesy of Dr. P.P. Liberski, Lodz, Poland.)

F

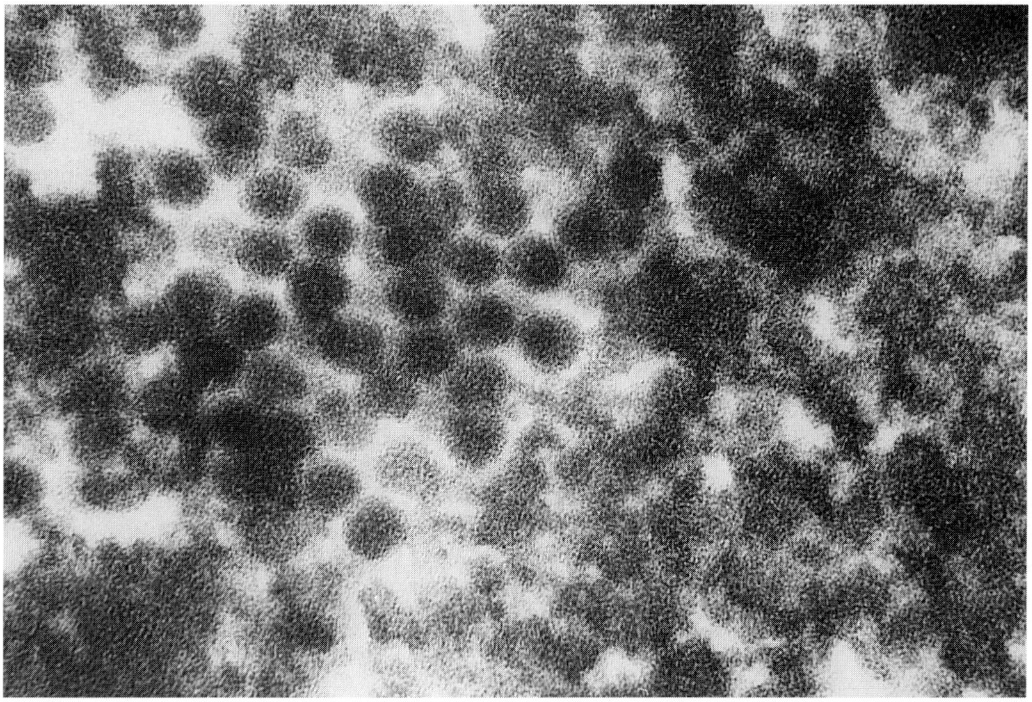

**Fig. 8-13, cont'd.** For legend see opposite page.

clei, with and without viral products (Fig. 8-13, *B*), are characteristic; however, they may be absent in lesions of recent vintage. Reactive or gemistocytic astrocytes are abundant, especially in more advanced lesions, and may contain viral products exclusively in peripheral parts of the cytoplasm but not in the nucleus (Fig. 8-13, *E*). There is a varying degree of inflammation, which may well be absent in the majority of cases. The cortex is involved to a much lesser degree, although many lesions favor the cortex-white matter junction. Rarely, the white matter of the spinal cord may be affected. The mechanism of virus-induced cell demise is yet unclear. Apoptosis of infected cells is a possibility; recently we found evidence for that when we studied AIDS brains by the in situ end-labeling technique. PML cells at the margin of a demyelinating lesion were strongly labeled,[30] indicating prominent DNA fragmentation.

PML lesions in AIDS usually are similar to those occurring with other basic diseases.[98,155,175] However, changes in AIDS may be more extensive, necrotizing, unilateral, or asymmetric, and may involve regions classically spared, such as the temporal lobes, basal ganglia, brainstem, or cerebellum. Inflammation is often mild or absent, and viral inclusions may be remarkably abundant.[2] Macrophages infiltrating demyelinating PML lesions may be infected by HIV-1.[155,172,182] In our autopsy series, four cases of PML had unusually extensive and necrotizing lesions infiltrated with abundant macrophages expressing HIV antigens. Combined antipapovavirus and anti-HIV ICC did not reveal cellular colocalization of JC and HIV virus in those cases. However, in another case of our biopsy series displaying a PML lesion infiltrated by HIV-infected macrophages, immunocytochemical double-labeling revealed colocalization of JC and HIV in a single macrophage.[74] The increase in damage to tissue in AIDS brains may be due to transactivation of one virus by the other.[155] JCV DNA may transactivate the HIV long terminal repeat sequence;[65] in contrast, the HIV-1 regulatory protein *tat* may enhance the JCV lytic cycle in glial cells by stimulating JCV gene expression.[165]

The diagnosis is done morphologically on biopsied brain tissue; ICC and ISH techniques or electron microscopy confirm the histologic diagnosis. Ultrastructurally, the virus particles are round (Fig. 8-13, *F*) or elongated and sometimes are arranged in crystalline arrays.

***BK polyoma virus.*** A case report identified disseminated infection with BKV in AIDS as the cause of a subacute meningoencephalitis with accentuation of the ventricular and meningeal surfaces of the brain. Besides distinctive cytopathic effects, the presence of intranuclear inclusions was a prominent histopathologic feature.[171]

**Flaviviruses.** Flaviviruses infect humans usually via mosquito or tick bites. The neuropathology of flavivirus encephalitis is not specific; it features all major elements of the spectrum of the encephalitic syndrome, with disseminated microglial nodules, gliosis, perivascular lymphocytic cuffing, and variable neuronal damage ranging from disseminated neuronophagia to large areas of necrosis. Because of this relatively unspecific morphology, virologic examination is required to establish an etiologic diagnosis.

**Diagnostic Hallmark:** ***Acute Encephalitis by Flaviviruses, Alphaviruses, Entero-Viruses***

- Disseminated microglial nodules and perivascular cuffing
- Mainly gray matter is involved, variable neuronal damage

***Central European/tick-borne encephalitis.*** Central European/tick-borne encephalitis (CEE/TBE), a disease that occurs in large parts of central Europe, Scandinavia, and Russia, is transmitted by bites of the tick *Ixodes ricinus*. Only a minority of infected persons develop neurologic signs and symptoms, and some of these have a severe encephalitis. Neuropathologic changes are typical of those of patchy polioencephalitis, which is seen in many acute viral encephalitides without distinct viral products. The disease is characterized by widespread perivascular and meningeal cuffing, reactive gliosis, and numerous microglial nodules (Fig. 8-14, *A*), which may include neuronophagia and coalesce to intensely infiltrated fields (Fig. 8-14, *B*). The cerebellum (Fig. 8-14, *C*), brainstem, and spinal cord (Fig. 8-14, *D*) tend to be most heavily affected; inflammation usually extends to the meninges and frequently to the spinal roots. The distribution of the lesions sometimes is similar to that of poliomyelitis; prominent involvement of the cerebellum in cases of CEE/TBE (Fig. 8-14, *C*) may help in the differentiation. Viral antigen can be readily detected in mouse brain experimentally infected with the CEE virus. I have tried unsuccessfully to visualize the antigen in human encephalitic autopsy brains; probably the antigen is cleared from brain or masked within a few days after

A

B

C

D

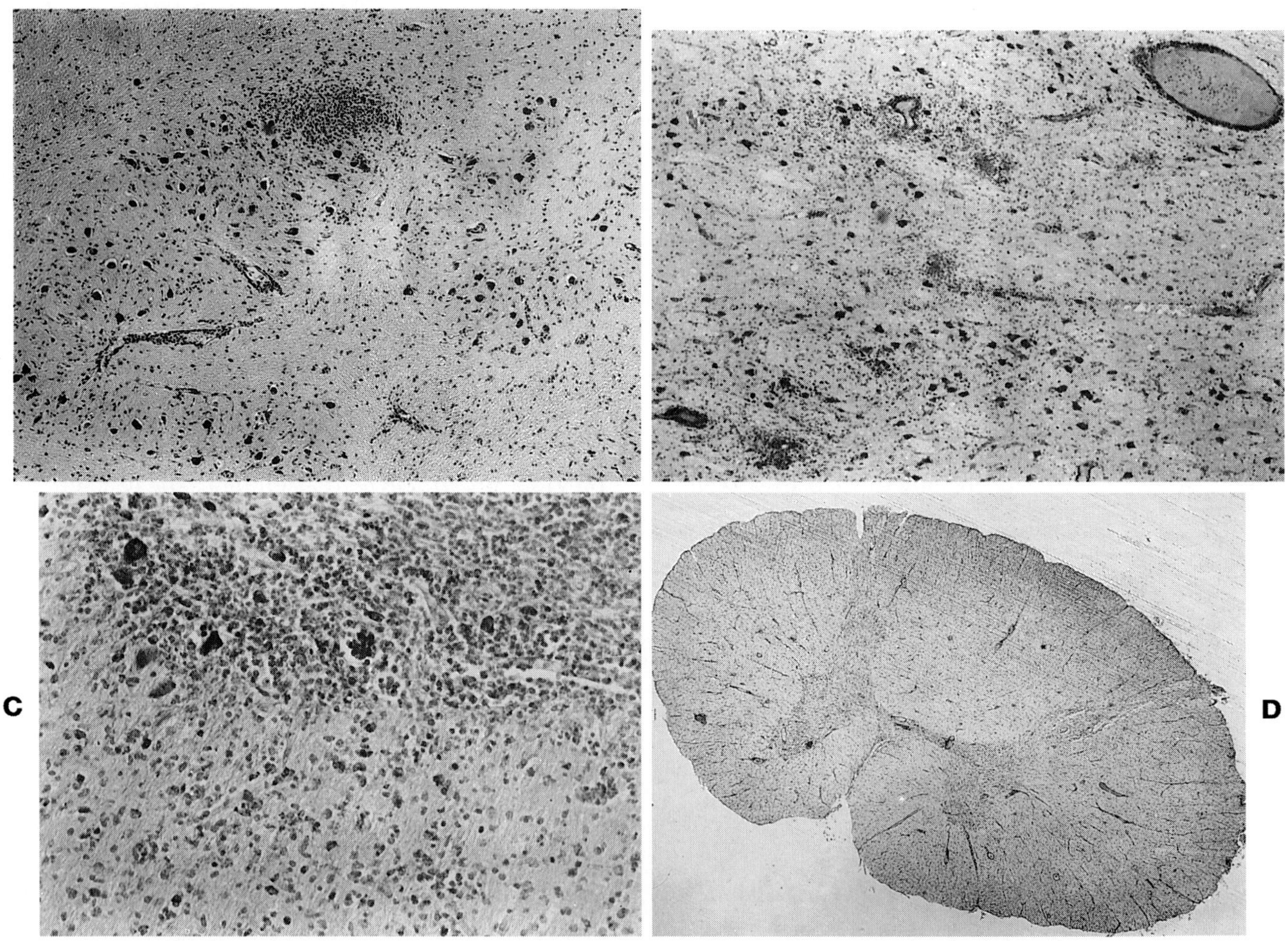

**Fig. 8-14.** Histology of central European/tickborne encephalitis (CEE/TBE) is characterized by perivascular cuffing, reactive gliosis and numerous microglial nodules (**A**) which may engulf central neuronophagia and coalesce to intensely infiltrated fields (**B**). **C**, The cerebellar cortex shows intense inflammation. **D**, The spinal cord has increased cellularity and perivascular cuffings. (All CV stain; **A**, **B** ×68; **C** ×150; **D** ×10.)

the development of encephalitis, so that it became undetectable in the specimens that I investigated; all samples originated from patients who had survived 2 weeks or longer.

***Japanese encephalitis.*** Neuropathologic features of Japanese encephalitis (JE) do not differ significantly from those seen in CEE/TBE. Viral antigen is progressively cleared in patients who survive 6 days or longer.[90] In one JE brain, neurons involved in neuronophagia were viral antigen positive; antigenic masses occasionally were encountered in the center of so-called acellular plaques.[86] Neurons with strong reactivity to viral antibodies were found sporadically in normal-appearing regions in the thalamus and cerebral cortex; viral antigens were demonstrable only in neurons and not in glial or vascular endothelial cells.[86] A recent study readily detected viral antigen in 11 of 13 brains; the topographic distribution of the tissue-associated antigen in the thalamus, hippocampus, substantia nigra, and medulla oblongata was thought to be the reason for the evolution of the sequelae commonly observed among survivors of JE.[53]

***St. Louis encephalitis.*** This acute type of encephalitis features no peculiarities different from those described for other flaviviruses. However, tissue necroses may be prominent in these encephalitides. Compared with WEE, inflammation was much more conspicuous and widespread in St. Louis encephalitis, whereas WEE had more extensive necroses.[102]

**Togaviruses.** Togaviruses include the mosquito-spread alphaviruses of Eastern (EEE), Western (WEE), and Venezuelan equine encephalitis (VEE), and rubellavirus. Alphaviruses cause acute encephalitis with neuropathologic features similar to those described in flavivirus encephalitis.

***Alphaviruses***

***Eastern equine encephalitis*** — The disease course is more fulminant in EEE than in WEE, and the neuropathologic changes are more acute and prominent. Brain swelling and polymorphonuclear leukocytes infiltration predominate in the acute stage, accompanied by areas of necrosis and acute vasculitis.[106] As in WEE, the lower parts of the spinal cord are generally spared. This may be important for differential diagnosis.[62]

***Western equine encephalitis*** — Western equine encephalitis (WEE) is rarely fatal; serious sequelae occasionally may be seen in infants.[89]

***Venezuelan equine encephalitis*** — Venezuelan equine encephalitis (VEE) may be severe in children. The neuropathologic features include relatively mild inflammation most prominent in the white matter and basal ganglia.[81]

***Rubella virus***

***Progressive rubella panencephalitis*** — Progressive rubella panencephalitis (PRPE) is a very rare late sequel of congenital[167] or childhood[168] rubella infection. The neuropathologic features resemble those of SSPE; however, inclusion bodies are absent and unique vascular changes with fibrinoid necrosis and mineral deposition have been described in some cases.[62,169]

**Paramyxoviruses**

***Measles virus.*** Encephalitis is a rare complication of measles virus (MV) infection. The clinical manifestations include these symptoms: (1) acute encephalitis; (2) subacute measles encephalitis in the immunosuppressed or measles inclusion body encephalopathy (MIBE); and (3) subacute sclerosing panencephalitis (SSPE).[132] Acute postmeasles encephalitis is an immune-mediated disorder characterized by extensive demyelination that typically occurs in the weeks following the rash and without local virus production.[62] In contrast, MIBE and SSPE are subacute or chronic complications of measles with latency and usually are characterized by abundant MV production in the brain. The seminal paper by Bouteille and co-workers demonstrated for the first time the pathognomonic 18-nm paramyxovirus nucleocapsids in brain samples from one case of SSPE.[18]

***Measles inclusion body encephalopathy*** — Patients with measles inclusion body encephalopathy (MIBE) or immunosuppressed patients with subacute productive MV encephalitis are usually undergoing cytotoxic treatment. These include, in particular, children with leukemia[60,161] who usually have a history of contact with measles or an actual attack from which they recover fully. Several months later, encephalitic signs, seizures, myoclonus, stupor, and coma develop. The histologic diagnostic features include eosinophilic intranuclear inclusion bodies in neurons and oligodendrocytes, as well as less distinct cytoplasmic inclusion (Fig. 8-15, *A*), and abundant MV antigen (Fig. 8-15, *C*) as in SSPE[33] but usually with much less inflammation or with none.[161] I have seen in one case very rare multinucleated giant cells in the brain with features similar to those of pulmonary Warthin-Finkelday cells (Fig. 8-15, *B*); another report confirms the rare occurrence of MV-induced fusion in brain cells.[138] Electron microscopy reveals the characteristic nuclear "smooth" (Fig. 8-15, *D*) and cytoplasmic "rough" paramyxovirus nucleocapsids.[161] Very rarely, subacute measles encephalitis develops in immunocompetent hosts; such cases might be considered as intermediary between acute [131]

Despite the ubiquity of MV infection, its complications in AIDS are exceptional. We recently observed productive MV encephalitis in a 15-year-old male he-

A
B
C

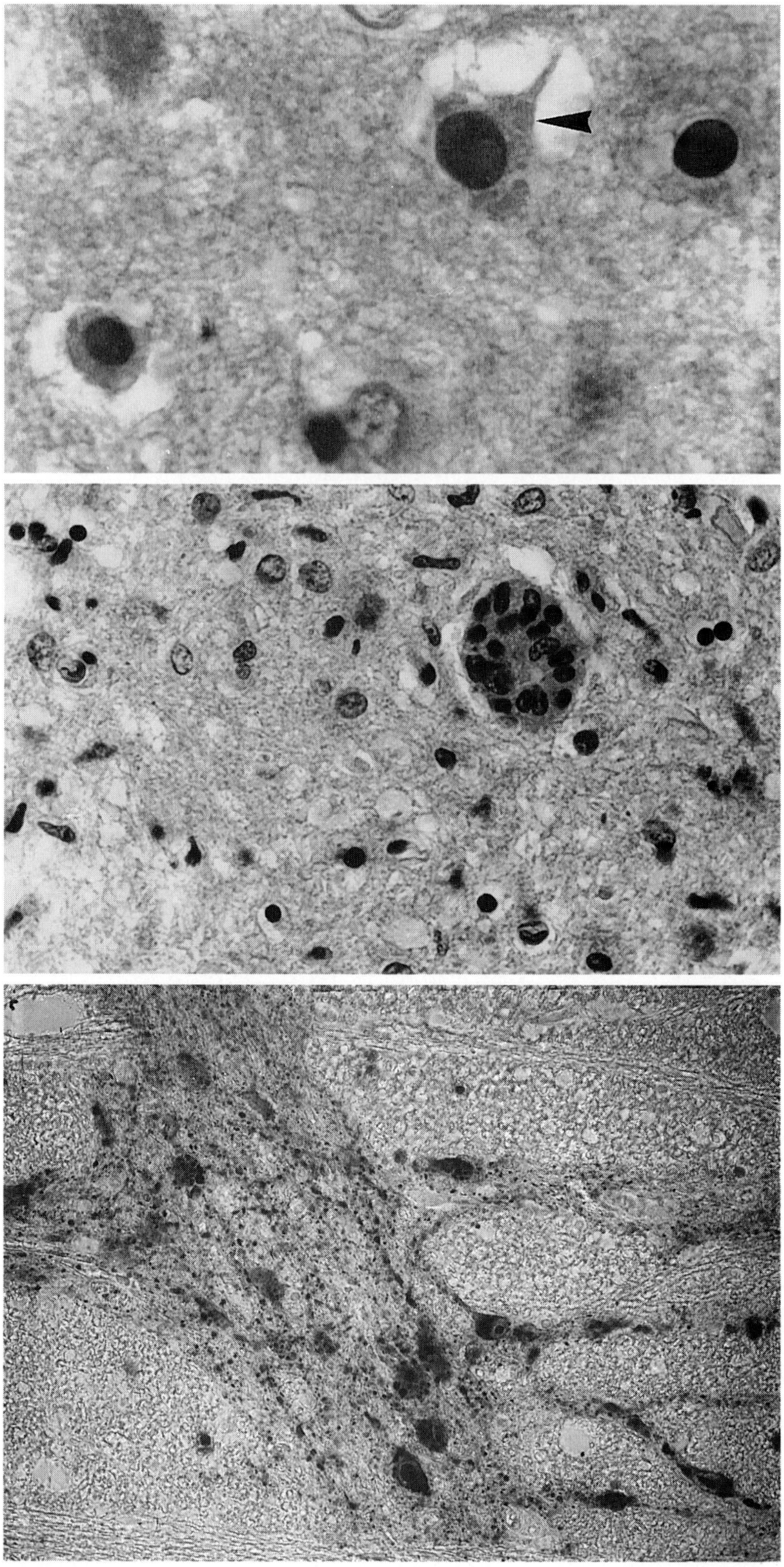

**Fig. 8-15.** Histology of measles inclusion body encephalopathy (MIBE) in the immunosuppressed (child with treated lymphoblastic leukemia). **A**, Densely eosinophilic inclusion bodies fill neuronal and glial nuclei. There are also indistinct cytoplasmic inclusion (*arrowhead*). **B**, A multinucleated giant cell in thalamic area with moderate gliosis. **C**, Abundant measles virus (MV) antigen mainly in neurons and their processes in the pons. **D**, Electron micrograph of helical MV nucleocapsids with an approximate diameter of 20nm in a neuronal nuclear inclusion body. (**A**, H&E; ×1200; **B**, H&E; ×480; **C**, ICC with anti-MV antiserum; ×250; **D**, ×315.) (**D**, Courtesy of Dr. P. P. Liberski, Lodz, Poland.)

D

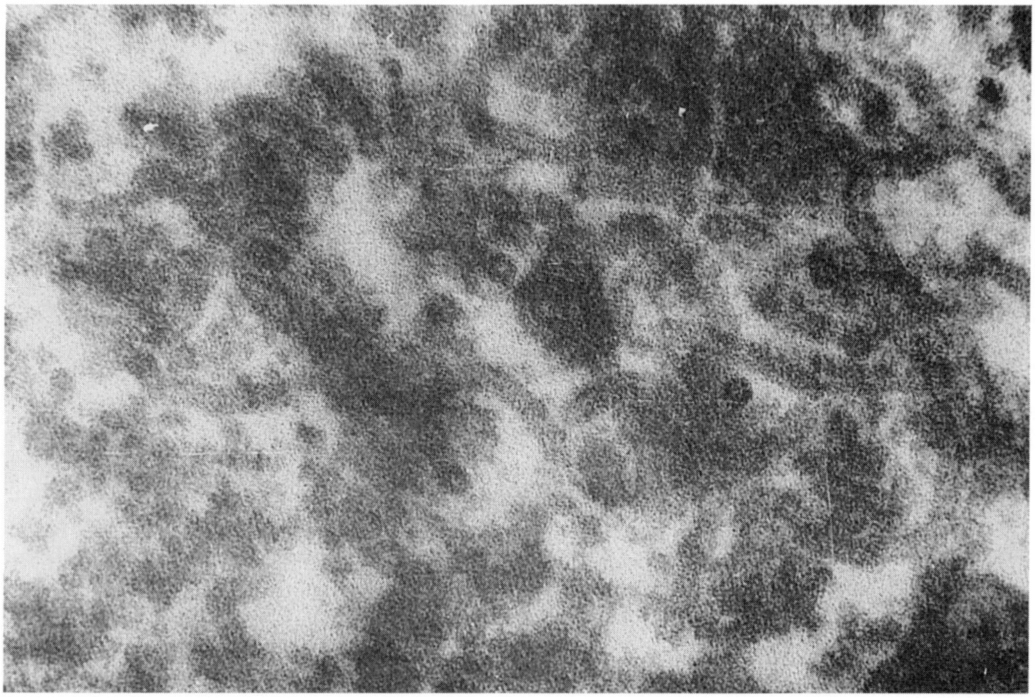

**Fig. 8-15, cont'd.** For legend see opposite page.

mophiliac patient with AIDS. Brain autopsy revealed significant diffuse gliosis and perivascular inflammatory infiltrates in gray and white matter with maximal involvement in the mesencephalon and diencephalon. Numerous cells had intranuclear and intracytoplasmic eosinophilic inclusions, which were strongly immunoreactive with an anti-MV antiserum and contained characteristic paramyxoviral nucleocapsids.[38] Previous reports have described measles virus in myelitis[159] and encephalitis[127] in AIDS, although in the latter report productive infection was not demonstrated. Thus subacute MV infection of the CNS has to be added to the range of viral complications of AIDS.

***Subacute sclerosing panencephalitis***—Subacute sclerosing panencephalitis (SSPE) is a late childhood, adolescent, or early adulthood complication of MV infection that most frequently occurred during infancy. Its neuropathologic features are characteristic and similar but not identical to those of MIBE. The very essence of the SSPE process is excessive local production of partly defective[160] measles virus in the brain, with an equally excessive antibody response.[29,33] However, expression of various MV proteins, especially of envelope and M proteins, is restricted in brain tissue.[104] Persistence in brain tissue of MV in SSPE is correlated with different defects of several genes that probably prevent assembly of fully functional MV particles.[12] Moreover, prominent hypermutation events in genes encoding the M protein were found to expand clonally throughout a SSPE brain,[11] strongly supporting the involvement of MV mutants in the pathogenesis of SSPE.

**Diagnostic Hallmark: *SSPE***

- Intranuclear (less conspicuous cytoplasmic) inclusion bodies
- Inflammation, gliosis, and tissue damage in gray and white matter

Most cases run a subacute to chronic course, but exceptionally features of a more acute encephalitis may be observed.[67,95] Macroscopically, the brain usually is atrophic (Fig. 8-16, *A*). Although SSPE was confusingly labeled as a "demyelinating" condition by some, the white matter is variably involved; frequently secondary, slight (Fig. 8-16, *B*) or even absent involvement may be observed in the white matter.[33] Histologically, diffuse panencephalitis involves both gray and white matter, featuring meningeal infiltration, perivascular cuffing, and intense cellularity (Fig. 8-17, *A*) by increase of astroglia and rod cells (Fig. 8-17, *B*). Diagnostic features are eosinophilic intranuclear (Fig. 8-17, *C*) and less conspicuous cytoplasmic inclusion bodies found mainly in neurons and oligodendroglia[50] (Table 8-2) and the presence of usually abundant MV antigen[33,99] (Fig. 8-18, *A*). Numerous plasmacytes produce abundant anti-MV immunoglobulins in CSF and perivascular spaces. Major viral cell targets are neurons and oligodendroglia, whereas astroglia usually are less involved,[33] one group reported also endothelial infec-

A

B

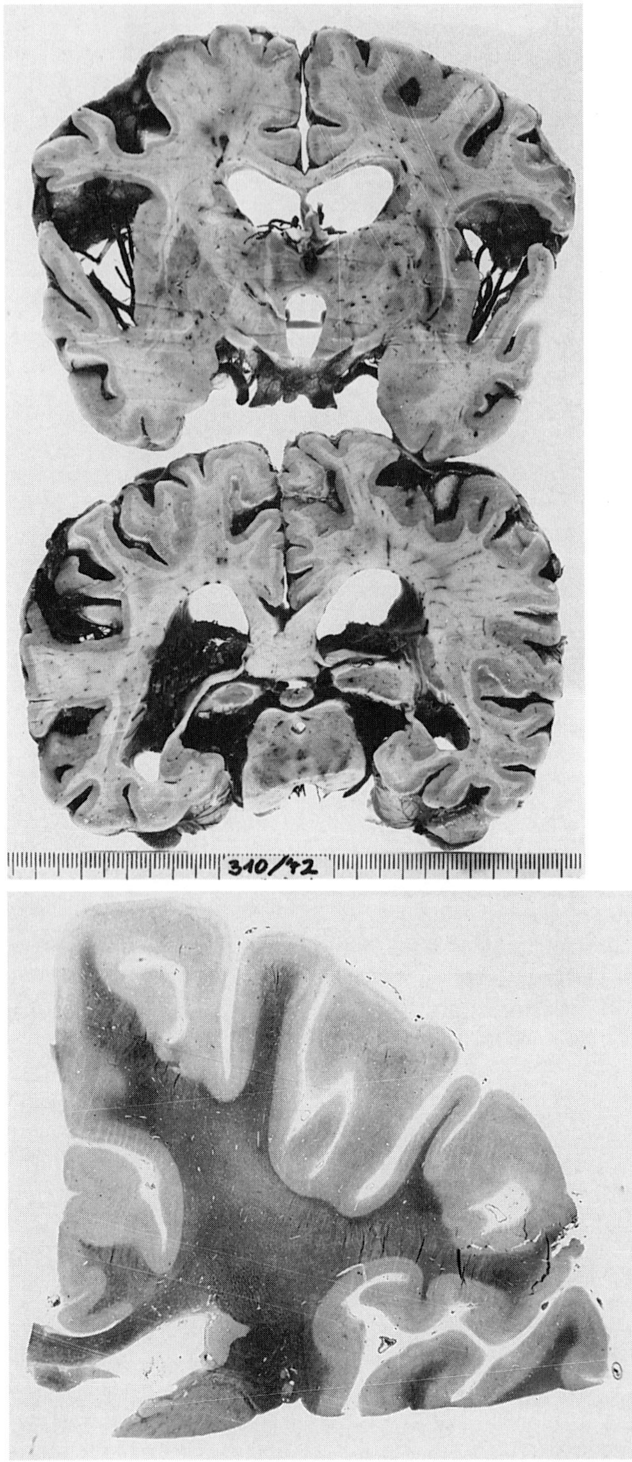


**Fig. 8-16.** Subacute sclerosing panencephalitis (SSPE), macroscopic aspect. **A**, Prominent diffuse brain atrophy in a 20-year-old female. **B**, Moderate cortical atrophy and slight white matter affection in a 12-year-old child. (LFB-NFR stain.)

tion.[96] Electron microscopy reveals nuclear inclusion bodies with the typical appearance of smooth paramyxovirus nucleocapsids with tubular structure.[18,56,83,99] MV antigens are especially abundant in neurons, where they decorate somata and processes in the neuropil up to long distances (Fig. 8-18, *B*). The endoplasmic reticulum (Nissl substance) is converted into a MV protein factory even when the nucleus does not, as yet, contain virus.[33] I found a significant inverse correlation between the amounts of MV antigens and the length of the clinical course, supporting an eventual burning out of the process to the extent that the virus may be completely eliminated from the brain in rare cases.[29] Neuronal neurofibrillary tangles may develop in SSPE as a late effect.

***Mumps virus.*** Neurologic complications of mumps are common and include lymphocytic meningitis and, more rarely, postinfectious/perivenular encephalitis. It is unclear whether direct virus production also occurs in the brain. Two cases of mumps encephalitis showed glial nodules in the cortex.[78] The ultrastructural study of a brain biopsy revealed, in addition to herpes virus particles, paramyxovirus-like particles in neurons and glial cells that were interpreted as mumps virus, as suggested by serologic study in serum and CSF.[146] However, "paramyxovirus like" nuclear changes have been reported in a variety of different conditions; most likely these are nonspecific chromatin changes[80] that require cautious interpretation.

### Rhabdoviruses

#### *Rabies*

**Diagnostic Hallmark: *Rabies***

- Cytoplasmic Negri bodies, best visible in large neurons (hippocampus, brainstem, Purkinje cells)
- Variable, frequently inconspicuous inflammation

Ample evidence demonstrates axoplasmic transport of the virus from the periphery to the CNS as well as within the CNS,[68] including transneuronal transfer.[170] The neuropathology and pathogenesis of rabies encephalitis was recently reviewed.[125] Inflammation is highly variable and inconspicuous in many cases. Immunocytochemical demonstration of viral antigens (Fig. 8-19, *A*) is a much more sensitive and easier diagnostic tool than searching for the pathognomonic neuronal cytoplasmic Negri bodies, which may be difficult to find in routine H&E-stained sections[36,112] (Fig. 8-19, *B*) but which lighten up brilliantly in immunomorphology (Fig. 8-19, *C*). Negri inclusion bodies have basophilic inner granules or sometimes a ringlike shape, in contrast with the smaller "lyssa bodies," which may in fact be early Negri bodies or products of nonviral

**A**

**B**

**C**

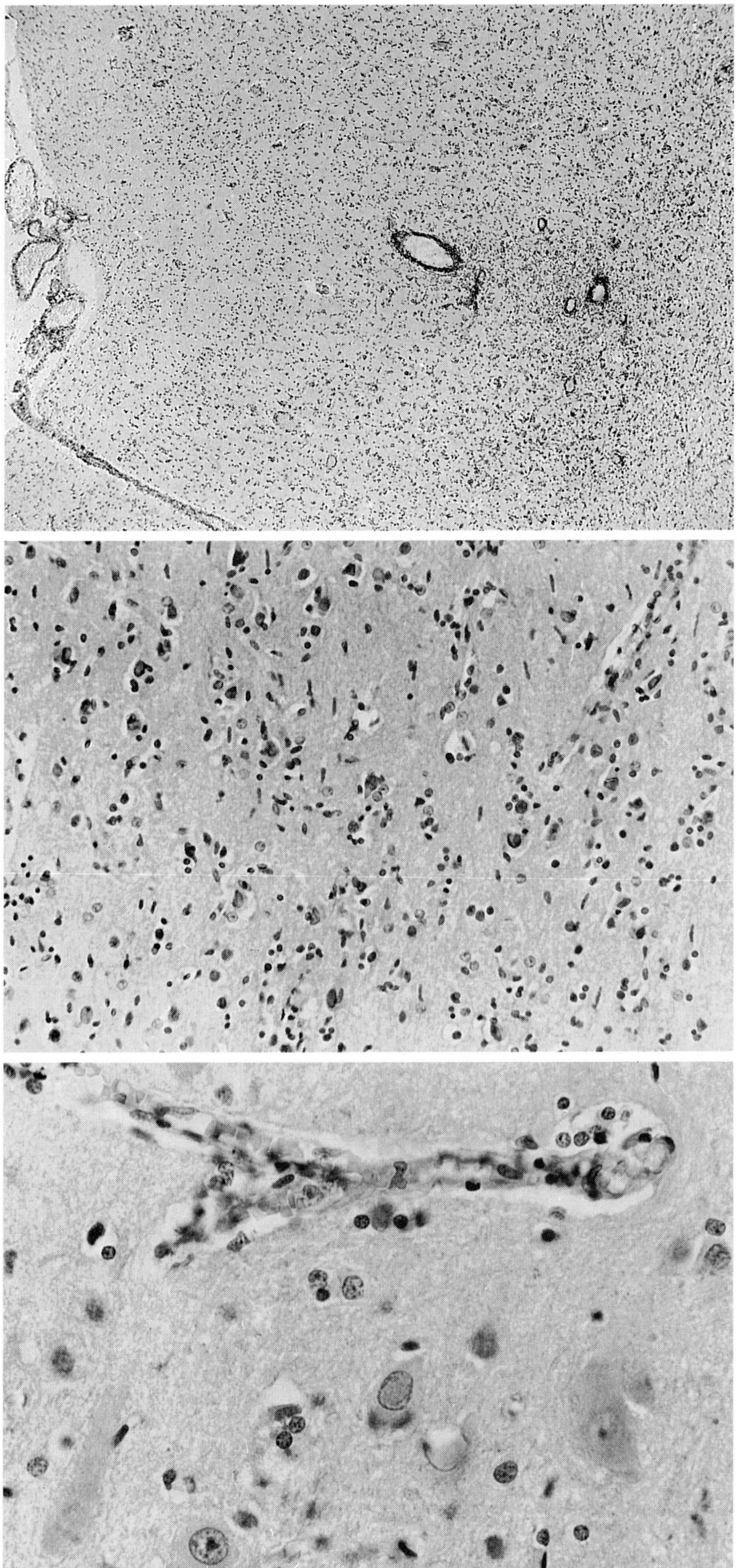

**Fig. 8-17.** Histology of SSPE. Cortex and white matter feature meningeal infiltration, perivascular cuffing, intense cellularity (**A**) by increase of astroglia and rod cells (**B**), and eosinophilic intranuclear inclusion bodies (**C**, center). (**A**, CV stain; ×40; **B**, H&E, ×200; **C**, H&E, ×400.)

A 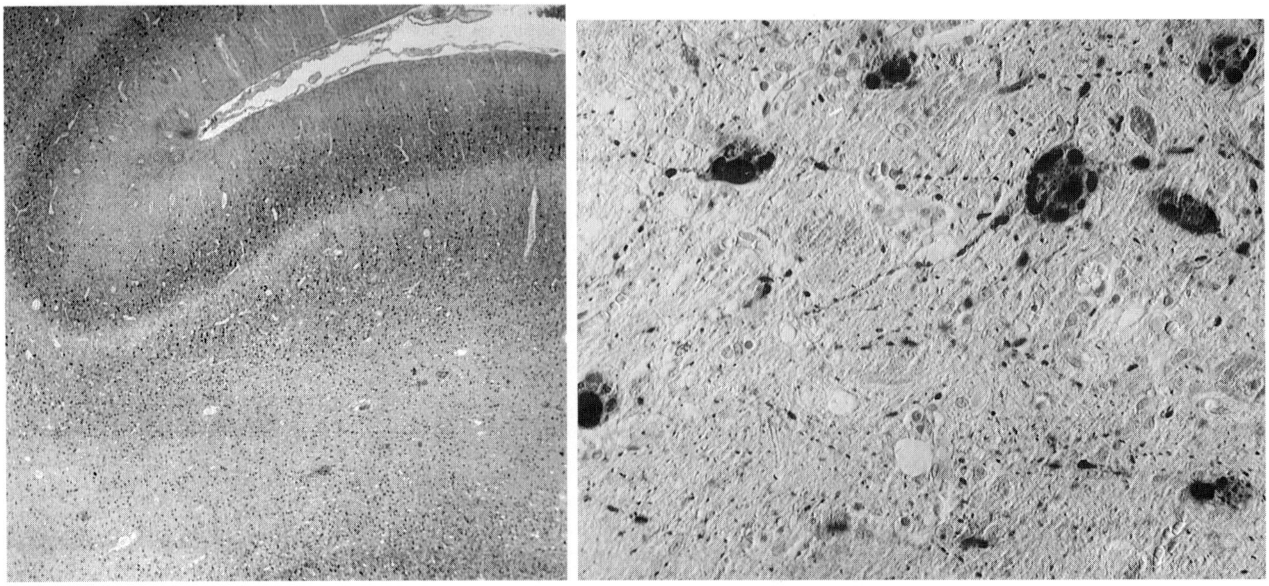 B

**Fig. 8-18.** ICC of SSPE. **A**, Numerous MV-producing cells in the cortex and subcortical white matter. **B**, Abundant MV antigen in neuronal nuclei, cytoplasm, and processes in the brainstem. (**A**, ICC with anti-MV antiserum, slight H counterstain; ×10; **B**, ICC with anti-MV antiserum, NICO; ×250.)

**Fig. 8-19.** Rabies. **A**, There is abundant viral antigen in cerebellar Purkinje's cells and their ascending dendrites in the molecular layer. (ICC with antirabies antiserum, slight H counterstain, ×63.) **B** and **C**, The same field of brainstem was stained with H&E (**B**) after performance of direct immunofluorescence with an antirabies antiserum-FITC conjugate (**C**). Negri bodies, sometimes circular, and smaller inclusions are much less prominent in the H&E stain than in immunomorphology. (**B** and **C** × 630.)

A 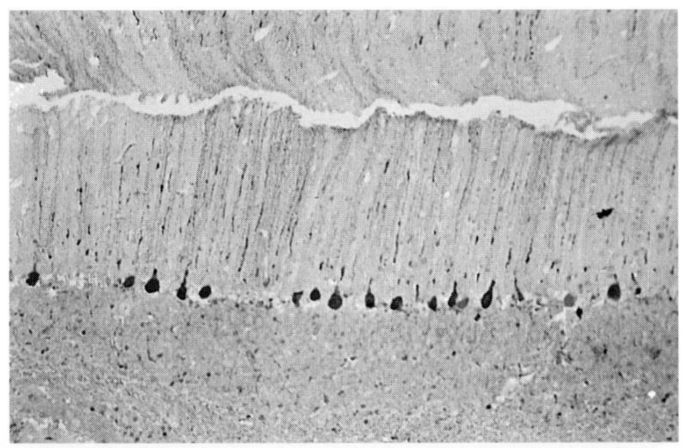

B 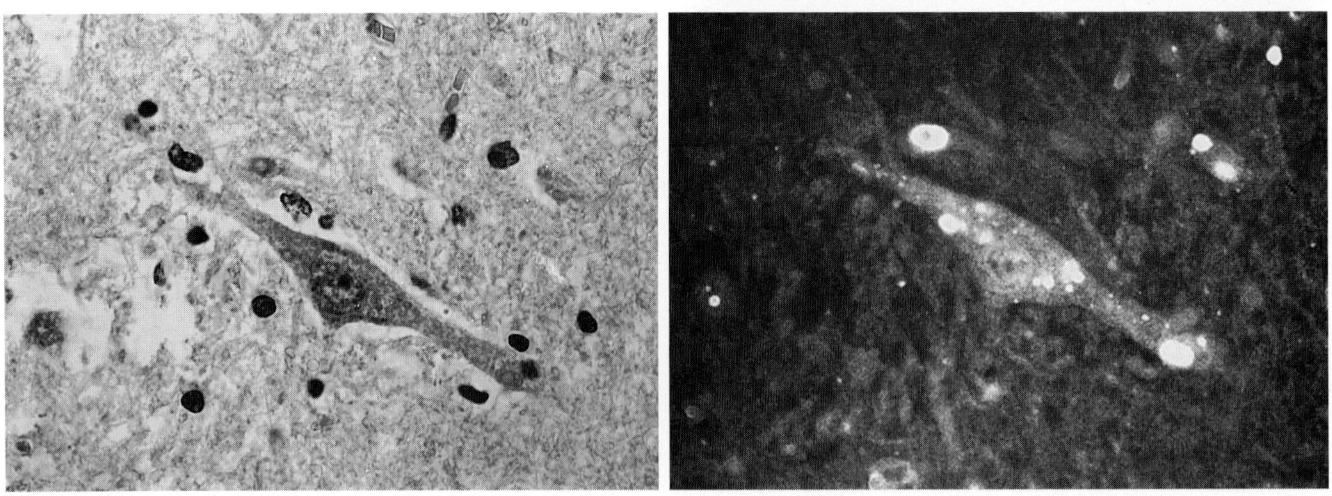 C degeneration.[164] Large pyramidal neurons of the hippocampus, temporal cortex, brainstem, and Purkinje's cells are best candidates for finding Negri bodies. Negri bodies may be quite pleomorphic and there may be differences in ultrastructure between those found in human brains and those seen in inoculated mice. Sometimes the typical bullet-shaped mature virions may not be seen in the granular matrix in human tissues but are readily visible in animal brains.[113] As routinely done for diagnosis of rabies on animal brains, tissue imprint preparations might give a quick diagnosis by immunofluorescence.[36] ICC on fixed brain samples has the same sensitivity and abolishes the need to handle highly infectious fresh tissue.[26] Neither viral antigen distribution nor inflammation parallels clinical presentations.[166] Virus genomic RNA and mRNA may be visualized by ISH on brain sections.[87]

**Arenaviruses**

***Lymphocytic choriomeningitis.*** The lymphocytic choriomeningitis (LCM) virus was the first virus isolated from aseptic meningitis in man. Signs of mild encephalitis are frequent, but fatal cases are very rare.[89]

**Retroviruses**

***Human immunodeficiency virus.*** Evidence accumulated for over a decade has identified human immunodeficiency virus (HIV) as a major pathogen for the CNS. This virus has emerged as the major paradigm for two important principles of viral processes in the CNS: (1) a novel restricted type of "neurotropism" that is complementary to classic viral encephalitis: HIV-1, although neuroinvasive and neurovirulent, does not appear to replicate in neural cells;[20,24] (2) a staged involvement of the nervous system with a massive viral onslaught occurs only in the final phase of the infection following prolonged latency.

The diagnostic neuropathology of AIDS is extensively covered in Chapter 9. Here, I will discuss only some general aspects of HIV and the diagnosis of HIV-specific neuropathology. The basic lesson on HIV and nervous system impairment may be summarized as follows:[22]

1. CNS involvement is staged: prominent CNS dysfunction usually occurs in the late (AIDS) stage of infection.
2. A single neuropathologic subset cannot explain all types of clinical dysfunction:
   - we do not deal here with a uniform disease
   - the monocausal approach is inappropriate.
3. Several pathogenetic factors (viral, systemic, and local) acting in concert lead to modulated neuropathology and clinical dysfunction: a pathogenetic system is operating.
4. Distinct pathologies need to be dissected in this system:
   - by careful clinical observation of differential presentation and course, response to distinct therapeutic approaches, and refined testing methods;
   - refined tissue analysis at biopsy and autopsy, and
   - ingenious experimental in vivo and in vitro modeling.

According to data derived mainly from CSF studies, HIV seems able to seed the CNS parenchyma during or shortly after the primary infection. The latent and persistently infected CNS cell reservoir is yet undefined. Whether, and how much, that putative reservoir contributes to late productive infection occurring in microglia/macrophages and resulting in HIV encephalitis (HIVE) or HIV leukoencephalopathy (HIVL), is unknown. Moreover, factors leading to the development of less conspicuous, morphologically unspecific "neuro(no)toxic" CNS pathology in vivo remain to be elucidated, especially their relevance to the clinical manifestations of cognitive impairment.[23] This is especially true for the prominent damage to the gray matter in many AIDS brains, including loss of cortical neurons,[94] which differs in extent between cortical regions[179] and may be the sole correlate of HIV-associated dementia.[71] Astroglial changes in the cerebral cortex of AIDS brains include hypertrophy and prominent GFAP reactivity by astrocytes that previously were of the protoplasmic type.[178] Early into the HIV pandemic, prominent damage to the white matter was recognized[97] and described in detail.[157] Frequently this leukoencephalopathy includes vacuolar myelin damage and post-BBB leakage, angiocentric foci,[157] reflecting the multitude of pathogenetic factors that co-orchestrate the complex scenario of brain damage in AIDS.[20]

It is useful to separate the disease entities of HIVE and HIVL as HIV-specific neuropathology from HIV-associated conditions in which the relationship with the virus is less clear. The frequency of HIV-specific and HIV-associated neuropathologic changes found at autopsy is summarized in Table 8-5. The considerable range observed among the various autopsy series probably reflects the influence of many factors, including age, gender, risk group, geographic factors, socioeconomic conditions, previous or present treatment, sample size, bias in sampling, and application of different diagnostic criteria. Apart from HIVE/HIVL, HIV products may be prominent also in lesions of purely degenerative, noninflammatory type, such as vacuolar myelopathy[34] and multifocal vacuolar leukoencephalopathy.[153] As is true of other viral infections, the depth of immunosuppression likely influences the features of the viral involvement of the CNS.

**Table 8-5.** Frequency of HIV-specific and HIV-associated CNS lesions in neuropathological AIDS autopsies

| Type of Lesion | Own series n | Own series % | All autopsy series[1] n | All autopsy series[1] % | All autopsy series[1] range in % |
|---|---|---|---|---|---|
| HIV-Specific lesions | 61/165 | 37 | 312/1450 | 21.5 | 11–40 |
| HIV encephalitis (HIVE) | 20/165 | 12 | 190/1198 | 16 | 11–28 |
| HIV leukoencephalopathy (HIVL) | 18/165 | 11 | 75/619 | 12 | 3–29 |
| HIVE combined with HIVL | 23/165 | 14 | 23/165 | 14[2] | — |
| HIV meningoventriculoencephalitis | 1/165 | 0.6 | 1/165 | 0.6[2] | — |
| HIV-Associated lesions | 76/165 | 46 | 76/165 | 46[2] | — |
| diffuse poliodystrophy (DPD) | 73/165 | 44 | 73/165 | 44[2] | — |
| lymphocytic meningitis | 7/165 | 4 | 7/165 | 4[2] | — |
| multifocal vacuolar leukoencephalopathy | 3/165 | 2 | 4/349 | 1 | 0.5–2 |
| VM[3] | 3/16 | 19 | 85/1118 | 8 | 0.5–30 |

Data from my series[21,31] and from a cumulative literature survey on major autopsy series.* Many brains had more than one type of pathology.
[1] For individual lesions, the total number evaluated varies because not all series cover all types of lesions or provide only ill-defined or lacking data on some lesion types.
[2] Data for this lesion are available only from my own series.
[3] Spinal cords were usually available for examination only in some selected cases of the respective series.
* See references 5, 43, 59, 70, 100, 101, 103, 114, 141, 145

**Table 8-6.** Neuropathologic diagnoses in 53 stereotaxic brain biopsies from 52 HIV-infected patients

| Type of lesion/ infectious agent | Biopsies n | Biopsies % |
|---|---|---|
| HIV encephalitis and HIV leukoencephalopathy | 1 | 2 |
| Malignant lymphoma | 10 | 19 |
| Toxoplasmosis | 15 | 28 |
| Progressive multifocal leukoencephalopathy | 17 | 32 |
| Aspergilloma | 1 | 2 |
| Tuberculoma | 1 | 2 |
| Necroses of undefined character | 8 | 15 |

Stereotactic brain biopsy is a highly accurate and safe diagnostic tool to ascertain the nature of cerebral lesions in AIDS patients, especially opportunistic infections and neoplasms.* Brain biopsy is usually undertaken to diagnose mass lesions that show poor clinical or radiologic responses to antitoxoplasma therapy. Table 8-6 lists the diagnoses found in stereotaxic brain biopsies of HIV-infected patients in Vienna.

Vast data are available about the CNS in HIV type 1 infection. As to the more recently described HIV type 2, information on associated nervous system pathology is scarce.[109] In our experience, the spectrum of HIV-2 related neuropathology is indistinguishable from that of HIV-1.[105]

* Refs. 3, 7, 42, 63, 91, 128, 140, 185.

### *HIV encephalitis/HIV leukoencephalopathy*

**Diagnostic Hallmark: *HIV Encephalitis/ Leukoencephalopathy***

- Multinucleated giant cells, perivascular or disseminated
- Disseminated microgranulomas or diffuse white matter damage

Macroscopically, HIVE and HIVL are not distinct; both are frequently associated with significant brain atrophy. Multinucleated giant cells (Fig. 8-20, *A*) of macrophage/microglial origin[24] have been established as the histologic hallmark of HIV-induced CNS pathology.[21,25,27] Individual neuropathologic features were defined in a consensus report,[39] exhaustively reviewed,[28] and illustrated[32] elsewhere. HIVE and HIVL represent the extremes of a wide neuropathologic spectrum.[21] Features of HIVE include multiple tiny focal lesions (Fig. 8-21, *A*) in the form of disseminated microgranulomas (Fig. 8-20, *B* and *C*) composed mainly of microglia and multinucleated cells with abundant HIV products (Fig. 8-22, *A* and *B*); these lesions are most prominent in basal ganglia, white matter (corpus callosum and anterior commissure), and brainstem (pons) (Table 8-1). HIVL is characterized by diffuse involvement of the white matter (Fig. 8-21, *B*) with myelin breakdown (evidenced by myelin ovoids), gliosis, and mononuclear as well as multinucleated macrophages; HIVL is thus more than mere "myelin pallor." Numerous diffusely disseminated microglial cells (Fig. 8-23, *A* and *B*) and macrophages (Fig. 8-23, *C*) are labeled for HIV products. In my autopsy series, about one third of HIV-specific neuropathology was diagnosed as

A
B
C

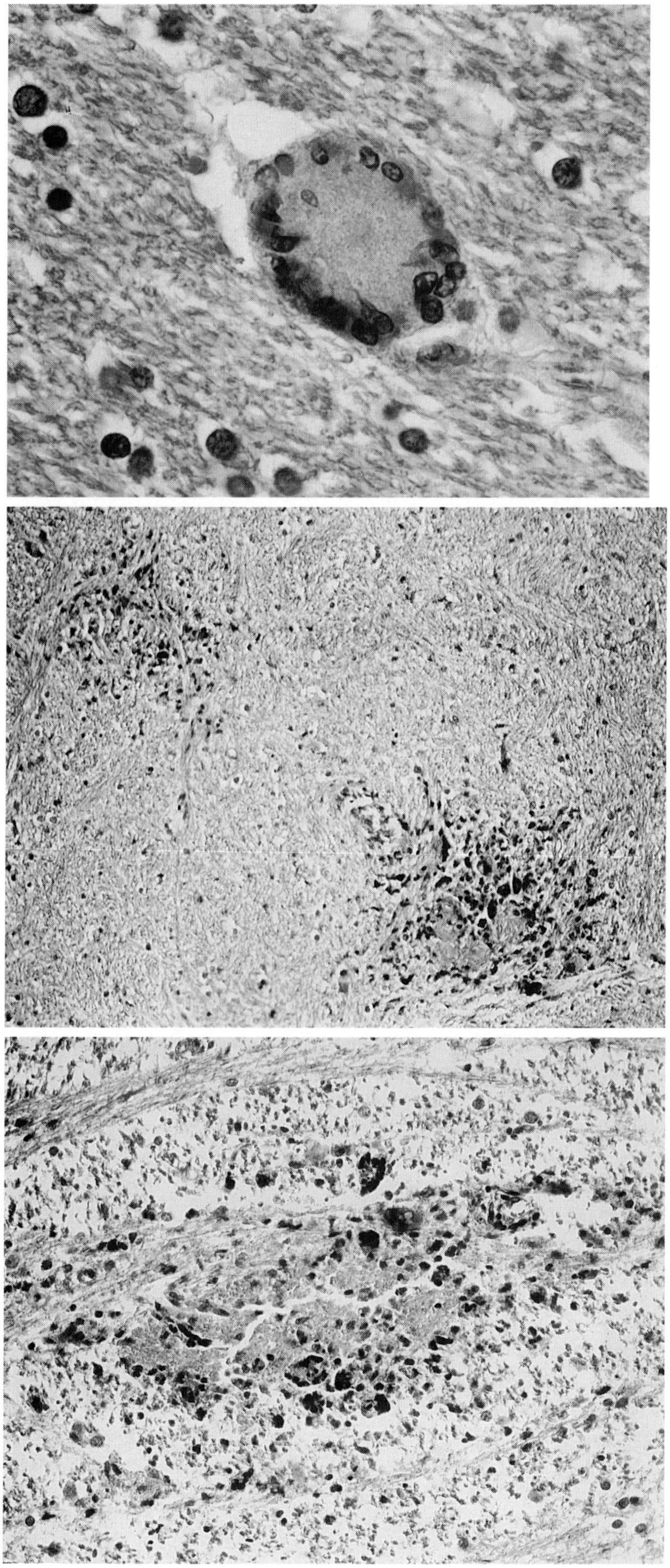

**Fig. 8-20.** Histology of HIV-specific pathology in the brain. **A**, A multinucleated giant cell in the white matter in HIVL. **B** (cerebral white matter) and **C** (pons), Typical microgranulomatous foci of HIVE feature microglia, macrophages and multinucleated giant cells; there may be occasional indistinct necrosis in the lesion center (**C**). (**A**, H&E; ×1.000; **B**, H&E; ×160; **C**, H&E; ×250.)

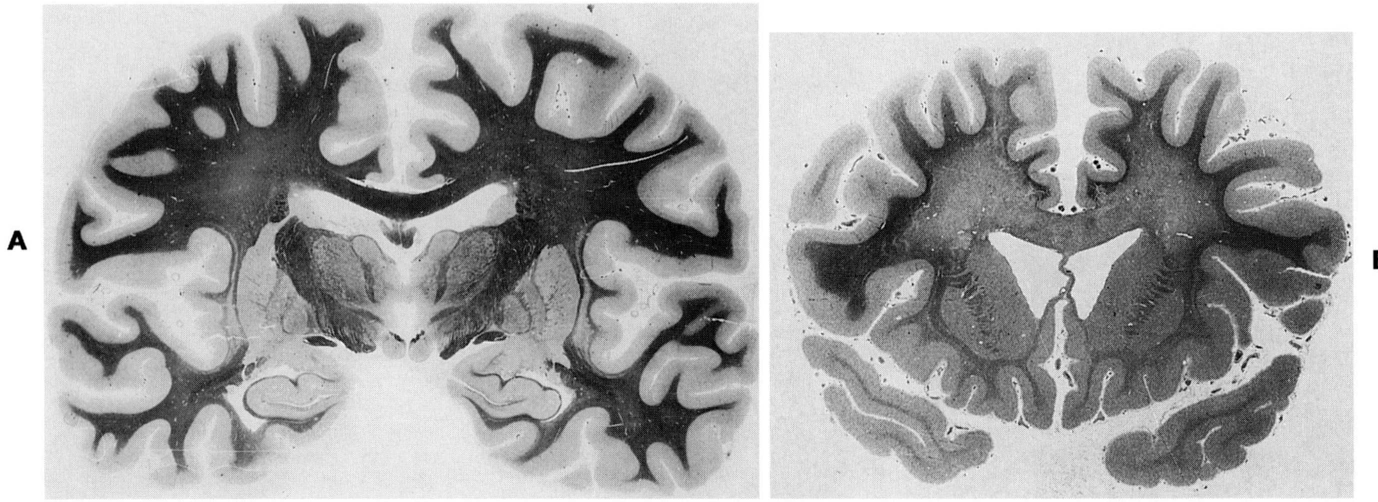


**Fig. 8-21.** Distribution of HIV-specific pathology in the brain. **A**, HIV encephalitis (HIVE) features innumerable tiny indistinct foci in centrum semiovale and internal capsule; there is slight indistinct pallor of the deep white matter. **B**, HIV leukoencephalopathy (HIVL) features prominent diffuse damage of deep white matter and corpus callosum. (LFB-NFR stain.)

HIVE, another third as HIVL, and the last third as a combination of both. The inflammatory changes of HIVE may spread to the ventricular walls and meninges where HIV antigens may be visualized within inflammatory infiltrates.[30]

Sensitive ICC and ISH techniques to detect HIV in brain tissue have contributed greatly to the characterization of these new types of neuropathology,[24,25] which are seen isolated, without any other type of CNS pathology, in 40% of my series of brains with HIV-specific neuropathology.[21] Both core and envelope HIV proteins are well detectable at cell membranes or within the cytoplasm of macrophages and microglial cells, including multinucleated giant cells.[24] Characteristic enveloped particles with conoid nucleoid are seen either in the cytoplasmic cisterns (Fig. 8-24, *A* and *B*) or at cell membranes.[31,118]

***Other HIV-associated neuropathologic syndromes***—In many brains of HIV-1 infected patients, the only histologic finding is the presence of gliomesenchymal nodules (GMN), giving a diagnosis of unspecified nodular encephalitis. These nodules, composed of lymphocytes, microglia, and macrophages, with adjacent reactive astrocytes, are scattered more widely in the gray than in the white matter[137] (Fig. 8-25). Nodular encephalitis in AIDS was described initially as "AIDS subacute encephalitis"[130] and frequently has been confused with HIVE. Nodular encephalitis of AIDS can be identified by the different distribution of foci (the cortex being preferentially involved), by the different composition of the nodules (more densely packed rounded cells in GMN vs. the usually looser arrangement of elongated microglia in HIVE[31]), and by the lack of multinucleated giant cells[39] and HIV antigens.[24] The most frequent cause of nodular encephalitis is CMV,[92] although only sporadic cytomegalic cells may be found within the nodules.[101] In some of our cases, numerous small samples did not reveal the infectious agent, whereas large sections demonstrated cytomegalic cells or other agents. In some cases, toxoplasma or HSV were the underlying cause of nodular encephalitis demonstrated by ICC or ISH.[31,152]

***Human T-cell leukemia/lymphoma virus I***

***HTLV-I-associated myelopathy/tropical spastic paraparesis***—HTLV-I-associated myelopathy/tropical spastic paraparesis (HAM/TSP) is caused by human T-cell lymphotropic virus type I (HTLV-I), which primarily infects T cells. However, HTLV-I appears to have a wide cellular spectrum of infectivity in human nervous tissues.[1] Nevertheless, the inflammatory demyelination characteristic of HAM/TSP has not been directly linked to the presence of the virus in CNS tissue. Thus, indirect mechanisms (e.g., cytokines) could be involved in demyelination and inflammation.[55] In contrast to the direct viral invasion, the CNS tissue damage appears to be heralded by the infiltration of helper/inducer T cells.[85] HTLV-I proviral DNA was detected only in the nucleus of infiltrating lymphocytes; proviral DNA was not amplified in any neural cells. This suggests that the demyelination of the spinal cord

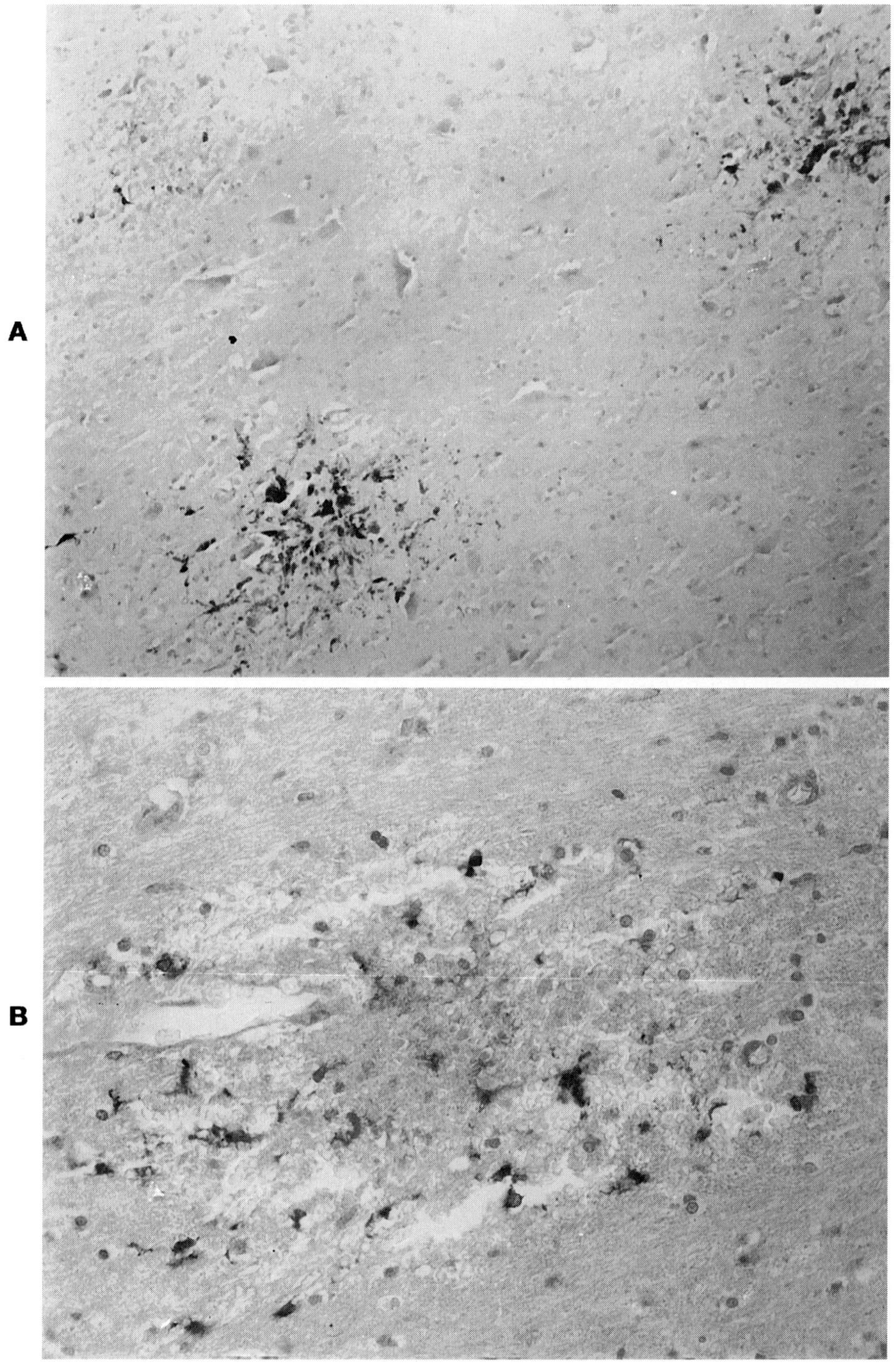


**Fig. 8-22.** ICC of HIVE. **A** and **B**, Numerous microglial cells in the lesions produce the HIV envelope protein. **A**, from same field as Fig. 8-20, **B**. (ICC with anti-gp41 antibody, slight H counterstain; **A** ×100; **B** ×250.)

by HTLV-I as a result of viral infection of oligodendrocytes or neuronal cells is unlikely.[76] Thus, the neuropathology of HAM/TSP suggests an immune-mediated disease rather than a productive viral infection. The lesions are restricted to the spinal cord and optic nerve, where demyelination, inflammation, and fiber loss are common features. Lymphocytes are seen close to nerve fibers, within which are changes resembling those seen in myelinated cultures of the central nervous system exposed to cytokines.[120] Autopsy in a case in which the disease existed for 28 years showed severely degenerated white matter; both the myelin and axons were equally lost and had been replaced by glial scars.[150]

**Picornaviruses**

***Poliomyelitis.*** Acute poliomyelitis of earlier endemic and later epidemic proportions has become rela-

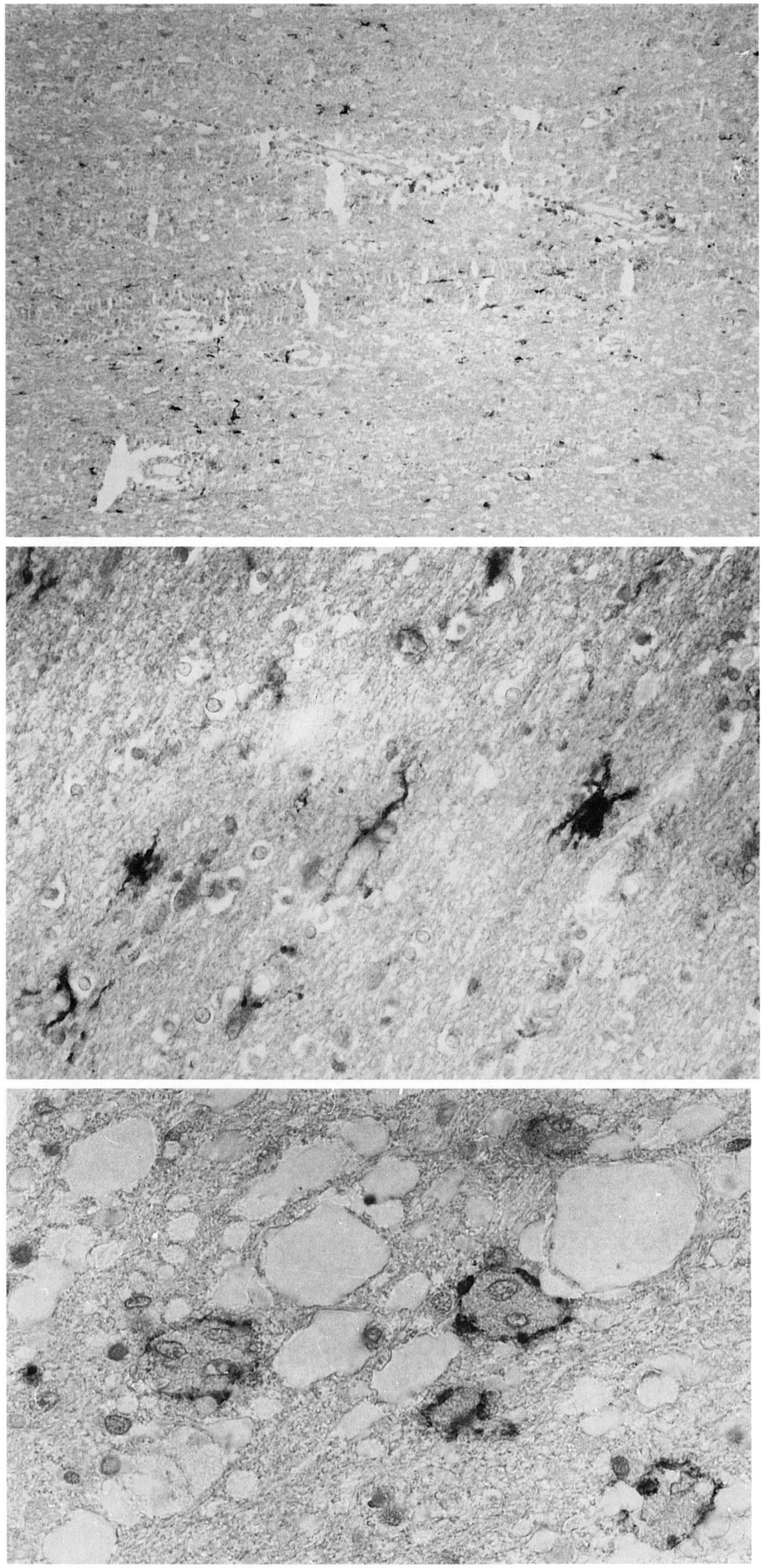

A

B

C

**Fig. 8-23.** ICC of HIVL. **A** and **B**, Numerous microglial cells are diffusely disseminated in the white matter and produce the HIV envelope protein. **C**, Multinucleate macrophages in vacuolar white matter damage express HIV core protein at the cytoplasmic membrane. (**A** and **B**, ICC with anti-gp41 antibody, slight H counterstain; A ×100; B × 400; **C**, ICC with anti-p24 antibody, slight H counterstain; ×630.)

A

B

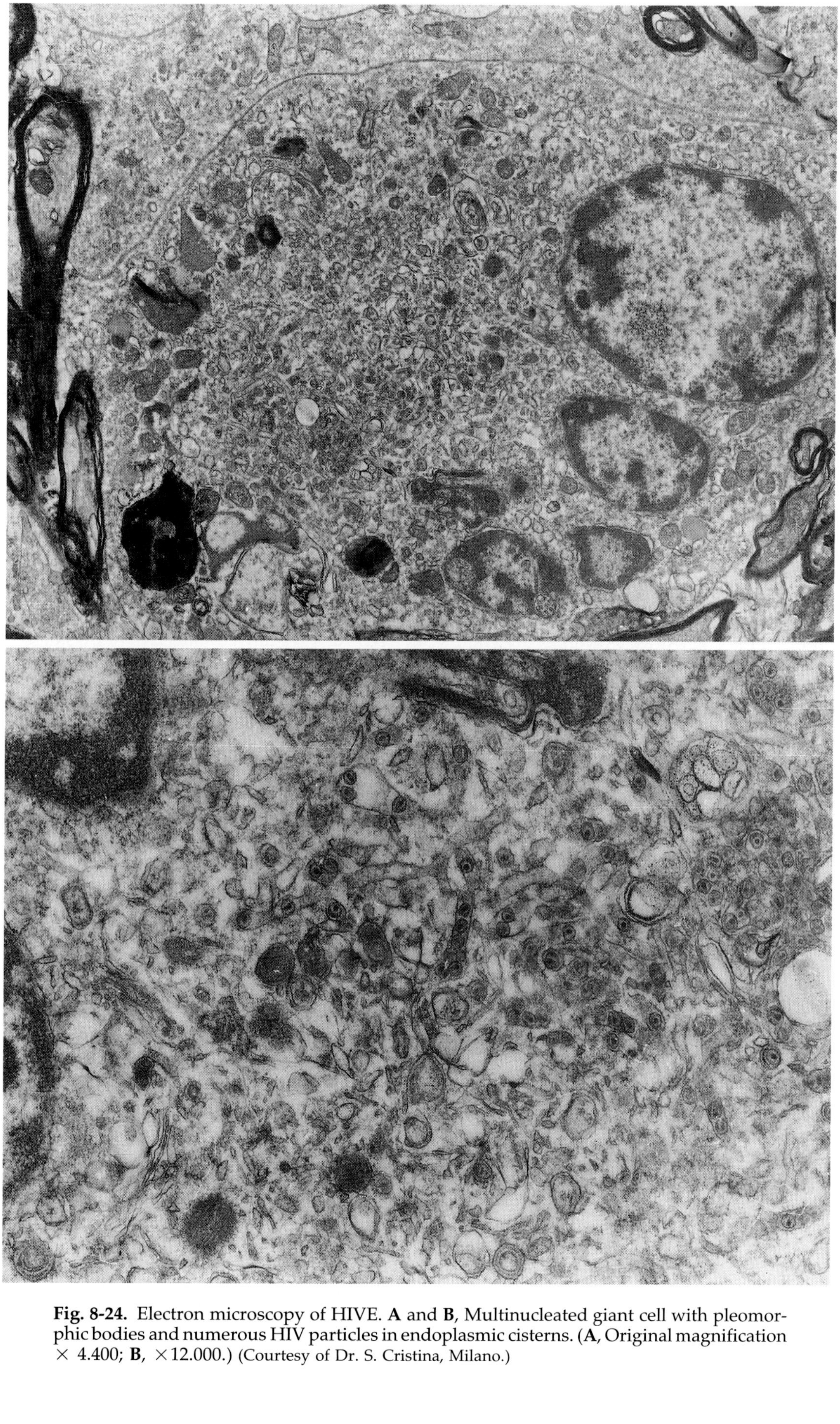

**Fig. 8-24.** Electron microscopy of HIVE. **A** and **B**, Multinucleated giant cell with pleomorphic bodies and numerous HIV particles in endoplasmic cisterns. (**A**, Original magnification × 4.400; **B**, ×12.000.) (Courtesy of Dr. S. Cristina, Milano.)

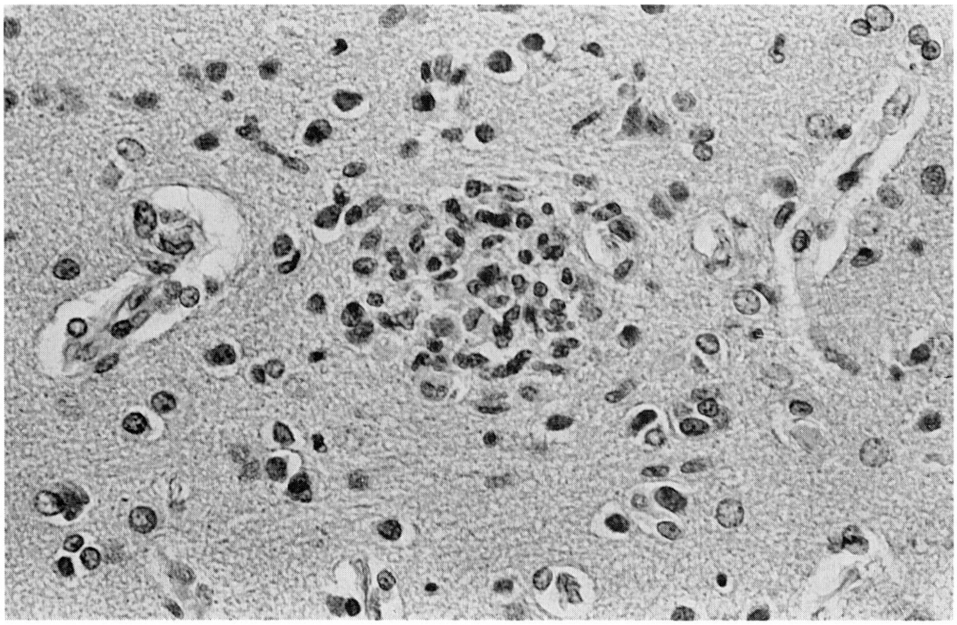

**Fig. 8-25.** Unspecified nodular encephalitis in AIDS. Cortical nodule comprises lymphocytes, macrophages, and microglial cells. (H&E, ×440.)

tively rare because of efficient vaccination campaigns. However, worsening economic and hygienic conditions in several parts of the world, as well as declining compliance for vaccination, favor a possible reemergence of poliomyelitis as one of the most devastating viral infections of the nervous system. The pathologic changes vary according to the stage of the disease; in most developed countries, residual damage may be seen at autopsy decades after acute disease. Macroscopically, anterior horns may show hemorrhagic necrosis in the acute stage and shrunken scarring in the residual state, when atrophy of the anterior roots also is prominent. Histologically, the acute disease features prominent infiltration of the spinal gray matter by granulocytes in the early days, and by lymphocytes with prominent neuronophagia of motoneurons and microglial nodules in subsequent days.[62] Perivascular lymphocyte and plasma cell cuffings become increasingly prominent. Motor nuclei of the brainstem also may be involved. In severe cases, lesions may be present throughout the neuraxis (Fig. 8-26), although the brunt of the injury always falls on spinal and medullar motoneurons. Depending on the stage of disease, skeletal muscle specimens feature denervation atrophy, frequently accompanied by prominent myopathic changes in the late stages of the disease.

Poliovirus antigen is detected only in nerve cells of the CNS; ultrastructurally, membrane-bound vesicles in the cytoplasm of the motoneuron closely correlate with virus multiplication, and damage of the nerve cell appears to be the result of direct invasion by the poliovirus.[79]

It has been suggested that late onset neurologic deterioration after acute poliomyelitis may be the result in some cases of persistent poliovirus infection of the CNS. CSF enteroviral RNA was detected in 3 of 24 patients with a clinical diagnosis of post-polio syndrome, but in none of 36 patients with stable poliomyelitis and in none of 36 patients with other neurologic conditions of noninfective origin. Moreover, enterovirus RNA was detected in tissue from the spinal cord from three patients with a history of paralytic poliomyelitis; thus, enteroviruses may persist in the CNS of man.[126] However, such possible virus persistence does not necessarily mean that the entire virus has a pathogenetic role in the post-polio syndrome. Some obscure type of "exhaustion" of the function of motoneurons at advanced age might lead to the seemingly new or progressive neurologic deficits among victims of juvenile poliomyelitis.

***Coxsackieviruses, echoviruses.*** Enteroviruses such as coxsackievirus or echoviruses rarely may cause acute poliomyelitis. However, these viruses more commonly are the cause of aseptic meningitis or acute nodular encephalitis in children; the latter is neuropathologically indistinguishable from the abnormalities seen in cases of infections with either flaviruses or alphaviruses.

## ACKNOWLEDGMENTS

The author is most grateful to Mrs. Helga Flicker for excellent technical assistance over many years, to Dr. J. A. Hainfellner for support with preparation of some figures and a literature survey, to Dr. S. Cristina, Milano, for providing Fig. 8-24, and to Professor PP Liberski, Lodz, Poland, for providing Figures 8-13, *F* and 8-15, *D*.

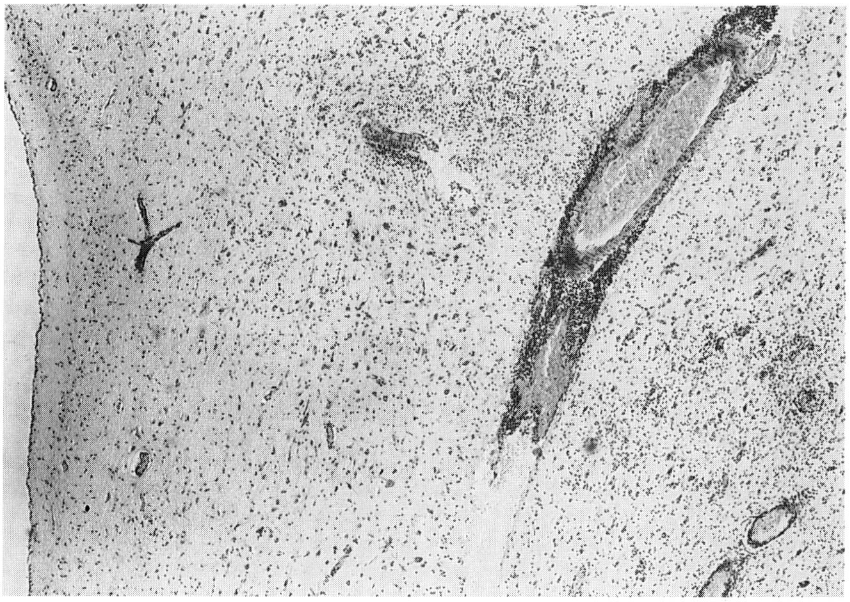

**Fig. 8-26.** Acute poliomyelitis. Prominent extension of inflammation from the spinal cord to the brain. Patchy cellular infiltration and perivascular cuffing in hypothalamus. (Cv stain, ×40.)

## REFERENCES


1. Akagi T, and others: Infectivity of human T-lymphotropic virus type I to human nervous tissue cells in vitro, Acta Neuropathol 84:147-152, 1992.
2. Aksamit AJ, and others: AIDS-associated progressive multifocal leukoencephalopathy (PML): comparison to non-AIDS PML with in situ hybridization and immunohistochemistry, Neurology 40:1073-1078, 1990.
3. Alesch F, Armbruster C, and Budka H: Diagnostic value of stereotactic biopsy of cerebral lesions in patients with AIDS, Acta Neurochir 134:214-219, 1995.
4. Amlie Lefond C, and others: The vasculopathy of varicella-zoster virus encephalitis, Ann Neurol 37:784-790, 1995.
5. Anders KH, and others: The neuropathology of AIDS: UCLA experience and review, Am J Pathol 124:537-558, 1986.
6. Anderson JR, and Field HJ: The distribution of herpes simplex type 1 antigen in mouse central nervous system after different routes of inoculation, J Neurol Sci 60:181-195, 1983.
7. Antinori A, and others: Primary central nervous system lymphoma and brain biopsy in AIDS, Lancet 341:1411-1412, 1993.
8. Aslanzadseh J, and others: A prospective study of the polymerase chain reaction for detection of herpes simplex virus in cerebrospinal fluid submitted to the clinical virological laboratory, Mol Cell Probes 6:367-373, 1992.
9. Åström KE, Mancall EL, and Richardson EP, Jr: Progressive multifocal leukoencephalopathy. A hitherto unrecognized complication of chronic lymphatic leukaemia and Hodgkin's disease, Brain 81:93-111, 1958.
10. Åström KE, and Stoner GL: Early pathological changes in progressive multifocal leukoencephalopathy: a report of two asymptomatic cases occurring prior to the AIDS epidemic, Acta Neuropathol 88:93-105, 1994.
11. Baczko K, and others: Clonal expansion of hypermutated measles virus in a SSPE brain, Virology 197:188-195, 1993.
12. Baczko K, and others: Expression of defective measles virus genes in brain tissues of patients with subacute sclerosing panencephalitis, J Virol 59:472-478, 1986.
13. Bale JF, Jr: Human cytomegalovirus infection and disorders of the nervous system, Arch Neurol 41:310-320, 1984.
14. Bashir R, and others: Expression of Epstein-Barr virus proteins in primary CNS lymphoma in AIDS patients, Neurology 43: 2358-2362, 1993.
15. Belec L, and others: Cytomegalovirus (CMV) encephalomyeloradiculitis and human immunodeficiency virus (HIV) encephalitis: presence of HIV and CMV co-infected multinucleated giant cells, Acta Neuropathol Berl 81:99-104, 1990.
16. Belec L, and others: Cytomegalovirus encephalopathy in an infant with congenital acquired immuno-deficiency syndrome, Neuropediatrics 21:124-129, 1990.
17. Berger JR, and others: Progressive multifocal leukoencephalopathy in HIV-1-infected children. AIDS 6:837-841, 1992.
18. Bouteille M, and others: Sur un cas d'encéphalite subaigue inclusions. Etude anatomoclinique et ultrastructurale, Rev Neurol 113:454-458, 1965.
19. Britton CB, and others: A new complication of AIDS: thoracic myelitis caused by herpes simplex virus, Neurology 35:1071-1074, 1985.
20. Budka H: Cerebral pathology in AIDS: a new nomenclature and pathogenetic concepts, Curr Opin Neurol Neurosurg 5:917-923, 1992.
21. Budka H: The definition of HIV-specific neuropathology, Acta Pathol Jpn 41:182-191, 1991.
22. Budka H: HIV-associated neuropathology. In Gendelman HE, Lipton S, Epstein L, and Swindells S, editors: Neurological and neuropsychiatric manifestations of HIV infection. New York, 1997, Chapman & Hall.
23. Budka H: HIV-related dementia: pathology and possible pathogenesis. In Scaravilli F, editor: The neuropathology of HIV infection. London, 1993, Springer.
24. Budka H: Human immunodeficiency virus (HIV) envelope and core proteins in CNS tissues of patients with the acquired immune deficiency syndrome (AIDS), Acta Neuropathol 79:611-619, 1990.
25. Budka H: Human immunodeficiency virus (HIV)-induced disease of the central nervous system: pathology and implications for pathogenesis, Acta Neuropathol 77:225-236, 1989.
26. Budka H: Immunohistological demonstration of serum proteins and structural and viral antigens in paraffin sections of nervous tissues, Ann N Y Acad Sci 420:176-184, 1983.
27. Budka H: Multinucleated giant cells in brain: a hallmark of the acquired immune deficiency syndrome (AIDS), Acta Neuropathol 69:253-258, 1986.
28. Budka H: Neuropathology of human immunodeficiency virus infection, Brain Pathol 1:163-175, 1991.

29. Budka H: Neuropathology of subacute sclerosing panencephalitis (SSPE). In Pantand B and Prabhakar S, editors: Subacute sclerosing panencephalitis. An update. Proc. 3rd International Symposium on SSPE. CMC Vellore, 1991 India.
30. Budka H: Pathology of virus infections in the central nervous system with long latency. In Kurata T and Amano T, editors: Latent infection of pathogens. Tokyo, 1995, Saikon Publishing.
31. Budka H, and others: Brain pathology induced by infection with the human immunodeficiency virus (HIV). A histological, immunocytochemical, and electron microscopical study of 100 autopsy cases, Acta Neuropathol 75:185-198, 1987.
32. Budka H and Gray F: HIV-induced central nervous system pathology. Lésions du système nerveux central liées au VIH. In Gray F, editor: Atlas of the neuropathology of HIV infection. Oxford, 1993, Oxford University Press.
33. Budka H, Lassmann H, and Popow Kraupp T: Measles virus antigen in panencephalitis. An immunomorphological study stressing dendritic involvement in SSPE, Acta Neuropathol 56: 52-62, 1982.
34. Budka H, Maier H, and Pohl P: Human immunodeficiency virus in vacuolar myelopathy of the acquired immunodeficiency syndrome. N Engl J Med 319:1667-1668, 1988.
35. Budka H, and Popow Kraupp T: Immunohistological studies in viral encephalitis, Acta Neuropathol Suppl 7:142-144, 1981.
36. Budka H, and Popow Kraupp T: Rabies and herpes simplex virus encephalitis. An immunohistological study on site and distribution of viral antigens, Virchows Arch Pathol Anat 390: 353-364, 1981.
37. Budka H, and Shah KV: Papovavirus antigens in paraffin sections of PML brains, Prog Clin Biol Res 105:299-309, 1983.
38. Budka H, and others: Subacute measles virus encephalitis: a new and fatal opportunistic infection in an AIDS patient, Neurology 46:586-587, 1996.
39. Budka H, and others: HIV-associated disease of the nervous system: review of nomenclature and proposal for neuropathology-based terminology, Brain Pathology 1:143-152, 1991.
40. Chang KL, and others: Brain lymphomas of immunocompetent and immunocompromised patients: study of the association with Epstein-Barr virus, Mod Pathol 6:427-432, 1993.
41. Chang Y, and others: Evolution of post-natal herpes simplex virus encephalitis to multicystic encephalopathy, Acta Neuropathol 80:666-670, 1990.
42. Chappell ET, Guthrie BL, and Orenstein J: The role of stereotactic biopsy in the management of HIV-related focal brain lesions, Neurosurgery 30:825-829, 1992.
43. Chimelli L, and others: Pathology of the central nervous system in patients infected with the human immunodeficiency virus (HIV): a report of 252 autopsy cases from Brazil, Neuropathol Appl Neurobiol 18:478-488, 1992.
44. Chrétien F, and others: Acute varicella-zoster virus ventriculitis and meningo-myelo-radiculitis in acquired immunodeficiency syndrome, Acta Neuropathol 86:659-665, 1993.
45. Cinque P, and others: Epstein-Barr virus DNA in cerebrospinal fluid from patients with AIDS-related primary lymphoma of the central nervous system, Lancet 342:398-401, 1993.
46. Cinque P, and others: Cytomegalovirus infection of the central nervous system in patients with AIDS: diagnosis by DNA amplification from cerebrospinal fluid. J Infect Dis 166:1408-1411, 1992.
47. Cohen JI, and Corey GR: Cytomegalovirus infection in the normal host, Medicine 64:100-114, 1985.
48. Coleman RM, and others: Determination of herpes simplex virus type-specific antibodies by enzyme-linked immunosorbent assay, J Clin Microbiol 18:287-291, 1983.
49. Cornford M, Said J, and Vinters H: Immunohistochemical localisation of human immunodeficiency virus (HIV) in central nervous system lymphoproliferative disorders of patients with AIDS, Mod Pathol 4:232-238, 1991.
50. Dawson JR: Cellular inclusions in cerebral lesions of lethargic encephalitis. Am J Pathol 9:7-15, 1933.
51. DeAngelis LM, and others: Epstein-Barr virus in acquired immune deficiency syndrome (AIDS) and non-AIDS primary central nervous system lymphoma, Cancer 70:1607-1611, 1992.
52. Deatly AM, and others: RNA from an immediate early region of the type 1 herpes simplex virus genome is present in the trigeminal ganglia of latently infected mice, Proc Natl Acad Sci USA 84:3204-3208, 1987.
53. Desai A, and others: Japanese encephalitis virus antigen in the human brain and its topographic distribution, Acta Neuropathol 89:368-373, 1995.
54. Devinsky O, and others: Herpes zoster myelitis, Brain 114:1181-1196, 1991.
55. Dhib Jalbut S, and others: Extracellular human T-cell lymphotropic virus type I Tax protein induces cytokine human microglial cells, Ann Neurol 36:787-790, 1994.
56. Dhib Jalbut S, and Liwnicz BH: Rapidly progressive subacute sclerosing panencephalitis: an ultrastructural and immunoperoxidase study, Eur Neurol 23:211-220, 1984.
57. Dix RD, and others: Herpes simplex virus type 2 encephalitis in two homosexual men with persistent lymphadenopathy, Ann Neurol 17:203-205, 1985.
58. Dörries K, and ter Meulen V: Detection of papovavirus JC in kidney tissue, J Med Virol 11:307-311, 1983.
59. Drlicek M, and others: Pathologie des Zentralnervensystems bei AIDS. Ein Überblick über 184 Patienten, Wien Klin Wochenschr 105:467-471, 1993.
60. Drysdale HC, and others: Measles inclusion-body encephalitis in a child with treated acute lymphoblastic leukaemia, J Clin Pathol 29:865-872, 1976.
61. Eidelberg D, and others: Thrombotic cerebral vasculopathy associated with herpes zoster, Ann Neurol 19:7-14, 1986.
62. Esiri MM, and Kennedy PGE: Viral diseases. In Adamsand JH and Duchen LW, editors: Greenfield's neuropathology. London, 1992, Edward Arnold.
63. Feiden W, and others: The stereotactic biopsy diagnosis of focal intracerebral lesions in AIDS patients, Acta Neurol Scand 87: 228-233, 1993.
64. Gelb LD: Varicella-zoster virus. In Fields BN and Knipe DM, editors: Virology, ed 2, vol 2, New York, 1990, Raven Press.
65. Gendelman HE, and others: Trans-activation of the human immunodeficiency virus long terminal repeat sequence by DNA viruses, Proc Natl Acad Sci USA 83:9759-9763, 1986.
66. Gilden DH, and others: Chronic progressive varicella-zoster virus encephalitis in an AIDS patient, Neurology 38:1150-1153, 1988.
67. Gilden DH, Rorke LB, and Tanaka R: Acute SSPE, Arch Neurol 32:644-646, 1975.
68. Gillet JP, Derer P, and Tsiang H: Axonal transport of rabies virus in the central nervous system of the rat, J Neuropathol Exp Neurol 45:619-634, 1986.
69. Gozlan J, and others: Rapid detection of cytomegalovirus DNA in cerebrospinal fluid of AIDS patients with neurologic disorders, J Infect Dis 166:1416-1421, 1992.
70. Gray F, and others: Etude neuropathologique de 135 cas adultes de syndrome d'immunodeficience acquisé (SIDA), Ann Pathol 11:236-247, 1991.
71. Gray F, and others: Prominent cortical atrophy with neuronal loss as correlate of human immunodeficiency virus encephalopathy, Acta Neuropathol 82:229-233, 1991.
72. Gray F, and others: Varicella-zoster virus encephalitis in acquired immunodeficiency syndrome: report of four cases, Neuropathol Appl Neurobiol 18:502-514, 1992.

73. Greenlee JE: Progressive multifocal leukoencephalopathy, Curr Clin Top Infect Dis 10:140-156, 1989.
74. Hainfellner JA, and Budka H: Neuropathology of human immunodeficiency virus related opportunistic infections and neoplasms, In Berger JR and Levy RM editors: AIDS and the nervous system, ed 2. Philadelphia, 1997 Lippincott-Raven Press.
75. Hamilton-Dutoit SJ, and others: AIDS-related lymphoma. Histopathology, immunophenotype, and association with Epstein-Barr virus as demonstrated by in situ nucleic acid hybridization, Am J Pathol 138:149-163, 1991.
76. Hara H, and others: Detection of human T lymphotrophic virus type I (HTLV-I) proviral DNA and analysis of T cell receptor V beta CDR3 sequences in spinal cord lesions of HTLV-I-associated myelopathy/tropical spastic paraparesis, J Exp Med 180: 831-839, 1994.
77. Harding B, and Baumer JA: Congenital varicella-zoster. A serologically proven case with necrotizing encephalitis and malformation, Acta Neuropathol 76:311-315, 1988.
78. Hart MN, and Earle KM: Haemorrhagic and perivenous encephalitis: a clinical-pathological review of 38 cases, J Neurol Neurosurg Psychiatry 38:585-591, 1975.
79. Hashimoto I, Hagiwara A, and Komatsu T: Ultrastructural studies on the pathogenesis of poliomyelitis in monkeys infected with poliovirus, Acta Neuropathol 64:53-60, 1984.
80. Hayano M, Sung JH, and Mastri AR: "Paramyxovirus-like" intranuclear inclusions occurring in the nervous system in diverse unrelated conditions, J Neuropathol Exp Neurol 35:287-294, 1976.
81. Haymaker W: Mosquito-borne encephalitides. In: van Bogaert, and others, editors: Encephalitides. Amsterdam, 1961, Elsevier.
82. Heilbronn R, and others: Human cytomegalovirus induces JC virus DNA replication in human fibroblasts, Proc Natl Acad Sci USA 90:11406-11410, 1993.
83. Hochberg FH, and others: Mononucleosis-associated subacute sclerosing panencephalitis, Acta Neuropathol 34:33-40, 1976.
84. Houff SA, and others: Involvement of JC-virus infected mononuclear cells from the bone marrow and spleen in the pathogenesis of progressive multifocal leukoencephalopathy, N Engl J Med 318:301-305, 1988.
85. Iwasaki Y, and others: Infiltration of helper/inducer T lymphocytes heralds central nervous system damage in human T-cell leukemia virus infection, Am J Pathol 140:1003-1008, 1992.
86. Iwasaki Y, and others: Immunohistochemical demonstration of viral antigens in Japanese encephalitis, Acta Neuropathol 70: 79-81, 1986.
87. Jackson AC, and Wunner WH: Detection of rabies virus genomic RNA and mRNA in mouse and human brains by using in situ hybridization, J Virol 65:2839-2844, 1991.
88. Jakobsen J, and others: Progressive multifocal leukoencephalopathy in a patient without other clinical manifestations of AIDS, Acta Neurol Scand 75:209-213, 1987.
89. Johnson RT: Viral diseases of the nervous system. New York, 1982, Raven Press.
90. Johnson RT, and others: Japanese encephalitis: immunocytochemical studies of viral antigen and inflammatory cells in fatal cases, Ann Neurol 18:567-573, 1985.
91. Kanavaros P, and others: Stereotactic biopsy diagnosis of primary non-Hodgkin's lymphoma of the central nervous system. A histological and immunohistochemical study, Pathol Res Pract 186:459-466, 1990.
92. Kato T, Hirano A, Llena JF, and Dembitzer HM: Neuropathology of acquired immune deficiency syndrome (AIDS) in 53 autopsy cases with particular emphasis on microglial nodules and multinucleated giant cells, Acta Neuropathol 73:287-294, 1987.
93. Kennedy PG, and others: Studies on the pathogenesis of neurological diseases associated with Varicella-Zoster virus, Neuropathol Appl Neurobiol 16:305-16, 1990.
94. Ketzler S, and others: Loss of neurons in the frontal cortex in AIDS brains, Acta Neuropathol 80:92-94, 1990.
95. Kim TM, and others: Delayed acute measles inclusion body encephalitis in a 9-year-old girl: ultrastructural, immunohistochemical, and in situ hybridization studies, Mod Pathol 5:348-352, 1992.
96. Kirk J, and others: Cerebral endothelial cell infection by measles virus in subacute sclerosing panencephalitis: ultrastructural and in situ hybridization evidence, Neuropathol Appl Neurobiol 17:289-297, 1991.
97. Kleihues P, and others: Progressive diffuse leukoencephalopathy in patients with acquired immune deficiency syndrome (AIDS), Acta Neuropathol 68:333-339, 1985.
98. Kuchelmeister K, and others: Progressive multifocal leukoencephalopathy (PML) in the acquired immunodeficiency syndrome (AIDS). A neuropathological autopsy study of 21 cases, Pathol Res Pract 189:163-173, 1993.
99. Kumanishi T, In S: SSPE: immunohistochemical demonstration of measles virus antigen(s) in paraffin sections, Acta Neuropathol 48:161-163, 1979.
100. Kure K, and others: Human immunodeficiency virus-1 infection of the nervous system: and autopsy study of 268 adult, pediatric, and fetal brains, Hum Pathol 22:700-710, 1991.
101. Lang W, and others: Neuropathology of the acquired immune deficiency syndrome (AIDS): a report of 135 consecutive autopsy cases from Switzerland, Acta Neuropathol 77:379-390, 1989.
102. Leech RW, and Harris JC: The neuropathology of Western equine and St. Louis encephalitis: a review of the 1975 North Dakota epidemic, J Neuropathol Exp Neurol 36:611, 1977.
103. Levy RM, Bredesen DE, and Rosenblum ML: Neurological manifestations of the acquired immunodeficiency syndrome (AIDS): experience at UCSF and review of the literature, J Neurosurg 62:475-495, 1985.
104. Liebert UG, and others: Restricted expression of measles virus proteins in brains from cases of subacute sclerosing panencephalitis, J Gen Virol 67:2435-2444, 1986.
105. Lima C, and others: The neuropathology of HIV-2 infection (abstr), Clin Neuropathol 11:277, 1992.
106. Lindenberg R, and Haymaker W: Tissue reactions in the gray matter of the central nervous system. In: Histology and Histopathology of the Nervous System. Edited by W Haymaker and RD Adams. Springfield, IL, 1982, Thomas.
107. Lipkin WI, Schneemann A, and Solbrig MV: Borna disease virus: implications for human neuropsychiatric illness. Trends Microbiol 3:64-9, 1995.
108. Loeber G, and Drries K: DNA rearrangements in organ-specific variants of polyomavirus JC strain GS, J Virol 62:1730-1735, 1988.
109. Lucas SB, and others: The mortality and pathology of HIV infection in a West African city, AIDS 7:1569-1579, 1993.
110. MacMahon EM, and others: Epstein-Barr virus in AIDS-related primary central nervous system lymphoma, Lancet 19:969-973, 1991.
111. Maier H, and others: Vacuolar myelopathy with multinucleated giant cells in the acquired immune deficiency syndrome (AIDS). Light and electron microscopic distribution of human immunodeficiency virus (HIV) antigens, Acta Neuropathol 78: 497-503, 1989.
112. Manghani DK, Dastur DK, and Budka H: Immunohistology and fine structure of viral material in the Negri bodies in human and experimental rabies, Neuropathology (Tokyo) Suppl 4:337-343, 1991.

113. Manghani DK, and others: Pleomorphism of fine structure of rabies virus in human and experimental brain, J Neurol Sci 75: 181-193, 1986.
114. Matthiessen L, and others: Neuropathology of the brain in 174 patients who died of AIDS in a Paris hospital 1982-1988, Ann Med Interne Paris 143:43-49, 1992.
115. Màzló M, Herndon RM: Progressive multifocal leukoencephalopathy: ultrastructural findings in two brain biopsies, Neuropathol Appl Neurol 3:323-339, 1977.
116. McArthur JC: Neurologic manifestations of AIDS, Medicine 66: 407-437, 1987.
117. McCormick WF, and others: Varicella-zoster encephalomyelitis: a morphologic and virologic study, Arch Neurol 21:559-570, 1969.
118. Meyenhofer MF, and others: Ultrastructural morphology and intracellular production of human immunodeficiency virus (HIV) in brain, J Neuropathol Exp Neurol 46:474-484, 1987.
119. Miller R, and others: Subacute radiculomyelopathy caused by cytomegalovirus in patients with AIDS, Neurology 38:242 (abstr), 1988.
120. Moore GR, and others: Tropical spastic paraparesis: a model of virus-induced, cytotoxic T-cell-mediated demyelination? Ann Neurol 26:523-530, 1989.
121. Moret H, and others: Virological diagnosis of progressive multifocal leukoencephalopathy: detection of JC virus DNA in cerebrospinal fluid and brain tissue of AIDS patients, J Clin Microbiol 31:3310-3313, 1993.
122. Morgello S: Epstein-Barr and human immunodeficiency viruses in acquired immunodeficiency syndrome-related primary central nervous system lymphoma, Am J Pathol 141:441-50, 1992.
123. Morgello S, and others: Varicella-zoster virus leukoencephalitis and cerebral vasculopathy, Arch Pathol Lab Med 112:173-177, 1988.
124. Morgello S, and others: Cytomegalovirus encephalitis in patients with acquired immunodeficiency syndrome: an autopsy study of 30 cases and a review of the literature, Hum Pathol 18:289-97, 1987.
125. Mrak RE, and Young L: Rabies encephalitis in humans: pathology, pathogenesis and pathophysiology, J Neuropathol Exp Neurol 53:1-10, 1994.
126. Muir P, and others: Evidence for persistent enterovirus infection of the central nervous system in patients with previous paralytic poliomyelitis, Ann NY Acad Sci 753:219-232, 1995.
127. Mustafa MM, and others: Subacute measles encephalitis in the young immunocompromised host: report of two cases diagnosed by polymerase chain reaction and treated with ribavirin and review of the literature, Clin Infect Dis 16:654-660, 1993.
128. Namiki TS, and others: Stereotaxic biopsy diagnosis of central nervous system lymphoma, Am J Clin Pathol 90:40-45, 1988.
129. Nicoll JA, and others: Autopsy findings in two cases of neonatal herpes simplex virus infection: detection of virus by immunohistochemistry, in situ hybridization and the polymerase chain reaction, Histopathology 24:257-264, 1994.
130. Nielsen SL, and others: Subacute encephalitis in acquired immune deficiency syndrome: a postmortem study, Am J Clin Pathol 82:678-682, 1984.
131. Nihei K, and others: Atypical subacute sclerosing panencephalitis, Acta Neuropathol 38:163-166, 1977.
132. Norrby E, and Oxman MN: Measles Virus. In Fields BN and Knipe DM editors: Fields virology, ed 2. New York, 1990, Raven Press.
133. Oksi J, and others: Fatal encephalitis caused by concomitant infection with tick-borne encephalitis virus and Borrelia burgdorferi, Clin Infect Dis 16:392-396, 1993.
134. Osamura T, and others: Isolation of adenovirus type 11 from the brain of a neonate with pneumonia and encephalitis, Eur J Pediatr 152:496-499, 1993.
135. Padgett BL, and Walker DL: Prevalence of antibodies in human sera against JC virus an isolate from a case of progressive multifocal leukoencephalopathy, J Infect Dis 127:467-470, 1973.
136. Padgett BL, and others: Cultivation of papova-like virus from human brain with progressive multifocal leucoencephalopathy, Lancet 1:1257-1260, 1971.
137. Patsouris E, and others: Cellular composition and distribution of gliomesenchymal nodules in the CNS of AIDS patients, Clin Neuropathol 12:130-137, 1993.
138. Paula Barbosa MM, and Cruz C: Nerve cell fusion in a case of subacute sclerosing panencephalitis, Ann Neurol 9:400-403, 1981.
139. Paulus W, and others: Human herpesvirus-6 and Epstein-Barr virus genome in primary cerebral lymphomas, Neurology 43: 1591-1593, 1993.
140. Pell MF, Thomas DG, and Whittle IR: Stereotactic biopsy of cerebral lesions in patients with AIDS, Br J Neurosurg 5:585-589, 1991.
141. Petito CK, and others: Neuropathology of acquired immunodeficiency syndrome (AIDS): an autopsy review, J Neuropathol Exp Neurol 45:635-646, 1986.
142. Pilz P, and Budka H: Herpes Zoster. Neuropathologische Befunde und Gedanken zur Pathogenese, Curr Top Neuropathol 7:119-127, 1982.
143. Puchhammer-Stöckl E, and others: Detection of varicella-zoster virus DNA by polymerase chain reaction in the cerebrospinal fluid of patients suffering from neurological complications associated with chicken pox or herpes zoster, J Clin Microbiol 29: 1513-1516, 1991.
144. Quinlivan EB, and others: Subclinical central nervous system infection with JC virus in patients with AIDS, J Infect Dis 166: 80-85, 1992.
145. Rhodes RH: Histopathology of the central nervous system in the acquired immunodeficiency syndrome, Hum Pathol 18:636-643, 1987.
146. Rio ME, and others: Double infection of the CNS with herpes simplex and mumps viruses. Serological and ultrastructural studies, Childs Nerv Syst 1:215-218, 1985.
147. Rosenblum MK: Bulbar encephalitis complicating trigeminal zoster in the acquired immune deficiency syndrome, Hum Pathol 20:292-295, 1989.
148. Rostad SW, and others: Transsynaptic spread of varicella zoster virus through the visual system: a mechanism of viral dissemination in the central nervous system, Hum Pathol 20:174-179, 1989.
149. Ryder JW, and others: Progressive encephalitis three months after resolution of cutaneous zoster in a patient with AIDS, Ann Neurol 19:182-188, 1986.
150. Sasaki S, and others: An autopsy case of human T lymphotropic virus type I-associated myelopathy (HAM) with a duration of 28 years, Acta Neuropathol 81:219-222, 1990.
151. Schmidbauer M, Budka H, and Ambros P: Comparison of in situ DNA hybridization (ISH) and immunocytochemistry for diagnosis of herpes simplex virus (HSV) encephalitis in tissue, Virchows Arch A Pathol Anat Histopathol 414:39-43, 1988.
152. Schmidbauer M, Budka H, and Ambros P: Herpes simplex virus (HSV) DNA in microglial nodular brainstem encephalitis, J Neuropathol Exp Neurol 48:645-652, 1989.
153. Schmidbauer M, and others: Multifocal vacuolar leucoencephalopathy: a distinct HIV-associated lesion of the brain, Neuropathol Appl Neurobiol 16:437-443, 1990.
154. Schmidbauer M, and others: Presence, distribution and spread of productive varicella zoster virus infection in nervous tissues, Brain 115:383-398, 1992.
155. Schmidbauer M, Budka H, and Shah KV: Progressive multifocal leukoencephalopathy (PML) in AIDS and in the pre-AIDS era. A neuropathological comparison using immunocytochemistry

and in situ DNA hybridization for virus detection, Acta Neuropathol 80:375-380, 1990.

156. Schmidbauer M, and others: Cytomegalovirus (CMV) disease of the brain in AIDS and connatal infection: a comparative study by histology, immunocytochemistry and in situ hybridization, Acta Neuropathol 79:286-293, 1989.
157. Schmidbauer M, and others: Morphological spectrum, distribution and clinical correlation of white matter lesions in AIDS brains, Neuropathol Appl Neurobiol 18:489-501, 1992.
158. Shah KV: Papovaviruses. In Fields BN editor: Virology. New York, 1985, Raven Press.
159. Sharer LR, and others: Spinal cord disease in children with HIV-1 infection: a combined molecular biological and neuropathological study, Neuropathol Appl Neurobiol 16:317-331, 1990.
160. Sidhu MS, and others: Defective measles virus in human subacute sclerosing panencephalitis brain, Virology 202:631-641, 1994.
161. Sluga E, and others: SSPE-like inclusion body disorder in treated childhood leukemia, Acta Neuropathol Suppl 6:267-272, 1975.
162. Spatz H: Encephalitis. In Bumke O, editor: Handbuch der Geisteskrankheiten. (vol XI, Part VII). Berlin, 1930 Springer.
163. Stark E, Haas J, and Schedel I: Diagnosis of cytomegalovirus infections of the nervous system by immunocytochemical demonstration of infected cells in cerebrospinal fluid, Eur J Med 2: 223-224, 1993.
164. Sung JH, and other: A case of human rabies and ultrastructure of the Negri body, J Neuropathol Exp Neurol 35:541-559, 1976.
165. Tada H, and others: Trans-activation of the JC virus late promoter by the tat protein of type 1 human immunodeficiency virus in glial cells, Proc Natl Acad Sci USA 87:3479-3483, 1990.
166. Tirawatnpong S, and others: Regional distribution of rabies viral antigen in central nervous system of human encephalitic and paralytic rabies, J Neurol Sci 92:91-99, 1989.
167. Townsend JJ, and others: Progressive rubella panencephalitis. Late onset after congenital rubella, N Engl J Med 292:990-993, 1975.
168. Townsend JJ, and others: Neuropathology of progressive rubella panencephalitis after childhood rubella, Neurology 32: 185-190, 1982.
169. Townsend JJ, Wolinsky JS, and Baringer JR: The neuropathology of progressive rubella panencephalitis of late onset, Brain 99:81-90, 1976.
170. Ugolini G: Specificity of rabies virus as a transneuronal tracer of motor networks: transfer from hypoglossal motoneurons to connected second-order and higher order central nervous system cell groups, J Comp Neurol 356:457-480, 1995.
171. Vallbracht A, and others: Disseminated BK type polyomavirus infection in an AIDS patient associated with central nervous system disease, Am J Pathol 143:29-39, 1993.
172. Vazeux R, and others: Severe encephalitis resulting from coinfections with HIV and JC virus, Neurology 40:944-948, 1990.
173. Vinters HV, and others: Necrotizing vasculitis of the nervous system in a patient with AIDS-related complex, Neuropathol Appl Neurobiol 14:417-24, 1988.
174. Vinters HV, and others: Cytomegalovirus in the nervous system of patients with the acquired immune deficiency syndrome, Brain 112:245-268, 1989.
175. von Einsiedel RW, and others: Progressive multifocal leukoencephalopathy in AIDS: a clinicopathologic study and review of the literature, J Neurol 240:391-406, 1993.
176. Warren KG, and others: Isolation of latent herpes simplex virus from the superior cervical and vagus ganglions of human beings, N Engl J Med 298:1068-1069, 1978.
177. Weber T, and others: Specific diagnosis of progressive multifocal leukoencephalopathy by polymerase chain reaction, J Infect Dis 169:1138-1141, 1993.
178. Weis S, Haug H, and Budka H: Astroglial changes in the cerebral cortex of AIDS brains: a morphometric and immunohistochemical investigation, Neuropathol Appl Neurobiol 19:329-335, 1993.
179. Weis S, Haug H, and Budka H: Neuronal damage in the cerebral cortex of AIDS brains: a morphometric study, Acta Neuropathol 85:185-189, 1993.
180. Weller TH: Varicella and herpes zoster: changing concepts of the natural history, control, and importance of a not-so-benign virus. Part 1, N Engl J Med 309:1362-1368, 1983.
181. Weller TH: Varicella and herpes zoster: changing concepts of the natural history, control, and importance of a not-so-benign virus. Part 2, N Engl J Med 309:1434-1440, 1983.
182. Wiley CA, and others: Human immunodeficiency virus (HIV) and JC virus in acquired immune deficiency syndrome (AIDS) patients with progressive multifocal leukoencephalopathy, Acta Neuropathol 76:338-346, 1988.
183. Wiley CA, and Nelson JA: Role of human immunodeficiency virus and cytomegalovirus in AIDS encephalitis, Am J Pathol 133:73-81, 1988.
184. Wiley CA, and others: Localization of cytomegalovirus proteins and genome during fulminant central nervous system infection in an AIDS patient, J Neuropathol Exp Neurol 45:127-139, 1986.
185. Zimmer C, and others: Stereotactic brain biopsy in AIDS, J Neurol 239:394-400, 1992.
186. Zu Rhein GM, and Chou SM: Particles resembling papova viruses in human cerebral demyelinating disease, Science 148: 1477-1479, 1965.

C • H • A • P • T • E • R

9

# AIDS and the Central Nervous System

Roy H. Rhodes



The major risk groups for the acquired immunodeficiency syndrome (AIDS) include homosexual males, intravenous drug abusers, individuals with multiple sexual contacts, and infants of mothers infected with the human immunodeficiency virus (HIV).[47,131,247] The diagnosis of AIDS is based on the generally accepted criteria proposed by the Centers for Disease Control (CDC),[37] keeping in mind that anatomic descriptions that follow are derived principally from symptomatic patients with high-stage clinical AIDS. The mean incubation period for the development of AIDS after infection with HIV is about 8 years in homosexual men and in recipients of blood containing HIV.[171,185] The mean incubation period in children is about 2 years,[47,171] and it is shorter for those children infected perinatally than for those infected by transfusion.[75] The HIV infection has a variable clinical course with a close relationship to the host's immune deficiency that is directly and indirectly affected by HIV itself.[142] Neurologic manifestations in HIV-infected individuals can be the initial or the only clinical finding,[138,176,203] but abnormalities in many systems are generally found before neurologic symptoms develop. The personal, national, and international impact of the AIDS epidemic is tremendous, and the acceleration of the case load observed yearly since AIDS was clearly identified in 1982 has been alarming.[23,47,58,80]

## HIV

HIV is in a retroviral subfamily characterized by a slow rate of infection and a small load of viral antigen that can be intracellular and hidden from immune surveillance. HIV can exist within the host cell as a persistent or latent infection that can be noncytopathic. The virus may avoid neutralizing antibodies by a high mutation rate in its envelope proteins, and these antibodies do not protect against infection or disease.[82,117,299] Retroviruses have two single-stranded RNA molecules with genes that include those designated as *gag* (encoding core proteins, i.e., *g*roup-specific *a*nti*g*ens), *pol* (encoding the RNA-dependent DNA *pol*ymerase, or reverse transcriptase), and *env* (encoding glycoproteins for the *env*elope of the nucleocapsid, i.e., the precursor gp160 that yields gp120 and gp41). Regulatory or accessory genes such as *tat, rev,* and *nef* (*ne*gative *f*actor, possibly regulating HIV-1 replication; formerly known as F/3′-*orf*) are becoming increasingly better known as their functions and diagnostic value are unraveled.[1,215,293] Reverse transcriptase allows the viral RNA to direct host transcription of viral DNA (thus a "retro" transcription names this viral family).[192,299] Antibodies, antigens, viral RNA, or proviral DNA may be detected in retroviral disease diagnosis.

HIV is about 70 to 160 nm in diameter, with a variably positioned dense nucleoid and a less dense shell. The retrovirus buds from intracellular membranes in monocyte/macrophages of the mononuclear phagocyte system and from cell surface membranes in monocyte/macrophages and T lymphocytes.[122,187,190,211] The entrance of the retrovirus into cells usually requires the CD4 cell-surface receptor protein.[76] CD4-positive cells include T4 lymphocytes,[322] part of the population of blood-borne monocytes and their differentiated form, the macrophage,[95] and some glial cells[40] and vascular endothelial cells.[252] The major route to infection of these cells by HIV is through receptor-mediated endocytosis.[216] It appears that some bone marrow,[83] lymph node,[130,174] and neural cells may not require this mode of viral attachment and penetration to become infected.[40,41,282] Viral fusion to plasma membranes may be an alternate route for infection.[16,174,284] Simple phagocytosis by macrophages destroys the infectivity of HIV.[216] The HIV envelope protein gp120 can itself inhibit T-cell responsiveness to antigens, probably by competitive inhibition with major histocompatibility complex antigen that binds to CD4 protein. Extracellular soluble gp120 may cause immunosuppression of uninfected CD4-positive cells through this mechanism because of the role of CD4 in immune responsiveness.[57] The Nef protein might act like a superantigen that nonspecifically promotes lymphocytic proliferation.[293] An infection expressing this early HIV protein could dysregulate the immune system, possibly resulting in chronic inflammatory cellular infiltration.

## GENERAL ASPECTS OF NERVOUS SYSTEM PATHOLOGY WITH HIV INFECTION

The pathology of the nervous system in AIDS is predominantly the pathology of an infectious disease, with overtones of apparent immunopathologic lesions.[247] In some AIDS patients the involvement of the nervous system may have an acute phase, appearing as an influenza- or mononucleosis-like illness with acute encephalopathy and neuritis,* while chronic nervous system involvement is more common. The brain weight in this condition may be lower than expected for a relatively young patient,[202,241] with gross thinning of the neocortical strip often being found.[73] The thickness and mean volume of the neocortex and the mean volume of the basal ganglia and white matter are actually reduced by over 10% in AIDS brains.[212] Central nervous system (CNS) lesions are reported in well over 50% of AIDS patients at autopsy. Many lesions carry nonspecific stigmata of a viral infection or possible hypersensitivity damage, while others have evidence of a specific etiologic agent, often an opportunist.† Monocyte/macrophages scattered or grouped around the microvasculature, in the parenchyma (Figs. 9-1 to 9-5), or in the subarachnoid space (Fig. 9-6) and gliomesenchymal cell nodules (microglial nodules or nodular encephalitis) are frequently seen (Figs. 9-7, 9-8). Multinucleated cells, including multinucleated giant cells, have been reported as a pathognomonic feature of HIV encephalitis in over 25% of AIDS cases at autopsy in several series (Figs. 9-2 to 9-5).‡ Demyelination and reactive astrocytosis are often seen (Fig. 9-9); occasionally arachnoidal fibrosis can be noted. Spongiform changes are usually confined to the white matter, but cortical spongiform changes have also been reported.[10,31,206,266]

---

* Refs. 33, 90, 120, 138, 224, 232.

† Refs. 5, 27, 31, 53, 66, 113, 114, 143, 161, 182, 198, 202, 205, 206, 222, 241, 247, 268, 270, 278.

‡ Refs. 30, 31, 112, 143, 202, 222, 247, 268, 270.

*Text continued on page 399.*

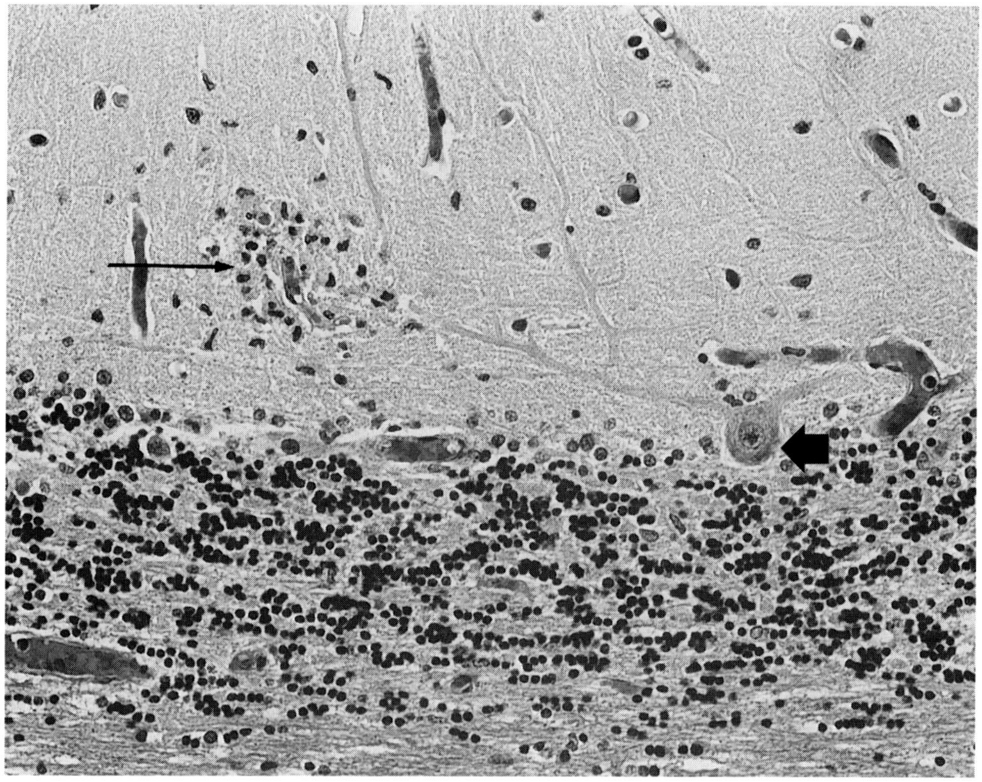

**Fig. 9-1.** Focal perivascular macrophages in the cerebellum. The pericapillary cluster of macrophages (*arrow*) is in an otherwise normal molecular layer of a folium. The Purkinje neuron (*arrowhead*) appears structurally intact, and the internal granule cell layer below is normal. (H&E; ×200.)

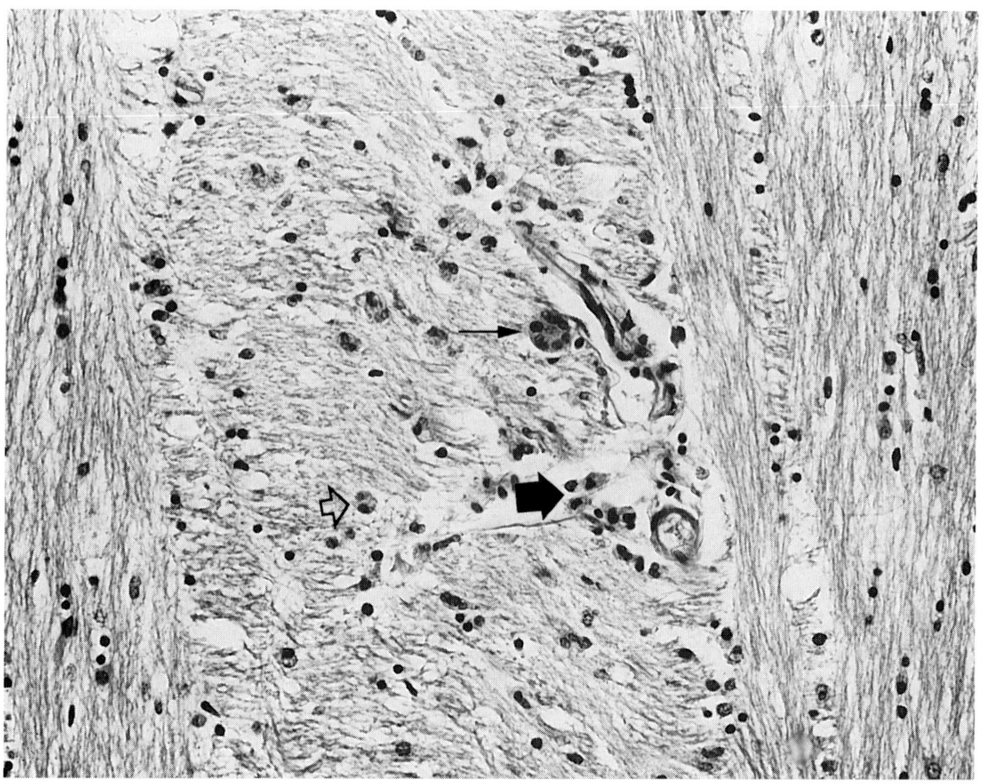

**Fig. 9-2.** Macrophages and multinucleated cells in the internal capsule of the cerebrum. Some macrophages are perivascular (*solid arrowhead*) and some are in the white matter (*open arrowhead*). A small to medium-size multinucleated cell (*arrow*) 25 μm in diameter is present. Lymphocytes, if present, are not easy to appreciate. (H&E; ×200.)

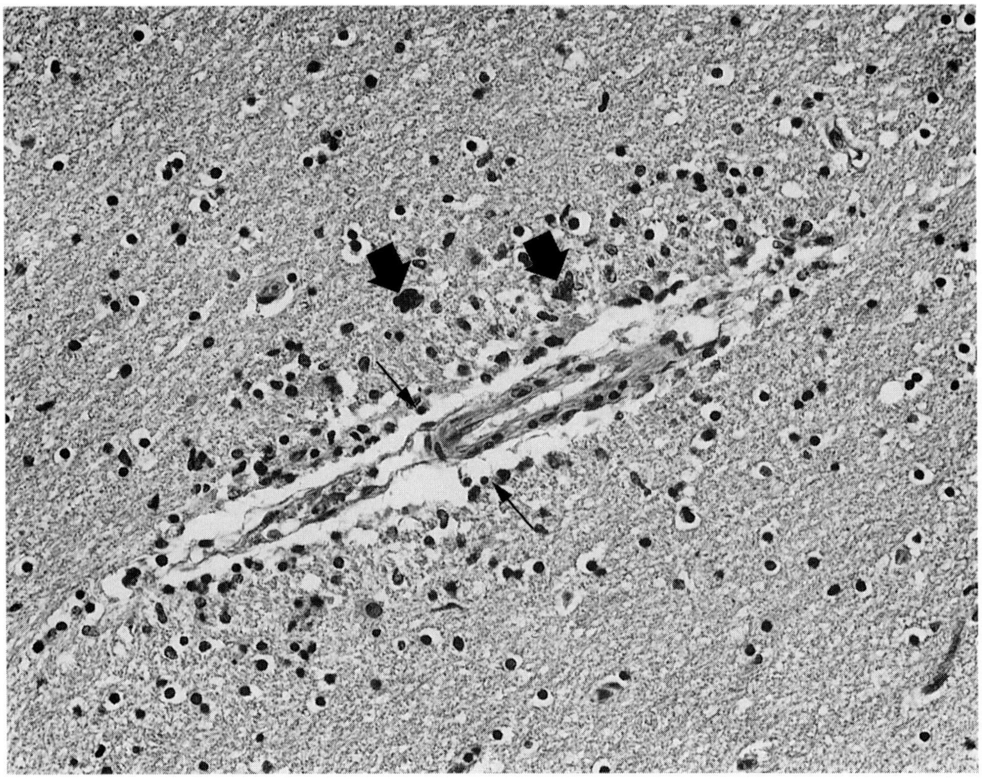

**Fig. 9-3.** Perivascular and parenchymal infiltration in the extreme capsule of the cerebrum (subcortical white matter of the insular cortex). A small blood vessel is surrounded by mononuclear cells that appear to be mostly monocyte/macrophages (*arrows*). A few small multinucleated cells with barely perceptible cytoplasm (*arrowheads*) are present. (H&E; ×200.)

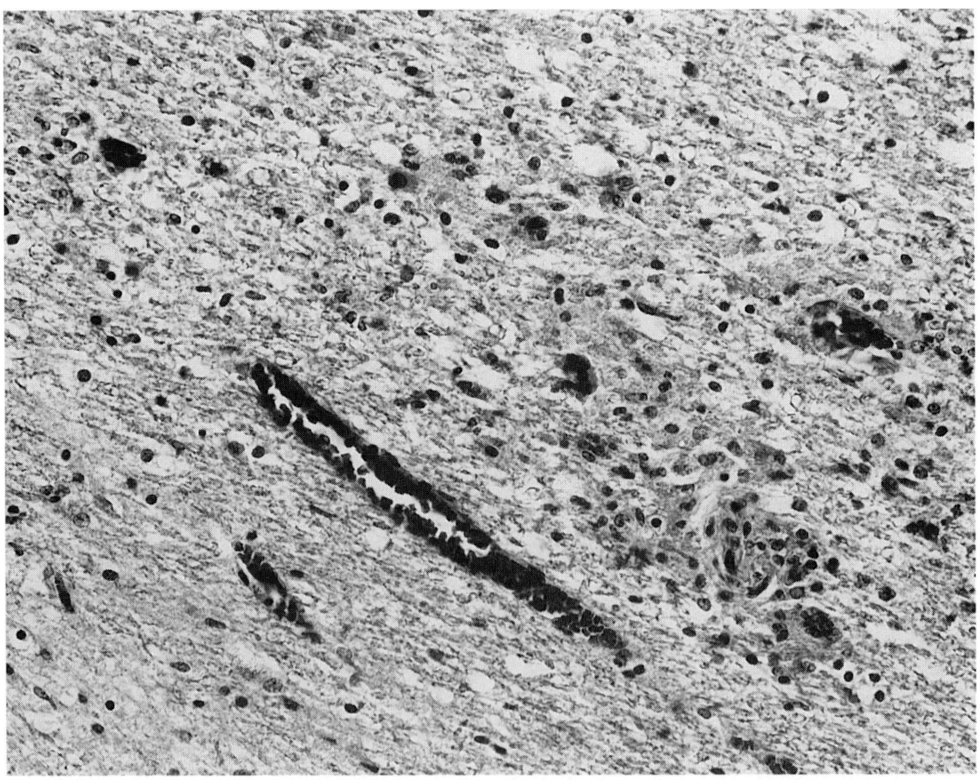

**Fig. 9-4.** Macrophages and multinucleated cells in cerebellar deep white matter. These cells tend to be near blood vessels, but there is significant infiltration into the parenchyma. (H&E; ×200.)

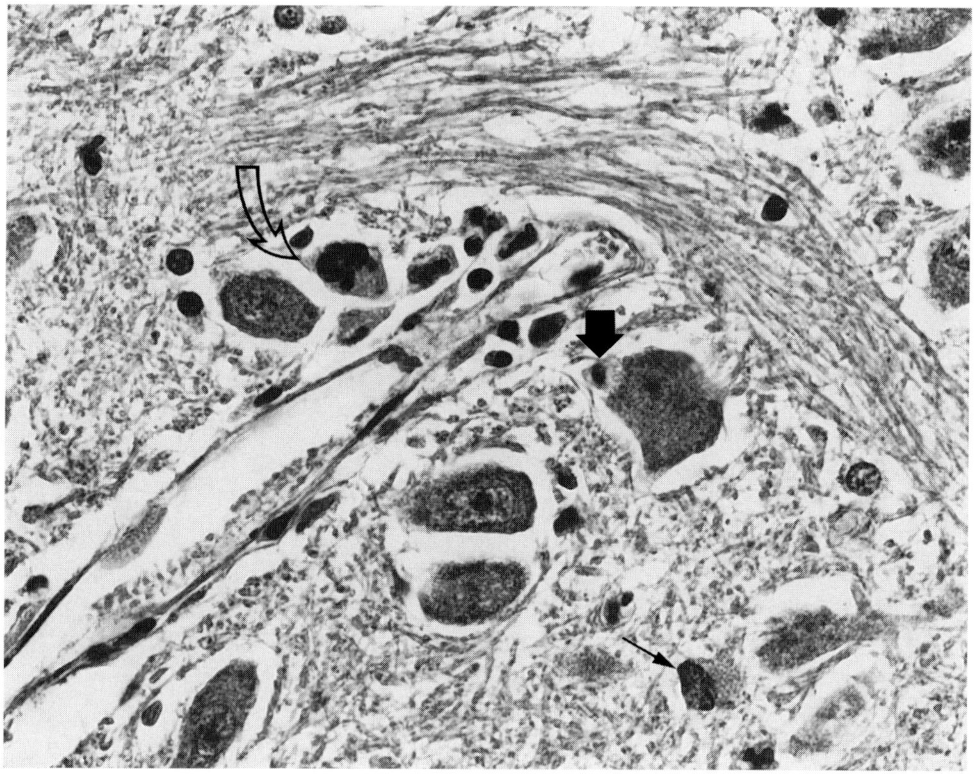

**Fig. 9-5.** Perivascular macrophages and multinucleated cells in the basis pontis. As in Figs. 9-1 and 9-2, there is little parenchymal alteration, and yet there are some perivascular macrophages and multinucleated cells (*open curved arrow*). However, a reactive astrocyte (*arrow*) can be seen in the parenchyma, and a mononuclear cell (*arrowhead*) has the appearance of reacting to a presumably damaged neuron. (H&E; ×500.)

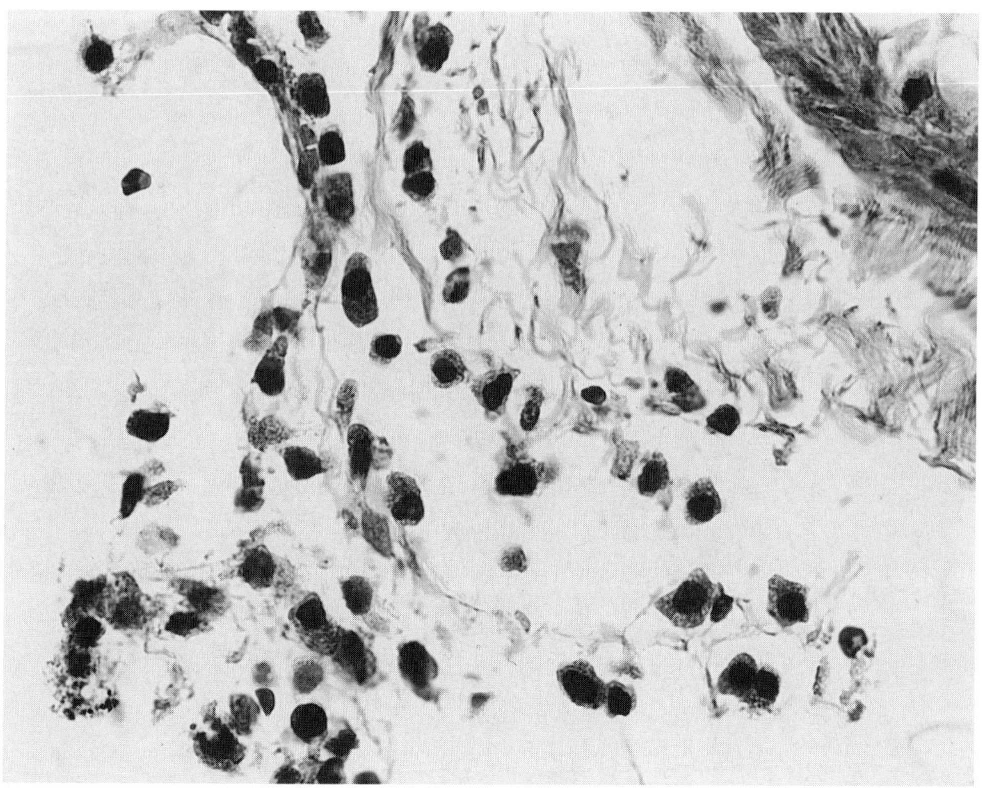

**Fig. 9-6.** Focal macrophages in the subarachnoid space. Such scattered groupings of monocyte/macrophages, sometimes including multinucleated cells, are commonly found in the absence of opportunistic infections in AIDS. (H&E; ×500.)

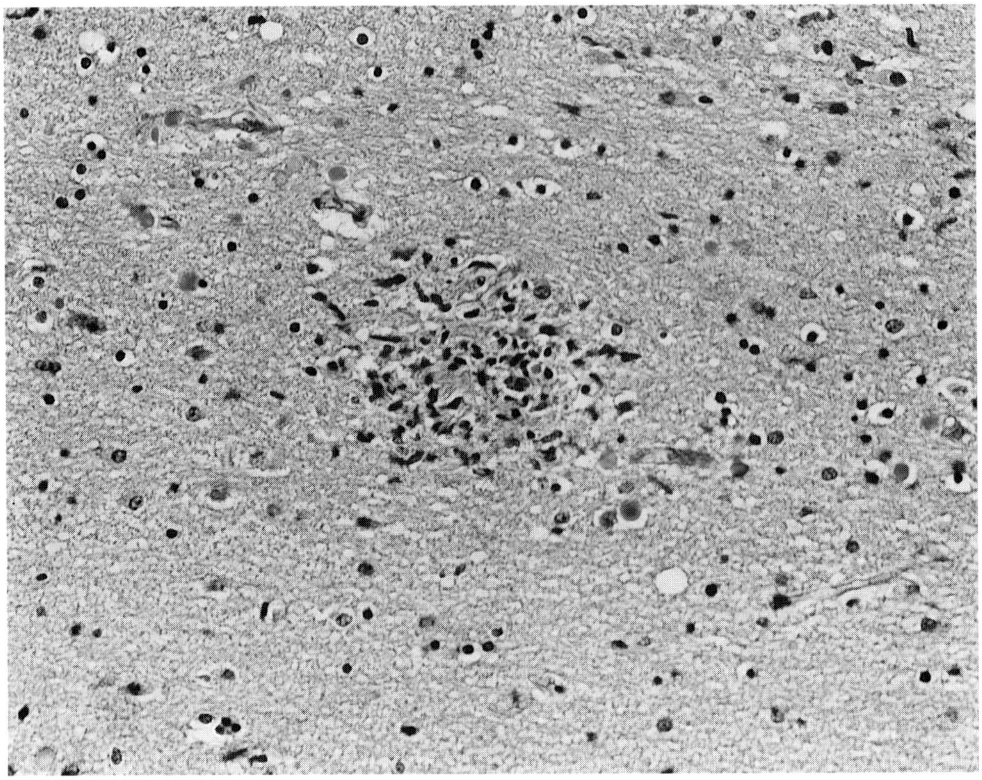

**Fig. 9-7.** A compact gliomesenchymal cell nodule in the hippocampus. The cellular nuclei form a heterogeneous population of shapes. (H&E; ×200.)

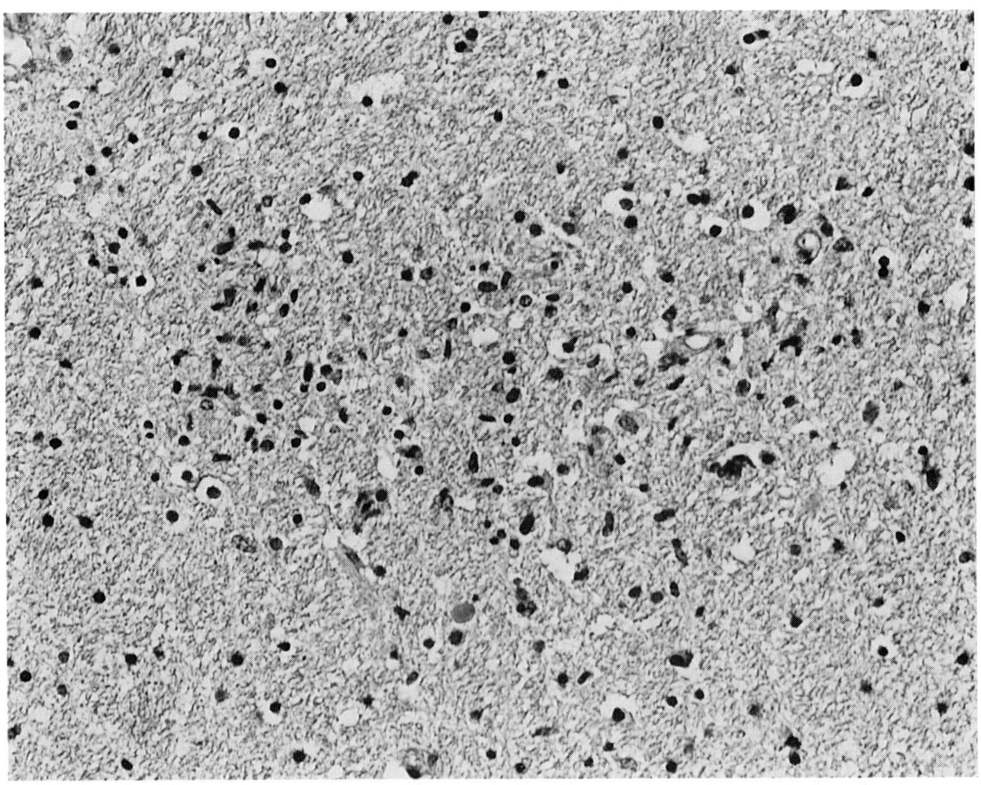

**Fig. 9-8.** A diffuse gliomesenchymal cell nodule in white matter of the temporal lobe. (H&E; ×200.)

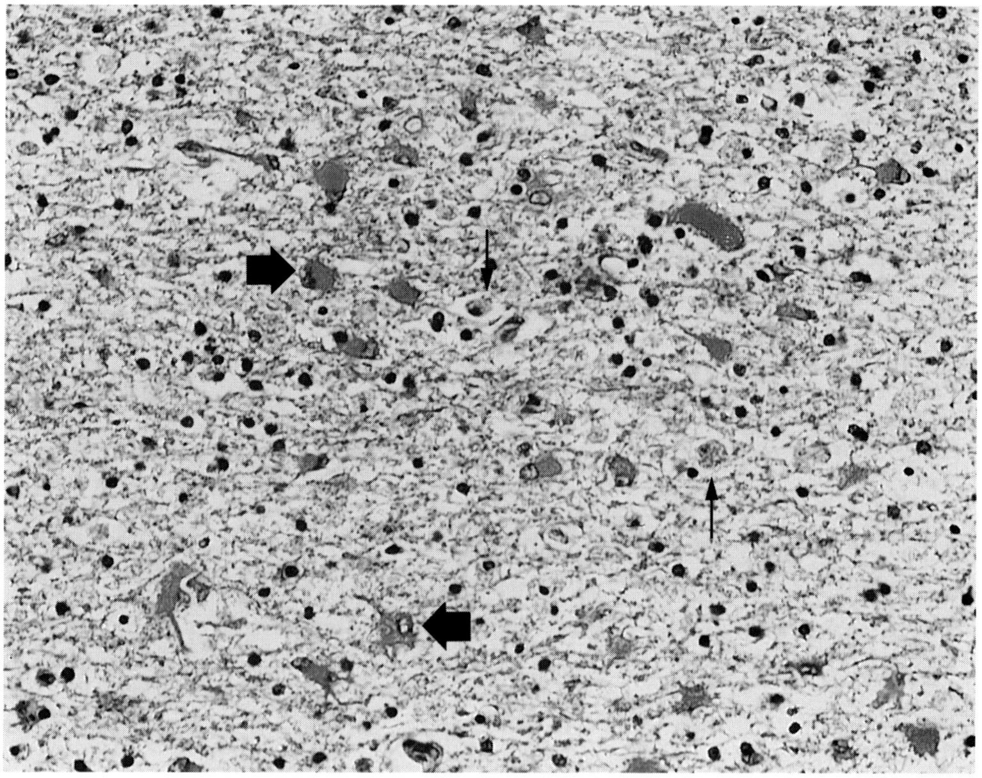

**Fig. 9-9.** Demyelination, macrophages, and reactive astrocytosis in white matter of the cingulate gyrus. Lesions of the frontal white matter such as this with variable numbers of macrophages (*arrows*) and reactive astrocytes (*arrowheads*) are common in AIDS; they may be as small as this microscopic field, or this same appearance can be found in a wide area of deep white matter. (H&E; ×200.)

Often very little chronic inflammation is seen in the CNS parenchyma; in most cases of clinical encephalopathy without opportunistic infections, relatively little inflammation is present in comparison with conditions such as herpes simplex encephalitis, post-measles encephalitis, or subacute sclerosing panencephalitis. An additional striking feature in AIDS is the relatively high incidence of primary CNS lymphomas.[205,222,247,278] A common but under-recognized finding is that of multifocal lesions discovered on microscopic examination of a grossly normal autopsy brain in an AIDS patient who had no neurologic complications.[155]

The linkage of HIV with AIDS and the isolation of the retrovirus from involved brain, spinal cord, peripheral nerve tissue, and cerebrospinal fluid (CSF) strongly implicate HIV as a direct or indirect cause of the nervous system lesions found in AIDS.* HIV-specific IgG is synthesized in the CNS in AIDS patients with neurologic symptoms.[107,108,243] This provides a further link between the retrovirus and the neurologic problems frequently observed in AIDS. Isolation of HIV or identification in the CNS by immunostaining or by in situ hybridization has been correlated with white matter pallor and gliosis and with chronic inflammatory foci, including monocyte/macrophages, multinucleated cells, and lymphocytes.*

* Refs. 53, 54, 89, 106–108, 120, 125, 137, 160, 163, 267, 271.

## GROSS CNS ASPECTS OF AIDS CASES

### Recommended HIV Neuropathology Autopsy Precautions and Technique

HIV can be recovered from blood, viscera, and bone in autopsies for at least several days after death. HIV has specifically *not* been recoverable from autopsy saw bone dust.[208] Careful autopsy technique, as traditionally practiced, poses no extra hazard from HIV to the pathologist or autopsy room personnel.[97,208] All personnel in the autopsy room for an AIDS autopsy should be gowned and double-gloved, wearing shoe covers, a hair cover, a mask, and a clear plastic face shield. The face shield need not always be down, but it protects against saw blades and fluid spray that can be hazardous during any autopsy. A separate isolation room with a turnover of at least 6 volumes of air per hour should be used to perform AIDS autopsies when available, but any autopsy room must be carefully cleaned with soap and water followed by bleach (diluted 1:10 with tap water)[96] after the autopsy is com-

* Refs. 31, 65, 89, 150, 177, 235, 249, 251, 256, 259, 285, 300, 308, 315, 318.

pleted, and the room should be considered contaminated for several hours until the air volume is fully replaced. A suction apparatus (industrial vacuum unit with a hose) can be attached to the bone saw near the blade to pick up particles; this instrument should be considered contaminated once it has been used.

The rule of thumb in handling AIDS autopsy material is to prepare a large number of sections from formalin-fixed brain and spinal cord tissue. The more sections reviewed, the more likely it is that lesions will be found. Focal lesions are not evenly spread throughout the CNS parenchyma. In our experience, increasing the number of tissue blocks and sections reviewed will increase the number and often the types of lesions identified in an AIDS case. Our minimum list of sections taken from coronal slices of cerebrum and cerebellum and from transverse slices of the brainstem and spinal cord includes:

1. *Frontal lobe.* A section with a small part of the genu or anterior body of the corpus callosum on one edge as a marker. The cingulate gyrus adjacent to the corpus callosum and abundant white matter of the subcortical region and corona radiata (deep white matter) are included. Small lesions are most likely to be seen in the *frontal white matter.*
2. *Basal ganglia and adjacent regions.* Including the mammillary body in one corner of the section allows easy reproducibility of the level taken to include hypothalamus, thalamus, internal capsule (where lesions similar to those in the frontal white matter can be found), lenticular nucleus (putamen and globus pallidus), claustrum, and insular cortex. For small, standard tissue cassettes, two sections will be needed. The lateral putamen, claustrum, and surrounding white matter frequently harbor microscopic lesions, and it is advisable to include them in each case.
3. *Temporal lobe.* The hippocampus is included medially, and as much medial, inferior, and inferolateral cortex and white matter as possible should be included. We prefer the temporal tissue adjacent to the lateral geniculate nucleus, both for reproducibility and for a level of the hippocampus that is easy to study.
4. *Occipital lobe.* The calcarine cortex is taken to include a landmark, but taking adequate white matter is the object.
5. *Cerebellum.* Sections should include folia of a lateral lobe (hemisphere) and the dentate nucleus.
6. *Midbrain.* A full cross section can show both cerebral peduncles, and two cassettes may be needed with the midbrain split down the midline.
7. *Pons.* A full cross section should include the basis pontis, with parts of the middle cerebellar peduncles and even the tegmentum trimmed away if necessary.
8. *Medulla.* A cross section of its widest part shows the most tissue.
9. *Spinal cord.* Sections of the cervical enlargement, midthoracic region, and lumber enlargement may show lesions with varying features. In patients with sensorimotor symptoms, the lesions could be located in the cerebrum, brainstem, or spinal cord; all of these regions are involved with great frequency.
10. *Abnormal areas* or areas under suspicion from clinical studies.

### Gross CNS Findings

There is no gross finding typical of AIDS in the brain, but even when an easily identified lesion is not present, small lesions can be noted on careful inspection in some cases. Atrophy is obvious when a large number of gyri have a neocortical strip that is only about 0.2 cm thick, but even milder cerebral atrophy can be diagnosed by computed tomography (CT) scans or magnetic resonance imaging (MRI).[110] Small, faint, round to irregular, white or yellow patches of coagulation necrosis in the cortical areas or white matter without appreciable softening or with a granular cut surface can be seen in areas of early toxoplasmic encephalitis (Fig. 9-10). Small holes close to one another, giving a soap bubble appearance, are classically although infrequently found in cryptococcal encephalitis (Fig. 9-11). Ventricular surface irregularities are sometimes caused by focal or extensive periventricular cytomegaloviral encephalitis (Fig. 9-12). An apparently minor irregularity of the ependymal surface anywhere in the ventricular system should be sectioned for microscopic study; it should be remembered that postmortem autolytic changes impart a similar appearance. Small depressed patches of subcortical white matter in the cerebrum should be studied in microscopic sections cut large enough to include overlying neocortex. These demyelinated patches might be part of a lesion that includes the gray matter, and it may not be possible to make a specific gross diagnosis. This general description includes some lesions of toxoplasmic encephalitis (Fig. 9-10), progressive multifocal leukoencephalopathy (PML) (Fig. 9-13), and herpetic encephalitis.[206,248,249] Cerebral lymphomas, although sometimes quite necrotic and hemorrhagic (Figs. 9-10, 9-14), may be difficult to see grossly, but CT and MRI films may identify areas from which samples should be taken. Widespread frontal periventricular densities in MRI studies for which no counterpart lesion exists on gross cut sections may be correlated with scattered gliomesenchymal cell nodules or small patches of demyelination in the white matter.[229] However, this find-

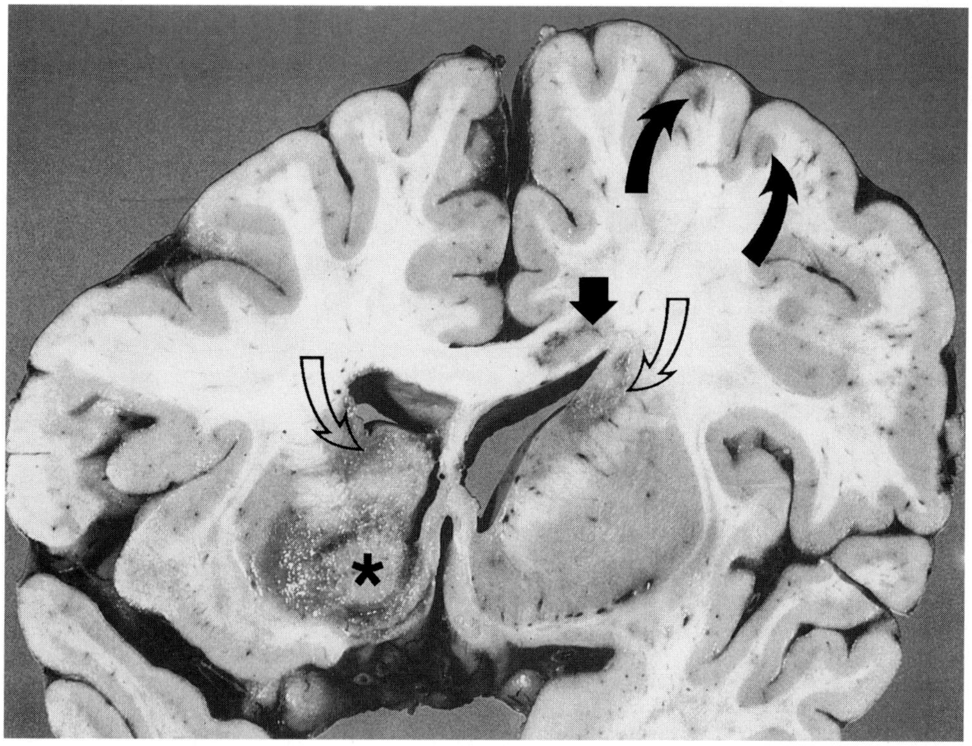

**Fig. 9-10.** The cerebrum from a case of multifocal primary lymphoma, toxoplasmic encephalitis, and progressive multifocal leukoencephalopathy, with a few microscopic foci of cytomegaloviral encephalitis. The small lesions at the gray-white junctions (*closed arrows*) and in the body of the corpus callosum (*arrowhead*) are typical of toxoplasmic involvement and have smooth cut surfaces. The small lesions at the junction of the neocortex and subcortical white matter resemble metastatic tumors. The granular-surfaced lesions in the caudate nuclei (*open arrows*) and the large lesion in the left corpus striatum (*) are irradiated, necrotic areas of lymphoma.

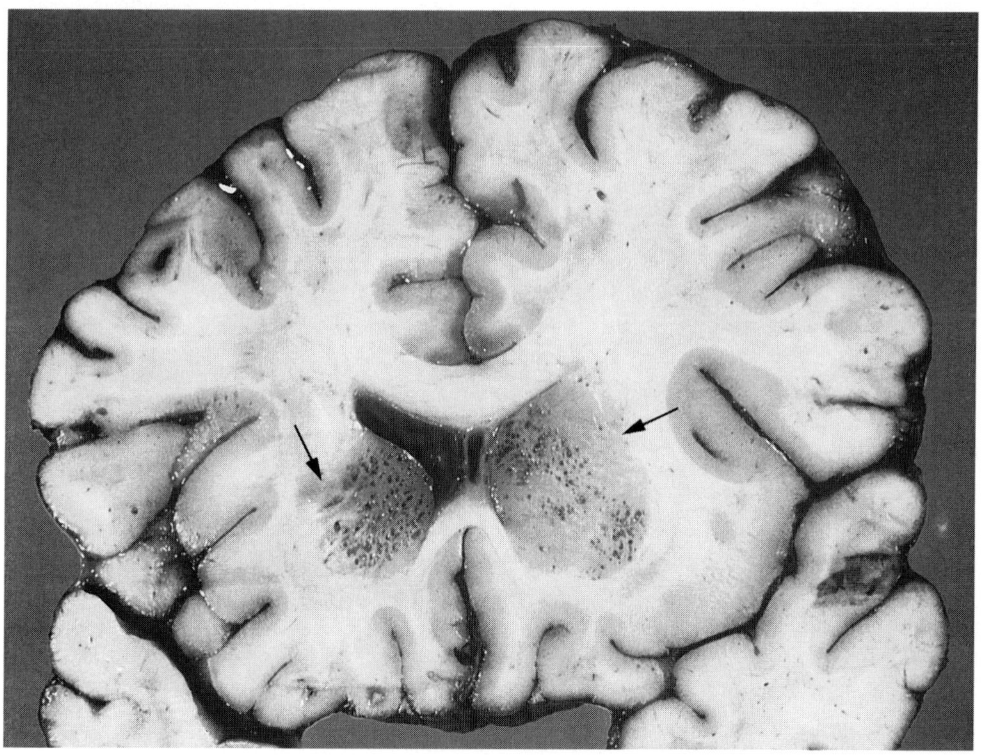

**Fig. 9-11.** A cerebrum with cryptococcal meningoencephalitis. The "soap-bubble" appearance of cryptococcal encephalitis is pronounced in the basal ganglia (*arrows*). These perivascular lesions extend into the brain from subarachnoid sleeves around penetrating blood vessels.

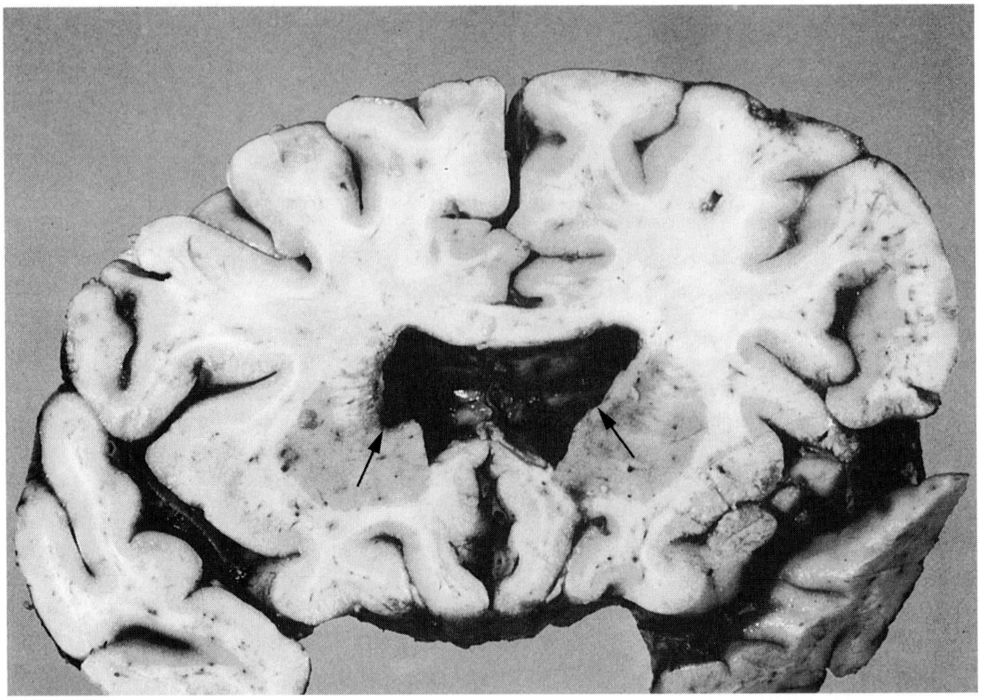

**Fig. 9-12.** Frontal lobes with periventricular cytomegaloviral encephalitis. The widened anterior horns of the lateral ventricles have irregular walls (*arrows*) as a result of necrosis from periventricular cytomegaloviral lesions.

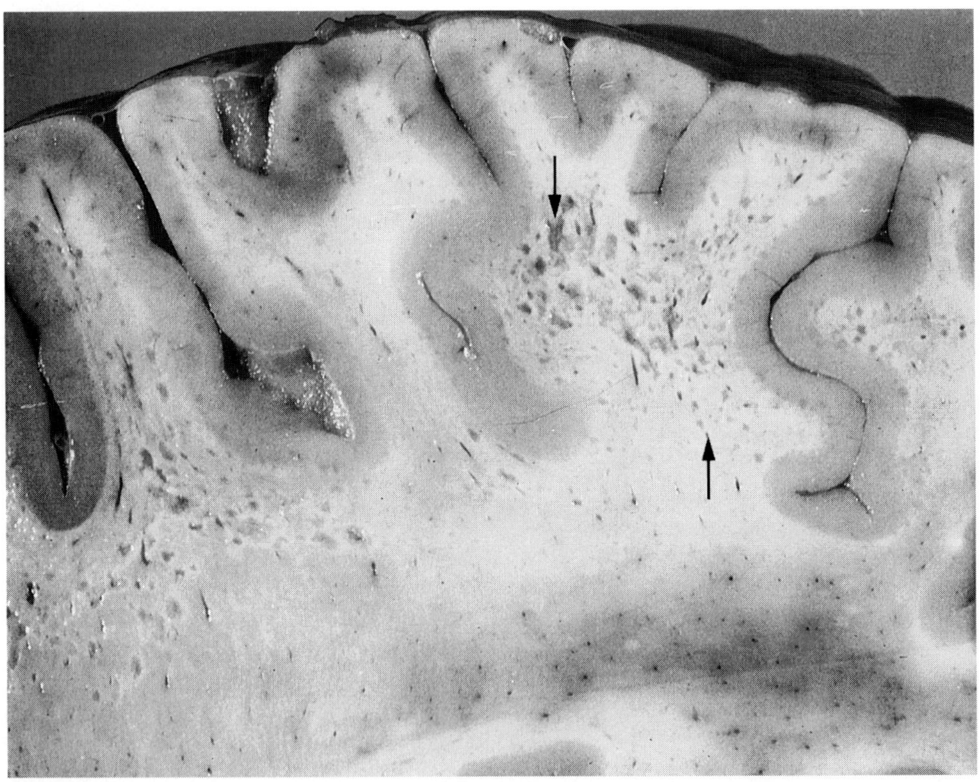

**Fig. 9-13.** White matter lesions typical of PML. The transversely sectioned hemisphere shows many small, slightly darkened, depressed lesions of demyelination (*arrows*).

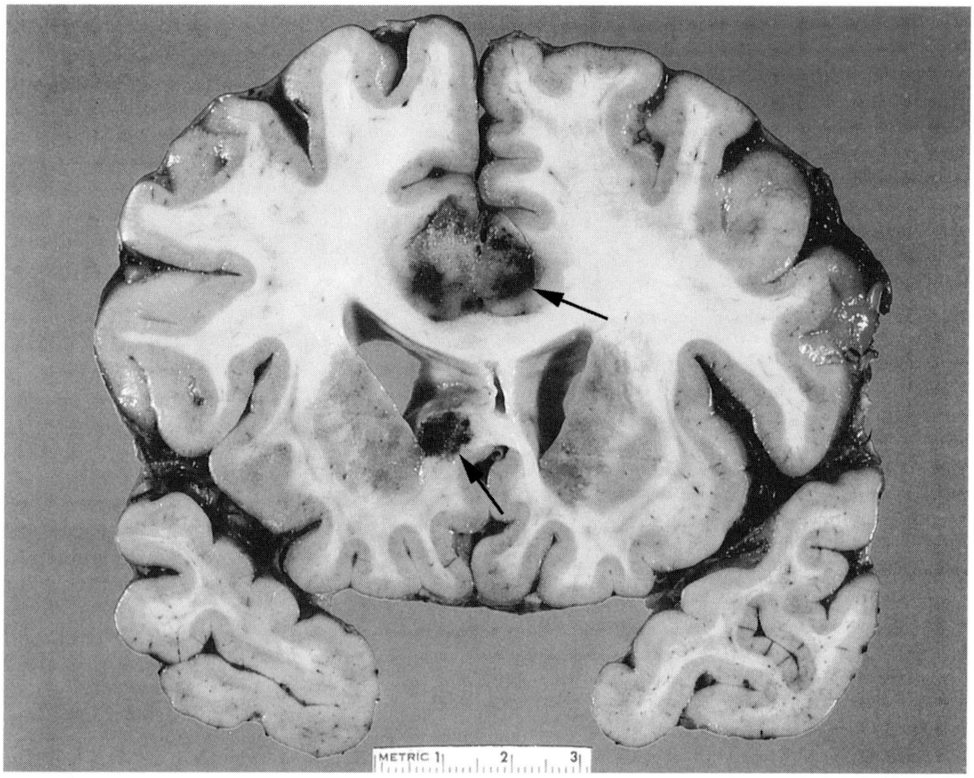


**Fig. 9-14.** A primary cerebral lymphoma. The tumor is multifocal and quite similar in appearance to toxoplasmosis. Typically, in cases such as this one in which a tumor can be easily localized grossly, findings differing from those of toxoplasmic encephalitis include areas of hemorrhage (*arrows*) and granular or irregular cut surfaces.

ing requires serial clinical studies because such frontal MRI findings can also be caused by small white matter infarcts;[179] the MRI abnormalities also can be found in brains without microscopic lesions.[289] The posterior columns of the spinal cord can be whiter than usual in tabes dorsalis. The posterior columns and lateral corticospinal tracts are pale white in advanced cases of vacuolar myelopathy.[250]

## HISTOPATHOLOGIC FEATURES OF THE CNS LESIONS ASSOCIATED WITH AIDS

The findings in 400 consecutive AIDS autopsies with CNS examination performed at the Los Angeles County General Hospital are categorized in Tables 9-1 through 9-7.[247]

### Infiltration of Monocyte/Macrophages and Multinucleated Cells, Inflammation, and Gliosis

A careful search of autopsy material obtained from the brains of patients with AIDS often reveals mononuclear cells typical of small macrophages. These cells are most commonly seen near small blood vessels in the cerebral white matter (Figs. 9-2, 9-3), subcortical nuclear masses, cerebellum (Figs. 9-1, 9-4), or brainstem (Fig. 9-5), and they can be found in scattered foci in the leptomeninges (Fig. 9-6) and spinal cord. The neocortex is often spared. Some of the perivascular macrophages are brown, and this pigment may be positive for PAS-stained material or iron.[202] The peculiar type of perivascular infiltration represented by small groups of slightly enlarged, often nonfoamy macrophages along with multinucleated cells is a hallmark of HIV encephalomyelitis, even more so than the simple presence of multinucleated giant cells. Although quite critical in making a histopathologic diagnosis, the perivascular macrophages are not a specific finding unless multinucleated cells are seen, and even then these findings cannot be considered pathognomonic of HIV encephalomyelitis. The perivascular macrophages in the absence of any tissue pallor or more specific signs of a lesion are strongly suggestive of HIV encephalomyelitis in and of themselves, but contributory data have to be used to confirm the diagnosis. There are usually few if any lymphocytes and no epithelioid cells in perivascular lesions containing giant cells. These perivascular lesions are quite different from the rare but striking lesions of noninfectious primary angiitis of the CNS in which giant cells are commonly found. An HIV-infected, non-AIDS case[320] and an AIDS case with primary angiitis of the CNS have been reported.[261]

**Table 9-1.** Inflammatory and reactive changes in the CNS in 400 AIDS autopsies*

| Change | Percentage of cases (%) |
|---|---|
| Gliomesenchymal cell nodules† | 36 |
| Cerebrum | 27 |
| Cerebellum | 11 |
| Brainstem | 21 |
| Spinal cord | 8 |
| Perivascular macrophages, multinucleated cells, or brown-pigmented macrophages | 19 |
| Spongiform white matter changes with macrophages, multinucleated cells, and astrogliosis (diffuse leukoencephalopathy)‡ | 8 |
| Focal necrosis with macrophages (necrotizing encephalitis) | 4 |
| Reactive astrocytes in white matter | 1 |
| Neocortical reactive astrocytosis | 4§ |
| Reactive astrocytosis in basal ganglia | 1 |

* Histopathologic findings in 400 consecutive examinations of the CNS in AIDS autopsies performed at the Los Angeles County General Hospital. Spinal cord was not examined in a few cases. Modified with permission from Rhodes RH: Histopathologic features in the central nervous system of 400 acquired immunodeficiency syndrome cases: implications of rates of occurrence, Hum Pathol 24: 1189–1198, 1993.

† Gliomesenchymal cell nodules containing identifiable opportunistic agents were not included in this category. Cytomegaloviral inclusions were found in 18 gliomesenchymal cell nodules from the entire group of 400 cases. Six additional nodules contained cells with intranuclear inclusions of uncertain type.

‡ Spongiform changes in the white matter are included in areas of demyelination.

§ This value is probably underestimated. Frequent enlarged glial nuclei were not classed as reactive unless an enlarged cytoplasm was easily seen in routine staining.

**Table 9-2.** Long-tract degeneration in the CNS in 400 AIDS autopsies*

| Change | Percentage of cases (%) |
|---|---|
| Cases with long tract degeneration in brain, apart from necrosis that may have locally included white matter long tracts | 15 |
| Bilateral spongiform changes of internal capsule with demyelination, macrophages, and gliosis | 4 |
| Also with associated bilateral wallerian degeneration of corticospinal tract | 1 |
| Also with associated wallerian degeneration of corticopontine tract | 1 |
| Spinal cord | 13 |
| Vacuolar myelopathy | 10 |
| Central spinal myelinolysis | 3 |
| Bilateral degeneration of corticospinal tract without other tract lesions | 2 |
| Bilateral wallerian degeneration of corticospinal tract and corticopontine tract | <1 |

* Histopathologic findings in 400 consecutive examinations of the CNS in AIDS autopsies at the Los Angeles County General Hospital. Modified with permission from Rhodes RH: Histopathologic features in the central nervous system of 400 acquired immunodeficiency syndrome cases: implications of rates of occurrence, Hum Pathol 24:1189–1198, 1993.

However, when found with an HIV infection, it is difficult to separate primary angiitis of the CNS from an infectious lesion. For instance, a patient with AIDS-related complex and apparent primary angiitis of the CNS without giant cells had intranuclear inclusions associated with the vascular lesions[302]; a viral vasculitis might also be considered in such cases.

Perivascular macrophages are found with half the frequency of gliomesenchymal cell nodules. There may be no other observable lesion in a section containing perivascular macrophages, and some of these macrophages and multinucleated cells can be immunostained to show a macrophage phenotype[95,150,235,318]; the cells can also be immunostained* or hybridized in situ for HIV markers.† This type of perivascular infiltration of mononuclear/multinucleated cells has been noted in the brain of some HIV-positive patients without CDC-defined AIDS, and it has been suggested that this histopathologic finding may be the earliest routinely detectable change in the development of HIV encephalitis.[156] Chronic perivasculitis, or perivenous encephalitis, consisting of partial or complete cuffing of venules by small round cells (Fig. 9-15), is frequently seen in AIDS or in an HIV infection before AIDS develops,[51,114] and it could be an early sign of hypersensitivity disease.[71] Lymphocytes infected with HIV are probably lysed too rapidly to be seen frequently in autopsy material,[130,308] but infected macrophages such as those found in the CNS can survive for extended periods of time.* T lymphocytes are, in fact, quite difficult to demonstrate in the parenchyma of AIDS brains, while CNS monocyte/macrophages can be double-labeled for one of their specific markers and for HIV protein with little difficulty.[310]

Relatively small, multinucleated cells were found in 28% of our first 200 autopsy cases, and multinucleated giant cells were seen in about 30% of the cases in which there were small multinucleated cells.[251] The smaller multinucleated cells may have five or ten nuclei in a

* Refs. 177, 235, 249, 250, 308, 318.

† Refs. 65, 95, 150, 256, 267, 315.

* Refs. 95, 121, 150, 152, 220.

**Table 9-3.** Vascular and hypoxic lesions in the CNS in 400 AIDS autopsies*

| Change | Percentage of cases (%) |
|---|---|
| Mixed acute and chronic perivasculitis | 2 |
| Cerebrum | 2 |
| Cerebellum | <1 |
| Brainstem | 1 |
| Chronic perivasculitis | 15 |
| Cerebrum | 10 |
| Cerebellum | 2 |
| Brainstem | 3 |
| Spinal cord | 1 |
| Spinal nerve roots | <1 |
| Mixed acute and chronic vasculitis | 2 |
| Cerebrum | 1 |
| Cerebellum | <1 |
| Brainstem | 1 |
| Chronic vasculitis | 7 |
| Cerebrum | 5 |
| Cerebellum | 2 |
| Brainstem | 3 |
| Spinal cord | 1 |
| Vascular malformation | 2 |
| Cerebral hypoxic nerve cell changes | 32 |
| Respirator brain | 6 |
| All infarcts | 9 |
| Recent | 6 |
| Healing | 4 |
| Healed | 2 |
| Cerebrovascular thromboembolism | 4 |
| Superior sagittal sinus thrombosis | <1 |
| Intracerebral hemorrhage/intraventricular hemorrhage (without tumor or inflammation) | 6 |
| Subarachnoid hemorrhage (without inflammation) | 4 |
| Perivascular petechial hemorrhages without inflammation | 2 |
| Perivascular petechial hemorrhages with scant acute inflammation | 2 |
| Intradural hemorrhage | 1 |

* Histopathologic findings in 400 consecutive examinations of the CNS in AIDS autopsies performed at the Los Angeles County General Hospital. Modified with permission from Rhodes RH: Histopathologic features in the central nervous system of 400 acquired immunodeficiency syndrome cases: implications of rates of occurrence, Hum Pathol 24:1189–1198, 1993.

cut section, but only a thin rim of cytoplasm is seen. They are roughly 20 to 30 $\mu$m in diameter (Figs. 9-2 to 9-5), while giant cells are generally over 50 $\mu$m across and contain abundant cytoplasm (Figs. 9-4, 9-5). Every intermediate size of multinucleated cell can be seen (Figs. 9-3, 9-4), and size has little significance. Multinucleation, or syncytial formation, is the histopathologic finding of importance in characterizing a case as one of possible—even probable—HIV encephali-

**Table 9-4.** Inflammatory/infectious lesions of uncertain etiology in the CNS in 400 AIDS autopsies*

| Change | Percentage of cases (%) |
|---|---|
| Acute and chronic leptomeningitis | 3 |
| Chronic leptomeningitis | 5 |
| Leptomeningeal macrophages (focal or multifocal) | 7 |
| Chronic leptomeningeal perivasculitis | 1 |
| Chronic leptomeningeal vasculitis | 3 |
| Chronic meningoencephalitis | 1 |
| Chronic encephalitis | 2 |
| Chronic radiculitis | <1 |
| Acute hemorrhagic leukoencephalitis | <1 |

* Histopathologic findings in 400 consecutive examinations of the CNS in AIDS autopsies performed at the Los Angeles County General Hospital. Modified with permission from Rhodes RH: Histopathologic features in the central nervous system of 400 acquired immunodeficiency syndrome cases: implications of rates of occurrence, Hum Pathol 24:1189–1198, 1993.

tis.[30,113,143,268] Many of the scattered parenchymal monocyte/macrophages contain no detectable retroviral antigen[308] or nucleic acid,[150] and this may indicate a low infection rate of these cells, an antigen or HIV genomic level too low to be detected,[267] expression of HIV genes or gene products that are not generally looked for,[259,292] overfixation,[105] or autolysis. Reports of HIV nucleic acid and protein localization in tissue sections suggest that more HIV early regulatory/accessory genes than structural genes are present and active in astrocytes and neurons, indicating a persistent or latent infection of the CNS parenchyma, while it is the structural genes and their protein products ("live" virus) that are found in infiltrating macrophages.[207,259,267] The amount of HIV protein that can be immunostained is low compared to other viral infections, and it becomes increasingly difficult to demonstrate when the tissue is overfixed in formalin.[105] Although HIV-labeled cells tend to be in the subcortical white matter,[259,292] glial cells in the neocortex can be reactive for HIV antigens.[89,249] Perineuronal cortical (Fig. 9-16) and interfascicular white matter glial cells that are HIV positive, although sometimes slightly shrunken, are normal or close enough to normal in appearance that they are not detectable as being altered on routine microscopic examination. Reactive gliosis, consisting of easily identified, swollen-bodied astrocytes in the gray and white matter, may accompany this otherwise silent glial cell HIV infection (Fig. 9-16),[249,251] and early HIV encephalitis could be one cause of gliosis without necrosis. These cellular findings may also be associated with small or large areas of evolving necrosis in the basal ganglia or in the subcortical or deep white matter (Figs.

**Table 9-5.** Infections with known or apparent etiology in the CNS in 400 AIDS autopsies*

| Infection | Percentage of cases (%) |
|---|---|
| Total cytomegalovirus | 8 |
| Focal in brain | 4 |
| Multifocal in brain | 2 |
| Multifocal in brain and spinal cord | 2 |
| Progressive multifocal leukoencephalopathy | 1 |
| Herpes simplex virus type 2 encephalitis | <1 |
| Total *cryptococcus* | 7 |
| Leptomeningitis | 2 |
| Meningoencephalitis | 5 |
| *Candida* encephalitis | 2 |
| *Coccidioides* encephalitis | <1 |
| *Histoplasma* meningoencephalitis | <1 |
| Total *Toxoplasma* | 9 |
| Focal encephalitis | 1 |
| Multifocal encephalitis | 7 |
| Encephalomyelitis | 1 |
| *Acanthamoeba castellanii* encephalitis | <1 |
| Meningovascular syphilis | <1 |
| Tabes dorsalis (with clinical syphilis) | <1 |
| Tuberculous meningoencephalitis | 1 |
| *Mycobacterium avium-intracellulare* vasculitis | 1 |
| Purulent leptomeningitis | 1 |
| Acute and chronic encephalitis/meningoencephalitis | 1 |
| Acute cerebritis | 1 |
| Acute focal myelitis | <1 |
| Microabscesses in brain | 2 |
| Microabscesses in spinal cord | 1 |
| Septic infarcts | 1 |
| Septic hemorrhages | <1 |
| Acute vasculitis in spinal cord | <1 |

* Histopathologic findings in 400 consecutive examinations of the CNS in AIDS autopsies performed at the Los Angeles County General Hospital Medical Center. Modified with permission from Rhodes RH: Histopathologic features in the central nervous system of 400 acquired immunodeficiency cases: implications of rates of occurrence, Hum Pathol 24:1189–1198, 1993.

**Table 9-6.** Tumors in the CNS in 400 AIDS autopsies*

| Tumor type | Percentage of cases (%) |
|---|---|
| Primary CNS lymphoma | 6 |
| Lymphoma metastatic to CNS | 2 |
| Glial hamartoma | <1 |

* Histopathologic findings in 400 consecutive examinations of the CNS in AIDS autopsies performed at the Los Angeles County General Hospital. Modified with permission from Rhodes RH: Histopathologic features in the central nervous system of 400 acquired immunodeficiency cases: implications of rates of occurrence. Hum Pathol 24:1189–1198, 1993.

**Table 9-7.** Miscellaneous findings in the CNS in 400 AIDS autopsies*

| Finding | Percentage of cases (%) |
|---|---|
| Granular ependymitis | 17 |
| Basal ganglia mineralization | 1 |
| Central chromatolysis and nuclear eccentricity in anterior horn cells of lumbar spinal cord | 1 |
| Subdural hematomas (acute or chronic) | 4 |
| Contusions | 2 |
| Total essentially normal CNS | 18 |
| No significant lesion | 6 |
| Essentially normal except for changes attributable to terminal hypoxia or foci of metastatic lymphoma | 12 |

* Histopathologic findings in 400 consecutive examinations of the CNS in AIDS autopsies performed at the Los Angeles County General Hospital. Modified with permission from Rhodes RH: Histopathologic features in the central nervous system of 400 acquired immunodeficiency cases: implications of rates of occurrence, Hum Pathol 24:1189–1198, 1993.

9-9, 9-17, 9-18). Relatively frequent findings of perivasculitis and vasculitis may be early or late signs of HIV encephalitis. Even before any histopathologic lesions are found in the brainstem, the polymerase chain reaction indicates that an HIV infection can be present there while it may be lacking in the cerebrum.[25] Opportunistic infections may either cause or contribute to some of the histopathologic findings of vascular, inflammatory, and necrotizing lesions in any given case.

Astrogliosis, one of the early signs of a CNS lesion in AIDS, could result from a subtle breakdown of the blood-brain barrier even before any cellular infiltration occurs,[159,231,246] from a response to a release of cytokines from infiltrating macrophages,[13,290] from toxicity from an HIV gene product such as gp120[219,234] or transactivator protein,[151] or from direct HIV infection.[259,292,318] Gliosis in the cerebral cortex in AIDS appears to be a hypertrophy through an increase in nuclear size and in the number of cytoplasmic intermediate filaments (making the cytoplasm of cortical protoplasmic astrocytes more eosinophilic and thereby more visible in routine stains), rather than an astrocytic hyperplasia since the actual number of astrocytes does not increase.[312] This same mechanism may operate in a frequently accompanying deep white matter gliosis, although when myelin loss and infiltration of macrophages accompany the white matter astrogliosis, a different pathogenesis or a more severe infectious, toxic, or immunopathologic stimulus is indicated.

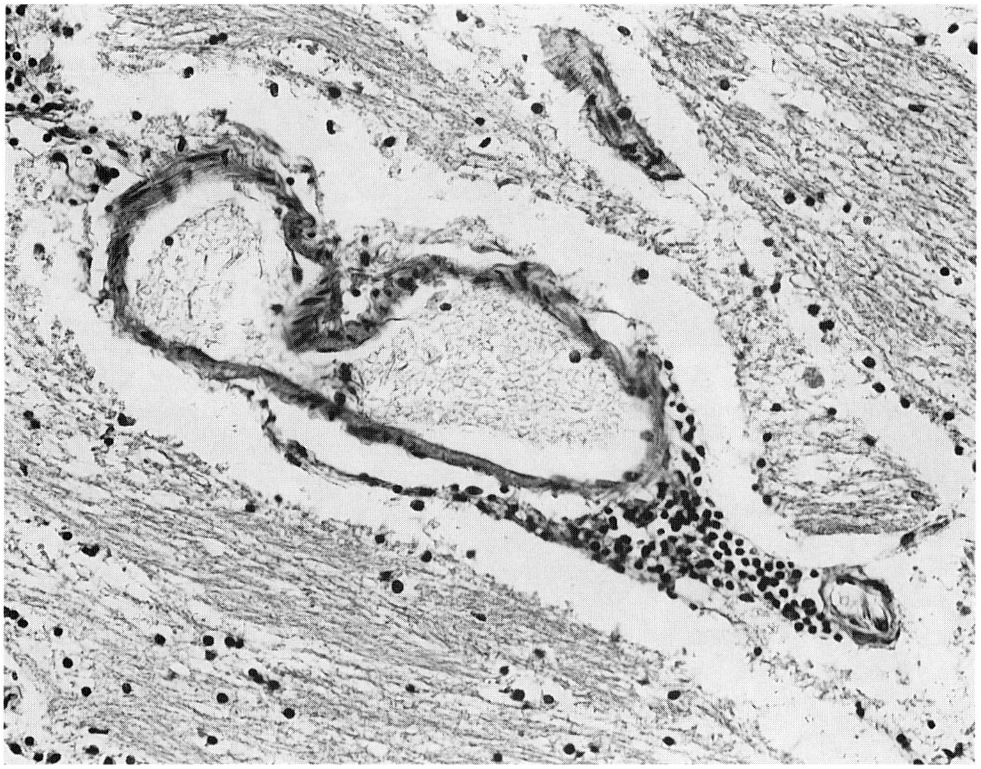

**Fig. 9-15.** Chronic perivasculitis in the internal capsule. There is lymphocytic infiltration around a cerebral vein. (H&E; ×200.)

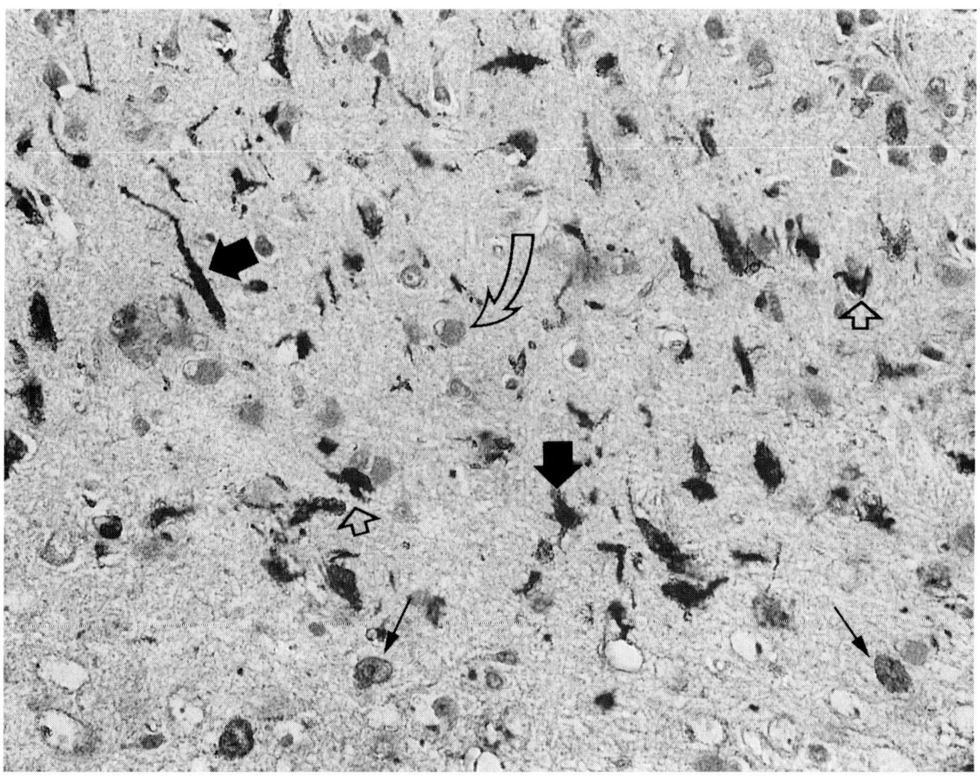

**Fig. 9-16.** HIV immunoreactivity at the junction of the neocortex and subcortex. The spongiform change in the white matter (*lower part of field*) is caused by PML. Macrophages (*closed arrows*) and glial cells (*closed arrowheads*) are immunoreactive for HIV. Some of the HIV-positive glial cells are perineuronal satellite cells (*open arrowheads*). The reactive astrocytes (*open curved arrow*) are not positive for HIV. (Anti-HIV rabbit antiserum #762; ×200.)

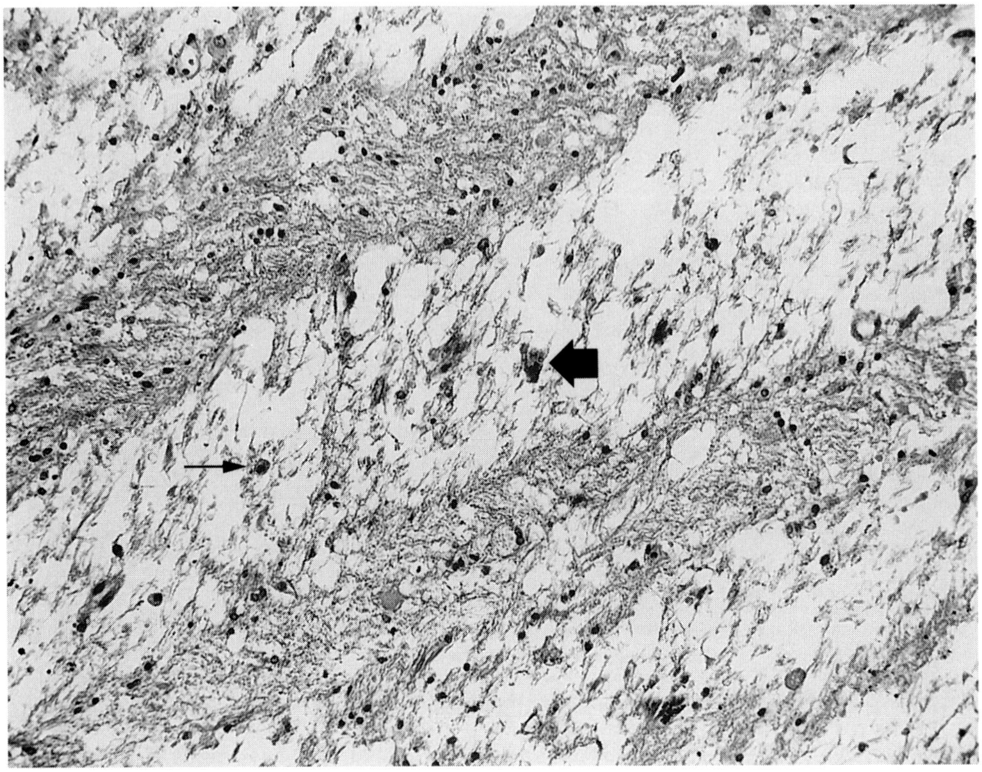

**Fig. 9-17.** Spongiform change and macrophages in the internal capsule. Similar spongiform alterations can be artificial but here macrophages (*arrow*) and multinucleated cells (*arrowhead*) are present, indicating tissue injury. (H&E; ×130.) (Reprinted with permission from Rhodes RH: Hum Pathol 18:636, 1987.)

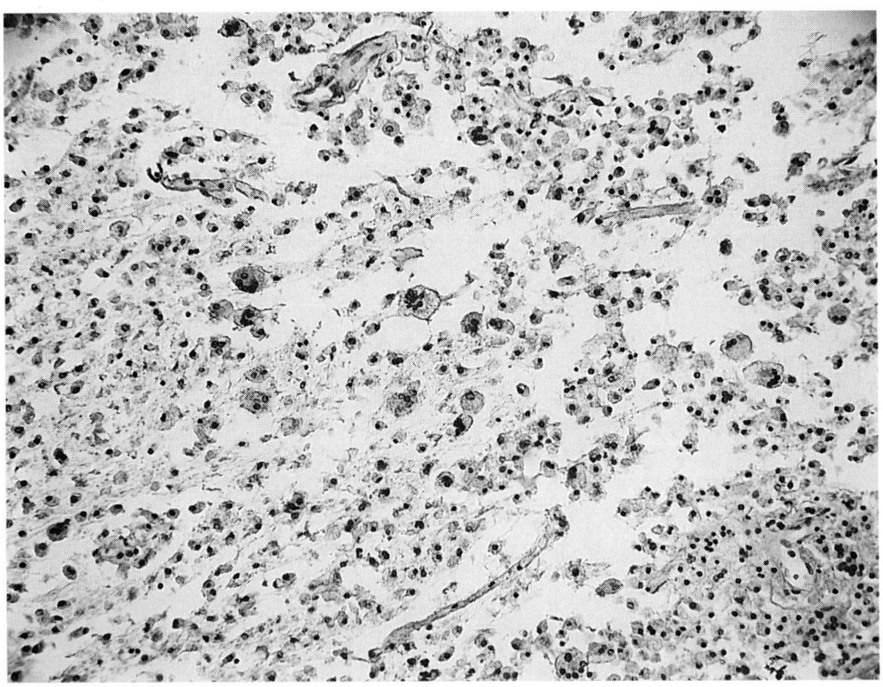

**Fig. 9-18.** Liquefactive necrosis with multinucleated giant cells in the internal capsule. This may be the eventual result of a lesion that begins as spongiform change or as coagulation necrosis. (H&E; ×130.) (Reprinted from Rhodes RH: Hum Pathol 18:636, 1987.)

### Demyelination in the CNS

Patches of spongiform demyelination with astrogliosis and foamy macrophages/multinucleated cells or areas of paravascular demyelination (in parenchyma around blood vessels; "perivascular" refers to the subarachnoid sheath surrounding blood vessels in the CNS) can be associated with clinical AIDS encephalopathy and with specific sensorimotor symptoms. Foci of white matter demyelination may appear on CT scans as low-density areas without enhancement or mass effect, while MRI can show progressive lesions on T2-weighted studies with high-intensity signals that tend to be near ventricles and in the corona radiata.[229] Films from a single study may show nonspecific alterations without demonstrating a progressive condition. Myelin loss (detected with a stain such as Luxol fast blue) is generally greater than loss of axons (seen with silver impregnation, e.g., Bodian or Bielschowsky's), but the tissue destruction can be severe enough to cause coagulation or cavitating necrosis (*necrotizing encephalitis*). These lesions are generally in the cerebral white matter, but a subset seems to have a predilection for the basis pontis.[6] The underlying mechanism associated with demyelination in AIDS is often not obvious, but mild astrocytosis and foamy macrophages or even multinucleated cells are generally found in the involved white matter (*diffuse leukoencephalopathy*), suggesting that demyelination can be a finding of direct HIV encephalitis (Figs. 9-9, 9-17, 9-18).[21] Because the white matter lesions could also be the result of opportunistic infections or hypersensitivity,* *demyelination is considered a nonspecific finding unless accompanied by an infectious agent in the tissue.* Regardless of the exciting phenomenon, demyelination in AIDS is peculiar in its frequency and in the common association with multinucleated cells in the absence of other recognized causes of granulomatous disease. Even when macrophages and multinucleated cells are present in the white matter, there can be few of these cells with little or no demyelination or few to many of these cells with extensive demyelination. The process of myelin destruction therefore may include toxic or humoral factors, but the source or sources remain unknown. Edema or postmortem changes might decrease the amount of myelin stained by traditional methods such as using Luxol fast blue stain, causing an apparent but fictitious "diffuse myelin pallor" in white matter areas devoid of any cellular "reaction" to myelin loss. The "pallor" is revealed as an artifact when immunostaining for myelin basic protein shows a normal myelin content in the same white matter area.[231]

Paravenular demyelination is sometimes accompanied by hemorrhage and scant acute inflammation. When the hemorrhages are large enough, the gross picture can resemble "brain purpura" of the type commonly seen in cases of fat embolism to the brain. The microscopic finding may include only erythrocytes around small venules, but a few scattered polymorphonuclear neutrophils are usually found (Fig. 9-19). When there are many acute inflammatory cells in the petechiae and thrombi in the venular lumen, the microscopic picture may resemble that of acute hemorrhagic leukoencephalitis.[2,237] Our patients with paravenular demyelination often had pneumonia, which is a common antecedent in acute hemorrhagic leukoencephalitis. However, AIDS patients commonly die with pneumonia,[148] and paravenular demyelination is uncommon in AIDS (Tables 9-3, 9-4). These paravenular lesions might be caused by direct damage to the endothelial cells or by damage to perivenular glial cells. The venular damage might be a hypersensitivity (autoimmune) phenomenon, or it may be more directly associated with HIV; HIV can be demonstrated by immunohistochemistry* and in situ hybridization in perivascular glial cells and in CNS endothelial cells.[256,315] It remains to be determined whether focal paravascular demyelination is related to the larger areas of demyelination described above.

Demyelination of long tracts can sometimes be traced from the cerebrum into the brainstem and spinal cord, or the spinal cord can be involved alone. Demyelination of ascending tracts in the spinal cord, particularly deep in the fasciculus gracilis in the medial part of the thoracic posterior columns, may be combined with motor-tract demyelination (Fig. 9-20). Demyelination limited to the gracile fasciculi, with prominence in upper rather than lower levels of the spinal cord, has been termed *central spinal myelinolysis.* This lesion can be found in a variety of patients, including some without AIDS.[141,239,250,324] Some AIDS patients have central spinal myelinolysis and demyelination of the internal capsules. Others have demyelination from the internal capsules into the frontopontine tracts in the midbrain or into the corticospinal tracts of the brainstem (Fig. 9-21) and spinal cord. Demyelination of the corticospinal tracts and posterior columns together forms the lesion complex termed *vacuolar myelopathy.*[221] The extent of demyelination may vary between the ascending and descending tracts. The general findings in HIV-associated vacuolar myelopathy are similar to those of avitaminosis $B_{12}$, including some cases with degeneration of the anterior or posterior spinocerebellar tracts, but histopathologic signs of HIV infection are also present, and serum levels of vitamin $B_{12}$ are normal when measured.[113,221,250] Spongiform change in the myelin sheath begins as intramyelinic

* Refs. 6, 102, 111, 112, 127, 132, 147, 237, 242, 247, 249, 251, 277.

* Refs. 235, 249, 276, 308, 315.

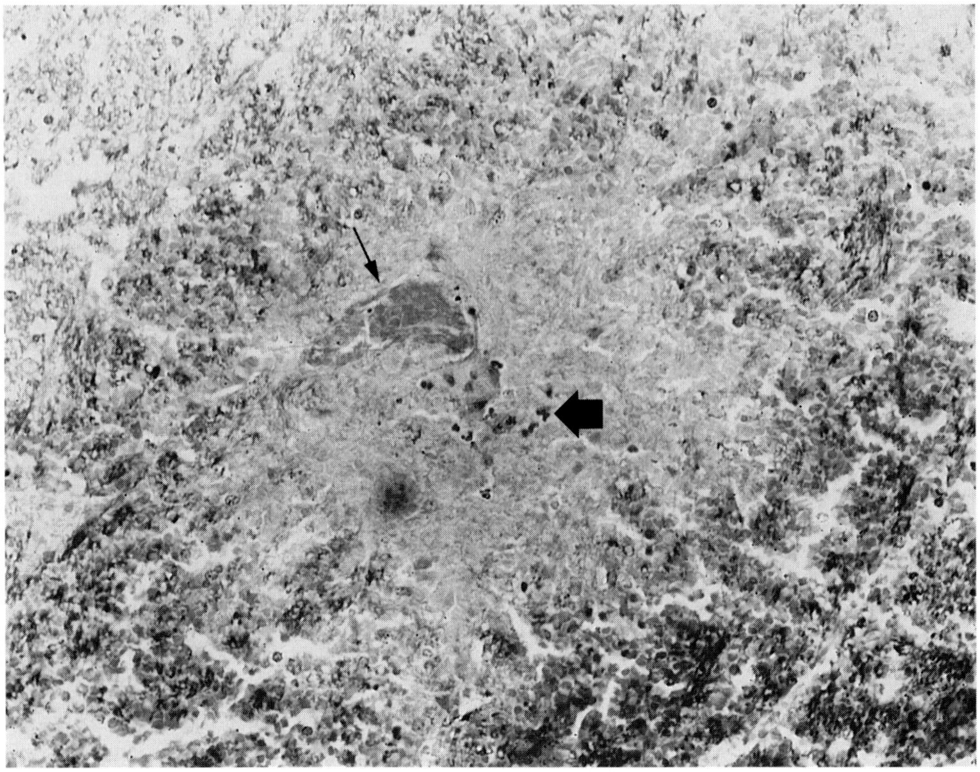

**Fig. 9-19.** Paravenular myelin loss and petechial hemorrhage in crus cerebri of the midbrain. A vein (*arrow*) is seen in a pale area of demyelination. Some acute inflammatory cells (*arrowhead*) are present in the demyelinated area. The dark staining around the demyelination is stained myelin. Red blood cells in the hemorrhage are pale or slightly darkened. (Luxol fast blue; ×200.)

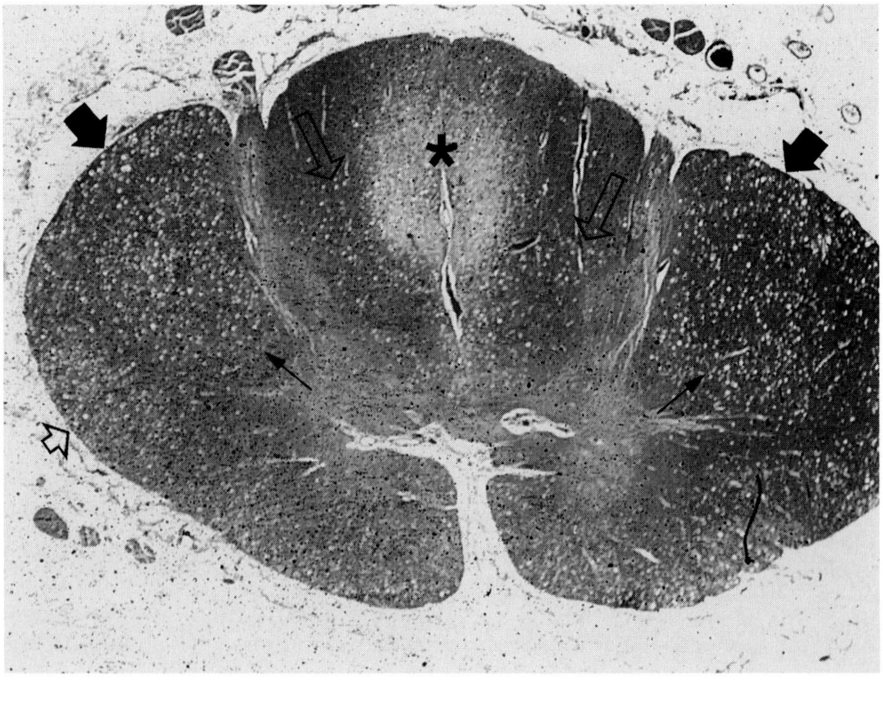

**Fig. 9-20.** Vacuolar myelopathy in the thoracic spinal cord. The middle part of each fasciculus gracilis (i.e., bilaterally along the median septum [*], deep to the pia mater, and not extending to the central canal area) shows pallor from severe demyelination. Lesser amounts of demyelination in the more laterally placed cuneate fasciculi of the posterior columns (*open arrows*), in the lateral corticospinal tracts (*black arrows*), and in the posterior (*closed arrowheads*) and anterior spinocerebellar tracts (*open arrowhead*) are visible because of the spongiform appearance of myelin swelling. (H&E; ×12.)

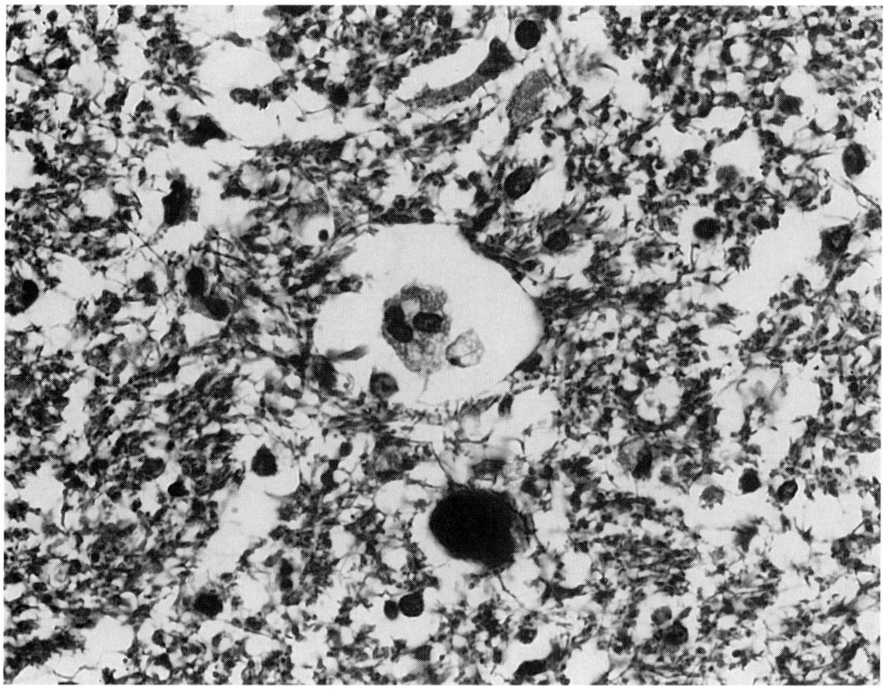

**Fig. 9-21.** Wallerian degeneration in a pyramid. A multinucleated cell is seen in a swollen myelin sheath in one of the corticospinal tracts in the medulla. (H&E; ×500.)

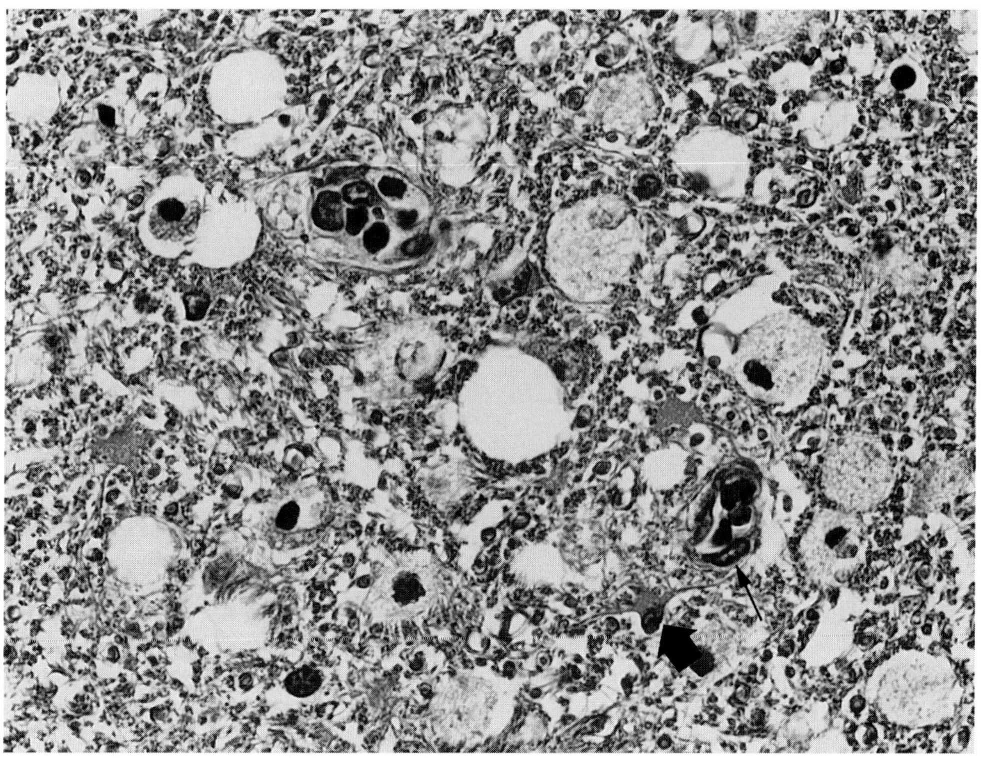

**Fig. 9-22.** Vacuolar myelopathy in a fasciculus gracilis of the cervical spinal cord. Foamy macrophages are found in most of the swollen myelin sheaths. Endothelial cell hypertrophy (*arrow*) is seen in the microvasculature. Reactive astrocytes are present (*arrowhead*). (H&E; ×500.)

edema,[221] and the myelin destruction is accompanied by foamy macrophages and reactive gliosis (Fig. 9-22). Demyelination may be slight or complete, but, as in the brain, myelin loss generally far exceeds axonal loss. The histopathologic distinction from tabes dorsalis might be difficult in a single tissue section; tabes generally begins in the posterior part of the lumbar gracile fasciculi, not centrally within these tracts in the middle and upper spinal cord, and tabes does not include gliomesenchymal cell nodules or multinucleated cells. Vacuolar myelopathy has been reported in 7[247] to 30% of AIDS cases,[202,221] and the myelin abnormality is held responsible for paresthesias, paraparesis, spasticity, incontinence, and ataxia. As with central spinal myelinolysis, vacuolar myelopathy is associated with multinucleated cell encephalitis. Some of the cytoplasm of spinal cord foamy macrophages, multinucleated giant cells, gliomesenchymal cell nodules, glial cells, or endothelial cells of capillaries and venules is immunoreactive for HIV proteins in most of our cases. Essentially, *HIV myelitis* has histopathologic findings similar to those in the brain of HIV-infected patients,[250] although not all investigators agree that the brain and spinal cord lesions are the same, even though both generally occur together.[22,119,223,255] The difference in perspective lies in the definition of HIV disease in the CNS. We use a definition that includes lesions directly or indirectly caused by HIV. Some of these lesions are difficult to classify by specific pathogenetic mechanisms, and indirectly-related lesions may not contain any multinucleated cells. However, the individual histopathologic lesions appear to be the same wherever they occur in the CNS (refer to the section on HIV Encephalomyelitis and HIV-Associated Encephalomyelitis in this chapter).

If all HIV-related lesions are considered, then at least two general mechanisms of tissue injury may cause cerebral and spinal cord damage. In both the brain and spinal cord, endothelial cell infection by HIV in susceptible long-tract regions might cause a leak in the blood-brain barrier,[250] or macrophages crossing the vessel walls may produce neurotoxic cytokines,[22] followed by serum exudation into the white matter, myelin degeneration, and spongiosis. Both mechanisms are likely to occur at the same time and in the same tissue areas. This could be the model of long-tract degeneration with little inflammation both in the brain and spinal cord, and a murine retroviral model with CNS endothelial cell infection accompanied by long-tract edema has been described.[225]

Vacuolar myelopathy might be confined to older children and adults with AIDS. Pediatric cases up to about 6 years of age reportedly have wallerian degeneration in the corticospinal tracts, with a predominance in the thoracic level or diffuse demyelination. However, the subacute combined degeneration (avitaminosis-$B_{12}$)-like picture of vacuolar myelopathy is lacking.[59]

### Gliomesenchymal Cell Nodules

Gliomesenchymal cell nodules (microglial nodules, nodular encephalitis) are collections of cells, presumed to originate from glial cells and hematogenous inflammatory cellular infiltrate, which are found apart from blood vessels in the CNS parenchyma. The cells in these nodules include those with round to oblong or elongated nuclei (denoting "rod" cells) and arciform nuclei (the classic "microglial" nucleus), and the cells have little identifiable cytoplasm. Acute inflammatory cells and reactive astrocytes with typical, enlarged eosinophilic cytoplasm can be seen, but these cells are rare. Too many acute inflammatory cells might be a clue to *Candida* encephalitis (demanding a fungal stain), toxoplasmic encephalitis, or early microabscess formation associated with bacterial cerebritis. Immunostaining can reveal HIV or cytomegaloviral antigens in some of these lesions. Gliomesenchymal cell nodules are found in over a third of all brains of AIDS victims (Table 9-1), but when present they only signify focal necrosis unless a specific cause can be assigned. Classically, gliomesenchymal cell nodules are the result of trauma or of encephalitis caused by viruses, rickettsiae, protozoa, fungi, or bacteria.[167] It is not known whether they form in different ways and from different cellular sources in reaction to different causes, but generally most of the cells in the nodules in HIV encephalomyelitis have little or no resemblance to the perivascular monocyte/macrophage infiltration found in many of the same cases. However, multinucleated cells can be found in gliomesenchymal cell nodules, even though typical foamy macrophages are not often recognized in these lesions. In cases in which multinucleated cells are present in the nodules, there is a strong tendency for many of the gliomesenchymal cell nodules to contain multinucleated cells. Macrophages/multinucleated cells that are near blood vessels and infiltrating into the parenchyma are infected by HIV or are a response to HIV, while gliomesenchymal cell nodules are foci of parenchymatous destruction that represent the limited ability of the CNS to form a chronic "inflammatory" response. Gliomesenchymal cell nodules in AIDS can be of the classical, small, compact type (Fig. 9-7), or they can be large and diffuse (Fig. 9-8). One or two may be found in a given case, in any of the sections, or many may be widely scattered throughout the CNS. Gliomesenchymal cell nodules are not of themselves diagnostic of AIDS. A few can be found with or without clinical correlation in an occasional patient who does not have AIDS. However, gliomesenchymal cell nodules correlate very highly with

HIV seropositivity and with signs of focal demyelination in CT scans.[229] These lesions are the most common to be found in an AIDS brain.[247]

### Granular Ependymitis

Granular ependymitis, a nonspecific loss of ependymal cells with subependymal gliosis, is seen fairly commonly in the brains of AIDS patients. This change of the ventricular lining can be seen in many normal people, especially in and near the anterior horns of the lateral ventricles.[289] It can be found adjacent to many periventricular lesions, including chronic encephalitis and primary lymphomas, and the adjacent ependyma may be involved in a cytomegaloviral infection.[17] Generally, no underlying lesion is found, although in other regions the brain may contain lesions typical of HIV encephalitis. Ependymal cells appear to be easily damaged, and they do not regenerate. Their focal loss is of no consequence, and the nonexudative manner of formation of granular ependymitis does not lead to ventricular obstruction.

### HIV Encephalomyelitis and HIV-Associated Encephalomyelitis

Lesions that seem to be a direct result of an HIV infection in the brain and spinal cord include: (1) perivascular and parenchymal macrophages/multinucleated cells and (2) gliomesenchymal cell nodules, and they are covered by the term HIV *encephalomyelitis.* In distinction, (1) diffuse leukoencephalopathy (demyelination with gliosis and macrophages, not simply "diffuse myelin pallor"), (2) necrotizing encephalitis (without a demonstrated opportunist), and (3) long-tract degeneration form a lesion group referred to as *HIV-associated encephalomyelitis.*[247] These "associated" lesions could be caused directly by HIV in some cases, yet essentially the same lesions can also be found in non-AIDS cases with immune system alterations.[250,277] The often extensive areas of diffuse leukoencephalopathy may be formed from perivascular foci of damage that coalesce.[263] Findings in individual cases can range from one focus of perivascular macrophages or one gliomesenchymal cell nodule to widespread findings of many of the lesions grouped here as HIV-related.

Gliomesenchymal cell nodules were seen in close to 50% of early AIDS cases, but in more recent cases these lesions have decreased, and there is a concomitant increase in the incidence of HIV-associated encephalomyelitis so that the sum of HIV-related lesions remains at a 50% incidence in autopsy cases. The microscopic gliomesenchymal cell nodules may either be incorporated into the larger destructive lesions of HIV-associated encephalomyelitis or the nodules may be early lesions that have healed by the time the patients die. Perivascular macrophages/multinucleated cells are found in about 20% of AIDS autopsies, both early and later in the AIDS epidemic, indicating that this likely reservoir of HIV infection has a constant and continuing presence in the CNS even with antiviral therapy.[247] Mean survival for the early AIDS cases (about 1982 to 1987) was about 1 year for all risk groups, but mean survival has increased since then to over 2 years for homosexual and bisexual males, while HIV-associated encephalomyelitis has also increased in these groups during this period. The longer survival may allow hypersensitivity phenomena or toxicity from HIV glycoproteins or infiltrating macrophages to enhance HIV-associated encephalomyelitis even if the HIV load in the CNS does not increase.[73,102,181,247]

## PITUITARY PATHOLOGY IN AIDS

There is a low incidence of incidental microadenomas (8–12%) and hyperplastic nodules in the anterior pituitary of AIDS patients that is the same as the incidence of these lesions in the general population of age-matched males. Infarcts are sometimes found, and these are not uncommon in other types of patients who, like terminal AIDS patients, have cerebral pathology with increased intracranial pressure that compromises the long portal vessels to the gland by direct pressure or through vasospasm.[295] Infections with opportunistic agents are seen in some cases, and they are generally only part of a systemic or CNS infection by the organism involved.[78,196,260]

## CLINICOPATHOLOGIC CORRELATIONS

### Adult AIDS Encephalopathy

A clinical picture of AIDS encephalopathy has been recognized since early in the AIDS epidemic. It was identified as the initial or only illness in some cases, and it may be seen in two thirds of those AIDS patients with neurologic complications.[163] Patients frequently complain of headaches, focal weakness, incoordination, confusion, mental slowness with forgetfulness, and loss of concentration (cognitive impairment). A blunted affect is fairly common. The patients can experience malaise, lethargy, loss of sex drive, and withdrawal from social and business contacts during the early stages of the lesions. There is a clinical depression that might be better characterized as psychomotor retardation.[278] Initial symptoms during the acute phase of an HIV infection sometimes occur with an influenza-like syndrome including fever, malaise, myalgias, arthralgias, and rash,[90,126] and acute encephalopathy will occasionally mark the onset of an HIV infection.[33] A mononucleosis-like illness with malaise and fever has also been described.[232] These acute symptoms usually resolve in a few days or weeks. Psychosis, hallucinations, and seizures are infrequent at the outset of the illness. The CSF may have mildly or moderately ele-

vated levels of white blood cells and protein and a mildly decreased level of glucose. Motor problems tend to occur later in the illness. Once the symptoms become severe, the patients become bedridden over weeks to months. Acute or chronic atypical meningitis without encephalopathy is described in some patients with chronic headaches, lymphocytic pleocytosis in the CSF, and often recovery of HIV from the CSF at the time of seroconversion.[125,126,163,201]

Neuropsychologic testing can reveal mild cognitive deficits (impaired abstracting ability, learning difficulties, and slowed speed of information processing) in a high percentage of asymptomatic patients with HIV seropositivity, in HIV-associated lymphadenopathy, in AIDS-related complex (minor systemic disease), or in AIDS.[110,230] Asymptomatic HIV-infected patients have a doubled rate of memory and dexterity problems compared to controls, while symptomatic patients have a quadrupled rate of cognitive problems pointing largely to frontal lobe deficits.[26] One cohort of presumably healthy, well-cared-for, HIV-positive subjects had no cognitive impairment demonstrated while they were asymptomatic until CSF abnormalities were identified.[103] It is at this point that a breakdown in the blood-brain barrier may exist in an HIV infection.[9,244] In some patient populations *all* individuals whose sera are positive for HIV antibodies may have antibodies to HIV in their CSF as well, and this is true for all clinical stages of HIV infection.[168]

The stereotyped progression of the constellation of *cognitive, behavioral, and sensorimotor impairment without impaired consciousness* in AIDS patients who do not have opportunistic infections or tumors in the CNS has been termed the AIDS-dementia complex, and more recently the *HIV-1 associated dementia complex.*[135] Patients may be alert late in the course of the disease. This clinical pattern has been compared to the subcortical dementia seen in Parkinson's disease (but without a resting tremor), Huntington's disease, and progressive supranuclear palsy. The onset of dementia is insidious or abrupt. The course may be steadily progressive or may fluctuate over a few months or more. Systemic disease usually does not seem sufficient to explain the neurologic problems, although symptoms and signs can alter with changes in systemic illness. Once severely demented, patients generally survive only a few months and die of aspiration pneumonia or a systemic opportunistic infection.* Mass lesions in the brain produce focal deficits or altered consciousness, and, of course, patients can have mixed symptoms and signs from involvement by several types of CNS lesions. When lethargy and coma develop, CNS or systemic lesions in addition to those of HIV encephalitis are present.[201,232] CT scans obtained late in the course of an HIV infection of the CNS often show enlarged ventricles and sulci as signs of parenchymal atrophy.[29] Examination of the brain after autopsy can show gliomesenchymal cell nodules, focal demyelination, macrophages around blood vessels or scattered in the white matter, small or enlarged multinucleated cells, astrocytosis, or opportunistic infections.* Patients with dementia are likely to have multinucleated cells in the brain[202] as well as a significant loss of neurons, but the neuronal loss may be found by quantitative measurement in areas lacking multinucleated macrophages or any inflammatory cells.[73]

* Refs. 66, 201, 203, 205, 278.

The progression of AIDS encephalopathy could depend in part on the social and hygienic practices of the patients as well as on the tropism of the retroviral strain. For instance, intravenous drug abusers are sometimes found to have a higher proportion of opportunistic infections and neurologic symptoms than are other risk groups, which probably indicates a greater degree of immune depression among them.[4,164] Stated in a more general way, *immune depression along with specific viral tropism seems to affect the progression of the neurologic symptoms and signs in AIDS encephalopathy.*[232,247]

Taken together, the evidence suggests that HIV causes the typical, progressive course of AIDS encephalopathy described here. The clinical use of the term HIV encephalitis may not be appropriate in some cases where lesions resulting in the major symptoms could be caused by opportunists that are not demonstrated until autopsy. It is true that the HIV infection is likely to underlie the pathologic condition of the CNS in HIV-infected individuals, and HIV is likely to be present in the brain in many of these patients at all stages of infection.[253,273] Although clinical symptoms and autopsy findings can suggest different substrates for encephalitis, the term HIV-1 associated dementia complex or AIDS encephalopathy is appropriate for clinical findings (1) to follow current usage, (2) because CNS lesions other than those directly related to HIV may only be found postmortem, and (3) because the major CNS lesions may result from the immunodeficient state itself as directly as from the systemic HIV infection.[247,277]

### Pediatric AIDS Encephalopathy

Congenital AIDS is clinically recognized by the age of 2 or 3 years.[75] A perinatal HIV infection is found in about one third of children born to seropositive mothers.[131] These infants may be symptom free, even though seropositive from maternal antibodies, and they may be seronegative by 2 years of age. Some HIV-infected infants may be seronegative while symptomatic because of hypogammaglobulinemia.[214] The lack

* Refs. 53, 90, 201, 202, 205, 206, 232, 247, 269, 278.

HIV seropositivity and with signs of focal demyelination in CT scans.[229] These lesions are the most common to be found in an AIDS brain.[247]

### Granular Ependymitis

Granular ependymitis, a nonspecific loss of ependymal cells with subependymal gliosis, is seen fairly commonly in the brains of AIDS patients. This change of the ventricular lining can be seen in many normal people, especially in and near the anterior horns of the lateral ventricles.[289] It can be found adjacent to many periventricular lesions, including chronic encephalitis and primary lymphomas, and the adjacent ependyma may be involved in a cytomegaloviral infection.[17] Generally, no underlying lesion is found, although in other regions the brain may contain lesions typical of HIV encephalitis. Ependymal cells appear to be easily damaged, and they do not regenerate. Their focal loss is of no consequence, and the nonexudative manner of formation of granular ependymitis does not lead to ventricular obstruction.

### HIV Encephalomyelitis and HIV-Associated Encephalomyelitis

Lesions that seem to be a direct result of an HIV infection in the brain and spinal cord include: (1) perivascular and parenchymal macrophages/multinucleated cells and (2) gliomesenchymal cell nodules, and they are covered by the term HIV *encephalomyelitis*. In distinction, (1) diffuse leukoencephalopathy (demyelination with gliosis and macrophages, not simply "diffuse myelin pallor"), (2) necrotizing encephalitis (without a demonstrated opportunist), and (3) long-tract degeneration form a lesion group referred to as *HIV-associated encephalomyelitis*.[247] These "associated" lesions could be caused directly by HIV in some cases, yet essentially the same lesions can also be found in non-AIDS cases with immune system alterations.[250,277] The often extensive areas of diffuse leukoencephalopathy may be formed from perivascular foci of damage that coalesce.[263] Findings in individual cases can range from one focus of perivascular macrophages or one gliomesenchymal cell nodule to widespread findings of many of the lesions grouped here as HIV-related.

Gliomesenchymal cell nodules were seen in close to 50% of early AIDS cases, but in more recent cases these lesions have decreased, and there is a concomitant increase in the incidence of HIV-associated encephalomyelitis so that the sum of HIV-related lesions remains at a 50% incidence in autopsy cases. The microscopic gliomesenchymal cell nodules may either be incorporated into the larger destructive lesions of HIV-associated encephalomyelitis or the nodules may be early lesions that have healed by the time the patients die. Perivascular macrophages/multinucleated cells are found in about 20% of AIDS autopsies, both early and later in the AIDS epidemic, indicating that this likely reservoir of HIV infection has a constant and continuing presence in the CNS even with antiviral therapy.[247] Mean survival for the early AIDS cases (about 1982 to 1987) was about 1 year for all risk groups, but mean survival has increased since then to over 2 years for homosexual and bisexual males, while HIV-associated encephalomyelitis has also increased in these groups during this period. The longer survival may allow hypersensitivity phenomena or toxicity from HIV glycoproteins or infiltrating macrophages to enhance HIV-associated encephalomyelitis even if the HIV load in the CNS does not increase.[73,102,181,247]

## PITUITARY PATHOLOGY IN AIDS

There is a low incidence of incidental microadenomas (8–12%) and hyperplastic nodules in the anterior pituitary of AIDS patients that is the same as the incidence of these lesions in the general population of age-matched males. Infarcts are sometimes found, and these are not uncommon in other types of patients who, like terminal AIDS patients, have cerebral pathology with increased intracranial pressure that compromises the long portal vessels to the gland by direct pressure or through vasospasm.[295] Infections with opportunistic agents are seen in some cases, and they are generally only part of a systemic or CNS infection by the organism involved.[78,196,260]

## CLINICOPATHOLOGIC CORRELATIONS

### Adult AIDS Encephalopathy

A clinical picture of AIDS encephalopathy has been recognized since early in the AIDS epidemic. It was identified as the initial or only illness in some cases, and it may be seen in two thirds of those AIDS patients with neurologic complications.[163] Patients frequently complain of headaches, focal weakness, incoordination, confusion, mental slowness with forgetfulness, and loss of concentration (cognitive impairment). A blunted affect is fairly common. The patients can experience malaise, lethargy, loss of sex drive, and withdrawal from social and business contacts during the early stages of the lesions. There is a clinical depression that might be better characterized as psychomotor retardation.[278] Initial symptoms during the acute phase of an HIV infection sometimes occur with an influenza-like syndrome including fever, malaise, myalgias, arthralgias, and rash,[90,126] and acute encephalopathy will occasionally mark the onset of an HIV infection.[33] A mononucleosis-like illness with malaise and fever has also been described.[232] These acute symptoms usually resolve in a few days or weeks. Psychosis, hallucinations, and seizures are infrequent at the outset of the illness. The CSF may have mildly or moderately ele-

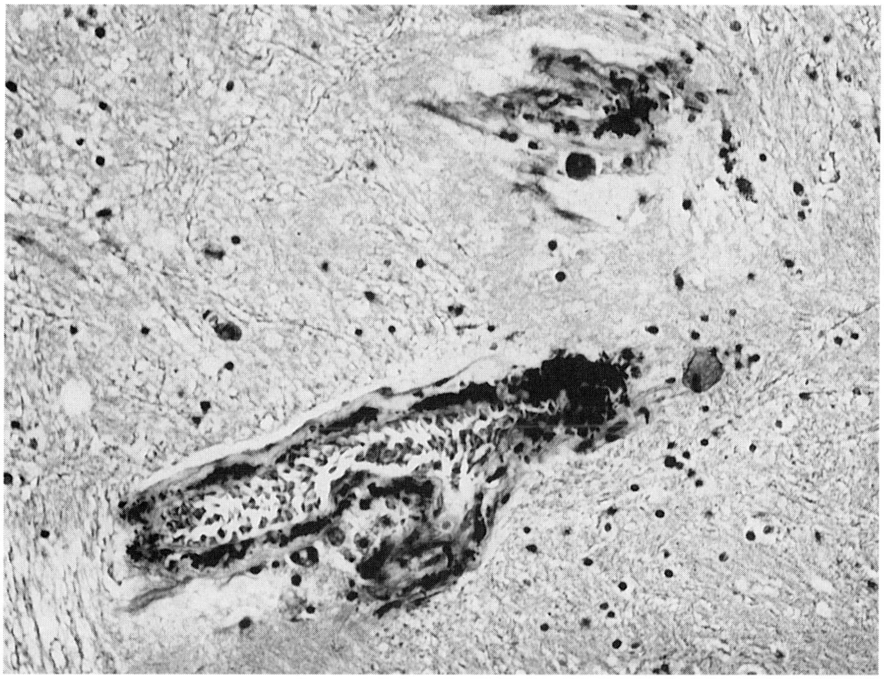

**Fig. 9-23.** Calcific vasculopathy in the globus pallidus. The walls of two blood vessels are darkened by calcium deposition. A few multinucleated cells are present. (H&E; ×200.)

of positive HIV serology findings is correlated with a poor outcome. The very sensitive polymerase chain reaction may demonstrate HIV genomic material in the peripheral white blood cells of some of these children by the time they are seronegative, and this will establish their HIV infection.[158] A perinatal infection has a more variable course and a more immediate poor outcome than one acquired later.[131] A dysmorphic syndrome described in some of these children includes growth failure, microcephaly, ocular hypertelorism, and other malformations.[178] Children receiving contaminated blood transfusions or those infected postnatally by breast milk as well as those with congenital HIV infections can have AIDS encephalopathy, often with long-tract signs and spasticity. Neurologic signs tend to worsen as the immunodeficient state worsens. Multinucleated cells, gliomesenchymal cell nodules, demyelination, white matter gliosis, chronic parenchymal inflammation, chronic vasculitis and perivasculitis, calcification of the basal ganglia, and calcific vasculopathy may be present. The vascular wall calcium salts are nonspecific, but they are associated with viral encephalitis in children (Fig. 9-23). The basal ganglia and white matter are affected more than the neocortex, just as in adult HIV encephalitis, but in children few opportunistic infections are found in the CNS. HIV has been isolated from the brain in some of these children.*

## AIDS Myelopathy/HIV Myelitis

Sensorimotor signs in AIDS might be similar to those in patients with tabes dorsalis or vitamin $B_{12}$ deficiency. An acute necrotizing myelitis associated with an infective process, described as early as 1955,[123] has a clinicopathologic resemblance to HIV myelitis, including a thoracic-level predominance and little inflammation in spongiform white matter that is filled with macrophages.[301] Influenza vaccination can be followed by this lesion.[111] Hereditary spastic paraplegia, also displaying a thoracic-level predominance, has chronic changes in the same sensorimotor systems of the spinal cord involved in the infectious and allergic conditions.[265] Vacuolar myelopathy can be seen in patients with a variety of apparently unrelated primary conditions in which immunostaining of the spinal cord is negative for HIV.[250] These factors suggest that at least some of the features described in clinical AIDS myelopathy and pathologically diagnosed HIV myelitis are related in a general way to a viral infection and possibly more specifically to allergic or toxic sequelae of an infection.

Perhaps the most surprising aspect of clinical AIDS myelopathy is the frequency of a sudden onset of symptoms and signs related to long tracts. Symptoms and signs of involvement of the corticospinal tract, posterior column, and cerebellar tracts are frequently described with concomitant onset or onset within a few days, and the clinically involved tracts tend to have vacuolar alterations and stigmata of HIV (i.e., gliomesenchymal cell nodules or multinucleated cells of various sizes). It is also surprising that these symptoms are often so clearly reported, since the patients are usually quite ill with multiple opportunistic infections. The systemic infections in fact often obscure the significance of the spinal cord symptoms in the clinical setting. Weakness, urinary incontinence, and progressive

* Refs. 18, 19, 66, 69, 134, 139, 214, 270.

paresis mark pyramidal tract lesions. Numbness of the distal extremities and decreased pinprick sensation are associated with posterior column lesions, while gait ataxia and loss of balance are correlated with involvement of the cerebellar tracts. The sensorimotor problems are often accompanied or followed by slowed speech and other signs of encephalitis. This is caused by the HIV encephalitis or HIV-associated encephalitis that usually accompanies HIV myelitis. Dementia and HIV myelitis are closely associated with each other and with cytomegaloviral infections and other opportunistic agents, and they are therefore associated with a low level of immune competence.[119,201,247,250] Marker studies for HIV nucleic acid and protein demonstrate the retrovirus in microvascular endothelial cells, perivascular and intramyelinic macrophages and multinucleated cells, gliomesenchymal cell nodules, and probably small glial cells in and near the spongiform tracts,[65,177,250] although HIV and immunopathologic mechanisms may combine in various degrees to form the full extent of the long tract lesions. There is one report of a patient with typical clinical AIDS encephalomyelopathy of sudden onset at the time of seroconversion for HIV antibody and with isolation of HIV from the blood and CSF.[55]

The following case illustrates the clinical presentation of AIDS encephalomyelopathy in a 27-year-old homosexual man. The patient had a headache, dizziness, malaise, and facial asymmetry and was unable to walk for 2 days before admission. Oral candidiasis was seen, and *Shigella sonnei* was cultured from the blood. He had lower extremity weakness and pain in the region of his middle back. He was lethargic, slow to respond to questions, and his speech was slow, but he was alert and well oriented. Physical examination showed mild neck stiffness, his lips were deviated to the right, and he had decreased sensation to pinprick at the T9 level on the right side, decreased position sensation and muscle strength of the lower extremities, and faulty finger-to-nose (cerebellar) coordination. The clinical impression was that he had a Brown-Séquard syndrome. Ten days after admission to the hospital he had bilateral Babinski's signs and was barely arousable. Ten days later his neurologic status had improved to the same level as on admission, but after another 2 weeks he was comatose. He died 11 weeks after admission. Autopsy revealed toxoplasmic encephalitis. There was myelin degeneration in the internal capsules in the cerebrum and in the posterior columns, lateral and anterior corticospinal tracts, and anterior spinocerebellar tracts in the spinal cord with HIV immunostained in several of these tracts. This case illustrates the sensory, pyramidal (corticospinal) tract, and cerebellar tract findings of HIV encephalomyelitis in a patient with multiple (including cerebral) opportunistic infections that clouded the meaning of the symptoms and signs until autopsy. The waxing and waning symptoms are reminiscent of multiple sclerosis, and they may well share, at least in part, an episodic, immunopathologic substrate.

### AIDS Retinopathy/Retinitis

Cytomegaloviral retinitis and toxoplasmic retinitis are often reported clinically. These agents need to be adequately demonstrated to substantiate the diagnosis.[201,278] Varicella-zoster virus was detected by immunostaining in a retinal biopsy specimen from an AIDS patient who suffered from cutaneous herpes zoster ophthalmicus and a newly detached retina.[38] HIV has been immunolocalized in retinal microvascular endothelial cells and retinal parenchymal cells, and it has been cultured along with cytomegalovirus from the retina in AIDS patients.[276]

Cotton-wool spots in the retina in some cases might be caused by HIV-induced ischemia.[226] Retinal microvasculopathy (cotton-wool spots or microhemorrhages) unrelated to opportunistic infections or neoplasms found in patients with AIDS-related systemic disease is not progressive or symptomatic.[84]

Visual system problems can be the result of lesions at any level from the eye to the brainstem. They are generally caused by opportunistic infections or lymphomas in AIDS patients, and the most common signs are those of central eye movement limitation.[145]

### AIDS-Associated Neuromuscular Diseases

Peripheral neuropathy or progressive polyneuritis is reported in as many as half of the patients with AIDS and AIDS-related complex in some series.* There can be a chronic distal symmetric polyneuropathy with predominant sensory loss, nerve deficits in several nerve distributions (mononeuritis multiplex), or an inflammatory neuropathy. In addition to sensory loss, there may be weakness, paralysis, painful dysesthesias, and depressed ankle jerks. Electromyography and nerve conduction velocity studies might show a distal sensorimotor neuropathy of a demyelinating type. This can begin early in an HIV infection, and it can be mild but slowly progressive[133]; nerve conduction abnormalities can be subclinical.[39] Cranial nerve involvement has been described. Recovery is sometimes seen spontaneously or after plasmapheresis; when recovery is not experienced there is axonal damage. Many patients with mononeuritis multiplex have a spontaneous recovery in weeks to months. The picture can resemble the Guillain-Barré syndrome (acute polyradiculoneuropathy),[11] but there is an increase of lymphocytes in the CSF in AIDS patients, and this clinical assessment is sometimes associated with a nerve root infection by cytomegalovirus.† On general

* Refs. 43, 50, 54, 201, 278, 280.

† Refs. 17, 64, 176, 274, 314.

grounds, the peripheral nerve inflammation and demyelination suggest that an immunopathologic lesion of some type, rather than or in addition to a direct infection, is occurring in at least some of these cases.[43,189] For instance, autoantibodies produced after an infection by cytomegalovirus can be associated with inflammation in the absence of the virus itself.[14]

HIV has been isolated from peripheral nerve, where it may have resided in infiltrating white blood cells or it may have been infecting cells of the nerve parenchyma; in either case it has the potential to cause the neuritis. There is often an associated dementia, and it is likely that HIV causes both CNS and peripheral nervous system infections, symptoms, and signs at the same time. The clinical impression may be, for instance, that leg weakness is more severe than can be accounted for from the peripheral neuropathy alone. Very likely, the associated CNS lesions enhance the findings elicited in peripheral nerve distributions.[118]

Peripheral nerves can have demyelination, axonopathy, chronic inflammation, an opportunistic virus (e.g., cytomegalovirus or varicella-zoster virus) or fungus, or metastatic lymphoma. The distal axonal degeneration might be a "dying-back" process related to metabolic or toxic problems.[36] Nerve or nerve root lesions may be responsible for an occasional finding of eccentric cellular nuclei and central chromatolysis in anterior motor neurons of the spinal cord. Damage to bodies of nerve cells in dorsal root ganglia could be responsible for some of the distal sensory abnormalities,* and a mild sensory ganglionitis may be common in AIDS.[72,321]

Myopathy seen in AIDS can be secondary to peripheral neuropathy or it can be inflammatory (polymyositis). Polymyositis can be the initial sign in AIDS. The etiology could be infective (retrovirus?) or autoimmune.[48,50,66,278] Rare neuromuscular diseases encountered in AIDS include type II muscle fiber atrophy, amyotrophic lateral sclerosis, and adult onset nemaline (rod) myopathy.[50]

### AIDS Autonomic Neuropathy

Autonomic nervous system dysfunction has been demonstrated in some HIV-positive patients with AIDS, generally in the absence of any peripheral neuropathy, by formal clinical testing of heart rate and blood pressure responses. Symptoms of postural hypotension and syncope have occurred. It has been suggested that features of AIDS such as diarrhea, disordered sweating, and impotence could result in part from autonomic dysfunction.[42,44,188] Sympathetic ganglia can contain HIV-infected macrophages that could play a central role in the autonomic dysfunction.[72]

* Refs. 8, 50, 66, 90, 175, 189.

## PATHOGENESIS OF HIV MENINGOENCEPHALOMYELITIS

### Immunologic Factors Affecting the CNS

The CNS is immunologically sequestered, in at least a limited sense. Once the blood-brain barrier is established in the newborn, CNS cells can differentiate in seclusion from the immune system, and lymphocytes cannot acquire tolerance to CNS self-antigens.[15] Access to the CNS parenchyma across the blood-brain barrier is limited by vascular endothelial cells. For access from blood vessels larger than capillaries, there is also a perivascular space, which is an extension of the subarachnoid space that must be traversed. The subarachnoid space drains by arterial lymphatics or lymphatic channels of craniospinal nerve sheaths into deep cervical lymph nodes.[45,313] This makes the perivascular space a route in the afferent limb of an immune response, while the blood vessel itself is part of the efferent limb. The white blood cells in the perivascular spaces have a normal turnover, bringing in more circulating monocytes than T cells.[157] It is from these perivascular spaces that white cell inflammatory infiltration of the CNS occurs. The macrophages can present antigens to the activated T cells also present there, and their cytokines activate the endothelium to produce adhesion molecules that attract an inflammatory cuff (chronic perivasculitis) consisting of some activated and many antigen-nonspecific lymphocytes. Activated T cells can enter the CNS without much restriction, although their migration is more commonly into perivascular spaces than into the parenchyma.[70,290] White cell cytokines such as interferon (IFN)-$\gamma$ and tumor necrosis factor (TNF)-$\alpha$ activate perivascular astrocytes, and the astrocytes in turn secrete chemokines (small cytokines such as TNF-$\alpha$ that mediate inflammation) with a gradient that is followed by perivascular lymphocytes into the CNS parenchyma.[290] TNF-$\alpha$ is also one of the messages giving rise to a leaky blood-brain barrier.[74]

The efferent limb of the immune system is represented in the CNS by macrophages, T cells, and B cells that remain for the most part in the perivascular spaces where they can form structures similar to lymphatic capillaries.[233] The perivascular space is therefore an immunologic space in which macrophages trap foreign antigens and present them to lymphocytes. Under immune stimulation the blood-brain barrier becomes more leaky, and serum proteins can upregulate major histocompatibility complex class II protein expression of newly recruited blood monocytes that can, as activated macrophages, help in the further progression of the immune response. The low number of lymphocytes normally found in the CNS perivascular spaces would allow low amplification of the immune response locally, but an effective amplification of the lymphocyte population would probably occur only after a response through a regional lymph node.[70,74] Such low initial local amplification would prevent the perivascular spaces from acting like "swollen glands" in the brain in the form of greatly enlarged, fluid-distended compartments when only a minor antigenic response is being made.

The CNS has a protective mechanism to rid itself very rapidly of infiltrating T cells so that destruction can be limited. Although the mechanism itself is obscure, T cells infiltrating a CNS lesion rapidly undergo programmed cell destruction (apoptosis) even though T cells in regional lymph nodes and other sites of the same subject do not. Clearing of CNS symptoms is found experimentally when the T cells are removed by apoptosis, and such removal does not require any further inflammatory infiltration to be achieved, thereby avoiding further "bystander damage" from reacting cells. Since the parenchymal T cells die (in perhaps 4 hours), no pseudolymphoid tissue aggregates form in the CNS, and only perivascular activated T cells remain.[264] These factors imply a suppressive environment for immune reactivity, but they can also allow self-stimulating cycles of immune responses that might be responsible for autodestructive CNS lesions,[74] perhaps leading to episodic CNS symptoms associated with cyclical HIV-related damage.

What is the immune reaction to an HIV infection in the CNS? It is no doubt quite complicated, but it may be reflected in part as the increased level of CSF cytokines found in symptomatic patients[91,218] and as the increase in CNS macrophages that can produce these cytokines.[247] Macrophages containing interleukin (IL)-1 and TNF-$\alpha$ can be found in degenerating white matter and may contribute to white matter lesions,[298] but astrocytes can also be stimulated to produce IL-1, IL-6, IFN, and TNF-$\alpha$.[165,186,207] Although CNS inflammation can be minor in AIDS, many astrocytes and possibly even oligodendrocytes and neurons might be infected by HIV.[207,259,292] Since both perivascular macrophages and astrocytes are producing TNF-$\alpha$ in activated, symptomatic, parenchymal HIV infection of the CNS,[207] the cytokine effects of TNF-$\alpha$ in altering the blood-brain barrier, hindering neuronal function, causing lysis of oligodendrocytes, and increasing HIV production in glial cells might explain many of the CNS findings.[74,291] A leaky blood-brain barrier would itself open up the CNS to toxic serum proteins as well as to T cells that might more easily explore the CNS for self-antigens (Fig. 9-24).[246,251,252]

### Development of HIV Meningoencephalomyelitis

There is no doubt that HIV can be identified in the CNS both early and late in the course of AIDS.[125,232] HIV can be isolated from the CSF early in an HIV infection,[183] and it is cultured more often in seropositive patients without AIDS than in seropositive patients with AIDS, indicating that more infectious retrovirus is present in the CNS early than is found later when neurologic complications appear.[244] It is not certain that the retroviral load is significantly increased as lesions and symptoms progress, although the brain is often the major site of HIV infection by the time of autopsy.[308] The high load of HIV DNA in the brain when histopathologic findings are minimal might be due to a persistent parenchymal HIV infection in which infectious virus production is minimal.[259,271] The early Nef proteins rather than core or envelope proteins are found in up to 20% of astrocytes using the polymerase chain reaction in situ hybridization method, suggesting a nonproductive (persistent) HIV infection,[259,292] and the Nef gene may restrict HIV structural protein production.[240] Nef protein has an external loop that functions as a superantigen, potentially attracting white cells into the CNS through the cascade producing the lymphocyte growth factor, IL-2.[86,293] This may be a cause of chronic perivasculitis, and it may allow CNS antigen sampling by activated T cells attracted in this manner to result in an autoaggressive immune attack on previously sequestered antigens in the white matter (Fig. 9-24).

The clinical findings may have little relationship to the morphologic findings until late in the disease. A discordance of symptoms and histologic lesions may also have a genetic basis in the host.[140] Early in the disease, there is no primary finding on CT scans of asymptomatic patients or of those with signs of encephalopathy.[229] Many seropositive patients, however, have a mild CSF pleocytosis or activated B lymphocytes that may be the earliest indication of a chronic HIV meningoencephalitis.[77] The viral load in the CNS may be considered to be relatively low, but with the use of the polymerase chain reaction HIV can be demonstrated in frozen brain tissue in cases with few[273] or no lesions as assessed in routine sections.[253] HIV proteins have been demonstrated immunohistochemically, and HIV nucleic acid has been localized by in situ hybridization in macrophages (including some in the leptomeninges), giant cells, astrocytes, and vascular endothelial cells, and in gliomesenchymal cell nodules in the CNS.* The HIV immunolocalized in perineuronal glial cells in the neocortex in our series and an identical finding reported elsewhere[285] suggest a possible indirect influence on neurons. The neurons in these neocortical areas appear normal morphologically (Fig. 9-16), but they could have been dysfunctional because of a persistent HIV infection of the neurons[207] or of their supportive glial cells† or through toxic actions of HIV proteins.[151,219,234] It is known that lymphocytic[116,220] and monocyte/macrophage functions de-

* Refs. 31, 65, 89, 150, 177, 235, 249, 251, 256, 259, 285, 292, 308, 314, 315, 318.

† Refs. 99, 249, 251, 259, 292.

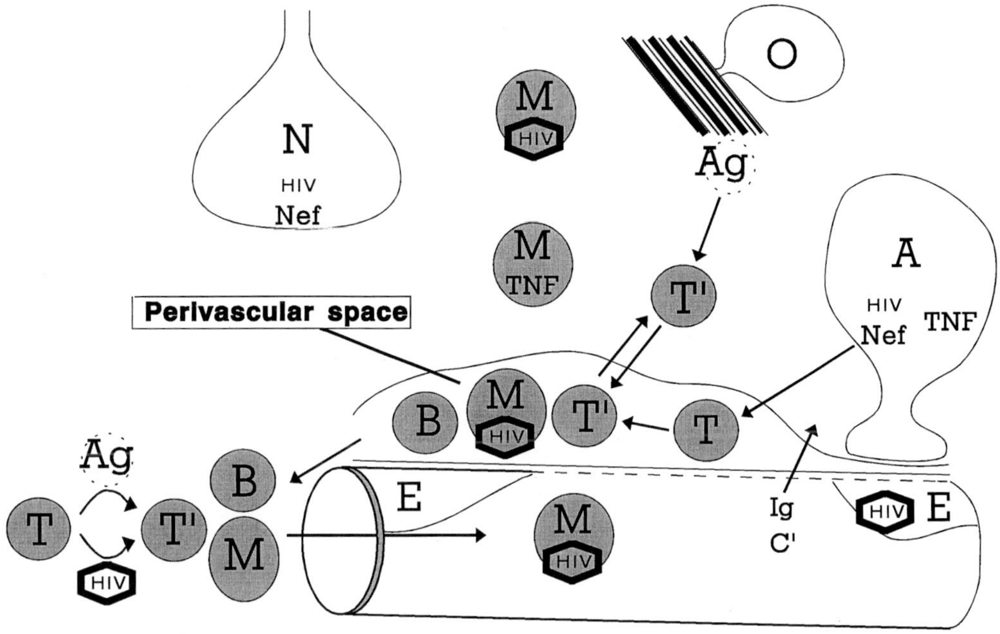


**Fig. 9-24.** Schematic representation of relationships that exist between CNS and immune system during HIV infection. T lymphocytes (*T*), activated T lymphocytes (*T'*), B lymphocytes (*B*), and macrophages (*M*) are systemic influences on the CNS infection by HIV (hexagons denote viral nucleocapsids), and they affect the CNS through blood vessels (*bottom of drawing*). There may be infected macrophages in the circulation (as well as infected lymphocytes), and endothelial cells (*E*) might be infected. The dotted line in the blood vessel wall indicates a leaky blood-brain barrier associated with the HIV infection. Serum proteins, including immunoglobulins (*Ig*) and complement components (*C'*), would enter the CNS parenchyma by crossing the vascular basement membrane, the perivascular space in which some white blood cells are in residence, and the astrocytic basement membrane (*basement membranes shown as thin, solid lines bounding perivascular space*). Turnover of macrophages from the circulation into the perivascular space includes HIV-infected cells, and these may remain as a perivascular reservoir of productive infection or the macrophages might enter the CNS parenchyma, where they presumably give rise to a mostly persistent infection (denoted by "HIV" without a nucleocapsid) of astrocytes (*A*) and neurons (*N*). Infected macrophages and astrocytes synthesize and secrete TNF-$\alpha$ (*TNF*) that further opens the blood-brain barrier and is toxic to the parenchyma, including oligodendrocytes (*O*). HIV Nef protein from infected neural cells may act as a superantigen to activate perivascular T cells that could, in turn, attract more inflammatory cells into the CNS. Activated T cells entering the CNS might also recognize myelin (*alternating lines associated with oligodendrocyte*) and other CNS components as "non-self," and through the afferent limb of the immune system a response might be generated to normal CNS components. Demyelination and other CNS damage might result from the response of the efferent limb of the immune system as well as from direct HIV infection and actions of resident perivascular white blood cells.

crease appreciably in an HIV infection;[257,307] that HIV-infected human glioma cells, which maintain their viability for months in culture, show subtle signs of degeneration;[56] and that astrocytic function can be decreased by a viral infection.[209] Thus HIV can harm some cells without killing them, probably in part by occupying a significant portion of the activity of the cellular protein synthesis machinery[281] and perhaps by existing in a persistent state. This parenchymal CNS infection by HIV appears to be nonproductive for the most part and restricted to early regulatory/accessory gene products, unlike the accompanying macrophage infection that routinely produces complete new virions.[95,259,292]

The CNS findings such as gliomesenchymal cell nodules and perivascular mononuclear cell cuffing can be considered nonspecific[113] unless marker studies for etiologic agents are successfully employed. Multinucleated giant cells in the absence of any other components of granulomatous inflammation might be the only relatively specific histopathologic finding in HIV meningoencephalomyelitis.[30,113,143,269] Subtle or significant demyelination might be another finding closely associated with HIV in the CNS.[31,247] We have found

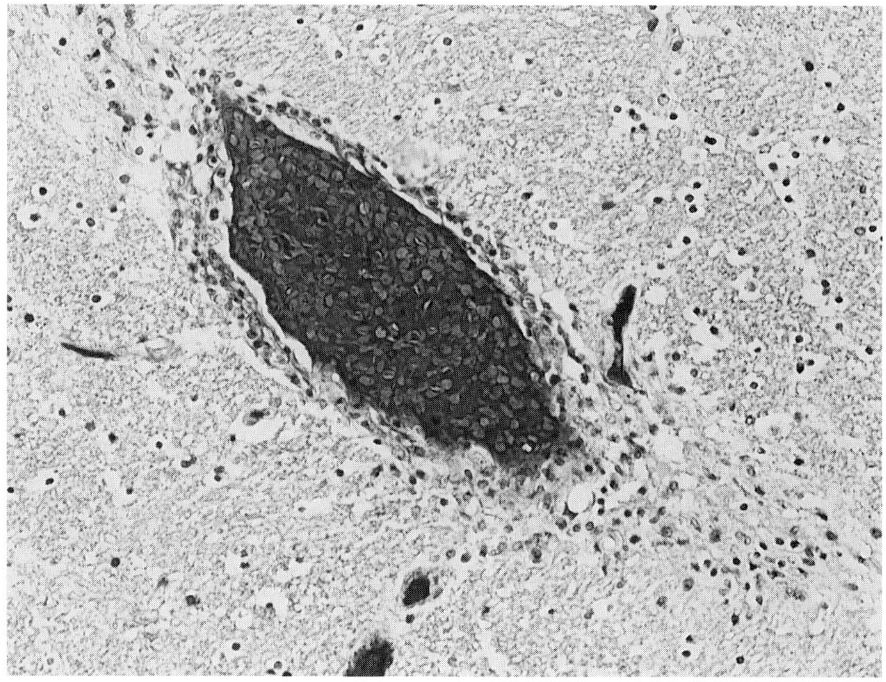

**Fig. 9-25.** Chronic vasculitis in periventricular white matter. The thin wall of a congested vein is infiltrated by lymphocytes. (H&E; ×200.)

demyelination associated with little reaction except for an occasional macrophage, yet demyelination can have many causes. Hypersensitivity phenomena, which are common in viral encephalitis[14,88,166] and identified in viral-associated peripheral neuropathy,[296] may also contribute to demyelination and other lesions found in the nervous system in AIDS. These lesions, like those associated with a direct infection, probably increase as immune competence decreases, with a morphologic correlation of clinical symptoms and signs often being seen late in the course of an HIV infection rather than early when the nervous system lesions are just developing.

Some speculation regarding possible hypersensitivity responses to the CNS is in order, particularly because of the relatively low retroviral structural protein load sometimes described in the CNS in the presence of widespread CNS lesions. The cells of the immune system share a variety of antigens with the nervous system.* The surfaces of T cells† and macrophages contain some epitopes also recognized as structural components of myelin.[283] Common viruses other than HIV with which an AIDS patient may be infected can contain myelin-like epitopes.[88,132] HIV itself has multiple peptide identities with normal human proteins.[252] Together, such normal and viral epitopes on the surfaces of T cells, macrophages, and perhaps glial cells and neurons may provide immunogens against which immune mechanisms are responding through the recognition of normal cells, myelin, and cell-surface viral protein as part of the immune target.[117,251,287] Once the blood-brain barrier is compromised, there may be inflammatory responses against the CNS target epitopes, against responding immunoglobulins that have regions resembling HIV,[173] and against lymphocytes that have epitopes with sequence identities to HIV.[311] An early sign of a breakdown of the blood-brain barrier could be gliosis alone,[159,318] while demyelination and advanced destruction of deep cerebral white matter may be the subsequent steps following a T-cell and macrophage autoaggressive response in AIDS.[129] Vasculitis (Fig. 9-25) and chronic perivasculitis (Fig. 9-15), commonly seen as early CNS findings in HIV infection,[51,114,159,184] could result from hypersensitivity responses as well as from toxicity to retroviral glycoproteins or a direct viral infection.

The extent of the involvement of the CNS by an HIV infection is not always clear after autopsy, even though HIV is the underlying cause of the pathologic condition. The term *AIDS encephalopathy* is clinically appropriate, but should not cause neglect of non-HIV lesions of the CNS that perhaps are amenable to therapy, while the term *HIV encephalitis* indicates that pathologic features of HIV are identified in brain tissue.

## OPPORTUNISTIC INFECTIONS

### Viral Meningoencephalomyelitis

**Progressive multifocal leukoencephalopathy (PML).** PML is a deep polyomaviral (a papovaviral genus) disease affecting the brain, and, considering its relatively infrequent occurrence in the past, it is seen

---

* Refs. 7, 49, 245, 288, 319.

† Refs. 12, 94, 199, 217, 309.

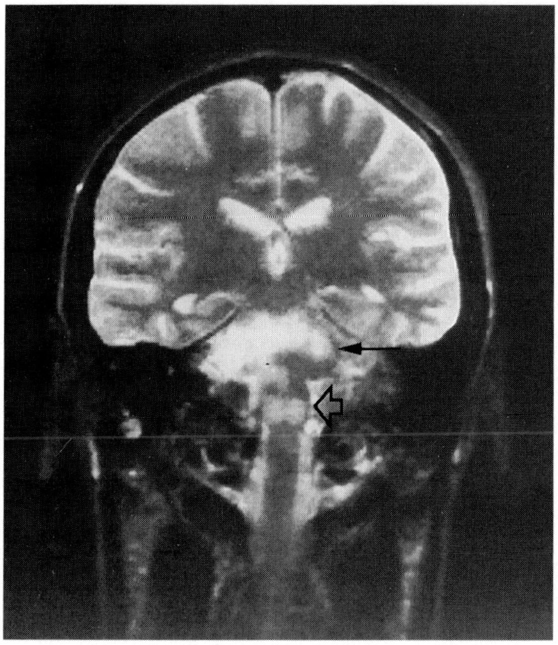

**Fig. 9-26.** A T2-weighted MRI of PML. Lesions are visible in the cerebellum (*arrow*) and brainstem (*arrowhead*).

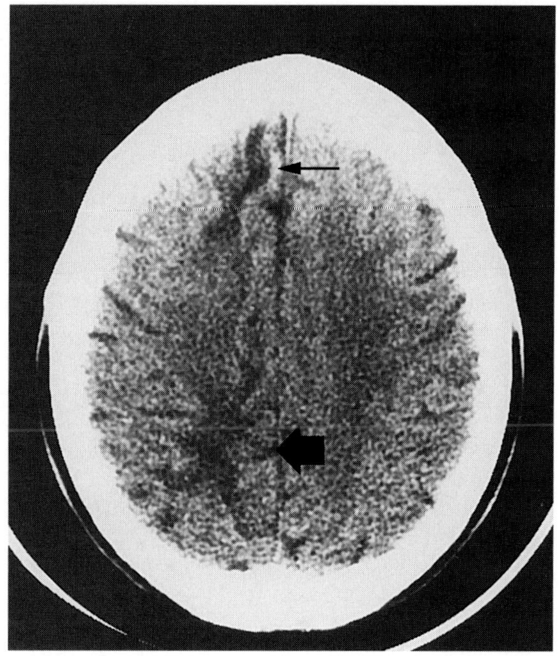

**Fig. 9-27.** A CT scan of PML. This noncontrast scan was the last of several taken in 14 months. The right frontal (*arrow*) and occipital (*arrowhead*) lucencies were diagnosed as infarcts because they lacked progression. This static picture is not a known feature of uncomplicated PML, but HIV was also found in these lesions.[249] The brain at autopsy is shown in Fig. 9-28.

with significant frequency in AIDS. Clinical presentation is varied. It may begin with mild cognitive changes, but it progresses over weeks to months, with multifocal signs that can include motor, sensory, and cerebellar systems. It ends with severe dementia in patients who are severely immunocompromised. PML can be the initial opportunistic infection in AIDS,[306] but associated clinical problems might obscure the diagnosis of PML until autopsy.* CT scans show low-density lesions in the white matter, hemorrhage, or a mass effect. There is a progression of the number, size, and lowered density of the lesions over weeks to months. MRI can localize small PML lesions more precisely by showing asymmetric, poorly marginated areas with increased T2-weighted intensity (Fig. 9-26), although the correct diagnosis might not be more readily made.[238] Two of our patients were diagnosed clinically as having strokes (Figs. 9-26 to 9-28).[87,249] Lymphomas may be multifocal, but they usually differ from PML by enhancing with contrast media.[67,153]

The lesions of PML classically are confined to the white matter and vary from small to large, with satellite formations but without cortical involvement. Lesioned areas are granular and depressed, with little to extensive necrosis (Fig. 9-13). There is a characteristic, diagnostic microscopic picture. Nuclei of oligodendrocytes are enlarged, deeply purple, have the appearance of ground glass, and are seen in areas of demyelination; there are foamy macrophages and often some bizarre astrocytes. The "ground glass" nuclei of the infected oligodendrocytes are several times the size of normal oligodendrocyte nuclei, forming a population of cells not seen in the normal brain tissue or in any other condition (Figs. 9-29, 9-30). The sharply demarcated lesions generally have much less axonal loss than myelin loss, but cavitating white matter necrosis can be prominent (Fig. 9-31). Classically, any cortical involvement is limited to gliosis and occasional viral inclusions in the deepest layers.[167,254]

Destruction of neocortex as well as of white matter is greater than usual in PML in AIDS patients (Figs. 9-32, 9-33),[249] and these cases are much more heavily infected with polyomavirus than brains in non-AIDS PML cases.[286] Both polyomavirus and HIV are often (if not usually) found together when PML is identified in AIDS,[249,317] possibly providing potentiating actions of dual destructive agents and enhanced activation of HIV replication known to be promoted by DNA viruses, particularly by JC polyomavirus.[98] Infected, infiltrating monocyte/macrophages could bring HIV into PML lesions, and PML could develop as a superinfection in areas of HIV encephalitis. Enlarged, pleomorphic astrocytes that are classically found in the white matter may also be seen in the gray matter. Hemorrhage can be encountered. The PML inclusions may be difficult to find, and in atypical cases immunostaining may only reveal them in occasional, widely scat-

* Refs. 20, 66, 154, 210, 249, 317.

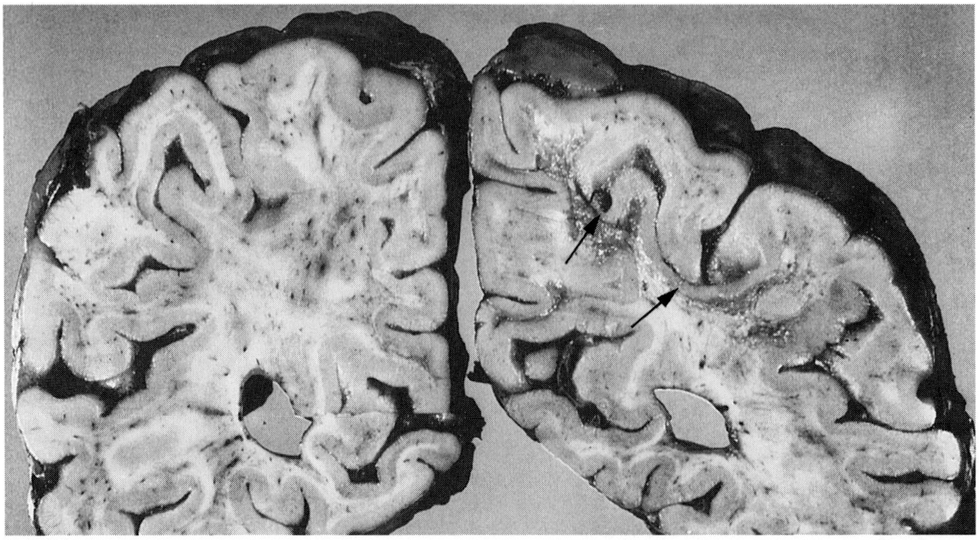

**Fig. 9-28.** Occipital lobes with PML and HIV encephalitis. Immunoreactivity for HIV and for the polyomaviral cause of PML were both demonstrated in the large lesion on the right.[249] Note the thin neocortical strip (*arrows*) in addition to the destruction and loss of white matter.

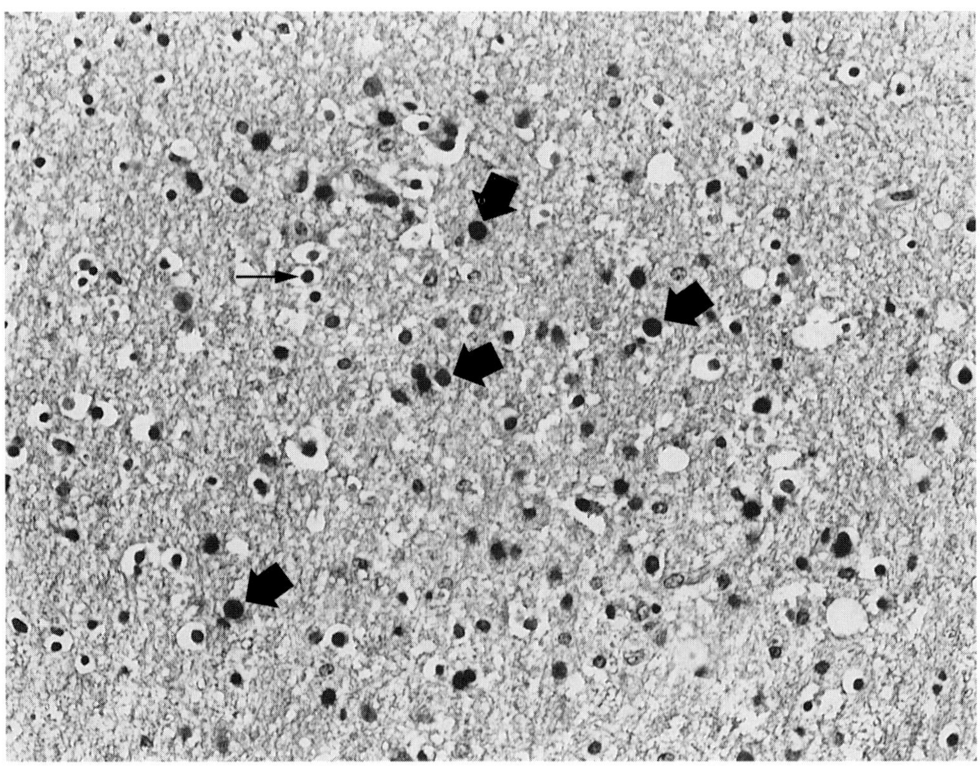

**Fig. 9-29.** Early PML in cerebral white matter. Normal-sized oligodendrocyte nuclei (*arrow*) are much smaller than oligodendrocyte nuclei that contain polyomaviral inclusions (*arrowheads*). (H&E; ×200.)

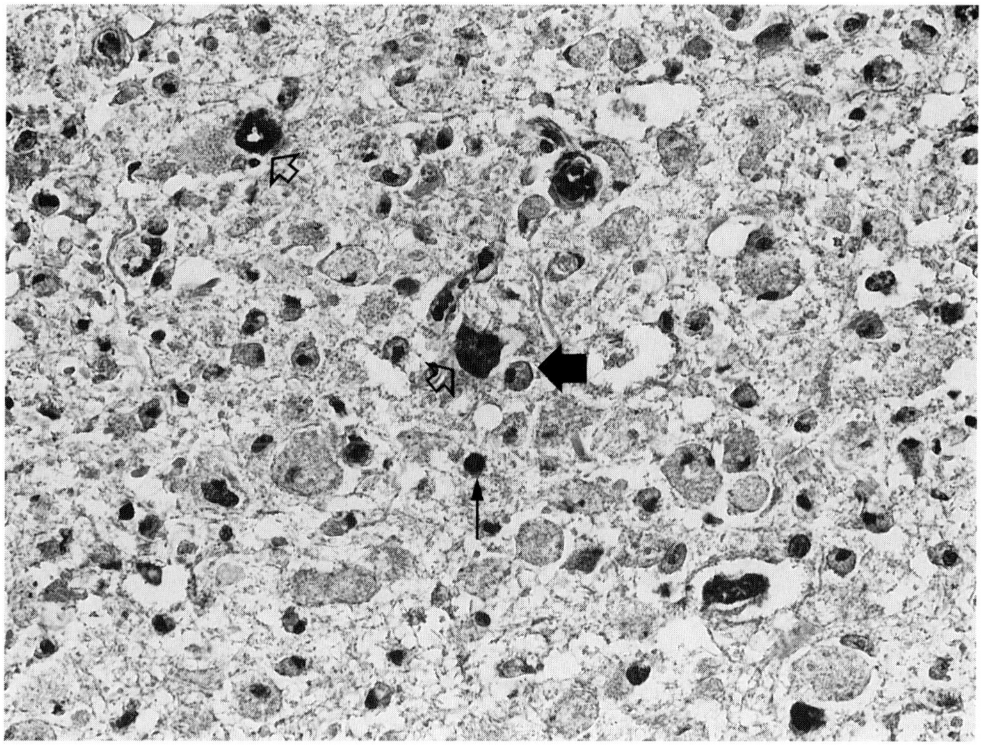

**Fig. 9-30.** Advanced necrotizing PML in cerebral white matter. Necrosis is almost complete, and few enlarged oligodendrocyte nuclei (*arrow*) remain. Macrophages (*closed arrowhead*) and astrocytes with bizarre nuclei (*open arrowheads*) can be seen. (H&E; ×200.)

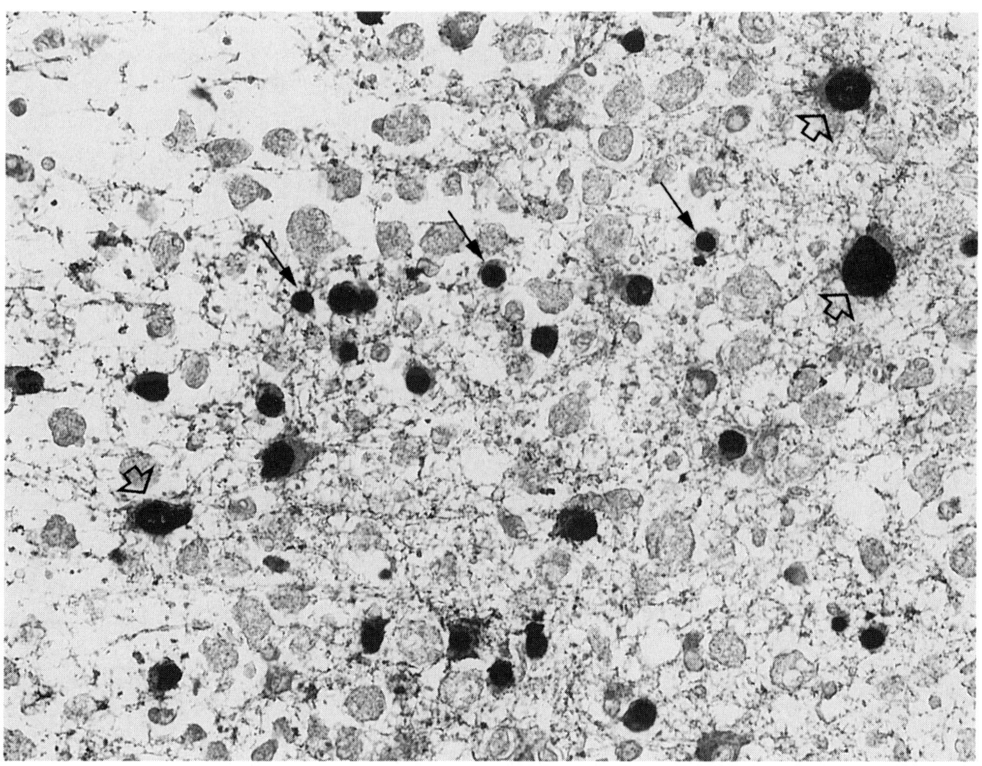

**Fig. 9-31.** Polyomaviral immunoreactivity in a partially cavitated PML lesion. Immunoreactive intranuclear viral inclusions in oligodendrocytes (*arrows*) and enlarged astrocytes (*open arrowheads*) are seen. The white matter is liquefied and filled with unstained macrophages, and the beginning of cavitation is evident. (Rabbit antiserum PML-Ab1; ×200.)

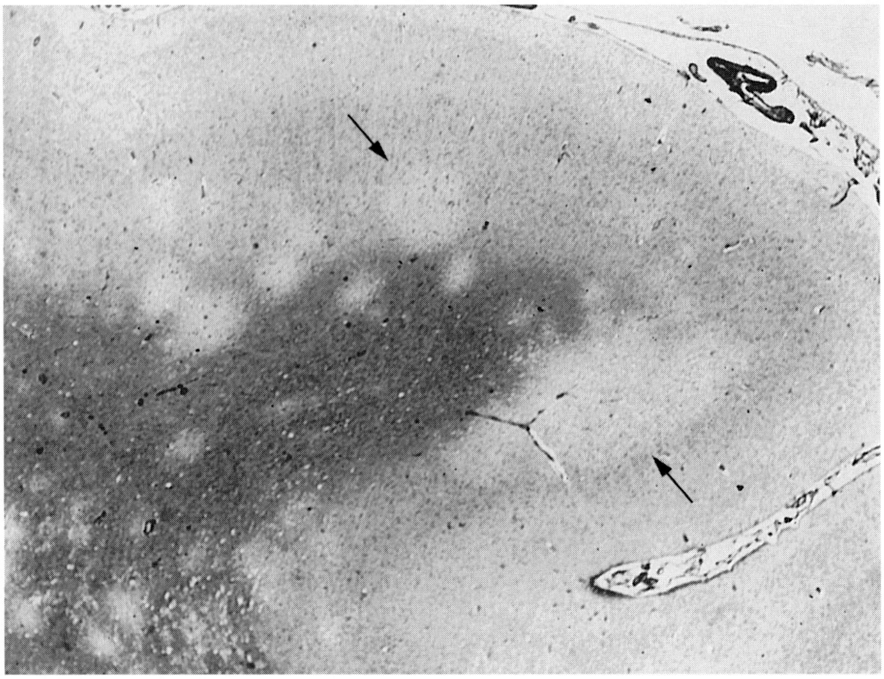

**Fig. 9-32.** Lesions in the cerebral cortex and subcortical white matter from a case of PML and HIV encephalitis. A stain for astrocytes shows many foci of pallor, indicating glial damage in the otherwise normally darkly stained white matter. These subcortical areas of pallor are typical PML lesions containing many infected oligodendrocytes. The pale lesions extending into the middle layers of the neocortex (*arrows*) are atypically extensive for PML, but not for PML in AIDS, and such cortical lesions can contain HIV (compare with Fig. 9-16). (Phosphotungstic acid-hematoxylin; ×12.)

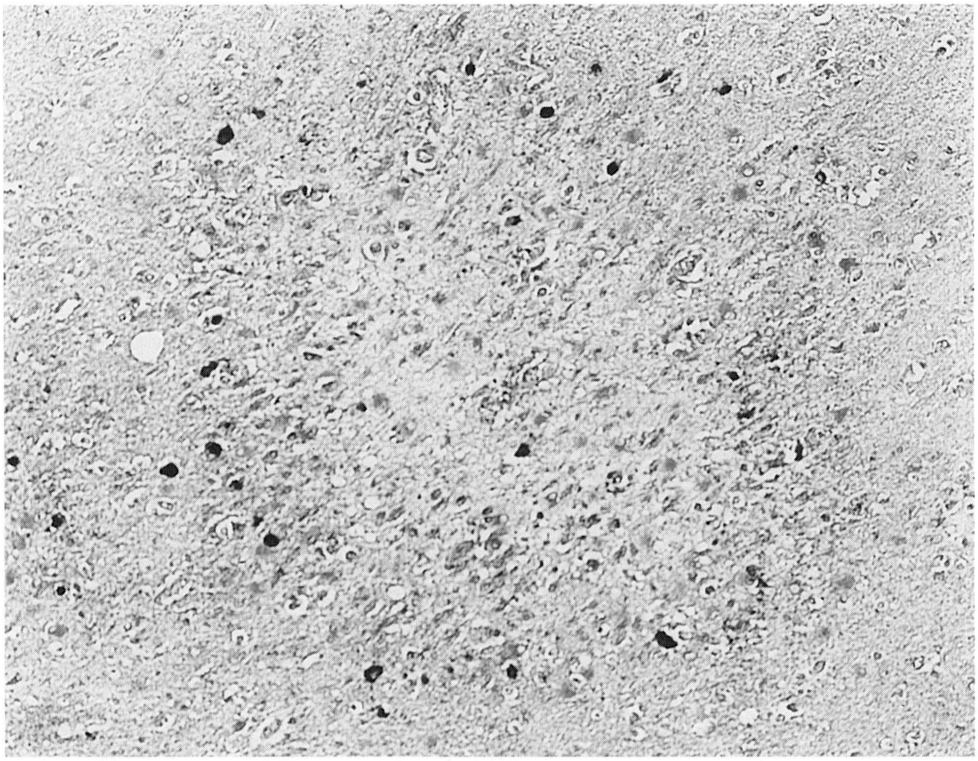

**Fig. 9-33.** An early PML lesion in the neocortex immunostained for polyomavirus. The pale lesion in the middle of the neocortex, from a case similar to the one in Fig. 9-32, has a few cells in it and at its edge is immunoreactive for polyomavirus. Polyomavirus is not found this far up into the neocortex in non-AIDS PML cases. It is within areas such as this focal lesion that neocortical immunostaining for HIV can sometimes be found (compare with Fig. 9-16). (Rabbit antiserum PML-Ab1; ×100.)

tered cells.[149] Immunoreactive PML inclusions in "burnt out" cases are only seen within the bizarre astrocytes that remain, while the infected oligodendrocytes have lysed and cannot be found. Spongiform alterations with demyelination and some necrosis (Figs. 9-9, 9-17, 9-18) and enlarged astrocytes can also be seen in HIV encephalitis (Figs. 9-5, 9-9), so that special studies (immunostaining, electron microscopy, or molecular biology techniques) are needed to demonstrate a combined polyomavirus-retrovirus encephalitis.

**Herpesviruses.** Systemic infections with *cytomegalovirus* are very common in AIDS patients,[148,236] and it is therefore no surprise that combinations of cytomegaloviral meningoencephalomyeloradiculitis are occasionally found.[247,303] The appearance of cytomegaloviral encephalitis on CT scans is varied, although periventricular enhancement is common, and MRI may show both periventricular lesions and leptomeningeal enhancement.[124] Radiologic findings may underestimate the extent of the lesions eventually found at autopsy.[228] Necrotizing lesions may be seen near the ventricles (Fig. 9-12), in the leptomeninges, beneath the pia mater on gyral surfaces, or elsewhere in the CNS. Cytomegaloviral vasculitis can be associated with cerebral infarcts in AIDS.[318] In one of our cases there was widespread parenchymal involvement of the occipital lobe that was diagnosed as an infarct with serial CT scans. It had the same gross appearance as one of the very destructive cases of PML (Fig. 9-34; cf., Fig. 9-28). Large intranuclear and cytoplasmic cytomegaloviral inclusions are present in ependymal cells and astrocytes (Fig. 9-35).[79] Neurons can contain immunoreactive cytomegalovirus.[252,318] Immunostaining can be positive in both the cytoplasmic and intranuclear inclusions with some monoclonal antibodies available. These inclusions are basophilic to a variable degree in routine stains. Multinucleated giant cells with cytomegaloviral inclusions (Fig. 9-36) might also be infected with HIV; and their infection with cytomegalovirus can be documented by in situ hybridization (Fig. 9-37).[79] Both HIV and cytomegaloviral markers can be present in the same cell.[204,276] Only an infrequent gliomesenchymal cell nodule contains cytomegaloviral inclusions in AIDS (Fig. 9-38; Table 9-1). However, reports of cytomegaloviral antigen in gliomesencyhymal cell nodules describe it from infrequent[267] to common (one third of cases),[318] while the same reports describe HIV immunoreactivity[318] or HIV gene detection at about 40% of cases.[267] Cytomegalovirus may promote HIV replication and HIV encephalitis even when the cytomegalovirus itself may be latent in the brain and can only be detected by the polymerase chain reaction.[247,253] Cytomegaloviral genomic material can be widespread in the CNS, but without inclusion-bearing cells and inflammation there is no morphologic sign of its presence.[314] The histologic detection of both types of viral encephalitides is probably a measure of the patient's poor immune status.[247]

*Herpes simplex virus type 1* (HSV-1) in the CNS is occasionally reported in AIDS. Typical HSV-1 encephalitis is characterized by hemorrhage and necrosis in

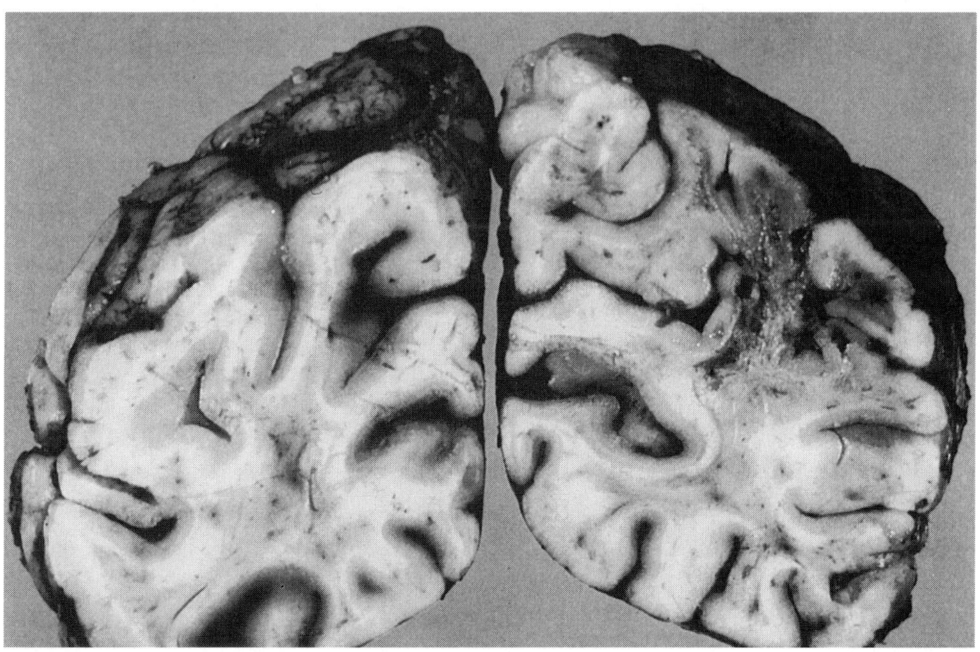

**Fig. 9-34.** Occipital lobes with cytomegaloviral encephalitis. The lesion on the right is similar to the PML lesion in Fig. 9-28, but here the cause is cytomegalovirus, and the neocortical destruction is more complete.

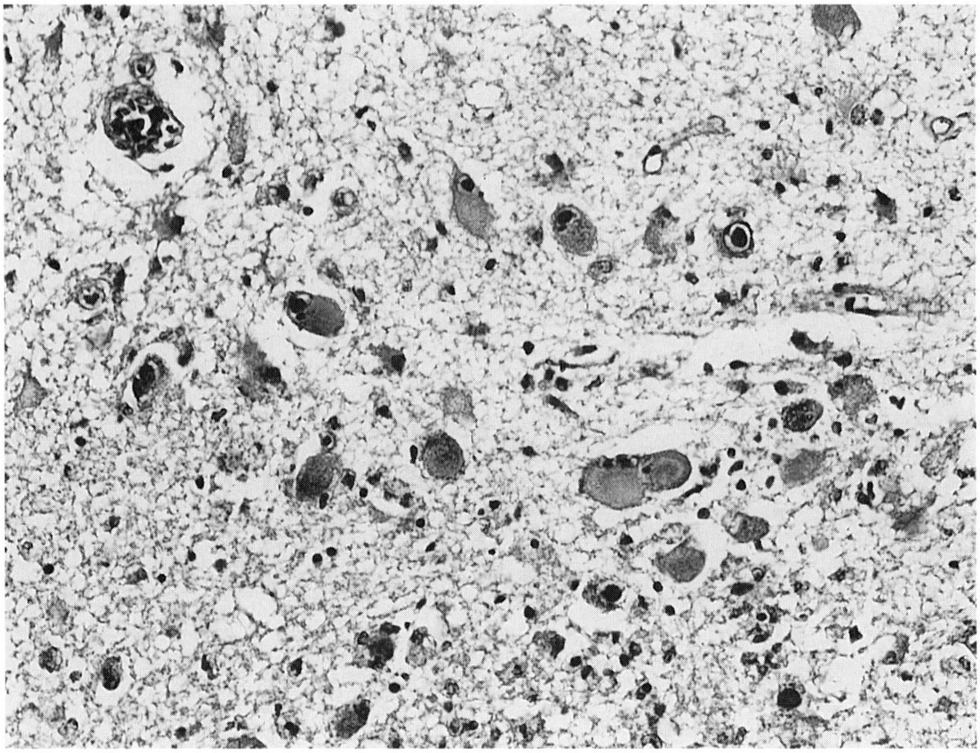

**Fig. 9-35.** Cytomegaloviral encephalitis. Astrocytes in the hippocampal white matter have cytomegaloviral intranuclear and cytoplasmic inclusions. (H&E; ×200.)

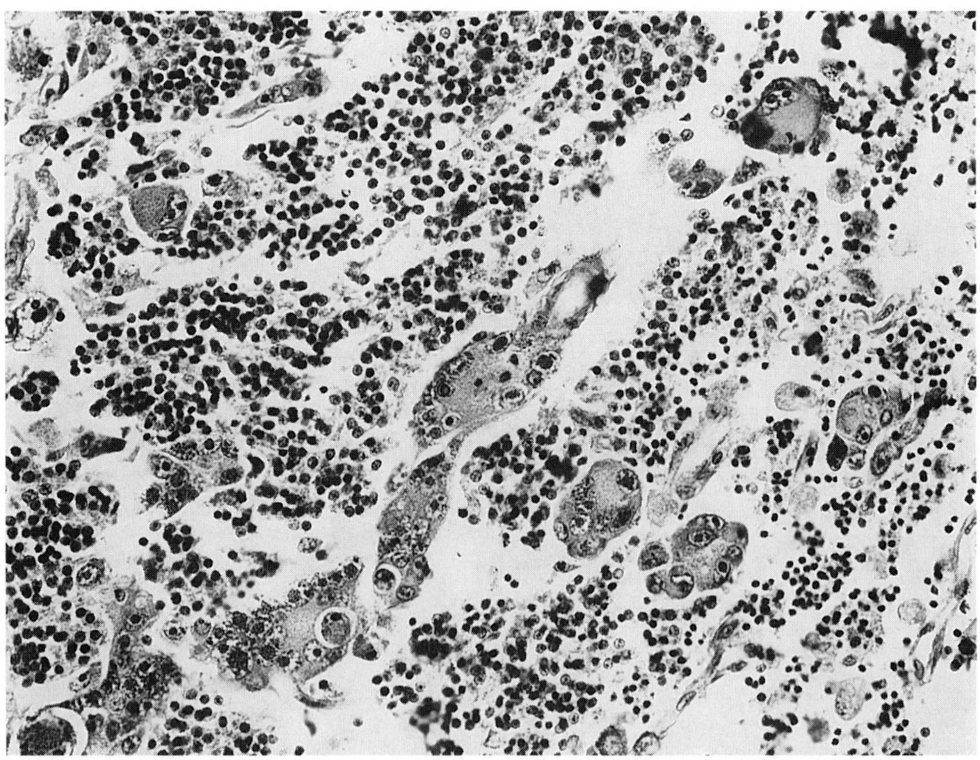

**Fig. 9-36.** Cytomegalovirus in multinucleated giant cells in the internal granule cell layer of the cerebellum. The infected giant cells have cytomegaloviral inclusions in most of their nuclei. The small cells constitute the normal cellular population in this cortical layer. (H&E; ×200.)

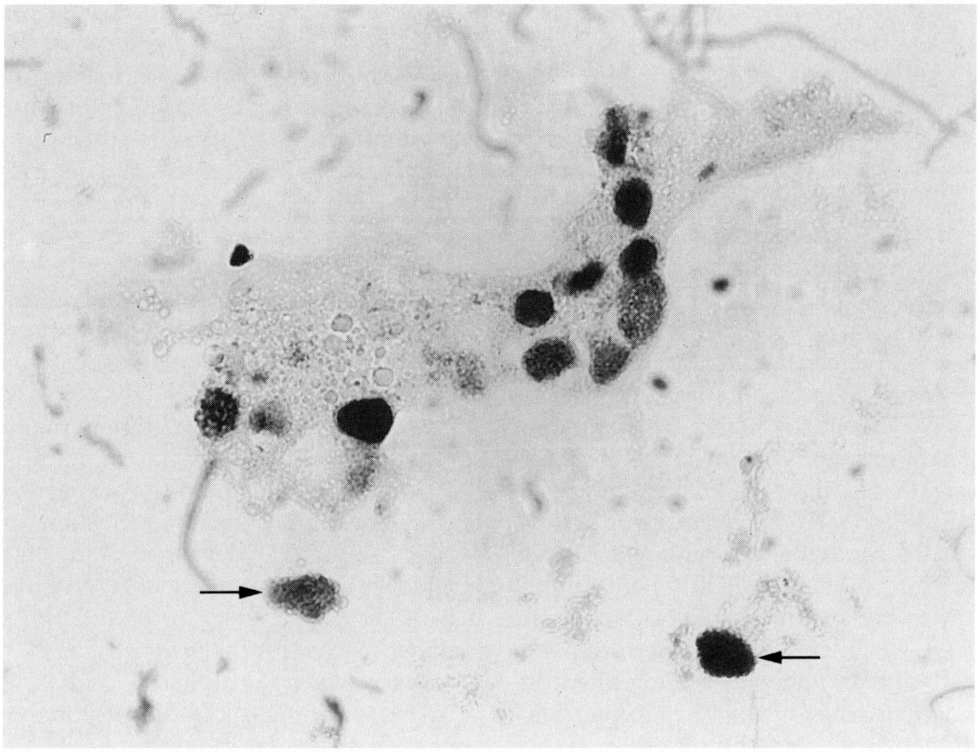

**Fig. 9-37.** In situ hybridization of cytomegaloviral DNA in a paraffin section of cerebral tissue. A multinucleated giant cell and two smaller cells (*arrows*) have dense marker signals in intranuclear inclusions in a liquefactive area of periventriculitis. (Oligonucleotide probe for cytomegalovirus, Enzo Diagnostics, with diaminobenzidine chromogen; ×500.)

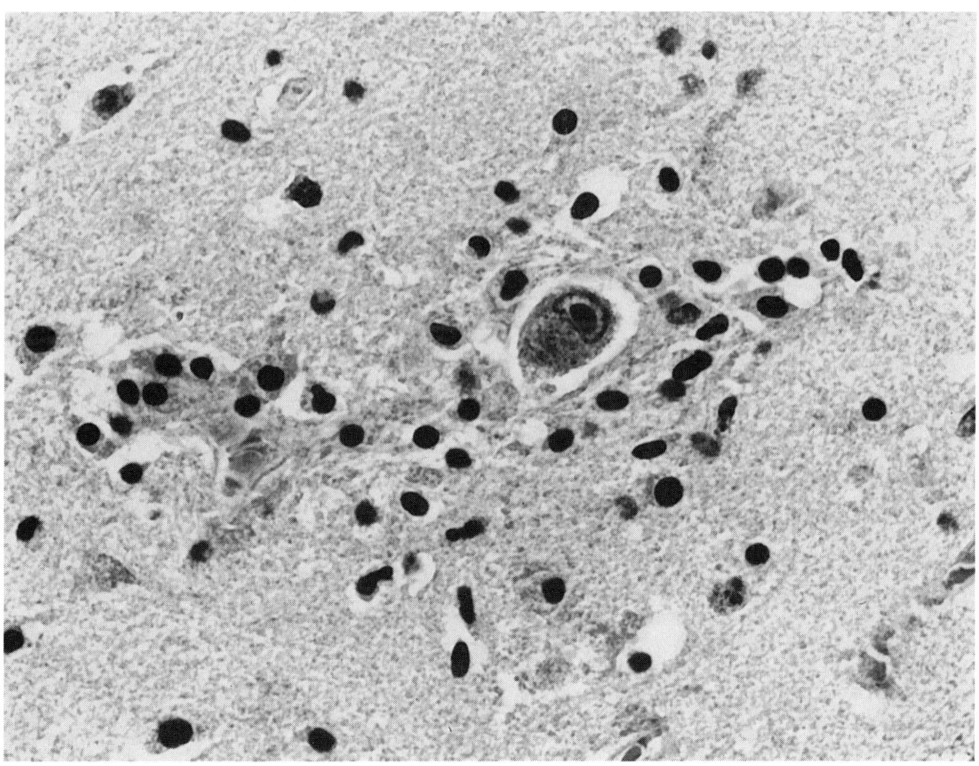

**Fig. 9-38.** Cytomegaloviral intranuclear and cytoplasmic inclusions in one cell within a gliomesenchymal cell nodule in the putamen. (H&E; ×500.)

the temporal lobes. *Varicella-zoster virus* and *herpes simplex virus type 2* have been identified in the CNS in AIDS patients at a much higher rate than in any non-AIDS population.[28,60,66,297] Varicella-zoster virus can cause demyelination and necrosis in the brain,[194] and occasionally it results in a noninflammatory[63] or granulomatous angiitis.[24]

Herpesviruses have been demonstrated in the brain of a few AIDS patients who had clinical and radiographic pictures corresponding to that of PML, but no evidence of PML was found at autopsy.[194,222,248,258] Although rare cases of herpetic meningoencephalitis may mimic PML very closely, CT scans in the herpetic disease more frequently show gray matter involvement, a mass effect, or hemorrhage. This rare type of *PML-like herpetic encephalitis* antedates the AIDS epidemic, most cases are caused by varicella-zoster virus, and it probably has included some cases of cytomegalovirus and HSV-1, differing from the usual HSV-1 encephalitis by lacking abundant hemorrhage. The characteristic lesions in these PML-like herpetic encephalitides have fairly discrete borders with liquefied centers filled by macrophages and involving mostly the deep white matter, but the full thickness of the neocortex can be liquefied in areas. Actual cavities several centimeters across can be formed, and a needle biopsy may retrieve only nondiagnostic tissue debris and macrophages. Acute and chronic vasculitis can be found in the parenchymal lesions and in the leptomeninges.[248]

We have seen some cases of encephalitis with necrosis (necrotizing encephalitis), with the etiology remaining undetermined, in which the lesions have predominantly white matter involvement but also include cortex. Intranuclear inclusions are lacking and immunostaining is negative for polyomavirus and herpesviruses. The histopathologic findings in these cases include focal spongiform change, demyelination in the white matter, areas of white-matter cavitation, and necrotizing panencephalitis (involvement of the gray and white matter) with vasculitis. The perivascular macrophages and gliomesenchymal cell nodules typical of HIV encephalitis can be found near the discrete lesions of demyelination and necrosis. In one of the cases viral inclusions were lacking and immunoreactive *Toxoplasma* cysts were found in a small part of a large lesion that was thought on gross examination to be PML or herpetic encephalitis (Fig. 9-39). This emphasizes the confusion that can exist in some AIDS cases in which multiple concomitant types of encephalitides so commonly occur. We have classified this type of necrotizing encephalitis as an HIV-associated lesion and have speculated that, as in other immunomodulated diseases, it might be caused by a severe hypersensitivity reaction.[247]

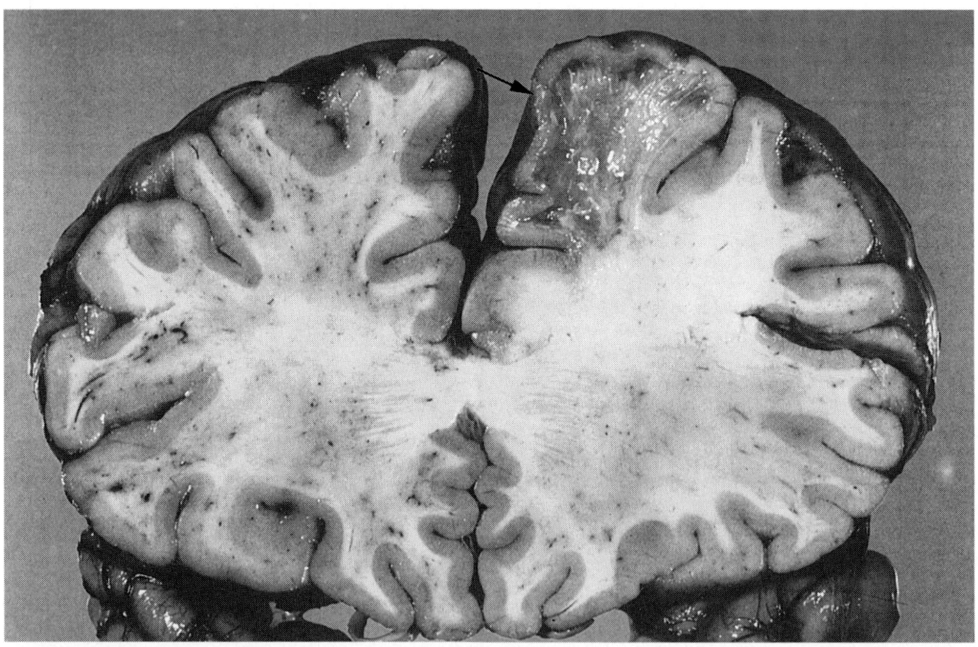

**Fig. 9-39.** Necrotizing encephalitis in a rostral view of the frontal lobes. The left superior frontal region has a distinct white matter lesion with depressed, demyelinated tissue and relative sparing of the overlying cortex (*arrow*). PML was suspected during the gross examination. No evidence of PML or herpetic encephalitis was found, and only one small area of the lesion had cysts immunoreactive for *Toxoplasma.* There was necrosis present with macrophages, but because of the lack of coagulation necrosis (compare with Figs. 9-10, 9-41, and 9-42) or extensive granulation tissue, it was uncertain whether the major portion of the lesion was caused by *Toxoplasma.*

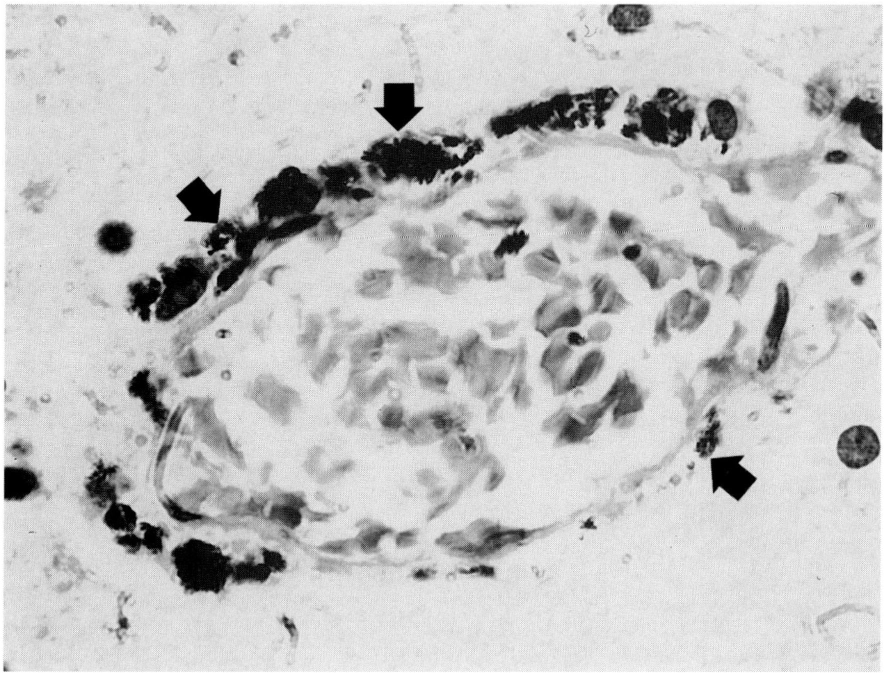

**Fig. 9-40.** *Mycobacterium avium-intracellulare* in a cerebral vascular wall. Large numbers of mycobacteria (*arrowheads*) are in cells of the vascular wall, and inflammation is virtually absent. (Acid-fast bacillus stain with hematoxylin counterstain; ×1000.)

Coinfection of cells (including neural cells) can occur with herpesviruses and HIV and the herpesviruses can stimulate a more rapid HIV replication and gene expression.* HIV may, in turn, enhance the production and cytopathology of herpesviruses.[275] Appropriate lesions should be examined for both types of viruses. Even though HSV-1 antigen is demonstrable or recoverable from the brain for only 2 or 3 weeks following encephalitis,[245] it might be demonstrated by the polymerase chain reaction in more chronic lesions.[115]

### Bacterial Leptomeningitis and Cerebritis

Purulent leptomeningitis, bacterial cerebritis, and abscesses, including tuberculous abscesses, are reported in AIDS.† *Mycobacterium avium-intracellulare* has been identified in the brains of AIDS patients. It may not be important as a CNS pathogen, and it seems to elicit little chronic inflammation even when it appears in cerebrovascular walls (Fig. 9-40). *Listeria monocytogenes* can cause leptomeningitis in AIDS,[109] and in our series there was one case with *Listeria*-associated meningoencephalitis and vasculitis. Whipple's disease of the nervous system has been reported in AIDS.[3,200] Bacterial infections of the nervous system, as might be expected, are often seen in patients with intravenous drug abuse as a risk factor.

### Protozoal Meningoencephalomyelitis

**Toxoplasmic meningoencephalomyelitis.** *Toxoplasma gondii* encephalitis is found in proportions varying from series to series of AIDS cases.* T4 lymphocytes and macrophages are part of the normal control mechanism for this organism,[32,305] perhaps explaining the presence of toxoplasmic infections as the immune status of AIDS patients is altered. The clinical picture can be that of a focal lesion with headaches and lethargy followed by progressive development of subacute meningoencephalitis, diffuse encephalopathy, or signs of a space-occupying mass.[66,169,170] The appearance of toxoplasmic lesions on CT scans is varied, but often there are many ringlike or solid, rounded, enhancing lesions scattered anywhere in the brain that resemble the findings with neoplasms (particularly lymphomas), PML, or abscesses.[67] Cortical toxoplasmic lesions can be suggestive of metastases (Fig. 9-10). Contrast enhancement around areas of necrosis can be very faint. The presence of small, slightly enhancing cortical lesions should increase suspicion of toxoplasmosis, and rising serum antibody titers should be sought. MRI defines the lesions better than CT.[238,323] The toxoplasmic lesions in sectioned brain specimens can be small or large and widespread. The smaller lesions are dark gray-white or yellow to yellow-tan, and they may be barely perceptible within the neocortex, at the cortical junction with the subcortical white matter, in the deep white matter, in the basal ganglia, or in the cerebellum, brainstem, or spinal cord. The smaller lesions usually have a smooth cut surface, and they can be located only by close attention to color changes and by extensive sampling of the gross specimen. The larger lesions may be either gray-white or yellow. They tend to be homogeneous because they consist of little

* Refs. 35, 52, 98, 128, 146, 172, 193, 195, 204, 213.

† Refs. 5, 198, 241, 247, 278.

* Refs. 5, 198, 205, 222, 241, 247, 278.

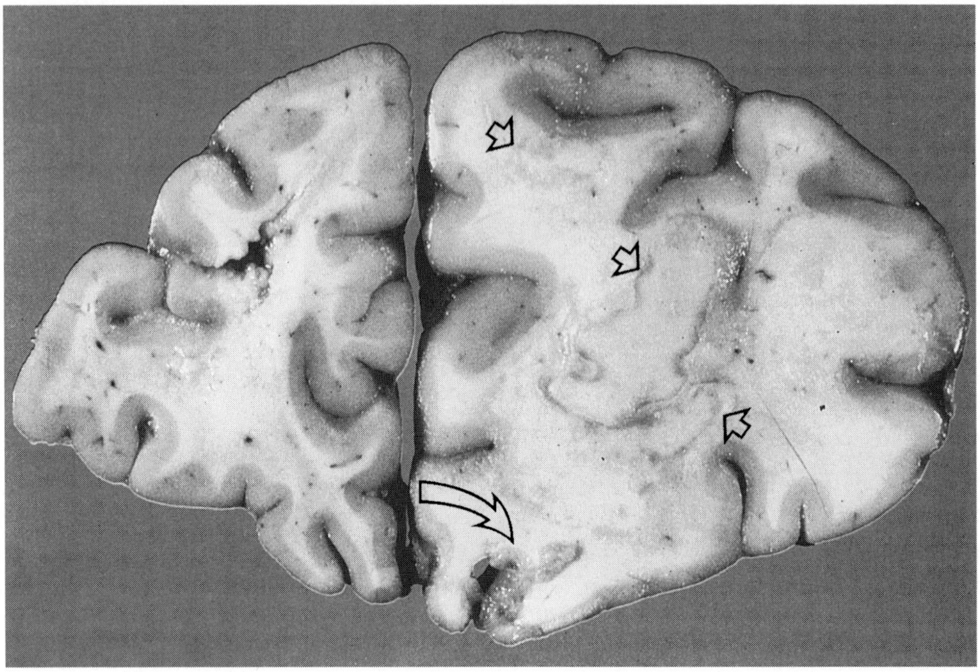

**Fig. 9-41.** Toxoplasmic encephalitis in the frontal lobes. The white matter of the right frontal lobe has large areas of coagulation necrosis with thin bands of granulation tissue (*open arrowheads*) separating areas of different degrees of destruction. Neocortical involvement is seen (*curved open arrow*). There is extensive infection of the white matter seen microscopically in both frontal lobes, including smooth and depressed areas and areas that grossly appear only edematous.

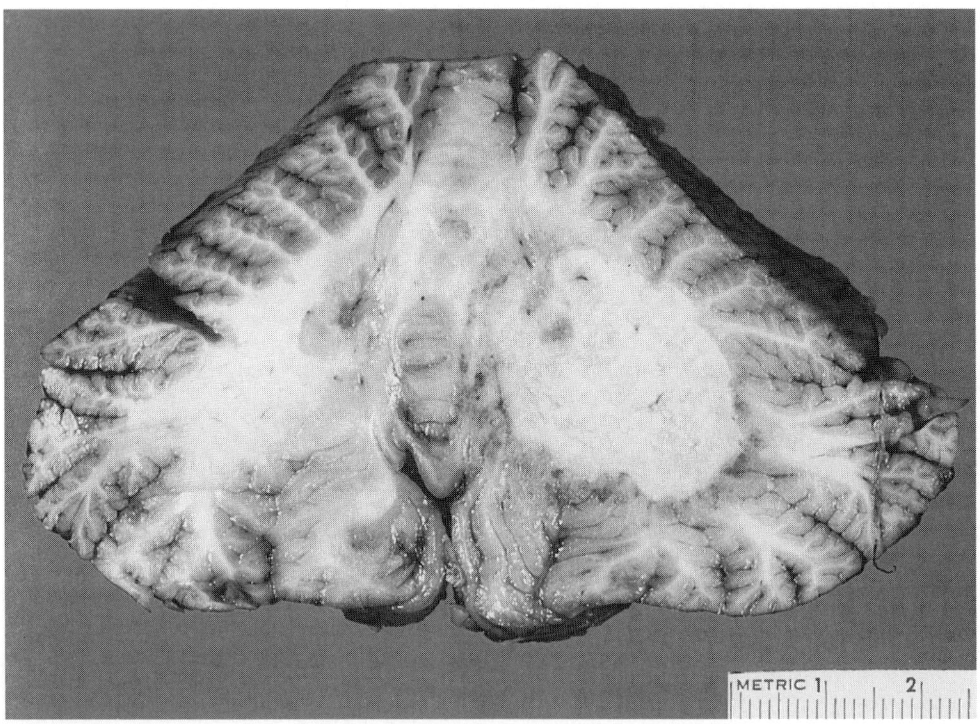


**Fig. 9-42.** Toxoplasmic encephalitis in the cerebellum. The large area of coagulation necrosis in the right lateral lobe has a thin capsule of granulation tissue around it. This homogeneous, starkly white lesion has an almost smooth cut surface and only mild softening. This is the typical appearance of many toxoplasmic lesions in the brain, but it is also the gross appearance of tuberculomas.

but coagulation necrosis. Large toxoplasmic lesions tend to soften, darken, and to have uneven cut surfaces when there is terminal, generalized cerebral infarction ("respirator brain"[197] or global ischemia[92]). Viable inflammatory cells and granulation tissue occur on the outer margins as a thin, partial capsule or as thin trabeculae or islands within the necrotic tissue (Figs. 9-10, 9-41, 9-42).

We have cut several brains in cases in which the clinical diagnosis was cerebral lymphoma, only to find *Toxoplasma* cysts but no tumor. This is a frequent occurrence,[62] and biopsy may not be completely satisfactory because both types of lesions, in addition to other types of lesions, can be present at the same site (Fig. 9-10).[162,249]

Encysted bradyzoites are found without accompanying inflammation until the wall of the *Toxoplasma* cyst ruptures (Figs. 9-43, 9-44). Often there is vasculitis with endothelial proliferation that is thought to be an allergic response. The individual, motile, free tissue tachyzoites (trophozoites) in fresh lesions are very destructive (Fig. 9-45), and a significant inflammatory response can develop against them. A cerebral biopsy

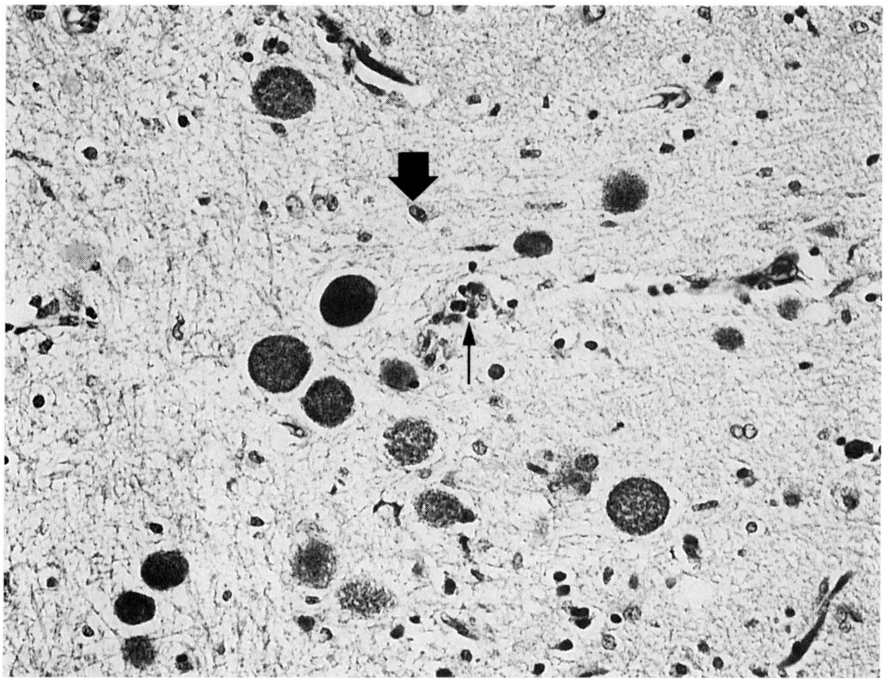

**Fig. 9-43.** Toxoplasmic encephalitis. Over a dozen unruptured *Toxoplasma* cysts are present, with only mild perivasculitis (*arrow*) and gliosis (*arrowhead*) seen. (H&E; ×200.)

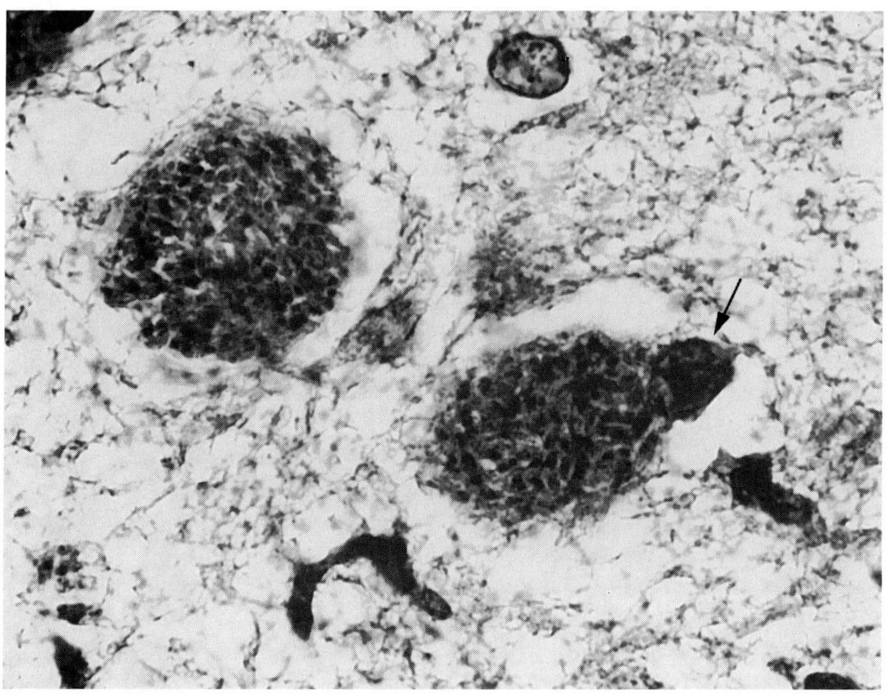

**Fig. 9-44.** Toxoplasmic encephalitis. Individual bradyzoites can be seen in these two parasitic cysts. The nucleus of a cell in which one of the cysts developed is still visible (*arrow*). (H&E; ×1000.)

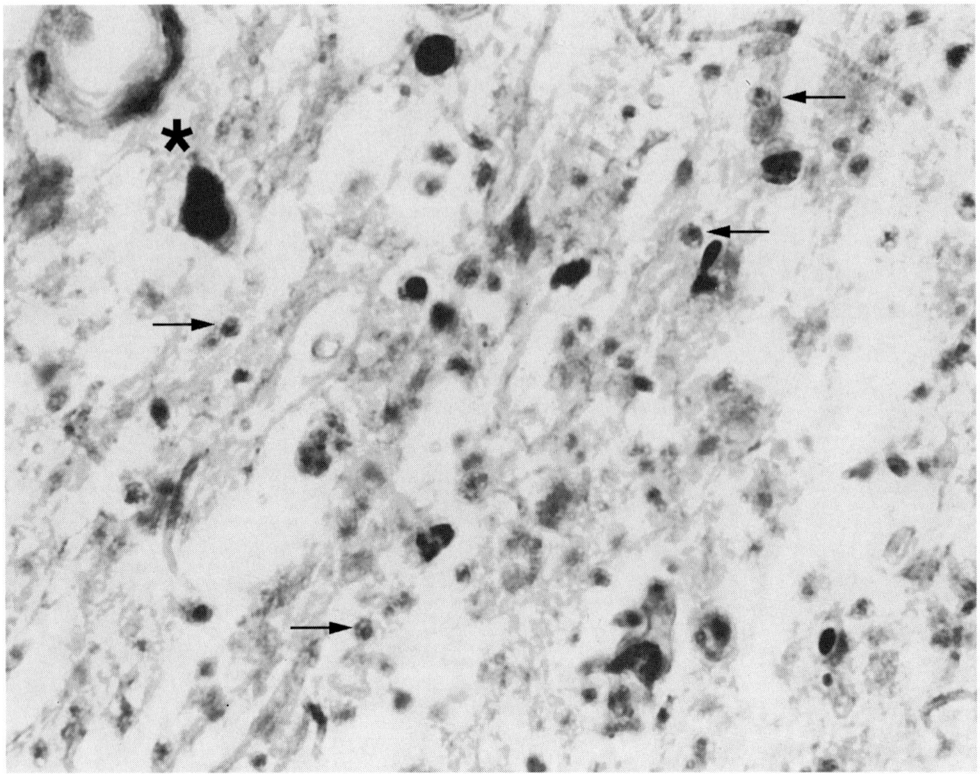

**Fig. 9-45.** Early toxoplasmic myelitis. Necrosis in the presence of free tissue tachyzoites (trophozoites) of *Toxoplasma gondii* (*arrows*) is found in the lumbar level of the spinal cord. The asterisk (*) lies between a small parasitic cyst containing bradyzoites that are too crowded to be seen individually and a venule with endothelial hyperplasia. (H&E; ×1000.)

specimen from a case of toxoplasmic encephalitis may show cysts, but often only necrotic debris or strikingly pleomorphic, mononuclear cellular infiltration and granulation tissue is recovered. An open excisional biopsy is more likely to yield positive results than a needle biopsy. If chemotherapy is begun without any biopsy or without a diagnostic biopsy, reevaluation for a biopsy in 10 days is recommended based on the clinical and radiographic response.[170] Clinical improvement and improvement apparent on CT scans correlate well in toxoplasmic encephalitis.[227]

*Toxoplasma* organisms cannot be differentiated in routine stains from the leishmanial form of *Trypanosoma cruzi* or from *Sarcocystis* or *Besnoitia* species,[85] but the latter organisms have not been reported in the CNS in AIDS. The ultrastructural appearance of *Toxoplasma* is characteristic,[100,272] but the method of choice for making the diagnosis is by immunostaining. The organisms may be very difficult to locate, however, and associated findings may provide a clue to the nature of the lesions even if a definitive diagnosis cannot be made. Early necrosis is associated with foamy macrophages, and encysted bradyzoites are generally present within small lesions where necrosis is minimal, and at the edge of lesions of any size that contain coagulation necrosis. Although toxoplasmic lesions that have not yet become coagulated are usually very small, extensive tissue destruction without coagulation necrosis is sometimes found. These large, noncoagulated lesions typically contain *Toxoplasma* cysts, including cysts that are still intracellular, and free tissue tachyzoites. The tachyzoites might be clearly delineated only following immunostaining. Granulation tissue surrounds the more chronic lesions, and cysts are not often found near these areas of granulation tissue (Fig. 9-46). The granulation tissue capsule of well-organized toxoplasmic lesions resembles a bacterial abscess wall, but the center is not filled with pus or lymphocytes. Rather, there is only coagulation necrosis and perhaps some foamy macrophages centrally, with viable cells being present in the outer margin or wall. Sometimes chronic inflammation and granulation tissue are poorly represented, and the lesions are almost liquefied centrally and contain poorly preserved macrophages and loose-appearing cellular debris. These bland-looking lesions, which range in size from very small to over 1 cm in diameter, are often called infarcts until the rare and often necrotic protozoal cysts are discovered. Much of the necrosis may indeed be caused by infarction, because vascular occlusion is fre-

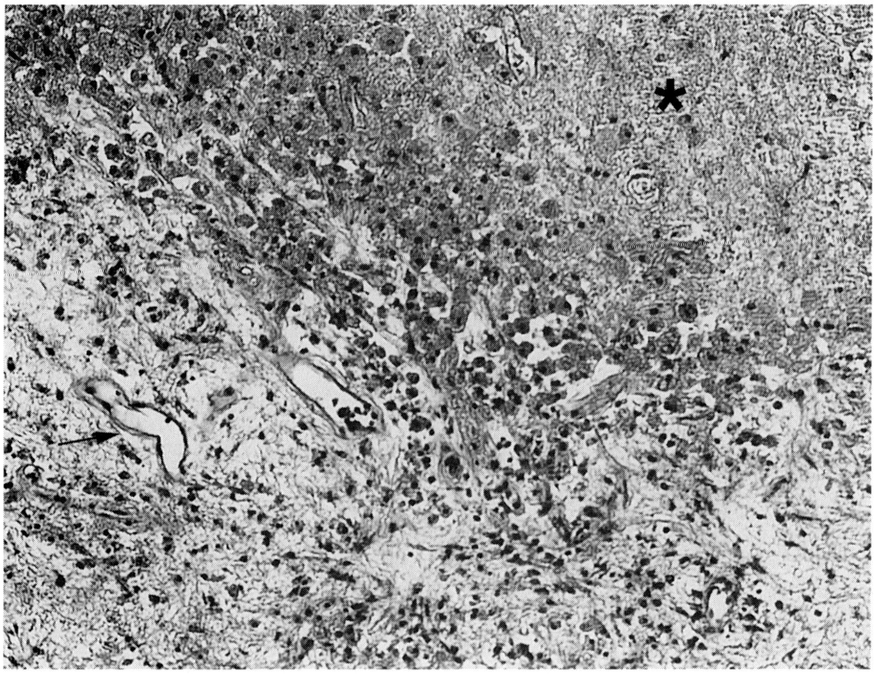

**Fig. 9-46.** Advanced toxoplasmic encephalitis. Coagulation necrosis (*) and granulation tissue with macrophages, multinucleated cells, and characteristic macrocapillaries (*arrow*) form most of this lesion. (H&E; ×100.)

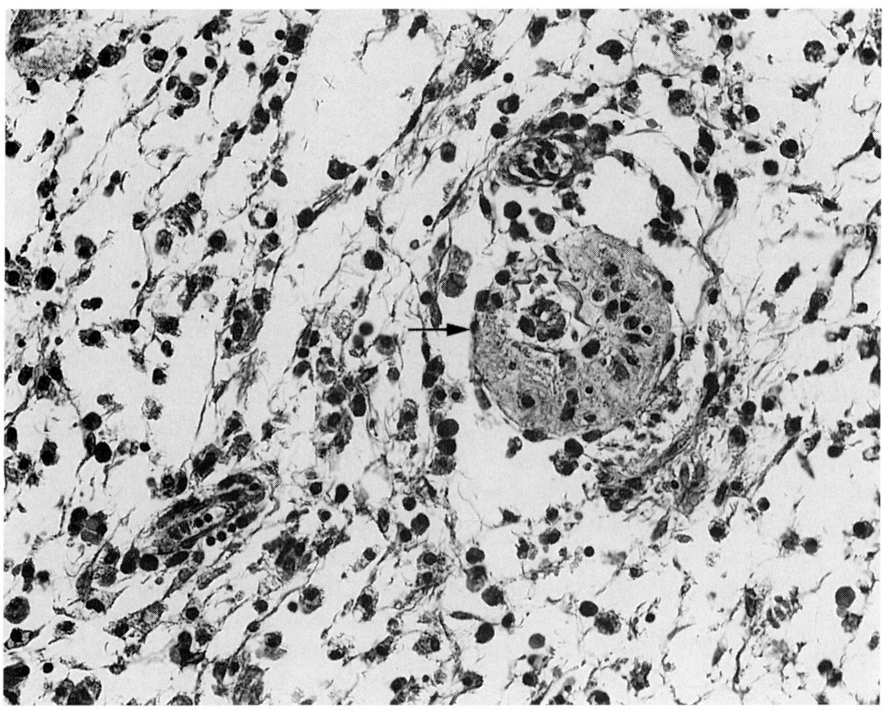

**Fig. 9-47.** Advanced toxoplasmic encephalitis with liquefactive necrosis. A thickened, occluded blood vessel (*arrow*) is seen in a liquefying area of coagulation necrosis. (H&E; ×200.)

quently found in toxoplasmic lesions (Fig. 9-47). Care should be exercised when parasitic cysts are not found because multifocal necrotizing encephalitis of unknown cause can be found in AIDS patients as well as in patients with other causes of immunodeficiency. These foci can be small, and like some small toxoplasmic infections they have pronounced spongiform change associated with necrotic cells, macrophages, mild gliosis, and calcium deposits.[6]

**Amebic meningoencephalitis.** *Acanthamoeba culbertsoni* has been identified in necrotic lesions in the brain of an AIDS patient. There was associated suppurative leptomeningitis, but the inflammation lacked a granulomatous component.[316] There is usually a lack of multinucleated giant cells in immunocompromised patients with this condition, although it is generally known as *granulomatous amebic encephalitis* (GAE). Impaired cell-mediated immunity or defects in the re-

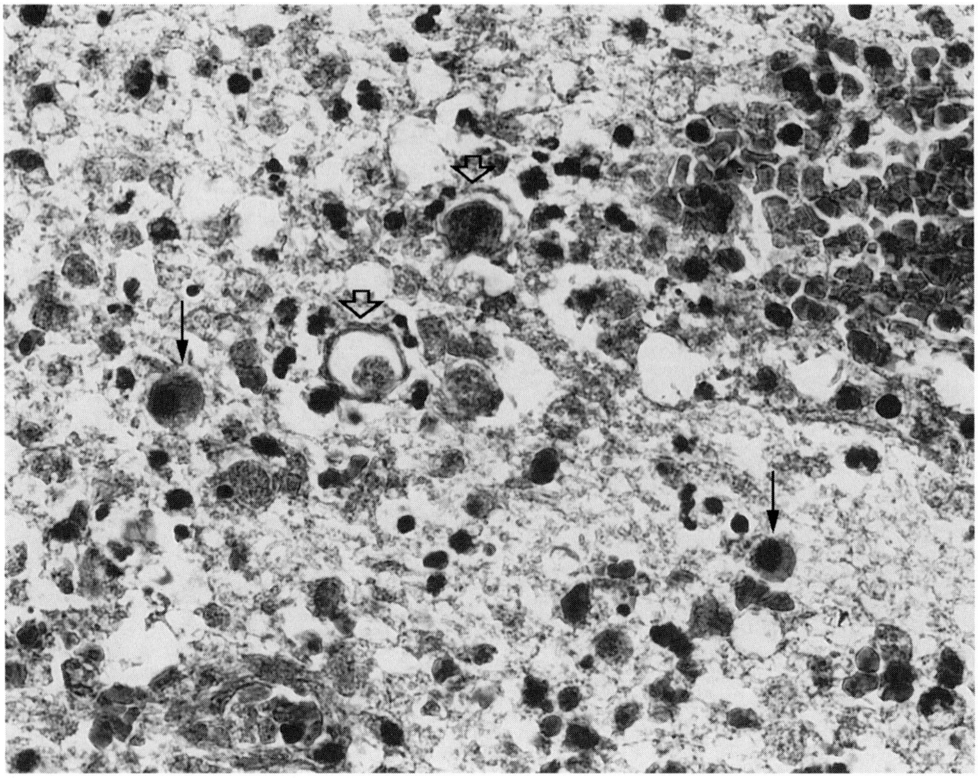

**Fig. 9-48.** Amebic encephalitis. Trophozoites (*arrows*) and cysts (*open arrowheads*) of *Acanthamoeba castellanii* were found in necrotic, hemorrhagic cerebral tissue. (H&E; ×500.)

sponse of macrophages may be responsible for this. About 30 of almost 100 GAE cases worldwide were found in AIDS patients.[180]

We have found trophozoites and cysts (12 to 30 $\mu$m) of *Acanthamoeba castellanii* in the brain of an AIDS patient within hemorrhagic, necrotic frontobasal cerebral lesions that include acute and chronic inflammation. Immunofluorescence staining for *Acanthamoeba* species was kindly performed in this case by Dr. Govinda S. Visvesvara of the Parasitic Diseases Branch at the Centers for Disease Control in Atlanta, Georgia. The trophozoites are difficult to recognize. The small, eccentric nuclei are inconspicuous except for a large nucleolus. The thick cyst wall, when present, contains a cell with the same inconspicuous nucleus (Figs. 9-48, 9-49). The cytoplasm is PAS-positive, although for *Acanthamoeba* this can be an inconstant feature. Such amebas tend to involve the frontobasal brain and could enter the blood vessels from the skin, nasal passages, or lungs.[304] In our case, no amebas were found in the lungs.

### Fungal Meningoencephalitis

Cryptococcal leptomeningitis and encephalitis, candidiasis, aspergillosis, histoplasmosis, nocardiosis, mucormycosis, and coccidioidomycosis are detected either as expected or unexpected gross and microscopic findings in the nervous system in cases of AIDS.* They may be only one of several infections in the tissue. The patients have a subacute or chronic meningitis with headaches and lethargy.[66] *Cryptococcus* organisms have no pathognomonic radiographic appearance, but an occasional cryptococcoma or cryptococcal leptomeningitis will enhance with contrast medium.[238] *Cryptococcus* often has a deficient capsule whenever it is found in AIDS, and granulomatous inflammation is not frequently seen in response to fungi in this disease. *Cryptococcus* organisms can hide unstained in macrophages that appear to have unusually large vacuoles containing the fungus. *Cryptococcus* usually takes up no stain (Fig. 9-50) but may take up some eosin, and *Candida* organisms are difficult to see but may take up some hematoxylin intermittently along the pseudohyphae. A fungal stain is always in order when the diagnosis of fungal meningoencephalitis is a possibility. Gliomesenchymal cell nodules containing a large amount of acute inflammatory cells should be stained for fungus because *Candida* organisms may well be harbored there. The cohabitation of retroviral particles and *Cryptococcus* organisms in a multinucleated giant cell has been documented.[113]

* Refs. 5, 46, 198, 241, 247, 269, 278.

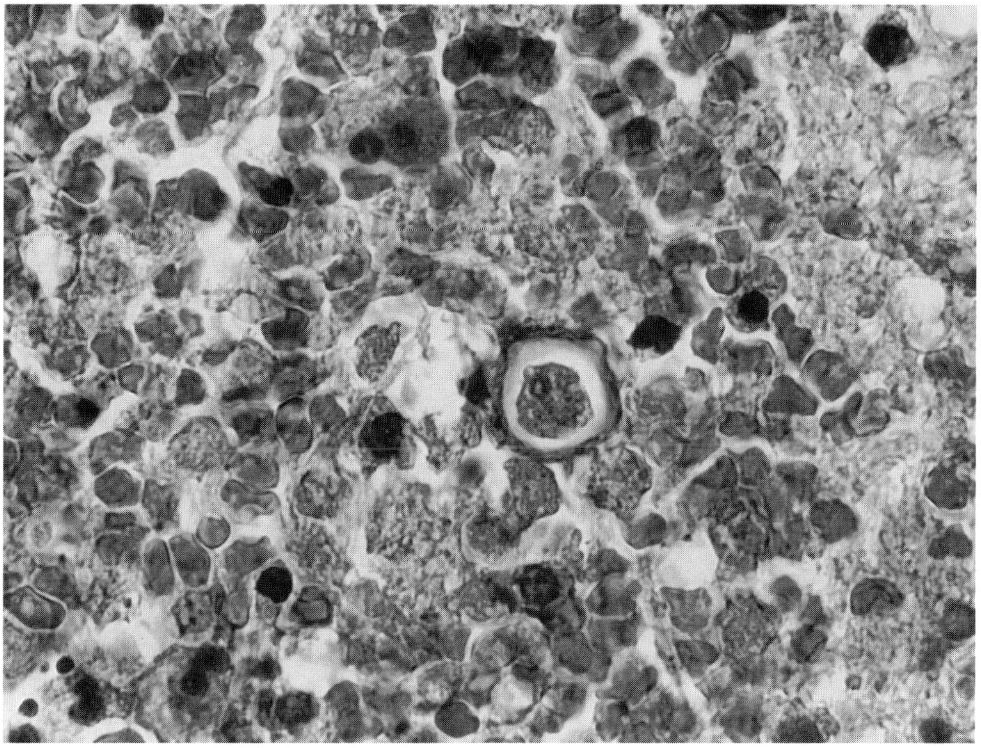

**Fig. 9-49.** Amebic encephalitis. An encysted ameba (*A. castellanii*) has a small, eccentric nucleus. The cyst wall has a characteristic woven appearance. (H&E; ×1000.)

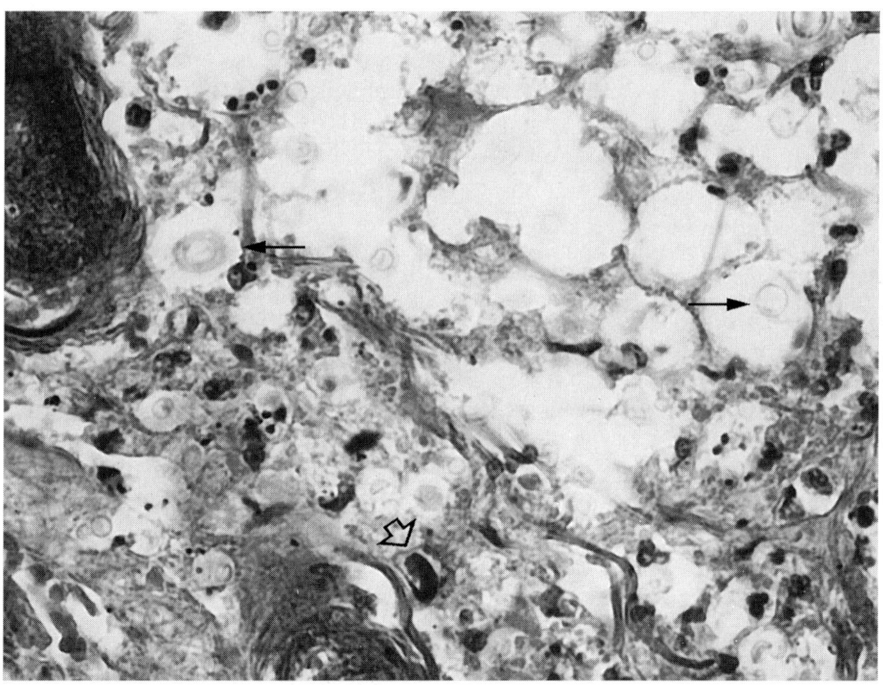

**Fig. 9-50.** Cryptococcal leptomeningitis. The fungi (*arrows*) are difficult to find because they do not stain well with routine stains. One of the cells in this region with a Cowdry type A intranuclear inclusion (*open arrowhead*) is seen, indicating that a viral meningitis is also present. (H&E; ×500.)

## SPIROCHETE INFECTIONS

### Neurosyphilis in AIDS

Syphilis is commonly found in homosexual males with AIDS as a sexually transmitted disease.[294] An HIV infection appears to alter the course of syphilis significantly, so that forms of neurosyphilis might be accelerated and respond poorly to conventional treatment.[136,144] Syphilitic optic neuritis in AIDS has been arrested clinically with penicillin treatment, but tissue examination has been unavailable.[34]

### Lyme Borreliosis in HIV Infection

An HIV-infected patient exposed to *Borrelia burgdorferi* through tick bites exhibited neurologic symptoms and signs typical of Lyme disease. After development of an annular, expanding cutaneous rash, he had slurred speech, facial weakness, and headache. There was an increase in lymphocytes and proteins in the CSF, and *B. burgdorferi* antigen and antibodies were detected in serum and CSF. This spirochete was the cause of neurologic disease unrelated to the HIV infection as far as could be demonstrated, and this case points out that Lyme disease should be considered in the differential diagnosis of neurologic disorders in endemic areas.[93]

## METAZOAL INFECTIONS

### Cysticercosis

Cysticercus, the larval form of the tapeworm *Taenia solium,* has been reported in the brain of an AIDS patient.[198] Cysticercus would be expected only in a patient who consumes contaminated pork or water. The hospital population from which our series of AIDS cases was taken has a relatively high incidence of CNS cysticercosis,[262] but there is no case involving an AIDS patient, either clinically or at autopsy.

### Lancet Liver Fluke Infection

*Dicrocoelium dendriticum,* a trematode carried from cattle and sheep to field ants, was found in a man with swollen lymph nodes who was infected by HIV. He had apparently contracted this parasitic disease from water contaminated by ants, and he was easily and successfully treated with praziquantel. It seemed likely that the HIV infection itself did not contribute to his parasitic disease.[61]

## HYPOXIC, HEMORRHAGIC, AND OTHER LESIONS

One of the most common autopsy findings in brains of AIDS victims is cerebral edema in the gross form of brain swelling. This is no doubt related to terminal events; the patients are often comatose and maintained on assisted ventilation. The microscopic findings related to hypoxia or small hemorrhages are those of "respirator-brain" changes[197] or "global ischemia" in such cases.[92] Hypoxic and hemorrhagic lesions in the brains of AIDS patients include hypoxic neuronal changes (cytoplasmic and nuclear shrinkage and darkening with loss of nuclear detail; nuclei in neocortical pyramidal neurons with a distinct triangular shape), infarcts, thromboemboli, subarachnoid hemorrhage, intracerebral hematomas (Fig. 9-51), and intraventricular hemorrhage.* The overall incidence of vascular complications has been low[66] but is increasing as patient survival increases with advances in treatment.[247] Acute necrotizing vasculitis is probably most commonly caused by a bacterial infection, and it is generally associated with sepsis and purulent leptomeningitis. Cytomegaloviral vasculitis causing cerebral infarcts has been noted.[318] Granulomatous arteritis can be caused by varicella-zoster virus,[24] which can infect the CNS in AIDS, while noninfectious primary angiitis of the CNS is also reported in HIV-infected patients.[261,320]

Calcific vasculopathy consisting of stainable calcium salts and some iron in small or medium sized blood vessel walls is found in some brains in AIDS patients. This change to the vessel wall is mostly found in the basal ganglia and mostly in pediatric AIDS patients (Fig. 9-23). It is not specific for AIDS, yet there is a known relationship to viral encephalitis.[270]

## NEOPLASMS

### Primary Lymphomas

The CNS in AIDS has the increased incidence of primary lymphomas known to be associated with immunodeficiency.† The symptoms are those of increased intracranial pressure: lethargy, confusion, and headache. In several of our cases the findings were microscopic and unexpected. Even in the usual symptomatic, multifocal cases, examination of the CSF might be diagnostic only if positive immunolabeling of tumor cells is obtained from large quantities of CSF.[279] CT scans of typical cases show isodense or hyperdense, homogeneous to ring-enhancing nodular masses or diffuse regions near a ventricle in the basal ganglia (Fig. 9-52; see also Fig. 9-10) or near the subarachnoid space. Enhancement with intravenous contrast medium differentiates a lymphoma from PML, yet only biopsy may differentiate a lymphoma from infections such as toxoplasmosis or from another type of tumor.[62,162,279] MRI is more sensitive but not more specific than CT.[238] The autopsy findings (Fig. 9-53; see also Fig. 9-14) correlate highly with the findings on CT scans, although microscopic studies often show further spread of tumor than is evident grossly.[279] In some cases, radiation treatment leaves no viable lymphoma, yet the CNS may have grave concomitant lesions of other types, so that no clinical improvement is seen (Fig. 9-10).

---

* Refs. 68, 156, 163, 191, 198, 205, 247, 270, 278.

† Refs. 198, 205, 241, 247, 278.

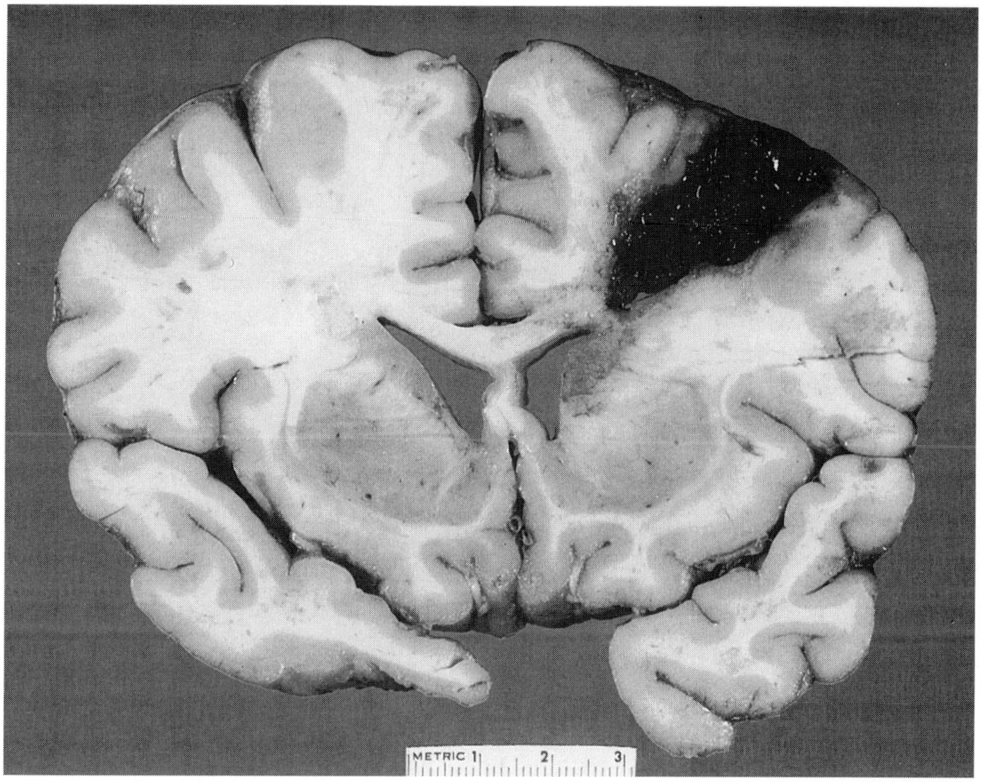


**Fig. 9-51.** A resolving cerebral lobar hemorrhage in a case of AIDS encephalitis. This brain has gliomesenchymal cell nodules and multinucleated giant cells identified microscopically. Large numbers of giant cells are crowded around blood vessels at the edges of the hematoma shown here. Are the giant cells part of a granulomatous reaction to hemorrhage, or are they part of a vasculopathy that caused the bleed?

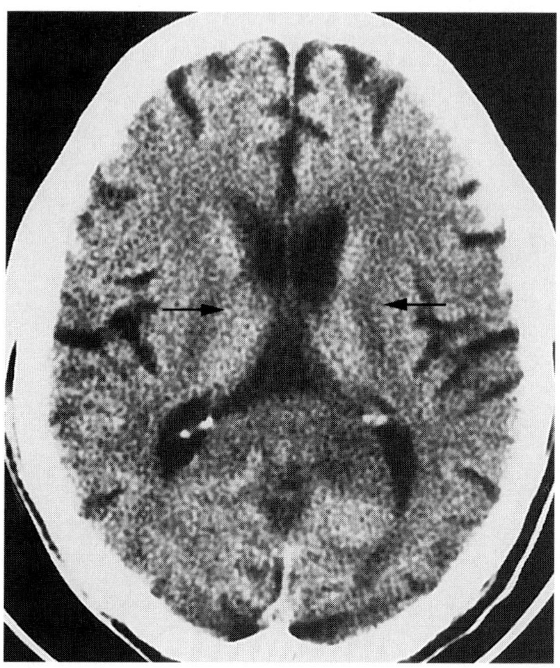

**Fig. 9-52.** A CT scan of a primary cerebral lymphoma. The basal ganglia-periventricular regions have densities resulting from lymphoma (*arrows*) thought clinically to be toxoplasmosis and not visible after autopsy when the brain was sectioned. The location and bilateral symmetry are more suggestive of lymphoma than of infection.

Primary lymphomas in the CNS usually originate from B lymphoid cells, with immunostaining commonly positive with any number of monoclonal antibodies that are reactive to B cells or with rabbit antisera for immunoglobulins.[245] The cases are usually of immunoblastic type, but small, noncleaved lymphomas have been reported.[101,279] Autolysis tends to yield a negative result with immunostaining. Some argue that primary CNS lymphoproliferative disorders are reactive rather than neoplastic.[245] These lesions are aggressive (Figs. 9-54 to 9-56) and rapidly fatal despite their morphologic or immunologic classification.[279] The tumors may enhance well in radiologic studies, but they may not be discernible grossly even when they are extensively infiltrating microscopically. This occurs because a mass effect is not always appreciated and the tumor blends imperceptibly with the surrounding edematous tissue. Lymphomas may involve the enlarged, edematous areas of deep white matter, with necrosis leaving parts of the tumor yellow; hemorrhagic areas may be present. Using CT scans as a guide has been very helpful in taking sections of the brain for microscopic study. The tumor replaces CNS tissue with wide infiltration, with the lymphoma cells spreading in perivascular spaces or infiltrating the parenchyma directly (Fig. 9-56). Involvement of vascular

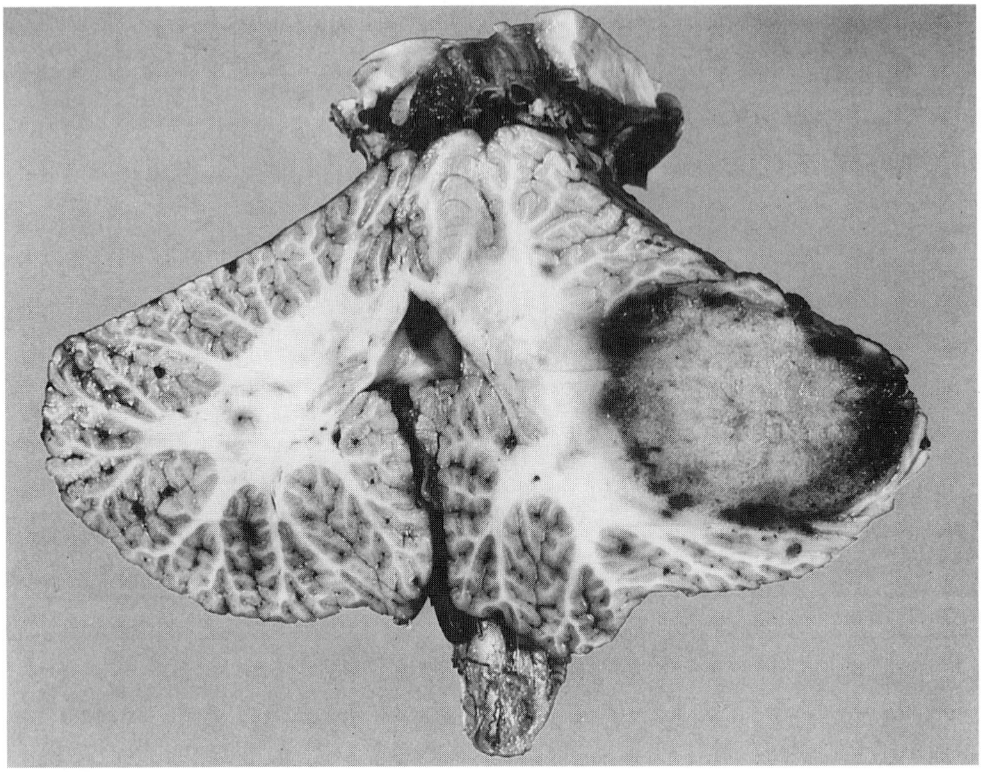

**Fig. 9-53.** A primary lymphoma in the cerebellum in the same brain as shown in Fig. 9-14. The large lymphomatous deposit demonstrates hemorrhage, a granular cut surface, and darkening. Compare with the lighter, homogeneous toxoplasmic lesion in Fig. 9-42.

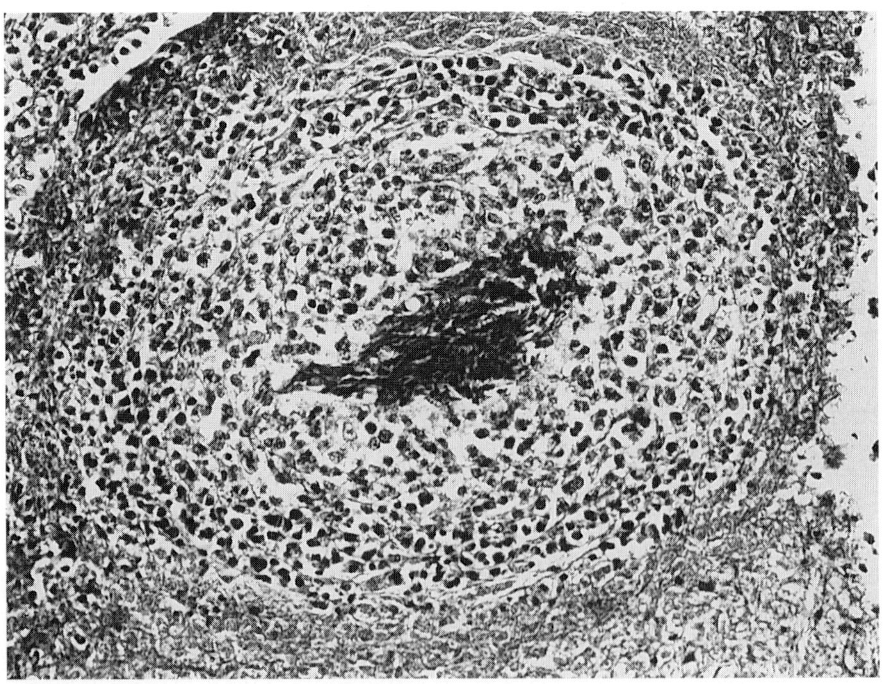

**Fig. 9-54.** Primary cerebral lymphoma. A vascular wall is completely infiltrated by lymphoma cells. (H&E; ×200.)

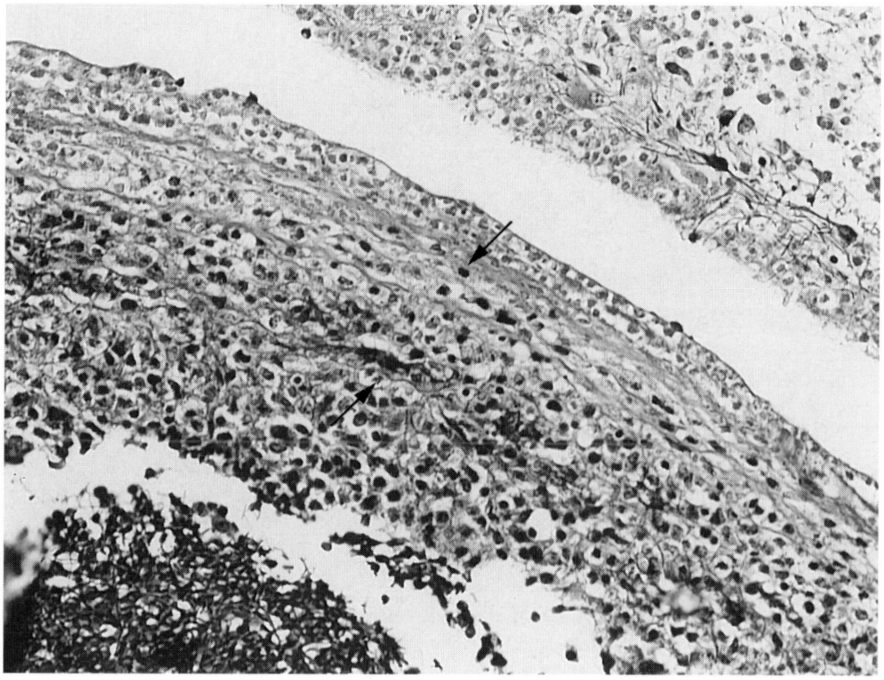

**Fig. 9-55.** Primary cerebral lymphoma. Another blood vessel from the same region as in Fig. 9-54 has mural tumor infiltration (*between arrows*). Here the vascular lumen also contains lymphoma, and centrally (*lower left*) the lumen contains a thrombus. (H&E; ×200.)

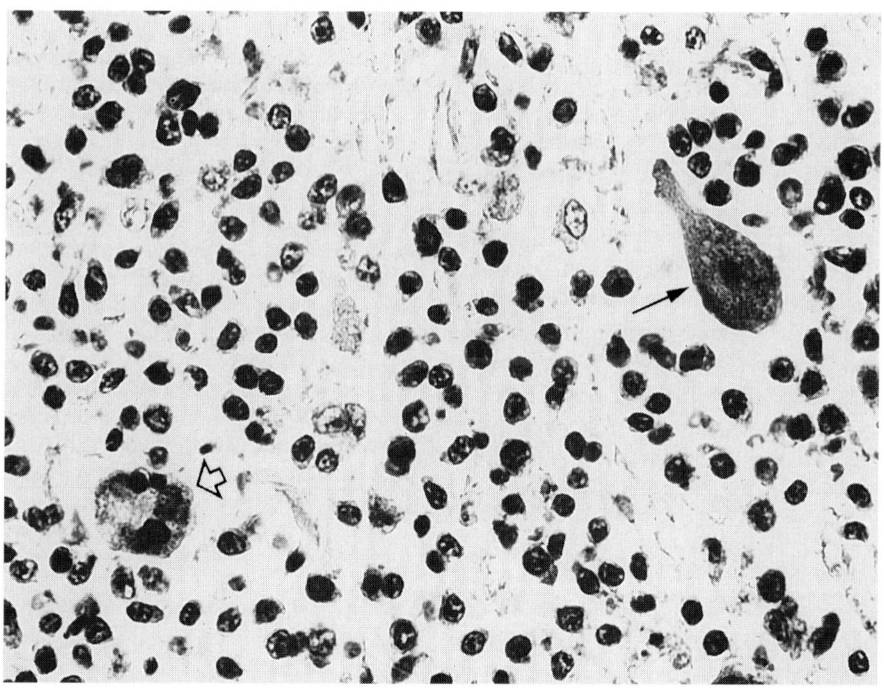

**Fig. 9-56.** Primary cerebral lymphoma. This pleomorphic B-cell tumor is from the case shown in Fig. 9-52. Infiltration is highlighted by the presence of a residual neocortical neuron (*arrow*). Multinucleated giant cells (*arrowhead*) are abundant in this tumor. (H&E; ×500.)

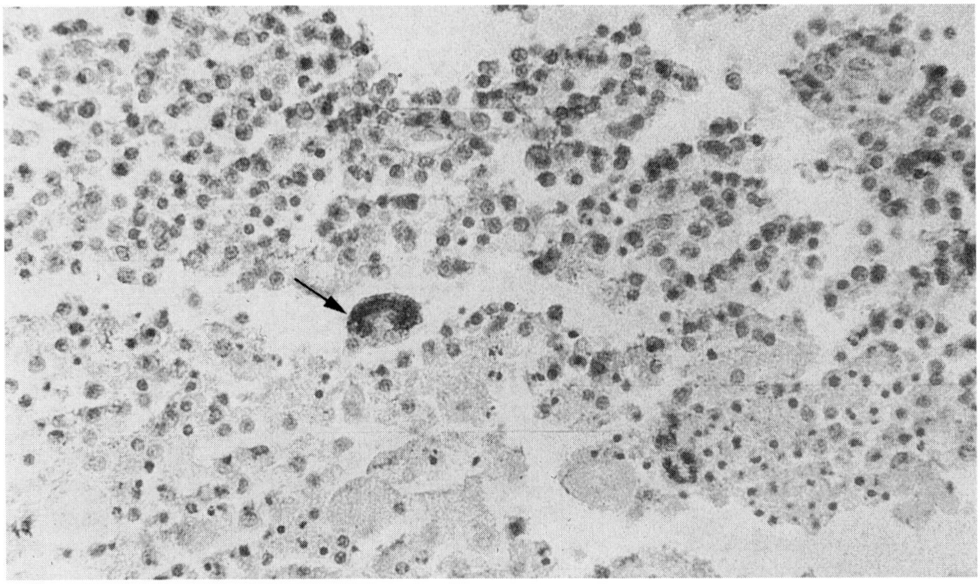

**Fig. 9-57.** An HIV determinant in primary cerebral lymphoma. A macrophage (*arrow*) within the lymphoma is immunoreactive for HIV core protein p24. (Mouse monoclonal anti-p24, DuPont-NEN Products; ×400.)

walls is exceptional (Figs. 9-54, 9-55). Peculiar to some cases is an inordinate number of macrophages and even multinucleated giant cells intermixed with lymphoma cells (Fig. 9-56). Some of the multinucleated cells in the lymphomas are immunoreactive for HIV antigens (Fig. 9-57).

### Metastatic Tumors

The two frequently occurring tumors of AIDS—Kaposi's sarcoma and systemic lymphoma—may be metastatic to the brain and meninges. Systemic lymphomas in AIDS patients metastasize to the leptomeninges, or even as small parenchymal masses. Several cases of CNS metastases from Kaposi's sarcoma have been reported.* There is nothing unusual about the appearance of the metastases on CT scans,[238] although, as expected, secondary tumors tend to be smaller than the primary tumors. The microscopic appearance of both Kaposi's sarcoma and the lymphomas is the same in the metastatic deposits as in the primary lesions.[206]

## ACKNOWLEDGMENT

Dr. Jerrold M. Ward of the Frederick Cancer Research Center, National Cancer Institute, performed the HIV immunostaining for this chapter, and we are greatly indebted to him for his efforts.

* Refs. 81, 104, 162, 163, 228.

## REFERENCES

1. Ahmad N, and Venkatesan S: *Nef* protein of HIV-1 is a transcriptional repressor of HIV-1 LTR, Science 241:1481-1485, 1988.
2. Allen IV, and Kirk J: Demyelinating diseases. In Adams JH, and Duchen LW, eds: Greenfield's Neuropathology, ed 5. New York, 1992, Oxford University Press.
3. Ambler MW, Homans AC, and O'Shea PA: An unusual central nervous system infection in a young immunocompromised host, Arch Pathol Lab Med 110:497-501, 1986.
4. Ambros RA, and others: The acquired immunodeficiency syndrome in intravenous drug abusers and patients with a sexual risk: clinical and postmortem comparisons, Hum Pathol 18: 1109-1114, 1987.
5. Anders KH, and others: The neuropathology of AIDS: UCLA experience and review, Am J Pathol 124:537-558, 1986.
6. Anders KH, and others: Multifocal necrotizing leukoencephalopathy with pontine predilection in immunosuppressed patients: a clinicopathologic review of 16 cases, Hum Pathol 24: 897-904, 1993.
7. Angeletti RH, and Hickey WF: A neuroendocrine marker in tissues of the immune system, Science 230:89-90, 1985.
8. Apostolski S, and others: The gp120 glycoprotein of human immunodeficiency virus type 1 binds to sensory ganglion neurons, Ann Neurol 34:855-863, 1993.
9. Appleman ME, and others: Cerebrospinal fluid abnormalities in patients without AIDS who are seropositive for the human immunodeficiency virus, J Infect Dis 158:193-199, 1988.
10. Artigas J, and others: Spongiform encephalopathy in AIDS dementia complex: report of five cases, J Acquir Immune Defic Syndr 2:374-381, 1989.
11. Asbury AK: Diagnostic considerations in Guillain-Barré syndrome, Ann Neurol 9(Suppl):1-5, 1981.
12. Baba H, and others: Characterization of the antigenic determinant on HSB-2 cells shared with myelin-associated glycoprotein (MAG) using monoclonal antibodies, J Neuroimmunol 13:89-97, 1986.

13. Balasingam V, and others: Reactive astrogliosis in the neonatal mouse brain and its modulation by cytokines, J Neurosci 14: 846-856, 1994.
14. Bartholomaeus WN, and others: Multiple autoantibodies following cytomegalovirus infection: virus distribution and specificity of autoantibodies, Immunology 64:397-405, 1988.
15. Bauer HC, and Hurtenbach U: Murine cortical brain cells are autoantigenic from a distinct developmental stage onwards, J Neuroimmunol 12:1-13, 1986.
16. Bedinger P, and others: Internalization of the human immunodeficiency virus does not require the cytoplasmic domain of CD4, Nature 334:162-165, 1988.
17. Behar R, Wiley C, and McCutchan JA: Cytomegalovirus polyradiculoneuropathy in acquired immune deficiency syndrome, Neurology 37:557-561, 1987.
18. Belman AL, and others: Neurological complications in infants and children with acquired immune deficiency syndrome, Ann Neurol 18:560-566, 1985.
19. Belman AL, and others: AIDS: calcification of the basal ganglia in infants and children, Neurology 36:1192-1199, 1986.
20. Berger JR, and others: Progressive multifocal leukoencephalopathy associated with human immunodeficiency virus infection: a review of the literature with a report of sixteen cases, Ann Intern Med 107:78-87, 1987.
21. Berger JR, and others: Relapsing and remitting human immunodeficiency virus-associated leukoencephalomyelopathy, Ann Neurol 31:34-38, 1992.
22. Bergmann M, and others: AIDS-myelopathy. A neuropathological study, Pathol Res Pract 189:58-65, 1993.
23. Bloom DE, and Carliner G: The economic impact of AIDS in the United States, Science 239:604-610, 1988.
24. Blue MC, and Rosenblum WI: Granulomatous angiitis of the brain with herpes zoster and varicella encephalitis, Arch Pathol Lab Med 107:126-128, 1983.
25. Bockstahler L, and others: Location of HIV genome in brains of AIDS patients. Abstract, Clin Neuropathol 12(suppl. 1):S1, 1993.
26. Bornstein RA, and others: Neuropsychological performance in symptomatic and asymptomatic HIV infection, AIDS 7:519-524, 1993.
27. Bredesen DE, Levy RM, and Rosenblum ML: The neurology of human immunodeficiency virus infection, Q J Med 68:665-677, 1988.
28. Britton CB, and others: A new complication of AIDS: thoracic myelitis caused by herpes simplex virus, Neurology 35:1071-1074, 1985.
29. Broderick DF, and others: White matter lesions and cerebral atrophy on MR images in patients with and without AIDS dementia complex, AJR 161:177-181, 1993.
30. Budka H: Multinucleated giant cells in brain: a hallmark of the acquired immune deficiency syndrome (AIDS), Acta Neuropathol (Berl) 69:253-258, 1986.
31. Budka H, and others: Brain pathology induced by infection with the human immunodeficiency virus (HIV). A histological, immunocytochemical, and electron microscopical study of 100 autopsy cases, Acta Neuropathol (Berl) 75:185-198, 1987.
32. Canessa A, and others: An in vitro model for *Toxoplasma* infection in man: interaction between $CD4^+$ monoclonal T cells and macrophages results in killing of trophozoites, J Immunol 140: 3580-3588, 1988.
33. Carne CA, and others: Acute encephalopathy coincident with seroconversion for anti-HTLV-III, Lancet 2:1206-1208, 1985.
34. Carter JB, Hamill RJ, and Matoba AY: Bilateral syphilitic optic neuritis in a patient with a positive test for HIV, Arch Ophthalmol 105:1485-1486, 1987.
35. Casareale D, and others: Cytomegalovirus enhances lysis of HIV-infected T lymphoblasts, Int J Cancer 44:124-130, 1989.
36. Cavanagh JB: The 'dying back' process. A common denominator in many naturally occurring and toxic neuropathies, Arch Pathol Lab Med 103:659-664, 1979.
37. Centers for Disease Control and Prevention: Revised classification system for HIV infection and expanded surveillance case definition for AIDS among adolescents and adults, MMWR 41 (no. RR-17), 1992.
38. Chambers RB, and others: Varicella-zoster retinitis in human immunodeficiency virus infection, Arch Ophthalmol 107:960-961, 1989.
39. Chavanet P, and others: Immune mechanisms in HIV-related neuropathies, Lancet 2:812-813, 1989.
40. Cheng-Mayer C, and others: Human immunodeficiency virus can productively infect cultured human glial cells, Proc Natl Acad Sci USA 84:3526-3530, 1987.
41. Chiodi F, and others: Infection of brain-derived cells with the human immunodeficiency virus, J Virol 61:1244-1247, 1987.
42. Cohen JA, and Laudenslager M: Autonomic nervous system involvement in patients with human immunodeficiency virus infection, Neurology 39:1111-1112, 1989.
43. Cornblath DR, and others: Inflammatory demyelinating peripheral neuropathies associated with human T-cell lymphotropic virus type III infection, Ann Neurol 21:32-40, 1987.
44. Craddock C, and others: Cardiorespiratory arrest and autonomic neuropathy in AIDS, Lancet 2:16-18, 1987.
45. Cserr HF, Harling-Berg CJ, and Knopf PM: Drainage of brain extracellular fluid into blood and deep cervical lymph and its immunological significance, Brain Pathol 2:269-276, 1992.
46. Cuadrado LM, and others: Cerebral mucormycosis in two cases of acquired immunodeficiency syndrome, Arch Neurol 45:109-111, 1988.
47. Curran JW, and others: Epidemiology of HIV infection and AIDS in the United States, Science 239:610-616, 1988.
48. Dalakas MC, and others: Polymyositis associated with AIDS retrovirus, JAMA 256:2381-2383, 1986.
49. Dalakas MC, and Trapp BD: Thymosin $\beta_4$ is a shared antigen between lymphoid cells and oligodendrocytes of normal human brain, Ann Neurol 19:349-355, 1986.
50. Dalakas MC, and Pezeshkpour GH: Neuromuscular diseases associated with human immunodeficiency virus infection, Ann Neurol 23 (Suppl):S38-S48, 1988.
51. Davis LE, and others: Early viral brain invasion in iatrogenic human immunodeficiency virus infection, Neurology 42:1736-1739, 1992.
52. Davis MG, and others: Immediate-early gene region of human cytomegalovirus trans-activates the promoter of human immunodeficiency virus, Proc Natl Acad Sci USA 84:8642-8646, 1987.
53. de la Monte SM, and others: Subacute encephalomyelitis of AIDS and its relation to HTLV-III infection, Neurology 37:562-569, 1987.
54. de la Monte SM, and others: Peripheral neuropathy in the acquired immunodeficiency syndrome, Ann Neurol 23:485-492, 1988.
55. Denning DW, and others: Acute myelopathy associated with primary infection with human immunodeficiency virus, Br Med J 294:143-144, 1987.
56. Dewhurst S, and others: Establishment of human glial cell lines chronically infected with the human immunodeficiency virus, Virology 162:151-159, 1988.
57. Diamond DC, and others: Inhibition of $CD4^+$ T cell function by the HIV envelope protein, gp120, J Immunol 141:3715-3717, 1988.
58. Dickens BM: Legal rights and duties in the AIDS epidemic, Science 239:580-586, 1988.

59. Dickson DW, and others: Spinal cord pathology in pediatric acquired immunodeficiency syndrome, Neurology 39:227-235, 1989.
60. Dix RD, and others: Herpes simplex virus type 2 encephalitis in two homosexual men with persistent lymphadenopathy, Ann Neurol 17:203-206, 1985.
61. Drabick JJ, and others: Dicroceliasis (lancet fluke disease) in an HIV seropositive man, JAMA 259:567-568, 1988.
62. Edwards KR, and Pendlebury WW: Central nervous system lymphomas versus toxoplasmosis in a patient with AIDS. Letter-to-the-editor, N Engl J Med 317:1540, 1987.
63. Eidelberg D, and others: Thrombotic cerebral vasculopathy associated with herpes zoster, Ann Neurol 19:7-14, 1986.
64. Eidelberg D, and others: Progressive polyradiculopathy in acquired immune deficiency syndrome, Neurology 36:912-916, 1986.
65. Eilbott DJ, and others: Human immunodeficiency virus type 1 in spinal cords of acquired immunodeficiency syndrome patients with myelopathy: expression and replication in macrophages, Proc Natl Acad Sci USA 86:3337-3341, 1989.
66. Elder GA, and Sever JL: Neurologic disorders associated with AIDS retroviral infection, Rev Infect Dis 10:286-302, 1988.
67. Elkin CM, and others: Intracranial lesions in the acquired immunodeficiency syndrome: radiological (computed tomographic) features, JAMA 253:393-396, 1985.
68. Engstrom JW, Lowenstein DH, and Bredesen DE: Cerebral infarctions and transient neurologic deficits associated with acquired immunodeficiency syndrome, Am J Med 86:528-532, 1989.
69. Epstein LG, and others: Neurologic manifestations of human immunodeficiency virus infection in children, Pediatrics 78:678-687, 1986.
70. Esiri MM, and Gay D: Immunological and neuropathological significance of the Virchow-Robin space, J Neurol Sci 100:3-8, 1990.
71. Esiri MM, and Kennedy PGE: Virus diseases. In Adams JH, and Duchen LW, editors: Greenfield's Neuropathology, ed 5. New York, 1992, Oxford University Press.
72. Esiri MM, Morris CS, and Millard PR: Sensory and sympathetic ganglia in HIV-1 infection: immunocytochemical demonstration of HIV-1 viral antigens, increased MHC class II antigen expression and mild reactive inflammation, J Neurol Sci 114: 178-187, 1993.
73. Everall I, Luthert P, and Lantos P: A review of neuronal damage in human immunodeficiency virus infection: its assessment, possible mechanism and relationship to dementia, J Neuropathol Exp Neurol 52:561-566, 1993.
74. Fabry Z, Raine CS, and Hart MN: Nervous tissue as an immune compartment: the dialect of the immune response in the CNS, Immunol Today 15:218-224, 1994.
75. Falloon J, and others: Human immunodeficiency virus infection in children, J Pediatr 114:1-30, 1989.
76. Fauci AS: The human immunodeficiency virus: infectivity and mechanisms of pathogenesis, Science 239:617-622, 1988.
77. Felgenhauer K, Lüer W, and Poser S: Chronic HIV encephalitis, J Neuroimmunol 20:141-144, 1988.
78. Ferreiro JA, and Vinters HV: Pathology of the pituitary gland in patients with the acquired immune deficiency syndrome (AIDS), Pathology 20:211-215, 1988.
79. Fiala M, and others: AIDS dementia complex complicated by cytomegalovirus encephalopathy, J Neurol 240:223-231, 1993.
80. Fineberg HV: Education to prevent AIDS: prospects and obstacles, Science 239:592-596, 1988.
81. Fischer P-A, and Enzensberger W: Neurological complications in AIDS, J Neurol 234:269-279, 1987.
82. Fisher AG, and others: Biologically diverse molecular variants within a single HIV-1 isolate, Nature 334:444-447, 1988.
83. Folks TM, and others: Infection and replication of HIV-1 in purified progenitor cells of normal human bone marrow, Science 242:919-922, 1988.
84. Freeman WR, and others: Prevalence and significance of acquired immunodeficiency syndrome-related retinal microvasculopathy, Am J Ophthalmol 107:229-235, 1989.
85. Frenkel JK: Toxoplasmosis. In Marcial-Rojas RA, editor: Pathology of Protozoal and Helminthic Diseases, with Clinical Correlation. Baltimore, 1971, Williams & Wilkins.
86. Freund J, and others: Stability and proteolytic domains of Nef protein from human immunodeficiency virus (HIV) type 1, Eur J Biochem 221:811-819, 1994.
87. Friedman DI, Keane JR, and Rhodes RH: When is a stroke not a stroke? Read before The Frank B. Walsh Society, 21st Annual Meeting, 10-11 February, Philadelphia, Pennsylvania, 1989.
88. Fujinami RS, and Oldstone MBA: Amino acid homology between the encephalitogenic site of myelin basic protein and virus: mechanism for autoimmunity, Science 230:1043-1045, 1985.
89. Gabuzda DH, and others: Immunohistochemical identification of HTLV-III antigen in brains of patients with AIDS, Ann Neurol 20:289-295, 1986.
90. Gabuzda DH, and Hirsch MS: Neurologic manifestations of infection with human immunodeficiency virus: clinical features and pathogenesis, Ann Intern Med 107:383-391, 1987.
91. Gallo P, and others: CSF cytokine detection in HIV-1-infected patients: correlation with neurologic disease and clinical utility. Abstract, Clin Neuropathol 12 (Suppl 1):S16, 1993.
92. Garcia JH, and Anderson ML: Circulatory disorders and their effects on the brain. In Davis RL, and Robertson DM editors: Textbook of Neuropathology, ed 2. Baltimore, 1991, Williams and Wilkins.
93. Garcia-Monco JC, and others: Lyme disease concurrent with human immunodeficiency virus infection, Am J Med 87:325-328, 1989.
94. Garson JA, and others: Monoclonal antibodies against human T lymphocytes label Purkinje neurones of many species, Nature 298:375-377, 1982.
95. Gartner S, and others: The role of mononuclear phagocytes in HTLV-III/LAV infection, Science 233:215-219, 1986.
96. Garza BW, and others: HIV-1 and bleach, J Acquir Immune Defic Syndr 7:169-170, 1994.
97. Geller SA: HIV and the autopsy. Editorial, Am J Clin Pathol 94:487-489, 1990.
98. Gendelman HE, and others: Trans-activation of the human immunodeficiency virus long terminal repeat sequence by DNA viruses, Proc Natl Acad Sci USA 83:9759-9763, 1986.
99. Genis P, and others: Cytokines and arachidonic metabolites produced during human immunodeficiency virus (HIV)-infected macrophage-astroglia interactions: implications for the neuropathogenesis of HIV disease, J Exp Med 176:1703-1718, 1992.
100. Ghatak NR, Poon TP, and Zimmerman HM: Toxoplasmosis of the central nervous system in the adult. A light and electron microscopic study of three cases, Arch Pathol 89:337-348, 1970.
101. Gill PS, and others: Primary central nervous system lymphoma in homosexual men: clinical, immunologic, and pathologic features, Am J Med 78:742-748, 1985.
102. Giulian D, and others: Reactive mononuclear phagocytes release neurotoxins after ischemic and traumatic injury to the central nervous system, J Neurosci Res 36:681-693, 1993.
103. Goethe KE, and others: Neuropsychological and neurological function of human immunodeficiency virus seropositive asymptomatic individuals, Arch Neurol 46:129-133, 1989.
104. Gorin FA, and others: Kaposi's sarcoma metastatic to the CNS, Arch Neurol 42:162-165, 1985.

105. Gosztonyi G: The rate of transcription and translation of HIV genes in HIV encephalitis. Abstract, Clin Neuropathol 12 (Suppl 1):S11, 1993.
106. Goudsmit J, and others: Expression of human immunodeficiency virus antigen (HIV-Ag) in serum and cerebrospinal fluid during acute and chronic infection, Lancet 2:177-180, 1986.
107. Goudsmit J, and others: Intrathecal synthesis of antibodies to HTLV-III in patients without AIDS or AIDS related complex, Br Med J 292:1231-1234, 1986.
108. Goudsmit J, and others: Intra-blood-brain barrier synthesis of human immunodeficiency virus antigen and antibody in humans and chimpanzees, Proc Natl Acad Sci USA 84:3876-3880, 1987.
109. Gould IA, Belok LC, and Handwerger S: *Listeria monocytogenes:* a rare cause of opportunistic infection in the acquired immunodeficiency syndrome (AIDS) and a new cause of meningitis in AIDS. A case report, AIDS Res 2:231-234, 1986.
110. Grant I, and others: Evidence for early central nervous system involvement in the acquired immunodeficiency syndrome (AIDS) and other human immunodeficiency virus (HIV) infections: studies with neurophysiologic testing and magnetic resonance imaging, Ann Intern Med 107:828-836, 1987.
111. Graus F, and others: Acute necrotic myelopathy associated with influenza vaccination, Lancet 1:1311-1312, 1987.
112. Gray F, and others: Leukoencephalopathy with multinucleated giant cells containing human immune deficiency virus-like particles and multiple opportunistic cerebral infections in one patient with AIDS, Acta Neuropathol (Berl) 73:99-104, 1987.
113. Gray F, and others: Pathology of the central nervous system in 40 cases of acquired immune deficiency syndrome (AIDS), Neuropathol Appl Neurobiol 14:365-380, 1988.
114. Gray F, and others: Early brain changes in HIV infection: neuropathological study of 11 HIV seropositive, non-AIDS cases, J Neuropathol Exp Neurol 51:177-185, 1992.
115. Gressens P, and others: Detection of viral DNA in neonatal herpes encephalitis autopsy tissues by solution-phase PCR: comparison with pathology and immunohistochemistry, Brain Pathol 3:237-250, 1993.
116. Gurley RJ, and others: CD4$^+$ lymphocyte function with early human immunodeficiency virus infection, Proc Natl Acad Sci USA 86:1993-1997, 1989.
117. Haase AT: Pathogenesis of lentivirus infections, Nature 322: 130-136, 1986.
118. Helweg-Larsen S, and others: Myelopathy in AIDS. A clinical and electrophysiological study of 23 Danish patients, Acta Neurol Scand 77:64-73, 1988.
119. Hénin D, and others: Neuropathology of the spinal cord in the acquired immunodeficiency syndrome, Hum Pathol 23:1106-1114, 1992.
120. Ho DD, and others: Isolation of HTLV-III from cerebrospinal fluid and neural tissues of patients with neurologic syndromes related to the acquired immunodeficiency syndrome, N Engl J Med 313:1493-1497, 1985.
121. Ho DD, Rota TR, and Hirsch MS: Infection of monocyte/macrophages by human T lymphotropic virus type III, J Clin Invest 77:1712-1715, 1986.
122. Hockley DJ, and others: Electron microscopy of human immunodeficiency virus, J Gen Virol 69:2455-2469, 1988.
123. Hoffman HL: Acute necrotic myelopathy, Brain 78:377-393, 1955.
124. Holland NR, and others: Cytomegalovirus encephalitis in acquired immunodeficiency syndrome (AIDS), Neurology 44: 507-514, 1994.
125. Hollander H, and Levy JA: Neurologic abnormalities and recovery of human immunodeficiency virus from cerebrospinal fluid, Ann Intern Med 106:692-695, 1987.
126. Hollander H, and Stringari S: Human immunodeficiency virus-associated meningitis: clinical course and correlations, Am J Med 83:813-816, 1987.
127. Horoupian DS, and others: Acquired immune deficiency syndrome and multiple tract degeneration in a homosexual man, Ann Neurol 15:502-505, 1984.
128. Horvat RT, Wood C, and Balachandran N: Transactivation of human immunodeficiency virus promotor by human herpesvirus 6, J Virol 63:970-973, 1989.
129. Houff SA: Neuroimmunology of human immunodeficiency virus infection. In Rosenblum RM, Levy RM, and Bredesen DE, editors: AIDS and the Nervous System. New York, 1988, Raven Press.
130. Hoxie JA, and others: Alteration in T4 (CD4) protein and mRNA synthesis in cells infected with HIV, Science 234:1123-1127, 1986.
131. Italian Multicentre Study: Epidemiology, clinical features, and prognostic factors of paediatric HIV infection, Lancet 2:1043-1045, 1988.
132. Jahnke U, Fischer EH, and Alvord EC Jr: Sequence homology between certain viral proteins and proteins related to encephalomyelitis and neuritis, Science 229:282-284, 1985.
133. Jakobsen J, and others: Progressive neurological dysfunction during latent HIV infection, Br Med J 299:225-228, 1989.
134. Janssen RS, and others: Human immunodeficiency virus (HIV) infection and the nervous system: report from the American Academy of Neurology AIDS Task Force, Neurology 39:119-122, 1989.
135. Janssen RS, and others: Nomenclature and research case definitions for neurologic manifestations of human immunodeficiency virus-type 1 (HIV-1) infection. Report of a Working Group of the American Academy of Neurology AIDS Task Force, Neurology 41:778-785, 1991.
136. Johns DR, Tierney M, Felsenstein D: Alteration in the natural history of neurosyphilis by concurrent infection with the human immunodeficiency virus, N Engl J Med 316:1569-1572, 1987.
137. Johnson RT, McArthur JC, and Narayan O: The neurobiology of human immunodeficiency virus infections, FASEB J 2:2970-2981, 1988.
138. Jones HR Jr, and others: Acute fulminating fatal leukoencephalopathy as the only manifestation of human immunodeficiency virus infection, Ann Neurol 23:519-522, 1988.
139. Joshi VV: Pathology of AIDS in children. In Rosen PP, Fechner RE, editors: Pathology Annual, vol. 24 (part 1). Norwalk, Connecticut, 1989, Appleton & Lange.
140. Källén B, and Nilsson O: Dissociation between histological and clinical signs of experimental auto-immune encephalomyelitis, Acta Pathol Microbiol Immunol Scand 94:159-164, 1986.
141. Kamin SS, and Petito CK: Idiopathic myelopathies with white matter vacuolation in non-acquired immunodeficiency syndrome patients, Hum Pathol 22:816-824, 1991.
142. Kaslow RA, and others: Infection with the human immunodeficiency virus: clinical manifestations and their relationship to immune deficiency: a report from the Multicenter AIDS Cohort Study, Ann Intern Med 107:474-480, 1987.
143. Kato T, and others: Neuropathology of acquired immune deficiency syndrome (AIDS) in 53 autopsy cases with particular emphasis on microglial nodules and multinucleated giant cells, Acta Neuropathol (Berl) 73:287-294, 1987.
144. Katz DA, and Berger JR: Neurosyphilis in acquired immunodeficiency syndrome, Arch Neurol 46:895-898, 1989.
145. Keane JR: Neuro-ophthalmologic signs of AIDS: 50 patients, Neurology 41:841-845, 1991.

146. Kenney S, and others: An Epstein-Barr virus immediate-early gene product trans-activates gene expression from the human immunodeficiency virus long terminal repeat, Proc Natl Acad Sci USA 85:1652-1656, 1988.
147. Khalili-Shirazi A, Gregson N, and Webb HE: Immunological relationship between a demyelinating RNA enveloped budding virus (Semliki Forest) and brain glycolipids, J Neurol Sci 76:91-103, 1986.
148. Klatt EC: Diagnostic findings in patients with acquired immune deficiency syndrome (AIDS), J Acquir Immune Defic Syndr 1: 459-465, 1988.
149. Kleihues P, and others: Progressive diffuse leukoencephalopathy in patients with acquired immune deficiency syndrome, Acta Neuropathol (Berl) 68:333-339, 1985.
150. Koenig S, and others: Detection of AIDS virus in macrophages in brain tissue from AIDS patients with encephalopathy, Science 233:1089-1093, 1986.
151. Kolson DL, and others: HIV-1 Tat alters normal organization of neurons and astrocytes in primary rodent brain cell cultures: RGD sequence dependence, AIDS Res Hum Retroviruses 9:677-685, 1993.
152. Koyanagi Y, and others: Cytokines alter production of HIV-1 from primary mononuclear phagocytes, Science 241:1673-1675, 1988.
153. Krupp LB, and others: Progressive multifocal leukoencephalopathy: clinical and radiographic features, Ann Neurol 17:344-349, 1985.
154. Kuchelmeister K, and others: Progressive multifocal leukoencephalopathy (PML) in the acquired immunodeficiency syndrome (AIDS): a neuropathological autopsy study of 21 cases, Pathol Res Pract 189:163-173, 1993.
155. Lantos PL, Tighe JR, and Bateman NT: Post-mortem neuropathological studies in AIDS, Lancet 2:1075-1076, 1988.
156. Lantos PL, and others: Neuropathology of the brain in HIV infection, Lancet 1:309-311, 1989.
157. Lassmann H, and others: Bone marrow derived elements and resident microglia in brain inflammation, Glia 7:19-24, 1993.
158. Laure F, and others: Detection of HIV1 DNA in infants and children by means of the polymerase chain reaction, Lancet 2: 538-541, 1988.
159. Lenhardt TM, Super MA, and Wiley CA: Neuropathological changes in an asymptomatic HIV seropositive man, Ann Neurol 23:209-210, 1988.
160. Levy JA, and others: Isolation of AIDS-associated retroviruses from cerebrospinal fluid and brain of patients with neurological symptoms, Lancet 2:586-588, 1985.
161. Levy RM, Bredesen DE, and Rosenblum ML: Neurological manifestations of the acquired immunodeficiency syndrome (AIDS): experience at UCSF and review of the literature, J Neurosurg 62:475-495, 1985.
162. Levy RM, Rosenbloom S, and Perrett LV: Neuroradiologic findings in AIDS: a review of 200 cases, AJR 147:977-983, 1986.
163. Levy RM, and Bredesen DE: Central nervous system dysfunction in acquired immunodeficiency syndrome, J Acquir Immune Defic Syndr 1:41-64, 1988.
164. Levy RM, and others: Neuroepidemiology of acquired immunodeficiency syndrome, J Acquir Immune Defic Syndr 1:31-40, 1988.
165. Lieberman AP, and others: Production of tumor necrosis factor and other cytokines by astrocytes stimulated with lipopolysaccharide or a neurotropic virus, Proc Natl Acad Sci USA 86:6348-6352, 1989.
166. Liebert UG, Linington C, and ter Meulen V: Induction of autoimmune reactions to myelin basic protein in measles virus encephalitis in Lewis rats, J Neuroimmunol 17:103-118, 1988.
167. Lindenberg R, and Haymaker W: Tissue reactions in the gray matter of the central nervous system. In Haymaker W, and Adams RD, eds: Histology and Histopathology of the Nervous System, vol. I. Springfield, Illinois, 1982, Charles C Thomas.
168. Lloyd A, and others: Antibodies to HIV are produced within the central nervous system of all subjects with all categories of HIV infection, Aust NZ J Med 18:854-860, 1988.
169. Luft BJ, and others: Toxoplasmic encephalitis in patients with acquired immune deficiency syndrome, JAMA 252:913-917, 1984.
170. Luft BJ, Remington JS: Toxoplasmic encephalitis, J Infect Dis 157:1-6, 1988.
171. Lui K-J, Darrow WW, and Rutherford GW III: A model-based estimate of the mean incubation period for AIDS in homosexual men, Science 240:1333-1335, 1988.
172. Lusso P, and others: Productive dual infection of human $CD4^+$ T lymphocytes by HIV-1 and HHV-6, Nature 337:370-373, 1989.
173. Maddon PJ, and others: The T4 gene encodes the AIDS virus receptor and is expressed in the immune system and the brain, Cell 47:333-348, 1986.
174. Maddon PJ, and others: HIV infection does not require endocytosis of its receptor, CD4, Cell 54:865-874, 1988.
175. Mah V, and others: Abnormalities of peripheral nerve in patients with human immunodeficiency virus infection, Ann Neurol 24:713-717, 1988.
176. Mahieux F, and others: Acute myeloradiculitis due to cytomegalovirus as the initial manifestation of AIDS, J Neurol Neurosurg Psychiatry 52:270-274, 1989.
177. Maier H, and others: Vacuolar myelopathy with multinucleated giant cells in the acquired immune deficiency syndrome (AIDS). Light and electron microscopic distribution of human immunodeficiency virus (HIV) antigens, Acta Neuropathol (Berl) 78:497-503, 1989.
178. Marion RW, and others: Human T-cell lymphotropic virus type III (HTLV-III) embryopathy: a new dysmorphic syndrome associated with intrauterine HTLV-III infection, Am J Dis Child 140: 638-640, 1986.
179. Marshall VG, and others: Deep white matter infarction: correlation of MR imaging and histopathologic findings, Radiology 167:517-522, 1988.
180. Martinez AJ, and Visvesvara GS: Free-living amebic infection in immuno-compromised patients. Abstract, Clin Neuropathol 12:257, 1993.
181. Masliah E, and others: Selective neuronal vulnerability in HIV encephalitis, J Neuropathol Exp Neurol 51:585-593, 1992.
182. McArthur JB: Neurologic manifestations of AIDS, Medicine (Baltimore) 66:407-437, 1987.
183. McArthur JC, and others: Cerebrospinal fluid abnormalities in homosexual men with and without neuropsychiatric findings, Ann Neurol 23 (Suppl):S34-S37, 1988.
184. McArthur JC, and others: Neuropathological changes in early HIV-1 dementia, Ann Neurol 26:681-684, 1989.
185. Medley GF, and others: The distribution of the incubation period for the acquired immunodeficiency syndrome (AIDS), Proc R Soc Lond B Biol Sci 233:367-377, 1988.
186. Merrill JE, and others: Induction of interleukin-1 and tumor necrosis factor alpha in brain cultures by human immunodeficiency virus type 1, J Virol 66:2217-2225, 1992.
187. Meyenhofer MF, and others: Ultrastructural morphology and intracellular production of human immunodeficiency virus (HIV) in brain, J Neuropathol Exp Neurol 46:474-484, 1987.
188. Miller RF, and Semple SJG: Autonomic neuropathy in AIDS, Lancet 2:343-344, 1987.
189. Miller RG, and others: Peripheral nervous system dysfunction in acquired immunodeficiency syndrome. In Rosenblum ML, Levy RM, and Bredesen DE, eds: AIDS and the Nervous System. New York, 1988, Raven Press.

190. Mirra SS, and del Rio C: The fine structure of acquired immunodeficiency syndrome encephalopathy, Arch Pathol Lab Med 113:858-865, 1989.
191. Mizusawa H, and others: Cerebrovascular lesions in acquired immune deficiency syndrome (AIDS), Acta Neuropathol (Berl) 76:451-457, 1988.
192. Moelling K: Gene products and replication mechanism of HIV. In Kubicki S, and others, editors: HIV and the Nervous System. Proceedings of the Symposium on Neurological Aspects in AIDS. Stuttgart, 1988, Gustav Fischer.
193. Montagnier L, and others: Adaptation of lymphadenopathy associated virus (LAV) to replication in EBV-transformed B lymphoblastoid cell lines, Science 225:63-66, 1984.
194. Morgello S, and others: Varicella-zoster virus leukoencephalitis and cerebral vasculopathy, Arch Pathol Lab Med 112:173-177, 1988.
195. Mosca JD, and others: Activation of human immunodeficiency virus by herpesvirus infection: identification of a region within the long terminal repeat that responds to a trans-acting factor encoded by herpes simplex virus 1, Proc Natl Acad Sci USA 84:7408-7412, 1987.
196. Mosca L, Costanzi G, and Antonacci C: Hypophyseal pathology in AIDS, Histol Histopathol 7:291-300, 1992.
197. Moseley JI, Molinari GF, and Walker AE: Respirator brain: report of a survey and review of current concepts, Arch Pathol Lab Med 100:61-64, 1976.
198. Moskowitz LB, and others: The neuropathology of acquired immune deficiency syndrome, Arch Pathol Lab Med 108:867-872, 1984.
199. Murray N, and Steck AJ: Indication of a possible role in a demyelinating neuropathy for an antigen shared between myelin and NK cells, Lancet 1:711-712, 1984.
200. Nath A, Jankovic J, and Pettigrew LC: Movement disorders and AIDS, Neurology 37:37-41, 1987.
201. Navia BA, Jordan BD, and Price RW: The AIDS dementia complex: I. Clinical features, Ann Neurol 19:517-524, 1986.
202. Navia BA, and others: The AIDS dementia complex: II. Neuropathology. Ann Neurol 19:525-535, 1986.
203. Navia BA, and Price RW: The acquired immunodeficiency syndrome dementia complex as the presenting or sole manifestation of human immunodeficiency virus infection, Arch Neurol 44:65-69, 1987.
204. Nelson JA, and others: HIV and HCMV coinfect brain cells in patients with AIDS, Virology 165:286-290, 1988.
205. Nielsen SL, and others: Subacute encephalitis in acquired immune deficiency syndrome: a postmortem study, Am J Clin Pathol 82:678-682, 1984.
206. Nielsen SL, and Davis RL: Neuropathology of acquired immunodeficiency syndrome. In Rosenblum M, Levy RM, and Bredesen DE, editors: AIDS and the Nervous System. New York, 1988, Raven Press.
207. Nuovo GJ, and others: *In situ* detection of polymerase chain reaction-amplified HIV-1 nucleic acids and tumor necrosis factor-$\alpha$ RNA in the central nervous system, Am J Pathol 144:659-666, 1994.
208. Nyberg M, Suni J, and Haltia M: Isolation of human immunodeficiency virus (HIV) at autopsy one to six days postmortem, Am J Clin Pathol 94:422-425, 1990.
209. Oldstone MBA, and others: Virus-induced alterations in homeostasis: alterations in differentiated functions of infected cells in vivo, Science 218:1125-1127, 1982.
210. Orenstein JM, and Jannotta F: Human immunodeficiency virus and papovavirus infections in acquired immunodeficiency syndrome: an ultrastructural study of three cases, Hum Pathol 19: 350-361, 1988.
211. Orenstein JM, and others: Cytoplasmic assembly and accumulation of human immunodeficiency virus types 1 and 2 in recombinant human colony-stimulating factor-1-treated human monocytes: an ultrastructural study, J Virol 62:2578-2586, 1988.
212. Oster S, and others: Cerebral atrophy in AIDS: a stereological study, Acta Neuropathol (Berl) 85:617-622, 1993.
213. Ostrove JM, and others: Activation of the human immunodeficiency virus by herpes simplex virus type 1, J Virol 61:3726-3732, 1987.
214. Pahwa R, Good RA, and Pahwa S: Prematurity, hypogammaglobulinemia, and neuropathology with human immunodeficiency virus (HIV) infection, Proc Natl Acad Sci USA 84:3826-3830, 1987.
215. Parmentier HK, and others: Epitopes of human immunodeficiency virus regulatory proteins *tat*, *nef*, and *rev* are expressed in normal human tissue, Am J Pathol 141:1209-1216, 1992.
216. Pauza CD, and Price TM: Human immunodeficiency virus infection of T cells and monocytes proceeds via receptor-mediated endocytosis, J Cell Biol 107:959-968, 1988.
217. Peault B, and others: Phylogenetically conserved antigen on nerve cells and lymphocytes resembles myelin-associated glycoprotein, Proc Natl Acad Sci USA 84:814-818, 1987.
218. Perrella O, and others: Cerebrospinal fluid cytokines in AIDS dementia complex, J Neurol 239:387-388, 1992.
219. Pert CB, and others: AIDS and its dementia as a neuropeptide disorder: role of VIP receptor blockade by human immunodeficiency virus envelope, Ann Neurol 23 (Suppl):S71-S73, 1988.
220. Petit AJC, and others: Decreased accessory cell function by human monocytic cells after infection with HIV, J Immunol 140: 1485-1489, 1988.
221. Petito CK, and others: Vacuolar myelopathy pathologically resembling subacute combined degeneration in patients with the acquired immunodeficiency syndrome, N Engl J Med 312:874-879, 1985.
222. Petito CK, and others: Neuropathology of acquired immunodeficiency syndrome (AIDS): an autopsy review, J Neuropathol Exp Neurol 45:635-646, 1986.
223. Petito CK, Vecchio D, and Chen Y-T: HIV antigen and DNA in AIDS spinal cords correlate with macrophage infiltration but not with vacuolar myelopathy J Neuropathol Exp Neurol 53: 86-94, 1994.
224. Piette AM, and others: Acute neuropathy coincident with seroconversion for anti-LAV/HTLV-III, Lancet 1:852, 1986.
225. Pitts OM, and others: Ultrastructural changes associated with retroviral replication in central nervous system capillary endothelial cells, Lab Invest 56:401-409, 1987.
226. Pomerantz RJ, and others: Infection of the retina by human immunodeficiency virus type I, N Engl J Med 317:1643-1647, 1987.
227. Post MJD, and others: Cranial CT in acquired immunodeficiency syndrome: spectrum of diseases and optimal contrast enhancement technique, AJR 145:929-940, 1985.
228. Post MJD, and others: Cytomegalic inclusion virus encephalitis in patients with AIDS: CT, clinical, and pathologic correlation, AJR 146:1229-1234, 1986.
229. Post MJD, and others: CT, MR, and pathology in HIV encephalitis and meningitis, AJR 151:373-380, 1988.
230. Poutiainen E, and others: Cognitive changes as early signs of HIV infection, Acta Neurol Scand 78:49-52, 1988.
231. Power C, and others: Cerebral white matter changes in acquired immunodeficiency syndrome dementia: alterations of the blood-brain barrier, Ann Neurol 34:339-350, 1993.
232. Price RW, and others: The brain in AIDS: central nervous system HIV-1 infection and AIDS dementia complex, Science 239: 586-592, 1988.
233. Prineas JW: Multiple sclerosis: presence of lymphatic capillaries and lymphoid tissue in the brain and spinal cord, Science 203: 1123-1125, 1979.

234. Pulliam L, and others: HIV-1 envelope gp120 alters astrocytes in human brain cultures, AIDS Res Hum Retroviruses 9:439-444, 1993.
235. Pumarola-Sune T, and others: HIV antigen in the brains of patients with the AIDS dementia complex, Ann Neurol 21:490-496, 1987.
236. Quinnan GV Jr, and others: Herpesvirus infections in the acquired immune deficiency syndrome, JAMA 252:72-77, 1984.
237. Raine CS: Demyelinating diseases. In Davis RL, and Robertson DM, editors: Textbook of Neuropathology, ed 2. Baltimore, 1991, Williams & Wilkins.
238. Ramsey RG, and Geremia GK: CNS complications of AIDS: CT and MR findings, AJR 151:449-454, 1988.
239. Rance NE, and others: Gracile tract degeneration in patients with sensory neuropathy and AIDS, Neurology 38:265-271, 1988.
240. Ranki A, and others: Antibodies to recombinant HIV-1 Nef protein detected in HIV-1 infection as well as in nonrisk individuals, J Acquir Immune Defic Syndr 3:348-355, 1990.
241. Reichert CM, and others: Autopsy pathology in the acquired immune deficiency syndrome, Am J Pathol 112:357-382, 1983.
242. Reik L Jr: Disseminated vasculomyelinopathy: an immune complex disease, Ann Neurol 7:291-296, 1980.
243. Resnick L, and others: Intra-blood-brain-barrier synthesis of HTLV-III-specific IgG in patients with neurologic symptoms associated with AIDS or AIDS-related complex, N Engl J Med 313:1498-1504, 1985.
244. Resnick L, and others: Early penetration of the blood-brain barrier by HIV, Neurology 38:9-14, 1988.
245. Rhodes RH: Diagnostic immunostaining of the nervous system. In Taylor CR, editor: Immunomicroscopy: A Diagnostic Tool for the Surgical Pathologist; Major Problems in Pathology; Vol 19. Philadelphia, 1986, WB Saunders.
246. Rhodes RH: Evidence of serum-protein leakage across the blood-brain barrier in the acquired immunodeficiency syndrome, J Neuropathol Exp Neurol 50:171-183, 1991.
247. Rhodes RH: Histopathologic features in the central nervous system of 400 acquired immunodeficiency syndrome cases: implications of rates of occurrence, Hum Pathol 24:1189-1198, 1993.
248. Rhodes RH, and others: Follow-up pathology of cranial CT: pitfalls in clinical-radiological evaluation, Ann Clin Lab Sci 17: 36-51, 1987.
249. Rhodes RH, and others: Progressive multifocal leukoencephalopathy and retroviral encephalitis in acquired immunodeficiency syndrome. Arch Pathol Lab Med 112:1207-1213, 1988.
250. Rhodes RH, and others: Immunohistochemical localization of human immunodeficiency viral antigens in formalin-fixed spinal cord with AIDS myelopathy, Clin Neuropathol 8:22-27, 1989.
251. Rhodes RH, and Ward JM: Immunohistochemistry of human immunodeficiency virus in the central nervous system and an hypothesis concerning the pathogenesis of AIDS meningoencephalomyelitis. In Rotterdam H, and others, editors: Progress in AIDS Pathology, vol. 1. Philadelphia, 1989, Field and Wood.
252. Rhodes RH, and Ward JM: AIDS meningoencephalomyelitis: pathogenesis and changing neuropathologic findings. In Rosen PP, and Fechner RE, editors: Pathology Annual, vol. 26, part 2. Norwalk, Connecticut, 1991, Appleton & Lange.
253. Rhodes RH, and others: Cytomegaloviral (CMV) and human immunodeficiency virus (HIV) coinfection of the brain in AIDS autopsies. Abstract. XII$^{th}$ International Congress of Neuropathology, Toronto, 18 - 23 September, 1994.
254. Richardson EP Jr, Webster H deF: Progressive multifocal leukoencephalopathy: its pathological features. In Sever JL, and Madden DL, editors: Progress in Clinical and Biological Research, vol. 105. Polyomaviruses and Human Neurological Disease. New York, 1983, Alan R Liss.
255. Rosenblum M, and others: Dissociation of AIDS-related vacuolar myelopathy and productive HIV-1 infection of the spinal cord, Neurology 39:892-896, 1989.
256. Rostad SW, and others: Human immunodeficiency virus (HIV) infection in brains with AIDS-related leukoencephalopathy, AIDS Res Hum Retroviruses 3:363-373, 1987.
257. Roy S, and others: Infection of human monocytes/macrophages by HIV-1: effect on secretion of IL-1 activity, Immunology 64: 233-239, 1988.
258. Ryder JW, and others: Progressive encephalitis three months after resolution of cutaneous zoster in a patient with AIDS, Ann Neurol 19:182-188, 1986.
259. Saito Y, and others: Overexpression of *nef* as a marker for restricted HIV-1 infection of astrocytes in postmortem pediatric central nervous tissues, Neurology 44:474-481, 1994.
260. Sano T, and others: Pituitary pathology in acquired immunodeficiency syndrome, Arch Pathol Lab Med 113:1066-1070, 1989.
261. Scaravilli F, and others: Chronic basal meningitis and vasculitis in acquired immunodeficiency syndrome: a possible role for human immunodeficiency virus, Arch Pathol Lab Med 113:192-195, 1989.
262. Scharf D: Neurocysticercosis: two hundred thirty-eight cases from a California hospital, Arch Neurol 45:777-780, 1988.
263. Schmidbauer M, and others: Morphological spectrum, distribution and clinical correlation of white matter lesions in AIDS brains, Neuropathol Appl Neurobiol 18:489-501, 1992.
264. Schmied M, and others: Apoptosis of T lymphocytes in experimental autoimmune encephalomyelitis: evidence for programmed cell death as a mechanism to control inflammation in the brain, Am J Pathol 143:446-452, 1993.
265. Schwarz GA, and Liu C-N: Hereditary (familial) spastic paraplegia: further clinical and pathologic observations, Arch Neurol Psychiatry 75:144-162, 1956.
266. Schwenk J, and others: Spongiform encephalopathy in a patient with acquired immune deficiency syndrome (AIDS), Acta Neuropathol (Berl) 74:389-392, 1987.
267. Shapshak P, and others: HIV-1 in postmortem brain tissue from patients with AIDS: a comparison of different detection techniques, AIDS 6:915-923, 1992.
268. Sharer LR, Cho E-S, and Epstein LG: Multinucleated giant cells and HTLV-III in AIDS encephalopathy, Hum Pathol 16:760, 1985.
269. Sharer LR, and Kapila R: Neuropathologic observations in acquired immunodeficiency syndrome (AIDS), Acta Neuropathol (Berl) 66:188-198, 1985.
270. Sharer LR, and others: Pathologic features of AIDS encephalopathy in children: evidence for LAV/HTLV-III infection of brain, Hum Pathol 17:271-284, 1986.
271. Shaw GM, and others: HTLV-III infection in brains of children and adults with AIDS encephalopathy, Science 227:177-182, 1985.
272. Sheffield HG, and Melton ML: The fine structure and reproduction of *Toxoplasma gondii*, J Parasitol 54:209-226, 1968.
273. Sinclair E, and others: Immunohistochemical changes and PCR detection of HIV provirus DNA in brains of asymptomatic HIV-positive patients, J Neuropathol Exp Neurol 53:43-50, 1994.
274. Singh BM, and others: Spinal cord syndromes in the acquired immune deficiency syndrome, Acta Neurol Scand 73:590-598, 1986.
275. Skolnik PR, Kosloff BR, and Hirsch MS: Bidirectional interactions between human immunodeficiency virus type 1 and cytomegalovirus, J Infect Dis 157:508-514, 1988.
276. Skolnik PR, and others: Dual infection of retina with human immunodeficiency virus type 1 and cytomegalovirus, Am J Ophthalmol 107:361-372, 1989.
277. Smith TW, De Girolami U, and Hickey WF: Neuropathology of immunosuppression, Brain Pathol 2:183-194, 1992.

278. Snider WD, and others: Neurological complications of acquired immune deficiency syndrome: analysis of 50 patients, Ann Neurol 14:403-418, 1983.
279. So YT, Beckstead JH, and Davis RL: Primary central nervous system lymphoma in acquired immune deficiency syndrome: a clinical and pathological study, Ann Neurol 20:566-572, 1986.
280. So YT, and others: Peripheral neuropathy associated with acquired immunodeficiency syndrome: prevalence and clinical features from a population-based survey, Arch Neurol 45:945-948, 1988.
281. Somasundaran M, and Robinson HL: Unexpectedly high levels of HIV-1 RNA and protein synthesis in a cytocidal infection, Science 242:1554-1557, 1988.
282. Srinivasan A, and others: Human immunodeficiency virus replication in human brain cells: brief report, Arch Virol 99:135-141, 1988.
283. Stefansson K, Reder AT, and Antel JP: An epitope shared by central nervous system myelin and peripheral blood macrophages, J Neuroimmunol 12:49-55, 1986.
284. Stein BS, and others: pH-Independent HIV entry into CD4-positive T cells via virus envelope fusion to the plasma membrane, Cell 49:659-668, 1987.
285. Stoler MH, and others: Human T-cell lymphotropic virus type III infection of the central nervous system: a preliminary in situ analysis, JAMA 256:2360-2364, 1986.
286. Stoner GL, and others: JC papovavirus large tumor (T)-antigen expression in brain tissue of acquired immune deficiency syndrome (AIDS) and non-AIDS patients with progressive multifocal leukoencephalopathy, Proc Natl Acad Sci USA 83:2271-2275, 1986.
287. Stricker RB, and others: An AIDS-related cytotoxic autoantibody reacts with a specific antigen on stimulated $CD4^+$ T cells, Nature 327:710-713, 1987.
288. Su TP, London ED, and Jaffe JH: Steroid binding at $\sigma$ receptors suggests a link between endocrine, nervous, and immune systems, Science 240:219-221, 1988.
289. Sze G, and others: Foci of MRI signal (pseudo lesions) anterior to the frontal horns: histologic correlations of a normal finding, AJR 147:331-337, 1986.
290. Tani M, and Ransohoff RM: Do chemokines mediate inflammatory cell invasion of the central nervous system parenchyma? Brain Pathol 4:135-143, 1994.
291. Tornatore C, and others: Persistent human immunodeficiency virus type 1 infection in human fetal glial cells reactivated by T-cell factor(s) or by the cytokines tumor necrosis factor alpha and interleukin-1 beta, J Virol 65:6094-6100, 1991.
292. Tornatore C, and others: HIV-1 infection of subcortical astrocytes in the pediatric central nervous system, Neurology 44: 481-487, 1994.
293. Torres BA, and Johnson HM: Identification of an HIV-1 Nef peptide that binds to HLA class II antigens, Biochem Biophys Res Commun 200:1059-1065, 1994.
294. Tramont EC: Syphilis in the AIDS era. Editorial, N Engl J Med 316:1600-1601, 1987.
295. Treip CS: The hypothalamus and pituitary gland. In Adams JA, Duchen LW, eds: Greenfield's Neuropathology, ed 5. New York, 1992, Oxford University Press.
296. Tsukada N, and others: Demyelinating neuropathy associated with hepatitis B virus infection—detection of immune complexes composed of hepatitis B virus surface antigen, J Neurol Sci 77:203-216, 1987.
297. Tucker T, and others: Cytomegalovirus and herpes simplex virus ascending myelitis in a patient with acquired immune deficiency syndrome, Ann Neurol 18:74-79, 1985.
298. Tyor WR, and others: Cytokine expression of macrophages in HIV-1-associated vacuolar myelopathy, Neurology 43:1002-1009, 1993.
299. Varmus H: Retroviruses, Science 240:1427-1435, 1988.
300. Vazeux R, and others: AIDS subacute encephalitis: identification of HIV-infected cells, Am J Pathol 126:403-410, 1987.
301. Veron JP, and others: Acute necrotic myelopathy, Eur Neurol 11:83-96, 1974.
302. Vinters HV, and others: Necrotizing vasculitis of the nervous system in a patient with AIDS-related complex, Neuropathol Appl Neurobiol 14:417-424, 1988.
303. Vinters HV, and others: Cytomegalovirus in the nervous system of patients with the acquired immune deficiency syndrome, Brain 112:245-268, 1989.
304. Visvesvara GS: Free-living pathogenic amoebae. In Lennette EH, and others, editors: Manual of Clinical Microbiology, ed 3. Washington, DC, 1980, American Society for Microbiology.
305. Vollmer TL, and others: Depletion of T-$4^+$ lymphocytes with monoclonal antibody reactivates toxoplasmosis in the central nervous system: a model of superinfection in AIDS, J Immunol 138:3737-3741, 1987.
306. von Einsiedel RW, and others: Progressive multifocal leukoencephalopathy in AIDS: a clinicopathologic study and review of the literature, J Neurol 240:391-406, 1993.
307. Wahl SM, and others: HIV-1 and its envelope glycoprotein down-regulate chemotactic ligand receptors and chemotactic function of peripheral blood monocytes, J Immunol 142:3553-3559, 1989.
308. Ward JM, and others: Immunohistochemical localization of human and simian immunodeficiency viral antigens in fixed tissue sections, Am J Pathol 127:199-205, 1987.
309. Webb M, and Barclay AN: Localisation of the MRC OX-2 glycoprotein on the surface of neurones, J Neurochem 43:1061-1067, 1984.
310. Weidenheim KM, Epshteyn I, and Lyman WD: Immunocytochemical identification of T-cells in HIV-1 encephalitis: implications for pathogenesis of CNS disease, Mod Pathol 6:167-174, 1993.
311. Weigent DA, and others: The HTLV-III envelope protein contains a hexapeptide homologous to a region of interleukin-2 that binds to the interleukin-2 receptor, Biochem Biophys Res Commun 139:367-374, 1986.
312. Weis S, Haug H, and Budka H: Astroglial changes in the cerebral cortex of AIDS brains: a morphometric and immunohistochemical investigation, Neuropathol Appl Neurobiol 19:329-335, 1993.
313. Weller RO, Kida S, and Zhang E-T: Pathways of fluid drainage from the brain—morphological aspects and immunological significance in rat and man, Brain Pathol 2:277-284, 1992.
314. Wiley CA, and others: Localization of cytomegalovirus proteins and genome during fulminant central nervous system infection in an AIDS patient, J Neuropathol Exp Neurol 45:127-139, 1986.
315. Wiley CA, and others: Cellular localization of human immunodeficiency virus infection within the brains of acquired immune deficiency syndrome patients, Proc Natl Acad Sci USA 83:7089-7093, 1986.
316. Wiley CA, and others: Acanthamoeba meningoencephalitis in a patient with AIDS, J Infect Dis 155:130-133, 1987.
317. Wiley CA, and others: Human immunodeficiency virus (HIV) and JC virus in acquired immune deficiency syndrome (AIDS) patients with progressive multifocal leukoencephalopathy, Acta Neuropathol (Berl) 76:338-346, 1988.
318. Wiley CA, and Nelson JA: Role of human immunodeficiency virus and cytomegalovirus in AIDS encephalitis, Am J Pathol 133:73-81, 1988.
319. Williams AF, and Gagnon J: Neuronal cell Thy-1 glycoprotein: homology with immunoglobulin, Science 216:696-703, 1982.
320. Yankner BA, and others: Cerebral granulomatous angiitis associated with isolation of human T-lymphotropic virus type III from the central nervous system, Ann Neurol 20:362-364, 1986.

321. Yoshioka M, and others: Expression of HIV-1 and interleukin-6 in lumbosacral dorsal root ganglia of patients with AIDS, Neurology 44:1120-1130, 1994.
322. Zagury D, and others: Long-term cultures of HTLV-III-infected T cells: a model of cytopathology of T-cell depletion in AIDS, Science 231:850-853, 1986.
323. Zee C-S, and others: MR imaging of cerebral toxoplasmosis: correlation of computed tomography and pathology, J Comput Assist Tomogr 9:797-799, 1985.
324. Zwick D, and Friede RL, Roessmann U: Central spinal myelinolysis, Neurology 35:891-893, 1985.

C • H • A • P • T • E • R

# 10

# *Transmissible Spongiform Encephalopathies (Prion Diseases)*

**Herbert Budka**



Transmissible spongiform encephalopathies (TSE), also called prion diseases, subacute spongiform encephalopathies, slow virus infections, unconventional slow virus diseases, or transmissible cerebral amyloidoses, were once largely neglected. These diseases were researched mainly by "scrapiologists," a small group of investigators who became fascinated by the predominant expression of TSE in animals. These diseases include scrapie in sheep and goats, which has been known for more than 250 years; transmissible encephalopathy in minks; chronic wasting disease in mule deer and elk; feline spongiform encephalopathy; exotic ungulate encephalopathy in zoo antelopes; and bovine spongiform encephalopathy (BSE). These diseases in different animal species were attributed to alimentary transmission from scrapie-contaminated foodstuffs. Manifestations of disease in humans, first reported 75 years ago, include Creutzfeldt-Jakob disease (CJD),[37,71] Gerstmann-Sträussler-Scheinker disease (GSS),[50,51] Kuru of the Fore people in Papua-New Guinea, and the newly described fatal familial insomnia (FFI).[49,93]

Most recently, research into these enigmatic diseases has become a "hot spot" in modern biomedicine. The reasons are twofold, one scientific and the other socioeconomic. First, these diseases are at the interface of heredity and infectivity, a unique situation and provocative new paradigm in biomedicine. A first stimulus originated with the experimental transmission of Kuru and CJD,[45] which thus became the first human neurodegenerative diseases with a proven infectious origin. This landmark was rightly honored by the Nobel prize for medicine and physiology in 1976. Moreover, if the "prion" ("proteinaceous infectious particle") hypothesis[106] on infectivity conferred by protein only proves to be correct, this concept will revolutionize basic biology. Pros and cons of the prion hypothesis were recently reviewed[83] and will not be reiterated here. Second, the emergence of the epidemic of BSE ("mad cow disease") in the UK raised significant economic and public health concerns about an eventual hazard for other species, including man. Until recently, however, there was no epidemiologic evidence for a link between BSE and CJD.[123] Nevertheless, three CJD deaths among UK farmers with BSE in their herds[114] were disturbing and were highly publicized by the mass media. Recent CJD cases in two UK teenagers[7,13] caused another media storm; however, four other cases in teenagers had been reported before the BSE epidemic.[7,13] Publicity "meltdown" occurred when a new CJD variant was recently described in the UK; its origin by transmission from BSE must be considered a possibility.[125a] A similar case was recently reported from France.[32a] Still more worrying, BSE transmitted to macaques exhibits similar, if not identical, clinicopathologic features of the new CJD variant.[82a] Validity and extent of a possible human BSE connection cannot be determined at time of this writing. In fact, there has been a definite increase in the incidence of diagnosed sporadic CJD both in the UK[123] and Austria[62]; in the latter, BSE has not been reported. In both countries, this rise was attributed to increased awareness, resulting in more diagnosed cases. Nevertheless, close surveillance of the CJD situation is indicated for years to come.

Research into TSE has intensified on a worldwide scale. Elegant disease modeling[31,68] has demonstrated a normal cell protein, the prion, or proteinase-resistant protein ($PrP^{c}$),[81] as a prerequisite for disease manifestation. Its abnormal isoform ($PrP^{CJD}$ or $PrP^{Scrapie(sc)}$) accumulates specifically in the whole group of disorders and copurifies with infectivity[105]; recently the abnormal protease-resistant isoform could be augmented in vitro.[77] Moreover, specific mutations and polymorphisms of the PrP-encoding gene PRNP associate with familial forms of CJD,[80] GSS,[20] and FFI.[93] PRNP codon 129 is important as a genetic susceptibility factor in sporadic[99] and iatrogenic[34] CJD as well as for determining clinical phenotypes in some,[49,55] but not all,[61] familial TSE. Most recently, PrP deposits were described in brains of patients with familial progressive subcortical gliosis (PSG).[102] It remains to be seen whether this signals the discovery of the newest prion disease; PSG will not be covered in this chapter.

The relation between the PRNP genotype and the varying clinicopathologic phenotype is one of the most fascinating but still enigmatic aspects of TSE. In GSS, the model of inherited prion diseases, factors other than hitherto known PRNP genotypes must be responsible for distinct phenotypes.[61] The distribution in brain of PrP concentrations as seen by Western blotting varies between sporadic/familial CJD and iatrogenic CJD/GSS and corresponds to the experimental transmission rates observed for each form of disease.[22] However, Western blotting revealed PrP only in 88% of successfully transmitted TSE cases.[19]

Because of the BSE epidemic and of the iatrogenic inoculation of CJD,[23] epidemiologic surveillance of CJD has intensified. National case registries and a respective European Union Biomed-1 Concerted Action (Project Leader: R.G. Will, Edinburgh, UK)[125] have been established. Definitive diagnosis of TSE is made by neuropathology, and a European Union Biomed-1 Concerted Action ("The human prion diseases: from neuropathology to pathobiology and molecular genetics") (Project Leader: H. Budka, Vienna, Austria) was started in late 1994 as a Europe-wide network of neuropathologic laboratories.[26,28] The project recently succeeded in defining neuropathologic diagnostic criteria for human TSE[29] based on an earlier proposal[27] and proposed a tissue handling protocol in these disorders.[30] In this chapter, I briefly cover clinical criteria for suspected CJD and then focus on the neuropathologic characteristics of human TSE, emphasizing the importance of immunocytochemistry for PrP. Finally, precautions and tissue handling in TSE are detailed as another important aspects pertinent to the diagnosis of these disorders.

## CLINICAL DIAGNOSIS OF CREUTZFELDT-JAKOB DISEASE

Suspicion of Creutzfeldt-Jakob disease (CJD) or other human TSE has important implications in clinical medicine, pathology, and neuropathology because specific precautions must be applied (see the discussion on precautions and tissue handling in suspected human spongiform encephalopathies, this chapter). Thus, a brief review of clinical criteria for CJD must be given in an article aimed at pathologists. Nevertheless, it is out of the scope of this report to elaborate in detail on clinical diagnosis. The following diagnostic criteria (see box on page 451), have been used successfully[4,39] by the EC Surveillance Group of Creutzfeldt-Jakob Disease in Europe (Project Leader: R.G. Will, Edinburgh).[125]

These criteria were established for epidemiologic surveillance and thus are considered as relatively broad, in order to avoid any significant loss of cases. However, when these criteria were applied retrospectively to our series of 79 CJD cases in Austria, 14% of neuropathologically and immunocytochemically confirmed cases did not meet clinical criteria for probable or possible CJD.[62] In comparison with Masters and colleagues' data,[91] which indicated a disease duration of 7 months, in Austria duration of disease was shorter, with a median of 4 months. In Austria, 76% of patients died within 6 months of onset.[62] In Masters and colleagues' series,[91] a considerable number of cases had long survival times, up to 55 months. Such long duration was very scarce in our series. One possible explanation for this difference is that we included only cases

**Diagnosis of Creutzfeldt-Jakob Disease**
*According to the EC Surveillance Group of Creutzfeldt-Jakob Disease in Europe (modified after Budka, and others[30])*

- Sporadic CJD
  - Definite CJD
    - Neuropathologic confirmation[27,29] and/or
    - Immunochemical confirmation-PrP positive (Western blot) and/or
    - Presence of scrapie-associated fibrils (SAF)
  - Probable CJD
    - Progressive dementia
    - Typical EEG
    - At least two out of four clinical features listed:
      - Myoclonus
      - Visual or cerebellar disturbance
      - Pyramidal/extrapyramidal dysfunction
      - Akinetic mutism
  - Possible CJD
    - Progressive dementia
    - No EEG or atypical EEG
    - At least two out of four clinical features listed:
      - Myoclonus
      - Visual or cerebellar disturbance
      - Pyramidal/extrapyramidal dysfunction
      - Akinetic mutism
    - Duration of less than 2 years
- Accidentally Transmitted CJD
  - Progressive cerebellar syndrome in a pituitary hormone recipient
  - Sporadic CJD with a recognized exposure risk (for example, dura mater transplant)
- Familial CJD
  - Definite or probable CJD plus definite or probable CJD in a first-degree relative
  - Neuropsychiatric disorder plus disease-specific PRNP mutation

confirmed by immunocytochemistry techniques and these were not available to Masters and co-workers. It is probable that some conditions of long duration are not true CJD. Some of our "CJD" cases diagnosed decades ago by neuropathologic means could not be confirmed by PrP immunocytochemistry.

The new CJD variant, recently described in the UK[125a] and France,[32a] is part of the CJD spectrum but has peculiar clinicopathologic features which deviate from classical CJD. However, all of the individual characteristics of this variant have also been found in other types of CJD, although infrequently; thus, it is the *peculiar combination of symptoms in an uncommon case cluster in time and place* that apparently has not been recognized previously.

The diagnostic neuropathologic features are described in the section on neuropathologic diagnosis of human spongiform encephalopathies. Unique clinical features of the new CDJ variant include the following:

- Age 41 or younger, including teenage cases
- Psychiatric presentation at onset, with subsequent development of cerebellar ataxia and only late cognitive impairment
- No typical EEG change (one exception in the French case)

## NEUROPATHOLOGIC DIAGNOSIS OF HUMAN SPONGIFORM ENCEPHALOPATHIES

Considerable advances have been made in clinical and laboratory techniques, infectivity studies, and the molecular biology and biochemistry of TSE in recent years. However, the definitive diagnosis of Creutzfeldt-Jakob disease (CJD) and other TSE relies on neuropathology. Neuropathologic diagnostic criteria and familiarity with the amazing spectrum of TSE features are prerequisites for research in and epidemiologic surveillance of these disorders. This becomes even more important in view of the steadily growing number of clinical and pathologic phenotypes. Moreover, other diseases, such as the recently reported chromosome 14-encoded Alzheimer's disease, are very similar to, if not indistinguishable from CJD in its clinical presentation.[63] Finally, we recently showed that 14% of neuropathologically confirmed CJD cases did not meet clinical diagnostic criteria of probable or possible CJD.[62] This further emphasizes the need for detailed neuropathologic assessment of these disorders.

The many historically described variants with different names are parts of this spectrum and were described in detail elsewhere.[84,109] The length of disease, the PRNP genotype,[15] and yet unidentified factors, including "strains" of the infectious agent, all influence pathology, resulting in considerable morphologic variation. The "prion" disease concept encompasses sporadic, inherited and infectious conditions.[107,118] It was recently proposed that the commonly used and historically entrenched disease names be replaced by the term "prion disease," with addition of the PRNP mutation site in the inherited conditions.[107] However, we believe it is still appropriate to retain the classic terminology, provided we can agree on accurate definitions of the terms. The main purpose of a consensus report[29] was to show that this can be done at the neuropathologic level when additional data are reasonably incorporated. Thus, these neuropathologic diagnostic criteria are detailed here. Nevertheless, it is not within the scope of this chapter to discuss in detail the relation between histopathologic and molecular genetic criteria. It must not be forgotten that a PRNP mutation is *not* synonymous with illness.

### The Role of Immunocytochemistry for PrP

Major characteristics of TSE are well appreciated by routine histopathology of the brain in most cases. However, immunocytochemistry for PrP has been recently added to classic histologic techniques and has rapidly evolved into a very useful diagnostic adjunct. Unfortunately, for diagnostic purposes it is at present a rather delicate procedure that requires an experienced laboratory. Another problem is that the available antibodies do not distinguish between the normal cellular $PrP^c$ and its pathologic isoform, $PrP^{Sc/CJD}$. Moreover, antibodies do not distinguish between PrP in nonfibrillated ("preamyloid") and fibrillated (amyloid) configurations. Western blotting, considered by many as the gold standard for the diagnosis of TSE, is done after treatment with proteinase K, so that only the protease-resistant $PrP^{Sc/CJD}$ is present. Pretreatment of paraffin sections before immunolabeling for PrP is mandatory and apparently this procedure destroys immunoreactivity with $PrP^c$. We and others[65] have not seen convincing labeling of normal brain with the procedures described below. However, we have seen some background staining, possibly reflecting $PrP^c$, when insufficient pretreatment or no pretreatment was performed or when antibodies were applied at high concentration.

Various pretreatment protocols for paraffin sections have been recommended, including formic acid and/or guanidine thiocyanate, hydrolytic or hydrated autoclaving, and microwave treatment.[9,112] Use of formic acid with guanidine thiocyanate and hydrolytic autoclaving was recommended as the most effective method.[65] Also a variety of antibodies have been used with varying results. In GSS, antibodies directed to epitopes spanning PrP residues 90-165 labeled amyloid cores best.[103] It is beyond the scope of this chapter to elaborate more on technical matters; however, see the box on this page for a simple protocol for PrP immunostaining that has proved reliable in our hands. Using this method, we have seen strong immunocytochemical signals, especially of the synaptic type. These are the most delicate and crucial structures to be labeled. In contrast, PrP plaques are nicely decorated, even with less sensitive methods. We had satisfactory results with the monoclonal anti-PrP antibody 3F4 and polyclonal rabbit antisera raised by Dr. H. Diringer, Berlin, and Drs. Kitamoto and Tateishi, Fukuoka, Japan. In our experience, hydrolytic autoclaving is not superior to hydrated autoclaving; although the overall signal might become stronger, the morphology deteriorates, and it becomes difficult to keep sections attached to the glass slide. Immunocytochemistry for PrP is most valuable, especially in histopathologically-atypical cases.[9,82] In our experience with 79 sporadic CJD cases in Austria, PrP immunocytochemistry enabled the diagnosis of two cases with nondiagnostic routine histopathology.[62] Similarly, nondiagnostic, nonspongiform pathology was seen in 2 out of 189 human TSE cases successfully transmitted experimentally at the NIH.[19]

**Protocol for PrP Immunostaining***

1. Hydrated autoclaving†
   —place deparaffinated sections in a metal jar filled with distilled water.
   —autoclave at 121°C for 30 minutes, then wash with phosphate-buffered saline (PBS).
2. Block endogenous peroxidase by immersing in 3% $H_2O_2$ in methanol for 10 minutes, then wash in PBS.
3. Block unspecific binding by covering sections with 10% fetal calf serum for 20 minutes.
4. Cover sections with anti-PrP antibody at optimized dilution‡ for 2 hours at room temperature or overnight at 4° C.
5. Continue with your most sensitive secondary immunostaining system for monoclonal or polyclonal antibodies, respectively.

* Protocols taken from the Institute of Neurology, Vienna, 1995.
† Alternative:
1. Hydrolytic autoclaving
   —place deparaffinated sections into metallic jar filled with 1–30 mmol HCl§
   —autoclave at 121°C for 30 minutes, then wash with phosphate-buffered saline (PBS)

‡ Determined by extensive testing for every antibody on known positive and negative control tissues.
§ In our experience, sections detach from the glass slide or disappear at concentrations higher than 5 mmol.

Another way to visualize PrP and to map its distribution is the "histoblot" (cryostat sections blotted onto nitrocellulose membranes, treated by proteolysis and immunostained). This "histoblot" yields impressive preparations in rodent brain[116] but is more difficult to apply on the much larger human brain. We made some preliminary histoblotting experiments on brains from Alzheimer and CJD patients, but found no definite advantage over immunostaining of large paraffin sections treated with hydrated autoclaving.[61]

### Neuropathologic Characteristics of Human Transmissible Spongiform Encephalopathies

**Creutzfeldt-Jakob disease.** Sporadic, iatrogenic, or familial forms of Creutzfeldt-Jakob disease (CJD) may be distinguished. The last have been associated with a variety of PRNP mutations. Sporadic and iatrogenic forms are tightly correlated to allelic homozygosity at PRNP codon 129.[16,99] At the neuropathologic level, however, these forms are not clearly distinct. However, cerebellar involvement is especially striking in iatrogenic cases associated with injections of pituitary gland extracts.[122]

Macroscopic inspection of the brain may show no obvious abnormality. More commonly there is cerebral

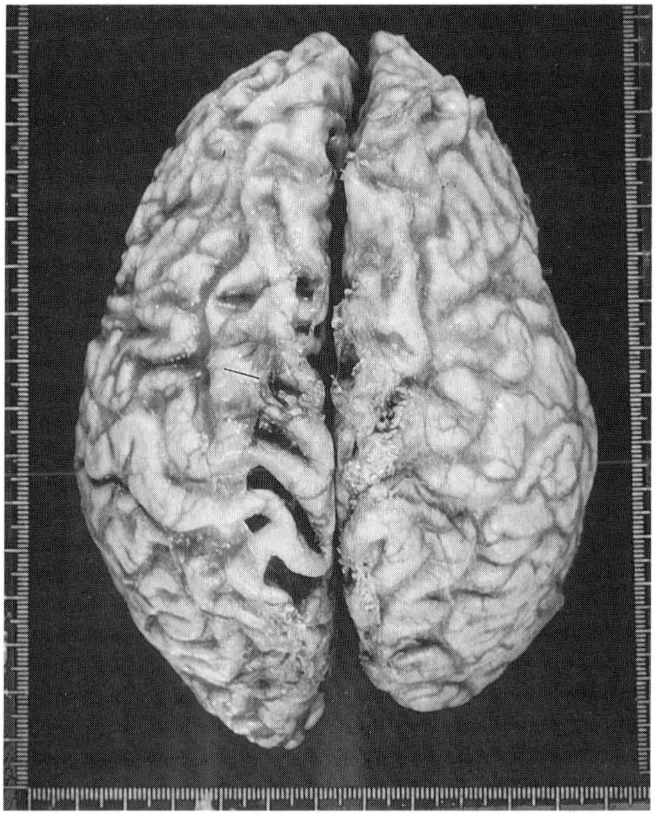

**Fig. 10-1.** Prominent diffuse atrophy of gyri with widening of sulci.

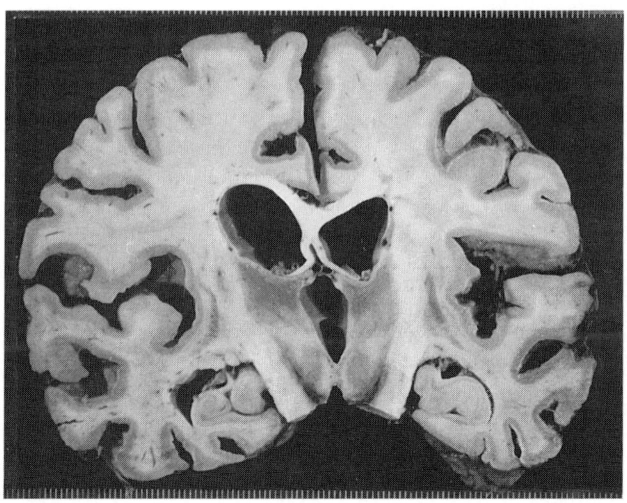

**Fig. 10-2.** Diffuse cortical and central atrophy with widening of ventricles and sulci. The hippocampus is well preserved.

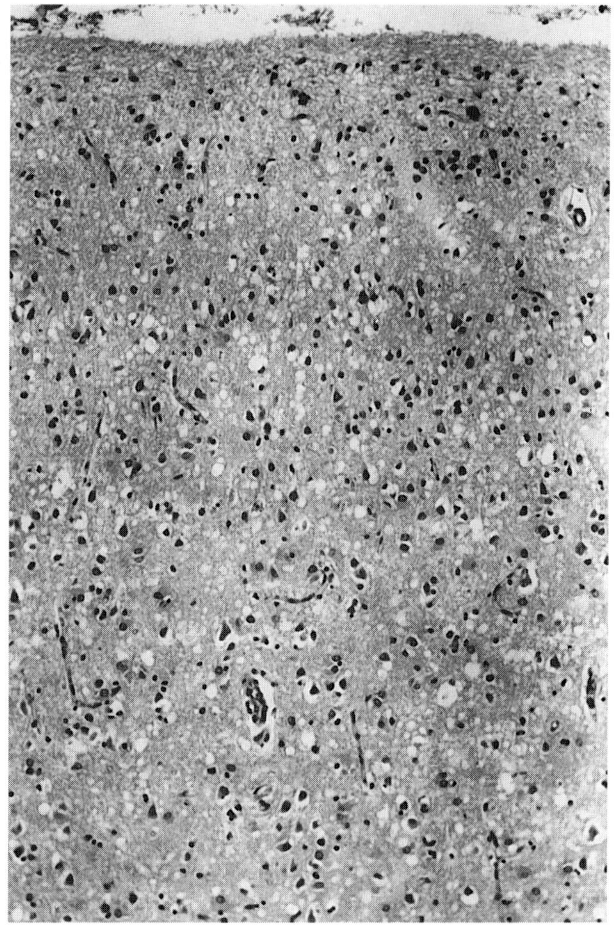

**Fig. 10-3.** Diffuse spongiform change in the cerebral cortex. Hematoxylin and eosin. (H&E; ×160.)

cortical atrophy that may be generalized (Figs. 10-1, 10-2) or that may show focal accentuation. The hippocampal formation is well preserved, even in cases of severe brain atrophy (Fig. 10-2). In addition to the classic diffuse pathology, regional involvement has been characterized as occipital,[66] striatal, thalamic, and cerebellar[25] variants.[109] Without PrP data, the crucial histopathologic feature is the classic triad of *spongiform change*[92] (Figs. 10-3 to 10-9) (definition and caveat discussed in box on page 456) neuronal loss (Fig. 10-10) (see also Figs. 10-4, 10-5, and 10-7), and astrocytosis (Figs. 10-10 to 10-15) (see also Fig. 10-4). All three features are highly variable. Very severe cortical damage of "burnt-out" cases may lack any specific feature (Fig. 10-16) and may be dominated by the nonspecific change of "status spongiosus" (Figs. 10-17, 10-18).[92] Especially in the early stage of the disease, microglial activation is prominent.[111] In the cerebellar cortex, "antler"-type dendritic hypertrophy and axonal torpedoes (Fig. 10-19) may occur. Neuroaxonal dystrophy may be widespread in some CJD brains.[89]

Spongiform change may vary greatly in severity and extent between affected gray matter parts. Most classic cases exhibit prominent diffuse histopathology in cerebral cortex (Figs. 10-3, 10-4) and subcortical gray matter and/or cerebellar cortex (Figs. 10-5, 10-7). Occasionally, diagnostic spongiform change may be confined to few focal areas (Figs. 10-8, 10-9), thus requiring detailed study of many tissue blocks. In some instances the

*Text continued on page 459.*

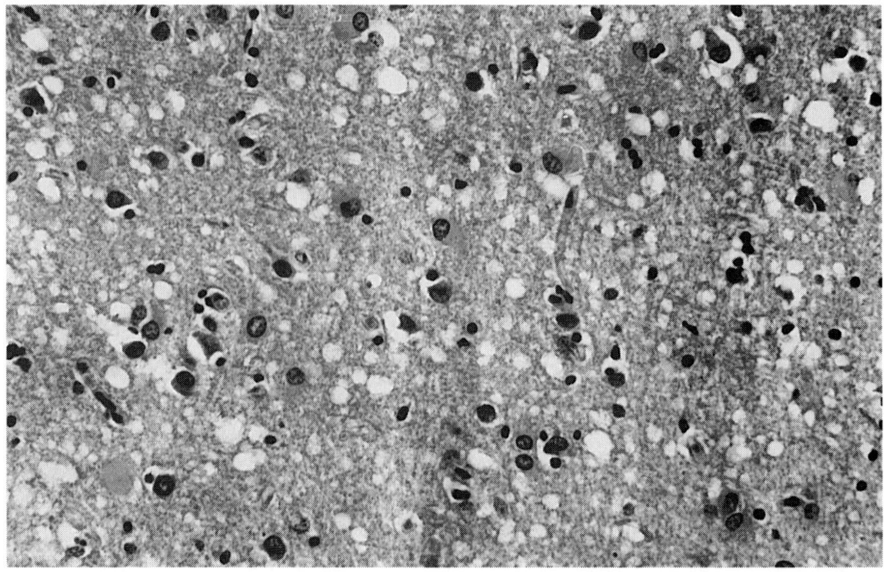

**Fig. 10-4.** Prominent spongiform change, neuronal loss, and reactive astrogliosis. (H&E; ×250.)

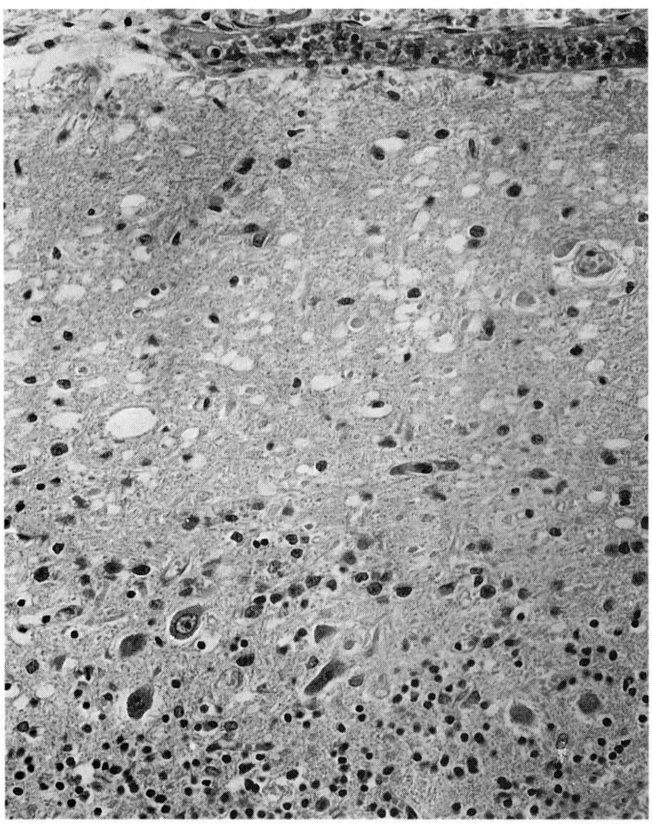

**Fig. 10-5.** Slight spongiform change of cerebellar molecular layer, prominent depletion of granule cell layer. (H&E; ×160.)

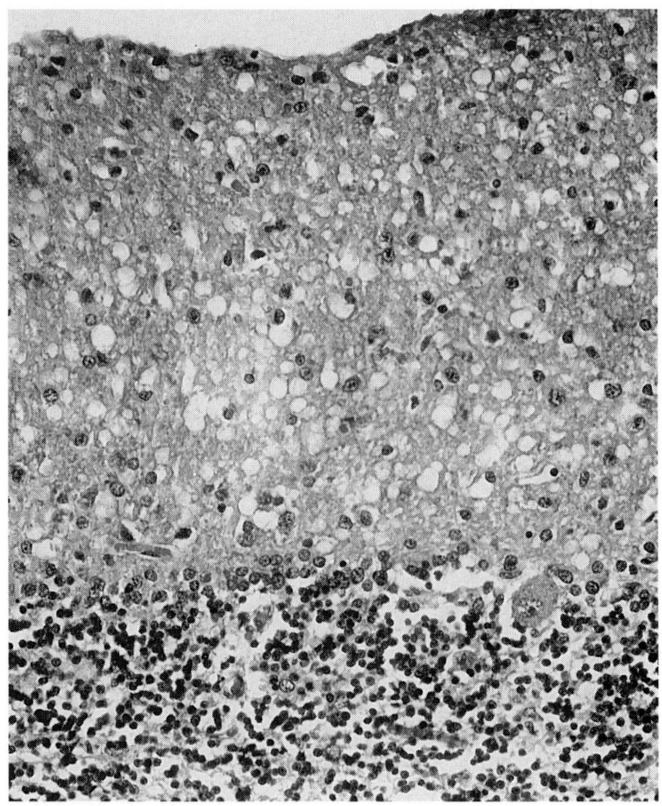

**Fig. 10-6.** Prominent spongiform change of cerebellar molecular layer. (H&E; ×250.)

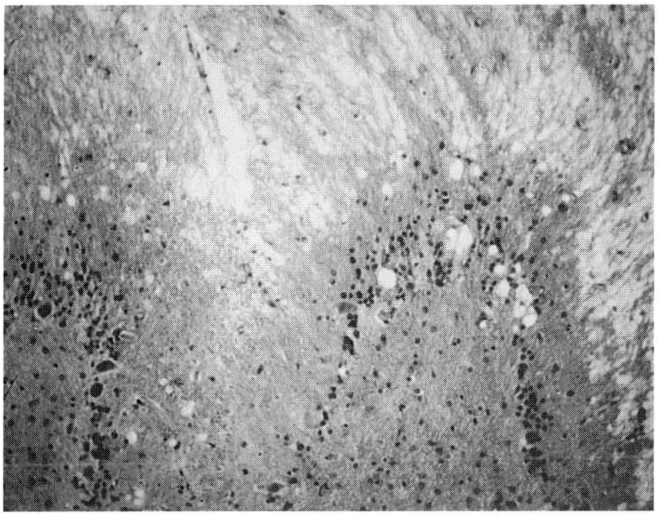

**Fig. 10-7.** Advanced spongiosis of cerebellar molecular layer, complete degeneration of granular layer. (H&E; ×78.)

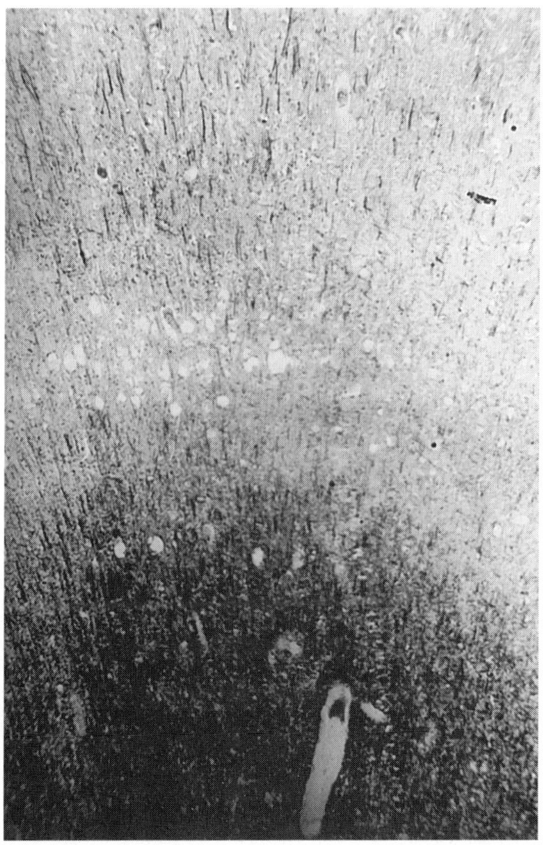

**Fig. 10-8.** Focal spongiform change in deep cortical layer. (Luxol fast blue; ×44.)

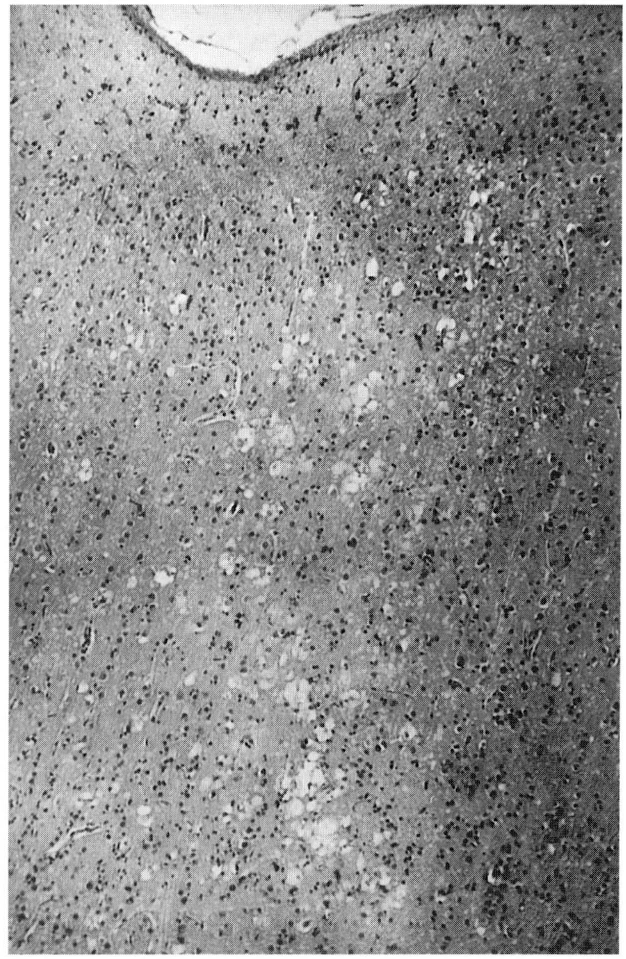

**Fig. 10-9.** Focal spongiform change in upper and deep cortical layers. (H&E; ×63.)

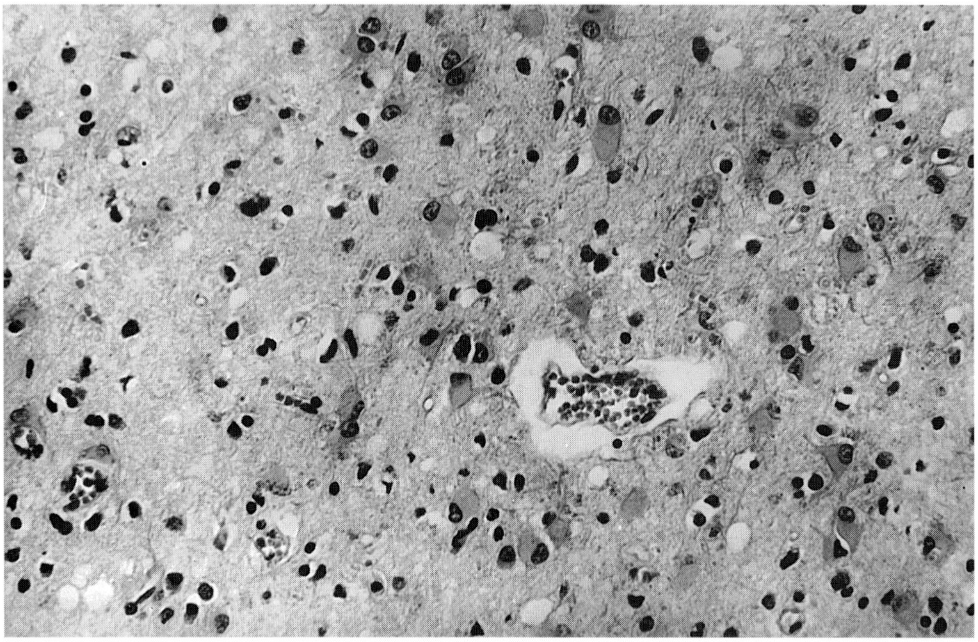

**Fig. 10-10.** Prominent gemistocytic astrocytosis and neuronal loss with slight spongiform change. (H&E; ×250.)

### Spongiform Change

Diffuse (Figs. 10-3 to 10-7) or focally clustered (morula-type) (Figs. 10-8, 10-9) small, round, or oval vacuoles in the neuropil of the whole depth (Fig. 10-3) or deep layers of the cerebral cortex (Fig. 10-8), in cerebellar cortex (predominantly in molecular layer [Figs. 10-5, 10-7]), or subcortical gray matter. The vacuoles may become confluent, resulting in a sievelike meshwork (Fig. 10-7).

*Caveat*: Nonspecific spongiosis

- Status spongiosus ("spongiform/spongy state")[92]—microcystic cavities of irregular shape in gliotic neuropil (Fig. 10-17) following extensive neuronal loss (including also lesions of "burnt-out" CJD, and dementia with neuronal loss but without PrP).[104]
- Changes similar to spongiform change may occur focally in the cerebral cortex in diffuse Lewy body disease or Alzheimer's disease.[64]
- Irregular "spongy" change occurring with brain edema and metabolic encephalopathies.
- Superficial "spongy" change in various processes including Pick's and Alzheimer's diseases and dementia lacking specific histologic features.
- Recent hypoxia/ischemia—perineuronal or perivascular vacuolation.
- Artifacts (fixation, paraffin embedding, section processing)—superficial cortical, perineuronal, perivascular, and perinuclear-oligodendroglial vacuolation (Fig. 10-18).

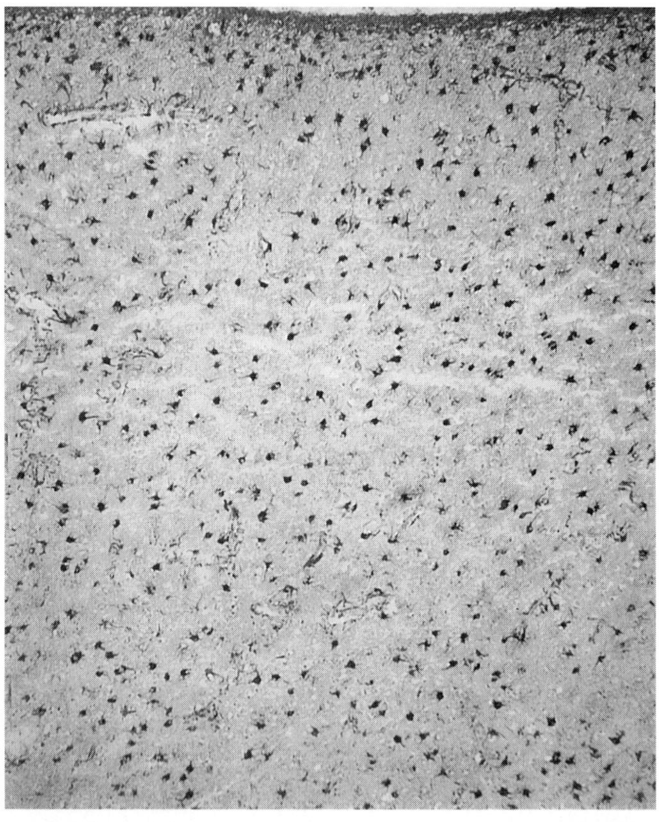

**Fig. 10-11.** Diffuse cortical astrogliosis. Immunocytochemistry (ICC) for glial fibrillary acidic protein (GFAP). (×63.)

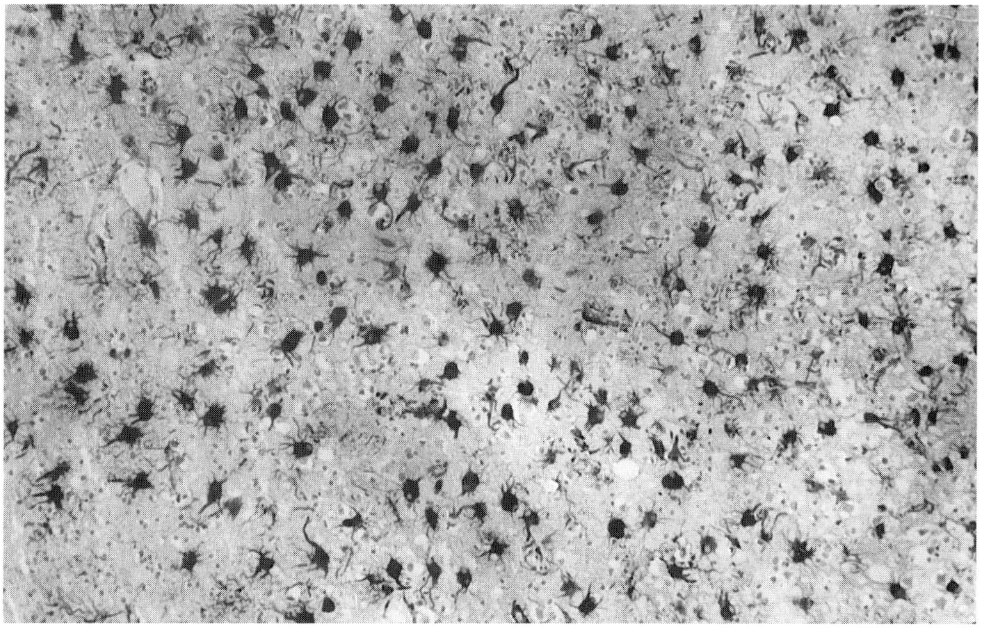

**Fig. 10-12.** Diffuse cortical astrogliosis (ICC for GFAP). (×150.)

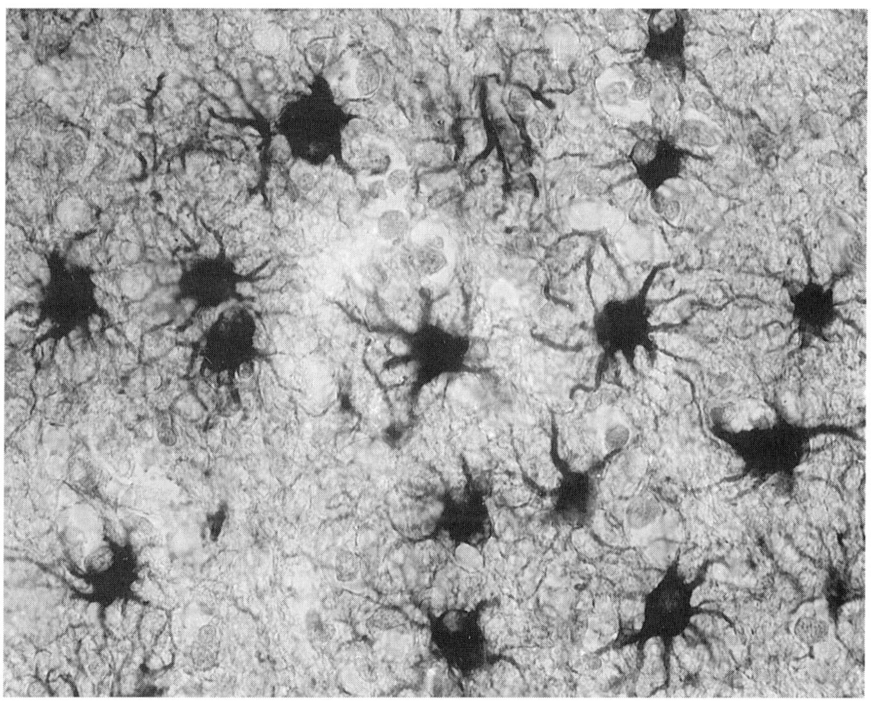

**Fig. 10-13.** Diffuse cortical astrogliosis (ICC for GFAP). (×400.)

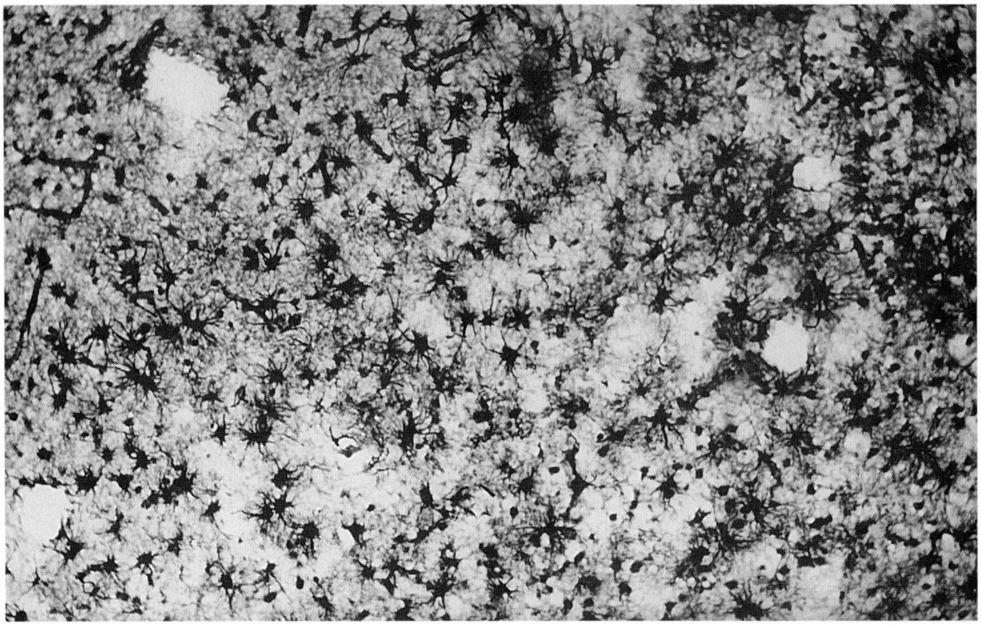

**Fig. 10-14.** Diffuse cortical astrogliosis. (Cajal's metallic impregnation for astroglia; ×150.)

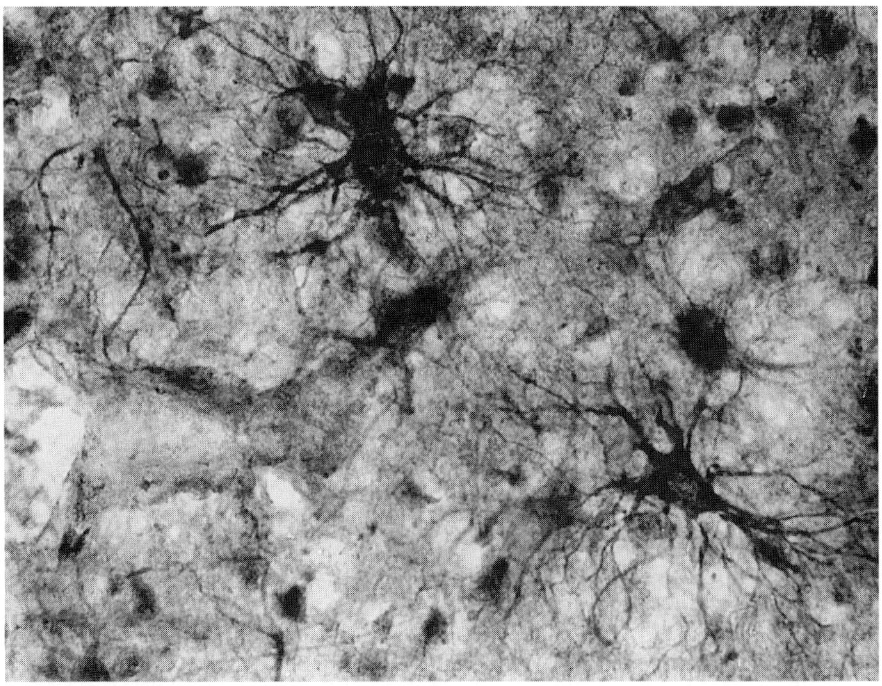

**Fig. 10-15.** Prominent hypertrophied astrocytes. (Cajal's metallic impregnation for astroglia; ×630.)

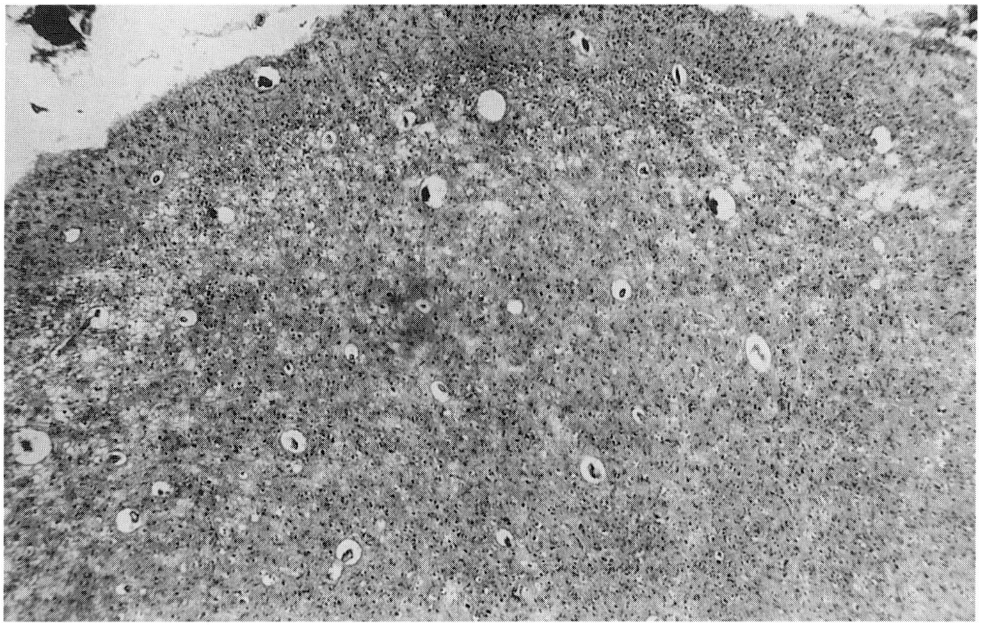

**Fig. 10-16.** Diffuse burnt-out cortical damage without specific features. (H&E; ×63.)

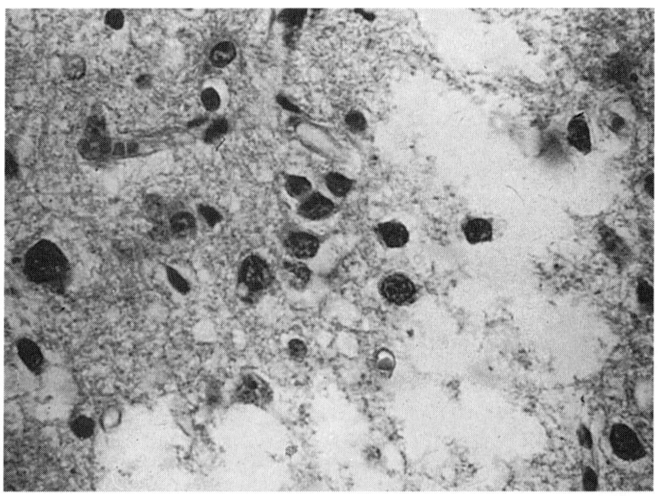

**Fig. 10-17.** "Spongiform state" with large irregular cavities. (H&E; ×335.)

spongiform change may be unilateral.[126] The vacuolation may involve all layers (Fig. 10-3) or only the deep layers of the cortex (Fig. 10-8). Vacuolation may be diffuse (Fig. 10-3) or focal (Figs. 10-8, 10-9) and affect subcortical gray matter and the cerebellar molecular layer (Figs. 10-5 to 10-7). Vacuolation restricted to superficial cortical layers usually is artifactual and samples from these cases have resulted in transmission of the disease.[84] According to some authors, the only constant location for spongiform change in CJD is the head of the caudate nucleus.[108] Occasional neurons may have vacuoles in their somata (Fig. 10-20) or may be ballooned by accumulated neurofilament proteins.[97] The granular cerebellar layer is frequently depleted (Figs. 10-5, 10-7). The "panencephalopathic" type of CJD may also reveal prominent damage in the white matter,[96] but this is rare outside of Japan. Meynert's basal nucleus may be variably affected,[5,32] either primarily or secondary to cortical neuronal loss. Spongiform change is rarely seen in the brain stem or spinal cord, although PrP accumulation can be demonstrated at these sites. The very existence of an "amyotrophic" type of CJD combining motor neuron loss with dementia remains to be proved; inoculations of tissues from such cases have not transmitted CJD.[110] While a significant portion of histopathologically typical TSE cases also did not transmit, including familial cases in 43%, absence of spongiform change was an almost 100% predictive indicator of nontransmissibility.[19]

Immunoreactivity for PrP is seen mainly in three patterns that may also overlap: plaque (Fig. 10-21), diffuse synaptic (Fig. 10-22), and patchy/perivacuolar (Figs. 10-23, 10-24) types. PrP immunoreactive amyloid plaques[75] occur in some 15% of CJD autopsies, usually as small to medium-size compact kuru type plaques with fringed outline. They also are usually stained with periodic acid-Schiff, Congo red (staining disappears after formic acid treatment), and alcian blue. Ubiquitin may be deposited around PrP plaques.[70,115] Kuru plaques of CJD are most frequent in the cerebellar cortex, where they usually are confined to the granular layer (Fig. 10-21). CJD and GSS may also show age-related Alzheimer-type senile plaques immunoreactive for the $\beta$-peptide, with or without co-localization of PrP deposits[95] and vascular $\beta$-peptide deposits.[57,69]

*Text continued on page 463.*

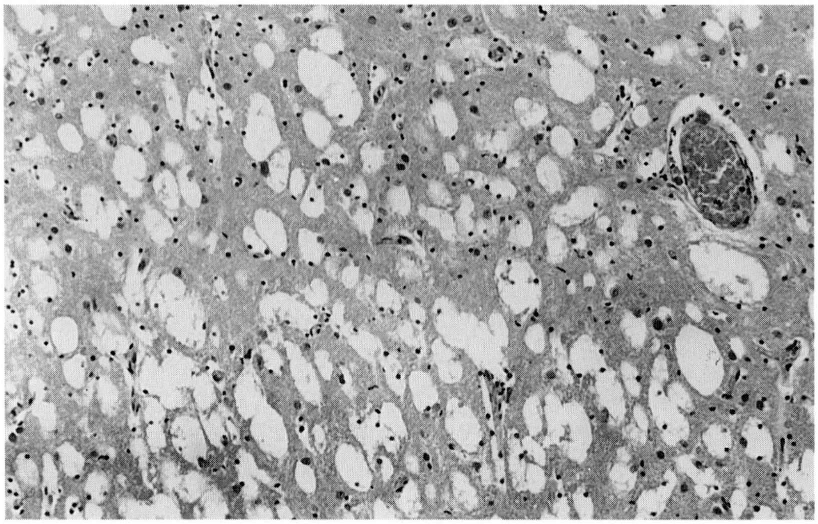

**Fig. 10-18.** Prominent artifactual perineuronal and perioligodendroglial vacuolization in putamen. (H&E; ×100.)

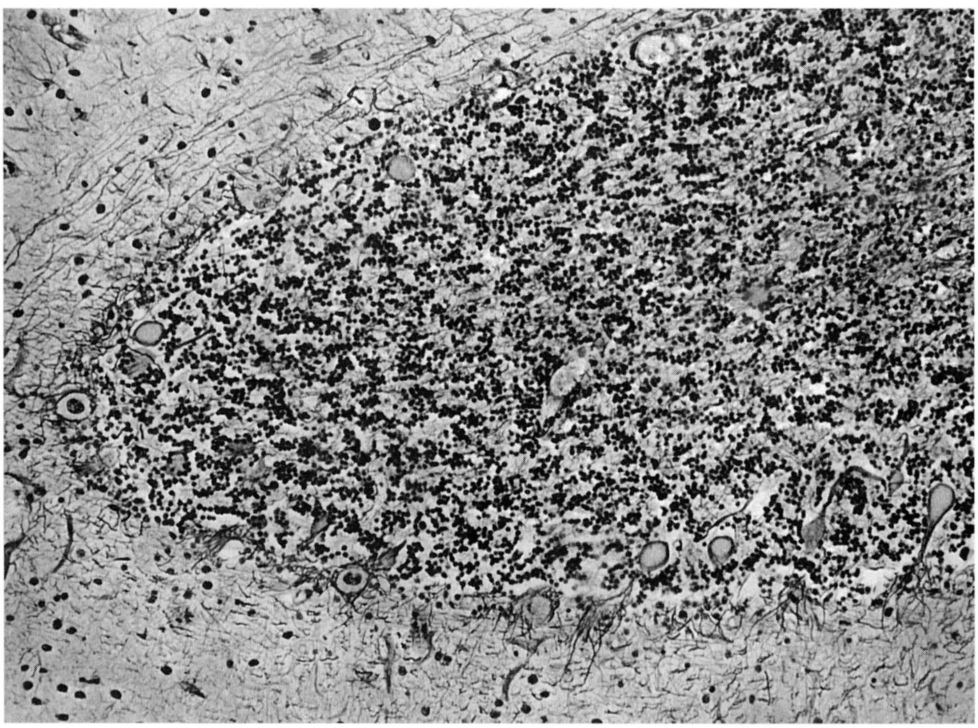

**Fig. 10-19.** Numerous axonal torpedoes in the granular layer of cerebellar cortex. (Bodian's silver impregnation; ×160.)

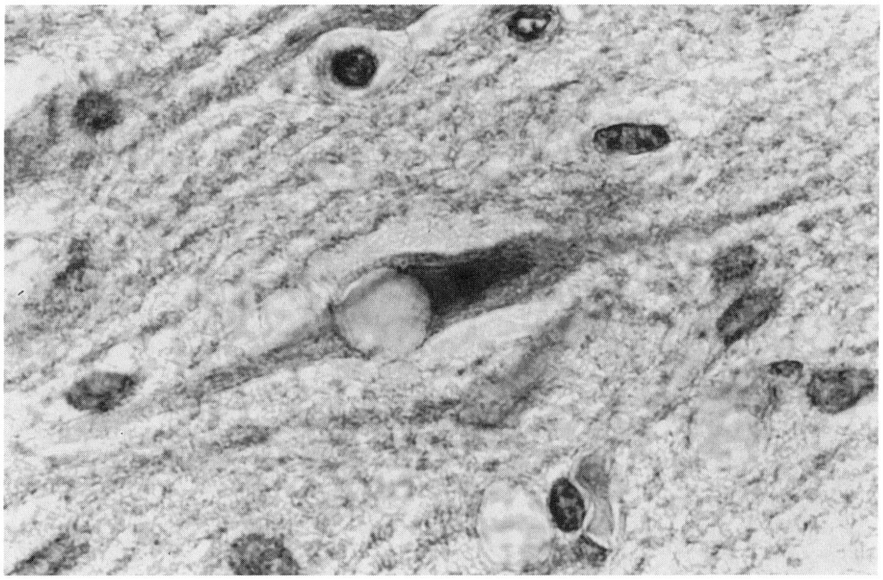

**Fig. 10-20.** Large intraneuronal vacuole. (H&E; ×400.)

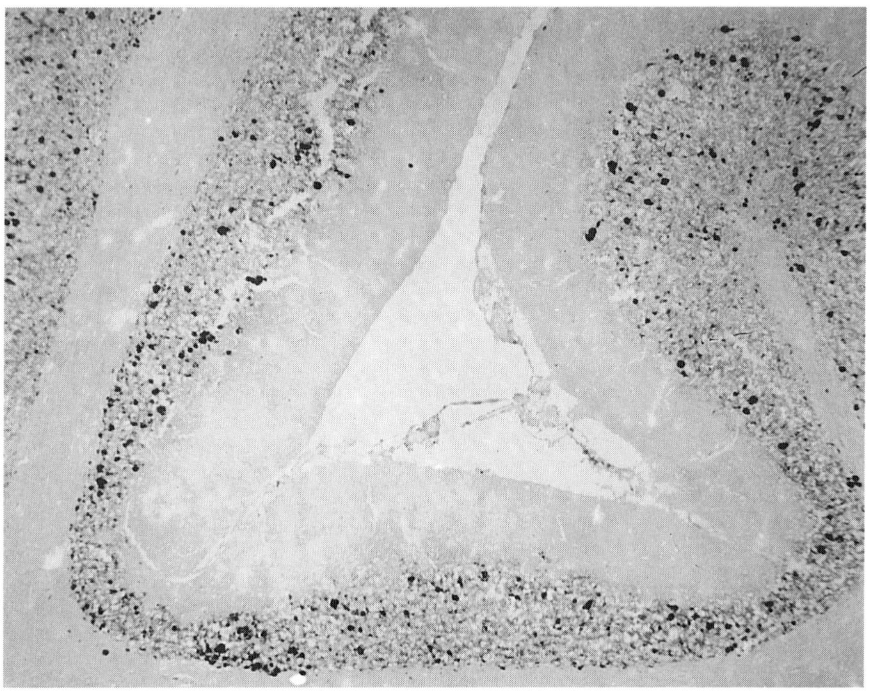

**Fig. 10-21.** Numerous small kuru-type plaques occupy predominantly the granular layer of the cerebellar cortex. ICC for the proteinase resistant/prion protein (PrP). (×63.)

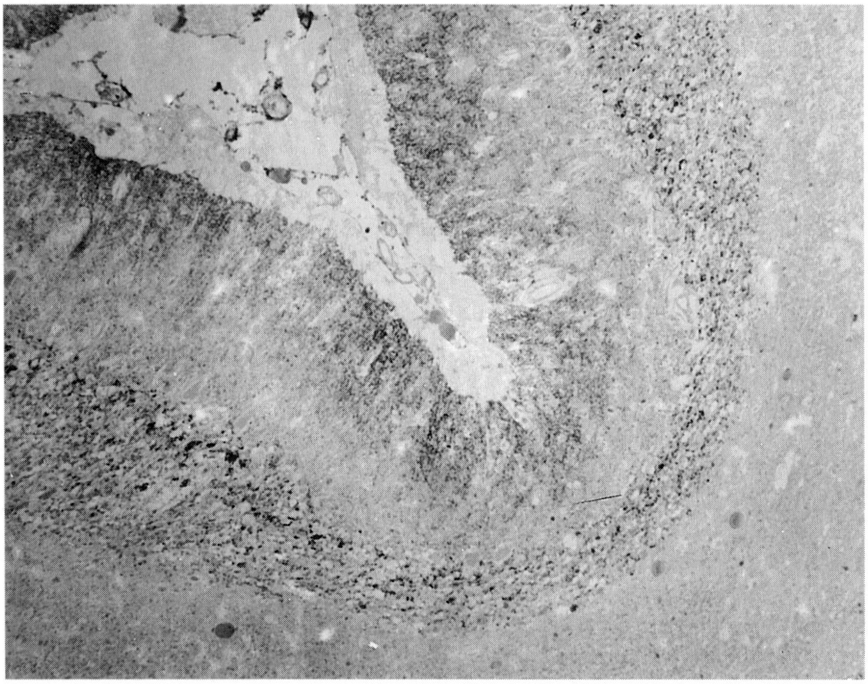

**Fig. 10-22.** Diffuse fine granular immunoreactivity of synaptic type in molecular and granular layers of the cerebellar cortex (ICC for PrP). (×100.)

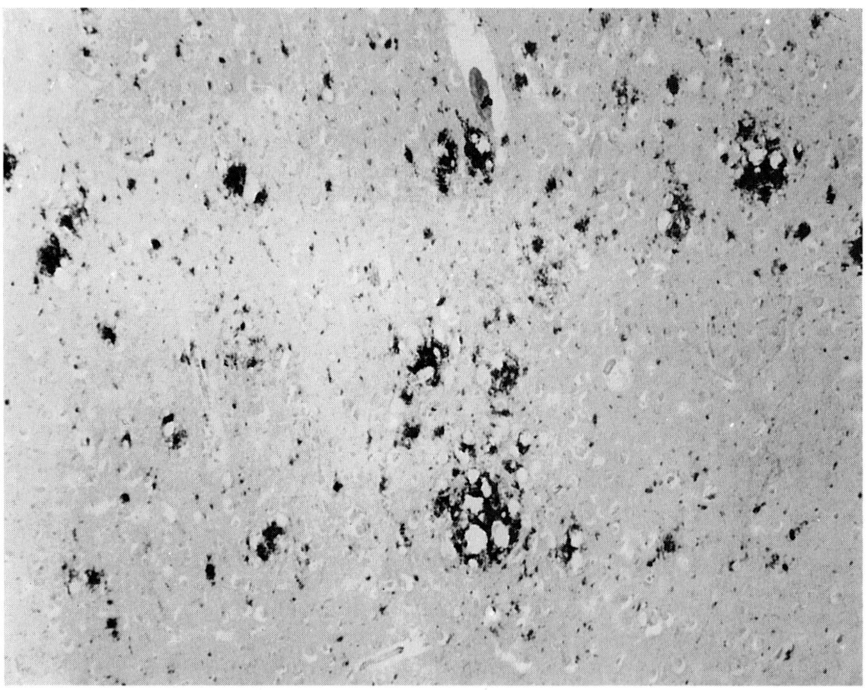

**Fig. 10-23.** Coarse perivacuolar and patchy PrP deposits (ICC for PrP). (×100.)

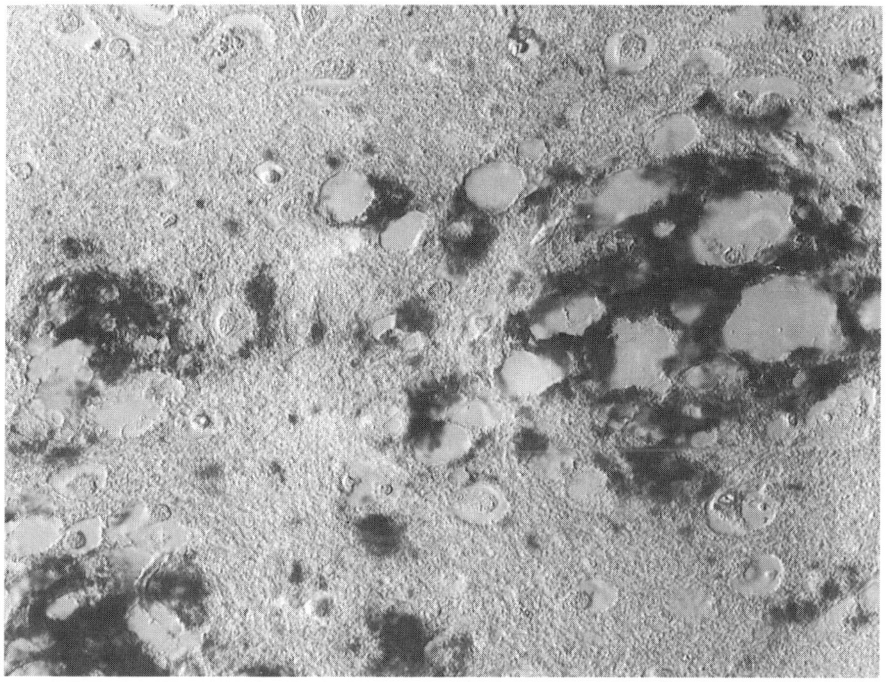

**Fig. 10-24.** Close relation of PrP deposits to large vacuoles (ICC for PrP). (×400.)

It is a matter of debate whether the coexistence of CJD with Alzheimer-type histopathology is just a chance finding or a "gray" area of overlapping pathologies with similar pathogenesis.[84] We observed prominent *β*/A4 immunoreactive plaques in 12.5% of our CJD brains,[84] including cases with prominent formation of neurofibrillary tangles in density higher than appropriate for the age (Fig. 10-25). The diffuse synaptic pattern usually shows abundant tiny immunolabeled dots throughout the neurophil, sometimes including coarser and bigger deposits (Fig. 10-22). In some brains, PrP immunoreactivity in the cerebral cortex is limited to only a few small dots or is even absent; however, the cerebellar cortex usually has more prominent immunoreactivity in these cases. In the cerebellar cortex, the granular layer is most frequently affected, with additional but variable fine stippling of the molecular layer (Fig. 10-22). In correlation with clinical, pathologic, and molecular genetic data, a PrP immunolabeling pattern was proposed to distinguish "plaque" and "synaptic/nonplaque" types of prion disease.[42,72-74]

Finally, many cases with prominent spongiform change exhibit a striking patchy deposition of PrP around the vacuoles (Figs. 10-23, 10-24). The submicroscopic structures involved in this type of PrP deposition (which usually is nonfibrillar) remain to be elucidated. Interestingly, ubiquitin is deposited in a similar pattern, suggesting accumulation of both proteins within lysosomes.[70] Cases may exhibit both "plaque" and "nonplaque" (synaptic, perivacuolar) staining patterns. As with the spongiform change, PrP deposition may be focal, thus again requiring immunostaining of several blocks in rare cases. In my experience, the correlation between PrP deposition and local histopathology is not clear-cut. In some cases the well-preserved hippocampus may harbor prominent deposition (Fig. 10-26), and abundant plaques may occupy otherwise intact tissue. In contrast, cases with prominent spongiform change frequently have abundant deposits. Early spongiform change seems to be more frequently associated with synaptic deposits, whereas coarse and prominent vacuolization accompanies patchy/perivacuolar deposits.

Peculiar tubulovesicular structures have been described as a specific ultrastructural marker of CJD and GSS, both in sporadic and experimental disease.[85-88] However, the diagnostic role of electron microscopy in these disorders has yet to be established.

Peculiar neuropathological features of the recently described new CJD variant[32a,125a] include the following:

- Abundant PrP *amyloid plaques* (well visible in H&E or PAS stains), characteristically surrounded by vacuoles ("florid" plaques)
- Spongiform change, gliosis and neuronal loss especially prominent in basal ganglia and thalamus
- Abundant PrP deposits including prominent "peri-

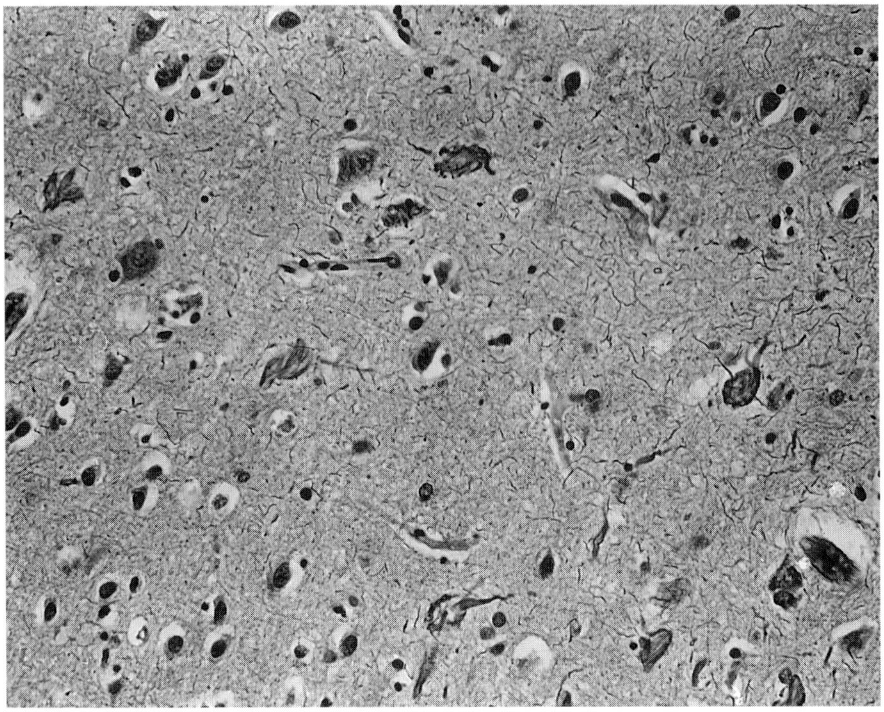

**Fig. 10-25.** 63-year-old CJD patient. Numerous neurofibrillary tangles in parahippocampal gyrus. (Bodian's silver impregnation; ×250.)

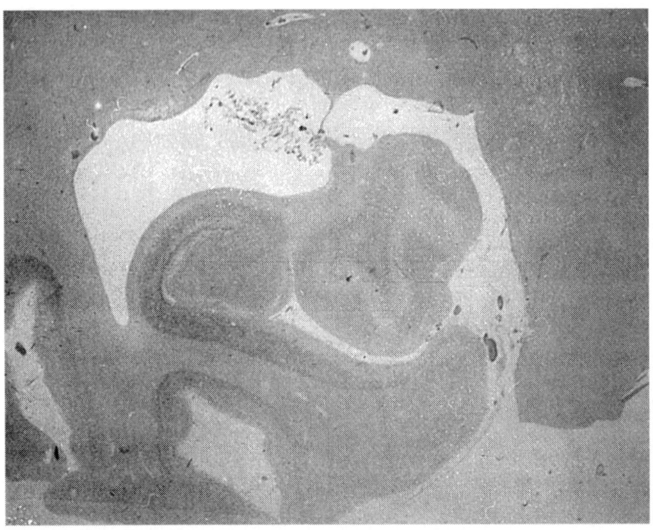

**Fig. 10-26.** Prominent PrP deposition in well-preserved pyramidal layer of hippocampus (ICC for PrP). (×6.)

cellular'' deposition in cerebral and cerebellar (especially in the molecular layer) cortex

For diagnosis of this variant, autopsy with neuropathological confirmation is mandatory. The abundant presence of ''florid'' plaques in brain appears to be the most distinctive diagnostic feature.

**Gerstmann-Sträussler-Scheinker disease (GSS).** The separation of GSS from familial CJD is debatable and may become conceptually difficult to maintain in the future. It was proposed that CJD with many PrP plaques should be categorized as GSS.[41] Such plaques are notably rare or absent in familial CJD.[67] However, large numbers of PrP plaques may exceptionally occur in sporadic CJD without PRNP mutation. According to the salient characteristics of most reports, GSS should be diagnosed at present only when the following features apply: a family with autosomal dominant inheritance; progressive ataxia and/or dementia; abundant PrP plaques of the multicentric type in the brain; and one of a variety of PRNP mutations.[44] The classic PRNP mutation of GSS is P102L, as seen in the original Gerstmann[79] and other families.

According to the clinical phenotype (ataxic and/or dementing),[67] the cerebellar and/or cerebral cortices are predominantly involved. The original Austrian GSS kindred has been shown recently to switch phenotypically from the classic ataxic type to CJD-like features. Pathologic features reflect this change as prominent telencephalic damage (Figs. 10-27 to 10-29) including pronounced spongiform change and prominent PrP deposition of the diffuse synaptic type (Fig. 10-30). The latter is less pronounced in the mid-cortical layers, resulting in a multilayered deposition pattern

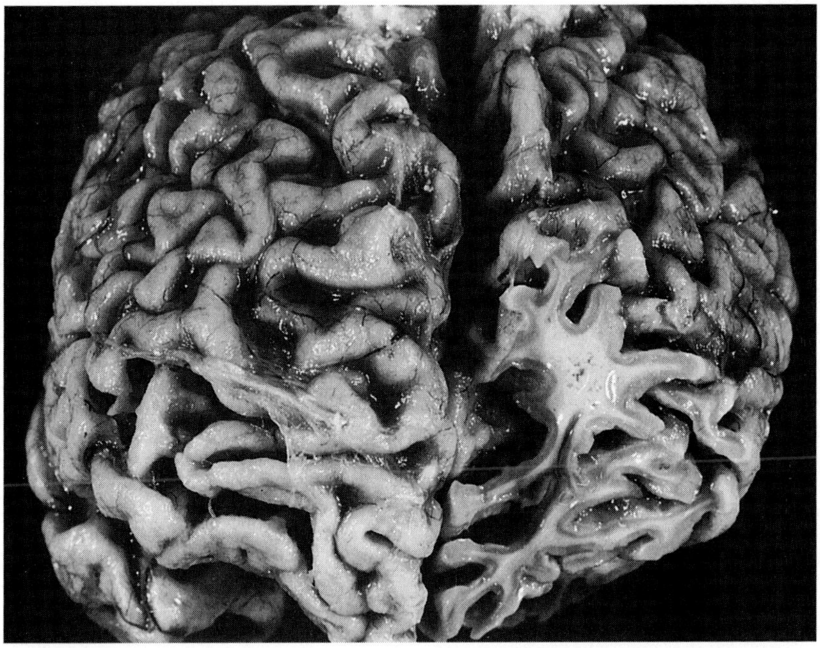

**Fig. 10-27.** Prominent gyral atrophy in recent GSS case of CJD-like phenotype.

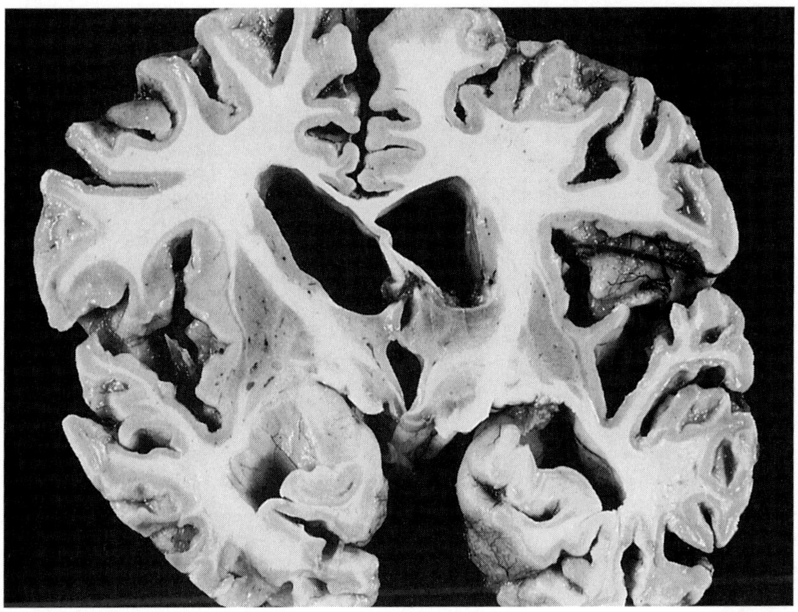

**Fig. 10-28.** Severe cortical atrophy with prominent widening of outer and inner CSF spaces.

(Fig. 10-31).[61] The CJD-like phenotype features a well-preserved cerebellar cortex (Fig. 10-32), despite abundant plaques there (Fig. 10-33). The spongiform change varies greatly in severity between cases and families, and may even be absent. PrP amyloid is the common denominator, most prominently in the form of multicentric plaques (Fig. 10-34). However, significant variability[52] may be seen, ranging from classic multicentric to compact Kuru-type plaques (Fig. 10-34), which may mimic senile plaques, "miniplaques," and "shapeless deposits."[12] In spastic-paraparetic GSS, the motor cortex may harbor large numbers of plaques. In the cerebellar cortex, the molecular layer contains most large plaques (Fig. 10-33), whereas in CJD plaques are smaller and usually occur in the granular layer. A dense glial fibrillary mesh entangles the plaques (Fig. 10-35). As in CJD with plaques, neuritic dystrophy reminiscent of that seen in Alzheimer's disease may be prominent around the plaques. Such dystrophy features accumulations of dystrophic organelles (Fig. 10-36), of phosphorylated neurofilament proteins,[61] and ubiquitin,[70] but not of paired helical filaments/tau pro-

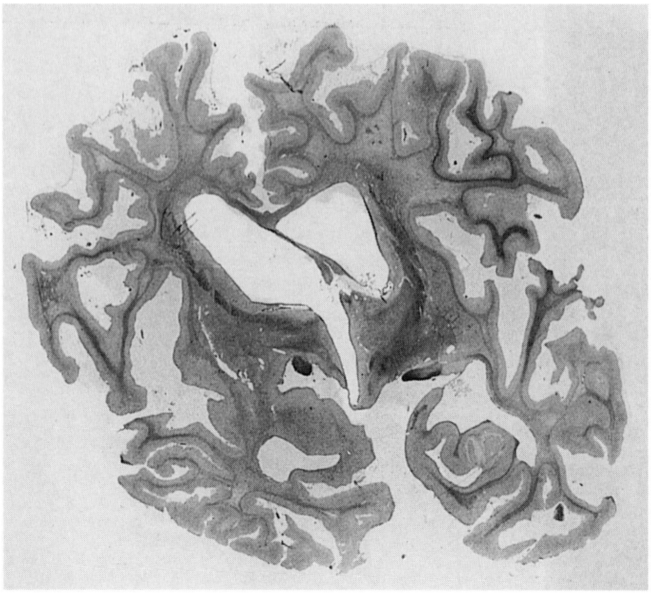

**Fig. 10-29.** Extreme cortical atrophy with prominent ventricular dilatation and secondary damage of white matter. (Luxol fast blue stain.)

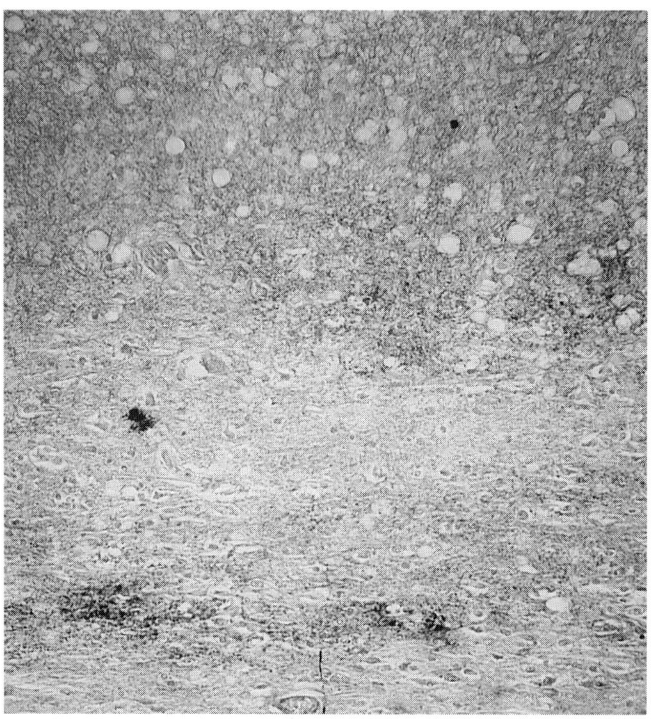

**Fig. 10-30.** Diffuse fine granular PrP deposition of synaptic type in cerebral cortex (*upper half*); few irregular plaques in cortex and subcortical white matter (ICC for PrP). (×160.)

tein.[61] However, some kindreds also have neurofibrillary tangles in the cerebral cortex[53,98] or throughout the neuraxis.[38] Another similarity with Alzheimer's disease is the prominent contribution of microglia to

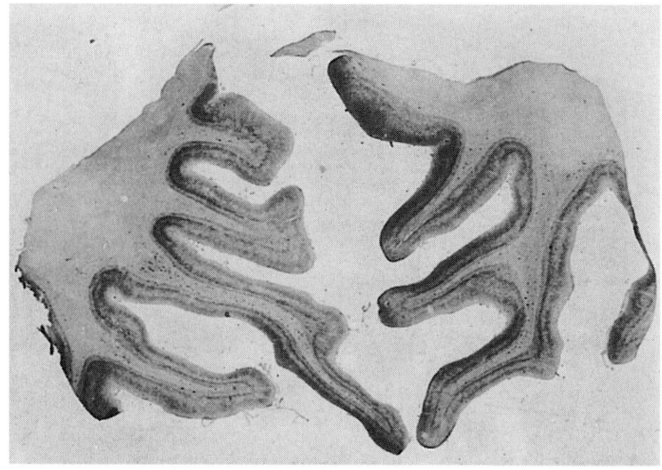

**Fig. 10-31.** Frontobasal gyri. Prominent diffuse bilayered PrP deposition in cortex.

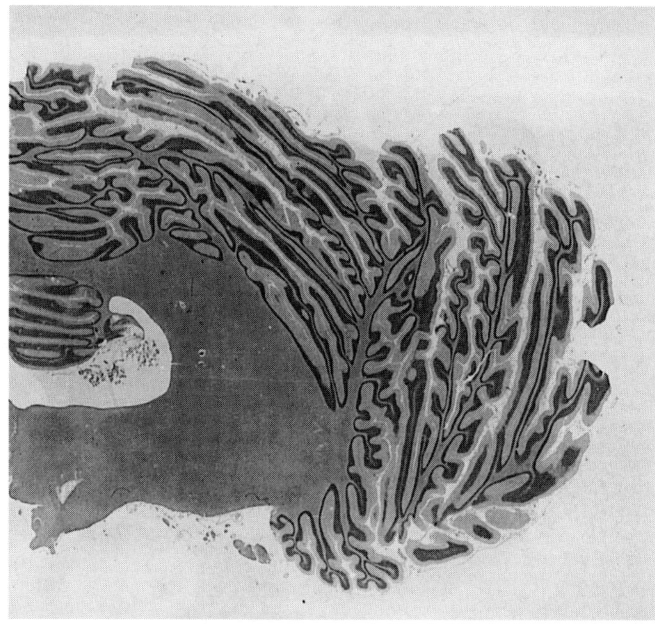

**Fig. 10-32.** Perfect preservation of cerebellar cortex in CJD-like GSS phenotype. (H&E; ×1.5.)

plaque formation.[6,59] In the Indiana GSS kindred, amyloid is exclusively labeled by an antiserum to residues 90-102 of PrP, whereas additional preamyloid deposits were labeled by antibodies against residues spanning the whole PrP molecule.[54]

**Familial fatal insomnia (FFI).** This newly described clinicopathologic phenotype has raised considerable interest, especially concerning the molecular and structural basis of sleep disorders, as evident from a recently published review.[58] According to molecular genetic data, this peculiar phenotype should be diagnosed only in a family member with the $PRNP^{178}$ muta-

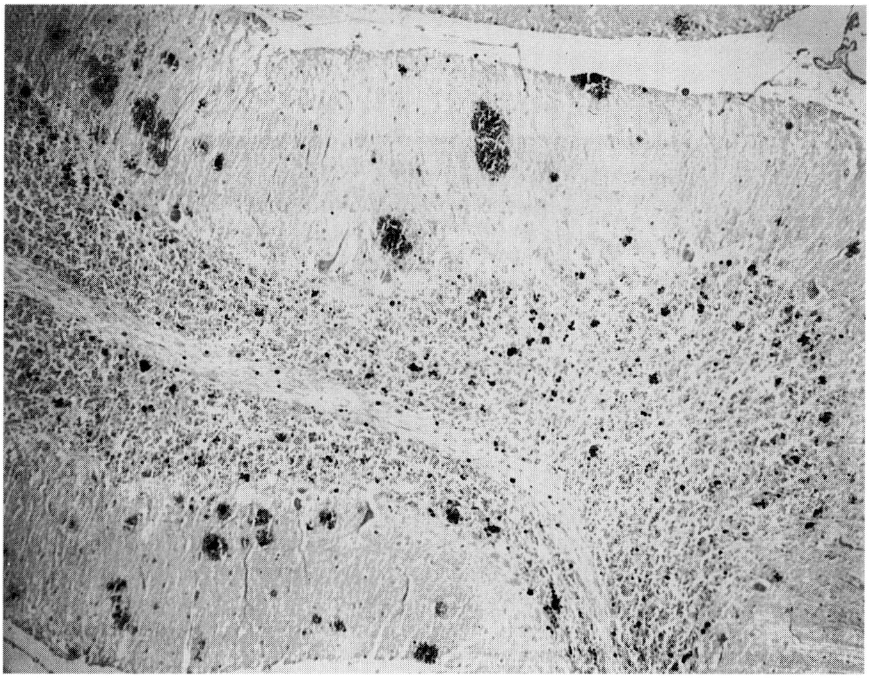

**Fig. 10-33.** Abundant PrP plaques in the cerebellar cortex. The largest plaques occupy the molecular layer, smaller plaques the granular layer (ICC for PrP). (×63.)

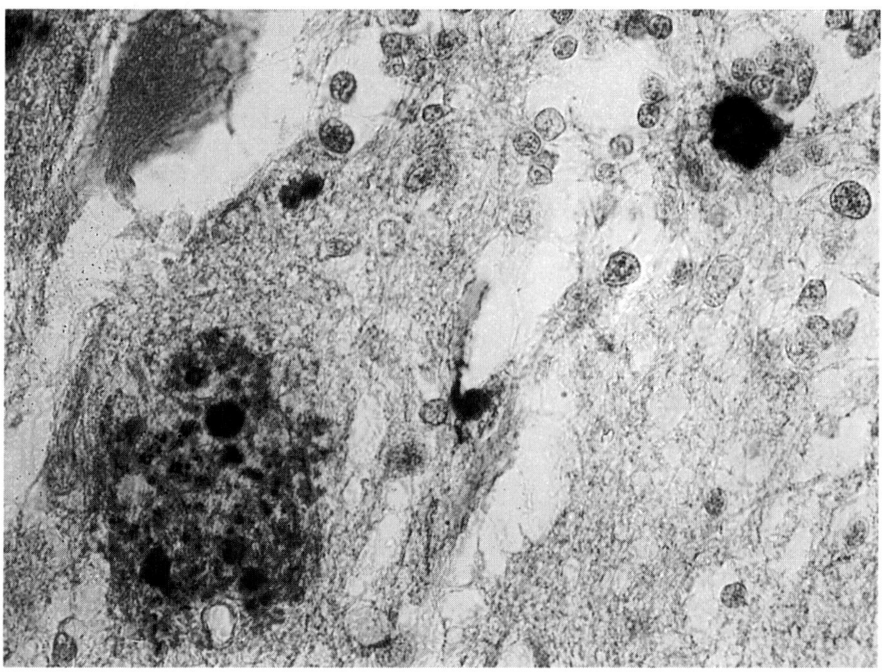

**Fig. 10-34.** A large multicentric PrP plaque and a small kuru plaque (ICC for PrP). (×630.)

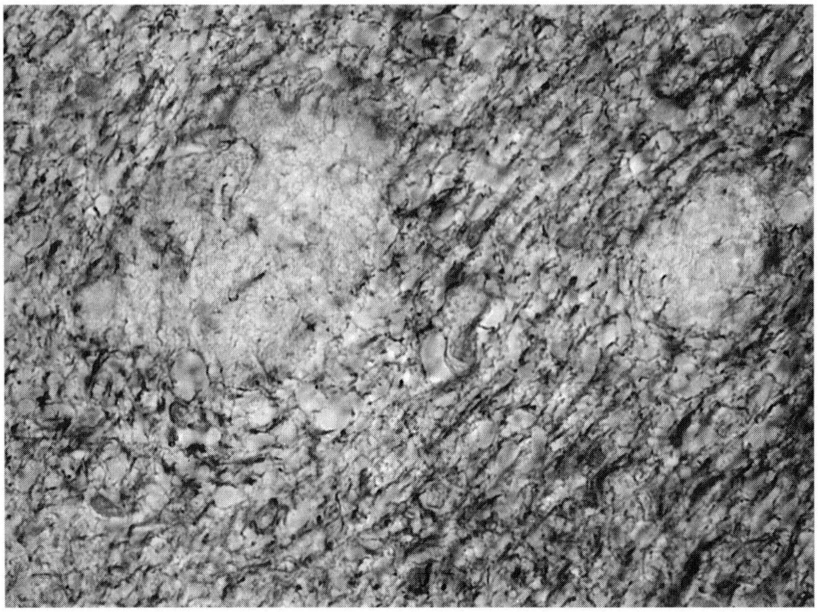

**Fig. 10-35.** Dense network of fibrillary astroglial processes around two plaques (ICC for GFAP). (×630.)

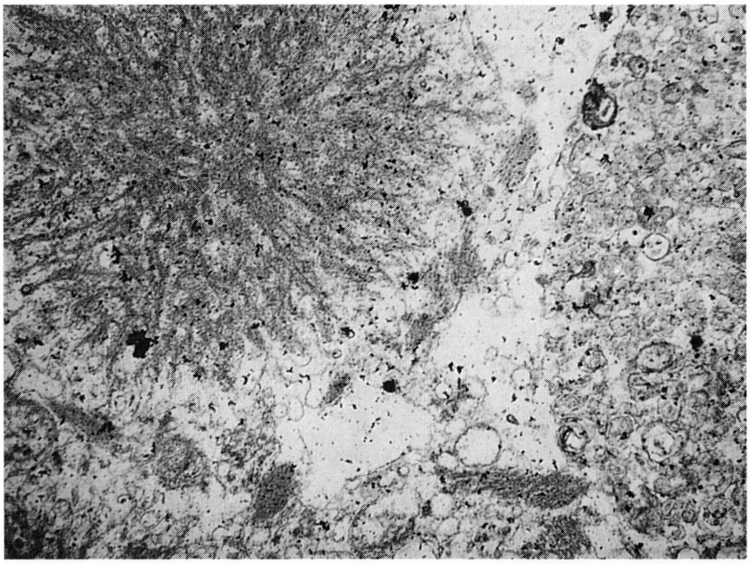

**Fig. 10-36.** Electron micrograph of dystrophic neurite (*at right*) next to amyloid star (*at left*). Cerebral cortex at autopsy, uranyl acetate, and lead citrate. (×10,000.)

tion combined with a methionine coding triplet at polymorphic codon 129.[55] Histopathology predominantly involves the thalamus, with neuronal loss and gliosis. Marked involvement of the anterior and dorsomedial nuclei is characteristic in FFI, in contrast to other types of thalamic degeneration.[90] Occasionally the cerebral cortex exhibits astrogliosis and/or mild spongiosis.[49] A spectrum of other abnormalities, including degeneration of the inferior olives as another characteristic feature, have been described in this rare disorder.[48] PrP deposition is restricted to subcortical structures in cases of short duration, but later appear to spread to neocortex and limbic structures.[100] Experimental transmission to mice was recently achieved.[117]

Apparent sporadic cases may show similar features, including highly focal cortical spongiform change[78]; however, without clearly diagnostic spongiform change, PrP examination and eventual molecular biologic studies are required for a definitive diagnosis.

**Kuru.** The discovery and scientific analysis of kuru are fascinating chapters of modern biomedicine. Hadlow recognized pathologic similarities with scrapie,[60] and the first successful transmission of a human neurodegenerative disease into other species followed.[46] Since the cessation of ritual cannibalism, the number of cases has dramatically declined. However, now, after decades, occasional cases of kuru still emerge. Clinically a cerebellar syndrome predominates.[47] While most neuropathologic features correspond to those of CJD with prominent spongiform change and numerous plaques,[76] kuru should be diagnosed only in members of the native population of Papua New Guinea.[27,29] In the one brain that I had the opportunity to examine immunocytochemically, PrP was deposited in synaptic distribution and in prominent plaques.

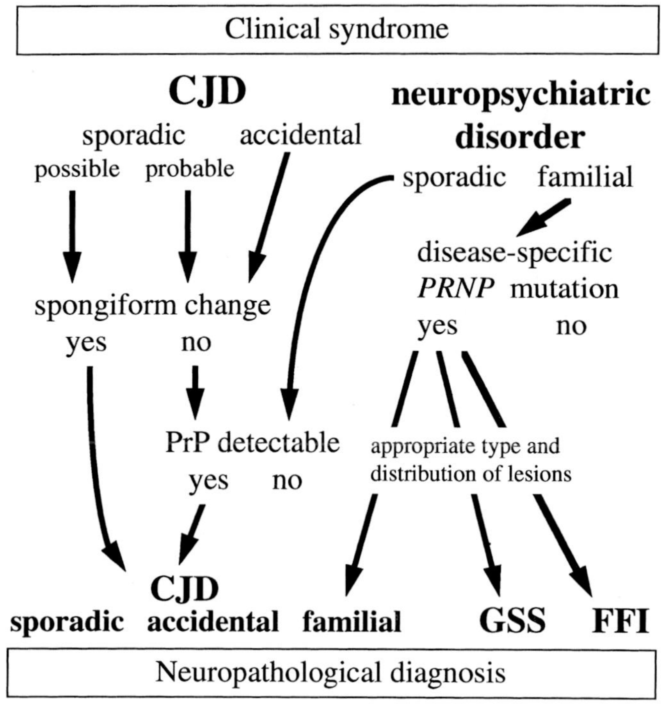


**Fig. 10-37.** Scheme summarizing diagnostic process from clinical syndrome to neuropathologic diagnosis of human TSE.

## Diagnostic Procedure

Ideally, available clinical information should allow a categorization of the clinical syndrome according to criteria given in the box on page 451. This is important for consideration of specific precautions to be taken for the performance of the autopsy (see discussion on precautions and tissue handling in suspected human spongiform encephalopathies, this chapter). Extensive sampling from various brain areas (minimum from frontal, temporal, and occipital lobes, basal ganglia, and cerebellum) is mandatory in every autopsy of suspected spongiform encephalopathy. Especially important is the comparison between cerebral and cerebellar involvement. However, one block of tissue with typical spongiform change and/or unambiguous PrP immunoreactivity should provide the definitive diagnosis. In nonspongiform histopathology, most frequently seen in familial disorders[19] in which molecular PRNP data also are required, detection of $PrP^{CJD}$ by immunocytochemistry or immunoblotting is mandatory for diagnosis. Familial conditions require molecular biologic analysis of PRNP. The diagnostic progression from clinical syndrome to neuropathologic diagnosis is summarized in the scheme shown in Figure 10-37.

Brain biopsies should be performed only if treatable alternatives to a diagnosis of spongiform encephalopathy are under serious consideration. However, brain biopsies have revealed diagnostic pathology in 95% of CJD patients confirmed by autopsy and experimental transmission.[19]

## Conclusion

Neuropathologic features in most cases of human prion diseases are well established in the context of clinical, epidemiologic, and molecular genetic data. It is thus possible to propose neuropathologic diagnostic criteria for the various types of prion diseases as summarized in the box on page 470. Very rare cases might not fit into this scheme ("prion dementia without characteristic pathology,"[33] "atypical dementias requiring further investigation,"[9] and "atypical forms of CJD"[109]). Then a diagnosis must be sought by additional techniques such as PrP immunoblotting, preparation of SAF, molecular biologic studies, or experimental transmission. As an example, entirely uncharacteristic brain pathology was described in familial presenile dementia with an insert PRNP mutation[33]; however, the significance of such molecular genetic aberration as disease precipitator has been questioned.[40,124] Given the rarity of such atypical histopathology as well as the absence of PrP in a spectrum of nonspongiform dementias,[21] there is no need to replace spongiform encephalopathy as a descriptive term for the whole group of disorders.

**Neuropathologic Diagnostic Criteria for Human Spongiform Encephalopathies (Modified after Budka, and others[29])**

1. Creutzfeldt-Jakob disease (CJD)—sporadic, iatrogenic (recognized risk), or familial (same disease in first-degree relative);
   Spongiform encephalopathy in cerebral and/or cerebellar cortex and/or subcortical gray matter; and/or
   Encephalopathy with PrP immunoreactivity (plaque and/or diffuse synaptic and/or patchy/perivacuolar types).
2. Gerstmann-Sträussler-Scheinker disease (GSS)—(in family with dominantly inherited progressive ataxia and/or dementia);
   Encephalo(myelo)pathy with multicentric PrP plaques.
3. Familial fatal insomnia (FFI) (in family with PRNP[178] mutation):
   Thalamic degeneration, with focal cerebral spongiform change.
4. Kuru—(in the native population of Papua New Guinea).

## PRECAUTIONS AND TISSUE HANDLING IN SUSPECTED HUMAN SPONGIFORM ENCEPHALOPATHIES

### Risk Assessment

Despite many sensational and intimidating reports in the mass media, TSE (prion diseases) are not contagious in the usual sense. Successful transmission requires both specific material (from or adjacent to CNS tissue) and specific modes (mainly penetrating contact with the recipient). As a result, these diseases are not easily acquired. Nevertheless, specific safety precautions are mandatory to avoid accidental transmission and, equally important and difficult, to decontaminate any infectivity. The recommendations given here are based on a recent consensus report.[30] However, safety guidelines vary between laboratories and countries and need to be continuously revised and updated as new scientific evidence emerges.[1–3]

Transmissible spongiform encephalopathies have been observed in health care workers.* However, there is no evidence that this professional group is at higher risk than other members of the population. Specifically, there is no proven case in which a TSE developed following contact with TSE patients. In contrast, it seems much more likely that other infections, e.g., tuberculosis, HIV, or hepatitis, might be contracted in the professional setting. It is somehow reassuring that numerous research laboratory personnel working with human and animal TSE have yet to experience a single case of accidentally transmitted disease.[14]

### Infectivity of Materials

Concerning infectivity, there is considerable lack of information on the human. Known human-to-human transmission in spongiform encephalopathies has been restricted to kuru in the formerly cannibalistic Fore population of Papua New Guinea and to accidental, iatrogenic inoculation with infected material (intracerebral EEG electrode, dura mater grafts, corneal transplants, and pituitary hormones derived from human glands). As a result, most data on potential infectivity in these diseases do not derive from transmission to humans, but rather from experimental CJD, scrapie, or BSE transmission to primates, rodents, or other species. However, CJD transmission by dural, corneal, and possibly hepatic[36] grafts requires exclusion of demented patients as potential donors of organs for transplantation.

Tissue and body fluids were classified into four classes of infectivity according to specific measures taken by the EU[43] to prevent spread of animal-derived disease:

- High infectivity: CNS tissues (brain, spinal cord) and adjacent tissues (eyes)
- Medium infectivity: lymphoid tissues (spleen, lymph nodes, tonsils), internal organs with lymphatic component (e.g., ileum, proximal colon), placenta, pituitary gland, dura mater, and CSF
- Low infectivity: peripheral nerves, bone marrow, liver, lung, pancreas, thymus
- No detectable infectivity: muscle, kidney, fat, bone, blood, milk, bile

(These classifications differ from those of the Advisory Committee on Dangerous Pathogens.)[3]

### The Autopsy

There is consensus that specific precautions should be taken for an autopsy performed on a patient with suspected TSE.[8,30,101] Because the procedures given below can be followed without imposing disproportionate hardship, there is no safety reason to refuse an autopsy on a patient with suspected transmissible spongiform encephalopathy. Moreover, obtaining an autopsy to establish a definite diagnosis is of utmost importance, not only for research into these enigmatic diseases, but also for epidemiologic and public health reasons. The risk of infection for the personnel can be thought of as lower than that in autopsies on patients with viral hepatitis or HIV infection. Precautions taken for such autopsies are more than adequate on patients with CJD. Decontamination of the autopsy material, however, requires specific measures. The following

* Refs. 10, 11, 56, 94, 113, 121.

protocol is kept as simple as possible; other and more detailed instructions may be found else where.[3,8,14,35,101]

The most important objective of the autopsy is to make possible a definitive diagnosis by neuropathology. It is thus sufficient, in most cases, to restrict the autopsy to removal of the brain. This can be done safely in any autopsy room and does not require special safety or containment facilities, provided that the following procedures[30] are correctly performed:

- The autopsy personnel should avoid accidental penetrating wounds by wearing protection gear as in other infectious autopsies (hepatitis, HIV infection, etc.), including safety gloves (e.g., Teflon-made from Spectra®, or metallic gloves) beneath rubber gloves, a disposable apron, and eye and mouth protection.
- Contamination of the autopsy table should be avoided by using a nonpermeable disposable plastic sheet or similar material.
- Removal of the brain: The head is positioned in the usual way, with a thick layer of cellulose sheets underneath. The skull should be opened with a mechanical (nonelectrical) hand saw, which is easier to decontaminate than an electrical saw. Before removal of the brain from the skull, it is strongly recommended that some parts of the brain be taken (recommended: apricot-sized pieces of cerebrum [preferentially from one pole] and of cerebellum) for freezing to be used in eventual further diagnostic procedures and research. This tissue must be put into two layers of small plastic bags and put into (and frozen within) a tightly-closing plastic container that is clearly marked. The brain is then removed from the skull in the usual way and put in a tight plastic container with buffered 4% formaldehyde solution for neuropathologic processing. Both the fixed brain and the fixative solution are still infectious and should be appropriately labeled. If desired, internal organs may be inspected and sampled in situ without removal from the body.
- After the autopsy is completed, the plastic and cellulose sheets are folded together and put into a container with other disposable infectious hospital waste material to be incinerated.
- All instruments (saw, knives, etc.) and contaminated surfaces must be decontaminated by the procedures given below.
- Accidents involving parenteral exposure to material or contaminated wastes from TSE should be recorded.[3]

## Neuropathology Service

Because neuropathologists and their staff work with TSE tissues containing the highest infectivity titers, they appear to be most at risk. However, this risk can be minimized by the following procedures:[30]

- The personnel should wear safety gloves; special care should be taken to avoid accidental penetrating wounds.
- The formaldehyde-fixed brain is processed on a table covered by a disposable plastic sheet and cut on layers of cellulose sheets (to be discarded by cremation with infectious hospital waste).
- To deactivate CJD infectivity,[24] it is recommended to soak the tissue blocks for histology in concentrated (95 to 100%) formic acid for 1 hour, followed by fresh formalin for at least 48 hours. However, this makes the tissue block brittle and more difficult to cut. Without this step, paraffin blocks may still be infectious.[18]
- All instruments and gloves that came into contact with potentially infectious material must be decontaminated. Instruments that were contaminated by formaldehyde-fixed, formic acid-untreated tissue are not decontaminated by autoclaving.[120] They should be immersed in 2N NaOH for 1 hour.
- Tissue remnants, cutting debris, and contaminated formaldehyde solution should be discarded within a plastic container to be cremated as infectious hospital waste.
- Accidents involving parenteral exposure to material or contaminated wastes from TSE should be recorded.[3]

## Decontamination

There is also consensus that appropriate decontamination measures must be followed for surfaces, instruments, gloves, and other devices that come in contact with tissue material and body fluids from patients with TSE.[8,30,101] Because conventional methods of sterilization and disinfection do not decontaminate the CJD infectious agent,[17] specific measures must be used. Unfortunately, however, there is no unanimity about optimal procedures.

- *Steam autoclaving* (glassware, instruments, safety gloves, etc.)

  134° C recommended for 1 hour.[3,35]

  *Comment:* Porous load is considered more effective than gravity displacement autoclaves.[3] The required time periods have been debated. For porous load autoclaving, only 18 min at 30 lbs psi, or six separate cycles for 3 min each at 30 lbs psi, have been recommended.[3] However, some laboratories recommend two cycles of autoclaving for 1 hour each, or autoclaving for at least 1 hour during or subsequent to soaking in NaOH (see below).
- *Chemical decontamination* of nonautoclavable materials and surfaces:

  2N NaOH (80 g per liter) for 1 hour; alternatively, 1N NaOH may be used for 2 hours.

  *Comment:* Some laboratories consider mere wiping off as sufficient for surfaces; others require more extensive washes. Do not use NaOH on aluminum material.

Alternatively, 5% NaOCl (at least 20,000 ppm free chloride, fresh solution) for 2 hours.

*Comment:* Very irritating and corrosive for steel. Some laboratories boil instruments or material in 3% SDS for at least 3 min as another option, either alone or in combination with autoclaving at 121 °C for 1 hour.[119]

## ACKNOWLEDGMENTS

This work was performed within the *European Union Biomed-1 Concerted Action, The human prion diseases: from neuropathology to pathobiology and molecular genetics* (Project Leader: H. Budka).

The author is grateful to the many clinical and neuropathologic colleagues who kindly provided tissue and other materials as important contributions to his work on TSE, to Ms. Flicker for excellent technical assistance, and to Dr. JA Hainfellner for support with a literature survey.

## REFERENCES

1. Advisory Committee on Dangerous Pathogens: Categorisation of pathogens according to hazard and categories of containment, ed 3 (interim issue). London, 1994, HMSO.
2. Advisory Committee on Dangerous Pathogens: Categorisation of pathogens according to hazard and categories of containment. ed 2, London, 1990, HMSO.
3. Advisory Committee on Dangerous Pathogens: Precautions for work with human and animal transmissible spongiform encephalopathies. London, 1994, HMSO.
4. Alperovitch A, and others: Incidence of Creutzfeldt-Jakob disease in Europe in 1993, Lancet 343:918, 1994.
5. Arendt T, Bigl V, and Arendt A: Neuron loss in the nucleus basalis of Meynert in Creutzfeldt-Jakob disease, Acta Neuropathol 65:85-88, 1984.
6. Barcikowska M, and others: Microglia is a component of the prion protein amyloid plaque in the Gerstmann-Sträussler-Scheinker syndrome, Acta Neuropathol 85:623-627, 1993.
7. Bateman D, and others: Sporadic Creutzfeldt-Jakob disease in a 18-year-old in the UK, Lancet 346:1155-1156, 1995.
8. Bell JE, and Ironside JW: How to tackle a possible Creutzfeldt-Jakob disease necropsy, J Clin Pathol 46:193-197, 1993.
9. Bell JE, and Ironside JW: Neuropathology of spongiform encephalopathies in humans, Br Med Bull 49:738-777, 1993.
10. Berger JR, and David NJ: CJD in health care workers, Neurology 43:2421, 1993.
11. Berger JR, and David NJ: Creutzfeldt-Jakob disease in a physician: a review of the disorder in health care workers, Neurology 43:205-206, 1993.
12. Boellaard JW, Doerr-Schott J, and Schlote W: Miniplaques and shapeless cerebral amyloid deposits in a case of Gerstmann-Sträussler-Scheinker's syndrome, Acta Neuropathol 86:532-535, 1993.
13. Britton TC, and others: Sporadic Creutzfeldt-Jakob disease in a 16-year-old in the UK, Lancet 346:1155, 1995.
14. Brown P: Guidelines for high risk autopsy cases: special precautions for Creutzfeldt-Jakob disease. In Autopsy performance and reporting, Northfield, Illinois, 1990, College of American Pathologists.
15. Brown P: The phenotypic expression of different mutations in transmissible human spongiform encephalopathy, Rev Neurol 148:317-327, 1992.
16. Brown P, and others: Iatrogenic Creutzfeldt-Jakob disease: an example of the interplay between ancient genes and modern medicine, Neurology 44:291-293, 1994.
17. Brown P, and others: Chemical disinfection of Creutzfeldt-Jakob disease virus, N Engl J Med 306:1279-1282, 1982.
18. Brown P, Gibbs CJ, and Gajdusek DC: Transmission of Creutzfeldt-Jakob disease from formalin-fixed, paraffin-embedded human brain tissue, N Engl J Med 315:1614-1615, 1986.
19. Brown P, and others: Human spongiform encephalopathy: the National Institutes of Health series of 300 cases of experimentally transmitted disease, Ann Neurol 35:513-529, 1994.
20. Brown P, Goldfarb LG, and Gajdusek DC: The new biology of spongiform encephalopathy: infectious amyloidoses with a genetic twist, Lancet 337:1019-1022, 1991.
21. Brown P, and others: Real and imagined clinicopathological limits of "prion dementia," Lancet 341:127-129, 1993.
22. Brown P, and others: Intracerebral distribution of infectious amyloid protein in spongiform encephalopathy, Ann Neurol 38:245-253, 1995.
23. Brown P, Preece MA, and Will RG: "Friendly fire" in medicine: hormones, homografts, and Creutzfeldt-Jakob disease, Lancet 340:24-27, 1992.
24. Brown P, Wolff A, and Gajdusek D: A simple and effective method for inactivating virus infectivity in formalin-fixed tissue samples from patients with Creutzfeldt-Jakob disease, Neurology 40:887-890, 1990.
25. Brownell B, and Oppenheimer D: An ataxic form of presenile polioencephalopathy (Creutzfeldt-Jakob disease), J Neurol Neurosurg Psychiatry 28:350-361, 1965.
26. Budka H: The human prion diseases: from neuropathology to pathobiology and molecular genetics. In Baert AE, and others: European Union Biomedical and Health Research. The Biomed-1 program, pp 513-514, Amsterdam, 1995, IOS Press.
27. Budka H: Neuropathological diagnostic criteria for Creutzfeldt-Jakob disease (CJD) and other human spongiform encephalopathies (prion diseases). In Cruz-Sanchez FF and others: Neuropathological diagnostic criteria for brain banking, pp 65-71 and 200-201, EU Biomedical and Health Research Series, Amsterdam, 1995, IOS Press.
28. Budka H: Prion diseases—from molecular biology to neuropathology, J Neuropathol Exp Neurol suppl:75S-76S, 1995.
29. Budka H, and others: Neuropathological diagnostic criteria for Creutzfeldt-Jakob disease (CJD) and other human spongiform encephalopathies (prion diseases), Brain Pathol 5:459-466, 1995.
30. Budka H, and others: Tissue handling in suspected Creutzfeldt-Jakob disease (CJD) and other human spongiform encephalopathies (prion diseases), Brain Pathol 5:319-322, 1995.
31. Büeler H, and others: Mice devoid of PrP are resistant to scrapie, Cell 73:1-20, 1993.
32. Cartier L, and others: The nucleus basalis of Meynert in 20 definite cases of Creutzfeldt-Jakob disease, J Neurol Neurosurg Psychiatry 52:304-309, 1989.

32a. Chazot G, and others: New variant of Creutzfeldt-Jakob disease in a 26-year-old French man, Lancet 347:1181, 1996.

33. Collinge J, and others: Prion dementia without characteristic pathology, Lancet 336:7-9, 1990.
34. Collinge J, Palmer MS, and Dryden AJ: Genetic predisposition to iatrogenic Creutzfeldt-Jakob disease, Lancet 337:1441-1442, 1991.
35. Committee on Health Care Issues ANA: Precautions in handling tissues, fluids, and other contaminated materials from patients with documented or suspected Creutzfeldt-Jakob disease, Ann Neurol 19:75-77, 1986.

36. Créange A, and others: Creutzfeldt-Jakob disease after liver transplantation, Ann Neurol 38:269-272, 1995.
37. Creutzfeldt HG: Über eine eigenartige herdförmige Erkrankung des Zentralnervensystems, Z Ges Neurol Psychiat 57:1-18, 1920.
38. de-Courten-Myers G, and Mandybur TI: Atypical Gerstmann-Sträussler syndrome or familial spinocerebellar ataxia and Alzheimer's disease? Neurology 37:269-275, 1987.
39. Delasnerie-Laupretre N, and others: Creutzfeldt-Jakob disease in Europe, Lancet 346:898, 1995.
40. Diringer H: Prion disease, Lancet 336:369, 1990.
41. Doh-ura K, and others: Creutzfeldt-Jakob disease patients with congophilic kuru plaques have the missense variant prion protein common to Gerstmann-Sträussler syndrome, Ann Neurol 27:121-126, 1990.
42. Doi Yi R, and others: Distribution of prion protein in German patients with Creutzfeldt-Jakob disease is different from that in Japanese patients, Acta Neuropathol Berl 87:481-483, 1994.
43. European Community: Guidelines for minimising the risk of transmission of agents causing spongiform encephalopathies via medicinal products. Document III/328/91-EN, 1991.
44. Farlow MR, and others: Gerstmann-Sträussler-Scheinker disease. In Vinken PJ, Bruyn GW, and Klawans HL, editors: Handbook of clinical neurology vol 16 (60), Amsterdam, 1991 Elsevier.
45. Gajdusek DC: Unconventional viruses and the origin and disappearance of kuru, Science 197:943-960, 1977.
46. Gajdusek DC, and Gibbs CJJ: Experimental transmission of kuru-like syndrome to chimpanzees, Nature 209:794-796, 1966.
47. Gajdusek DC, and Zigas V: Degenerative disease of the central nervous system in New Guinea: the endemic occurrence of kuru in the native population, N Engl J Med 257:974-978, 1957.
48. Gambetti P, and others: Fatal familial insomnia. A prion disease with distinctive histopathological and genotypic features. In Guilleminault C and others: Fatal familial insomnia. Inherited prion diseases, sleep, and the thalamus, New York, 1994, Raven Press.
49. Gambetti P, and others: Fatal familial insomnia and familial Creutzfeldt-Jakob disease: clinical, pathological and molecular features, Brain Pathol 5:43-51, 1995.
50. Gerstmann J: Über ein noch nicht beschriebenes Reflexphänomen bei einer Erkrankung des zerebellären Systems, Wien Med Wochenschr 78:906-908, 1928.
51. Gerstmann J, Sträussler E, and Scheinker I: Über eine eigenartige hereditär-familiäre Erkrankung des Zentralnervensystems. Zugleich ein Beitrag zur Frage des vorzeitigen lokalen Alterns, Z Neurol 154:736-762, 1936.
52. Ghetti B, and others: Gerstmann-Sträussler-Scheinker disease and the Indiana kindred, Brain Pathol 5:61-75, 1995.
53. Ghetti B, and others: Gerstmann-Sträussler-Scheinker disease. II. Neurofibrillary tangles and plaques with PrP-amyloid coexist in an affected family, Neurology 39:1453-1461, 1989.
54. Giaccone G, and others: Prion protein preamyloid and amyloid deposits in Gerstmann-Sträussler-Scheinker disease, Indiana kindred, Proc Natl Acad Sci USA 89:9349-9353, 1992.
55. Goldfarb LG, and others: Fatal familial insomnia and familial Creutzfeldt-Jakob disease: disease phenotype determined by a DNA polymorphism, Science 258:806-808, 1992.
56. Gorman DG, and others: Creutzfeldt-Jakob disease in a pathologist, Neurology 42:463, 1992.
57. Gray F, and others: Creutzfeldt-Jakob disease and cerebral amyloid angiopathy, Acta Neuropathol Berl 88:106-111, 1994.
58. Guilleminault C, and others: Fatal familial insomnia. Inherited prion diseases, sleep, and the thalamus, New York 1994, Raven Press.
59. Guiroy DC, and others: Relationship of microglia and scrapie amyloid-immunoreactive plaques in kuru, Creutzfeldt-Jakob disease and Gerstmann-Sträussler syndrome, Acta Neuropathol Berl 87:526-530, 1994.
60. Hadlow WJ: Scrapie and kuru, Lancet II: 289-290, 1959.
61. Hainfellner JA, and others: The original Gerstmann-Sträussler-Scheinker family of Austria: divergent clinicopathological phenotypes but constant PrP genotype, Brain Pathol 5: 201–211, 1995.
62. Hainfellner JA, and others: Creutzfeldt-Jakob disease in Austria, J Neurol Neurosurg Psychiat, 61:139-142, 1996.
63. Haltia M, and others: Chromosome 14-encoded Alzheimer's disease: genetic and clinicopathological description, Ann Neurol 36:362-367, 1994.
64. Hansen LA, and others: A neuropathological subset of Alzheimer's disease with concomitant Lewy body disease and spongiform change, Acta Neuropathol 78:194-201, 1989.
65. Hayward PAR, Bell JE, Ironside JW: Prion protein immunocytochemistry: reliable protocols for the investigation of Creutzfeldt-Jakob disease, Neuropathol Appl Neurobiol 20:375-383, 1994.
66. Heidenhain A: Klinische und anatomische Untersuchungen über eine eigenartige Erkrankung des Zentralnervensystems im Praesenium, Z Ges Neurol Psychiatr, 118:49-114, 1929.
67. Hsiao KK, Prusiner SB: Inherited human prion diseases, Neurology 40:1820-1827, 1990.
68. Hsiao KK, and others: Spontaneous neurodegeneration in transgenic mice with mutant prion protein, Science 250:1587-1590, 1990.
69. Ikeda S, and others: Gerstmann-Sträussler-Scheinker disease showing b-protein type cerebellar and cerebral amyloid angiopathy, Acta Neuropathol 88:262-266, 1994.
70. Ironside JW, and others: Ubiquitin immunocytochemistry in human spongiform encephalopathies, Neuropathol Appl Neurobiol 19:134-140, 1993.
71. Jakob A: Über eigenartige Erkrankungen des Zentralnervensystems mit bemerkenswertem anatomischem Befunde (spastische Pseudosklerose—Encephalomyelopathie mit disseminierten Degenerationsherden), Dtsch Z Nervenheilk 70:132-146, 1921.
72. Kitamoto T, Doh-ura K, and Tateishi J: Primary structure of prion protein influences clinical and pathological aspects of Creutzfeldt-Jakob disease. In Corain B: Alzheimer's disease: advances in clinical and basic research. Chichester, 1993, John Wiley & Sons.
73. Kitamoto T, and others: Abnormal isoform of prion proteins accumulates in the synaptic structures of the central nervous system in patients with Creutzfeldt-Jakob disease, Am J Pathol 140:1285-1294, 1992.
74. Kitamoto T, and Tateishi J: Human prion diseases with variant prion protein, Phil Trans R Soc Lond B 343:391-398, 1994.
75. Kitamoto T, and Tateishi J: Immunohistochemical confirmation of Creutzfeldt-Jakob disease with a long clinical course with amyloid plaque core antibodies, Am J Pathol 131:435-443, 1988.
76. Klatzo I, Gajdusek DC, and Zigas V: Pathology of kuru, Lab Invest 8:799-847, 1959.
77. Kocisko DA, and others: Cell-free formation of protease-resistant prion protein, Nature 370:471-474, 1994.
78. Kornfeld M, and Seelinger DF: Pure thalamic dementia with a single focus of spongiform change in cerebral cortex, Clin Neuropathol 13:77-81, 1994.
79. Kretzschmar HA, and others: Prion protein mutation in a family first reported by Gerstmann, Sträussler, and Scheinker, Lancet 337:1160, 1991.
80. Kretzschmar HA, Neumann M, and Stavrou D: Codon 178 mutation of the human prion protein gene in a German family (Backer family): sequencing data from 72-year-old celloidin-embedded brain tissue, Acta Neuropathol 89:96-98, 1995.
81. Kretzschmar HA, and others: Molecular cloning of a human prion protein cDNA, DNA 5:315-324, 1986.

82. Lantos PL, and others: Prion protein immunocytochemistry helps to establish the true incidence of prion diseases, Neurosci Lett 147:67-71, 1992.
82a. Lasmezas CI, and others: BSE transmission to macaques, Nature 381:743-744, 1996.
83. Liberski PP: Prions, beta-sheets and transmissible dementias: is there still something missing? Acta Neuropathol 90:113-125, 1995.
84. Liberski PP, and Budka H: An overview of neuropathology of the slow unconventional virus infections. In Liberski PP, editor: Light and electron microscopic neuropathology of slow virus disorders. Boca Raton, FL, 1993, CRC Press.
85. Liberski PP, and Budka H: Tubulovesicular structures in Gerstmann-Sträussler-Scheinker disease, Acta Neuropathol 88:491-492, 1994.
86. Liberski PP, and others: Tubulovesicular structures in Creutzfeldt-Jakob disease, Acta Neuropathol 84:238-243, 1992.
87. Liberski PP, and others: Tubulovesicular structures in human and experimental Creutzfeldt-Jakob disease, Eur J Epidemiol 7:551-555, 1991.
88. Liberski PP, and others: Tubulovesicular structures. In Liberski PP: Light and electron microscopic neuropathology of slow virus disorders, Boca Raton, FL, 1993, CRC Press.
89. Liberski PP, and others: Neuroaxonal dystrophy in unconventional slow virus disease. In Liberski PP: Light and electron microscopic neuropathology of slow virus disorders, Boca Raton, FL, 1993, CRC Press.
90. Martin J-J: Thalamic degenerations. In Vinken PJ, Bruyn GW: Handbook of clinical neurology, vol 21, Amsterdam, 1975, North-Holland.
91. Masters CL, and others: Creutzfeldt-Jakob disease: patterns of worldwide occurrence and the significance of familial and sporadic clustering, Ann Neurol 5:177-188, 1979.
92. Masters CL, and Richardson EPJ: Subacute spongiform encephalopathy (Creutzfeldt-Jakob disease). The nature and progression of spongiform change, Brain 101:333-344, 1978.
93. Medori R, and others: Fatal familial insomnia is a prion disease with a mutation at codon 178 of the prion gene, N Engl J Med 326:444-449, 1992.
94. Miller D: Creutzfeldt-Jakob disease in histopathology technicians, N Engl J Med 318:853-854, 1988.
95. Miyazono M, and others: Colocalization of prion protein and b protein in the same amyloid plaques in patients with Gerstmann-Sträussler syndrome, Acta Neuropathol 83:333-339, 1992.
96. Mizutani T, and others: Panencephalopathic type of Creutzfeldt-Jakob disease: primary involvement of the cerebral white matter, J Neurol Neurosurg Psychiatry 44:103-115, 1981.
97. Nakazato Y, and others: Swollen cortical neurons in Creutzfeldt-Jakob disease contain a phosphorylated neurofilament epitope, J Neuropathol Exp Neurol 49:197-205, 1990.
98. Nochlin D, and others: Familial dementia with PrP-positive amyloid plaques: a variant of Gerstmann-Sträussler syndrome, Neurology 39:910-918, 1989.
99. Palmer MS, and others: Homozygous prion protein genotype predisposes to sporadic Creutzfeldt-Jakob disease, Nature 352: 340-342, 1991.
100. Parchi P, and others: Regional distribution of protease-resistant prion protein in fatal familial insomnia, Ann Neurol 38: 21-29, 1995.
101. Peiffer J: Umgang mit Gewebe von Patienten mit Verdacht auf Creutzfeldt-Jakob'scher Krankheit, Pathologe 14:355, 1993.
102. Petersen RB, and others: Familial progressive subcortical gliosis: presence of prions and linkage to chromosome 17, Neurology 45:1062-1067, 1995.
103. Piccardo P, and others: Gerstmann-Sträussler-Scheinker disease (PRNP P102L): amyloid deposits are best recognized by antibodies directed to epitopes in PrP region 90-165, J Neuropathol Exp Neurol 54:790-801, 1995.
104. Pollanen MS, Bergeron C, and Weyer L: Absence of protease-resistant prion protein in dementia characterized by neuronal loss and status spongiosus, Acta Neuropathol 86:515-517, 1993.
105. Prusiner SB: Molecular biology of prion diseases, Science 252: 1515-1522, 1991.
106. Prusiner SB: Novel proteinaceous infectious particles cause scrapie. Science 216:136-144, 1982.
107. Prusiner SB, and Hsiao KK: Human prion diseases, Ann Neurol 35:385-395, 1994.
108. Ribadeau-Dumas JL, and Escourolle R: The Creutzfeldt-Jakob syndrome: a neuropathological and electron microscopic study. In Subirana A, Espalader JM, editors: Neurology, Amsterdam, 1974, Elsevier.
109. Richardson EP Jr, and Masters CL: The nosology of Creutzfeldt-Jakob disease and conditions related to the accumulation of $PrP^{CJD}$ in the nervous system, Brain Pathol 5:33-41, 1995.
110. Salazar AM, and others: Syndromes of amyotrophic lateral sclerosis and dementia: relation to transmissible Creutzfeldt-Jakob disease, Ann Neurol 14:17-26, 1983.
111. Sasaki A, Hirato J, and Nakazato Y: Immunohistochemical study of microglia in the Creutzfeldt-Jakob diseased brain, Acta Neuropathol 86:337-344, 1993.
112. Shin R, and others: Hydrated autoclave pretreatment enhances tau immunoreactivity in formalin-fixed normal and Alzheimer's disease brain tissues, Lab Invest 64:693-702, 1991.
113. Sitwell L, and others: Creutzfeldt-Jakob disease in histopathology technicians, N Engl J Med 318:854, 1988.
114. Smith PEM, and others: Creutzfeldt-Jakob disease in a dairy farmer, Lancet 346:898, 1995.
115. Suenaga T, and others: Ubiquitin immunoreactivity in Kuru plaques in Creutzfeldt-Jakob disease, Ann Neurol 28:174-177, 1990.
116. Taraboulos A, and others: Regional mapping of prion proteins in brain, Proc Natl Acad Sci USA 89:7620-7624, 1992.
117. Tateishi J, and others: First experimental transmission of fatal familial insomnia, Nature 376:434-435, 1995.
118. Tateishi J, and Kitamoto T: Inherited prion diseases and transmission to rodents, Brain Pathol 5:53-59, 1995.
119. Tateishi J, Tashima T, and Kitamoto T: Practical methods for chemical inactivation of Creutzfeldt-Jakob disease pathogen, Microbiol Immunol 35:163-166, 1991.
120. Taylor DM, and McConnell I: Autoclaving does not decontaminate formol-fixed scrapie tissues, Lancet 1:1463-1464, 1988.
121. Weber T, and others: Transmission of Creutzfeldt-Jakob disease by handling of dura mater, Lancet 341:123-124, 1993.
122. Weller RO, Steart PV, and Powell-Jackson JD: Pathology of Creutzfeldt-Jakob disease associated with pituitary-derived human growth hormone administration, Neuropathol Appl Neurobiol 12:117-129, 1986.
123. Will RG: Epidemiology of CJD in the UK. International Symposium: epidemiology, biochemistry and molecular biology. Göttingen, 1995, Medien in der Medizin.
124. Will RG: Prion disease, Lancet 336:369, 1990.
125. Will RG: Surveillance of Creutzfeldt-Jakob disease in the European Community. In Baert AE, and others: European Union biomedical and health research. The biomed-1 programme, Amsterdam, 1995, IOS Press.
125a. Will RG, and others: A new variant of Creutzfeldt-Jakob disease in the UK, Lancet 347:921-925, 1996.
126. Yamanouchi H, Budka H, and Vass KS: Unilateral Creutzfeldt-Jakob disease, Neurology 36:1517-1520, 1986.

C • H • A • P • T • E • R

# 11

# *Forensic Neuropathology*

**Jan E. Leestma**



As western societies become more complex, their legal systems share this complexity. A natural extension of these phenomena can be seen in the demand for increasingly detailed and sophisticated information within the legal system for medical, scientific, and technologic information. Included in this development is the demand and appreciation for neuropathologic information and expertise. More than ever, neuropathologists now are asked in legal proceedings to render opinions and expert testimony on neuropathologic issues. Forensic pathology in large urban areas is practiced in special facilities that often are physically and administratively separate from hospital-based training facilities and therefore are not readily accessible to resident trainees. It is difficult for pathologists in training to be exposed to the fascinating and instructive material found at a medical examiner's/coroner's facilities at a time when the need for such knowledge is increasing.

Forensic neuropathology is rapidly becoming a special field, one that deserves study by all pathologists. This chapter reviews major issues of forensic neuropathology and illustrates the importance of this information to the forensic exercise. This review is necessarily incomplete and covers only basic aspects of the field. The reader who requires more complete information is encouraged to consult the cited references, a monograph devoted entirely to this subject,[219] and a chapter devoted to forensic issues in the pediatric population.[218]

## FORENSIC ISSUES IN NEUROPATHOLOGY

### Interactions with the Legal System

All physicians including pathologists and neuropathologists may be called upon to render service to the legal system.[64,151,318] Such service may take the form of formal or informal consultations regarding various disease processes, their course, etiology, appearance and pathology, and prognosis. Procedures may range from examination of tissues and organs from an autopsy or microscopic slides to examination of photographs, medical records, or physical evidence. The product of this consultation may or may not result in formal testimony in depositions of discovery or at trial or hearings.[89] Forensic neuropathologic practice includes diagnosis of a basic disease process, but more often involves a determination of the duration or age of lesions and processes, identifying complicating, contributing, or unrelated pathologic processes, determination of mechanisms involved in various conditions, and clinical-circumstantial-pathologic correlations.

For most physicians, discussions between colleagues over these very same issues will take a different form and have a different outcome than when these discussions occur against a forensic backdrop. In the context of forensics different conventions are operative. The consulting party (attorney, judge, or jury) may have but slight understanding of the subject matter and insufficient background against which to interpret information and comments. In formal legal proceedings, all statements are made under oath and are officially recorded. The resulting record may become a public document. The manner of communicating a diagnosis or professional opinion is often precisely defined, and cannot encompass the element of doubt often expressed between colleagues or employed in a typical differential diagnosis.[89] In legal proceedings, opinions are expected to be "black or white." The physician expert is often asked to state an opinion or to present a diagnosis that is "more likely than not" to be so. Or the physician must provide an opinion that represents one's "best medical and surgical certainty."[88,360] Doubt, in the usual medical sense, is neither understood nor accepted. Often, opinions are challenged on the basis of "possibility" of an alternative interpretation. In these circumstances one must freely admit that many alternatives are possible, but may not have a high probability of being true. For an expert to be drawn into quantifying the veracity of an opinion by the use of percentages of certainty can be a dangerous trap. In most civil legal actions, all the system demands is the well-considered opinion of a given expert within a framework of "more likely than not" or "to a reasonable degree of medical (pathologic) certainty" in responding to questions. Wordings of this context of certainty can vary between jurisdictions and with the nature of the case, but each implies that the expert must be at least 51% sure of his/her opinion. In criminal matters a more exacting standard of certainty is implied, since the trier of fact (judge or jury) must weigh the totality of the evidence and convict only if they find the defendant to be guilty "beyond a reasonable shadow of doubt." This does not mean that the expert must be as certain or play the role of judge. It only means that some greater degree of certainty than 51% may be called for. In this situation, and others, it is required that the expert say if he/she has no opinion or simply does not know the answer. Failure to do so may violate the oath taken at the start of testimony.

A particularly instructive forensic exercise is the practice of being asked to state the basis for an opinion. This forces the physician expert to think logically, to examine premises, to understand fully the basic processes (anatomy, physiology, pathology), and to express clearly and concisely the intellectual path taken to reach a given opinion.

Physicians may become involved in a forensic issue by virtue of their involvement in the management, treatment, or diagnosis of a case. In such instances the physician may be subject to subpoena. This is a legal summons, carrying penalties for noncompliance that directs the material witness to be present at a given time and place, to provide certain relevant materials and records, and to be prepared to answer questions under oath.

In other circumstances the physician may be a purely voluntary participant in a legal proceeding by serving as an expert on behalf of one party or another, either by way of a background consultant or with the full intention of offering testimony as an expert. This will generally require that the individual be "qualified" as an expert by the retaining attorney.

Beyond informal interactions[216] between a retained witness and an attorney are two legal proceedings that have their own characteristics: the discovery deposition, and the interrogatory process (the trial). Before the trial or deposition, written questions may be submitted to a prospective witness by opposing counsel. Discovery depositions are legal proceedings in which a witness is questioned (examined), under oath, usually by opposing counsel, with a court reporter preparing a verbatim transcript. Depositions enable opposing counsel to learn what the expert will say at trial and the basis for this testimony. Questions almost always include a review of the qualifications; training and experience of the witnesses that would qualify them as experts; the opinions to be expressed and the basis for them; and the materials and information relied upon to render the opinions.

During depositions, objections may be made by retaining counsel as to what has been asked. Since no judge is present to mediate such objections, they are noted for the record and answered anyway. All statements made in discovery deposition are admissible in court and, if at variance with later testimony, may be used to discredit or impeach the witness. Therefore, it is vital to prepare adequately for a deposition to ensure that a question is properly understood, and that the answers reflect the true opinion of the expert. Depositions may be recorded on videotape for later use at trial in lieu of an in-person appearance by the witness.

The most formal of legal proceedings is a trial,

where one may be called to testify either as a material witness or as a voluntary expert. These proceedings are conducted before a judge who rules on points of law. Trials can involve either a judge as the trier of fact (bench trial) or a jury as the trier of fact. The number of jurors can vary from 6 to 12 or more. At criminal trials, the prosecution presents its case first, calling witnesses and questioning them under oath. Afterwards, the defense has the opportunity to cross-examine the witnesses. In civil trials the plaintiff occupies an analogous position to the prosecution, and the questioning flows as above.

A number of excellent books, monographs, and other publications provide detailed information about appropriate conduct in court and with attorneys, basic aspects of malpractice litigation, and related matters.[64,151,167,219]

### The Forensic Neuropathologic Examination

Just as a forensic autopsy differs from the standard hospital autopsy examination, the forensic neuropathologic examination serves special functions.[47,87,219] The information sought in the forensic autopsy pertains to facts that will determine *cause* and *manner* of death. Cause of death is (are) the condition(s) leading to death. Establishing the manner of death is peculiar to the forensic environment and involves assigning the death to one of five categories: accident; natural; homicide; suicide; undetermined. These determinations generally are made by the primary forensic pathologist, and rarely by the neuropathologist. The significance of this latter determination is largely legal, having to do with what comes later (an indictment for murder, payment of double indemnity awards, cancellation of insurance and other benefits, or further investigation).[13] To some degree, the forensic neuropathologic examination also embodies these two qualities (cause and manner). Several portions of this chapter deal with these special applications of the neuropathologic examination. These include determination of likelihood of willful versus accidental head and brain trauma, falls versus blows, accidents versus willful injury in infants and children (child abuse), functional state of the brain, behavioral ramifications of brain lesions, epilepsy and behavior, aging and dating of processes, and clinical-pathological correlations, reconstruction of events and processes.

A number of general principles should be considered. The examination will likely answer questions at issue or anticipated to be issues. Evidence will be preserved by means of appropriate diagrams; drawings; photographs; preserved materials; histologic and electron microscopic; toxicologic and other examinations. The "chain of evidence" and "chain of custody" will be preserved;[253] and a complete and appropriate neuropathologic report will be issued.[219]

Generally, the neuropathologic examination will include careful documentation of the nature of surface injuries (if any) on the face, head, scalp, neck, back, and extremities as well as their photographic preservation. Relationship to medical interventions (such as needle punctures) and apparent injuries or bruises is very important. This evidence can be more fully evaluated later when complete information regarding the case is available. Tissues from cutaneous or missile gunshot wounds may be cut out, fixed, and preserved for later analysis. When the scalp is reflected, careful documentation of the nature, appearance, and extent of subgaleal hemorrhages must be made. This provides vital correlative information when evaluating injuries to the skull and brain in light of other evidence.

After the scalp is reflected, careful inspection of the skull includes percussion of the intact cranium in search of possible fractures. Fractures must be diagrammatically or photographically documented and correlated with possible impact points on the scalp. The skull cap and brain are removed and the basal dura stripped; the base of the skull then carefully examined. This will allow discovery of fracture lines, infections extending from sinuses, and other lesions.

The brain should be removed with great care, avoiding the introduction of artifacts. This is especially critical in infants and newborns in whom the brain is soft and easily fragmented. Brain removal methods adequate for specific conditions are described in detail elsewhere.[76,163,186,219,266] Extreme care should be exercised not to distort the brainstem when removing the brain. This can introduce troublesome and confusing artifacts that could interfere with adequate interpretation. Once the brain is removed, it should be manipulated as little as possible before it is fixed. If, however, immediate information is needed or if a specimen is required for toxicologic or other study, a single coronal cut may be made through the mamillary bodies. After a specimen is obtained for toxicologic study, for example, the sections should be placed cut face down, in a sufficiently large container filled with formalin. Another option is to make a single midsagittal cut, dividing the brain into two equal halves. The disadvantage of this cut is that midline structures and brainstem may be distorted. This can be avoided if the brainstem and cerebellum are separated at the midbrain level by a single, fan-shaped cut made with a scalpel blade through the upper pons or lower midbrain.

Exceptions to fixing the brain immediately after removal include the presence of subarachnoid caused by hemorrhage, which might be a ruptured aneurysm; the need for bacteriologic or virologic cultures; or the need for electron microscopic or chemical analysis. In these instances only the required regions are sampled, whereas the remainder of the specimen can be fixed in formalin according to standard methods. In the case of an acute subarachnoid hemorrhage that probably originated from a ruptured aneurysm, the basal arachnoid membrane is carefully stripped and the blood is flushed away under a gentle jet of cold water. This permits a much easier identification of an aneurysm than if the blood is allowed to harden under fixation. Most aneurysms are located within a centimeter or so of the circle of Willis, so disruption of the brain parenchyma to expose the major branches of the circle of Willis is not required.

The dura from the skull (vertex and base) should be included with the brain specimen; this is especially desirable when extraparenchymal hematomas are present. Histologic sections of these blood clots will be valuable and at times crucial when questions of aging and dating of lesions are at issue. Likewise, removal of the spinal cord is especially desirable in cases of alleged child abuse or head and neck trauma. In general, the posterior approach to removing the cord is more instructive and revealing than is the anterior approach. This is especially true in cases of suspected child abuse when "whiplash-shaking" is to be considered.[219,266] The posterior approach allows observation of epidural cervical or upper thoracic hemorrhages that might be missed by another removal method. In some cases it is useful to preserve all or portions of the spine. Many techniques for doing this are detailed elsewhere.[186,266,359]

In cases of severe ischemic brain injury,[104,108] sometimes referred to as "respirator brain,"[256] in which the intracranial contents are mushy or frankly liquified, these specimens, distorted as they are, must be preserved because they can yield surprisingly useful information.

In cases of suspected fatal child abuse[327] the eyes and a portion of the optic nerve and sheath should be removed. This usually can be accomplished after the brain has been taken out by removing the orbital roofs and the eyes. The eyes should be fixed whole in formalin and then sectioned, usually by making two anterior-posterior cuts with a sharp razor blade at the limbus so that there are two concave tops or sides of the globe and one block that includes the optic nerve head and the uvea. This is usually the most important and useful block to be examined. Trauma cases require an examination that adequately demonstrates the lesions. Proper examination of gunshot and missile wounds requires cutting the brain in the plane(s) of wound tracks, sometimes in order to recover projectiles. Cutting the brain in the planes employed in MRI or CT scans obtained in life may be the most appropriate way of sectioning the brain. Special neuropathologic examinations often are needed for the brains of infants and children. Specific suggestions regarding these and other examinations are discussed below in relation to specific conditions; moreover, several excellent papers and other sources of information regarding methodology of brain examination are available.[76,186] Documentation of lesions and their location is very important. Photography is always best, but good drawings or sketches of brain outlines may suffice. Identification of the case number and date of examination always should be included in the photographs.

The microscopic examination of the nervous system in the forensic situation, although not radically different from that practiced in other circumstances, tends to be goal-directed. The forensic examination must display the lesions of interest and provide information about the subject's age and the duration of the processes observed. Two recent monographs may be useful in completing this endeavor.[12,169] Aging and dating are more common issues in the forensic examination than in the hospital autopsy, since they may have evidentiary importance in relation to a possible criminal act or accident. Unfortunately, reliable information to aid in the determination of the age of scalp, subgaleal, brain, and dural hemorrhages is scanty and often very old.[205,257,258]

When the neuropathologic examination is completed it is often necessary to render a formal report. However, in many civil cases, the expert is specifically asked *not* to make a written report, but instead to communicate the findings verbally. In such instances, the existence of a written report usually means that opposing counsel will eventually have access to it, and could use information in the report at trial if later opinions differed from those expressed in trial. At other times a report may serve to bring a case to settlement before trial. When a written report is rendered it usually is appropriate to begin with a recitation of what was examined and how the evidence was obtained. This should be followed by gross and microscopic descriptions that avoid conclusions. Generally it is appropriate to list the diagnoses and the interpretation of these findings. Naturally the report should be complete and error-free; errors and omissions can prove embarrassing and confusing at trial. Expert witnesses should bear in mind that their entire work product, including notes, drawings, business records, and correspondence with counsel are discoverable at deposition time and at trial. When reviewing microscopic slides it is advisable to photocopy the slides examined or to take photomicrographs of important regions on the slide so that the microslides or items contained in them can be identified subsequently. This is especially important when slides cannot be retained in one's possession.

A key element of a forensic examination includes preserving the "chain of possession" of the evidence.[47,87,253] The essence here is that the material examined actually represents that related to the case at hand and is not mixed up with some other case. This can be resolved by making sure that appropriate identification labels are affixed to specimens, tissues, paraffin blocks, slides, and photographs. Documents must establish the identity of each person who had possession of a piece of evidence (a bullet, for example), when they had it, and how it was secured from tampering or substitution. This may be necessary to ensure that the evidence provided has not been mixed with materials from another case and can be traced back to the case at hand. It is highly advisable to keep receipts when materials are received or given to another person, and to make sure that the identity of materials and their continuity of possession are maintained.

### Forensic Aspects of General Neuropathology

**Intracranial causes of death.** Most cases brought to the attention of the medical examiner/coroner fall into one of the following categories. (1) The death either occurred outside the care or observation of a physician or there is no one who can or will execute a death certificate. (2) The death occurred under suspicious circumstances (in an accident, probable suicide, involved foul play, occurred in jail or prison, or within 24 hours of admission to a hospital [including death during surgery or childbirth]). About two-thirds of all deaths called to the attention of the medical examiner are caused by "natural" disease processes. About 10% of these are sudden and unexpected. The remaining one-third are the result of homicide, suicide, accident, or of undetermined cause.[13]

The cause and sometimes the manner of death may be found in the central nervous system (CNS), especially when no obvious anatomic cause is found in the general autopsy, and when someone dies unexpectedly. Most sudden and unexpected deaths are caused by diseases that involve the heart and lungs (sudden fatal arrhythmia with or without myocardial infarction, pulmonary embolism, ruptured aortic aneurysm, aspiration of food or vomitus, pneumonia).[198,199] Other common causes are gastrointestinal hemorrhage and sepsis. Comparatively few sudden or unexpected deaths are associated with intracranial processes.[69] Among these, the most common causes of death are such circulatory catastrophes as ruptured intracranial aneurysm, intracerebral hemorrhage, ruptured vascular malformation, and brainstem infarction. Deaths also are associated with epileptic seizures. In the latter instance deaths are truly sudden; in most other circumstances, several hours must elapse between the precipative event (such as a stroke) and death. This is true even in cases of massive intracerebral hemorrhage. Fatal intracranial hemorrhages occurring at night in the absence of a witness may appear to be sudden, but are actually unexpected. Other intracranial causes of death involve undocumented head trauma (epidural, subdural, or intracerebral hemorrhage), bleeding tumors of the brain, ruptured brain abscess, sudden intracranial decompensation associated with chronic subdural hemorrhage, obstruction to the flow of cerebrospinal fluid (CSF) as a consequence of bleeding or edema, as in unrecognized brain tumors (colloid cysts of the third ventricle, subependymoma of the aqueduct, cerebellar astrocytomas, and other tumors).[69,155,219]

**Intracranial pressure and volume.** The intracranial and intraspinal spaces constitute a dynamic system of real and potential spaces that maintain a constant intracranial physical environment. Alterations within this system must be recognized if one is to understand and analyze head trauma, toxic states, intracranial hemorrhage, and cerebral edema as well as obstructions to the CSF flow.

Cerebrospinal fluid is produced by the choroid plexuses of the lateral and fourth ventricles at a rate of about 0.4 ml/minute. About 70% of the 120 to 150 ml of CSF in the normal adult is contained within the cerebral ventricles; the remainder is distributed to the spinal sac, various cisterns, and the surface of the brain.[95,179] The volume of the CSF is pressure related and, in response to pressure rises, the fluid can be driven out (reabsorbed by arachnoid granulations along the superior sagittal sinus, and by dural sheaths at the roots of spinal nerves), and by bulk flow across the ependyma into the brain's extracellular compartment. The intraventricular pressure is a function of the rate of secretion of CSF and the rate of its outflow, which occurs via bulk flow into the extracellular space of the brain, through the ependyma and by direct passage through the foramina of Munro, cerebral aqueduct, foramina of Luschka and Magendie in the cerebellum, the impedance offered by the subarachnoid space, the reabsorptive potential of the arachnoid villi and dural sheaths, the rate of leakage of water from brain vessels into the extracellular space, and the volume of the brain (cells, vessels, water). Volumetric changes in any one of these compartments can raise or lower intracranial pressure.[307] Of vital importance is the brain-vessel interface or blood-brain barrier. The barrier function is subserved by the brain capillary network, which is sealed by very tight intercellular junctions (zonulae occludentia), a vascular basement membrane, and an investing layer of astroglial foot processes.

Interference by physical or chemical means with the blood-brain barrier causes water to be retained in the brain's extracellular spaces producing one form of edema. Astroglia have a limited ability to compensate for this water retention which remains contained within cells (brain swelling or "dry" edema). This state has been referred to as "dry" edema because although the area may swell, its cut surface appears dry. In uncompensated edema, astroglia may rupture or may not absorb extracellular water, which beads on the cut sur-

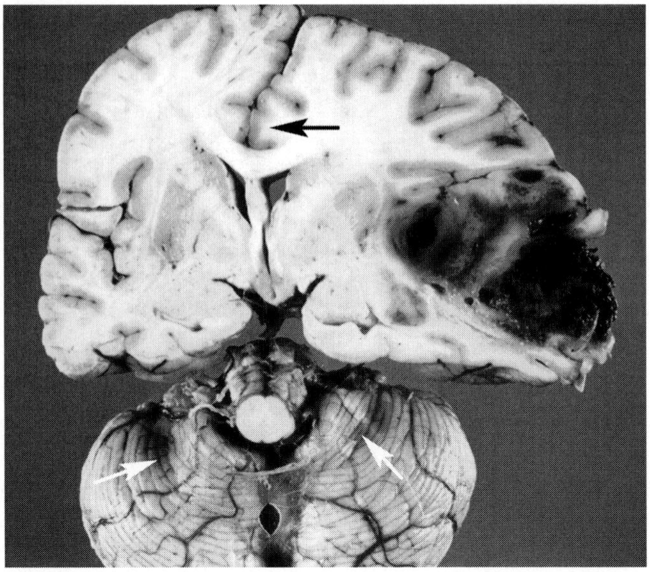

**Fig. 11-1.** This coronal section of brain and a basal view of the cerebellum illustrate a major shift of cerebral midline structures producing a transfalcial herniation (*dark arrow*) caused by a hemorrhage into a previously undiscovered metastatic brain tumor. This mass lesion also produced a prominent cerebellar tonsillar herniation with obvious circular impression at its base (*white arrows*).

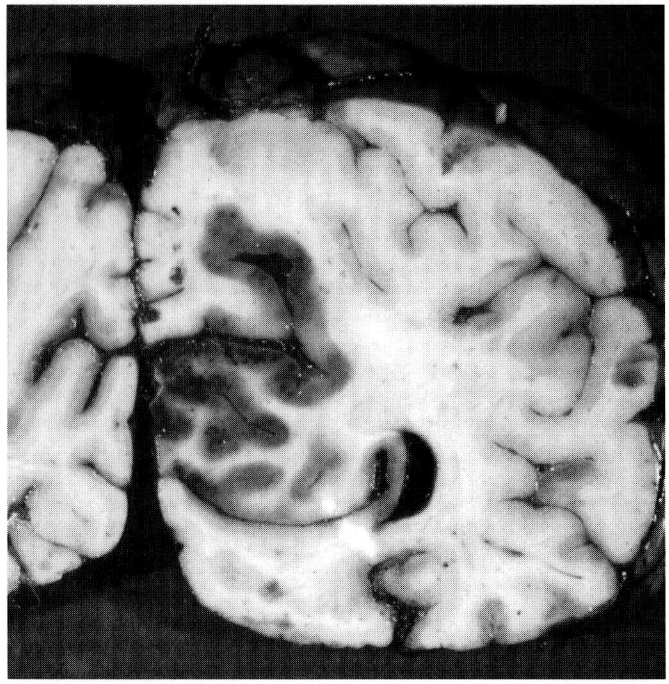

**Fig. 11-2.** This coronal section of the occipital lobes reveals a right-sided hemorrhagic infarction caused by herniation-compression of the branches of the right posterior cerebral arteries that nourished the midline cortex, which includes Brodmann Area 17, the primary visual cortex. If this patient had survived the large acute subdural hematoma that was present, a left homonymous hemianopsia would have resulted.

face of the brain like perspiration even in the freshly cut and fixed brain. A yellowish or slightly creamy color can be noted in the area and is visible microscopically as vacuoles or bubbles. Brain edema can be caused by a multitude of pathologic processes: hypoxia; ischemia; acidosis; hypoglycemia; toxic drugs, industrial compounds, alcohols and solvents; physical injury; heat or cold; inflammatory processes; and neoplasms.[219] Brain edema can occur rapidly and unexpectedly, alone or in combination with other intracranial masses, and may cause death rapidly or may produce brain death (discussed later in this chapter).

A common pathologic consequence of brain swelling, edema, or any enlarging mass lesion is the physical displacement of a portion of the brain to an adjacent compartment—the process of herniation.

Herniation occurs by rearrangement or absorption of CSF, which fills the ventricles and overlies the brain surfaces. Cerebellar tonsillar and uncinate herniations are two of the more common types. Here the cerebellar tonsils flow into the foramen magnum and show a typical circular grooving at the base of the cerebellum (Fig. 11-1). This form of herniation exerts pressure on the lower brainstem and leads to progressive disorders of consciousness and ventilation, which may lead to coma and death. The mesial temporal lobes (or unci) may flow toward the midline and posterior fossa, impinge on the tentorial edge, and compress the third cranial nerve. These events may be followed by decrease in the level of consciousness, loss of the "doll's eye" phenomenon, and eventual development of "Duret hemorrhages" in the brainstem.[280] Extensive transtentorial or uncinate herniation may extend a pressure groove far enough posteriorly so that branches of the posterior cerebral artery are compressed. This may lead to hemorrhagic infarction (Fig. 11-2) of the medial occipital lobe, or may affect the midbrain to the point that the cerebral aqueduct is compressed (further raising intracranial pressure). This process may blend with tonsillar herniation to produce a Duret hemorrhage (Fig. 11-3). Such herniations usually are homolateral; that is, a right uncinate herniation usually is accompanied by right tonsillar herniation.

Duret hemorrhages are secondary events that follow the unilateral or asymmetric and rapid expansion of lesions in the supratentorial compartment. These hemorrhages occur along the midline of the pons and midbrain and may fan out into the tegmentum to produce a Rorschach-like ink blot pattern of hemorrhage. The lesions frequently destroy much of the reticular activating formation and the medial longitudinal fasciculus, resulting in a deeply comatose, nonbreathing patient who may not recover consciousness, will show absence of doll's eye movements, and will probably

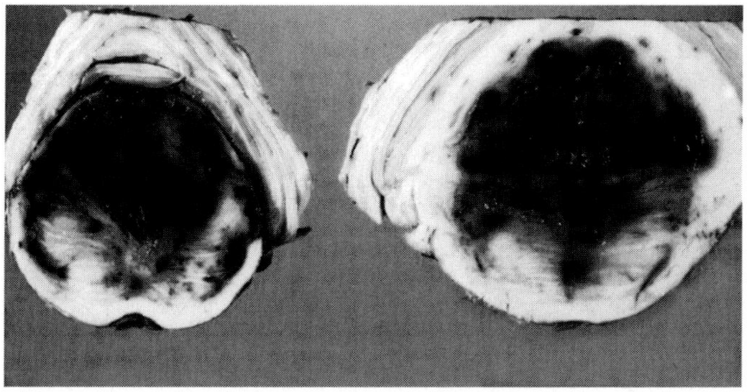

**Fig. 11-3.** These two cross sections of the pons illustrate typical Duret hemorrhages that occurred after an acute "hypertensive" hemorrhage in the right lateral ganglionic region.

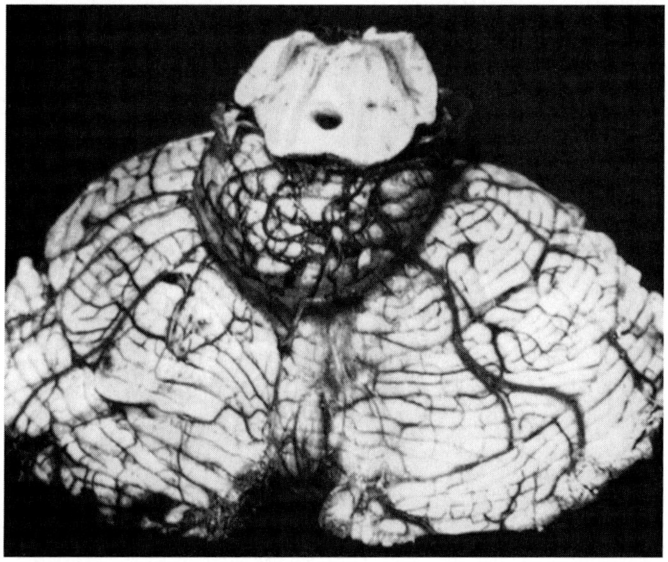

**Fig. 11-4.** This view of the rostral surface of the cerebellum and the midbrain illustrates an "upward" transtentorial herniation that occurred in conjunction with a left acute "hypertensive" cerebellar hemorrhage.

die a "brain" death. These lesions do not extend into the medulla because the vascular supply to this structure is separate from that of the tegmentum of the midbrain and pons.

Other forms of brain herniation include transfalcial, across midline herniations (Fig. 11-1), and herniation of middle fossa structures into the anterior fossa or vice versa. The cerebellum also may herniate upward through the tentorial notch (Fig. 11-4) when the expanding process affects mainly the posterior fossa.[63] Such herniations are life-threatening. Herniated brain tissue may compress blood vessels and produce infarctions that usually are hemorrhagic; this further increases the mass effect and may cause additional herniation.

Hydrocephalus is equivalent to CSF volume in excess of normal. This process is most commonly caused by some disorder of CSF flow or reabsorption; only rarely is it caused by excessive fluid production, as in the case of or choroid plexus papilloma. Hydrocephalus is commonly classified as being *communicating* (nonobstructive) or *noncommunicating* (obstructive).[95,307] In the former instance there is an uncoupling between production of CSF and its absorption, in the absence of physical obstruction to the CSF flow. Net reabsorption may be decreased because of scarring or dysfunction of the arachnoid villi (usually secondary to the effects of subarachnoid hemorrhage or inflammation), or there may be a separate or coexistent increased impediment to flow over the surface of the brain because of a scarred or narrowed subarachnoid space following meningitis, subarachnoid hemorrhage, or some other poorly understood reason.[182] The conditions of deficient reabsorption or increased resistance to flow may be intermittent and may result in no sustained increased CSF pressure; yet such conditions still may produce enlargement of the ventricles (so-called normal or low pressure hydrocephalus). The ventricular chambers are often symmetrically enlarged in *communicating* (nonobstructive) hydrocephalus. In congenital hydrocephalus the head may be grossly enlarged and the cortex/white matter reduced to a thin mantle because of the malleable skull. In adult hydrocephalus, the ventricles enlarge to a certain limit, at which time the septum pellucidum is fenestrated. Eventually sufficient CSF pressure develops to cause severe neurologic symptoms or death. Patients may survive for years with what appears to be static hydrocephalic conditions, and then may suddenly decompensate when the fragile balance of accommodation is upset. Among these patients, events such as an episode of trivial head trauma may trigger rapid decompensation and death.

In *obstructive* (noncommunicating) hydrocephalus tumors or neoplasms create a physical barrier to CSF flow, usually within the brain. This can occur within the lateral ventricular chambers (hemorrhage, infection, tumor), at the foramina of Monro (colloid cysts, various tumors), at the cerebral aqueduct (inflammation-infection, glial scarring, tumor, cyst or hemorrhage), within the fourth ventricle (tumor, infection, hemorrhage), or at the lateral foramina of Luschka or the midline foramen of Magendie (tumor, infection). Depending on the site and nature of the obstruction, the proximal CSF-filled chamber(s) will become progressively dilated.[215] Other chambers will be normal in size. Limitations to the extent of these enlargements are imposed by the ability of the brain to move, shift, and accommodate the enlarging lesion. Several cases of unexpected death secondary to sudden obstructions to CSF flow have been reported.[155,215,219]

A form of ventricular dilatation unrelated to alteration of CSF flow and attributed to loss of brain tissue with a compensating replacement with fluid is called hydrocephalus *ex-vacuo*. Large brain infarctions or other destructive processes that markedly reduce the cerebral volume are accompanied by ventricular dilatation of the ex-vacuo type.

The ependymal cells in hydrocephalus become very flat and lose their cilia; total or focal loss of ependymal cell lining, and several forms of reaction of the subependyma glia (tanycytes) also are common. Subependymal reactions range from the formation of a mat of proliferated fibrillary glia beneath the ependyma to the appearance of nodular "bales" of proliferated glia that rise above the ependymal surface in the form of granular ependymitis. The subependymal glia may proliferate over the damaged or fragmented ependymal cell layer, trapping ependymal remnants beneath a carpet of glial fibers.

The subependymal region and adjacent white matter may become vacuolated in acute hydrocephalus. Eventually if this process becomes chronic, gliosis of deep white matter and cavitary spaces (pseudoventricles) may develop. In cases of longstanding hydrocephalus, a steady state is reached (arrested hydrocephalus) in which an equilibrium between production and absorption of CSF is achieved. Determining the cause of acute or chronic hydrocephalus may require careful gross and histologic examination of the cerebellar foramina. The continuity and dimensions of the fourth ventricle, the cerebral aqueduct, the foramina of Monro, and other ventricular chambers must be noted. The arachnoid villi examination may reveal extensive fibrosis or some other abnormalities. Examining the arachnoid in different locations may reveal pia-arachnoid adhesions and obliteration of the subarachnoid space.

**Brain death and the "respirator" brain.** With advances in the ability to maintain vital signs in a comatose, nonbreathing individual, definitions of death and viability have become important medical, ethical, and legal issues.[8,29,348] The importance of these definitions is apparent in head trauma victims who are respirator-dependent and whose organs may be considered for donation and transplantation, and in brain-damaged individuals who remain in coma for extended periods, as in the case of Karen Ann Quinlan.[114,183,184]

The criteria that should be employed in declaring "brain death" and terminating "life" support are discussed in detail elsewhere.[86] The stringency of criteria varies widely in the United States and in the rest of the world. Broadly speaking, the brain is thought to have died when individuals in coma are not able to breathe on their own, when drug intoxication and hypothermia have been ruled out, and when some measure(s) of the loss of cerebral physiologic activity has been documented for a sufficient period. This has been accomplished by performing, a few hours apart, two or more electroencephalograms that show "electrocerebral silence" or loss of other physiologic activity as defined in several works on the subject.[137,154,348] Cerebral blood flow measurements also can be employed to determine the absence of circulation to the brain.[7,221,348] In addition to or, in some circumstances, in place of the above tests, demonstrating lack of brainstem function is an acceptable type of "brain death." This is not universally accepted, however.[310,348]

***Illustrative Case 1:*** *An individual was shot in the head with a pistol loaded with .22 caliber "short" ammunition. The victim was brought to a hospital emergency room in ventilatory arrest and was placed on a respirator. Later, the victim was transferred to another hospital where death was declared and the kidneys and other organs removed for transplantation. A review of the record revealed that at least five different dates and times of death had been recorded.*

*The medical evidence in the case did not demonstrate classic "respirator" brain alterations, and the possibility existed, although small, that the normal criteria for brain death were not present at the time death was first declared by the emergency room personnel. The gunshot wound involved one frontal lobe, and there was no major hemorrhage. Such a wound would not generally be considered fatal.*

*There are multiple issues in this case. All are contentious and carry significant legal and financial consequences. The neuropathologic information in this case was of paramount importance. The issues: Was a "respirator brain" present or not? Was the gunshot wound likely to be or to have been fatal? If the wound was not fatal, what brought about death? If prevailing criteria for brain death were not followed, would the result for the victim have been the same or not? The answers to these questions are not clear.*

All of these issues have been amply discussed in numerous publications, for example the excellent monograph by Walker,[348] the collaborative study of brain death conducted by the National Institutes of Health,[56] and several other publications.[29,154,212,219,256]

The mechanisms behind the death of the brain (Fig. 11-5) always involve massive circulatory or metabolic embarrassment, which at some point also involves increased intracranial pressure.[30,95,108,348,349] Common circumstances that lead to brain death include circulatory shock in connection with cardiorespiratory arrest; shock and hypoxemia as seen in drowning, asphyxiation, and various toxic states; and processes that increase intracranial pressure beyond the point at which perfusion of the brain is inadequate. Such circumstances include rapidly enlarging intracranial lesions, as in traumatic cerebral edema, acute epidural or subdural hemorrhage, intracerebral hemorrhage, large brain infarctions, hemorrhage within a tumor, sudden obstruction or decompensated obstruction of CSF flow, or combinations of the above.

As with most intracranial processes, the degree of compensation in relation to circulation and intracranial

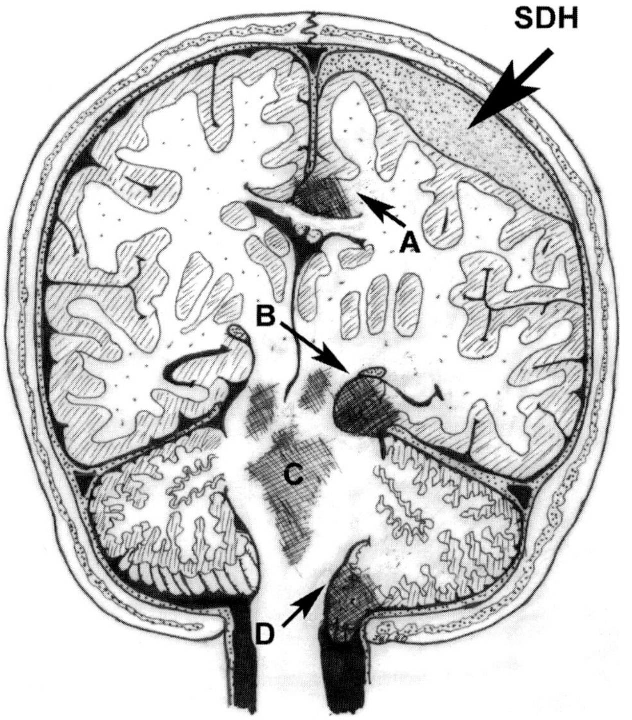


**Fig. 11-5.** This diagram illustrates the sequential events and mechanisms that lead to brain "death" and the "respirator" brain. The upper portion of the diagram continues in a circular fashion until no more space can be gained by reabsorption of CSF, then the process enters the lower part of the diagram, which also may cycle until cerebral circulatory arrest has occurred. After stasis of circulation has been in place for a period of time, the "no reflow" phenomenon occurs, in which, regardless of what corrective actions are taken, cerebral perfusion can no longer occur.

pressure/volume relationships may be slight. Intracranial pressure may vary significantly as a result of compensatory mechanisms. There may be a decrease in perfusion pressure, leading to brain ischemia and eventually to brain edema that further increases intracranial pressure. Pressure may rise sufficiently to impair venous drainage, causing a further rise that eventually may approach mean arterial pressure and lead to serious embarrassment of cerebral circulation. When this condition persists for more than several minutes, many neurons are irreversibly injured.

The end-point of this process is global cerebral *ischemia*[108] as demonstrated by angiography, bolus scintigraphy, or other means of estimating cerebral blood flow.[7,56,221,310,348] At this point the brain becomes electrically silent (electrocerebral silence—flat EEG). This state usually is irreversible and constitutes what has become known as "brain death." From this point on the brain disintegrates, and in the course of about 12 hours (while "life" support systems are operating) begins to take on the gross appearance of the "respirator" brain.[212,349] Typically at this time the brain is dusky in color and congested. The brainstem and cerebellum are softer than other parts of the brain. Ventricles are usually compressed. The gray-white matter junction becomes blurred, may become pink, and the basal ganglia may be softer than the surrounding tissue. The cortex may fall away from the subcortical white matter. The cerebellum is usually soft, gray, and even liquified. The same is true for the core of the upper brainstem and the pituitary gland. The spinal cord, in contrast, has a normal appearance and texture.[108,212,256]

When these ischemic brain changes are advanced (more than 24 hours after cerebral circulatory arrest and electrocerebral silence), the brain becomes exceedingly soft and may crumble or disintegrate when removed for examination. The brainstem and cerebellum may be virtually liquified. Sloughed fragments of cerebellar cortex may be found in the subarachnoid space along the lower brainstem and around the spinal cord, even at the level of the lumbar sac. When the brain may be liquified it is important to examine it both in situ and after the liquified tissue has been fixed. In some cases it is possible to obtain meaningful histologic information: at times a thin rim of the molecular layer may be preserved. In the typical "respirator" brain, all cellular elements will stain poorly and there will be excessive preparation artifacts (cracks, splits, pericellular spaces, perivascular spaces, variable staining). These changes are typical of totally ischemic tissues, are not specific for "respirator" brains, and generally are not a reliable measure of the severity of injury or duration of the process. An appreciation of the extent of injury is much more reliable on gross inspection than by microscopic examination.[168] The interval between removal of "life" support and performance of the autopsy is not a factor in the development or extent of "respirator" brain changes, nor is the interval of delay in refrigeration of the body.[177,212]

Not every case of "respirator" brain will show the same changes at the same times. Factors responsible include: variations in the progression of the process that led to the "respirator" brain and the influence of therapy; duration and severity of circulatory arrest (complete, as in cardiac standstill, or partial, as in severe hypotension); severity of increase in intracranial pressure; the presence of intracranial hemorrhage; the anatomic condition of the large vessels; body temperature; and serum glucose. The waxing and waning character of intracranial pressure caused by compensatory mechanisms may allow pressures to rise and fall several times, perhaps sequentially damaging the microcirculation until finally the no-reflow phenomenon occurs.[83,168] This will be reflected in the appearance of the brain at autopsy, with some portions showing more advanced ischemic changes than others. When brain bleeding is the cause of increased intracranial pressure, the added presence of blood pigments and components seems to accelerate the structural changes and gross appearance of the "respirator" brain. The previous state of health and the acuteness of a cerebral catastrophe also may have some effect on the rapidity of "respirator" brain development.[229,230] When a previously healthy individual suffers a sudden cardiac event that produces severe cerebral ischemia and is resuscitated but remains in a coma, visible advanced ischemic brain changes may be present even before 12 hours have elapsed. In such cases the distribution of "red" neurons can be even more striking than if the individual had been ill for some time or than if the genesis of the comatose state, including the rate at which blood pressure declined, had been more gradual. The dying individual appears to derive some "protective" effect, from the progression of the ischemic changes. The reasons for this are not clear, but Lindenberg has discussed extensively this issue.[229,230]

**Persistent vegetative state.** Another group of conditions can induce various degrees of brain damage that lead to a state of diminished consciousness or persistent coma. These individuals have been in coma and have been maintained on ventilatory support, yet altered but physiologic brain electrical activity continues. Some of these patients can be weaned from the respirator and are able to breathe on their own. Between 10,000 and 25,000 individuals of all ages apparently exist in a persistently vegetative state (PVS) in the United States. They consume vast amounts of health care resources.[184] The ethical, moral and fiscal quandaries raised by their limbo-like state have not been resolved.

Individuals in a vegetative coma can vary greatly in their clinical appearance.[184,280] Many may appear to be asleep or to be awake with no response to their environment (coma vigil). A pattern of waking-sleeping cycles[154] can be shown by electrophysiologic monitoring. The individual may make pseudopurposeful movements, phonate by groaning or screaming, smile or grimace, or even shed tears. These phenomena may be misinterpreted by laymen and some medical personnel as evidence of consciousness, but have no basis in conscious action.[184,280,348] Pseudopurposeful actions long have posed a conundrum from the neurophysiologic and anatomic points of view: the issues they raise go to the core of the physiology and philosophical definition of human consciousness.[62,184]

Results of a careful study of the brains of victims in a vegetative state have been published.[184] These authors review both cases of their own and those of others and their findings emphasize that no single lesion is responsible for all cases of PVS. Rather, multiple lesions that diffusely involve the cerebral cortex, the cerebral white matter and deeper nuclei (thalamus and basal ganglia), and the hippocampal formation, cerebellum, and brainstem usually are present. These multiple lesions must effectively disrupt the normal communicative pathways between the brainstem-diencephalon reticular formations and the thalamus/basal ganglia and the cerebral cortex, which together are required for consciousness.

Victims of PVS come to this state most commonly as a result of traumatic injuries to the brain (falls, blows, missile injuries) and by global processes such as hypoxia/ischemia in connection with drowning, carbon monoxide intoxication, asphyxia, cardiac arrest, drug overdoses, and toxic agents. Some have degenerative disorders such as Parkinson's, Huntington's, or Jakob-Creutzfeldt diseases; others have metabolic-storage diseases or suffer from congenital conditions such as brain malformations or "cerebral palsy."

The forensic issues surrounding such cases are many, but only some of them potentially involve the neuropathologist. These questions revolve around the type and locations of lesions, their causes, and their consequences. The most difficult questions involve interpretations and judgments about the subject's state of awareness and perception as they may relate to suffering. Observed pseudopurposeful actions may be emotionally devastating to attending family members (crying, moaning, grimacing, etc.) and may provide an impetus to pursue litigation that has at its premise presumably conscious pain and suffering on the part of the victim. The best general interpretation is that PVS victims are "locked out."[184] They are permanently separated from the external world, existing only at a basal, vegetative, automatic, or reflex level, in spite of appearances to the contrary. It is obvious that a full understanding of the physiology, anatomy, and neurobiology of consciousness does not exist.

**Epilepsy and epilepsy related deaths.** Although there are many types of "seizures," not all of them reflect an epileptic state. Epilepsy is defined as "a chronic brain disorder of various etiologies characterized by recurrent seizures due to excessive discharge of cerebral neurons."[111] The two key points are that the disorder is electrophysiologic and chronic. Febrile seizures and others that are sporadic or occasional should not be considered epilepsy.

Epileptic seizures have been classified in a number of different ways, but the International League Against Epilepsy[281] has promulgated a classification that recognizes three major categories: (1) focal, partial or local seizures; (2) generalized convulsive or nonconvulsive seizures; and (3) unclassified seizures. In the first category, the disturbances are focal, at least initially, as in the typical Jacksonian seizure. The second category would include all generalized seizures such as absence (petit mal), generalized tonic-clonic (grand mal), and others. The third group would include complex seizure disorders that do not fit into either of the other two categories.

Epilepsy affects all societies with varying prevalence. In Scandinavian countries the prevalence is about 11/100,000 persons; in the United States it is 30 to 54/100,000 persons; and in Great Britain it is 30 to 70/100,000 persons. The incidence of epilepsy is highest in the under 4-year-old age group, it then falls steadily until about age 30 years, when it levels off at about one fourth the incidence in the youngest age group. Most new cases of epilepsy are diagnosed among men younger than 20 years.[220,365] The percentage of a given population suffering from epilepsy is between 1 and 2%.[176,220,277] This translates into 3 to 6 million persons in the United States alone.

A number of forensic issues arise in connection with persons suffering from epilepsy. These range from seizure-related accidents in the workplace and elsewhere, sometimes with fatal consequences for the affected individual or others. The neuropathologist occassionally is asked to determine whether a seizure disorder is likely to have been present on the basis of the postmortem examination of the brain or whether epilepsy might have been related to death. Often, the answers to these questions are inconclusive.

Epileptic conditions may cause death in several ways: status epilepticus; sudden seizure-associated cardiac or respiratory mediated death; death due to accident; death due to suicide.[210,220,240] Status epilepticus is a condition in which seizure activity of any type persists for lengthy periods. The consequences of status epileptus depend on the type of seizure activity and its duration. In generalized tonic-clonic status, the risk of death may be 10% to 20% or higher, depending on the underlying cause of the seizures and the age and physical condition of the victim. Death may be the consequence of cerebral edema, increased intracranial pressure, and global cerebral ischemia. The mechanism of death in status epilepticus is not fully understood but, in part, is the result of systemic exhaustion, which can be prevented by curarization.[240] Several processes affect the brain metabolism during status. These include initial increases followed by decreases in cerebral blood flow, oxygenation and metabolism.[196] Dysfunctions of energy metabolism and the production of arachidonic acid metabolites (eicosanoids) may act as inflammatory mediators (prostaglandins, leukotrienes, and others) and have profound effects on cerebral vascular tone and on neuronal function.[17,25,160,196,242] If status is incompletely or inappropriately treated, the end result is damage or death to affected neurons by several mechanisms, which include altered energy and membrane function, acidosis, and ischemia.[160]

The brains of individuals dying in status epilepticus are edematous and may show "respirator" (ischemic) brain changes. Edema and ischemic neuronal damage reflected on the eosinophilic ("red") staining of neurons in the hippocampus, striatum, globus pallidus, dentate nuclei, and Purkinje cells of the cerebellum, as well as in the large neurons of the cerebral cortex.

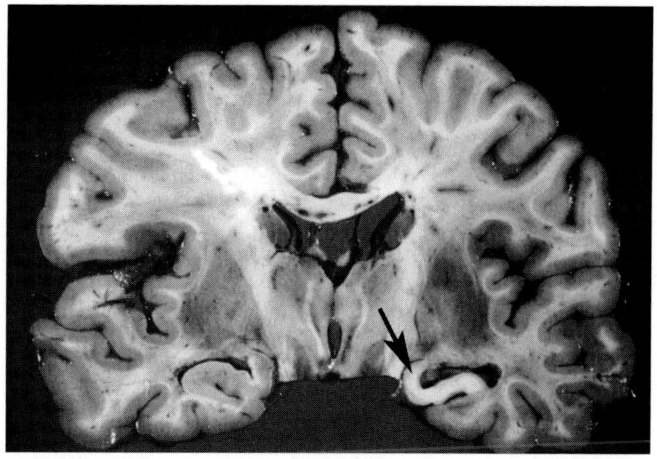

**Fig. 11-6.** This coronal section of the brain illustrates a sclerotic Ammon's horn of the hippocampus (*arrow*) in an individual who suffered from chronic, intractable epileptic seizures and was found dead in bed. Autopsy revealed no anatomic cause of death. Such cases are typical for so-called SUDEP (sudden unexpected death in epilepsy) deaths.

These changes are not diagnostic of status and can be seen in hypoxia, ischemia, toxic states, and some viral infections. A period of perfusion (survival) is required before "red" neurons become visible. In most cases, 8 to 12 hours are required, but in certain instances as little as 1 or 2 hours may be sufficient to induce the histologic change.[32,219,303] In time these dead neurons will either be "reabsorbed" or converted into mineralized (ferruginated) neuron ghosts. No obvious lesions are found in the brains of epileptics who never experienced status, although one of the most common (about 10% of cases) is "hippocampal sclerosis" (Fig. 11-6) or evidence for chronic damage with gliosis of the CA-1 (Ammon's horn) region of the hippocampus.[60,248] Some epileptics may show concomitant atrophy of the cerebellum.[219,220]

Epileptic individuals may experience seizures at work, while driving an automobile or some other conveyance, or while swimming, diving, or bathing. Should death occur during these circumstances, it is often difficult unequivocally to correlate a seizure with a fatal injury unless there is a witness to the event. At autopsy, one may discover Ammon's horn sclerosis, ectopic gray matter, a cortical malformation, small tumor, or one of the many other lesions associated with an epileptogenic focus. Subsidiary information may reveal that the individuals were known epileptics who had anticonvulsant medication in their possession, or had a positive toxicologic test for such a drug at autopsy. Because death supervenes in a matter of minutes, structural brain changes related to the act of dying may be absent.

A phenomenon often referred to as SUDEP (Sudden Unexpected Death in Epilepsy) has been re-

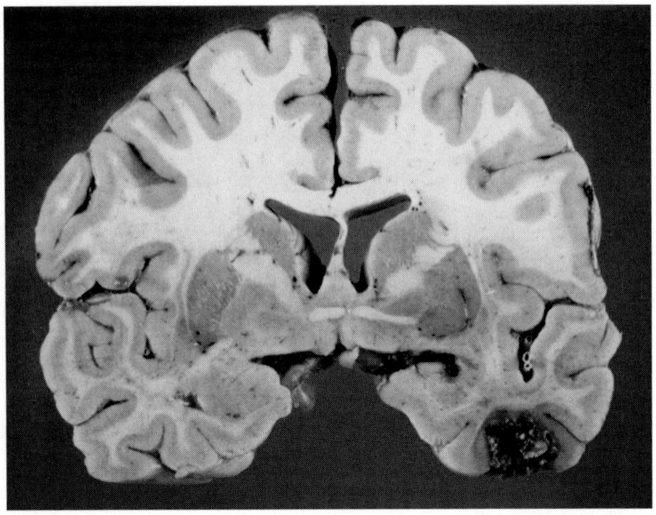

**Fig. 11-7.** This coronal section of the brain illustrates a relatively small cryptic arterio-venous malformation of the right inferior temporal lobe. This lesion, never diagnosed in life, caused focal (temporal lobe) and generalized seizures in this individual. Death was sudden and unexpected with no anatomic cause of death; an apparent so-called SUDEP death.

ported[99,214, 217,326] in which presumably healthy individuals who suffer from epilepsy die suddenly and unexpectedly. A study of several hundred of such cases[217] revealed that the average victim is between 30 and 40 years of age, is more likely to be black than white, male than female, and to have had epilepsy for 5 or more years. Often these victims had relatively infrequent seizures of the generalized tonic-clonic (grand mal) variety, tended to abuse alcohol, and had some sort of structural lesion in the brain likely to be responsible for the seizure disorder (Fig. 11-7). Most die at the onset, in the course of, or upon awakening from sleep, usually in bed, or in places in the home that suggest approximation with sleep. In one study of SUDEP most male victims had heavier than expected hearts, lungs and livers, and lighter than expected brains. Their lungs often showed high protein content pulmonary edema.[325] In the rare instances in which victims of SUDEP were observed during their fatal seizure, only about one half showed a typical tonic-clonic seizure, and many showed only rigidity or simply fell to the floor without obvious signs of a seizure. Resuscitation attempts are usually fruitless, even by trained personnel, for reasons that are unclear. When resuscitation and restoration of normal heart beat is accomplished, most "survivors" remain comatose and ultimately die a brain death while on a respirator. In these cases it is assumed that too long a time elapsed between cessation or ineffective heart beat and its restoration such that the brain suffered global hypoxia/ischemia.

The foregoing characteristics of the SUDEP phenomenon should not be employed to "prove" that a given individual died as the result of SUDEP. The logical trap of such an exercise, often indulged in by attorneys, is that when cases are selected on the basis of (1) sudden or unexpected death, (2) a history of epilepsy, and (3) no adequate anatomic cause of death at autopsy, there are certain associated observations in this population which, when increasingly present, tend to solidify the diagnosis. To attempt to reverse the reasoning process in which these associated observations become predictive of SUDEP in the absence of a history of epilepsy is spurious and has not been tested. No study has yet been done in which the basis of selection for correlation with SUDEP rested on race, age, gender, presence or absence of epilepsy, compliance with medication, past medical history, or any other variable.

The pathogenesis of SUDEP is not known, but death may be mediated by seizure-related autonomic discharges to the heart[209,210] alone or in combination with neurogenically mediated pulmonary edema and heart failure.[325,217] Important risk factors are the prevalence of epileptogenic lesions, usually old traumatic contusions at the base of the brain, probable alcohol withdrawal, and lack of therapeutic blood levels of anticonvulsants. Experimentally induced ictal and subictal electrical brain discharges can result in "lock-step" parasympathetic and sympathetic impulses to the heart which can cause arrhythmias.[209,210] These studies may provide some support for the mechanism of SUDEP syndrome in man.

There may be one case of SUDEP for each 1500 to 1800 epileptic individuals,[214,217] but the risk of sudden death for the typical SUDEP victim (30 to 40 years of age, male, and likely to have epilepsy secondary to a demonstrable lesion in the brain) may be as high as one in 50.[217] Data from a large epilepsy center in the United Kingdom suggest that the incidence of SUDEP-epileptics whose seizures are not under control in spite of medication may be one in 200.[35] From another study[211] in a therapeutic trial of a new anticonvulsant medication, Lamotrigine (Lamictal) the incidence of SUDEP-3480 patients who received either the medication or a placebo was between 2.5 and 3.5 deaths per 1000 patient years of "exposure." These figures compare favorably with previously reported statistics of 0.5 to 5 deaths per 1000 patient years.

**Forensic aspects of vascular disease.** In most cases examined by forensic pathologists the individual died of a natural disease process most likely related to some aspect of circulatory disease.[198,199] Cardiovascular disease is the most common cause of unexpected and probably sudden death (death in minutes); cerebral vascular diseases (strokes) are important, since they occur suddenly and unexpectedly but most strokes take hours or days before they become fatal. The most common and important cerebrovascular conditions are subarachnoid hemorrhage secondary to rupture of an intracranial aneurysm, intracerebral associated with hemorrhages (especially those involving the brainstem, or cerebellum), rupture of a vascular anomaly, and, less commonly, brainstem infarction.[5,104,105] The latter may cause a sudden and severe neurologic deficit but usually does not cause death until 2 to 3 days later.

***Spontaneous subarachnoid hemorrhage.*** Only 5% of unexpected deaths in a large autopsy series were associated with subarachnoid hemorrhage but in over 25% of cases in which the cause of death was an intracranial process subarachnoid hemorrhage played a central role.[198,199,233] In the analysis and examination of such cases when the cause of death is not known, it is vital to obtain historical information about the circumstances of death. Did the final event occur suddenly and was it witnessed (at dinner, at rest, at work or during strenuous exercise, stress, or during sexual activity)? Was trauma involved? Was medical treatment or chiropractic manipulation involved? What underlying medical conditions existed? Was the victim taking any medication (anti-hypertensive medication, anticoagulants, other)? Answers to these questions can focus the inquiry and avoid time-consuming examinations. If death occurred during normal activity or sleep one must, on the basis of statistical probabilities, suspect a ruptured aneurysm and perform an appropriate search of the circle of Willis vessels for the affected vessel; in 90% of instances, saccular aneurysms exist at a distance covered by a 2-cm radius of the internal carotid arteries. Ruptured aneurysms that cause lethal hemorrhage are most commonly located near the bifurcation of the internal carotid artery and its immediate anastomoses.[219,233] It is much easier to uncover an aneurysm when the blood is fresh than after it has been fixed and hardened. Most ruptured aneurysms are likely to measure more than 5 mm in diameter. If the fundus or dome of the aneurysm is directed of apposed to the brain, a "jet" lesion may carry blood into the brain parenchyma and the ventricles. This may give the false impression of another cause for the hemorrhage.

Most aneurysms develop at branching points of arteries. It is frequently asserted that some activity the individual was engaged in may have been responsible for the rupture. Such assertions cannot be proved in most instances; moreover, about 36% of ruptures occur during sleep, 32% have no known association with any obvious activity, and only 12% occur in association with lifting or straining. Only a few instances have been positively associated with traumatic events or with emotional strain.[219,233] Ruptured aneurysms may be found in individuals who appear to die in traffic accidents, apparently accidental falls, and in other circumstances where a different cause of death is initially suspected. In these cases, the rupture of the aneurysm may have preceded and caused the subsequent accident or trauma. This circumstance may have legal implications for the beneficiary of an insurance policy where double indemnity payment for accidental rather than natural death is at issue. Rupture of an aneurysm may be the cause of an accident, but not necessarily the cause of death, if other injuries are sufficient to produce death. One would have to take into consideration the natural course of a primary subarachnoid hemorrhage (associated with aneurysm rupture) and the probability that the ruptured aneurysm could have been successfully treated before coming to some opinion as to whether a given death was an accident caused by a natural disease process or otherwise.[219]

Intracerebral hemorrhages once caused about 25% of all "strokes," but this percentage has decreased steadily, possibly as a result of effective control of hypertension.[33,104,105,191] Spontaneous intracerebral hemorrhages are forensically important in the same context as subarachnoid hemorrhages. The most significant issue to be investigated in analyzing any intracerebral hemorrhage is: Does it have the location typical for a "hypertensive" hemorrhage? The most common location for such a hemorrhage is in the putamen-external capsule region. Less common are hemorrhages in the region of the dentate nuclei of the cerebellum and in the base of the pons.[94,104] In areas peripheral to the hemorrhage, and in the homotopic anatomic structures, there is evidence of arteriolar disease, including hemosiderin-laden macrophages at the site of previous small hemorrhages.[93,104,105,239] Microaneurysmal structures, "bleeding globes," recent hemorrhages, or other evidence of chronic disease may be visible.[93,97] A history of arterial hypertension is not always discovered or known, but evidence of increased weight of the heart (in the absence of valvular disease) and sclerosis of the renal arterioles may support a presumption of hypertension.

A recently recognized cause of intracerebral hemorrhage is exposure to "crack" cocaine.[65,190] Arteriovenous malformations and other vascular anomalies can cause sudden death with either intracerebral or subarachnoid hemorrhage. The natural history of the various vascular malformations is discussed in Chapter 6 and elsewhere.[104,233]

Other causes of fatal intracerebral, intraventricular, and subarachnoid hemorrhages include disorders of coagulation or blood dyscrasias (anticoagulant medication, hemophilia, or other bleeding disorders, leukemia), lupus erythematosus, cerebral amyloid angiopathy (congophilic angiopathy) in the elderly, reactions due to therapeutic or illicit drug use,[171,180,237] or spontaneous hemorrhage into a tumor.

Any intracerebral hemorrhage may cause death. The precise mechanisms are not always clear but probably involve: (1) the sudden increase in volume with attendant acute increased intracranial pressure; (2)

local expanding effect of the hemorrhage, especially on vital brainstem or ventricular structures; (3) direct or indirect effect of extravascular blood (release of vasoactive inflammatory mediators, calcium and potassium disequilibrium); (4) release of neurotransmitter substances; (5) interference with CSF flow and reabsorption, causing increased intracranial pressure.[104,219] Regardless of the type of the hemorrhage, the interval from inception of the process to death may be several hours or days.

A relatively common forensic issue concerning intracerebral hemorrhage is the phenomenon of "delayed posttraumatic apoplexy."[13,17,229,231,255] This phenomenon classically was applied to cases in which there had been an episode of head trauma, and some days or weeks later the individual suffered an intracerebral hemorrhage. At contention is the connection between the trauma and the belated hemorrhage, which in most cases is circumstantial and rarely provable. An interval of 1 to 2 weeks usually is observed between trauma and hemorrhage. The hemorrhage can occur anywhere in the brain, generally not at the surface in a contusion, but can include hemorrhage in the subarachnoid space only. Numerous possibilities for etiology include subclinical shearing injury to vessels damaged by vascular disease, at sites of cryptic vascular anomalies, within the brain substance, or to vessels of the circle of Willis by medial or intimal tearing.*

***Cerebral ischemia and infarction.*** Most ischemic strokes have few forensic implications because they are recognized as naturally occurring processes that do not kill unexpectedly. A few exceptions are the alleged correlations between the use of oral contraceptive agents and stroke, stroke due to neck trauma or chiropractic manipulation, vascular injury in connection with an intravascular procedure, or strangulation or ligature injuries to the neck.

Since the introduction of oral contraceptive agents (OCs) several epidemiologic studies have analyzed statistical correlations between the ingestion of OCs and cerebral thromboembolism and venous thrombosis.† Reviews of the methodology of these studies concluded that most could not imply causality of stroke.[291] Prospective and better controlled, yet still flawed, studies showed no statistical correlation between oral contraceptive use and stroke.[101] After nearly 20 years of various epidemiologic studies that utilized a variety of methods, a causative relationship has not been demonstrated. *The Physicians' Desk Reference*[278] and package inserts for OCs list among adverse or potentially adverse reactions to these drugs allegations of stroke and venous thromboembolic phenomena. Dissenting or critical references are not allowed by the Food and Drug Administration of the U.S. federal government. The justification for this censorship is that prescribing physicians must at least be warned of *possible, not proved* adverse reactions against which they must weigh the potential risks and benefits to a given patient.

Considerable confusion to this issue has been added through several papers by Irey and others[161,162] who assert that oral contraceptives produce specific intimal proliferative lesions that may cause strokes. These studies suffer from the same difficulty as the epidemiologic studies in controlling causative influences and implying causality from a small sample using naturally occurring human material. Although the suspicion lingers that oral contraceptive agents are responsible for some strokes, young individuals and even infants were known to suffer strokes before the introduction of these drugs.[168,241,309]

Injuries to the neck, whether in conjunction with an accident, attempted chiropractic[31,66,77,150,305] or other manipulation of the neck for therapeutic purposes, or with an act of violence (strangulation, hanging, "karate" blows, etc.) can produce vascular injury to cervical vessels with immediate or belated thrombosis, embolism, infarction, or ischemia.[193,194] The most common neck vascular injury is to the vertebral arteries. About 30% of individuals possess only one vertebral artery (usually the right); thus occlusion or interference with vertebral circulation can be catastrophic. If the cervical spine is rotated forcefully with or without tractive force, one or both vertebral arteries may be compressed, stretched, or sheared.[313] This may produce rupture of the vessel, or it may induce an intimal injury where a thrombus or dissection may form and produce embolization or occlusion at a later time.[145,308] Krauland[194] points out that in case of trauma to the neck, longitudinal opening of the vessels at autopsy will regularly demonstrate intimal tears, thrombosis, or chronic reaction processes, including pseudoaneurysm. The consequences of such injury may be embolic infarction of the cerebellum,[145] portions of the brainstem, or posterior cerebral artery circulation. Thromboemboli may enter the basilar artery and obstruct the mesencephalic arteries with resultant ischemia of the upper midbrain and diencephalon.[184,280]

***Illustrative Case 2:*** *A 30-year-old woman suffered a brainstem stroke mostly involving the lower pons. She was "locked-in" for a period of time and eventually died. She had allegedly been taking oral contraceptive pills for some years, but also had used a variety of other medications, including a "diet" pill that contained thyroid extract, digitalis, and amphetamines. Postmortem examination revealed a scarred, calcified, and virtually obliterated vertebral artery on one side and a central pontine infarction appropriate for the duration of the survival. There was essentially no other cerebral vascular disease nor was there significant coronary or other arteriosclerosis present. Questioning family and*

---

* Refs. 66, 193, 194, 219, 228, 231.

† Refs. 158, 172, 297, 300, 337-339.

*friends of the victim revealed that several weeks before her "stroke" the victim had been hit in the posterior-lateral neck with the edge of a hand ("karate" blow) by an estranged boyfriend. She had suffered pain and some dizziness but no loss of consciousness at the time and did not seek medical attention. It was thought that the neck injury had damaged her vertebral artery, producing an intimal injury that ultimately dissected slightly and then thrombosed and embolized to her pons.*

Vascular mediated injury can occur to the spine in association with spinal trauma, malposition at surgery or during sleep or intoxication. It is also seen in association with spinal or retroperitoneal surgery, portacaval shunting, and in chronic liver disease (so-called Zieve's syndrome).[78,232] Presumably most of these conditions involve interruption or embarrassment of the spinal arterial circulation, probably the anterior spinal arterial system. There are several sites in the cord where end-arterial territories (watersheds) exist. During arterial hypotension or other circulatory embarrassments these sites (defined in Chapter 6) are vulnerable to ischemic injury, which may lead to the clinical syndrome of transverse myelopathy.

***Brain purpura and microembolization.*** A number of conditions are associated with multiple, punctate hemorrhagic lesions, or petechiae, usually confined to the white matter. Many of these have forensic implications.[219] The differential diagnosis of multiple or diffuse petechial lesions includes: disseminated intravascular coagulopathy; embolism by: fat, amniotic fluid, foreign material (polyvinyl alcohol, oil, barium, and adulterants) and rarely, air; viral and rickettsial encephalitis and bacterial sepsis; carbon monoxide intoxication; asphyxia; diffuse cerebral trauma; Shwartzman reactions (hemorrhagic encephalitis) and immune-mediated responses; cerebral malaria; toxins and venoms.*

With or without gross evidence of the fact, cerebral fat embolization probably occurs far more commonly than is recognized. The classic syndrome of fat embolization consists of progressive pulmonary insufficiency and encephalopathy occurring about 12 hours or more after a major episode of trauma, most commonly with but sometimes without skeletal fracture(s).[24] Such patients after appearing to be well suddenly deteriorate, sometimes experiencing multiple organ failure. Fat embolization usually does not occur from the dislodgement of fat from bones or soft tissues, but rather from in-situ precipitation of fatty acids in the blood due to the influence of inflammatory mediators, eicosanoids, which may alter plasma lipoproteins that keep plasma fats in fine emulsion.[24] The nature of the neurologic manifestations of fat embolization may be diffuse, producing a fatal encephalopathy, or focal and more subtle, in which confusion or delirium, seizures, paralysis, and other rather nonspecific symptoms may occur. CT imaging studies may not reveal any abnormality, but MRI examination may disclose multiple foci of hyperintensity.[84,153,166]

Autopsy examination of individuals who die shortly after fat embolism may show brain petechiae; at these sites as well in samples of the lung Oil Red O positive material is demonstrable in the lumina of small vessels. In nonacute cases, the fatty emboli will have dissolved, leaving no evidence of their presence. Gross examination of the brain in such patients may reveal nothing but microscopic examination may show perivascular areas of demyelination in cerebral, cerebellar white matter or within the brainstem.[345] These findings often correlate with the clinical picture of posttraumatic coma or dementia. In cases in which manifestations of cerebral fat embolization result in a protracted postconcussive syndrome, behavioral pathology, memory disturbances, confusion or other symptoms, white matter demyelination or perivascular injury may be demonstrable (Fig. 11-8). The perivascular capillary lesions including perivascular rarefaction of myelin, siderophages, and gliosis have been produced experimentally.[46]

The forensic implications of fat embolization fall primarily into the following areas: its sudden occurrence many hours or days after trauma, with catastrophic and often fatal consequences; the chronic consequences to the long term survival and quality of life of the individual; unrecognized cases of posttraumatic syndromes (dementia, depression, and psychosis). In the first instance, legal actions have been brought against physicians for allegedly failing to recognize or treat fat embolization acutely or for the apparent failure of treatment protocols in a badly injured person who appeared to be doing well and then deteriorated. In these

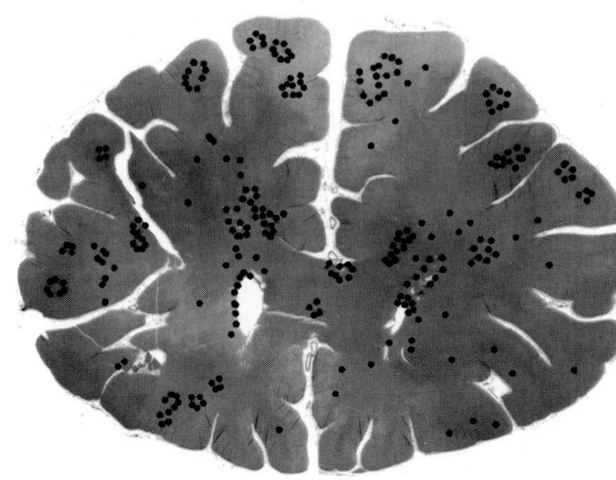

**Fig. 11-8.** This H&E stained macro section of the frontal lobe of the brain illustrates the distribution of small destructive perivascular lesions that were interpreted as having been due to fat embolization. Note the subcortical and deep white matter distribution of the lesions.

* Refs. 106, 125, 219, 236, 245, 247, 252.

cases, demonstration of fat emboli at autopsy will be important and may explain deterioration and death, for even when fat embolization is recognized, its treatment often is unsuccessful.[24,153] In those who survive, the legal question may relate to the prognosis for an individual who is encephalopathic or in coma. In most of these cases a pathologist is not able to provide expert testimony to help resolve the issue on survival or quality of life. In the latter instances, in which an individual suffers a debilitating brain-related problem following trauma, fat embolization may provide a causal basis for the illness. The following example is illustrative of such an instance.

***Illustrative Case 3:*** *A healthy, nonhypertensive 45-year-old man was injured in an automobile accident in which he suffered numerous lacerations and bruises about the head and shoulders and was apparently rendered unconscious for a time after the accident. The patient was admitted briefly to a local hospital and was treated symptomatically after CT scans and other studies were essentially negative. He apparently did not suffer a skull fracture and appeared to be doing well except for a headache. Approximately 2 days after returning home the patient experienced confusion and disorientation for which treatment was not sought. In the 2 years that followed the accident the patient experienced continued lapses of memory, periods of confusion, difficulties in performing mundane tasks (tying tie or shoe laces, using a manual transmission automobile), outbursts of temper, and difficulty at work. He experienced depressive episodes and during one of these hanged himself. Autopsy revealed numerous sutured lacerations, no skull fracture, no subdural hematoma, and no apparent cerebral injury. Microscopic examination using standard as well as large "window-pane" sections revealed countless small subcortical and deeper white matter perivascular lesions that resembled lacunae, in which capillaries showed prior injury, rarefaction of myelin, and residual siderophages and gliosis. The neuropathologic interpretation was that this man suffered posttraumatic fat embolization that was not recognized and that caused the residual cognitive and behavioral symptoms that ended with his suicide (Fig. 11-8).*

**Forensic aspects of brain neoplasia.** As with vascular disease, forensic aspects of brain neoplasms are infrequent concerns. Such circumstances involve previously unappreciated brain tumors that cause unexpected deaths, accidents and injuries that are alleged to produce behavioral abnormalities or that become the subject of medical malpractice litigation for failure to diagnose and treat. Brain neoplasms, primary or secondary, are not rare incidental findings at hospital autopsies or in forensic pathologic material. The largest series of these types of cases was reported by Huntington.[155]

***Illustrative Case 4:*** *A middle-aged man had suffered for several years from headaches that were ascribed to tension and work pressure. He was discovered to be hypertensive and this was treated, but his headaches continued intermittently and were not responsive. Since this case occurred before CT scanners were prevalent, an arteriogram was done that showed enlarged ventricles but no mass lesions. Before any treatment or further diagnostic studies could be performed, the man died suddenly after a bout of nausea and vomiting. Autopsy revealed a subependymoma about 5 mm in diameter filling the cerebral aqueduct, and there was moderately severe obstructive hydrocephalus.*

***Illustrative Case 5:*** *Charles Whitman, a 25-year-old University of Texas student, after shooting his wife and mother, ascended a tall building at the center of the campus in Austin, in August of 1966 and, armed with several rifles and other weapons, proceeded to shoot scores of people. He killed 12 before he was shot to death by police.*[262-265] *His autopsy was performed at a State Mental Hospital by a pathologist untrained in forensic methods who allegedly found a "vascular" mass deep in Whitman's brain and suggested that this mass may have caused his irrational and violent behavior. Because of the furor over this case, which propeled it into the realm of folk legend, the Governor of Texas, John Connally (himself a victim of an assassin's attempt 3 years before), empaneled a group of experts to determine the facts of the case. Upon careful examination of the brain, which had not been retained or photographed, but had been placed within the body cavity and buried with the body, missile wounds were found but no residual tumor was noted. Considerable portions of the brain had been lost. The "vascular" mass was found only in one paraffin block supplied by the hospital pathologist who performed the autopsy. This mass was a sample of a glioblastoma multiforme, but little normal tissue remained in the margins to accurately localize the lesion. No conclusion could be drawn about any influence this alleged tumor might have had on Whitman's behavior. Nevertheless, an interaction has been assumed or alleged frequently in the media since 1966 whenever similar violent multiple homicides are perpetrated.*[219]

This case illustrates the harm and confusion that can result from an incomplete or improper forensic neuropathologic examination. The deficiencies in this case were incomplete description of wounds, the specimen and its lesions; lack of proper preservation of physical evidence; lack of photographs or other objective materials; precipitate and ill-founded release of information to the media; failure to consult with appropriate experts; and an inadequate report. Many guides to proper procedure can be found in several forensic pathology monographs and texts.[47,70,71,83]

Occasionally, forensic issues arise conserning a possible etiologic link between traumatic injuries, exposure to toxic or carcinogenic agents, or exposure to electromagnetic fields and the development of a brain neoplasm. These are interesting and confusing issues for which confident answers are only rarely available. This issue of head injuries as causes of brain tumors has been discussed at length by many authors.[18,75,219] The following criteria for probable causality seem sensible:

1. The site of injury should correspond to the site of the tumor in the brain. 2. The traumatic injury should be sufficiently severe and not incidental (possibly open brain injury). 3. The area where the injury occurred should be shown free of tumor at the time of the injury. 4. The time interval between injury and tumor discovery must be sufficiently long to be appropriate for tumorigenesis (probably years). 5. There must be continuity in the pathologic changes of the injured areas in the brain with the tumor. 6. There must be histologic proof for a diagnosis of neoplasm. These criteria are rarely met, but provocative cases have been reported.[219]

On the question of environmental toxins as etiologic agents for brain tumors, many have been proposed, but little has been proved. If there is a link between environmental exposure to a carcinogen and a brain tumor, the toxin most likely acts transplacentally in much the same manner as does the experimental administration of the nitrosoureas to pregnant animals,[170,188,323] and affects the offspring rather than the exposed individual.

A number of allegations have claimed that exposure to electromagnetic fields or radiation may cause or promote growth of a tumor de novo or promote dedifferentiation if a tumor already was present. The circumstances of greatest interest are exposures to the fields that surround electrical transmission lines, transformers, or other major power sources. It also has been alleged that low-power sources, such as electric blankets and some household appliances may be hazardous and perhaps cause brain neoplasms.[223,328] Another cause of brain and other tumors alleged by various individuals, and at the same time denied vociferously, is exposure to radio frequency electromagnetic energy, particularly in the microwave spectrum used by cellular telephones, police radar guns, and similar devices. Most alleged cases are anecdotal and sometimes compelling, but causality cannot be proved until far more rigorous data are collected. By the same token, allegations of complete safety cannot be accepted without the same rigorous data collection and statistical analysis. Thus the questions remain open.

**Forensic aspects of infectious/inflammatory diseases.** Infectious or inflammatory diseases of the nervous system occasionally have medical-legal or public health import. Examples are proper diagnosis of contagious nervous system infections (the equine encephalitides and other arbovirus infections, meningococcal and other meningitides, polio, AIDS, rabies), Creutzfeld-Jakob disease (CJ disease) and mode of acquisition; pathogenesis and pathology of alleged operatively-acquired infections; analysis of inoculation and vaccination reactions affecting the nervous system (DPT vaccination, measles vaccination); allergic conditions possibly caused by exogenous agents or drugs; Guillain-Barrĕ syndrome; postinfectious encephalomyelitis. The complexity in these conditions is not in their diagnosis but in such peripheral issues as mode of infection or acquisition, age and duration of processes, effects on function, and prognosis and outcome.

***Illustrative Case 6:*** *A 3-month-old infant who by all measures was normal received a routine DPT inoculation. The child suffered a febrile reaction to the injection and was irritable. A few days later the infant experienced a seizure and showed some lethargy and over the next several weeks and months, failed to develop, worsened neurologically, became vegetative, and died several months later. Imaging studies had demonstrated a destructive nonspecific white matter process. At autopsy the classic findings of Alexander's disease were noted. Since the etiology of Alexander's disease is not known, but suspected of being inherited, it is unlikely that the DPT injection had any causal relationship; however, the question of irritating and hastening or unmasking the underlying Alexander's disease remains open.*

Several reports have been published of individuals who apparently were inoculated or contaminated with Creutzfeldt-Jakob infected material and subsequently developed the disease. The first of these cases involved a recipient of a corneal graft obtained from a patient dying of C-J disease.[219] Other cases have involved inoculation, presumably by depth electrodes that had been sterilized by formalin vapor after having been used on a C-J patient. The injection of human pituitary pooled extracts of growth hormone has been abandoned because of the infection of one or more individuals by C-J disease, presumed to have come from this extract.[261] Most recently an individual apparently contracted C-J after receiving a cadaveric dural graft during a neurosurgical procedure.[280,356] These cases clearly have forensic importance and constitute a warning and a responsibility of preventing other occurrences. Neuropathologists can be key persons in education and in preventing similar situations when they have special knowledge of importance to others.[34]

A classic forensic dilemma with neuropathologic impact was illustrated by the problem of fatal so-called "swimming hole" encephalitis in the southeastern United States during the 1950s and 1960s. Typical histories were those of individuals who, after having swum in fresh-water pools, where water often was stagnant in the summer, developed classic signs of meningitis and encephalitis and died within a few days. Autopsies showed a hemorrhagic and necrotizing meningoencephalitis. The organisms responsible had a strikingly similar appearance to macrophages, but were, in fact, free-living amoebae of the *Naeglaria* or *Hartmanella* species, clustered about blood vessels in the brain.[49,50]

## Forensic Aspects of Perinatal/Pediatric Neuropathology

Most of the forensic applications in this age group center about congenital anomalies and the pathologic conditions of the perinatal period. Child abuse is discussed separately later in this chapter.

The incidence of fatal developmental anomalies of the brain such as anencephaly[204]: varies enormously from country to country (between 1 and 7:100,000 births) but nonfatal anomalies are common.[201,219] The type of anomaly observed is not so much a function of the precise etiology of the anomaly but of the time during neural development when the agent affects the brain. The outcome is directly related to interference with individual development processes. Time tables for the various developmental events may be found in texts on embryology, brain development, perinatal pathology, and other sources.[117,118,342]

Defects of neuronal migration include heterotopias and ectopias of gray matter (Fig. 11-9) lobar and gyral anomalies, and such cortical anomalies as lissencephaly, macrogyria or pachygyria, micropolygyria and micropolygyria, or combinations of all of these, as well as disorders of lobe formation (holoprosencephaly and related conditions). These various anomalies often occur in combination and often are associated with such other anomalies as agenesis of the corpus callosum, porencephaly, schizencephaly, and others.[100] Survivors often are mentally subnormal, but may not be. When these defects are present in a viable individual they usually lead to seizures, which may be the main forensic aspect of these cases, although allegations of medical mismanagement, in utero trauma, and side effects of drugs may be made under circumstances of potential litigation. Usually only theoretic implications of external events are possible, and since most events that might cause these anomalies occur well before fetal viability, obstetricians are rarely deemed culpable for their occurrence. The following case history illustrates the forensic neuropathologic aspects of one case in which a neuronal migration anomaly was involved.

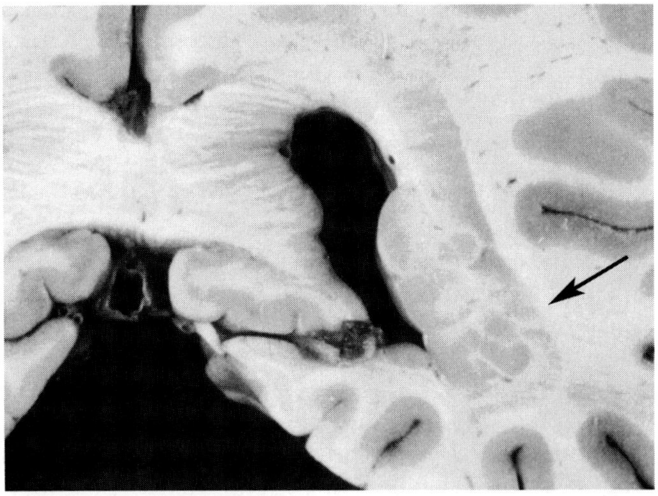

**Fig. 11-9.** This selected field of a coronal section of the posterior portion of the brain illustrates a complex island of ectopic gray matter protruding into the right lateral ventricle. Such ectopias may be associated with epilepsy of focal or generalized types. This particular individual, a young female, died as a result of status epilepticus. Such lesions have been found in victims of single car accidents, having presumably suffered a seizure with loss of control of the vehicle. Such an instance is described in Illustrative Case 7.

***Illustrative Case 7:*** *A teenage girl was killed in an accident when the car she was driving veered off the road and struck an abutment. The girl died from multiple trauma. No mechanical fault was discovered in her car. No stress imprint of the brake pedal or accelerator pads were found on the soles of her shoes. A witness reported that the car drifted off the roadway and that the driver made no attempt to stop. She was reported to have been looking straight ahead when the accident occurred. Neuropathologic examination revealed ectopic gray matter and an anomalous hippocampal formation in one temporal lobe. Retrospective investigation revealed that the girl's classmates at school jokingly referred to her as "old dreamy" (or similar nicknames) because she was often observed out of contact and staring ahead while in class. Although there was no history of medical diagnosis or treatment, it appears likely that the girl suffered from absence seizures (petit mal epilepsy). It is possible that the head lamps of approaching cars, shuttered by a barrier between highway lanes may have produced an epileptogenic photic stimulation, triggering an absence attack in the girl as she drove her car that evening.*

In two major morphologic anomalies of the cerebellum no known cause has been demonstrated, but either can have forensic neuropathologic consequences. These are the Dandy-Walker and the Arnold-Chiari malformations. The former consists of agenesis of the ventral cerebellar vermis with formation of a large cyst over the defect. The Arnold-Chiari malformation often is associated with hydrocephalus, platybasia, spina bifida, and myelomeningocele.[100,219,235] The forensic implications of these anomalies rest with lack of recognition of their existence or with a mistaken diagnosis; sometimes unexpected death occurs in connection with them.

***Illustrative Case 8:*** *A 35-year-old man, a known wheelchair-bound chronic alcoholic and derelict, was found in ex-*

*tremis on a sidewalk near his residence. According to the press, a taxi driver with whom the man was riding threw him from his cab and beat him the day before. Apparently the man had spent the night beside the sidewalk, but this was not considered unusual by his neighbors. Eventually the man died without regaining consciousness. Autopsy revealed no signs of a significant beating, only trauma on the lower extremities. Neuropathologic examination revealed a greatly enlarged head circumference, a contusion near the occiput, no skull fracture, a Dandy-Walker malformation with advanced hydrocephalus, and bilateral chronic subdural hematomas (none with current bleeding Fig. 11-10). This man had not had infantile paralysis; rather, he suffered from a congenital malformation of the brain. He had clearly sustained multiple episodes of head trauma. His death was likely due to increased intracranial pressure, chronic hydrocephalus, chronic subdural hematoma, recent intoxication, and mild head trauma resulting in brainstem compression by herniated brain tissues.*

Severe destructive processes in the infant brain such as hydranencephaly and porencephaly may have many causes, usually thought to be circulatory in origin, in which an intrauterine brain infarction has occurred, leaving either a cavity in the brain or nearly complete destruction of the cerebrum.[235,336] Occasionally abnormal or atretic vessels may be discovered, but infectious causes for these anomalies also are found. The most common infectious cause is toxoplasmosis, transplacentally acquired. These cases can have forensic implications, mostly because of allegations of responsible causality.

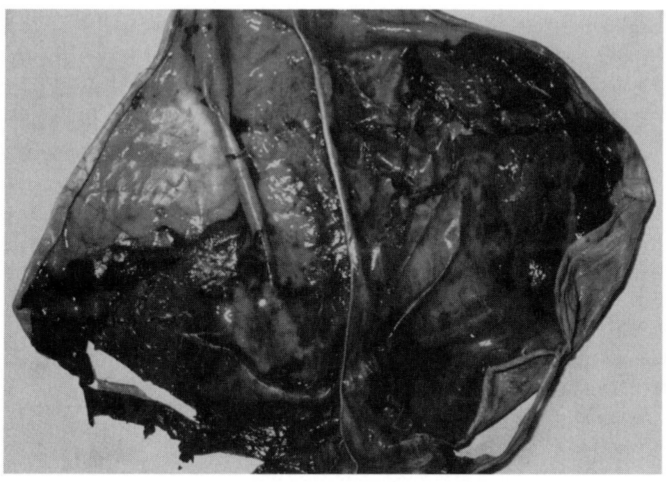

**Fig. 11-10.** This photograph of the underside of the cerebral dura shows a diffuse chronic and focally acute subdural hematoma (see Illustrative Case 8). The head was much larger than normal owing to the chronic hydrocephalus this victim suffered, hence the dura was at least three times the normal size. There were no large cyst or clot collections. No significant mass effects were observed caused by the extensive system of hematoma membranes. (Courtesy of the Office of the Medical Examiner, Cook County, Illinois.)

Cerebral palsy and perinatal brain injury can have great forensic implications, especially in view of the epidemic of current malpractice actions against obstetricians in which allegations of improper prenatal and perinatal medical management are made.[156,157,333] The focal point of these cases involves expert judgment, and often testimony, regarding the temporal genesis and etiology of cerebral palsy. There is often precious little objective research evidence available for aging and dating perinatal acquired lesions and their cause.[219]

During the process of birth the neonate is almost certainly hypoxic for a time before the establishment of respiration after birth,[202] and many infants suffer from neonatal jaundice.[110] It appears that the gray matter of the perinatal infant's brain is more resilient to hypoxemia than is the white matter. This thesis is supported by the pathologic changes observed in infants who died after experiencing a difficult or prolonged birth and who experience difficulty in breathing at birth, as reflected by an Apgar score of 5 or less at birth and for many minutes thereafter. It is presumed, perhaps erroneously, that white matter lesions are due to the difficult birth and not to some preexisting or coexistent condition.[81] These lesions, in the premature infant, can take the form of periventricular hemorrhages, and liquefactive changes in the periventricular white matter, which also can be seen in term infants when circumstances are severe. The magnitude and phase of these changes depends on the age of the infant and their duration before death.[15,100,117,118,359]

Periventricular-subependymal hemorrhages usually are related to prematurity, hypoxia and acidosis, and microcirculatory abnormalities.[100,276] In older infants, these changes may be seen in conjunction with other ischemic/hypoxic lesions. Cavitary white matter lesions are more prone to occur in term or near-term infants and may coexist with hemorrhagic lesions. The etiology, pathogenesis, and time of occurrence of these lesions and other causes of perinatal intraventricular and subarachnoid hemorrhage are controversial.[100,113,336,359] Perhaps the thesis that the neonatal cortex is preserved during hypoxia is more apparent than real. The cortex may appear to be grossly preserved, but microscopically there may be profound neuronal loss and glial replacement. The basal ganglia also may appear intact but are firm and rubbery to the touch, even in the unfixed brain. Sometimes these changes are associated with hyperbilirubinema (kernicterus), especially in the premature infant.[110,366] Microscopically there may be severe neuronal loss and gliosis in the basal ganglia, which also may affect the brainstem.[356] Often the lower brainstem is fairly preserved, and the spinal cord, apart from descending degeneration in the corticospinal tracts and other major descending pathways, is essentially normal. Even when these lesions are especially severe, such infants may be kept alive for years, although in a vegetative state.

Damage to the basal ganglia is said to be absolutely indicative of damage remote from birth (well beyond the possibility of intervention by the obstetrician) and is the basis for the clinical state known as "cerebral palsy."[333] There are many difficulties with such an absolutist opinion. Basal ganglia, cortex, and white matter vulnerability are relative, not absolute in terms of time. Numerous factors can influence the existence of lesions and their proportionality in relation to other damage in the brain.[110] These include: the relative proportion of hypoxia to preserved blood flow (hypoxic hypoxia versus ischemic hypoxia);[208] the degree of acidosis and electrolyte abnormality; the etiology of the process of ischemia and/or hypoxia; state of maturity of the individual, and of cerebral microvascular responses; other conditions such as congenital CNS, cardiac, renal, or pulmonary anomalies; the competence and physiology of the placenta; various maternal factors such as diabetes, toxicity, metabolic abnormality, presence of drugs. Most of these factors are essentially unknowable even at the time they occur, much less in retrospect from the viewpoint of the pathologist.

"Cerebral palsy" (C-P) is a general term used to describe infants and children who have suffered some form of congenital (intrauterine) or perinatally acquired injury to the brain that results in permanent, nonprogressive brain malfunction. Many C-P children have movement disorders (spasticity, dystonia, athetoid-choreiform movements) but have normal intelligence. Some are mentally retarded or totally disabled. Others may suffer from hypotonia and paralysis, with or without mental impairment. An important aspect of C-P is that once the abnormalities become apparent during development they do not tend to progress. The neuropathologic appearance of C-P brains varies enormously. Some brains appear grossly normal and show abnormality only after intense studies; others have grossly visible lesions. In this latter category are infants who have cortical malformations (gyral anomalies, ectopias and heterotopias, porencephaly and schizencephaly), lytic lesions of the white matter, so-called état marbre (marbled brain) of the thalamus and basal ganglia or combinations of these. Clinical pathologic correlations between symptoms and lesions is difficult at best, as are pronouncements regarding etiology or time of occurrence.[81] Well-prepared and analytical case reports are scanty; however, numerous references and individual observations seem to indicate that the perinatal period (a few weeks before and a few weeks after birth) is the time when most C-P brain lesions have their genesis.[156,157]

The prevailing prejudice is that hypoxia/ischemia is the leading cause of C-P.[322] Whether all lesions must occur at the same time is far from clear. For instance, a neurologically compromised fetus (because of an earlier event or chronic in utero condition) may experience difficulty adjusting to existence outside the uterus and may, therefore, be incapable of an appropriate respiratory drive and/or circulatory adjustment. Such an infant will necessarily display a lower than normal Apgar score. This difficulty may impose further injury on an already damaged CNS, which acts as a multiplier of the final neurologic state. To gain knowledge about the intrauterine status of the fetus, some have suggested that perinatal ultrasound imaging of the fetal brain may resolve the question of "before or after" casualty in C-P.[275]

Although there is no consistent etiology for all cases of C-P, a number of factors and conditions correlate significantly with its development. The Apgar score is said to be a good predictor of C-P, but this is not the case. Apgar scores alone, have no predictive value unless the infant maintains a score below 3 for 10 minutes or longer after birth.[260] In contrast, when the selecting variable is C-P, a high degree of correlation with low Apgar scores is demonstrable. When a group of high-risk babies who suffered severe respiratory depression for 20 or more minutes after birth were followed, about 50% of such infants died. However, 75% of the survivors apparently were normal thereafter, and no means was discovered to determine which infant in the surviving group would develop neurologic sequelae.[274,275]

It is now clear that a C-P outcome is multifactorial. Statistically significant risk factors include prematurity and/or birth weight below 2500 g, twin gestations (with or without twin-twin transfusion), a complicated delivery including breech presentation and nuchal cord, use of obstetric forceps, persistent Apgar scores below 5, neonatal seizures, extremes of maternal age, incidence of previous maternal spontaneous abortion and stillbirths, major placental pathology, chorioamnionitis, and intrauterine exposure to drugs and toxic substances.[259] When all these and some other risk factors were applied to a test population, a "high-risk" group was identified of which 5% of cases resulted in 34% of the C-P outcomes, yet two-thirds of the C-P population did not come from this group, and 97% of high-risk babies did not suffer from C-P.[259] Regardless of all efforts to develop reliable predictors of C-P, no rigid, universally accepted standard has been found. In spite of advances in obstetric practice the incidence of C-P remains relatively constant, and in more than two-thirds of all C-P children no obvious risk factor or causal circumstance can be identified. The impact of "bad baby" litigation on the practice of obstetrics has been significant in the United States and has prompted a major increase in cesarian deliveries over standard spontaneous vaginal deliveries under the mistaken notion that cerebral palsy can be prevented. In spite of radical rises in cesarian sections, the C-P rate has remained unchanged at between 1.4 to 2.9 cases per 100 live births.[83,91,304]

Congenitally acquired infections may have considerable impact on the ability of the infant or fetal brain to develop properly. Examples of transplacentally acquired infections with significant neurodevelopmental effects are toxoplasmosis, cytomegalovirus, rubella, mumps, herpes simplex, HIV, syphilis, and probably others. Bacterial infections are important in the pathogenesis and etiology of meningitis. In the neonatal and perinatal period, the coliform organisms are chiefly responsible, causing meningitis at a level of about 4 per 10,000 live births.[26] Neonatal meningitis is nearly always fatal after several days, and may be caused or contributed to by unclean, unattended, or improper delivery. Most cases are caused by infection of the umbilical veins and may accompany premature rupture of the fetal membranes, endometritis, chorioamnionitis, and other regional septic conditions. When infants grow older, especially when the titers of maternal antibodies declined in upper airway, *hemophilus influenzae* may become the chief cause of meningitis. This form of meningitis when recognized and treated is rarely fatal and leaves few sequelae.[26,219]

### Forensic Aspects of Neurotoxicology

The fields of toxicology and neurotoxicology are broad and complex, and one of the fastest growing fields of specialization in toxicology has been neurotoxicology. All aspects of neurotoxicology as they relate to forensic science cannot be considered in this chapter, but notable examples of toxic conditions with historical and current import will be reviewed. More complete treatment of the general field can be found in several excellent monographs.[44,72,165,294,316]

Toxins affecting the nervous system can be classified several ways,[219,316] by chemical type, structure, or class; by the organs they affect or even the cellular organelles or biochemical processes with which they interfere; by the symptoms or diseases they produce; by the cellular processes affected; and by whether they are fatal or not. From a neuropathologic point of view it is convenient to consider toxins in terms of the diseases and effects they produce. Certain toxins in the pregnant animal or human produce developmental defects or neoplasms in the offspring. These teratogens have great value in the experimental laboratory, but also have considerable impact on federal regulations that govern testing, safety, and ultimate licensing and approval of drugs, foods, dyes, chemicals, insecticides, and medical devices. In large measure these regulations were influenced by the limb agenesis (phocomelia) that affected the infants of mothers who took thalidomide in Europe and the United States in the early 1960s.[96] Thalidomide babies are still born in Brazil, a country where this drug apparently is distributed without obvious warnings against its use during pregnancy. The profound neurotoxic effect on infants caused by the maternal use of alcohol, cocaine, and other drugs has led to the enforced labeling of beverages, active public awareness and educational programs, and the drafting and enforcement of special applications to the child abuse and neglect laws when mothers knowingly and willfully damage their babies during pregnancy by harmful behavior. Neuropathologists have played a significant role in understanding the mechanisms by which alcohol and cocaine affect unborn babies.[51,68,134] Other examples of neuroteratology involve the maternal use of anticonvulsants such as phenytoin (Dilantin) and the exposure to mercury and other heavy metals as typified by the Minamata Bay disaster in Japan.[200,316] In animals, neuroteratogens may also be oncogenic (especially the nitrosourea compounds), but no such role for these or other compounds has been proved in humans.[170,316,323]

A number of neurotoxic compounds produce cerebral edema. The heavy metals (lead, mercury, tin, nickel, cobalt) may damage the blood-brain barrier and ionic membrane pump systems.[316] A classic example of metallic poisoning occurred in France in the 1950s, when more than 100 people lost their lives to malignant cerebral edema after ingesting a medicinal preparation (Stalinon) that contained diethyl tin. Fortunately, this compound is no longer available, and rapid public awareness prevented more fatalities. The alkyl tins were utilized extensively in experimental laboratories to better understand this unusual form of edema.[296,330] Various hydrocarbons including the alcohols can have fatal effects when ingested or inhaled in sufficient quantity. Among the alcohols, ethyl alcohol is probably the most common cause of fatal cerebral edema. Ingestion of methanol and isopropanol also may produce fatal intoxication by cerebral edema and profound acidosis.[47,219]

Several toxic substances affect intracellular transport, specifically neuroplasmic (axonal) transport mechanisms, often in different ways. Typical of these agents are the "mitotic spindle inhibitors" such as colchicine, vinblastine, vincristine, griseofulvin, and podophyllotoxin.[243] These compounds bind tenaciously to tubulin and apparently depolymerize neurotubule.[312] Other agents, such as IDPN and the hexacarbons (2,5 hexanedione, hexane, methylbutyl ketone, cyclohexanone), as well as aluminum salts, acrylamide monomer, and fluororganic compounds bind to or somehow alter neurofilaments, inhibiting their interactions and disrupting axonal transport.[316] Drugs such as Adriamycin and other chemotherapeutic agents may also have effects on neural transport and may induce either CNS effects or peripheral neuropathies.[299]

A neuropathy known as "dying back" neuropathy appears to result from a toxic effect by such agents as acrylamide monomer and phosphocresols on the synesthetic and transport mechanisms of the neuronal soma. The effect of the intoxication is observed strikingly at the distal axonal process, perhaps a meter away in an extremity.[287] Industrial exposure, the intentional use of various compounds for intoxication by "sniffing," therapeutic misadventures occasioned by inappropriate routes or sites of administration, and simple complications of therapy provide fertile ground for pathologic effects and the possibility of involvement in a forensic situation, litigative or otherwise.

Some toxic compounds have their effect on the myelin sheath, central or peripheral. Examples of peripheral myelin toxicity include lead, various organometallic compounds, nitrous oxide, diphtheria toxin, and many others. Centrally active toxins include carbon monoxide, cyanide, hexachlorophene, lead and probably organic mercury compounds, and possibly some alcohols.[316] The effects are not always confined to the myelin sheath, and eventually the toxins affect axons as well. The consequences of such intoxications in the peripheral nervous system are neuropathic processes that may involve several cycles of demyelination and remyelination, resulting in a hypertrophic type of neuropathy.[38,197] The shortening or alteration of internodal length almost uniformly produces prolonged nerve conduction times and motor weakness or paralysis or paresthesias and sensory loss (Chapter 17). Centrally, loss of myelination can produce encephalopathy, weakness, aphasias, dementia, blindness, paralysis, ataxia, and behavioral symptoms. Although not exogenously a toxic state, dehydration and acidosis and too rapid replacement of blood electrolytes, particularly sodium, may result in diffuse white matter damage and death.[93,130] Another example is the occasional disastrous interaction between radiation therapy and methotrexate on deep cerebral white matter.[10] Still another is the delayed toxic effect of carbon monoxide intoxication on white matter.[207] All these situations can have forensic and potentially litigative possibilities in which the neuropathologist may be called upon to diagnose or otherwise render an opinion. These processes are discussed in detail elsewhere in this textbook and in other work.[72,216,294,316]

Several toxins and toxic states affect neural transmission, either at the neural membrane or synapse, or by an indirect effect on neural transmitter substances. Examples are marine and animal toxins such as tetrodotoxin, ciguatoxin, batrachotoxin, bombesin, and various spider and snake venoms.[216,238] Microbiologic toxins such as botulinus toxin, tetanus toxin, and diphtheria toxin are well known in the neurotoxicologic literature and have been well studied.[316] Various chemical toxins such as the organic phosphates and alkaloids are well known as potent neurotoxins. The former are potent "nerve" gases and insecticides that occasionally produce industrial illness and fatalities.[72] The narcotic alkaloids are not only drugs of abuse but one of these, MPTP (an analog of meperidine), produces a clinical syndrome virtually identical to Parkinson's disease. This compound when taken by any route is metabolized by monoamine oxidase containing cells (usually pigmented nuclei such as the substantia nigra) to a toxic intermediate that kills the cells, thus depriving their connections of dopamine. In this instance the nigral-striatal pathway is damaged and an akinetic parkinsonian syndrome develops rapidly. This phenomenon has delivered into the hands of the experimental neurobiologist an excellent experimental model for parkinsonism.[39,206]

**Ethyl alcohol.** There is probably no more important neurotoxin than ethanol with respect to the spectrum of neuropathology and other organ damage it produces and the sheer numbers of individuals affected by ethyl alcohol. The basis for its effects on the nervous system are still not understood nor fully appreciated.

Acute alcohol intoxication usually is willful, but can be accidental (e.g., by inhaling alcohol-containing vapors or fumes or unknowingly consuming alcohol in the forms of "spiked" beverages, or medicines).[47] The most common effect is known to virtually everyone: a sense of giddiness, elevation or depression of mood, excitation or suppression of activity, loss of coordination together with inability to think clearly, and eventually a stuporous and lethargic state or nausea and vomiting followed hours later by an unhappy, post-toxic state (the "hangover"). In most cases this intoxicated state is self-limited and abates over 12 to 24 hours. In most legal jurisdictions, worldwide, the toxicologic definitions of alcohol intoxication range from any detectable blood level of ethanol, to 50 or 100 mg/dl, at which level the individual is considered legally drunk and thus incapable of operating a motor- or self-propelled vehicle. The penalties for operating a vehicle when intoxicated vary widely, from virtually none to a fine, loss of one's driver's license, imprisonment, and even imposition of the death penalty in some Muslim countries.[216] Acute ethanol intoxication rarely involves a neuropathologist. An exception is an incident in a which a child or young adult unknowingly or accidentally rapidly consumes a large amount of alcohol. Stupor and coma may occur rapidly and be so severe that respiratory failure and death ensue. In such cases, severe cerebral edema often is present, which in combination with neural depression, probably is responsible for the fatal result. Fatality in a neophyte is not always well correlated with blood levels of alcohol.

Chronic alcohol use and abuse may lead to a broad

spectrum of directly-related neurologic disease.[140,332] These include: Wernicke-Korsakoff syndrome; alcoholic cerebellar degeneration; central pontine myelinolysis; alcoholic neuropathy; alcoholic myopathy; chronic brain syndrome; Marchiafava-Bignami syndrome; alcoholic withdrawal seizures and delirium tremens; fetal alcohol syndrome. Neuropathologic conditions related to alcohol include cerebral, spinal, and multiple trauma; transverse myelopathy; associated and accidental poisoning with lead, methanol, propanol and ethylene glycol; hepatic failure and encephalopathy; homicide and suicide; seizure deaths; and nutritional disorders.

*Wernicke's disease* is not always secondary to alcohol abuse, but in most cases the syndrome is associated with chronic alcohol abuse.[41,292] The clinical syndrome is highly variable, showing the classic features of Korsakoff syndrome (delusions, confabulation, hallucinations) alone or with disorientation, confusion, agitation, memory disturbances, ataxia, and nystagmus, oculomotor and/or trochlear nerve dysfunction or coma. A brownish discoloration or hemorrhagic necrosis of the mamillary bodies at times involving portions of the hypothalamus, the periaqueductal regions and tectal region of the midbrain, and about the fourth ventricle in the cerebellum and pons are common findings. The optic chiasm and anterior commissures also may be affected. Preservation of small neurons and many axons may be noted in affected structures. Usually there is prominence of small capillaries and products of hemorrhage (siderophages, reactive gliosis, inflammation). The pathogenesis of the lesions probably involves direct toxic and genetically mediated effects on utilization or metabolism mediated by thiamine in the glycolytic pathway. Serotoninergic neurons are selectively injured in the process.[140,141,341]

*Alcoholic cerebellar degeneration* was defined by Victor and co-workers.[340] Fifty of their own cases were compared with 60 others culled from the medical literature. Most victims of this condition are middle-aged men who have abused alcohol for many years and generally have other alcohol-related conditions such as delirium tremens, Wernicke-Korsakoff disease, neuropathy, or an encephalopathy. The syndrome can be insidious and progressive or nonprogressive, or it can be more abrupt of onset. Not all affected individuals show improvement on cessation of alcohol intake. Symptoms involve ataxia, stumbling, and lack of upper extremity coordination with or without intention tremor. Difficulty in speech and articulation as well as nystagmus also may be part of the syndrome. Atrophy of the rostral vermis of the cerebellum alone or in combination with a wider area of atrophy of the superior surface of the cerebellum is the most common feature. Here folial atrophy usually is striking, with loss of Purkinje cells and granular cells. There may be atrophy of the inferior olivary nuclei and other nuclei, but the dentate nuclei and other parts of the spinocerebellar system usually are spared. This pattern is not observed in any other form of cerebellar atrophy, inherited or acquired. The etiology of the process is not known, although some suggest that repeated bouts of posterior fossa edema in connection with alcohol intoxication results in pressure-ischemia of the rostral cerebellum.

*Central pontine myelinolysis,* like Wernicke's disease, is not seen exclusively in alcoholics, but can be seen in nonalcoholic liver disease, poor nutrition, severe dehydration followed by too-rapid rehydration (hyponatremia), and other cases of severe and/or chronic metabolic abnormality.[6,130] The disease is rarely suspected and diagnosed in life, and may be associated with other alcohol-related conditions. Symptoms include quadriplegia, pseudobulbar palsy, and ocular movement abnormalities as a result of damage to the medial longitudinal fasciculus. The lesion usually is located in the center of the pons at the junction with the pontine tegmentum, and it usually consists of a diamond-shaped gray or brownish abnormality in which the main pathologic change is loss of myelinated fibers with preservation of neurons. Chronic lesions may show necrosis of other elements and some degree of inflammation and gliosis. Comparable lesions may be seen in the medulla, cerebellum, cerebrum, or in other areas where there is myelin loss but neurons are preserved.[90] Most of these regions are circumscribed and show no pattern suggestive of multiple sclerosis.[285]

*Marchiafava-Bignami disease*[189] is an exceedingly rare condition reported mostly in Europe in heavy wine drinkers. The lesion consists of coagulative necrosis of midline structures and commissures of the brain (such as the corpus callosum) as well as of the deep white matter. Gray matter areas usually are spared. The etiology of this obscure condition is not known.

*Alcoholic neuropathy, myopathy, and myelopathy* may be primarily vitamin deficiency related, most often thiamine[140,316] deficiency or interference with the action of thiamine. In most cases other stigmata of alcohol-induced pathology are present in the nervous system. In some cases pernicious anemia ($B_{12}$ and folic acid deficiency) may be the appropriate etiology for the conditions observed. The pathology of alcoholic myopathy is related to rhabdomyolysis perhaps secondary to severe metabolic abnormality and hypokalemia from prolonged vomiting and electrolyte loss, cold injury from exposure, consumption of substitutes for alcohol, and rhabdomyolysis associated with seizures, delirium tremens, or agitation.

The teratogenic and developmental effects of alcohol have become widely appreciated in recent years. As a result, printed warnings on alcohol-containing products and widespread publicity concerning the risks of consumption of alcohol by pregnant women are required by law in many states. The level of fetal tolerance for alcohol appears to be very low, and normal social drinking may have measurable effects on behavior and learning abilities of exposed children. In more severe cases a typical external appearance has become recognized in alcohol-affected babies. The typical affected baby may be of low birth weight and have slitlike eyes with a birdlike flattened face.[174,175] Psychomotor development in affected children is slow, and they may show features typical of alcohol withdrawal including seizures and delirium tremens. Most such children display learning and behavioral abnormalities. In some infants whose mothers abused several drugs including cocaine, other abnormalities may be seen. It may be difficult to isolate the effects of alcohol from those of other substances to which the child was exposed. Either obvious or subtle changes in the brain including a small cerebrum or cerebellum, disorders of neuronal migration (ectopias and heterotopias, cortical abnormalities, sulcal maldevelopment), porencephaly, Arnold-Chiari and Dandy-Walker malformations, and closure defects (myelomeningocele and anencephaly) have been noted in this syndrome. The literature on this devastating and common syndrome demonstrates that much of this same pathology and more subtle dendritic and cortical organizational defects[124,138,174,175] can be induced in experimental animals exposed to alcohol at a very young age.

**Carbon monoxide.** Carbon monoxide intoxication is a frequent cause of death by accident or suicide.[47,122] The classical postmortem "cherry red" color of the skin is well known, but the spectrum of neuropathologic changes is not as well known. Carbon monoxide exposure occurs in almost any closed space where a gasoline or other internal combustion engine or a heating device that relies upon combustion (kerosene or gasoline heater, fireplace or furnace) operates with inadequate ventilation. Any combustion process in which carbon is burned inevitably will produce carbon monoxide, which combines tenaciously with hemoglobin when inhaled. Carbon monoxide is colorless and odorless; thus, no warning other than some form of intoxication is possible. When the ambient atmosphere contains as little as 1 part of CO per 10,000 parts of air, an individual can accumulate at least 10% carboxymethemoglobin in the blood in a very short time. This level of CO may be symptomless (especially in cigarette smokers) or produce headache and malaise. This level, however, can have significant cardiovascular effects in anyone with emphysema and/or coronary artery disease. When CO levels rise to 20% to 30%, headache and nausea usually appear. At levels of 30% to 40% carboxymethemoglobin in the blood, confusion and disorientation develop. If this level of intoxication persists for an hour or longer, sequelae may persist. Older or debilitated persons can die from this level of intoxication. At levels over 40% delirium and coma are common, and permanent sequelae are typical. At levels of 60% or higher almost all survivors will have neurologic deficits. When the ambient concentration of CO is high (1:1000 or more) one can inspire a fatal level of CO very quickly. Even when the victim breathes pure oxygen it may take many hours to restore normal hemoglobin levels. Treatment often involves the use of hyperbaric oxygen in order to "blow-off" CO as rapidly as possible.[47,72,122,207]

Comparatively little change in the brain (cherry red color, congestion, edema) may exist in individuals who die acutely of CO poisoning. When exposure has been severe and the individual survives for some hours or days, the brain may no longer show the "cherry red" color. Edema may or may not be present, but there may be evident discoloration and necrosis of the basal ganglia (caudate, putamen, globus pallidus) (Fig. 11-11) hippocampus, and cerebellar cortex. This "selective" vulnerability parallels that seen in global brain ischemia. In individuals who have had a longer exposure to moderate levels of CO and who have remained unconscious for a long period of time, the brain may show a "late" degeneration of the white matter, which can develop after an apparent recovery. This phenomenon, called "Grinker's myelinopathy," appears to be the result of a delayed effect on white matter veins leading to congestive necrosis that affects the centrum semiovale (Fig. 11-12) and the cerebellar white matter but spares the subcortical "U" fibers.[129,219,286] The mechanisms involved in this curious injury are not fully understood but have been duplicated in the experimental laboratory.[286]

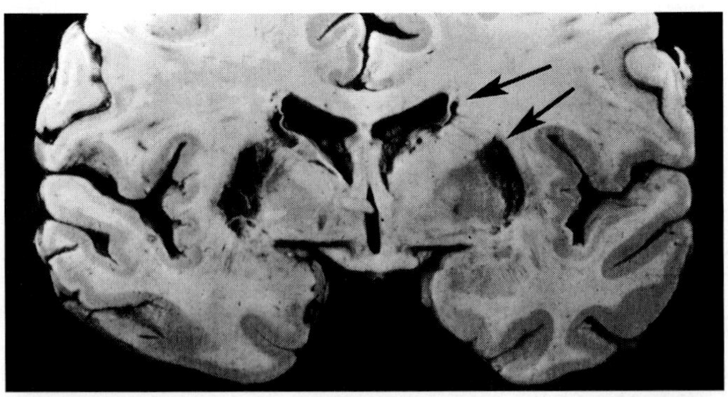

**Fig. 11-11.** This coronal section of the brain illustrates longstanding, cystic necrosis of the corpora striata (caudate-putamen) *(arrows)* in this individual who survived a major exposure to carbon monoxide in a fire. The individual was severely compromised and essentially lived a very limited existence for several years after fire.

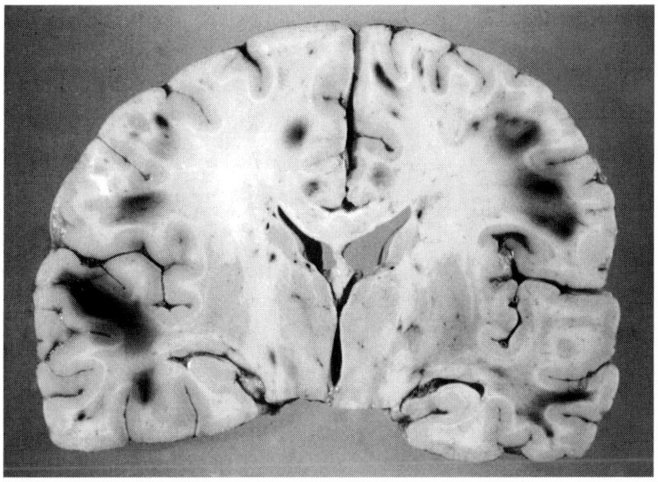

**Fig. 11-12.** This coronal section of the brain illustrates many subcortical hemorrhagic lesions and a generalized pallor, edema of the white matter, and prominence of the subcortical "U" fibers due to acute carbon monoxide intoxication due to a faulty furnace. This individual survived several weeks in hospital without regaining consciousness and then suddenly experienced neurological deterioration and death. This case illustrates the early phase of Grinker's myelinopathy. (Courtesy of the Office of the Medical Examiner, Cook County, Illinois.)

### Forensic Aspects of Hypoxia-Anoxia

Ischemic-hypoxic damage to the brain is so common that virtually every autopsy brain has some degree of damage due to deprivation of circulation and/or oxygenation of the blood, probably as a reflection of the process of dying, during which blood pressure drops or respiration declines inexorably.[108] The chief forensic aspects of these phenomena center about aging and dating of the processes and their etiology in relation to death or debilitating conditions. Ischemia-hypoxemia can occur alone or in combination with some disorder of blood flow or with hypoglycemia. The effects on the brain often are considered identical, but probably are more analogous than identical. In general, hypoxemia alone with adequate circulation is less damaging than is coexistent circulatory failure. This may be due to the relative lack of accumulation of lactic acid and other products of metabolism with an intact circulation. The effects of one without the other may be seen in strangulation, hanging, and asphyxial conditions. Hypoglycemia without hypoxia exists when excessive amounts of insulin are administered, although eventually hypoxia secondary to respiratory failure ensues. The effects on the brain of these conditions follow patterns of "selective vulnerability," extensively described elsewhere.[32,303] The areas most sensitive to ischemic/hypoxic injury are the Sommer's sector of the hippocampus, the cerebellar Purkinje cells, the large neurons of the globus pallidus, caudate nucleus and putamen, the dentate nucleus of the cerebellum, large neurons of the middle laminae of the cerebral cortex, and neurons of the brainstem reticular formation. Less sensitive neuronal populations are those located in the thalamus, brainstem and spinal cord.

The pathologic changes of hypoxia, ischemia, and hypoglycemia are first visible microscopically as eosinophilia and blurring of neuronal profiles. Such "red" neurons are fatally damaged cells that eventually fade away, usually within 2 weeks' time.[54] It is generally believed that about 6 to 12 hours of survival are required for these cells to reach the stage of obvious shrinkage and tinctorial change, but many factors influence the development and course of this important cellular change as well as the interval required for its appearance; many of these factors have forensic importance. Lindenberg[229,230] has suggested that the previous "health" of the individual and the acuteness of the injury may in some way affect the neuronal damage.

Personal observations in experimental and human case material suggest that fewer than 12 hours are needed for the appearance of "red" neurons. The process of eosinophilic cellular injury is not uniform, is gradual in its evolution, and is subject to many variables. In its earliest form, the neuron may swell and appear "cloudy," as described by Cajal.[289] After this, neurons begin to shrink and gradually change their tinctorial characteristics to a purple color and then to progressively more obvious shades of orange to red. In the process the nucleus loses its distinct margins and chromatin pattern and nucleolus until it adopts a dark purple color (pyknosis). The process may take a day or less in the case of Purkinje cells, but as much as 2 weeks in large cortical neurons and brainstem neurons.

Perhaps the most rapid evolution of "red" neurons in response to hypoxia/ischemia can be seen in hippocampal "slice" preparations of rat brain. In these preparations, "red" neurons can be seen in the center of the slice about 30 minutes to an hour after the "injury." In an experimental model of focal brain ischemia in rats significant numbers of "red" neurons are not detectable until 4 to 6 hours after the arterial occlusion.[107]

The time of the hypoxic/ischemic events and the time of the postmortem examination have been well documented in some instances. Such instances involve anesthetic mishaps, instances of severe blood loss with delay in replacement, surgical vascular occlusion, drowning, and asphyxial events. In such cases "red" neurons in the most vulnerable populations (Ammon's horn of the hippocampus; middle laminae of cerebral cortex; and cerebellar Purkinje cells) have been detected as early as 1 to 2 hours after the injury. The following case illustrates some of the issues involved in interpretation of ischemic-hypoxic change.

***Illustrative Case 9:*** *A teenage boy was found dead in bed by his father. The autopsy appeared initially unreveal-*

*ing, and toxicologic examination also was unrevealing. The brain showed moderate edema and "red" neurons in areas known to be vulnerable to hypoxia (Ammon's horn of the hippocampus, Purkinje cells, larger cortical neurons). These findings indicated that an ischemic-hypoxic insult had been followed by a period of several hours during which circulation was preserved. Examination of photographs of the body revealed faint marks around the neck which could have been produced by a padded ligature. Investigators were instructed to reinterview the father, who admitted that he had found his son nude and unconscious, hanging by a rope. It was immediately apparent to the investigators that the young man had been the victim of an autoerotic asphyxial accident.[47] The father had, out of embarrassment, cut his unconscious son down and placed him in bed in the hope that he would revive. The period of time that elapsed between his discovery and his calling the rescue squad was about 3 hours. By that time the victim was dead.*

It appears that a period of hypoxia and a short period of survival in a previously healthy young person can result in "red" neurons sooner than is generally expected. The forensic implications of this case analysis were significant. Cause of death was determined, and the manner of death, which could have been homicide, suicide, natural, or undetermined, was deemed to have been accidental.

When there is prolonged survival after an ischemic-hypoxic event the changes in the brain may be invisible grossly, although when there is diffuse neuronal loss but not cortical necrosis, affected areas such as the brainstem and basal ganglia may feel rubbery after fixation. More commonly when there is severe hypoxia with survival of a few days or more, varying degrees of necrosis can be observed in the cerebral cortex (laminar and pseudolaminar necrosis) and hippocampus, and in the globus pallidus or the corpus striatum (caudate and putamen). After prolonged survival, the cortex and basal ganglia may be shrunken and cavitary. The cerebellum may be shrunken and rubbery. Microscopic examination usually will reveal replacement gliosis, cavitation, occasional microhemorrhages, and often remnants of dead neurons. In these severe cases, global ischemic injury (respirator brain) also may exist, but is a late phenomenon and can be distinguished from prior damage.[216] In the case of typical ischemic infarction, the degradative and reactive processes progress through a number of stages well chronicled by Garcia[109] and Chuaqui, and others.[54]

## NEUROTRAUMA

Traumatic physical injury to the nervous system probably is the most common and important pathologic condition encountered in the forensic autopsy. The spectrum of conditions and their pathogenesis and pathology are broad and complex. Ample opportunities exist for forensic correlations and interpretations. There is also much that is imperfectly understood.

Traumatic injury to the nervous system should be thought of as a dynamic process.[1–4] Immediately after trauma, the injured parts of the brain, spinal cord, and nerve (unless physically disrupted) rarely show any sign of injury either grossly or by ordinary light microscopy. Following trauma to the head there may be total loss of neurologic function due to "neural shock," which has no morphologic representation and probably involves disruption of membrane ionic channels, especially fluxes of calcium.[20,133] Ultrastructurally and biochemically there may be very early abnormalities, including breakage of neuronal microtubules and other cytoskeletal structures, calcium activation of neutral proteases, and alterations in mitochondrial function and neuroplasmic function.[20,21,185] Neural capillaries are frequently injured, but do not show this injury immediately. It may be 30 minutes or more before the earliest gross or microscopic abnormalities are evident. Edema and slight congestion would be observed first. Later the "vascular" phase of the injury becomes evident: increased congestion, microcirculatory failure, early hemorrhage, and increased edema. The area of injury expands progressively over the next 24 or more hours, at which time the lesion is mostly hemorrhagic, highly congested, and softened. This process continues until the necrosis with progressive softening appears. This coagulative-liquefactive effect peaks about 7 to 10 days after the injury. Macrophages and capillary proliferative reaction are much in evidence, and the eventual process of clearing the dead material is well under way. At 10 to 14 days glial reactions are in evidence and continue for months or years as the inflammatory phase subsides.[20,21,128]

Each phase of physical injury has elements that are self-limited and at least potentially reversible and other elements that are not. Furthermore, each phase carries with it real or potential sources of further injury separate from the original injury. Such secondary events include edema and other vascular-mediated phenomena, and release of such cellular products as neurotransmitter substances, cytokines, vasoactive and inflammatory mediators, calcium, potassium, and other electrolytes. Systemic factors also can affect local cellular and tissue repair reactions. These include hypoxia, acidosis, ischemia, toxic states, fever, development of hydrocephalus, infection, multiple organ failure, blood loss, and interactive effects of drugs and therapeutic agents. This "cascade" of the neurotraumatic lesion has been illustrated by Grcevic and others.[21,126,127,347] The practical significance of these phenomena in a forensic sense is that it is possible, within variable limits of confidence, to age and date traumatic lesions and place them within a causal context to external events.

### Cranial Trauma in the Adult

The effects of trauma to the head in the adult usually are quite different from those seen in an infant or

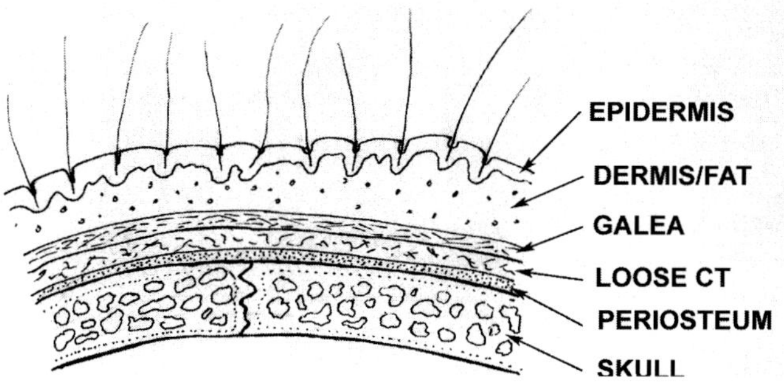


**Fig. 11-13.** This illustration depicts the structure of the scalp. When the scalp is reflected at autopsy, especially in adults, all layers are usually automatically separated from the skull. However, in infants, only the upper three layers come away. Evidence of impacts (hemorrhages) will be seen at least in the inner portion of the scalp, which has peeled away, and may also be seen in any portions of the subgaleal connective tissues that remain adherent to the skull.

young child, and thus will be discussed separately here. Biomechanically and anatomically the adult brain is protected by a thick, five-layered scalp,[362] ossified and fused cranial bones, and an elastic and tough meningeal covering. Moreover, the brain is suspended in a layer of cerebrospinal fluid.

**The scalp and its injuries.** The scalp thickness is greatest near the occiput, where it may measure 1 cm or more. It is thickest in males and thinnest in females, especially aged ones (Fig. 11-13). Impacts to the head are cushioned by the scalp, and in one series of experiments it took 1/10th the force to fracture the skull with the scalp removed as when it was covered.[131] Thus the scalp provides a significant absorber of kinetic energy that otherwise would be transmitted to affect deeper structures. The scalp is quite elastic and can deform or elongate more than one half its length. Impacts to the scalp may or may not be visible externally, although if enough vessels are broken a "goose egg" may appear in minutes, which will turn blue if the bleeding is superficial. If the hemorrhages are deeper, discoloration may only appear as any accumulated blood diffuses along fascial planes and is broken down. Only general measures of age can be inferred from the change in color of a bruise from blue to purple, to red, to orange to yellow.[47,122,267] Inferences about the extent and duration of sub-scalp hemorrhages are notoriously unreliable.[205] In many instances impressive subgaleal bleeding may not be visible from a surface view.

If an impacting surface or object has a pattern on its surface or a characteristic edge, these may imprint the scalp and leave a so-called "pattern injury," which may give a clue about the type of object or surface that caused the injury and may correlate with a weapon or object found at the scene.[47,122,317] The existence of "pattern" injuries has been known to forensic scientists for at least a century and forms an important chain of evidence that can play a major role in the prosecution and defense of criminal and other cases.

Typical examples of "pattern" injuries are crescent shaped marks caused by blows with a hammer; double inverted "Y" shaped lacerations caused by blows with heavy cylindrical objects; a circular bruise with or without a central stellate laceration caused by impact with an unyielding flat surface by the rounded cranium; grip mark and finger nail imprints caused by violent gripping of an extremity or the neck by an assailant; imprints of surface structures of an object in the skin, such as a file or crosshatched gun butt and a braided leather whip; imprint of the muzzle of a pistol held in contact with the skin at the time of discharge; imprints on the skin of the wadding carried with pellets in shotgun wounds; bite marks and tooth imprints on the skin. Many additional examples are amply illustrated in forensic pathology texts.*

Surface inspection at autopsy is not sufficient to discover subgaleal injuries; thus the scalp must be peeled back from the cranium during autopsy. This will reveal impact sites and give a truer measure of severity and age of the impact than can be appreciated externally. These subgaleal hemorrhages must be documented by drawing, verbal description, and photographs. Correlation with deeper injuries and external evidence may spell the difference between a correct or incorrect analysis of a case. After several days, subgaleal hemorrhages (bruises) display the same change of color as the more superficial bruises, and may remain evident grossly and microscopically for months as a yellow/orange or brown local stain.

**The skull and its injuries.** The skull becomes ossified and its sutures completely fused at about the age of 5 or 6 years. For all purposes it becomes biomechanically an adult skull by this time or before.[131,324] The bones of the skull are diploic with a marrow cavity in the middle; the outer layer of bone is about twice as thick as the inner layer. The skull bone is thickest at the occiput and frontal pole and thinnest in the temporal region. Black males tend to have thicker skulls than do caucasians. Women, Asians, and children tend to have the thinnest skulls. The skull appears rigid but is quite flexible and elastic, and as a result it deforms considerably on impact. The ability of the skull to deform and to "spring back" absorbs considerable force of impact, but injury to the underlying brain can be induced by propagating undissipated force waves into the brain tissue. The skull fractures after its elastic-deformational limit has been exceeded. Skull fractures are clas-

* Refs. 47, 55, 70, 87, 88, 317, 324.

sified in many ways but essentially fall into one of the following groups as outlined by Gurdjian.[131] (1) Linear fracture of calvaria or base. (2) Basilar fracture. (3) Depressed fracture. (4) Comminuted fracture of calvaria or base. (5) Diastatic fracture. (6) Expressed fracture. (7) Stellate fracture. (8) Multiple fractures. (9) Combinations of these.

Linear fractures, as their name implies, are single and straight. They usually are located in the parietal region over the convexity of the skull or through the base of the skull.[85,149] Linear fractures account for 70% or more of skull fractures. The fracture line emanates from the point of impact and extends in the direction of the impact toward weaker bony areas. The extent of the fracture is highly variable and is related to the forces involved in the impact. The fracture may involve only one level of the skull or both; it may course for a few or many centimeters, and occasionally the fractures branch. Fractures of the linear type are most commonly associated with falls or accidents; fractures that are simple and narrow (less than 2 mm) portend less serious injuries than those that are complex and wide. Fractures may be seen in imaging studies but are regularly missed clinically and radiographically. It is essential that the skull be percussed at autopsy to determine if there is a "cracked pot" sound, and to strip the dura from the vertex as well as the base to demonstrate fracture lines in suspicious cases. Basilar fractures may pass through sinuses or the petrous bone, may lead to CSF rhinorrhea or otorrhea, and may be the route of entry of infection. In infants and children, when obvious accidental trauma has been eliminated, anything but a simple, narrow, linear, parietal skull fracture is deemed child abuse until proved otherwise.[146,250]

Basilar skull fractures can be simple, narrow, and linear and can result from frontal or lateral blows. When more complex and wider-spaced they usually are caused by occipital impact. A particularly helpful sign, visible at the autopsy table in a basilar skull fracture is the Battle's sign.[244] This clinical sign is bilateral mastoid or ear hematomas in the absence of obvious impacts to these structures. The cause of Battle's sign is a fracture hemorrhage with dissection in fascial planes about the mastoid and ear. It should be obvious that proper examination of basilar fractures requires that the basal dura be stripped. As with any fracture, a diagram or photograph to preserve evidence is required. Basilar skull fractures classically produce fracture contusions in the overlying brain, sometimes coinciding quite precisely with the fracture line. With occipital impacts and basilar skull fractures a backward or occipital fall is most common, but forceful blows with very heavy objects such as baseball bats or "2 × 4s" also can produce these injuries. CSF leaks and meningitis are typical complications of basilar skull fractures.[219,244]

Depressed fractures may be caused by blows (typically with hammers and other heavy objects) or falls (swimming pool impacts). Because of the nature of these fractures and the common accompaniment of subdural and epidural hematomas, they may be life-threatening unless treated promptly. A special case of a depressed skull fracture is the "stellate" fracture, which usually is caused by a heavy impact on a pointed object or by an edged or small-surfaced object such as a hammer, pick, or the edge of a brick. The impact point is the nexus of the stellate fracture. Comminuted and multiple fractures usually result from massive impacts (blows or falls) where the skull is fragmented and probably driven into the brain or pushed under an adjacent rim of bone. Often these fractures occur with open brain injuries, as seen with multiple hammer blows, in explosions, and in high velocity missile and gunshot wounds. Their seriousness is in keeping with the violent forces involved. Expressed fractures occur when a portion of the fractured bone is elevated away from the normal curvature of the skull, usually by bullets or missiles.

Diastatic fractures develop when fracture lines follow the skull sutures and separation of the bony plates of the skull occurs (Fig. 11-14) Great force is required to produce such a fracture, even though at times it may be alleged that such fractures in an adult may be secondary to brain swelling. Massive violent blows or instances in which an individual is thrown from a vehicle and strikes the pavement are typical circumstances.

**The dura and its injuries.** The dura mater is the periosteum of the inner surface of the skull and exists as a single, though layered, membranous structure that in the intact meninges blends imperceptibly with the arachnoidal membrane, forming the "roof" of the sub-

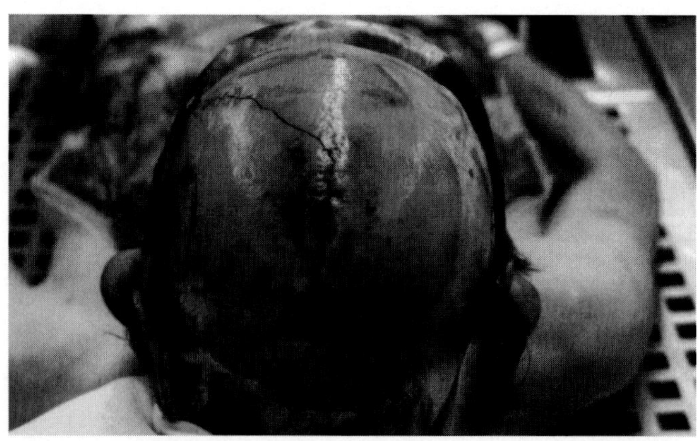

**Fig. 11-14.** Extensive, complex-diastatic skull fracture in an individual who was struck with a heavy object near the top of the head. The fracture was associated with a sizeable acute subdural hematoma (not shown), which was the cause of death.

arachnoid space. These "two" membranes are easily separated by physical forces.[301,302] The dura is a double-layered dense fibrous connective tissue membrane that has a parchment-like character and appearance. It encloses the brain and spinal cord and encloses venous sinuses and invests the spinal nerve roots. Specializations of the dura-arachnoid, the arachnoidal villi (granulations) and dural sheaths, act as the reabsorbing surface for CSF. Traumatic injury may manifest itself by epidural hemorrhage, subdural hemorrhage, subarachnoid hemorrhage, or combinations of these.

Epidural hemorrhage is almost always due to trauma and is almost always an acute process. However, instances of delayed hemorrhage can occur.[219] Bleeding usually is secondary to laceration or injury of branches of the middle meningeal artery in connection with a skull fracture in the frontotemporal region, but can occur elsewhere when the skull is indented or deformed, but not fractured, especially in a young child. In this instance a branch or region of the middle meningeal artery may be avulsed and bleed. Occasionally epidural hemorrhages follow lacerating injuries of a venous sinus or emissary vein and may accumulate in the posterior fossa, where they are especially dangerous.[254] Accumulation of blood may be slower and the course less acute with venous bleeding than when an artery is torn. Epidural hematomas are usually one-sided on the lateral portion of the head, and on the same side as a fracture, but contrecoup examples have been reported. Epidural hematomas may occur in the posterior fossa or spinal canal, but in these locations may have presentations different from the classic supratentorial epidural hemorrhage.[53,246]

The basic consequence of epidural hemorrhage is a rapidly expanding volume within the intracranial compartment that cannot be compensated by pressure absorption of CSF. Following trauma and unconsciousness the victim may awaken but later become unconscious again ("lucid" interval).[57,295] This interval is highly variable, but the shorter the interval the more ominous the situation, because it is an indicator of the rapidity of hematoma accumulation and the need for prompt surgical evacuation. Delays in recognition of an acute epidural or acute subdural hematoma and delays in their treatment are the most important and preventable factor in death of head trauma victims who are able to talk during their lucid interval. These issues, of course, have forensic import. The general mortality of acute epidural hemorrhages is age-related: about 11% less than age 20, 18% to 40% in the 20 to 40 year group, and 25% to 29% in the over 40 year age group. The gross appearance of an epidural hemorrhage is usually that of a fresh (liquid or clotted) hematoma, usually with a skull fracture, which pushes the dura inward and indents the brain. The volume of such hematomas often exceeds 100 ml and results in severe brain distortion and herniation. Duret hemorrhages are common. The increase in intracranial pressure may lead to global ischemia (respirator brain). Organization or expansion of epidural hemorrhages, other than those occurring after surgery, are uncommon.[251]

Subdural hematomas are more common than epidural hemorrhages and have much greater pathologic and forensic importance, largely because they can be subtle, chronic, unappreciated, missed entirely, and may cause death. Subdural hemorrhages can be traumatic or nontraumatic, acute, subacute, or chronic. Subdural hematomas have certain important age relationships. When they occur at a young age they are most likely caused by significant trauma; in older age groups they may occur in the absence of significant trauma.[152] The basic condition is an accumulation of blood at the interface between arachnoid and dura, usually of venous origin. Cortical veins as they drain the surface of the brain must cross the subarachnoid space to enter the dural sinuses. When the brain is subjected to "high strain" acceleration or deceleration, these "bridging" veins may be torn or broken, sometimes taking with them a small cuff of arachnoid membrane, thus allowing venous blood and CSF to mix, sometimes producing a small amount of subarachnoid hemorrhage as well. The biomechanics of traumatic acute subdural hematomas have been carefully studied, and many important parameters of injury have been defined.[113] Once a bridging vein has been broken, blood can accumulate rapidly, apace with that seen in epidural hematomas, especially if a small accompanying cortical artery is injured as well. Subdural hemorrhages also can accumulate in an incremental and slow fashion, showing almost no symptoms until compensation is no longer effective. Subdural hematomas usually are unilateral and are found in at least 30% of serious head injuries.[92,113,363]

Following trauma, there may or may not be a loss of consciousness, or a skull fracture along with the subdural hemorrhage. There is often a "lucid" interval that may last several hours or longer before a sufficient volume of blood accumulates (additive to any volumetric brain swelling effect) to exceed the compensating pressure-mediated exit of CSF. When the compensatory equilibrium is insufficient to accommodate the increasing mass of the hematoma and its associated edema if the brain is injured, intracranial pressure rises and neurologic symptoms including coma develop. Mortality rates for acute subdural hematomas are on a par with epidural hematomas.[319] Fifty percent of subdural hematomas are discovered and removed surgically within 24 hours of occurrence, and another 20% are operated upon within 48 hours of occurrence. The remaining 30% are either self-limited or undiscovered initially but are discovered later as a subacute or chronic subdural hematoma. Not all subdural hematomas, even when discovered, are operated upon, but all, once discovered, should be monitored for changes that might indicate a need for surgical intervention. All forms of subdural hematoma cause potentially preventable deaths and significant morbidity.[295]

Acute subdural hematomas usually are laterally placed, but blood can accumulate interhemispherically along the falx, at the base of the skull, in the posterior fossa, diffusely, or along the spinal canal (comparatively rare). Grossly the acute subdural clot (Fig. 11-15) may be jelly-like or liquified and usually is dark red or almost black. Within a few days, the color turns brownish, and layering or margination of some of the components of the hematoma will be evident. It may be difficult on the basis of an evacuated specimen to determine whether the hematoma represents an acute hemorrhage into a more chronic hematoma or an acute hematoma.[219]

Most acute hematomas contain preserved red blood cells and no organizing membrane formation. After 2 to 3 days many red blood cells progressively lose their tinctorial characteristics and begin to lose their sharp, rounded features (laking). As they do this it is possible to detect products of hemoglobin digestion (hemosiderin) with Prussian blue iron stains, perhaps as early as 3 or 4 days after the injury. With time the quantity and ease of detection of hemosiderin increase, then, over many weeks or months, it is removed. Some residual hemosiderin may remain for years following injury.

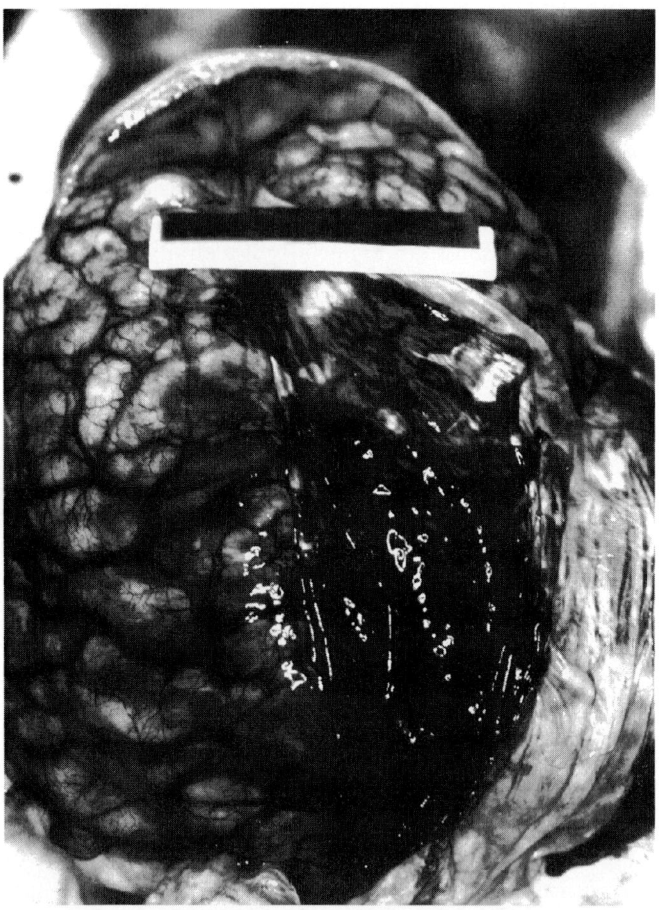

Fig. 11-15. Typical appearance of an acute subdural hematoma that happens to be in a fatally abused and apparently shaken infant. Smaller focal collections of blood near the midline represent collections of blood from traumatized bridging veins.

Precise definition of an acute subdural hematoma becomes less and less possible with each day that elapses; about 7 to 10 days after inception, the hematoma should be considered a subacute subdural hemorrhage, which has its own characteristics and importance.[257,258]

Acute subdural hematomas cause death and morbidity in the same manner as do acute epidural hemorrhages—by their expanding volumetric effects, which exceed the ability of the brain to accommodate, and by causing herniations. Since these lesions evolve at varying speeds, CT imaging methods may fail to detect a very acute process when it is minimal; unless the image is taken at a time when the hematoma has evolved, CT may give the false impression of normal. The "missed" subdural hemorrhage is a common feature of forensic cases.

Subacute subdural hematomas are those that have had the time to begin the processes unique to hemorrhages in the subdural space, evolution and chronicity.[45] (Fig. 11-16). Blood in the subdural compartment incites a cellular proliferative response in the former dura-arachnoid "border zone" on the arachnoidal side of the clot. These fibroblastic cells proliferate rapidly and carry with them fine capillaries that spread gradu-

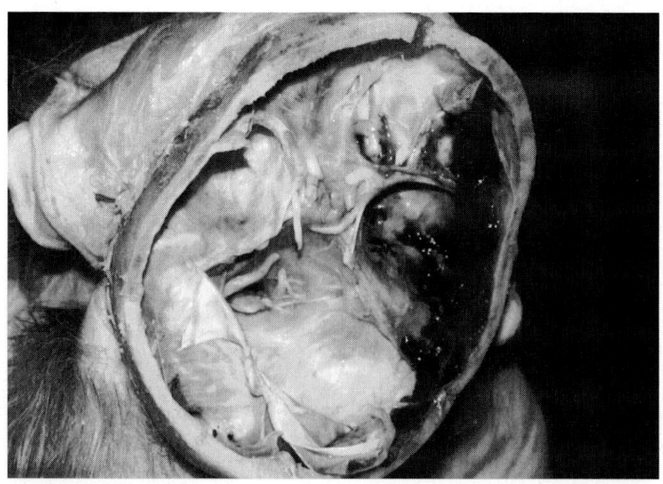

Fig. 11-16. A subacute-chronic subdural hematoma on the right side of the skull in an elderly victim of a beating that occurred during a home invasion. The hematoma has a membrane and the colors of the hematoma (though not well-illustrated here) show a spectrum of black-red to yellow-orange.

ally around the edges of the clot and totally invest it with a cellular and then a collagenous membrane. The accumulation of this membrane and other cellular reactive changes makes possible the aging and dating of subdural hemorrhages. Unfortunately no modern study exists that takes into account variations due to individual age, interventional therapy, and other factors in the time-development of the chronic subdural hematoma. The only studies to have approached this, upon which most forensic pathologists have to rely, are those of Merritt and Munro dating from the 1930.[257,258] These are summarized in Table 11-1.[219]

When a subdural blood clot becomes totally invested with a fibrovascular membrane it becomes a chronic subdural hematoma. This lesion is capable of expanding its volume, thus producing symptoms and consequences that can prove fatal and that can have forensic importance. Volumetric expansion of the hematoma occurs through the ruptures of capillaries in the investing membrane by repeated trauma, by influence of medication (anticoagulation), disorders of blood coagulation, or seemingly in the absence of a precipitating cause. During membrane investment there may be few if any symptoms, but suddenly these may become more serious and even life-threatening. Symptoms are determined by the volumetric increase in the hematoma, which in combination with other volume expanding processes (cerebral edema or intracerebral hemorrhage) exceeds the ability of compensatory mechanisms to maintain volume-pressure relationships inside the skull. Herniation then occurs. The following case illustrates this phenomenon.

***Illustrative Case 10:*** *A 35-year-old laborer fell backward, striking his head. He was briefly unconscious and suffered from a headache, neck pain, and symptoms of a mild concussion for some days afterward. Medical examination was within normal limits. Over the next 2 weeks the man complained of increasing headaches, which became refractory to pain medication. He sought the advice of a physician who ordered no laboratory or imaging tests and told him to return the following week. On the way back to his home the man experienced nausea and vomiting and became stuporous, complaining bitterly of agonizing headache. Upon re-*

**Table 11-1.** Aging and Dating of Subdural Hematomas

| Interval | Clot | Dural side | Arachnoid side |
|---|---|---|---|
| 24 hr | Intact RBCs | Thin layer fibrin | Thin layer fibrin |
| 36 hr | Intact RBCs | Early fibroblastic activity | Thin layer fibrin |
| 4 days | Loss of RBC sharp contour and variability of staining | 2–4 layers of fibroblasts | Thin layer fibrin |
| 5 days | Loss of RBC sharp contour and variability of staining | 3–5 layers of fibroblasts. First siderophages appear at edges of the clot | Thin layer fibrin |
| 7–8 days | Laked RBCs, clot liquefies, fibroblasts enter clot | 12–14 layers of fibroblasts; neomembrane visible grossly when clot scraped away | Thin layer fibrin |
| 11 days | Broken up into islands by capillaries and fibroblasts and thick strands of fibrin | Fibroblasts migrate around the edges of the clot | Siderophages are visible on arachnoid side |
| 15–17 days | Most original RBCs lysed. Capillary formation obvious | Membrane $\frac{1}{2}$ to $\frac{1}{3}$ dural thickness | Variably thin, earliest complete neomembrane. Clot may be completely enveloped |
| 18–26 days | Clot completely liquefied. Larger vessels permeate clot. | Membrane same thickness as dura. Siderophages in membranes | Membrane up to $\frac{1}{2}$ dural thickness. Siderophages in membranes |
| 27–36 days | Large capillaries | Well-formed membrane | Well-formed membrane |
| 1–3 months | Giant capillaries, secondary bleeding and fresh RBCs | Hyalinization of membranes less cellular, more collagen | Hyalinization of membranes, less cellular, more collagen. Nearly thickness of dura. |
| 3–6 months | No original RBCs and only focal rebleeding | Hyalinized neomembrane | Hyalinized neomembrane |
| >1 year | No RBCs | Resembles dura | Resembles dura |

(The data in this table were excerpted from the seminal papers by Munro and Merritt[257,258] and appeared originally in Forensic Neuropathology, Raven Press, 1988.[219] Used with permission.)

*turn to the physician's office he was referred to a nearby hospital, but it was several hours before the on-call physician came to the hospital, at which time the man was comatose and hemiplegic. An emergency craniotomy revealed a large subdural hemorrhage which was removed. The man, however, remained hemiplegic, aphasic, and severely compromised neurologically, requiring chronic nursing home care with little hope for recovery. Pathologic examination of the evacuated clot revealed a subacute subdural hemorrhage with portions showing membranous organization and others showing acute bleeding.*

Chronic subdural hematomas are hemorrhages that become enclosed by an organizing membrane over a period of about 14 days. Chronic hematomas in the young usually are traumatic in origin, but may develop in the elderly without any obvious traumatic event; these hemorrhages can occur in conjunction with dialysis and dehydration.[16,192,363] This may be due to the fact that bridging veins in the elderly are longer and possibly more stretched because of cerebral atrophy and are thus more vulnerable to tearing especially when the brain suddenly shrinks during dialysis or in any relatively sudden fluid shift. Nontraumatic events such as meningitis in infants can split the dura-arachnoid and lead to a subdural fluid collection that is in many ways indistinguishable from a chronic subdural hematoma. This is referred to as subdural hygroma.[119,159] The investing membrane of the chronic hematoma or hygroma allows the enclosed blood to liquify and for the hematoma to enlarge, often to many times its original size. This tendency for progressive enlargement is characteristic of this lesion. Compared with subacute subdural hemorrhage, the chronic subdural hemorrhage may be silent until its volume either suddenly changes or a critical juncture in volume compensation by the brain is reached (Fig. 11-17) Most chronic subdural hemorrhages become symptomatic within 3 months of their inception. The aging and evolution of the organization process is tabulated in Table 11-1. Like the subacute subdural hemorrhage, the chronic lesion also shows a tendency to bleed spontaneously and may enlarge suddenly after a period of relative quiescence: Presumably, the enlargement is secondary to liquefaction of blood and the creation of a hyperosmolar state inside the hematoma that draws water across its semipermeable membrane thus expanding itself. This expansion may tear the delicate capillaries in the wall.[119,192] However, this theory has been discredited because hyperosmolality of the hematoma fluid.[123,354,355] A more acceptable theory is that the volume of a subdural hemorrhage increases because of spontaneous rupture of capillaries in the neomembrane[354,355] and because fibrinolytic and anticoagulant substances are present in the liquified clot fluid. It is curious that this process appears to occur nowhere else in the body. Numerous theories have attempted to explain this phenomenon.[164,351] The gross appearances of the chronic subdural hemorrhage depend on the thickness of its investing membrane which can range from that of a few cell layers of fibroblasts to a very thick leathery membrane, thicker than the normal dura.

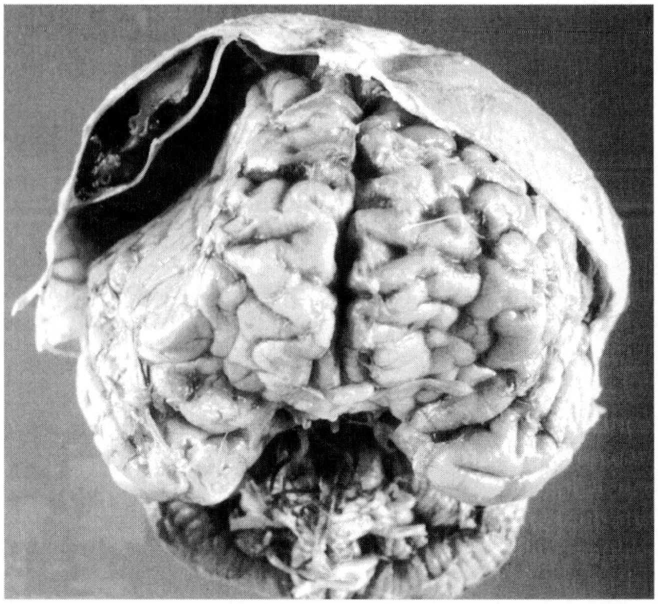

**Fig. 11-17.** A chronic subdural hematoma with a very thick wall (equal in thickness to the dura) probably of months' duration. The hematoma indents the brain and contains recent clotted blood in the cavity, which does not necessarily imply repeated trauma. Rather, the natural evolution of such lesions is characterized by repeated hemorrhages. The indentation of the brain, even if the hematoma were to be removed, might not fully expand to a normal cortical shape.

***Illustrative Case 11:*** *An active and healthy elderly man fell on an icy sidewalk and struck his head. He experienced no unconsciousness and other than disorientation for a brief period showed no ill effects from his fall. A visit to his physician revealed nothing of note. Over the next 3 months he began to show signs of forgetfulness and aged visibly. A neurologist found him to be demented, ataxic, and incontinent of urine. A CT scan revealed a large membranous subdural hematoma, which upon surgical removal measured in excess of 125 ml. Following surgery the man regained his mental capacities and became the active, healthy man he had been before his fall.*

Sometimes in connection with removal or drainage of a large chronic subdural hematoma, following decompression, secondary hemorrhage may occur in the brain beneath the former site of the hematoma.

**Cerebral injury.** Traumatic injury to the head can be associated with injuries to the scalp, skull, meninges, spine, and spinal cord as well as with skeletal and visceral trauma. Brain injury is rarely simple and focal. Brain trauma can be thought of as a "virus" that affects the brain.[126,127] Trauma can produce obvious focal and recognizable lesions that give the impression of only a local injury, but actually injuries are more disseminated or diffuse. Studies indicate that there is probably *no* insignificant brain injury. Whenever anyone receives an impact to the head, by fall or blow, brain tissue is damaged and this damage is detectable by cognitional neuropsychologic testing, often many months after injury.[11,79,122] Furthermore, when trauma occurs again, before full recovery, the effect may be more than additive. The implications of this information on professional boxing have led to increasing pressure to abandon this activity as a legitimate sport.[59,61]

Many theories seek to explain observed phenomena that only recently have begun to yield to experimental studies. The following represents a greatly simplified review of mechanisms involved in the production of the major types of brain injuries and their functional and forensic pathologic significance.

The most typical brain injury following an impact is the cerebral contusion (bruise). Contusions may occur on the surface of the brain beneath the site of impact (so-called "coup" lesion) characteristic of an inflicted blow, at a location at or near the surface of the brain 180° away on a straight line opposite the site of impact (so-called "contrecoup" lesion) characteristic of a fall impact, or between the site of impact and the opposite surface in such brain structures as the white matter, corpus callosum periventricular region, and the upper brainstem (so-called "intermediary coup,"[225,228,231] inner cerebral trauma,[126,127,219] diffuse axonal injury).[2,3] Another form of contusion is the so-called "gliding" contusion or "fracture" contusion.[225,226] The former is found on the inferior surface of the brain in the orbital lobes and in the inferior temporal lobes where there are bony ridges. Fracture contusions are found over regions where the skull has been fractured. Still another form of brain contusion is that seen in young infants, the contusional tear that occurs in the subcortical white matter.[226a]

The *contusion* is a microvascular hemorrhagic lesion in which varying amounts of damage to neural structures occur and become necrotic with time.[3,269] This is especially true of surface contusions (coup, contrecoup, gliding and fracture contusions). All surface contusions are relatively superficial, involving mostly the cerebral cortex. When fresh, contusions have a hemorrhagic, often shaggy appearance. Old contusions show a focal or serpentine course, usually following the crowns of the gyri and sparing the sulci. Contusive lesions usually are brown, orange, or yellow and have a sunken appearance (so-called plaques jeaune or état vermoulou), and their age can be estimated both grossly and microscopically.[269] Contusions do not conform to a vascular territorial and thus can be differentiated from infarcts. The mechanisms involved in the production of contusions remain controversial, even after more than 200 years of scientific argument and experiment.* Various forms of contusions may occur under differing circumstances and have differing mechanisms.

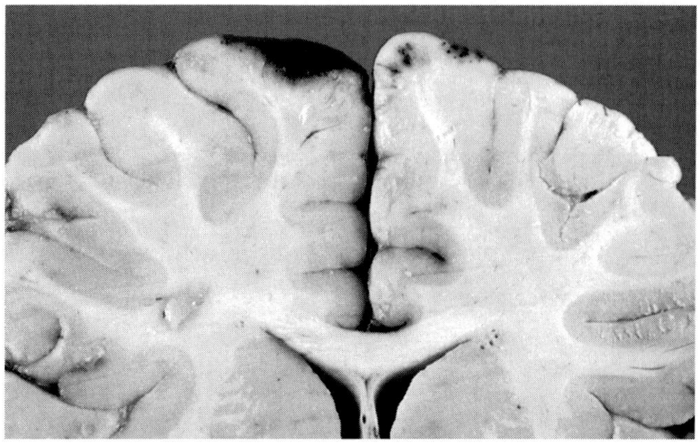

**Fig. 11-18.** This coronal section of the brain illustrates a typical "coup" contusion at the vertex of the brain caused by a blow. On the left, the lesion is cone shaped and hemorrhagic and on the right, away somewhat from the force of the blow, the lesion is less well-formed. Most contusions, coup or contrecoup, are superficial even though they do not appear so externally.

***Coup contusions*** Brain contusions that follow simple blows to the head (so-called "coup" contusions), occur beneath the site of impact (Fig. 11-18) except when the impacting object has nearly the same or greater mass than the head. In the latter circumstance, the blows may produce contrecoup contusions (fall-like blows) alone or in combination with coup contusions. Based on clinical observations and experimental studies,[131,219,225,271,288] coup contusions are known to be more common when a blow fractures the skull than when it does not. In-bending and subsequent out-bending (and perhaps oscillation) of the skull certainly alter the underlying ambient tissue pressures. These pressures also result in shear forces transmitted to the underlying brain that dampen out with increasing distance from the axis of the impact and with increasing depth in the brain. Greater shear forces involve the subjacent brain when the skull fractures (especially if the fracture is depressed) than when the skull is not fractured. Shear forces may be intense in other portions of the brain, however. The coup contusion is probably a product of both sudden pressure phenomena and shear forces, and also of the oscillating character of both.[147,148,344]

In the case of pressure phenomena, with in-bending of the skull the local pressure increases suddenly, but upon release and out-bending (present even when the skull fractures), the pressure becomes negative with respect to the static condition and may fall to only a

* Refs. 121, 147, 148, 225, 334, 335, 344.

few psi, a level that may be below the vapor pressure of water as well as dissolved gases in blood and tissues at 37° C, thus causing an evanescent cavitation or gas bubble to form in either the tissues or in small blood vessels in the region. This sudden volumetric change will stretch or break endothelial cells and capillaries, and probably will damage the blood-brain barrier (astrocytic foot processes and other components).[131,282,283,288] If fragments of fractured bone are driven into the brain, shear forces may cause a tear in the brain, with attendant capillary and neuropil disruption (so-called fracture contusion). Initially, the contusion may be invisible even microscopically, but it expands and becomes more obviously a bruise and then a hemorrhage after several hours. This phenomenon has considerable forensic importance in attempts to determine the time of injury in relation to circumstances and other evidence.[269]

***Contrecoup contusions.*** In the case of contusions that develop after fall-type injuries to the head, the accelerating head impacts a floor or other similar large mass. In this circumstance, with or without skull fracture, contusions usually are seen at a location opposite the impact site, on the surface of the brain (the contrecoup phenomenon) (Fig. 11-19). Other lesions, visible or not, almost always occur in deeper structures, also opposite the impact site and perhaps in between.[282] This seeming enigma has baffled scientists and physicians for more than two centuries. As with the case of coup contusions, many clinical observations, experiments, and model studies have been employed to understand the phenomenon.[67,147,148,225,271] Probably most theories for contrecoup contusions capture some element of the truth, as pointed out by Holbourn,[147,148] Ommaya,[271] Dawson and others.[67,225,334] Many of the same theories that attempt to explain the pathogenesis of coup contusions can apply to contrecoup contusions.

When the head accelerates toward the impact surface (the floor in the case of fall from the standing position), the fall is most likely to occur backward owing to the relative inability of man to compensate correctly and automatically from such a vulnerable position. By the time the occiput strikes the floor, the brain has accelerated only slightly behind the skull, perhaps allowing time for a greater cushion of CSF to form on the most dependent part of the head and a lesser cushion to exist at the most distant part of the head. In any case, at impact, the skull will in-bend against a downward moving brain, producing a relatively sudden high pressure at the impact site. Opposite this location, 180° away, the brain is moving away from the overlying skull toward the floor, while the overlying skull, once impact has occurred, may also be rebounding away from the brain, relatively speaking. At the brain-inner skull interface, the pressure will be much lower than normal, and, as in the previously discussed mechanism

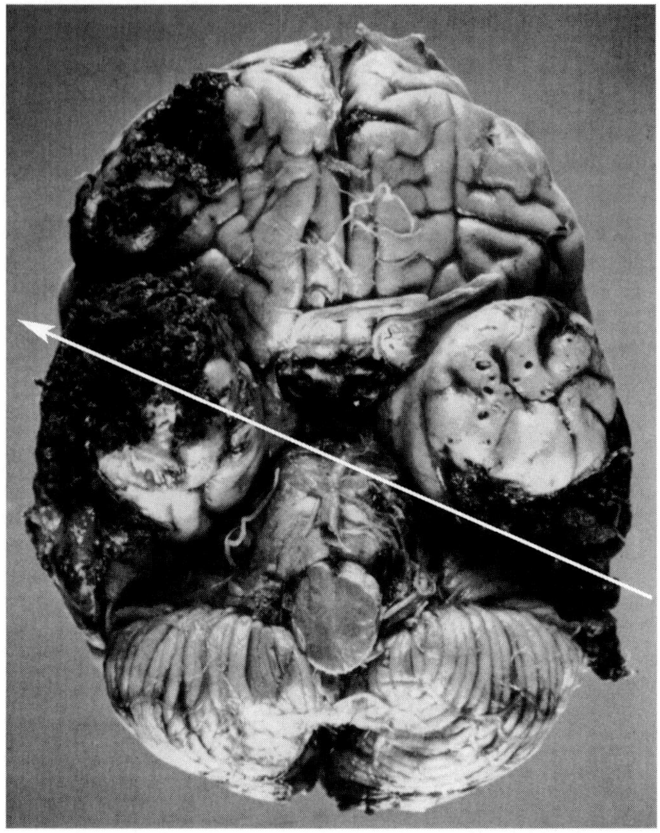

**Fig. 11-19.** This basal view of the brain illustrates the contrecoup phenomenon. This individual sustained a fall, striking the left posterior temporal-parietal region and causing an extensive basilar skull fracture. The direction of forces is illustrated by the white arrow. Almost exactly opposite in the brain is a wide area of contusions which represent contrecoup contusions. Also present are probably some "gliding" contusions of the under surface of the frontal and temporal lobes. Additionally there is a contusion near the side of impact which is a "fracture" contusion caused by the ragged edges of the petrous bone broken during the impact.

of coup contusion, may be lower than the vapor pressure of blood, tissue water, and dissolved gases, thus allowing a cavitation gas bubble to form in capillaries and possibly in the neuropil. This sudden volumetric expansion injures capillaries and surrounding tissues and leads to focal hemorrhage and eventual edema and necrosis. At the site of impact, the negative pressure rebound wave may be dampened and may not be sufficient to permit cavitation and injuries due to this process.[131] In support of this theory are the experiments in which animals whose calvaria were replaced with transparent plastic skull caps were filmed during impacts. At the sites opposite major impacts, momentary cavitations were demonstrated.[288] Other experiments have demonstrated the pressure phenomena described above.[131]

In forward falls, contrecoup brain injuries are relatively uncommon, because the individual can raise the arms to cushion impact and because of the impact-absorbing anterior facial structures, which dissipate the kinetic energy of the fall. When falls are lateral, contrecoup contusions are regularly observed over the opposite hemisphere. In instances where the vertex of the head is the primary impact site, contrecoup contusions can be observed at the base of the brain.

***Combination coup/contrecoup contusions.*** There are circumstances in which blows by heavy objects such as a baseball bat, brick, or heavy club, duplicate the forces and accelerations experienced in falls, producing patterns of brain injury like those seen in fall (contrecoup contusions), like a blow (coup contusions), or some of both.[225, 229] Differentiation in a forensic situation between a blow and a fall usually involves analysis and interpretation of all available information: witness accounts; circumstantial information and evidence; physical evidence; general autopsy and clinical information; sites of external trauma and impacts; sites of subgaleal hemorrhages; locations and course of skull fractures; patterns of injury on the surface of the brain.

***Illustrative Case 12:*** *A woman was found dead in the remains of a building where an explosion and fire had occurred. Gas fittings in the basement of the building had been removed, and the remains of a pipe bomb and a timer were found near the body. It was noted at autopsy that one of the victim's arms had been avulsed, and there were no other fatal injuries in the noncranial structures. In spite of the fire, there was no carbon monoxide in the blood of the victim and no evidence of soot in the respiratory tract. Furthermore, extensive injuries to the face appeared to be unrelated to the bomb blast and showed evidence of bleeding into tissues as well as prominent "black" eyes. There was a depressed skull fracture on the top of the head and an irregular laceration of the overlying scalp, well away from the damages inflicted by the bomb. There was a small subdural hematoma and probable coup or fracture contusions below the fracture. Contusions at the base of the temporal and frontal lobes were interpreted as contrecoup contusions from a massive blow with a very heavy object.*

*Interpretation of these findings indicated that the woman had most likely been beaten or killed by beating before the explosion, in which case she could not have set the bomb herself. This implicated her common law husband, who was the beneficiary of insurance policies on the building and on her life. One of the crucial issues in the case was the fact that brain contusions and subdural hemorrhages require time to develop and do not occur postmortem except in very rare circumstances.*

***Inner cerebral traumatic lesions.*** Some damage to the deeper structures and white matter of the brain accompanies almost all cases of head trauma. "Inner cerebral" trauma, intermediary coup, or diffuse axonal injury, which may accompany forceful blows or falls, are produced in deep brain structures by shearing torsional-rotational forces.* Experiments have shown that the brain, because of its gelatin-like consistency can vibrate and wobble inside the intact cranial compartment, and these movements make portions of the brain move in opposing directions.[147,148,288] Where particular strains occur depends on the sites of impact and the underlying brain structure. In a large series of fatal head injuries most impacts that occurred in motor vehicle collisions involved primarily anterior/posterior/vertex impacts rather than lateral impacts.[127] Most lesions, in addition to the expected superficial contusions, were found in relatively constant locations in the brain parenchyma. These locations, depicted in Fig. 11-20, are found in the periventricular region (margins of the lateral ventricles, corpus callosum, septum), in the centrum ovale beneath the superior frontal gyrus, and in the perihippocampal region, as well as in the upper brainstem.

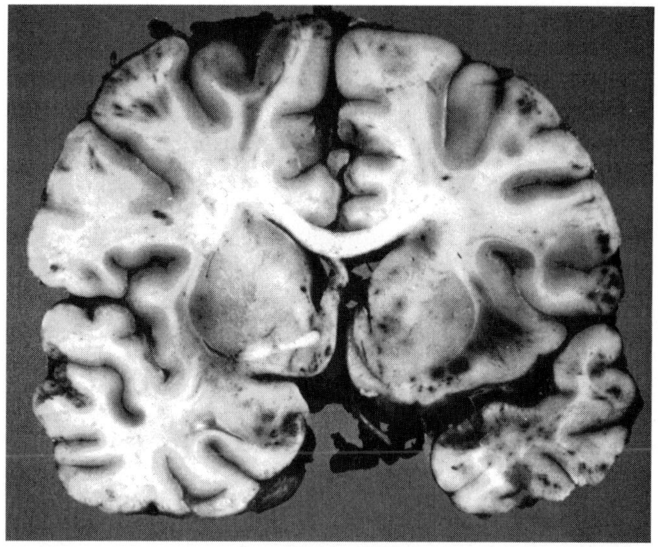

**Fig. 11-20.** This coronal section of a brain of a traffic accident victim who sustained a complex pattern of trauma with multiple cranial impacts illustrates diffuse cerebral injury (diffuse axonal injury). Numerous ball and streak hemorrhages are noted mostly beneath the cortical mantle in the white matter. Though not illustrated here, there are often hemorrhages in the corpus callosum in such cases.

In cases of inner cerebral trauma, diffuse axonal injury or intermediary coup conditions, the nonhemorrhagic multiple lesions are visible only many days after the impact and then usually only microscopically. These regions of injury appear to have a central zone of damage that gradually diminishes away from the "epicenter." At the epicenter only swollen and ballooned axons (axonal injury) and some local edema may be seen within an hour or two after the injury.[2,3,282,284] Later, the epicenter becomes hemorrhagic and necrotic (so-called "ball" and "streak" hemor-

* Refs. 126, 127, 147, 148, 222, 224, 320, 321, 344.

rhages). Away from the necrotic center a zone of damage can be seen where varying degrees of axonal ballooning, edema, myelin loss, and other reactive processes appear.[2,3,126,147] Survival of various neural elements may be possible in this zone. The degree and extent of damage are determined by a large number of primary and secondary factors, which form a "cascade." These include: blood-brain barrier damage,[282,283] release or activation of proteolytic enzymes and neurotransmitters,[20] microcirculatory and autoregulatory dysfunctions, vessel damage,[225,304] regional swelling and brain herniation, and systemic alterations that affect brain function. Among these latter we include the degree of hypoxia, acidosis, blood pressure level, effectiveness of respiration and gas exchange, electrolyte balance, hemostasis, presence of infection or sepsis, nutrition, and several other factors including fat embolization.

The changes observed across an inner brain traumatic lesion are constantly changing and probably continue to evolve for years. Injured areas may show ballooned axons at the margins of the lesion for many months. Areas where axons have been damaged will display myelin pallor, glial nodular scarring, and other reactions. These phenomena have been described by several authors.[2,3,228,320,321]

***Gliding and fracture contusions.*** A pattern of contusions may occur on the orbital surfaces of the inferior frontal lobes and over the inferior surface of the temporal lobes that may be different from the frontal and temporal lobe tip contrecoup contusions observed in most cases of severe closed head trauma.[225,228,343] These contusions are thought to represent injuries to the brain surface produced by bony ridges as the brain moves or glides over them. The mechanism of these contusions probably can be explained using the same model employed for coup and contrecoup contusions.

***Contusional tears.*** Lindenberg and Freytag[225] described lesions in the brains of infants and children who had suffered major head trauma in which, instead of surface contusions, there were small slitlike hemorrhagic lesions immediately beneath the cortical ribbon (Fig. 11-21). These lesions were found most commonly in the frontal portions of the brain below the superior frontal convolutions, orbital cortex, and in the anterior temporal lobe and insular cortex.[219] The fresh lesions will show slit hemorrhages and the old ones may show only an orange or yellow slitlike space or scar beneath the cortex. Contusional tears are thought to occur because the infant skull is malleable and does not allow sufficient low pressures to develop to produce a typical contusion upon impact; rather, the cortex may "creep" away from the subcortical white matter and create a shearing bleeding lesion. The time course and aging/dating parameters described by Lindenberg and Freytag[227] are especially valuable in the analysis of child abuse cases.

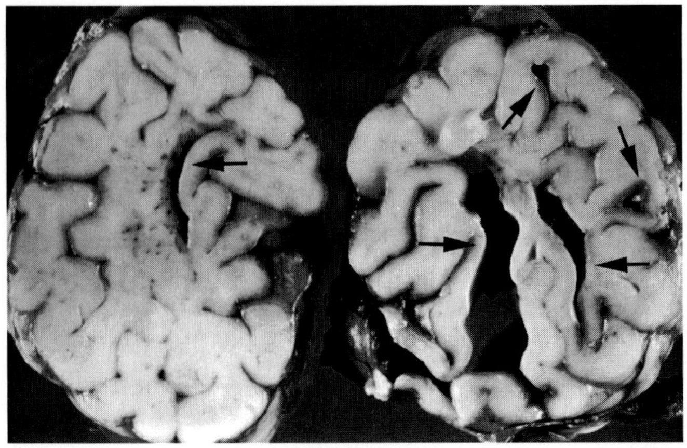

**Fig. 11-21.** This coronal section of the brain of an infant who was fatally abused illustrates multiple contusional tears *(arrows)* which occur as slits, with and without hemorrhage, in the immediate subcortical white matter. Such lesions are typical after effects of blows or other major impacts in infants with a soft, malleable skulls instead of the cortical contusions that would occur if the skull were ossified.

These lesions often are not properly appreciated by most pathologists and may be called malformational lesions or the results of birth trauma. The following case history offers many of these issues of interpretation.

***Illustrative Case 13:*** *A woman was charged with homicide in the deaths of two of her children. The deaths of both babies were virtually identical. Within a few days of bringing each infant home after birth, the mother reported that the babies would experience periods of fussiness, vomiting, apnea, and apparent seizures. On numerous visits to hospitals, bruises were noted, but no one suspected child abuse. Both babies died at about 3 months of age, both with seizures, low body weight, developmental arrest, and autopsy findings that included multiple fractures of long bones, ribs, and skull. The brains were reduced to a walnut-like shrunken state, with many layers of subdural hematoma membranes and a cavitary brown cortical surface. The subcortical regions on both hemispheres showed many brown-orange slitlike spaces that initially were interpreted as probably being the result of birth trauma or congenital in nature.*

*Examination of the birth records revealed normal term infants with normal Apgar scores and no record of difficulty during delivery, nor of instrumentation having been employed. In the course of the lengthy trial of the mother, former family physicians recounted their examinations. A pattern of abuse emerged that correlated with the lesions observed at autopsy and with the allegation that the mother had been brutally beating her babies almost from the time of birth until they died. The original autopsy examinations failed to interpret the findings properly and to declare them for what they were.*

***Brainstem trauma.*** Traumatic injury to the brainstem almost always accompanies any episode of major closed head injury in which inner cerebral trauma occurs. This injury is the consequence of torsional-rotational shear forces that impact the upper brainstem by virtue of its location and relatively fixed position in relation to the overlying cerebral hemisphere.[59,126] This vulnerability is illustrated by the types of blows that are required to render someone unconscious, usually those in which the head is accelerated and the neck is twisted forcefully.[328] Blows to a fixed-immobilized head require great force to produce unconsciousness, whereas much less is required when the head is moveable.[2,3,125,126] Small punctate hemorrhages may be seen in the upper brainstem in fatal head injuries, these being distinguishable from herniation hemorrhages of Duret.[219] These lesions interrupt and disrupt the reticular formation of the upper brainstem, causing unconsciousness and prolonged coma. Damage to the reticular formation probably accounts for many of the disturbances of consciousness that plague the recovering head trauma victim. Other lesions in the brainstem may account for instances of posttraumatic parkinsonism,[59,329] in which the nigral-striatal pathway is damaged.

Brainstem injury that probably results from hyperextension or rotational injuries to the neck are pontomedullary Fig. 11-22 and cervical-medullary avulsions or tears, which have been described by several authors.[213,219,226,279] Such lesions usually cause instant death but survivors have been reported.[226] The lesion is a physical tear or complete separation between pons and medulla or between medulla and cervical cord. The lesions usually are associated with "ring" fractures of the base of the skull and fracture-dislocations of the upper cervical spine. In most cases, the injury is sustained when victims are struck from behind by vehicles or while riding in a motor vehicle involved in either a head-on or rear-end collision that produces severe "whiplash." There may or may not be significant hemorrhage at the tear.

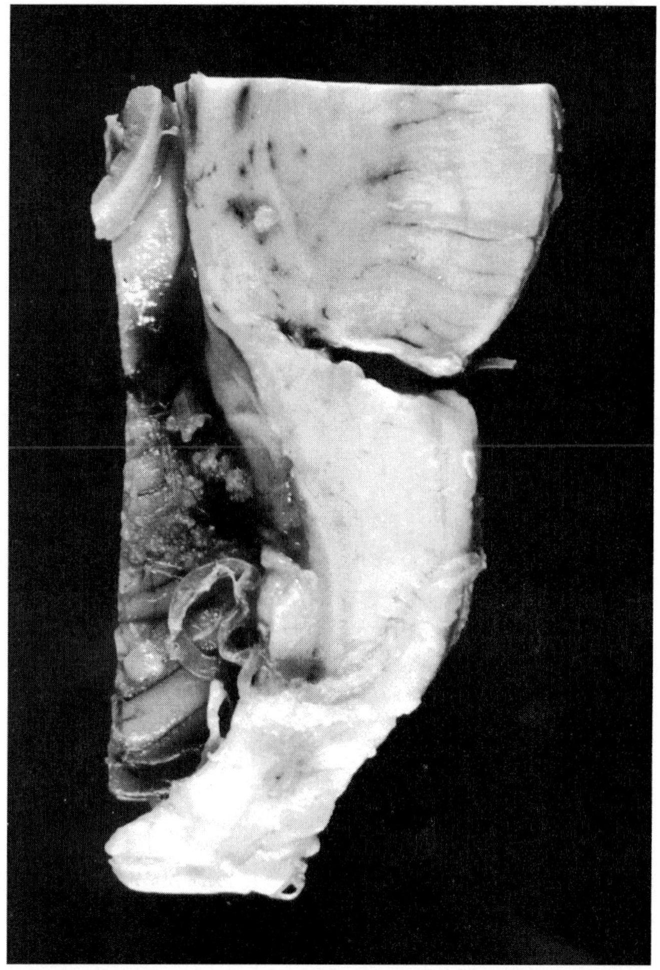

**Fig. 11-22.** This midline section of the brainstem illustrates a typical ponto-medullary avulsion-tear associated with a small puddle of blood in the 4th ventricle. This lesion is due to hyperextension injury of the neck which is usually associated with high cervical fractures/dislocations and often "ring" fractures of the skull base. Such injuries characteristically result from posterior impacts to pedestrians by vehicles. Most such injuries are immediately fatal.

## Spinal Cord Trauma

Injuries to the spinal cord have been documented since antiquity and have had forensic importance for nearly as long.[21] Cord injuries have differing pathogenesis depending on the level of involvement in the spine and the etiology. These injuries can occur against in a healthy spine or a diseased one; as the result of accident; following attempts at suicide; after the willful actions of another including missile and gunshot injuries; in the course of medical and chiropractic treatment;[31,77] or as the result of natural disease processes.[232] Owing to the breadth and complexity of the subject, only a brief review of spinal cord injury will be attempted here.

Accidental injury to the spine is common in most westernized nations, with at least 50% occurring in connection with motor vehicle accidents,[21] usually automobiles, but percentagewise motorcycle and bicycle accidents are probably more common. Injury during sports activities accounts for much of the remainder of accidentally spine injuries. Industrial and other accidents, usually falls or crush injuries, comprise the rest. Between 50% and 70% of victims become quadriplegic and 30% to 50% become paraplegic as the result of their injuries. About one half of the cases in any category are complete cord lesions.[128]

Injuries to the cervical spine are almost always caused by hyperextension or hyperflexion, which is more likely to injure the middle or lower cervical cord than the upper portions. This is because there is more space about the cord in the upper cervical canal to accommodate fractures, dislocations, and subluxations of the spine than at lower levels. Some upper cervical fractures, in spite of their radiographic appearances, only occasionally involve spinal cord injury (Jefferson's and "hangman's" fractures).[112] Some especially violent forms of "whiplash" to the neck may result in true avulsion of the cervical cord from the medulla,[213,226] however, most upper spinal cord injuries do not occur as the result of immediate physical transection of the cord, even though the clinical symptomatology is that of complete transection due to immediate neural shock. In most cases the cord is concussed or squeezed for a brief period during the traumatic episode; persistent compression may be secondary to bone fragments or an unstable spine. In cases of spondylitis, spinal stenosis, scoliosis, spondylolisthesis, or other spine disorders, the normal perispinal spaces are markedly reduced, making severe injuries possible in less traumatic circumstances than would otherwise be the case. Injury to the cervical, thoracic or lumbar cord can occur in conjunction with spinal disk or other surgical procedures. It is often impossible in the immediate post-trauma period to determine the true extent of the underlying cord damage. This is explained by the neural shock, which may take many days or weeks to wear off. Injury to the upper portion of the cervical cord is more ominous because the ability to breathe may be impaired. The significance of lower injury rests with the amount of arm and lower cord function maintained, including the degree of bladder function that is preserved.

Injuries to the thoracic spine and lumbar spine are less common because of the mechanical support of the spine in these locations by the rib cage and pelvis. Injuries in these locations are more commonly due to crushing, compression injury, and missile or gunshot wounds than to simple impacts. A variety of medical and surgical conditions also may contribute to thoracic and lumbar cord injuries. These include inadvertent interruption of blood supply to the cord (radicular arteries) in the course of aortic aneurysm repair, portocaval shunting,[78] and in the course of thoracic and lumbar spinal surgery for disk disease.[103] Transverse myelopathy or myelitis can occur spontaneously, perhaps as a result of minor trauma in a patient with spinal stenosis, following malpositioning at surgery or while the victim is intoxicated.[232]

The processes involved in the evolution of the traumatic spinal cord injury have been the subject of considerable observation and experimentation.[128,358] The earliest events probably involve interruption of the cytoskeleton (microtubules and neurofilaments) of the axon,[185] damage to the axonal membrane ion channel function (may explain neural shock), and possibly injury to the vascular endothelium. Chemical events may include calcium activation of neural proteases, neurotransmitter and inflammatory mediator responses, and generation of oxygen free radicals.[20,21] The next phase of injury is mostly confined to the gray matter of the cord and consists of the "microvascular phase" expressed as vascular congestion and edema, which appears 20 to 30 minutes after concussion.[347,358] This process becomes more obvious about 4 hours after injury when the gray matter is severely affected and the surrounding tracts of the cord become edematous. By 8 to 24 hours after impact, the whole surface of the cord at the level of injury may show hemorrhage and early necrosis (Fig. 11-23). Over the succeeding weeks, the cord undergoes breakdown as macrophages are activated and remove dead matter; several months after injury, the typical cord lesion is fusiform in shape, tapering off both cranially and caudally away from the most severely injured segment, where the cord may be totally necrotic and reduced to a small thread. Rostral to the injury there will be changes of ascending degeneration (demyelination of sensory tracts, particularly the dorsal columns). Caudal to the injury there will be descending degeneration of tracts, most notably the corticospinal tracts.

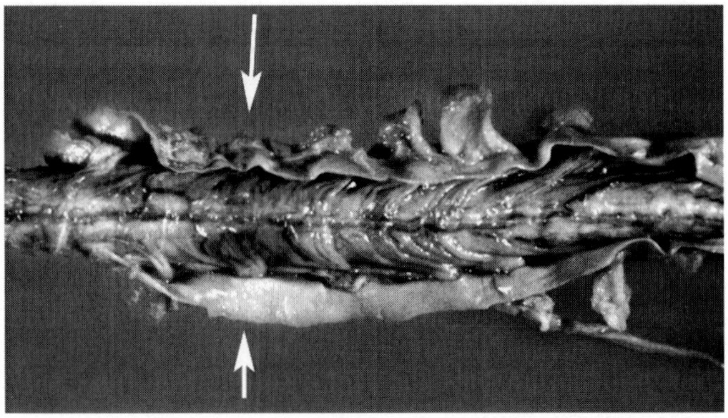

**Fig. 11-23.** Portion of the upper cervical spinal cord from an individual who suffered a fracture-dislocation of the cervical spine after a shallow water diving accident. A segmental area of contusion *(arrows)* caused quadriplegia and respiratory compromise. The victim lived only a few days following the accident. This appearance is typical for an acute spinal cord injury of this duration.

Of forensic import in spinal cord injury cases are often etiologic and mechanistic analyses of injuries and confirmation of processes observed at autopsy. This is especially true in cases of therapeutic misadventure or alleged chiropractic injury.[77,103,173,293,306] Such cases require a careful autopsy examination including removal of the portion of the spine segment in question for later radiography and dissection. The same is true for gunshot and missile wound cases in which recovery of a projectile may provide vital evidence for the legal proceedings. In this instance great care must be exercised in recovering bullets so that rifling grooves are not damaged by metal forceps, saws, or pliers.[71,88,219] Physical objects of evidence must be properly labeled, identified, described and securely stored in an appropriate manner so that the chain of custody of the evidence is preserved.[87,253]

### Pediatric Head Trauma and Neuropathology of Child Abuse

The phenomenon of child abuse is tragic. There are no more difficult and challenging cases that can regularly involve a coroner/medical examiner, prosecuting or defense attorney, or neuropathologist. The victim can communicate only through the physical evidence in his/her body. Secondly, the perpetrator, usually a parent, often provides a plausible explanation for the events that led to the death and may offer the ultimate picture of innocence, including appropriate grief and mourning. An accusation of possible child abuse is a damning allegation and crowning insult under these circumstances, and the fear of being wrong often restrains medical personnel from offering firm opinions. The same is true of police, prosecutors, coroners, and others. Fortunately, in most American states, child abuse reporting laws protect those who report suspicions to the appropriate government agency. Furthermore, in most states, failure to report suspicions may be punishable and open to civil action.[52,98,102] The civic and professional duties of physicians is to report such suspicions for proper investigation by vested authority.[142]

The "battered baby" is a true clinical, pathologic, and sociologic syndrome, consisting of a constellation of regularly observed phenomena and findings in all three areas.[143,327] From a sociologic point of view, the abused child exists within a family that usually is dysfunctional, regardless of socioeconomic status. Marital discord is common, and families are often disrupted. A personal history of abuse often can be elicited from one or both caretakers of the victim. More than one child may have been abused in the past. A history of sudden infant death syndrome (SIDS) is not uncommon. From a clinical point of view, it is common for the victim to have been examined by several physicians for accidents, falls, and other injuries. Victims may show signs of neglect, psychomotor retardation, and failure to thrive. The spectrum of injuries can be amazing and may include multiple fractures of differing ages involving long bones, ribs, skull, and pelvis.[42,143,181] There may be evidence of multiple burns, cuts, lacerations, bruises, and scars, but there may be no marks whatever on the child. The spectrum of neural injury may also be wide, including skull fractures (old and new), subdural and epidural hematomas (acute and chronic), brain contusions and tears, intracerebral hemorrhages and hydrocephalus as well as cervical and other spine injuries.[219] The correct interpretation of these injuries for what they are, willfully acquired physical trauma, is often difficult and demands great care.[187] Many comprehensive works on child abuse have been published.[52,143,219,327]

**Neuropathologic examination in child abuse.** Up to 75% of all fatal child abuse cases involve some form of cerebral injury; thus the neuropathologic examination often is vital.[27,58] The proper analysis of a child abuse fatality begins before the autopsy with an examination of the medical records, information about the alleged circumstances of the death based on police reports, interviews by social agencies, and statements by hospital personnel. The external surface of the body must be examined for wounds, bruises, scars, marks, and evidence of medical treatment, all of which should be photographed. The eyes should be examined externally and if possible by ophthalmoscope. The anal and genital areas should be examined for evidence of possible injury or sexual activity in accordance with procedures described elsewhere.[25,327] It is advisable that the body be radiographed to search for any fractures. The pathologist must examine the body cavities for fractures, injuries and lesions. The scalp and galea must be carefully examined for bruises and lesions, which should be photographed and documented as well as sampled histologically. The spine should be examined posteriorly, with an incision running from the occiput to the sacrum, and the soft tissues of the neck inspected for hemorrhage. The laminae should be opened and the spine exposed. The cord should be examined for epidural hemorrhage and then removed and fixed. The skull should be percussed before opening to avoid missing a subtle fracture. Once removed, any collections of blood must be documented and histologic samples taken. The brain should be carefully removed and fixed before cutting, and the dura should be stripped from both the vertex and the base of the skull to permit examination and inspection of the skull base. The eyes should be carefully removed to permit detection of injuries and preretinal hemorrhages.

When the brain is sectioned after fixation, all lesions (congenital or acquired) must be documented (preferably photographed) and then sampled histologically to permit proper analysis and dating of the lesions. Appropriate toxicologic studies also should be carried out. More detailed and specific guidelines for postmortem examination of suspected abuse victims can be found elsewhere.*

***Analysis of neuropathologic findings.*** Aging and dating of lesions and their proper documentation are crucial in child abuse cases. Bruises of the scalp must be correlated with underlying lesions in galea, skull, and brain. Precise aging of bruises is difficult and inexact.[361] All lesions must be examined for plausibility

* Refs. 44, 186, 219, 267, 298, 357, 361.

within the context of the allegations of circumstance by the possible perpetrator. Herein lies the most difficult task for the pathologist. Perpetrators consistently provide "stories" to explain the victim's injuries.[28,136] The following case history is illustrative.

**Illustrative Case 14:** *A 4-month-old baby was brought dead to an emergency room by the mother who reported that the baby had become unresponsive and blue after he had fallen from a table to a kitchen floor while his diaper was being changed. There was no record of the child having visited the hospital before. There were numerous bruises on the child's head, trunk, and legs. The autopsy revealed a separated linear skull fracture on the back of the head, an acute subdural hematoma, severe cerebral edema, and evidence of several previously fractured and healing ribs. The bruises on the trunk and legs and the injuries described above could not be the result of the simple fall described by the mother. It was likely that someone had swung the child by the trunk and/or legs against a wall, floor, or other immobile object. The manner of death was homicide and the cause of death was craniocerebral injury.*

*The mother confessed to having injured her crying child in just the manner described. This phenomenon is not rare.*[136]

### Scalp Injuries

Infant skin is more flexible than the adult's and may not show obvious changes after impact, especially if the blows are against a flat or somewhat soft surface. Also, bruises may appear not as black-and-blue marks but as erythematous areas, making recognition difficult. Aging and dating skin lesions is an imperfect procedures and one must not be overly confident with one's ability to attach an age or cause to an external bruise.[121,205,267,361] Subgaleal hemorrhages not visible externally can become apparent after resecting the scalp (Fig. 11-24, *A* to *D*). These lesions provide important correlations for sites of impact and must be noted.

### Skull Injuries

In the course of their everyday lives children fall from common objects and playthings but rarely fracture their skulls.[23,249,314] Generally skull fractures occurs only in connection with falls from 20 feet or more, in vehicular or pedestrian accidents, or when the child is physically injured by another person (abused). Several studies[136,144,146,195,250] indicate that when high falls and vehicular accidents have been ruled out and when the "story" that accompanies a child with anything but a narrow, simple, linear parietal skull fracture and the fall was from 3 or 4 feet (from most common tables and beds), child abuse has occurred until proved otherwise! The authors of these studies stress that any multiple, complex, depressed, comminuted, growing, basilar, or any skull fracture associated with underlying intracranial injury in a young child must be suspected of being the result of willful injury (Fig. 11-25).

The data supporting these assertions involve more than 1000 cases and come from several sources and perspectives. Helfer and others,[144] collected incident reports from hospitals in which infants or children fell from their beds or were dropped by personnel from heights averaging about 36 inches or more (90 to 150 cm) usually on a noncarpeted floor. Eighty-five such cases were collected between 1969 and 1975 among children under 5 years of age. Of these 85 cases, 57 showed no injury, 17 had small cuts or abrasions or bloody noses, 20 had a bruise, and only one child who fell from a gurney sustained a simple, linear skull fracture without unconsciousness or any neurologic complications. Histories of 176 other infants who were brought to a hospital emergency room were thoroughly investigated. None had any record or evidence of previous abuse, and most were brought for examination by anxious parents following reported falls to the floor from sofas, tables, chairs, and beds. Of the 176, only 37 suffered minor injuries. Only six children with more serious injuries: three clavicular fractures; two simple, narrow, linear uncomplicated skull fractures; and one fractured humerus. The two children with skull fractures had no subdural hemorrhages and no neurologic symptoms. A study reported by Kravitz and others[195] in which 536 cases were analyzed yielded an even lower incidence of serious injury in similar cases.

Particularly telling is the study of Hahn and others[136] who reported that, from 621 cases admitted to a children's hospital for falls, 77 children suffered serious and often multiple injuries. 126 cerebral injuries (average of 1.6 per patient) were found in this group. Skull fractures and subdural hematomas were found in 55% of these, and despite the initial "story" of an innocent fall, injuries in all cases were eventually shown to be the result of child abuse.

The prevailing evidence is that when children innocently fall from common household objects to the floor, carpeted or not, only a very small percentage will sustain a serious injury of any sort, much less one with any neurologic consequence. When young children experience serious head injury, more likely than not, and by some considerable margin, they have been injured willfully by someone else.[73] The magnitude of forces that must be employed to cause neurologic damage is based on eventual confessions of perpetrators and on other evidence such as that gained by noting the types of injuries sustained by children. Falls from such heights as fourth story windows to the pavement below (30 to 35 feet) carry an incidence of serious or fatal injury of only 2% to 20%.[314,350] It is only when falls reach or exceed five stories that a lethal dose (L.D.) 50% occurs. Therefore, it is reasonable to conclude that

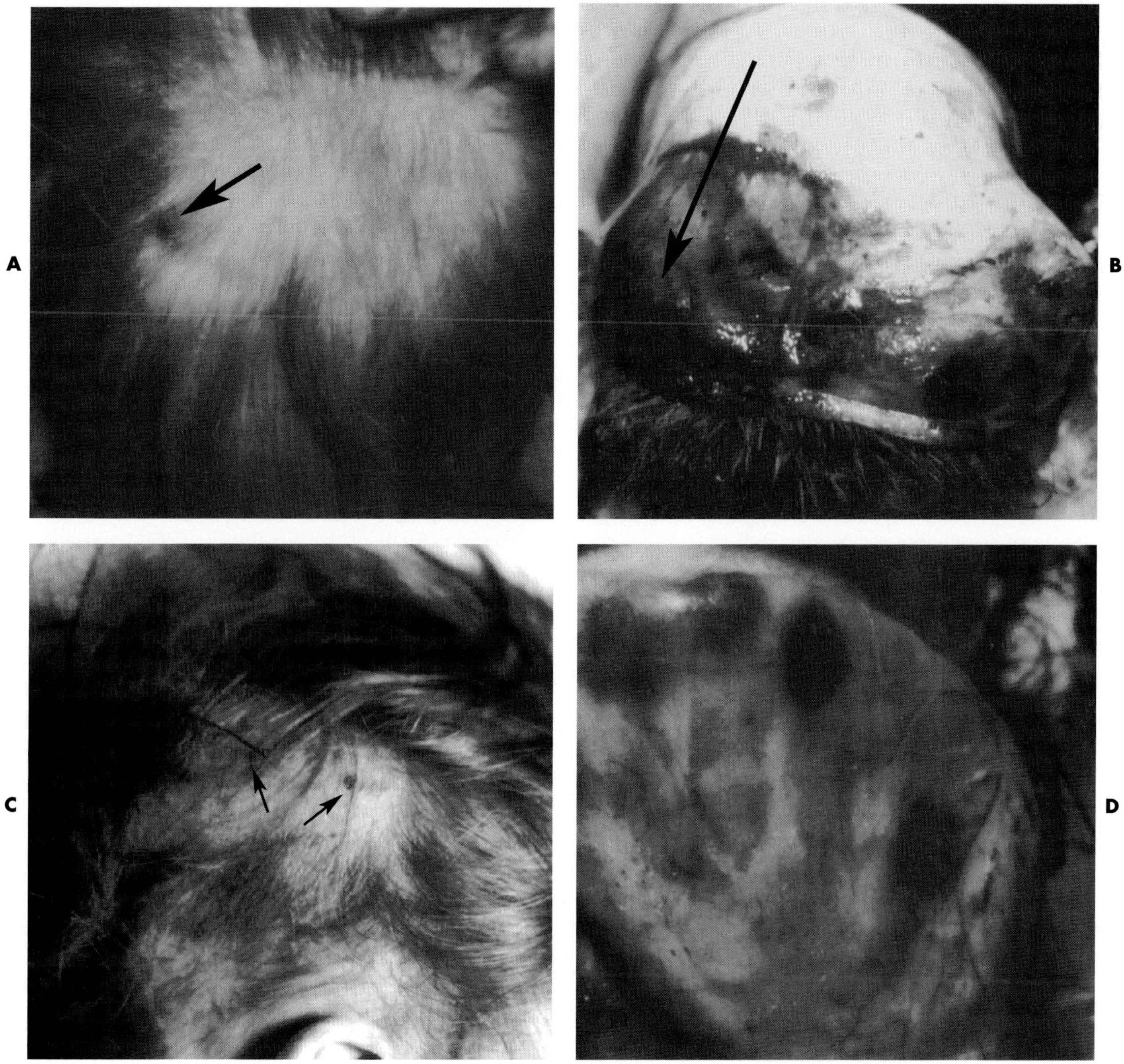

**Fig. 11-24.** These photographs taken at autopsy of a 12-month-old infant who was fatally abused, illustrate the disparity between the appearance of surface injuries and those in the subgaleal tissues. **A**, This photograph of the scalp of the vertex of the head illustrates a rather ill-defined, obvious bruise with possible abrasion *(arrow)* to the left of the shaved area and a much less distinct, roughly circular bruise that includes the abrasion. **B**, This photograph of the reflected scalp illustrates a rather extensive and very obvious subgaleal hematoma *(arrow)* of circular shape that corresponds to the indistinct circular bruise seen externally in **A**. **C**, This photograph of the shaved scalp over the right ear in the same infant reveals, again, a rather indistinct bruise-abrasion *(arrow)* but little else. **D**, This photograph of the reflected scalp beneath the external lesion at left, reveals not one but four rather linear hemorrhages which suggest the imprint of fingers or knuckles or may be the result of multiple blows which were not apparent externally.

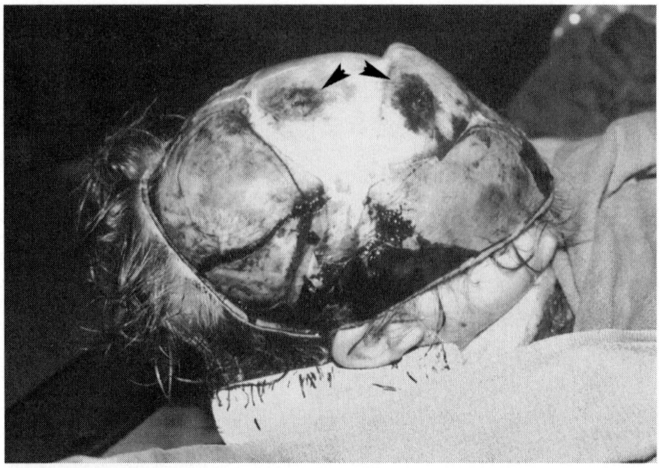

**Fig. 11-25.** A fatally abused two-year-old child suffered from a complex, stellate, and widely separated fracture associated with an obvious subgaleal hematoma. One must also appreciate the difference between iatrogenic and true traumatic injuries. As illustrated here *(arrowheads)* an intracranial pressure monitor/burr hole has produced a hemorrhage that might be misinterpreted as part of the original pathology. Fractures such as those shown are generally regarded, in the absence of a well-documented accidental incident, as evidence of willful injury. However, accidental injury, especially with a fully ossified skull, cannot be ruled out in the absence of other information.

forces equivalent to a fall from about 20 feet or more are required to produce the head injuries regularly observed in fatal child abuse. These injuries most commonly are produced by swinging the child against a wall, the floor, or an object of furniture, by stomping on the child, or by striking its head with a large and heavy object. An appreciation of the magnitude of forces required to injure a child fatally weighed against the "story" of the accused, usually is not lost on juries or judges involved in trying such cases.

As is often the case, the literature can be quite helpful but also controversial. The neuropathologic literature about child abuse head injury is no exception. Of particular concern is the controversial paper of Weber,[352] which often is cited in legal trials to support the claim that innocent falls from low height can fracture the skull. This particular study, done in Germany, reported the results of experiments in which the cadavers of infants were dropped onto floors of various compositions from an average height of 82 cm (about 3 feet). Weber reported that all the cadavers sustained skull fractures as proved by autopsy. The results are remarkable when compared with studies in live children cited above, and one can only wonder at the experimental design and the results that came from a cadaver study that provided little other information upon which to judge the merit of the work.

Another report, that of Aoki and Masuzawa,[14] is similarly confusing. In this study, conducted in Japan, 26 cases of acute subdural hemorrhages in infants were reported to have occurred in connection with minimal head trauma, apparently without loss of consciousness or cerebral contusions. The reported circumstances in which most of the children sustained their injuries were falls from a bed and falls from a sitting position or while being held onto a fiber tatami floor mat. The interval between alleged falls and unconsciousness or convulsion was generally 15 minutes or less, and some occurred within as little as 1 minute. All subdural hemorrhages were evacuated surgically. Of further note is that 100% of the infants had retinal and preretinal hemorrhages. The authors cite several other publications in the Japanese literature of similar reports. The conclusion often ascribed to this paper, but not stated in it, is that innocent and benign falls onto even soft surfaces can produce the picture of the whiplash-shaking syndrome, casting doubt on the phenomenon of the "shaken baby syndrome" and its cause.

A major difficulty with this paper is that the cases were non-fatally injured children, and only a token mention is made of the possibility of child abuse as a cause in these cases, with no attempt being made to investigate for this possibility. It is possible that child abuse in Japan is not widely recognized nor accepted, as was the case in the United States before 1960.[143] The coexistence of intracranial hemorrhage and retinal hemorrhages in 100% of cases, strongly suggests willful rather than accidental injury in these children.

**Malignant cerebral edema.** Most children under the age of 5 years who suffer head injury will experience some degree of cerebral edema that may become uncontrollable and fatal. The degree of edema may be out of proportion to the magnitude of the injury and external evidence of trauma. This syndrome may develop at varying intervals after injury during which the child may appear essentially normal or only slightly irritable, then become comatose.[36,311,315,331,367] The following is an example of the condition.

***Illustrative Case 15:*** *A 12-month-old child fell from a window on the fifth floor of a tenement to the sidewalk below. The child was dazed but not unconscious when found and apparently had suffered only a bloody nose and various scrapes and cuts. In the emergency room, a skull radiograph and an examination revealed no significant findings. Some 8 hours later, the child was returned by rescue squad ambulance to the hospital in coma after having been found nonbreathing, apparently asleep in its crib. The child died 2 days later with a "respirator" brain due to massively increased intracranial pressure. At autopsy, only a subgaleal bruise was found near the top of the forehead; no subdural or intracerebral hemorrhage was noted. There was a previously unappreciated linear fracture of the clavicle.*

The mechanism for immediate or delayed massive cerebral edema in children is not known; however, it may be explained, at least superficially, by the fact that the child's brain reacts differently than does the adult's to the effects of head trauma.[9,36,37,278a,346] Perhaps autoregulation of cerebral microcirculation in the child accounts for their response of increased cerebral blood flow as opposed to the adult, in whom decreased cerebral blood flow occurs with concussive injury.[273,278a] The biomechanical differences of less myelin and greater percentage of the brain being water also may play a role in these differences.

***Whiplash shaking syndrome.*** First formally reported by Guthkelch[132] and Caffey,[41,43] the so-called "whiplash-shaking" or "shaken baby" syndrome consists of fatal or nonfatal subdural hemorrhages, retinal hemorrhages, and brain swelling with or without apparent external injury or skull fracture in apparently abused children. The condition was first seen in fatally injured infants, but death does not necessarily occur. Investigation of the phenomenon has shown that vigorous shaking of infants by caretakers is a common, highly dangerous practice.[37,41,43] Other workers report that a considerable percentage of mental retardation and visual difficulties in children may be associated with shaking injury among those who survive.[41,43,139]

The whiplash-shaking syndrome apparently results when a young child is shaken by holding the thorax, shoulders, or abdomen. This shaking must be done by an individual much larger than the child, usually an adult, in order to achieve sufficient acceleration of the body of the child. During the shaking, it is assumed that the head can be whipped back and forth because of the relative inability of the infant to control its neck muscles and because of the relatively large mass of the head in relation to body.[135] This mechanical instability perhaps explains why whiplash-shaking deaths are uncommon in children older than 1 year.

Intraocular hemorrhages, often observed in these cases, probably develop rapidly but may continue to evolve for hours after the injury. The ocular hemorrhages reported in shaking deaths include hemorrhagic retinal separations (subretinal hemorrhage), preretinal hemorrhages, subhyaloid, vitreous or anterior segment hemorrhages, and hemorrhage into the optic nerve and sheath.[82,139,268] Suggested mechanisms for the intraocular hemorrhages associated with shaking are that venous engorgement of the eye occurs with high G accelerations, which may lead to vessel rupture. Further elevated venous pressures may be produced by tightly gripping the thorax of the infant, thus impeding venous return and producing a sort of Valsalva condition (Purtscher's retinopathy). The precise mechanism is not known, however.[115,203,234] When there has been accompanying battering of the infant, there may be ecchymoses in the orbit, conjunctival hemorrhage, hyphema, and corneal or ocular lacerations or ruptures probably unrelated to shaking. The specificity of each of these forms of hemorrhage for shaking deaths as opposed to other or collateral causes is a subject of controversy. Clearly not all hemorrhages in infants are the result of shaking; some may be caused by blood dyscrasia, the trauma of birth, increased intracranial pressure, venous engorgement, and other causes.[203,268] Nevertheless, according to Eisenbrey,[80] ". . . retinal hemorrhages in a child under four years of age should strongly suggest the possibility of battering (child abuse and whiplash shaking)." In a traumatized child with multiple injuries and an inconsistent history, the presence of retinal hemorrhages is highly suggestive of battering.[40] Others take a much more critical view of the specificity of retinal hemorrhages.[19,120,178,187,353]

It is often alleged by a parent or attorneys that a child was shaken in an effort to revive it after breathing stopped and the child turned blue. They claim that this effort produced the findings seen at autopsy. This allegation is difficult to interpret but in the face of other evidence of abuse, it is appropriate to discount it.[48] This issue is especially difficult in so-called "near-miss" sudden infant death cases or in cases of aspiration in which shaking may have been involved in attempts at resuscitation.

Significant cerebral edema usually is evident, and most infants who are alive at the time of admission to the hospital but are in coma will die with "respirator" brain changes. The mechanism of death is probably first and foremost the increased intracranial pressure caused by contusional or concussional cerebral edema and only secondarily the result of the mass effect of subdural and/or subarachnoid hemorrhage, which may be minimal. The phenomenon of "malignant" cerebral edema is discussed above.

With respect to subdural hematomas (which often are midline in location) among infants injured by shaking, the experimental work of Ommaya and others,[113,270,272] provides some understanding that movements of the brain and tearing of dural bridging veins occur during rapid angular acceleration-deceleration of the head on the neck in the range of 40,000 radians/sec$^2$ with a pulse duration of greater than 10 msec, will regularly produce subdural hemorrhages in the paramedian location as well as concussive syndromes and brain swelling. Of particular importance in these observations, carried out in rhesus monkeys, was that physical impact on the head was not required. This particular point has recently been challenged in the work of Duhaime and others[74] who constructed a model of a 1-month-old baby implanted with mechanical sensors. This model was then vigorously shaken by lab workers with and without impacts. Without impacts is was possible only to reach angular accelerations of somewhat under 1200 radians/sec$^2$ and G forces of only about 9 Gs. On the other hand, when the model head was shaken with impact, the G forces rose to about 428 Gs and angular accelerations reached more than 50,000 radians/sec$^2$, close to the level of acceleration observed in the animal studies.[270,272] The conclusion, based on the experiment was that impacts were required to produce subdural hemorrhages in the shaken baby syndrome.

There have been many criticisms of this work, among them: assumptions made in connection with the construction of the model; the surfaces against which the model was impacted; and the basic biomechanical data which is available on young infants to which the model is compared. Additionally, confessions and witness accounts have been obtained that confirm that shaken infants who subsequently died show classic ocular and intracerebral hemorrhages had no evidence of impact.[37,73,74,135] Duhaime and others,[74] however reviewed 48 cases of whiplash shaking deaths and noted that 37.5% of these cases lacked evidence of impact, yet displayed the classical neuropathologic findings of the other cases.

Many aspects of the whiplash shaking syndrome must be appreciated and taken into account before applying this diagnosis. In most cases, there will be evidence of an impact on the head, suggested by an externally or internally visible bruise (which may be subtle). About 25% of cases will show skull fractures, and perhaps 50% or more will show evidence of soft tissue hemorrhage in the paracervical muscles and/or epidural space of the cervical cord.[135,219] Furthermore, more often than not there will be other signs of abuse injury or evidence of previous intracranial or intraocular injury.[139,203] These observations clearly place whiplash-shaking within the context of the child abuse syndrome.

Many controversies about the "natural history" of the shaken baby find their way into the courtroom. Chief among these is the issue of a "latent" period between the shaking/trauma and the time the child decompensates and dies. Some experts maintain vociferously that once a child is shaken it becomes immediately unconscious and tends to remain that way until it experiences respiratory arrest and dies, within 20 to 30 minutes or an hour or two later. Such a view is extreme and is not supported by the facts. Obviously this is the case with some shaken infants, but not all.

Quite clearly, some infants are shaken and injured because of shaking but do not die.[41,116,364] These are the infants who may never be recognized as having been abused but may or may not suffer such sequelae of this abuse as mental subnormality, seizure disorders, perceptual and cognitive difficulties, and visual deficits. No one knows how severely they were shaken or otherwise injured, nor does anyone know what happened in connection with their injuries. Did they become unconscious and then awaken? What were they like until they recovered? No one knows how many such children fall into this category of recovered or missed abuse.

Also quite clearly there must be children, like adults, who are rendered unconscious, then regain some measure of consciousness, but are then overtaken by evolving intracranial space-occupying processes such as epidural or subdural hematomas, or cerebral edema, become unconscious again, and perhaps go on to die. Again, no one knows what percentage of shaken infants fall into this category. Another controversy that surrounds such infants is what they are like during the "lucid" interval? Anecdotal cases seem to indicate that there is a spectrum of behavior during an alleged "lucid" period. This ranges from extreme stupor and lethargy to a child who behaves apparently normally, even feeding and appearing to play. Other children will be irritable and whiny, may vomit, and may or may not feed, or may display variations of behaviors before apparently falling into coma and eventual respiratory arrest.[116]

Well-collected and reliable data to answer these questions are not available.

## MISSILE AND GUNSHOT WOUNDS

The injury produced by any object striking the head is a function of the kinetic energy (KE) of the object, which is determined by the velocity (v) of the object and its mass (m), summarized by the following equation: $KE = mv^2/2$. One further factor is the area of the impacting object and its angular relationship to the object it strikes. At collision the object will begin to dissipate its kinetic energy and will cease motion only when this process has been completed. Kinetic energy can be dissipated by transfer of momentum to another object (the head or brain); physical disruption, bending, breaking or penetration of the object (scalp, skull, brain); or dissipation as heat (vaporization of tissue fluids). These components each have neuropathologic consequences when missiles strike the head.

Most civilian missile injuries are caused by firearms, specifically handguns, which are a leading cause of death by suicide, homicide, and to a lesser degree by accident. The functioning of firearms is a science all its own and cannot be reviewed in anything but a superficial manner here. The interested reader is referred to the many excellent chapters and monographs for more information.[45,71,88,122,317]

Basically a firearm consists of a structure for holding the cartridge and bullet, a mechanism for firing the cartridge and channeling the bullet through a steel barrel that releases the bullet at high velocity in a parabolic course. The cartridge usually is constructed of brass or some other metal and contains a primer, a charge of explosive powder, and a bullet pushed into the end of the cartridge. The primer, when struck by the firing pin of the weapon, ignites itself, and the explosive powder contained in the cartridge drives the bullet into the barrel of the gun by the gaseous products of combustion, which follow the bullet down and out the barrel. The barrel usually contains spiral rifling grooves that cause the bullet to spin on exit, stabilizing its course by gyroscopic action. The bullet follows a parabolic course out of the barrel, first rising slightly then falling until it either strikes a target or falls to earth. The cartridge, ejected or retained in the weapon now contains an imprint of the firing pin which usually is unique and can be employed for evidentiary purposes in connecting the cartridge with the weapon. Furthermore, the bullet, having passed along the rifling grooves of the barrel also bears marks unique to the weapon from which it came. These also can be used for evidentiary purposes. For this reason, recovery of bullets from victims, especially if a weapon exists, is of vital importance in tying the bullet to a possible perpetrator. Special care must be exercised, therefore, when bullets are recovered at autopsy or at surgery to preserve the delicate rifling grooves in the bullet. No pliers or toothed forceps should be used to handle the projectile. Furthermore, connection of the bullet with the victim and with whomever has had possession of it is vital in guaranteeing that this bullet came from a specific victim and could not have been substituted or mixed up with another case (the chain of custody and evidence).[71]

The shotgun is another type of firearm. In this instance the cartridge usually has a metal base containing a primer, and a paper or plastic casing into which a powder charge is placed, followed by paper or plastic "wadding" and a charge of lead or steel shot. The size of the shot is variable, ranging from small (bird shot) to larger pellets ("buck" shot). Most shotguns have a smooth bore (don't possess rifling grooves) and control the spread of the shot by "choking" the end of the barrel with a device that narrows the lumen and extends the range of clustered shot. Some shotgun shells contain solid projectiles that possess rifling (rifled slugs, sabot rounds). These projectiles may have a range of 100 yards.

The entrance wound in tissue caused by a bullet may have several characteristics that can give vital information about the circumstances of the case. Owing to the explosion of gases and unburnt powder and carbon particles from the barrel of the gun, if the gun (depending on its caliber and nature of the cartridge) had been within a foot or two of the skin, it will leave a residue of particles in the skin (tattooing/sooting); thus, if this is found, some measure of the distance of the shot can be inferred. The type of powder in the propellant also can be deduced from the appearance of unburnt residues in or on the skin. By the same token if the gun barrel had been pressed against the skin at discharge, the gases and unburnt power released will tear the skin and balloon the subcutaneous tissues, causing an imprint of the barrel on the skin, a stellate entrance wound, and deposition of soot and particles deep in the wound.[317] The size of the entrance wound may bear little relation to the caliber of the bullet and mistakes are often made in estimating the caliber of a projectile only on the basis of its wound.

Many special characteristics of bullet wounds provide important forensic information to the knowledgeable expert. Similarly, at the skull, if the projectile should penetrate it, there are typical interactions of the projectile with the bone. For example, the bone will be torn away so that the inner table of the skull shows internal beveling, angulating away from the path of the bullet while the outer table of the skull is cleanly punctured, identifying it as the site of entrance. If the bullet has sufficient energy to exit the skull, the opposite is true. The inner table shows a clean and sharp edge; the outer table shows external beveling at an angle away from the axis of the bullet.[219] The exit wound may be larger than the site of entrance owing to expansion and mushrooming of the bullet. Estimation of the size or caliber of the bullet from its entrance or exit wound is often imprecise and should be avoided.[71,88] Shotgun wounds may be misinterpreted as being due to a bullet.

As a missile passes into tissue, especially the gelatin-like brain, the shock wave of the bullet creates a cavity in the brain tissue hundreds or thousands of times the volume of the bullet. This cavity lasts some milliseconds before collapsing; its size is a function of the velocity other than the mass of the bullet.[219,317] It is this transient cavity that probably causes most damage to tissues, including the brain. This expanding cavity is responsible for fractures of long bones when only the soft tissues have been penetrated by modern military rifle rounds. The pressures of the cavity may cause rupture and cause a virtual explosion of the head in some instances. Curiously, gunshot wounds to the head often do not produce massive hemorrhage, even when large vessels have been transected. In fact the margins of the bullet track (Fig. 11-26) often appear pale, with only the immediate walls showing hemorrhage.[228,231] This has been interpreted as the result of the cautery-like action of heat generated by the passage of the bullet. In spite of the great forces involved in gunshot wounds to the brain, many are not immediately fatal, unless they involve the brainstem or deep nuclear structures. There have been instances in which multiple self-inflicted gunshot wounds to the brain have occurred before death finally occurs.[71] The factors determining whether a wound is or will be fatal include: destruction of vital neural centers; degree of bleeding; degree of cerebral edema; mass of destroyed tissue; and late effects of infection and neurologic deficit.

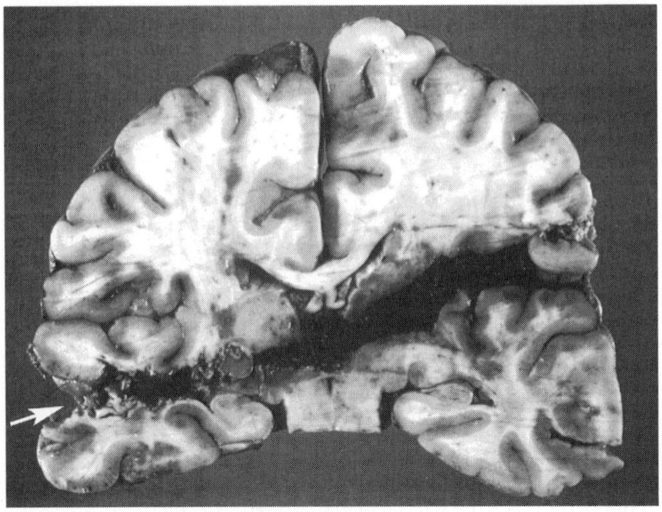

**Fig. 11-26.** Coronal section of the brain, the wound track from a self inflicted gunshot with a .38 caliber pistol. At the left *(arrow)* is the entrance wound cavity, which is somewhat smaller in diameter and extent than the exit track at the right. The track is filled with hemorrhage but outside the track the hemorrhage is minimal, a typical feature of such wounds.

Bullets that lack sufficient kinetic energy to exit the skull may rest within the brain, not always in a straight line with the entrance wound. The wound track sometimes takes a downward parabolic course or a course governed by fragmentation of the bullet or its having struck a bony surface that caused a ricochet. At times a bullet may carom around the inside of the skull and rest at completely unexpected locations on the surface of the brain.[231,317] Quite often bone fragments from the skull are driven into the brain and cause their own "missile" tracks. Fluoroscopy or radiography can be quite helpful in locating projectiles and missile fragments and facilitating their recovery for evidentiary purposes.

Bullets retained in the brain or not removed because of technical difficulty almost invariably elicit foreign-body reaction and may act as an epileptogenic focus. Infection in connection with projectile wounds of the brain is surprisingly much less common than might be expected. Neuropathologic findings away from the wound track in the brain in gunshot wounds include diffuse axonal injuries, contrecoup contusions, and satellite hemorrhages. Contrecoup contusions, which require some period of survival and vital signs to evolve, appear in the temporal and frontal lobe tips, orbital surface (gliding contusions), near the entrance wound, and often near the cerebellar tonsils or within the brain (corpus callosum, periventricular regions, upper brainstem). These disseminated deep injuries produce cerebral edema, prolonged coma, and belated death. Occasionally it is possible to observe so-called "blow-out" or contrecoup fractures of the orbital or cribriform plates. This presumably occurs because of tremendously high pressures of the cavity of passage of the bullet, which ruptures these very thin portions of the calvarium.

Neuropathologic examination of cerebral gunshot wounds usually involves cutting the brain in nonstandard ways, generally along the track(s) of the bullet(s) so that one can determine the structures through which the projectile(s) passed. This is sometimes important in the analysis of multiple wounds where the ability of the individual to function during the altercation might be important.[317]

The locations of gunshot wounds often give clues as to manner of death.[47,71,317] For example, suicide wounds typically are of the contact type in the temporal region (in relation to the handedness of the individual) or in the mouth, again with angulation typical for the victim's handedness. Homicidal wounds can be of the contact or noncontact type and may occur in places not reachable or not commonly employed in suicides. There may be "defense" wounds on the hand or arm.

Proper recovery and preservation of bullets and other projectiles have been mentioned above, mostly in connection with autopsy recovery; however, the pathologist often is in the position of receiving bullets as surgical specimens in ordinary hospital practice. It is vital that these objects be treated with care, properly labeled, and stored appropriately, because they may constitute important legal evidence.

## REFERENCES


1. Adams JH, and others: Deep intracerebral (basal gaglia) hematomas in fatal non-missile head injury in man, J Neurol Neurosurg Psychiatry 49:1039-1043, 1986.
2. Adams JH, and others: Diffuse axonal injury due to nonmissile head injury in humans: an analysis of 45 cases, Ann Neurol 12: 557-563, 1982.
3. Adams JH, and others: Diffuse brain damage of immediate impact type, Brain 100:489-502, 1977.
4. Adams JH, and others: The contusion index: a quantitative approach to cerebral contusions in head injury. Neuropathol Appl Neurobiol 6:319-324, 1980.
5. Adams RD, and Fisher CM: Pathology of cerebral arterial occlusion. In Fields WS, editor: Pathogenesis and Treatment of Cerebrovascular Disease, Springfield, Illinois, 1961, Charles C Thomas.
6. Adams RD, Victor M, and Mancall EL: Central pontine myelinolysis, Arch Neurol Psych 81:154-172, 1959.
7. Adelstein W: Confirmation of brain death using 99m Tc HM-PAO, J Neurosci Nurs 26:118-120, 1994.
8. Ad Hoc Committee of the Harvard Medical School: A definition of irreversible coma: Report of the Ad Hoc Committee of the Harvard Medical School to examine the definition of brain death. JAMA 237:337-340, 1968.
9. Aldrich EF, and others: Diffuse brain swelling in severely head-injured children. A report from the NIH Traumatic Coma Data Bank, J Neurosurg 76:450-454, 1992.
10. Allen JC, and others: Leukoencephalopathy following high-dose IV methotrexate chemotherapy with leucovorin rescue. Cancer Treat Rep 64:1261-1273, 1980.

11. Alves WM, and Jane JA: Mild brain injury: damage and outcome. In Becker DP, and Povlishock JT, editors: Central Nervous System Trauma Status Report—1985, Volume 31. Nat Inst Neurol Communic Dis Stroke, 1987.
12. Andrews JM, and Schumann GB: Neurocytopathology, Baltimore, 1992, Williams & Wilkins.
13. Annual Report. Office of The Medical Examiner, Cook County, Chicago, Illinois, 1977–1979.
14. Aoki N, and Masuzawa H: Infantile acute subdural hematoma. Clinical analysis of 26 cases, J Neurosurg 61:273-280, 1984.
15. Armstrong DL, and Norman MG: Periventricular leukomalacia in neonates: complications and sequelae, Arch Dis Child 49: 367-375, 1974.
16. Aronson SM, and Okazaki H: A study of some factors modifying response of cerebral tissue to subdural hematomata, J Neurosurg 20:89-93, 1963.
17. Auer RN, and Siesjo BK: Biological differences between ischemia, hypoglycemia, and epilepsy, Ann Neurol 24:699-707, 1988.
18. Auster LS: The role of trauma in oncogenesis. A juridical consideration, JAMA 175:946-950, 1961.
19. Bacon CJ, Sayer GC, and Howe JW: Extensive retinal haemorrhages in infancy—an innocent cause, Br Med J 1:281, 1978.
20. Balentine JD, and others: Calcium and the pathogenesis of spinal cord injury, In Dacey RG Jr, editor; Trauma of the Central Nervous System, New York, 1985, Raven Press.
21. Balentine JD: Impact injuries of the spine and spinal cord. In Leestma JE, editor: Forensic Neuropathology, New York, 1988, Raven Press.
22. Baratham G, and Dennyson WG: Delayed traumatic intracerebral hemorrhage, J Neurol Neurosurg Psychiatry 35:698-706, 1972.
23. Barlow B, and others: Ten years of experience with falls from height in children, J Pediatr Surg 18:509-511, 1983.
24. Batra P: The fat embolism syndrome, J Thorac Imaging 2:12-17, 1987.
25. Bazan NG, and others: The accumulation of free arachidonic acid, diacylglycerols, prostaglandins, and lipoxygenase reaction products in the brain during experimental epilepsy, Adv Neurol 44:879-902, 1986.
26. Bell WE, and McCormick WF: Neurologic infections in children, Philadelphia, 1975, WB Saunders.
27. Benzel EC, and Hadden TA: Neurologic manifestations of child abuse, South Med J 82:1347-1351, 1989.
28. Billmire E, and Myers PA: Serious head injury in infants: accident or abuse? Pediatrics 75:340-342, 1985.
29. Black PM: Brain death. N Engl J Med 299:338-344, 393-402, 1978.
30. Bontross AR, and Henry CE: Electrocerebral silence associated with adequate spontaneous ventilation in a case of fat embolism. A clinical and medicolegal dilemma, Arch Neurol 39:314-316, 1982.
31. Braun IF, and others: Brain stem infarction due to chiropractic manipulation of the cervical spine, South Med J 76:1507-1510, 1983.
32. Brierley JB, and Graham DI: Hypoxia and vascular disorders of the central nervous system, In Adams JH, Corsellis JAN, and Duchen LW, editors: Greenfield's Neuropathology, ed 4, New York, 1984, John Wiley.
33. Broderick JP, and others: Incidence rates of stroke in the eighties: the end of the decline in stroke? Stroke 20:577-582, 1989.
34. Brown P, and others: Chemical disinfection of Creutzfeldt-Jakob disease virus, N Engl J Med 306:1279-1282, 1982.
35. Brown S: Personal communication, The David Lewis Centre, Cheshire, England, 1994.
36. Bruce DA, and others: Diffuse cerebral swelling following head injuries in children the syndrome of "malignant brain edema," J Neurosurg 54:170-178, 1981.
37. Bruce DA, and Zimmerman RA: Shaken impact syndrome, Pediatr Ann 18:482-494, 1989.
38. Buchthal F, and Behse F: Electrophysiology and nerve biopsy in men exposed to lead, Br J Ind Med 36:135-147, 1979.
39. Burns RS, and others: The clinical syndrome of striatal dopamine deficiency induced by 1-methyl-4-phenyl-1,2,3,6-tetrahydropyridine (MPTP), N Engl J Med 312:1418-1421, 1985.
40. Buys YM, and others: Retinal findings after trauma in infants and young children, Ophthalmology 99:1718-1723, 1992.
41. Caffey J: The whiplash shaken infant syndrome. Manual shaking by the extremities with whiplash-induced intracranial and intraocular bleeding, linked with residual permanent brain damage and mental retardation, Pediatrics 4:396-403, 1974.
42. Caffey J: Multiple fractures of long bones of children suffering from subdural hematoma, Am J Radiol 56:163-173, 1946.
43. Caffey J: On the theory and practice of shaking infants, Am J Dis Child 124:161-169, 1972.
44. Cameron JM, and Rae LJ: Atlas of the battered child. Edinburgh, 1975, Churchill-Livingstone.
45. Cameron M: Subacute and chronic subdural hematoma, J Neurol Neurosurg Psychiatry 41:834-839, 1978.
46. Cammermeyer J: Cerebral fat embolism with focal siderosis and pericapillary hemorrhages after intraperitoneal injection of oil in cats terminally fixed by perfusion, Exp Neurol 55:690-708, 1977.
47. Camps FE, and others: Gradwohl's Legal Medicine, ed 3. Chicago, 1976, John Wright-Year Book Medical Publishers.
48. Carter JE, and McCormick AQ: Whiplash shaking syndrome: retinal hemorrhages and computerized axial tomography of the brain, Child Abuse Negl 7:279-286, 1983.
49. Carter RF: Primary amoebic meningo-encephalitis: clinical, pathological and epidemiological features of six fatal cases, J Pathol Bacteriol 96:1-25, 1968.
50. Carter RF, and others: A fatal case of meningoencephalitis due to free-living amoeba of uncertain identity-probably acanthamoeba sp, Pathology 13:51-68, 1981.
51. Chasnoff IJ, and others: Cocaine and pregnancy: clinical and toxicological implications for the neonate, Clin Chem 35:1276-1278, 1989.
52. Children's Bureau: Child Abuse and Neglect: State Reporting Laws. DHEW, Washington, 1979.
53. Choux M, Lena G, and Genitori L: Intracranial hematomas. In Raimondi AJ, Choux M, and Genitori L, editors: Head injuries in the newborn and infant. New York, 1986, Springer-Verlag.
54. Chuaqui R, and Tapia J: Histologic assessment of the age of recent brain infarcts in man, J Neuropathol Exp Neurol 52:481-489, 1993.
55. Clark DH: Practical forensic odontology, Oxford, 1992, Wright.
56. Collaborative Study on Brain Death: An appraisal of the criteria of cerebral death: a summary statement. JAMA 237:982-986, 1977.
57. Cooper PR: Delayed brain injury: secondary insults. In Becker DP, and Povlishock JT, editors: Central nervous system trauma status report—1985, Volume 31. Bethesda, Maryland, 1987, Nat Inst Neurol Communic Dis Stroke, 1987.
58. Copeland AR: Homicide in childhood. The Metro-Dade County experience from 1956 to 1982, Am J Forensic Med Pathol 6:21-24, 1985.
59. Corsellis J, Bruton C, and Freeman-Browne D: The aftermath of boxing. Psychol Med 3:270-303, 1973.
60. Corsellis JAN: The incidence of Ammon's horn sclerosis, Brain 80:193-208, 1957.
61. Council on Scientific Affairs: Brain injury in boxing, JAMA 249: 254-257, 1983.
62. Crick F, and Koch C: Towards a neurobiological theory of consciousness, Semin Neurosci 2:263-275, 1990.
63. Cuneo RA, and others: Upward transtentorial herniation. Arch Neurol 36:618-622, 1979.

64. Curran WJ: Tracy's the doctor as a witness. Philadelphia, 1965, WB Saunders.
65. Daras M, and other: Neurovascular complications of cocaine, Acta Neurol Scand 90:1214-1129, 1994.
66. Davidson KD, Weiford ED, and Dixon GD: Traumatic vertebral artery pseudoaneurysm following chiropractic manipulation, Radiology 115:651-652, 1975.
67. Dawson SL, and others: The contrecoup phenomenon. Reappraisal of a classic problem, Hum Pathol 11:155-166, 1980.
68. Day NL, and others: Prenatal exposure to alcohol: effect on infant growth and morphologic characteristics, Pediatrics 84: 536-541, 1989.
69. De Villiers J: Unexpected natural death of cerebral origin in medicolegal practice, Forensic Sci 5:11-19, 1975.
70. DiMaio DJ, and DiMaio VJM: Forensic pathology. New York, 1989, Elsevier.
71. DiMaio VJM: Gunshot wounds. Practical aspects of firearms, ballistics, and forensic techniques. New York, 1985, Elsevier.
72. Doull J, Klaassen CD, and Amdur MO, editors: Casarett and Doull's toxicology. The basic science of poisons, ed 2, New York, 1980, Macmillan.
73. Duhaime AC and others: Head injury in very young children: mechanisms, injury types, and ophthalmologic findings in 100 hospitalized patients; younger than 2 years of age. Pediatrics 90:179-185, 1992.
74. Duhaime AC, and others: The shaken baby syndrome. A clinical, pathological, and biomechanical study. J Neurosurg 66:409-415, 1987.
75. Dunsmore RH, and Roberts M: Trauma as a cause of brain tumor. A medicolegal dilemma, Conn Med 38:521-523, 1974.
76. Earle KM: Examination of the brain (necropsy technique). American Registry of Pathology, AFIP, Washington, D.C.
77. Easton JD, and Sherman DG: Cervical manipulation and stroke, Stroke 8:594-597, 1977.
78. Ebel W, Hegewald G, and Heese R: The Zieve syndrome, Z Gesamte Int Med 27:805-808, 1972.
79. Eisenberg HM: Outcome after head injury: general considerations and neurobehavioral recovery. Part I: General considerations. In Becker DP, and Povlishock JT, editors: Central nervous system trauma status report—1985, Bethesda, Maryland, 1987, Nat Inst Neurol Communic Dis Stroke.
80. Eisenbrey AB: Retinal hemorrhages in the battered child, Childs Brain 5:40-44, 1979.
81. Ellenberg JH, and Nelson KB: Cluster of perinatal events identifying infants at high risk for death or disability, J Pediatr 113: 546-552, 1988.
82. Elner SG, and others: Ocular and associated systemic findings in suspected child abuse. A necropsy study, Arch Ophthalmol 108:1094-1101, 1990.
83. Emond A, Golding J, and Peckham C: Cerebral palsy in two national cohort studies, Arch Dis Child 64:848-852, 1989.
84. Erdem E, and others: Cerebral fat embolism studied with MRI and SPECT. Neuroradiology 35:199-201, 1993.
85. Evans JP: Initial clinical appraisal, grading, classification of craniocerebral trauma. In Caveness WE, and Walker AE, editors: Head injury. Conference proceedings. Philadelphia, 1966, JB Lippincott.
86. Farrell MM, and Levin DL: Brain death in the pediatric patient: historical, sociological, medical, religious, cultural, legal and ethical considerations. Crit Care Med 21:1951-1965, 1993.
87. Fatteh A: Handbook of forensic pathology, Philadelphia, 1973, JB Lippincott.
88. Fatteh A: Medicolegal investigation of gunshot wounds, Philadelphia, 1976, JB Lippincott.
89. Federal Rules. Civil Procedure. St. Paul, Minnesota, 1986, West Publishing Co.
90. Feigin I, and others: Degeneration of white matter in hypoxia, acidosis, and edema, J Neuropathol Exp Neurol 32:125-143, 1973.
91. Feldman GB, and Freiman JA: Prophylactic caesarian section at term? N Engl J Med 312:1264-1267, 1985.
92. Fell DA, and others: Acute subdural hematomas. Review of 144 cases, J Neurosurg 42:37-42, 1975.
93. Fisher CM: Lacunes: small, deep cerebral infarcts, Neurology 15:774-784, 1965.
94. Fisher CM, and others: Acute hypertensive cerebellar hemorrhage: diagnosis and surgical treatment, J Nerv Ment Dis 140: 38-57, 1965.
95. Fishman RA: The cerebrospinal fluid in diseases of the nervous system, ed 2. Philadelphia, 1992, WB Saunders.
96. Florence AL: Is Thalidomide to blame? Br Med J 2:1954, 1960.
97. Forbus WD: On the origin of miliary aneurysms of the superficial cerebral arteries. Bull Johns Hopkins Hosp 47:239-284, 1930.
98. Fraser S: A glance at the past, a gaze at the present, a glimpse at the future: a critical analysis of the development of child abuse reporting statutes, Chicago Kent Law J 54:641-686, 1978.
99. Freytag E, and Lindenberg R: 294 medicolegal autopsies in epileptics, Arch Pathol 78:274-286, 1964.
100. Friede RL: Developmental neuropathology, ed 2. New York, 1989, Springer-Verlag.
101. Fuertes de La Haba A, and others: Deaths among users of oral and non-oral contraceptives, Obstet Gynecol 36:597-602, 1970.
102. Gall D, and Weil B: Confidentiality and the obligation to report child abuse. Case for discussion, Prog Clin Biol Res 139:47-48, 1983.
103. Gambee MJ: Vertebral artery thrombosis after spinal injury: case report, Paraplegia 24:350-357, 1986.
104. Garcia JH, and Anderson ML: Circulatory disorders and their effects on the brain. In Davis RL, and Robertson DM, editors: Textbook of neuropathology, ed 3 Baltimore, 1996, Williams & Wilkins.
105. Garcia JH, and others: Arterial hypertension injures brain capillaries. Definition of the lesions. Possible pathogenesis, Stroke 12:410-413, 1981.
106. Garcia JH, and others: Arterial air embolism: structural effects on the gerbil brain, Stroke 12:414-421, 1981.
107. Garcia JH, Liu KF, and Ho KL: Neuronal necrosis after middle cerebral artery occlusion in Wistar rats progresses at different time intervals in the caudoputamen and the cortex, Stroke 26: 636-642, 1995.
108. Garcia JH: Morphology of global cerebral ischemia, Crit Care Med 16:979-987, 1988.
109. Garcia JH: The evolution of brain infarcts. A review, J Neuropathol Exp Neurol 51:387-393, 1992.
110. Gartner LM, and others: Kernicterus: high incidence in premature infants with low serum bilirubin concentrations, Pediatrics 45:906-917, 1970.
111. Gastaut H: Dictionary of epilepsy, Geneva, 1973, World Health Organization.
112. Gehweiler JA Jr, Osborne RL Jr, and Becker RF: The radiology of vertebral trauma. Philadelphia, 1980, WB Saunders.
113. Gennarelli TA, and Thibault LE: Biomechanics of acute subdural hematoma. J Trauma 22:680-686, 1982.
114. Gianelli DM: Karen Ann Quinlan's family remembers, Am Med News December 15 1989, pp 9, 33.
115. Giangiacomo J, and others: Sequential cranial computed tomography in infants with retinal hemorrhages, Ophthalmology 95: 295-199, 1988.
116. Gilles EE: Abusive head injury in children: a review, Western State Univ Law Rev 20:335-378, 1993.
117. Gilles FH, Lenton A, and Dooling EC: The developing human brain: growth and epidemiologic neuropathology. Littleton, Massachusetts, 1983, John Wright.
118. Gilles FH: Perinatal neuropathology. In Davis RL, and Robert-

son DM, editors: Textbook of neuropathology, Baltimore, 1985, Williams & Wilkins.
119. Gitlin D: Pathogenesis of subdural collections of fluid, Pediatrics 16:345-352, 1955.
120. Goetting MG, and Sowa B: Retinal hemorrhage after cardiopulmonary resuscitation in children: an etiologic reevaluation, Pediatrics 85:585-588, 1990.
121. Goggio AI: The mechanism of contrecoup injury, J Neurol Neurosurg Psychiatry 4:11-22, 1941.
122. Gonzales TA, and others: Legal medicine and toxicology. New York, 1954, Appleton-Century-Crofts.
123. Goodell CL, and Mealey J Jr: Pathogenesis of chronic subdural hematoma: experimental studies. Arch Neurol 8:429-437, 1941.
124. Graff RNR, and others: Brain atrophy and neuropsychological impairment in young alcoholics, J Stud Alcohol 43:859-868, 1983.
125. Graham DI, Behan PO, and More IA: Brain damage complicating septic shock. Acute hemorrhagic leucoencephalitis as a complication of the generalized Schwartzman reaction, J Neurol Neurosurg Psychiatry 42:19-28, 1979.
126. Grcevic N: The concept of inner cerebral trauma, Scand J Rehabil Med Suppl 17:25-31, 1988.
127. Grcevic N: Topography and pathogenic mechanisms of lesion in the "inner cerebral trauma," Rad Jazu (J Yugosl Acad Sci) 402:265-402, 1982.
128. Green BA, Klose KJ, Goldberg ML: Clinical and research considerations in spinal cord injury. In Becker DP, and Povlishock JT, editors: Central nervous system trauma status report—1985, Volume 31, Bethesda, Maryland, 1987, Nat Inst Neurol Communic Dis Stroke.
129. Grinker RR: Parkinsonism following carbon monoxide poisoning, J Nerv Ment Dis 64:18-28, 1926.
130. Gross SG, and Bell RD: Central pontine myelinolysis and rapid correction of hyponatremia. Tex Med 78:59-60, 1982.
131. Gurdjian ES: Impact head injury. Mechanistic, clinical and preventive correlations, Springfield, Illinois, 1975, Charles C Thomas.
132. Guthkelch AN: Infantile subdural haematoma and its relationship to whiplash injuries, Br Med J 2:421-431, 1971.
133. Guttman L: Spinal shock. In Vinken PJ, and Bruyn GW, editors: Handbook of clinical neurology, volume 25, New York, 1976, Elsevier-North Holland.
134. Hadeed AJ, and Siegel SR: Maternal cocaine use during pregnancy: effect on the newborn infant, Pediatrics 84:201-210, 1989.
135. Hadley MN, and others: The infant whiplash-shake injury syndrome: a clinical and pathological study, Neurosurgery 24:536-540, 1989.
136. Hahn YS, Raimondi AJ, and McLone DG: Traumatic mechanisms of head injury in child abuse, Childs Brain 10:229-241, 1983.
137. Halevy A, and Brody B: Brain death: reconciling definitions, criteria, and tests, Ann Intern Med 119:519-525, 1993.
138. Hammer RP Jr, and Scheibel AB: Morphologic evidence for a delay of neuronal maturation in fetal alcohol exposure, Exp Neurol 74:587-597, 1981.
139. Harley RD: Ocular manifestations of child abuse, J Pediatr Ophthalmol Strabismus 17:5-13, 1980.
140. Harper C: The incidence of Wernicke's encephalopathy in Australia—a neuropathological study of 131 cases, J Neurol Neurosurg Psychiatry 46:593-598, 1983.
141. Harper C: Neuropathology of brain damage caused by alcohol, Med J Aust 2:276-282, 1982.
142. Helfer RE: The responsibility and role of the physician. In Helfer RE, and Kempe CH, editors: The battered child, Chicago, 1974, University of Chicago Press.
143. Helfer RE, and Kempe CH: The Battered Child. Chicago, 1974, University of Chicago Press.
144. Helfer RE, Slovis TL, and Black M: Injuries resulting when small children fall out of bed, Pediatrics 60:533-535, 1977.
145. Heros RC: Cerebellar infarction resulting from traumatic occlusion of a vertebral artery: case report, J Neurosurg 51:111-113, 1979.
146. Hobbs CJ: Skull fracture and the diagnosis of abuse, Arch Dis Chil 59:246-252, 1984.
147. Holbourn AHS: Mechanics of head injuries, Lancet 2:438-441, 1943.
148. Holbourn AHS: The mechanics of brain injuries, Br Med Bull 3:147-149, 1945.
149. Hooper R: Patterns of acute head injury Baltimore, 1969, Williams & Wilkins.
150. Horn SW: The "locked-in" syndrome following chiropractic manipulation of the cervical spine, Ann Emerg Med 12:648-650, 1983.
151. Horsley JE, and Carlova J: Testifying in court, ed 2. Oradell, New Jersey, 1983, Medical Economics Books.
152. Howard MA, and others: Acute subdural hematomas: an age-dependent clinical entity, J Neurosurg 71:858-863, 1989.
153. Hsu DR, Chao EK, and Shih CH: Post-traumatic fat embolism syndrome—a 10 year retrospective study in Chang Gung Memorial Hospital, Chang Keng I Hsueh, 113:86-95, 1990.
154. Hughes JR, Boshes B, and Leestma J: Electroclinical and pathologic correlations in comatose patients, Clin Electroencephalogr 7:13-30, 1976.
155. Huntington HW Jr, and others: Discovery of fatal primary intracranial neoplasms at medicolegal autopsies, Cancer 18:117-127, 1965.
156. Illingworth RS: A paediatrician asks—why is it called birth injury? Br J Obstet Gynaecol 192:122-130, 1985.
157. Illingworth RS: Why blame the obstetrician? A review, Br Med J 1:797-801, 1979.
158. Illis L, and others: Oral contraceptives and cerebral arterial occlusion, Br Med J 5471:1164-1166, 1965.
159. Ingraham FD, and Heyl LH: Subdural hematoma in infancy and childhood, JAMA 112:198-204, 1939.
160. Ingvar M, Folbegrova J, and Siesjo BK: Metabolic alterations underlying the development of hypermetabolic necrosis in the substantia nigra in status epilepticus, J Cereb Blood Flow Metab 7:103-108, 1987.
161. Irey NS, McAllister HA, and Henry JM: Oral contraceptives and stroke in young women: a clinicopathologic correlation, Neurology 28:1216-1219, 1978.
162. Irey NS, and Norris HJ: Intimal vascular lesions associated with female reproductive steroids, Arch Pathol 96:227-234, 1973.
163. Isaacson G: Postmortem examination of infant brains. Techniques for removal, fixation, and sectioning, Arch Pathol Lab Med 108:80-91, 1984.
164. Ito H, Komai T, and Yamamoto S: Fibrinolytic enzyme in the lining walls of chronic subdural hematoma, J Neurosurg 48:197-200, 1978.
165. Jacobs JM, and LeQuesne PM: Toxic disorders of the nervous system. In Adams JH, Corsellis JAN, and Duchen LW, editors: Greenfield's neuropathology, ed 4. New York, 1984, John Wiley.
166. Jacobson DM, Terrence CF, and Reinmuth OM: The neurologic manifestations of fat embolism. Neurology 36:847-851, 1986.
167. James AE Jr: Legal medicine with special reference to diagnostic imaging, Baltimore, 1980, Urban & Schwarzenburg.
168. Janaki S, and others: Stroke in the young: a four year study, 1968 to 1972, Stroke 6:318-320, 1975.
169. Janssen W: Forensic histopathology. Berlin, 1984, Springer-Verlag.
170. Jänisch W, and Schreiber D: Experimental tumors of the central nervous system, Kalamazoo, Michigan, 1977, Upjohn Co.
171. Jellinger K: Cerebrovascular amyloidosis with cerebral hemorrhage, J Neurol 214:195-206, 1977.

172. Jennett WB, and Cross JN: Influence of pregnancy and oral contraception on the incidence of stroke in women of childbearing age, Lancet 1:1019-1023, 1967.
173. Jentzen JM, Amatuzio J, and Peterson GF: Complications of cervical manipulation: a case report of fatal brain stem infarct with review of the mechanisms and predisposing factors, J Forensic Sci 32:1089-1094, 1987.
174. Jones KL, and Smith DW: Recognition of the fetal alcohol syndrome in early infancy, Lancet 2:999-1001, 1973.
175. Jones KL, and others: Patterns of malformations in offspring of chronic alcoholic mothers, Lancet 1:1267-1271, 1973.
176. Juul-Jensen P, and Foldspang A: Natural history of epileptic seizures, Epilepsia 24:2297-3112, 1983.
177. Kalimo H, and others: Cellular and subcellular alterations of human CNS: studies utilizing in situ perfusion-fixation in immediate autopsies. Arch Pathol 97:352-359, 1974.
178. Kanter RK: Retinal hemorrhage after cardiopulmonary resuscitation or child abuse, J Pediatr 108:430-432, 1986.
179. Katzman R, and Pappius HM: Brain electrolytes and fluid metabolism, Baltimore, 1973, Williams & Wilkins.
180. Kelly MA, Gorelik PB, and Mirza D: The role of drugs in the etiology of stroke, Clin Neuropharmacol 15:249-275, 1992.
181. Kempe CH, and others: The battered child syndrome, JAMA 181:17-24, 1962.
182. Kennady JC: Investigations of the early fate and removal of subarachnoid blood, Pac Med Surg 75:163-168, 1967.
183. Kinney HC, and others: Neuropathologic findings in the brain of Karen Ann Quinlan: the role of the thalamus in the persistent vegetative state, N Engl J Med 330:1469-1475, 1994.
184. Kinney HC, and Samuels MA: Neuropathology of the persistent vegetative state. A review, J Neuropathol Exp Neurol 53:548-558, 1994.
185. Kirkpatrick JB, and others: In vitro simulation of neural trauma by laser, J Neuropathol Exp Neurol 44:268-284, 1985.
186. Kirkpatrick JB: Forensic considerations in examining the brain, Semin Diagn Pathol 1:98-113, 1985.
187. Kirschner RH, and Stein RJ: The mistaken diagnosis of child abuse. A form of medical abuse? Am J Dis Child 139:873-875, 1985.
188. Kleihues P, Aguzzi A, and Wiestler OD: Cellular and molecular aspects of neurocarcinogenesis. Toxicol Pathol 18:193-203, 1990.
189. Koeppen AH, and Barron KD: Marchiafava-Bignami disease. Neurology 28:290-294, 1978.
190. Konzen JP, Levine SR, and Garcia JH: Vasospasm and thrombus formation as possible mechanisms of stroke related to alkaloidal cocaine, Stroke 26:1114-1118, 1995.
191. Kotila M: Declining incidence and mortality of stroke? Stroke 15:255-259, 1984.
192. Krauland W: The traumatic subarachnoidal hemorrhage, Z Rechtsmed 87:205-215, 1981.
193. Krauland W: ÜDer de Quellen des akuten und chronischen subduralen Hämatomas. Stuttgart, 1961, Thieme.
194. Krauland W: Verletzungen der intrakraniellen Schlagadern, Berlin, 1982, Springer-Verlag.
195. Kravitz H, and others: Accidental falls from elevated surfaces in infants from birth to one year of age. Pediatrics (suppl) 44: 869-876, 1969.
196. Kreisman NR, Sick TJ, and Rosenthal M: Importance of vascular responses in determining cortical oxygenation during recurrent paroxysmal events of varying duration and frequency of repetition, J Cereb Blood Flow Metab 3:330-338, 1983.
197. Krigman MR, Bouldin TW, and Mushak P: Lead. In Spencer PS, and Schaumburg HH, editors: Experimental and Clinical Neurotoxicology, Baltimore, 1980. Williams & Wilkins.
198. Kuller L, Lilienfeld A, and Fisher R: An epidemiological study of sudden and unexpected deaths in adults, Medicine 46:341-361, 1967.
199. Kuller L: Sudden and unexpected non-traumatic death in adults: a review of epidemiological and clinical studies, J Chron Dis 19:1165-1192, 1966.
200. Kurland LT, Faro SN, and Seidler H: Minamata disease, World Neurol 1:370-395, 1960.
201. Kurtzke JF, Golderg ID, and Kurland LT: The distribution of deaths from congenital malformations of the nervous system, Neurology 23:483-496, 1973.
202. Lagercrantz H, and Slotkin TA: The "stress" of being born. Sci Am 254:922-998, 1986.
203. Lambert SR, Johnson TE, and Hoyt CS: Optic nerve sheath and retinal hemorrhages associated with the shaken baby syndrome, Arch Ophthalmol 104:1509-1512, 1986.
204. Lamire RJ, Beckwith JB, and Warkany J: Anencephaly. New York, 1978, Raven Press.
205. Langlois NEI, and Gresham GA: The aging of bruises: a review and study of the colour changes with time, Forensic Sci Int 50: 227-238, 1991.
206. Langston JW: MPTP neurotoxicity: an overview and characterization of phases of toxicity, Life Sci 36:201-206, 1985.
207. LaPresle J, and Fardeau M: The central nervous system and carbon monoxide poisoning; II. Anatomical study of brain lesions following intoxication with carbon monoxide (22 cases), Prog Brain Res 24:31-74, 1967.
208. Larroche JC: Lesions of the ischaemic type, mainly arterial. In: Developmental pathology of the neonate. Amsterdam, 1977, Excerpta Medica.
209. Lathers CM, Schraeder PL, and Weiner FL: Synchronization of cardiac autonomic neural discharge with epileptogenic activity: the lock step phenomenon, Electroencephalogr Clin Neurophysiol 67:247-259, 1987.
210. Lathers CM, and Schraeder PL: Sudden death in epileptic persons: occurrence and possible causes. New York, 1990, Marcel Dekker.
211. Leestma JE, and others: Sudden unexplained death in epilepsy (SUDEP) in the Lamotrigine clinical development program. Epilepsia (in press, 1997).
212. Leestma JE, Hughes JR, and Diamond ER: Temporal correlates in brain death. EEG and clinical relationships to the respirator brain, Arch Neurol 41:147-152, 1984.
213. Leestma JE, Kalelkar MB, and Teas SS: Ponto-medullary avulsion associated with cervical hyperextension. In Adams JH, editor: Trauma and regeneration. Acta Neurochir (Suppl) 32:69-73, 1983.
214. Leestma JE, and others: Sudden unexpected death associated with seizures; analysis of 66 cases. Epilepsia 25:84-88, 1984.
215. Leestma JE, and Konakci Y: Sudden unexpected death caused by neuroepithelial (colloid) cyst of the third ventricle, J Forensic Sci 26:486-491, 1981.
216. Leestma JE, and Magee DJ: Pathology and neuropathology in the forensic setting. In Leestma JE, editor: Forensic neuropathology, New York, 1988, Raven Press.
217. Leestma JE, and others: A prospective study on sudden unexpected death in epilepsy, Ann Neurol 26:195-203, 1989.
218. Leestma JE: Forensic neuropathology. In Duckett S, editor: Pediatric neuropathology, Baltimore, 1995, Williams & Wilkins.
219. Leestma JE: Forensic neuropathology, New York, 1988, Raven Press.
220. Leestma JE: Natural history of epilepsy. In Lathers CM, and Schraeder PL, editors: Sudden death in epileptic persons: occurrence and possible causes, New York, 1990, Marcel Dekker.
221. Lemmon GW, and others: Determination of brain death with use of color duplex scanning in the intensive care unit setting, Arch Surg 11130:517-520, 1995.
222. Levin HS: Outcome after head injury: general considerations and neurobehavioral recovery. Part II: Neurobehavioral recovery. In Becker DP, and Povlishock JT, editors: Central nervous

system trauma status report—1985, Volume 31, Bethesda, Maryland, 1987, Nat Inst Neurol Communic Dis Stroke.

223. Lin RS, and others: Occupational exposure to electromagenntic fields and the occurrence of brain tumors. An analysis of possible associations, J Occup Med 27:413-419, 1985.
224. Lindenberg R: Compression of brain arteries as pathogenetic factor for tissue necrosis and their areas of predilection, J Neuropathol Exp Neurol 14:223-243, 1955.
225. Lindenberg R, and Freytag E: The mechanism of cerebral contusions, a pathologic-anatomic study, Arch Pathol 69:440-469, 1960.
226. Lindenberg R, and Freytag E: Brainstem lesions characteristic of traumatic hyperextension of the head, Arch Pathol 90:509-515, 1973.

226a. Lindenberg R, and Freytag E: Morphology of brain lesions from blunt trauma in early infancy, Arch Pathol 87:298-305, 1969.

227. Lindenberg R, and Freytag E: Morphology of cortical contusions, Arch Pathol 63:23-42, 1957.
228. Lindenberg R, and Freytag E: Trauma of the meninges and brain. In Minckler J, editor: Pathology of the nervous system, vol 2, New York, 1971, McGraw-Hill.
229. Lindenberg R: Systemic oxygen deficiencies: the respirator brain. In Minckler J, editor: Pathology of the nervous system, New York, 1971, McGraw-Hill.
230. Lindenberg RL: Anoxia does not produce brain damage, Japan J Legal Med 36:38-57, 1981.
231. Lindenberg RL: Mechanical injuries of brain and meninges. In Spitz WU, and Fisher RS, editors: Medicolegal investigation of death. Guidelines for the application of pathology to crime investigation, Springfield, Illinois, 1974, Charles C Thomas.
232. Lipton HL, and Teasdale RD: Acute transverse myelopathy in adults. A follow-up study, Arch Neurol 28:252-257, 1973.
233. Locksley HB: Natural history of subarachnoid hemorrhage: intracranial aneurysms and arteriovenous malformations. Based on 6368 cases in the cooperative study. In Sahs AL, and others, editors: Intracranial aneurysms and subarachnoid hemorrhage. A cooperative study, Philadelphia, 1969, JB Lippincott.
234. Ludwig S: Shaken baby syndrome. A review of 20 cases. Ann Emerg Med 13:104-107, 1984.
235. Ludwin SK, and Norman MG: Congenital malformations of the nervous system. In Davis RL, and Robertson DM, editors: Textbook of neuropathology, Baltimore, 1985, Williams & Wilkins.
236. Majak M, Majak J, and Papierz W: Morphological changes in the brains of female patients who died in connection with pregnancy or delivery, Acta Neuropathol (suppl) 7:375-380, 1981.
237. Mandybur TI, Stephen RD, and Bates MB: Fatal massive intracerebral hemorrhage complicating cerebral amyloid angiopathy, Arch Neurol 35:246-248, 1978.
238. Maretic Z: Some clinical and epidemiological problems of venom poisoning today. Toxicon 20:345-348, 1982.
239. Margolis G: The vascular changes and pathogenesis of hypertensive intracranial hemorrhage. In: Cerebrovascular disease, ARNMD Vol XLI, Baltimore, 1969, Williams & Wilkins.
240. Marsden CD, and Reynolds EH: Neurology. In Laidlaw J, and Richens A, editors: A Textbook of Epilepsy, ed 2 Edinburgh, 1982, Churchill-Livingstone.
241. Matsumoto N, and others: Natural history of stroke in Rochester, Minnesota, 1955 through 1969: an extension of a previous study, 1945 through 1954, Stroke 4:20-29, 1973.
242. McCandless DW, and others: Status epilepticus-induced changes in primate cortical energy metabolism, Am J Physiol 251:C774-779, 1986.
243. McClure WO: Effect of drugs upon axoplasmic transport, Adv Pharmacol Chemother 10:185-200, 1975.
244. McCormick WF: Pathology of closed head injury. In Wilkins RH, and Rengachary SS, editors: Neurosurgery, New York, 1985, McGraw-Hill.
245. McDowell FH: Cerebral embolism. In Vinken PJ, and Bruyn GW, editors: Handbook of clinical neurology. Vascular diseases of the nervous system, vol. II. Amsterdam, 1972, Elsevier-North Holland. pp 386-414.
246. McKissock W, and others: Extradural hematoma: observations on 125 cases, Lancet 2:167-172, 1960.
247. McNamara JJ, and others: Lipid metabolism after trauma. Role in the pathogenesis of fat embolism. J Trauma 63:968-972, 1972.
248. Meldrum BS, and Corsellis JAN: Epilepsy. In Adams JH, Corsellis JAN, and Duchen LW, editors: Greenfield's neuropathology, ed 4 New York, 1984, John Wiley.
249. Meller JL, and Shermeta DW: Falls in urban children. A problem revisited, Am J Dis Child 141:1271-1275, 1987.
250. Merten DF and Osborne DRS: Craniocerebral trauma in the child abuse syndrome, Pediatr Annu 12:882-887, 1983.
251. Milo R, Razon N, and Schiffer J: Delayed epidural hematoma. Review, Acta Neurochir 84:13-23, 1987.
252. Minna JD, Robboy SJ, and Colman RW: Disseminated intravascular coagulation in man, Springfield, 1974, Charles C Thomas.
253. Moenssens AA, Moses RE, and Inbau FE: Scientific evidence in criminal cases. Mineola, New York, 1973, The Foundation Press.
254. Mori K, and others: Epidural hematomas of the posterior fossa in children, Childs Brain 10:130-140, 1983.
255. Morin MA, and Pitts FW: Delayed apoplexy following head injury ("traumatische Spat-Apoplexie"). J Neurosurg 33:542-547, 1970.
256. Moseley JI, Molinari GF, and Walker AE: Respirator brain: report of a survey and review of the current concepts. Arch Pathol Lab Med 100:61-64, 1976.
257. Munro D: The diagnosis and treatment of subdural hematomata, N Engl J Med 210:1145-1160, 1934.
258. Munro D, and Merritt HH: Surgical pathology of subdural hematoma. Based on a study of one hundred and five cases, Arch Neurol Psychiatry 35:64-78, 1936.
259. Nelson KD, and Ellenberg JH: Intrapartum events and cerebral palsy. In Kubli F, and others, editors: Perinatal events and brain damage in surviving children. Berlin, 1988, Springer-Verlag.
260. Nelson KD, and Ellenberg JH: Apgar scores as predictors of chronic neurologic disability, Pediatrics 68:38-44, 1981.
261. New MI, and others: Preclinical Creutzfeldt-Jakob disease discovered at autopsy in a human growth hormone recipient, Neurology 38:1133-1134, 1988.
262. New York Times, August 2, 1966.
263. New York Times, August 3, 1966.
264. New York Times, September 9, 1966.
265. New York Times, August 7, 1966.
266. Norman MG, and others: The postmortem examination on the abused child. Pathological, radiographic, and legal aspects, Perspect Pediatr Pathol 8:313-343, 1984.
267. Nosek-Cenkowska B, and others: Bleeding/bruising symptomatology in children with and without bleeding disorders, Thromb Haemost 65:237-241, 1991.
268. Ober RR: Hemorrhagic retinopathy in infancy: a clinicopathologic report. J Pediatr Ophthalmol Strabismus 17:17-20, 1980.
269. Oehmichen M, and Raff G: Timing of cortical contusion. Correlation between histomorphologic alterations and post-traumatic interval. Z Rechtsmed 84:79-94, 1980.
270. Ommaya AK, Faas F, and Yarnell P: Whiplash injury and brain damage. An experimental study. JAMA 204:285-289, 1968.
271. Ommaya AK, Grubb RL Jr, and Naumann RA: Coup and contre-coup injury. Observations on the mechanics of visible brain injuries in the rhesus monkey. J Neurosurg 35:503-516, 1971.
272. Ommaya AK, and Yarnell P: Subdural hematoma after whiplash injury, Lancet 2:237, 1969.

273. Overgaard J, and Tweed WA: Cerebral circulation after head injury. Part I. Cerebral blood flow and its regulation after closed head injury with emphasis on clinical correlations, J Neurosurg 41:532-541, 1974.
274. Paneth N, and Stark RI: Cerebral palsy and mental retardation in relation to indicators of perinatal asphyxia. An epidemiologic overview, Am J Obstet Gynecol 147:960-966, 1983.
275. Paneth N: The causes of cerebral palsy. Recent evidence, Clin Invest Med 16:95-102, 1993.
276. Pasternak JF, and others: Regional cerebral blood flow in the beagle puppy model of neonatal intraventricular hemorrhage: studies during systemic hypertension, Neurology 33:559-566, 1983.
277. Penry JK: Epilepsy. The Eighth International Symposium. New York, 1977, Raven Press.
278. Physicians' Desk Reference. Oradell, NJ, 1990, Medical Economics Co.
278a. Pickels W: Acute general edema of the brain in children with head injuries. N Engl J Med 242:607-610, 1950.
279. Pilz P, Strohecker J, and Grobovschek M: Survival after traumatic ponto-medullary tear. J Neurol Neurosurg Psychiatry 45: 422-427, 1982.
280. Plum F, and Posner JB: The diagnosis of stupor and coma, ed 3 Philadelphia, 1982, FA Davis.
281. Porter RJ: Epilepsy. 100 elementary principles. Philadelphia, 1960, WB Saunders.
282. Povlishock JT, and others: The morphopathologic substrates of concussion, Acta Neuropathol 47:1-11, 1979.
283. Povlishock JT, and others: Vascular permeability alterations to horseradish peroxidase in experimental brain injury, Brain Res 153:223-39, 1978.
284. Povlishock JT, and others: Axonal change in minor head injury, J Neuropathol Exp Neurol 42:225-242, 1983.
285. Powers JM, and McKeever PE: Central pontine myelinolysis. An ultrastructural and elemental study. J Neurol Sci 29:65-81, 1976.
286. Preziosi TJ, and others: An experimental investigation in animals of the functional and morphologic effects of single and repeated exposures to high and low concentrations of carbon monoxide, Ann NY Acad Sci 174:369-384, 1970.
287. Prineas J: The pathogenesis of dying-back polyneuropathies. I. An ultrastructural study of experimental tri-orth-cresyl phosphate intoxication in the cat, J Neuropathol Exp Neurol 28:571-597, 1969.
288. Pudenz RH, and Shelden CH: The Lucite calvarium—a method for direct observation of the brain, J Neurosurg 3:487-505, 1946.
289. Ramon y Cajal S: Degeneration and regeneration of the nervous system. May RM, editor and translator. London, 1968, Hafner.
290. Rappaport EB: Iatrogenic Creutzfeldt-Jakob disease, Neurology 37:1520-1522, 1987.
291. Realini JP, and Goldsieher JW: Oral contraceptives and cardiovascular disease: a critique of the epidemiologic studies, Am J Obstet Gynecol 152:729-798, 1985.
292. Reuler JB, Girard DE, and Cooney TG: Current concepts—Wernicke's encephalopathy, N Engl J Med 312:1035-1038, 1985.
293. Rinsky LA: A cervical spinal cord injury following chiropractic manipulation, Paraplegia 13:223-227, 1976.
294. Roizin L, Shiraki H, and Grcevic N, editors: Neurotoxicology. New York, 1977, Raven Press.
295. Rose J, Valtonen S, and Jennett B: Avoidable factors contributing to death after head injury, Br Med J 2:615-618, 1977.
296. Rouzaud M, and Lutier J: Oedeme subaigue cerébromeninge dué à une intoxication d'actualité. Presse Med 62:1075, 1954.
297. Royal College of General Practitioners Oral Contraceptive Study. Further analysis of mortality in oral contraceptive users, Lancet 1:541-546, 1981.
298. Rudelli R, Byrne J, and Wisniewski HM: A technique for fetal brain removal, Arch Pathol Lab Med 107:144-146, 1981.
299. Sahenk Z, and Mendell JR: Analysis of fast axoplasmic transport in nerve ligation and adriamycin-induced neuronal perikaryon lesions. Brain Res 171:414-453, 1979.
300. Sartwell PE, and others: Thromboembolism and oral contraceptives: an epidemiologic case-controlled study, Am J Epidemiol 90:365-380, 1969.
301. Schachenmayr W, and Friede RL: The origin of subdural neomembranes. I. Fine structure of the dura-arachnoid interface in man, Am J Pathol 92:53-68, 1978.
302. Schachenmayr W, Friede RL: The origin of subdural neomembranes. II. Fine structure of neomembranes, Am J Pathol 92:69-79, 1978.
303. Schade JP, and McMenemey WH: Selective vulnerability of the brain in hypoxemia, Philadelphia, 1963, FA Davis.
304. Scheller JM, and Nelson KB: Does caesarian delivery prevent cerebral palsy or other neurologic problems of childhood? Obstet Gynecol 83:624-630, 1994.
305. Schellhas KP, and others: Vertebrobasilar injuries following cervical manipulation, JAMA 244:1450-1453, 1980.
306. Schmidley JW, and Koch T: The non-cerebrovascular complications of chiropractic manipulation, Neurology 34:684-685, 1984.
307. Schmidley JW: Cerebrospinal fluid, blood-brain barrier, and brain edema. In Pearlman AL, and Collins RC, editors: Neurological pathophysiology, ed 3, New York, 1984, Oxford University Press.
308. Schmitt HP: Ruptures and thromboses of the vertebral artery following closed mechanical injuries, Schweiz Arch Neurol Neurochir Psychiatr 119:363-379, 1976.
309. Schoenberg BS, and others: Strokes in women of childbearing age. A populations study, Neurology 20:181, 189, 1970.
310. Schwarz G, and others: Brain death: timing of apnea testing in primary brain stem lesion, Int Care Med 18:315-316, 1992.
311. Shapiro K: Head injury in children. In Becker DP, and Povlishock JT, editors: Central nervous system trauma status report—1985, Volume 31, Bethesda, Maryland, 1987, Nat Inst Neurol Communic Dis Stroke.
312. Shelanski ML, and Wisniewski H: Neurofibrillary degeneration induced by vincristine therapy, Arch Neurol 20:199-206, 1969.
313. Sherman DG, Hart RG, and Easton JD: Abrupt change in head position and cerebral infarction, Stroke 12:2-6, 1981.
314. Smith MD, Burrington JD, and Woolf AD: Injuries in children sustained in free falls: an analysis of 66 cases, J Trauma 15:987-991.
315. Snoek JW, Minderhoud JM, and Wilmink JT: Delayed deterioration following mild head injury in children, Brain 107:15-36, 1984.
316. Spencer PS, and Schaumberg HH. Experimental and clinical neurotoxicology. Baltimore, 1980, Williams & Wilkins.
317. Spitz WU, and Fisher RS: Medicolegal investigation of death. Guidelines for the application of pathology to crime investigation. Springfield, Illinois, 1973, Charles C Thomas.
318. Stetler JC, and Moritz AR: Doctor and patient and the law. St. Louis, 1962, CV Mosby.
319. Stone JL, and others: Subdural hematomas. I. Acute subdural hematoma: progress in definition, clinical pathology, and therapy, Surg Neurol 19:216-231, 1983.
320. Strich S: Lesions in the cerebral hemispheres after blunt head trauma, J Clin Pathol (suppl) 23:166-171, 1970.
321. Strich S: Shearing of nerve fibers as a cause of brain damage due to head injury. Lancet 2:443-448, 1961.
322. Sunshine P: Epidemiology of perinatal asphyxia. In Stevenson DI, and Sunshine P, editors: Fetal and neonatal brain injury. Mechanisms, management and the risks of practice. Philadelphia, 1989, BC Decker.
323. Swenberg JA, and others: Quantitative aspects of transplacental tumor induction with ethylnitrosourea in rats, Cancer Res 32: 2656-2660, 1972.

324. Tedeschi CG, Eckert WG, and Tedeschi LG: Forensic medicine: a study in trauma and environmental hazards. Philadelphia, 1977, WB Saunders.
325. Terrence CF, Rao GR, and Perper JA: Neurogenic pulmonary edema in unexpected unexplained death of epileptic patients, Ann Neurol 9:458-464, 1981.
326. Terrence CF, Wisotskey HM, and Perper JA: Unexpected unexplained death in epileptic patients, Neurology 25:594-598, 1975.
327. The Task Force for the Study of Non-accidental Injuries and Child Deaths: Protocol for child death autopsies. Illinois Dept Child Fam Services, Chicago, 1987.
328. Thomas TL, and others: Brain tumor mortality risk among men with electrical and electronics jobs. A case control study, J Natl Cancer Inst 79:233-238, 1987.
329. Tomlinson BE: Brain-stem lesions after head injury, J Clin Pathol (suppl 4) 23:154-165, 1970.
330. Torack RM, Terry RD, and Zimmerman HM: The fine structure of cerebral fluid accumulation; II. Swelling produced by triethyltin poisoning and its comparison with that in the human brain, Am J Pathol 36:273-287, 1960.
331. Tornheim PA: Traumatic edema in head injury. In Becker DP, and Pavlishock JT, editors: Central nervous system trauma status report–1985, volume 31, Bethesda, Maryland, 1987, Nat Inst Neurol Communic Dis Stroke.
332. Torvik A, Lindboe CF, and Rogde S: Brain lesions in alcoholics. A neuropathological study with clinical correlations, J Neurol Sci 56:233-248, 1982.
333. Towbin A: Obstetric malpractice litigation. The pathologist's view, Am J Obstet Gynecol 155:927-935, 1986.
334. Unterharnscheidt F: Neuropathology of rhesus monkeys undergoing $-G_x$ impact acceleration. In Ewing CL, and others, editors: Impact injury of the head and spine, Springfield, IL, 1983, Charles C Thomas.
335. Unterharnscheidt F, and Sellier K: Mechanics and pathomorphology of closed brain injuries. In Caveness WS, and Walker AE, editors: Head injury. Conference proceedings, Philadelphia, 1966, JB Lippincott.
336. Urich H: Malformations of the nervous system, perinatal damage and related conditions in early life. In Blackwood W, Corsellis N, editors: Greenfield's neuropathology, London 1976, Edward Arnold.
337. Vessey MP: Oral contraception and thromboembolic disease, Am Heart J 78:285-286, 1969.
338. Vessey MP, and Doll R: Investigation of relation between use of oral contraception and thromboembolic disease. A further report, Br Med J 2:651-657, 1968.
339. Vessey MP, McPherson K, and Johnson B: Mortality among women participating in the Oxford/Family Planning Association contraceptive study, Lancet 2:731-733, 1977.
340. Victor M, Adams R, and Mancall EL: A restricted form of cerebellar cortical degeneration occurring in alcoholic patients, Arch Neurol 1:579-688, 1959.
341. Victor M, Adams RD, and Collins GH: The Wernicke-Korsakov syndrome: a clinical pathological study of 245 patients, 82 with post-mortem examinations. Oxford, 1971, Blackwell.
342. Vinken PJ, and Bruyn GW: Congenital malformations of the brain and skull. Handbook of neurology, Amsterdam, 1977, Elsevier-North Holland.
343. Voigt E, and Löwenhielm P: "Gliding contusions" des Grosshirns, Hefte Unfallheilk 117:329-335, 1974.
344. Voigt GE, Löwenhielm CG, and Ljung CB: Rotational cerebral injuries near the superior margin of the brain, Acta Neuropathol 39:201-209, 1977.
345. von Hochsteter AR, and Friede RL: Residual lesions of cerebral fat embolism, J Neurol 216:227-233, 1977.
346. Waga S, Tochio H, and Sakakura M: Traumatic cerebral swelling developing within 30 minutes after injury, Surg Neurol 11: 191-193, 1979.
347. Wagner FC Jr, Dohrmann GJ, and Bucy PC: Histopathology of transitory traumatic paraplegia in the monkey, J Neurosurg 35: 272-276, 1971.
348. Walker AE: Cerebral death, ed 2. Baltimore, 1981, Urban & Schwarzenberg.
349. Walker AE, Diamond EL, and Moseley J: The neuropathological findings in irreversible coma: a critque of the "respirator" brain, J Neuropathol Exp Neurol 34:296-323, 1975.
350. Warner KG, and Demling RH: The pathophysiology of free-fall injury, Ann Emerg Med 15:1088-1093, 1986.
351. Watanabe S, Shimada H, and Ishii S: Production of clinical form of chronic subdural hematoma in experimental animals, J Neurosurg 37:552-561, 1972.
352. Weber W: Experimentelle Untersuchungen zu Schädelbruchverletzungen des Säuglings. Rechtsmed 92:87-94, 1984.
353. Weedn VW, Mansour AM, and Nichols MM: Retinal hemorrhage in an infant after cardiopulmonary resuscitation, Am J Forensic Med Pathol 11:79-82, 1990.
354. Weir B: The osmolality of subdural hematoma fluid. J Neurosurg 34:528-533, 1971.
355. Weir B, and Gordon P: Factors affecting coagulation: fibrinolysis in chronic subdural fluid collections. J Neurosurg 58:242-245, 1983.
356. Weller RO: Iatrogenic transmission of Creutzfeldt-Jakob disease. Psychol Med 19:1-4, 1989.
357. Weston JT: The pathology of child abuse. In Helfer RE, and Kempe CH, editors: The battered child, Chicago, 1968, University of Chicago Press.
358. White RJ, and others: Spinal cord injury: sequential morphology and hypothermic stabilization. Surg Forum 20:432-434, 1969.
359. Wigglesworth JS: Perinatal pathology. Philadelphia, 1986, WB Saunders.
360. Wigmore, JH: Evidence in trials at common law. Boston, 1974, Little, Brown.
361. Wilson EF: Estimation of the age of cutaneous contusions in child abuse. Pediatrics 60:750-752, 1977.
362. Woodburne RT: Essentials of human anatomy, ed 4. New York, 1983, Oxford University Press.
363. Yamashima T, and Friede RL: Why do bridging veins rupture into the virtual subdural space? J Neurol Neurosurg Psychiatry 47:121-127, 1984.
364. Zepp F, and others: Battered child syndrome: cerebral ultrasound and CT findings after vigorous shaking. Neuropediatrics 23:188-191, 1992.
365. Zielinski JJ: Epidemiology. In Laidlaw J, and Richens A, editors: A textbook of epilepsy, Edinburgh, 1982, Churchill-Livingstone.
366. Zimmerman HM, and Yannet H: Kernicterus jaundice of the nuclear masses of the brain. Am J Dis Child 45:740-759, 1933.
367. Zimmerman RA, and others: Computed tomography of pediatric head trauma: acute general cerebral swelling. Radiology 126: 403-408, 1978.

C · H · A · P · T · E · R

# 12

# *Microscopic Criteria to Determine Gestational Age of the Fetal and Neonatal Brain*

**Harvey B. Sarnat**



The weight and gross anatomic features of the developing brain change in a predictable sequence that correlates with gestational age in the normal fetus and premature infant. External morphologic criteria also predict gestational age within a 2-week period at autopsy. These include the closure of the operculum to cover the insula, the closely time-linked formation of gyri and sulci of the cerebral cortex, and the size of the cerebellum relative to surrounding structures.

Histologic criteria are equally useful in estimating gestational age in brains of fetuses, preterm and term neonates, and postmature infants, using sections stained with simple histologic stains such as hematoxylin-eosin or cresyl violet. Special histochemical and immunocytochemical stains add another dimension of precision to this correlation, but the present chapter will focus on maturational features detected by ordinary histologic examination.

Several specific parts of the brain are particularly useful in determining maturation or gestational age. Structures that undergo development very early in ontogenesis, such as the nuclei of the brainstem, are not as helpful for this purpose. Processes such as myelination of the subcortical white matter or of the corpus callosum also are not helpful in the perinatal period because of their later postnatal development. Structures that undergo major morphologic change during the second half of gestation are ideal for estimating gestational age in the fetus and neonate.

## HISTOLOGIC REGIONS OF THE BRAIN USEFUL FOR ESTIMATING GESTATIONAL AGE

### Cerebellum

Because of its clearly defined histologic features, limited number of neuronal types, and morphologic development, the cerebellar cortex was recognized early in the 20th century as one of the easiest and most reliable structures of the brain to demonstrate predictable maturational changes that correlate with gestational age.* These early observations have been reconfirmed and expanded by modern neuroembryologists, and the growth parameters and histologic progression of development, both prenatally and postnatally, continue to provide objective estimation of gestational age.†

**External granular layer.** The external granular layer (EGL) consists of premigratory granule cells that spread out over the surface of the entire cerebellar cortex at the eighth week of gestation (stage 23) from a different germinal plate of the rhombic lip than gives origin to Purkinje cells and neurons of the deep cerebellar nuclei. The superficial part of the EGL is a proliferative zone of neuroepithelial cells still undergoing active mitosis; these cells have dark, round nuclei and sparse cytoplasm. The inner half of the EGL is composed of postmitotic premigratory neuroblasts with elongated nuclei or a spindle shape; they exhibit less densely compacted chromatin (Figs. 12-1 to 12-4). EGL neuroblasts migrate through the molecular and Purkinje cell layers of the cerebellar cortex, guided by radial glial fibers of the Bergmann cells, whose cell bodies reside in the Purkinje cell layer, to reach the internal granular layer, where they join previously migrated EGL cells to complete their maturation as granule neurons and form synaptic "glomeruli."

The thickness of the EGL is approximately the same as that of the molecular zone underlying it and does not change appreciably between 24 weeks' gestation and the second to fourth postnatal months, when it decreases rapidly in size.[15] It is about six to eight cells thick during this time, but at 4 to 6 months it is two cells thick, and by 9 months it forms a continuous single cell layer over the cerebellar surface (Fig. 12-5). It then becomes discontinuous, and by 12 months of age only occasional isolated premigratory EGL cells remain over the lateral hemispheres of the cerebellum. The EGL over the vermis disappears earlier, varying from 4 to 12 months.[5,15] There is much more age variance in the timing of complete disappearance of the EGL than in the timing of its involution between 2 and 4 months of postnatal life.[15] Premature birth does not affect the rate of involution of the EGL in healthy infants, so that adjusted gestational age or "conceptional age" should always be considered.

The internal granular layer remains sparsely populated with cells, and its margin with the deep white matter indistinct, until about 32 weeks' gestation in the cerebellar hemispheres; in the vermis, the increase in cellular density begins at 30 weeks, and by 36 weeks the internal granular layer is sharply demarcated from the core white matter of each folium.[15]

The bipolar shape of external granule cells is best appreciated in sagittal or parasagittal sections of the cerebellum because of their uniform orientation; in transverse sections they appear round and are more difficult to distinguish from the less mature EGL cells in the outer proliferative zone. During actual migration through the molecular layer, the spindle-shaped granule cells become reoriented with their long axis perpendicular to the cerebellar surface and may be identified as bipolar cells in any plane of section.[41]

**Lamina dissecans.** This transitory fetal zone interposed between Purkinje cells and the internal granular layers forms at about 21 weeks and persists only until 32 weeks' gestation (Fig. 12-1). It consists of thick preterminal axonal segments.[36] It appears in histologic sections as a cell-sparse, amorphous eosinophilic lamina and temporarily creates a five-layered cerebellar cortex (EGL, molecular layer, Purkinje cell layer, lamina dissecans, internal granular layer) that makes the fetal cerebellum appear more complex than the simpler three-layered adult cerebellar cortex. It is a reliable marker of this 11-week period in gestation.

**Purkinje cell morphology.** In the term neonate, as in the adult, Purkinje cells are easy to identify by their distinctive size, shape, and position within the folium. Purkinje cells in the vermis begin their growth at about 25 weeks' gestation and, in the cerebellar hemispheres, at about 33 weeks; prior to those times, the Purkinje cells have sparse cytoplasm and only rudimentary dendritic arborization, and are difficult to distinguish histologically from surrounding cells (Fig. 12-1).[15,51] Development of the internal granular layer starts considerably earlier than does the growth of Purkinje dendrites in the molecular layer, though the axons of granule cells that form the parallel fibers of the molecular layer are extended *before* the migration of granule cells from the EGL through the molecular layer.[1,48] At 25 weeks' gestation, Purkinje cells are not yet neatly aligned as a single row of cells in the folium, but rather as a row two to four cells thick; by 32 weeks a continuous single row of Purkinje cells is seen.

**Neuroepithelial cell rests.** Clusters of undifferentiated neuroepithelial cells often are found in the deep

* Refs. 5, 6, 9, 13, 14, 20, 43.

† Refs. 15, 16, 32, 36, 40, 51.

A

B

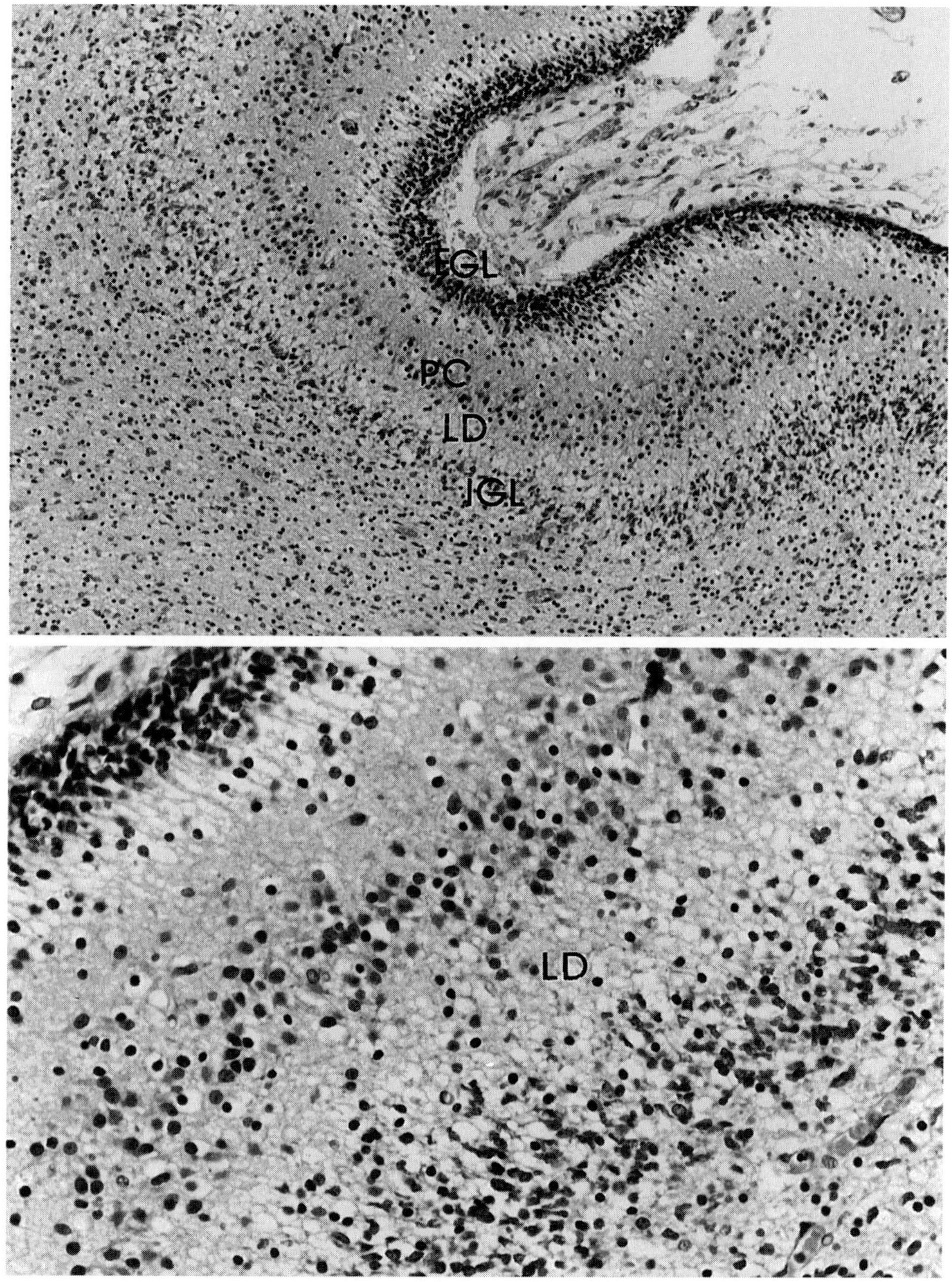


**Fig. 12-1.** Cerebellar cortex of lateral hemisphere of a fetus of 23 weeks' gestation. Purkinje cells (PC) have little cytoplasm and lack their characteristic mature morphology. The internal granular layer (IGL) is sparsely populated and not demarcated from the underlying white matter. The external granular layer (EGL) of premigratory neuroblasts is prominent. The lamina dissecans (LD) is a cell-sparse lamina between the PC layer and the IGL and persists only until 32 weeks' gestation. (**A**, H&E; ×100; **B**, H&E; ×250.)

cerebellar white matter of the vermis, in or near the midline at midgestation; these disappear by 28 weeks' gestation and are rare after that age.[16,40] They should not be confused with pathologic heterotopia. It is uncertain how these persistent primitive neural cells differentiate and where they go.

## Subpial Granular Layer of Cerebral Cortex

The subpial granular layer of the cerebral cortex arises as columns of neuroectodermal cells from the subventricular zone of the hippocampus and forms a thin layer at the surface of the archicortex at 12 weeks' gestation.[8] These cells rapidly spread over the neocor-

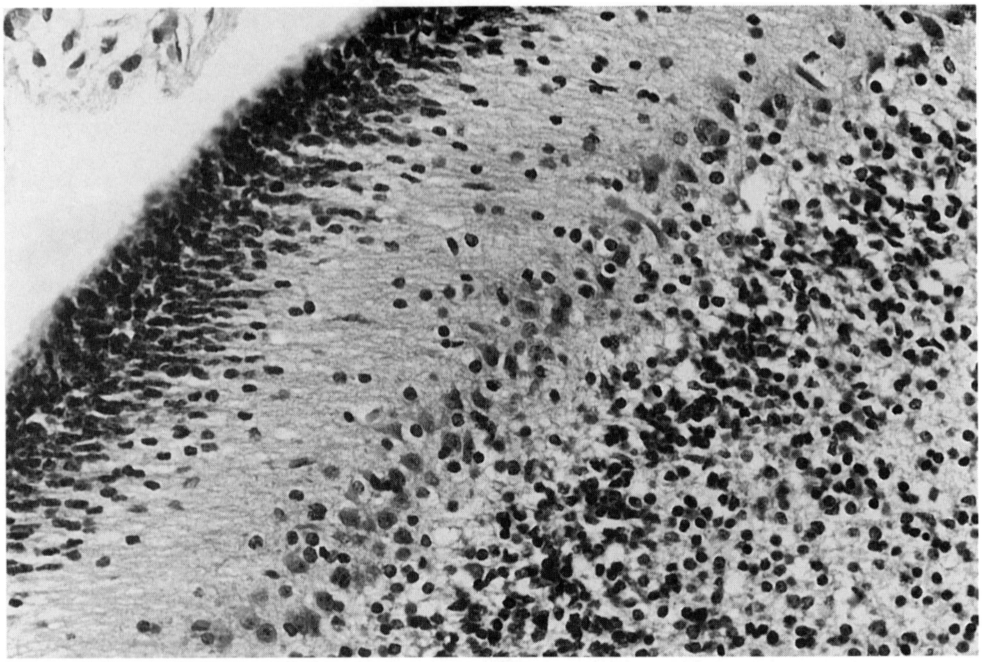

**Fig. 12-2.** Cerebellar cortex of lateral hemisphere at 28 weeks' gestation. Active migration of external granule cells is seen in the molecular layer. Purkinje cells still have sparse cytoplasm but are showing early cytologic distinction. The IGL remains sparsely populated. The lamina dissecans is still present. (H&E; ×250.)

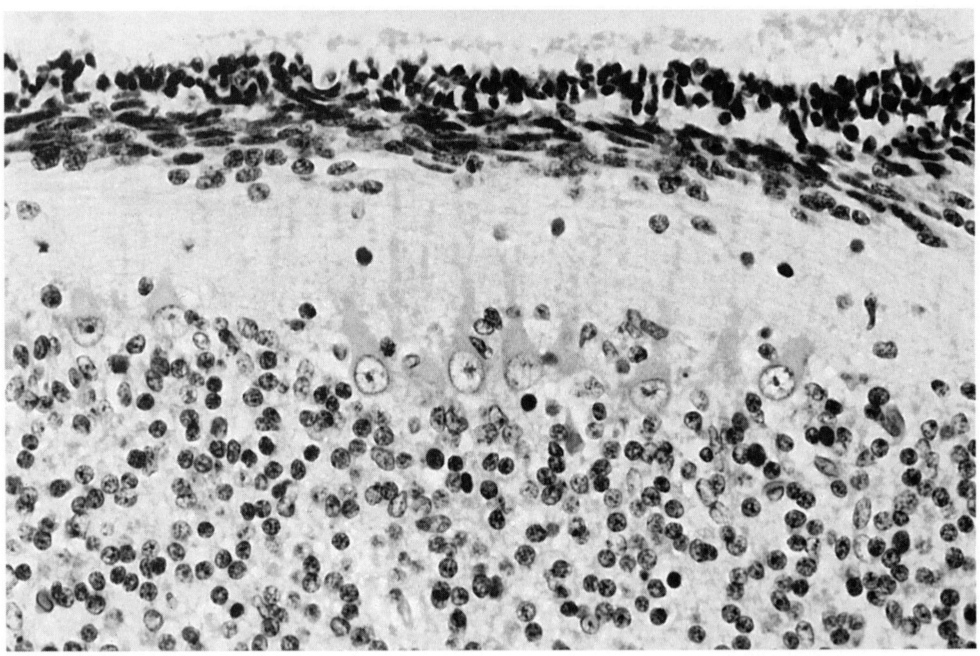

**Fig. 12-3.** Sagittal section of cerebellar vermis at 36 weeks' gestation. The EGL is divided into an outer half of proliferative undifferentiated cells with round nuclei and an inner half of postmitotic, premigratory spindle-shaped neuroblasts, some of which are migrating through the molecular layer. Purkinje cells have more abundant cytoplasm than before 32 weeks and are easily identified. The IGL is still not highly cellular. The lamina dissecans is no longer present. (H&E; ×250.)

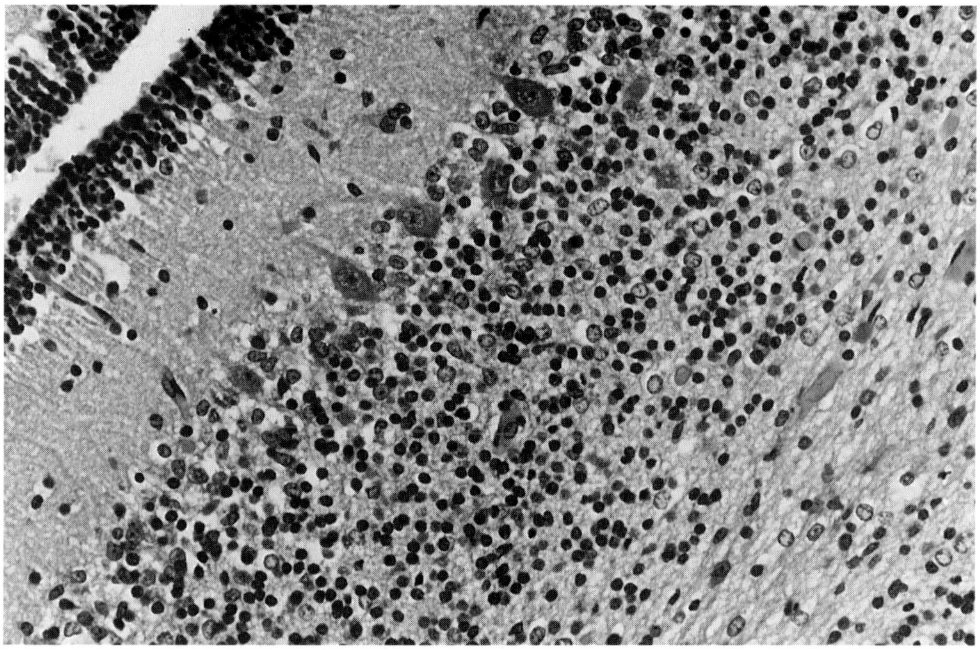

**Fig. 12-4.** Cerebellar cortex, lateral hemisphere, of a term neonate. The EGL is still quite thick, but the IGL also is highly cellular and well demarcated from the white matter. Synaptic glomeruli are forming. Purkinje cells are large and have abundant cytoplasm and prominent basal dendritic trunks. (H&E; ×250.)

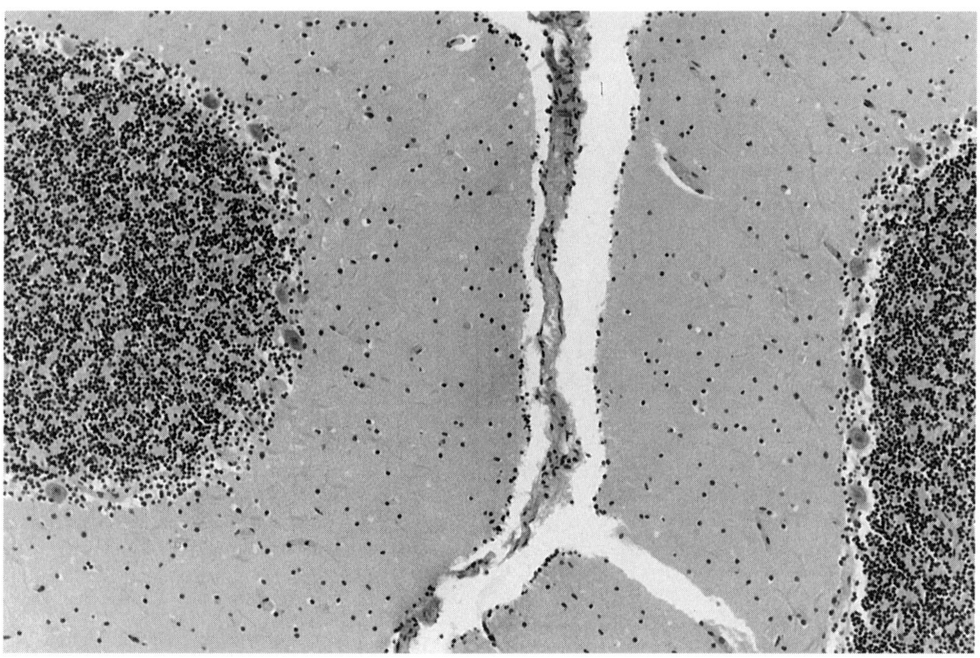

**Fig. 12-5.** Cerebellar cortex, lateral hemisphere, of a 6-month-old infant born at 32 weeks' gestation, adjusted age of 9 months. The EGL is a continuous layer only one cell thick, identical to the expected finding in a 9-month-old infant born at term. Purkinje cells are large and appear mature. The IGL is densely cellular with granule cells and synaptic glomeruli. (H&E; ×100.)

A

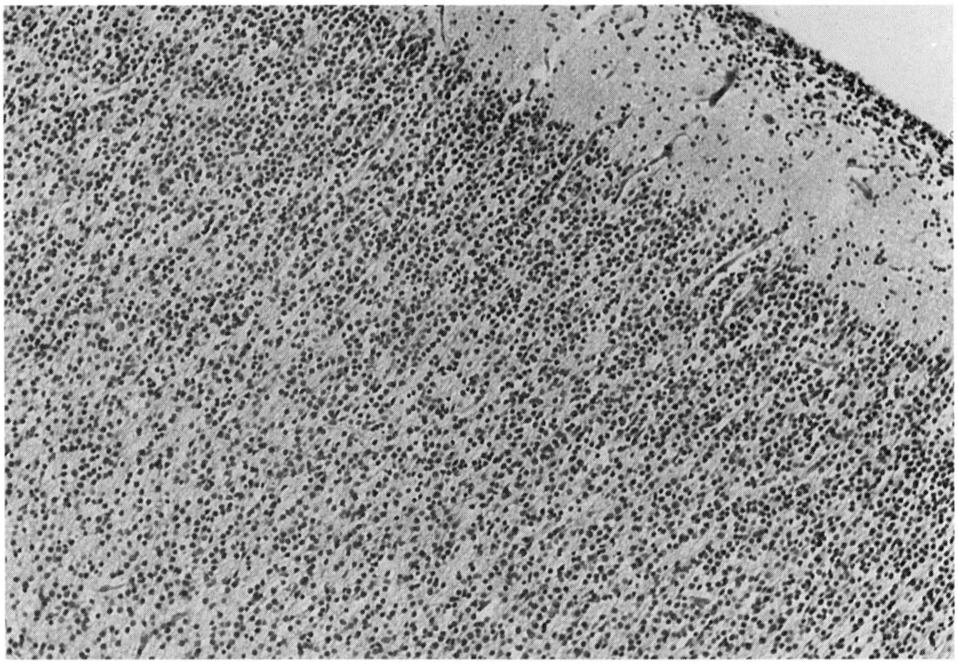

B

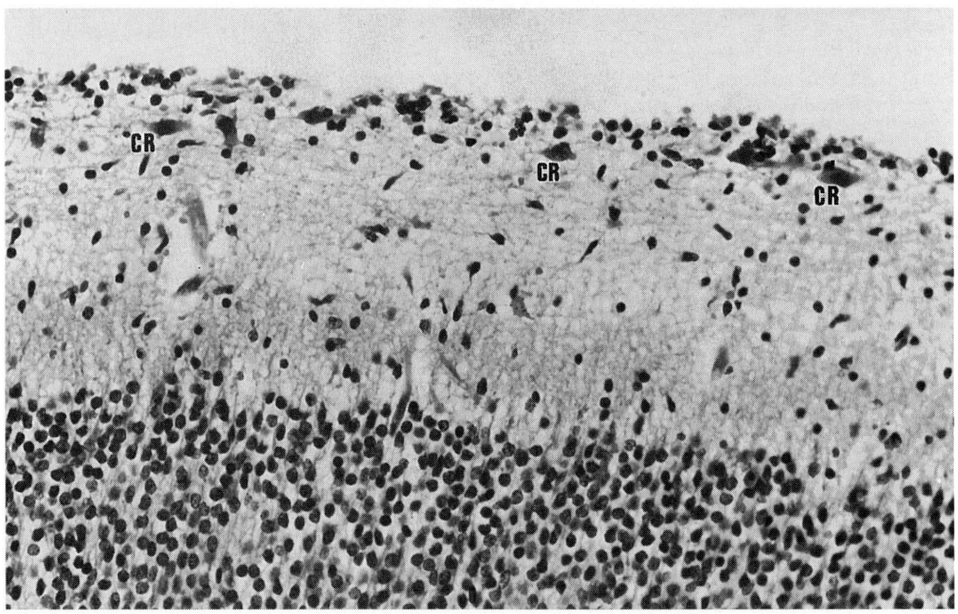


**Fig. 12-6.** Frontal cortex of a preterm infant of 27 weeks' gestation, demonstrating subpial granular layer at the surface. These cells are glial, unlike the premigratory neuroblasts of the external granular layer of the cerebellum. Cajal-Retzius neurons (CR) are seen in the molecular layer. Neurons of the cortical plate are uniform small cells but early lamination is beginning. (**A**, H&E; ×100; **B**, H&E; ×250.)

tex in a predictable sequence to cover the entire convexity of the cerebral hemispheres between the sixteenth and eighteenth weeks of gestation, reaching the greatest thickness of the layer at 22 weeks (Fig. 12-6).[16] Unlike the external granular layer of the cerebellum, which is composed of primordial neurons, subpial granular cells are glial in nature and eventually become mature astrocytes. Subsequent involution of this layer results from migration of the cells into the cerebral cortex, where they no longer are distinguished from other astrocytes. By term, only remnants of this once prominent layer persist, confined to the inferior termporal and frontal orbital surfaces, the last sites from which they disappear.[8]

### Cortical Plate

The cortical plate begins forming with the first wave of radial migration of neuroblasts from the germinal matrix at about 8 weeks' gestation. It forms within the marginal zone, which is then divided into the molecular layer superficially and the subplate zone deep to the cortical plate. The molecular layer becomes layer 1 of the mature cortex; the subplate zone is transitory and becomes incorporated into layer 6 in midgestation. Successive migrations add cells to the cortical plate. Later arrivals remain at the surface of the cortical plate, so that the deepest layers are the earliest migrations, creating an "inside-out" arrangement of the neocortex relative to migratory sequences. In the three-layered paleocortex of the hippocampus, by contrast, the most superficial layer is the earliest to migrate.

By midgestation, the cortical plate is a solid band of homogeneous-appearing, tightly packed cells in a layer about 40 cells thick. Definite laminae cannot yet be distinguished by cell type, cell size, or laminated architecture. The earliest distinction of layers is detected in the motor cortex of the frontal lobe at about 22 weeks, but definite lamination is not generally appreciated histologically until 24 weeks in other areas, and the distinctive six layers are not easily discerned until 32 weeks.

Cajal-Retzius cells (Fig. 12-6) are neurons in the fetal molecular zone and represent the earliest neurons of the future cerebral cortex, being present in the plexiform marginal zone before the first wave of radial migrations is initiated.[12,29,36,40] These bipolar neurons extend their long axons parallel to the cerebral surface and their large dendrites horizontally from the opposite pole.[29,30] Axonal collaterals penetrate the early cortical plate to form synapses with the early migrating neurons that will form layer 6, creating the first intrinsic cortical synaptic circuit. Cajal-Retzius neurons produce both acetylcholine and gamma aminobutyric acid (GABA), and immunocytochemical features suggest that they represent a heterogeneous population.[22,40]

Cajal-Retzius neurons may be demonstrated in the molecular zone of the neocortex throughout most of gestation, but begin to degenerate and decrease in number after 32 weeks as more complex synaptic circuits develop.[11] By term, only a few scattered Cajal-Retzius cells may still be seen.[40]

### Hippocampus

Early stages of hippocampal development are helpful for dating embryonic and early fetal brains. The hippocampal formation, Ammon's horn, and dentate gyrus are the first regions of the forebrain cortex to differentiate, developing within the dorsomedial wall of the cerebral hemisphere adjacent to the lamina terminalis, at about stage 16 (9 mm crown-rump length; 37 postovulatory days).[21,28,33] The hippocampus proper or Ammon's horn precedes, but the dentate gyrus follows, the formation of the olfactory bulbs[21]; the neurohypophysis develops at this same time.[33] The hippocampal formation later rotates into a more ventromedial position with the formation of the lateral ventricles and corpus callosum. At 70 postovulatory days (144 mm), the best developed region of the hippocampal formation is seen in the temporal lobe rather than over the diencephalon; the dorsomedial hippocampus undergoes regressive changes with the development of the corpus callosum at this same time.[28] As the dentate gyrus continues to roll in, the interlocking of it with the hippocampus occurs between 70 and 100 days (112 and 143 mm), thereby establishing the mature relations. Remnants of the early hippocampal formation in the adult brain are the indusium griseum just above the corpus callosum and the septohippocampal nucleus just below it.[28]

At 9 weeks' gestation, the hippocampal region consists of four layers: a ventricular zone of undifferentiated neuroepithelium, an intermediate zone, a homogeneous-appearing hippocampal plate composed of bipolar neurons, and a wide marginal zone; at 15 to 19 weeks individual subfields may be distinguished. A distal-to-proximal gradient of architectural and neuronal morphologic maturity is seen, with the subiculum appearing more advanced in development than the ammonic subfields; the dentate gyrus is the least mature and assumes a mature cytoarchitecture only after 34 weeks.[2]

The characteristic "seahorse" shape of the hippocampus becomes evident at 14 to 15 weeks' gestation.[26] Neurons of the CA2 region mature earliest, followed by those of the endplate; in term neonates these neurons have vesicular nuclei, whereas those in Sommer's sector still retain an immature neuroblastic morphology.[16] The maturation of the cells in Sommer's sector progresses from the outside inward. The mature adult profile is not achieved until the second year, so that normal immaturity of neurons in Sommer's sector in term infants should not be confused with perinatal hypoxic/ischemic lesions.[16] Karyometric studies of the growth in size of granule cells in the dentate gyrus of the rat demonstrate three gradients of development: external-to-internal, suprapyramidal-to-infrapyramidal, and caudal-to-rostral.[34] Similar gradients are seen in the perinatal human dentate gyrus.

### Thalamus and Basal Ganglia

The thalamus is formed by the germinal matrix of the walls of the third ventricle, except for the pulvinar, which arises from the ganglionic eminence.[37] Migration to the thalamus and depletion of this germinal matrix are completed early in fetal life, by 9.5 weeks. By 24 weeks' gestation, all nuclear groups in the thalamus may be identified histologically.[10]

Neurons of the globus pallidus mature at 24 weeks' gestation; striatal neurons are still neuroblasts at that time. Large cells of the putamen and caudate nucleus are distinguished at 28 to 30 weeks' gestation, and often appear chromatolytic as a normal stage of maturation; small cells of the corpus striatum remain immature as small, dark, round neuroblasts with sparse cytoplasm until 33 to 36 weeks' gestation, but are well differentiated by 38 weeks.[16]

### Subventricular Germinal Matrix

The "germinal matrix" is composed of postmitotic, premigratory cells of the subventricular zone of the forebrain (see Fig. 2-12). These small, dark, round cells with sparse cytoplasm appear histologically uniform, though their fate and later differentiation may be at least partially predetermined. They migrate outward to the cortical plate in waves along radial glial cell processes that extend to the pial surface, but later retract as the radial glial cell is transformed into a mature astrocyte. Most germinal matrix cells form cortical neurons during the migration period of 8 to 16 weeks; from 16 to 24 weeks the ratio shifts; and after 24 weeks the great majority become glial cells. The traditional term *germinal matrix* is not favored by modern neuroembryologists because it has been applied to encompass both the ventricular zone of neuroepithelium and the subventricular zone of postmitotic neuroblasts and glioblasts as well as the intercellular vascular channels and matrix proteins. However, it is still widely used by clinicians and pathologists because it identifies in two words a distinct population of fetal neural cells in a specified location.

The thickness of the germinal matrix correlates with gestational age, but similar sites should be compared. Three good sites to examine the thickness of the germinal matrix are: (1) lateral to the frontal horn of the lateral ventricle, over the head of the caudate nucleus; (2) the neocortical (ventrolateral) side of the temporal horn; and (3) the lateral wall of the occipital horn.

The germinal matrix regresses as cells migrate away. Mitotic activity in the neuroepithelium ceases with the differentiation of an ependyma (see below), so that no new cells are added to the germinal matrix in regions where an ependyma is formed at the ventricular surface. Waves of migratory neuroblasts and glioblasts form a transient laminar appearance of the subcortical white matter (Fig. 2-12). This pattern persists longest in the occipital lobe.

Term infants have only scattered islands of remaining germinal matrix cells in the periventricular region, except for a thicker cushion between the thalamus and head of the caudate nucleus. This final cushion frag-

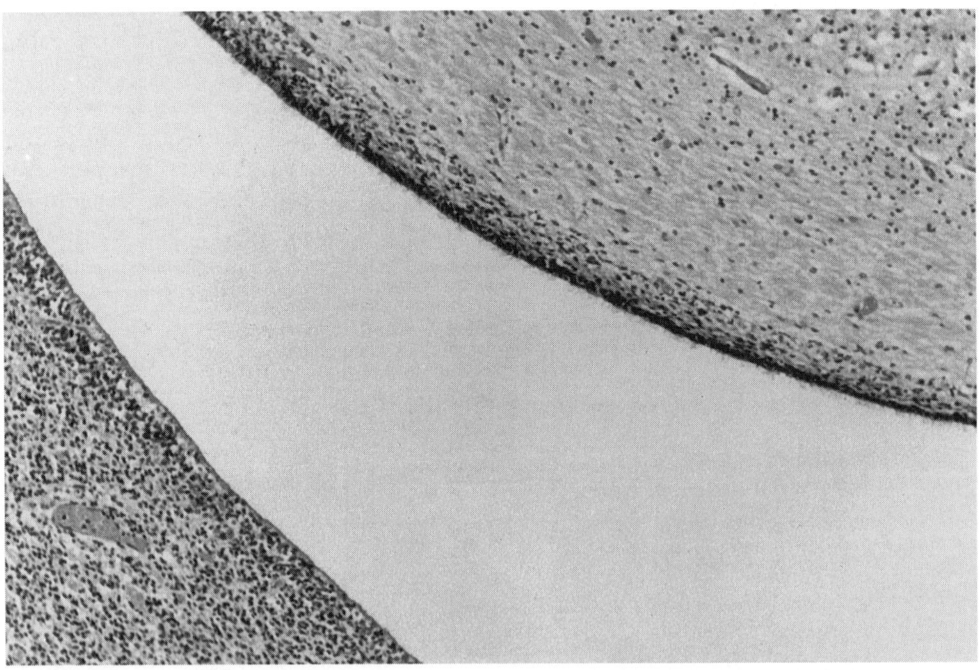

**Fig. 12-7.** Temporal horn of lateral ventricle of a 20-week human fetus. The ependyma is differentiated on the hippocampal side, but not yet on the neocortical side, where a prominent cellular neuroepithelium is still present. Glial fibrillary acidic protein (GFAP) confirmed that the cells lining the hippocampal side are ependymal and that those lining the other are not (not shown); GFAP is expressed in ependymal cells only in fetal life, not postnatally. (H&E; ×100.)

ments during the first three postnatal months and nearly disappears by one year of age; small nests of germinal matrix cells also occur basally around the frontal horn and occipital horn in term neonates.[16]

### Ependyma

The fetal ependyma is a key structure involved in many developmental processes of the CNS, such as axonal growth cone guidance. The differentiation of an ependyma at the ventricular surface signals the termination of mitotic activity of the neuroepithelium at that site, hence it is advantageous to the fetus to postpone ependymal formation as long as possible to allow all necessary mitotic cycles to be completed.[40]

The ependyma differentiates in a precisely timed spatial sequence that begins at 4 weeks' gestation with the notochordal induction of the floor plate ependyma in the ventral midline of the future spinal cord and brainstem, before closure of the neural tube. The final regions of the lateral ventricles to be lined by ependyma are in the temporal and occipital horns and are delayed until as late as 22 weeks' gestation (Fig. 12-7).[41]

## MYELIN STAINS

Myelination is poorly discerned by H&E. The next stage of precision beyond ordinary histology in estimating gestational age by light microscopy of the CNS is to apply special stains for myelin. Myelination cycles occur in a precise spatial and temporal sequence in the various tracts and white matter regions of the brain and spinal cord, and it is feasible to demonstrate myelination in most histopathology laboratories. Myelination is an especially important index of maturation because it can be compared with the degree of myelination demonstrated during life by magnetic resonance imaging (MRI). The timing of myelination sequences differs between MRI and tissue demonstration at autopsy by special stains because of the greater sensitivity of the latter, allowing earlier detection.

Sensitivity also is a factor in the selection of the histochemical stain. The traditional myelin stain for developmental studies is luxol fast blue,[7,17,19,38,50] requiring overnight incubation, and usually counterstained with cresyl violet (Klüver-Barrera method), periodic acid-Schiff (PAS) reaction, or H&E. Myelin appears blue. A more recent and somewhat more sensitive technique is the use of gallocyanin stains, such as the Lapham technique, to metachromatically stain myelin phospholipids red. The most sensitive methods for myelination rely on immunocytochemical demonstration of antibodies against myelin basic protein or one of the transient fetal forms of myelin, myelin-associated glycoprotein, or proteolipid protein.[6a,47] Immunoreactiv-

**Table 12-1.** Myelination cycles of the human central nervous system*

| Pathway | Begins | Completed |
|---|---|---|
| Spinal motor roots | 16 weeks | 42 weeks |
| Spinal sensory roots | 20 weeks | 5 months |
| Cranial motor nerves III, IV, V, VI | 20 weeks | 28 weeks |
| Ventral commissure, spinal cord | 24 weeks | 4 months |
| Dorsal columns, spinal cord | 28 weeks | 36 weeks |
| Medial longitudinal fasciculus | 24 weeks | 28 weeks |
| Habenulopeduncular tract | 28 weeks | 34 weeks |
| Acoustic nerve | 24 weeks | 36 weeks |
| Trapezoid body and lateral lemniscus | 25 weeks | 36 weeks |
| Acoustic radiations (thalamocortical) | 40 weeks | 3 years |
| Inferior cerebellar peduncle (inner part) | 26 weeks | 36 weeks |
| Inferior cerebellar peduncle (outer part) | 32 weeks | 4 months |
| Middle cerebellar peduncle | 42 weeks | 3 years |
| Superior cerebellar peduncle | 28 weeks | 6 months |
| Medial lemniscus | 32 weeks | 12 months |
| Optic nerve | 38 weeks | 6 months |
| Optic radiations | 40 weeks | 6 months |
| Ansa lenticularis | 28 weeks | 8 months |
| Fornix | 2 months | 2 years |
| Mammillothalamic tract | 8 months | 6 years |
| Thalamocortical radiations | 2 months | 7 years |
| Corticospinal tract | 38 weeks | 2 years |
| Corpus callosum | 2 months | 14 years |
| Intracortical association fibers (frontotemporal and frontoparietal) | 3 months | 32 years |

* Myelination determined by light microscopy using luxol fast blue stain. Gestational age stated in weeks; Postnatal age stated in months and years. Reproduced with permission from Sarnat HB: Cerebral Dysgenesis. Embryology and Clinical Expression. New York, 1992, Oxford University Press.

ity is usually reserved for investigative use rather than clinical diagnostic purposes, however, because of the greater technical complexity and expense. Other research tools sometimes employed to study myelin development are phase contrast microscopy[31] and biochemical analysis of myelin lipids and proteins.[25]

Table 12-1 provides a summary of myelination cycles in the prenatal and postnatal human brain, as determined by luxol fast blue stain of formalin-fixed, paraffin-embedded sections taken at autopsy. In some sites, such as the dorsal roots and medial longitudinal fasciculus, myelination begins as early as 24 weeks' gestation. Myelination of the human brain is not completed until adult life,[38,40] though very late myelination requires further study.

## HISTOCHEMICAL AND IMMUNOCYTOCHEMICAL STUDIES

Precision of determination of gestational age may be greatly enhanced by the application of special histochemical and immunocytochemical stains. Because such studies often require technical preparations not readily available in most standard histopathology laboratories, they are beyond the scope of this chapter and will not be discussed in detail. However, a brief general discussion and a few select examples are offered to emphasize a potential of estimating maturation of CNS tissues even more precisely than can be done by ordinary histologic techniques.

Many standard histochemical techniques have the disadvantage of requiring frozen, unfixed sections, hence special preparation in advance. However, they may have applications in determining maturation. Examples are Sudan stains and oil red O for showing "myelination gliosis" in white matter; sudanophilic deposits of lipid are a product of active myelination but not of completed myelination.[27] Mitochondrial "oxidative" enzymatic stains, such as succinic dehydrogenase, malic dehydrogenase, isocitric dehydrogenase, and others of the tricarboxylic Krebs cycle, as well as cytochrome oxidase and nicotinamide adenine dinucleotide tetrazolium reductase (NADH-TR) are useful for demonstrating zones of synapse formation, because both axonal terminals and postsynaptic end plates have high concentrations of mitochondria. Synaptogenesis of axodendritic synapses in particular is well demonstrated, as in the glomeruli of the internal granular layer of the cerebellum or of the olfactory bulb, in the hippocampus, in the molecular layer of the cerebral cortex, or in the reticular nuclei of the brainstem.

Some standard histochemical stains may be applied to formalin-fixed, paraffin-embedded sections of brain tissue, and may be applied to the question of estimating gestational age. Acridine orange (AO) forms highly fluorescent complexes with nucleic acids, with different wavelengths of absorption of ultraviolet light and emission of visible light. Thus, AO-DNA complexes are perceived as yellow and AO-RNA complexes are orange-red in the fluorescence microscope. The proliferation of ribosomes in neurons signals a stage of maturation beyond the neuroblast and is correlated with the initiation of production and secretion of neurotransmitters and the enzymes associated with their biosynthesis and degradation. AO fluorochrome thus demonstrates a predictable sequence of neuronal maturation in the CNS and may be correlated with gestational age.[42] AO also may be applied to frozen sections.

Acid phosphatase, a lysosomal enzyme, may be demonstrated in frozen or paraffin sections and viewed with an ordinary light microscope. It is a useful stain for demonstrating cells undergoing apoptosis, programmed cell death, as a physiologic maturational process.

Immunocytochemical (ICC) stains generally may be applied to formalin-fixed, paraffin sections and may be prepared either for immunofluorescence or for viewing in the light microscope by biotin-avidin or immunoperoxidase methods. Some techniques require special fixatives other than formalin, and therefore must be planned prospectively rather than decided retrospectively. The number of specific monoclonal antibodies available is prodigious and growing daily. An example of the application of ICC to the determination of maturation is the demonstration in the cerebellar cortex of class III $\beta$-tubulin isotypes and calbindin-D expression in distinct neuronal types during fetal life.[24] Immunocytochemical demonstration of MAP (microtubule-associated proteins) antibodies in the cerebellar vermis shows regional differences between the various lobules of the timing of Purkinje cell dendritic outgrowth.[18] MAPs and various neurofilament proteins of different molecular weights and degrees of phosphorylation are useful in demonstrating maturational changes in neurons of the human hippocampus, using formalin-fixed, paraffin-embedded sections.[18]

Other immunocytochemical neuronal markers also exhibit predictable appearances at critical stages of neuronal maturation, usually corresponding to the beginning of transmitter biosynthesis. Examples include chromatogranin in monoamine-producing cells; synaptophysin, which denotes the presence of synaptic vesicles; and the glycolytic enzyme "neuron-specific" enolase. A newly demonstrated marker of neuronal nuclei, NeuN, also shows immunocytochemical expression as the neuron matures. It does not identify glial cells, ependymal cells, endothelial cells, or any other cells in the brain nor does it show immunoreactivity with certain specific neuronal types, such as cerebellar Purkinje cells, olfactory bulb mitral cells, retinal photoreceptor cells, and sympathetic ganglion cells; the reason for its specificity is uncertain.[49]

## GOLGI IMPREGNATIONS

Heavy metal impregnations of neurons are somewhat capricious but provide excellent detail at the light microscopic level of dendritic arborizations and spines. Golgi techniques were extensively used by Cajal to describe this aspect of cerebral maturation, and he correlated dendritic branching in various regions of the brain with maturational age[9]; the techniques continue to have an important place in classic neuroembryology and developmental neuropathology.[23,35] The rapid silver Golgi method is more reliable than the Golgi-Cox method, substituting mercury for silver in demonstrating immature dendrites. However, Golgi-Cox often is preferred for mature cerebral tissue, despite a long period of impregnation for weeks or months. Golgi stains are not a tool for the standard histopathology laboratory, and their interpretation also requires some experience. They do demonstrate that in human neocortex, dendritic branching begins earlier and continues to be more advanced in layer 5 than in layer 3.[4] The development of visual (striate) cortex lags behind that of the motor cortex and hippocampus by 4 to 6 weeks.[4,46] The auditory cortex (superior temporal gyrus) shows a pattern of dendritic arborization similar to that of visual and motor cortices, but also somewhat earlier.[45]

## ELECTRON MICROSCOPY

Transmission electron microscopy (EM) provides ultrastructural details about organelles that correlate with the development of neurotransmitter biosyntheses, synaptogenesis, and myelination beyond the resolution of the light microscope, and may be combined with some immunocytochemical stains for subcellular localization. EM has an application for documenting maturation in experimental animals, but has little place in human diagnostic neuropathology for this purpose because autopsy tissues are affected by autolytic changes that may be confused with physiologic or pathologic features.

## IN SITU HYBRIDIZATION

In situ hybridization is a molecular genetic technique for demonstrating the expression of gene products in tissue sections, and thus achieving precise histologic localization as with immunocytochemistry. Some homeotic genes of early neural tube segmentation also mediate the differentiation of specific neural cell types and maintain their identity in adult life. For example, in the cerebellum *Pax-6* is expressed by granule cells, *Pax-3* with Bergmann glial cells, and *Wnt-3* with fetal Purkinje cells.[39,45] The molecular genetic approach to cell identity promises much precise information about maturation of the nervous system and, though presently strictly an investigative approach, might eventually find a more routine application in determining early gestational ages more precisely than any other method.

## REFERENCES


1. Altman J: Postnatal development of the cerebellar cortex in the rat. I. The external germinal layer and transitional molecular layer, J Comp Neurol 145:353-397, 1972.
2. Arnold SE, and Trojanowski JQ: Human fetal hippocampal development: I. cytoarchitecture, myeloarchitecture and neuronal morphologic features, J Comp Neurol 367:274-292, 1996.
3. Arnold SE, and Trojanowski JQ: Human fetal hippocampal development: II. the neuronal cytoskeleton, J Comp Neurol 367: 293-307, 1996.
4. Becker LE, and others: Dendritic development in human occipital cortical neurons, Dev Brain Res 3:117-124, 1984.
5. Berliner K: Beiträge zur Histologie und Entwicklung des Kleinhirnes, Arch mikr Anat 66:220-270, 1905.
6. Biach P: Zur normalen und pathologischen Anatomie der aüsseren Körnerschicht des Kleinhirnes, Arb Neurol Inst Univ Wien 18:13-30, 1909.

6a. Bodhireddy SR, and others: Immunohistochemical detection of myelin basic protein is a sensitive marker of myelination in second trimester human fetal spinal cord, J Neuropathol Exp Neurol 53:144-149, 1994.

7. Brody BA, and others: Sequence of central nervous system myelination in human infancy. I. an autopsy study of myelination, J Neuropathol Exp Neurol 46:283-301, 1987.
8. Brun A: The subpial granular layer of the foetal cerebral cortex in man. Its ontogeny and significance in cortical malformations, Acta Pathol Microbiol Scand 179 (suppl), 1965.
9. Cajal, S de Ramón y: Histologie du système nerveux central de l'homme et des vértébrés, Paris, 1909-1911 Maloine.
10. Dekaban A: Human thalamus. An anatomical, developmental and pathological study. II. Development of the human thalamic nuclei, J Comp Neurol 100:63-97, 1954.
11. Derer P, and Derer M: Cajal-Retzius cell ontogenesis and death in mouse brain visualized with horseradish peroxidase and electron microscopy, Neuroscience 36:839-856, 1990.
12. Duckett S, and Pearse AGE: The cells of Cajal-Retzius in the developing human brain, J Anat 102:183-187, 1968.
13. Dunn HL: The growth of the central nervous system in the human fetus as expressed by graphic analysis and empirical formulae, J Comp Neurol 33:405-491, 1921.
14. Ellis RS: Norms for some structural changes in the human cerebellum from birth to old age, J Comp Neurol 32:1-35, 1992.
15. Friede RL: Dating the development of human cerebellum, Acta Neuropathol 23:48-58, 1973.
16. Friede RL: Developmental Neuropathology, ed 2. Berlin, 1989, Springer-Verlag.
17. Gilles FH: Myelination in the neonatal brain, Hum Pathol 7:244-248, 1976.
18. Goodlett CR, Hamre KM, and West JR: Regional differences in the timing of dendritic outgrowth of Purkinje cells in the vermal cerebellum demonstrated by MAP2 immunocytochemistry, Dev Brain Res 53:131-134, 1990.
19. Hasegawa M, and others: Development of myelination in the human fetal and infant cerebrum: a myelin basic protein immunohistochemical study, Brain Dev 14:1-6, 1992.
20. Hayashi M: Einige wichtige Tatsachen aus der ontogenetischen Entwicklung des menschlichen Kleinhirnes, Dtsch Z Nervenheilk 81:74-82, 1924.
21. Humphrey T: The development of the human hippocampal fissure, J Anat 101:655-676, 1967.
22. Huntley GW, and Jones EG: Cajal-Retzius neurons in developing monkey neocortex show immunoreactivity to calcium binding proteins, J Neurocytol 19:200-219, 1990.

23. Jagadha V, and Becker LE: Dendritic pathology: an overview of Golgi studies in man, Can J Neurol Sci 16:41-50, 1989.
24. Katsetos CD, and others: Differential localization of class III $\beta$-tubulin isotype and calbindin-D28k defines distinct neuronal types in the developing human cerebellar cortex, J Neuropathol Exp Neurol 52:655-666, 1993.
25. Kinney HC, and others: Myelination in the developing human brain: biochemical correlates, Neurochem Res 19:983-996, 1994.
26. Larroche J-C: Developmental Pathology of the Neonate, Amsterdam, 1977, Excerpta Medica.
27. Leech RW, and Alvord EC Jr: Glial fatty metamorphosis: an abnormal response of premyelin glia frequently accompanying leukomalacia, Am J Pathol 74:603-612, 1974.
28. Lemire RJ, and others: Normal and abnormal development of the human nervous system, Hagerstown, Maryland, 1975, Harper & Row.
29. Marín-Padilla M: Prenatal and early postnatal ontogenesis of the human motor cortex. A Golgi study. I. The sequential development of the cortical layers, Brain Res 23:167-183, 1970.
30. Marín-Padilla M: Dual origin of the mammalian neocortex and evolution of the cortical plate, Anat Embryol 152:109-126, 1978.
31. Miklossy J, Van der Loos H: The long-distance effects of brain lessions: visualization of myelinated pathways in the human brain using polarizing and fluorescence microscopy, J Neuropathol Exp Neurol 50:1-15, 1991.
32. Norman MG, and others: Congenital malformations of the brain. Pathological, Embryological, Clinical, Radiological and Genetic Aspects, New York, 1995, Oxford University Press.
33. O'Rahilly R, and Müller F: The embryonic human brain. An atlas of developmental stages, New York, 1994, Wiley-Liss.
34. Pérez-Delgado MM, and others: Postnatal development of the dentate gyrus: a karyometric and topographic study, Acta Anat 144:160-166, 1992.
35. Purpura DP: Dendritic differentiation in human cerebral cortex. Normal and aberrant developmental patterns, Adv Neurol 12: 91-116, 1975.
36. Rakic P, and Sidman RL: Histogenesis of cortical layers in human cerebellum, particularly the lamina dissecans, J Comp Neurol 139:473-500, 1970.
37. Rakic P, and Sidman RL: Telencephalic origin of pulvinar neurons in the fetal human brain, Z Anat Entwicklungsgesch 129: 53-82, 1969.
38. Rorke LB, and Riggs HE: Myelination in the Brain in the Newborn, Philadelphia, 1969, JB Lippincott.
39. Salinas PC, and others: Maintenance of Wnt-3 expression in Purkinje cells of the mouse cerebellum depends on interactions with granule cells, Development 120:1277-1286, 1994.
40. Sarnat HB: Cerebral dysgenesis. Embryology and Clinical Expression, New York, 1992, Oxford University Press.
41. Sarnat HB: Regional differentiation of the human fetal ependyma: immunocytochemical markers, J Neuropathol Exp Neurol 51:58-75, 1992.
42. Sarnat HB: Repartition de l'ARN au cours de la migration neuronale dans les cerveaux normaux et dysplastiques en développement chez l'homme: étude a l'acridine-orange, Rev Neurol (Paris) 145:127-133, 1989.
43. Scammon RE, Dunn HL: On the growth of the human cerebellum in early life, Proc Soc Exp Biol NY 21:217-221, 1924.
44. Seldon HL: Structure of human auditory cortex. I. Cytoarchitectonics and dendritic distributions; Brain Res 229:277-294, 1981.
45. Stoykova A, and Gruss P: Roles of *Pax* genes in developing and adult brain as suggested by expression patterns, J Neurosci 14: 1395-1412, 1994.
46. Takashima S, and others: Morphology of the developing visual cortex of the human infant. A quantitative and qualitative Golgi study, J Neuropathol Exp Neurol 39:487-501, 1980.
47. Weidenheim KM, and others: Temporal and spatial expression of major myelin proteins in the human fetal spinal cord during the second trimester, J Neuropathol Exp Neurol 55:734-745, 1996.
48. West MJ, and Del Cerro M: Early formation of synapses in the molecular layer of the fetal rat cerebellum, J Comp Neurol 165: 137-160, 1975.
49. Wolf HK, and others: NeuN: a useful neuronal marker for diagnostic histopathology, J Histochem Cytochem 44:1167-1171, 1996.
50. Yakovlev PI, Lecours A-R: The myelination cycles of regional maturation of the brain. In Minkowski A: Regional development of the brain in early life, Philadelphia, 1967, FA Davis.
51. Zecevic N, and Rakic P: Differentiation of Purkinje cells and their relationship to other components of developing cerebellar cortex in man, J Comp Neurol 167:27-48, 1976.

C • H • A • P • T • E • R

# 13

# *Perinatal Hypoxic/Ischemic Encephalopathy: Neuropathological Features*

**Harvey B. Sarnat**



Hypoxic/ischemic encephalopathy (HIE) is the most frequent cause of neurologic disease in neonates at all gestational ages. The complications of HIE and its clinical expression vary greatly with gestational age at birth and with conceptional age (gestational age + postnatal chronologic age) owing to many factors, including the state of development of collateral circulation and the vascular bed for perfusion of the brain, maturation of autoregulation of cerebral blood flow, and differing metabolic demands of immature and mature cells. Nevertheless, the fundamental impairment of neuronal and glial metabolism is a constant feature.

Many complex factors induce cellular death in hypoxic/ischemic encephalopathy: impairment of energy-production mechanisms utilizing adenosine triphosphate (ATP); calcium influx; lactic acidosis; loss of transmembranous ion exchange through ion channels; and damage by free radical formation and neurotoxic excitatory amino acid release. All of these phenomena contribute to failure of the neuronal resting membrane potential, inhibition of RNA transcription, and a cascade of degenerative changes in the neuron.[156] Some metabolic factors may affect immature and mature neurons differently. The induction of immediate early genes in the neonatal brain may be of particular importance, particularly of c-*fos* and c-*jun* and their transcription products that encode proteins that regulate events in apoptosis.[4,53,86] In addition, c-*fos* expression associated with ischemic neuronal death appears to induce basic fibroblast growth factor, which in turn stimulates both glial cell proliferation and angiogenesis in the CNS.[21,75] Other neurotrophic factors also may play a role both in cell death of neurons and in the responses of non-neuronal cells to the brain tissue injury. Immature astrocytes die much earlier than do mature astrocytes when deprived of substrates such as sugars, amino acids, and lipids, in the presence of oxygen, a feature perhaps related to the ability of the cell to scavenge free radicals.[58] Substrates are depleted more rapidly in the immature brain than in the adult because of smaller stores and generally higher metabolic rate.

In the human clinical situation, it is difficult if not impossible to isolate hypoxic and ischemic insults, but these may be analyzed independently in animals under controlled experimental conditions. It is clear from such studies that ischemia rather than hypoxia is responsible for most of the tissue injury and impairment of cellular function.[156] Hypoglycemia also often accompanies hypoxic/ischemic insults in human neonates; it would seem to make little difference whether oxygen or glucose becomes the limiting substrate of aerobic metabolism, but a major difference is the severe lactic acidosis induced by ischemia but not by hypoglycemia.[8]

The arterial blood supply of the brain is unlike most other organs; rather than a large central hilar artery feeding multiple radiating branches, the major cerebral vessels (anterior, middle, and posterior cerebral arteries) surround the brain and give origin to branches at right angles that penetrate the cerebrum and extend toward the ventricles, supplying the cerebral cortex, the subcortical white matter, and the deep gray matter nuclei, such as the thalamus and corpus striatum.[28,91,145,155] Arterial blood flow is therefore centripetal rather than centrifugal. Collateral circulation between the penetrating cerebral vessels is poorly developed until near term and, in the infant of less than 35 weeks' gestation, vessels supplying the subcortical white matter are essentially end-arterioles. The periventricular region, including the germinal matrix, is the last zone to receive blood flow from these long arterioles from the surface of the cortex, and deep sites are the first to suffer poor perfusion if flow is reduced, as might occur during periods of systemic hypotension or decreased cardiac output. Furthermore, only the deep white matter, thalamus, and basal ganglia rely on a single arterial source in the adult as well as in the neonate, rendering these vascular territories at even greater risk for infarction.[83] Edema may result from ischemia or from circulatory disturbances of deep venous drainage, further diminishing perfusion by arterial blood and contributing to infarction.[88]

Arteries and veins are difficult to distinguish in the fetal brain because thick muscular arterial walls are not yet well developed. A second centrifugal circulation oriented away from the ventricles and toward the cortical surface was thought to represent another vascular system of the fetal brain,[29,145,155] but these vessels are now recognized as veins rather than arteries.[61,81,100] Interpretations of periventricular infarcts or hemorrhages based on the premise that these vessels are arterial and form boundary zones with the centripetal arteries therefore require revision.

Despite the common clinical association of HIE with autonomic instability and respiratory insufficiency, intrapartum anoxia or "birth asphyxia" has been greatly overstated as an etiologic factor in cerebral palsy.* Much of this exaggeration has come not from the medical profession or the basic neuroscience community, but rather from the legal establishment. Litigation continues to allege negligence of delivery procedures causing brain damage. Some is justified; most is not.

The following discussion is a survey of histopathologic changes in the CNS of preterm and term infants who have suffered insufficient oxygen or circulatory disturbances in the perinatal period that resulted in the general condition known as HIE. Infarcts of the neonatal brain may or may not be hemorrhagic, but both categories are topographically unique to the immature brain and unlike strokes in the adult. Experimental nodules of HIE in the immature rat show a sequence of neuropathologic changes similar to those demonstrated in human neonates.[153]

## ISCHEMIC INFARCTS OF THE CEREBRAL WHITE MATTER

The cerebral white matter receives the brunt of most hypoxic-ischemic lesions of the fetal and neonatal brain at all gestational ages, but the distribution of lesions differs between the preterm and term or near-term infant. The principal cerebral white matter lesion of infants of less than 35 weeks' gestation is termed *periventricular leukomalacia*; after 35 weeks, *subcortical leukomalacia* is the predominant lesion. Both are potentially devastating to neurologic development and cause long-term neurologic disabilities that often are not yet clinically evident in the neonatal period. In most cases, fetal distress, intrapartum asphyxia, or neonatal HIE are symptomatic. However, in infants of advanced gestational age, common signs that can be semiquantitatively graded include muscle tone, reflexes, autonomic impairment, and levels of consciousness. EEG activity adds another parameter, but the

* Refs. 15, 49, 62, 87, 90, 92, 112, 141, 148.

presence or absence of seizures denotes neither severity of the insult nor prognosis.[38,129,159]

### Periventricular Leukomalacia

The term *periventricular leukomalacia* (PVL) was coined by Banker and Larroche in their now classic 1962 paper that offered the first modern, detailed description of white matter degeneration in neonates exposed to hypoxic-ischemic insults in fetal life, during labor and delivery, or in the early postnatal period.[11] Subsequent objections have been voiced to this term on the bases that many of the lesions are deep within the subcortical white matter and are not confined to a periventricular distribution and that much of the subependymal cerebral parenchyma is not white but gray matter, such as the thalamus, caudate nucleus, and even the densely cellular germinal matrix of the immature brain. Nevertheless, the earliest lesions detected by ultrasonography in the living patient are periventricular in location, and the term has been embraced by neonatologists and radiologists and is firmly entrenched in the literature. To challenge such a universally understood term would not serve the cause of scientific communication between pathologists and our clinical and radiologic colleagues and, despite its technical shortcomings, PVL may be used if defined.

The periventricular regions, particularly of the lateral and third ventricles, are selectively vulnerable to ischemic injury, leading to frank infarction and subsequent cavitation and gliosis (Fig. 13-1). Periventricular leukomalacia is a lesion that often accompanies and sometimes precedes germinal matrix hemorrhage (see below), but the pathogenesis of the two differs and they are not a progressive continuum. PVL is probably the most common neuropathologic finding in the preterm neonatal brain. Regardless of whether it is accompanied by hemorrhage, PVL is readily detected by ultrasound imaging in the fetus prenatally as well as in the neonate after delivery, and accounts for considerable clinical morbidity later, particularly spastic diplegia (i.e., "cerebral palsy"). The pathologist therefore is often asked to make correlations at autopsy with imaging diagnoses of periventricular lesions, not only in neonates but also in older children who were born prematurely or suffered perinatal difficulties.

The periventricular regions of the fetal brain are highly cellular because the subventricular zone is the source of neuronal and glial precursor cells before they migrate to their mature cortical and subcortical sites (Fig. 13-2). Prior to the differentiation of an ependyma, the ventricular wall is a pseudostratified columnar epithelium of undifferentiated neuroepithelial cells with nuclei that move to-and-fro in synchrony with mitotic cycles, within thin bipolar radial cytoplasmic processes that span the brain from the ventricular to the pial surfaces. Mitotic activity occurs mainly at the ventricular surface; with the differentiation of the ependyma, this process is arrested, leaving the subventricular zone filled with postmitotic, premigratory neuroblasts and glioblasts that represent the "germinal matrix." The

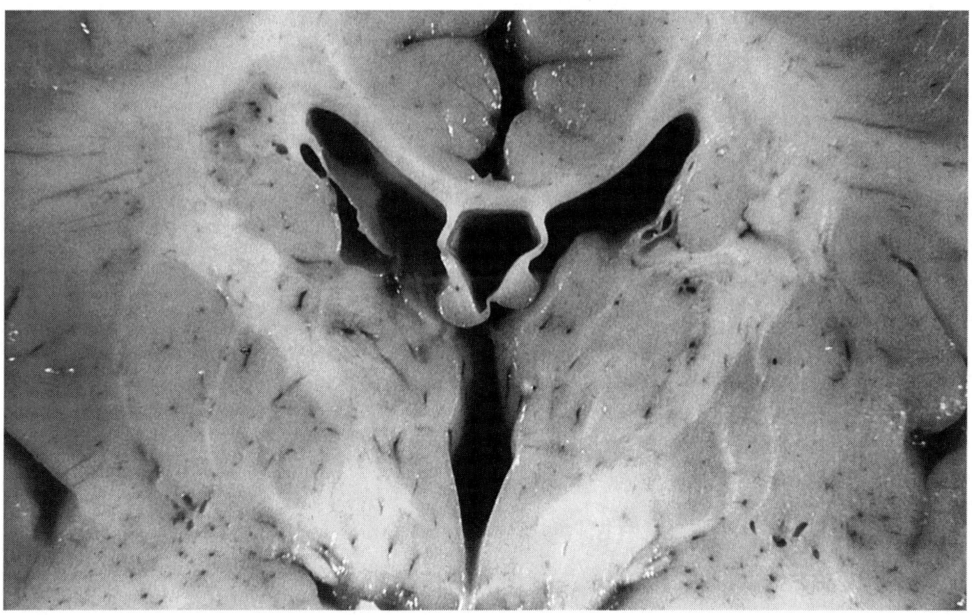

**Fig. 13-1.** Subependymal pseudocysts as a result of periventricular leukomalacia around the frontal horns of the lateral ventricles, in a coronal section of brain at the level of the corpus striatum. A large cavum septi pellucidi and moderate ventriculomegaly are evident. The corpus callosum is thin but myelinated. The patient was 6 years old at the time of death and had been born prematurely at 30 weeks.

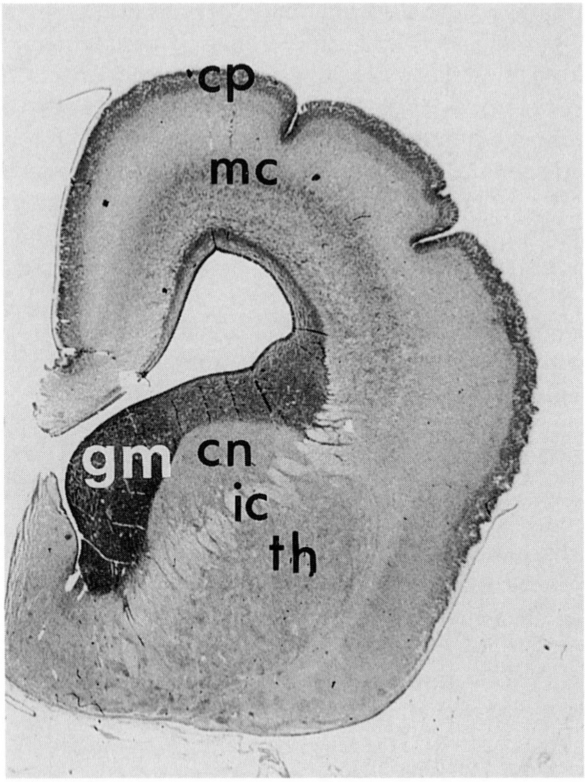


**Fig. 13-2.** Coronal section of one cerebral hemisphere of a 20-week human fetus to show highly cellular periventricular germinal matrix (*gm*) of premigratory neuroblasts and glioblasts and wave of migrating cells (*mc*) that are mostly glioblasts at this age, within the deep subcortical white matter. The cortical plate (*cp*) is at the surface, and only a few sulci are beginning to form. *cn*, head of the caudate nucleus; *ic*, anterior limb of internal capsule; *th*, thalamus. (H&E; ×16.)

ependyma differentiates in the human fetus in a precise temporal and spatial sequence, beginning with the floor plate of the neural tube at 4 weeks' gestation and finishing with the final lining of the lateral ventricular surface at about 22 weeks' gestation.[47,123–125] The germinal matrix is perfused by thin-walled vascular channels of various sizes that are neither mature capillaries nor venules and arterioles. As the germinal matrix is depopulated by migration of its cells, the subventricular zone becomes incorporated into the white matter or into deep gray matter such as the caudate nucleus.

Periventricular leukomalacia occurs mainly around the lateral ventricles, and the most frequent site is around the occipital horns and parietal regions of preterm infants.[46,70,133] The loss of white matter in the posterior half of the cerebral hemispheres may lead to dilatation of the occipital horns and relatively less or no dilatation of the frontal and temporal horns. It represents an acquired cause of *colpocephaly* not due to agenesis of the corpus callosum or primary dysgenesis.[64,123]

Leech and Alvord,[70] Grunnet,[50] and Shuman and Selednik[133] found a much more widespread topography of lesions in the subcortical white matter of preterm infants than had originally been described in a periventricular distribution by Banker and Larroche.[11] Several patterns of white matter necrosis were recognized, in addition to the periventricular lesions that were reconfirmed. Some deep white matter lesions were small, focal infarcts; others were linear and formed concentric lines of degeneration parallel to the ventricular wall; still others were long streaks of necrosis radiating from the angles of the ventricles toward the cortex. Leech and Alvord pointed out that these various lesions often coexisted but were of different ages, the more peripheral ones being more recent and usually less extensive.[70]

Many infants who have suffered severe hypoxic-ischemic insults die with terminal sepsis in addition, and a question of whether some bacterial endotoxin might play a role in the pathogenesis of white matter lesions has been posed. However, endotoxic damage probably is not a major factor. Most neuropathologic lesions are not terminal agonal changes.

A precursor protein of $\beta$-amyloid is expressed early in axon swellings (i.e., spheroids) around zones of PVL and may be demonstrated immunocytochemically in early (but not in chronic) stages of cavitation.[5] This membrane glycoprotein is encoded by a gene on chromosome 21 and is strongly expressed in Down syndrome and in adults with Alzheimer's disease; it also is described in adult brains in regions of recent cerebral infarction.

A unique feature of periventricular and deep white matter infarcts of the immature brain is that such lesions may interrupt radial glial fibers so that migrating neuroblasts and glioblasts cannot reach their final destinations in the cerebral cortex, even if the migratory cells themselves escape the zone of infarction.[120,126] This situation can lead to focal cortical dysplasias that might later become epileptic foci or that might be expressed as other neurologic deficits referable to the involved region of cortex.

### Subcortical Leukomalacia

Takashima and associates recognized a distinctive topography of white matter infarcts in the term and near-term neonate that differs from the more periventricular distribution of lesions in the younger preterm infant.[142] These lesions in the older fetuses and neonates predominate just beneath the cerebral cortex and especially at the depths of sulci. It is their location rather than unique histopathologic features that distinguishes these subcortical lesions.

The explanation of subcortical leukomalacia was postulated by Takashima and associates to be related to less vascular, hence more vulnerable, zones created by progressive gyration of the cerebral cortex in late gestation, causing medullary and subcortical arterioles supplying the white matter to curve around the depths of sulci.[142] However, Kuban and Gilles pointed out the increased number of short, penetrating vessels and that the many lateral and acute angle branches that join nearby trunks to supply these subcortical regions make the hypothesis less tenable.[61] Also, term neonates often show a parasagittal distribution of infarction involving the watershed zone between the anterior and middle cerebral artery distribution characteristically seen in adult brains and cortical gray matter as well as white matter.[71,97,161]

Azzarelli and co-workers correlated the zones of infarction in the white matter of term neonatal brains in infants suffering perinatal hypoxia with areas of primary myelination.[9,10] Active myelination is associated with a high rate of metabolic activity of oligodendrocytes and of fibrillary astrocytes in the region as well as proliferation of the developing capillary network. These all contribute to a high metabolic rate and selective vulnerability to insults such as ischemia, hypoxia, or lactic acidosis because of the high rates of oxygen and glucose utilization, and cellular enzymatic activity for this metabolism and for the synthesis of myelin proteins. Regions of the neonatal white matter suffering the most damage are those showing the highest levels of glucose utilization by positron emission tomography (PET).[23]

Subcortical leukomalacia is not confined to the immediate zone beneath the deepest layer of cerebral cortex, but often extends into the white matter; additional isolated lesions deep in the subcortical white matter also occur. Coagulative necrosis also is not always confined to the centrum semiovale, but may involve the axes of individual cerebral gyri, while leaving the gray matter cortex of the gyri relatively spared.[25]

### Nonhemorrhagic Histopathologic Changes in White Matter of Preterm and Term Neonates

The historical aspects of the elucidation of white matter damage in the neonatal brain are described well by Paneth and associates.[100] The first description may have been made by Virchow himself,[157] but the first modern systematic description of the sequence of white matter changes and reactive cellular responses must be credited to Banker and Larroche, who also documented for the first time that premature infants were more severely affected than term neonates by similar insults.[11] Subsequent investigations by other developmental neuropathologists confirmed and expanded their meticulous observations.*

The fundamental features of white matter infarcts in neonatal brains are similar to white matter infarcts at any age, but the distribution of the lesions is unique, and immature features, such as radial glial fibers, incompletely migrated neural cells, unmyelinated or actively myelinating axons, and an immature vascular bed, all confer special identity to and unique functional consequences of neonatal infarcts. The sequence of histopathologic changes is summarized in Table 13-1.

**Table 13-1.** Histopathologic changes of infarction in the periventricular and subcortical white matter of preterm and term neonates

| | |
|---|---|
| **Early phase (first 24 hours)** | |
| 3 hours | Microglial accumulation at the periphery of the zone of infarction |
| 6 hours | Coagulation necrosis; pallor with histologic stains; retraction balls of swollen and degenerating axons |
| 8 hours | Astrocytic degeneration within the zone of necrosis: karyorrhexis; pyknosis; clasmatodendrosis |
| 12 hours | Reactive astrocytes mixed with microglial cells at the margins of zones of infarction |
| 24 hours | Endothelial cell hyperplasia at margin of infarct |
| **Intermediate phase (1 day to 2 weeks)** | |
| 1–3 days | Prominent endothelial swelling |
| 5 days | Macrophages appear in the zone of infarction to phagocytose myelin precursor lipids and cellular debris |
| 7 days | Neovascular proliferation |
| 8–12 days | Subependymal and deep white matter microcysts and small cavities; ependymal cell loss (may be minimal) |
| 14 days | Zones of infarction and cavities filled with macrophages; glial proliferation at periphery |
| **Late phase (weeks to months)** | |
| 2–24 weeks | White matter atrophy; gliosis; cavitation and macroscopic pseudocyst formation; subependymal glial nodules; mineralization of walls of cysts; multicystic encephalomalacia |

The earliest histologically detectable lesion is an accumulation of microglial cells at the periphery of a zone of infarction as early as 3 hours after the insult; coagulative necrosis is seen at 6 hours as a subtle region of pallor with hematoxylin and eosin stain, containing *retraction balls* and *clubs*—rounded or club-shaped structures staining red with eosin or PAS representing retracted and swollen axons undergoing degeneration. Astrocytic degeneration is detected at 8 hours as karyorrhexis, nuclear and cellular pyknosis, and fragmentation of cytoplasmic processes, called *clasmatodendrosis*.[159] These microscopic features indicate astrocytic death, but astrocytes injured by ischemia but still viable also become globular and show retraction of their processes, well demonstrated by GFAP immunoreactivity (Fig. 13-3).[35,120] By 3 to 5 days, white mat-

* Refs. 39, 73, 80, 102, 103, 116, 123, 145, 151.

A

B

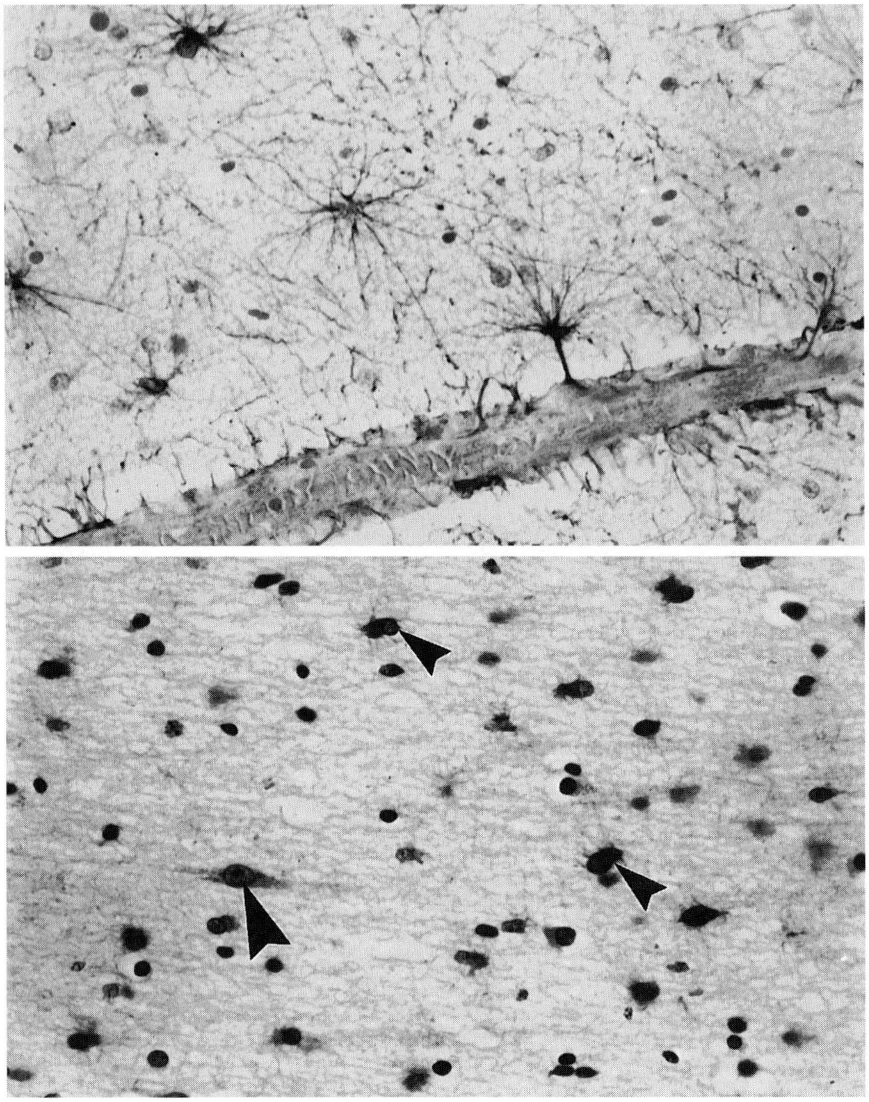

**Fig. 13-3.** **A**, Normal white matter of a term neonate, showing normal fibrillary astrocytes with delicate processes, some with end-feet on thin-walled blood vessels. **B**, After an hypoxic/ischemic insult, the processes of white matter astrocytes retract as short stumps (*small arrowheads*). A displaced neuron is seen (*large arrowhead*). Glial fibrillary acidic protein. (**B**, ×250.)

ter astrocytes reform short, stellate cytoplasmic processes, and at 5 to 7 days these processes elongate and interdigitate to form a meshwork or "gliotic scar."[113] Astrocytes are interspersed with earlier-appearing microglia within 12 hours after the ischemic injury. The injured fetal brain is capable of mobilizing reactive glia as early as 20 weeks' gestation.[113]

Macrophages swollen with lipoid material are observed after 5 days in the periphery of and within the zone of infarction. The lipids they phagocytose are not myelin breakdown products as in the adult brain, but rather are mainly sudanophilic myelin precursors.[69] Macrophages persist for several weeks and disappear after all necrotic debris is removed.

Endothelial cell swelling and hyperplasia may be detected at 24 hours after an ischemic insult, but neovascular proliferation and numerous reticuloendothelial cells do not become prominent until 5 to 7 days.[35]

Late changes in white matter infarcts in neonatal brain after several weeks or months include cavitation with loculated pseudocysts surrounded by gemistocytic astrocytes and lined by glial processes from the periphery (Figs. 13-4, 13-5). Dystrophic calcifications sometimes form in the walls of such cysts (Fig. 13-6). These are mainly mineralized remnants of degenerated axons.[39] Such calcifications may be detected by computed tomography in the living patient if the aggregate is large enough (Fig. 13-7).

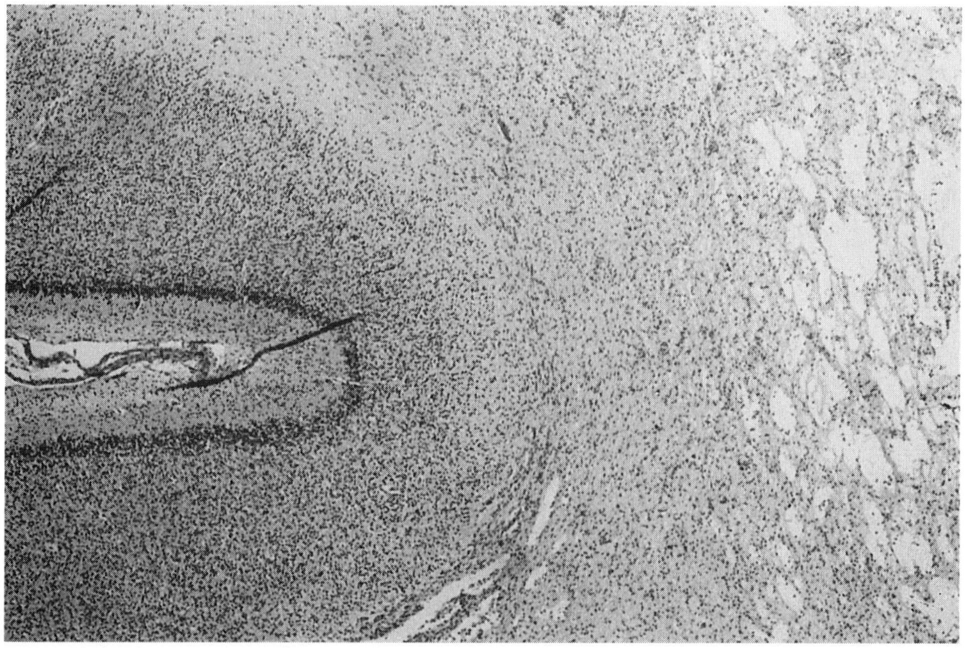

**Fig. 13-4.** Deep white matter infarction with preservation of the cortical gray matter in a preterm infant. Cavitation and gliosis indicate a chronic stage of evolution of this lesion, weeks to months after the insult. (H&E; ×40.)

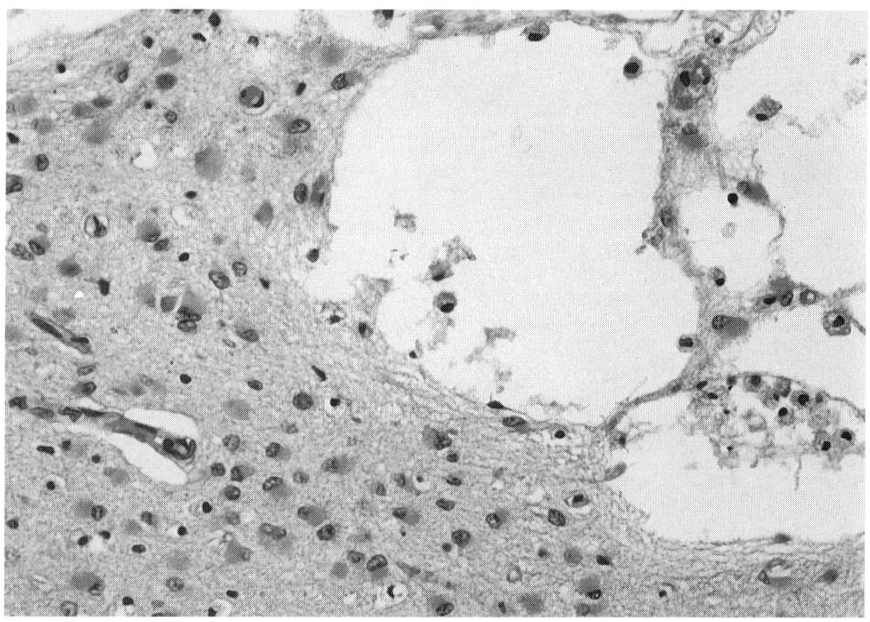

**Fig. 13-5.** Cavitation or pseudocysts of the subcortical white matter of a neonate with hypoxic/ischemic encephalopathy in the subacute to chronic phases, 7 weeks after a cardiopulmonary arrest. Many gemistocytic astrocytes are seen in the parenchyma around the cyst. A few macrophages persist within the cavity. The pseudocysts are not lined by epithelium. Delicate trabeculae of gliotic tissue traverse and subdivide the cavity. (H&E; ×250.)

A

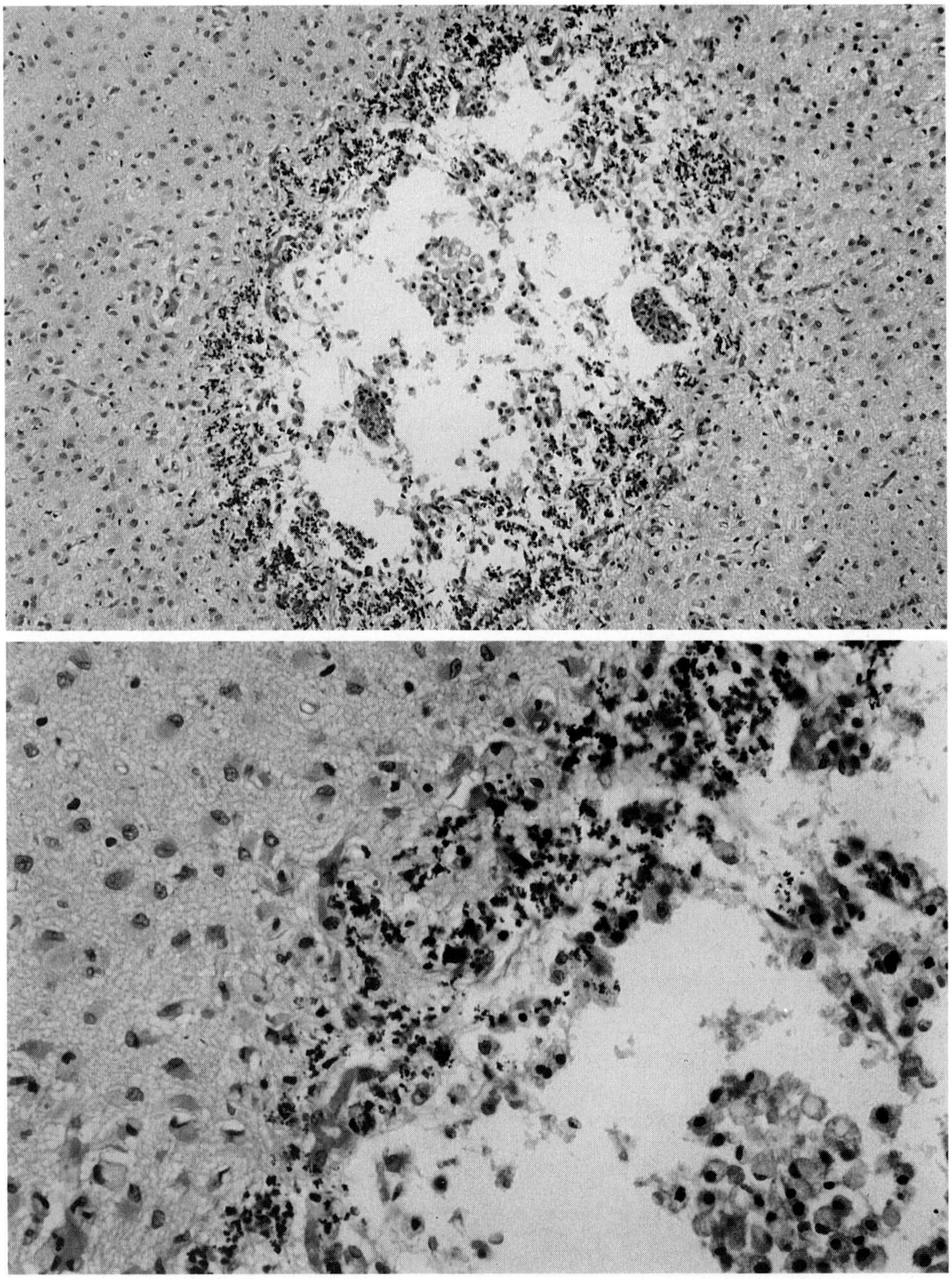

B

**Fig. 13-6.** Pseudocyst from another part of the subcortical white matter of the same brain as shown in Fig. 13-5. In addition to gemistocytes and macrophages, calcifications are already beginning to form at the margins of the pseudocysts, the so-called "dystrophic calcifications" of old perinatal infarcts sometimes identified in CT imaging studies (Fig. 13-7). (**A**, H&E; ×100; **B**, H&E; ×400.)

Periventricular leukomalacia is marked by a band of subependymal gliosis (Fig. 13-8). Discontinuities or gaps in the overlying ependyma are filled by astrocytes and their processes. The gliosis may be focally so intense that glial nodules are formed that protrude into the ventricular lumen, either beneath the intact surface ependyma or within the gaps. If initially covered by ependyma, the ependymal cells at the apex of large nodules become atrophic and eventually disappear (Fig. 13-9).[128] The subependymal gliosis may entrap ependymal cells, and clusters of these cells form subventricular rosettes (Fig. 13-10).[128] Larger areas of subventricular infarction may form subependymal pseudocysts.[66] A *pseudocyst* is a cavity lacking an epithelial lining. Because simple epithelia cannot be discerned by imaging, radiologists tend to call these cavitations

*Text continues on page 552.*

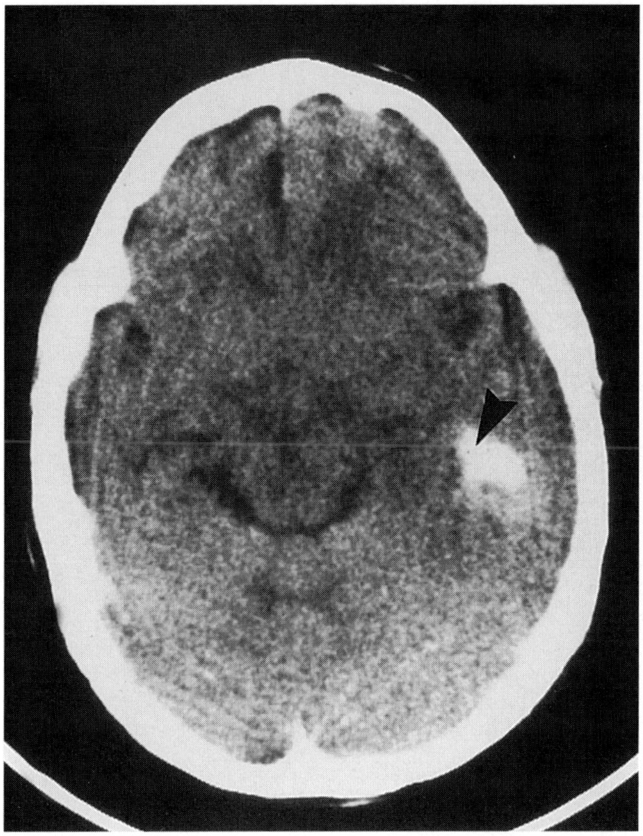

**Fig. 13-7.** Unenhanced CT scan of a 16-month-old boy with dystrophic calcification in the left temporal lobe (*arrowhead*) secondary to deep white matter infarction in the neonatal period. The child had been born prematurely at 27 weeks' gestation.

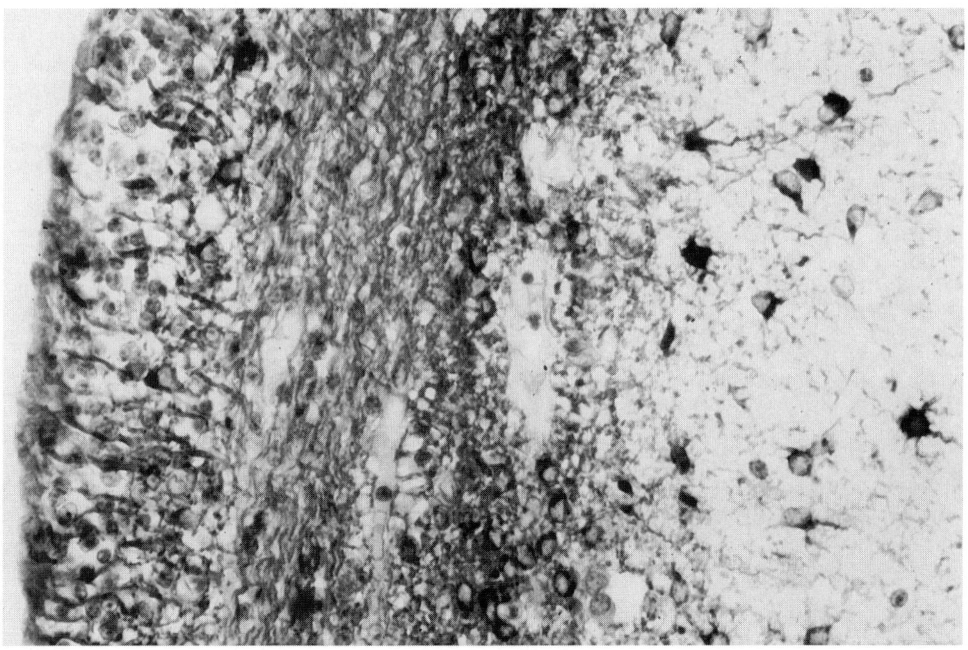

**Fig. 13-8.** Zone of dense gliosis in periventricular region of a 9-week-old infant born at 30 weeks' gestation. Periventricular leukomalacia was demonstrated by cranial ultrasound during life. A broad band of glial fibers is seen in the subventricular zone over the head of the caudate nucleus. Many ependymal cells still show basal processes, a mild delay in maturation. Radial glial fibers are not demonstrated, but the white matter superficial to the periventricular region shows mature astrocytes with processes. Glial fibrillary acidic protein. (×400.)

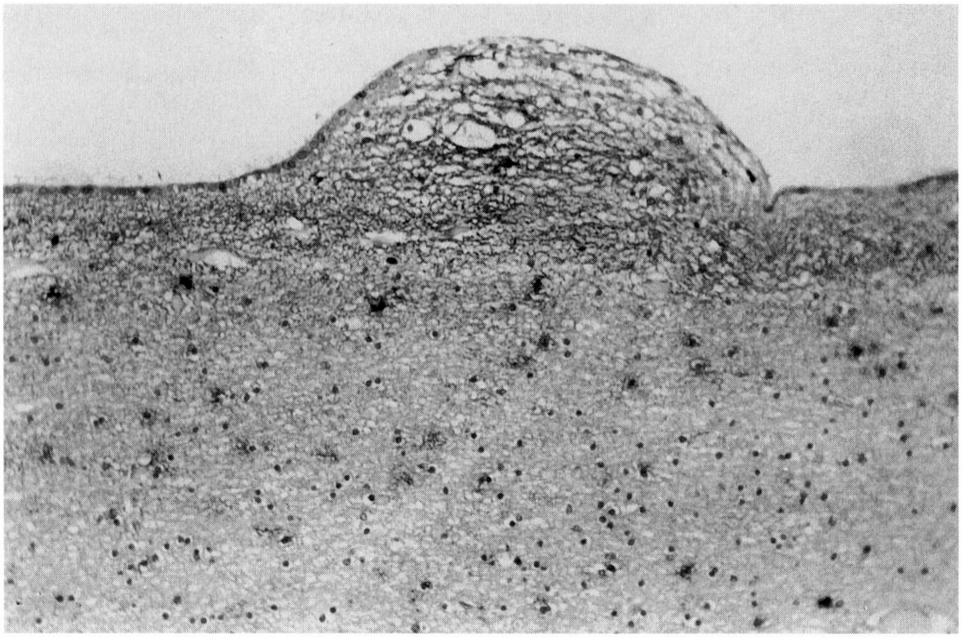

**Fig. 13-9.** Subependymal gliosis and a large glial nodule protruding into the lateral ventricle in an infant of 6 months who was born prematurely and had periventricular leukomalacia. The ependyma is flattened and atrophic and disappears from the apex of the nodule. (H&E; ×250.)

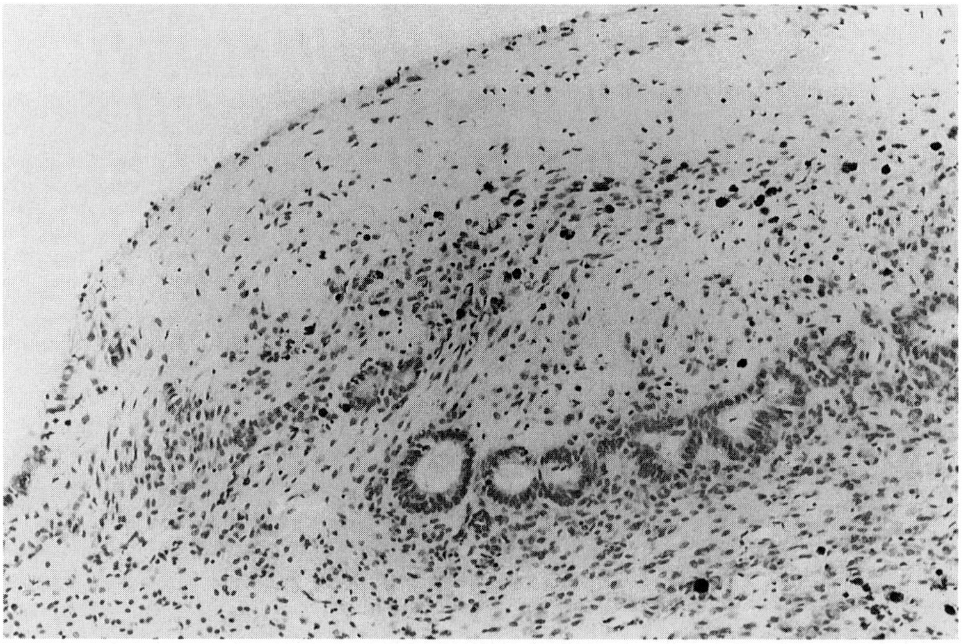

**Fig. 13-10.** Subventricular ependymal rosettes formed by gliotic overgrowth of periventricular region, burying islands of surface ependymal cells that then form tubular structures or "rosettes." These heterotopic ependymal cells are common in end-stages of healed periventricular leukomalacia. (H&E; ×100.)

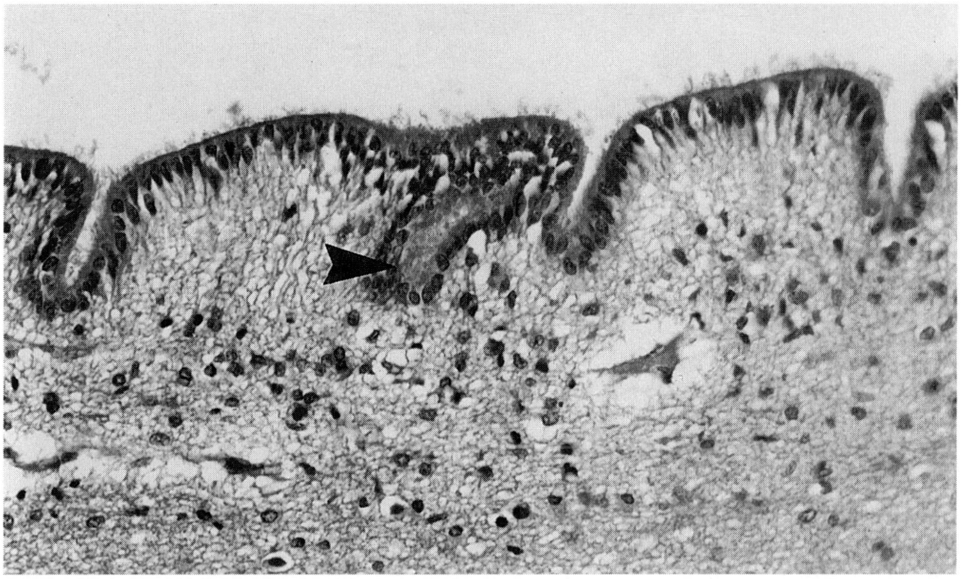

**Fig. 13-11.** Ependymal diverticulum becoming separated beneath the ventricular surface (*arrowhead*) to form a true cyst, unlike the more common pseudocysts that are not lined by an epithelium. Mild gliosis also is seen in this zone of mild periventricular leukomalacia. (H&E; ×250.)

**A**

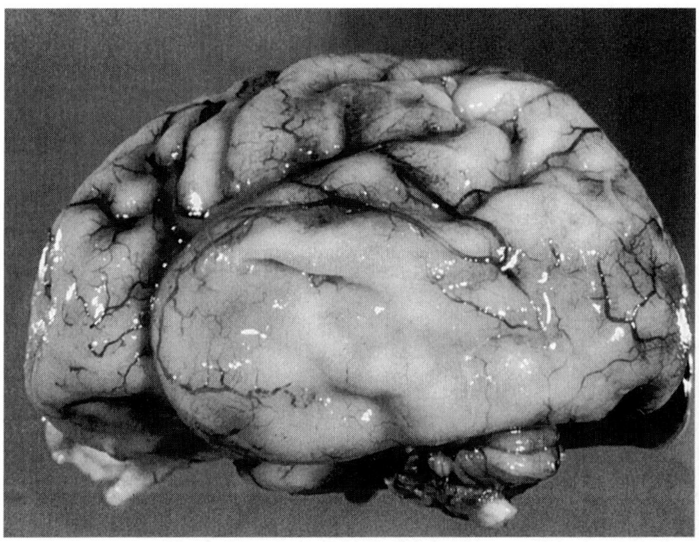

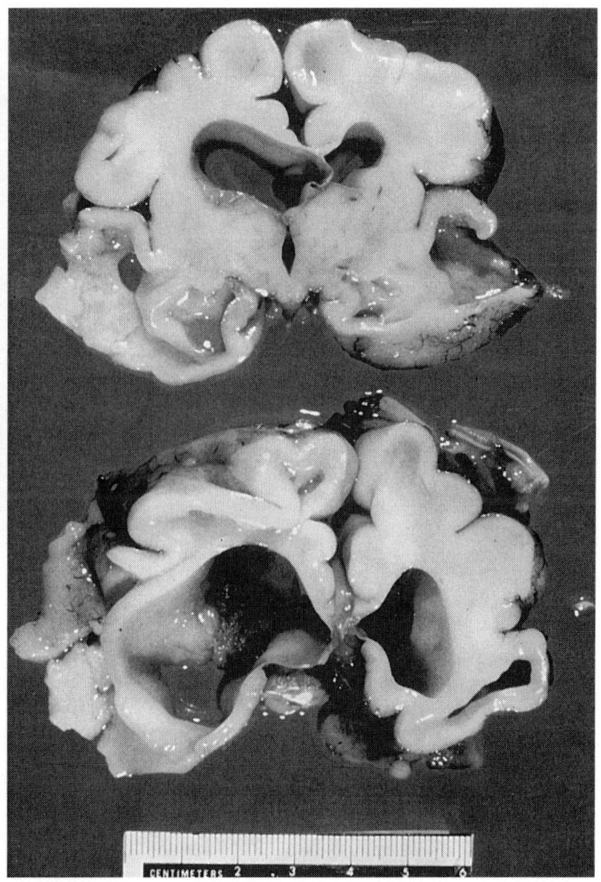

**B**

**Fig. 13-12. A**, Lateral aspect of the left cerebral hemisphere; **B**, coronal sections of the brain of a stillborn full-term fetus who suffered prolonged ischemia for several weeks in utero. The temporal lobe is swollen and softened, and shows loss of the convolutional pattern. Severe cortical atrophy and liquefactive necrosis of the white matter are present.

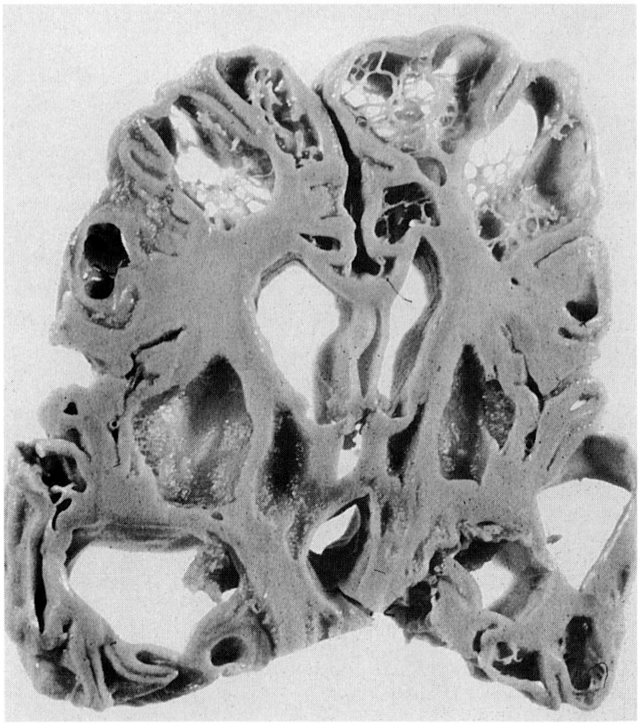

**Fig. 13-13.** Coronal section of the cerebral hemispheres of a 38-week neonate showing multicystic encephalomalacia. The multiple loculated cysts traversed by their glial trabeculae are the result of intrauterine infarcts. The ventricular system and basic architecture of the brain is well formed. (Courtesy of Dr. M.G. Netsky. Reproduced with permission from Sarnat HB: Cerebral dysgenesis. Embryology and clinical expression, New York, 1992, Oxford University Press.)

*cysts* or periventricular *cystic* leukomalacia. The only true cysts in the subventricular zone are loculated ependymal rosettes that form as diverticuli from the ventricular surface and become "pinched off," losing their continuity with the overlying surface ependyma (Fig. 13-11).[128]

The condition characterized by multiple loculated cavities separated by trabeculae of glial tissue without neurons is termed *multicystic encephalomalacia* and is a late or final stage in the evolution of extensive white matter necrosis, usually accompanied by severe gray matter changes as well (Figs. 13-12 to 13-15). If both cerebral hemispheres are destroyed by carotid occlusions at midgestation, leaving only a small amount of residual supratentorial cerebral tissue in the posterior cerebral artery territory, *hydranencephaly* results and must be distinguished from end-stage fetal hydrocephalus. Multiple micropseudocysts sometimes do not coalesce to create large cavitations; they eventually collapse and leave *white matter atrophy*. The cerebral cortex surrounding the depths of sulci in such cases almost reaches the ependymal surface because of the loss of white matter, and the brain grossly appears small and underweight with a normal pattern of convolutions. Laminar necrosis of the cerebral cortex in the neonate is unusual and primarily involves layer 3, but more commonly all layers become necrotic with loss of architecture and total or near-total disappearance of neurons (Fig. 13-15).

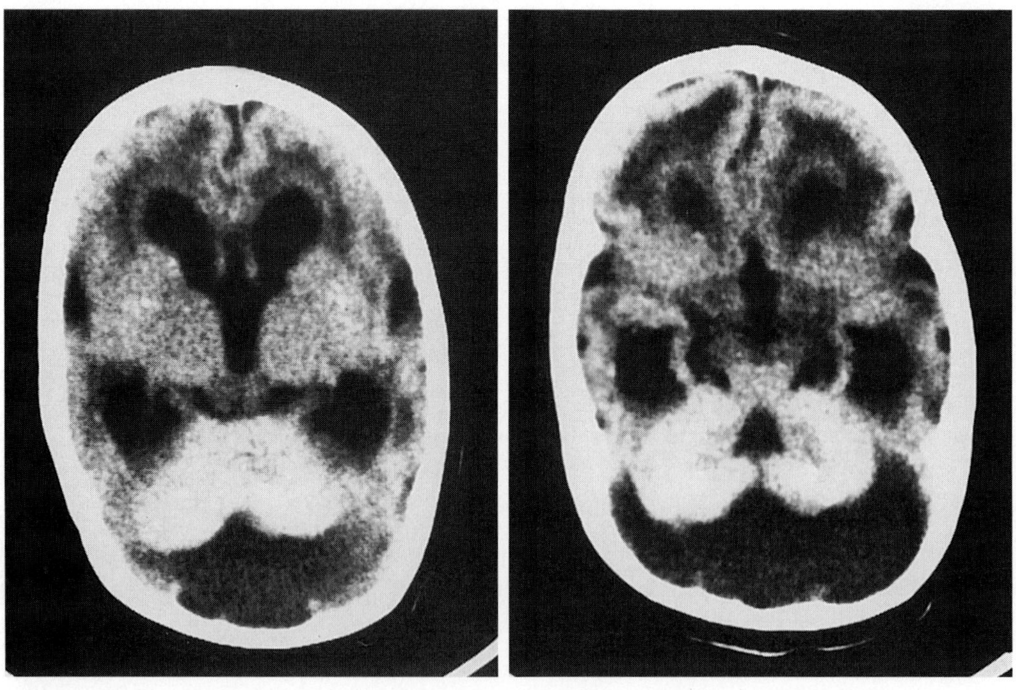

**Fig. 13-14.** Unenhanced CT images in two axial planes of a term neonate with extensive white matter necrosis and early stages in the formation of multicystic encephalomalacia, secondary to prolonged fetal distress and ischemic injury.

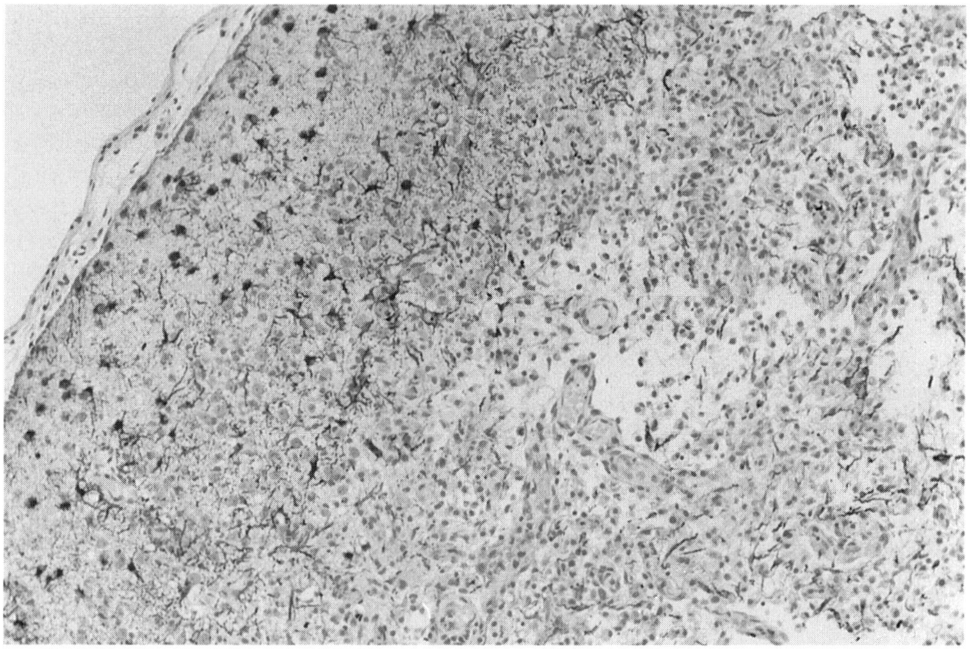

**Fig. 13-15.** Extensive encephalomalacia of the neonatal cerebrum 18 days after a severe ischemic episode. Histologically, extensive white matter necrosis and replacement by sheets of macrophages and pseudocysts are seen. The gray matter of the cortex no longer exhibits recognizable laminated architecture because of complete neuronal loss and gliosis. Glial fibrillary acidic protein. (×40.)

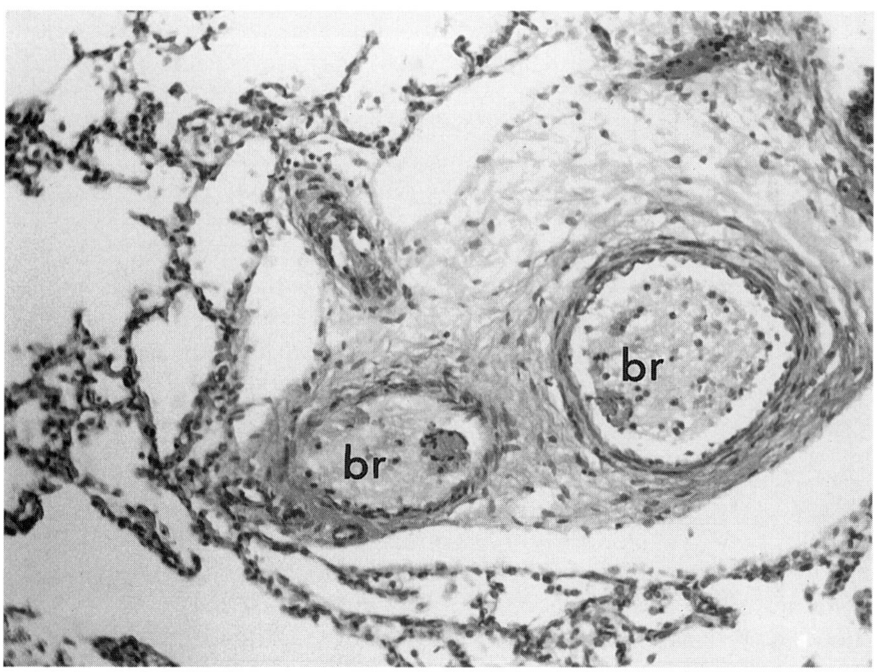


**Fig. 13-16.** Emboli of necrotic brain fragments (*br*) within arterioles of the lung in a term neonate with extensive ischemic encephalomalacia. The embolized cerebral tissue still demonstrated GFAP immunoreactivity of astrocytes (not shown). This complication of embolic brain to the lung may aggravate respiratory distress and cause further hypoxemia. (H&E; × 250.)

Infarcted, necrotic brain fragments sometimes become dislodged and pass down into the spinal subarachnoid space. They may even enter blood vessels and be carried as emboli to distant parts of the body, particularly the lungs (Fig. 13-16).

Transforming growth factor-alpha (TGF-$\alpha$) has been implicated in stimulating the proliferation of subependymal astrocytes and the synthesis of GFAP in those cells in the neonatal mouse brain.[163] Other trophic factors also might be released in response to ischemia and initiate or mediate reactive gliosis. The ependyma itself is surprisingly resistant to hypoxia and ischemia, and often survives at the ventricular surface despite extensive periventricular leukomalacia.[128] Ependymal cells do not regenerate,[128] but some subventricular undifferentiated glioblasts or stem cells might become new ependymal cells.[84]

Another unique feature of perinatal white matter infarcts is the appearance of amphophilic extracellular globules near capillaries and venules, probably proteinaceous material escaping from damaged endothelium. This finding and the mixture of both hypertrophic reactive astrocytes and degenerating glial cells in the same region is characteristic of actively myelinating white matter, and is seen neither in areas that have not yet begun myelination nor in areas that are fully myelinated.[74,157] It may be related to the increased metabolic rate of myelinating tissue.[74] In chronic stages, delayed myelination may be demonstrated by MRI and neuropathologically in regions of white matter gliosis.[56] This phenomenon may result from the diversion of glial stem cells into reactive astrocytes, reducing the population of oligodendrocytes available to synthesize myelin.[140] Morphometric examination of myelination and ferritin-containing oligodendrocytes reveals normal development in the non-necrotic and nongliotic cerebral white matter of brains with focal PVL.[56] Myelination is not affected in all cases of chronic perinatal hypoxia, as in infants with prolonged respiratory distress requiring ventilator support.[17] In other cases, however, damage to oligodendrocytes during ischemia of periventricular and subcortical white matter in fetuses and neonates may lead to delayed or reduced myelination.[143]

In sum, the sequence of changes is coagulation necrosis and microglial mobilization early; reactive gliosis, macrophagic infiltration, and neovascularity in the intermediate phase; and cavitation, white matter atrophy, gliosis, and mineralization in the late phase (see Table 13-1).

## HEMORRHAGIC INFARCTS OF THE CEREBRAL WHITE MATTER

### Germinal Matrix Hemorrhages (GMH)

The *germinal matrix* is a traditional, though not entirely accurate, term applied to the densely cellular layer of small, round, dark cells with large round nuclei and sparse cytoplasm that occupies much of the subventricular zone (Fig. 13-2). These cells are postmitotic, premigratory neuroepithelial cells that have undergone their last mitosis before the differentiation of the ependyma at the ventricular surface of the lateral ventricles.[125,137]

The neuroepithelial cells of the germinal matrix are undifferentiated neuroblasts and glioblasts. The majority become neurons of the cerebral cortex during the first half of gestation, and nearly all become protoplasmic astrocytes in the cortex during the second half of gestation, though a few neuronal precursors are still migrating until at least 34 weeks' gestation. In late gestation some become oligodendrocytes of the subcortical white matter. The only differentiated cells of the germinal matrix are the cell bodies of radial glia that guide migratory cells to the cortex and the endothelial cells of thin, fragile vascular channels. Whether germinal matrix cells are preprogrammed to differentiate as specific cell types or retain a plasticity to differentiate in another direction if different synaptic input, ischemia, or other pathologic conditions occur is still an unresolved issue. Evidence is available to support each of these two opposing hypotheses; but this topic is beyond the scope of the present chapter.

At midgestation, the germinal matrix is a thick layer of periventricular cells beneath the head and body of the caudate nucleus. It gradually thins and disappears by about 34 weeks' gestation as its cells progressively migrate toward the cerebral cortex. At term a few scattered premigratory germinal matrix cells may be demonstrated beneath the ependyma, but these no longer are numerous enough to form a layer.

**Vascular perfusion of the germinal matrix.** The "capillary bed" of the germinal matrix consists of thin-walled sinuses that are neither mature capillaries nor venules and lack the muscular walls and collagenous adventitia of arterioles. They are variable in size; most are equal in size or smaller than capillaries and others are large enough to appear as sinusoids coursing through the highly cellular germinal matrix.[51] Anastomoses are few. The arterial supply of these vascular channels over the head and body of the caudate nucleus is provided by Heubner's artery (the recurrent or medial striate artery that is the large first branch of the anterior cerebral artery just beyond the anterior communicating artery), a branch of the lateral striate artery (from the middle cerebral artery), and the anterior choroidal artery, the latter a more prominent and relatively larger vessel in the fetus than in the adult and usually a direct branch of the internal carotid artery. Leptomeningeal vessels penetrate the brain to supply blood to the germinal matrix caudal to the thalamus and deep telencephalic nuclei.[91] Microangiography confirms only a rudimentary vascular bed in the germinal matrix.[146] Arterial blood flow through the germinal matrix is low in beagle pups[104] and presumably also in premature human infants. The venous drainage is through the internal cerebral veins and great vein of Galen into the straight sinus and is better developed than is the microcirculation within the germinal matrix.

The "capillary unit" of germinal matrix microvascular channels is developed by midgestation to consist of the endothelial cell, pericyte, basal lamina (basement membrane), and astrocytic end-foot.[68,103,106] The end-feet of polymorphous astrocytes are in a constant state of remodeling.[103] These vessels still differ, however, from mature capillaries; the endothelial cell is thinner and has fewer cytoplasmic organelles such as vacuoles, pinocytotic vesicles, microvilli, and the rodshaped bodies believed to be related to thromboplastic and clotting activity. The vascular channels of the germinal matrix enter large venous branches at right angles. In the fetal baboon, radial glial cells contribute end-feet to the walls of the vascular channels, and the basal lamina is continuous and well-formed, as in the human.[13] In the rabbit, by contrast, ultrastructural studies reveal that processes of the germinal matrix cells themselves rather than astrocytes form end-feet on the vascular wall, and the basal lamina is thin, discontinuous, and of low electron density.[139]

**Hemorrhagic infarction of the germinal matrix and intraventricular hemorrhages (IVH).** Periventricular leukomalacia is usually ischemic infarction with coagulative necrosis, but microscopic perivascular hemorrhages accompany PVL in about 25% of cases.[7] Frank hemorrhage into the germinal matrix is a distinct lesion and one of the most common of the premature infant brain (Fig. 13-17). It accounts for a high proportion of neurologic disability in survivors, and represents a major cause of death in intensive care nurseries.

The first autopsy description of a cerebral hemorrhage in a newborn infant was published by Thomas Willis in 1667,[165] the same author who described the anastomotic circle at the base of the brain. Several early 19th-century French physicians also provided descriptions of neonatal intracerebral hemorrhages, the most notable of which is that of Cruveilhier, which was complete with an illustration of an IVH in a preterm infant.[24] Details of these early reports and a reproduction of Cruveilhier's drawing are provided by Paneth and associates.[100]

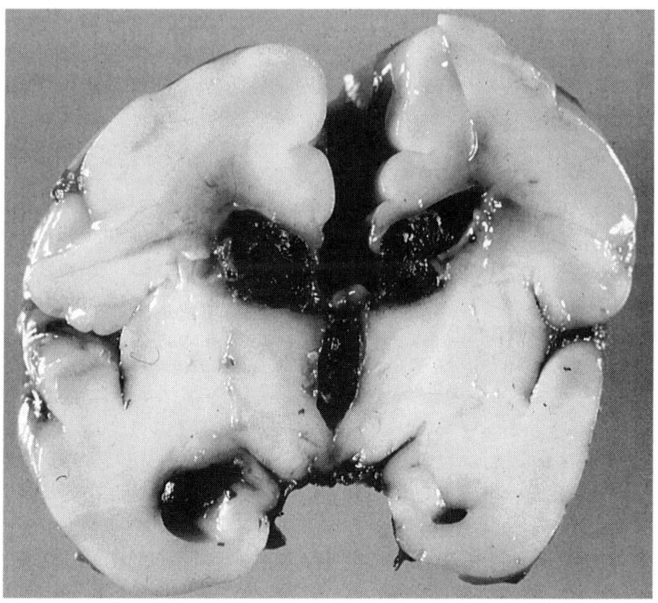

**Fig. 13-17.** Coronal section of the brain at autopsy of a 26-week preterm infant with grade 3 intraventricular hemorrhage by cranial ultrasound. Blood fills and dilates the entire ventricular system but does not infiltrate the cerebral parenchyma beyond the periventricular region.

The clinical grading system of IVH in the preterm infant widely used in intensive care nurseries is based on noninvasive examination of the brain by ultrasound echoes detected through the anterior fontanelle. Four grades of hemorrhage are recognized by ultrasonographic criteria and usually are regarded by clinicians as progressive stages of the same process; neuropathologic correlation with each of these grades confirms that this assumption is indeed the case for grades 1 through 3; however, grade 4 hemorrhages are different in character from the others and have a different pathogenesis.

Ultrasonography is used in the preterm infant as the principal imaging technique for good reasons: (1) it can be performed at the bedside and does not require moving unstable patients; (2) it requires no anesthesia; (3) it involves no x-rays or other radiation risks; (4) it can be repeated weekly, daily, or as often as necessary to provide serial data on the evolution of the changes; (5) it provides good visualization of the size of the lateral and third ventricles, demonstrates periventricular leukomalacia, hemorrhages, and cavitations, and can detect midline defects of cerebral development such as holoprosencephaly and agenesis of the corpus callosum; and (6) it can provide dynamic real-time examination of the brain, including pulsations. The disadvantages of ultrasonography are: (1) the resolution is not as good as with CT or MR imaging; and (2) it does not provide reliable visualization of peripheral parts of the cerebral hemispheres, including the cerebral cortex and extraaxial spaces, or of infratentorial structures. The routine use of serial real-time ultrasound scanning has permitted the development of a time scale to characterize the temporal evolution of histopathologic reactions to hemorrhage in the premature human brain.[26]

The four grades of IVH standardized by ultrasonographic criteria in the living infant are: *grade 1*: small focal subependymal hemorrhages that do not extend into the lateral ventricle; *grade 2*: subependymal hemorrhage that extends into the lateral ventricle locally but does not dilate the ventricular system; *grade 3*: more extensive hemorrhage within the germinal matrix; blood fills the ventricular system and causes generalized dilatation; and *grade 4*: intraparenchymal hemorrhage outside the germinal matrix, involving the subcortical white matter and even the gray matter of the cerebral cortex or deep telencephalic nuclei and thala-

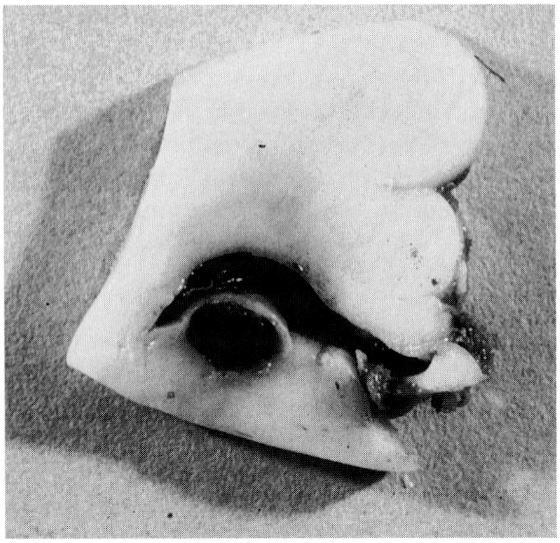

**Fig. 13-18.** A subependymal germinal matrix hemorrhage that has broken through the thin ependymal epithelium into the lateral ventricle of a 32-week preterm infant.

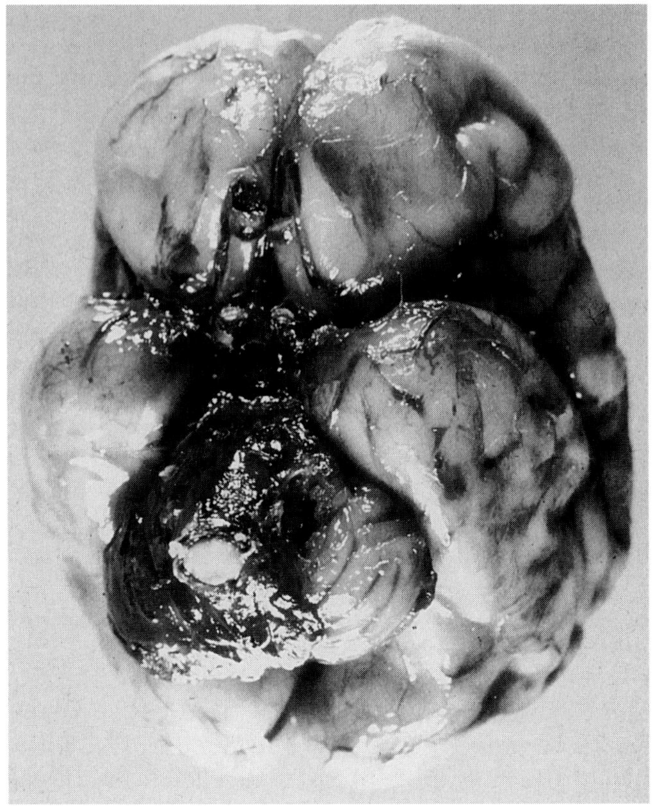

**Fig. 13-19.** Ventral aspect of the brain of a 33-week preterm infant with intraventricular hemorrhage originating in the germinal matrix over the head of the caudate nucleus. Blood passes through the ventricular system and enters the subarachnoid space through the foramina of Magendie and Luschka to surround the brainstem and ventral surface of the cerebellum. It obscures the cranial nerves.

mus. Grade 4 hemorrhage is nearly always accompanied by intraventricular hemorrhage and ventricular dilatation, as in grade 3.

Subependymal and intraventricular hemorrhages are not the natural progression of periventricular leukomalacia, and the two lesions are different. Periventricular leukomalacia is essentially ischemic infarction and coagulative necrosis. Hemorrhage may occur in zones of periventricular leukomalacia, but usually does not. Hemorrhage generally occurs spontaneously in previously intact and histologically normal germinal matrix.

Over 90% of GMH occurs over the head of the caudate nucleus adjacent to the foramen of Monro (Fig. 13-18).[72] This site, near the stria terminalis, was first noted to be the origin of most GMH by Ruckensteiner and Zöllner in 1929,[118] and their careful observations have been reconfirmed by many later neuropathologists. Additional sites are the roof of the temporal horn and along the occipital horn of the lateral ventricle; these posterior zones are the most frequent sites of nonhemorrhagic PVL. GMH often begin in multiple subependymal foci and are bilateral in about half the cases.[32] Blood easily ruptures through the thin ependyma and into the ventricle. Large hemorrhages may dissect beyond the limits of the germinal matrix and into the head of the caudate nucleus or into the deep subcortical white matter, but other factors are more important in white matter hemorrhagic infarcts or "grade 4 IVH," as discussed below. IVH also may originate independently from the tela choroidea or choroid plexus in preterm infants,[67,111] but these origins are a more common cause of IVH in the term neonate (see below).

Small amounts of intraventricular blood usually remain in the liquid state, but large hemorrhages form clots and thrombotic casts of the ventricles. Blood is carried by the normal CSF circulation to be redistributed to the third ventricle and through the cerebral aqueduct into the fourth ventricle, from which it then passes through the foramina of Magendie and Luschka to enter the subarachnoid space of the posterior fossa and surround the cerebellum and brainstem (Fig. 13-19). It then filters down the spinal subarachnoid space, where it may be detected by lumbar puncture. Eventually the blood circulates over the convexities of the cerebral hemispheres.

Since the germinal matrix is a transitory structure that essentially disappears by 35 weeks' gestation, hemorrhages into it are strictly a disorder of premature infants; most at risk are those at less than 30 weeks' gestation or weighing less than 1500 g.

GMH are most commonly a postnatal event; only 5% of such hemorrhages begin prenatally.[26] The peak occurrence is 48 to 72 hours after birth. However, such hemorrhages may begin in utero if fetal distress has occurred, and even stillborns may be shown at autopsy to have suffered GMH, not always as a terminal event, as demonstrated by macrophages, hemosiderin, and reactive gliosis, documenting that the hemorrhages occurred at least 7 to 14 days earlier. Autopsies of infants who have survived several weeks postnatally may show several subependymal hemorrhages of different ages, denoting recurrent events.

In chronic states, the histopathologic lesions of mild (grades 1 and 2) periventricular hemorrhages are similar to those described in PVL earlier in this chapter except that hemosiderin persists as a marker of the previous blood, free in the parenchyma or in macrophages and astrocytes.[12] However, hemosiderin often is cleared completely in chronic states from premature brains, a major difference from adult brains in which iron pigment persists for years after an intracerebral hemorrhage, in macrophages and especially in astrocytes.[26] Early reactions by macrophages occur at about the same rate in the premature brain as in the adult with intracerebral hemorrhage, but the routine transfer of iron from macrophages to astrocytes is much slower.[26] Oligodendrocytes also contain cytoplasmic deposits of ferritin in sites of old hemorrhage.[56] Hemosiderin may be present in ependymal cells also but is minimal. Grossly, the normal glistening white ventricular surface becomes yellow, splotched, and less shiny because of hemosiderin deposited by intraventricular blood.

**Pathogenesis of GMH.** The cause of GMH is still a much debated topic. Predisposing conditions include hypoxia, ischemia, hypercapnia, acidosis, and especially episodes of systemic hypotension. Respiratory distress syndrome and dependence on mechanical ventilation are important related conditions. The lack of autoregulation of cerebral blood flow in the immature brain of preterm infants is probably a major contributory factor.[76,107] Neither the critical closing pressure of premature cerebral circulation nor the resistance area product correlates with pH, $pCO_2$, or hematocrit, but mean arterial pressure is important.[99] Placental abruption and placenta previa are not directly associated with GMH. Mode of delivery, by vertex, breech, or cesarean section, does not appear either to predispose to or protect from subsequent GMH.

The likely cascade of events leading to GMH is that hypoxia and lactic acidosis, induced by transient systemic hypotension, damage the delicate endothelial cells of the microcirculation. When normal systemic blood pressure and flow are restored, the damaged endothelium of the thin vascular channels ruptures and hemorrhage occurs. More mature endothelial cells in the cerebral cortex are more resistant and better survive these transient ischemic conditions. The right angle junctions where germinal matrix vessels enter venous branches are common sites of rupture in GMH.[54] Deposits of fibrin and small thrombi often precede or accompany such hemorrhages.[67] The principal tributaries of the internal cerebral veins (i.e., thalamostriate, terminal, frontal, septal, and choroidal veins) become severely dilated. Electron microscopy reveals swollen glial end-feet, indistinct basal laminae, and extravasation of blood through widened endothelial cell junctions of germinal matrix vessels.[68]

The density of small vascular channels progressively increases in the normal neuroepithelium surrounding the lateral ventricles from 8 to 18 weeks' gestation; thereafter, the number of vascular lumina per unit of surface area decreases, an inverse contrast with the proliferation of capillaries in the cortical plate in the second half of gestation.[68] The germinal matrix may therefore ironically be more resistant to ischemic injury and hemorrhage during the first half of gestation because of relatively greater perfusion than during the second half, when the vascular channels are involuting.

Metabolic endotoxins, such as occur with bacterial sepsis or with the accumulation of ammonia, may contribute additional insults to the endothelium. The role of such endogenous hormones as prostaglandins is uncertain. Indomethacin, a potent inhibitor of prostaglandin synthetase, is commonly administered to preterm infants to induce closure of a patent ductus arteriosus, and may additionally inhibit platelet aggregation. However, no association is demonstrated between the use of this drug and the occurrence or size of GMH.[77]

In sum, GMH occurs when the structural integrity of the endothelium of the thin vascular channels is compromised by factors leading to transient decreased perfusion pressure followed by restoration of normal intravascular blood pressure and flow. Junction points where these vascular channels enter small veins at right angles are the most likely sites of rupture with reperfusion.

### Subcortical White Matter Hemorrhagic Infarcts

The *grade 4 intraventricular hemorrhage "with parenchymal involvement"* is not merely an "extension" of grade 3 as the sonographic grading scale implies, but rather is distinct in pathogenesis from GMH. Nevertheless it usually coexists and most often occurs on the same side as a large GMH.[100] Deep white matter hemorrhagic infarcts often begin as linear hemorrhagic streaks radiating outward from the angles of the frontal and occipital horns of the lateral ventricles, parallel to the distribution of the medullary veins.[7,39,48,100,160] These fan-shaped hemorrhages with the apex toward the angle of the lateral ventricle suggest that venous compression by a large GMH might initiate the sequence of events leading to large hemorrhagic infarcts of the deep white matter.[48,100] Postmortem cerebrovascular injection studies support this interpretation and

A B

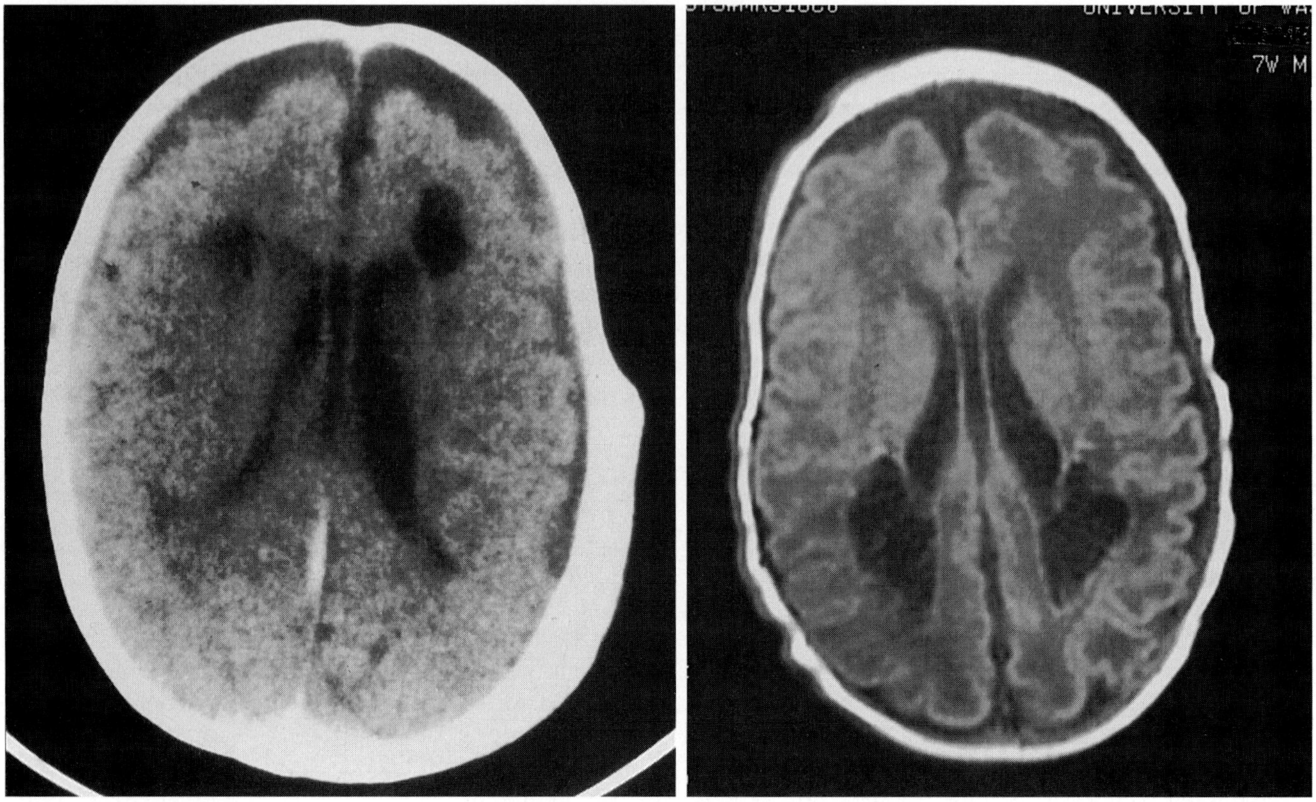

**Fig. 13-20.** Bilateral white matter cavitations at the angles of the **A**, frontal horns and **B**, occipital horns of the lateral ventricles in two infants born prematurely who had periventricular leukomalacia and grade 4 intraventricular hemorrhages in the first postnatal week. These are the most common sites of white matter hemorrhages, perhaps because of compression of fanlike, converging deep medullary veins by germinal matrix hemorrhages. A large midline cavum vergae is an incidental finding in both cases. (**A**, CT scan with contrast; **B**, MRI, T1-weighted sequence.)

demonstrate the fan-shaped topography of medullary veins in preterm infant brains without hemorrhages.[144] In chronic stages, symmetric cystic infarcts at the angles of the frontal and occipital horns of the ventricles denote earlier hemorrhagic infarction of the white matter in that location (Fig. 13-20). These "grade 4 intraventricular hemorrhages" are, therefore, often complications of GMH resulting from venous obstruction, but are not simple extravasations of blood dissecting beyond the confines of the germinal matrix.[100,160] Some deep white matter hemorrhages become so extensive that they destroy most of the hemisphere. Towbin proposed major venous thromboses as the basis of GMH and IVH in preterm infants,[150] but thrombosis of large venous sinuses is rare.

A less common pattern is diffuse hemorrhagic infarction of the centrum semiovale that extends into the white matter cores of gyri (Fig. 13-21).

### Supratentorial Hemorrhages in the Full-Term Neonate

After 35 weeks' gestation, germinal matrix hemorrhage no longer can be implicated as a cause of intraventricular hemorrhage, and bleeding within a ventricle is rare in the term infant. Birth trauma from a difficult delivery and molding of the head commonly results in subarachnoid bleeding from the tearing of the small veins that traverse the leptomeninges or subdural hematoma, and contusions of the cortical surface may be hemorrhagic by causing thrombosis of small cortical veins. However, intraventricular hemorrhage is uncommon and nearly always is accompanied by extensive multiple hemorrhagic infarcts throughout the brain (Fig. 13-22). Bleeding disorders such as X-linked factor VIII hemophilia, low platelet count due to disseminated intravascular coagulation, and vitamin K deficiency may present with intracerebral and intraventricular hemorrhage, but also are rare conditions. Hypoxia/ischemia per se, even under conditions of acidosis and systemic hypotension, generally should not be regarded as causes of spontaneous periventricular or intraventricular hemorrhage in the term neonate. In a majority of cases, no etiology of intraventricular or intracranial hemorrhage in the term infant is demonstrated.[14]

Cryptic hemangiomas of the choroid plexus are fre-

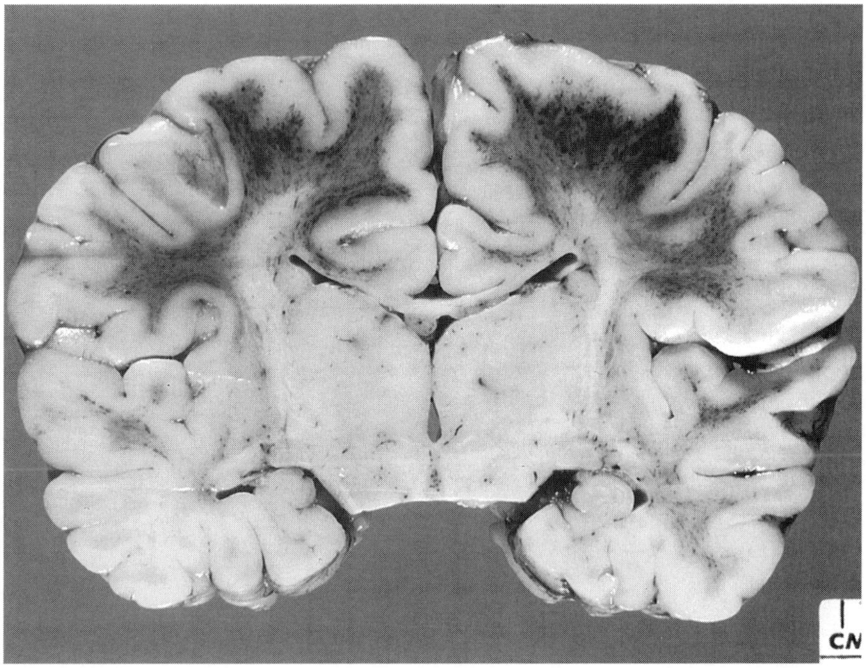


**Fig. 13-21.** Uncommon pattern of diffuse hemorrhagic leukoencephalopathy in an infant born at 41 weeks' gestation and who lived 3 days after severe fetal distress, meconium aspiration, respiratory failure, and seizures. Extensive hemorrhagic infarction involves the centrum semiovale symmetrically and extends into the white matter cores of gyri, but selectively spares gray matter, including the cerebral cortex, thalamus, and basal ganglia. Except for subacute ischemic neuronal changes, the brainstem and cerebellum were not involved.

A

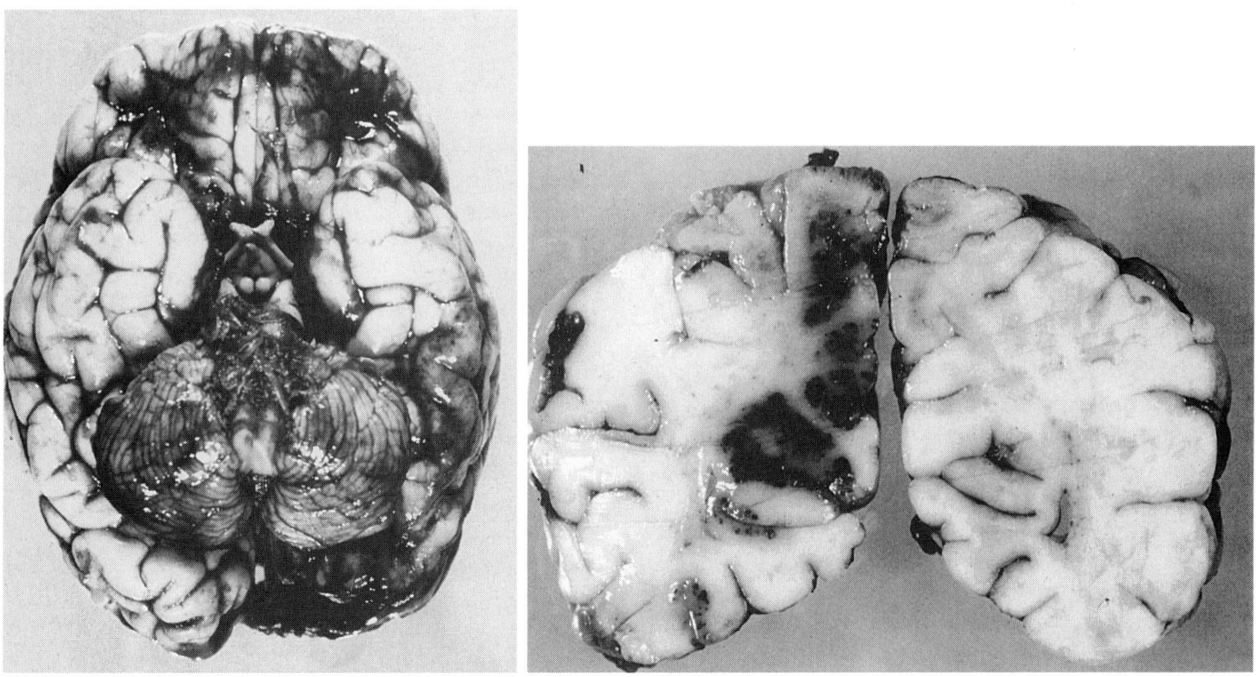

B

**Fig. 13-22.** **A**, Ventral aspect and **B**, coronal section of the brain of a term neonate delivered by midforceps extraction, who suffered extensive birth trauma to the head. Multiple hemorrhagic contusions of the brain are seen, and the left occipital pole is infarcted and shrunken. The right parasagittal hemorrhages seen in the coronal section are the result of contusions from pressure against the falx cerebri during delivery of the head. (Courtesy of Dr. N.B. Rewcastle.)

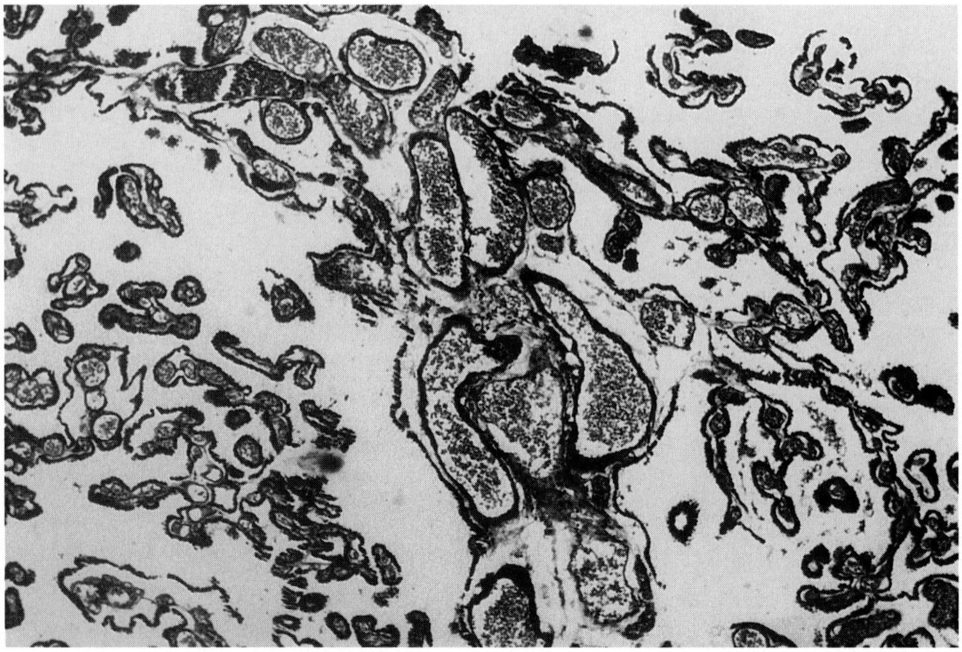

**Fig. 13-23.** Unruptured cryptic hemangioma of the choroid plexus of the lateral ventricle in a full-term neonate. The thin-walled dilated vascular channels are only partially covered by epithelium and are surrounded by fronds of normal choroid plexus. Rupture of such vascular malformations may be a common cause of spontaneous intraventricular hemorrhage in the term neonate. (Verhoeff-van Gieson stain; ×250.)

quently undetected because most remain asymptomatic and do not rupture to cause hemorrhage (Fig. 13-23);[30] the choroid plexus is often not routinely examined in neonatal brains at autopsy in infants dying of causes other than intracerebral hemorrhage, but this lesion is much more common than is generally recognized and may be a frequent cause of spontaneous intraventricular hemorrhage in the term neonate. The incidence of choroid plexus hemangioma is unknown because the great majority of them are small, do not rupture, and remain asymptomatic. Hemangiomas most often involve the choroid plexi of the lateral ventricles and consist of a largely cavernous angioma with thin-walled anastomosing channels of various sizes, usually not lined externally by choroid epithelium. Fronds of normal choroid plexus are adjacent to or mixed with angioma (Fig. 13-23). Endothelial cell proliferation is seen. Because the choroid plexus normally is a highly vascular structure, it may be difficult or impossible to distinguish normal choroid plexus from one containing this vascular malformation by contrast-enhanced CT or MR scans, unless it ruptures (Fig. 13-24). Choroid plexus often becomes highly congested as a terminal event and should not be confused with angioma. Hemorrhages originating in choroid plexus hemangiomas may destroy the original vascular malformation, but evidence of a few remaining pathologic vessels sometimes is found at the margins. Choroid plexus hemorrhages in full-term neonates are sometimes attributed to hypoxia,[31,63] but a small hemangioma may have been present as a precondition and the role of hypoxia is uncertain.

Primary thalamic hemorrhages occur rarely in term neonates (Fig. 13-25),[60,154] and striatal hemorrhages are equally uncommon (Fig. 13-26).[60] Such hemorrhages usually remain focal within the parenchyma and often are bilateral, but occasionally they rupture into the third or a lateral ventricle.[114] In some cases they are attributed to microangiomatosis[3] but also have been described after severe hypoxic insults. Excitotoxins also have been implicated in the pathogenesis of infantile striatal necrosis,[117] but the evidence is poorly documented. Thalamic and striatal hemorrhages may be detected during life by cranial ultrasound, CT, and MR.[158]

The vein of Galen "aneurysm" is really an arteriovenous malformation and usually does not rupture into the quadrigeminal cistern above the midbrain or into the ventricular system, though it does produce hydrocephalus by compressing the cerebral aqueduct and cardiac failure by creating a massive arteriovenous fistula.

### Posterior Fossa Hemorrhages

In preterm infants of less than 35 weeks' gestation, extravascular blood in the posterior fossa is usually

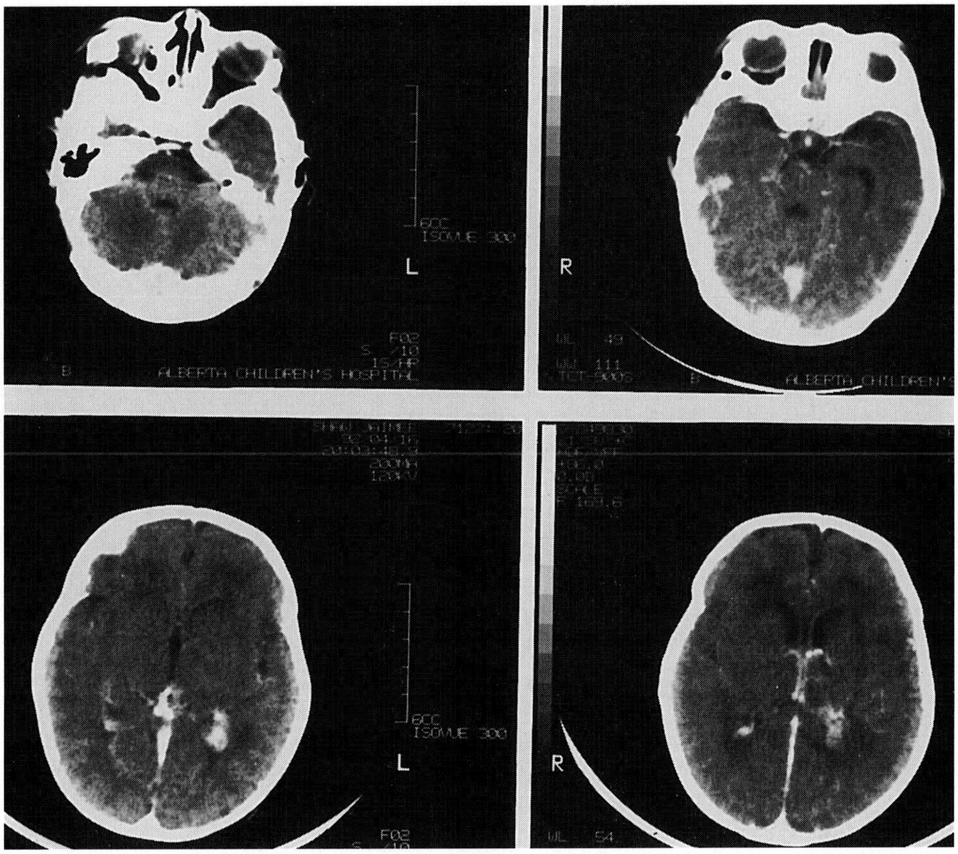


**Fig. 13-24.** Contrast-enhanced CT scan of a term neonate with a cryptic hemangioma of the choroid plexus in the left lateral ventricle.

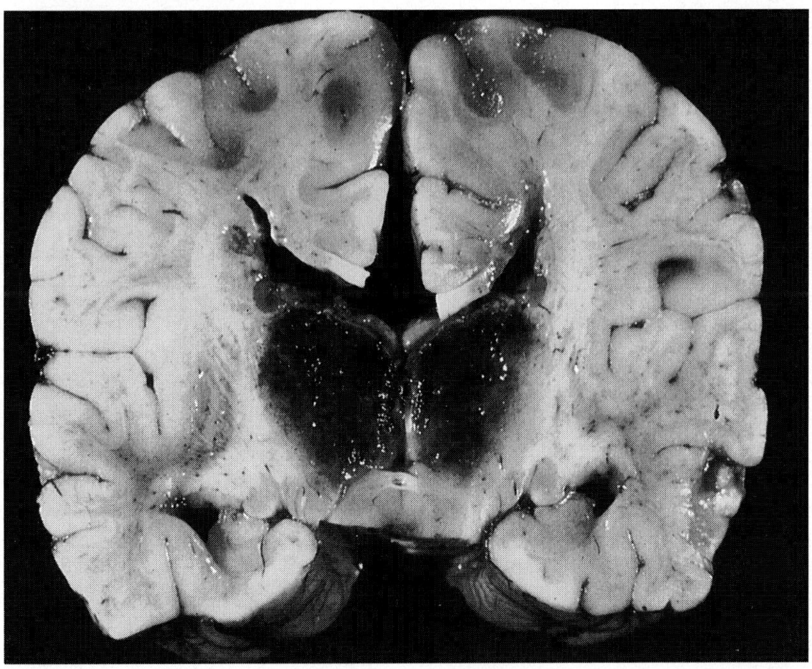

**Fig. 13-25.** Gross coronal section of brain disclosing bilateral symmetric thalamic hemorrhages and bilateral infarcts in the territory of the anterior cerebral arteries, involving the parasagittal cerebral cortex in a full-term infant with severe birth asphyxia. The corpus callosum was intact and artifactually severed.

A

B

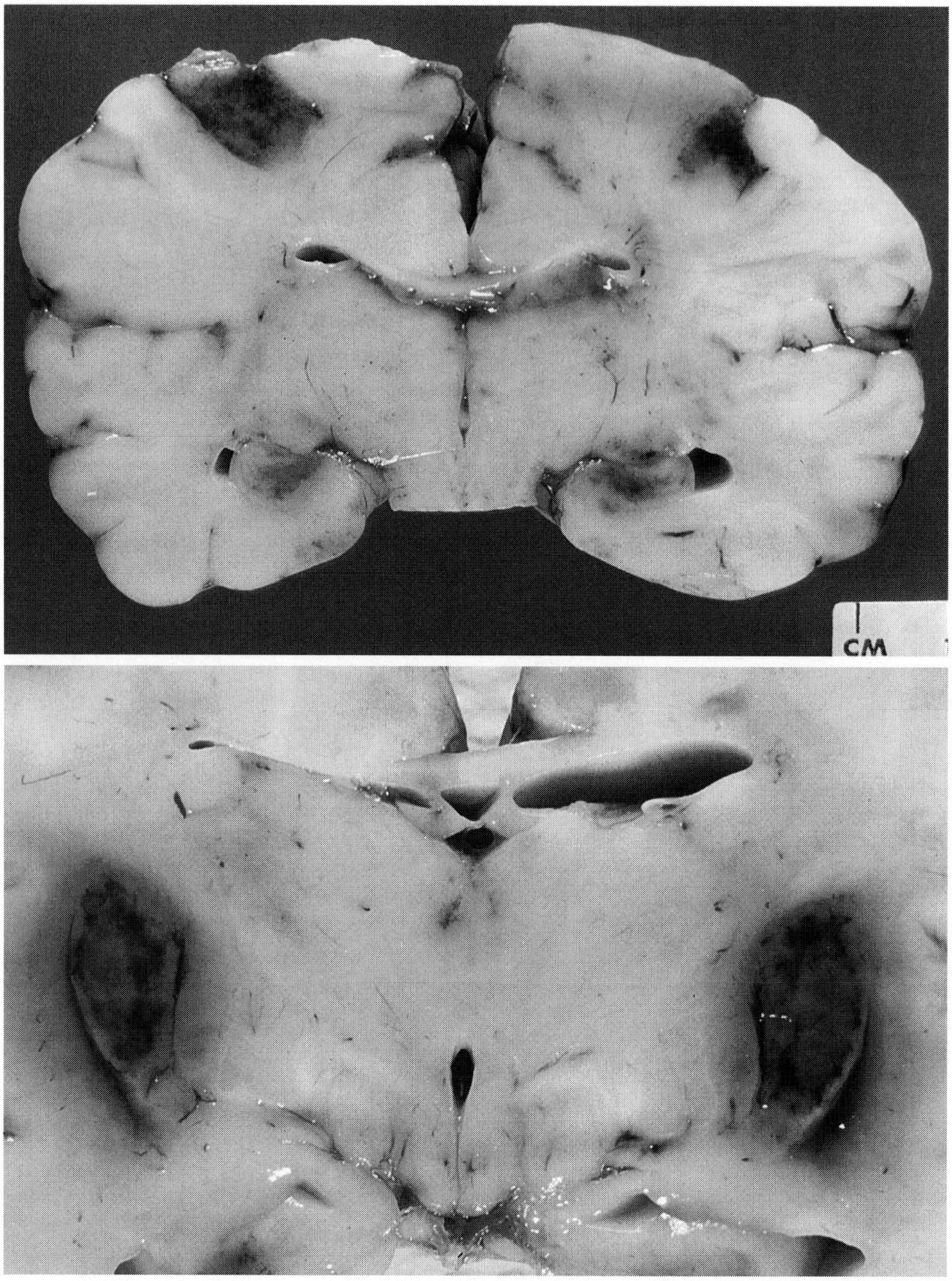


**Fig. 13-26.** Two coronal sections of brain of a full-term neonate with **A**, bilateral watershed infarcts in the zones between the territories of the anterior and middle cerebral arteries and of the middle and posterior cerebral arteries, including the hippocampi; and **B**, symmetric hemorrhagic infarcts of the putamen.

secondary to GMH with extension into a lateral ventricle, but the blood remains confined to the fourth ventricle and subarachnoid spaces around the brainstem and cerebellum and does not involve the parenchyma. In full-term or near-term neonates, posterior fossa hemorrhages are nearly always traumatic in origin and result from tentorial tears associated with molding of the head at the time of delivery (Fig. 13-27). Large intracerebellar hematomas may compress the fourth ventricle and obstruct the flow of CSF.[110,115]

The external granular layer of the cerebellar cortex at times develops spontaneous hemorrhage following hypoxia or systemic hypotension and essentially behaves similar to the germinal matrix of the supratentorial periventricular regions. Immature vasculature of the external granular layer is similar to that of the ger-

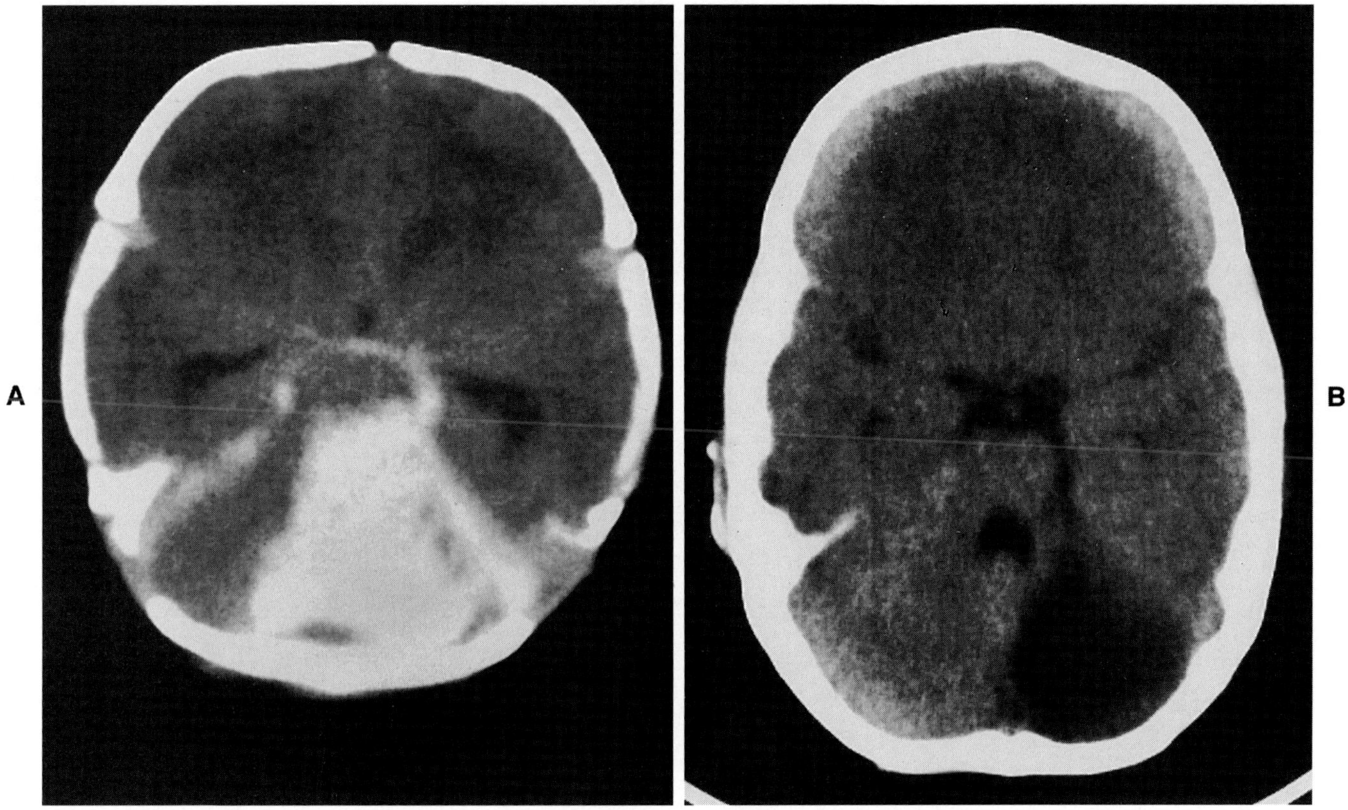

Fig. 13-27. Unenhanced computed axial tomography of an infant at age **A**, 1 day and **B**, 11 months who suffered a traumatic cerebellar hemorrhage at birth due to a tentorial tear at the time of delivery. A large hemorrhagic infarct involves the left cerebellar hemisphere and vermis (**A**), and in chronic stages leaves a cavity filled with CSF in communication with the subarachnoid space of the posterior fossa. This type of cerebellar hemorrhage is not due to perinatal hypoxic/ischemic encephalopathy.

minal matrix but, unlike the germinal matrix, the external granular layer is still prominent at term, and hypoxic/ischemic encephalopathy may induce hemorrhage in that structure beyond 35 weeks' gestation. However, it occurs more frequently in preterm than in term neonates. These hemorrhages are usually small and focal, but may become massive.[52] They usually occur in the cerebellar hemispheres rather than the vermis, perhaps only because the surface of the lateral hemispheres is so much larger than that of the vermis.

## BRAINSTEM AND SPINAL CORD LESIONS

The brainstem is often regarded as more resistant to hypoxic/ischemic injury than is the supratentorial white or gray matter.[36] This traditional view is only partially correct, but the basilar artery in the neonate has much less dense sympathetic innervation than do supratentorial arteries such as the anterior cerebral artery. Hence vasoconstriction is a less prominent response to hypoxia and induces less ischemia.[132] Both preterm and term infants who have suffered severe ischemic insults may develop microinfarcts of the brainstem (Fig. 13-28). These are usually symmetric and involve both gray matter nuclei and adjacent white matter tracts, but gray matter is more focally involved, probably because of its higher metabolic rate. The lesions may involve the inferior or superior colliculi almost selectively,[39] or at times infarction occurs in the segmental reticular core of the brainstem[1,45] or in the periaqueductal gray matter of the midbrain.[9,39] Multiple symmetric lesions of the brainstem tegmentum extending from the midbrain to the caudal medulla oblongata are seen as microscopic foci of infarction.[71,130] Prenatal HIE occasionally results in extensive destructive lesions of the thalamus, basal ganglia, brainstem tegmentum, and spinal cord, but with little involvement of the cerebral cortex.[89] Most brainstem ischemic infarcts are accompanied by extensive cerebral cortical lesions as well, however.

Neuronal degeneration without frank tissue infarction occurs in the basis pontis and is known as *pontosubicular degeneration* (discussed later in this chapter). Cholinergic neurons, such as those of the pedunculo-

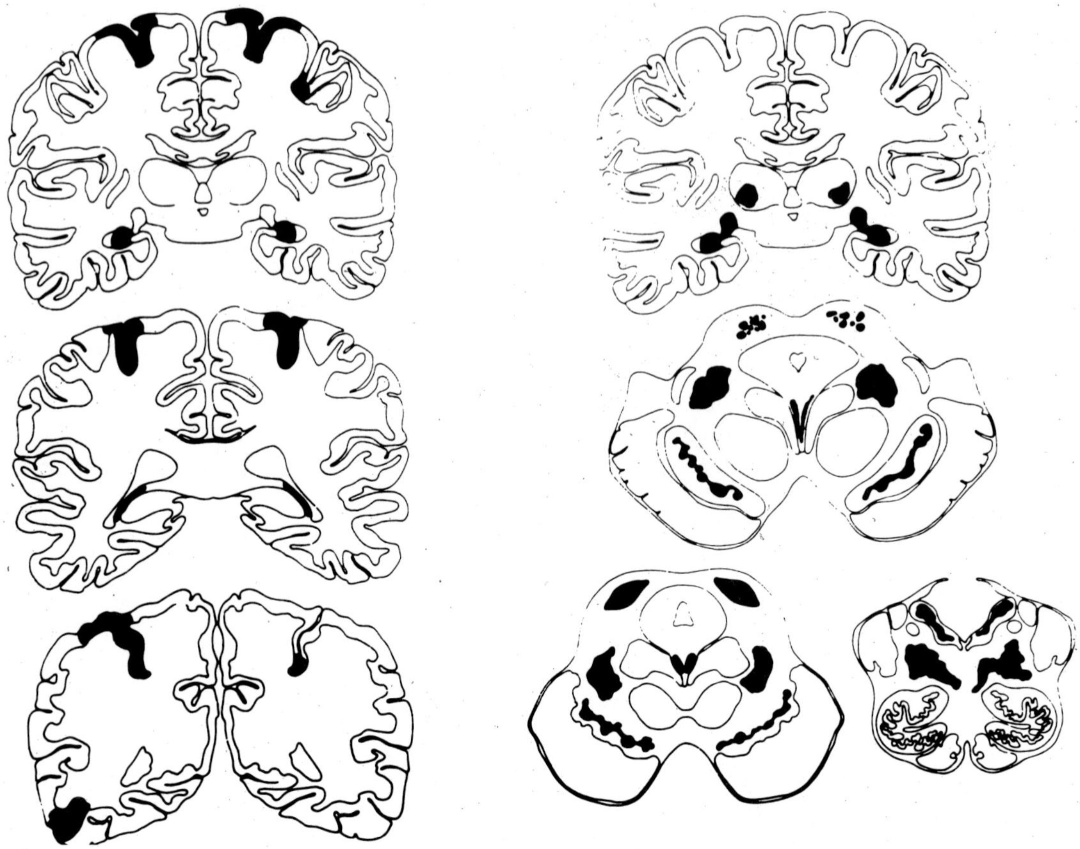

**Fig. 13-28.** Drawing of coronal sections of neonatal term infant brain to show two patterns of symmetrical cerebral infarction: the three illustrations on the left denote watershed zone infarcts in the cerebrum; the drawings on the right indicate symmetric infarcts in the tegmentum of the brainstem and deep in the thalamus. (Reproduced with permission of the American Medical Association from Leech RW, Alvord EC Jr: Anoxic-ischemic encephalopathy in the human neonatal period: the significance of brainstem involvement, Arch Neurol 34:109-113, 1977.)

pontine nucleus and dorsolateral tegmental nucleus, may be selectively vulnerable to hypoxia in the neonate.[147] Motor neurons also are cholinergic and show marked hypoxic chromatolysis.

In nonhuman primates, brainstem and thalamic infarcts appear to be more strongly correlated with sudden total asphyxia, whereas cerebral cortical lesions are associated with more gradual hypoxic/ischemic insults, but neither is absolute.[18]

Focal lesions may involve cranial nerve nuclei, such as the hypoglossal nucleus or the intramedullary course of its nerve, causing atrophy and fasciculations of the tongue that may be misinterpreted clinically as a sign of infantile spinal muscular atrophy (Werdnig-Hoffmann disease). Möbius syndrome is often attributed to congenital aplasia of the abducens and facial nuclei, but usually is the result of symmetric perinatal infarcts in the tegmentum at the pontomedullary junction; months or years later, mineralized old infarcted tissue is demonstrated in and around these cranial nerve nuclei at autopsy (Fig. 13-29).[55,152]

Feeding and swallowing difficulties in neonates who have suffered hypoxia usually are transient, but persistent dysphagia might be secondary to symmetric brainstem infarcts involving the nucleus ambiguus and dorsal motor nucleus of the vagus. Such microscopic lesions might be too small to demonstrate by MRI during life.

Fewer lesions are seen in the spinal cord than in the cerebrum or brainstem in infants exposed to hypoxic/ischemic insults, but symmetric microinfarcts, core lesions, and focal degenerative changes of neurons occur as in the brainstem. Motor neurons often show central chromatolysis after an hypoxic insult in the term neonatal spinal cord, well demonstrated by acridine orange fluorochrome, which shows the distribution of ribosomes; as the motor neuron recovers, a perinuclear ring of RNA fluorescence is seen by contrast with the

A

B

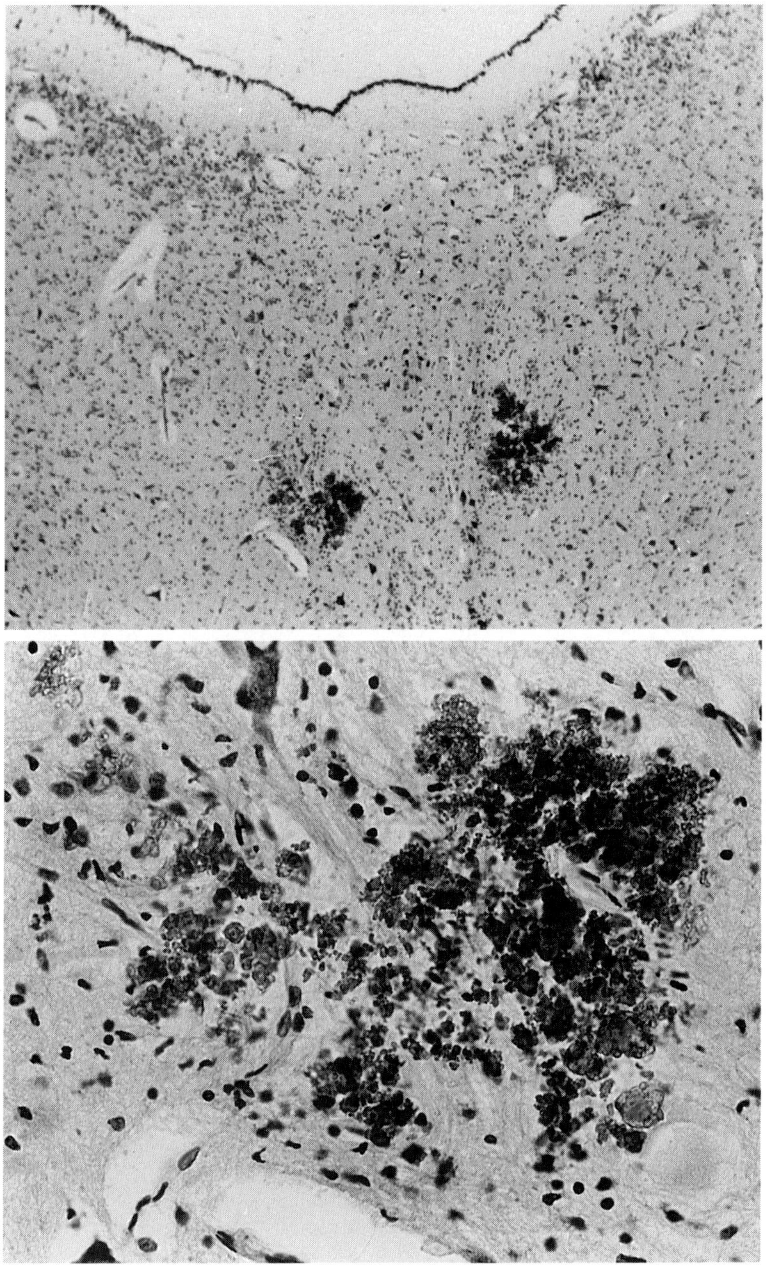

**Fig. 13-29.** Calcified neurons of the facial nuclei in a child with Möbius syndrome. This condition represents old infarction in utero rather than a congenital absence of the nucleus. (**A**, H&E; ×40; **B**, H&E; ×250.)

peripheral or centrifugal redistribution of ribosomes that occurs with chromatolysis as an acute or subacute injury.[121] However, early damage to the Golgi apparatus may be a more important marker of lethal neuronal injury than ribosomal release (i.e., degranulation) of the endoplasmic reticulum.[109]

## CEREBELLAR LESIONS

The deep cerebellar white matter may show microinfarcts similar to those of the brainstem and deep cerebral white matter, but usually they are smaller and sparser than the supratentorial lesions in both preterm and term infants. Large infarcts also occur, but usually are old pseudocysts from cerebellar hemorrhages due to birth trauma (Fig. 13-30). The presence of hemosiderin discloses the previous blood. Purkinje cell loss is more extensive than granule cell loss in the cerebellar cortex, but the external granule cell layer of premigratory granule cells may show cellular degeneration. Multiple focal microinfarcts resembling embolic phenomena also are seen in the cerebellar cortex and may later appear first as microglial nodules or macrophages and then as zones of gliosis and of disorganized lamination in the vicinity because of the involvement of Bergmann glial guides of migratory external granule cells (Fig. 13-31). Bergmann cells later proliferate as a

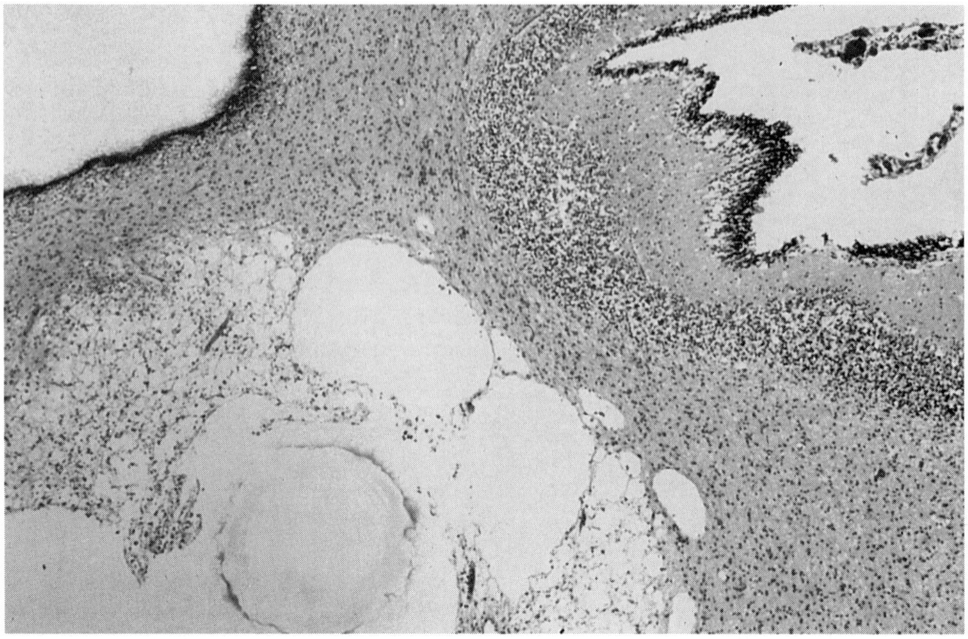

**Fig. 13-30.** Cavitation in the deep white matter of cerebellum in a 4-month-old infant who suffered extensive cerebral and cerebellar white matter spongy degeneration secondary to ischemia. The child was born at 34 weeks' gestation.

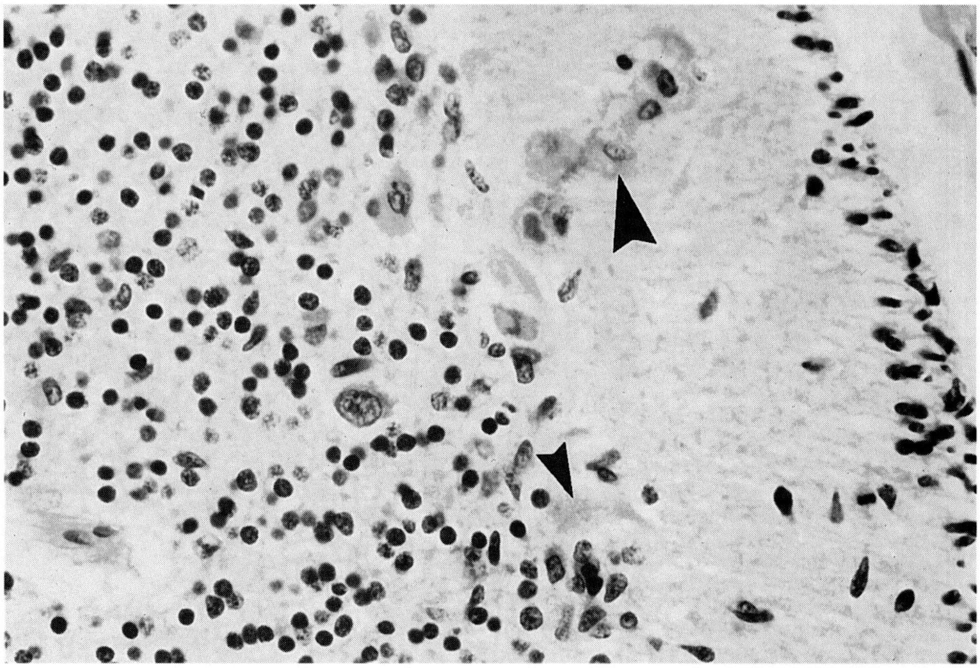

**Fig. 13-31.** Cerebellar cortex of a term infant 7 weeks after a cardiopulmonary arrest. There is a severe loss of Purkinje cells, with ghosts remaining (*small arrowhead*), partial depletion of the internal and especially of the external granular layers, and foci of macrophages in the molecular layer (*large arrowhead*).

reactive response or as a part of generalized gliosis during repair. Transsynaptic degeneration of cerebellar Purkinje cells in the hemisphere contralateral to an infarcted inferior olivary nucleus occurs in preterm infants.[59]

Neonatal asphyxia in the mouse reduces the number of granule cells more than Purkinje cells,[166] unlike the human situation, although occasionally lysis of granule cells is seen in adults as well as in neonates following severe anoxia, a histopathologic condition known as *état glacé* and not due to postmortem autolysis. In the neonatal rat, hypoxia inhibits proliferative activity of stem cells of the external granular layer and also retards the sprouting of dendrites and the growth of axons; the net result is a small, atrophic or hypoplastic cerebellum.[167]

## GRAY MATTER LESIONS

Several unique distribution patterns of gray matter injury occur in the preterm and term neonatal brain after hypoxic/ischemic insults that are not found in the mature brain after similar exposure. By contrast with white matter lesions that consist largely of infarcts or fields of necrosis involving all types of cells, cell processes, and blood vessels, gray matter lesions often are *selective neuronal necrosis,* in which neurons are destroyed but glial cells and vascular structures in the field are spared. This type of injury is seen in the cerebral cortex and in the deep forebrain gray matter structures such as the thalamus and corpus striatum. Dying neurons have shrunken nuclei with condensed chromatin that stains darkly; eosinophilic, amorphous cytoplasm; and indistinct cell membranes. Pale "ghost cells" with loss of staining qualities of both nuclei and cytoplasm are a stage just preceding total disappearance, with or without a microglial nodule or astrocytic proliferation in its place. Some neurons calcify (Fig. 13-32), and the excessive entry of calcium ions through the NMDA receptor is thought to be the major cause of glutamate toxicity.[34] It might also be a clue to the pathogenesis of such mineralized dead neurons.

### Pontosubicular Degeneration

One unique topology of neuronal degeneration follows hypoxia or ischemia in the neonatal brain, selectively involving the pontine nuclei of the basis pontis and the subiculum of the hippocampal complex. The selective vulnerability of these neurons is not always obvious because hypoxic changes are usually detected also in the gray matter of the cerebral cortex, thalamus, and cerebellum, especially involving granule cells, and widespread white matter infarcts also are evident.* Pontosubicular necrosis more frequently stands out as selectively severe involvement in preterm infants of 29 weeks' gestation or more and in term neonates. Extremely premature infants of 28 weeks' gestation or less have such equally extensive neuronal degeneration throughout the brain that the pontosubicular degeneration is not as conspicuous.[135,136] Nevertheless, this distribution pattern in the pons and subiculum is

* Refs. 2, 40, 44, 53, 67, 102, 116, 135, 136, 138, 149.

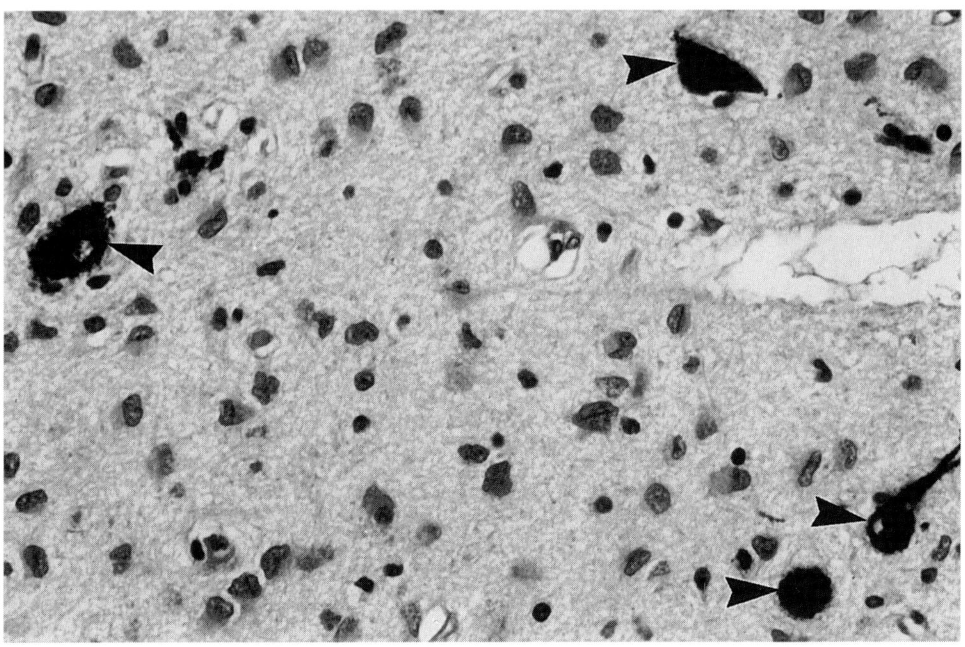

**Fig. 13-32.** Calcified neurons (*arrowheads*) in the thalamus of a 7-week-old infant born at near-term, who suffered fetal distress in the last week before delivery. (H&E; ×400.)

seen only rarely in the adult brain, although it is reported occasionally.[108]

Hyperoxemia in the presence of acidosis and hypoxia is described in some infants with the speculation that oxygen toxicity plays a role in the pathogenesis of pontosubicular degeneration,[2] but these cases represent a small minority. Pontine neurons exhibiting karyorrhexis exhibit immunoreactivity to ferritin if accompanied by spongy changes and gliosis, suggesting that iron is released to the damaged pontine nuclei.[98] In situ DNA fragmentation studies confirm the morphologic sequence of changes in subicular and basis pontis neurons that indicate apoptosis rather than frank necrosis as the mechanism of cellular death.[19] Experimental ischemia in the infant rodent brain produces similar nuclear DNA fragmentation.[37,93] Apolipoprotein E, implicated in neuronal regeneration, is probably synthesized by astrocytes and taken up by neurons during membrane remodeling during early responses to cerebral hypoxic/ischemic insults in pontosubicular degeneration.[6]

Pontosubicular necrosis has been described in stillborn fetuses, indicating that the lesions may result from intrauterine fetal distress and are not necessarily acquired intrapartum or postpartum.[82,134] Congenital heart disease was present in 12 of 65 neonates with pontosubicular degeneration.[82] The time interval between the hypoxic/ischemic insult and the onset of histologically evident pontosubicular necrosis is probably within 2 days, but the most obvious lesions require a week to evolve. Gliosis begins within 2 days, but healed gliosis is not complete for several weeks to many months.

Microscopic features are karyorrhexis, either scattered or involving most of the pontine neurons, with or without microcystic degeneration of the white matter neuropil. Large cavities and infarcts do not occur. Cytoplasmic eosinophilia in neurons not yet showing nuclear changes indicates an earlier stage of hypoxic injury. Chromatolysis may precede neuronal death (Fig. 13-33). Gliosis develops quickly, and gemistocytes often are seen side by side with degenerating neurons.[116] Larger zones of necrosis are infiltrated by macrophages within several days. The middle cerebellar peduncle, composed of axons of basis pontis neurons, shows degeneration due to axonal loss and, if the infant is old enough to have myelin in this white matter, sudanophilic degeneration products are demonstrated. This is not a prominent feature, however, because myelination of the middle cerebellar peduncle does not normally begin until 42 weeks' gestation and is not completed until 3 years of age.[123]

Neurons of the pontine tegmentum are generally well preserved, in contrast with those of the basis pontis. Symmetric microinfarcts of the tegmentum occasionally are demonstrated, however.[71,130] The subiculum is more severely involved than are the CA1 to CA4 zones of the Ammon's horn or the dentate gyrus of the hippocampus, a striking contrast with the usual distribution of lesions in the mature hippocampal complex after acute hypoxic/ischemic insults or in chronic mesial temporal lobe sclerosis in older children and adults with epilepsy. However, a 22-week stillborn fetus showed severe neuronal karyorrhexis in Sommer's sector, with preservation of neurons in the adjacent subiculum.[42] In the neonatal pig exposed to transient HIE, selective vulnerability of the small cells of the inner granule cell layer of the dentate gyrus of the hippocampus occurs.[59]

In most series, between 6% and 16% of infants born before 38 weeks' gestation who died in the first postnatal month had pontosubicular necrosis,[2,100,116] but some authors, reporting a prevalence of as much as 59% in a series of 96 preterm infants, suggest that it is the most common brain lesion of preterm neonates, exceeding even germinal matrix hemorrhages.[136]

### Status Marmoratus

This uncommon neuropathologic sequela to perinatal hypoxic/ischemic encephalopathy occurs in term neonates and sometimes in infants who suffer asphyxia as late as 3 months postnatally.[78] The name means "marbled state" because of the gross appearance of the cut surface of the thalamus and basal ganglia as a coarsely streaked or patchy interwoven pattern. Microscopically, hypermyelinated fibers are seen[116]; ultrastructural studies demonstrate that these fibers are actually myelinated astrocytic processes rather than axons.[16] The only other part of the brain in which hypermyelinated glial fibers occasionally occur is at the depth of sulci in ulegyria (see below),[134] but not in other regions of the cerebral cortex or in the brainstem or cerebellum. The early speculation that status marmoratus was a result of inflammation[78] has not been confirmed, but the reason why oligodendrocytes respond to hypoxia by ensheathing astrocytic processes in such selective areas of the brain and in such a narrowly restricted age group remains speculative. Middle cerebral artery occlusion in the adult rat produces infarction earlier in the corpus striatum than in the cerebral cortex, but hypermyelination does not occur even with incomplete coagulative necrosis.[43]

### Ulegyria

This uncommon hypoxic/ischemic lesion of late preterm and term infants consists of necrosis of neurons of the cerebral cortex in the depths of sulci, with relative sparing of those in the crowns of gyri and a demarcated transition from normal to abnormal cortical laminae about two thirds of the distance into the sulcus along the side of the gyrus.[96,97] *Ulegyria* originates etymologically from the Greek *oule,* meaning "see," and *gyros,*

A

B

C

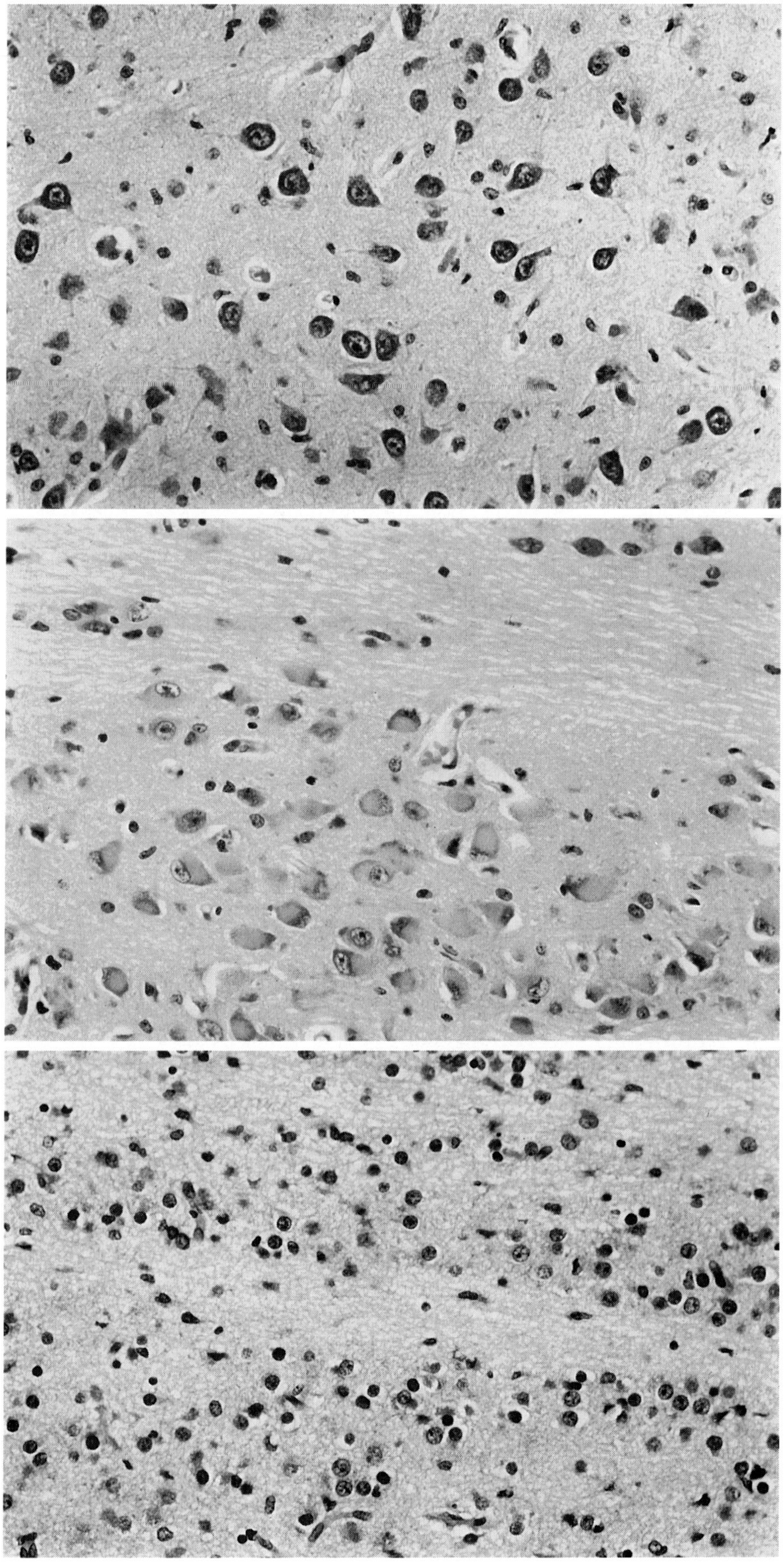

**Fig. 13-33.** Pontine nuclei of the basis pontis in three full-term neonates: **A**, normal; **B**, chromatolysis of neurons at an early stage of hypoxic injury; **C**, degenerating and dead neurons with dark, shrunken nuclei and reactive gliosis in pontosubicular degeneration in an infant who lived a week after severe birth asphyxia. (H&E; ×250.)

meaning "ring." Grossly, the gyri appear shrunken or mushroom-shaped and may be confused with polymicrogyria as a developmental defect. Acute microscopic changes include pallor and vacuolation of the cortical layers, followed by neuronal loss, massive increase of glial cells and fibers, abundant macrophages, and vascular proliferation. Laminar necrosis, mainly of layer 3, may occur, or the laminar structure of the cortex may be lost entirely. The adjacent white matter shows irregular patches of incomplete necrosis. Later, coarse, abnormally oriented bundles of myelinated fibers traverse the gliotic tissue, but the myelin sheaths enclose astrocytic processes as well as axons.[16]

Ulegyria most commonly occurs in major arterial border areas or watershed zones, in a parasagittal distribution in the venous drainage territory of the superior sagittal sinus, or within the territory of a major cerebral artery. It may be bilateral or confined to one hemisphere. The deepest layers of cortex at the depths of sulci and the U-fibers of the white matter just beneath these zones have interdigitating branches of adjacent arterioles that provide collateral circulation if one vessel becomes occluded, but these branches do not protect the territory supplied in the event of generalized reduced blood flow.[83] The perisulcal topography of the necrosis is probably related to reduced perfusion from hypotension that may preferentially damage the deep sulcal cortex further if sulcal venous drainage is impaired by compression of the stems of veins that ascend between gyri edematous from preceding hypoxic episodes.[96] Deep white matter infarcts often are associated. Ulegyria is not a hemorrhagic lesion, and hemosiderin is not demonstrated in old lesions.

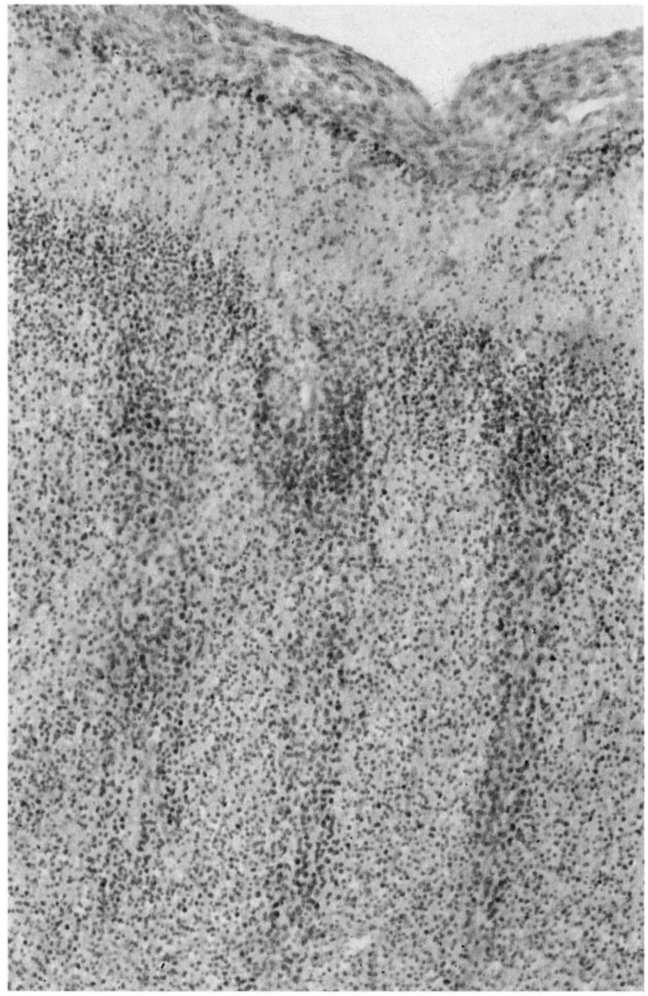

**Fig. 13-34.** Columnar infarcts in the cerebral cortex of a 29-week preterm infant who lived 3 months. This unique pattern of watershed infarction occurs exclusively in immature brains after systemic hypotension. Columns of preserved cortex around arterioles that penetrate the cortex perpendicular to its surface alternate with columns of infarcted tissue between arterioles. The leptomeninges over the cortex in this case are thickened from meningitis. (H&E; ×100.)

### Watershed Infarcts of the Cerebral Cortex

A unique pattern of watershed zone infarction is found in the cerebral cortex of preterm infants and at no other age. Alternating columns of necrosis and preserved cortex, perpendicular to the pial surface, involve all cortical layers (Fig. 13-34). These columns of infarcted cortex are watershed zones between branches of meningeal arterioles that penetrate the cerebral cortex and supply exclusive local perfusion of surrounding tissue, but have few anastomoses and thus provide meager collateral microcirculation. During the last 6 weeks of gestation, the proliferating capillary network of the intracortical circulation replaces the isolated penetrating arterioles so that columnar infarcts no longer occur in term or near-term neonates. After about 34 weeks' gestation, poor perfusion of the cerebral cortex in states of systemic hypotension yields adult-type watershed zone infarcts in the territories bordering the blood supply of major cerebral arteries—between the anterior and middle cerebral artery circulations and between the middle and posterior cerebral territories (Figs. 13-26 and 13-28).

### Damage to the External Glial Limiting Membrane

An external glial limiting membrane over the neocortex is maintained throughout development as well as throughout postnatal life.[103,123] It consists of glial end-feet with closely apposed tight junctions, covered by a basal lamina and intimately associated with the internal lamella of the pia mater. Entering capillaries and arterioles penetrate the membrane at specific sites early in development. After neuroblast and glioblast migrations are complete, the radial glia retract their processes; their end-feet at the cortical surface are replaced by those of additional layer 1 astrocytes, thus preserving the structural integrity of the external glial limiting membrane.[79,80,103]

Edema in HIE causes separation of the external glial limiting membrane from the underlying cortex, elongation of perforating capillaries, and swelling of end-feet.[103] Local rupture of the membrane and of perforating capillaries causes discontinuities and small subpial hemorrhages. The involved sites become filled with microglial cells and circulating macrophages, and the damaged radial glial fibers sprout numerous regenerative end-feet to reestablish the integrity of the external glial limiting membrane. Small foci may heal without residual gliosis or architectural damage, but larger pial disruptions require extensive revascularization and scarring, both glial and fibroblastic, that could disrupt underlying cortical architecture.[103,123,130] Sites of rupture of the external glial limiting membrane in fetal life followed by regeneration of terminal ends of radial glial fibers also sometimes produce subsequent overmigration beyond the surface of the cortex, resulting in glioneuronal heterotopia in the leptomeninges.[20,103,123]

Subpial gliosis may occur with or without apparent breaks in the external glial limiting membrane or may accompany extensive white matter lesions as the only gray matter involvement.

Hemorrhagic lesions of the neocortex in preterm and term neonates are usually confined to the subpial region and molecular zone (layer 1), although the underlying neuronal architecture also may be altered; damage to the external limiting membrane and rupture of small pial vessels is the probable pathogenesis.[80b]

## TERRITORIAL INFARCTS OF MAJOR CEREBRAL ARTERIES

Infarcts demarcating the territories of major cerebral arteries are more common in term infants than in prematures. The immature brain has rich vascular anastomoses between arteries supplying the meninges and the major cerebral arteries; these prominent anastomoses regress with maturation and have nearly disappeared by term. Nevertheless, territorial infarcts also occur at times in preterm infant brains, and the distinction by gestational age is not absolute. In term neonates, infarcts occur more commonly in the territories of the anterior and middle cerebral arteries than in that of the posterior cerebral, and rarely in the distribution of the vertebrobasilar circulation. A dense sympathetic innervation of the major vessels arising from the carotid artery, less dense autonomic fibers of the posterior cerebral artery, and only sparse sympathetic nerve fibers to the basilar artery may explain the greater potential for vasospasm and territorial infarction in supratentorial arterial territories, with relative preservation of the brainstem and cerebellum in asphyxiated neonates.[132]

The most frequent causes of major cerebral arterial occlusions and infarction in term neonates are birth trauma and contusion, sepsis and meningitis, disseminated intravascular coagulation, and polycythemia. Embolic occlusions of major cerebral vessels may occur in some congenital cardiac malformations. Maternal diabetes mellitus is associated with a higher incidence of major vascular thromboses. Developmental anomalies of the vessels are an uncommon cause, but stenosis of the supraclinoid portion of the internal carotid artery and deficiencies of the internal elastic membrane may lead to closure of the lumen in the neonatal period or months or years later. This stenosis without early occlusion may lead to the condition known as "moyamoya," probably a reactive proliferation of small vessels distal to the carotid narrowing within the deep nuclei of gray matter. Arteriovenous malformations usually cause hemorrhagic rather than coagulative infarcts. Hypercoagulable states, such as circulating antiphospholipid antibodies or deficiencies of protein C or S, are rare causes of major cerebrovascular thromboses in neonates.

*Extracorporeal membrane oxygenation (ECMO)* is a method for providing oxygen to the blood for a temporary period when pulmonary disease prevents adequate gas exchange. It is an increasingly important life-support system for neonates to prevent brain damage from the hypoxia of persistent pulmonary hypertension, atelectasis, pneumothorax, diaphragmatic hernia with pulmonary compression, and other transient but potentially fatal neonatal pulmonary conditions. To perform this modified cardiopulmonary bypass, the right common carotid artery and jugular vein are catheterized and tied off, and gas exchange occurs across an artificial membrane that substitutes for alveoli. Most neonates tolerate the right carotid ligation well because of adequate collateral circulation through the circle of Willis, but some infants suffer massive cerebral infarcts, usually coagulative but sometimes hemorrhagic, because of the heparinization required during the procedure. Cerebral infarction usually corresponds to the territory of a major cerebral artery, most commonly the middle or anterior cerebral (Fig. 13-35), and it may be extensive, bilateral, and lead to multicystic encephalomalacia if the patient survives. Infarcts may occur in the hemisphere ipsilateral to the carotid ligation; at times they paradoxically occur in the contralateral hemisphere from emboli or because of a "steal" phenomenon with shunting of blood from the left to the right side of the brain. Asymmetries in cerebral blood flow have been demonstrated during life by ultrasound Doppler study in preterm infants with periventricular leukomalacia,[85] and these pre-existing

A

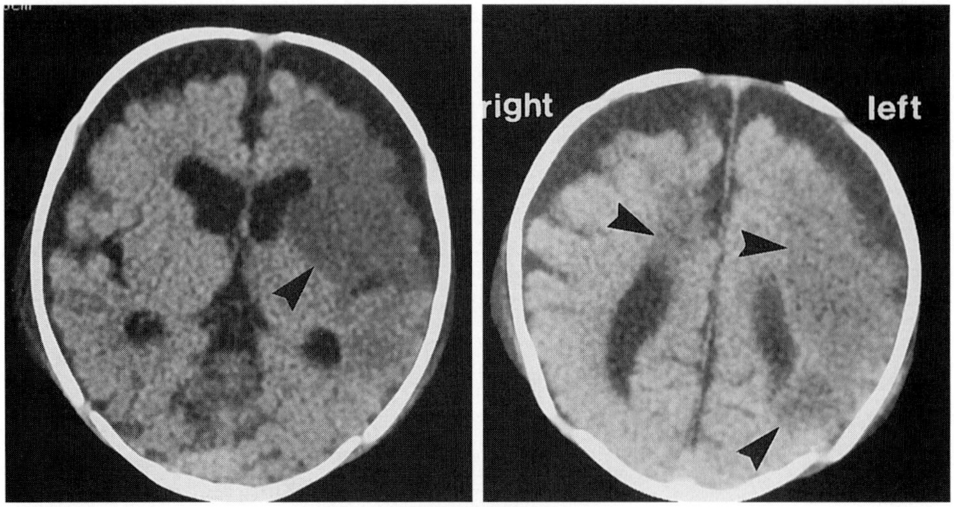


B

C

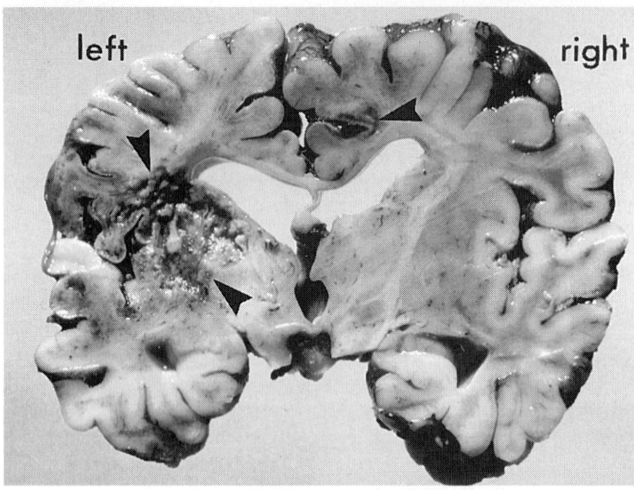


**Fig. 13-35.** Territorial infarcts in the distribution of the left middle cerebral and right anterior cerebral arteries (*arrowheads*) in a 6-week-old infant born at 26 weeks' gestation. These infarcts are a complication of ECMO therapy requiring catheterization and ligation of the right internal carotid artery and jugular vein. **A, B**, Two axial planes of computed tomographic imaging without enhancement. **C**, Coronal sections of cerebral hemispheres at autopsy showing recent infarcts in the distributions identified in the CT images. The infarcts do not involve the entire territories of either the left middle or right exterior cerebral arteries; these major arteries were patent, and their branches had thrombosed or contained emboli. The infant died 13 days after the strokes. **D**, Microscopic examination disclosed congested leptomeninges and infarction of the cerebral cortex, with replacement of necrotic cerebral tissue by cavitation and macrophages in both gray and white matter. (**D** H&E; ×100.)

D

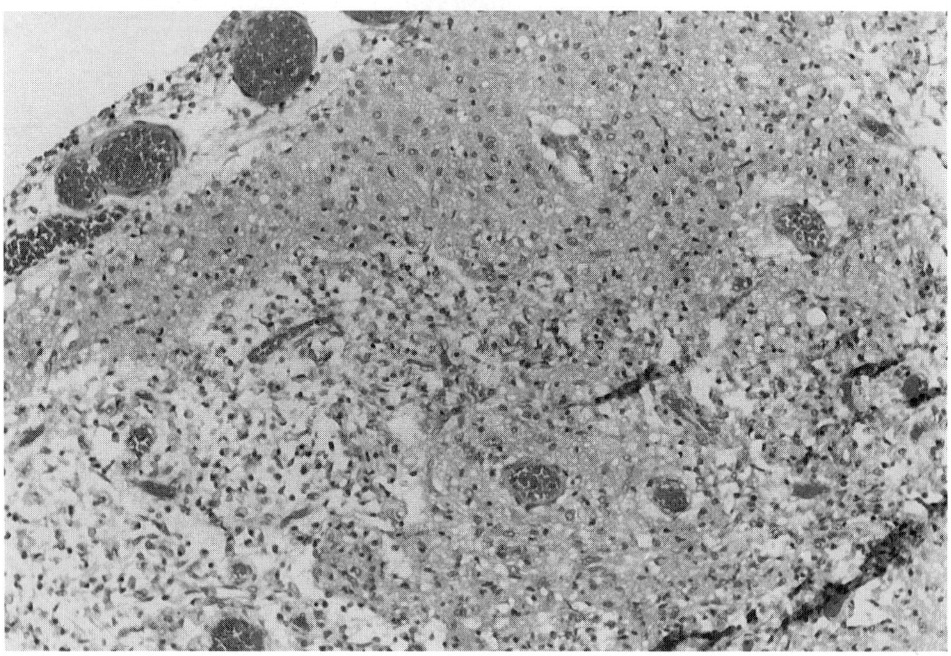

asymmetries also may contribute to the laterality of the territorial infarcts during ECMO therapy. Neuropathologic findings are not distinctive from other causes of territorial infarctions, but also include PVL and intracerebral hemorrhages in about half the cases.[57,162]

The common placental circulation of monozygotic twins may lead to ischemic cerebral injury and infarction secondary to twin-to-twin transfusion in middle to late gestation or exsanguination injury to the survivor in the event of co-twin demise at near-term; infarcts are usually territorial; even multicystic encephalomalacia may result.[164]

Simple hypoxic/ischemic encephalopathy superimposed on an otherwise normal brain often is listed in textbooks as a cause of major arterial occlusions in the CNS, but is rare or does not occur.

The end result of middle cerebral artery occlusion is classic porencephaly, a large cavitary lesion of brain in the territory of that vessel, the void being filled with CSF and communicating with the lateral ventricle. Although imaging studies usually suggest that the cavity communicates with the subarachnoid space as well, careful postmortem examination usually discloses preservation of the thin pial membrane, which depends on the intact leptomeningeal circulation rather than the cerebral arterial perfusion as its source. Anterior and posterior cerebral infarcts also may lead to porencephaly, but are less common.

At 6 to 8 weeks' gestation, the direction of flow in the developing basilar artery is rostrocaudal from the carotid circulation through a series of transitory fetal communicating vessels, the paired trigeminal, otic, and hypoglossal arteries. The vertebral arteries develop later than do the carotids, but when these vessels finally form and become connected with the caudal end of the basilar artery, the direction of basilar flow is reversed and becomes caudorostral, as in the adult. Occasionally, the change is delayed by a few weeks in some fetuses. Carotid occlusions in such cases at 10 to 16 weeks' gestation may result in infarcts in the territories of the posterior cerebral and superior cerebellar arteries on the ipsilateral side, as well as in the expected middle cerebral territory.

## VENOUS THROMBOSES

The thrombosis of the superior sagittal sinus leads to infarction in a parasagittal distribution. However, it is distinguished from territorial infarction from occlusion of the anterior cerebral artery by its bilateral symmetry and by the hemorrhagic rather than coagulative or liquefactive character of the infarct. The etiology is nearly always either infection, such as generalized sepsis or meningitis, or dehydration. Birth trauma is a rare cause. Disseminated intravascular coagulation is another cause, but usually is a complication of sepsis. Thrombi may extend to other sinuses, but begin in a transverse sinus or the straight sinus in only a minority. Subdural hematoma may be a complication of sagittal sinus thrombosis.

The thrombosis of a major venous sinus results in vascular congestion intracranially, in the external carotid artery distribution in the face and scalp, and in the retina. If the infant survives, recanalization of the thrombus begins within 1 to 2 weeks and in most cases eventually restores adequate venous return. Treatment of major venous sinus thrombosis consists of good hydration, appropriate antibiotic treatment of infection, and heparinization. The administration of heparin carries a risk of more extensive intracerebral hemorrhage, but in most cases is well tolerated and effectively stops the propagation of the thrombus.

Small cortical vein thromboses in term neonates usually result from traumatic delivery and cerebral contusion. They are focal, often microscopic infarcts that are difficult to detect by imaging; only rarely does the opportunity for neuropathologic confirmation present itself. In chronic cases, the hallmarks are focal zones of disrupted cortical architecture, neuronal loss, and gliosis without cavitation, often accompanied by telltale hemosiderin deposits. Clinically, such events may be silent or are detected, early or late, as focal epileptiform discharges on EEG that may remain subclinical or become expressed as seizures.

## SECONDARY CEREBRAL MALFORMATIONS RESULTING FROM PERINATAL INFARCTS

Ischemia of the immature brain not only causes neuronal loss and impairs synaptogenesis and myelination, but also may result in secondary focal dysplasias by interfering with developmental processes not yet complete. Subcortical infarcts may damage the delicate radial glial fibers that guide neuroblasts and glioblasts in their migration from the subventricular zone to the cerebral cortex (Fig. 13-36). Cells thus arrested in migration complete their maturation in situ and form subcortical heterotopia, unable to establish their intended synaptic relations.[94,95,123] The regressing stumps of radial glial fibers often can still be recognized within hemorrhagic zones in the deep white matter.[103]

Focal areas of abnormal cortical lamination may be microscopic in size and below the limits of resolution of present-day imaging techniques, but may generate seizures and may be detected by electroencephalography (EEG). Because of the vulnerability to vascular injury of the external glial limiting membrane formed by glial end-feet and the pia mater, some focal zones of abnormal cortical lamination are associated with breaks in this membrane.[103] Discontinuities in the pia caused by ischemic injury, contusion, and subarach-

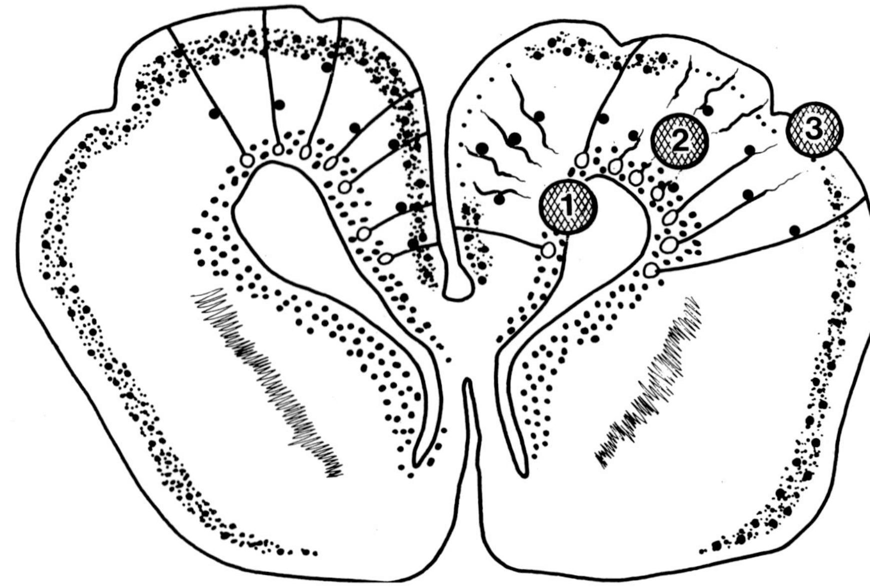


**Fig. 13-36.** Drawing of a coronal section of the cerebral hemispheres of a preterm infant to illustrate three possible sites where hypoxic/ischemic lesions might disrupt radial glial cells or their fibers to interrupt neuroblast and glioblast migration, which causes subcortical heterotopia and focal dysplasias of the cerebral cortex as secondary malformations not of genetic origin: (1) in the periventricular region, such as PVL or GMH; (2) in the deep subcortical white matter, such as either ischemic or hemorrhagic infarcts; and (3) at the pial surface, where injury might cause retraction of radial glial end-feet, as with contusions at delivery, subarachnoid hemorrhages, or neonatal meningitis. (Reproduced with permission from Sarnat HB: Cerebral dysgenesis. Embryology and clinical expression, New York, 1992, Oxford University Press.)

noid hemorrhage account for *glioneuronal heterotopia*, small nodules of disorganized neural tissue in the leptomeninges connected to the cortex by a stalk; these heterotopia result from overmigration in the absence of a limiting membrane, when injured radial glial fibers regenerate.[20,22,103,123] If the heterotopia of neurons and glial cells become detached by regression or loss of the stalk, the isolated islands of gray matter entirely surrounded by leptomeninges are then *ectopic*.[127]

## CLINICAL SEQUELAE OF PERINATAL HYPOXIC/ISCHEMIC ENCEPHALOPATHY

The clinical sequelae of hypoxic/ischemic encephalopathy in the preterm infant are predictably related to the white matter lesions primarily, but neuronal loss and gliosis in the gray matter of the cerebral cortex bilaterally are later expressed as mental retardation, delayed language acquisition, and perceptual disturbances.

Periventricular leukomalacia (PVL) of limited extent does not necessarily produce clinically evident deficits. Extensive PVL in the occipital and posterior temporal regions may involve the optic radiations (i.e., the geniculocalcarine tract) and produce cortical blindness. Hearing, by contrast, is rarely impaired by PVL. The most constant and predictable correlate of PVL in later infancy and childhood, however, is *spastic diplegia*, i.e., "cerebral palsy." Lesions over the head and body of the caudate nucleus are very near to the internal capsule; hence, corticospinal and corticobulbar axons are exposed to ischemia and sometimes infarction. Deep lesions in the subcortical white matter of the centrum semiovale also involve these fibers more proximally, as the corona radiata. As with the neuropathologic lesions, the residual clinical motor deficit often is asymmetric. Spastic diplegia often cannot yet be detected in the term and especially the preterm neonate, and the infant may appear to have a deceptively "normal" clinical neurologic examination or may show only vague, nonspecific signs such as hypotonia. Hemiparesis is rarely evident in the neonatal period.

Corticospinal tract deficits in neonates differ from those of the mature nervous system. Alterations of muscle tone and posture are seen in term neonates because of a loss of antagonistic balance between bulbospinal or "subcorticospinal" pathways and the corticospinal pathway; subcorticospinal pathways mainly subserve proximal extension and distal flexion, and the CST subserves proximal flexion and distal flexion.[122] Extensive destruction of the cortex or CST, usually bilaterally, with preservation of brainstem function, therefore results in overaction of the axial and limb girdle extensors and of distal flexors—opisthotonus or arching of the back, extension of hips and shoulders, and tightly adducted thumbs and flexed fingers, wrists, and toes.[122] This "decorticate posturing" does not necessarily denote irreversible brain damage, as it may be a transitory impairment of neuronal function with potential survival and recovery of neurons following hypoxic insults.

Corticobulbar tract involvement is expressed as pseudobulbar palsy, suprasegmental facial paresis, and often strabismus. Esotropia is more common than exotropia and may be noted early, progressing in infancy from an intermittent to a constant inturning of an eye. Treatment by an ophthalmologist is required to prevent *amblyopia ex anopsia*, permanent visual loss not related to anatomic destruction of visual pathways as in occipital PVL. *Dysphagia*, poor suck, feeding and swallowing difficulties, and incoordination usually reflect corticobulbar tract involvement and impairment of tactile reflexes,[122] but also may be symptomatic of structural lesions in the brainstem. *Nystagmus* and cranial nerve palsies are other signs of brainstem involvement rather than of suprasegmental lesions. *Apnea* and other respiratory irregularities not related to pulmonary dysfunction are serious and potentially life-threatening signs that suggest brainstem disease.

Cerebellar lesions are difficult to detect in neonates and young infants and may be expressed only as diffuse muscular hypotonia, a nonspecific sign. As the child matures, truncal titubation, ataxia, and other clinical cerebellar deficits become apparent and sometimes are associated with spasticity as "ataxic cerebral palsy." Lesions of the corpus striatum similarly may appear later as dyskinesias or movement disorders, with or without an additional spastic component. Hypotonia may predominate over spasticity in the presence of either cerebellar or basal ganglionic lesions, or both alterations of muscle tone may coexist.

Extensive PVL and grade 3 intraventricular hemorrhage are nearly always followed by permanent motor sequelae, whether they occur together or separately. Parenchymal infarction beyond the limits of the germinal matrix, whether coagulative or hemorrhagic (i.e., "grade 4"), is always predictive of irreversible brain damage with later clinical manifestations. Mental deficiency depends upon gray matter involvement of the cortex *bilaterally* or extensive bilateral subcortical white matter infarcts; even large lesions such as porencephaly due to middle cerebral artery occlusion do not necessarily result in mental retardation if confined to one cerebral hemisphere.

White matter lesions including PVL are not in themselves epileptogenic. Seizures denote cerebral cortical, i.e., gray matter, disease but do not necessarily indicate an irreversible anatomic lesion; they sometimes are an expression of what is clinically called "neuronal irritability," a consequence of subarachnoid hemorrhage, transient ischemic impairment of synaptic function or of neurotransmitter synthesis, release of transmitters as a sudden bolus, electrolyte disturbances, hypoglycemia, or other metabolic stresses. Ischemia impairs energy production by the $Na^+/K^+$ ATPase pump, resulting in an unstable resting membrane potential and a decreased threshold for neuronal membrane depolarization. Seizures may occur in utero in distressed fetuses. Segmental myoclonus usually indicates brainstem or spinal cord dysfunction rather than epileptic activity of cerebral cortical origin.

Finally, ischemic impairment of the hypothalamus may result in subacute, inappropriate secretion of antidiuretic hormone (ADH) and diabetes insipidus; clinically there may be poor body temperature regulation and extreme fevers with trivial viral illnesses and neuroendocrine dysfunctions, including either precocious or delayed onset of puberty.

**Posthemorrhagic Hydrocephalus**

Hydrocephalus is a major complication of grade 3 intraventricular hemorrhage, occurring in about 60% of infants. Even small, local, grade 2 hemorrhages may occasionally be situated to compress a foramen of Monro, but this obstruction is usually transitory and brief. Posthemorrhagic hydrocephalus may be divided into early and late phases, with different mechanisms of pathogenesis.

Early phase hydrocephalus occurs within hours or days after the hemorrhage and is due to direct mechanical obstruction of CSF pathways by blood or thrombus. The most frequent site of obstruction is the cerebral aqueduct, even though the aqueduct in preterm infants of 26 to 30 weeks, who are at highest risk for GMH, is relatively larger than at term. The obstruction often is temporary and resolves within days as the thrombus lyses, the lumen of the aqueduct again becomes patent, and the normal flow of CSF resumes. Larroche had earlier postulated that red blood cells clogging the pacchionian granulations, particularly in the basal cisterns, caused the hydrocephalus,[65] but this probably is not the only mechanism.

Late-phase hydrocephalus may appear to be a recurrence of early-phase hydrocephalus, delayed for weeks or months, or may occur even if neonatal hydrocephalus was not an early complication. Late-phase hydrocephalus is an insidious process that is slowly progressive over several weeks or months, is compensated for or may appear "arrested" for a time, and often does not become overtly symptomatic or cause a rapid increase in head circumference until the second half of the first year of life. The obstruction is believed to be a defect in the absorption of CSF by the pacchionian granulations of the meninges, the final site of CSF circulation and well distal to the aqueductal or other intraventricular sites of early phase hydrocephalus. Older classifications would have considered late-phase a "communicating" hydrocephalus. The previous neonatal IVH extends into the subarachnoid space and stimulates fibroblastic activity and fibrosis of these absorptive surfaces of the pacchionian granulations. However, this process is gradual, hence the delay in onset of intracranial hypertension.

The clinical diagnosis of posthemorrhagic hydrocephalus is not always easy. Ventriculomegaly and increasing head circumference do not always coincide and, because young infants can split sutures and bulge the fontanelles, they may be able to compensate for the increased intracranial pressure by increasing their intracranial and intraventricular volumes and thus redistribute the force over a larger surface area. When compensation no longer is possible or the augmentation of intracranial pressure is too rapid, the clinical signs of hydrocephalus appear: lethargy, vomiting, high-pitched cry, overactive or clonic tendon stretch reflexes, and decorticate or even decerebrate posturing.

Histopathologically, ventriculomegaly causes ependymal tears and discontinuities, followed by gliosis and especially glial nodule formation at the ventricular surfaces. The gliosis sometimes overgrows the remaining surface ependyma and buries patches, clusters, and rosettes of ependymal cells beneath the ventricular surface. The ependyma does not proliferate or regenerate, no mitotic activity is seen in ependymal cells, and proliferating cell nuclear antigens demonstrate no immunoreactivity.[128] Gliosis is generally evident throughout the subventricular zone, but probably represents reaction to periventricular leukomalacia or germinal matrix hemorrhage more than reaction to hydrocephalus itself. By 2 weeks of age in preterm infants dying with posthemorrhagic hydrocephalus, hemosiderin deposits are demonstrated in the ventricular walls, and nodular gliosis, ependymal cell loss, and subventricular ependymal rosettes are seen.[12,41] Ferritin-positive glia are increased in the molecular layer, and diffuse gliosis of the cerebellar cortex and white matter is found, with loss of Purkinje's cells and of inferior olivary neurons. These changes correlate well with the presence of cerebellar subarachnoid hemorrhage, but not with pontosubicular degeneration.[41]

Moderate to severe ventriculomegaly due to increased intraventricular pressure stretches the white matter fiber tracts and in time may cause them to atrophy; radial glial fibers also are stretched in preterm infants, but this stretching does not cause frank necrosis of axons or of radial glia. Only when the hydrocephalus becomes so extreme that the intracranial pressure exceeds the perfusion pressure of the cerebrovascular system does infarction occur. Cerebral tissue is quite compressible, and the thickness of the cerebral mantle often is surprisingly restored after a shunt is installed to relieve the pressure, even after dramatic thinning as seen by serial imaging studies. The changes in the cortical gray matter are minimal and related more to conditions such as hypoxia that contributed to the IVH than to the hydrocephalus itself. If untreated, there may be slow neuronal loss and mild gliosis, but these sequelae are subtle. In experimental obstructive hydrocephalus in the neonatal kitten, however, white matter changes are similar to those of periventricular leukomalacia, suggesting that ischemia plays a role. Extracellular edema and axonal damage are evident within days of the onset of hydrocephalus and are followed by reactive gliosis, white matter atrophy and, in some animals, cavitation of the white matter.[27]

Finally, ventriculomegaly secondary to cerebral atrophy, i.e., "hydrocephalus-ex-vacuo," often is misinterpreted as pressure hydrocephalus. White matter damage in particular results in dilatation of the lateral ventricles, whereas selective damage of the cerebral cortical gray matter does not appreciably affect ventricular size.[100,101] A good correlation is demonstrated between ultrasonographic indication of ventricular enlargement and the postmortem demonstration of leukomalacia.[63] For a given head circumference, the lateral ventricular area is larger in infants with ventriculomegaly secondary to white matter degeneration than in infants with posthemorrhagic pressure hydrocephalus.[119] Irregularities of ventricular margins and walls are a sign of ventriculomegaly secondary to atrophy and closely associated with clinical disabilities.[105] Among children with shunts, a higher incidence of long-term sequelae occurs when lack of ventricular decompression is noted immediately after insertion of the shunt, suggesting that loss of brain tissue already has occurred before shunting, even when the shunt is inserted early.[131] Investigators also found that the outcome of infants with severe posthemorrhagic hydrocephalus does not differ from that of infants in whom the progression of hydrocephalus becomes spontaneously arrested or who improve before the hydrocephalus becomes severe.[33]

Nonsurgical approaches to the treatment of posthemorrhagic hydrocephalus have included the use of carbonic anhydrase inhibitors such as acetazolamide and inhibitors of the $Na^+/K^+$ ATPase energy pump, such as ouabain and digoxin, to attempt to decrease the secretion of CSF by choroid plexus and ependymal cells. However, success has been very modest, and only a minority of patients show improvement in intracranial hypertension. For small premature infants in particular, such medical approaches might be at least a temporizing treatment until they have grown enough to tolerate a shunt. The pharmacologic control of CSF production and resorption by new investigational drugs remains the most promising hope for the treatment of posthemorrhagic hydrocephalus in infancy, and neuropathology is a key element in finding a solution.

## REFERENCES


1. Adams RD, Prod'hom LS, and Rabinowicz T: Intrauterine brain death. Neuroaxial reticular core necrosis, Acta Neuropathol 40: 41-49, 1977.
2. Ahdab-Barmada M, Moossy J, and Painter M: Pontosubicular necrosis and hyperoxemia, Pediatrics 66:840-847, 1980.
3. Alonso A, and others: Spontaneous hematomas caused by microangiomatosis of the basal ganglia, Child Brain 11:202-211, 1984.
4. An G, and others: Expression of c-*fos* and c-*jun* family genes after focal cerebral ischemia, Ann Neurol 33:457-464, 1993.
5. Arai Y, and others: Expression of $\beta$-amyloid precursor protein in axons of periventricular leukomalacia brains, Pediatr Neurol 13:161-163, 1995.
6. Arai Y, and others: Transient expression of apoplipoprotein-E in neonates with pontosubicular neuron necrosis, Acta Neuropathol 91:396-399, 1996.
7. Armstrong D, and Norman MG: Periventricular leukomalacia in neonates: complication and sequelae, Arch Dis Child 49:367-375, 1974.

8. Auer RN, and Siesjö BK: Biological differences between ischemia, hypoglycemia and epilepsy, Ann Neurol 24:699-707, 1988.
9. Azzarelli B, and others: Hypoxic-ischemic encephalopathy in areas of primary myelination: A neuroimaging and PET study, Pediatr Neurol 14:108–116, 1996.
10. Azzarelli B, Meade P, and Muller J: Hypoxic lesions in areas of primary myelination. A distinct pattern in cerebral palsy, Child Brain 7:132-145, 1980.
11. Banker BQ, and Larroche J-C: Periventricular leukomalacia of infancy: a form of neonatal anoxic encephalopathy, Arch Neurol 7:386-410, 1962.
12. Barth PG, and others: On the relationship between germinal layer haemorrhage and telencephalic leucoencephalopathy in the preterm infant, Neuropädiatrie 11:17-26, 1980.
13. Bass T, and others: Radial glial interaction with cerebral germinal matrix capillaries in the fetal baboon, Exp Neurol 118: 126-132, 1992.
14. Bergman I, and others: Intracerebral hemorrhage in the full-term neonatal infant, Pediatrics 75:488-496, 1985.
15. Blair E, and Stanley FJ: Intrapartum asphyxia: a rare cause of cerebral palsy, J Pediatr 112:515-519, 1988.
16. Borit A, and Herndon RM: The fine structure of plaques fibromyéliniques in ulegyria and status marmoratus, Acta Neuropathol 14:304-308, 1970.
17. Brand MM, and Bignami A: The effects of chronic hypoxia on the neonatal and infantile brain, Brain 92:233-254, 1969.
18. Brann AW, and Myers RE: Central nervous system findings in the newborn monkey following severe in utero partial asphyxia, Neurology 25:327-338, 1975.
19. Brück Y, and others: Evidence for neuronal apoptosis in pontosubicular neuron necrosis, Neuropathol Appl Neurobiol 22:23-29, 1996.
20. Brun A: Marginal glioneuronal heterotopia of the central nervous system, Acta Pathol Microbiol Scand 65:221-233, 1965.
21. Chen HH, Chien C-H, and Liu HM: Correlation between angiogenesis and basic fibroblast growth factor expression in experimental brain infarct, Stroke 25:1651-1657, 1994.
22. Choi BH, and Matthias SC: Cortical dysplasia associated with massive extopic of neurons and glial cells within the subarachnoid space, Acta Neuropathol 73:105-109, 1987.
23. Chugani HT: Positron emission tomography scanning: applications in newborns, Clin Perinatol 20:395-409, 1993.
24. Cruveilheir J: Anatomie Pathologique du Corpus Humain, ou Descriptions avec Figures Litographiées, des Diverses Altérations Morbides dont le Corps Humain est Susceptible. Tome Premier, Livre XV. L'apoplexie des Enfants Nouveau-nés Paris, 1829-1835, JB Ballière.
25. Dambska M, Laure-Kamionowska M, and Schmidt-Sidor B: Early and late neuropathological changes in perinatal white matter damage, J Child Neurol 4:291-298, 1989.
26. Darrow VC, and others: Histological evolution of the reactions to hemorrhage in the premature human infant's brain, Am J Pathol 130:44-58, 1988.
27. Del Bigio MR, and others: Acute and chronic cerebral white matter damage in neonatal hydrocephalus, Can J Neurol Sci 21:299-305, 1994.
28. DeReuck J: The human periventricular arterial blood supply and the anatomy of cerebral infarctions, Eur Neurol 5:321-334, 1971.
29. DeReuck J, Chattha AS, and Richardson EP Jr: Pathogenesis and evolution of periventricular leukomalacia in infancy, Arch Neurol 27:229-236, 1972.
30. Doe FD, Shuangshoti S, and Netsky MG: Cryptic hemangioma of the choroid plexus, Neurology 12:1232-1239, 1972.
31. Donat JF, and others: Intraventricular hemorrhages in full-term and premature infants, Mayo Clin Proc 53:437-441, 1978.
32. Donn SM, and Bowers RA: Unilateral germinal matrix hemorrhage in the newborn, J Ultrasound Med 4:251-253, 1985.
33. Dykes FD, and others: Posthemorrhagic hydrocephalus in high-risk preterm infants: natural history, management and long-term outcome, J Pediatr 114:611-618, 1989.
34. Eimerl S, and Schramm M: The quantity of calcium that appears to induce neuronal death, J Neurochem 62:1223-1226, 1994.
35. Ellis WG, Goetzman BW, and Lindenberg JA: Neuropathologic documentation of prenatal brain damage, Am J Dis Child 142: 858-866, 1988.
36. Fazekas JF, Alexander FAD, and Himwich HE: Tolerance of newborn to anoxia, Am J Physiol 134:281-287, 1941.
37. Ferrer I, and others: Evidence of nuclear DNA fragmentation following hypoxia-ischemia in the infant rat brain, and transient forebrain ischemia in the adult gerbil, Brain Pathol 4:115-122, 1994.
38. Finer NN, and others: Hypoxic-ischemic encephalopathy in term neonates: perinatal factors and outcome, J Pediatr 98:112-117, 1981.
39. Friede RL: Developmental neuropathology, ed 2. Berlin, 1989, Springer-Verlag.
40. Friede RL: Ponto-subicular lesions in perinatal anoxia, Arch Pathol Lab Med 94:343-354, 1972.
41. Fukumizu M, Takashima S, and Becker LE: Neonatal posthemorrhagic hydrocephalus: neuropathologic and immunohistochemical studies, Pediatr Neurol 13:230-234, 1995.
42. Galloway PG, and Roessmann U: Neuronal karyorrhexis in Sommer's sector in a 22-week stillborn, Acta Neuropathol 70: 343-344, 1986.
43. García JH, Liu K-F, and Ho K-L: Neuronal necrosis after middle cerebral artery occlusion in Wistar rats progresses at different time intervals in the caudal putamen and the cortex, Stroke 26: 636-643, 1995.
44. García JH, and Pantoni L: Strokes in childhood, Semin Pediatr Neurol 2:180-191, 1995.
45. Gilles FH: Hypotensive brain stem necrosis. Selective symmetrical necrosis of tegmental neuronal aggregates following cardiac arrest, Arch Pathol Lab Med 88:32-41, 1969.
46. Gilles FH, and Murphy SF: Perinatal telencephalic leucoencephalopathy, J Neurol Neurosurg Psychiatry 32:404-413, 1969.
47. Gould SJ, Howard S, and Papadaki L: The development of ependyma in the human fetal brain. An immunohistological and electron microscopic study, Dev Brain Res 55:255-267, 1990.
48. Gould SJ, and others: Periventricular intraparenchymal cerebral hemorrhage in preterm infants: the role of venous infarction, J Pathol 151:197-202, 1987.
49. Grant A, and others: Cerebral palsy among children born during the Dublin randomised trial of intrapartum monitoring, Lancet 2:1233-1236, 1989.
50. Grunnet ML: Periventricular leukomalacia complex, Arch Pathol Lab Med 103:6-10, 1979.
51. Grunnet ML: Morphometry of blood vessels in the cortex and germinal plate of premature neonates, Pediatr Neurol 5:12-16, 1989.
52. Grunnet ML, and Shields WD: Cerebellar hemorrhage in the premature infant, J Pediatr 88:605-608, 1976.
53. Gubits RM, and others: Immediate early gene induction after neonatal hypoxia-ischemia, Mol Brain Res 18:228-238, 1993.
54. Hambleton G, and Wigglesworth JS: Origin of intraventricular haemorrhage in the preterm infant, Arch Dis Child 51:651-659, 1976.
55. Hotchkiss MG, and others: Bilateral Duane's retraction syndrome. A clinico-pathologic case report, Arch Ophthalmol 98: 870-874, 1980.
56. Iida K, Takashima S, and Ueda K: Immunohistochemical study of myelination and oligodendrocyte in infants with periventricular leukomalacia, Pediatr Neurol 13:296-304, 1995.

57. Jarjour IT, and Ahdab-Barmada M: Cerebrovascular lesions in infants and children dying after extracorporeal membrane oxygenation, Pediatr Neurol 10:13-19, 1994.
58. Juurlink BHJ, Hertz L, and Yager JY: Astrocyte maturation and susceptibility to ischaemia or substrate deprivation. Neuroreport 3:1135-1137, 1992.
59. Kamei A, and others: Immunohistochemical demonstration of olivocerebellar transneuronal degeneration in neonates, Brain Dev 19:in press, 1996.
60. Kotagal S, and others: Symmetrical bithalamic and striatal hemorrhage following perinatal hypoxia in a term infant, J Comput Assist Tomogr 7:353-355, 1983.
61. Kuban KCK, and Gilles FH: Human telencephalic angiogenesis, Ann Neurol 17:539-548, 1985.
62. Kuban KCK, and Leviton A: The epidemiology of cerebral palsy, N Engl J Med 330:188-195, 1994.
63. Lacey DJ, and Teryslan K: Intraventricular hemorrhage in full-term neonates, Dev Med Child Neurol 24:332-337, 1982.
64. Landman J, and others: Radiological colpocephaly: a congenital malformation or the result of intrauterine and perinatal brain damage? Brain Dev 11:313-316, 1989.
65. Larroche J-C: Post-haemorrhagic hydrocephalus in infancy: anatomical study, Biol Neonate 20:287-299, 1972.
66. Larroche J-C: Subependymal pseudo-cysts in the newborn, Biol Neonate 21:170-183, 1972.
67. Larroche J-C: Developmental pathology of the neonate. Amsterdam, 1977, Excerpta Medica.
68. Larroche J-C: Structure of the capillaries of the subependymal matrix in the developing human brain, 1988.
69. Leech RW, and Alvord EC Jr: Glial fatty metamorphosis: an abnormal response of premyelin glia frequently accompanying leukomalacia, Am J Pathol 74:603-612, 1974.
70. Leech RW, and Alvord EC Jr: Morphological variations in periventricular leukomalacia, Am J Pathol 74:591-602, 1974.
71. Leech RW, and Alvord EC Jr: Anoxic-ischemic encephalopathy in the human neonatal period—the significance of brainstem involvement, Arch Neurol 34:109-113, 1977.
72. Leech RW, and Kohnen P: Subependymal and intraventricular hemorrhage in the newborn, Am J Pathol 77:465-475, 1974.
73. Leech RW, Olson MI, and Alvord EC Jr: Neuropathologic features of idiopathic respiratory distress syndrome, Arch Pathol Lab Med 103:341-343, 1979.
74. Leviton A, and Gilles FH: Acquired perinatal leukoencephalopathy, Ann Neurol 16:1-8, 1984.
75. Liu HM, and Chen HH: c-fos protein expression and ischemic changes in neurons vulnerable to ischemia/hypoxia, correlated with basic fibroblast growth factor immunoreactivity, J Neuropathol Exp Neurol 53:598-605, 1994.
76. Lou HC: Hypoxic-hemodynamic pathogenesis of brain lesions in the newborn, Brain Dev 16:423-431, 1994.
77. Maker P, and others: Does indomethacin cause extension of intracranial hemorrhage: a preliminary study, Pediatrics 75: 497-500, 1985.
78. Malamud N: Status marmoratus: a form of cerebral palsy following either birth injury or inflammation of the central nervous system, J Pediatr 37:610-619, 1960.
79. Marín-Padilla M: Prenatal development of fibrous (white matter), protoplasmic (gray matter) and layer 1 astrocytes in the human cerebral cortex: a Golgi study, J Comp Neurol 358:1-19, 1995.
80. Marín-Padilla M: Review of perinatal brain damage, repair, and neurologic sequelae in the prematurely born infant, Int Pediatr 10 (suppl):26-33, 1995.
80b. Marín-Padilla M: Developmental neuropathology and impact of perinatal brain damage, hemorrhagic lesions of the neocortex, Neuropathol Exp Neurol 55:758–773, 1996.
81. Mayer PL, and Kier EL: The controversies of the periventricular white matter circulation: a review of the anatomic literature, Am J Neuroradiol 12:223-228, 1991.
82. Mito T, and others: Clinicopathological study of pontosubicular necrosis, Neuropediatrics 24:204-207, 1993.
83. Moody DM, Bell MA, and Challa VR: Features of the cerebral vascular pattern that predict vulnerability to perfusion or oxygenation deficiency: an anatomic study, Am J Neuroradiol 11: 431-439, 1991.
84. Morshead CM, and others: Neural stem cell in the adult mammalian forebrain: a relatively quiescent subpopulation of subependymal cells, Neuron 13:1071-1082, 1994.
85. Mullaart RA, and others: Asymmetry of the cerebral blood flow: an ultrasound doppler study in preterm newborns, Pediatr Neurol 13:319-322, 1995.
86. Munell F, and others: Localization of c-fos, c-jun, and hsp70 mRNA expression in brain after neonatal hypoxia-ischemia, Dev Brain Res 77:111-121, 1994.
87. Naeye RL, and others: Origins of cerebral palsy, Am J Dis Child 143:1154-1161, 1989.
88. Nakamura Y, Okudera T, and Hashimoto T: Vascular architecture in white matter of neonates: its relationship to periventricular leukomalacia, J Neuropathol Exp Neurol 53:582-589, 1994.
89. Natsume J, and others: Clinical, neurophysiologic, and neuropathological features of an infant with brain damage of total asphyxia type (Myers), Pediatr Neurol 13:61-64, 1995.
90. Nelson KB, and Ellenberg JH: Antecedents of cerebral palsy. Multivariate analysis of risk, N Engl J Med 315:81-96, 1986.
91. Nelson MD, Gonzáles-Gómez I, and Gilles FH: The search for human telencephalic ventriculofugal arteries, Am J Neuroradiol 12:215-222, 1991.
92. Nelson KB, and Leviton A: How much of neonatal encephalopathy is due to birth asphyxia? Am J Dis Child 145:1325-1331, 1991.
93. Nitatori T, and others: Delayed neuronal death in the CA1 pyramidal cell layer of the gerbil hippocampus following transient ischemia is apoptosis, J Neurosci 15:1001-1011, 1995.
94. Norman MG, and others: Congenital malformations of the brain, New York, 1995, Oxford University Press.
95. Norman MG: Bilateral encephaloclastic lesions in a 26-week gestation fetus: effect on neuronal migration, Can J Neurol Sci 7:191-194, 1980.
96. Norman MG: On the morphogenesis of ulegyria, Acta Neuropathol 53:331-332, 1981.
97. Norman RM: Patterns of symmetrical brain damage. In Selective vulnerability of the brain to hypoxemia. Oxford, UK, 1963, Blackwell.
98. Ozawa H, and others: Ferritin immunohistochemical study on pontine nuclei from infants with pontosubicular neuron necrosis, Brain Dev 17:20-23, 1995.
99. Panerai RB, and others: Estimation of critical closing pressure in the cerebral circulation of newborns, Neuropediatrics 26:168-173, 1995.
100. Paneth N, and others: Brain damage in the preterm infant. London, 1994, MacKeith Press and Cambridge University Press.
101. Paneth N, and others: White matter necrosis in very low birth weight infants: neuropathologic and ultrasonographic findings in 22 infants surviving six days or more, J Pediatr 116:975-984, 1990.
102. Pape KE, and Wigglesworth JS: Haemorrhage, ischaemia and the perinatal brain, Clinics in Developmental Medicine, No. 69/70, London, 1979, Spastics International Medical Publications.
103. Pape KE, and Wigglesworth JS: Perinatal Brain Lesions, Oxford, 1988, Blackwell Scientific Press.

104. Pasternak JF, and others: Regional blood flow in the newborn beagle pup: the germinal matrix is a 'low-flow' structure, Pediatr Res 16:499-503, 1982.
105. Pellicer A, and others: Natural history of ventricular dilatation in preterm infants: prognostic significance, Pediatr Neurol 9: 108-114, 1993.
106. Povlishock JT, Martinez AJ, and Moossy J: The fine structure of blood vessels of the telecephalic germinal matrix in the human fetus, Am J Anat 149:439-452, 1977.
107. Pryds O: Control of cerebral circulation in the high-risk neonate, Ann Neurol 30:321-329, 1991.
108. Pullicino P, and others: Pontine ischemic rarefaction, Ann Neurol 37:460-466, 1995.
109. Rafols JA, and others: Global brain ischemia and reperfusion: Golgi apparatus ultrastructure in neurons selectively vulnerable to death, Acta Neuropathol 90:17-30, 1995.
110. Ravenal SD: Posterior fossa hemorrhage in the term newborn: report of two cases, Pediatrics 64:39-42, 1979.
111. Reeder JD, Kaude JV, and Setzer CS: Choroid plexus hemorrhage in premature neonates: recognition by sonography, Am J Neuroradiol 3:619-622, 1982.
112. Riikonen R, and others: Changing pattern of cerebral palsy in the southwest region of Finland, Acta Paediatr Scand 78:581-587, 1989.
113. Roessmann U, and Gambetti P: Pathological reaction of astrocytes in perinatal brain injury: immunohistochemical study, Acta Neuropathol 70:302-307, 1986.
114. Roland EH, Flodmark O, and Hill A: Thalamic hemorrhage with intraventricular hemorrhage in the full-term newborn, Pediatrics 85:737-742, 1990.
115. Rom S, Serfontein GL, and Humphreys RP: Intracerebulbar hematoma in the neonate, J Pediatr 93:486-488, 1978.
116. Rorke LB: Pathology of perinatal brain injury, New York, 1982, Raven Press.
117. Röyttä M, and others: Infantile bilateral striatal necrosis. Clinical and morphologic report of a case and a review of the literature, Acta Neuropathol 55:97-103, 1981.
118. Ruckensteiner E, and Zöllner F: Über die Blutungen im Gebiete der Vena terminalis bei Neugeborenen, Frankfurt Z f Pathol 37: 568-578, 1929.
119. Saliba E, and others: Area of lateral ventricles measured on cranial ultrasonography in preterm infants: association with outcome, Arch Dis Child 65:1033-1037, 1990.
120. Sarnat HB: Disturbances of late neuronal migrations in the perinatal period, Am J Dis Child 141:969-980, 1987.
121. Sarnat HB: Hypoxic alterations of neonatal neurons. An acridine orange fluorochromic study of nucleic acids, Brain Dev 9: 43-47, 1987.
122. Sarnat HB: Do the corticospinal and corticobulbar tracts mediate functions in the human newborn? Can J Neurol Sci 16: 157-160, 1989.
123. Sarnat HB: Cerebral dysgenesis. Embryology and clinical expression, New York, 1992, Oxford University Press.
124. Sarnat HB: Regional differentiation of the human fetal ependyma: immunocytochemical markers, J Neuropathol Exp Neurol 51:58-75, 1992.
125. Sarnat HB: Role of human fetal ependyma, Pediatr Neurol 8: 163-178, 1992.
126. Sarnat HB: Impairment of late neuroblast migrations by ischemia. In Lou HC, Greisen G, Larsen JF, editors: Brain lesions in the newborn. Hypoxic and haemodynamic pathogenesis, Copenhagen, 1994, Munksgaard.
127. Sarnat HB: Ectopic or heterotopic? An appeal for semantic precision in describing developmental disorders of the nervous system, Pediatr Neurol 13:178-179, 1995.
128. Sarnat HB: Ependymal reaction to injury. A review, J Neuropathol Exp Neurol 54:1-15, 1995.
129. Sarnat HB, Sarnat MS: Neonatal encephalopathy following fetal distress. A clinical and electroencephalographic study, Arch Neurol 33:696-705, 1976.
130. Schneider H, and others: Anoxic encephalopathy with predominant involvement of basal ganglia, brain stem and spinal cord in the perinatal period, Acta Neuropathol 32:287-298, 1975.
131. Shankaran S, and others: Outcome after posthemorrhagic ventriculomegaly in comparison with mild hemorrhage without ventriculomegaly, J Pediatr 114:109-114, 1989.
132. Sheth RD, and others: Differential involvement of the brain in neonatal asphyxia. A pathogenic explanation, J Child Neurol 10:464-466, 1995.
133. Shuman RM, and Selednik LJ: Periventricular leukomalacia: a one-year autopsy study, Arch Neurol 37:231-235, 1980.
134. Skullerud K, and Skjaeraasen J: Clinicopathological study of germinal matrix hemorrhage, pontosubicular necrosis and periventricular leukomalacia in stillborn, Child Nerv Syst 4:88-91, 1988.
135. Skullerud K, Torvik A, and Skaare-Botner L: Progressive degeneration of the cerebral cortex in infancy, Acta Neuropathol 24: 153-160, 1973.
136. Skullerud K, and Westre B: Frequency and prognostic significance of germinal matrix hemorrhage, periventricular leukomalacia and pontosubicular necrosis in preterm infants, Acta Neuropathol 70:257-261, 1986.
137. Smart IHM: Proliferative characteristics of the ependymal layer during the early development of the spinal cord in the mouse, J Anat 111:365-380, 1972.
138. Sohma O, and others: The prenatal age critical for the development of the pontosubicular necrosis, Acta Neuropathol 90:7-10, 1995.
139. Sotrel A, and Lorenzo AV: Ultrastructure of blood vessels in the ganglionic eminence of premature rabbits with spontaneous germinal matrix hemorrhages, J Neuropathol Exp Neurol 48: 462-482, 1989.
140. Squier M, and Keeling JW: The incidence of prenatal brain injury, Neuropathol Appl Neurobiol 17:29-38, 1991.
141. Sugimoto T, and others: When do brain abnormalities in cerebral palsy occur? An MRI study, Dev Med Child Neurol 37: 285-292, 1995.
142. Takashima S, Armstrong DL, and Becker LE: Subcortical leukomalacia, Arch Neurol 35:470-472, 1978.
143. Takashima S, Iida K, and Deguchi K: Periventricular leukomalacia, glial development and myelination, Early Hum Dev 43: 177-184, 1995.
144. Takashima S, Mito T, and Ando Y: Pathogenesis of periventricular white matter hemorrhages in preterm infants, Brain Dev 8:25-30, 1986.
145. Takashima S, and Tanaka K: Development of cerebrovascular architecture and its relationship to periventricular leukomalacia, Arch Neurol 35:11-16, 1978.
146. Takashima S, and Tanaka K: Microangiography and vascular permeability of the subependymal matrix in the premature infant, Can J Neurol Sci 5:45-50, 1978.
147. Tanaka H, and others: Effects of neonatal hypoxia on brainstem cholinergic neurons: pedunculopontine nucleus and laterodorsal tegmental nucleus, Brain Dev 17:264-270, 1995.
148. Torfs CP, and others: Prenatal and perinatal factors in the etiology of cerebral palsy, J Pediatr 116:615-619, 1990.
149. Torvik A, and others: Affection of the hippocampal granule cells in pontosubicular necrosis, Acta Neuropathol 83:535-537, 1992.

150. Towbin A: Cerebral intraventricular hemorrhage and subependymal matrix infarction in the fetus and premature newborn, Am J Pathol 52:121-134, 1968.
151. Towbin A: Cerebral hypoxic damage in fetus and newborn, Arch Neurol 20:35-43, 1969.
152. Towfighi J, and others: Möbius syndrome. Neuropathologic observations, Acta Neuropathol 48:11-17, 1979.
153. Towfighi J, and others: Temporal evolution of neuropathologic changes in an immature rat model of cerebral hypoxia: a light microscopic study, Acta Neuropathol 90:375-386, 1995.
154. Trounce JQ, and others: Primary thalamic hemorrhage in the newborn: a new clinical entity, Lancet 1:190-192, 1985.
155. Van den Bergh R: Centrifugal elements in the vascular pattern of the deep intracerebral blood supply, Angiology 20:88-94, 1969.
156. Vannucci RC: Heterogeneity of hypoxic-ischemic thresholds in experimental animals. In Lou HC, Larsen JF, Thaysen JH, editors: Brain lesions in the newborn: Hypoxic and haemodynamic pathogenesis, Copenhagen, 1994, Munksgaard.
157. Virchow R: Zur Pathologischen Anatomie des Gehirns: I. Congenitale Encephalitis und Myelitis, Virch Arch 38:129-142, 1867.
158. Voit T, Lemburg P, Stork W: NMR studies in thalamic-striatal necrosis, Lancet 2:445, 1985.
159. Volpe JJ: Neurology of the newborn, ed. 3, Philadelphia, 1995, WB Saunders.
160. Volpe JJ: Intraventricular hemorrhage in the premature infant: current concepts, Part 1, Ann Neurol 25:3-11, 1989.
161. Volpe JJ, and Pasternack JF: Parasagittal cerebral injury in neonatal hypoxic-ischemic encephalopathy. Clinical and neuroradiologic features, J Pediatr 91:472-476, 1977.
162. Weber TR, and others: A clinical-pathological study of nonsurvivors of newborn ECMO, J Pediatr Surg 28:135-137, 1993.
163. Weickert CS, and Blum M: Striatal TGG-$\alpha$: postnatal developmental expression and evidence for a role in the proliferation of subependymal cells, Dev Brain Res 86:203-216, 1995.
164. Weig SG, and others: Patterns of cerebral injury and clinical presentation in the vascular disruptive syndrome of monozygotic twins, Pediatr Neurol 13:279-285, 1995.
165. Willis T: Pathologiae cerebri et nervosi generis specimen. In Quo agitur de morbis convulsives et de scorbuto, 1667, Oxford.
166. Yoshioka H, and others: Granule cell deficit in the mouse cerebellum after total asphyxia, Ann Neurol 19:356-359, 1986.
167. Yu MC, Yu W-HA: Effect of hypoxia on cerebellar development: morphologic and radioautographic studies, Exp Neurol 70:652-664, 1980.

C • H • A • P • T • E • R

# 14

# *Neurodegenerative Diseases: Biopsy Diagnosis in Children*

**Hans H. Goebel**



In 1983, the authors of a seminal review produced a 2 ⅔-page table of "well over 600 disorders and variants which were considered to be neurodegenerative diseases of infancy and childhood."[57] This list included such diverse conditions as alcoholic encephalopathy, kuru, rabies, and status marmoratus. Obviously, the diagnostic recognition of neurodegenerative diseases in children (NDIC) should use the entire armamentarium available to the pediatric neurologist including collaboration with neuroradiology, neurogenetics, neurochemistry, neurophysiology, and neuropathology. The neuropathologist at the autopsy often may be the ultimate diagnostician of many neurodegenerative diseases in children. However, even then, the diagnosis of an individual child's neurodegenerative disease may not be successful. This is because many NDIC lack morphologic features that are disease specific.

Conversely, although many of these disorders are chronically progressive and ultimately fatal, nosologic diagnosis is to be sought and may even be mandatory to separate treatable from untreatable conditions, for genetic counseling and for eventual prenatal diagnosis. Sometimes the physician can only provide a diagnosis and thus remove uncertainties and unwarranted expectations, assuring the parents that everything possible was done for their child.

Among the many NDIC only a small minority may be successfully diagnosed by means of a biopsy.[72,73] Diagnostic accuracy is enhanced when the biopsy is done at the major site of the neurodegenerative disease. Usually this can be achieved only if (1) the disease process can be recognized on morphologic grounds and (2) the tissue is a amenable to biopsy without major risk, that is, when the NDIC involves tissues outside the central nervous system (CNS). Brain biopsy carries a high surgical hazard, and many cerebral subcortical areas are entirely inaccessible to biopsy. Therefore, brain biopsy is performed rarely for diagnostic purposes.

Among the NDIC there are, however, groups of disorders and individual conditions that may be successfully diagnosed by extracerebral biopsy. This cohort is limited to two categories. The first includes multiorgan disorders that affect the central nervous system and extracerebral organs/tissues by the same morphologic process. These multiorgan disorders are also called multisystem diseases, although this appears to be a misnomer. Not a multitude of systems, but rather a multitude of organs—or even a single system—may be affected; that is, single systems of mitochondria, of lysosomes, or of peroxisomes, respectively. These groups of neurodegenerative conditions are marked by morphologic abnormalities both inside and outside the nervous system, the mitochondrial, lysosomal, and peroxisomal disorders. The former are also called mitochondrial encephalomyopathies. Certain disorders of carbohydrate metabolism not marked by lysosomal storage also belong to this group. The neuronal ceroid lipofuscinoses (NCL) are another important group of these pediatric conditions. Defects in several classes of intermediate filaments, for example, vimentin, glial fibrillary acidic protein, and neurofilaments, provide the basis for the ubiquitous giant axonal neuropathy (GAN) that involves the central (CNS) and peripheral nervous system (PNS) as well as non-neural cell types.

The second major category includes disorders that affect both the CNS and the PNS and are recognized by biopsy of tissues that contain nerves, both myelinated and unmyelinated. Examples of these disorders are the lysosomal and peroxisomal leukodystrophies and the neuroaxonal dystrophies.

Many conditions diagnosable by extracerebral biopsy are neurometabolic disorders with known enzyme deficiencies,[158a] and these also can be recognized by biochemical examination. Indeed, biochemical confirmation of a morphologic diagnosis is mandatory. The NDIC that lend themselves to diagnostic examination by biopsy are nonmetabolic; others are metabolic types. In the former group, morphologic investigation by electron microscopy is essential for in vivo diagnosis. These are the true NDIC—in the metabolic group, morphologic examination is ancillary.

The indispensable diagnostic tool for investigating biopsied tissues morphologically is the electron microscope.[158a] Histology, enzyme histochemistry, and immunohistochemistry are of limited value. Electron microscopy is time-consuming and requires specially trained personnel, and thus is rather expensive. In contrast, few pediatric and neuropediatric neurodegenerative disorders can be diagnosed by extracerebral biopsy; therefore, their recognition requires experience that usually is commensurate with the number of specimens studied and diseases encountered. For these two reasons few pathologists have experience and regularly have dealt with biopsied tissues of NDIC. One purpose of this chapter is to share my experience with others and in this manner augment the cohort of pathologists engaged in the biopsy diagnosis of these NDIC.

Retrospective analysis of pertinent reports on morphologic data obtained by biopsy in NDIC reveals that hardly any unequivocally recognizable new disorders have been discovered by extracerebral biopsies within the last 15 years. Thus, the catalogue of conditions diagnosed by extracerebral biopsy has remained unchanged since the early 1980s. Only clinical variants have been added recently. Conversely, the spectrum of tissues available by diagnostic biopsy has been enlarged slightly by examining prenatal tissues, including amniotic fluid cells, chorion, fetal skin, and fetal lymphocytes.

## ORGANS AND TISSUES SUITABLE FOR DIAGNOSTIC BIOPSY (Table 14-1)

Two general types of biopsies may be performed, curative and diagnostic. The former attempts to combine cure and diagnosis, whereas the latter is intended to provide a diagnosis with or without subsequent therapy. Thus, criteria for diagnostic biopsy may be more limited.

In neurodegenerative diseases of the central nervous system, an ideal target for diagnostic biopsy would be the CNS itself. Two conditions must be met to render a brain biopsy successful: an accessible target and morphologic expression of the suspected disorder. Few CNS disorders express pathognomonic morphologic features. For many of the neurodegenerative disorders listed by Dyken and Krawiecki,[57] there are no morphologic identifiers, even at autopsy. Other groups may show sets of findings demonstrable only at autopsy, e.g., motor neuron diseases. Diagnostic brain biopsy has therefore become obsolete because of limited access to the tissue targets, usually the cerebral cortex, the immediate subcortical white matter and, perhaps, the cerebellar cortex. Modern stereotactic techniques theoretically allow the neurosurgeon to biopsy almost any target in the CNS, including the basal ganglia in Hallervorden-Spatz disease. However, very few neurodegenerative diseases have morphologic features that are disease-specific and that can be recognized by biopsy: approximately only 20 of the conditions listed by Dyken and Krawiecki do fulfill such criteria.[57] Furthermore, the increased diagnostic reliability of biochemical assays and recent molecular ge-

**Table 14-1.** Diagnostic suitability of tissues to biopsy in NDIC

| Disease | Skin | Conjunctiva | Lymphocytes | Muscle | Nerve | Rectum | Brain |
|---|---|---|---|---|---|---|---|
| Vacuolar lysosomal diseases (MPS, ML, oligosaccharidoses) | + + | + | + + | + | + | + | ? |
| Neuronal intranuclear hyaline inclusion disease | ? | − | − | + | − | + + | + |
| Avacuolar lysosomal disorders | | | | | | | |
| GM$_1$-Gangliosidosis | + + | + | + | + | + | + + | + + |
| GM$_2$-Gangliosidosis | +* | +* | − | ? | − | + + | + + |
| Farber disease | + + | − | − | ? | − | + + | + + |
| Fabry disease | + + | + | + | + | + | + | + |
| Niemann-Pick disease | + + | + | + | + | + | + + | + + |
| Gaucher disease | − | − | − | − | − | + | + |
| Metachromatic leukodystrophy | ? | + | − | ? | + + | + | + + |
| Globoid cell leukodystrophy | + | + | − | ? | + + | + | + + |
| Type II glycogenosis | + | + | + | + + | + | + | + |
| Peroxisomal diseases | | | | | | | |
| Adrenoleukodystrophy | +* | + | − | ? | + + | + | + + |
| Polyglucosan diseases | | | | | | | |
| Lafora disease | + + | − | − | + | − | + | + + |
| Type IV glycogenosis | + | − | − | + + | − | + | ? |
| Polyglucosan myopathy | ? | − | − | + + | + + | ? | ? |
| Childhood neuronal ceroid-lipofuscinoses | + + | + | + + | + + | + | + + | + + |
| Giant axonal neuropathy | + + | + + | − | ? | + + | + + | + + |
| Carbohydrate-deficient glycoprotein syndrome | | ? | | | ? | | |
| Mitochondrial encephalomyopathies | ? | ? | − | + + | ? | − | + |
| Rett syndrome | ? | ? | − | − | − | − | − |
| Neuroaxonal dystrophies | | | | | | | |
| infantile | + + | + + | − | ? | + | + + | + + |
| juvenile | ? | ? | − | ? | + | ? | ? |

+ + = very suitable; + = suitable; ? = questionable; − = unsuitable; *where nerves present in biopsy specimen.

netic methods also have made brain biopsy outmoded. During the era of diagnostic brain biopsy, largely the two decades of the 1960s and 1970s, it became possible to study extensively the ultrastructure of the diseased human brain, but today these types of biopsies are restricted to instances of neoplastic disease and trauma.

The only neurodegenerative disease in children that requires brain biopsy for recognition is Alexander's disease, which is marked by demyelination and formation of Rosenthal fibers in the cerebral cortex. Subcortical subtypes of Alexander's disease usually develop later in childhood and adulthood, manifesting themselves in the brainstem[78] and the spinal cord. Another disorder that might require brain biopsy for antemortem diagnosis is Creutzfeldt-Jakob disease, which rarely occurs in children, showing sponginess of the cerebral cortex and increased deposition of prion protein that can be recognized by immunohistochemistry, as discussed in Chapter 10.

Formation of disease-specific morphologic features in and around neuronal perikarya in certain lysosomal disorders and in infantile neuroaxonal dystrophy, respectively, prompted studies on extracerebral tissues that also contain nerve cells—the intestine, especially the rectum. Rectal biopsy was the next evolutionary step in the diagnosis by biopsy of NDIC.[3,20,21,23,176] Two types of lysosomal disorders may be recognized in rectal biopsies or in other parts of the intestine, e.g., the appendix—(1) those affecting neurons only, largely GM$_2$-gangliosidosis of the infantile or Tay-Sachs type, and (2) those affecting neurons and other cell types, the sphingolipidoses, mucopolysaccharidoses, and oligosaccharidoses, and NCL. Because of the scarcity of myelinated (preganglionic autonomic) axons in intestinal nerve farcides, biopsy in search of a lysosomal leukodystrophy, often is futile. Rectal biopsy has only slightly greater diagnostic value than brain biopsy. Recently, however, it was established that neuronal intranuclear hyaline inclusion disease[89] can be diagnosed by rectal biopsy. Recognition of these neuronal diseases requires full thickness sections of the rectal wall to obtain neurons of the myenteric plexus, a requirement not satisfied by suction biopsy.[1] Rectal biopsy by suction has been recommended, even in recent years in a limited number of diseases.[160] An occasional report[185] still refers to diagnostic rectal biopsy findings in disorders that can be recognized by other means, e.g., biochemistry or noncerebral, nonrectal biopsies.

Examination of rectal tissues also may reveal nonspecific abnormalities in axons, for example, enlargement by nonspecific dense bodies in several lysosomal diseases[1] including infantile $GM_2$-gangliosidosis or mucopolysaccharidosis III.

Because PNS structures are present in the intestine, neuroaxonal dystrophy[76] and giant axonal neuropathy (GAN) can be recognized by biopsy. Rectal biopsy data are not available on hereditary sensory neuropathy IV, a congenital PNS disorder marked by absence of unmyelinated axons in somatic peripheral nerves including sudomotor sympathetic axons,[77] but intestinal dysfunction is not known.

Visceral organs other than intestine are of very limited value for diagnostic biopsy in NDIC. Certain lysosomal diseases manifest themselves in liver, but also in organs more easily accessible to biopsy. Only certain forms of Gaucher disease are best recognized morphologically by biopsy of liver or spleen. Several clinical types of Niemann-Pick disease seriously affect the liver. Conversely, in certain peroxisomal disorders, a reliable diagnosis may be achieved only by biopsy of the liver, where presence or absence of peroxisomes or variations in their size can be determined.

Skeletal muscle, which makes up some 30% to 40% of total body mass and represents the largest organ, may yield diagnostic information in a number of NDIC, both metabolic and nonmetabolic. When considering muscle as a diagnostic target one has to bear in mind that in addition to the skeletal muscle fibers, other types of cells are encountered in a biopsied muscle sample. Mural cells of vessels, fibroblasts, macrophages, and occasionally nerve fascicles with myelinated and unmyelinated axons, and neuromuscular junctions may be found by chance or by intentional biopsy. During motor point biopsy, a small transversely running band of increased connective tissue at the mid-belly of the biceps muscle may be recognizable to the naked eye; similar findings are seen in very short muscles, such as the intercostal or peroneus brevis muscles. Facial[168] and extraocular muscles are rich in motor endplates, but hardly represent a target of diagnostic biopsy.

Skeletal muscle biopsy is essential in mitochondrial encephalomyopathies, which are part of the spectrum of mitochondrial disorders and mitochondrial myopathies. Details concerning diagnostic suitability of skeletal muscle and the mitochondrial disorders are covered in Chapter 17. The ubiquity of lysosomal disease-specific residual bodies in type II glycogenosis and in the childhood forms of neuronal ceroid-lipofuscinoses makes skeletal muscle a reliable target to biopsy,[36] even though this procedure is more invasive than biopsies of skin, conjunctiva, and circulating lymphocytes. Accretions of lysosomal glycogen and NCL-specific lipopigments, respectively, allow screening for increased activity of acid phosphatase, the marker enzyme of the lysosomal compartment, and for autofluorescence when NCL is suspected. Mucolipidosis IV also manifests itself in skeletal muscle[80] by increased phosphatase activity. Other disorders in which autofluorescent acid phosphatase-active lipopigments accrue are different forms of vitamin E deficiency, both secondary and primary, which often give clinical evidence of spinocerebellar degeneration.[28] Lafora disease and type IV glycogenosis can be recognized by the sarcoplasmic formation of fibrillar glycogen. The presence of other mesenchymal cytologic elements also permits group diagnosis of vacuolar lysosomal diseases and those avacuolar lysosomal disorders that particularly affect vessel walls, e.g., Fabry disease and Niemann-Pick disease. When nerve fascicles are encountered in a muscle biopsy, the diagnostician should recall their involvement in disorders that affect primarily peripheral nerve fibers and their Schwann cells, such as metabolic leukodystrophies, infantile neuroaxonal dystrophy, or giant axonal neuropathy.

Skin is now the preferred tissue for diagnostic biopsy in NDIC.[39,53,134] It is the second most easily retrievable tissue, after circulating lymphocytes, and has the further advantage of providing fibroblasts for tissue culture and subsequent biochemical studies. Skin contains a wealth of diversified mesenchymal, epithelial, and neuroectodermal cells. Skin biopsy provides diagnostic information on lysosomal disorders including the NCL, on the neuroaxonal dystrophies, on certain polyglucosan disorders, on GAN, and on certain peroxisomal disorders, adrenoleukodystrophy and adrenomyeloneuropathy. The diagnostic yield from biopsied skin depends considerably on the extent of the specimen. A superficial biopsy containing only epidermis and a few vessels gives little information.[107] Sweat gland epithelial cells should always be incorporated in the removed dermal tissue.

Some morphologic features encountered in the epithelial cells of eccrine sweat gland are normal constituents, such as membrane-bound vacuoles as precursors to secretory granules, membrane-bound nonvacuolar inclusions in ducts (Fig. 14-1), and lipopigments of different size and form. Epithelial cells of apocrine sweat glands also may contain physiologic inclusions, which are not to be confused with disease-related inclusions. Likewise, accumulation of lipopigments in epithelial cells of eccrine sweat gland of healthy individuals may vary considerably as to frequency, size, and shape. Other cells of the skin have physiologic inclusions that are ultrastructurally conspicuous. Among these are melanocytes (melanosomes) and melanosome-containing macrophages, Langerhans cells (Birbeck granules), mast cells (granules), basophilic or eosinophilic granulocytes, and nonspecific macrophages[174] or undulating tubules in endothelial cells in dermatomyositis or human immunodeficiency virus (HIV) infection (Fig. 14-1). Likewise, solid solitary lipopigment granules or pigment granules with fingerprint profiles have been seen in two siblings whose NCL began in adolescence.[69] Under favorable circumstances, normal nerve fascicles may be present or even abundant in the skin biopsy, allowing recognition of myelin-related lysosomal disorders, e.g., metachromatic and globoid cell leukodystrophies as well as adrenoleukodystrophy.[137,139] Sebaceous gland epithelial cells and hair follicles are of no diagnostic help, but smooth muscle cells and mural cells of dermal vessels are. The endings of somatic sensory and autonomic nerves of the skin lend themselves to easy diagnosis of infantile neuroaxonal dystrophy, which preferentially affects terminal segments of axons. Lipopigments may be encountered normally in Schwann cells, more often of unmyelinated than of myelinated axons.

Conjunctiva is another tissue that some favored for biopsy[9,146] because its richness in nerves facilitates recognition of nerve-related conditions.[137] In this context, one wonders whether other neuropathies may express morphological abnormalities in skin (and conjunctiva) to a degree that identifying these changes allows recognition of pathologic findings or even a particular disease process. This diagnostic aspect has not been satisfactorily investigated. In hereditary sensory and

A

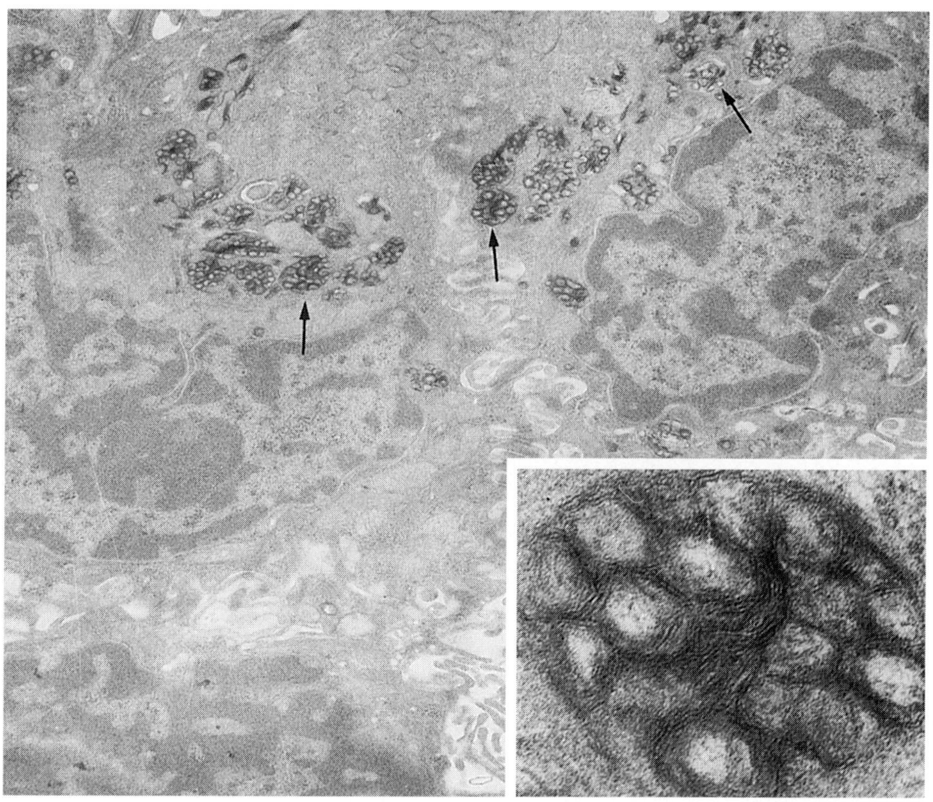

**Fig. 14-1.** Nonspecific inclusions in skin. **A**, Inclusions (*arrows*) in eccrine sweat gland epithelial cells. **B**, Aggregates of undulating tubules/ tubuloreticular structures (*arrows*) in an endothelial cell, dermatomyositis. **C**, Mast cell: several inclusions with curved lamellae, occasionally confused with fingerprint bodies. (**A**, ×19,950; **Inset**, ×125,000; **B**, ×47,500; **C**, ×85,000.).

*Continued.*

B

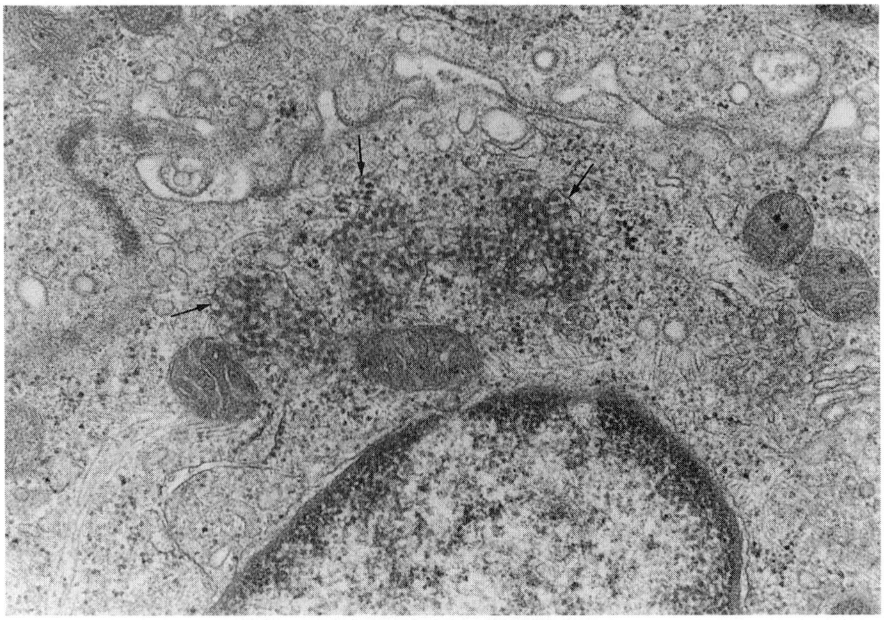

C

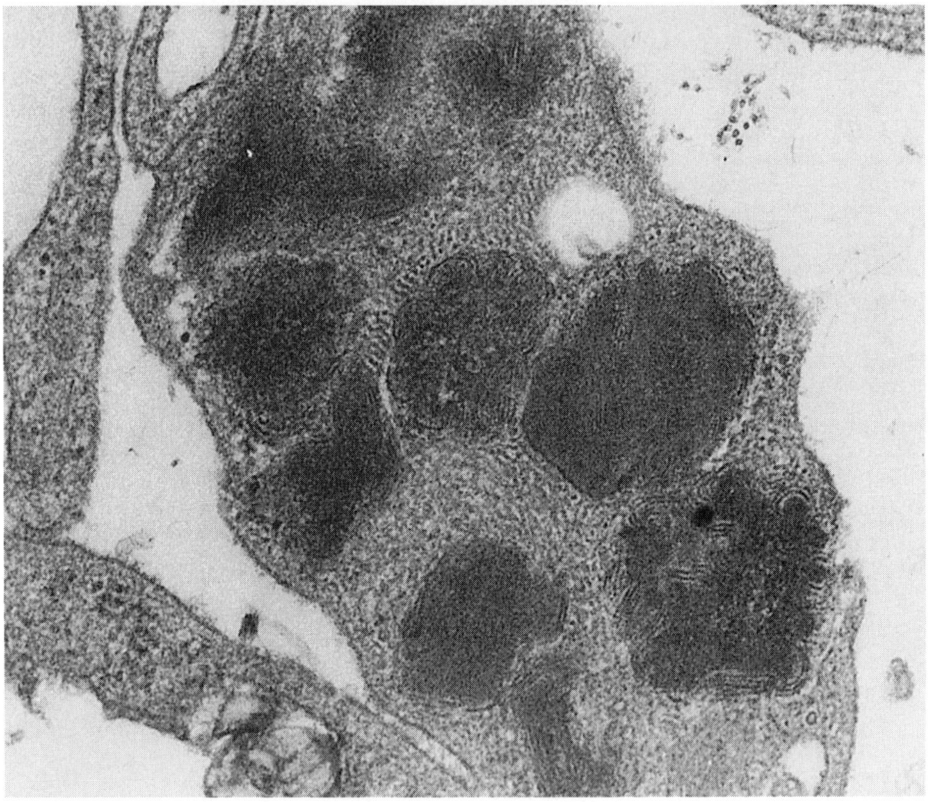

**Fig. 14-1, cont'd.** For legend see previous page.

autonomic neuropathy type IV, characterized by loss of pain sensation,[77] only a few Schwann cells without terminal axons were identified close to the epithelial cells of sweat glands.[121] This may indicate a lack of terminal axons about sweat gland epithelial cells that parallels the lack of unmyelinated axons within peripheral nerves and the inability to sweat; that is, congenital absence of sudomotor unmyelinated nerve fibers. Leukodystrophies marked by disease-specific morphologic features, i.e., lysosomal metachromatic[66] and Krabbe's globoid cell leukodystrophies[84] and peroxisomal adrenoleukodystrophy,[139] may be diagnosed by biopsy in skin (and conjunctiva) as described below. As quantitative data on cytologic components of dermal nerve fascicles and of terminal nerve areas are largely unavailable, the incidence of abnormalities of the PNS lacking disease-specific features, as seen in various hereditary motor and sensory neuropathies as well as hereditary sensory and autonomic neuropathies and other hereditary neuropathies, may be difficult to determine. Thus, skin biopsy in children (and adults) has not yet replaced peripheral nerve biopsy and the diagnostic work-up of childhood neuropathies. These disorders are covered in depth in Chapter 18.

Finally, circulating lymphocytes are the easiest source of cells in certain morphologic diagnoses,[52,53,102,133,203] but studying these cells usually requires isolation by differential centrifugation and immediate fixation, unlike a buffy coat preparation, which consists of all types of white blood cells. Circulating lymphocytes also manifest disease-specific pathology, but only in a limited number of NDIC, e.g., in lysosomal conditions. Lymphocytes, in these diseases, may show vacuolar or avacuolar lysosomes, the latter are especially common in infantile and late-infantile NCL. Retrieval and isolation of circulating lymphocytes for adequate electron microscopic examination may be unsatisfactory when lymphocytes cannot be separated from other cells, especially thrombocytes, or when the sampled lymphocytes are few. At least 100 lymphocytes should be screened for disease-specific lysosomal residual bodies, vacuolar or avacuolar. We prefer 200 lymphocytes altogether, 100 in each of two separate specimens, to ascertain the findings. The ratio of affected circulating lymphocytes for each patient, each disease, and each tissue of examination may thus be determined.[113] Bone marrow may provide results identical to those furnished by examination of circulating leukocytes, but also may harbor additional abnormal, larger histiocytic cells, the Gaucher cells, the Niemann-Pick cells, and the sea-blue histiocytes.

Possibly because of their surgical and diagnostic experience, some diagnosticians prefer certain tissues to others, e.g., rectal tissues versus nonrectal tissue, conjunctiva versus skin, circulating blood cells versus skin.

## NON-METABOLIC DISEASES

### The Neuronal Ceroid-Lipofuscinoses

The neuronal ceroid-lipofuscinoses (NCL) (Figs. 14-2 to 14-5) are among the most frequent NDIC. They are autosomal, recessively inherited, and uniformly fatal in childhood or adolescence. A causative biochemical defect has not been discovered in patients with NCL. There are several clinical forms–infantile NCL, late infantile NCL, early juvenile NCL, juvenile NCL, and, in adolescents and adults, protracted juvenile NCL and adult NCL. Respective abnormal genes have been mapped to chromosome 1 for infantile NCL, to chromosome 13 for a variant of late infantile NCL, and to chromosome 16 for juvenile NCL.

Apart from variable loss of neurons, which is especially apparent in the cerebral and cerebellar cortices, NCL are marked by ubiquitous accumulation of abnormal lipopigments that differ ultrastructurally among the clinical subtypes. This nosologic hallmark of NCL, the ubiquitous lipopigments, makes possible the diagnosis of NCL by biopsy of extracerebral tissues; the lack of a reliable biochemical diagnostic test and the necessity to recognize NCL by electron microscopy make biopsies essential.

The simplest, most reliable way to diagnose NCL is through the electron microscopic study of circulating lymphocytes.[101,170,205,207,208] The procedures to obtain circulating lymphocytes are easy. When blood is drawn for various examinations, blood cells may be available only when serum is needed for chemical investigations. Therefore, lymphocytes may become repeatedly available from the same patient.[113] Moreover, the ultrastructural features of different NCL lipopigments closely correlate with the various clinical subtypes (Fig. 14-2). Finally, isolated lymphocytes, easily allow quantitation of the pathologic process. The disadvantage of the procedure is that lymphocytes must be isolated by differential centrifugation, a technique not available in every hospital. Another disadvantage is that the number of lipopigment-carrying lymphocytes is often small; therefore, pigment-containing cells might be missed. Furthermore, the preservation of lymphocytes is sometimes inadequate to permit recognition of nonvacuolar lipopigments; this is especially true when recognition of cytologic details is insufficient.

Circulating lymphocytes contain granular lipopigments in infantile NCL (Fig. 14-2, *A*), curvilinear bodies in late infantile NCL (Fig. 14-2, *B*), compact, usually solitary lipopigments with fingerprint profiles in early juvenile[112] and juvenile[69] NCL (Fig. 14-2, *C*), and fingerprint profiles within membrane-bound, lysosomal vacuoles in juvenile NCL (Fig. 14-2, *D* and *E*). Fingerprint profiles are rare, while empty membrane-bound vacuoles abound in juvenile NCL. Accumulation of lipopigments affects both B and T cells[24] and subsets

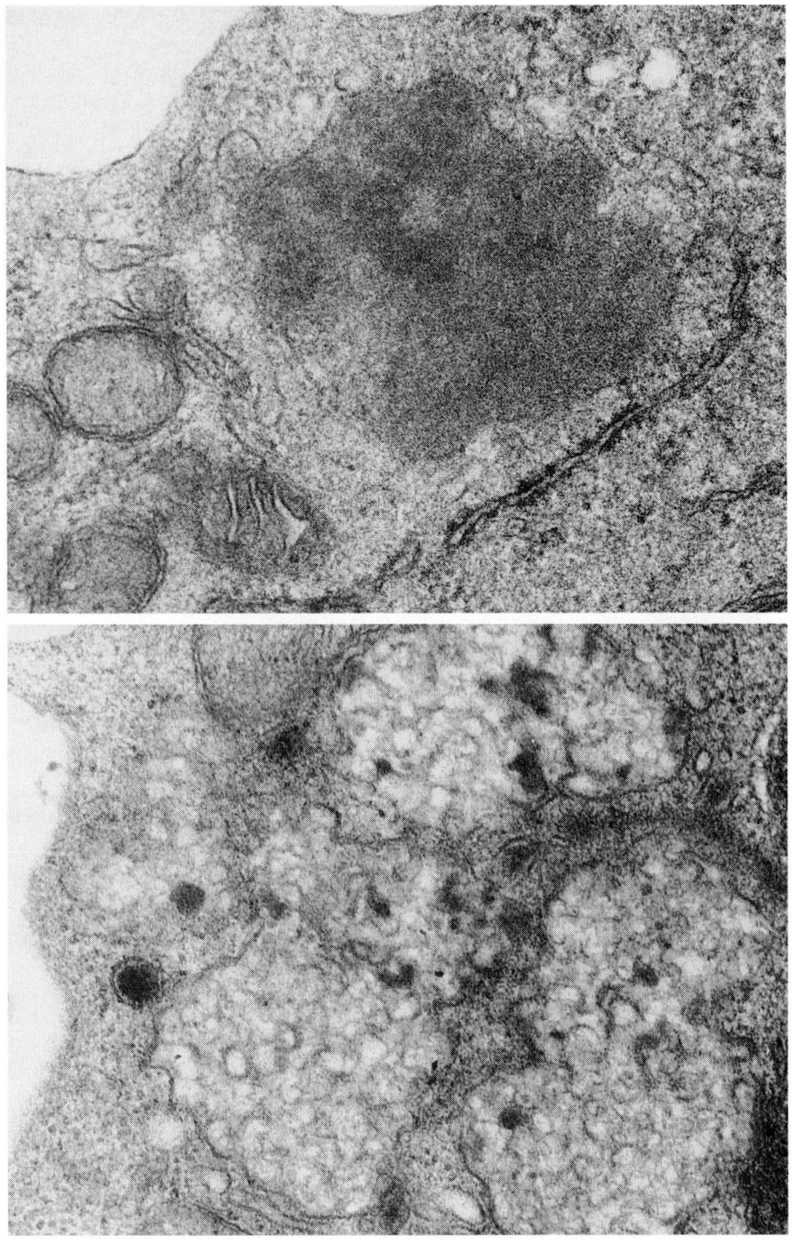

**Fig. 14-2.** Circulating lymphocytes in different forms of neuronal ceroid-lipofuscinosis with different types of lipopigments. **A**, Granular body, infantile form. **B**, Curvilinear bodies, late-infantile form.

of T cells.[111] Whether lymphocytes harbor abnormal lipopigments in protracted juvenile NCL or adult NCL is unknown, but lymphocytes from NCL heterozygotes do not show any morphologic abnormalities.[26]

The tissue most widely used for diagnosis of NCL is skin[205] (Fig. 14-4, *B* and *C*). Granular lipopigments in infantile NCL and curvilinear bodies containing fingerprint profiles, may be found in the epithelial cells of eccrine sweat glands (but not in sebaceous gland epithelial cells), as well as in smooth muscle cells of the arrectores pilorum bundles, and in mural cells of dermal vessels, both in endothelial cells and pericytes. In a few cases of juvenile NCL, vacuoles with fingerprints can be found in eccrine sweat gland epithelial cells. Abnormal NCL lipopigments are more frequent in eccrine sweat gland epithelial cells than in smooth muscle cells or in vascular mural cells. Therefore, a skin specimen without eccrine sweat glands may be inadequate for diagnosis. The epidermis may rarely contain abnormal lipopigments.[107] Therefore, a superficial skin specimen containing only epidermis usually is inappropriate for detailed electron microscopic examination. Epithelial cells of hair bulbs and surrounding hair shafts also are inadequate for electron microscopic study.

Umyelinated terminal axons may occasionally appear considerably expanded by mitochondria and dense bodies (possibly degenerated mitochondria)

C

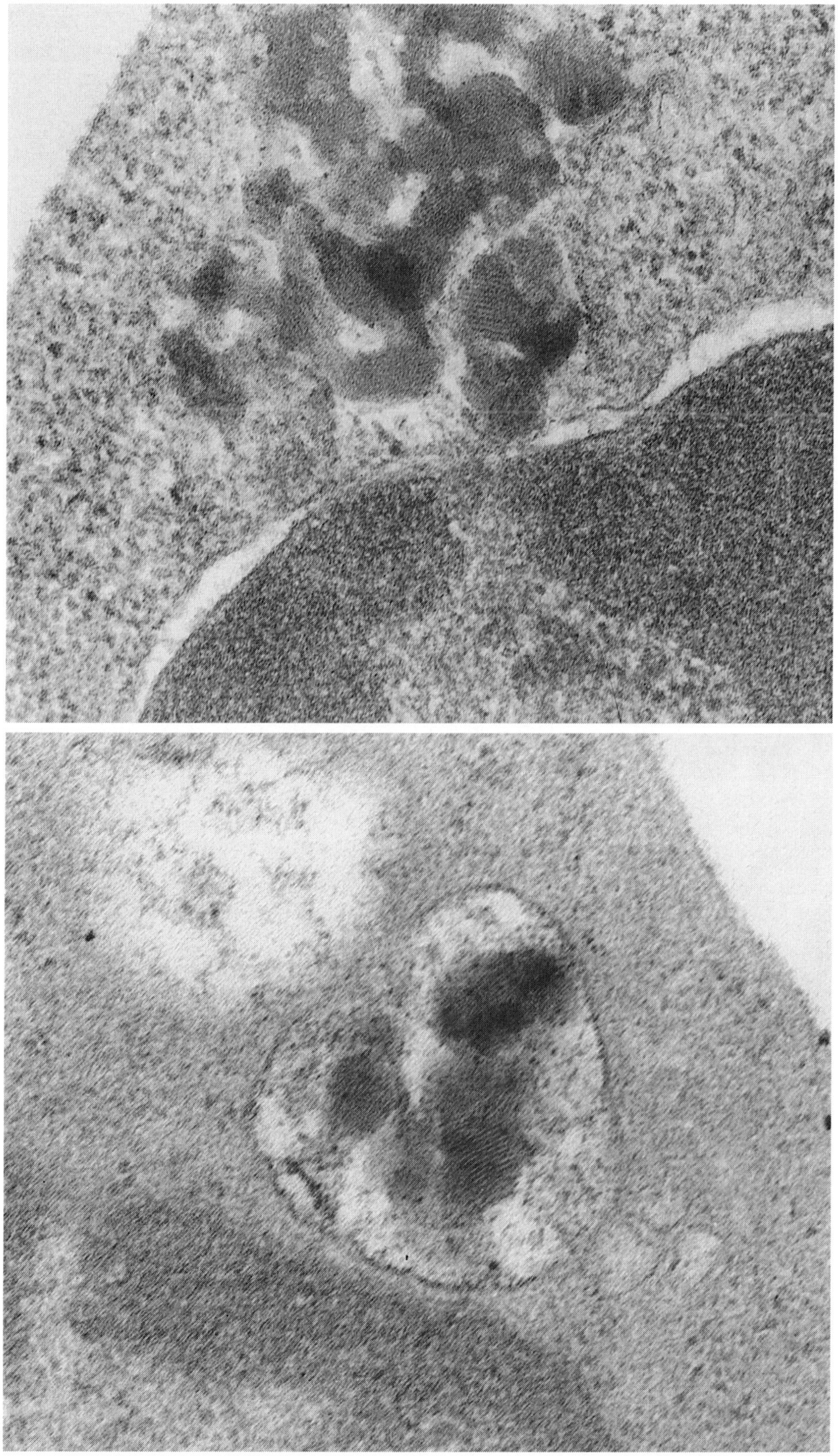

D

**Fig. 14-2, cont'd.** **C**, Nonvacuolar fingerprint complex, early-juvenile form. **D**, Lysosomal vacuole with fingerprint profiles, juvenile form. (**A**, ×103,850; **B**, ×81,200; **C**, ×112,500; **D**, ×102,000).

A

B

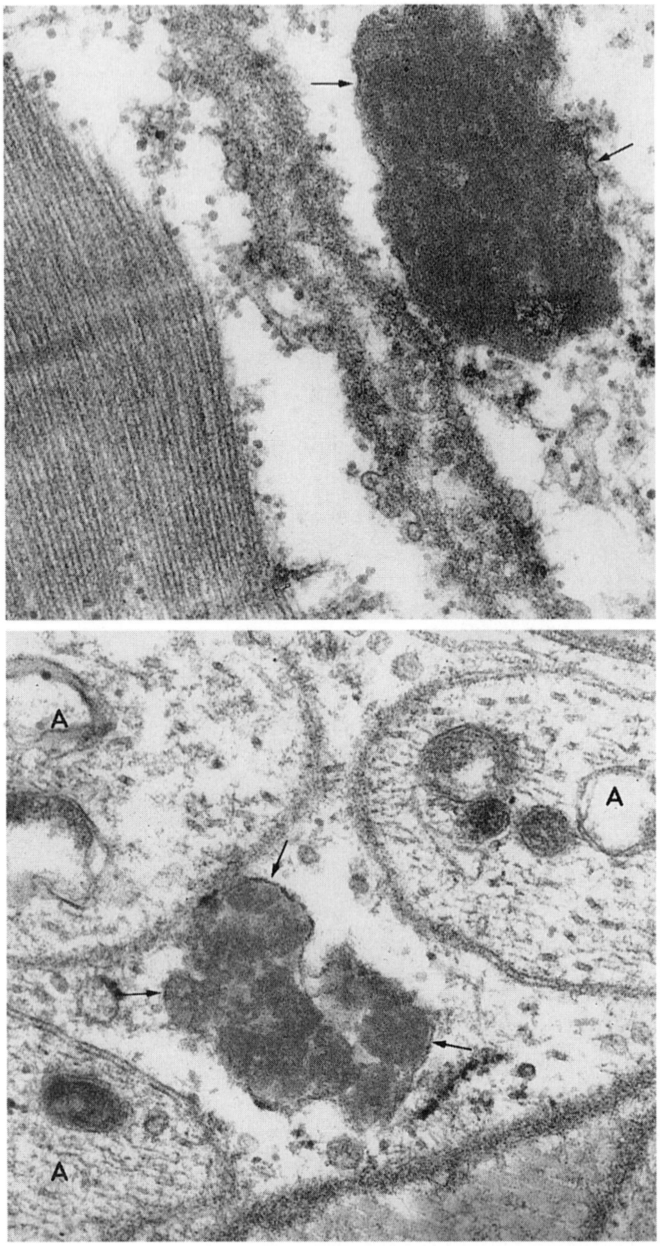


**Fig. 14-3.** Infantile neuronal ceroid lipofuscinosis. 2-year-old boy. **A**, Skeletal muscle. A single membrane-bound (*arrows*) finely granular lipopigment granule in the subsarcolemmal region. Some artificial sacroplasmic swelling makes this granule more conspicuous. **B**, Sural nerve. A membrane-bound (*arrows*) granular lipopigment in a Schwann cell harboring unmyelinated axons (*A*). (**A**, ×75,000; **B**, ×62,500.)

while NCL-specific lipopigments are absent. The NCL share this nonspecific expansion of terminal unmyelinated axons with other lysosomal diseases.[54,197] This phenomenon is poorly understood; one possible explanation is that the respective neuronal perikarya harbor disease-specific lysosomal residual bodies that impede axonal transport and result in nonspecific accumulation of mitochondria and other intraaxonal contents at the turning point of the anterograde and retrograde axonal transport systems. NCL-specific lipopigments may be encountered, however, in Schwann cells—more often in those of unmyelinated axons than in Schwann cells of myelinated axons.[75]

In conjunctiva, NCL-specific lipopigments may be encountered in mural vascular cells (Fig. 14-4, *D*) and in Schwann cells, but not in epithelial cells.

Other tissues that contain NCL-specific lipopigments are intestine (rectum[171] and appendix[38]), liver, skeletal muscle,[74] (Figs. 14-3, *A*, 14-4, *A*, 14-5), peripheral nerve[75] (Fig. 14-3, *B*), bone marrow,[64] and kidney.[48] Epithelial cells of the renal tubules containing NCL-specific lipopigments may be released into the urine. Lipopigments may then be freed from disintegrating epithelial cells and may be detected in the urinary sediment.[47,55,70] Examination of fetal tissues for the prenatal diagnosis of NCL is covered below in this chapter.

Curvilinear bodies, not related to NCL, may be encountered within skeletal muscle in chloroquine-induced myopathy and cardiomyopathy.[11] The term "curvilinear" has been applied to various ultrastructural features, quite different from NCL; for example, lamellar profiles in adrenoleukodystrophy,[95,183] inclusions in histiocytes of Farber disease (also called "Farber bodies"),[165] an individual, unexplained finding have all been called curvilinear.[159] Fingerprint profiles, usually solitary, may at times be seen within membrane-bound lysosomal vacuoles in certain mucopolysaccharidoses[79] (Fig. 14-6).

### Neuroaxonal Dystrophies

The neuroaxonal dystrophies (NAD), a group of progressive neurodegenerative disorders, are still incompletely and unsatisfactorily classified.[68] Among these, Seitelberger disease, i.e., infantile NAD (INAD) (Fig. 14-7), and Hallervorden-Spatz disease (HSD) are the two best known. Their clinical symptomatology is largely neurological and is associated with enlarged axons, often called spheroids, either located in the cortex and subcortically (INAD) or exclusively in subcortical structures (other NADs). HSD is also marked by abnormal pigmentation of basal ganglia. Both autosomal-recessive inheritance (INAD) and sporadic occurrence (other NADs) have been recorded in these diseases. Enzyme deficiencies have not been demonstrated in these patients; abnormal genes have not been mapped, and the cause of the NAD is still unknown. NCL has been on occasions clinically confused with INAD.[32]

In the context of this topic, however, the involvement of the PNS in NAD is important in the diagnosis. INAD was originally diagnosed by brain biopsy, through the identification of enlarged synaptic complexes in the cerebral cortex associated with abnormal cisternal profiles, organelles, and dense bodies. How-

*Text continues on page 595.*

A

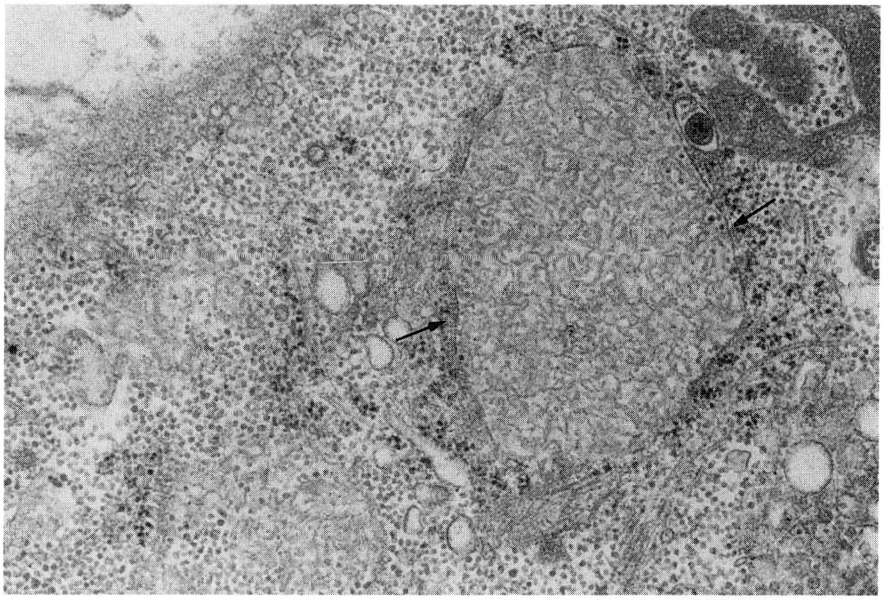

B

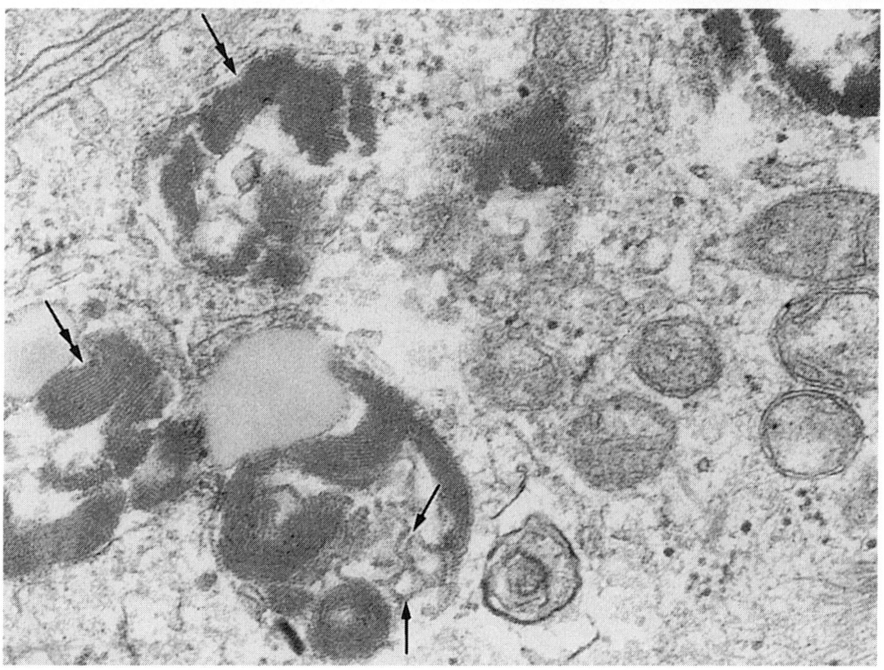

**Fig. 14-4.** Late-infantile neuronal ceroid-lipofuscinosis. 5-year-old boy. **A**, A membrane-bound curvilinear body (*arrows*) is located subsarcolemmally in a muscle fiber skeletal muscle. **B**, Membrane-bound lipopigments in a sweat gland epithelial cell contain curvilinear profiles (*arrows*) and fingerprint profiles (*double arrows*). *Continued.*

C

D

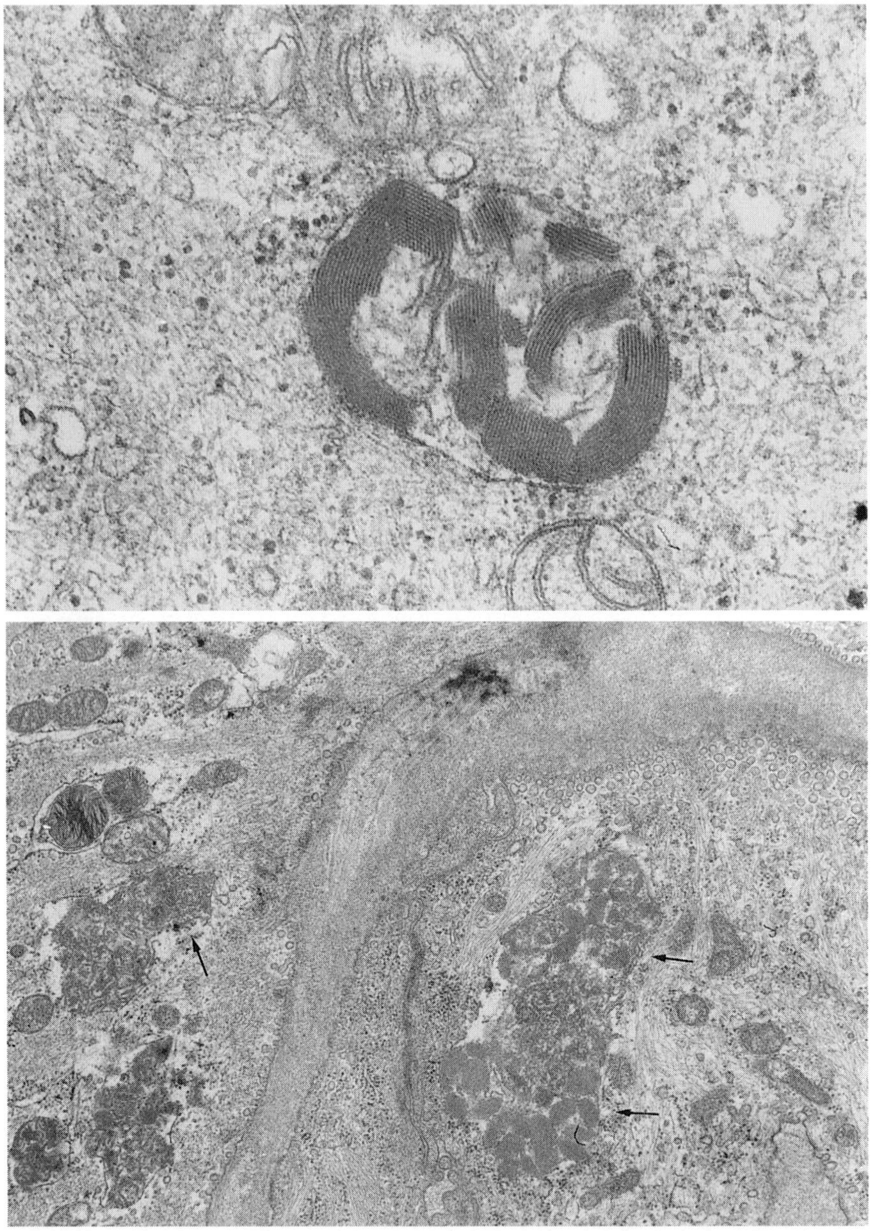

**Fig. 14-4, cont'd. C**, At higher magnification, a membrane-bound lipopigment contains numerous fingerprint profiles. **D**, Conjunctiva. Several lipopigment inclusions (*arrows*) in mural cells of a conjunctival vessel. (**A**, ×65,000; **B**, ×66,500; **C**, ×85,000; **D**, ×27,300.)

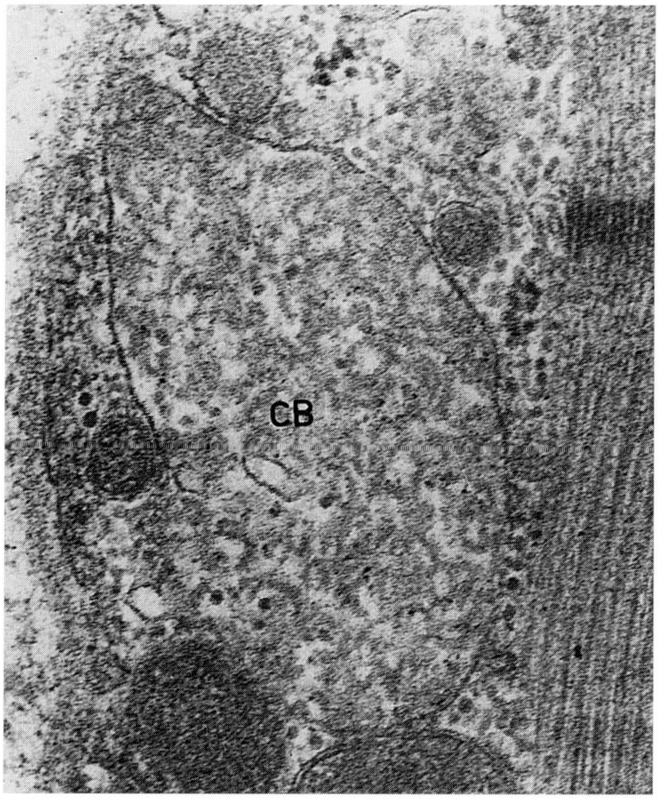


**Fig. 14-5.** Neuronal ceroid-lipofuscinosis. Skeletal muscle. A membrane-bound curvilinear (CB) body can indicate both juvenile and late-infantile NCL. (×85,000.)

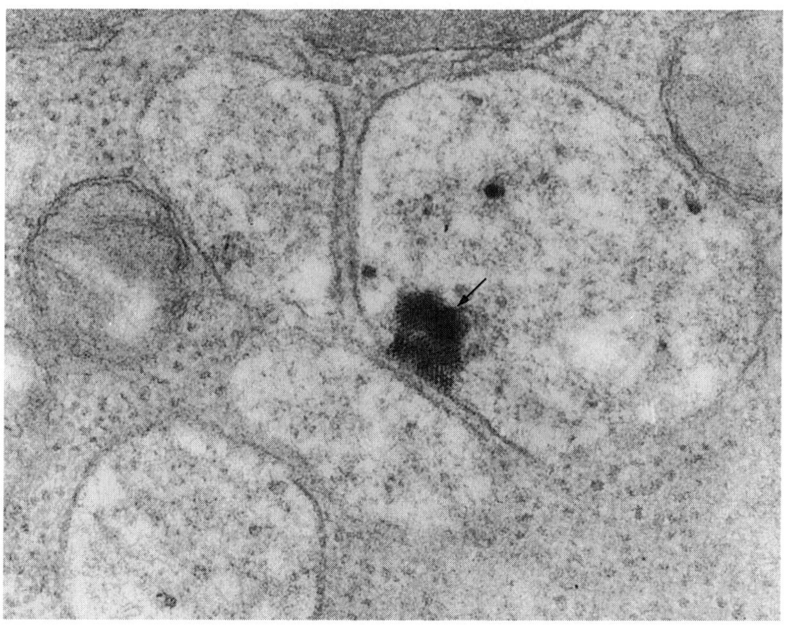

**Fig. 14-6.** Mucopolysaccharidosis II. Within one membrane-bound vacuole of a small aggregate of vacuoles a distinct electron-dense inclusion with fingerprint appearance (*arrow*) is apparent in a circulating lymphocyte. (×74,400.)

A

B

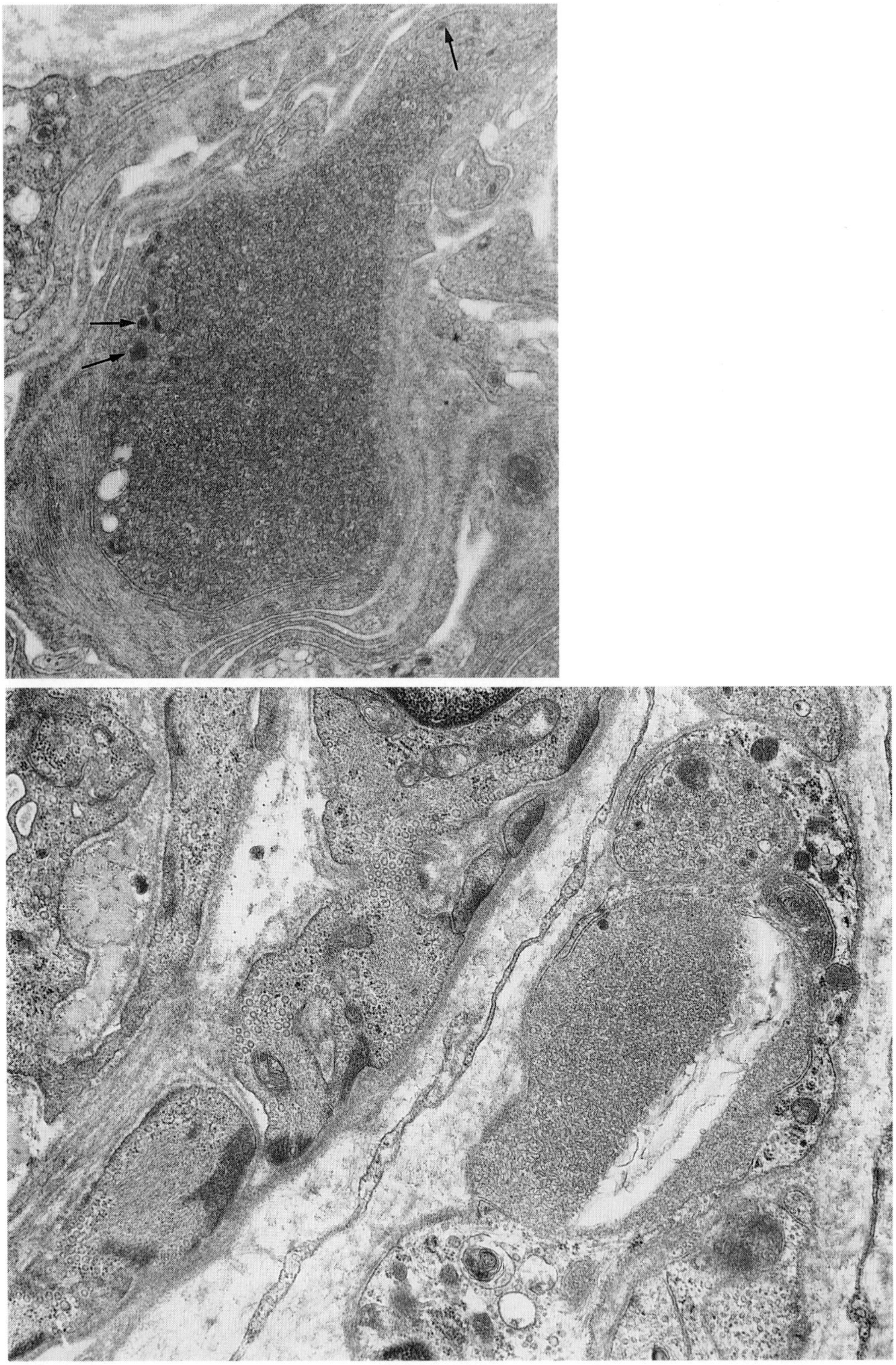

**Fig. 14-7.** Infantile neuroaxonal dystrophy. **A**, Rectum.[76] An enlarged axon contains cisternal profiles and marginal (*arrows*) dense core vesicles. **B**, Skin. Enlarged unmyelinated axons close to a dermal vessel with enlarged cisternal profiles and a large cleft. (**A** ×24,000; **B**, ×22,750.)

ever, cerebrocortical biopsy would not be helpful in other forms of NAD. Moreover, in noninfantile NAD, axons often contain spheroids replete with other organelles, and dense bodies, possibly derived from degenerated mitochondria; these spheroids are not pathognomonic aggregates of cisternal profiles. The typical ultrastructural features of INAD have been variably termed vesicular-tubular profiles, tubulogranular profiles, or membranotubular profiles.[204] The origin of these tubulomembranous profiles is still unknown. Enzyme and immunohistochemical data that might further characterize these structures are not available. The widespread involvement of peripheral nerve fibers by axonal enlargement and the ubiquitous presence of nerve fibers, especially terminal ones, in virtually every region of the body make INAD another multiorgan disorder—and thus INAD is a disease accessible to extracerebral diagnostic biopsy. The historic evolution in the diagnosis of INAD by biopsy resembles that of lysosomal disorders, particularly the NCL. Hence, following the era of brain biopsy, rectal biopsy was introduced. These biopsies revealed highly enlarged synaptic contacts in rectal tissue[76] (Fig. 14-7, *A*), that were also found in juvenile NAD (JNAD).[170]

Subsequently, skeletal muscle[143,196] and conjunctiva[8,60,138] became targets for biopsy. The muscle sample must contain motor endplates for diagnosis of NAD, and these often are absent or hard to find.[196] In this context, one needs to remember that whether the peripheral nerves are myelinated or unmyelinated is not diagnostically meaningful in biopsied conjunctiva,[45] but what counts is the status of the terminal axons. For this reason, peripheral nerve biopsies are not consistently rewarding.[136,211]

Today, the most reliable tissue for the diagnosis of INAD is the skin, where terminal axons may be seen lying free in the dermis or abutting the basal layers of the epidermis and other epithelial structures, e.g., sweat glands. The perivascular tissues of the dermal vessels (Fig. 14-7, *B*) and the smooth muscle cells of the arrectores pilorum muscle are additional sites of INAD pathology.

Unmyelinated axons that may on occasion be recognized in semi-thin sections tend to be considerably expanded by cisternal profiles. The frequent presence of empty or dense core vesicles in expanded axons attests to the distant site of the pathologic process close to or at the synaptic region. Often, a peculiar wedge-shaped cleft also may be present in a tubulomembranous axonal meshwork. Occasionally, only a sector rather than the entire cross-sectioned axoplasm, is filled with cisternal profiles that form circumscribed aggregates. Then, INAD may be difficult to detect and a second biopsy of the skin may be required. Thus, absence of INAD-specific features does not rule out this disease. These findings pertain to classic INAD. The PNS may show typical features in noninfantile forms of NAD,[124] but this seems to be very rare.[170]

In addition to pathognomonic intraaxonal pathology, specific inclusions have been observed in Schwann cells[204,211] and other endoneurial cells.[204] Occasionally, features of INAD and GAN, may coexist in the same biopsy.

Another nonspecific abnormality indicative of PNS involvement in NAD is neurogenic atrophy of skeletal muscle fibers, detectable by both muscle biopsy[124] and electromyography.

### Neuronal Intranuclear Hyaline Inclusion Disease

An unusual multiorgan disorder that affects both adults and children[175] has a progressive neurodegenerative character and is called neuronal intranuclear hyaline inclusion disease (NIHID). The main cellular abnormality consists of innumerable intranuclear inclusions, sometimes slightly larger than nucleoli (Fig. 14-8). They are found in neurons of the CNS and the PNS, but also have been reported in cardiac myocytes, adrenal medulla, skeletal muscle fiber nuclei,[186] and intestinal neurons (Fig. 14-8). This latter observation makes rectal biopsy a suitable procedure for possible antemortem diagnosis.[89] The intranuclear inclusions consist of haphazardly branched filaments 8 to 12 nm thick. In skeletal muscle, however, these intranuclear inclusions are of the tubulofilamentous type, measuring 15 to 20 nm, and resembles those seen in inclusion body myositis.[186] The tubulofilamentous inclusions within neuronal nuclei measure 10 to 20 nm in diameter. Whether NIHID is a single entity or represents a group of similar conditions remains to be seen. Clinical symptoms vary considerably, and include patients that mimic the symptoms of Friedreich ataxia, Parkinson disease, olivopontocerebellar atrophy, $GM_2$-gangliosidosis, or INAD.[175] The nature of the disease may be further clarified when the origin and pathogenesis of the intraneuronal inclusions are better understood. The neuronal intranuclear inclusions have not been characterized immunohistochemically, even after application of antibodies against neurofilaments and glial fibrillary acidic protein (GFAP),[175] vimentin, and cytokeratin.[65] In the PNS, intranuclear filaments have been demonstrated only in the spinal ganglia neurons, but not in Schwann cells; therefore, evidence for involvement of skin and peripheral nerves does not exist. To date, only rectal biopsy seems to allow antemortem diagnosis.

### Giant Axonal Neuropathy

Giant axonal neuropathy (GAN) (Fig. 14-9), another autosomal-recessive hereditary progressive disease that affects both the CNS and the PNS,[184] is an example of a multiorgan disease for two reasons: (1) it affects

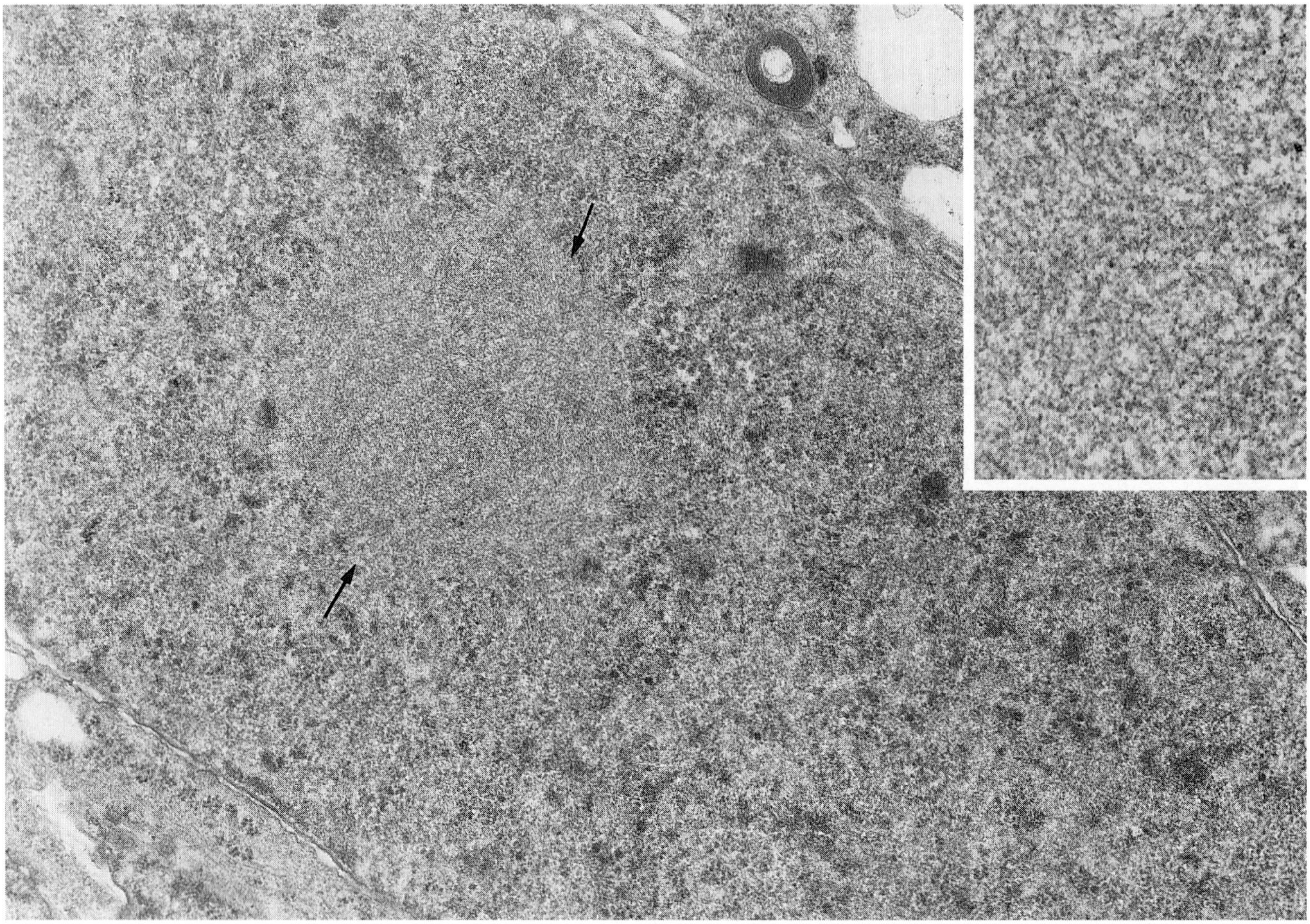

**Fig. 14-8.** Neuronal intranuclear inclusion disease. 15-year-old boy.[89] Rectum. Ill-defined round aggregate (*arrows*) of filaments within neuronal nucleus. Inset, Haphazardly arranged filaments of higher magnification. (×23,207; **Inset**, ×70,272.) (Courtesy of Prof. J. Mikol, Paris.)

the PNS; and (2) it is characterized by accumulation of intermediate filaments present in different cell types[115] of different organs. In GAN, neurofilaments collect within axons; vimentin-reactive intermediate filaments in fibroblasts, endoneurial cells, and Schwann cells; and glial fibrillary acidic protein-reactive filaments in astrocytes.

Although peripheral nerves may be biopsied with rewarding results and may demonstrate enlarged axons (Fig. 14-9, *A*), the physiologic presence of nerve fascicles in skin (and conjunctiva) and the accretion of intermediate filaments within other skin cell types make skin (Fig. 14-9, *B*) a good target for diagnostic biopsy. However, biopsy studies of skin in GAN have not been reported, and my own search for GAN-typical findings in one skin specimen of a young boy afflicted with GAN[179] was not successful. Since GAN is a very rare disease, however, the entire spectrum of dermal (and conjunctival) manifestations of GAN may not yet have been explored and elucidated. Bundles of intermediate filaments may often be seen in mesenchymal cells of the skin as a feature of unknown, but nonspecific, conditions.

### Polyglucosan Diseases

Polyglucosan diseases are a clinically and biochemically heterogeneous group of disorders marked by the intracellular formation of filamentous material of glycogen nature, usually forming inclusion bodies, that is, polyglucosan bodies (Figs. 14-10, 14-11). These inclusions usually are not membrane-bound. Some polyglucosan disorders are clinically different forms of type IV glycogenosis caused by a defect of the brancher enzyme. Infantile, juvenile (Fig. 14-10), and adult forms of type V glycogenosis have been described, the infantile form affecting not only the skeletal muscle, but also liver and brain. The juvenile form affects both skeletal and cardiac muscle,[162] and an adult form seems to affect skeletal muscle exclusively.

A classic neurodegenerative disease of childhood that is marked by polyglucosan inclusion bodies is Lafora disease (Fig. 14-11), which is autosomal-reces-

A

B

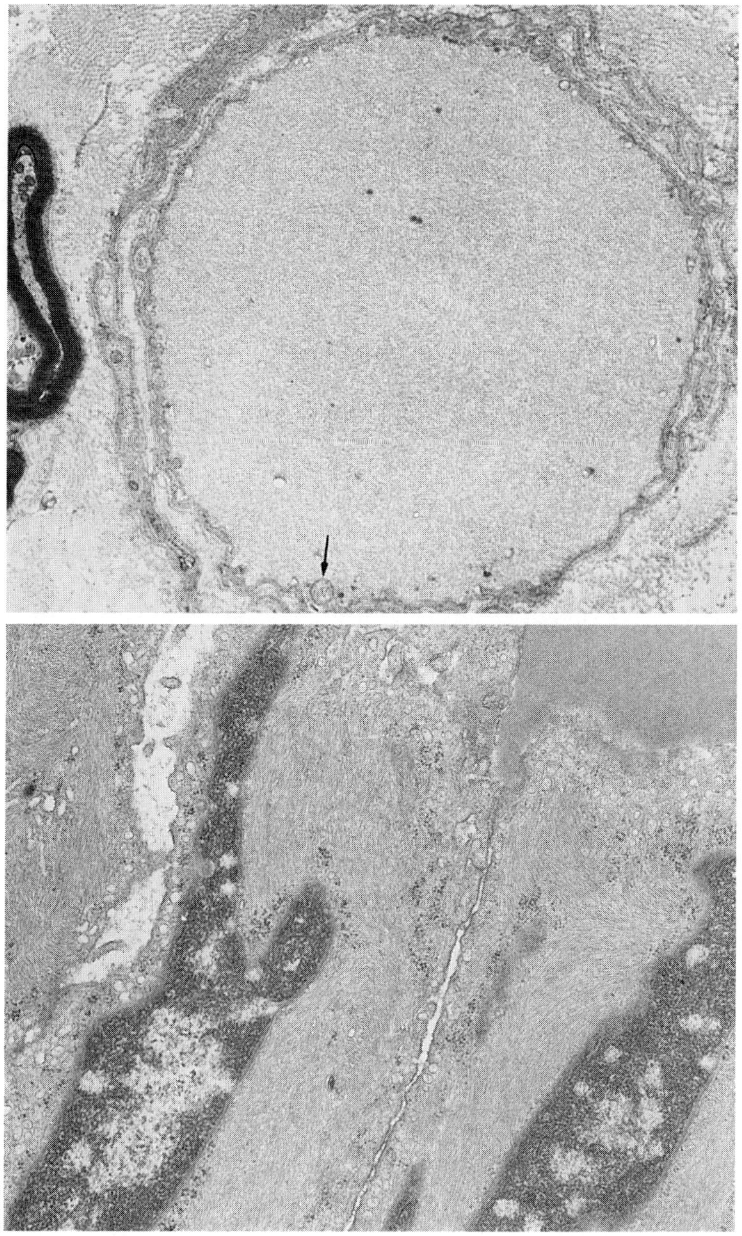

**Fig. 14-9.** Giant axonal neuropathy. 11-year-old Persian boy.[179] **A**, Sural nerve. Enlarged axon without myelin sheaths, it is replete with neurofilaments and a marginal mitochondrium (*arrow*), but devoid of neurotubules. **B**, Skin. Endothelial cells of a small dermal vessel contain densely packed filaments. (**A**, ×8750; **B**, ×27,300.)

sively inherited, but lacks a known gene or enzyme defect. Polyglucosan filaments make up the Lafora bodies, which are seen as intraneuronal inclusions in cortical and subcortical neurons of the CNS. In addition, similar filamentous polyglucosan material also may be present in ductal cells of eccrine sweat gland epithelial cells[35,81,100,200] (Fig. 14-11, *D*), especially in duct cells of axillary apocrine sweat glands,[30,31] making skin a target tissue for pathologic diagnosis. Likewise, filamentous material may be found in smooth muscle cells (Fig. 14-11, *E*) in striated muscle fibers[37,81,100,147] (Fig. 14-11, *B*). In skeletal muscle and liver (Fig. 14-11, *A*), however, this material has been encountered within membrane-bound compartments[81] (Fig. 14-11, *B* and *C*), where apparently it is of lysosomal character because it may be associated with lipopigments (Fig. 14-11, *B*) and the muscle fibers may show increased acid phosphatase activity. The clinical form of myoclonus epilepsy related to the term "Unverricht-Lundberg (or Baltic) type," however, is not marked by formation of polyglucosan material at all; therefore, this disease is not a polyglucosan disorder.

Lafora disease is a member of the clinically and nosologically heterogeneous group of myoclonus epilepsies. Other members of this group that occur in childhood and are marked by disease-specific features are: (1) mitochondrial encephalomyopathy MERRF (myoclonus epilepsy and ragged red fibers), which can also be recognized in skeletal muscle; and (2) late-infantile NCL, which also is marked by an increase of acid phos-

A

B

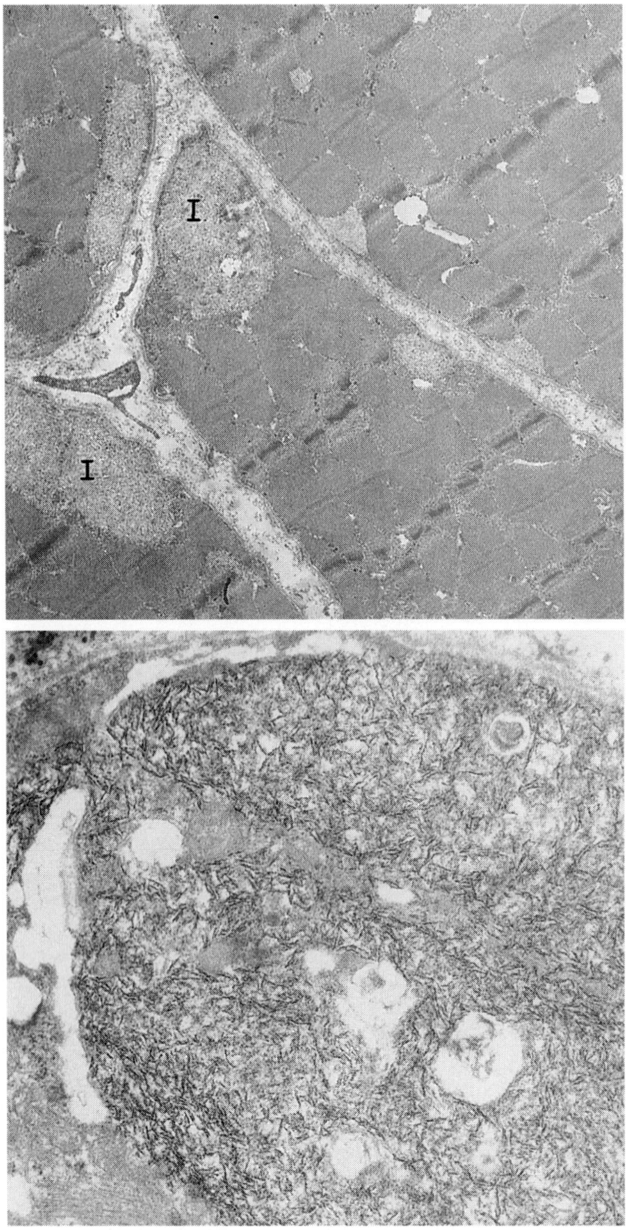


**Fig. 14-10.** Polyglucosan inclusions. 6-year-old boy, type IV glycogenosis. Skeletal muscle. **A**, Several peripherally located sharply demarcated inclusions (*I*). **B**, At higher magnification, these inclusions consist of randomly arranged short filaments. (**A**, ×10,360; **B**, ×28,600.)

phatase activity in skeletal muscle fibers, and curvilinear bodies of the lipopigment type.

### Rett Syndrome

Until recently, Rett syndrome, a slowly progressive neurologic disease of young girls, was thought to be a disorder of developmental arrest[15] without consistent and diagnostically reliable pathologic evidence in extracerebral tissues. However, recent examination of conjunctiva, skeletal muscle, and perivascular capillaries in two biopsy specimens taken at different times from the same young girl with clinical Rett syndrome[51] revealed extracellular periendothelial and intraendothelial homogeneous electron-dense non-membrane-bound deposits. Except for these two instances in a single patient, however, such largely extracellular deposits of obscure origin and composition, have not been encountered again. Thus, their diagnostic value in Rett syndrome awaits confirmation.

## NEUROMETABOLIC DISEASES

Metabolic conditions affecting the CNS may be classified as congenital or hereditary, inborn errors of metabolism, and acquired ones. The latter forms, such as hepatic, uremic, and endocrinologic encephalopathies, produce scant lesions in the CNS and none outside the CNS. Therefore, only hereditary forms of neurometabolic diseases will be considered here.

In general, morphologic in vivo diagnosis of a CNS-related neurometabolic disease always remains incomplete in the absence of biochemical investigation. Thus, when one suspects a neurometabolic CNS disorder, a biopsy may serve two purposes; retrieval of tissue for direct biochemical analysis or culturing of fibroblasts, and samples for morphologic investigation. Morphologic examination requires immediate tissue fixation, especially when electron microscopy is planned, whereas biochemical investigation requires immediate freezing of the tissue or immediate transfer into a sterile culture medium.

The hereditary neurometabolic disorders of the CNS comprise a heterogeneous group that may be divided into two major subgroups: (1) those producing lesions in the CNS only, such as the disorders of amino acid metabolism; and (2) those affecting both the CNS and extraneural tissues. Classic single-organelle multiorgan disorders belong to this category, namely the lysosomal diseases, the mitochondrial diseases, and the peroxisomal diseases. These three groups of single-organelle multiorgan diseases have different connotations for the morphologist. The lysosomal diseases are diagnosed by intralysosomal metabolic compounds that have a very typical ultrastructure. The ultrastructure and its underlying lysosomal disease are often closely correlated with a precise lysosomal enzyme defect: there is a correlation between chemical defects and morphology. Mitochondrial disorders can be recognized by the morphologist only when abnormally structured mitochondria are present. However, individual mitochondriopathies, marked by different mitochondrial and nuclear gene defects and respective biochemical enzyme deficiencies, cannot be individually identified by ultrastructural findings of mitochondria. The pathology of the peroxisomes exists largely in the liver and kidney, whereas typical inclusions, not situated in the peroxisomal compartment, may represent diagnostic hallmarks, e.g., in adrenoleukodystrophy.

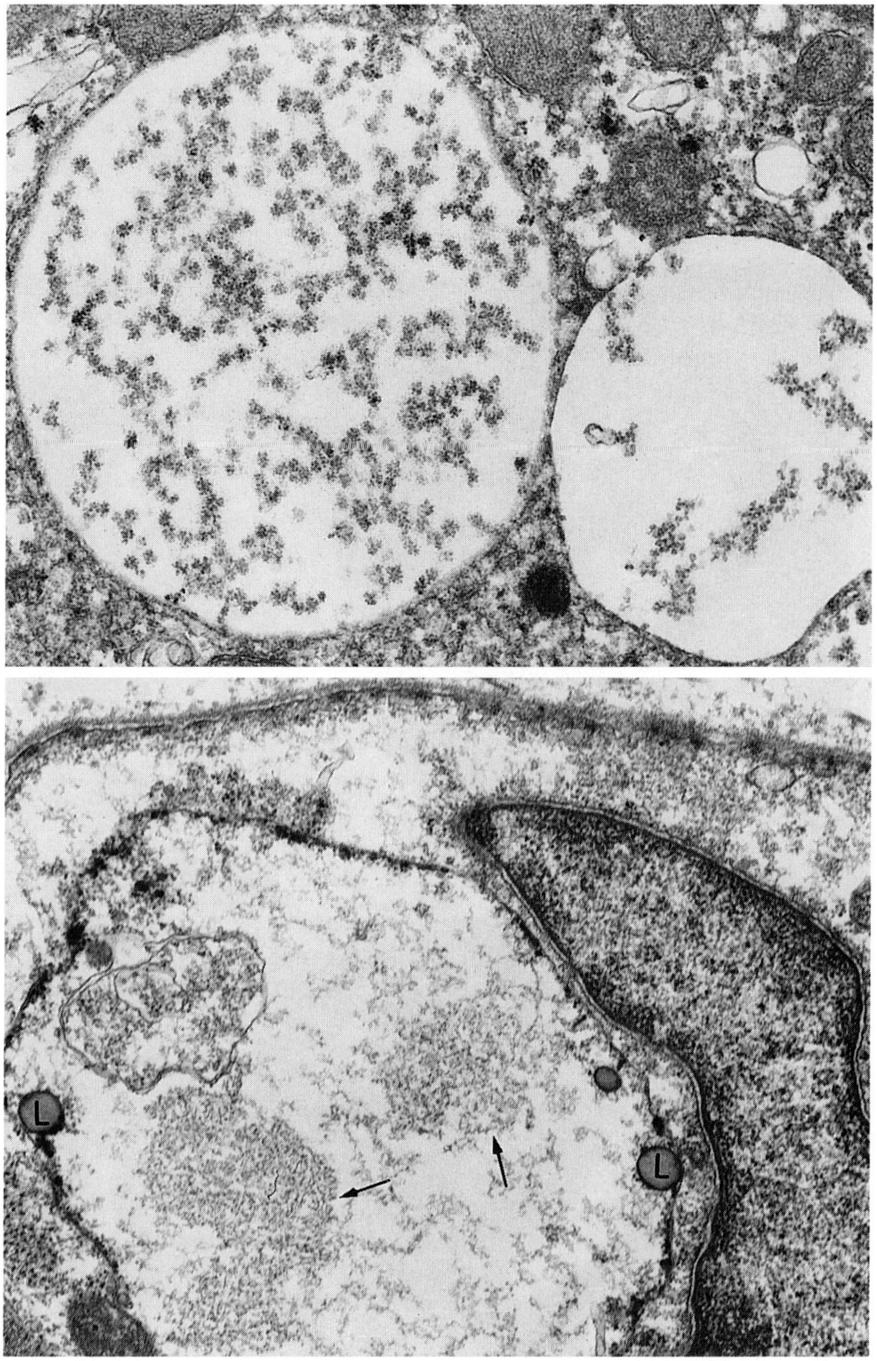


**Fig. 14-11.** Lafora disease. 14-year-old girl.[81] **A**, Liver. Membrane-bound vacuoles contain particulate glycogen in hepatocytes. **B**, Skeletal muscle. Subsarcolemmal membrane-bound vacuoles with lipid (*L*) droplet and finely fibrillar glycogen (*arrows*). *Continued.*

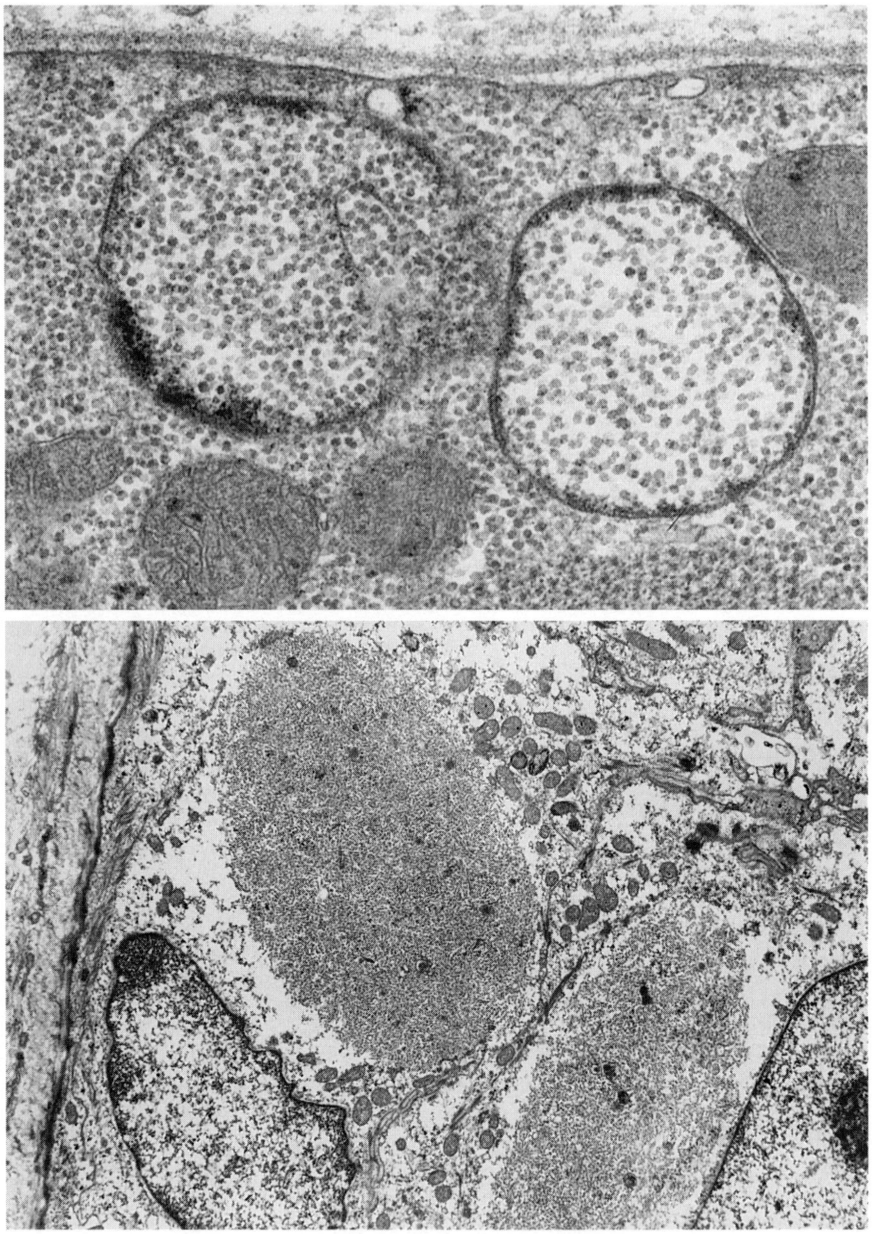


**Fig. 14-11, cont'd.** **C**, Subsarcolemmal membrane-bound inclusions that contain particulate glycogen, but no fibrils. **D**, Skin. Large fibrillar non-membrane-bound inclusions in ductal sweat gland epithelial cells.

E

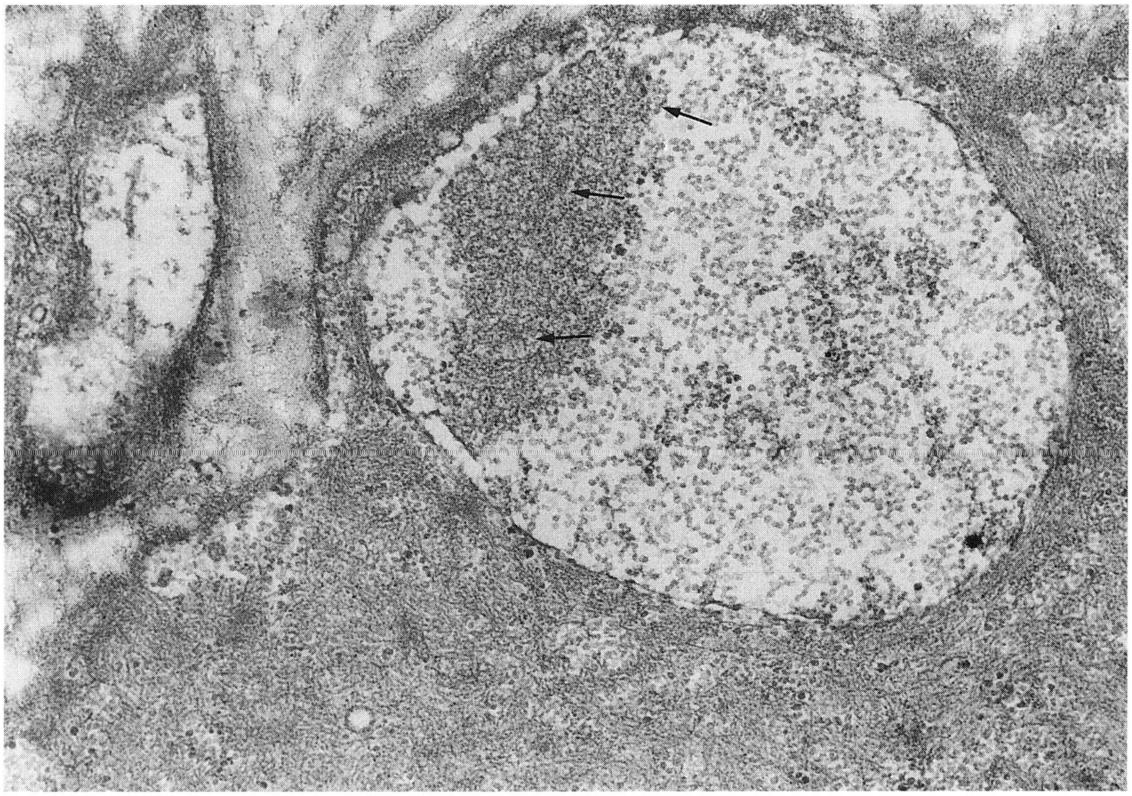

**Fig. 14-11, cont'd.** **E,** A membrane-bound vacuole contains particulate and fibrillar (*arrows*) glycogen, smooth muscle cell. (**A,** ×42,000; **B,** ×27,500; **C,** ×180,000; **D,** ×11,700; **E,** ×47,500.)

**Lysosomal Diseases**

Lysosomal diseases affect the catabolism of complex lipids (the sphingolipidoses) and of glycoproteins (the mucopolysaccharidoses, mucolipidoses, and oligosaccharidoses, and type II glycogenoses). These diseases are not completely synonymous with "storage" disorders,[135] but the group includes many of them; they also have been dubbed "thesaurismoses" or "thesauropathies."

The characteristic ultrastructural hallmarks of lysosomal diseases are the lysosomal residual bodies, which contain disease-specific and metabolism-specific compounds that accumulate because of respective inherited (chiefly autosomal-recessive, occasionally X-linked recessive) lysosomal enzyme defects. Thus, there is an increase in size and number of lysosomes, resulting in enlargement of the cell or "storage." These are the classic storage disorders or thesaurismopathies.

Lysosomal disorders also can be grouped as nonvacuolar and vacuolar disorders. Tissues, organs, and cell types affected in a particular lysosomal disease depend on the biochemical role of the respective substrate in the lysosomal metabolism of these tissues or cell types. Hexosaminidase A deficiency, resulting in $GM_2$-gangliosidosis, especially in Tay-Sachs disease, is one of the typical neuronal lysosomal disorders, whereas hexosaminidase A and B defects or Sandhoff disease, affect many cell types in addition to neurons.

In autosomal recessively inherited lysosomal enzyme deficiencies, to which most of the lysosomal disorders belong, heterozygotes do not form morphologically evident disease-specific lysosomal residual bodies. Thus, electron microscopy and other morphologic investigations cannot contribute to the recognition of the heterozygous state. However, these methods can identify with very low lysosomal enzyme deficiency that are destined to become diseased later. Biochemical examinations are essential and useful, but there is still a need for morphologic diagnostic study of a lysosomal disease. Selected tissues of heterozygotes (females) in X-linked recessive lysosomopathies, e.g., MPS II (Fabry disease), may show disease-specific lysosomal residual bodies.

**Avacuolar lysosomal disorders.** Avacuolar conditions in lysosomal disorders are diagnostically important for two reasons: (1) the nonvacuolar lysosomal residual bodies can hardly be recognized by light microscopy; and (2) their ultrastructure often appears disease-specific, for example, membranous cytoplasmic bodies in gangliosidoses and prismatic and tufaceous lamellar bodies in metachromatic leukodystrophy. Therefore, electron-microscopic examination is mandatory when these entities are part of the differential diagnosis.

***The sphingolipidoses.*** The sphingolipidoses are the most important group of disorders characterized by lysomal defects and cellular storage because sphingolipids play an essential biochemical role in the physiologic metabolism of nerve and glial cells. Sphingolipidoses that affect the CNS fall into two categories: (1) those largely affecting neurons, the lysosomal poliodystrophies; and (2) those largely affecting oligodendrocytes and myelin, the lysosomal leukodystrophies. Because of the role of sphingolipid metabolism within the lysosome involving specific lysosomal hydrolases, individual sphingolipidoses show ultrastructurally characteristic lysosomes. Incompletely metabolized lysosomal sphingolipids form different—and often characteristic, ultrastructural features. Knowledge of these features and their recognition are important for the neuropathologist.[2,182]

***Gangliosidoses.*** The gangliosidoses are classified as $GM_1$-gangliosidoses (secondary to a deficiency of $\beta$-galactosidase) and $GM_2$-gangliosidoses (based on deficiencies of hexosaminidases A and B, or their activator protein). The former enzyme defect results in the formation of both nonvacuolar and vacuolar giant lysosomes, the latter lysosomal enzyme defects induce formation of nonvacuolar lysosomal residual bodies only.

***$GM_1$-gangliosidoses*** — The $GM_1$-gangliosidoses (Fig. 14-12), classified as infantile or generalized severe type (I) and juvenile or mild type (II), are caused by a deficiency of the lysosomal enzyme $\beta$-galactosidase. This enzyme normally catabolizes $GM_1$-ganglioside and oligosaccharides. Abnormal lysosomes in $GM_1$-gangliosidoses are seen in two types. A nonvacuolar form of a membranous cytoplasmic or some other lamellar type may be found in neurons, including those of the myenteric plexus, and in Schwann cells. The other, a vacuolar type, is ubiquitously distributed in parenchymal cells of viscera, mesenchymal cells including fibroblasts (Fig. 14-12, *C*), mural vascular cells (Fig. 14-12, *D*), smooth muscle cells (Fig. 14-12, *E*), and circulating lymphocytes (Fig. 14-12, *A*). $\beta$-galactosidase deficiency or $GM_1$-gangliosidosis is an example of how one enzyme catabolizes two different classes of chemical compounds, leading to the creation of two different classes of lysosomal residual bodies, the nonvacuolar membranous cytoplasmic and lamellar lysosomes as well as the vacuolar lysosomes. Rarely, lysosomal storage in dermal vessels may amount to an angiokeratoma corporis diffusum.[16] In Kupffer cells of the liver[67,132] and splenic macrophages,[181] the lysosomes display tubular structures. Similar lysosomal vacuoles may be present in skeletal muscle fibers, interstitial vessels, and Schwann cells of skeletal muscle and peripheral nerves, respectively.[142]

***$GM_2$-gangliosidoses*** — $GM_2$-gangliosidoses are lysosomal disorders (Fig. 14-13) characterized by a deficiency of hexosaminidase A (Tay-Sachs disease) and B variants, by deficiencies of hexosaminidases A and B (Sandhoff disease), or by deficiency of an activator protein. Hexosaminidase A deficiency, the classic type being Tay-Sachs disease, is largely an intraneuronal lysosomal storage disorder; its diagnosis requires mor-

A

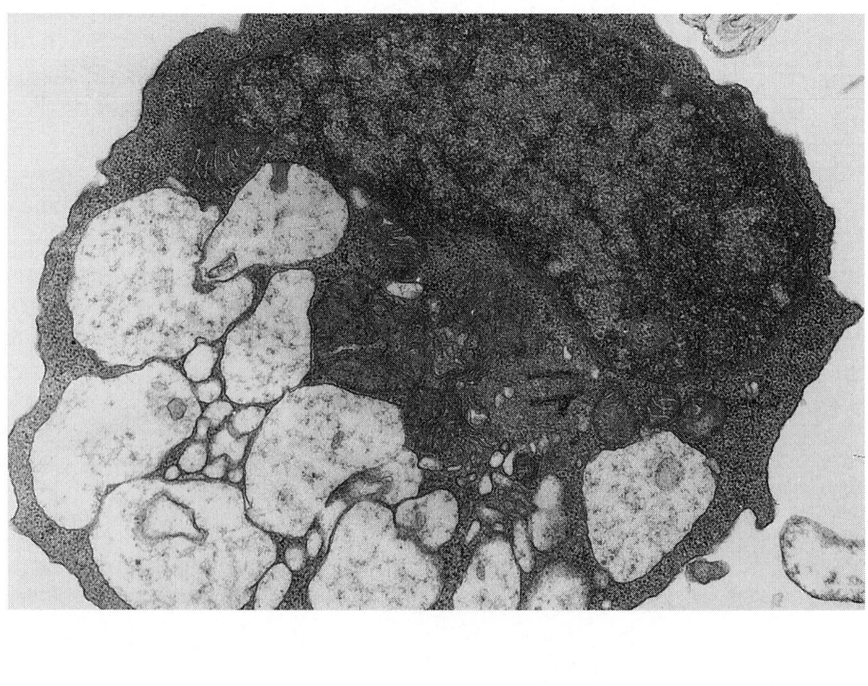

**Fig. 14-12.** $GM_1$-gangliosidosis. 4-month-old boy, severely reduced $\beta$-galactosidase activity, type I, in cultured fibroblasts. Circulating lymphocytes. **A**, Numerous membrane-bound vacuoles. **B**, Membrane-bound vacuoles in another cell contain dense spheroid inclusions (*arrows*). Skin. 2-year-old boy, severely reduced $\beta$-galactosidase activity, type II. **C**, Numerous membrane-bound vacuoles in a dermal fibroblast. **D**, Numerous membrane bound vacuoles in endothelial cells of a dermal capillary (C) (×11,250). **E**, Several membrane-bound vacuoles in a dermal smooth muscle cell. (**A**, ×26,400; **B**, ×19,600; **C**, ×14,800; **D**, ×11,250; **E**, ×22,750.)

B

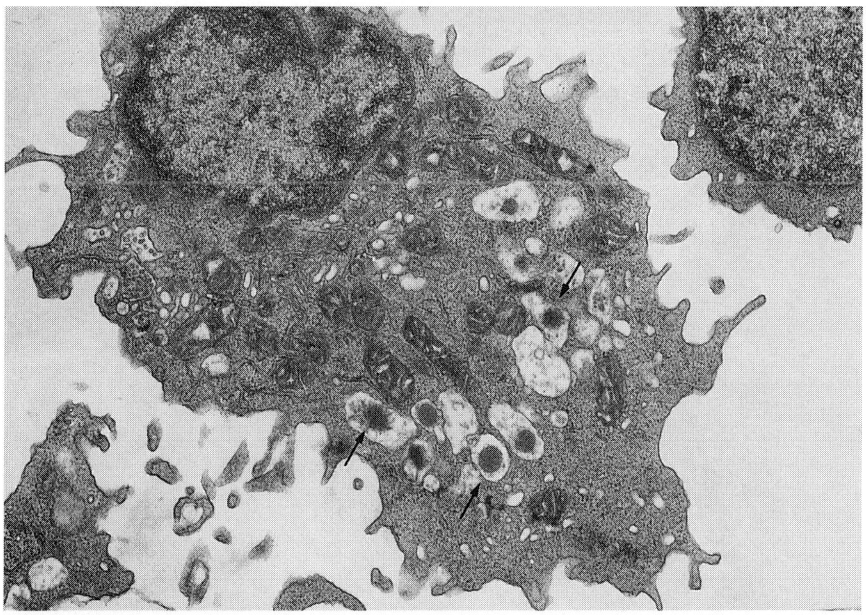

C

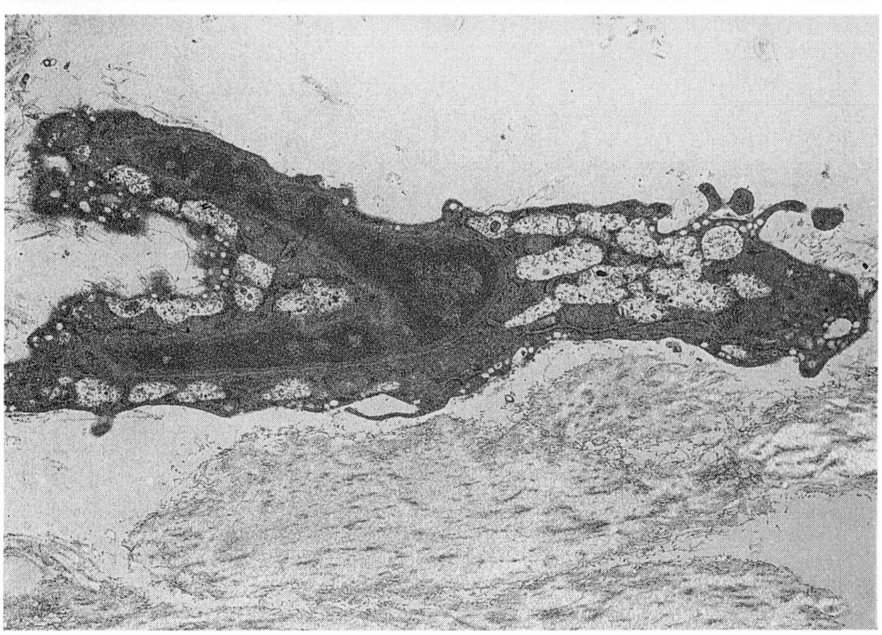

**Fig. 14-12, cont'd.** For legend see opposite page.

D

E

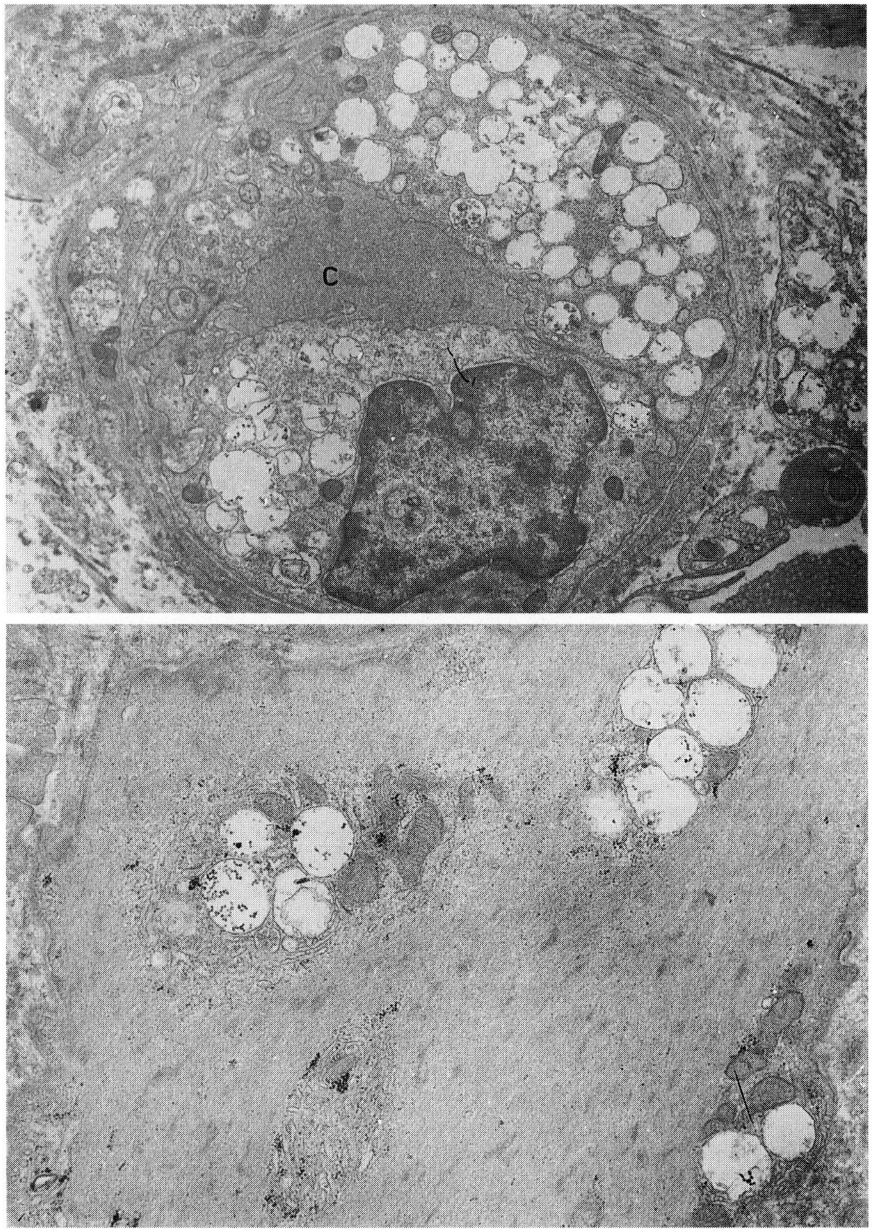


**Fig. 14-12, cont'd.** For legend see page 602.

phological recognition of nerve cells. Before the biochemical era of diagnosis brain biopsy used regularly to diagnose Tay-Sachs disease, revealed the presence of typical membranous cytoplasmic bodies. Subsequently, similar lysosomal accretions were recognized in nerve cells of the rectum. Enlarged axons also were observed in the myenteric neurons,[1] and similarly enlarged axons, containing mitochondria, dense bodies, and some membranous cytoplasmic bodies, also were observed in the skin[54] (Fig. 14-13, *A* to *C*). Skin is a useful tissue for the study of $GM_2$-gangliosidosis of the hexosaminidase A deficiency type, but only when axons, usually in the terminal area, are carefully studied. Tay-Sachs disease occurs frequently in Jewish patients; other forms of hexosaminidase A deficiency are seen in non-Jewish patients. Recognition of conspicuously enlarged axons in skin and conjunctiva, together with characteristic membranous cytoplasmic bodies in an affected child,[187] may result in identification of variants of hexosaminidase A deficiency.[27,83]

In Sandhoff disease, the same enlarged axons may be observed in skin,[129] but other cell types such as mural cells of dermal vessels (Fig. 14-13, *D*), Schwann cells, sweat gland epithelial cells, and smooth muscle cells of arrectores pilorum muscle cells also are affected. The latter inclusions are often partly vacuolar and filled with membranes, but these are not of the membranous cytoplasmic body type. Thus, the more widespread occurrence and the different ultrastructure of lysosomal residual bodies in Sandhoff disease dis-

A

B

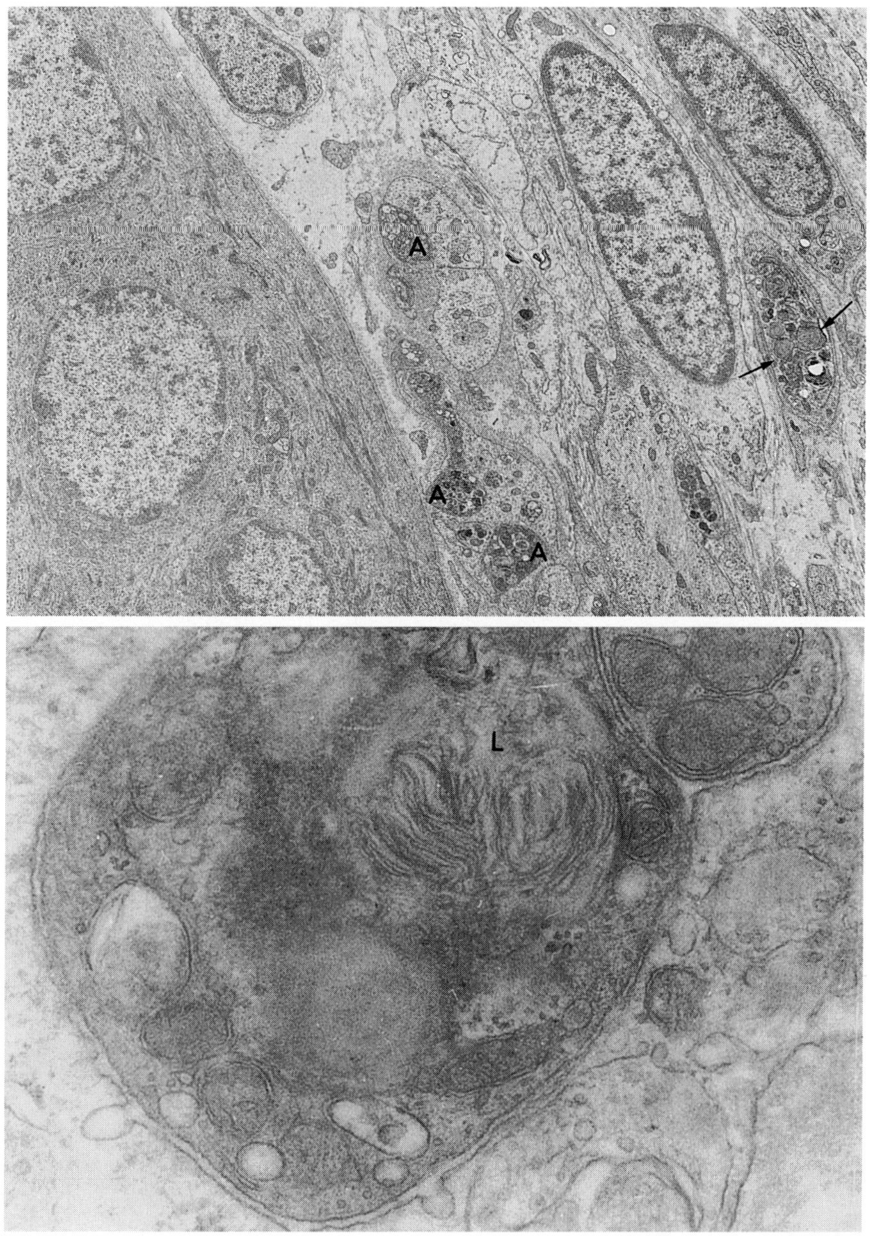


**Fig. 14-13.** $GM_2$-gangliosidosis. 2-year-old Turkish boy with severe hexosaminidase A deficiency.[27] Skin. **A**, Numerous subepithelial axons (*A*) are enlarged, some containing membranous cytoplasmic bodies (*arrows*). **B**, Lamellar (*L*) bodies in an unmyelinated axon.

*Continued.*

C

D

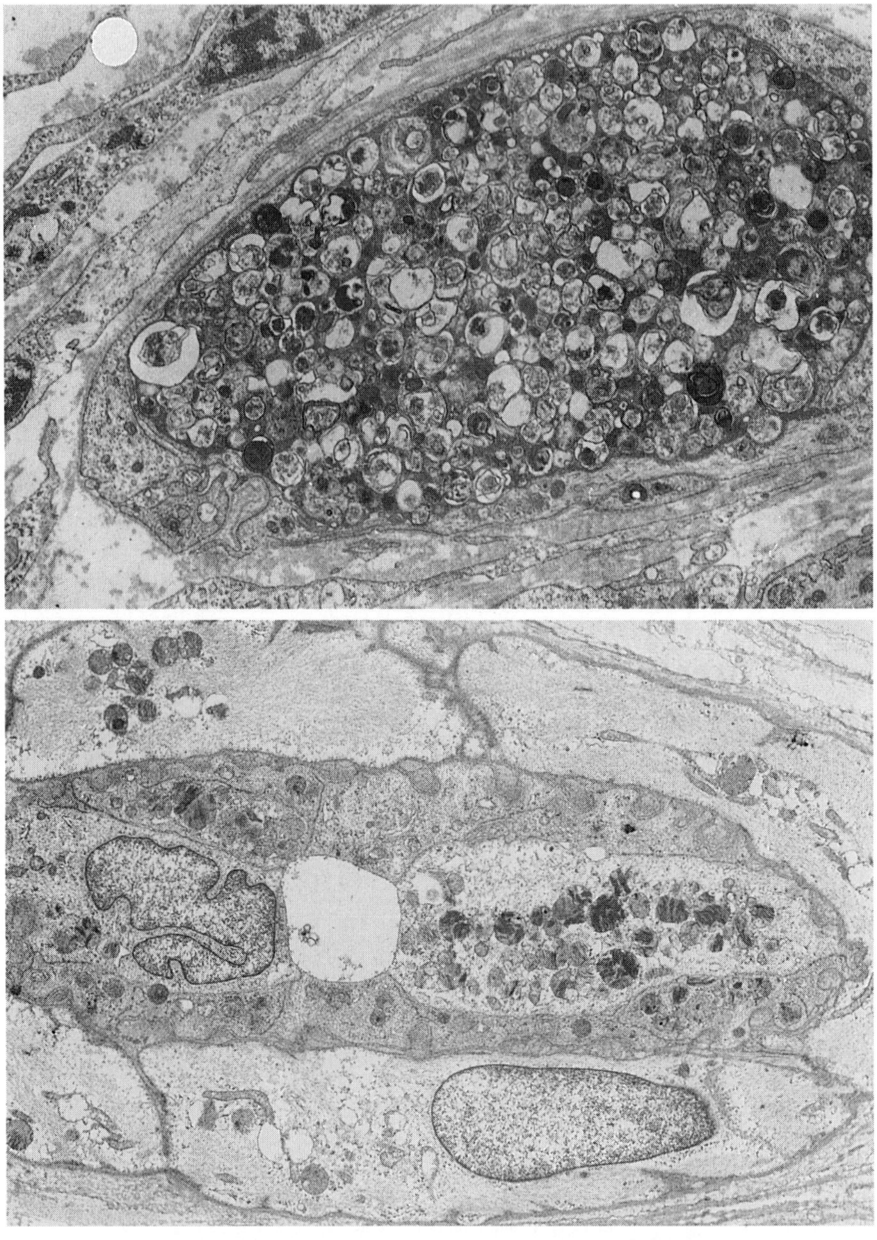

**Fig. 14-13, cont'd. C**, An unmyelinated axon is enlarged by innumerable light and dense bodies, a nonspecific feature. **D**, In hexosaminidases A and B deficiencies (Sandhoff disease), mural vascular cells also show lysosomal aggregation: 22-month-old girl, 1% of normal hexosaminidase A and B activities in cultured fibroblasts. (**A**, ×7600; **B**, ×104,400; **C**, ×19,720; **D**, ×7750.)

tinguish this condition from the more limited ultrastructural pathology seen in Tay-Sachs disease and its variants. Whether visceral organs and skin or conjunctiva are affected in the AB variant of GM-2 gangliosidosis (which is due to a defect of an activator protein) is not known, possibly because this variant is infrequent and is correctly diagnosed only by biochemical studies. In late-onset $GM_2$-gangliosidoses, characterized by partial or profound deficiency of hexosaminidase A, lysosomal storage also seems to be confined to the neuronal compartment; thus outside the brain it is detectable only in rectal biopsies.[22] Whether dermal axons are enlarged is not known. Enlarged axons also may be encountered in the skin in partial juvenile or adult hexosaminidase A-deficient $GM_2$-gangliosidoses.

***Farber Disease (Ceramidosis).*** Farber disease (Ceramidosis) lysosomal disorder (Fig. 14-14) characterized by storage of the simplest type of sphingolipid, ceramide, which consists of the alcohol sphingosin and a fatty acid—but no additional components, especially no sugar moieties. The autosomal recessively inherited defect is that of ceramidase, which affects children in different clinical forms. Lysosomal accretion is widespread, affecting neuroectodermal, mesenchymal, and epithelial cells of the nervous system, visceral organs, and subcutaneous regions. Therefore, skin biopsy is useful in the diagnosis as it may show different types of lysosomal residual bodies. The so-called "Farber bodies," granulomas containing swollen histiocytes, are hallmarks of this disease. Membrane-bound large lysosomes of varying shapes contain curved tubular profiles, sometimes misleadingly called curvilinear profiles making up "curvilinear" or "Farber" bodies[165] (because they are different from curvilinear profiles and curvilinear bodies in childhood NCL). A better appellation may be curved tubular profiles[29,212] (Fig. 14-14, *A*). Lamellar bodies (Fig. 14-14, *B*), often resembling zebra bodies, are encountered in epithelial cells, in both the epidermis[29] and the sweat glands.[212] A third group of inclusions does not display any particular fine structure, but appears rather empty, showing a "needle"- or "banana"-like shape; these inclusions are prominent in Schwann cells of myelinated axons,[29,195,212] and often resemble those seen in Schwann cells in Krabbe's globoid cell leukodystrophy. Circulating lymphocytes do not contain abnormal lysosomal residual bodies.[29] Ultrastructural abnormalities typical of the disease have not been observed in the conjunctiva, but rather vacuolar membrane-bound inclusions in mesenchymal cells, epithelial cells, and macrophages, lacking the typical Farber bodies.[213]

Ceramidosis is a characteristic example of how a metabolic defect of a single metabolite, ceramide, can induce different ultrastructural abnormalities in different types of cells. Thus, not only the metabolite, but also the cell type may determine ultrastructural phenotypical changes.

***Fabry Disease.*** Fabry disease (Fig. 14-15), or angiokeratoma corporis diffusum, is a lysosomal storage disorder in which there is accumulation of dihexoside and trihexoside ceramides based on an X-linked deficiency of the lysosomal trihexoside ceramidase or $\alpha$-galactosidase. This is often, but not always, marked by small angiomatous-type lesions of the skin and conjunctiva. With angiokeratomata, the clinical features relate to vessels in skin and kidney. Thus, Fabry disease may not be considered a true neurodegenerative disease of children, but rather a vascular disorder. Although clinical symptoms may commence in childhood or adolescence, often they progress to clinical manifestations only in adulthood. Mesenchymal, epithelial, and neuroectodermal tissue components are affected, most prominently the mural cells of vessels, especially endothelial cells. Smooth muscle cells and pericytes also are affected. The lysosomal residual bodies appear as lamellar bodies and as zebra bodies, and sometimes also are called fingerprint profiles and even curvilinear profiles.[155] These are, in their fine structure, mostly similar to the curved profiles seen in histiocytes in Farber disease. The endothelial cells also may show large, almost giant inclusions protruding into the capillary lumina. These have been described as "sunburstlike"[33] and atypical ultrastructure.[59]

Skin biopsies (Fig. 14-15, *A* and *B*) provide an ideal way to document the homozygous and heterozygous states of Fabry disease. Not only vascular cells are affected, but also smooth muscle cells of the pili arrectorum muscles and sweat gland epithelial cells,[63] fibroblasts, and cellular components of dermal nerve fascicles, especially perineurial cells.[33] Schwann cells of myelinated and unmyelinated nerve fibers also may be affected, but this may be more prominent in peripheral nerve biopsy specimens.[172] Axons, especially of the unmyelinated type may be mildly enlarged by increased numbers of mitochondria and dense bodies.[33,150] A membrane-bound lamellar inclusion may be present in the axoplasm in some cases.[172] Similar inclusions have been found within striated muscle fibers.[172,188] In addition, intramuscular vessel walls may show marked effects of lysosomal storage. Findings similar to those seen in skin may be demonstrated in conjunctiva.

The peripheral nerve may show loss of unmyelinated axons, with sprouting, loss of small myelinated fibers,[150,172] and even loss of large myelinated axons.[155] Preferential loss of small myelinated and unmyelinated axons is the result of preferential loss of small neuronal perikarya in spinal ganglia.[150] This loss may result from lysosomal storage, which could be demonstrated in surviving neuronal perikarya.[150]

A

B

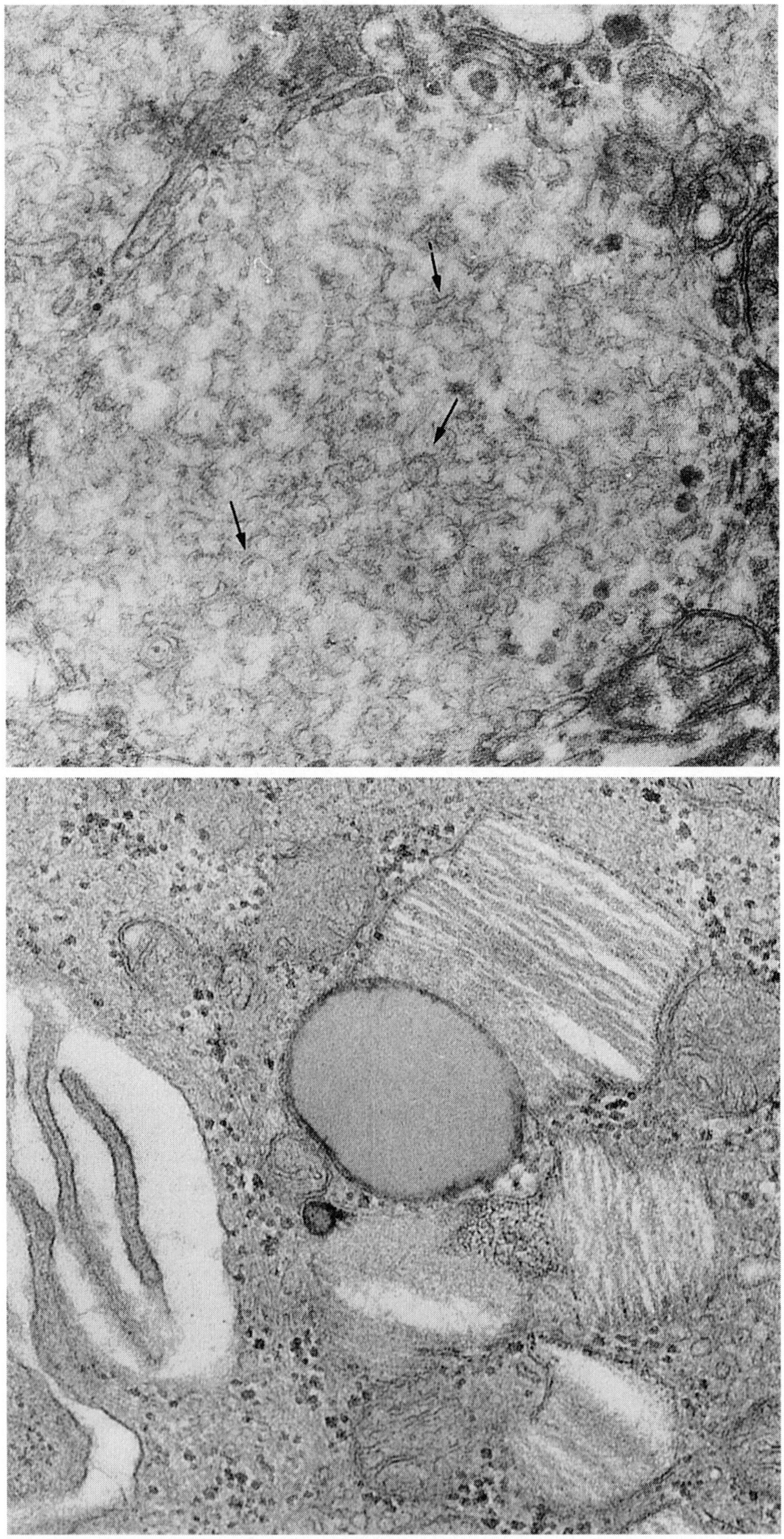

**Fig. 14-14.** Farber disease. 20-month-old girl with 0-activity in cultured fibroblasts of acid ceramidase.[29] **A**, A dermal histiocyte contains a membrane-bound lysosome with curved profiles (*arrows*). **B**, Membrane-bound lamellar bodies in a sweat gland epithelial cell. (**A**, ×66,960; **B**, ×55,000.)

A

B

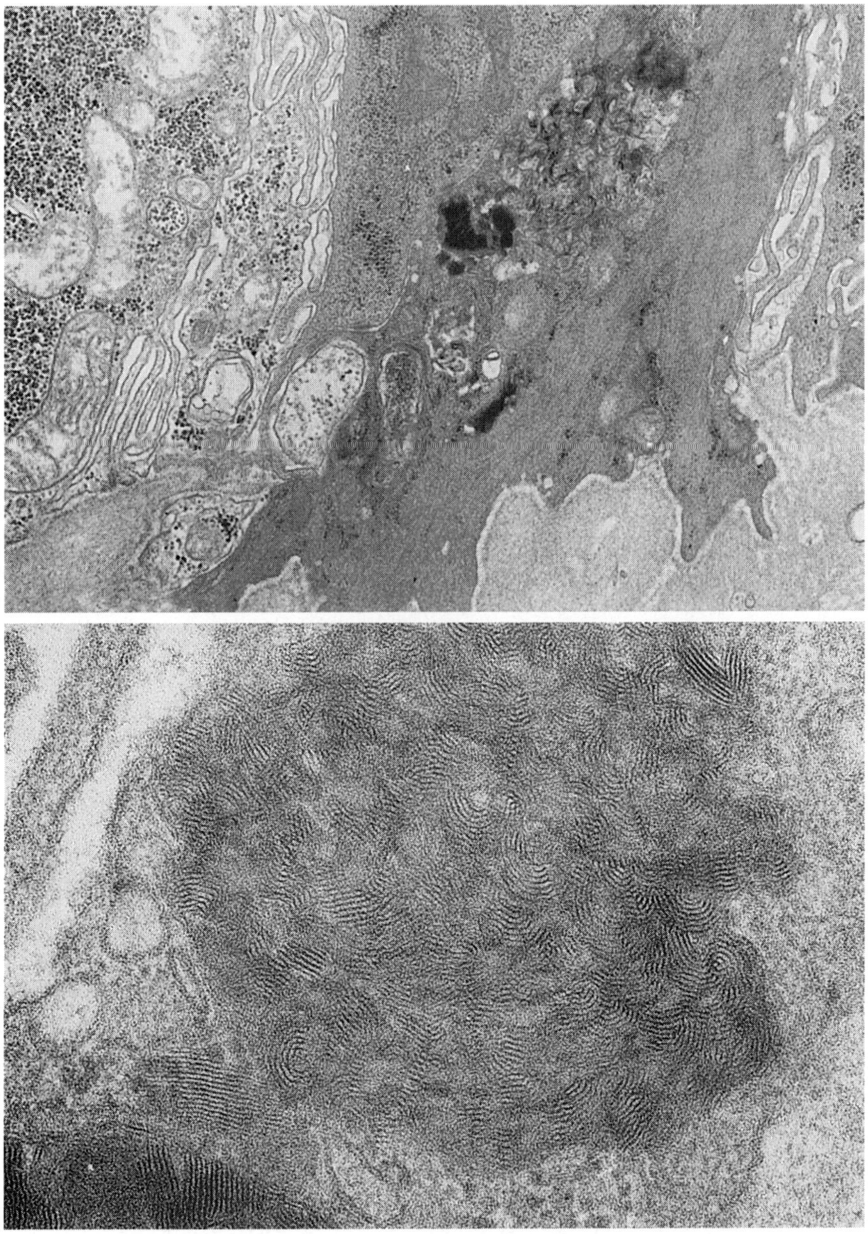

**Fig. 14-15.** Fabry disease. 23-year-old female carrier, $\alpha$-galactosidase activity in cultured fibroblasts reduced to some 50% of normal control. Skin. **A**, A myoepithelial cell of a sweat gland contains a large lamellar lysosomal body. **B**, At high magnification, circular and straight parallel lamellae in a Fabry body are obvious. (**A**, ×30,030; **B**, ×180,000.)

***Niemann-Pick Diseases—Sphingomyelinoses.*** Niemann-Pick disease (NPD) (Fig. 14-16) encompassses a group of lysosomal disorders marked by the abnormal accumulation of sphingomyelin in various cell types and organs. These disorders appear in different biochemical and clinical forms. Types A and B, also called NPD I, are secondary to an autosomal-recessively inherited defect of sphingomyelinase; types C, D, and E, also called NPD II, show normal or slightly reduced activities of sphingomyelinase. Different entities commencing at different ages show a wide spectrum of clinical symptoms, but hepatosplenomegaly and foam cells in the bone marrow (dubbed Niemann-Pick cells or sea-blue histiocytes) are common to all clinical forms. Lysosomal storage is widespread, affecting mesenchymal, epithelial, and neuroectodermal cells, although varying in degree and distribution among the different biochemical and clinical forms. The etiology of NPD type C remains unclear, although intracellular cholesterol transport has been found defective.

Types A and B, NPD I, and types C-E, NPD II, belong to seemingly different nosologic categories, NPD I being lysosomal sphingomyelinoses, and NPD II (or at least its type C) being a cholesterol lipidosis; however of these processes the ultrastructural changes are identical. Recognition of widespread lysosomal storage in NPD has finally made biopsy of the liver, the most prominently affected organ, obsolete. Niemann-Pick cells can be seen in bone marrow, and circulating lymphocytes (Fig. 14-16, *A*) may be conspicuously in-

A

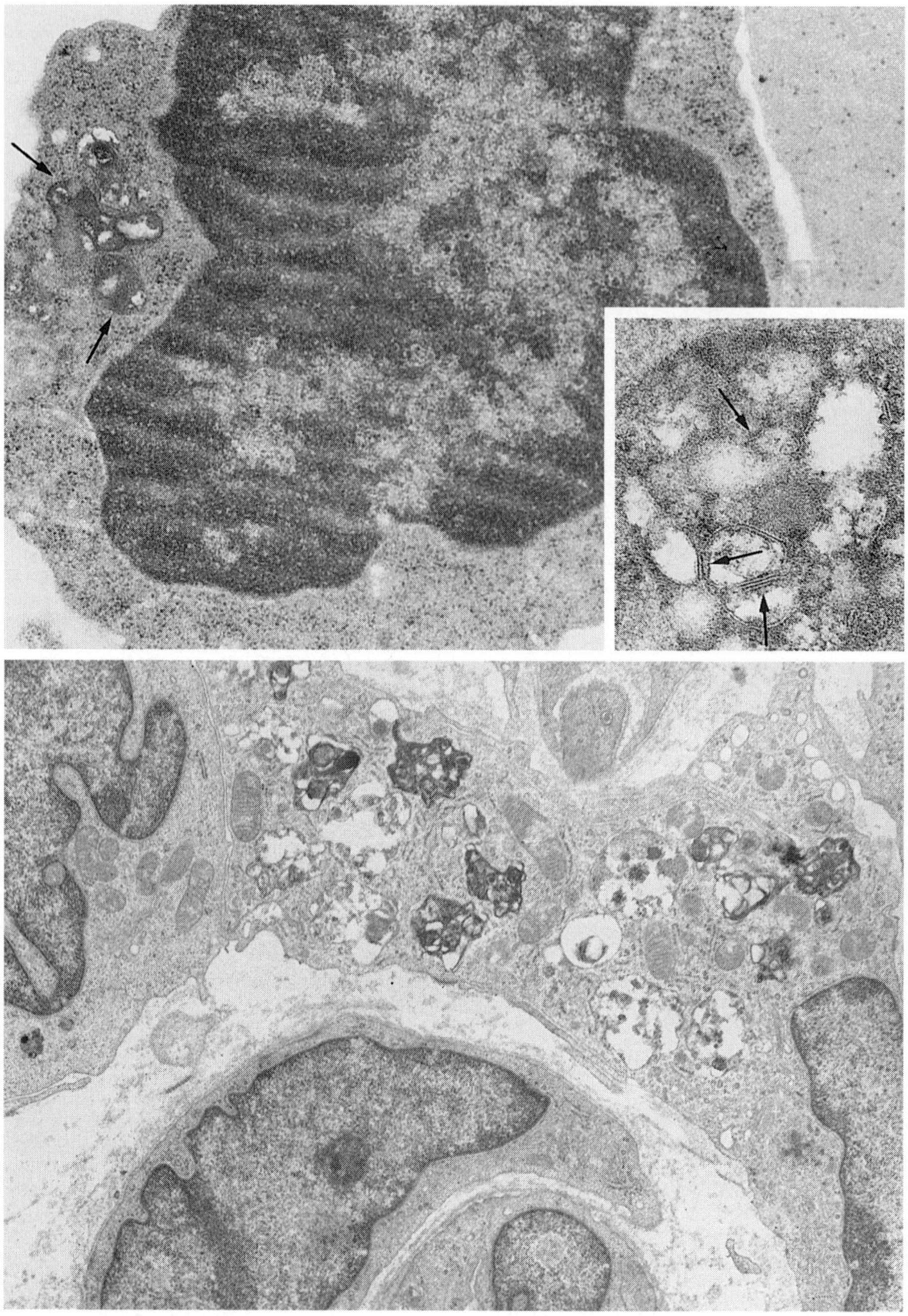

B

**Fig. 14-16.** Niemann-Pick disease. 6-year-old girl. **A**, Circulating lymphocyte. Several partly dense, partly light irregular inclusions (*arrows*). Inset. A complex body contains several lamellae (*arrows*). Skin. **B**, Mesenchymal cells around a dermal vessel contain innumerable irregular partly electron-dense, partly electron-lucent inclusions. **C**, Typical lysosomal inclusion (*arrows*) in a sweat gland epithelial cell. **D**, Largely vacuolar inclusions, membrane-bound, with some irregular electron-dense material (*arrows*) in a Schwann cell of a myelinated axon. **E**, An enlarged axon within the epidermis is filled with innumerable dense bodies, a nonspecific feature in many lysosomal disorders. (**A**, ×31,850; **Inset**, ×92,200; **B**, ×11,250; **C**, ×53,200; **D**, ×37,500; **E**, ×14,250.)

C

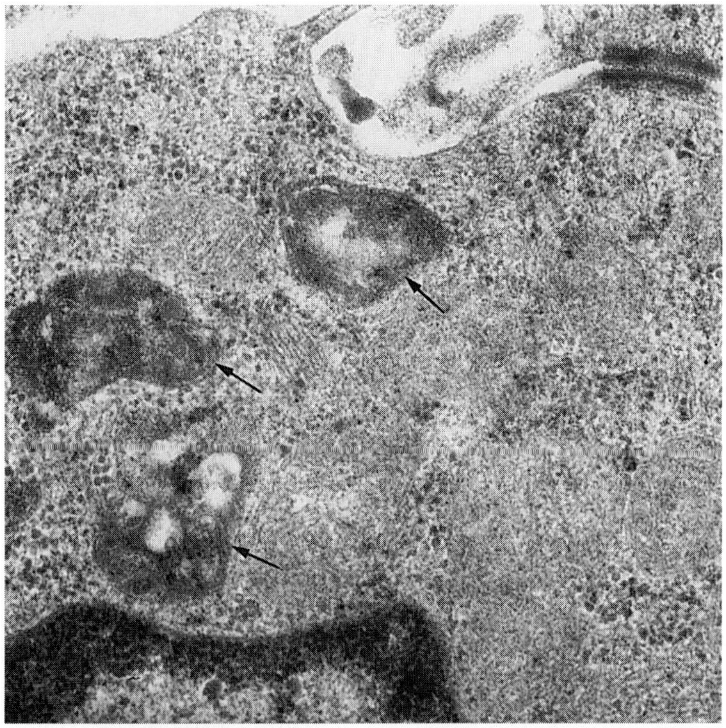

D

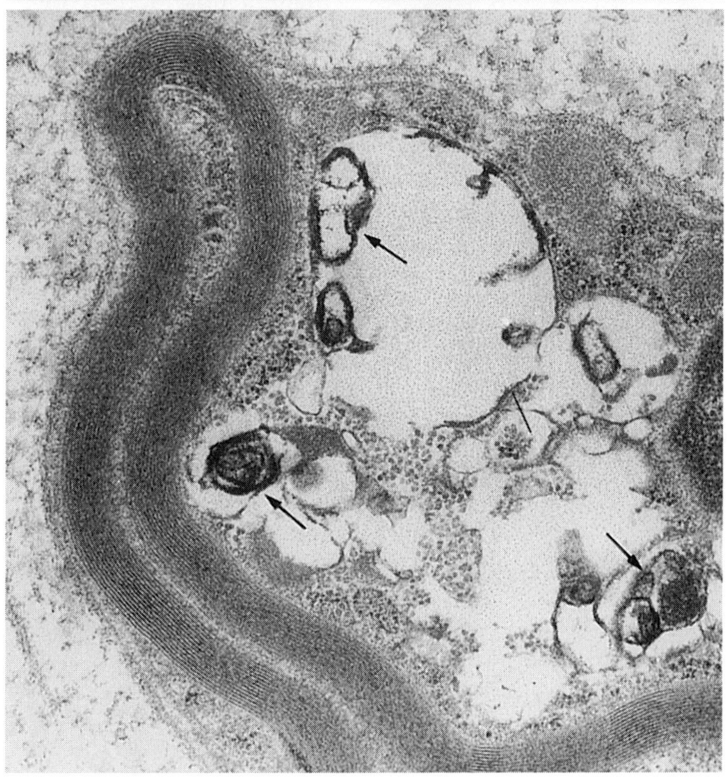

**Fig. 14-16, cont'd.** For legend see opposite page.

volved.[123] Circulating monocytes, are much less affected.[123,194] Because of its availability, skin biopsy (Fig. 14-16, *B* to *E*) is most helpful; numerous cell types are affected (mesenchymal, epithelial, and neuroectodermal) (Fig. 14-16, *B* to *D*). Similarly, conjunctiva is suitable for diagnosis.[10] Ultrastructural differential diagnostic criteria among the three different types A, B, and C have been invoked in conjunctival biopsy specimens,[125] but these differences are quantitative, not qualitative, and therefore not applicable in an individual patient's tissue study.

The ultrastructure of the lysosomal residual bodies consists of lamellar profiles, granular material, and electron-lucent empty areas, randomly admixed within the same lysosomal residual body. The lamellae within lysosomes are arranged in stacks or circles. Lysosomal residual bodies vary considerably in size and shape, and sometimes approach giant dimensions. Random admixture of electron-lucent and electron-dense, amorphous, or lamellar components is the ultrastructural hallmark of lysosomal storage in NPD. Lysosomal storage may be observed in Schwann cells of both unmyelinated[194] and myelinated axons. However, in the latter compartment, myelin debris, possibly from demyelination, may also be present; then, features of primary lysosomal storage and demyelination cannot always be easily distinguished.[94,96] Differences in structural abnormalities between dermal nerve fascicles and fascicles of biopsied peripheral nerves are only of quantitative nature. Likewise, axons, largely of the unmyelinated type, are frequently expanded by dense bodies and inclusions similar to lysosomal residual bodies (Fig. 14-16, *E*). This accumulation of dense bodies is considered a nonspecific feature in many lysosomal disorders.[197] The finding of curvilinear bodies in endoneurial and endothelial cells of NPD type C[96] seems to be an extremely rare feature in my experience—an illustration figure[96] is reproduced at too low magnification to be convincing.

E

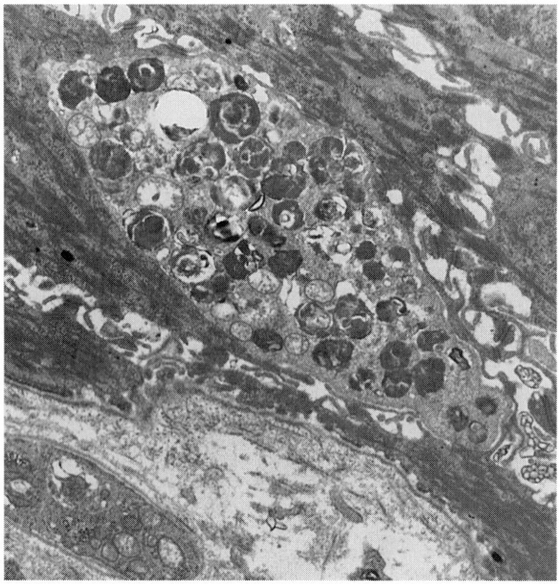

**Fig. 14-16, cont'd.** For legend see page 610.

***Gaucher Disease.*** Gaucher disease is a classic lysosomal disease (Fig. 14-17) marked by lysosomal storage of glucosyl ceramide/glucocerebroside secondary to lysosomal deficiency of acid $\beta$-glucosidase. The disease is characterized clinically by hepatosplenomegaly and morphologically by the Gaucher cell, a monocyte-turned-macrophage with typical needlelike inclusions that somewhat resemble the inclusions of galactocerebroside in globoid cell leukodystrophy (Krabbe's disease), an ultrastructural and biochemical, but not clinical, "sister" disorder. However, apart from the most frequent non-neuronopathic form, the classic Gaucher disease (type I), there are two neuronopathic forms, a severe or infantile one (type II) and a milder form with

A

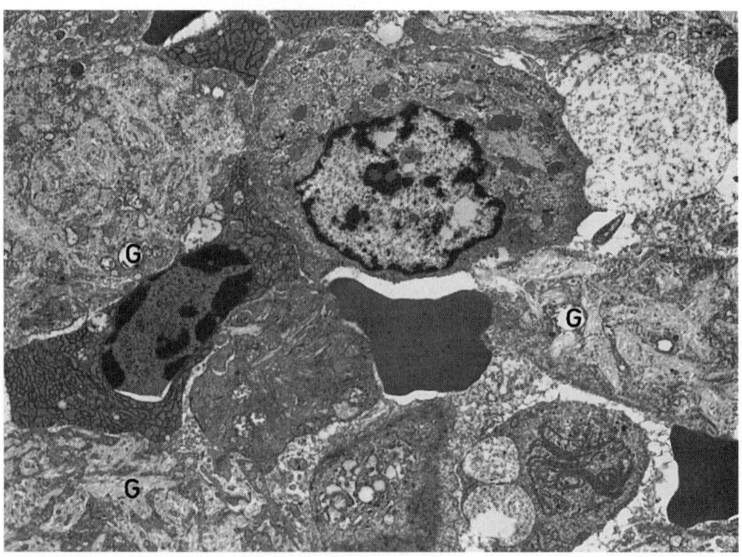


**Fig. 14-17.** Gaucher disease. Spleen. **A**, Numerous Gaucher cells (*G*) among erythrocytes and other splenic cells. **B**, Tubular profiles (*T*) surrounded by a limiting membrane (*arrows*) form the characteristic ultrastructural features of the Gaucher cell and of Gaucher disease. Bone marrow. **C**, Gaucher cell. (**A**, ×5700; **B**, ×24,000; **C**, 91,200.)

B

C

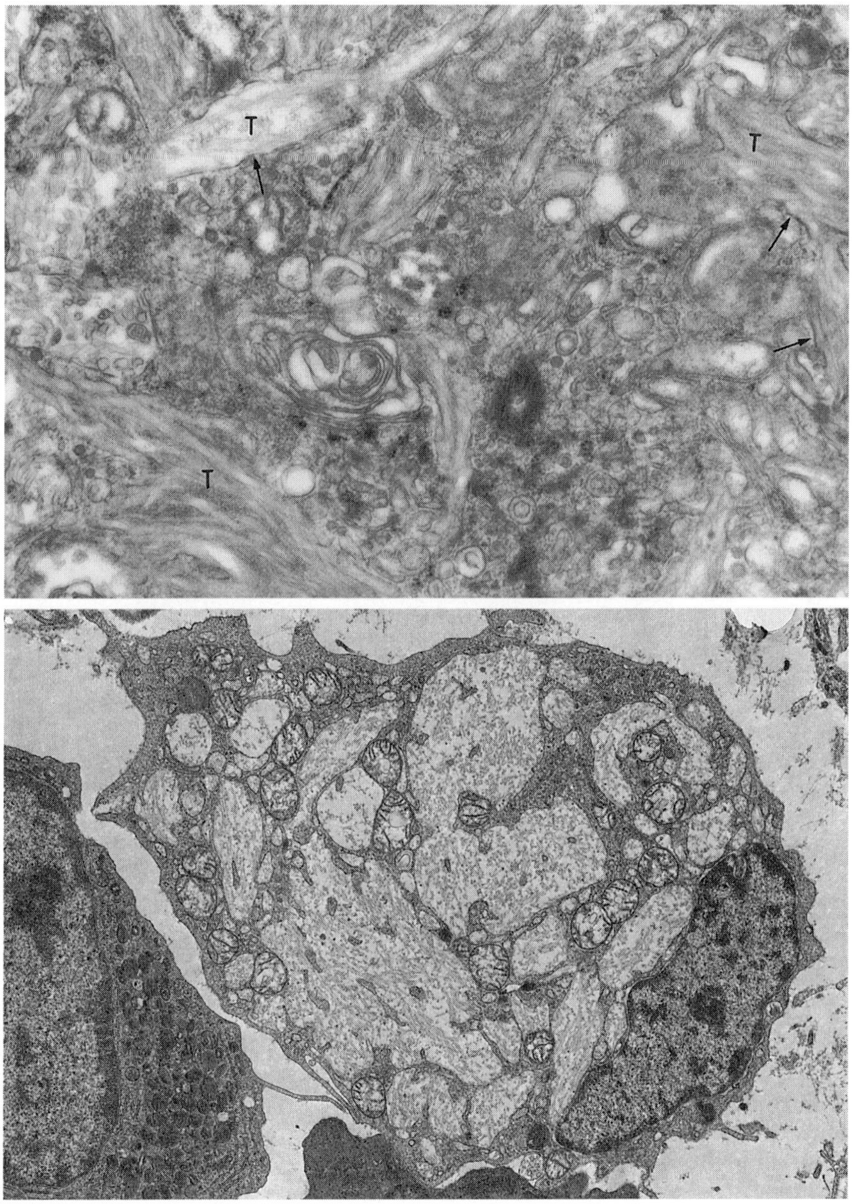


**Fig. 14-17, cont'd.** For legend see opposite page.

later onset (type III). Because the CNS is affected in both of these childhood neuronopathic types II and III, with Gaucher-type cells in the perivascular spaces of the CNS[42,110] and some intraneuronal formation of needle-like lamellae,[42] similar morphologic features may be expected to develop in neurons of the PNS, e.g., the rectal myenteric plexus. Thus, rectal biopsy may contribute to the diagnosis of neuronopathic forms II and III of Gaucher disease in those cases in which acid $\beta$-glucosidase levels have not been determined. However, the spectrum of extracerebral and extrahepatic morphologic diagnosis of the neuronopathic types II and III of Gaucher disease has hardly been explored. Involvement of rectal neurons in types II and III of Gaucher disease may only be inferred from involvement of CNS neurons.

**Lysosomal leukodystrophies.** The leukodystrophies are progressive degenerative or metabolic disorders of the myelin sheaths. Some of these affect the central myelin, e.g., Pelizaeus-Merzbacher disease. These diseases are caused by deficiencies of protein components of either the central or the peripheral myelin. Examples include the central PLP/DM20 myelin protein, which is defective in Pelizaeus-Merzbacher disease, a central nonlysosomal leukodystrophy (Chapter 16), and the peripheral P-0 myelin protein, defective in hereditary motor and sensory neuropathies (HMSN I), now called CMT I B. Metabolic leukodystrophies are unrelated to myelin protein defects, but are marked by ubiquitous metabolic defects that affect both the central and the peripheral myelin.

A

B

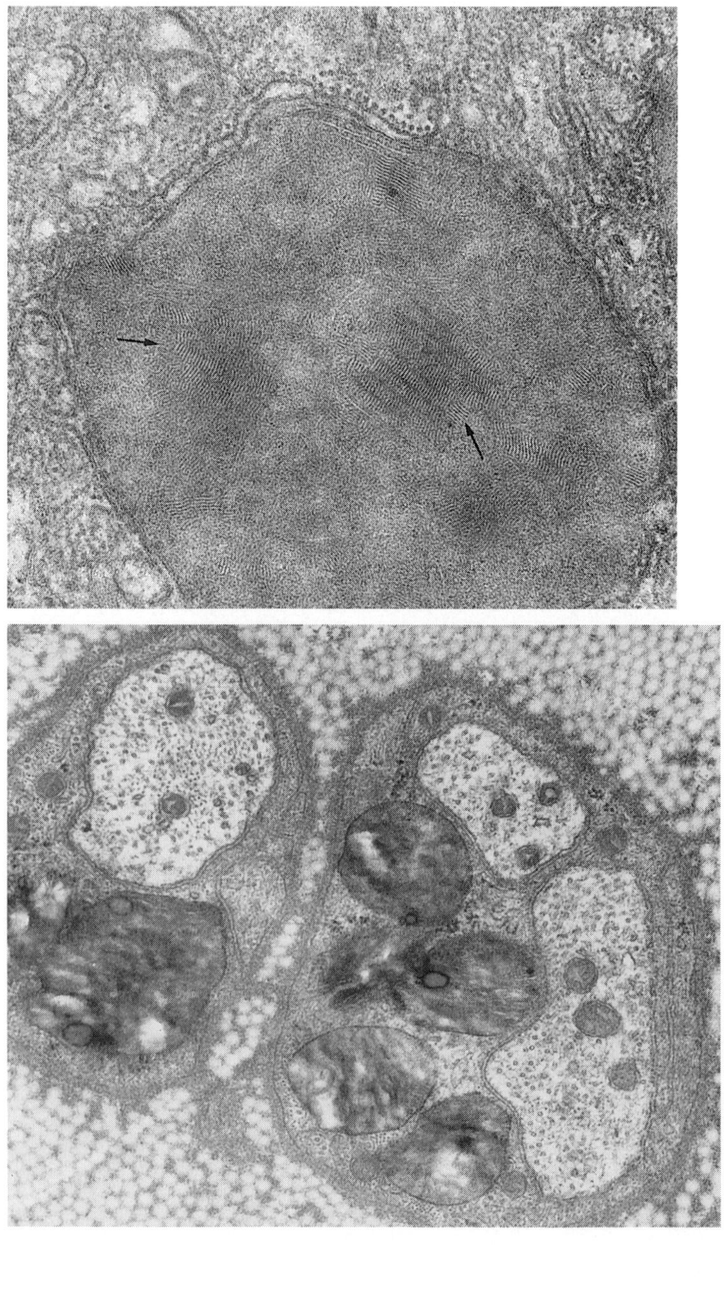

**Fig. 14-18.** Metachromatic leukodystrophy. 2.25-year-old boy, arylsulfatase-A activity absent in circulating leukocytes. Sural nerve. **A**, Typical membrane-bound lamellar body with prismatic or herringbone structures (*arrows*). **B**, Schwann cells of primarily unmyelinated axons also harbor membrane-bound lamellar inclusions. (**A**, ×142,500; **B**, 37,400.)

Among these metabolic leukodystrophies are two lysosomal disorders: metachromatic leukodystrophy and globoid cell or Krabbe's leukodystrophy, and several peroxisomal disorders, the adrenoleukodystrophies. Because the neuropathologic lesions are related to the myelin sheaths, peripheral nerves or dermal and conjunctival nerve fascicles are suitable for examination, provided that they include myelinated nerve fibers. Biopsies of these peripheral nerve-containing tissues are informative, less because of the demyelinating process, which is nonspecific, than because of the presence of disease-characteristic inclusions in Schwann cells and endoneurial macrophages. The subsequent loss of myelinated fibers may be obvious in biopsied peripheral nerves, but not in dermal or conjunctival nerve fascicles. Quantitative controls for dermal or conjunctival tissues do not exist.

### Metachromatic Leukodystrophy (MLD)

MLD (Fig. 14-18) is caused by an autosomal recessively inherited defect of the lysosomal enzyme arylsulfatase-A. The disorder appears clinically in late-infantile, juvenile, and adult forms. Apart from evidence of the demyelinating polyneuropathy, details of which are described in Chapter 18, characteristic lysosomal residual bodies appear in Schwann cells of myelinated axons. Lamellar inclusions often take the forms of so-called tufaceous or tuff stone bodies and herring-bone or prismatic inclusions (Fig. 14-18, *A*). These inclusions must be sufficiently abundant in the respective Schwann cells of myelinated axons before they can be detected in dermal or conjunctival nerve fascicles,[66] as a result they are seldom seen in biopsied skin. Lysosomal residual bodies are also seen in Schwann cells of unmyelinated axons, and frequently in neuronal penkanya. Lysosomal storage does not affect other dermal and conjunctival cells in MLD and for this reason biopsies of skin and conjunctiva are not particularly helpful. Occasionally, conjunctival epithelial cells and stromal fibroblasts may contain vacuolar lysosomes, as seen in mucopolysaccharidosis (MPS).[126]

Mucosulfatidosis, an autosomal-recessive lysosomal condition, involves multiple sulfatase deficiencies. The disease combines morphologic features of MLD and MPS, e.g., MLD-specific lysosomal inclusions in Schwann cells of conjunctival myelinated axons and MPS-typical lysosomal vacuoles with some amorphous finely granular content in conjunctival epithelial and fibroblastic cells.[126] Sometimes, the MPS-like vacuolar lysosomal component may be present in biopsied conjunctiva.[93]

### Globoid Cell (GCL) or Krabbe's Leukodystrophy

This lysosomal leukodystrophy (Figs. 14-19, 14-20) is caused by an autosomal recessively inherited defect of lysosomal galactocerebrosidase. The infantile form is most frequent, but forms with later onset also have been described.[84] In addition to the demyelinating process, needlelike inclusions are encountered in Schwann cells of myelinated axons. In late onset forms of the disease the ultrastructural inclusion patterns may deviate from the classic ultrastructural pattern[84] (Fig. 14-20, *A*). Unlike MLD, the epithelial cells of eccrine sweat glands also contain accreted needlelike structures in biopsies of GCL[58,85] (Figs. 14-19, 14-20). Also unlike MLD, skin biopsy may prove to be a helpful diagnostic procedure in GCL.

### Vacuolar Lysosomal Disorders

A biochemically similar group of lysosomal disorders is marked by membrane-bound lysosomal vacuoles. In this group are the mucopolysaccharidoses (MPS)[19,50,133,145] (Fig. 14-21), certain mucolipidoses (types I[41], Fig. 14-22) or sialidosis[127] and II[118,140] (Fig. 14-23), and certain oligosaccharidoses, such as $\alpha$- and $\beta$-mannosidosesl;[97] fucosidosis;[103] aspartylglucosaminuria, and sialic acid disorders such as sialidosis, galactosialidosis, siluria; and sialic storage disorders including Salla disease.[209] Mesenchymal cells, including circulating lymphocytes (Figs. 14-21, 14-23), fibroblasts (Fig. 14-23), and mural cells of vessels contain lysosomal vacuoles. Nonmesenchymal cells such as sweat gland epithelial cells also may show lysosomal vacuoles. In circulating lymphocytes, these vacuoles often appear as aggregates. Although their content is largely watery, some granular, amorphous, fuzzy, and even lamellar material may be enclosed (Figs. 14-21, 14-22). In certain MPS additional inclusions within the lysosomal vacuoles of circulating lymphocytes have a granular matrix with some parallel fingerprint-type lamellae[79] (see Fig. 14-6).

Upon encountering membrane-bound vacuoles that must be differentiated from swollen preexisting organelles, especially mitochondria with disrupted cristae, the examiner can only diagnose a vacuolar lysosomal disorder, rather than a nosologically defined lysosomal entity.

Type IV mucolipidosis (Fig. 14-24), however, is marked not only by lysosomal vacuoles, but also by avacuolar lysosomes of a lamellar type. These may be encountered in Schwann cells, circulating lymphocytes,[80] and other cells.[62,163]

### Glycogenoses

The glycogenoses can be considered as NDIC only within limits. One of these disorders is infantile type IV glycogenosis (Anderson disease), which is caused by a defect of the brancher enzyme. The patients can present with neurologic symptoms, but some of the symptoms actually are induced by concurrent hepatic involvement. The other one is type II glycogenosis.

Type IV glycogenosis is marked not only by particu-

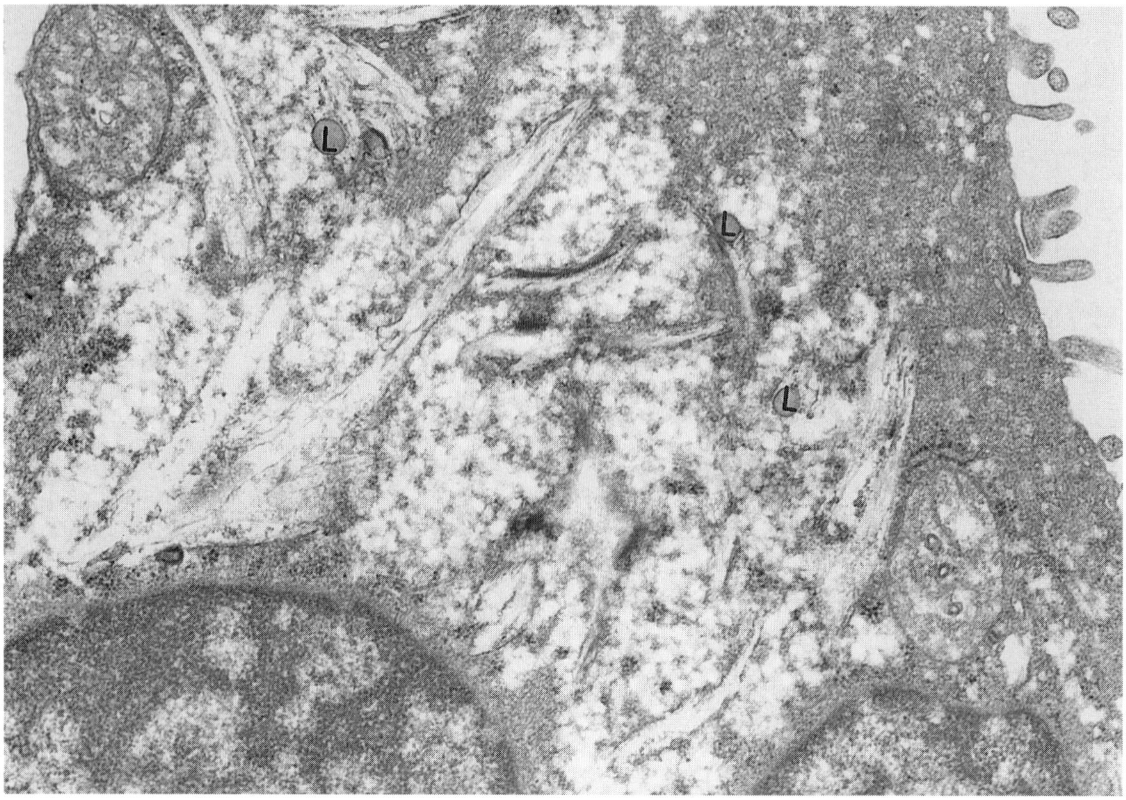

**Fig. 14-19.** Krabbe's globoid cell leukodystrophy. 6-month-old girl, very reduced cerebroside $\beta$-galactosidase activity in leukocytes. Skin. Typical needlelike inclusions within a sweat gland epithelial cell, often in conjunction with lipid droplets (*L*). ($\times$30,800.)

late, but also by fibrillar glycogen, the nature of which can be demonstrated with silver proteinate.[187] Such fibrillar glycogen is found in both skeletal muscle fibers and in epithelial cells of eccrine sweat glands. In juvenile type IV glycogenosis, skeletal muscle, skin, and other tissues such as the appendix[162] show fibrillar glycogen; in adult type IV glycogenosis, this typical fibrillar glycogen can be demonstrated only in skeletal muscle fibers.

Type II glycogenosis, which is the result of a deficiency of the lysosomal enzyme acid maltase, is characterized by ubiquitous accumulations of lysosomal glycogen. These deposits can be seen in neurons and Schwann cells as well as in skeletal muscle fibers, in epithelial and mesenchymal cells of the skin, and in circulating lymphocytes (Fig. 14-25). When the specimen preservation is inadequate, e.g., because of delayed fixation, lysosomes may appear to be vacuolar, thus obscuring the true nature of the lysosomal pathology. A different disorder, still nosologically enigmatic, is "lysosomal glycogen storage disease without acid maltase deficiency,"[46] also termed Danon's disease.[189] In this disease, membrane-bound glycogen and other vacuoles are seen in muscle fibers, but apparently not in other cell types. This condition may not be a lysosomal disorder at all.

Tissues from other glycogenoses can show various enzymatic deficiencies in skeletal muscle fibers and hepatocytes, with increased cytoplasmic particulate glycogen, but these conditions are not NDIC. However, in type III glycogenosis (again not a neurodegenerative disease), in which the debrancher enzyme is deficient, cytoplasmic particulate glycogen accumulates not only in skeletal muscle fibers but also in smooth muscle cells and in epithelial and myoepithelial cells of eccrine sweat glands.[164]

### Vitamin E Deficiency

Vitamin E deficiency is usually associated with diseases of the gastrointestinal tract, such as biliary cirrhosis and malabsorption syndromes. This vitamin deficiency also occurs in A-$\beta$ lipoproteinemia or Bassen-Kornzweig syndrome. However, there seems to be a primary disorder as well, a slowly progressive neurologic disease marked by clinical and morphologic symptoms of spinocerebellar degeneration. Mutations in the $\alpha$-tocopherol transfer protein, the gene of which maps to chromosome 8q13[153] result in vitamin E defi-

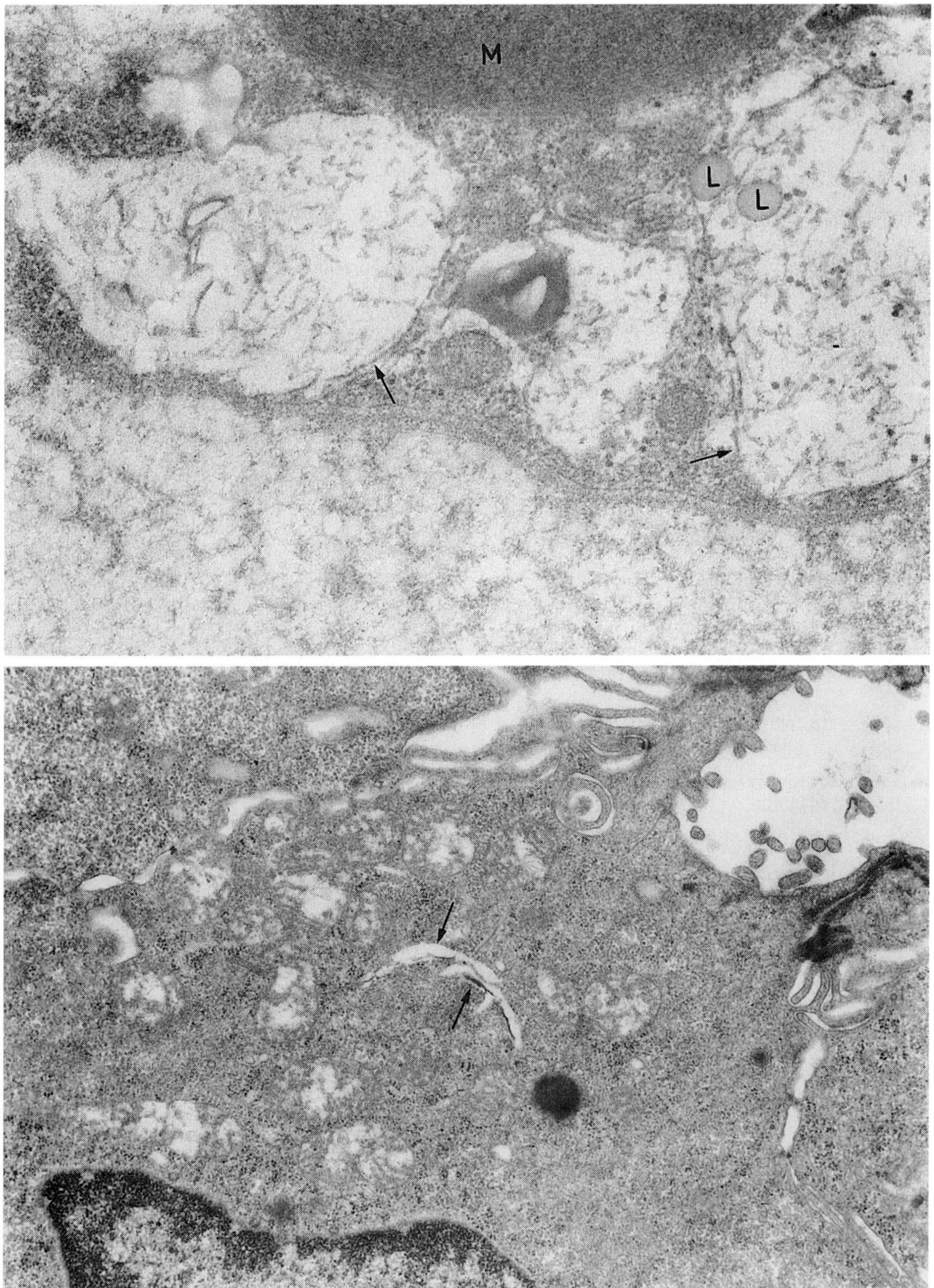


**Fig. 14-20.** Late-onset Krabbe's globoid cell leukodystrophy. 12-year-old girl, cerebroside $\beta$-galactosidase activity reduced to 10% in cultured skin fibroblasts.[84] Skin. **A**, Large membrane-bound (*arrows*) vacuoles with widely dispersed lamellae and two lipid (*L*) droplets in a Schwann cell of a myelinated (*M*) fiber, dermal nerve fascicle. **B**, Needlelike inclusions (*arrows*) in a sweat gland epithelial cell. **C**, Macrophage with large complex lysosomal inclusion. (**A**, ×55,000; **B**, ×30,940; **C**, ×17,292.) *Continued.*

C

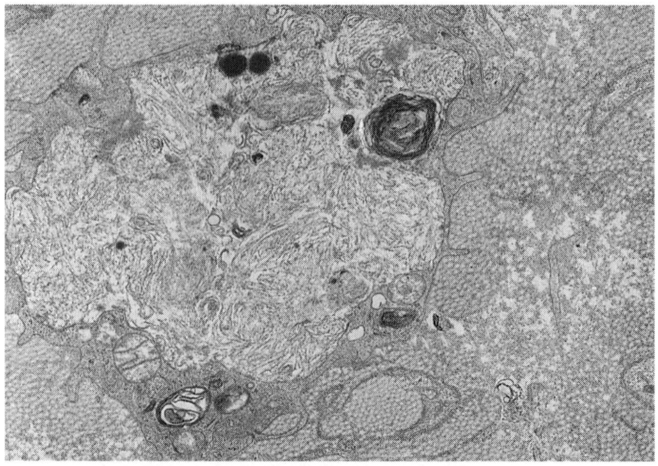

**Fig. 14-20, cont'd.** For legend see previous page.

ciency and represent a nosologic entity within the spectrum of "idiopathic" vitamin E deficiency. Both in primary and secondary vitamin E deficiencies, accumulation of finely granular membrane-bound autofluorescent lipopigments with increased acid phosphatase activity may be observed in muscle fibers[147a] and Schwann cells[28] of peripheral nerves. The complete morphologic spectrum of abnormal lipopigment formation in biopsy-accessible tissues is not known. The lipopigments encountered in vitamin E deficiency are different from those seen in NCL and from regular lipofuscin, in that in vitamin E deficiency the opaque lipid droplets are usually absent and the granular matrix is much finer than in the other two conditions. Our own observations on skin and lymphocytes of one patient did not reveal the characteristic lipopigments of vitamin E deficiency in dermal and lymphocytic cells[28]. Because vitamin E deficiency is a treatable disease, its recognition in respective biopsy specimens is of utmost importance. Clinical symptoms in our patient[28] have not progressed over the past 15 years since the time when vitamin E was prescribed.

### Peroxisomal Disorders

Peroxisomal disorders are enzymatic deficiencies that may be inherited autosomal- or X-linked recessively. They arise from defective peroxisomes and can be divided into three groups:[198] (1) peroxisomes are absent, therefore all their enzymes are absent; (2) multiple enzymes are deficient; and (3) single enzymes are deficient. Most of these peroxisomal disorders become clinically manifest early in life; some occur prenatally, combining developmental and progressively degenerative aspects, e.g., Zellweger disease. Others develop later in life, e.g., adrenomyeloneuropathy. Because peroxisomes are ultrastructurally most easily recognizable in liver[49,99,157] and kidney, biopsies of these organs offer the best diagnostic assistance. The morphologist thus must be familiar with the structure, size, and number of peroxisomes to render a useful diagnosis, which then must be confirmed biochemically. Small slitlike or needlelike lamellar inclusions can be seen in Schwann cells of myelinated fibers in adrenoleukodystrophy,[137] adrenomyeloneuropathy,[106] and neonatal adrenoleukodystrophy and in histiocytes.[183] Therefore, peripheral nerve, skin, conjunctiva, and rectal[183] biopsies may all be helpful in the diagnosis of these conditions.

### Mitochondrial Encephalomyopathies (MEM)

The concept of mitochondrial disease was ushered in by morphologists who encountered abnormally structured mitochondria on electron microscopic examination of skeletal muscle fibers. However, diagnosis of this extremely diverse group of diseases is now based on biochemical and genetic criteria. The spectrum of MEM is so heterogeneous and its boundaries are so ill-defined that morphologists now contribute less to the recognition of these diseases than in the past. There are MEM without abnormal mitochondria in skeletal muscle. Further, abnormal mitochondria in skeletal muscle do not necessarily indicate an MEM, because abnormally structured mitochondria may be encountered in such unrelated conditions as acid maltase deficiency, inclusion body myositis, polyglucosan body myopathy, polymyositis, and oculopharyngeal muscular dystrophy. Abnormal mitochondria also are seen in other neuromuscular or non-neuromuscular conditions as a nonspecific or fortuitously associated phenomenon. Unfortunately, the ultrastructure of abnormal mitochondria does not allow distinction between MEM and non-MEM. The tissue where abnormal mitochondria most frequently are present and where their presence is more meaningful is skeletal muscle. Abnormal mitochondria are also visible in liver biopsies but their significance at this site is less

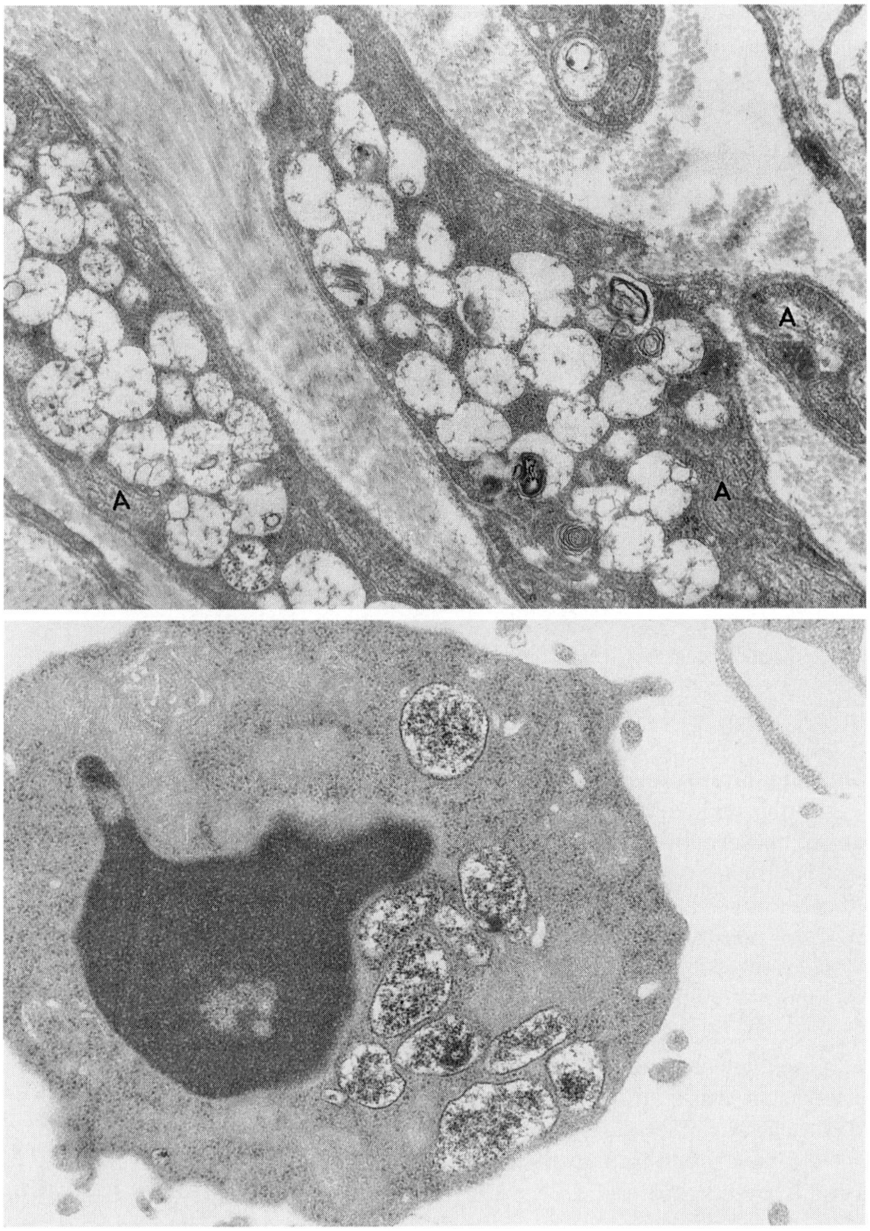


**Fig. 14-21.** Mucopolysaccharidosis III A (Sanfilippo). A 6-year-old girl with sulfamatase activity in cultured fibroblasts of less than 5% of normal control. **A**, Skin. Several Schwann cells of unmyelinated axons (*A*) are filled with numerous membrane-bound lysosomal vacuoles. **B**, A circulating lymphocyte contains several membrane-bound inclusions, partly vacuolar, partly filled with amorphous material. (**A**, ×23,660; **B**, ×37,400.)

clear than in muscle fibers because liver biopsies are not a common procedure in the diagnostic regimen for MEM.

Because encountering abnormal mitochondria does not identify a particular type of MEM, only basic principles are elaborated here.

The light microscopic hallmark of mitochondrial abnormalities is the ragged red fiber. This may be associated with an increased activity of oxidative enzymes, e.g., cytochrome-C oxidase, succinate dehydrogenase, NADH tetrazolium reductase, and menadione-linked $\alpha$-glycerophosphate dehydrogenase. Even in myoadenylate deaminase preparations, ragged red fibers may be clearly visible. The ultrastructural features of mitochondrial abnormalities are: (1) increased numbers of mitochondria, formerly termed pleoconial mitochon-

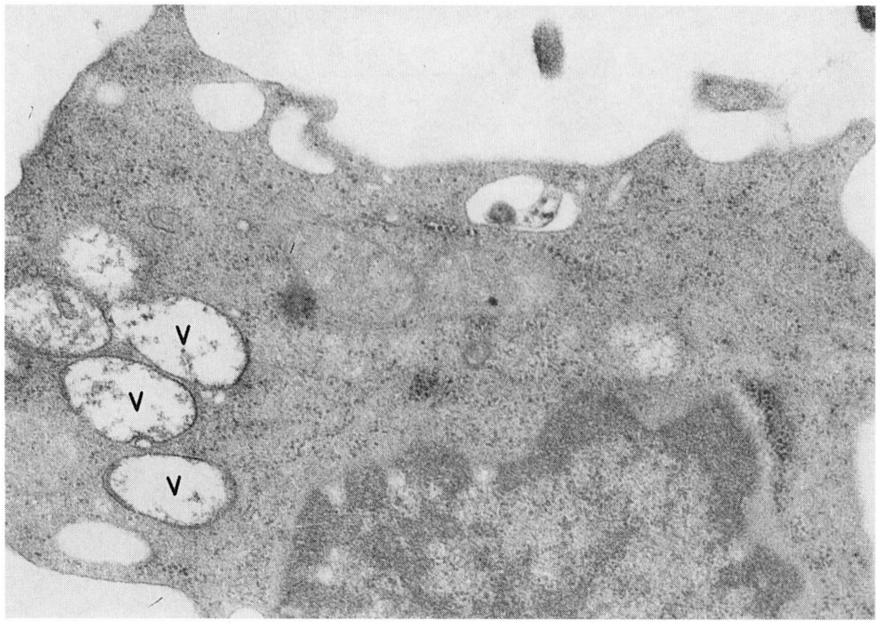


**Fig. 14-22.** Mucolipidosis I (Sialidosis). Circulating lymphocyte. An aggregate of membrane-bound vacuoles (*V*) with some amorphous material. (×46,500.)

drial myopathy; (2) enlarged mitochondria, emphasized by the term megaconial mitochondrial myopathy; and (3) an abnormal pattern of cristae, usually having a circular rather than the usual ladder-type pattern. Inclusions may be homogeneous and electron-dense; they may be opaque, possibly because of their lipid content; they may be numerous, small and particulate, representing glycogen; and they may be of a crystalloid nature. Intramitochondrial crystals belong to two types, one seen in the intracisternal matrix, type I, the other located between the inner and outer membrane, type II.[178] Intramitochondrial crystals of type I are thought to develop in type I myofibers; intramitochondrial crystals of type II are encountered in type II muscle fibers.[177]

Abnormal mitochondria occasionally have been observed in cells other than skeletal muscle fibers, but not with the same frequency.[9,34,108] Therefore, finding abnormal mitochondria in cells and tissues other than skeletal muscle has even less diagnostic value than finding few abnormal mitochondria in skeletal muscle fibers. Mitochondrial structural abnormalities has been encountered in mural cells of vessels equivalent to those seen in cerebral vessels. Although it is known that MEM may induce a mild neuropathy, best recognized by loss of axons, and primary demyelination,[82] abnormally structured mitochondria are an occasional feature in peripheral nerve.[166] The wealth of structurally abnormal mitochondria seen in skeletal muscle fibers, however, has never been encountered in peripheral nerve biopsies or in other tissue samples from children with neurodegenerative disorders (skin, conjunctiva, rectum, lymphocytes). A mildly structurally abnormal mitochondrion has been encountered in eccrine sweat gland epithelial cells,[144] but the infrequency of the observations make this an unreliable diagnostic feature.

### Carbohydrate–Deficient Glycoprotein Syndrome (CDG Syndrome)

The CDG syndrome is a recessive neurodegenerative multi-organ disorder affecting children's CNS and PNS as well as visceral organs. The biochemical defect is not yet completely known. Defective transfer of increased arylsulfatase A activity has been shown in patients' sera. Biopsy studies of the peripheral nerve[149] and the liver[44] have revealed, by electron microscopy, lamellar and multi-vacuolar inclusions in Schwann cells and hepatocytes,[104] having ultrastructural features sometimes similar to those of Niemann-Pick disease, and compact fibrillar inclusions in fibroblasts. Thus, dermal and conjunctival nerve fascicles may show similar lesions. Variants II and III of this CDG syndrome, which lack peripheral nerve involvement, have been described.[105] The inclusions within Schwann cells, fibroblasts, and hepatocytes are considered lysosomes, but lysosomal enzyme deficiencies are not known.

## PRENATAL DIAGNOSIS

The spectrum of prenatal diagnosis[4,156,173] has been widened considerably through the use of ultrasonography to detect malformations, karyotyping to ascertain chromosomal anomalies,[61,98] biochemical analysis to

A

B

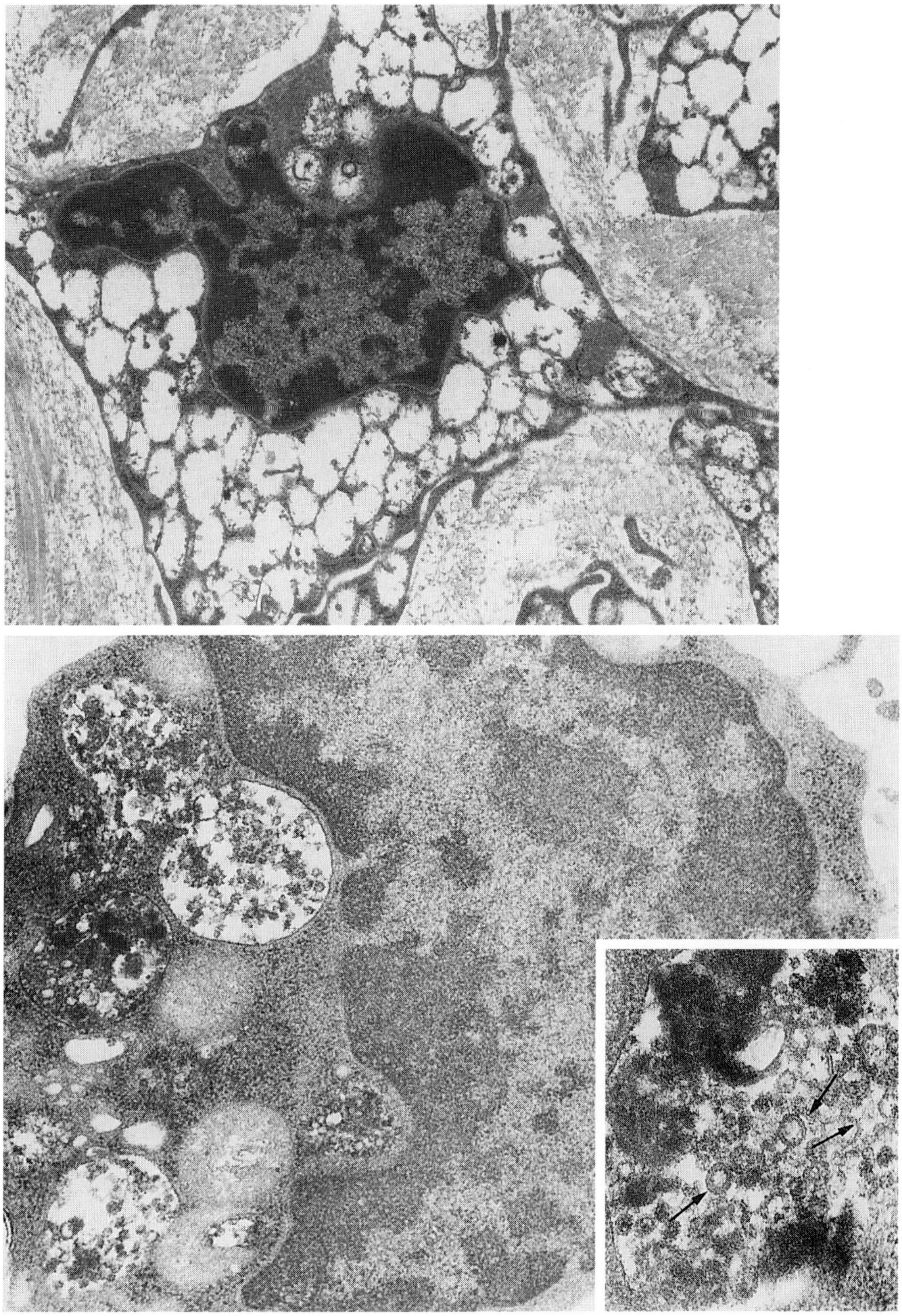

**Fig. 14-23.** Mucolipidosis II. **A**, Skin. Numerous fibroblasts, replete with often coalescing vacuoles. **B**, Circulating lymphocyte. Several membrane-bound, occasionally confluent inclusions, partly vacuolar, partly filled with amorphous material. Inset, At higher magnification, one such membrane-bound vacuole contains amorphous granular electron-dense material and ring and curved structures (*arrows*). (**A**, ×17,100; **B**, ×32,050; **Inset**, ×57,000.)

A

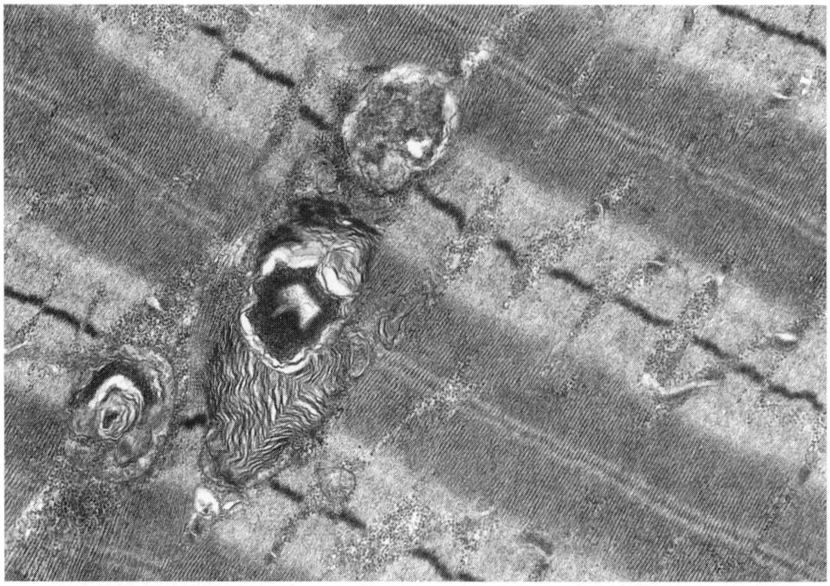

B

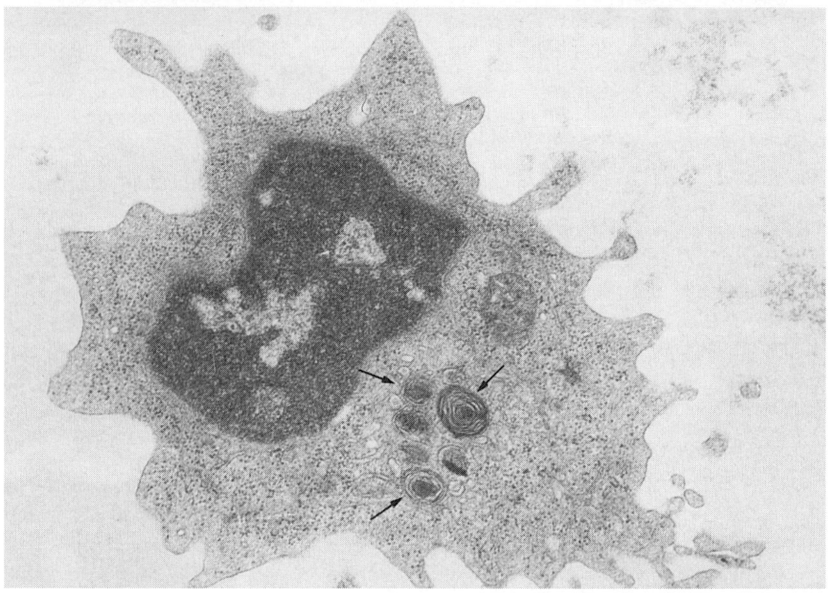

**Fig. 14-24.** Mucolipidosis type IV. 14-year-old girl.[80] **A**, Skeletal muscle. A large laminated body in the center of a muscle fiber. **B**, Circulating lymphocyte. Several small lamellar bodies (*arrows*) in a lymphocyte. (**A**, ×26,400; **B**, ×22,000.)

identify enzyme defects,* and molecular genetic techniques. However, the morphologic approach to prenatal diagnosis remains rather limited,[109,148,152,210] because such diagnosis aims at recognizing a fatal disease. Diagnostic targets may be amniotic cells,[88,148,180] chorionic villi[4,199] (including their cultured cells), and fetal tissues, particularly skin.[5,6,13] The number of disorders recognizable from available fetal tissues is low.

Morphologic prenatal studies must meet two prerequisites. (1) Lack of a universally applicable prenatal screening method (such as karyotyping in mothers older than 35 years) except for well-defined disorders already known in the family or frequent in certain groups such as Ashkenazi Jews who have a high rate of heterozygosity for Tay-Sachs disease. Here, unlike regular diagnostic approaches in which a previously unknown disease process is to be looked for, the disease suspected in utero has already been documented in the family.

(2) The disease sought for must have unique morphological characteristics—and the abnormality must be present in the fetal tissue at the time the biopsy is performed. The state of fetal development is particularly important in the skin, as this is a frequent source of prenatal biopsy.

The diagnostic preparation of fetal tissues does not

* Refs. 18, 90, 114, 154, 191, 202.

A

B

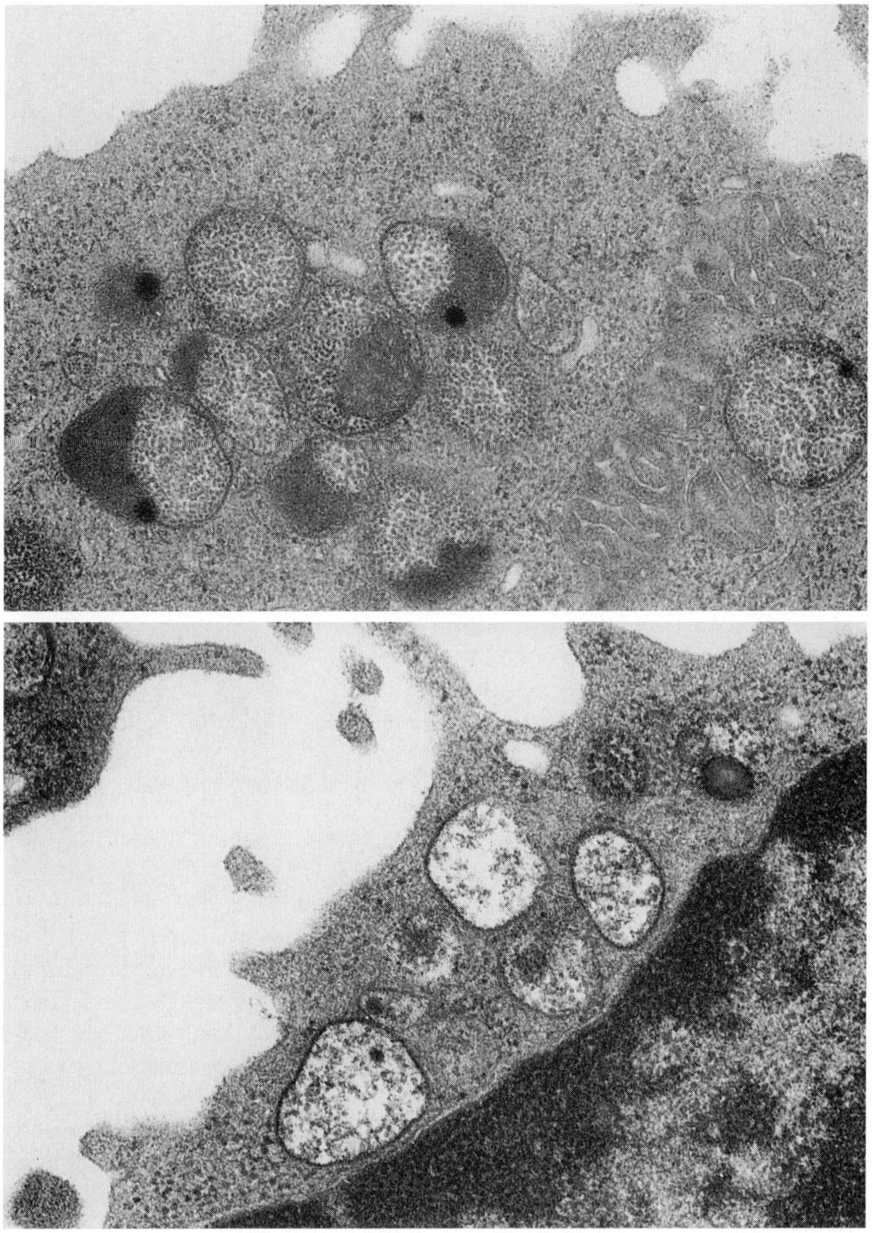

**Fig. 14-25.** Juvenile type II glycogenosis. 17-year-old girl, acid maltase deficiency. Circulating lymphocytes: **A**, Membrane-bound lysosomes contain granular matrix and particulate glycogen. **B**, In this lymphocyte, the membrane-bound lysosomes are largely vacuolar. (**A**, ×68,400; **B**, ×66,500.)

differ from that of other tissues, but the procedures pose additional difficulties because of: (1) smallness of the sample, especially when dealing with circulating fetal blood cells (a microtechnique has been employed requiring only 50 $\mu$l of fetal blood)[117] and (2) the time factor.

Electron microscopic embedding techniques are often modified for fast diagnostic study. Finally, if the suspected disease is confirmed, and if termination of the pregnancy is requested by the parents, this must occur within a limited period of time. Therefore, diagnostic electron microscopy of prenatal tissues may considerably disrupt the normal routine flow of laboratory work.

Only very few NDIC can be diagnosed prenatally by morphologic methods. However, lysosomal enzyme deficiencies, always recognized by biochemical analysis of fetal cells, may require morphologic confirmation should biochemical data be equivocal. Apart from these disorders, only NCL, Chediak-Higashi syndrome,[120] and possibly infantile neuroaxonal dystrophy can be recognized in tissues obtained before birth.

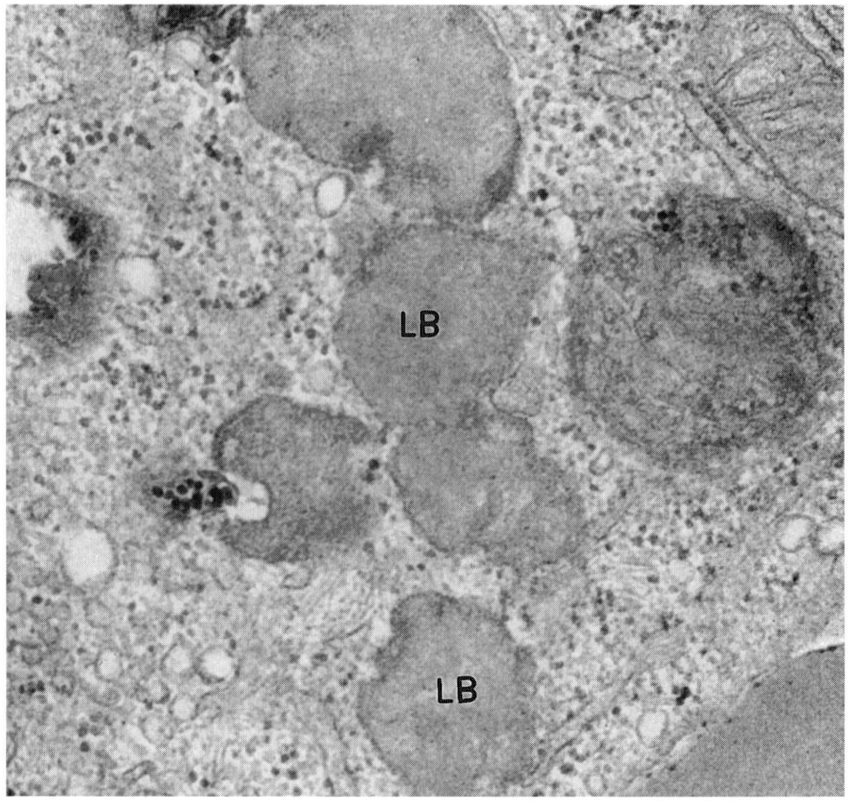


**Fig. 14-26.** Prenatal electron microscopic diagnosis. Several granular lipopigment bodies (*LB*) in an endothelial cell of a stromal chorion blood vessel. Fetal infantile neuronal ceroid-lipofuscinosis. (×63,800.)

Chorionic tissue is usually obtained at the ninth to eleventh week of gestation. At that time, granular lipopigments of infantile NCL may be present in endothelial cells (Fig. 14-26), but not in other chorionic cells.[86,161] Late-infantile form of NCL has not been recognized in chorionic tissue. Other lysosomal diseases, usually of the vacuolar type, may manifest themselves not only in endothelial cells but also in fibroblasts and trophoblasts of chorionic villi. These lysosomal disorders include type II glycogenosis.[120]

Uncultured amniotic cells, usually collected several weeks after a chorionic biopsy, may show curvilinear bodies typical of late-infantile NCL.[40,130,131] Granular lipopigments of infantile NCL may be present in amniotic cells.

Juvenile NCL has been documented by electron microscopy, in chorion,[144a] and in trophoblasts.[43] Genetic markers, for infantile and juvenile NCL, associated with the respective abnormal genes on chromosomes 1 and 16, may support or provide the diagnosis.[190,193]

If NCL is not recognized after the study of chorionic tissue and amniocytes, examination of circulating fetal lymphocytes is warranted because NCL lipopigments have been documented in fetal lymphocytes.[40] This approach has been attempted in juvenile NCL, including skin biopsy, but such evaluation has resulted in completely negative findings.[116] It is not known whether lysosomal vacuoles occur in fetal circulating lymphocytes in juvenile NCL. Finally, fetal skin and other tissues may be biopsied to document prenatal NCL,[40] but that procedure has not been successful. Lysosomal vacuoles of $GM_1$-gangliosidosis have been documented in fetal circulating lymphocytes.[120] Lysosomal diseases marked by lysosomal vacuoles, such as sialic acid disease, also may be demonstrated in chorionic cells.[120]

Because infantile neuroaxonal dystrophy (INAD) is a condition characterized by typically enlarged terminal axons, including those in skin, prenatal diagnosis by fetal skin biopsy is possible. Unmyelinated nerves are present in skin at 21 weeks' gestation. However, successful prenatal diagnosis of INAD has not been reported. Another condition that can be prenatally diagnosed by skin biopsy is Lafora disease; this is because sweat gland epithelial cells harbor typical nonmembrane-bound fibrillar inclusions. Eccrine sweat glands, however, are not fully developed before weeks 24 to 26 of gestation.[7]

Any neurodegenerative disease diagnosed prenatally that results in termination of the pregnancy requires confirmation of the diagnosis in the aborted tissues. This has been accomplished in cases of infantile NCL[71,161] and late-infantile NCL,[40] but apparently not in juvenile NCL.[119] Granular lipopigments of infantile NCL have been documented in cerebellar tissue,[161] liver,[71] and skeletal muscle,[86] and curvilinear profiles of late-infantile NCL have been seen in several tissues.[40]

Numerous lysosomal diseases have been morphologically documented in aborted fetal tissues, confirming previous biochemical analyses by demonstrating the disease-specific lysosomal inclusions, e.g., globoid cell[158] and metachromatic[201] leukodystrophies, mucolipidosis II,[12] and mucopolysaccharidosis II.[141]

## EXTRACEREBRAL BIOPSY IN ADULT NEURODEGENERATIVE AND NEUROMETABOLIC DISEASES

Although this chapter deals with pediatric neurodegenerative and neurometabolic diseases, a brief note concerning similar disorders in adults and their diagnosis by extracerebral biopsy may be germane. Neurodegenerative and neurometabolic disorders of adults that are diagnosable by biopsy fall into three categories:

(1) Adult forms that express structural abnormalities similar to their equivalent childhood forms, e.g., type II glycogenosis, certain mucopolysaccharidoses, and others. Included in this category are patients whose disorder began in childhood, but in whom the disease diagnosis had been delayed.

(2) Adult forms of NDIC have extracerebral morphologic expressions different from those of their childhood counterparts. Little information is available concerning the spectrum of organs amenable to biopsy. Late-onset $GM_2$-gangliosidosis has been recognized as a form of spinal muscular atrophy, biopsy findings but the spinal cord are not available. Another such disorder is adult neuronal ceroid-lipofuscinosis (Kufs' disease). This condition appears to be clinically and morphologically different from the childhood forms, e.g., the retinal atrophy of childhood NCL is not a feature of adult NCL. Accretion of extracerebral NCL-specific lipopigments in adult NCL has been occasionally reported.[17,192,206] The spectrum of lipopigments in adult NCL is largely unknown; this includes the lipopigments of aging and those of nonspecific disorders, including several primary diseases of the skin. The appearance of fingerprint profiles, indistinguishable from those encountered in childhood NCL, may pose a diagnostic dilemma in a demented patient.[57] Recognizing fingerprint profiles in sweat gland epithelial cells alone has not been considered sufficient evidence of NCL because the same profiles also may occur in MELAS (mitochondrial encephalopathy, lactic acidosis, and stroke) (Carpenter, personal communication, 1993). Morphologic evidence of noninfantile neuroaxonal dystrophies outside the CNS, has been encountered in a few individuals.[124]

(3) The third category of conditions includes adult neurodegenerative and neurometabolic disorders that have no childhood counterpart, e.g., Huntington chorea, Parkinson disease, Alzheimer disease, and others. Diagnostic morphologic features specific of those disorders have not been encountered in any of them. "CADASIL" (cerebral autosomal-dominant arteriopathy with subcortical infarcts and leukoencephalopathy) may be identified through granular deposits in the tunica media of vessels of the sural nerve.[167] Similar mural vascular deposits may be observed in other easily accessible extracerebral tissues, e.g., skin and skeletal muscle (Fig. 14-27).

## PITFALLS IN DIAGNOSTIC EVALUATION

The misdiagnosis of NDIC in biopsied tissue may have several grave consequences: delaying the final diagnosis; making the diagnosis at autopsy only; inadequate family counseling; lack of genetic counseling and, worst of all, omission of the prenatal diagnosis.

One cause of misdiagnosis is that the disease does not manifest morphologically in the biopsied and examined tissue, as occurs with Gaucher disease in skin and mitochondrial encephalomyopathies in circulating lymphocytes. Second, a disease that usually manifests itself in biopsied tissue may not be recognizable because the patient is too young or the biopsied sample too small. NCL may not be diagnosed in 15% of first skin biopsies.[206] Infantile neuroaxonal dystrophy falls in the same category. Another cause of misdiagnosis may be insufficient contrast of fixed circulating lymphocytes.

False-positive results may be equally disastrous because they delay a correct diagnosis. The most dire consequence, false prenatal diagnosis, may cause unnecessary anxiety or may cause a delay or omission of therapy.

There are two types of false-positive results. (1) Abnormal nonspecific non-NDIC-related structures, such as undulating tubules or tubuloreticular structures[91,92,128,151] may be misinterpreted. There may be confusion with physiologic cellular constituents,[174] such as certain inclusions in epithelial cells of sweat gland ducts (Fig. 14-1), Gall bodies (Fig. 14-28, *B*) parallel tubular arrays[25] (Fig. 14-28, *A*), and other inclusions (Figs. 14-29, 14-30). Even fragments of a mitotic figure (Fig. 14-28, *C*) in circulating lymphocytes and cell-specific inclusions in mast cells (Fig. 14-1, *C*) have been confused with fingerprint bodies and thus mistaken for neuronal ceroid-lipofuscinosis. Nonspecific lysosomal inclusions, e.g., in mucosal macrophages of a rectal biopsy and pi granules in Schwann cells of myelinated axons often closely resemble lamellar inclusions of sphingolipidoses, particularly of metachromatic leukodystrophy.

Abnormal inclusions, often of lysosomal nature, can be drug-induced rather than disease-related. Certain amphiphilic cationic psychotropic drugs[56] may form abnormal lysosomal residual bodies in a variety of tis-

A

B

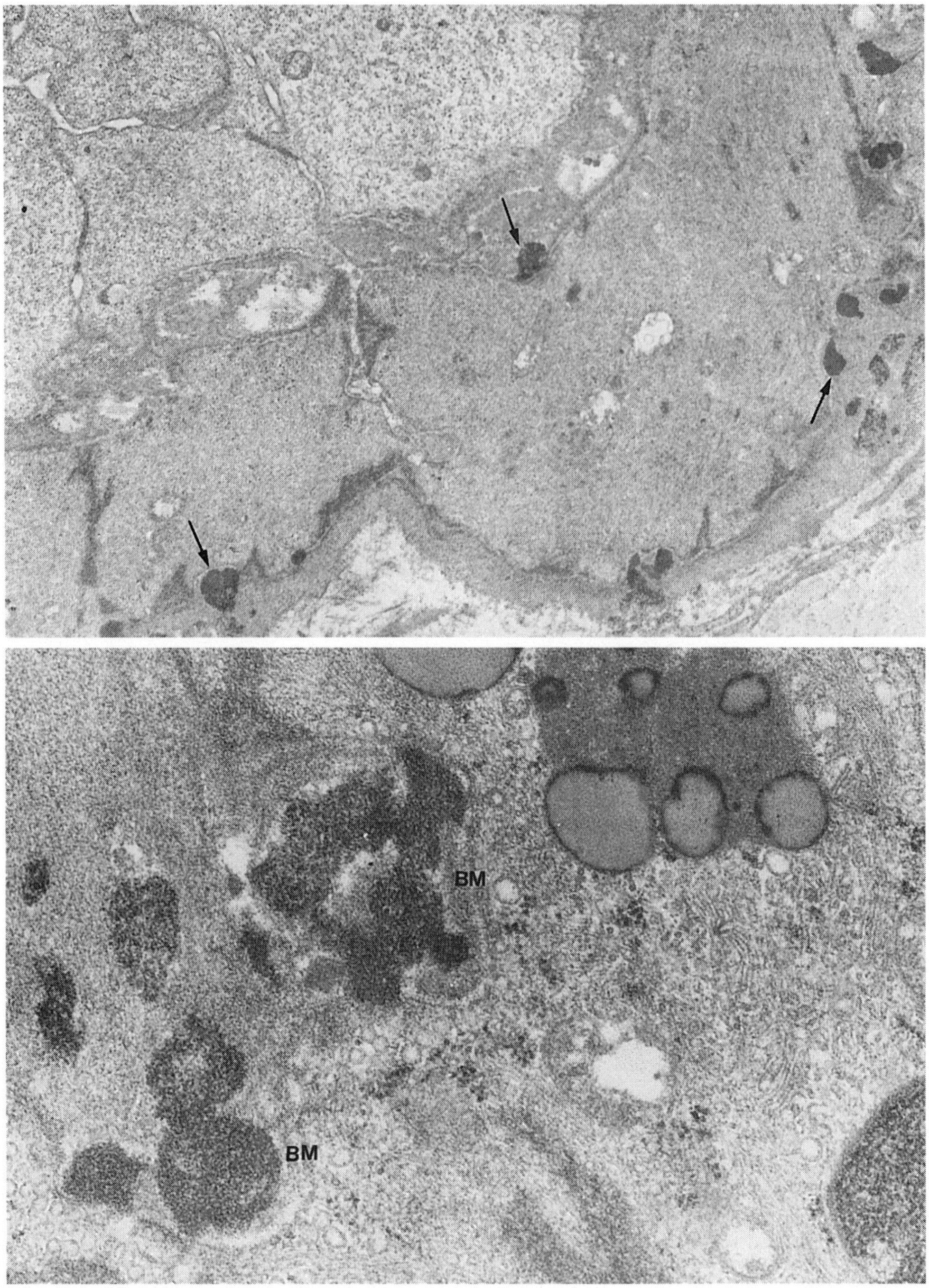


**Fig. 14-27.** Cerebral autosomal-dominant arteriopathy with subcortical infarcts and leukoencephalopathy. 53-year-old woman whose sister, father, and paternal grandfather are also said to be affected. Skeletal muscle. **A**, Numerous electron-dense granular aggregates within the basement membrane of smooth muscle cells (*arrows*). **B**, At higher magnification, both the granularity of the deposits and their relation to the basement membrane (*BM*) are apparent. (**A**, 11,914; **B**, ×44,550.)

A

B

C

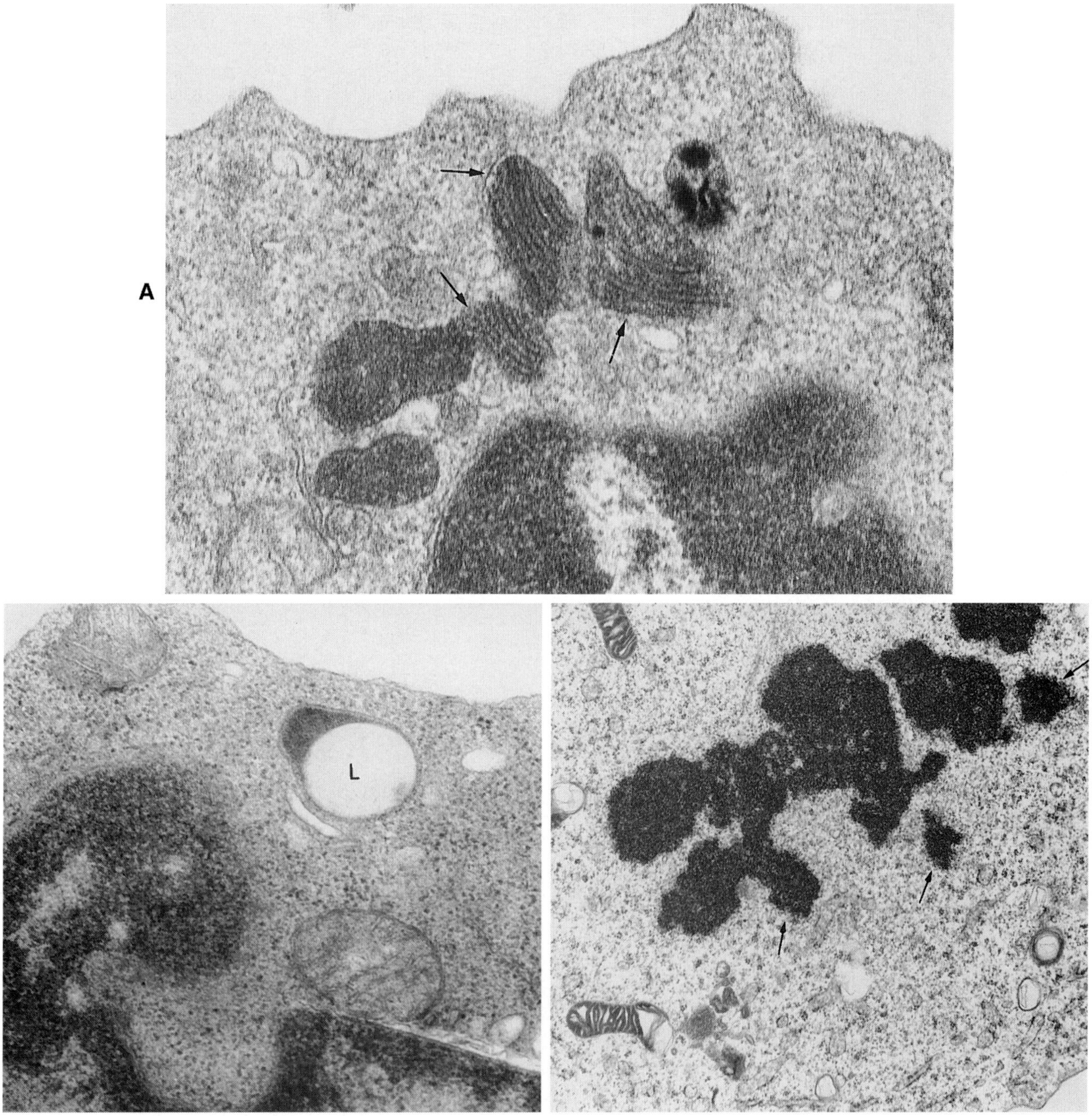


**Fig. 14-28.** Nonspecific inclusions in circulating lymphocytes. **A**, Parallel tubular assays, membrane-bound (*arrows*), no evidence of lysosomal storage. **B**, A Gall body consists of a lipid (*L*) component and a peripheral granular component, both membrane-bound. **C**, Nuclear fragments (*arrows*) of a mitotic figure. (**A**, 200,000; **B**, ×63,800; **C**, ×23,660.)

sues and cells. Chloroquine induces curvilinear bodies.[11] Although many reports are based on experimental studies, drug-induced lysosomal residual bodies occasionally may be encountered in human biopsy specimens (Fig. 14-31, *A*). The entire spectrum of both ultrastructure and distribution of drug-induced inclusions is not known. Drugs that induce formation of lysosomal residual bodies often are prescribed over many years for chronic diseases; since most NDIC also are chronic disorders, often requiring psychotropic medication, the occurrence of drug-related abnormal inclusions in biopsy specimens may create another reasons for misinterpretation and misdiagnosis.

Spurious vacuolation (Fig. 14-31, *B*) may develop secondary to delayed fixation. This usually affects mitochondria, but may be seen in other structures,

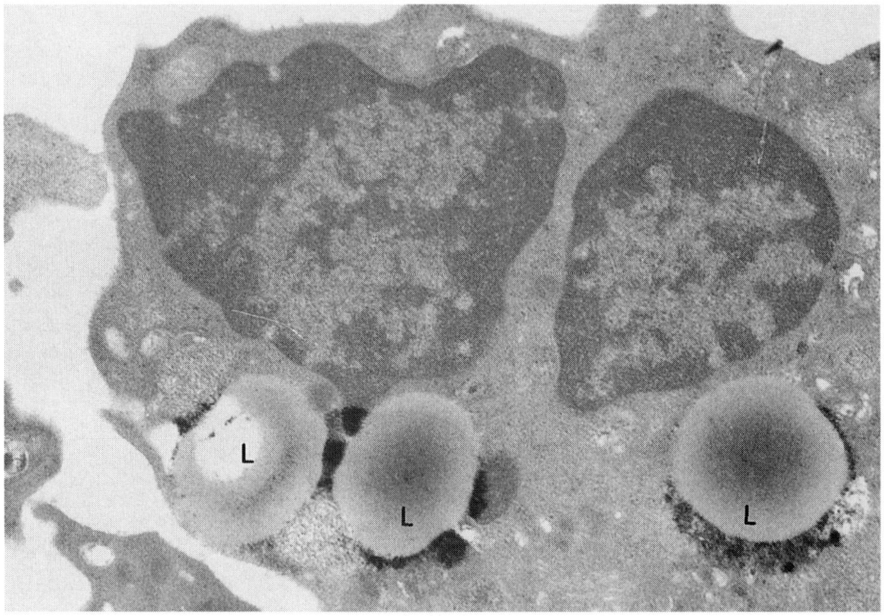

**Fig. 14-29.** Specific, but nonlysosomal inclusions. Several lipid (*L*) droplets in a circulating lymphocyte; Jordan anomaly associated with lipid myopathy. (×27,360.)

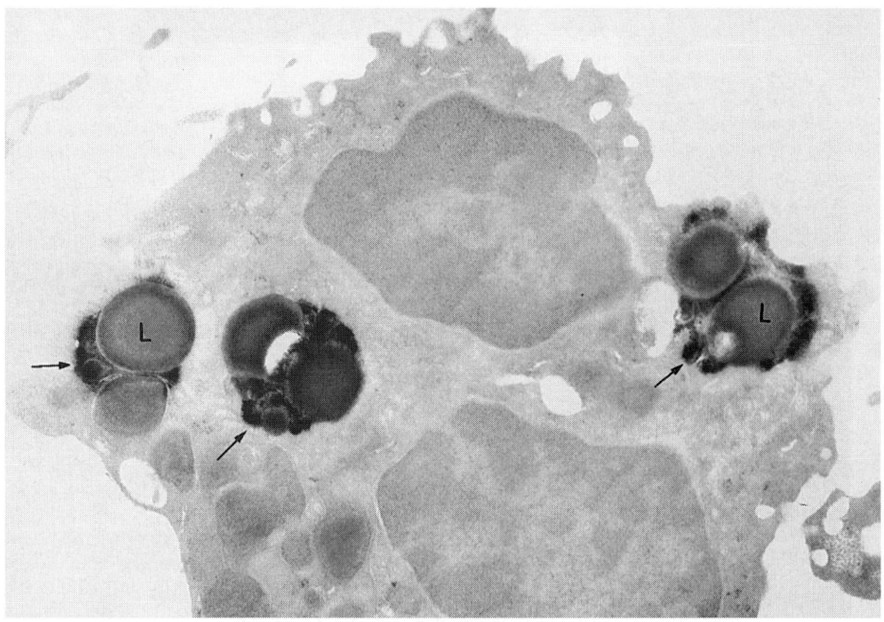

**Fig. 14-30.** Unknown inclusions. Black pigment inclusions (*arrows*) of unknown connotation (in a black person) containing some very dark lipid (*L*) droplets. (×32,400.)

e.g., the endoplasmic reticulum, the Golgi apparatus, or the nuclear envelope. Such artificial swelling of preexisting organelles may be mistaken for true vacuolation lysosomal. The remnants of ruptured cristae vacuolation usually help the recognition of swollen mitochondria. This is one of the reasons why I consider a diagnostic workup of an NDIC (within the context of this chapter) incomplete without proper electron microscopic examination.

## NON-ELECTRON MICROSCOPIC TECHNIQUES

It has been made abundantly clear that electron microscopy is the main technique employed in extracerebral (and cerebral) biopsy examination in NDIC.[158a] The dominance of the electron microscope has led to the general abandonment of conventional histologic techniques. Electron microscopy emphasizes not only precise identification of abnormal structures, but also their submicroscopic size. This renders the histologic study almost obsolete. Conventional histology may be occasionally helpful, e.g., allowing recognition of a neuron that has ballooned from lysosomal neuronal storage, or permitting identification of a large inclusion in neuronal intranuclear hyaline inclusion disease (NIHID).

Enzyme histochemistry is usually applied to muscle specimens, and may be useful when dealing with rag-

A

B

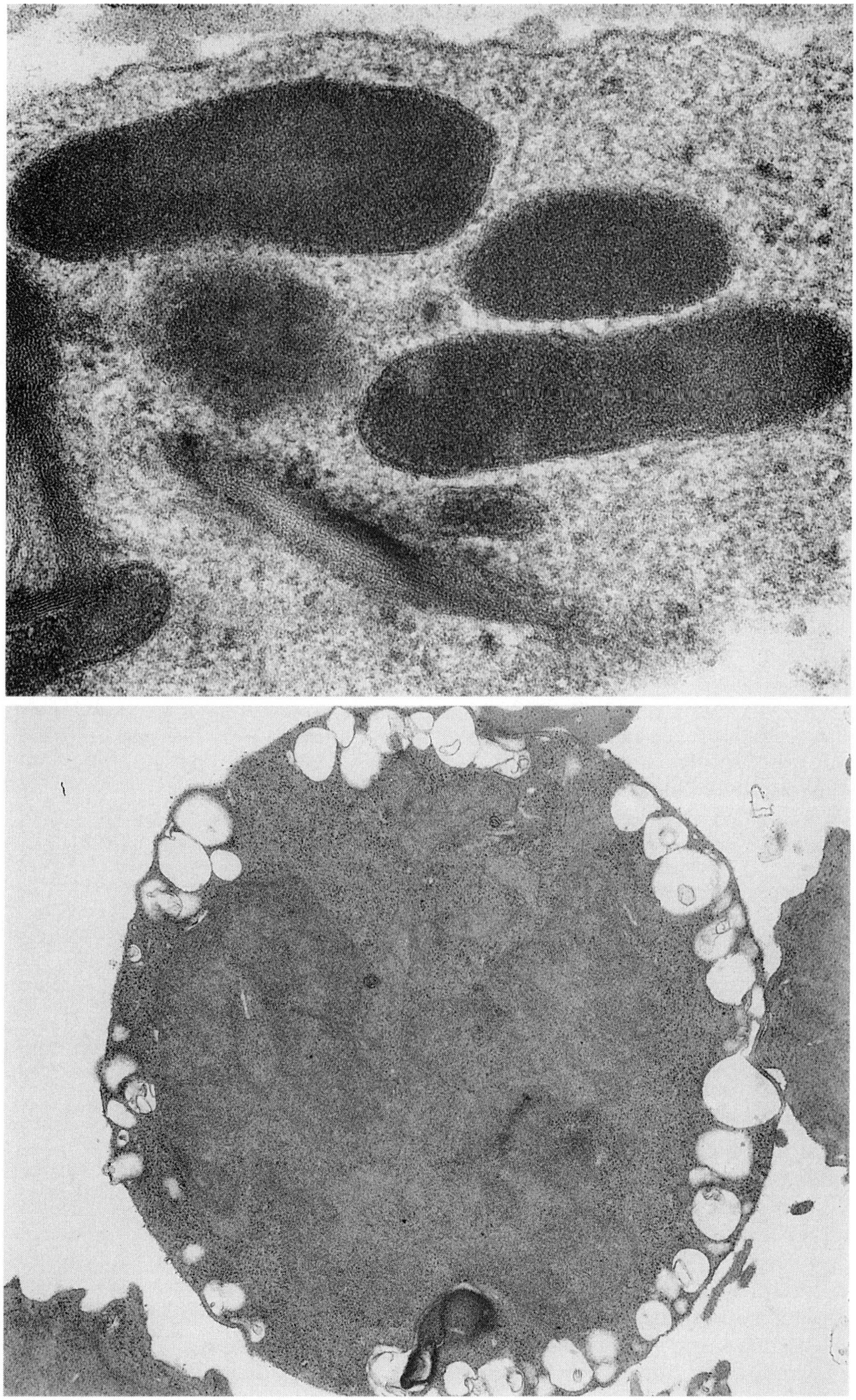

**Fig. 14-31. A**, Drug-induced lysosomal storage. Several membrane-bound irregular inclusions due to amiodarone treatment. **B**, Artifacts. Numerous vacuoles arranged in a beadlike peripheral fashion of a circulating lymphocyte; note little contrast of cytologic structures. (**A**, 119,000; **B**, ×22,750.)

ged red fibers of encephalomyopathies or certain lysosomal diseases that manifest in muscle by increased activity of the lysosomal marker enzyme acid phosphatase, type II glycogenosis, the neuronal ceroid-lipofuscinoses, vitamin E deficiency, and mucolipidosis IV. Autofluorescence of certain lysosomal lipopigments, again seen in NCL and vitamin E deficiency, is another characteristic but minimally helpful application of fluorescence microscopy. Immunohistochemistry has not gained a role in the diagnostic examination of NDIC although the lack of cytochrome-C oxidase protein, elucidated by negative antibody reaction in cytochrome-C oxidase deficiency has been documented. Antibodies against lipopigments in NCL, the subunit C in late-infantile and juvenile NCL, and other antibodies against the saponins in infantile NCL, have been reported. In view of the not completely clarified nosologic specificity of the subunit C and the saponins in NCL, widespread diagnostic application of these antibodies may never develop.

As tissue must be embedded in resins for electron microscopy, usually Epon or Araldite, semithin sections can serve only to select areas suitable for ultrathin sections; however, they also may indicate morphologic lesions to be confirmed later by electron microscopy, e.g., lysosomal vacuolation, enlarged or ballooned neurons in lysosomal neuronal storage, giant axons, neuroaxonal dystrophic spheroids, and polyglucosan bodies. Thus, of the non-electron microscopic techniques, histology of plastic embedded material seems to be the most rewarding of those mentioned.

### Preparation of the Biopsy Specimens and Artifacts

Evaluation of 1-$\mu$m plastic sections can be useful for identifying target tissues and target cell types, rather than for identifying lesions. Often a lack of contrast makes recognition of avacuolar lysosomal inclusions impossible. Thus, the physician doing the biopsy must be informed or aware of the special features of electron microscopy. The smallness of the specimens may mean that a second sample is needed.

When enzyme histochemistry of muscle tissue is required, proper preparation of tissue becomes even more important. When prenatal diagnosis is desired, the time factor in preparation and tissue examination may be crucial. Application of shortened embedding techniques for electron microscopy may be necessary to speed up tissue preparation. Hence, the physician who requests an electron microscopic study of his patient's circulating lymphocytes ought to insure that suitable facilities for preparation are available at or around the site and time of blood retrieval.

Lymphocytes should be isolated before fixation and right after removal of noncoagulated blood; heparinized blood should not be sent across considerable distances. Nonisolated, nonfixed lymphocytes become autolysed; nonisolated fixed lymphocytes cannot be isolated after fixation.

### Additional Ancillary Nonmorphologic Techniques to Arrive at a Correct Final Diagnosis

In addition to the complete clinical investigation, imaging studies form part of a thorough diagnostic work-up and can provide important diagnostic clues. Radiographs of bones in MPS and related disorders, computed tomography, and magnetic resonance imaging in primary brain disorders, as well as sonography are all useful. Electrophysiology studies, e.g., evoked potentials, nerve conduction studies, and electromyography, are especially helpful in evaluating disease of the peripheral nervous system. Electroretinography is useful in retinopathies, a component of as well as NCL in other NDIC. Biochemical studies are indispensable for recognizing the neurometabolic conditions among NDIC, the lysosomal, mitochondrial, and peroxisomal disorders. Recent molecular genetic techniques may reveal defects in both the mitochondrial and nuclear genomes, such as deletions of the mitochondrial genome in mitochondrial encephalomyopathies or mutations in lysosomal diseases. Thus, the triad of morphology, biochemistry, and genetics forms the basis of a correct and final diagnosis of an NDIC. However, the individual components of this triad differ in diagnostic significance according to the individual NDIC clinically suspected, i.e., morphology in nonmetabolic NDIC, biochemistry in neurometabolic NDIC, and genetics in mitochondrial encephalomyopathies.

## ACKNOWLEDGMENTS

I am grateful for substantial collaboration by Mrs. Irene Warlo (electron microscopy), Mr. Walter Meffer (photography), and Mrs. Astrid Wöber (editorial assistance).

Support by the European Commission (Contract No. BMH4–CT95–0563) is also gratefully acknowledged.

## REFERENCES

1. Adachi M, Volk BW, Schneck L, and Torii J: Fine structure of the myenteric plexus in various lipidoses, Arch Pathol 87:228-241, 1969.
2. Adachi M, Schneck L, and Volk BW: Progress in investigations of sphingolipidoses, Acta Neuropathol (Berl) 43:1-18, 1978.
3. Andermann F, Fawcett J, Owen HF: The role of rectal biopsy in neuropathological diagnosis, Trans Am Neurol Assoc 89:40-44, 1964.
4. Anderson JC, and others: Outcome of 1500 consecutive chorionic villus samplings, Med J Aust 155:657-661, 1991.
5. Anton-Lamprecht I, and others: Prenatal diagnosis of epidermolysis bullosa dystrophica Hallopeau-Siemens with electron microscopy of fetal skin, Lancet 2:1077-1081, 1981.
6. Anton-Lamprecht I: Genetically induced abnormalities of epidermal differentiation and ultrastructure in ichthyoses and epidermolyses: pathologenesis, heterogeneity, fetal manifestation, and prenatal diagnosis, J Invest Dermatol 81:149-155, 1983.

7. Anton-Lamprecht I, Arnold M-L, and Holbrook KA: Methodology in sampling of fetal skin and pitfalls in the interpretation of fetal skin biopsy specimens, Semin Dermatol 3:203-215, 1984.
8. Arsénio-Nunes ML, and Goutières F: Diagnosis of infantile neuroaxonal dystrophy by conjunctival biopsy, J Neurol Neurosurg Psychiatry 41:511-515, 1978.
9. Arsénio-Nunes ML, Goutières F, and Aicardi J: An ultramicroscopic study of skin and conjunctival biopsies in chronic neurological disorders of childhood, Ann Neurol 9:163-173, 1981.
10. Arsénio-Nunes ML, and Goutières F: Morphological diagnosis of Niemann-Pick disease type C by skin and conjunctival biopsies, Acta Neuropathol (Berl) Suppl VII:204-207, 1981.
11. August C, and others: Histological and ultrastructural findings in chloroquine-induced cardiomyopathy, J Mol Med 73:73-77, 1995.
12. Aula P, and others: Prenatal diagnosis and fetal pathology of I-cell disease (mucolipidosis type II). J Pediatr 87:221-226, 1975.
13. Bakharev VA, and others: Fetal skin biopsy in prenatal diagnosis of some genodermatoses, Prenat Diagn 10:1-12, 1990.
14. Begeer JH, and others: Infantile neuroaxonal dystrophy and giant axonal neuropathy: are they related? Ann Neurol 6:540-548, 1979.
15. Belichenko PV, Oldfors A, Hagberg B, and Dahlström A: Rett syndrome: 3-D confocal microscopy of cortical pyramidal dendrites and afferents, Neuro Report 5:1509-1513, 1994.
16. Beratis NG, Varvarigou-Frimas A, Beratis S, and Sklower SL: Angiokeratoma corporis diffusum in $GM_1$ gangliosidosis, Type 1, Clin Genet 36:59-64, 1989.
17. Berkovic SF, and others: Kufs' disease: a critical reappraisal, Brain 111:27-62, 1988.
18. Besley GTN, Young EP, Fensom AH, and Cooper A: First trimester diagnosis of inherited metabolic disease: experience in the UK, J Inher Metab Dis 14:128-133, 1991.
19. Bioulac P, Mercier M, Beylot C, and Fontan D: The diagnosis of mucopolysaccharidoses by electron microscopy of skin biopsies, J Cutan Pathol 2:179-190, 1975.
20. Bodian M, and Lake BD: The rectal approach to neuropathology, Br J Surg 50:702-714, 1963.
21. Brett EM, and Berry CL: Value of rectal biopsy in paediatric neurology: report of 165 biopsies, Br Med J 3:400-403, 1967.
22. Brett EM, and others: Late onset $GM_2$-gangliosidosis, Arch Dis Child 48:775–785, 1973.
23. Brett EM, and Lake BD: Reassessment of rectal approach to neuropathology in childhood, Arch Dis Child 50:753-762, 1975.
24. Brück W, Goebel HH, and Dienes P: B and T lymphocytes are affected in lysosomal disorders—an immunoelectron microscopic study, Neuropathol Appl Neurobiol 17:219-222, 1991.
25. Brunning RD, and Parkin J: Ultrastructural studies of parallel tubular arrays in human lymphocytes, Am J Pathol 78:59-70, 1975.
26. Bürrig KF, Schwendemann G, and Löhler J: Lack of structural abnormalities in lymphocytes from heterozygotes of juvenile type of generalized ceroilipofuscinosis. A light and electron microscopic study, Neuropediatrics 13:216-218, 1982.
27. Burck U, and others: Ultrastructural pathology of skin biopsy and fibroblast enzyme studies in a case of $GM_2$-gangliosidosis with deficient hexosaminidase A and thermolabile hexosaminidase B, Neuropädiatrie 11:161-176, 1980.
28. Burck U, and others: Neuromyopathy and vitamine E deficiency in man, Neuropediatrics 12:267-278, 1981.
29. Burck U, and others: A case of lipogranulomatosis Farber: some clinical and ultrastructural aspects, Eur J Pediatr 143:203-208, 1985.
30. Busard HLSM, and others: Lafora's disease, Arch Neurol 43: 296-299, 1986.
31. Busard HLSM, and others: Axilla skin biopsy: a reliable test for the diagnosis of Lafora's disease, Ann Neurol 21:599-601, 1987.
32. Butzer JF, Schochet SS Jr, and Bell WE: Infantile neuroaxonal dystrophy. (An electron microscopic study of a case clinically resembling neuronal ceroidlipofuscinosis.) Acta Neuropathol (Berl) 31:35-43, 1975.
33. Cable WJL, Dvorak AM, Osage JE, and Kolodny EH: Fabry disease: significance of ultrastructural localization of lipid inclusions in dermal nerves, Neurology 32:347-353, 1982.
34. Carpenter S: Skin biopsy for diagnosis of hereditary neurologic metabolic disease, Arch Dermatol 123:1618-1621, 1987.
35. Carpenter S, and Karpati G: Sweat gland duct cells in Lafora disease: diagnosis by skin biopsy, Neurology 31:1564-1568, 1981.
36. Carpenter S, and Karpati G: Lysosomal storage in human skeletal muscle, Hum Pathol 17:683-703, 1986.
37. Carpenter S, and others: Lafora's disease: peroxisomal storage in skeletal muscle, Neurology 24:531-538, 1974.
38. Carpenter S, and others: The ultrastructural characteristics of the abnormal cytosomes in Batten-Kufs' disease, Brain 100:137-156, 1977.
39. Ceuterick C, and Martin JJ: Electron microscopic features of skin in neurometabolic disorders, J Neurol Sci 112:15-29, 1992.
40. Chow CW, Borg J, Billson VR, and Lake BD: Fetal tissue involvement in the late infantile type of neuronal ceroid lipofuscinosis, Prenat Diagn 13:833-841, 1993.
41. Cibis GW, Harris DJ, Chapman AL, and Tripathi RC: Mucolipidosis I, Arch Ophthalmol 101:933-939, 1983.
42. Conradi NG, and others: Neuropathology of the Norrbottnian type of Gaucher disease, Acta Neuropathol (Berl) 65:99-109, 1984.
43. Conradi NG, and others: First-trimester diagnosis of juvenile neuronal ceroid lipofuscinosis by demonstration of fingerprint inclusions in chorionic villi, Prenat Diagn 9:283-287, 1989.
44. Conradi N, and others: Liver pathology in the carbohydrate-deficient glycoprotein syndrome, Acta Paediatr Scand Suppl 375:50-54, 1991.
45. Crisci C, and others: Is conjunctival biopsy useful for diagnosis of neuroaxonal dystrophy? Ann Neurol 26:691, 1989.
46. Danon MJ, and others: Lysosomal glycogen storage disease with normal acid maltase, Neurology 31:51-57, 1981.
47. de Baecque C: Diagnosis of neuronal ceroid lipofuscinosis by electron microscopy of urinary sediment, N Engl J Med 292: 1408, 1975.
48. de Baecque CM, Pollack MA, and Suzuki K: Late infantile neuronal storage disease with curvilinear bodies, Arch Pathol Lab Med 100:139-144, 1976.
49. De Craemer D, and others: Very large peroxisomes in distinct peroxisomal disorders (rhizomelic chondrodysplasia punctata and acyl-CoA oxidase deficiency): novel data, Virchows Arch [A] 419:523-525, 1991.
50. de Kremer RD, and others: Mucopolysaccharidosis type VII ($\beta$-glucuronidase deficiency): a chronic variant with an oligosymptomatic severe skeletal dysplasia, Am J Med Genet 44:145-152, 1992.
51. Dieler R, Schröder JM, and Reddemann K: Electron-dense lipidic capillary deposits in Rett syndrome, Acta Neuropathol (Berl) 79:573-578, 1990.
52. Dolman CL: Diagnosis of neurometabolic disorders by examination of skin biopsies and lymphocytes, Diagn Pathol 1:82-97, 1984.
53. Dolman CL, MacLeod PM, and Chang E: Skin punch biopsies and lymphocytes in the diagnosis of lipidoses, J Can Neurol Sci 2:67-73, 1975.
54. Dolman CL, MacLeod PM, and Chang E: Fine structure of cutaneous nerves in ganglioside storage disease, J Neurol Neurosurg Psychiatry 40:588-594, 1977.
55. Dolman CL, McLeod PM, and Chang EC: Lymphocytes and urine in ceroid lipofuscinosis, Arch Pathol Lab Med 104:487-490, 1980.

56. Drenckhahn D, and Lüllmann-Rauch R: Experimental myopathy induced by amphiphilic cationic compounds including several psychotropic drugs, Neuroscience 4:549-562, 1979.
57. Dyken P, and Krawiecki N: Neurodegenerative diseases of infancy and childhood, Ann Neurol 13:351-364, 1983.
58. Elleder M: Eccrine gland involvement in Krabbe's disease, Virchows Arch A 421:351-354, 1992.
59. Elleder M, and others: An atypical ultrastructural pattern in Fabry's disease: a study on its nature and incidence in 7 cases, Ultrastruct Pathol 14:467-474, 1990.
60. Ferrer I, and others: Diagnosis of infantile neuro-axonal dystrophy by conjunctival biopsy, Neuropediatrics 14:53-55, 1983.
61. Finikiotis G, Callen D, Langlois SLeP, and Jones WR: Prenatal diagnosis. (A preliminary study of first-trimester chorionic villous biopsy.) Med J Aust 142:299-300, 1985.
62. Folkerth RD, and others: Mucolipidosis IV: morphology and histochemistry of an autopsy case, J Neuropathol Exp Neurol 54:154-164, 1995.
63. Fukuhara N, Suzuki M, Fujita N, and Tsubaki T: Fabry's disease on the mechanism of the peripheral nerve involvement, Acta Neuropathol (Berl) 33:9-21, 1975.
64. Gadoth N, O'Croinin P, and Butler IJ: Bone marrow in the Batten-Vogt syndrome, J Neurol Sci 25:197-203, 1975.
65. Garen PD, Powers JM, Young GF, and Lee V: Neuronal intranuclear hyaline inclusion disease in a nine year old, Acta Neuropathol (Berl) 70:327-332, 1986.
66. Gebhart W, Lassmann H, and Niebauer G: Demonstration of specific storage material within cutaneous nerves in metachromatic leukodystrophy, J Cutan Pathol 5:5-14, 1978.
67. Gilbert EF, and others: Generalized gangliosidosis type II (juvenile $GM_1$ gangliosidosis), Z Kinderheilk 120:151-180, 1975.
68. Gilman S, and Barrett RE: Hallervorden-Spatz disease and infantile neuroaxonal dystrophy, J Neurol Sci 19:189-205, 1973.
69. Goebel HH: Fingerprint inclusions in non-vacuolated lymphocytes in juvenile neuronal ceroid-lipofuscinosis, Clin Neuropathol 4:210-213, 1985.
70. Goebel HH: Neuronal ceroid-lipofuscinoses: the current status, Brain Dev 14:203-211, 1992.
71. Goebel HH: Prenatal ultrastructural diagnosis in the neuronal ceroid-lipofuscinoses, Pathol Res Pract 190:728-733, 1994.
72. Goebel HH, and Warlo I: Biopsy studies in neurodegenerative diseases of childhood: part I, Barrow Neurological Institute Quarterly 6: No 1, 19-27, 1990.
73. Goebel HH, and Warlo I: Biopsy studies in neurodegenerative diseases of childhood: part II, Barrow Neurological Institute Quarterly 6: No 2, 24-30, 1990.
74. Goebel HH, Zeman W, and Pilz H: Significance of muscle biopsies in neuronal ceroid-lipofuscinoses, J Neurol Neurosurg Psychiatry 38:985-993, 1975.
75. Goebel HH, Zeman W, and Pilz H: Ultrastructural investigations of peripheral nerves in neuronal ceroid-lipofuscinosis, J Neurol 213:295-303, 1976.
76. Goebel HH, Kohlschütter A, and Schulte FJ: Rectal biopsy findings in infantile neuroaxonal dystrophy, Neuropediatrics 11: 388-392, 1980.
77. Goebel HH, Veit S, and Dyck PJ: Confirmation of virtual unmyelinated fiber absence in hereditary sensory neuropathy type IV, J Neuropathol Exp Neurol 39:670-675, 1980.
78. Goebel HH, Bode G, Caesar R, and Kohlschütter A: Bulbar palsy with Rosenthal fiber formation in the medulla of a 15-year-old girl. Localized form of Alexander's disease? Neuropediatrics 12:382-404, 1981.
79. Goebel HH, and others: Fingerprint profiles in lymphocytic vacuoles of mucopolysaccharidoses I-H, III-A, and III-B, Acta Neuropathol (Berl) 55:247-249, 1981.
80. Goebel HH, Kohlschütter A, and Lenard HG: Morphologic and chemical biopsy findings in mucolipidosis IV, Clin Neuropathol 1:73-82, 1982.
81. Goebel HH, and others: Lafora's disease: biopsy and autopsy studies, Clin Neuropathol 7:167, 1988 (abstract).
82. Goebel HH, and others: Sural nerve biopsy studies in Leigh's subacute necrotizing encephalomyelopathy, Muscle Nerve 9: 165-173, 1986.
83. Goebel HH, Stolte G, Kustermann-Kuhn B, and Harzer K: B1-variant of $GM_2$-gangliosidosis in a 12-year-old patient, Pediatr Res 25:89-93, 1989.
84. Goebel HH, and others: Late-onset globoid cell leukodystrophy: unusual ultrastructural pathology and subtotal $\beta$-galactocerebrosidase deficiency, J Child Neurol 5:299-307, 1990.
85. Goebel HH, Kimura S, Harzer K, and Klein H: Ultrastructural pathology of eccrine sweat gland epithelial cells in globoid cell leukodystrophy, J Child Neurol 8:171-174, 1993.
86. Goebel HH, and others: Prenatal diagnosis of infantile neuronal ceroid-lipofuscinosis: a combined electron microscopic and molecular genetic approach, Brain Dev 17:83-88, 1995.
87. Goebel HH, Warlo I, Klockgether T, and Harzer K: Significance of lipopigments with fingerprint profiles in eccrine sweat gland epithelial cells, Am J Med Genet 57:187-190, 1995.
88. Gosden CM: Amniotic fluid cell types and culture, Br Med Bull 39:348-354, 1983.
89. Goutiéres F, Mikol J, Aicardi J: Neuronal intranuclear inclusion disease in a child: diagnosis by rectal biopsy, Ann Neurol 27: 103-106, 1990.
90. Grebner EE, and Jackson LG: Prenatal diagnosis for Tay-Sachs disease using chorionic villus sampling, Prenat Diagn 5:313-320, 1985.
91. Grimley PM, Decker JL, Michelitch HJ, and Frantz MM: Abnormal structures in circulating lymphocytes from patients with systemic lupus erythematosus and related diseases, Arthritis Rheum 16:313-323, 1973.
92. Grimley PM, and others: Tubuloreticular inclusions in peripheral blood mononuclear cells related to systemic therapy with $\alpha$-interferon, Lab Invest 52:638-649, 1985.
93. Guerra WF, and others: Multiple sulfatase deficiency: clinical, neuropathological, ultrastructural and biochemical studies, J Neuropathol Exp Neurol 49:406-423, 1990.
94. Gumbinas M, Larsen M, and Mei Liu H: Peripheral neuropathy in classic Niemann-Pick disease: ultrastructure of nerves and skeletal muscles, Neurology 25:107-113, 1975.
95. Haas JE, Johnson ES, and Farrell DL: Neonatal-onset adrenoleukodystrophy in a girl, Ann Neurol 12:449-457, 1982.
96. Hahn AF, and others: Nerve biopsy findings in Niemann-Pick type II (NPC), Acta Neuropathol (Berl) 87:149-154, 1994.
97. Halperin JJ, and others: Communicating hydrocephalus and lysosomal inclusions in mannosidosis, Arch Neurol 41:777-779, 1984.
98. Hogge WA, Schonberg SA, and Golbus MS: Prenatal diagnosis by chorionic villus sampling: lessons of the first 600 cases, Prenat Diagn 5:393-400, 1985.
99. Hughes JL, and others: Pathology of hepatic peroxisomes and mitochondria in patients with peroxisomal disorders, Virchows Arch A 416:255-264, 1990.
100. Iannaccone S, and others: Early detection of skin and muscular involvement in Lafora disease, J Neurol 238:217-220, 1991.
101. Ikeda K, and Goebel HH: Ultrastructural pathology of lymphocytes in neuronal ceroid-lipofuscinoses, Brain Dev 1:285-292, 1979.
102. Ikeda K, Goebel HH, Burck U, and Kohlschütter A: Ultrastructural pathology of human lymphocytes in lysosomal disorders: a contribution to their morphological diagnosis, Eur J Pediatr 138:179-185, 1982.
103. Ikeda S, and others: Adult fucosidosis: histochemical and ultrastructural studies of rectal mucosa biopsy, Neurology 34:451-456, 1984.
104. Jaeken J, Carchon H, and Stibler H: The carbohydrate-deficient

glycoprotein syndromes: pre-Golgi and Golgi disorders? Glycobiology 3:423-428, 1993.

105. Jaeken J, and others: (Short Report). Carbohydrate-deficient glycoprotein syndrome type II, J Inher Metab Dis 16:1041, 1993.
106. Julien J, and others: Adrenomyeloneuropathy: demonstration of inclusions at the level of the peripheral nerve, Eur Neurol 20:367-373, 1981.
107. Kaesgen U, and Goebel HH: Intraepidermal morphologic manifestations in lysosomal diseases, Brain Dev 11:338-341, 1989.
108. Karpati G, Carpenter S, Larbrisseau A, and Lafontaine R: The Kearns-Shy syndrome: a multisystem disease with mitochondrial abnormality demonstrated in skeletal muscle and skin, J Neurol Sci 19:133-151, 1973.
109. Kaufmann P, Stark J, and Stegner HE: The villous stroma of the human placenta, Cell Tissue Res 177:106-121, 1977.
110. Kaye EM, Ullman MD, Wilson ER, and Barranger JA: Type 2 and type 3 Gaucher disease: a morphological and biochemical study, Ann Neurol 20:223-230, 1986.
111. Kieseier BC, and Goebel HH: Characterization of T-cell subclasses and NK-cells in lysosomal disorders by immuno-electron microscopy, Neuropathol Appl Neurobiol 20:604-608, 1994.
112. Kimura S, and Goebel HH: Electron microscopic studies on skin and lymphocytes in early juvenile neuronal ceroid-lipofuscinosis, Brain Dev 9:576-580, 1987.
113. Kimura S, and Goebel HH: Light and electron microscopic study of juvenile neuronal cerod-lipofuscinosis lymphocytes, Pediatr Neurol 4:148-152, 1988.
114. Kleijer WJ: First-trimester diagnosis of genetic metabolic disorders, Contrib Gynecol Obstet 15:80-89, 1986.
115. Koch T, Schult P, Williams R, and Lampert P: Giant axonal neuropathy: a childhood disorder of microfilaments, Ann Neurol 1:438-451, 1977.
116. Kohlschütter A, and others: Probable exclusion of juvenile neuronal ceroid lipofuscinosis in a fetus at risk: an interim report, Prenat Diagn 9:289-292, 1989.
117. Kohlschütter A, and others: Infantile cardiomyopathy and neuromyopathy with $\beta$-galactosidase deficiency, Eur J Pediatr 139: 75-81, 1982.
118. Kula RW, Shafiq SA, Sher JH, and Qazi QH: I-Cell disease (mucolipidosis II), J Neurol Sci 63:75-84, 1984.
119. Lake BD: Morphological approaches to the prenatal diagnosis of late-infantile and juvenile Batten disease, J Inher Metab Dis 16:345-348, 1993.
120. Lake BD: Histopathological investigation of prenatal tissue samples (excluding skin). In Reed GB, Claireaux AE, Cockburn F, editors: Diseases of the fetus and newborn. London, 1995, Chapman & Hall.
121. Langer J, Goebel HH, and Veit S: Eccrine sweat glands are not innervated in hereditary sensory neuropathy type IV, Acta Neuropathol (Berl) 54:199-202, 1981.
122. Laplante P, and others: A progressive neurological syndrome associated with an isolated vitamin E deficiency, Can J Neurol Sci 11:561-564, 1984.
123. Lazarus SS, Vethamany VG, Schneck L, and Volk BW: Fine structure and histochemistry of peripheral blood cells in Niemann-Pick disease, Lab Invest 17:155-170, 1967.
124. Lehmann J, and Goebel HH: Intermediäre generalisierte Form der neuroaxonalen Dystrophie-licht-und elektronenmikroskopische Befunde, Acta Histochem 42:311-318, 1992.
125. Libert J, and Danis P: Differential diagnosis of type A, B and C Niemann-Pick disease by conjunctival biopsy, J Submicrosc Cytol 11:143-157, 1979.
126. Libert J, and others: Ocular findings in metachromatic leukodystrophy, Arch Ophthalmol 97:1495-1504, 1979.
127. Loonen MCB, Reuser AJJ, Visser P, and Arts WFM: Combined sialidase (neuraminidase) and $\beta$-galactosidase deficiency. Clinical, morphological and enzymological observations in a patient, Clin Genet 26:139-149, 1984.
128. Luu J, and others: Tubuloreticular structures and cylindrical confronting cisternae., Hum Pathol 20:617-627, 1989.
129. MacLeod PM, and others: Progressive cerebellar ataxia, spasticity, psychomotor retardation, and hexosaminidase deficiency in a 10-year-old child: juvenile Sandhoff disease, Neurology 27: 571-573, 1977.
130. MacLeod PM, and others: Prenatal diagnosis of neuronal ceroid-lipofuscinoses, Am J Med Genet 22:781-789, 1985.
131. MacLeod PM, Nag S, and Berry C: Ultrastructural studies as a method of prenatal diagnosis of neuronal ceroid-lipofuscinosis, Am J Med Genet 5:93-97, 1988.
132. Mamelle J-C, and others: Etude clinique, ultrastructurale et biochimique d'un cas de gangliosidose à $GM_1$ de type 2, Arch Fr Pediatr 32:925-940, 1975.
133. Markesbery WR, Robinson RO, Falace PV, and Frye MD: Mucopolysaccharidoses: ultrastructure of leukocyte inclusions, Ann Neurol 8:332-336, 1980.
134. Martin JJ, and Ceuterick C: Morphological study of skin biopsy specimens: a contribution to the diagnosis of metabolic disorders with involvement of the nervous system, J Neurol Neurosurg Psychiatry 41:232-248, 1978.
135. Martin JJ, and Ceuterick C: The contribution of pathology to the study of storage disorders, Path Res Pract 183:375-385, 1988.
136. Martin JJ, and Martin L: Infantile neuroaxonal dystrophy. (Ultrastructural study of the peripheral nerves and of the motor end plates), Eur Neurol 8:239-250, 1972.
137. Martin JJ, Ceuterick C, Martin L, and Libert J: Skin and conjunctival biopsies in adrenoleukodystrophy, Acta Neuropathol (Berl) 38:247-250, 1977.
138. Martin JJ, and others: Skin and conjunctival biopsies in infantile neuroaxonal dystrophy, Acta Neuropathol (Berl) 45:247-251, 1979.
139. Martin JJ, Ceuterick C, and Libert J: Skin and conjunctival nerve biopsies in adrenoleukodystrophy and its variants, Ann Neurol 8:291-295, 1980.
140. Martin JJ, Leroy JG, van Eygen M, and Ceuterick C: I-Cell disease, Acta Neuropathol (Berl) 64:234-242, 1984.
141. Meier C, Wiesmann U, Herschkowitz N, and Bischoff A: Morphological observations in the nervous system of prenatal mucopolysaccharidosis II (M Hunter), Acta Neuropathol (Berl) 48: 139-143, 1979.
142. Mihatsch MJ, and others: $G_{M1}$-gangliosidosis. Part II: morphological aspects and review of the literature, Helv Paediatr Acta 28:521-542, 1973.
143. Miike T, Ohtani Y, Nishiyama S, and Matsuda I: Pathology of skeletal muscle and intramuscular nerves in infantile neuroaxonal dystrophy, Acta Neuropathol (Berl) 69:117-123, 1986.
144. Mori K, and others: Renal and skin involvement in a patient with complete Kearns-Sayre syndrome, Am J Med Genet 38: 583-587, 1991.

144a. Munroe PB, and others: Prenatal diagnosis of Batten's disease, Lancet 347:1014–1015, 1996.

145. Murata F, Wohltman H, Spicer SS, and Nagata T: Fine structural and ultracytochemical studies on the lymphocytes in three types of genetic mucopolysaccharidoses, Virchows Arch B 25: 61-73, 1977.
146. Navarro C, and Sancho S: Valor de la biopsia de piel y conjuntiva en el diagnóstico de las enfermedades lisosomales de depósito, Patologia 21:1-6, 1988.
147. Neville HE, Brooke MH, and Austin JH: Studies in myoclonus epilepsy (Lafora body form), Arch Neurol 30:466-474, 1974.

147a. Neville HE, and others: Ultrastructural and histochemical abnormalities of skeletal muscle in patients with chronic vitamin E deficiency, Neurology 33:483-488, 1983.

148. Nieland ML, Parmley TH, and Woodruff JD: Ultrastructural

observations on amniotic fluid cells, Am J Obstet Gynecol 108: 1030-1042, 1970.

149. Nordborg C, Hagberg B, and Kristiansson B: Sural nerve pathology in the carbohydrate-deficient glycoprotein syndrome, Acta Paediatr Scand Suppl 375:39-49, 1991.
150. Ohnishi A, and Dyck PJ: Loss of small peripheral sensory neurons in Fabry disease, Arch Neurol 31:120-127, 1974.
151. Orenstein JM, Simon GL, Kessler CM, and Schulof RS: Ultrastructural markers in circulating lymphocytes of subjects at risk for AIDS, J Clin Pathol 84:603-609, 1985.
152. Ornoy A, Sekeles E, Cohen R, and Kohn G: Electron microscopy of cultured skin fibroblasts and amniotic fluid cells in the diagnosis of hereditary storage diseases, Monogr Hum Genet 10: 32-39, 1978.
153. Ouahchi K, and others: Ataxia with isolated vitamin E deficiency is caused by mutations in the $\alpha$-tocopherol transfer protein. Nature Genet 9:141-145, 1995.
154. Pannone N, Gatti R, Lombardo C, and Di Natale P: Prenatal diagnosis of Hunter syndrome using chorionic villi, Prenat Diagn 6:207-210, 1986.
155. Pellissier JF, and others: Morphological and biochemical changes in muscle and peripheral nerve in Fabry's disease, Muscle Nerve 4:381-387, 1981.
156. Platt LD, and Carlson DE: Prenatal diagnosis—when and how? N Engl J Med 327:636-638, 1992.
157. Poll-The BT, and others: A new peroxisomal disorder with enlarged peroxisomes and a specific deficiency of acyl-CoA oxidase (pseudo-neonatal adrenoleukodystrophy), Am J Hum Genet 42:422-434, 1988.
158. Pollanen MS, and Brody BA: Fetal globoid cell leukodystrophy, Arch Pathol Lab Med 114:213-216, 1990.
158a. Prasad A, Kaye EM, and Alroy J: Electron microscopic examination of skin biopsy as a cost-effective tool in diagnosis of lysosomal storage diseases, J Child Neurol 11:301–308, 1996.
159. Probst A, Ulrich J, Kaeser HE, and Heitz P: Scapulo-peroneal muscular atrophy, Eur Neurol 16:181-196, 1982.
160. Rapola J, Santavuori P, and Savilahti E: Suction biopsy of rectal mucosa in the diagnosis of infantile and juvenile types of neuronal ceroid lipofuscinoses, Hum Pathol 15:352-360, 1984.
161. Rapola J, Salonen R, Ämmälä P, and Santavuori P: Prenatal diagnosis of infantile neuronal ceroid-lipofuscinosis, INCL: morphological aspects, J Inher Metab Dis 16:349-352, 1993.
162. Reusche E, and others: A mild juvenile variant of type IV glycogenosis, Brain Dev 14:36-43, 1992.
163. Riedel KG, and others: Ocular abnormalities in mucolipodosis IV, Am J Ophthalmol 99:125-136, 1985.
164. Sancho S, and others: Skin biopsy findings in glycogenosis III: clinical, biochemical, and electrophysiological correlations, Ann Neurol 27:480-486, 1990.
165. Schmoeckel C: Subtle clues to diagnosis of skin diseases by electron microscopy, Am J Dermatol 2:153-156, 1980.
166. Schröder JM: Neuropathy associated with mitochondrial disorders, Brain Pathol 3:177-190, 1993.
167. Schröder JM, Sellhaus B, and Jörg J: Identification of the characteristic vascular changes in a sural nerve biopsy of a case with cerebral autosomal dominant arteriopathy with subcortical infarcts and leukoencephalopathy (CADASIL), Acta Neuropathol (Berl) 89:116-121, 1995.
168. Schwarting S, Schröder M, Stennert E, and Goebel HH: Enzyme histochemical and histographic data on normal human facial muscles, ORL J 44:51-59, 1982.
169. Schwendemann G: Lymphocyte inclusions in the juvenile type of generalized ceroid-lipofuscinosis, Acta Neuropathol (Berl) 36:327-338, 1976.
170. Schwendemann G, and others: Diagnosis of juvenile-adult form of neuroaxonal dystrophy by electron microscopy of rectum and skin biopsy, J Neurol Neurosurg Psychiatry 50:818-821, 1987.
171. Schwendemann G, and others: Juvenile type of generalized ceroid-lipofuscinosis (Spielmeyer-Sjögren syndrome), Neuropädiatrie 9:28-48, 1978.
171a. Sewell AC, and others: The spectrum of free neuraminic acid storage disease in childhood: clinical, morphological and biochemical observations in three non-Finnish patients, Am J Med Genet 63:203–208, 1996.
172. Sima AAF, and Robertson DM: Involvement of peripheral nerve and muscle in Fabry's disease, Arch Neurol 35:291-301, 1978.
173. Simoni G, and others: Diagnostic application of first trimester trophoblast sampling in 100 pregnancies, Hum Genet 66:252-259, 1984.
174. Sipe JC, and O'Brien JS: Ultrastructure of skin biopsy specimens in lysosomal storage diseases: common sources of error in diagnosis, Clin Genet 15:118-125, 1979.
175. Sloane AE, and others: Neuronal intranuclear hyaline inclusion disease with progressive cerebellar ataxia, Pediatr Neurol 10: 61-66, 1994.
176. Smith P, Dickson JAS, and Lake BD: Rectal biopsy in the diagnosis of neurological disease in childhood, Br J Surg 63:313-316, 1976.
177. Stadhouders AM, Mitochondrial ultrastructural changes in muscular diseases. In Busch HFM, Jennekens FGI, Scholte HR, editors: Mitochondria and muscular diseases. Beetsterzwaag/ The Netherlands, 1981, Mefar b.v.
178. Stadhouders AM, and Sengers RCA: Morphological observations in skeletal muscle from patients with a mitochondrial myopathy, J Inher Metab Dis 10 (Suppl 1):62-80, 1987.
179. Stollhoff K, Albani M, and Goebel HH: Giant axonal neuropathy and leukodystrophy, Pediatr Neurol 7:69-71, 1991.
180. Sutherland GR, Brock DJH, and Scrimgeour JB: Amniotic fluid macrophages and the antenatal diagnosis of anencephaly and spina bifida, J Med Genet 12:135-137, 1975.
181. Suzuki K, Suzuki K, and Chen GC: Morphological, histochemical and biochemical studies on a case of systemic late infantile lipidosis (generalized gangliosidosis), J Neuropathol Exp Neurol 27:15-38, 1968.
182. Takahashi K, and Naito M: Lipid storage disease: part II. Ultrastructural pathology of lipid storage cells in sphingolipidoses, Acta Pathol Jpn 35:385-408, 1985.
183. Tanaka K, and others: Electronmicroscopic study on biopsied rectal mucosa in adrenoleukodystrophy, Neurology 37:1012-1015, 1987.
184. Tandan R, and others: Childhood giant axonal neuropathy, J Neurol Sci 82:205-228, 1987.
185. Taniike M, and others: Ultrastructural pathology of rectum and skin biopsy specimens in lysosomal storage diseases, Acta Histochem Cytochem 23:81-92, 1990.
186. Tateishi J, and others: Intranuclear inclusions in muscle, nervous tissue, and adrenal gland, Acta Neuropathol (Berl) 63:24-32, 1984.
187. Thiéry J-P: Mise en évidence des polysaccharides sur coupes fines en microscopie électronique, J Microsc (Paris) 6:987-1018, 1967.
188. Tomé FMS, Fardeau M, and Lenoir G: Ultrastructure of muscle and sensory nerve in Fabry's disease, Acta Neuropathol (Berl) 38:187-194, 1977.
189. Usuki F, and others: Morphologic findings in biopsied skeletal muscle and cultured fibroblasts from a female patient with Danon's disease (lysosomal glycogen storage disease without acid maltase deficiency), J Neurol Sci 127:54-60, 1994.
190. Uvebrant P, and others: Successful DNA-based prenatal exclusion of juvenile neuronal ceroid lipofuscinosis, Clin Neuropathol 3:165, 1992.
191. Vanier MT, Boue J, and Dumez Y: Niemann-Pick disease type B: first-trimester prenatal diagnosis on chorionic villi and bio-

chemical study of a foetus at 12 weeks of development, Clin Genet 28:348-354, 1985.

192. Vercruyssen A, and others: Adult ceroid-lipofuscinosis: diagnostic value of biopsies and of neurophysiological investigations, J Neurol Neurosurg Psychiatry 45:1056-1059, 1982.
193. Vesa J, and others: A single PCR marker in strong allelic association with the infantile form of neuronal ceroid lipofuscinosis facilitates reliable prenatal diagnostics and disease carrier identification, Eur J Hum Genet 1:125-132, 1993.
194. Vethamany VG, Welch JP, and Vethamany SK: Type D Niemann-Pick disease (Nova Scotia variant), Arch Pathol 93:537-543, 1972.
195. Vital C, Battin J, Rivel J, and Hehunstre JP: Aspects ultrastructuraux des lésions du nerf périphérique dans un cas de maladie de Farber, Rev Neurol (Paris) 132:419-423, 1976.
196. Wakai S, and others: Infantile neuroaxonal dystrophy: axonal changes in biopsied muscle tissue, Pediatr Neurol 9:309-311, 1993.
197. Walter S, and Goebel HH: Ultrastructural pathology of dermal axons and Schwann cells in lysosomal diseases, Acta Neuropathol (Berl) 76:489-495, 1988.
198. Wanders RJA, and others: Peroxisomal disorders in neurology, J Neurol Sci 88:1-39, 1988.
199. Watters PA, and Stewart L: Chorionic biopsy for prenatal diagnosis. (An investigative study of 110 cases.) Med J Aust 144:64-67, 1986.
200. White JW, Jr. and Gomez MR: Diagnosis of Lafora disease by skin biopsy, J Cutan Pathol 15:171-175, 1988.
201. Wiesmann UN, and others: Prenatal metachromatic leukodystrophy, Helv Paediatr Acta 30:31-42, 1975.
202. Winchester B: Prenatal diagnosis of enzyme defects, Arch Dis Child 65:59-67, 1990.
203. Wisniewski K: The diagnostic value of ultrastructural studies of skin-punch biopsies and buffy coat for the early diagnosis of some neurodegenerative diseases, Ann NY Acad Sci 447:285-311, 1986.
204. Wisniewski K, and Wisniewski HM: Diagnosis of infantile neuroaxonal dystrophy by skin biopsy, Ann Neurol 7:377-379, 1980.
205. Wisniewski KE, Rapin I, and Heaney-Kieras J: Clinico-pathological variability in the childhood neuronal ceroid-lipofuscinoses and new observations on glycoprotein abnormalities, Am J Med Genet Suppl 5:27-46, 1988.
206. Wisniewski KE, Kida E, Patxot OF, and Connell F: Variability in the clinical and pathological findings in the neuronal ceroid-lipofuscinoses, Am J Med Genet 42:525-532, 1992.
207. Witzleben CL: Lymphocyte inclusions in late-onset amaurotic idiocy, Neurology 22:1075-1078, 1972.
208. Witzleben CL, and others: Ultrastructural studies in late-onset amaurotic idiocy: Lymphocyte inclusions as a diagnostic marker, J Pediatr 79:285-293, 1971.
209. Wolburg-Buchholz K, and others: Familial lysosomal storage disease with generalized vacuolization and sialic aciduria. Sporadic Salla disease, Neuropediatrics 16:67-75, 1985.
210. Wyatt PR, and Cox DM: Utilization of electron microscopy in the prenatal diagnosis of genetic disease, Hum Hered 27:22-37, 1977.
211. Yagishita S, and others: Infantile neuroaxonal dystrophy, Acta Neuropathol (Berl) 41:257-259, 1978.
212. Zappatini-Tommasi L, Dumontel C, Guibaud P, and Girod C: Farber disease: an ultrastructural study, Virchows Arch A 420: 281-290, 1992.
213. Zarbin MA, Green WR, Moser HW, and Morton SJ: Farber's disease. Light and electron microscopic study of the eye, Arch Ophthalmol 103:73-80, 1985.

C • H • A • P • T • E • R

# 15

# *Dementias and Other Neurodegenerative Diseases*

**Anders A.F. Sima**
**Constance D'Amato**

**Neurodegenerative Disorders with Dementias**
**Cortical Dementias**
- Alzheimer's Disease
- Diffuse Lewy Body Disease
- Pick's Disease
- Cortical-Basal Ganglionic Degeneration
- Progressive Subcortical Gliosis
- Chromosome 17-Linked Dementia
- Mesolimbocortical Dementia

**Subcortical Dementias**
- Huntington's Disease
- Progressive Supranuclear Palsy
- Amyotrophic Lateral Sclerosis
- Parkinson's Disease
- Hallervorden-Spatz Syndrome

Neurodegenerative disorders, particularly those associated with dementia, have received increased general awareness over the last decade. The greater number of elderly people in Western societies susceptible to these disorders has led to new socioeconomic concerns and heavier demands on social and medical resources. Because the potentially beneficial effects of interventional pharmacologic treatments are greater early in the disease processes, there exists a growing demand for precision in early diagnosis. Better understanding of genetic linkages and specific predisposing genetic defects in several dementing disorders is likely to increase the knowledge of underlying disease mechanisms. Over the last several years we have witnessed the delineation of numerous previously unrecognized degenerative and dementing entities that occur both sporadically or as chromosome-linked familial disorders.

At times it is extremely difficult to diagnose these disorders accurately on clinical grounds alone. Therefore to provide accurate diagnoses neuropathologists must be cognizant of the clinical features of each case. Moreover, the interpretation of the brain tissue samples is greatly aided by functional imaging (e.g., PET) and the analysis of psychometric characteristics. The elucidation of clinicopathologic correlates, of predisposing genetic features, and of pathophysiologic mechanisms will become essential prior to the design of specific therapies.

This chapter will not provide an overall comprehensive listing of all disorders in this rapidly evolving field. Instead we describe the pathologic characteristics of common disorders. For the less common disorders we emphasize the histopathologic findings (or lack thereof) that set these entities apart from the more common classic dementias.

**Table 15-1.** Neurodegenerative disorders with dementia

| Cortical dementias | Subcortical dementias |
|---|---|
| • Alzheimer's disease<br>• Diffuse Lewy body disease<br>• Pick's disease<br>• Cortical basal ganglionic degeneration<br>• Progressive subcortical gliosis<br>• Chromosome 17-linked dementia<br>• Mesocorticolimbic dementia | • Huntington's disease<br>• Progressive supranuclear palsy<br>• Parkinson's disease<br>• ALS with dementia<br>• Hallervorden-Spatz disease |

## NEURODEGENERATIVE DISORDERS WITH DEMENTIAS

A wide variety of dementias are associated with degenerative changes of the cerebral cortex and subcortical nuclei. Although there often is involvement of both cerebral cortex and subcortical nuclei in various disorders, it is helpful to group these diseases according to the localization of the major degenerative processes into cortical and subcortical dementias (Table 15-1). In addition to degenerative processes of unknown etiology, dementia may be associated with several cerebrovascular disorders, such as congophilic angiopathy, or cerebral infection and inflammation, such as Creutzfeldt-Jakob disease, HIV infection, or multiple sclerosis. These nondegenerative dementing disorders are discussed elsewhere in this textbook.

## CORTICAL DEMENTIAS

### Alzheimer's Disease

Alzheimer's disease (AD) is the most common dementing disorder, accounting for about 60% of all dementias. The prevalence in the United States is approximately 10% in persons over 65 years, and increases to 50% in those over 85 years.[24,91] The disease was first described by Alois Alzheimer in 1907[4] and since has become almost synonymous with senile dementia. Most AD cases are sporadic. Familial AD occurs in approximately 10% of cases[25] with an autosomal dominant inheritance, which may be linked to chromosome 21[135] or chromosome 14.[69] Familial cases generally show a younger age of onset and a more rapid course.[62,103] The traditional division between presenile- (early) and senile- (late) onset of AD with distinctions in aphasia and apraxia syndromes and extrapyramidal signs[126] has not been supported by recent epidemiologic studies of sporadic AD.[77] However, it should be mentioned that both clinical and pathologic deviations from the classic form of AD are common, although they may fulfill existing clinical[5] and pathologic[64] criteria for the diagnosis of AD. It is not known whether they represent extremes of the same disorder or distinct diseases with different etiologies.

**Clinical features and natural course of Alzheimer's disease.** The spectrum of symptoms and signs displayed by AD patients probably reflects the widespread and sometimes varied pathologic involvement of cerebral cortex and subcortical nuclei. The early cognitive impairments consist of poor recall of new information, difficulty in finding words (dysnomia),[18] and visuospatial impairment resulting in misplacing objects or getting lost and not finding the way home.[10] Remote memories are relatively well preserved. Early behavioral signs may include delusions, insomnia, and depression. Neurologic findings consist of frontal release signs, presence of primitive reflexes, and impaired graphesthesia.[32] As the disease progresses, remote memory becomes increasingly affected, as do language skills, with nonconfluent speech, poor comprehension, and impaired repetition. Behavior may become agitated or aggressive. Signs of extrapyramidal involvement and gait disorders commonly develop. In the late stage of AD, recent and remote memory is severely impaired and patients may become almost mute, with completely obliterated visuospatial cognition.[93] They become incontinent and develop loss of gait and rigidity. The disease has an insidious onset during which the patient may be aware of the cognitive impairments. AD usually has a relentless course, and the late stage develops 5 to 10 years after the first presentation.

Magnetic resonance imaging (MRI) shows marked reduction in brain volume with diffuse symmetric cortical atrophy, particularly of the frontal and parietal lobes, and marked ventricular dilatation secondary to loss of white matter (hydrocephalus ex vacuo). MRI does not distinguish AD from other entities with generalized cerebral atrophy.[21,26] Positron emission tomography (PET) employing $^{15}O_2$-labeled tracers reveals decreased oxygen metabolism and blood flow, particularly of the temporal and parietal lobes, whereas the frontal lobes appear to be affected only at late stages.[31] A similar pattern is seen in fluorodeoxyglucose PET scans. In late stages of the disease the posterior cingulate gyrus is affected, with sparing of the anterior cingulate.[2,21,121] This may be helpful in distinguishing AD from diffuse Lewy body disease.[2] (See below.)

**Gross changes in Alzheimer's disease.** The most striking gross finding is the marked loss of cerebral tissue and the corresponding reduction in brain weight. Exterior inspection reveals marked gyral atrophy of the temporal, frontal, and parietal regions. The meninges are often thickened, particularly along the superior sagittal sinus. The subarachnoid space is generous, often with pooling of CSF. Coronal sections emphasize the frontal and temporal atrophy with widening of the sulci (Fig. 15-1). The ventricles are symmetrically enlarged, with marked atrophy of the white matter and thinning of the corpus callosum. Inspection of the hippocampal formation on coronal section will show generalized and often marked atrophy. Subcortical structures such as basal ganglia and thalami often appear small, although less strikingly so compared with the cortical mantle and underlying white matter.

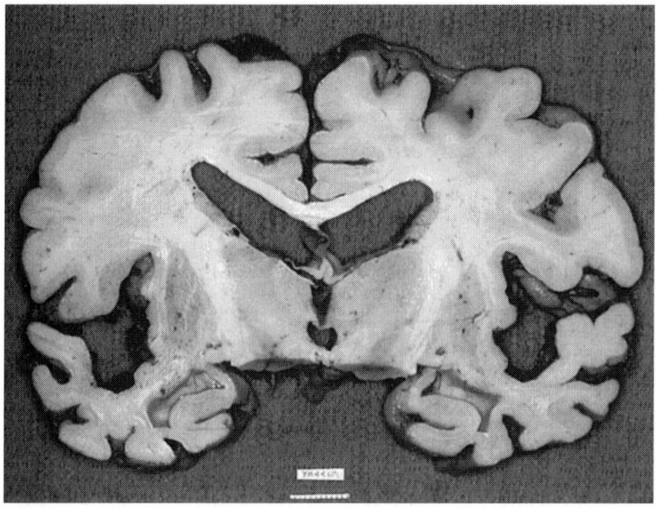

**Fig. 15-1.** Coronal section of a brain with AD. Marked atrophy of the temporal lobes and widening of the lateral ventricles are apparent.

**Histologic changes in Alzheimer's disease.** The histologic hallmarks of AD consist of neurofibrillary tangles (NFT) and senile plaques (SP) (Fig. 15-2). These changes are often associated with neuronal loss and gliosis of the cerebral cortex. NFT consist of cytoplasmic argyrophilic fibrillary bundles, which are easily demonstrated using conventional silver staining techniques, such as Bielschowsky's modified silver technique or the more sensitive Gallyas silver technique. NFT are flame-shaped or globose structures of abnormal filaments of the perinuclear cytoplasm. They are particularly numerous, although not restricted to the pyramidal cells of $CA_1$ (Fig. 15-3), subiculum of the hippocampus, and entorhinal cortex. Also the neurons in layers III and V of the association cortices, amygdala, substantia innominata, and the raphe nuclear complexes of the brainstem contain NFT. Extracellular NFT, also called ghost tangles, are commonly seen in hippocampus, entorhinal cortex (Fig. 15-4), and substantia innominata, reflecting neuronal degeneration and loss, as well as the inertness of NFT in the neuropil. NFT stain positively for various isoforms of the tau protein,[66,74] phosphorylated epitopes of the 150 and 200 kD neurofilaments,[139] MAP-2, $\beta$-amyloid, and ubiquitin[90] (Fig. 15-5), but not for tubulin. Ultrastructurally, NFT consist of paired helical filaments, each measuring 10 nm with a helical periodicity of 80 nm. They consist of protofilaments that differ from normal neurofilaments.[154]

SP are heterogeneous rounded structures composed of degenerating neurites, extracellular amyloid fibrils, and reactive microglia and astrocytes. Several subtypes of SP can be distinguished and probably represent different stages in the development of SP. Diffuse

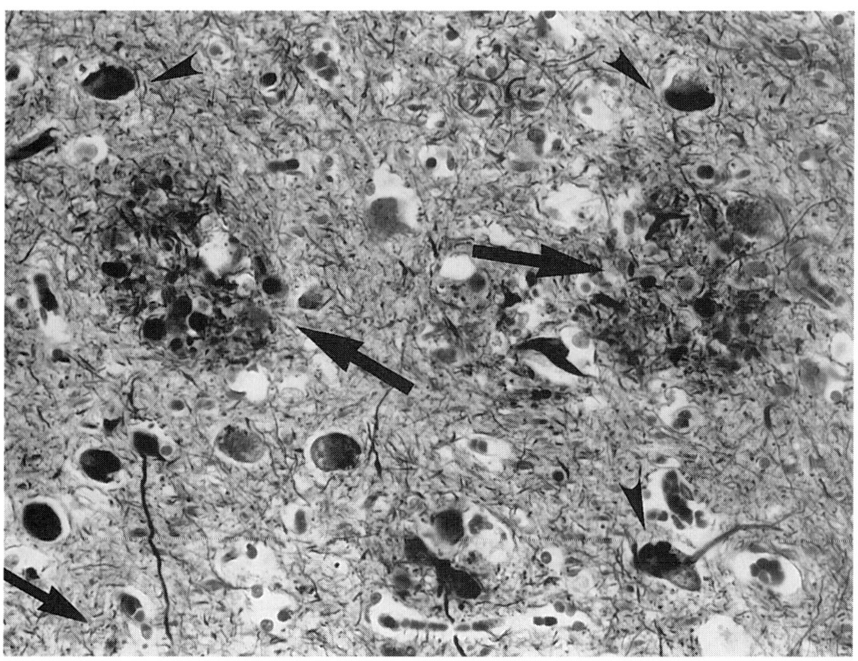

**Fig. 15-2.** Section of the entorhinal cortex showing two senile plaques (*arrows*) and neurons containing neurofibrillary tangles (*arrowheads*). (Bielschowsky's silver stain; ×330.)

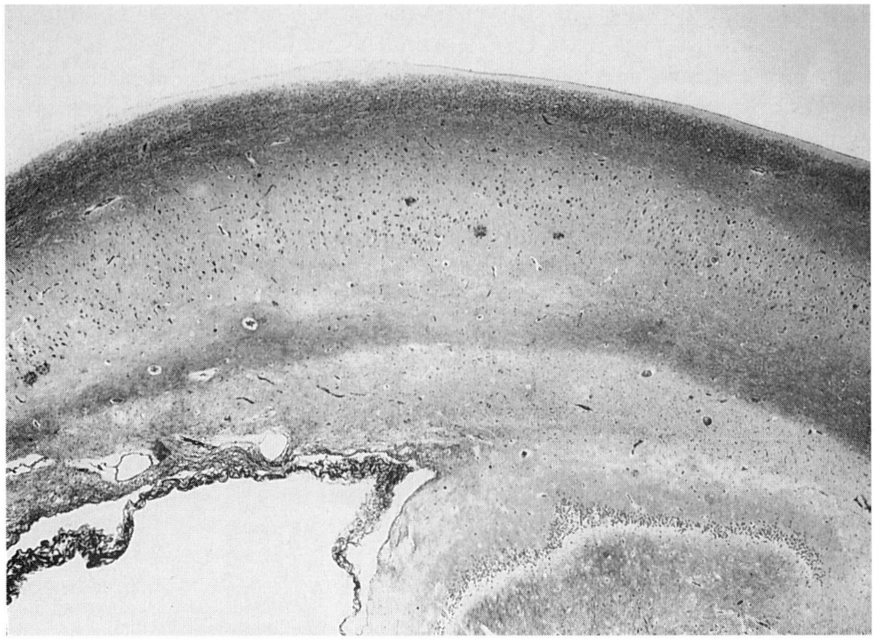

**Fig. 15-3.** Low magnification view of sectors $CA_1$ and $CA_2$ of the hippocampus showing multiple neurofibrillary tangles. (Bielschowsky's silver stain; ×21.)

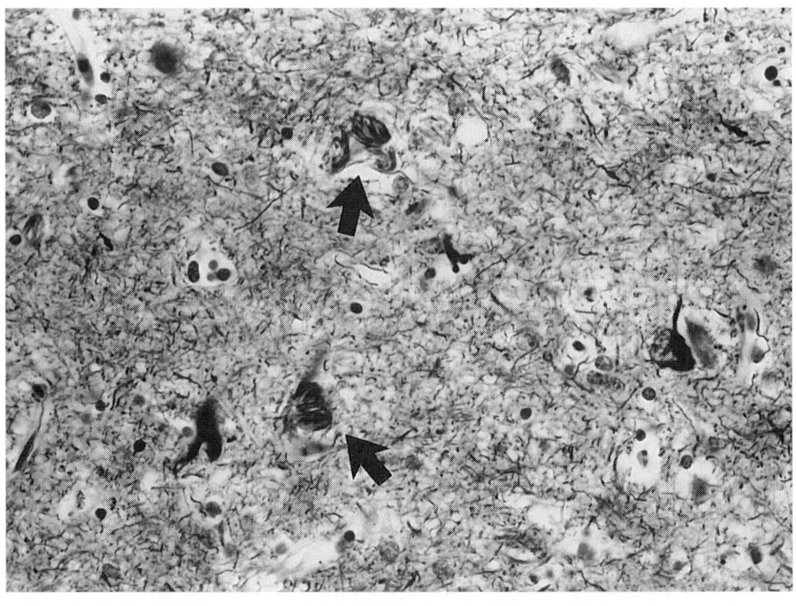

**Fig. 15-4.** Ghost tangles free in the neuropil (*arrow*) are commonly seen in the substantia innominata and the entorhinal cortex. (Bielschowsky's silver stain; ×330.)

plaques consist of deposits of amorphous β-amyloid immunoreactive clusters in the neuropil in the cerebral cortex, and also may be seen in the cerebellar cortex. Primitive plaques consists of diffusely dispersed amyloid fibrils and swollen dystrophic neurites. Mature plaques show a compact central amyloid core surrounded by a ring of dystrophic neurites (Fig. 15-6). Finally, burned-out plaques consist of a stellate amyloid core without dystrophic neurites. The dystrophic neurites contributing to the SP appearance with silver impregnations contain paired helical filaments identical to those of NFT. In addition, SP also show microglial and reactive astrocytes. The dystrophic neurites of SP contain different neuropeptides and synthetic enzymes for neurotransmitters and therefore originate from a variety of neuronal populations.[106] SP in AD are markedly increased in both archicortical and neocortical areas, and their density serves as an objective criterion for the histopathologic diagnosis of definite AD. SPs tend to be most frequent in the entorhinal, the parietal, and, surprisingly, in the visual association cortex, as well as in the amygdala.

A consensus panel sponsored by the National Institute on Aging has set forth histopathologic criteria for the diagnosis of AD based mainly on the number of SP in the four most severely affected areas of the brain.[64] Since both NFT and SP are found in small but increasing numbers in nondemented aged persons, the

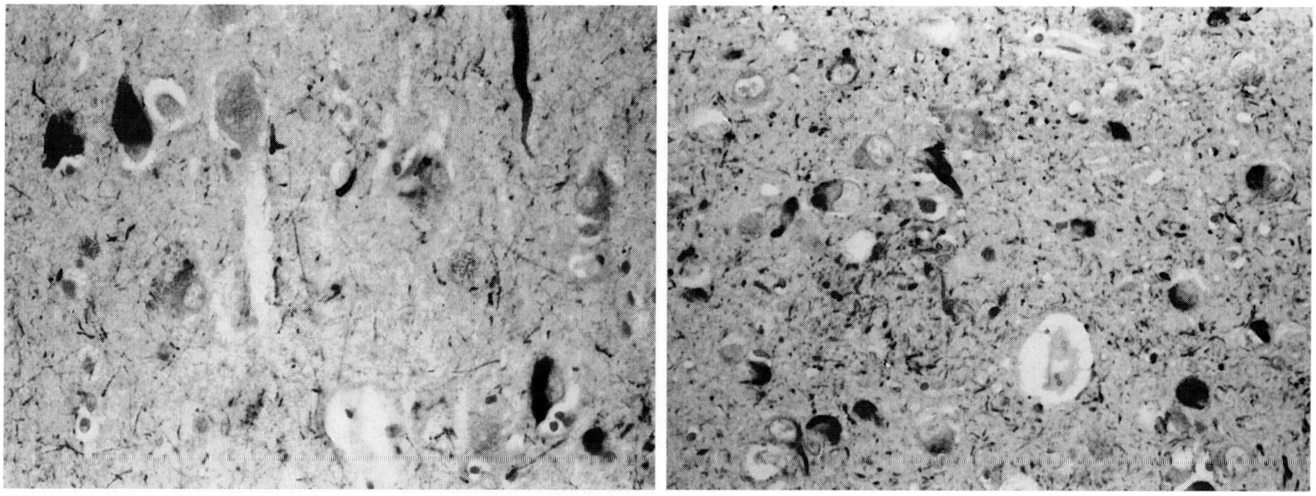


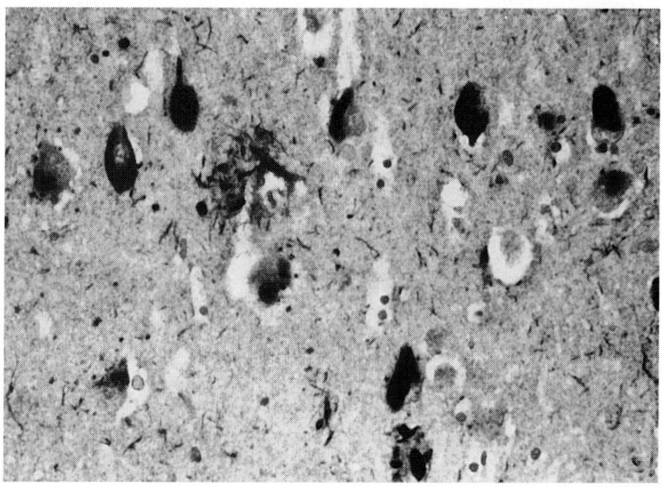


**Fig. 15-5.** Neurofibrillary tangles staining positive with antibodies directed against **A,** phosphorylated neurofilament; **B,** tau-protein; and **C,** ubiquitin. In **C,** altered neurites of a senile plaque also stain positive with anti-ubiquitin. (×330.)

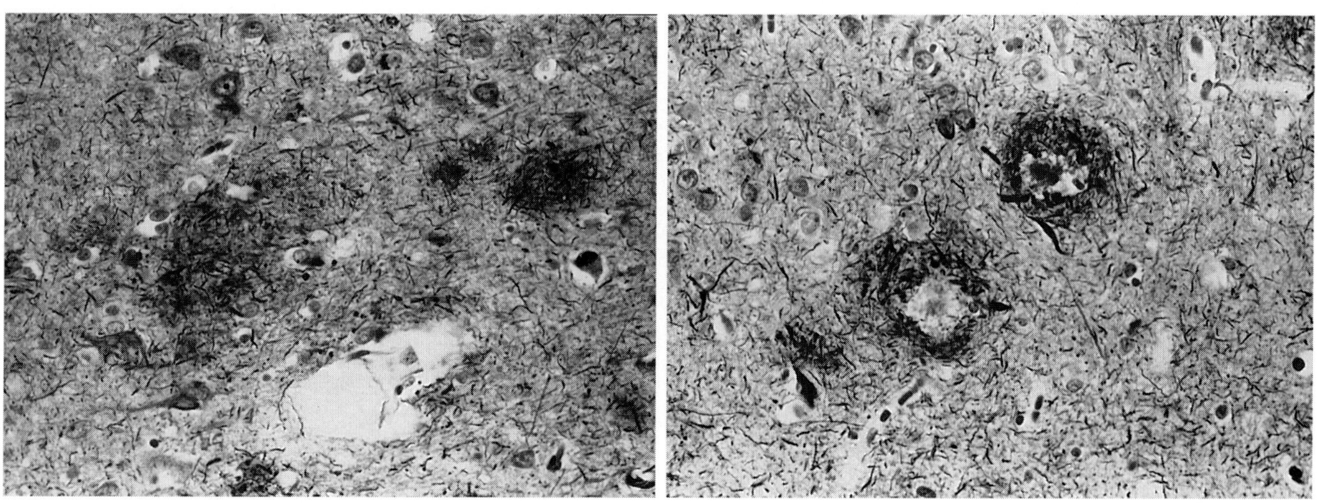


**Fig. 15-6. A,** Primitive plaques composed of silver positive neurites. **B,** Mature plaques display amyloid core. (Bielschowsky's silver stain, ×330.)

criteria for the diagnosis of AD are age-dependent. A firm diagnosis of AD can be established according to patient age as follows: <50 years of age, SP and NFT exceed 2 to 5 per ×200 field in neocortex; 50 to 65 years of age, SP exceeds 8 per ×200 field in four areas; age 66–75, SP are >10 per ×200 field; older than 75 years, SP should exceed 15 per ×200 field for the firm diagnosis of AD.[64] A similar but semiquantitative and hence less objective scoring system for the diagnosis of AD has been proposed by CERAD.[89]

The presence of NFT and SP is often associated with severe neuronal loss and gliosis. This is pronounced in the entorhinal, parietal, and supraorbital frontal cortex and may be associated with spongiform change, particularly prominent in layers I and II (Fig. 15-7). Severe involvement of the entorhinal cortex often is associated with marked degeneration and gliosis of the perforant tract. Furthermore, hippocampus exhibits profound neuronal loss in the $CA_1$ and in the subiculum. Of subcortical structures, amygdala and ventral hypothalamus often are severely affected by neuronal loss and gliosis. Milder but at times severe degeneration also affects the anteroventral striatum, including the nucleus accumbens, substantia innominata (particularly the basal nucleus of Meynert), and the anterior and dorsomedial nuclei of the thalamus.

Additional characteristic histopathologic features of AD, which however are not used as criteria for diagnosis, consist of neuropil threads (Fig. 15-8), Hirano bodies, granulovacuolar degeneration (Fig. 15-9), and accompanying congophilic angiopathy (Fig. 15-10). Neuropil threads consist of degenerated neurites which, in sections immunostained for tau or ubiquitin, show a widespread distribution in cerebral cortex and the most severely affected areas of hippocampus. They consist mainly of straight filaments with the same immunocytochemical profile as NFT, except for β-amyloid, which is negative in neuropil threads. Hirano bodies are rodlike highly eosinophilic cytoplasmic inclusions of the pyramidal cells of hippocampus (Fig. 15-9). Ultrastructurally, Hirano bodies consist of crystalloid arranagements of 10-nm filaments, which, like NFT, also may be found free in the neuropil. Granulovacuoles also are characteristic of the pyramidal cell

**Fig. 15-7.** Low magnification of the entorhinal cortex in AD showing astrogliosis, particularly noticeable in the superficial cortical layers (I to III). Spongiform change in layers I and II is also visible. (PTAH stain; ×42.)

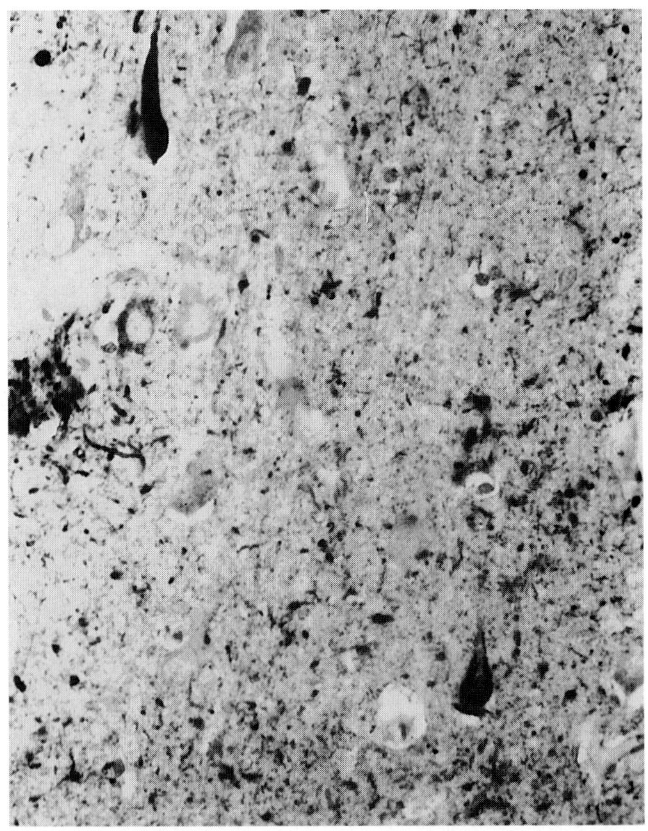

**Fig. 15-8.** Entorhinal cortex stained with anti-ubiquitin antisera. Note two positively stained neurofibrillary tangles. Numerous positively stained threads and granules are seen. (×330).

neurons of the hippocampus, which may contain up to a dozen small vacuoles with an argyrophilic dense particle in their centers (Fig. 15-9). The granular material has tubulin-like immunoreactivity.[112]

Deposition of $\beta$A4 amyloid protein in meningeal and intraparenchymal arteries and arterioles is common in AD. Vascular amyloid deposition also is seen in normal aging. Congophilic angiopathy is more common in occipital and parietal lobes than in more rostral parts of the cerebrum. The vessel walls are thickened and acellular and show the presence of amyloid with the appropriate stains (Fig. 15-10). Although the amyloid found in both SP and NFT as well as in the cerebral vessels originates from the transmembranous preamyloid molecule, each of these amyloids represents different splicing products.[82,117] A role for amyloid in the progression of AD has not been substantiated.

**Etiologic considerations.** The etiology of AD is unknown. In recent years important strides have been made, particularly with respect to familial AD, which often begins in the third to the fifth decade as an autosomal dominant disorder with very high penetrance. Three genes have been identified among these families: the amyloid precursor protein on chromosome 21; presenilin I on chromosome 14; and presenilin II on chromosome 1.[122] Interestingly, within these genotypes the phenotypic expressions of both the clinical picture and the neuropathologic findings appear to be relatively consistent.[69] However, the AD that occurs late in life appears to be much more complex. Recent data suggest an association between the apo-E $\epsilon 4$ allele and late-onset AD in 20% to 40% of cases. However, this association is a weak one, since patients with this allele may never develop the disorder; conversely, patients lacking the allele do develop AD.[58,86] The apo-E $\epsilon 4$ has been associated with more widespread vascular amyloid deposition and a higher number of amyloid plaques in AD.[124] However, significant variations exist in the association between apo-E $\epsilon 4$ and AD among

A B C

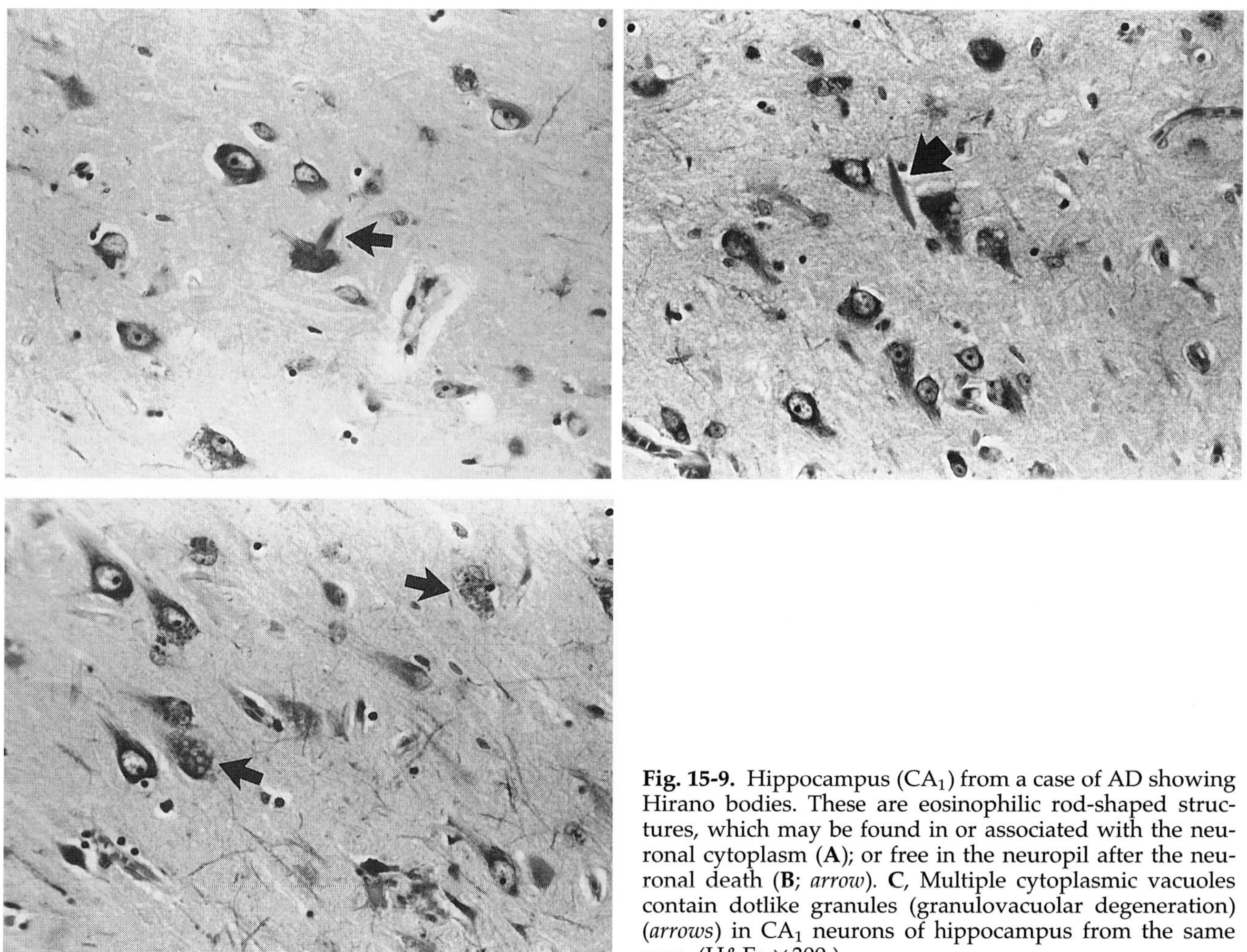

**Fig. 15-9.** Hippocampus ($CA_1$) from a case of AD showing Hirano bodies. These are eosinophilic rod-shaped structures, which may be found in or associated with the neuronal cytoplasm (**A**); or free in the neuropil after the neuronal death (**B**; *arrow*). **C**, Multiple cytoplasmic vacuoles contain dotlike granules (granulovacuolar degeneration) (*arrows*) in $CA_1$ neurons of hippocampus from the same case. (H&E; ×300.)

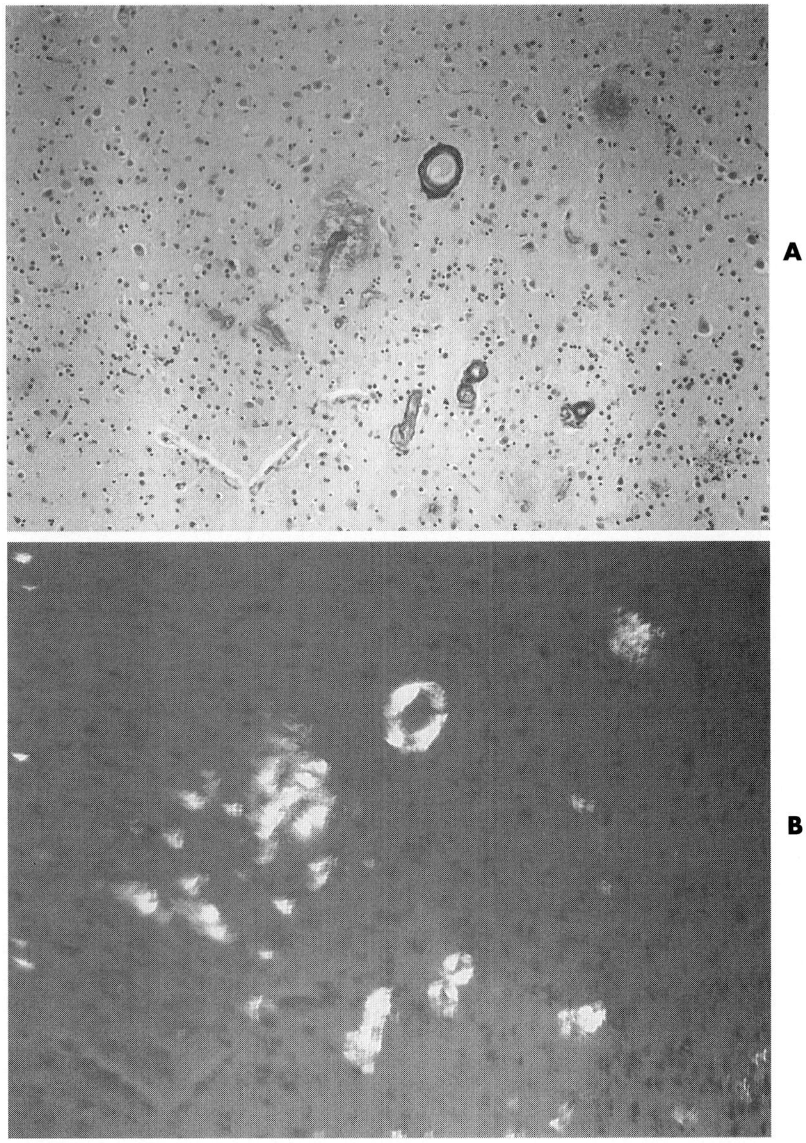


**Fig. 15-10.** Congophilic angiopathy, consisting of amyloid deposition in intracerebral vessel walls, is common in AD. **A**, Amyloid stains brightly red with congo-red. **B**, Amyloid shows birefringence in polarized light. (×83.)

various ethnic groups.[81] Other genes and environmental risk factors may likely interact with apo-E ϵ4 or may in themselves show, when identified, stronger associations with the development of late-onset AD. Finally we suggest that once the multigenetic background to AD is unraveled, the heterogeneous pathology often encountered in this disorder may become understandable.

### Diffuse Lewy Body Disease

Diffuse Lewy body disease (DLBD) is a recently recognized entity. The first systematic descriptions occurred in the mid to late 1980s.[22,35,129] DLBD is now recognized as the second most common degenerative type of dementia; it accounts for 25% to 30% of all dementias[14,107] and occurs in two forms. One consists pathologically of cortical and subcortical Lewy bodies with an insufficient number of NFT and SP for the diagnosis of concomitant AD. A second form shows cortical and subcortical inclusion Lewy bodies and a sufficient number of NFT and SP for the diagnosis of AD; hence, a pure form of DLBD exists as well as a combined form with AD.[22,50] In a series of 54 cases of DLBD examined at the Michigan Alzheimer Disease Research Center between the years 1991 and 1995, approximately 30% showed, on neuropathologic examination, the pure form of DLBD; 70% showed combined pathology with AD (Sima, unpublished data).

The clinical symptoms of the disorder start at an earlier age than pure AD, not uncommonly in the early 60s.[22,50] The disease may start with cognitive impairments, features shared with AD, such as gradual onset and progressive memory loss, disorientation, and impaired language and visuospatial skills[49,50] with subsequent development of extrapyramidal symptoms, often without resting tremor.[49] Clinically these cases are often classified as AD with extrapyramidal signs. Conversely the extrapyramidal signs may be the presenting complaints, with subsequent gradual development of cognitive impairments.[22,87] These cases clinically often are referred to as Parkinson's disease with dementia. Although no systematic study has been undertaken with respect to clinical responses to levodopa treatment in DLBD, the general consensus is that the signs and symptoms of DLBD respond only modestly or not at all to substitution therapy.[50,87] Some authors have emphasized that fluctuations in cognitive function over short time spans and such psychiatric features as delusions and hallucinations are more common in DLBD than in pure AD.[107] Familial forms of DLBD have not been reported.

In view of the interest in developing experimental therapies for AD and the difficulty in distinguishing DLBD from AD on clinical grounds, attempts have been made to apply objective measures for the early clinical separation of these two entities. We have reported that $^{18}$F-2-fluoro-deoxy-D-glucose PET scans reveal some distinguishing features between AD and DLBD.[2] Although no differences were found with respect to glucose metabolism in parietal, frontal, or temporal lobes, patients with DLBD have significantly reduced glucose utilization of the primary visual and occipital association cortices, which is not seen in AD. In addition, the anterior cingulate gyrus is more severely affected in patients with DLBD than it is among those diagnosed with AD.

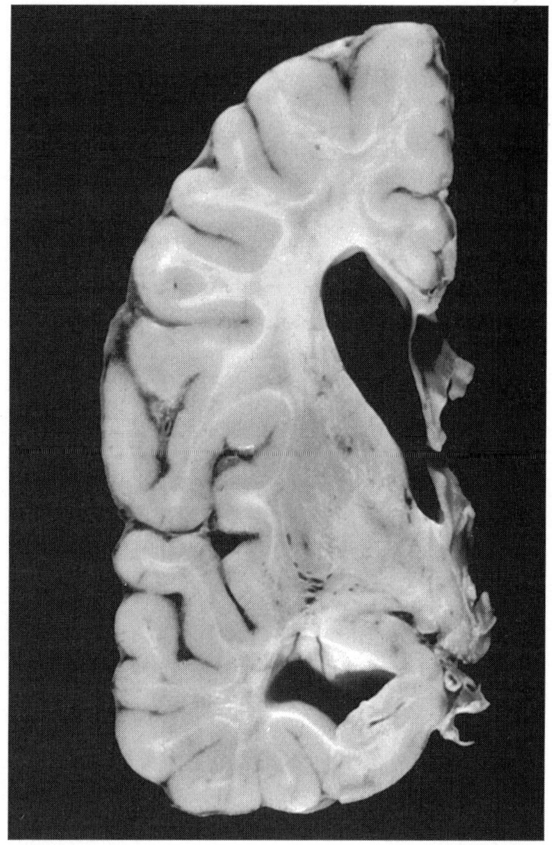

**Fig. 15-11.** Coronal sections through one hemisphere of a case with combined DLBD and AD showing mild ventricular dilatation. Compare with the more severe atrophy seen in AD (Fig 15-1.).

**Gross findings in diffuse Lewy body disease.** External inspection of the brain shows no, or only mild, generalized cerebral astrophy, even in cases of combined DLBD and AD (Fig. 15-11). On coronal sections there may be minimal generalized cortical and white matter atrophy, generally not exceeding that noticed in brains from nondemented patients of comparable age. The most striking gross finding is the depigmentation of the substantia nigra (Fig. 15-12), which is commonly more pronounced in the medial aspects of the nuclei in contrast to idiopathic Parkinson's disease, in which depigmentation is more severe in the lateral aspects of the substantia nigra. The hippocampi may show modest atrophy, but usually this is not striking.

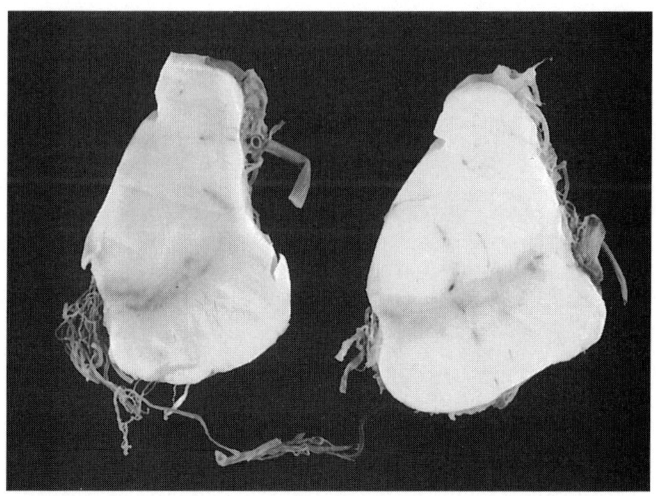

**Fig. 15-12.** Sections from the midbrain showing depigmentation of the substantia nigra in a 68-year-old case of DLBD (*right*), compared with an age-matched control case (*left*).

**Histopathologic findings in DLBD.** The characteristic histopathologic feature in DLBD is the presence of cortical or immature inclusion Lewy bodies in the cerebral cortex, which can be recognized by conventional hematoxylin-eosin (H&E) stain (Fig. 15-13) but which are more readily apparent in sections immunostained for ubiquitin[20,22,76] (Fig. 15-14). The cerebral Lewy bodies differ from the classic Lewy bodies of Parkinson's disease in that they lack the characteristic dense central core and halo. In DLBD the inclusions are usually round eosinophilic bodies (occasionally oblong) that meld in with the less eosinophilic neuronal

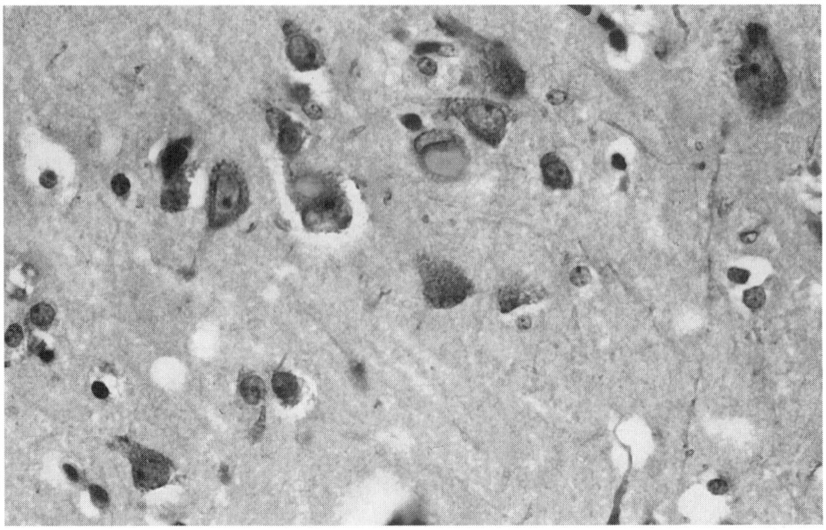

**Fig. 15-13.** Entorhinal cortex in a case of pure DLBD. Cerebral Lewy bodies are homogeneous round cytoplasmic inclusions. (H&E; ×330.)

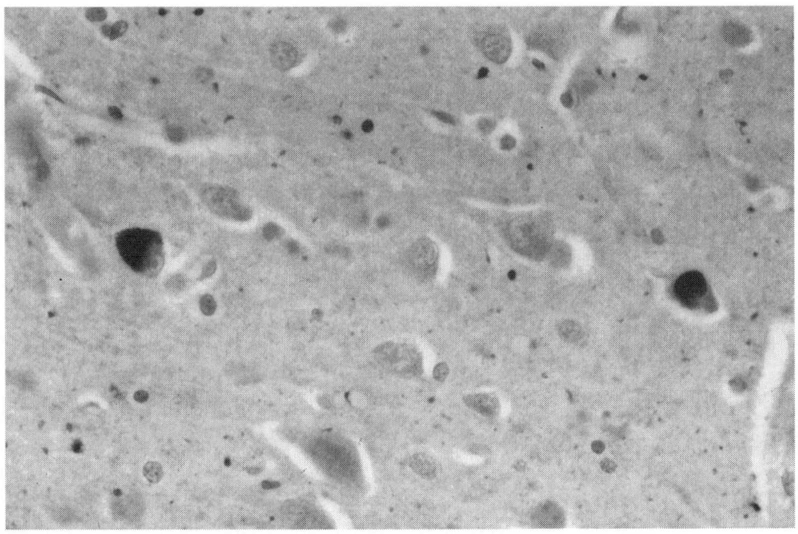

**Fig. 15-14.** Insular cortex from a case of pure DLBD stained with anti-ubiquitin immunostain demonstrating positively stained Lewy bodies. (×330.)

cytoplasm. These cytoplasmic inclusions often are present in several adjacent neurons, forming clusters of affected neurons most commonly seen in the V and II layers of affected cortices.[22] Ultrastructurally, the inclusions consist of accumulations of neurofilaments that are arranged in a less orderly radial fashion (Fig. 15-15) than in classic Lewy bodies of idiopathic Parkinson's disease.[22] Cortical Lewy bodies are most commonly encountered in the entorhinal, anterior cingulate, and insular cortices.[20,129] The neuronal inclusions are also common in the amygdala, particularly in the central nucleus and the medial cortical complex of the nucleus. Affected cortical areas often show only mild or modest neuronal loss and gliosis as well as occasional so-called ballooned neurons containing extended cytoplasm that stains positive for tau and phosphorylated neurofilaments.[20] The presence of "threads" and "granules" that stain positive for ubiquitin is a common accompaniment in the superficial layers of affected cortices. Cerebral Lewy bodies also may be found in the prefrontal cortex, visual association cortex, and motor cortex, but at these locations the inclusions are less numerous. Lewy bodies may be rarely found in pyramidal cells of the subiculum and in the granule cells of the dentate fascia.

The substantia nigra exhibits a severe decrease in the number of pigmented neurons, particularly in the ventral tegmental area (Fig. 15-16) and the medial aspects of the nucleus.[22,129] Neuronal loss also may be pronounced in the medial and lateral aspects. Substantia nigra contains classic Lewy bodies as well as immature Lewy bodies of the cortical type. Lewy bodies of both types also may be found in locus ceruleus and in substantia innominata, where substantial neuronal loss may be noted.[22]

The severity of neuronal loss in the basal nucleus of

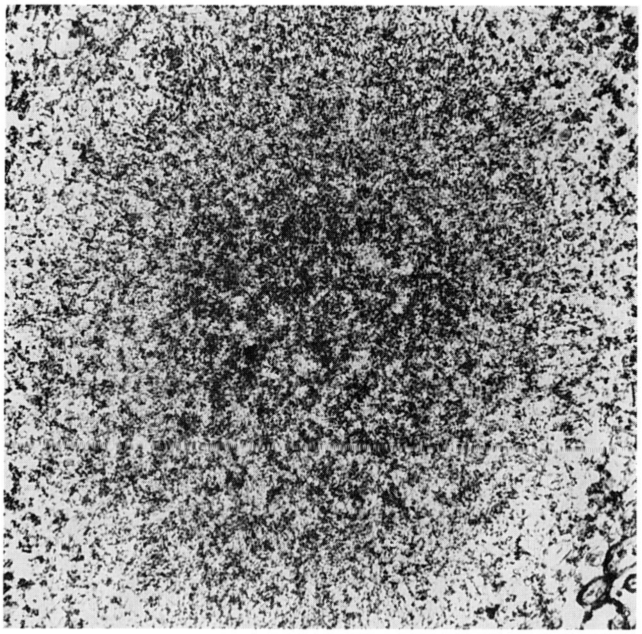

**Fig. 15-15.** Electronmicrograph showing a cerebral Lewy body in DLBD. Somewhat irregularly arranged neurofilaments are visible. (×21,000.)

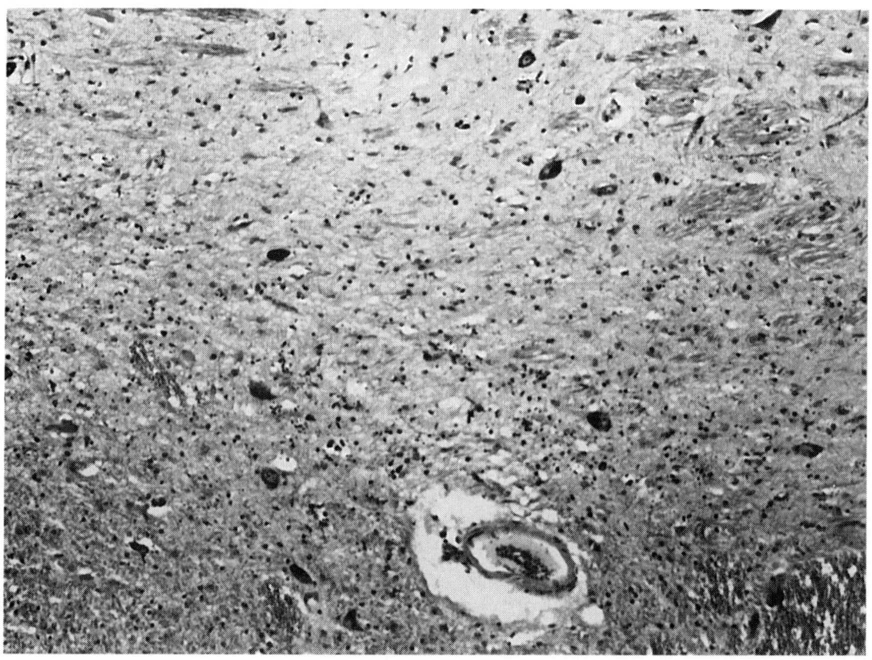

**Fig. 15-16.** Ventral tegmental area of the substantia nigra in a case of combined DLBD and AD showing marked loss of pigmented neurons and astrogliosis. (PTAH; ×83.)

Meynert is similar in both pure DLBD and the combined form of DLBD and AD. Mild to moderate neuronal loss of pyramidal cells affects the hippocampus; this is most severe in $CA_4$ and less so in $CA_3$ to $CA_1$. Apart from the severe involvement of the amygdala, DLBD is characterized by notable neuronal loss and gliosis of the anterior ventral striatum, including the nucleus accumbens.

As mentioned above, in the pure form of DLBD, NFT and SP of the Alzheimer type are rare and their numbers usually do not exceed those typical of normal aging. For the diagnosis of the combined form of DLBD and AD the density of SP should meet the criteria set forth by Khachaturian.[64] Although present in numbers sufficient for the diagnosis of AD, NFT and SP rarely are not found in the high numbers characteristic of the severe cases of pure AD.[50,58]

**Pathophysiologic considerations.** DLBD has both clinical and neuropathologic aspects in common with both idiopathic Parkinson's disease and AD. The density of Lewy bodies in the cerebral cortex of patients with DLBD correlates with the severity of dementia.[87] Furthermore, the fairly typical distribution of Lewy bodies in the cerebral cortex corresponds roughly to the mesocortical dopaminergic projections originating from the ventral tegmentum, which is significantly affected in DLBD. Thus, the dementia seen in DLBD may represent a mesocortical dopaminergic defect.[22] In addition, cholinergic cortical projections originating from the nucleus basalis of Meynert are involved in both the pure and mixed forms of DLBD,[105,129] although these projections usually are not involved to the extent seen in pure AD. Hence, injury to these projections may contribute to the global dementia, as in AD.

The substantia nigra pathology in DLBD is interesting in view of the extrapyramidal symptoms exhibited by these patients as well as in patients with pure idiopathic Parkinson's disease. The nigral neuronal loss in Parkinson's disease affects mainly the lateral part of the nucleus that projects to the striatum. Therefore, Parkinson's disease and DLBD may represent the two extremes of the same disease process, affecting, in one case, mainly the lateral aspect of substantia nigra (Parkinson's disease), and in DLBD mainly its medial ventral tegmental part. These questions have not yet been addressed by analyses of large numbers of cases; answers to these and similar questions could shed some light on common pathophysiologic mechanisms in these entities.

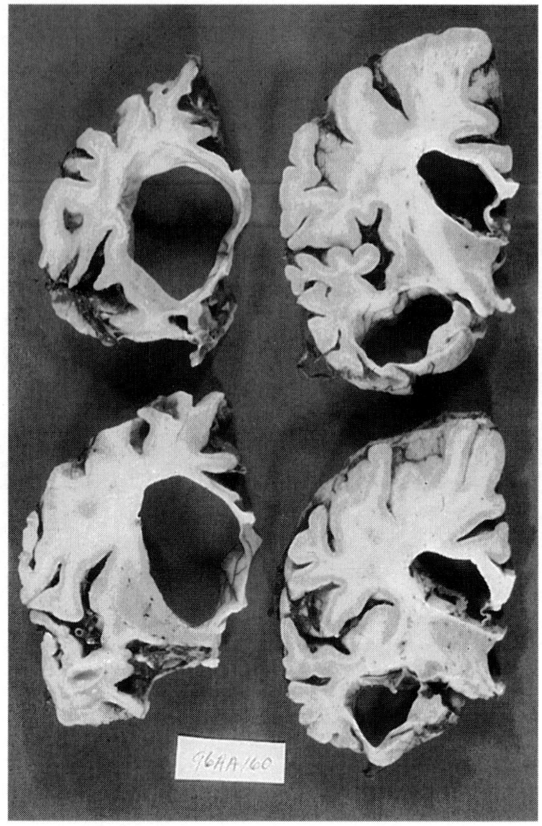

Fig. 15-17. Coronal brain sections from a patient with Pick's disease. There is profound atrophy of the frontal and temporal lobes with "knife-sharp" gyri.

## Pick's Disease

This rare dementing disorder was first described by Pick in 1906.[110] The symptoms become manifest in middle age or later, and the disease shows a variable progression ranging from 1 to 10 years. Women are slightly more affected than men in a 5 to 4 ratio.[144] Familial forms of the disorder are common.[123,132,136] In the early stages of the disease there are signs of frontal lobe involvement with intellectual decline. This usually is followed by the appearance of disorientation, bizarre behavior, dysphasia, dyslexia, and dyspraxia; eventually, patients may become mute. Motor dysfunction including gait disturbances is common in advanced stages of the illness, which culminates in global dementia.

**Gross findings.** There is profound cortical atrophy, often more severe in the frontal and temporal lobes (Fig. 15-17). Characteristically the two posterior thirds of the superior temporal lobe are spared from atrophy. The cerebral atrophy is accompanied by marked dilatation of the ventricular system.[92] Severe atrophy of the caudate nucleus often is present. The frontal and temporal atrophy may at times show some asymmetry between hemispheres.[144] The parietal and occipital lobes are rarely atrophic.

**Histopathologic changes.** The hallmark is profound cortical atrophy with decreased numbers of neurons and gliosis in the affected lobes. This is commonly associated with a spongiform change in the superficial layers of affected cortices (Fig. 15-18). Large, swollen, ballooned neurons or Pick cells are common in cerebral cortex and affected subcortical structures (see below). Individual neuronal perikarya display eosinophilic cytoplasm with the nucleus displaced to one side (Fig. 15-19). These neurons stain positive for ubiquitin, tau, and phosphorylated neurofilaments. It should be stressed that ballooned neurons are not specific for Pick's disease because neurons with the same appearance can be seen in a number of other degenerative disorders, including AD. Of subcortical nuclei the caudate nucleus is often most severely involved, with marked neuronal loss and gliosis. The putamen, globus pallidus, and thalamus usually are mildly atrophic. Neuronal loss and gliosis without preference to any specific area may exist in the hippocampus. Nucleus basalis of Meynert is not involved in Pick's disease. Moderate neuronal loss and gliosis may exist in the pars compacta of the substantia nigra.[39]

Preserved neurons of affected areas of the cortex

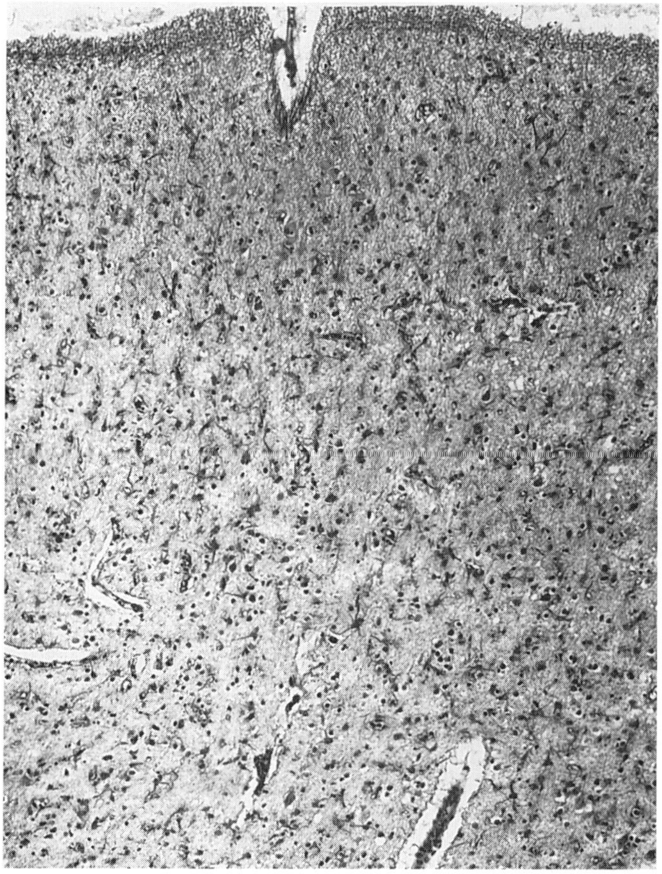

**Fig. 15-18.** Frontal cortex in Pick's disease. There is profound pancortical neuronal loss and marked gliosis. Mild spongiform change in the superficial cortical layers is also visible. (PTAH; ×21.)

and subcortical structures often demonstrate argyrophilic rounded inclusions or Pick inclusion bodies (Fig. 15-20). In classic Pick's disease these are characteristically present in the granule cells of the dentate fascia of the hippocampus (Fig. 15-21). The immunocytochemical profile of Pick bodies is similar to that of NFTs in AD.[92] Ultrastructurally, Pick bodies consist of haphazardly arranged fibrils, amorphous granular material, and tubules.[92]

The histopathologic diagnosis of Pick's disease may be difficult because of its close resemblance to cortical-basal ganglionic degeneration.[39] The distinguishing features include absence of Pick bodies, noninvolvement of hippocampus, and severe degeneration of the substantia nigra in cortical-basal ganglionic degeneration (Table 15-2).

The etiology of Pick's disease is unknown, and genetic linkages have not been identified in familial cases.

### Cortical-Basal Ganglionic Degeneration

Cortical-basal ganglionic degeneration (CBGD) is a relatively rare sporadic disorder that starts insidiously, usually in the sixth decade of life, and spans a course of 5 to 10 years. The clinical presentation and course of the disease are characterized by asymmetry of symptoms and signs. The presenting symptoms commonly are motor difficulties accompanied by rigidity, tremor, and focal reflex myoclonus[70] starting in one upper limb and gradually involving the contralateral and lower limbs. Apraxia and language disturbances often are prominent in established cases. Other symptoms include alien limb phenomenon[9] and oculomotor impairment. Cognitive functions may be preserved for several months; therafter, global dementia commonly ensues.

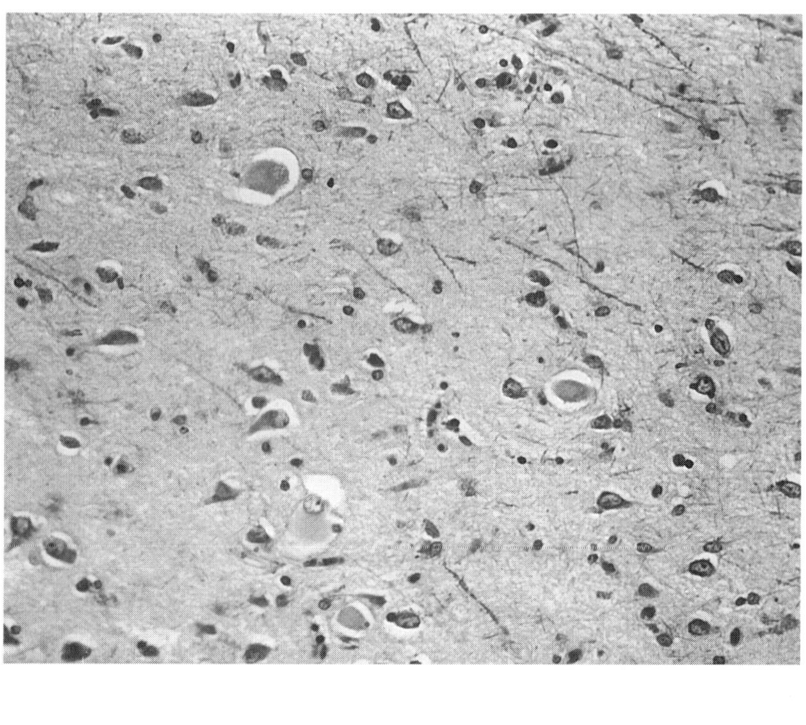

**Fig. 15-19.** Sample from the frontal cortex showing three ballooned neurons in Pick's disease. (H&E; ×83.)

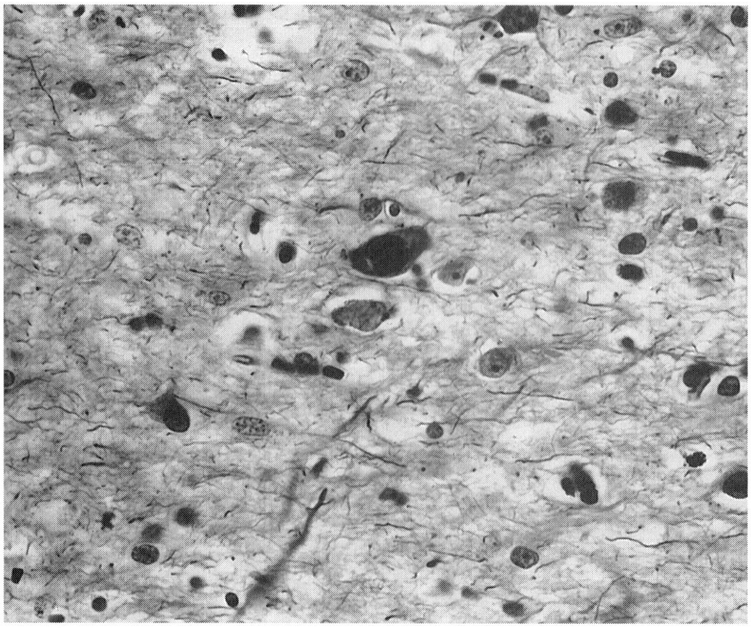

**Fig. 15-20.** Temporal cortex stained with Bielschowsky's silver stain showing an intracytoplasmic Pick's body. (×330.)

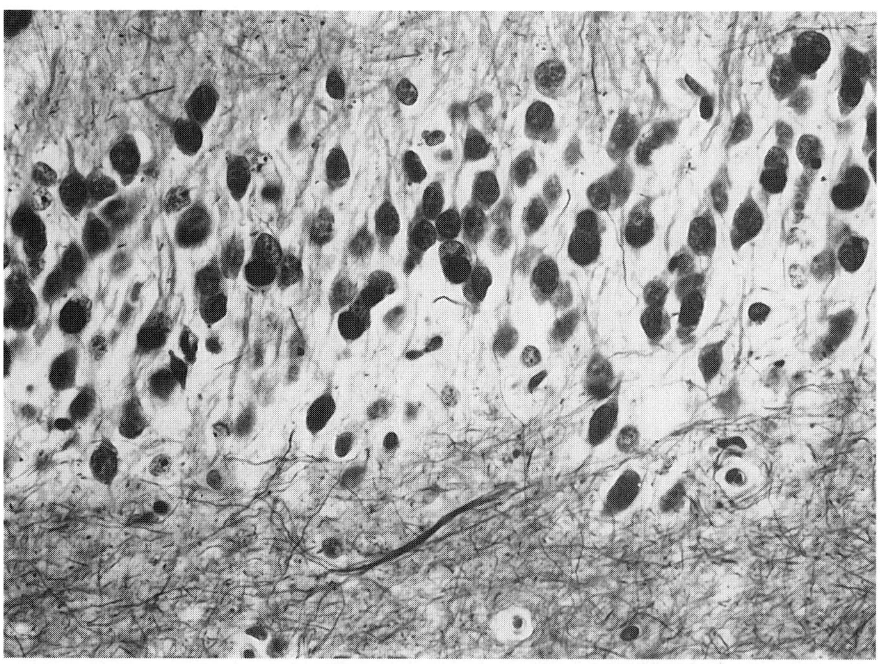

**Fig. 15-21.** Fascia dentata of the hippocampus in Pick's disease showing multiple silver positive inclusions in the granule cells. (Bielschowsky's silver stain; ×330.)

**Table 15-2.** Pathologic characteristics that may help in the differential diagnosis of cortical dementias

| Entity | Cortical degeneration (neuronal loss/ gliosis) | Substantia nigra (neuronal loss) | Basal ganglia (neuronal loss + gliosis) | Hippo-campus | Thalamus | Inclusions | |
|---|---|---|---|---|---|---|---|
| | | | | | | Neuronal | Glial |
| Alzheimer's disease | + + (temporo-parietal) | + | + + + + | + | + | Neurofibrillary tangles | absent |
| Diffuse Lewy body disease | (+) (selective) | + + | + | + | 0 | Lewy bodies | absent |
| Pick's disease | + + + (frontotemporal) | 0 | + + | + | + | Pick bodies | absent |
| Cortical basal ganglionic degeneration | + + (asymmetric) | + + + | + + + (asymmetric) | + | + | Basophilic inclusions (substania nigra) | present |
| Progressive subcortical gliosis | + (patchy) | + + | + + | + + | + + | 0 | absent |
| Chromosome 17-linked dementia | + + (selective) | + + + | + + | + | + | Neurofibrillary tangle-like inclusions | present |
| Mesocorticolimbic dementia | + + (selective) | + + + | + + | + + | 0 | 0 | absent |

0—Normal; +—Mild; + +—Moderate; + + +—Severe changes

Imaging studies often reveal frontoparietal atrophy, commonly asymmetric, and associated hemiatrophy of midbrain and pons.[116] PET glucose utilization scans show corresponding changes and decreased glucose metabolism of the thalamus and hippocampus.[23]

**Neuropathology.** Brain weight usually is substantially reduced. The characteristic gross findings consist of asymmetric atrophy, particularly of the frontal and parietal regions. In coronal sections there is thinning of the corpus callosum and atrophy of centrum semiovale.[78] Lateral thalamic nuclei and basal ganglia may show gross atrophy. Apart from the profound cortical atrophy, depigmentation of the substantia nigra probably is the most characteristic gross finding in cases of CBGD.

The affected areas of the cerebral cortex show marked decrease in the number of neurons and gliosis that commonly involves the entire thickness of the cortex (Fig. 15-22). Swollen ballooned (achromatic) neurons are abundant. In severely degenerated parts of the cortex, the superficial layers may display spongiform change. Within affected cortical areas the severity of the degenerative changes may vary from one microscopic field to another.[70] Substantia nigra exhibits severe loss of pigmented neurons (Fig. 15-23) in the pars compacta, sometimes with relative sparing of the medial portion.[115] Basal ganglia and striatum often are involved in the degenerative process; the putamen usually is more severely affected than the globus pallidus or caudate nucleus. Thalamic involvement usu-

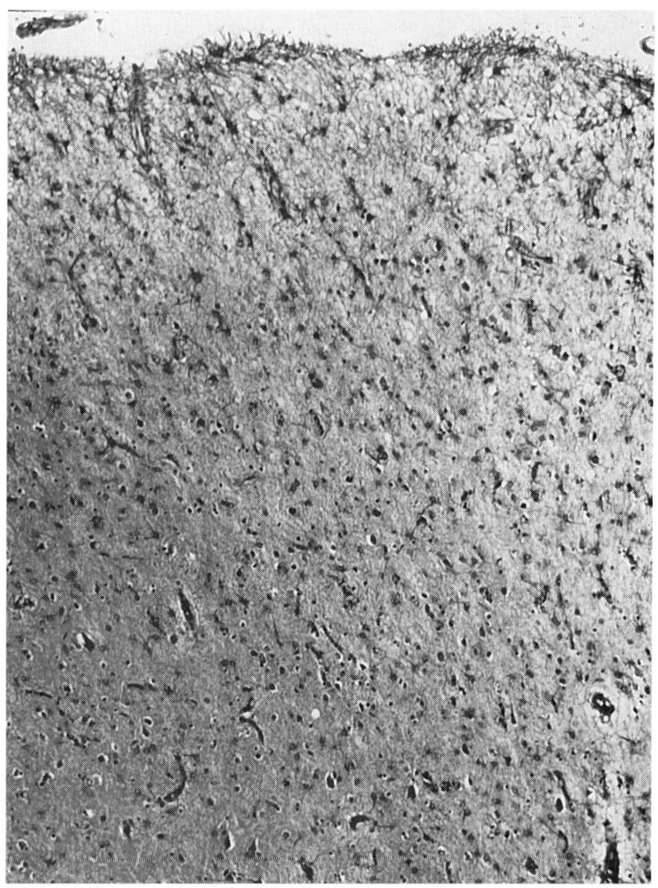

**Fig. 15-22.** Parietal cortex from a case with cortical-basal ganglionic degeneration showing severe neuronal loss and gliosis. (PTAH; ×21.)

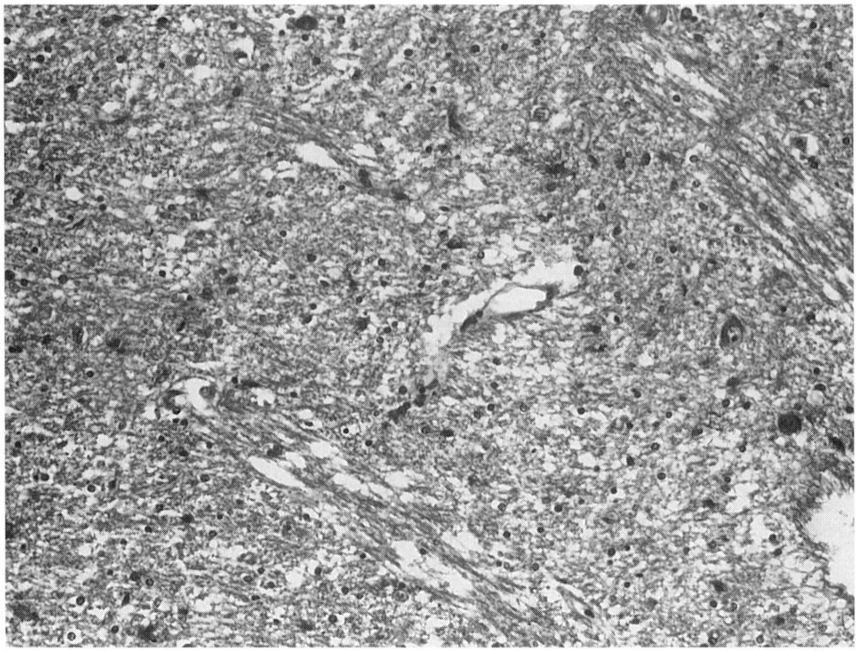

**Fig. 15-23.** Substantia nigra showing severe neuronal loss and gliosis in cortical-basal ganglionic degeneration. (PTAH; ×83.)

ally is more pronounced in the lateral nuclei.[39] The white matter underlying affected cortices shows rarefaction with myelin pallor and axonal loss. Other nuclei that may be involved, albeit to a lesser extent, include the claustrum, the red nucleus, and the subthalamic nucleus. The hippocampus characteristically is devoid of degenerative structural changes. Typical basophilic (or corticobasal) inclusions,[39] most commonly encountered in substanti nigra (Fig. 15-24), locus ceruleus, and raphe nuclei, are one of the hallmarks of CBGD. Ballooned neurons are positive for antibodies to phosphorylated 160 and 200 kD neurofilaments.[70] Furthermore, cytoplasmic inclusions in glial cells immunopositive for tau protein have been reported in multiple system atrophy.[102] Pick bodies are not part of CBGD, and their absence may be helpful in the sometimes difficult differential diagnosis between CBGD and Pick's disease (Table 15-2).

### Progressive Subcortical Gliosis

Progressive subcortical gliosis (PSG), a rare dementing neurodegenerative disorder that occurs both sporadically and in familial forms,[7,65,125,146] was first described by Neumann.[95,96] The disorder has a relatively early onset (between 40 and 60 years of age) and a course that varies between 4 and 6 years. The early symptoms consist of loss of language comprehension and speech agnosia followed by dementia.

The brain weight is moderately decreased with frontoparietal and temporal atrophy with sparing of the inferior temporal gyrus and hippocampus. The pathologic hallmark of PSG is gliosis in the subcortical white matter, usually most severe in the frontal lobes (Fig. 15-24), that is variably asymmetric.[109,146] The gliosis,

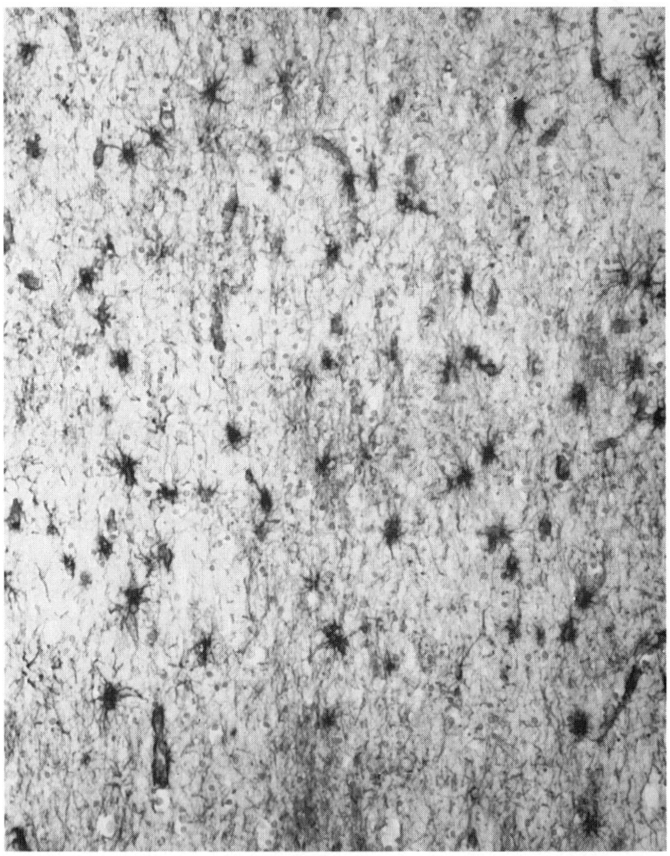

**Fig. 15-24.** Deep frontal cortex and immediate subcortical area demonstrating astrogliosis in a case of PSG. (GFAP-immunostain; ×83.)

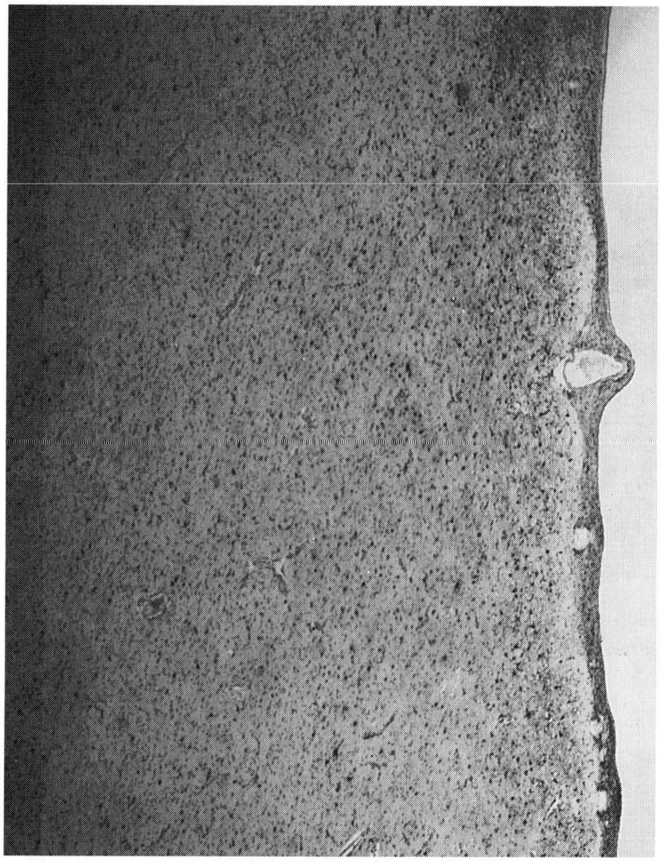

**Fig. 15-25.** Histology sample from the head of the caudate nucleus in a case of PSG, showing diffuse astrogliosis. (GFAP-immunostain; ×21.)

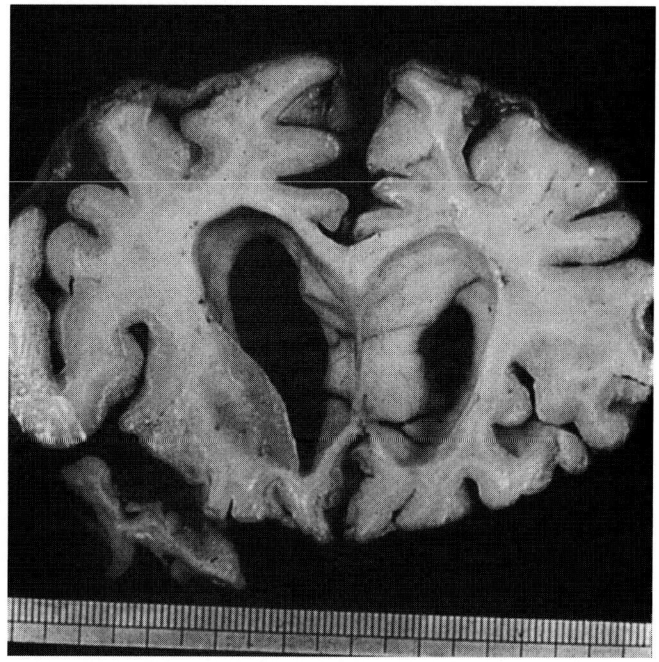

**Fig. 15-26.** Coronal section through the anterior frontal lobe in a case with chromosome 17-linked dementia. Moderate generalized atrophy and marked atrophy of the anterior cingulate are visible.

which may extend into the deeper cortical layers, is diffuse. The astrocytes often show abundant cytoplasm and may attain a gemistocytic-like character. The neuronal loss is mild relative to the extent of gliosis (Fig. 15-25). PSG often is accompanied by severe involvement of the substantia nigra, whereas the hippocampus is spared from the degenerative process. The involvement of striatum is mild or moderate, with the caudate nucleus usually being more severely affected (Fig. 15-25). The thalamus also may show marked neuronal loss. Characteristic neuronal or glial inclusions have not been demonstrated in PSG (Table 15-2). Petersen and co-authors[109] reported two kindreds with familial PSG, originally described by Lanska and associates,[71] that showed proteinase K-resistant PrP and that appeared to be allelic to chromosome 17.

### Chromosome 17-Linked Dementia

A recently described entity with circumscribed cortical degeneration occurring in a large kinship of Irish descent has been linked to chromosome 17.[80,128,151] The symptoms develop in the mid-40s and include personality and behavioral changes and disinhibition manifested as a Klüver-Bucy-like syndrome.[80] Memory eventually becomes affected, with preservation of orientation and speech until late in the disease. Extrapyramidal symptoms are part of the disease.

The brain weight varies from 950 to 1300 g. There is gyral atrophy of anterior and inferior temporal lobes, the prefrontal areas, and anterior cingulate gyrus. Hippocampus is normal in size. Substantia nigra is severely depigmented. Affected cortices show decreased number of neurons, particularly of layers I to III and VI. Characteristically, the affected cortical regions such as the anterior cingulate gyrus are sharply demarcated vis à vis uninvolved neighboring gyri (Fig. 15-26). Neuronal loss is pronounced in the substantia nigra as well as in the putamen and the caudate. The involvement of thalamus is mild. Characteristic changes of chromosome 17-linked dementia include the presence of lattice-like neuronal inclusions that are particularly prominent in the brainstem nuclei[130] (Fig. 15-27). The inclusions show positive immunoreaction for phosphorylated 150/200 neurofilament and ubiquitin, but react negatively with tau and $\beta$-amyloid. Glial cytoplasmic inclusions, similar to those originally described in multiple system atrophy,[130] also are present in PSG (Fig. 15-28). Protease-resistant prion protein has not been identified in dementias linked with chromosome 17.

As in other familial dementing disorders there appear to exist sporadic forms of PSG with pathologic and clinical phenotypes similar to the familial type of dementia linked to chromosome 17.[128] However, these

A

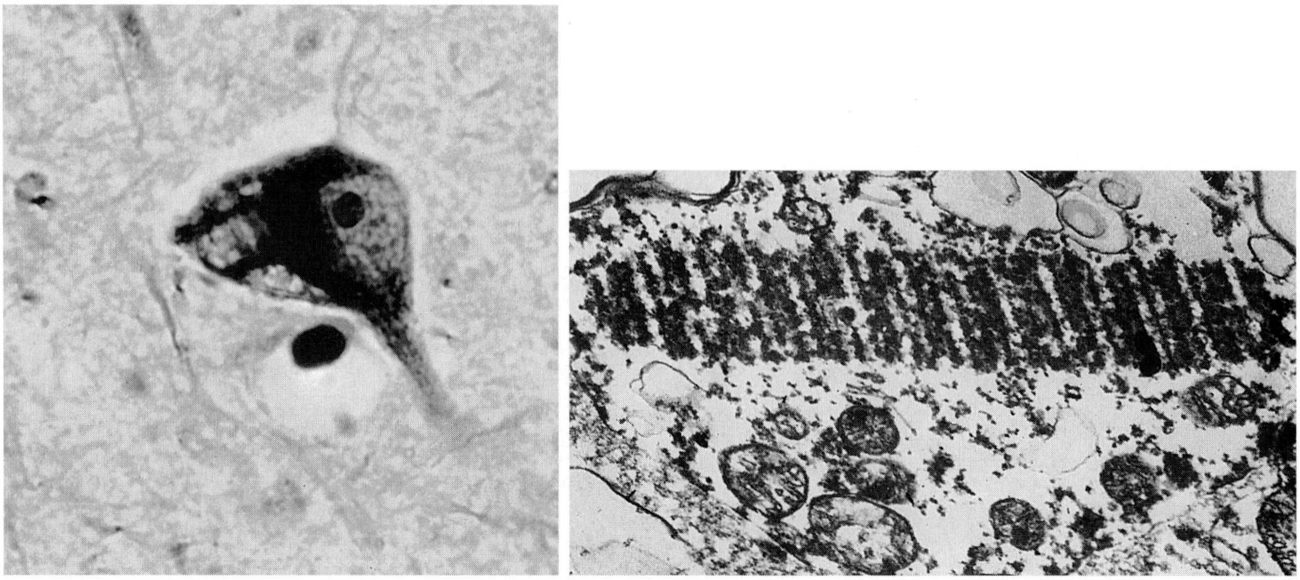

B

**Fig. 15-27.** Argyrophilic neuronal inclusion in chromosome 17-linked dementia. The inclusions are made of lattice-like crystalloid structures. (**A**; Bielschowsky's silver stain; ×1040; **B**; ×11,400.)

A

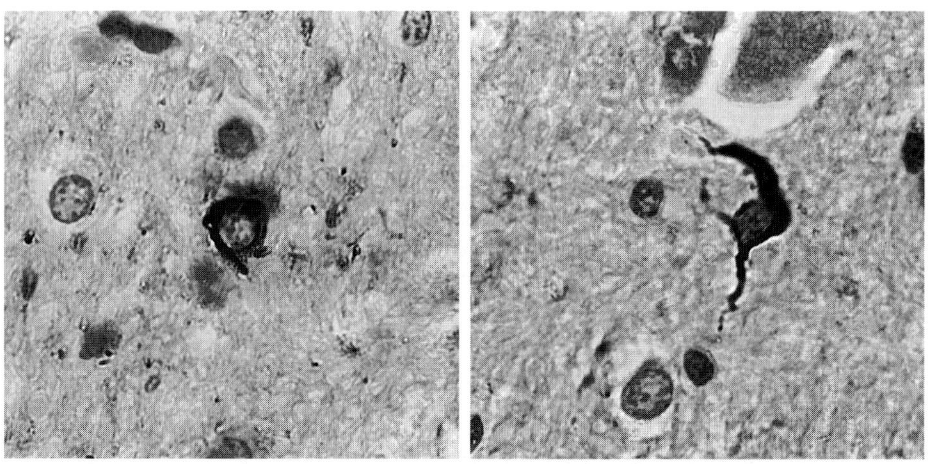

B

**Fig. 15-28.** Micrographs of cytoplasmic glial inclusions in a case with chromosome 17-linked dementia, immunostained with anti-ubiquitin (**A**) and with anti-tau (**B**).

cases show milder involvement of substantia nigra and lack the neuronal and glial inclusions.[128] Prion protein has not been identified in sporadic cases. For differential diagnosis see Table 15-2.

### Mesolimbocortical Dementia

A total of 12 cases of mesolimbocortical dementia (MLCD) have been described.[131,142,143,147] There is a wide range of age of onset (48 to 87 years) and duration of the disease (3 to 26 years). There is no evidence of familial MLCD. The defining clinical feature is dementia, often accompanied or preceded by parkinsonian symptoms or psychiatric and behavioral changes.

At autopsy, the brains of patients with MLCD have shown varying degrees of atrophy involving the medial temporal lobe, the hippocampus, the supraorbital cortex, and the anterior cingulate gyrus.[131,143] Microscopic examination reveals a striking neuronal loss of substantia nigra, particularly of the ventral tegmental area (Fig. 15-29).[131,143] The neurons of the locus ceruleus usually are less involved.

These changes are accompanied by decreased numbers of neurons and gliosis of the entorhinal cortex, anterior cingulate, and supraorbital cortex, often in a sharply demarcated fashion similar to the pathology described in chromosome 17-linked dementia[130] and progressive limbic sclerosis.[128] Marked degeneration

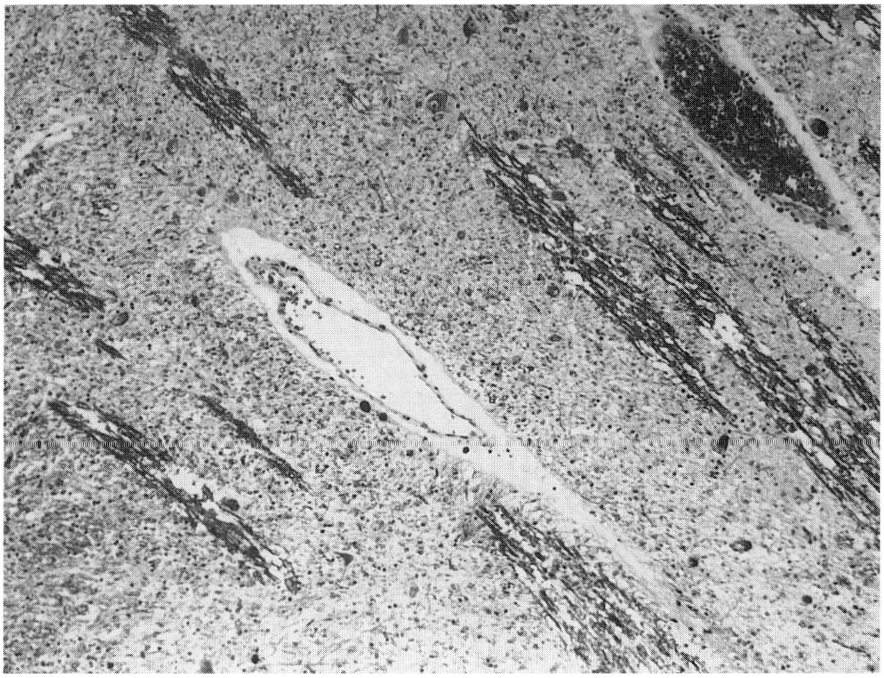

**Fig. 15-29.** Marked loss of pigmented neurons in the medial aspect of the substantia nigra in MLCD. (H&E/LFB; ×21.)

of the perforant tract (Fig. 15-30) and of CA4, CA1, and subiculum (Fig. 15-31) is also visible in the hippocampus (Fig. 15-32). The involvement of subcortical nuclei is usually relatively mild, with rostral caudate being most severely affected by neuronal loss.[131,142] While NFT and ballooned neurons have been identified in some cases, the numbers are scarce. Lewy bodies have not been described in MLCD.

## SUBCORTICAL DEMENTIAS

### Huntington's Disease

Huntington's disease (HD) is an autosomal dominant disorder with full penetrance.[45] The disease is linked to the short arm of chromosome 4, with a variable number of trinucleotide repeats constituting an insertion mutation. The number of repeats gives rise to anticipation: the higher the number of nucleotide repeats, the earlier the onset of disease and the more rapid its course.[57] Within a given kinship the number of repeats may vary widely, even within the same sibship; this gives rise to marked heterogeneity as to onset and course of the disease within the same family.[57,140]

One of the first symptoms is the loss of fast saccadic eye movement.[17] Hyperkinetic chorea follows, progressing to disabling and involuntary violent movements of the limbs. As the disorder progresses, dystonia becomes prominent, with rigidity and bradykinesia.[104] Cognitive impairment, an important feature of HD, often is evident early on by psychometric testing and progresses as the disease advances.[6] Early impairment is seen as an inability to perform complex tasks, and both immediate and remote recall become

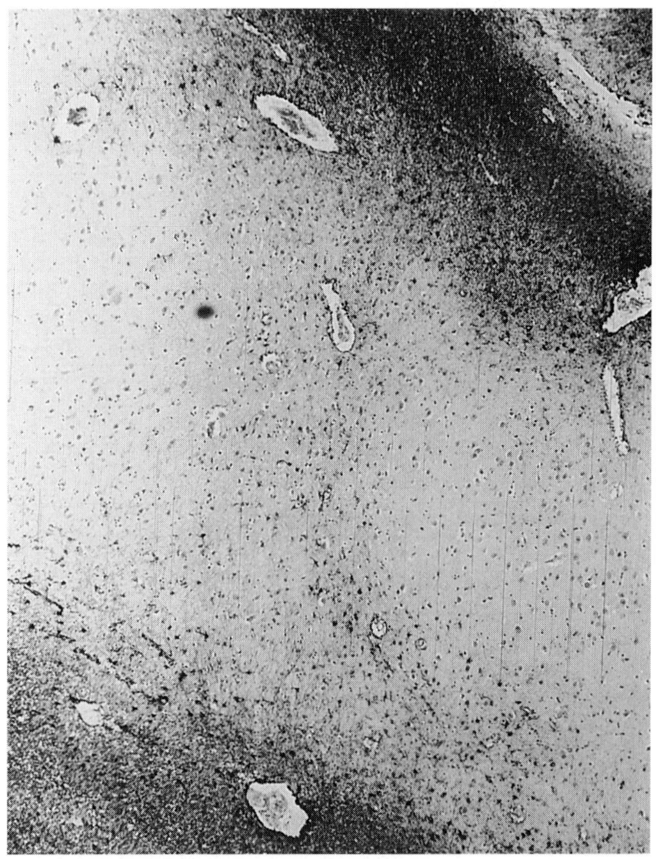

**Fig. 15-30.** Photomicrograph of the subiculum showing degeneration and astrogliosis of the perforant tract in MLCD. (GFAP immunostain; ×21.)

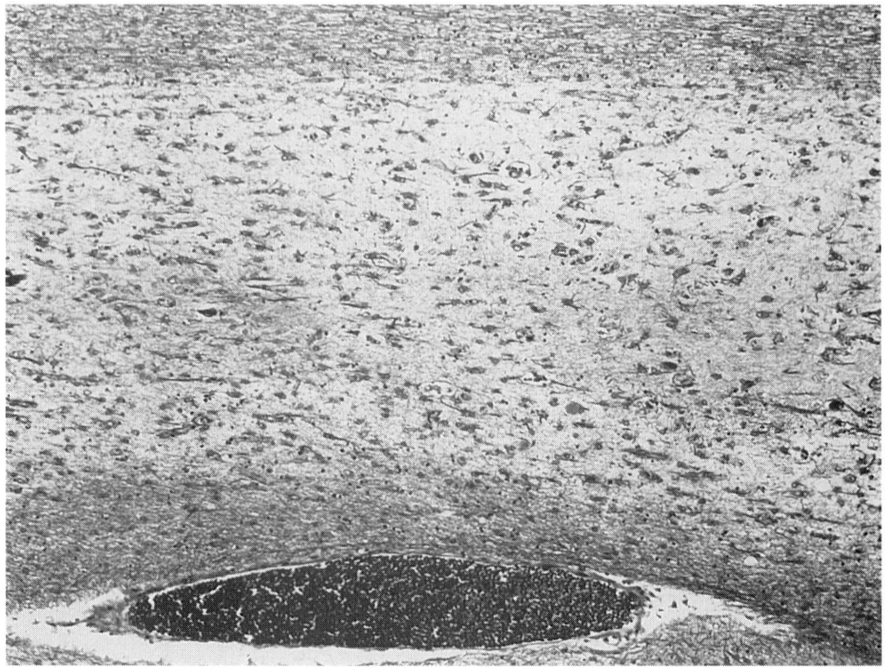

**Fig. 15-31.** Subiculum, from the same case shown in Fig. 15-30, showing marked neuronal loss and dense gliosis. (PTAH; ×41.)

deficient. Hence the cognitive impairment in HD differs from that of the "cortical" dementias, and is believed to be related to the basal ganglia pathology.[6,8] A large percentage of HD patients develop psychiatric symptoms including unipolar or bipolar depressive disorders or sometimes schizophrenia-like disturbances.[29]

In severe cases of HD the brain weight may be reduced by 20% to 30%. Mild cortical atrophy may exist. The main pathology is found in the caudate nucleus, which may be reduced to a thin discolored rim of paraventricular gray matter (Fig. 15-32). The involvement of putamen and globus pallidus is usually milder. The pathology in basal ganglia consists of neuronal loss that particularly affects small spiny neurons; this is accompanied by dense gliosis (Fig. 15-33).[42]

The degenerative process tends to start in the tail of the caudate nucleus. In the head and body of the caudate nucleus the medial aspects are most severely involved by the degenerative process, whereas the dorsal aspects of the nucleus tend to be more severely affected in the putamen. The hypothalamus may display severe changes, including neuronal loss and gliosis, whereas changes in the thalamus are mild. Substantia nigra may undergo up to 40% loss of pigmented neurons; this is believed to be a primary effect, rather than transsynaptic degeneration secondary to the profound changes in the basal ganglia.[101] In addition, degeneration and gliosis may affect the tectal midbrain and periaqueductal gray matter as may the inferior olivary nuclei and the dentate nuclei of the cerebellum, although the changes in the latter two sites usually are mild. Based

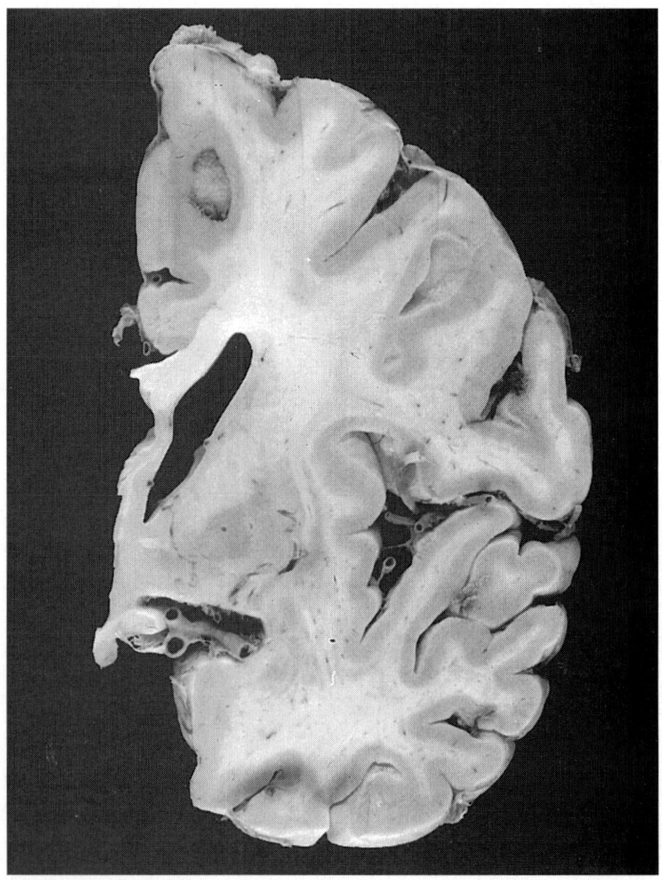

**Fig. 15-32.** Coronal section at the level of the head of the caudate nucleus in Huntington's disease. There is marked atrophy of the caudate nucleus.

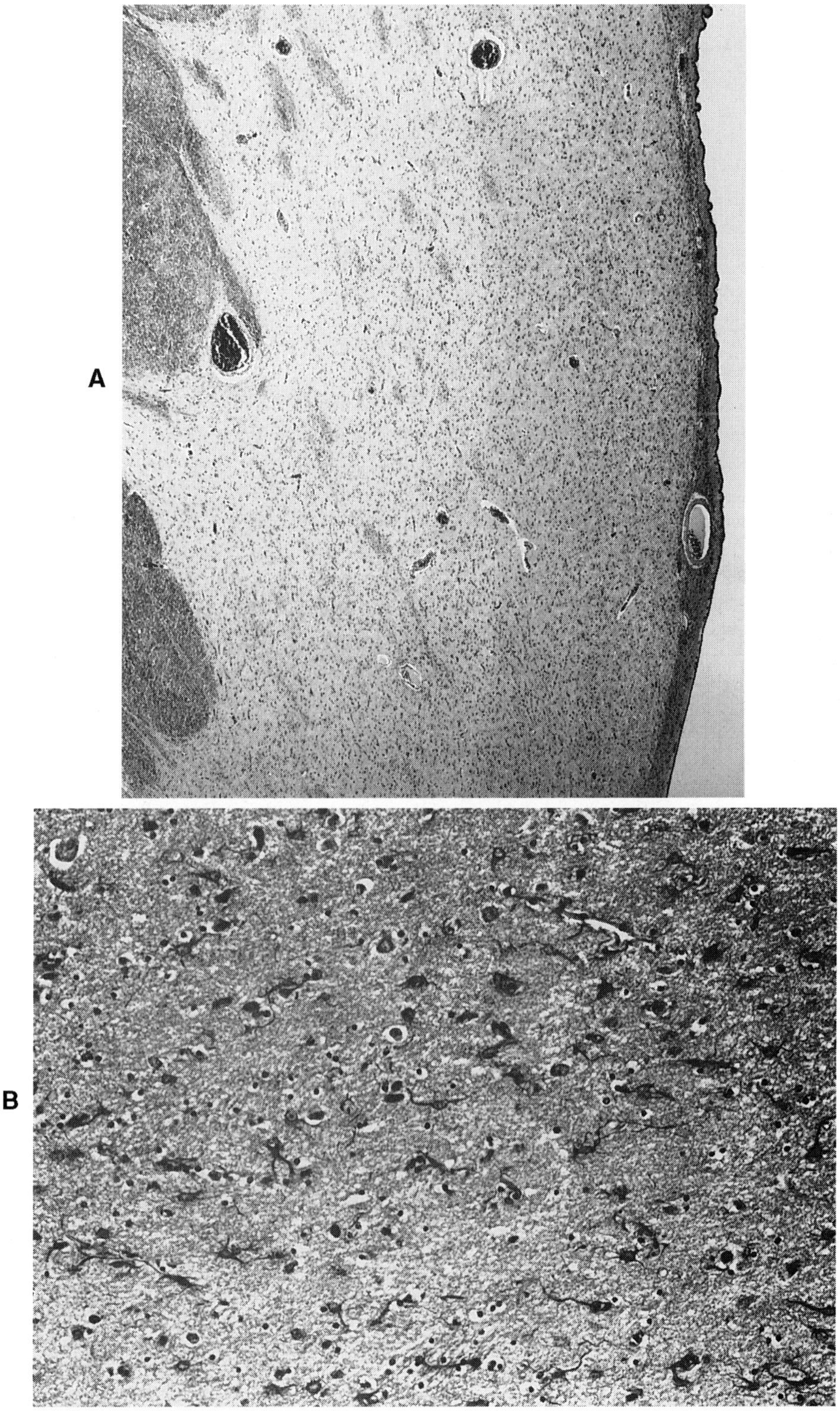


**Fig. 15-33.** **A**, Low magnification of the head of the caudate nucleus in Huntington's disease showing neuronal loss and gliosis. **B**, Higher magnification showing dense isomorphic astrogliosis. (**A**, H&R/LFB; ×21; **B**, PTAH; ×330.)

on the severity of basal ganglia atrophy, the severity of HD has been classified as ranging between 0 (normal) and grade 4 (profound atrophy of caudate, putamen, and internal capsule).[148]

The cerebral cortex may exhibit mild neuronal loss, particularly pronounced among pyramidal cells of layers III and V of the frontal cortex.[134] These changes correlate with decreased cortical glucose utilization in HD.[85]

The striatal pathology corresponds to a marked depletion of $\gamma$-amino-butyric acid (GABA), that are the primary efferent neurons of the striatum.[3] In addition, several neuropeptides, including substance P, cholecystokinin, and enkephalins also are decreased in the striatum of HD patients.[84]

Much attention has been paid to glutamate, a neuronal excitotoxin, and its potential role in the pathogenesis of HD. For reviews on this topic the reader is referred to in reviews by Greenamyre and Shoulson.[43,44]

### Progressive Supranuclear Palsy

Progressive supranuclear palsy (PSP) was recognized as a distinct neurodegenerative entity by Steel, Richardson, and Olszewski in 1963.[138] Most cases of PSP are sporadic, and the onset in most patients is after age 55 years with an even sex distribution. Familial cases of PSP have been reported.[11,155]

The initial symptoms are extrapyramidal, with postural instability, bradykinesia, and rigidity; tremor is rare.[59,67] These symptoms often lead to the misdiagnosis of Parkinson's disease. A typical feature of PSP is neck dystonia, often followed by dystonia of the limbs.[114] Corticospinal and corticobulbar abnormalities are common, leading to dysarthria and dysphagia.[41,138] Another manifestation of PSP is emotional incontinence. Neuroophthalmic abnormalities are the clinical hallmark of PSP although sometimes these symptoms develop late in the disease. The most characteristic deficit is supranuclear gaze palsy;[40] downgaze is most severely affected, and this is followed by limitations in upward gaze and lateral gaze.[40] Cognitive dysfunction in PSP has been associated with the subcortical pathology characteristic of this disorder and consists of depression, apathy, impaired executive function, and visuospatial disturbances.[1] Some authors[59] have suggested that the perceived cognitive dysfunction among patients with PSP can be explained by the neuroophthalmic impairments.

Frontal lobe dysfunction in patients with PSP, such as impaired verbal fluency, forced grasping, and recall impairment, has been described in recent studies.[111]

A

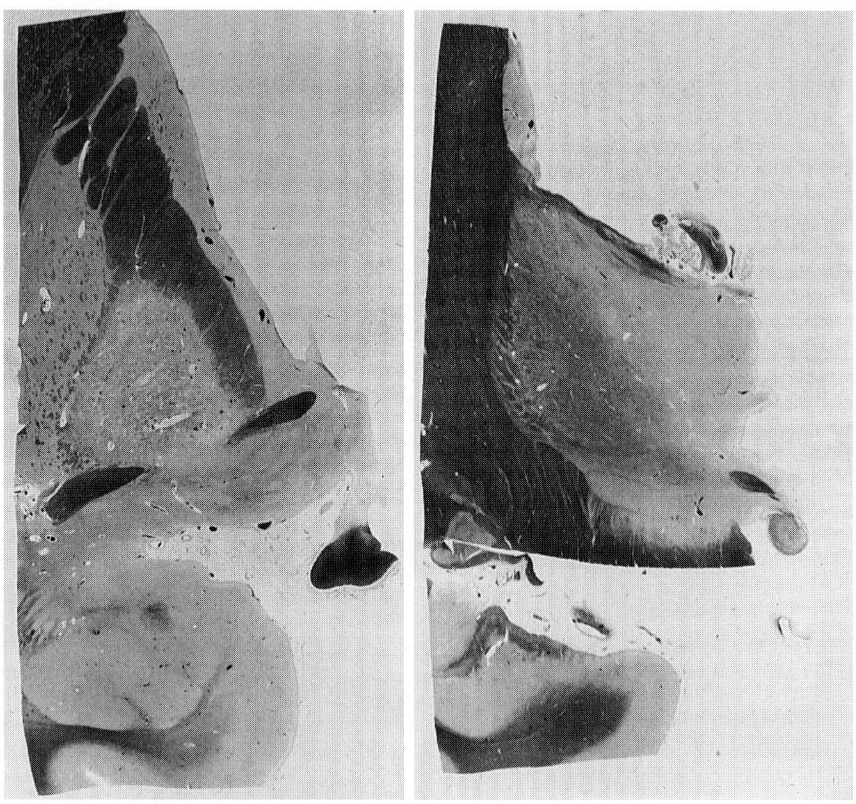

B

**Fig. 15-34.** Basal ganglia in a case of PSP showing moderate atrophy of the globus pallidus (**A**) and subthalamic nucleus (**B**). (H&E/LFB; ×21.)

Both glucose utilization PET scans[30] and detailed neuropathologic examination of 20 cases of PSP (Sima and Foster, unpublished data) support the concept that frontal lobe pathology is a contributing factor to the cognitive dysfunction in PSP.

**Neuropathology of PSP.** On gross inspection there is atrophy of the midbrain and pontine tegmentum. The substantia nigra is depigmented. Coronal sections may reveal mild ventricular and aqueductal dilatation and discoloration and atrophy of the globus pallidus (Fig. 15-34) and the subthalamic nucleus. The cerebral cortex usually is well preserved.[19,72,137,138]

The histopathologic findings consist of NFTs (Fig. 15-35), neuronal loss, and gliosis. The most severely affected nuclei include pars compacta of the substantia nigra, periaqueductal gray matter, subthalamic nucleus, and globus pallidus. Other nuclei commonly involved are the dentate nucleus of the cerebellum, the inferior olivary nucleus, and the anterior thalamic nuclei.[19,72,137] The hippocampus usually is not affected, but may show some neuronal loss and gliosis of CA4. Involvements of amygdala, substantia innominata, and dorsomedial thalamus are usually mild. The changes in cerebral cortex are mild or absent; when present these changes are most notable in the frontal cortex.

The NFT in PSP have been described as globose and composed of 15-nm straight filaments; therefore, these are different from the NFTs of AD and those found in normal aging (Fig. 15-36). NFTs in PSP are easily recognized by conventional silver impregnations. Like the NFTs in AD they stain immunocytochemically with antibodies directed against tau, ubiquitin, and Alz-50, although stainability with the latter two may be weak.[79] The frequency of NFT in the affected nuclei correlates poorly with the severity of neuronal loss. NFTs occasionally are found in the cerebral cortex in PSP, and usually are of the AD type. However, individual cases meeting the diagnostic criteria for both AD and PSP have been reported.[34] A consistent finding in PSP is the presence of tau-positive neuropil threads and astrocytic tangle-like inclusions. However, these findings are not specific for PSP, as both have been observed in cases of corticobasal ganglionic degeneration and postencephalitic Parkinson's disease.[28] There appears to be a close correlation between the density of tau-positive threads and the neuronal loss in affected nuclei (Sima and co-workers, unpublished data). Tau-positive astrocytic tangles are frequent in affected subcortical nuclei, but are found rarely in the cerebral cortex in PSP.

The severity of pathologic changes in PSP correlates poorly with disease duration, and the distribution of these changes may vary from case to case. This led Houw and co-workers[55] to propose pathologic criteria for typical and atypical PSP based on the number of tangles in specific nuclei. However, these criteria have not proved useful, since atypical PSP as defined by Houw and associates probably represent more severe cases of otherwise clinically and pathologically typical PSP.

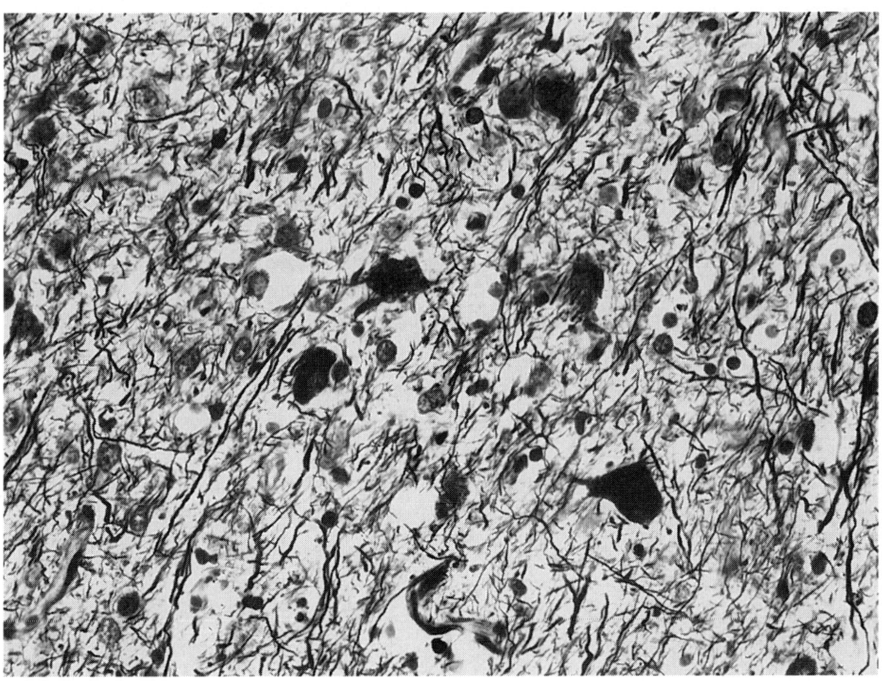

**Fig. 15-35.** Neurofibrillary tangles in the subthalamic nucleus in PSP. (Bielschowsky's silver stain; ×330.)

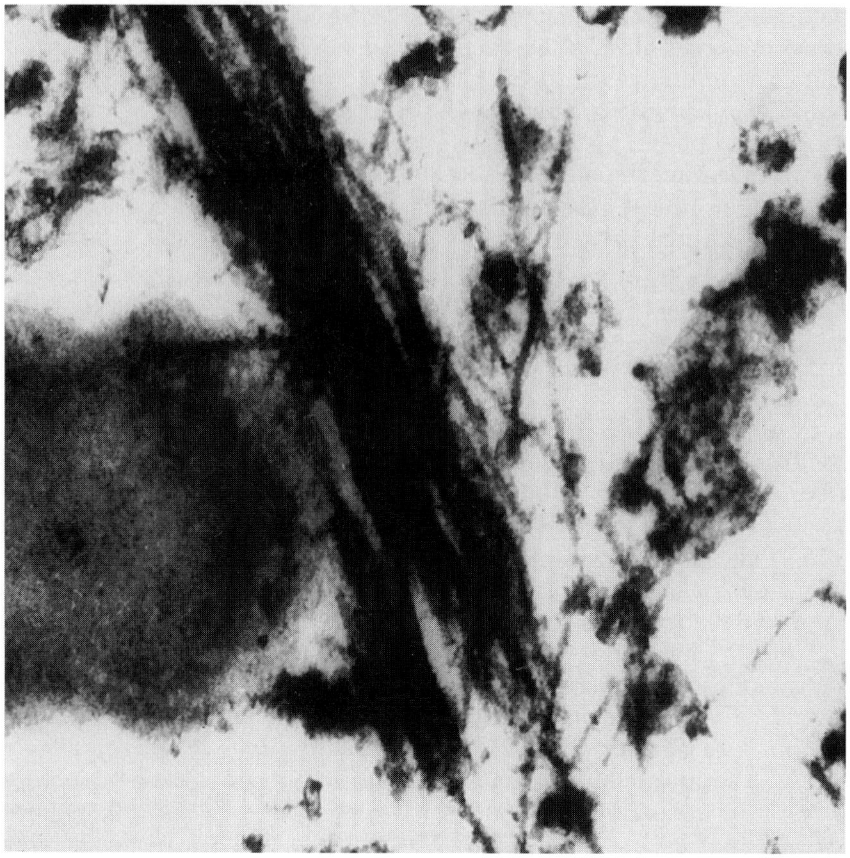

**Fig. 15-36.** Electronmicrograph of neurofibrillary tangle in PSP. The tangles consist of straight filaments each measuring approximately 15 nm in diameter. (×98,000.)

The etiology of PSP is unknown. Neurochemical studies have revealed major defects in both dopamine levels and cholinergic activity. However, the distribution of these changes in PSP differs significantly from that found in both Parkinson's disease and AD, respectively. For an update on the neurochemistry in PSP, the reader is recommended the review by Cardoso and Jankovic.[15]

### Amyotrophic Lateral Sclerosis

Amyotrophic lateral sclerosis (ALS) or motor neuron disease is a progressive, ultimately fatal disease with degeneration of motor neurons of the brain, brainstem, and spinal cord. Familial forms of ALS account for approximately 10% of cases. The incidence of sporadic ALS peaks between 50 and 70 years, whereas familial forms became manifest at a later age. Familial ALS is linked to chromosome 21 q.[127] The phenotypic expression of familial ALS may vary widely within the same kinship.[127,145] Classic ALS is commonly associated with dementia and parkinsonian symptoms. This constellation of the clinical features appears to be more common among the familial cases.

A rare type of ALS, called Kennedy's syndrome, has, in addition to the classic motor deficits, hypogonadism and gynecomastia.[73] ALS is insidious in onset; weakness often starts in the hands, then spreads to the proximal arm muscles and the legs. Early in the course of the disease the weakness may be asymmetric. Sometimes the symptoms may start in the lower limbs. Cranial symptoms usually are restricted to dysphagia and dysarthria. The rate of progression and the duration of symptoms vary between 6 months and 25 years.[73] The mean duration of ALS is approximately 4 years.

**Pathogenesis.** Familial chromosome 21-linked ALS is associated with a mutation of the gene encoding for Cu/Zn superoxide dismutase; this would suggest that defects in scavenging of free radicals may play a pathogenetic role in ALS.[119] In the X-linked Kennedy's syndrome a mutation of the androgen receptor gene has been demonstrated;[133] the mutation consists of an enlarged repeat of CAG.

Specific pathogenetic mechanisms have not been identified in most cases of sporadic ALS, although several as yet inconclusive mechanisms have been suggested. Altered levels of excitatory amino acids have been reported in the brain, spinal cord, and CSF.[83,120]

Immunologic mechanisms linked to the higher incidence of monoclonal gammopathies in ALS[156] are an alternative suggestion to explain the pathogenesis of motor neuron degeneration. Other abnormalities in ALS include antiganglioside antibodies.[108] It is doubtful that these mechanisms are primary factors in the genesis of this disease. More likely, these abnormalities reflect secondary phenomena occurring during the evolution of the disease process. A variety of environmental factors such as viral infections and exposure to toxic substances have been suggested in the pathogenesis of ALS.

**Pathology of ALS and ALS dementia.** Classic ALS is characterized by selective degeneration of upper and lower somatic motor neurons (Fig. 15-37) with sparing of the Onuf's nucleus of the sacral cord and the oculomotor neurons of the brainstem. Involvement of the neurons in the Clark's column is common.[152] These changes are accompanied by degeneration of the corticospinal tracts (Fig. 15-38), anterior spinal roots, and peripheral motor nerve fibers. Skeletal muscles show the characteristics of neurogenetic myopathy with group fiber atrophy and, in severe cases, marked replacement of the muscle fibers by fibrous and adipose tissue. However the pathology is not confined to the motor systems only. In advanced cases of ALS, subcortical nuclei may show neuronal loss and gliosis; this tends to be particularly noticeable in the red nucleus, substantia nigra, globus pallidus, thalamus, subthalamic nuclei, and the dentate nucleus of the cerebellum.[12,56] These changes may be accompanied by degeneration of the dorsal columns of the spinal cord, medial lemniscus, central tegmental tract, and spinocerebellar pathways.[51] Extramotor involvement, except for degeneration of the dorsal columns, appears to be more common in advanced cases and is different in nonfamilial and familial ALS.

A characteristic but not specific histopathologic feature of ALS is the presence of Bunina bodies.[13,16] These are small eosinophilic cytoplasmic granular inclusions that often are accompanied by larger, ubiquitin-positive cytoplasmic inclusions. Both types of inclusions have been seen in the anterior horn cells. Sometimes ubiquitin-positive grains also are present; this tends to be particularly true in the motor neurons of the anterior horn.[94]

The incidence of AD or Parkinson's disease in ALS patients or their family members appears to be higher than would be expected in the general population.[118] The reason for this is unknown.

ALS with dementia shows the same pathology seen in classic ALS but in this variant there is additional involvement of the frontotemporal cortex. This dementia of frontal lobe type (DFLT)[94] is accompanied by severe neuronal loss, gliosis, and spongy degeneration of the frontotemporal and at times the parietal and entorhinal cortices. This degenerative process appears to affect more severely layers II and III of neocortical areas and is accompanied by subcortical gliosis. These changes often are associated with severe degeneration, of the substantia nigra; basal ganglia, thalamus, and subthalamus also may be involved. Ubiquitin-positive inclusions in the granule cells of the fascia dentata and the superficial layers of the frontotemporal cortex have been demonstrated in ALS with DFLT.[98,150] In such situations the cortical pathology may be difficult to separate from the changes considered typical of Pick's disease.

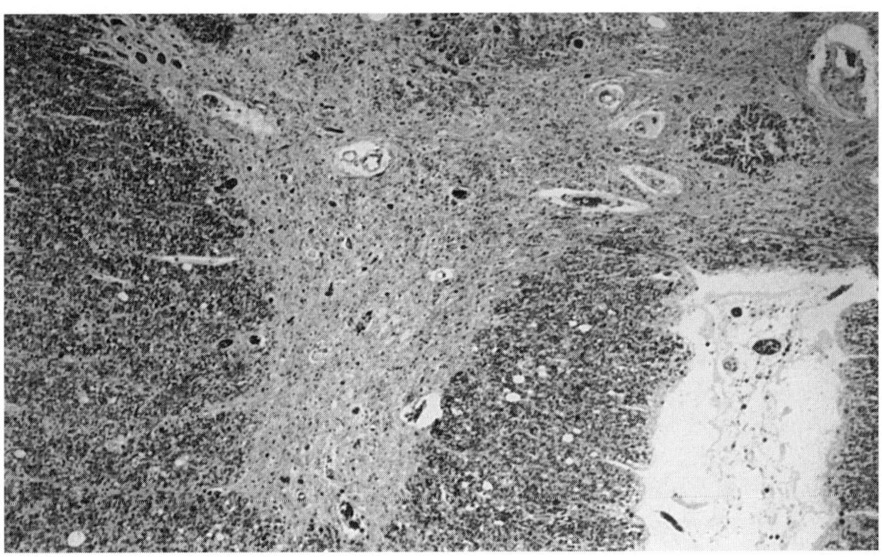

**Fig. 15-37.** Ventral horn of the thoracic cord in ALS showing loss of anterior horn cells. (H&E/LFB; ×21.)

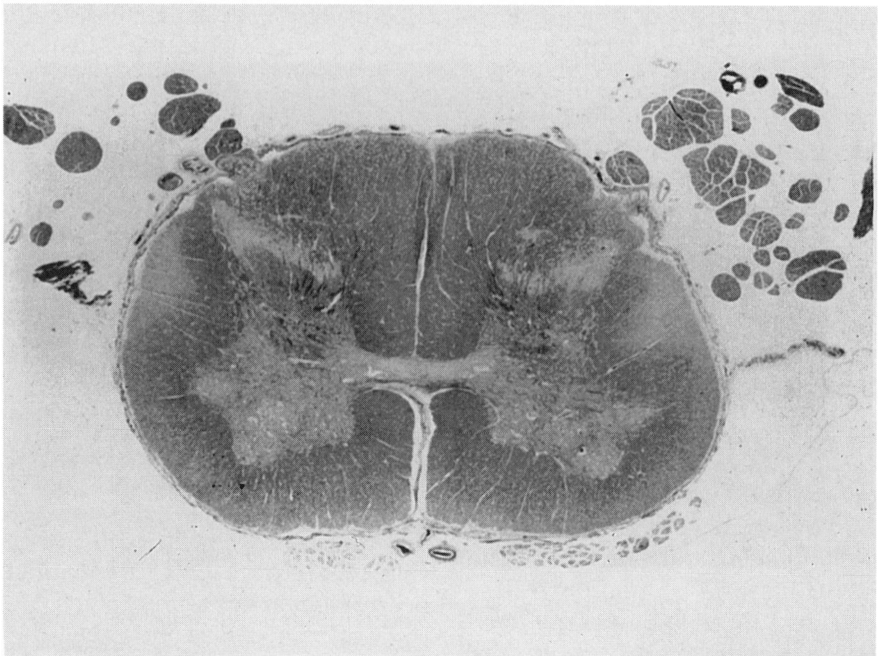

**Fig. 15-38.** Transverse section of the lumbar cord in ALS demonstrating degeneration of the lateral corticospinal tracts. Also there is marked atrophy of the anterior roots compared with the normal dorsal roots. (H&E/LFB; ×14.)

## Parkinson's Disease

Parkinson's disease (PD) is clinically characterized by resting tremor, muscular rigidity, bradykinesia, postural instability, and gait disturbance. Tremor is the most common presenting symptom and usually involves one upper limb that soon spreads to the contralateral upper limb and lower limbs.[39,46] PD often is divided into idiopathic Parkinson's disease and atypical Parkinson's disease (AP). These two forms of PD may be distinguished on high-strength T2-weighted MRI because of the characteristic and marked hypointensity of putamen in AP that does not exist in idiopathic PD.[100] Patients with AP usually have a more rapid progression of symptoms. Secondary PD is the result of destructive lesions in the basal ganglia, whether they are infarcts, neoplasms, or infectious processes. PD is a disorder of the elderly, with a prevalence rate of 1% in persons 60 years and older that increases to 2.6% in those over 85 years.[68] The mean age of onset is the early 60s. Considerable heterogeneity in the clinical picture and in the response to treatment has been noted by several authors.

Dementia in PD patients is approximately four times more common than in the non-PD population.[88] Dementia appears to be particularly common in patients with late-onset PD, and in patients with AD and rapid progression.[53] Patients with PD often have symptoms of autonomic dysfunction characterized by a slow, low-volume speech. The major underlying pathophysiology of PD is degeneration of pigmented neurons in the substantia nigra and striatal dopamine deficiency.[54] Drug-induced parkinsonism is a well known consequence of having postsynaptic dopamine receptors blocked by tranquilizing drugs.

**Pathology of PD.** The pathologic hallmark of PD is neuronal loss and gliosis of the substantia nigra and pars compacta and the presence of Lewy bodies. These are eosinophilic cytoplasmic inclusions exhibiting a dense central core and a pale concentric halo that separates the inclusion from the cytoplasm (Fig. 15-39).[37,60] The loss of pigmented nigral neurons often is accentuated by the presence of melanin pigment in the neuropil; this often is referred to as "pigment incontinence." The most severe changes affect the lateroventral part of substantia nigra, whose main projections contact neurons of the dorsolateral putamen. This nucleus also shows the most severe dopamine depletion in PD.[63] Other structures involved in PD include the locus ceruleus, nucleus basalis of Meynert, dorsal motor nucleus of vagus, the intermediolateral column of the spinal cord, and vertebral sympathetic ganglia; neurons at each of these sites also may contain classic Lewy bodies.[60] Neuronal loss in varying degrees and usually mild gliosis may affect these anatomical sites.

The characteristic Lewy bodies are easily detected in eosin-hematoxylin stained sections but can be accen-

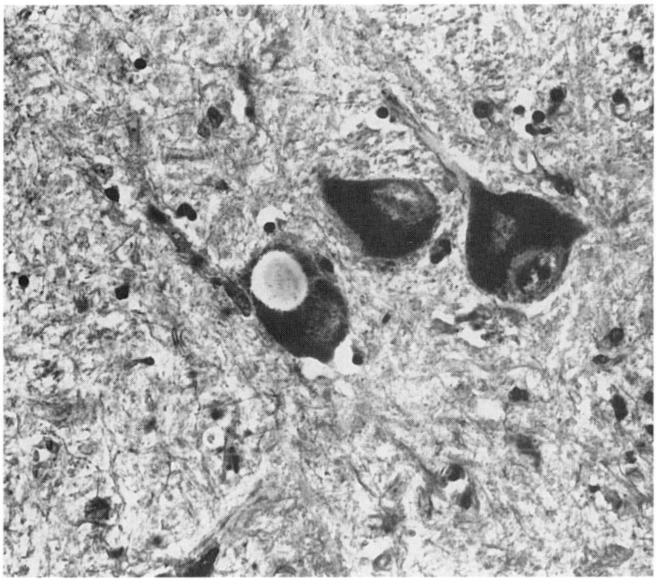

**Fig. 15-39.** Pigmented neurons of the substantia nigra with a classic Lewy body showing a dark center and a lighter halo. (H&E/LFB; ×330.)

tuated with immunostains for ubiquitin or phosphorylated neurofilaments. Ultrastructurally the inclusion bodies consist of radially arranged neurofilaments more densely packed at the center (Fig. 15-40); this accounts for the appearance of the dense eosinophilic core in light-microscopy.

Patients with AP, who make up about 25% of those with PD, often show more widespread degenerative changes than patients with idiopathic PD. These changes usually involve the striatum, thalamus, subthalamic nucleus, hypothalamus, amygdala, and to some extent the cerebral cortex.[38]

The dementia that commonly accompanies PD has not been well explained. Some authors suggest that this syndrome may be caused by subcortical degeneration specifically involving the caudate nucleus; this type of dementia is more common in cases of AP. Furthermore, AD may occur concomitantly with PD, and the possibility of adding DLBD to the diagnosis of PD also should be kept in mind. The possible pathophysiologic relationships between PD and DLBD have been discussed previously in the diffuse Lewy body disease section of this chapter.

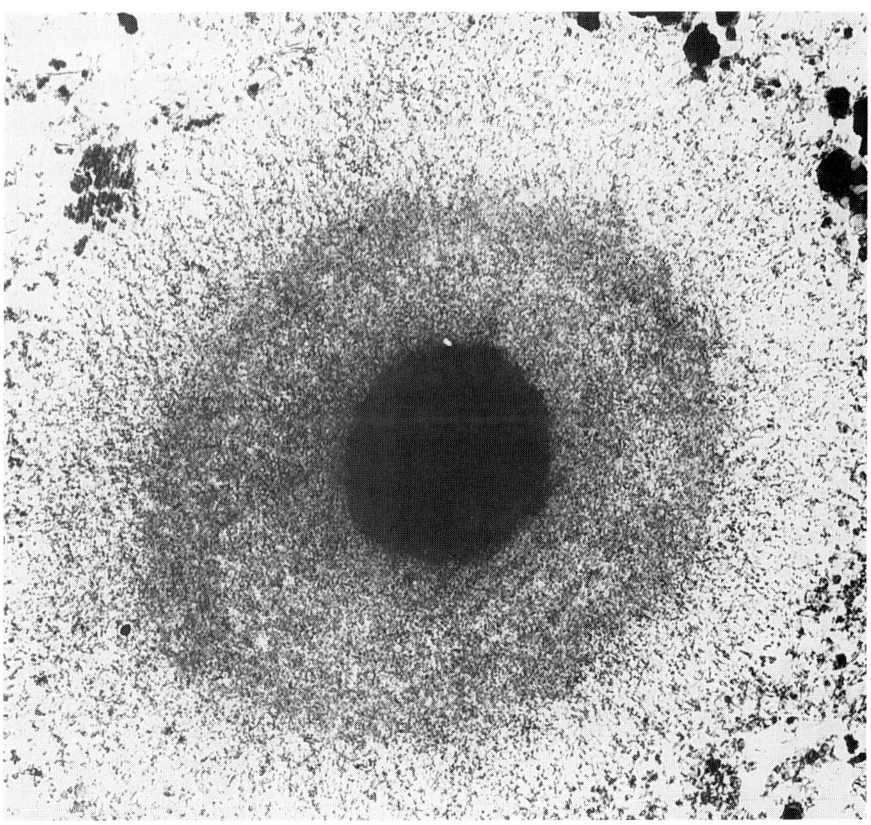

**Fig. 15-40.** Electronmicrograph of a classic Lewy body in Parkinson's disease. The dense core and the light peripheral halo are made of radially oriented neurofilaments. (×28,000.)

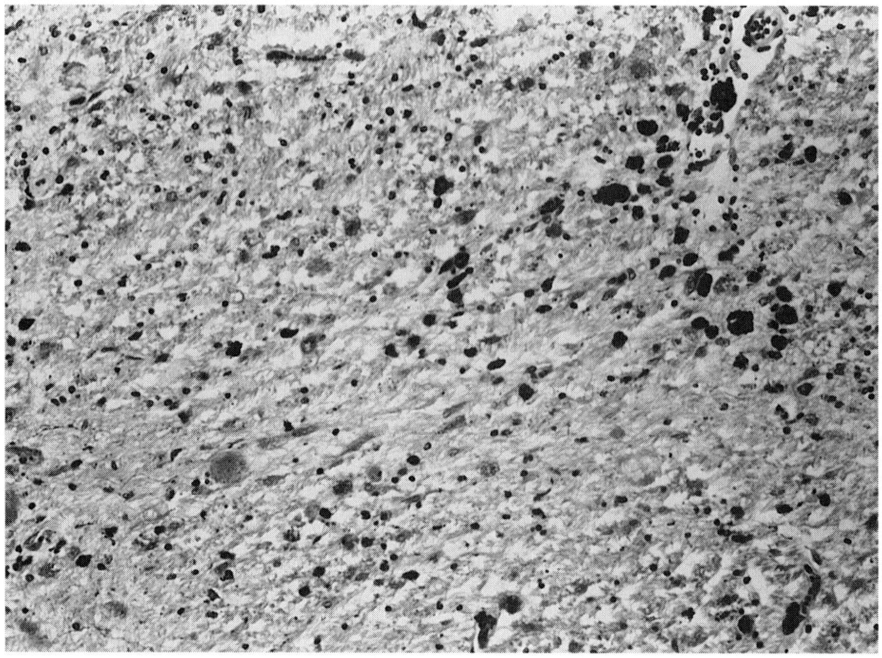

**Fig. 15-41.** Photomicrograph of the globus pallidus in Hallervorden-Spatz disease showing hyperpigmentation and axonal spheroids. (H&E/LFB; ×165.)

### Hallervorden-Spatz Syndrome

Hallervorden-Spatz syndrome (HSS) is a rare disorder characterized by extrapyramidal symptoms that include rigidity, dystonia, choreoathetosis, tremor, signs of corticospinal disease, and dementia. HSS occurs both in a familial form, as an autosomal recessive trait, and sporadically.[99] The age of onset of disease varies, and this has led to the separation of juvenile and late-onset forms.[113,153]

The typical neuropathologic features of HSS include atrophy and brownish discoloration of the globus pallidus that is particularly prominent in the mesial segment of the nucleus. This is accompanied by degeneration of the substantia nigra (pars reticularis). Diffuse neuronal loss, gliosis, and abundant axonal spheroids in the globus pallidus, substantia nigra, and to a lesser extent in the accessory cuneate nucleus of the medulla, are the characteristic microscopic changes.[47] These changes are associated with accumulation of large amounts of pigment in macrophages, astrocytes, or extracellularly in the neuropil (Fig. 15-41). The pigment is composed of neuromelanin, ceroid lipofuscin, and iron. Iron salts also may be found within neurons.[141]

The juvenile and late-onset forms of HSS have similar pathology, although axonal spheroids are more widespread in the juvenile form.[153]

No specific gene locus has been identified in familial cases. The pathogenesis of HSS is not known. The characteristic deposition of iron has recently drawn attention to the formation of free radical formation as a possible mechanism of neuronal death.[48]

### REFERENCES


1. Albert LM, Feldman RG, and Willis AL: The "subcortical dementia" of progressive supranuclear palsy, J Neurol Neurosurg Psychiatry 37:121-130, 1974.
2. Albin RL, and others: Fluoro-deoxyglucose positron emission tomography in diffuse Lewy body disease, Neurology 47: 462–466, 1996.
3. Albin RL, Young AB, and Penney JB: The functional anatomy of basal ganglia disorders, Trends Neurosci 12:366-375, 1989.
4. Alzheimer A: Über eine eigenartige Erkrankung der Hirnrinde, Zentralbl Nervenheilk Psychiatr (Leipzig) 30:177-179, 1907.
5. American Psychiatric Association: Diagnostic and Statistical Manual of Mental Disorders, ed 3, Washington, DC, 1987, American Psychiatric Association.
6. Bamford KA, and others: Clinical-pathological correlations in Huntington's disease: a neuropsychological and computed tomography study, Neurology 39:796-801, 1980.
7. Bergmann M, Gullotta F, and Weitbrecht WU: Progressive subkortikale Gliose, Fortschr Neurol Psychiatr 59:328-334, 1991.
8. Brandt J, Folstein SE, and Folstein MF: Differential cognitive impairment in Alzheimer's and Huntington's disease, Ann Neurol 23:555-561, 1988.
9. Brion S, and Jedynak CP: Troubles du transfert interhemispherique (callosal disconnection), Rev Neurol 126:257-266, 1972.
10. Brouwers P, and others: Differential perceptual-spatial impairment in Huntington's and Alzheimer's dementias, Arch Neurol 41:1073-1076, 1984.
11. Brown J, and others: Familial progressive supranuclear palsy, J Neurol Neurosurg Psychiatry 56:473-476, 1993.
12. Brownell B, Oppenheimer DR, and Hughes TJ: The central nervous system in motor neuron disease, J Neurol Neurosurg Psychiatry 33:338-357, 1970.

13. Bunina TL: On intracellular inclusions in familial amyotrophic lateral sclerosis, Zh Nevropatol Psikhiatr Im S S Korsakova 62: 1293-1299, 1962.
14. Byrne J, and others: Diffuse Lewy body disease. Clinical features in 15 cases, J Neurol Neurosurg Psychiatry 52:709-717, 1989.
15. Cardoso F, and Jancovic J: Progressive supranuclear palsy. In Calne DB, editor: Neurodengenerative Diseases. Philadelphia, 1994, WB Saunders.
16. Chou SM: Pathognomy of intraneuronal inclusions in ALS. In Tsubaki T and Toyokura Y, editors: Amyotrophic Lateral Sclerosis. Tokyo, 1979, Tokyo University Press.
17. Collewijn H, and others: Oculomotor defects in patients with Huntington's disease and their offspring, J Neurol Sci 86:307-320, 1988.
18. Cummings JL, and others: Aphasia in dementia of the Alzheimer type, Neurology 35:394-397, 1985.
19. Daniel SE, de Bruin VMS, and Lees AJ: The clinical and pathological spectrum of Steele-Richardson-Olszewski syndrome (progressive supranuclear palsy): a reappraisal, Brain 118:759-770, 1995.
20. Dickson DW, and others: Diffuse Lewy body disease: neuropathological and biochemical studies of six patients, Acta Neuropathol 75:8-15, 1987.
21. Drayer BP: Imaging of the aging brain: Part II. Pathologic conditions, Radiology 166:797-806, 1988.
22. Eggertson DE, and Sima AAF: Dementia with cerebral Lewy bodies—a mesocortical dopaminergic defect? Arch Neurol 43: 524-532, 1986.
23. Eidelberg D, and others: The metabolic landscape of corticobasal ganglionic degeneration. Regional asymmetries studied with positron emission tomography, J Neurol Neurosurg Psychiatry 54:856-862, 1991.
24. Evans DA, and others: Prevalence of Alzheimer's disease in a community population of older persons, JAMA 262:2551-2556, 1989.
25. Farrer LA, and others: Assessment of genetic risk for Alzheimer's disease among first-degree relatives, Ann Neurol 25:485-493, 1989.
26. Fazekas F, and others: MR signal abnormalities at 1.5 T in Alzheimer's dementia and normal aging, Am J Neuroradiol 8: 421-426, 1987.
27. Fearnley J, and Lees A: Pathology of Parkinson's disease. In Calne DB editor: Neurodegenerative Diseases. Philadelphia, 1994, WB Saunders.
28. Feavy MB, Mattiace LA, and Dickson DW: Neuropathologic overlap of progressive supranuclear palsy, Pick's disease and corticobasal degeneration, J Neuropathol Exp Neurol 55:53-67, 1996.
29. Folstein S: Huntington's disease: a disorder of families. Baltimore, 1989, Johns Hopkins Press.
30. Foster NL, and others: Cerebral hypometabolism in progressive supranuclear palsy studied with positron emission tomography, Ann Neurol 24:399-406, 1988.
31. Frackowiak RSJ, and others: Regional cerebral oxygen supply and utilization in dementia. A clinical and physiological study with oxygen-15 and positron tomography, Brain 104:753-778, 1981.
32. Galasko D, and others: The mini-mental state examination in the early diagnosis of Alzheimer's disease, Arch Neurol 47:49-52, 1990.
33. Gallyas F: Silver staining of Alzheimer's neurofibrillary changes by means of physical development, Acta Morphol Hung 19:1-8, 1971.
34. Gearing M, and others: Progressive supranuclear palsy: neuropathologic and clinical heterogeneity, Neurology 44:1015-1024, 1994.
35. Gibb RG, Esiri MM, and Lees AJ: Clinical and pathological features of diffuse cortical Lewy body disease (Lewy body dementia), Brain 110:1131-1153, 1985.
36. Gibb WAG: Neuropathology of the substantia nigra, Eur Neurol 31 (suppl 1): 48-59, 1991.
37. Gibb WRG: Neuropathology of Parkinson's disease and related syndromes, Neurol Clin 10:361-376, 1992.
38. Gibb WRG, and Lees AJ: A comparison of clinical and pathological features of young- and old-onset Parkinson's disease, Neurology 38:1402-1406, 1988.
39. Gibbs NRG, Luthert PJ, and Marsden CD: Corticobasal degeneration, Brain 112:1171-1182, 1989.
40. Golbe LI, and Davis PH: Progressive supranuclear palsy. In Jankovic J and Tolosa E, editors: Parkinson's Disease and Movement Disorders, ed 2. Baltimore, 1990, Williams & Wilkins.
41. Golbe LI, and others: Prevalence and natural history of progressive supranuclear palsy, Neurology 38:1031-1034, 1988.
42. Graveland GA, Williams RS, and DiFiglia M: Evidence of degenerative and regenerative changes in neostriatal spiny neurons in Huntington's disease, Science 227:770-773, 1985.
43. Greenamyre JT: The role of glutamate in neurotransmission and neurologic disease, Neurobiol Aging 10:593-602, 1989.
44. Greenamyre JT, and Shoulson I: Huntington's disease. In Calne DB, editor: Neurodegenerative Diseases. Philadelphia, 1994, WB Saunders.
45. Gusella JF, and others: A polymorphic DNA marker linked to Huntington's disease, Nature 306:234-238, 1983.
46. Hallett M: Differential diagnosis in tremor. In Vinken PJ, Bruyn GW, and Klawaus HL, editors: Handbook of Clinical Neurology, ed 49. New York, 1986, Elsevier.
47. Hallevorden J, and Spatz H: Eigenartige Erkrankung im extrapyramidalen System mit besonderer Beteiligung des Globus pallidus und der Substantia nigra, Z Ges Neurol Psychiatr 79: 254-302, 1924.
48. Halliwell B, Gutteridge JMC, and Gross CE: Free radicals, antioxidants and human disease. Where are we now? J Lab Clin Med 119:598-620, 1992.
49. Hansen L, and others: The Lewy variant of Alzheimer's disease. A clinical and pathological entity, Neurology 40:1-8, 1990.
50. Hansen LA, and Galasko D: Lewy body disease, Curr Opin Neurol Neurosurg 5:889-894, 1992.
51. Hayashi H, and Kato S: Total manifestations of amyotrophic lateral sclerosis (ALS) in the totally locked in state, J Neurol Sci 93:19-35, 1989.
52. Henderson AS, and others: Apolipoprotein E allele ε4, dementia and cognitive decline in a population sample, Lancet 346:1387-1390, 1995.
53. Hietanen M, and Teräväinen H: The effect of age of disease onset on neuropsychological performance in Parkinson's disease, J Neurol Neurosurg Psychiatry 51:244-249, 1988.
54. Hornykiewicz O, and Kish SJ: Biochemical pathophysiology of Parkinson's disease. In Yahr MD, and Bergmann KJ, editors: Parkinson's Disease. Advances in Neurology, Vol 45. New York, 1986, Raven Press.
55. Houw JJ, and others: Preliminary NINDS neuropathologic criteria for Steele-Richardson-Olszewski syndrome (progressive supranuclear palsy), Neurology 44:2015-2019, 1994.
56. Hughes TJ: Pathology of amyotrophic lateral sclerosis. In Rowland EP, editor: Human Motor Neuron Diseases. Advances in Neurology, Vol 36. New York, 1982, Raven Press.
57. The Huntington's Disease Collaborative Research Group: A novel gene containing a trinucleotide repeat that is expanded and unstable on Huntington's disease chromosomes, Cell 72: 971-983, 1993.
58. Ince P, and others: Quantitative neuropathological study of Alzheimer type pathology in the hippocampus. Comparison of

senile dementia of Alzheimer type, senile dementia of Lewy body type, Parkinson's disease and nondemented elderly control patients, J Neurol Sci 106:142-152, 1991.

59. Jankovic J, and others: Progressive supranuclear palsy: motor, neurobehavioral, and neuroophthalmic findings. In Streifer MB, and others, editors: Parkinson's Disease: Anatomy, Pathology and Therapy. Advances in Neurology, Vol 53. New York, 1990, Raven Press.
60. Jellinger K: The pathology of parkinsonism. In Marsden CD and Fahn S, editors: Movement disorders 2. London, 1987, Butterworths.
61. Jellinger K: Neuropathological substrate of dementia in Parkinson's disease, Ann Neurol 28:723-724, 1990.
62. Karlinsky H, and others: A family with multiple instances of definite, probable and possible early-onset Alzheimer's disease, Br J Psychiatry 159:524-530, 1991.
63. Kish SJ, Shannak K, and Hornykiewicz O: Uneven pattern of dopamine loss in the striatum of patients with idiopathic Parkinson's disease: pathophysiologic and clinical implications, N Engl J Med 318:876-880, 1988.
64. Khachaturian ZS: Diagnosis of Alzheimer's disease. Arch Neurol 42:1097-1105, 1985.
65. Khoubesserian P, and others: Démence familiale de type Neumann (gliose sous corticale), Rev Neurol (Paris) 141:706-712, 1985.
66. Kosik KS, Joachim CL, and Selkoe DJ: The microtubule-associated protein tau ($\tau$) is a major antigenic component of paired helical filaments in Alzheimer's disease, Proc Natl Acad Sci USA 83:4044-4048, 1986.
67. Kristensen MO: Progressive supranuclear palsy—20 years later, Acta Neurol Scand 71:177-189, 1985.
68. Kurland LT: Epidemiology: incidence, geographic distribution, and genetic considerations. In Fields WS, editor: Pathogenesis and Treatment of Parkinsonism. Springfield, IL, 1958, Charles C Thomas.
69. Lampe TH, and others: Phenotype of chromosome 14-linked familial Alzheimer's disease in a large kindred, Ann Neurol 36: 368-378, 1994.
70. Lang AE, Riley DE, and Bergeron C: Cortical-basal ganglionic degeneration. In Calne DB, Neurodegenerative Diseases. Philadelphia, 1994, WB Saunders.
71. Lanska DJ, and others: Familial progressive subcortical gliosis, Neurology 44:1633-1643, 1994.
72. Lantos PL: The neuropathology of progressive supranuclear palsy, J Neural Transm Suppl. 42:137-152, 1994.
73. LaSpada AR, and others: Androgen receptor gene mutations in X-linked spinal and bulbar muscular atrophy, Nature 352: 77-79, 1991.
74. Lee VMY, and others: A68: a major subunit of paired helical filaments and derivatized forms of normal tau, Science 251:675-678, 1991.
75. Leigh PN, and others: Ubiquitin deposits in anterior horn cells in motor neuron disease, Neurosci Lett 93:197-203, 1988.
76. Lennox G, and others: Diffuse Lewy body disease: correlative neuropathology using anti-ubiquitin immunocytochemistry, J Neurol Neurosurg Psychiatry 52:1236-1247, 1989.
77. Liebson E, and Albert ML: Cognitive changes in dementia of the Alzheimer type. In Calne DB, editor: Neurodegenerative Diseases. Philadelphia, 1994, WB Saunders.
78. Lippa CF, Smith TW, and Fontneu N: Cortico-nigral degeneration with neural achromasia, J Neurol Sci 98:301-310, 1990.
79. Love S, and others: Alz-50, ubiquitin and tau immunoreactivity of neurofibrillary tangles, Pick bodies and Lewy bodies, J Neuropathol Exp Neurol 47:393-405, 1988.
80. Lynch T, and others: Clinical characteristics of a family with chromosome-17-linked disinhibition-dementia-parkinsonism-amyotrophy complex, Neurology 44:1878-1884, 1994.
81. Maestre G, and others: Apolipoprotein E and Alzheimer's disease: ethnic variation in genotypic risks, Ann Neurol 37:254-259, 1995.
82. Maggio JE, and Mantyh PW: Brain amyloid—a physiochemical perspective, Brain Pathol 6:147-162, 1996.
83. Malessa S, and others: Amyotrophic lateral sclerosis: glutamate dehydrogenase and transmitter amino acids in the spinal cord, J Neurol Neurosurg Psychiatry 54:984-988, 1991.
84. Martin JB, and Gusella JF: Huntington's disease: pathogenesis and management, N Engl J Med 315:1267-1276, 1986.
85. Martin WRW, and others: Cortical glucose metabolism in Huntington's disease, Neurology 42:223-229, 1992.
86. Mayeux R: Understanding Alzheimer's disease: expect more genes and other things, Ann Neurol 39:689-690, 1996 (editorial).
87. McKeith IG, and others: Lewy body dementia—diagnosis and treatment, Br J Psychiatry 167:709-711, 1995 (editorial).
88. Mindham RHS, Ahmed SWA, and Clough CG: A controlled study of dementia in Parkinson's disease, J Neurol Neurosurg Psychiatry 45:969-974, 1982.
89. Mirra SS, and others: The consortium to establish a registry for Alzheimer's disease (CERAD). Part II: Standardization of the neuropathologic assessment of Alzheimer's disease, Neurology 41:479-486, 1991.
90. Mori H, Kondo J, and Ihara Y: Ubiquitin is a component of paired helical filaments in Alzheimer's disease, Science 325: 1641-1644, 1987.
91. Mortimer JA, Shuman LM, and French LR: Epidemiology of dementing illness. In Mortimer JA, and Shuman LM, editors: Epidemiology of Dementia. Oxford, 1981, Oxford University Press.
92. Munoz-Garcia D, and Ludwin SK: Classic and generalized variants of Pick's disease: a clinicopathologic, ultrastructural and immunocytochemical comparative study, Ann Neurol 16:467-480, 1984.
93. Murdock BE, and Chenerey HJ: Language disorders in dementia of the Alzheimer type, Brain Lang 31:122-137, 1987.
94. Neary D, and others: Frontal lobe dementia and motor neuron disease, J Neurol Neurosurg Psychiatry 53:23-32, 1990.
95. Neumann MA: Pick's disease, J Neuropathol Exp Neurol 8:255-282, 1949.
96. Neumann MA, and Cohn R: Progressive subcortical gliosis, a rare form of pre-senile dementia, Brain 90:405-427, 1967.
97. Norris FH Jr: Adult progressive muscular atrophy and hereditary spinal muscular atrophies, Handb Clin Neurol 59:13-34, 1991.
98. Okamoto K, and others: New ubiquitin-positive intraneuronal inclusions in the extra-motor cortices of patients with ALS, Neurosci-Lett 129:233-236, 1991.
99. Olanow CW: Hallervorden-Spatz syndrome: an iron storage disease. In Calne DB, editor: Neurodegenerative Diseases. Philadelphia, 1994, WB Saunders.
100. Olanow CW, and Hauser RA: Magnetic resonance imaging in neurodengenerative diseases. In Calne DB, editor: Neurodegenerative Diseases. Philadelphia, 1994, WB Saunders.
101. Oyanagi K, and others: A quantitative investigation of the substantia nigra in Huntington's disease, Ann Neurol 26:13-19, 1989.
102. Papp Mi, Khan JE, and Lantos PL: Glial cytoplasmic inclusions in the CNS of patients with multiple system atrophy (striatonigral degeneration, olivopontocerebellar atrophy and Shy-Drager syndrome), J Neurol Sci 94:79-100, 1989.
103. Patel SV: A family with Alzheimer's disease, Br J Psychiatry 155:405-408, 1989.
104. Penney JB, and others: Huntington's disease in Venezuela: 7 years of follow-up on symptomatic and asymptomatic individuals, Mov Disord 5:93-99, 1990.

105. Perry EK, and others: Topography, extent and clinical relevance of neurochemical deficits in dementia of Lewy body type, Parkinson's disease and Alzheimer's disease, Ann NY Acad Sci 640:197-202, 1991.
106. Perry EK, and Perry PH: New insights into the nature of senile (Alzheimer type) plaques, Trends Neurosci 8:301-303, 1985.
107. Perry PH, and others: Senile dementia of Lewy body type, J Neurol Sci 95:119-139, 1990.
108. Pestrouk A, and others: Patterns of serum IgM antibodies to GM, and $GD_{1a}$ gangiosides in amyotrophic lateral sclerosis, Ann Neurol 25:98-102, 1989.
109. Petersen RB, and others: Familial progressive subcortical gliosis: presence of prions and linkage to chromosome 17, Neurology 45:1062-1067, 1995.
110. Pick A. Ueber einen weiteren Symptomenkomplex im Rahmen der Dementia senilis bedingt durch umschriebene stärkere Hirnatrophie (gemischte Apraxie), Monatschr f Phychiatrie u Neurologie 19:97-108, 1906.
111. Pillon B, and others: Severity and specificity of cognitive impairment in Alzheimer's, Huntington's and Parkinson's disease and progressive supranuclear palsy, Neurology 41:634-643, 1991.
112. Price DL, and others: Aggregation of tubulin in neurons in Alzheimer's disease, J Neuropathol Exp Neurol 44:366, 1985.
113. Rabinowicz T, and Wildi E: Spastic amaurotic axonal idiocy: a familial juvenile form of a lipoglyco-protidic thesaurismosis including a pallidal siderosis. In Cummings JN, editor: Cerebral Lipidosis. Springfield, IL, 1957, Charles C Thomas.
114. Rafal RD, and Friedman JH: Limb dystonia in progressive supranuclear palsy, Neurology 37:1546-1549, 1987.
115. Reibeiz JJ, Kalodny EH, and Richardson EP: Corticodentatonigral degeneration with neuronal achromasia, Arch Neurol 18: 20-33, 1968.
116. Riley DE, and others: Cortical-basal ganglionic degeneration, Neurology 40:1203-1212, 1990.
117. Roher AE, and others: $\beta$-amyloid (1-42) is a major component of cerebrovascular amyloid deposits: implications for the pathology of Alzheimer's disease, Proc Natl Acad Sci USA 90: 10836-10840, 1993.
118. Rowland LP: Natural history and clinical features of amyotrophic lateral sclerosis and related motor neuron diseases. In Calne DB, editor: Neurodengenerative Diseases. Philadelphia, 1994, WB Saunders.
119. Rosen DR, and others: Mutations in Cu/Zn superoxide dismutase gene are associated with familial amyotrophic lateral sclerosis, Nature 362:59-62, 1993.
120. Rothstein JD, and others: Abnormal excitatory amino acid metabolism in amyotrophic lateral sclerosis, Ann Neurol 28:18-25, 1990.
121. Salmon E, and Franck G: Positron emission tomographic study in Alzheimer's disease and Pick's disease, Arch Gerontol Geriatr 1:241-247, 1989.
122. Schellenberg GD: Progress in Alzheimer's disease genetics, Curr Opin Neurol 8:262-267, 1995.
123. Schenk VWD: Re-examination of a family with Pick's disease, Ann Hum Genet 23:325-333, 1959.
124. Schmechel DE, and others: Increased amyloid $\beta$-peptide deposition as a consequence of apolipoprotein E genotype in late-onset Alzheimer's disease, Proc Natl Acad Sci USA 90:9649-9653, 1993.
125. Seitelberger F: Präsenile gliale Dystrophie, Acta Neuropath (Berlin) Suppl 4:109-118, 1968.
126. Selzer B, and Sherwin I: A comparison of clinical features in early- and late-onset primary degenerative dementia, Arch Neurol 40:143-146, 1983.
127. Siddique T, and others: Linkage analysis in familial amyotrophic lateral sclerosis, Neurology 39:919-926, 1989.
128. Sima AAF, and others: Primary limbic lobe gliosis: familial and sporadic cases, Brain Pathol 4:538, 1994.
129. Sima AAF, and others: Lewy body dementia without Alzheimer changes, Can Neurol Sci 13:490-497, 1986.
130. Sima AAF, and others: The neuropathology of chromosome 17-linked dementia, Ann Neurol 39:734-743, 1996.
131. Sima AAF, and others: Mesolimbocortical dementia: DLBD without Lewy bodies or a separate entity? J Neuropathol Exp Neurol 55:609, 1996.
132. Sjögren T, Sjögren H, and Lindgren A: Morbus Alzheimer and morbus Pick. Genetic, chemical and pathoanatomic studies, Acta Psychiatr Neurol Scand Suppl 74:189–192, 1952.
133. Sobue G, and others: X-linked bulbospinal neuronopathy. A clinicopathological study, Brain 112:209-232, 1989.
134. Sotrel A, and others: Morphometric analysis of the prefrontal cortex in Huntington's disease, Neurology 41:1117-1123, 1991.
135. St. George-Hyslop PH, and others: The genetic defect causing familial Alzheimer's disease maps on chromosome 21, Science 235:885-890, 1987.
136. Stater E, and Cowie V: The genetics of mental disorders. London, 1971, Oxford University Press.
137. Steele JC: Progressive supranuclear palsy, Brain 95:693-704, 1972.
138. Steele JC, Richardson JC, and Olszewski J: Progressive supranuclear palsy: a heterogeneous degeneration involving the brain stem, basal ganglia and cerebellum with vertical gaze and pseudobulbar palsy, medial dystonia and dementia, Arch Neurol 2: 473-486, 1964.
139. Sternberger NH, Sternberger LA and Ulrich J: Aberrant neurofilament phosphorylation in Alzheimer disease, Proc Natl Acad Sci USA 82:4274-4276, 1985.
140. Strong TV, and others: Widespread expression of the human and rat Huntington's disease gene in brain and non-neural tissue, Nature Genet 5:259-265, 1993.
141. Szanto J, and Gallyas F: A study of iron metabolism in neuropsychiatric patients. Hallervorden Spatz disease, Arch Neurol 14:438-442, 1966.
142. Torack RM, and Morris JC. Mesolimbocortical dementia. A clinicopathologic case study of a putative disorder, Arch Neurol 43:1074-1078, 1986.
143. Torack RM, and Morris JC. The association of ventral tegmental area histopathology with adult dementia, Arch Neurol 45:497-501, 1988.
144. van Mansvelt J: Pick's disease. A syndrome of lobar cerebral atrophy, Thesis, Enschede, Netherlands, 1954.
145. Veltema AN, Ross RAC, and Bruyn GW: Autosomal dominant adult amyotrophic lateral sclerosis, J Neurol Sci 97:93-115, 1990.
146. Verity A, and Wechsler AF: Progressive subcortical gliosis of Neumann: a clinicopathologic study of two cases with review, Arch Gerontol Geriatr 6:245-261, 1987.
147. Verity MA, Roitberg B, and Kepes JJ: Mesolimbocortical dementia, clinicopathological studies in two cases, J Neurol Neurosurg Psychiatry 53:492-495, 1990.
148. Vonsattel JP, and others: Neuropathologic classification of Huntington's disease, J Neuropathol Exp Neurol 44:559-577, 1985.
149. Wakabayashi K, and others: Corticobasal degeneration: etiopathological significance of the cytoskeletal alterations, Acta Neuropathol (Berlin) 87:545-553, 1994.
150. Wightman G, and others: Hippocampal and neocortical ubiquitin-immunoreactive inclusions in amyotrophic lateral sclerosis with dementia, Neurosci Lett 139:269-274, 1992.
151. Wilhelmsen KC, and others: Localization of disinhibition-dementia-parkinsonism-amyotrophy complex (DDPAC) to 17 q 21-22, Am J Hum Genet 55:1159-1165, 1994.
152. Williams C, and others: Degeneration of spinocerebellar neurons in amyotrophic lateral sclerosis, Ann Neurol 27:215-225, 1990.

153. Williamson K, and others: Neuroaxonal dystrophy in young adults. A clinicopathological study of two unrelated cases, Ann Neurol 11:335-343, 1982.
154. Wisniewski HM, and Weu GY: Substructure of paired helical filaments from Alzheimer's disease neurofibrillary tangles, Acta Neuropathol 66:173-176, 1985.
155. de Yébenes JG, and others: Familial progressive supranuclear palsy. Description of a pediagree and review of the literature, Brain 118:1095-1103, 1995.
156. Younger DS, and others: Motor neuron disease and ALS: Relation of high CSF protein content to paraproteinemia and clinical syndromes, Neurology 40:595-599, 1990.

C • H • A • P • T • E • R

# 16

# *Demyelinating Disorders and Leukodystrophies*

**Kinuko Suzuki**



Myelin is a membranous structure formed by an extended and modified plasma membrane of the myelin forming cells: oligodendrocytes in the central nervous system (CNS), and Schwann cells in the peripheral nervous system (PNS). Myelin wraps itself spirally around the axon to form its sheath and functions as an electric insulator that facilitates axonal conduction. Thus, myelin is an important component of nerve fibers in both the CNS and the PNS; destruction of myelin, aberrant formation, or absence of myelin causes serious neurologic disease. In this chapter, the basic morphology and biochemistry of myelin are reviewed briefly, and the neuropathologic features of common myelin disorders are described. Emphasis is placed on the identification of practical diagnostic features. Clinical features of these diseases and other laboratory information, including abnormalities visible on computerized tomography (CT) or magnetic resonance imaging (MRI), are also included where deemed appropriate.

## MORPHOLOGY AND CHEMICAL COMPOSITION OF MYELIN

Myelin is formed by oligodendrocytes in the CNS and by Schwann cells in the PNS. A predominant element of the white matter in the CNS is the myelin sheath, which comprises approximately 50% of the total dry weight of the adult human brain. Diseases affecting myelin, therefore, are diseases almost exclusively involving the white matter of the brain. The structure as well as the chemical composition of myelin in the CNS and PNS differ significantly from one another. Therefore, most acquired demyelinating diseases affecting the CNS do not involve the PNS, while diseases caused by genetic defects in myelin forming cells usually affect both the CNS and the PNS. With routine hematoxylin and eosin stain (H&E), myelin appears pale pink or lightly eosinophilic, and myelin pathology may not be easily appreciated. However, by replacing hematoxylin with solochrome in routine sections (solochrome and eosin stain) white matter can be differentially stained with pale blue color, and white matter lesions will be better appreciated. Many stains are specific for myelin, and individual laboratories usually have their own preferences. Commonly used myelin stains are listed in Table 16-1. In our institution, the myelin stain most commonly used on paraffin sections is Luxol fast blue stain counterstained with periodic acid Schiff stain (LFB-PAS). With LFB-PAS stain, the myelin in the CNS stains light greenish-blue; PNS myelin stains purplish blue.

Myelinated fibers are segmentally arranged by myelin internodes separated at the nodes of Ranvier. In the PNS one Schwann cell myelinates one myelin internode, while in the CNS one oligodendrocyte myelinates 30 to 50 internodes. At the light microscopic level, the node of Ranvier and the Schmidt-Lantermann incisure are easily recognized in large myelinated fibers in the PNS but not in the CNS. As a rule, myelin sheaths are thicker in the PNS than in the CNS when compared with axons of the same caliber. Myelin has a characteristic ultrastructural feature, a lamellar structure composed of alternating dark and less-dark lines (protein layers) separated by unstained zones (the lipid hydrocarbon chains). The less-dark, or intraperiod line represents the closely apposed outer protein coat of the plasma membrane of the myelin forming cell (oligodendrocyte or Schwann cell). In well-prepared electron micrographs, two plasma membranes (double intraperiod lines) are recognizable. The dark, or major period, line is the fused, inner protein coat of the plasma membrane. In certain pathologic conditions, e.g., Canavan disease or central pontine myelinolysis, the intraperiod lines split to form vacuoles, giving the white matter a spongy appearance in light microscopy.

**Table 16-1.** Stains commonly used for the investigation of myelin disorders

| Stain | Comments |
|---|---|
| 1. Solochrome & Eosin (P) | Myelin is stained pale blue in eosinophilic background. Good as an overall routine stain. |
| 2. Luxol Fast Blue (LFB) (P) | |
| A. LFB & PAS | CNS myelin is stained greenish-blue; PNS myelin is stained purplish blue. Thus, a good stain for differentiation of CNS and PNS myelin on sections. |
| B. LFB & cresyl violet (Kluver-Barrera) | Stain Nissl substance and cellular nuclei blue in addition to myelin. Good as combined stain for neuron and myelin. |
| 3. Other myelin stains<br>Heidenhain (P), (C)<br>Kulschitzky (C)<br>Loyez (P), (F), (C)<br>Weigert (C)<br>Weigert-Pal (C)<br>Weil (P), (F), (C),<br>Woelcke (P), (F), (C)<br>Spielmeyer (F) | These methods are used to stain myelin exclusively. Black to dark blue myelin stain provides good contrast for demonstration of demyelinating lesions. However, these methods are time-consuming in practice. |
| 4. Marchi (F) | Used for demonstration of early stage of myelin degeneration. Degenerating myelin stains as black deposits. |
| 5. Oil red-O & Sudan IV (F) | Used for demonstration of lipid macrophages in demyelinating lesions. Macrophages stain brilliant red. |
| 6. Immunocytochemistry for myelin proteins (P), (F) (MBP, PLP, MAG, and others) | |

P—Paraffin; F—Frozen; C—Celloidin sections. Technical details of most of these stains are described in the manual published by Armed Forces Institute of Pathology (AFIP).[103,108] For selected stains, however, the reader is advised to refer to the original references.[18,19,65,103,108,135]

Myelin contains high proportions of lipids (70 to 85%) and relatively low proportions of proteins (15 to 30%). The major myelin lipids are cholesterol, phospholipid, and galactolipid (cerebroside and sulfatide). Among these lipids, cerebroside (galactocerebroside) is the most typical lipid of myelin, and the concentration of cerebroside in the brain is directly proportional to the amount of myelin present. Proteolipid protein (PLP) and myelin basic protein (MBP) are the major CNS myelin proteins, making up 60 to 80% of the total. PNS myelin does not contain PLP, and the content of MBP is low (5 to 18%). More than one half of the PNS myelin protein is a protein named $P_0$. Myelin associated glycoprotein (MAG) is present in both CNS and PNS myelin and MAG plays an important role in the interaction between axon and myelin forming cells. For further information on the morphology, biochemistry, and molecular basis of the myelin structure, the readers are referred to other publications.[43,110,116,138,151]

## DEFINITION AND CLASSIFICATION OF MYELIN DISORDERS

Myelin disorders described in this chapter are defined as disorders caused by the degeneration of myelin sheaths, either as a primary event or as a result of the degeneration or dysfunction of the myelin forming cells. Therefore, myelin disintegration secondary to axonal injury (wallerian degeneration) is excluded. Traditionally, myelin disorders are classified into two large groups: demyelinating disorders (acquired myelin diseases) and leukodystrophies (genetic myelin diseases). Demyelinating disorders are further subclassified into immune-mediated (or inflammatory), viral, and toxic types of demyelination. Leukodystrophies are diseases associated with genetic defects in myelination (dysmyelinating disease). Most leukodystrophies are characterized by demyelination with the exception of Pelizaeus-Merzbacher disease and possibly Alexander disease. The following box outlines the tentative classification of the diseases described in this chapter.

**Classification of Myelin Disorders**

- A. Demyelinating disorders
  - I. Immune-mediated (or inflammatory) demyelination
    - Multiple sclerosis (MS)
    - Variants of MS
      - Benign or subclinical MS
      - Acute MS
        - Marburg type
        - Schilder type
        - Balò type
      - Neuromyelitis optica (Devic type)
    - Acute disseminated (postinfectious) encephalomyelitis (ADEM)
    - Acute hemorrhagic leukoencephalitis (AHL)
  - II. Viral demyelinating disorder
    - Progressive multifocal leukoencephalitis (PML)
  - III. Toxic demyelinating and/or degenerative white matter disorders
    - Central pontine myelinolysis (CPM)
    - Marchiafava-Bignami disease (MB)
    - Solvent vapor abuse leukoencephalopathy (SVAL)
    - Necrotizing leukoencephalopathy following chemotherapy
    - Postradiation white matter injury
  - IV. Chronic progressive subcortical demyelination (Binswanger disease) and leuko-araiosis.
- B. Inherited metabolic diseases affecting white matter (leukodystrophies)
  - I. Metachromatic leukodystrophy (MLD)
    - Arylsulfatase pseudodeficiency
    - Activator protein deficiency
    - Multiple sulfatase deficiency (mucosulfatidosis)
  - II. Krabbe disease, globoid cell leukodystrophy (GLD)
  - III. Adrenoleukodystrophy (ALD) and adrenomyeloneuropathy (AMN)
  - IV. Sudanophilic (orthochromatic) leukodystrophy (SL)
  - V. Spongy degeneration of the CNS in infancy, van Bogaert and Bertrand type (Canavan disease)
  - VI. Alexander disease
  - VII. Pelizaeus-Merzbacher disease (PMD)
  - VIII. Autosomal dominant-adult onset leukodystrophy

## IMMUNE-MEDIATED (INFLAMMATORY) DEMYELINATION

### Multiple Sclerosis

In general terms, multiple sclerosis (MS) is considered a demyelinating disease of adults with onset of symptoms between 14 and 45 years of age.[163] The peak onset of MS occurs in the early or mid-twenties. However, MS has been reported in early childhood (even before the age of 3 years)[64,69,114] and in individuals over 45.[104,124] In older MS patients, spondylitic myelopathy is the clinical variant most often seen. While the cause and pathogenesis of MS are unknown, the current leading hypothesis is that autoimmunity to CNS antigens is triggered by environmental factors (viral infection, for example) in genetically susceptible individuals and that the immune response leads to demyelination. Thus, the diagnosis is made clinically by applying established criteria,[141] but laboratory tests are very useful to confirm or establish the diagnosis. The test with the highest sensitivity in the diagnosis of MS is magnetic resonance imaging (MRI) of the brain.[125,134,182] The brain MRI is abnormal in over 95% of patients with a definite clinical diagnosis of MS[131] (Figs. 16-1 to 16-5).

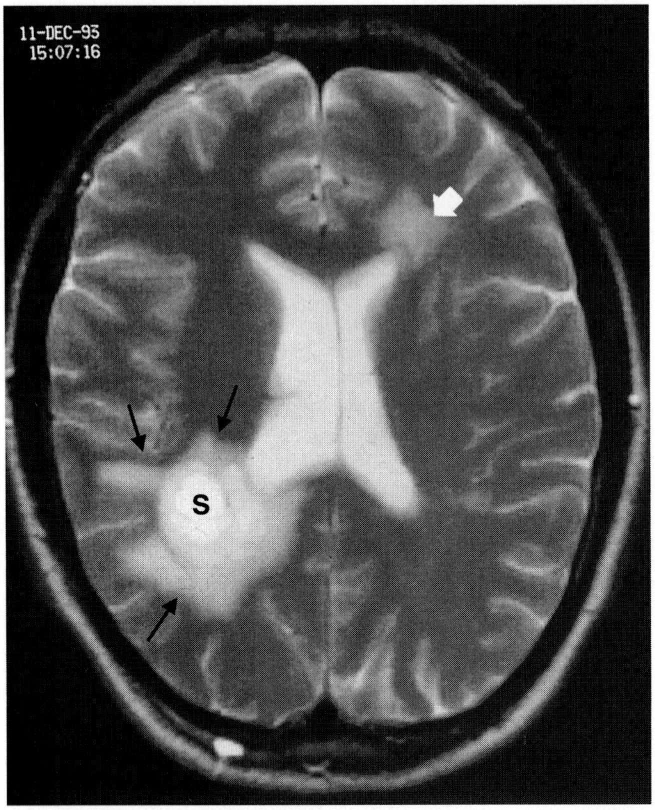


**Fig. 16-1.** Axial MRI T2-weighted image in a 33-year-old man with new onset of seizures. A hyperintense lesion (S) is surrounded by vasogenic edema (*arrows*) in the right forceps major. A second and less well defined lesion (*open arrow*) is present in the left forceps minor. The lesions are atypical in location and configuration for multiple sclerosis and may be confused with neoplastic metastases. The lesions enhanced after contrast administration. (Courtesy of Dr. Mauricio Castillo, University of North Carolina at Chapel Hill.)

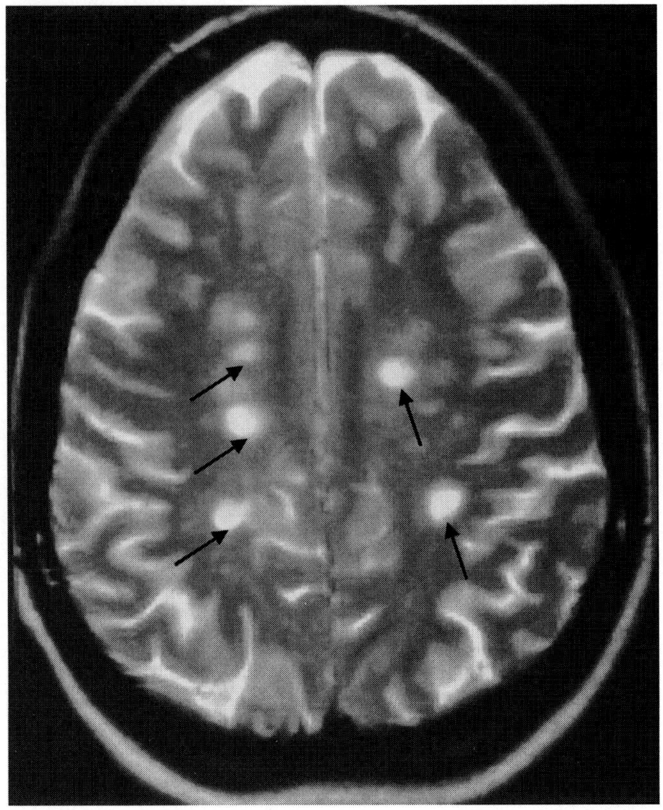

**Fig. 16-2.** Axial MRI T2-weighted image in a 27-year-old woman with known multiple sclerosis. These white matter lesions (*arrows*) are bright, have minimal surrounding edema, are ovoid in shape, and are oriented perpendicular to the long axis of the lateral ventricle. These features are typical for demyelinating plaques. (Courtesy of Dr. Mauricio Castillo, University of North Carolina at Chapel Hill.)

The second best test to diagnose MS is the CSF detection of oligoclonal IgG bands by isoelectric focusing.[8] The neuropathology of MS has been described in several textbooks of neurology and neuropathology.* Therefore, the emphasis in this chapter will be on the diagnostic features of MS. Those interested in experimental and/or more investigative aspects of MS are encouraged to consult these references.

**Macroscopic appearance of brain and spinal cord in MS.** On external examination of fixed brains autopsy, the cerebrum and cerebellum of patients with MS usually do not reveal specific abnormalities. However, mild cortical atrophy with a widening of the cerebral sulci and fibrotic leptomeninges may be present. Irregular gray patches representing areas of demyelination can be appreciated on the ventral surface of the pons, medulla, dorsal surface of the corpus callosum, optic nerve and chiasm, and along the length of the spinal cord, where white matter is covered only by the pia. If the demyelinating areas (plaques) are extensive, these areas may be recognized as gray, shrunken, and firm areas on external inspection. On cut sections the plaques appear as areas or foci of gray discoloration of variable size and shape that involve both gray and white matter. Certain areas such as the periventricular regions, especially those near the lateral angles and around the posterior horns of the lateral ventricle in the cerebrum, often are preferentially and symmetrically affected (Fig. 16-6). As a result, the ventricles may appear enlarged (hydrocephalus ex vacuo). Long-standing chronic plaques in the white matter are sharply demarcated from the surrounding normal white matter. Smaller plaques in the white matter may be confused with invaginated segments of the cerebral cortex. Because of the gray-brown color of the cerebral cortex, basal ganglia, and thalamus in the fixed brain, MS plaques at these locations, particularly small ones, may be difficult to detect. Recent or active plaques are slightly granular, usually yellowish-white (rather than

* Refs. 5, 6, 130, 144, 145, 150, 152.

A

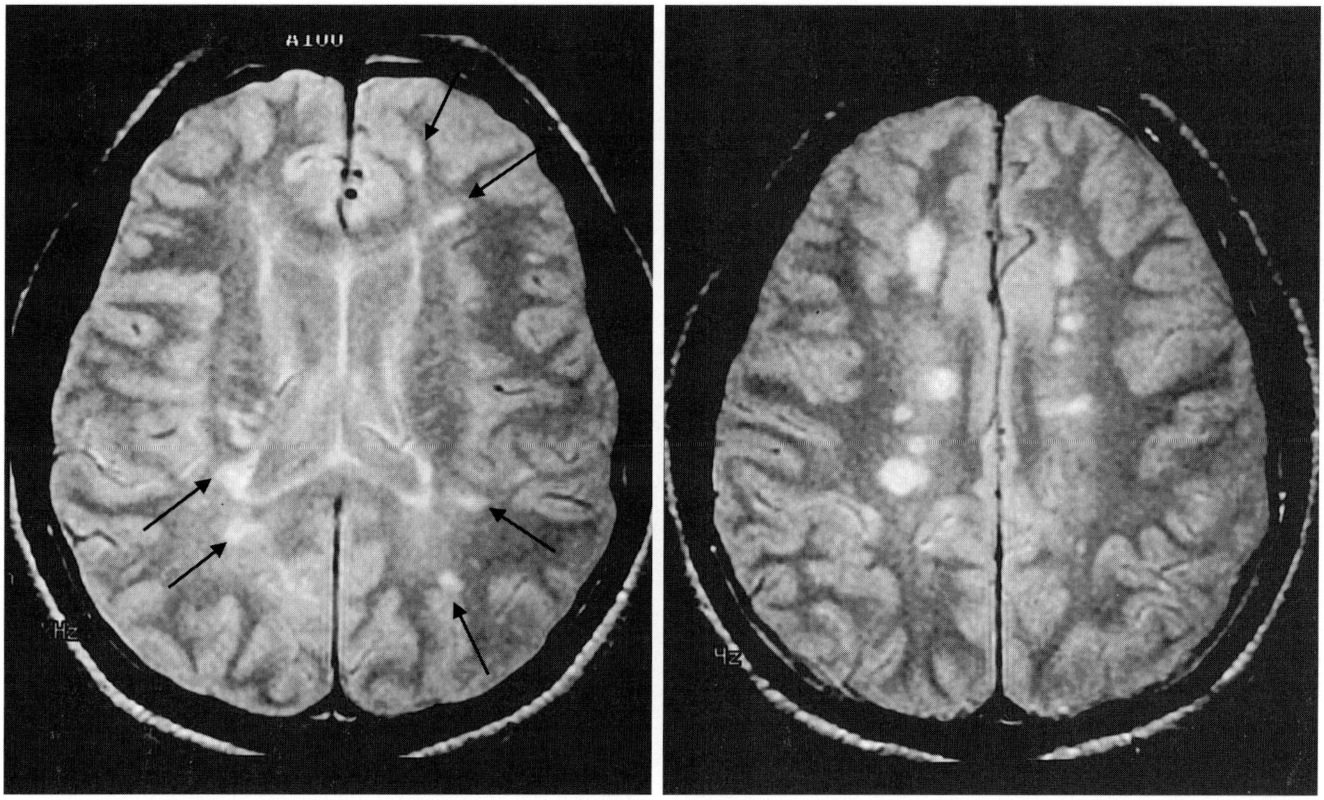

B

**Fig. 16-3. A**, Axial proton density weighted image in a 33-year-old man with multiple sclerosis. Multiple, small high signal intensity lesions are visible in the white matter (*arrows*). **B**, Axial proton density weighted image above lateral ventricles shows additional, multiple high signal intensity white matter lesions. (Courtesy of Dr. Richard Silbergleit, Henry Ford Hospital and Medical Center.)

gray), and not well demarcated (Fig. 16-7). Some of the fresh resolving lesions of MS may be indistinguishable from normal white matter. Plaques containing large numbers of foamy macrophages have a characteristic chalky white appearance.

Demyelinating lesions occasionally have been reported in the PNS, mostly in the spinal roots; these lesions may be invisible in acute MS and are considered rare in chronic MS. However, Thomas and coworkers[181] reported chronic demyelinating peripheral neuropathy in six patients with a syndrome having clinical and CT or MRI features of chronic MS. These authors reviewed publications reporting cases in which there was CNS and PNS demyelination. In some cases, the typical feature of hypertrophic polyneuropathy, an "onion bulb" formation, the result of multiple layers of Schwann cells wrapped around axons, has been found in the spinal roots and sometimes even within the plaques of MS.[169]

**Microscopic features of MS.** Histologic features characteristic of MS include scattered foci of demyelination and variable degrees of gliosis. Demyelinating areas (plaques) can be recognized easily in routine preparations stained with H&E. However, specific stains for myelin and axons are required for the diagnosis of MS since these staining methods clearly demonstrate areas devoid of myelin where the axons remain intact (Fig. 16-8). Acute infarcts in the white matter may mimic MS plaques on histology preparations stained for myelin. However, unlike the lesions of MS, axons together with myelin are injured in infarcts. MS plaques usually are subclassified into active (or acute) and inactive (or chronic) plaques.

The active plaque is the site where the demyelinating process is in progress. The active plaque tends to be smaller than the inactive plaque; the lesion is intensively cellular, with increased numbers of microglia/macrophages and astrocytes (Fig. 16-9). Macrophages often show foamy cytoplasm containing fragments of disintegrating myelin; this feature may be recognized readily in myelin stains or by immunocytochemistry with antibodies specific for myelin proteins (such as MBP or MAG).[78] In fresh-frozen tissues, the lipid content within these macrophages is well demonstrated with Oil red-O or Sudan IV stain (Fig. 16-10). These

*Text continued on page 677.*

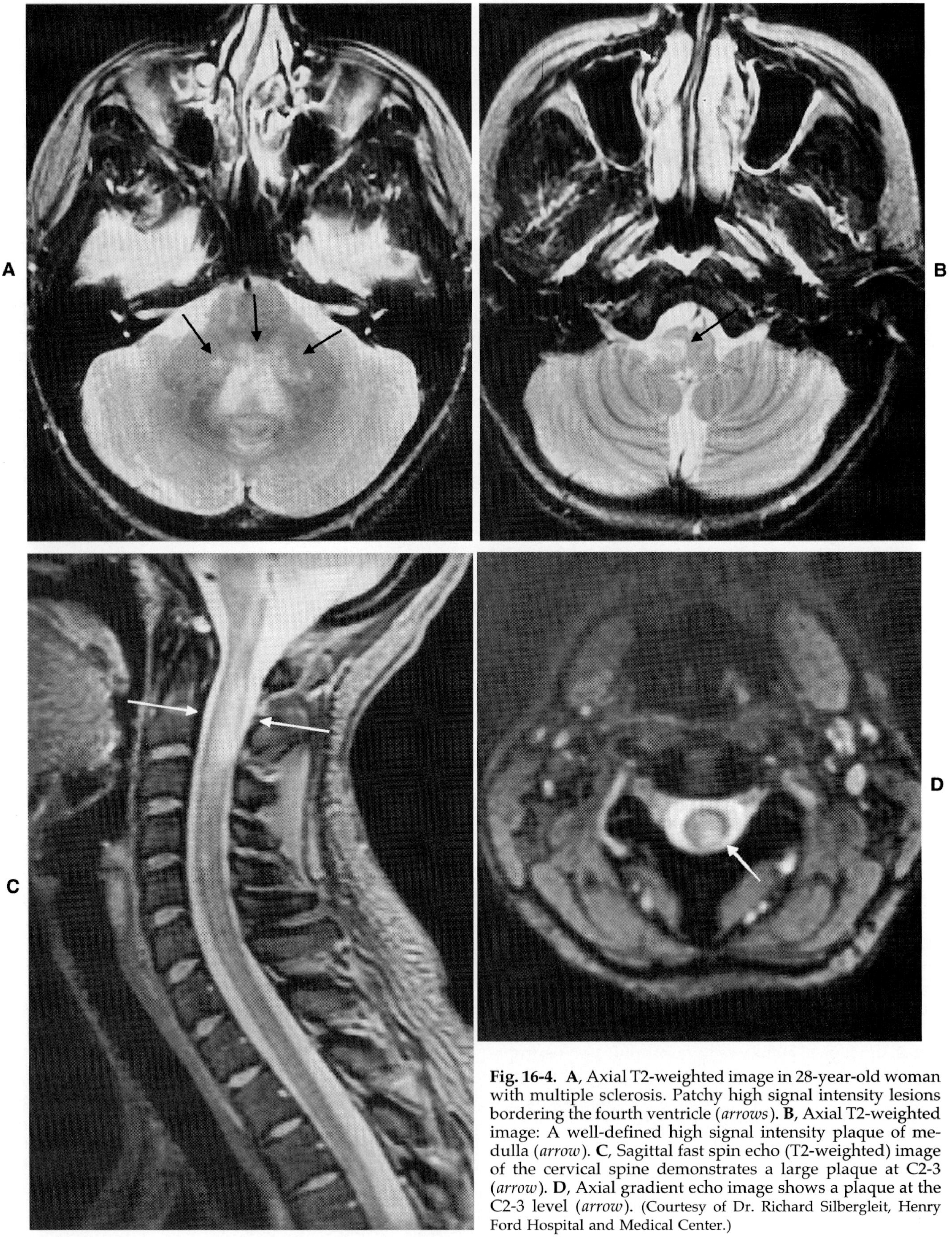


**Fig. 16-4.** **A**, Axial T2-weighted image in 28-year-old woman with multiple sclerosis. Patchy high signal intensity lesions bordering the fourth ventricle (*arrows*). **B**, Axial T2-weighted image: A well-defined high signal intensity plaque of medulla (*arrow*). **C**, Sagittal fast spin echo (T2-weighted) image of the cervical spine demonstrates a large plaque at C2-3 (*arrow*). **D**, Axial gradient echo image shows a plaque at the C2-3 level (*arrow*). (Courtesy of Dr. Richard Silbergleit, Henry Ford Hospital and Medical Center.)

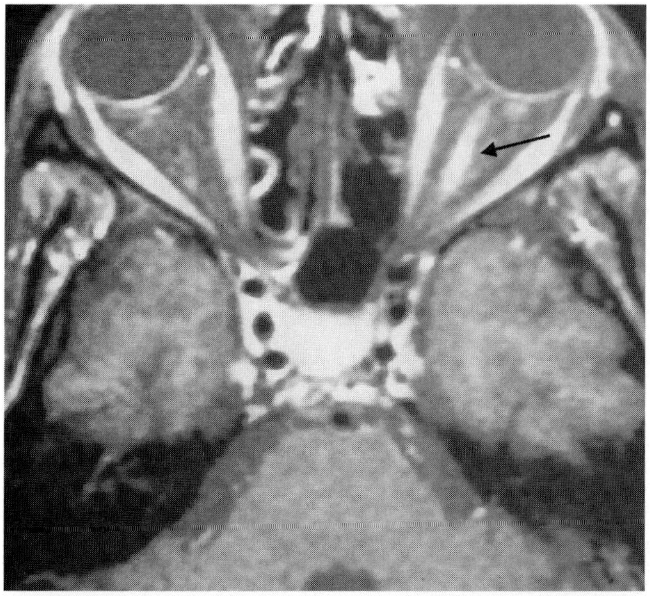

**Fig. 16-5.** 39-year-old woman with multiple sclerosis and optic neuritis. Axial T1-weighted image of the orbit with fat suppression after gadolinium administration shows pathologic enhancement of the left optic nerve (*arrow*). (Courtesy of Dr. Richard Silbergleit, Henry Ford Hospital and Medical Center.)

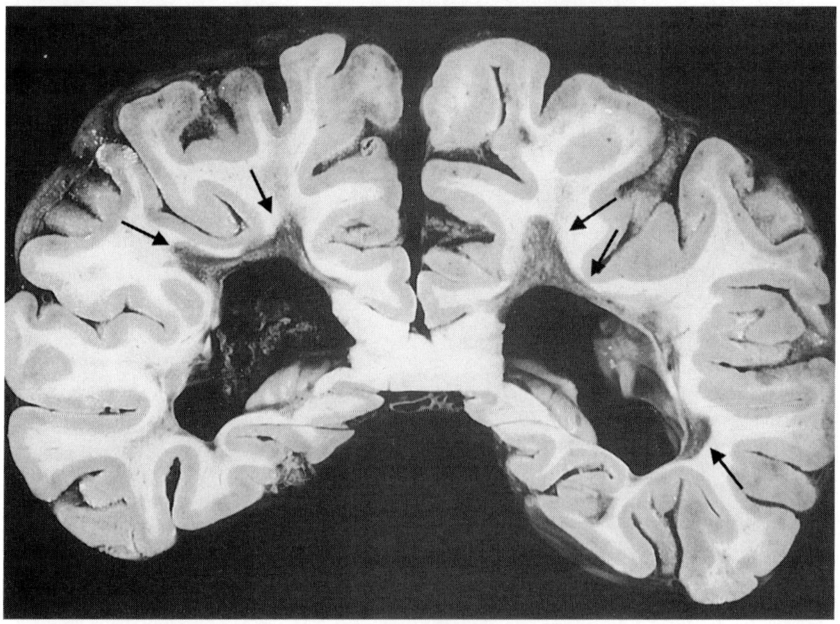

**Fig. 16-6.** Chronic or old demyelinating plaques of MS around the posterior horns of the markedly dilated lateral ventricles. The plaques are sharply demarcated from the normal white matter, gray-discolored, and shrunken (*arrows*).

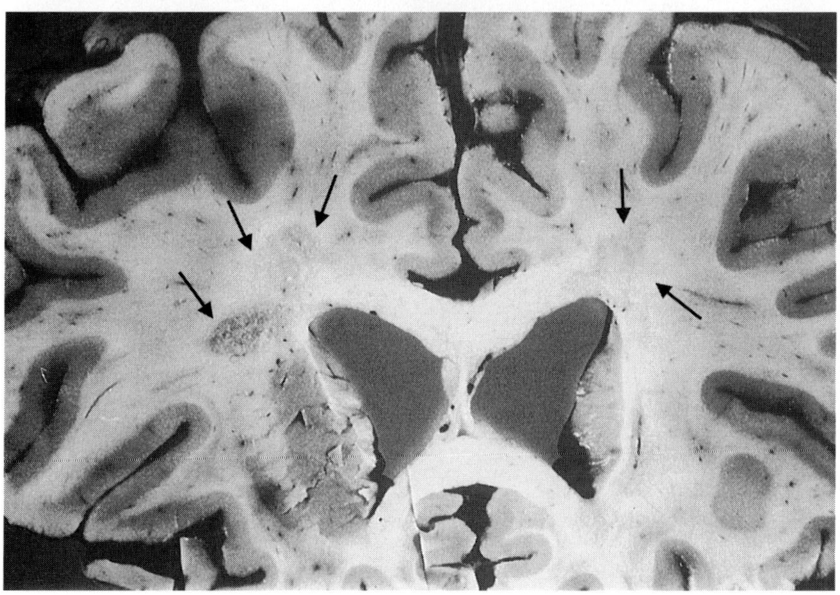

**Fig. 16-7.** Acute (active) demyelinating plaques of MS have ill-defined borders and are granular in appearance (*arrows*).

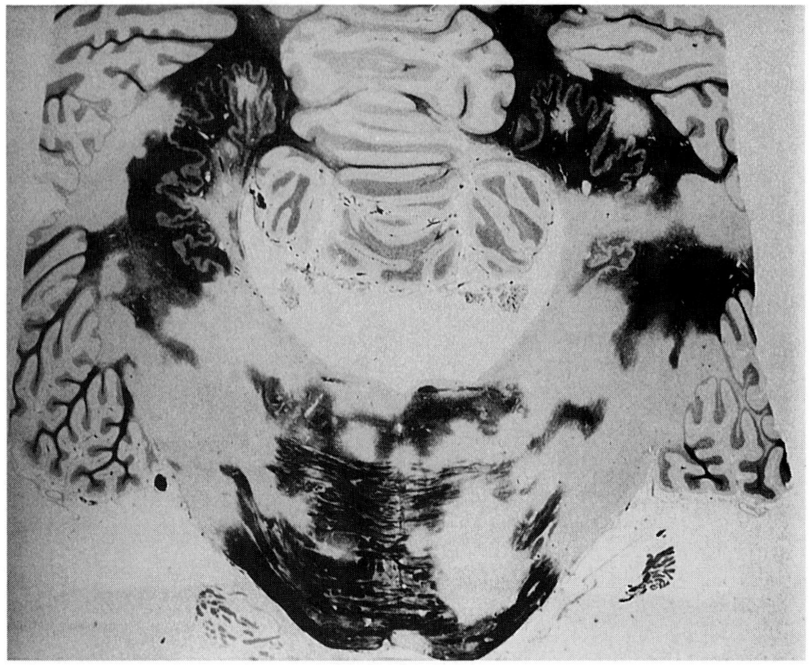

**Fig. 16-8.** A myelin stained section of the pons and cerebellum shows well demarcated plaques of MS.

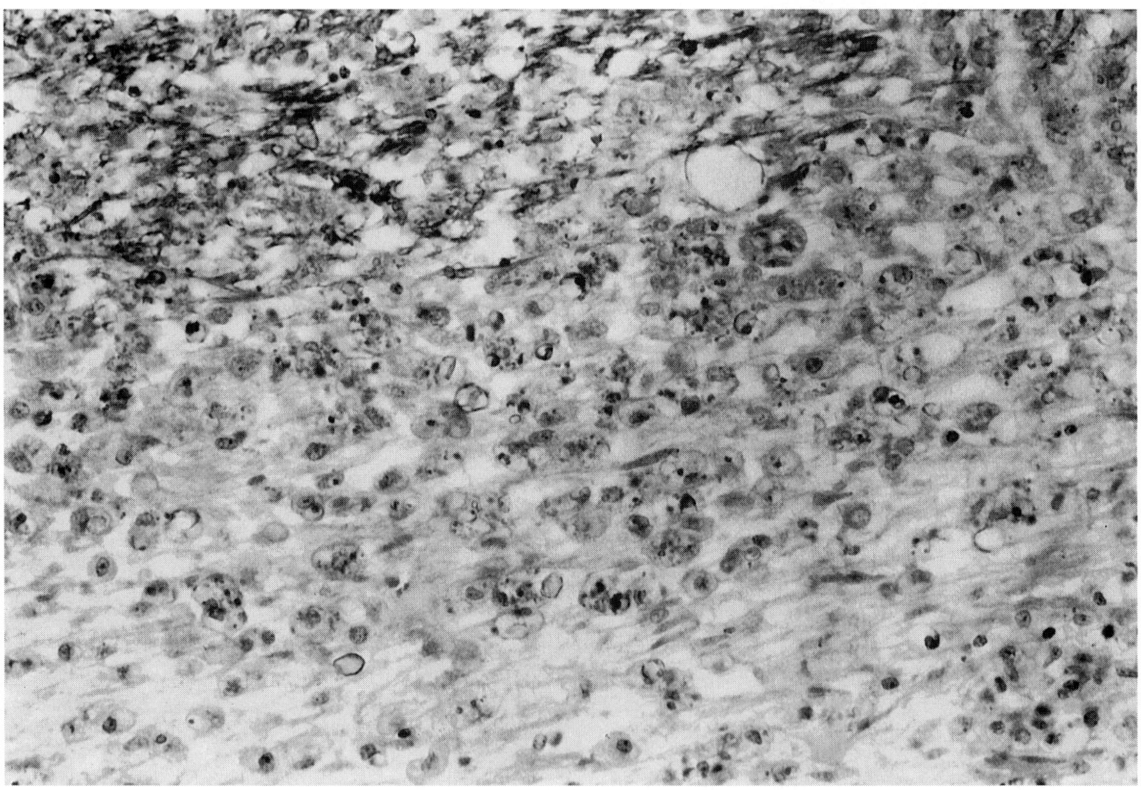

**Fig. 16-9.** Active plaque of MS shows abundant lipid-laden macrophages. (LFB-PAS; ×150.)

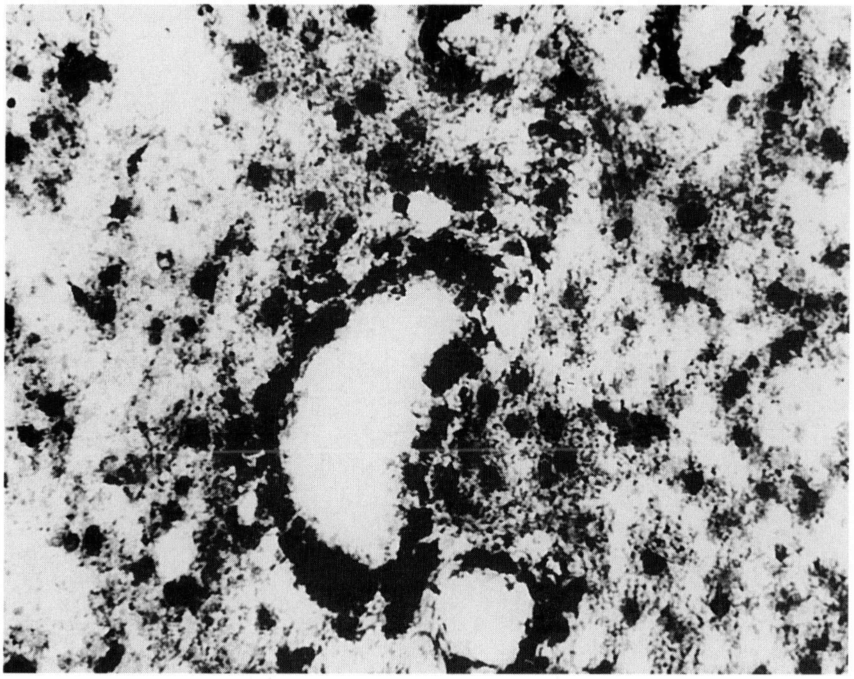

**Fig. 16-10.** Foamy macrophages in MS plaque contain Oil red-O positive lipid droplets in the cytoplasm. (Oil red O stain; ×150.)

macrophages are of heterogeneous lineage and express various macrophage markers. Some microglia and a subpopulation of macrophages within the plaques express human leukocyte antigen (HLA) class II.[122] Astrocytes are reactive and display an enlarged eosinophilic cytoplasm with conspicuous processes. Oligodendrocytes appear well preserved by light microscopy; however, subtle changes such as widening of inner myelin lamellae and degeneration of the inner glial loops can be demonstrated at the ulrastructional level as early abnormalities.[156] In actively demyelinating lesions, oligodendrocytes proliferate, and a close topographic association is observed between oligodendrocytes and hypertrophic astrocytes. Morphologically intact oligodendrocytes occasionally are visible within the astrocyte cytoplasm.[54,149,195] This phenomenon might be akin to emperipolesis, a term describing the presence of lymphocytes within a neoplastic cell.[74] However, it is by no means specific to MS and has been observed in a variety of pathologic conditions affecting white matter.[195]

Perivascular inflammatory infiltrates of variable intensity and composed mostly of lymphocytes and macrophages are seen in the plaques as well as in the adjacent brain tissue (Fig. 16-11). Most lymphocytes are T cells; plasma cells are infrequently present as well. Axons remain intact, although some may show irregular beadlike swellings. When demyelinating plaques involve the gray matter, neuronal perikarya are intact (Fig. 16-12) but some may show chromatolytic changes. Interstitial edema is often associated with active plaques.

Inactive (chronic) plaques usually have a sharp margin between the plaque and the normally myelinated white matter (Fig. 16-8); inactive plaques are less cellular than active plaques and contain more plasma cells than do the acute lesions. Oligodendrocytes are present in various numbers in MS plaques of patients who die shortly after disease onset or during early exacerbation of chronic MS.[27,148,153] During early exacerbation, selective demyelination may be associated with well preserved oligodendrocytes and remyelination. In inactive lesions that are examined long after the onset of the disease, extensive demyelination usually is accompanied by a marked decrease in the number of oligodendrocytes and sparse remyelination.[132] Chronic inactive plaques are gliotic with increased density of glial fibers, but unlike the reactive form seen in active plaques, the astrocytes cytoplasm is not conspicuous. Inactive plaques demonstrate intense immunoreactivity to glial fibrillary acidic protein (GFAP). On occasion, numerous Rosenthal fibers may be seen within these plaques. As a rule, axons are preserved in MS plaques but their number may be reduced. Large chronic plaques, particularly those located in the spinal cord, may be associated with wallerian degeneration in the adjacent nerve fiber tract. Thinly myelinated nerve fibers indicative of remyelination also may be detected at the periphery of these inactive plaques. In the spinal cord and brainstem, plaques may be remyelinated by peripheral myelin forming cells, Schwann cells.[51,52,126] On occasion, demyelinated areas may remyelinate and convert into partially remyelinated plaques known as shadow plaques[115,146]; also, new active demyelinating

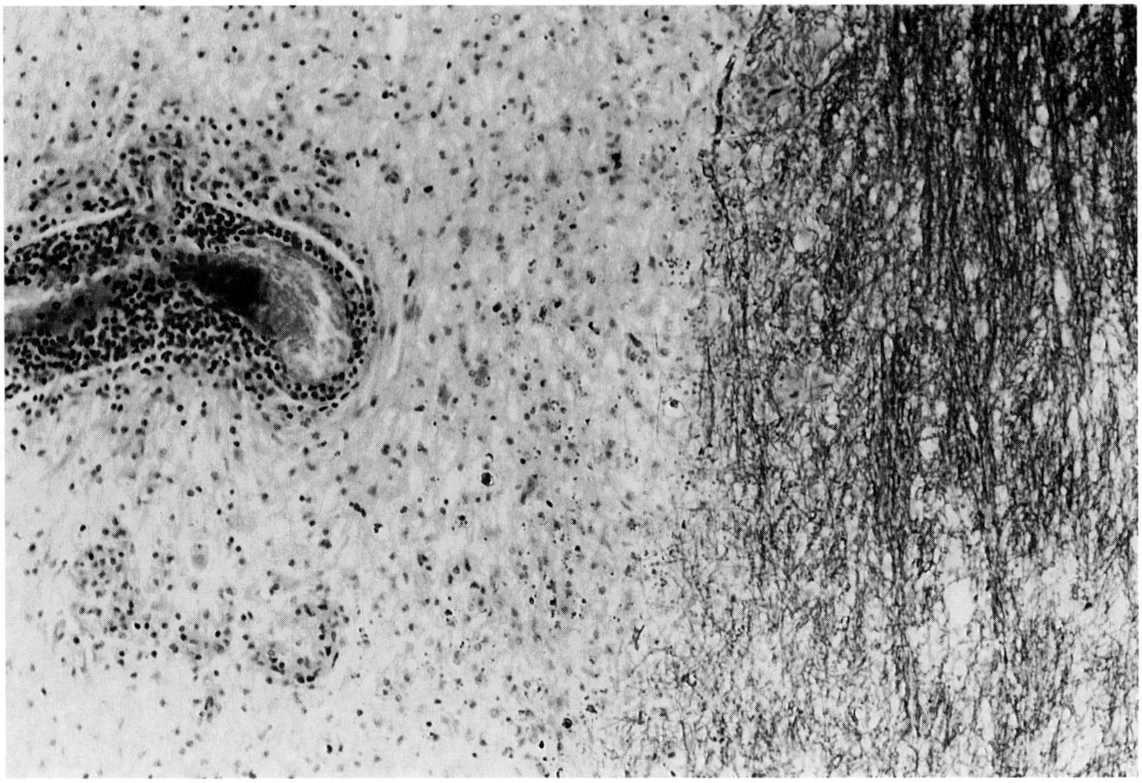

**Fig. 16-11.** Perivascular cuffs of mononuclear inflammatory cells in an active demyelinating MS plaque. (LFB-PAS; ×60.)

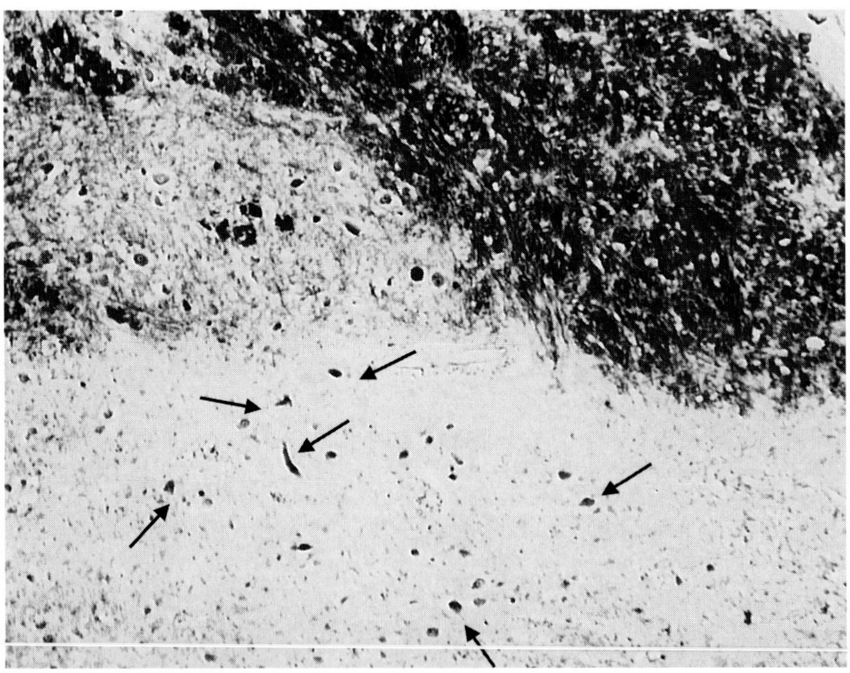

**Fig. 16-12.** Well-preserved neurons (*arrows*) within a sharply demarcated plaque of MS. (Myelin stain [Heidenhain]; ×60.)

lesions may be located within or may overlap remyelinated shadow plaques.[147]

These features of myelin pathology in MS correlate well with MR and CT images. In general, the lesions with more inflammatory components (thus acute) and increased vascular permeability are demonstrable with gadolinium-diethylenetriamine pentaacetic acid (Gd-DTPA)-enhanced magnetic resonance imaging (MRI)[85,121,155] (Figs. 16-1 to 16-3). Serial Gd-DTPA-enhanced MRI studies have shown breakdown of the blood-brain barrier (BBB) in new lesions in 90% of patients with relapsing MS.[58] Clinically silent plaques can be demonstrated by MRI in patients with relapsing-remitting MS. Thus, MRI may be useful to monitor the effectiveness of experimental therapies.[112]

### Variants of MS

***Benign (or subclinical) MS.*** Old, inactive plaques may be found unexpectedly in the brains of asymptomatic individuals who died of other causes. In some of these cases, it appears, the disease processes remitted prematurely after one or a few mild clinical episodes; in others, there may not have been any clinical signs or symptoms of disease. These plaques usually are small in size and few in number. Histologically they are hypocellular and gliotic; therefore, they are classified as inactive or chronic plaques.[53,106,139] Plaquelike lesions with Gd-DTPA-enhanced MRI have been detected in persons free of obvious clinical symptoms; therefore, the incidence of subclinical MS may be higher than the numbers of the symptomatic population would indicate.

***Acute multiple sclerosis.*** MS is in most cases a slowly progressive disease, but rapidly progressive forms also have been reported.[81,113] Acute MS has been called Marburg type after the author who first described it.[107] The acute disease usually affects young individuals and is characterized by rapid deterioration and death within a year of onset. In these cases, destruction of myelin and oligodendrocytes, axonal disintegration, and perivascular inflammatory infiltrates may be very extensive and often are associated with marked edema. In some cases of acute MS, there may be widespread areas of demyelination with axonal damage and destruction of oligodendrocytes and astrocytes involving both cerebral hemispheres. This form is more common among children (known as Schilder type[167]) and must be differentiated from leukodystrophy. The white matter lesions in leukodystrophies are usually symmetric and spare subcortical U-fibers; this topographic pattern does not exist in the Schilder type of acute MS. The clinical onset is also acute, and the course is fulminant in the Balò variant of MS.[16,17,115,196] In this type of MS, the lesions consist of alternating zones of normal and demyelinated white matter arranged in concentric patterns. Large demyelinating lesions frequently involve the frontal white matter, but may be found anywhere in the neuroaxis including the brainstem and spinal cord (Figs. 16-13, 16-14). Concentric patterns of demyelination may be found in the lesions of the Marburg type of acute MS. Also, typical demyelinating plaques of MS can be found in the brain of patients with the Balò type of demyelination, suggesting that the Balò type is a subtype of MS. Within the areas of demyelination, axons are relatively well preserved, but extensive inflammatory infiltrates, hypertrophic astrocytes, and decreased numbers of oligodendrocytes are also apparent. As noted in active plaques of MS, hypertrophic astrocytes often contain oligodendrocytes within their perikarya, a feature resembling emperipolesis.[74] The Balò type of MS appears to be more common in China and the Philippines where the incidence of the classic type of MS with remission is low. The clinical course of concentric

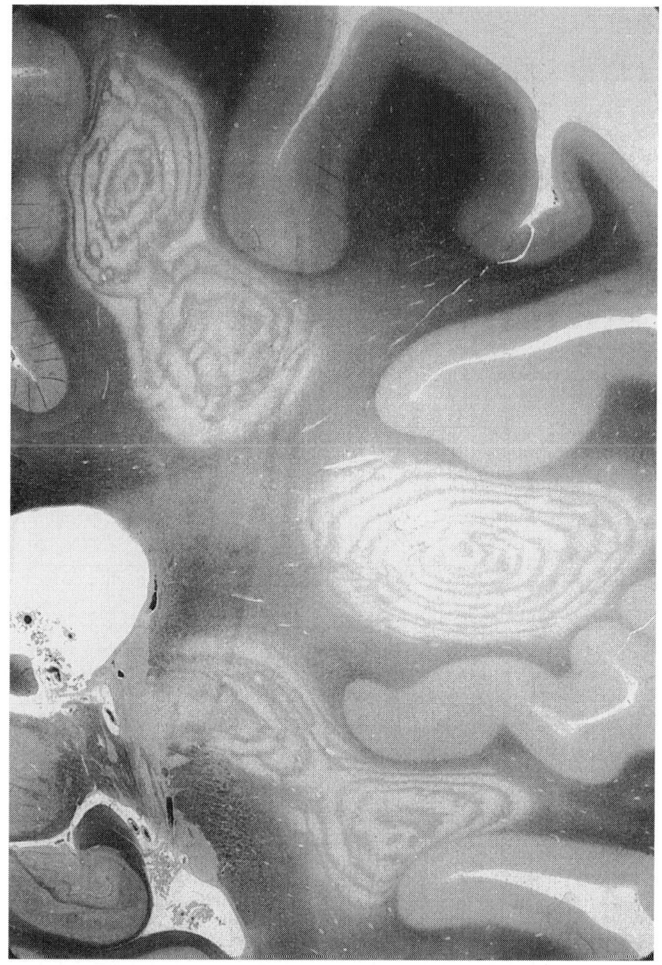

**Fig. 16-13.** Balò type of concentric demyelination in the cerebral white matter. (From Yao D-L, and others: Concentric sclerosis (Balò): morphometric and in situ hybridization study of lesions in six patients, Ann Neurol 35:18, 1994, reproduced with publisher's permission.)

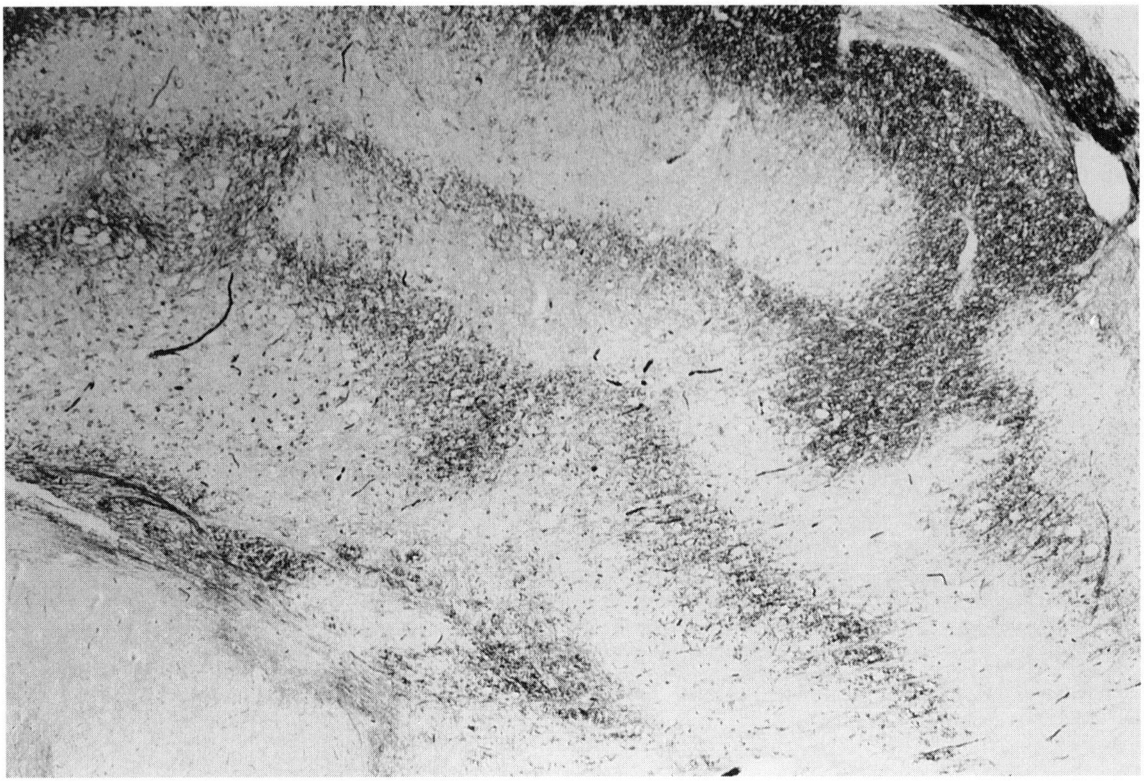

**Fig. 16-14.** Alternating bands of myelinated and demyelinated white matter in Balò type of MS. (Myelin stain [Heidenhain]; ×30.)

sclerosis is very rapid, and the duration of the disease in six patients reported by Yao and associates[196] ranged from 15 to 100 days. The disease often becomes manifest during the second and third decades of life, although onset among older patients also has been recorded.[140]

***Neuromyelitis optica, Devic type.*** In this type of MS, visual symptoms and signs of spinal cord involvement occur within a few days or weeks of each other; the structural changes are characterized by partial or total demyelination of the optic nerves and spinal cord (the upper thoracic spinal cord is most frequently involved).[40] In some cases, the optic nerve and spinal cord lesions may include destruction of neurons and axons, with formation of cavities (Figs. 16-15, 16-16). The areas of extensive demyelination located at the periphery of the spinal cord may be remyelinated by Schwann cells, and this may be associated with accumulation of Rosenthal fibers and fibrillary gliosis. Additional plaques of demyelination may be found in the cerebrum, cerebellum, and brainstem.[36] Neuromyelitis optica appears to be more common among Chinese and Japanese patients than among Europeans or Americans.[77]

**Diagnostic difficulties in MS.** Diagnostic problems or difficulties rarely exist in most cases of MS; the brain of patients who die after a remittent clinical course typical of MS readily shows chronic or inactive plaques that may be admixed with more recent or active plaques. The diagnosis of acute MS with a rapid progressive course may sometimes present challenging difficulties particularly when it is based on small biopsies. Many of these patients have symptoms similar to those of brain or spinal cord tumors. CT or MRI studies are often interpreted as having features consistent with those of a tumor (see Fig. 16-1). The tissue is very cellular in active plaques of acute MS, and numerous reactive astrocytes with abundant cytoplasm and foamy macrophages are present. These astrocytes may have hyperchromatic, bizarre nuclei, and some may contain mitotic figures; foci of necrosis may be encountered occasionally. Therefore, these lesions can be mistaken for a high-grade astrocytoma. An infectious disease may be suggested by inflammatory infiltrates that are extensive. In contrast with chronic or inactive MS plaques, the margins of the active plaques are not always well demarcated because of the ongoing demyelination and associated edema. The presence of numerous foamy macrophages is an uncommon feature of astrocytomas, although clusters of macrophages can be found in some tumors,[89] especially when surgery at the same site preceded the current biopsy. Detection of well-preserved axons in areas of hypercellularity is

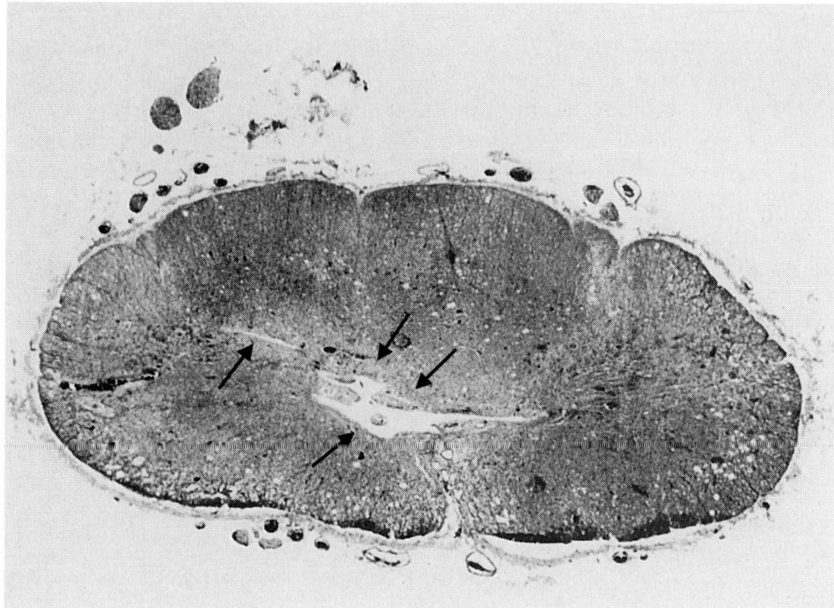

**Fig. 16-15.** Devic type of MS. Extensive degeneration results in cavitary changes (*arrows*) in the spinal cord. (LFB-PAS; ×8.)

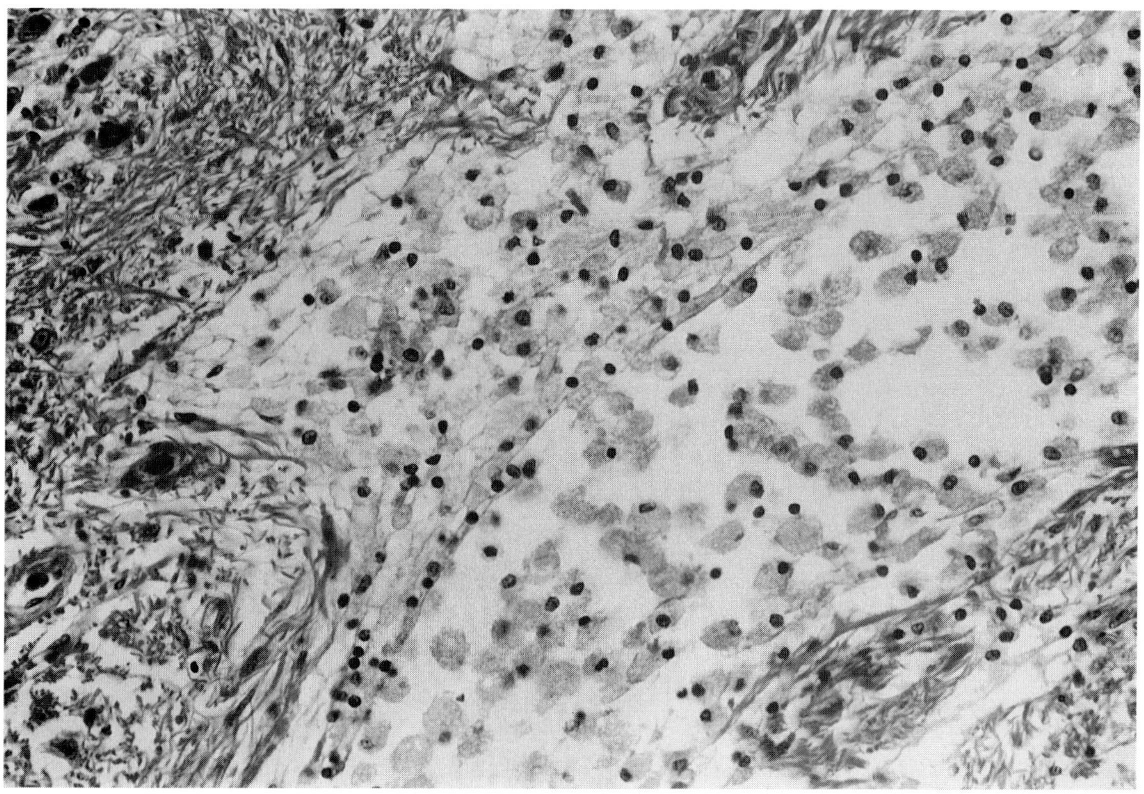

**Fig. 16-16.** Numerous macrophages in the cavity shown in Fig. 16-15. (×150.)

crucial to establish the diagnosis of MS, and well-demarcated margins may be detectable in sufficiently large specimens. The presence of many foamy macrophages in CSF samples may help establish the diagnosis.[75,88,121,201] More helpful in reaching a correct diagnosis of MS are the presence of multiple, similar-looking lesions, and either drastically rapid growth or resolution of lesions in neuroimaging studies. However, a rare topographic coexistence of a glioma and a MS plaque has been well documented in a few cases.[7,162]

## OTHER IMMUNE-MEDIATED DEMYELINATING DISORDERS

### Acute Disseminated (Postinfectious) Encephalomyelitis

Acute disseminated encephalomyelitis (ADEM) is thought to be an autoimmune disorder that usually follows either viral infections (measles, mumps, chickenpox, rubella, and whooping cough) of childhood, or immunizations. The clinical features of ADEM include the sudden onset of neurologic symptoms, usually 5 to 14 days after the clinical onset of the initial infection or immunization. Symptoms are those of widespread CNS involvement, including coma or drowsiness and seizures. ADEM is a monophasic illness; prognosis is favorable in most patients, but death occurs in approximately 10% of cases, usually during the acute phase. Pleocytosis usually is detected in the CSF together with oligoclonal IgG bands, but, unlike MS, oligoclonal bands usually do not persist. In most ADEM patients, MRI demonstrates multifocal asymmetric white matter lesions in the brain that are indistinguishable from those seen in MS. However, if a gadolinium-DTPA-enhanced MRI shows a mixture of enhancing and nonenhancing lesions, the diagnosis is more likely to be MS rather than ADEM. This is because ADEM usually is a monophasic disease, and all lesions are likely to be in the acute phase and display enhancement. Some MRI abnormalities may persist in patients with ADEM despite full clinical recovery.[90] Grossly, the brain and spinal cord may look entirely normal or may show congestion and edema. Histologically, dense inflammatory infiltrates are seen around veins and venules. Both gray and white matter are involved by the inflammatory process. In the early stages, most inflammatory cells are polymorphonuclear leukocytes, but lymphocytes become the predominant cell type in the later stages, at which time perivascular demyelination associated with foamy macrophages and activated microglia as well as reactive astrocytes may become conspicuous. In almost all cases of ADEM, narrow zones of subpial demyelination are visible in the spinal cord and brainstem[5,152] (Fig. 16-17).

### Acute Hemorrhagic Leukoencephalitis

Most cases of acute hemorrhagic leukoencephalitis (AHL) occur in individuals under the age of 30 and are characterized by the abrupt onset of encephalitis-like features with fever and coma. Death usually supervenes within a few days.[76] In some cases the onset of the neurologic symptoms is preceded by nonspecific upper respiratory infection. Increased protein content and high cell counts, mostly polymorphonuclear leukocytes, as well as red blood cells and breakdown products of hemoglobin, may be detected in the CSF. Within a day or so after the onset of the neurologic symtpoms, CT shows a localized lesion in the white matter of the cerebral hemispheres, where increased absorption coefficient corresponds to the site of pathology. Contrast "enhancement" reflects abnormal permeability of damaged blood vessels. The clinical symptoms of herpes simplex encephalitis (HSE) may be similar to those of AHL, but the CT in patients with

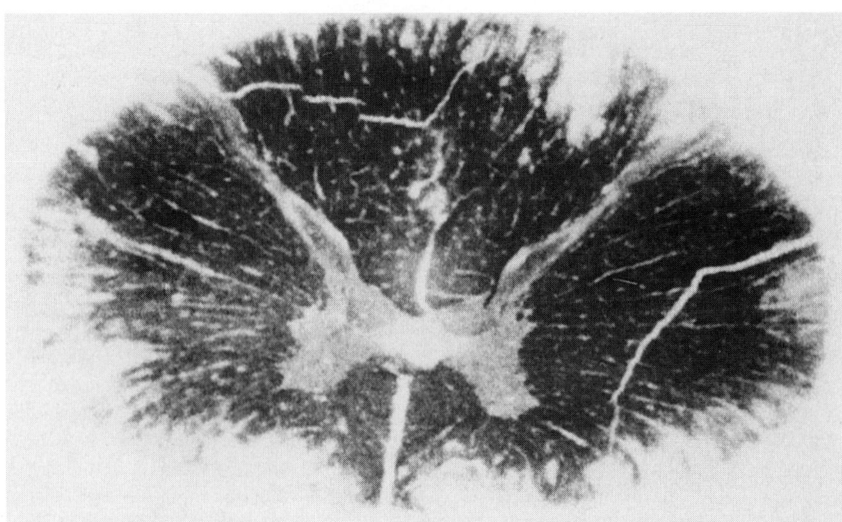

**Fig. 16-17.** Spinal cord from a patient with ADEM, showing multiple demyelinating lesions in a subpial location. (Myelin stain [Woelcke]; ×10.)

viral infections usually is normal in the early stages; CT changes in these patients usually appear 3 to 11 days after the onset of clinical symptoms.[158,190]

AHL may be preceded by upper respiratory tract infection, drug therapy, and various diseases of an allergic nature such as glomerulonephritis.[60] Grossly, the brain and spinal cord are soft and swollen. Multiple petechiae are seen, mostly in the cerebral and cerebellar white matter, brainstem, and spinal cord. Some confluent large hemorrhagic lesions may be seen unilaterally (Fig. 16-18), although as a rule the brain hemorrhages are multiple, small, and symmetric. Under the microscope, "ball" and "ring" hemorrhages are detected around thrombosed blood vessels that show mural fibrinoid necrosis; most of these are veins, and a few are arteries (Fig. 16-19). In addition, there are massive perivascular infiltrates of polymorphonuclear leukocytes associated with edema, demyelination, and some axonal loss. In addition to the hemorrhages, multiple small foci of perivascular demyelination, similar to those of ADEM, usually are found in the nonhemorrhagic white matter (Fig. 16-20). In the advanced stages of ADEM, lymphocytes and macrophages also participate in the perivascular infiltrates.[59,70] Cerebral ma-

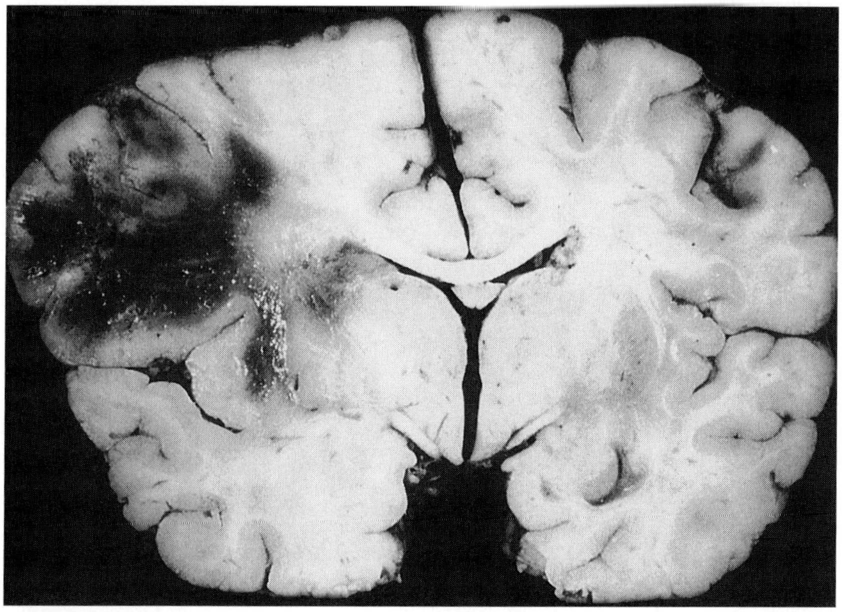

**Fig. 16-18.** Coronal section of the cerebrum from a patient who died with AHL. In addition to multiple small foci of hemorrhage, a large intracerebral hemorrhage is visible in the parietal white matter.

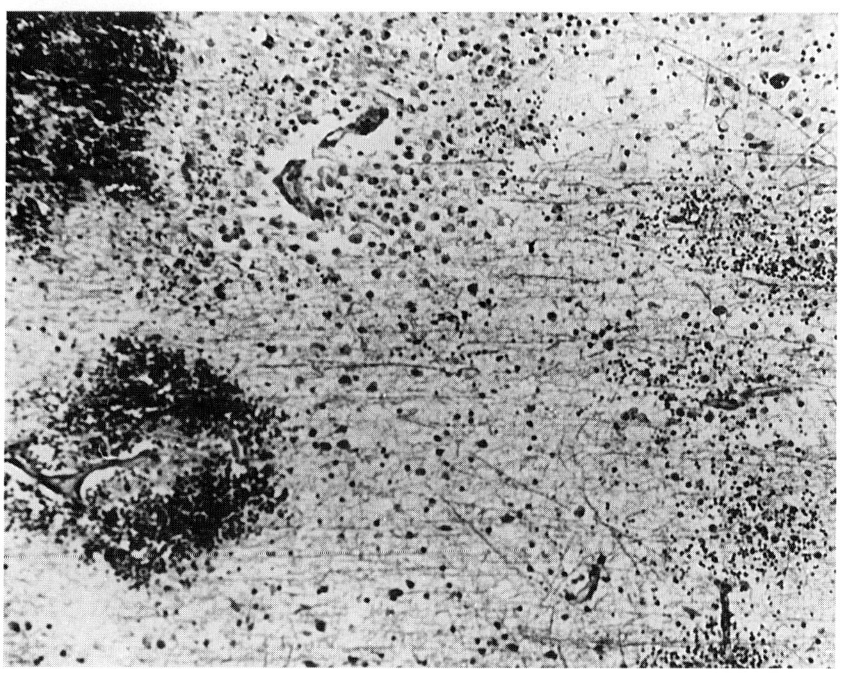

**Fig. 16-19.** Microscopic features of AHL: perivascular cuffs of inflammatory cells, and ring hemorrhages. (Solochrone-eosin; ×60.)

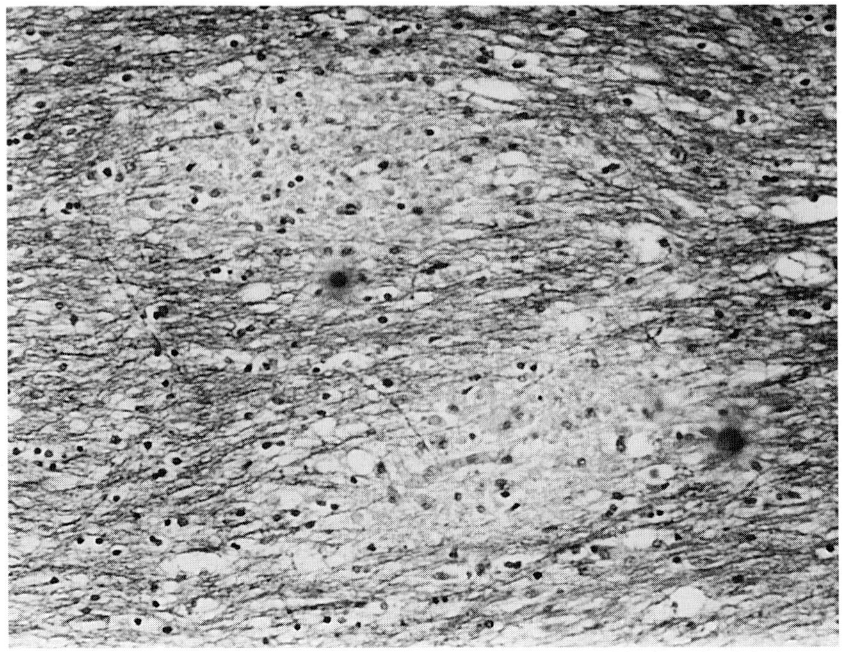

**Fig. 16-20.** Focal perivascular demyelination in the corpus callosum from the case shown in Fig. 16-18. (Solochrone-eosin; ×60.)

laria and to some extent fat embolism to the brain may mimic the histopathology of AHL. Although there are some clinical similarities between herpetic encephalitis and AHL, the histologic features of herpes simplex encephalitis clearly differ from those of AHL, in that the former affects predominantly the cortex while the white matter is the major site of the pathology in AHL. Identification of intranuclear viral inclusion bodies (Cowdry type A) is one of the features that supports the diagnosis of HSE.

## VIRAL DEMYELINATING DISORDERS

Subacute or chronic viral infections of the CNS are known to cause primary injury to the cerebral white matter. The details of the diagnostic features of viral infections of the CNS are described in Chapter 8; therefore, the description here is limited to one of the most common viral demyelinating diseases, progressive multifocal leukoencephalopathy.

### Progressive Multifocal Leukoencephalopathy

Progressive multifocal leukoencephalopathy (PML) is a demyelinating disease caused by a papova virus infection of glial cells, most notably the oligodendrocyte. Most cases of PML are caused by the JC strain; a few cases have been attributed to infection by the SV-40 strain.[13,203] A few years ago PML was a rare disease affecting immunocompromised patients, in particular recipients of organ transplants. Nowadays, PML is a common complication of AIDS,[100] and as a result the disease has become commonly diagnosed in surgical pathology as well as in autopsy specimens. Most cases of PML are found in AIDS patients who exhibit relatively typical neuroimaging features; the ultimate di-

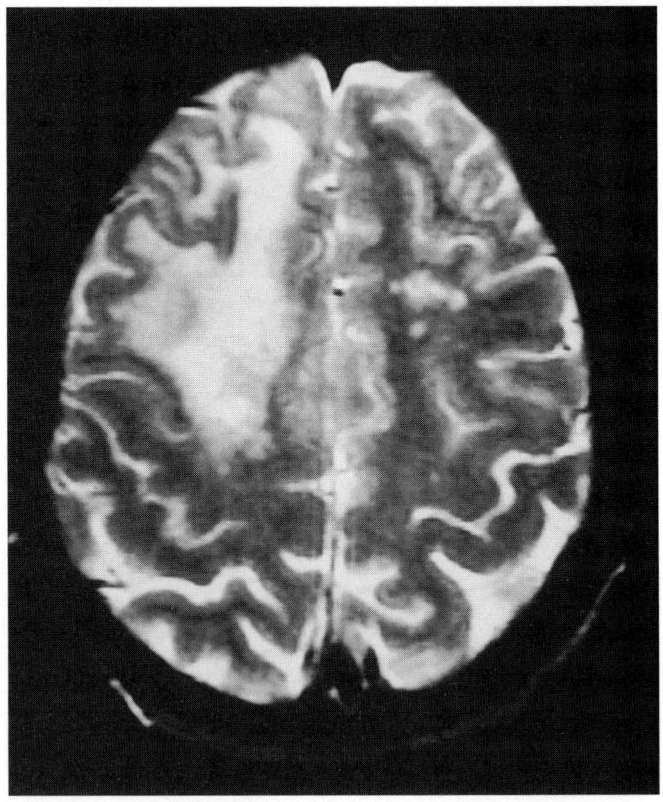

**Fig. 16-21.** 37-year-old man with AIDS and progressive multifocal leukoencephalopathy. Axial T2-weighted image above the level of the lateral ventricles shows a large, high signal intensity lesion in the deep white matter of the right cerebral hemisphere without mass effect. (Courtesy of Dr. Richard Silbergleit, Henry Ford Hospital and Medical Center.)

agnosis of PML requires microscopic evaluation of brain tissues. There are no serologic methods to confirm the diagnosis of PML.

On CT, the PML lesions are hypodense without significant enhancement, edema, or displacement of neighboring structures. On MRI the lesions are hyperintense; on T2-weighted sequences and on T1-weighted sequences the PML lesions fluctuate between low intensity and isointensity. Most PML lesions are located in the subcortical white matter, are usually multiple, and progressively involve deeper white matter tracts[91] (Fig. 16-21).

Grossly, the brain may be completely normal on external examination. On sections, the typical lesions of PML are represented by multiple relatively small foci of demyelination, which appear gray on brain tissues fixed in formalin. In some instances, these foci become confluent, forming large areas of gray-discolored demyelination reminiscent of plaques of MS. These lesions typically involve subcortical white matter, but the large lesions may involve both the cerebral cortex and deep white matter. Some lesions may have yellow discoloration and become either necrotic or cavitary (Fig. 16-22). The cerebellum and brainstem are involved less frequently than the cerebrum. Foci of demyelination (Fig. 16-23) can be easily identified, even in routine H&E preparations, because less eosinophilic sites of hypercellularity where reactive astrocytes, microglia and macrophages, may be abundant. Perivascular inflammatory infiltrates, mostly composed of lymphocytes, may be present, but usually are sparse. The nuclei of some of the reactive astrocytes are large

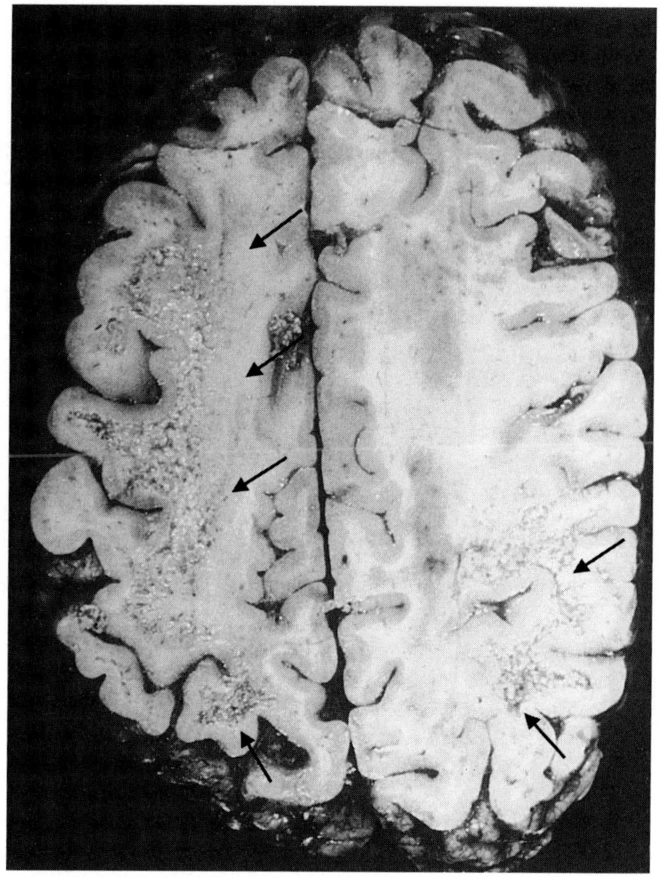

**Fig. 16-22.** Confluent, large demyelinating lesion of PML in the cerebral white matter shows granular appearance (*arrows*).

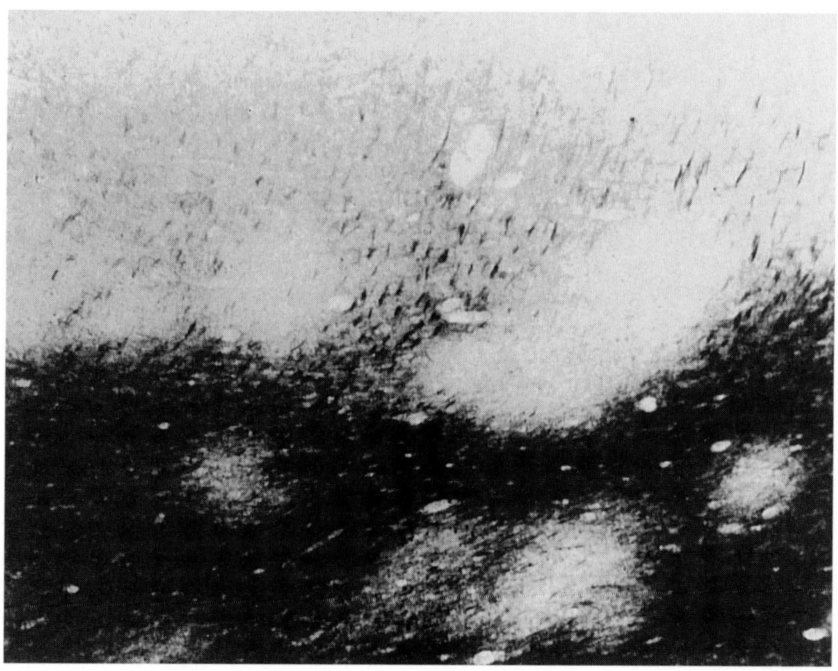

**Fig. 16-23.** Multiple foci of demyelination in PML. (Myelin stain [Woelcke]; ×30.)

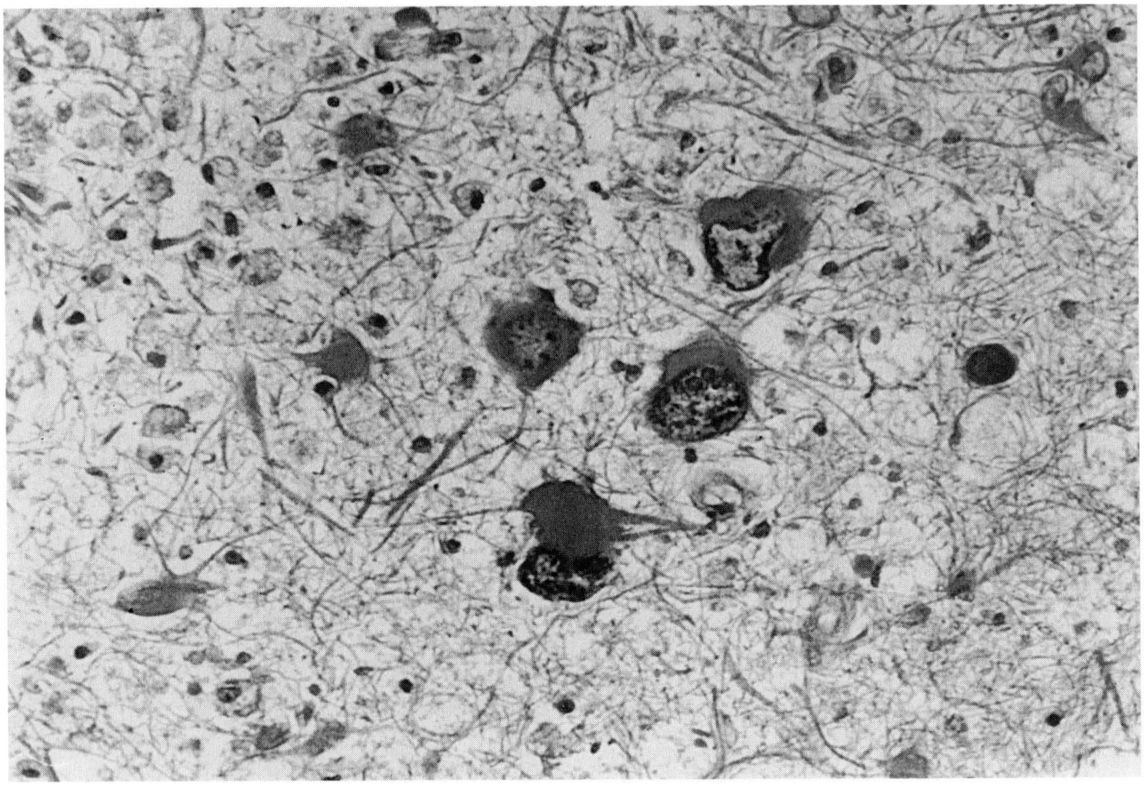

**Fig. 16-24.** Astrocytes with bizarre nuclei (Alzheimer type I) within the demyelinating lesion of PML. (H&E; ×300.)

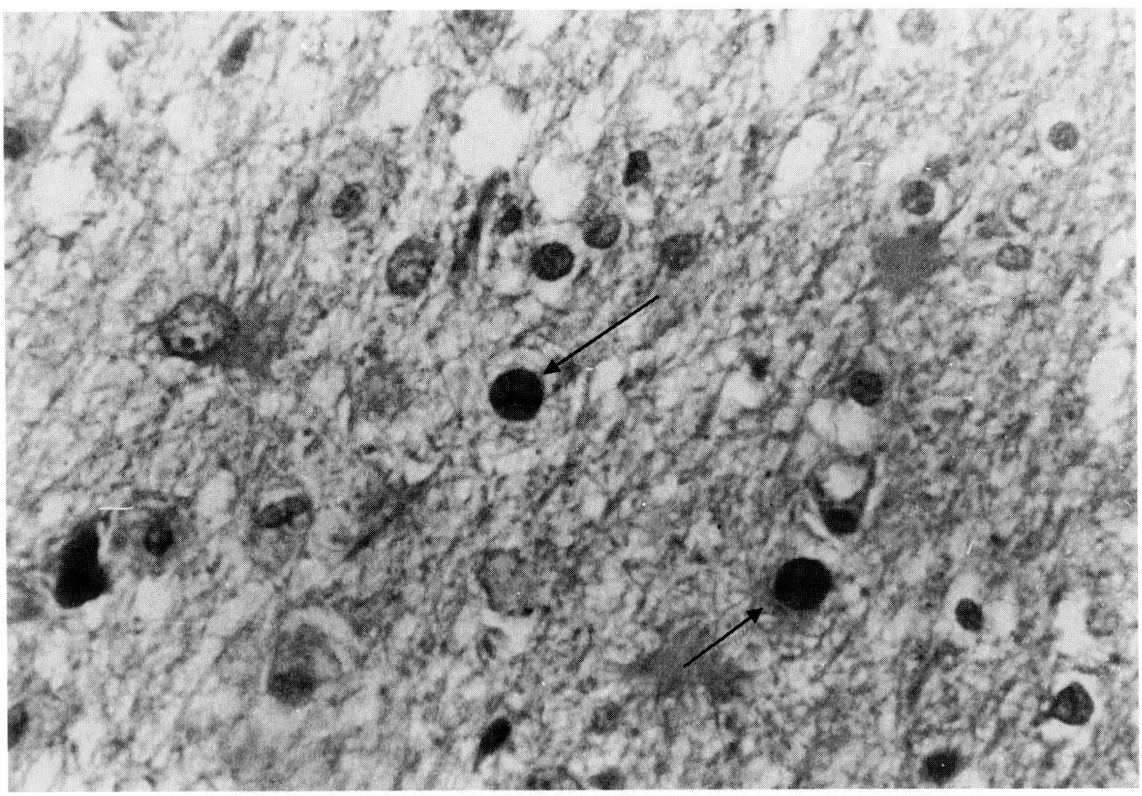

**Fig. 16-25.** Oligodendrocytes with enlarged hyperchromatic nuclei (*arrows*) at the periphery of a demyelinating lesion of PML. (H&E; ×300.)

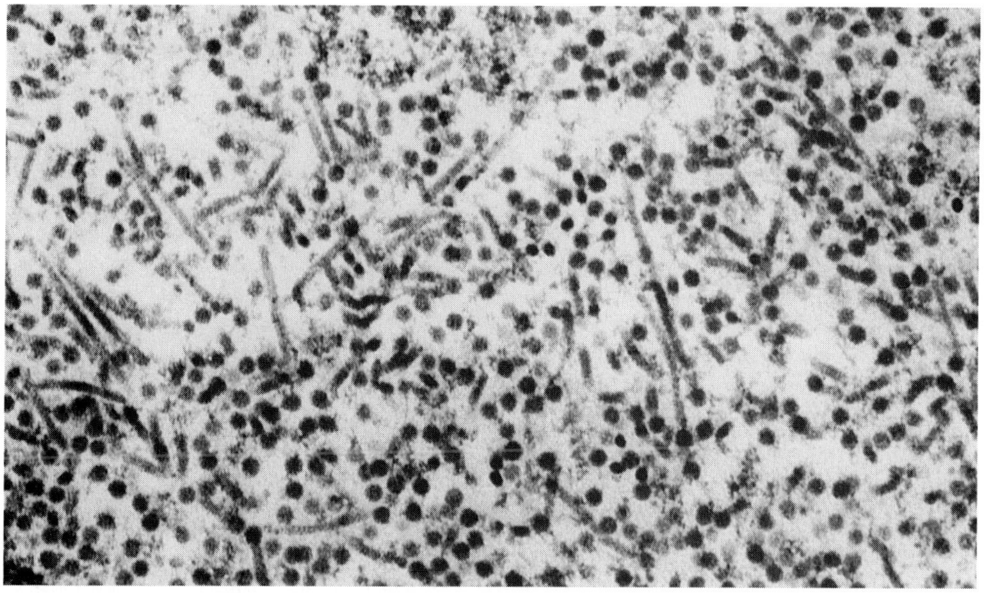

**Fig. 16-26.** Electron micrograph of virions within the enlarged nucleus of an oligodendrocyte, in a case of PML. (×60,000.)

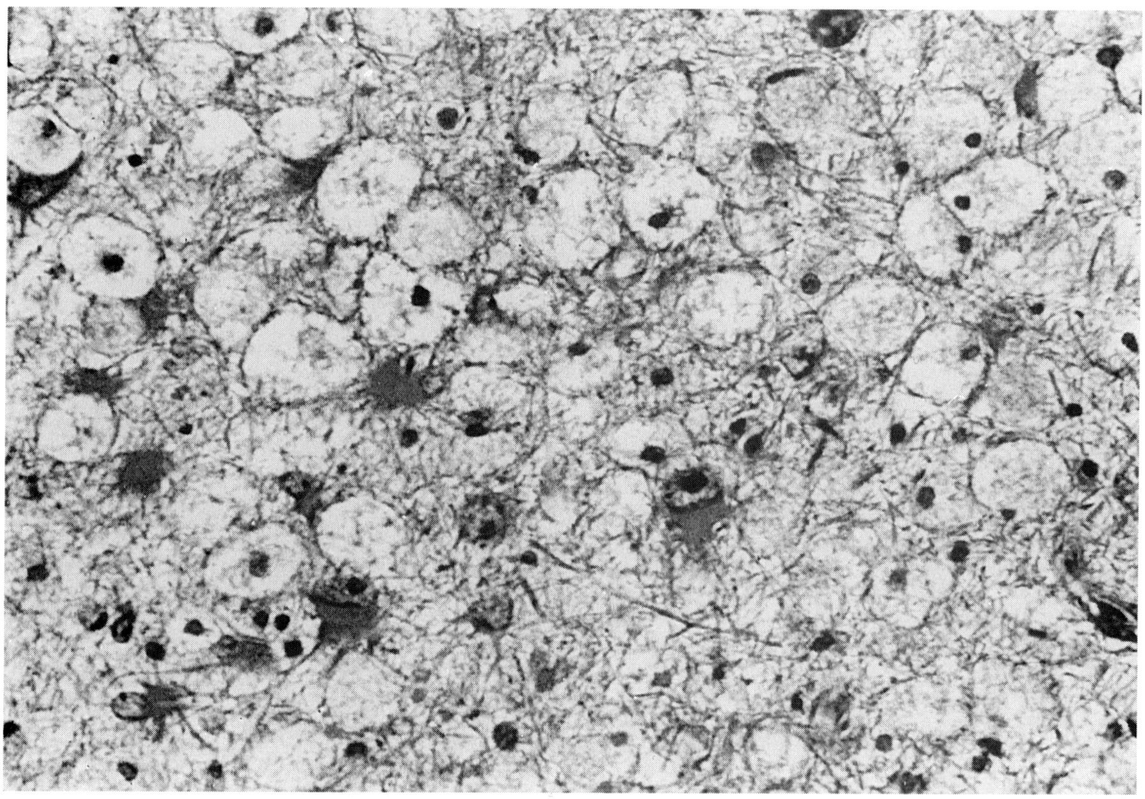

**Fig. 16-27.** Demyelinating lesion of PML: numerous reactive astrocytes and foamy macrophages. (H&E; ×300.)

and exhibit bizarre chromatin patterns (Fig. 16-24), suggestive of neoplastic astrocytes (Alzheimer type I astrocytes). Oligodendrocytes with enlarged homogeneously basophilic nuclei are well recognized in the peripheral regions of these sites of demyelination (Fig. 16-25). Electron microscopic examination has revealed abundant virions filling the entire nucleus of these oligodendrocytes (Fig. 16-26). The viral antigen in these nuclei, and to some extent in the cytoplasm of oligodendrocytes and astrocytes, can be demonstrated by immunocytochemical methods. In situ hybridization with JC virus DNA probe identifies the infected cells more precisely.[4] The histologic features of the PML lesion differ depending on the stage of the disease. In the early stage, only scattered, reactive astrocytes may be visible in foci of the white matter, where myelin sheaths may be still preserved. In areas where the lesions become confluent, the tissues may be densely infiltrated with reactive astrocytes that alternate with areas of necrosis where foamy macrophages occupy most of the lesion (Fig. 16-27). At these sites only the edge of the lesion may have oligodendrocytes containing the characteristic nuclear inclusion bodies. These regional differences sometimes create a diagnostic difficulty because the biopsied tissue may not include all the components of the lesion. The JC strain of the human papova virus that causes PML is highly oncogenic in experimental animals. However, occurrence of gliomas in the demyelinating lesion of PML appears to be a rare event. Only two instances of multiple glioma occurring in patients with PML have been reported.[33,172]

## TOXIC DEMYELINATING AND/OR DEGENERATIVE WHITE MATTER DISORDERS

### Central Pontine Myelinolysis

Central pontine myelinolysis (CPM) was originally described as a neurologic complication occurring in patients with chronic alcoholism and malnutrition.[2] CPM is now thought to be caused by a rapid correction of serum electrolyte imbalances, resulting in rapid or excessive rise in serum sodium in hyponatremic patients,[123] and thus CPM is associated with a variety of underlying diseases.[46] In most cases localizing signs indicative of a pontine location were present clinically. A typical lesion in the center of the pontine base and also some extrapontine lesions can be demonstrated on MRI[186] (Fig. 16-28). On gross examination of the brain, gray areas of demyelination are seen in the central portion of the base of the upper and middle pons. The size of the lesion is variable. In some cases, similar demyelinating sites can be found in other regions of the CNS; these include the striatum, the lateral geniculate body, and the internal and external capsules, among others (extrapontine myelinolysis).[57,193]

The histologic features are typical of demyelination (Fig. 16-29), with myelin disintegration accompanied by infiltration of foamy macrophages. Axons and neuronal perikarya are structurally intact. A decreased number of oligodendrocytes associated with reactive astrocytosis are additional features. In some chronic, inactive lesions of CPM, fibrillary gliosis may be the only recognizable abnormality at the pontine base.

### Marchiafava-Bignami Disease

Marchiafava-Bignami disease (MB) is a rare disease that originally was described in poorly nourished Italian men addicted to drinking crude red wine. Marchiafava and co-workers interpreted the lesion involving the corpus callosum (typical of this disorder) as a primary demyelinating lesion similar to MS.[109] The disease is characterized by a focal area of demyelination associated with some loss of axons involving the midlayers of the body of corpus callosum (Fig. 16-30). Additional myelin injury may be found in other symmetric pathways such as the optic chiasm, the anterior commissure, the hippocampal commissure, and the middle cerebellar peduncles. The lesions are bilaterally symmetric when demyelination involves the centrum semiovale. In some cases, however, cavitary necrosis with many macrophages is found in the center of the corpus callosum. The coexistence of Wernicke's encephalopathy and pellagra has been well documented in some patients with MB.[92,96] In the past, the diagnosis of MB was possible only at postmortem examination of the brain; recently, several cases have been diagnosed by either CT or MRI.[25,30,34,87]

### Solvent Vapor Abuse Leukoencephalopathy

Toluene (methyl benzene) is one of the most widely used and abused organic solvent. Chronic abusers inhale vapors from such toluene-containing products as spray paint, lacquer thinner, glues, and adhesives. These individuals develop neurologic symptoms characterized by severe cognitive impairment, cerebellar ataxia, corticospinal tract dysfunction, oculomotor abnormalities, tremor, deafness, and hyposmia.[73,98] The MRI of patients with neurologic symptoms show: (1) diffuse cerebral, cerebellar, and brainstem atrophy with increased ventricular size; (2) loss of differentiation between the gray and white matter throughout the CNS on the T2-weighted sequences; and (3) increased periventricular white matter signal intensity on T2-weighted images.[157] In such patients the brain is diffusely atrophic and the white matter shows a grossly mottled appearance with grayish patchy discoloration. Histology sections of the cerebral white matter stained with H&E show uneven pale areas where loss of myelin is clearly demonstrable. Macrophages containing coarse PAS-positive granules are scattered or clustered around the blood vessels in these demyelinated areas (Fig. 16-31). These changes also may be found in the

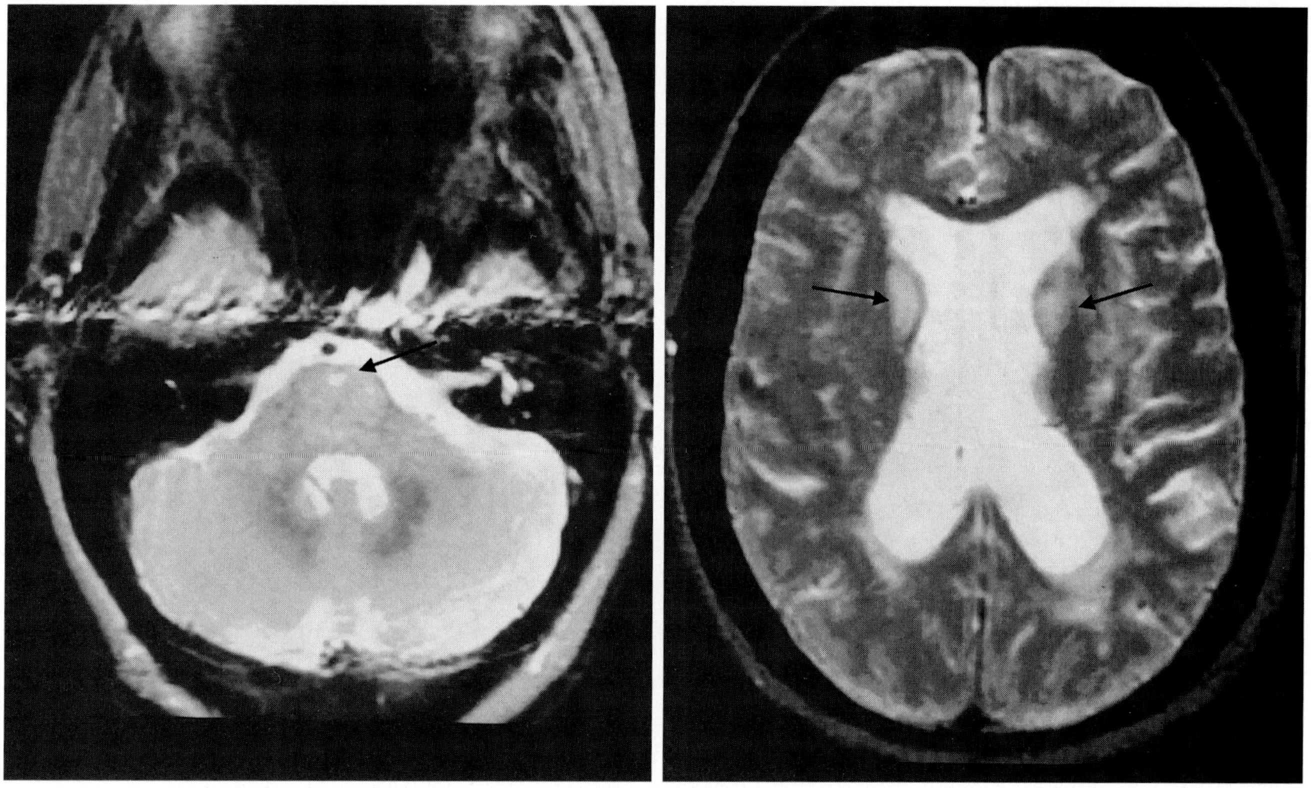


**Fig. 16-28.** 61-year-old man with osmotic myelinolysis. **A**, Axial T2-weighted image at level of pons shows patchy high signal intensity (central pontine myelinolysis; *arrow*). **B**, Axial T2-weighted image at the level of the lateral ventricles shows high signal intensity in the caudate nuclei (extrapontine myelinolysis) (*arrows*). (Courtesy of Dr. Richard Silbergleit, Henry Ford Hospital and Medical Center.)

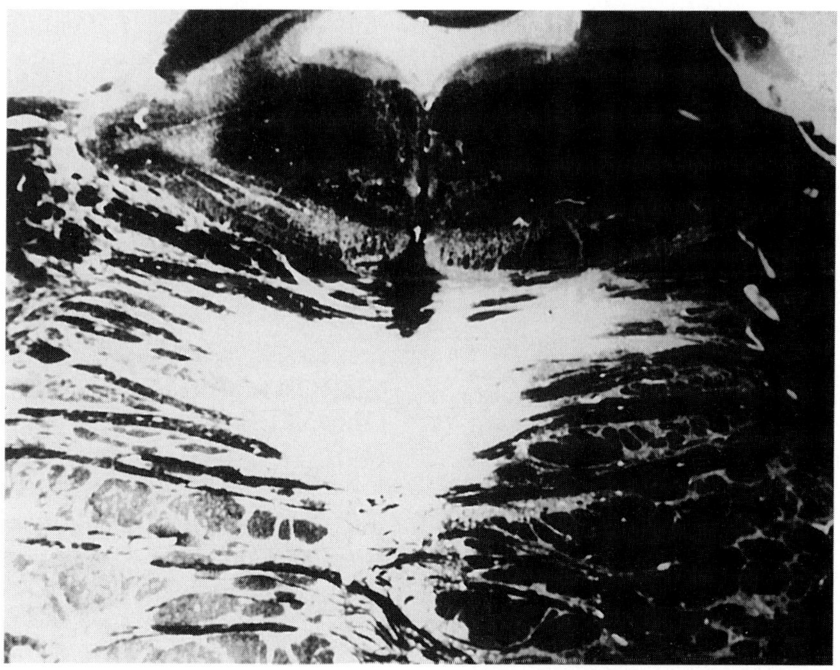

**Fig. 16-29.** Pons showing well-demarcated demyelinating lesion near the midline (center) of the pontine base in a case of CPM. (Myelin stain [Woelcke]; ×10.)

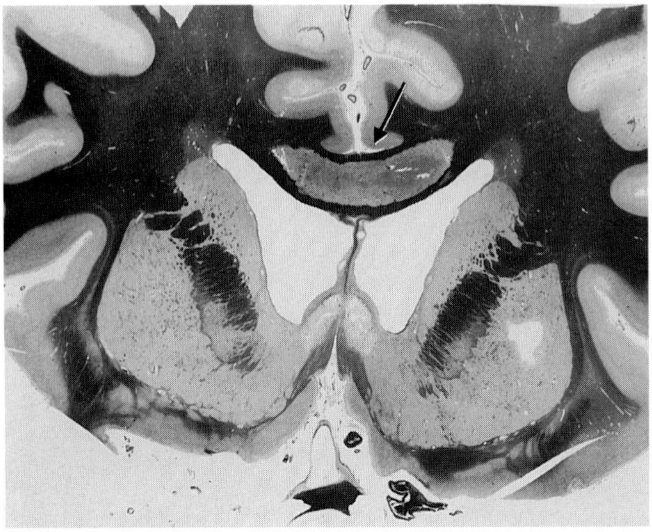

**Fig. 16-30.** Coronal section of the cerebrum showing a demyelinating lesion in the corpus callosum (*arrow*). (From Kosaka K, and others: A non-alcoholic Japanese patient with Wernicke's encephalopathy and Morchiafava-Bignami disease, Clin Neuropathol 6:231, 1984, reproduced with publisher's permission).

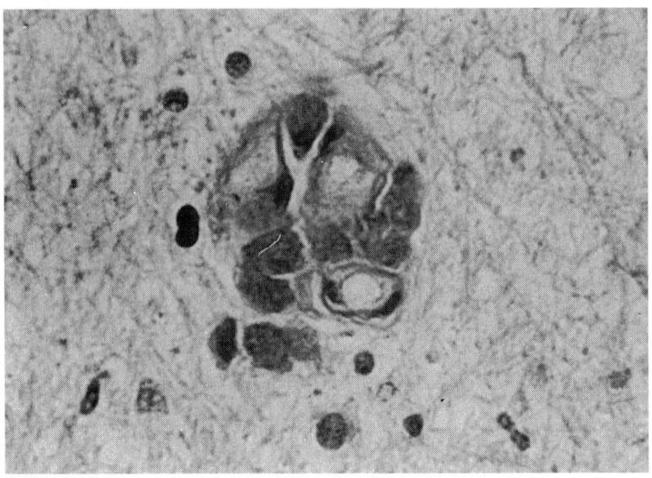

**Fig. 16-31.** PAS-positive macrophages are conspicuously clustered around a blood vessel in the white matter in a case of SVAL. (LFB-PAS; ×300.)

brainstem. The histologic features of demyelination and lamellar intracytoplasmic inclusions contained in these macrophages are similar to those of adrenoleukodystrophy (ALD) (see Fig. 16-51). Unlike ALD, however, there are no significant monoclear cell infiltrates in the areas of demyelination, and the adrenal glands and testes are normal in patients with solvent vapor abuse leukoencephalopathy (SVAL).[95]

### Necrotizing Leukoencephalopathy Following Chemotherapy

This condition was first described in patients who received intrathecal methotrexate for the treatment of childhood leukemia;[84] subsequently, this leukoencephalopathy was diagnosed in patients who received treatment with other types of chemotherapeutic agents, with or without associated irradiation.[99,159] The combination of chemotherapy and irradiation markedly increases the incidence of this type of brain injury. Impaired mental function, confusion, and learning difficulties are some of the prominent symptoms. The gross and microscopic features of the lesion are those of disseminated foci of coagulative necrosis. At these foci there is severe loss of myelin, decreased number of oligodendrocytes, and axonal degeneration with minimal tissue breakdown accompanied by necrosis. Inflammatory cellular infiltrates and macrophages are rare. Small blood vessel walls exhibit fibrinoid necrosis, and parenchymatous fibrin extravasation also may be present. In chronic lesions, there is a variable degree of fibrillary gliosis, and scattered foci of calcification may be seen.[160]

### Postradiation White Matter Injury

Cerebral radiation injury has been classified according to time of appearance of symptoms after tumor irradiation. Acute injury occurs in the form of transient worsening of symptoms during or shortly after radiation therapy to brain tumors. Late radiation injury usually occurs over several months after therapy, and may appear either as a focal lesion or as diffuse white matter injury. On MRI the latter form of this lesion appears as a diffusely increased signal in the deep periventricular white matter on T2-weighted images. The prominent clinical features of such diffuse white matter injury include impairment of mental function, personality changes, impairment of memory, confusion, learning difficulties, and dementia. Diffuse white matter changes reflect a wide spectrum of pathology ranging from frank edema to necrosis. Visible CT contrast enhancement is usually associated with necrosis. Vascular changes such as hyalinization and fibrinoid necrosis of arterioles are characteristic features of radiation injury. Vascular proliferation resembling that seen in malignant glioma can be seen, in particular in the acute phase of radiation-induced necrosis.[29,185]

## CHRONIC PROGRESSIVE SUBCORTICAL DEMYELINATION (BINSWANGER DISEASE) AND LEUKO-ARAIOSIS

"Binswanger disease" is a designation attached by some authors to a rare condition that may be prone to affect patients with systematic hypertension. The leukoencephalopathy is characterized by rarefaction of the subcortical white matter. The cortex and subcortical U-fibers are intact, but the deep cerebral white matter shows vacuolation accompanied by a decreased number of myelinated fibers. In the areas involved, sclerotic changes of the blood vessels, of the type found in hypertensive patients, are common.[129] This poorly-

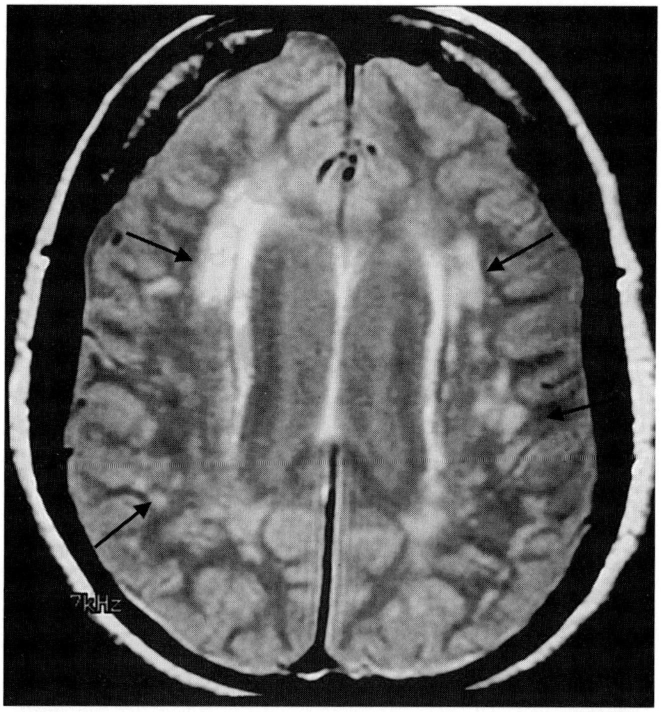


**Fig. 16-32.** Leuko-araiosis in a 68-year-old woman. Axial proton density weighted image at the level of the lateral ventricles shows both confluent and nonconfluent increased signal intensity in the deep white matter (*arrows*). (Courtesy of Dr. Richard Silbergleit, Henry Ford Hospital and Medical Center.)

defined neuropathologic entity may be identified by appropriate neuroimaging methods.[133]

The term leuko-araiosis (white matter rarefaction in Greek) designates the CT or MRI findings of white matter alterations. On CT, leuko-araiosis appears as either patchy or diffuse ill-defined nonenhancing hyperdensity involving the periventricular or deep white matter. Leuko-araiosis may be seen in many persons, especially the elderly, who may or may not have specific signs and symptoms of neuropsychiatric disease.[66] Leuko-araiosis is not found in those under 30 to 45 years, and becomes a frequent finding after the ages of 60 to 70. Leuko-araiosis has been found in about 46% of patients with Alzheimer's disease. Leuko-araiosis is thought to be related to risk factors associated with reduced cerebral blood flow to the subcortical white matter. On MRI, leuko-araiosis is demonstrated as white matter hyperintensity in T2-weighted spin-echo sequences (Fig. 16-32). Some white matter alterations are clearly age-related, but others are caused by a range of white matter lesions including small infarcts, plaques of demyelination, and incomplete infarctions. In some cases, well-defined histopathologic lesions could not be demonstrated at sites where CT or MRI changes were apparent.[26,50,189] For more details and discussion on the subject of leuko-araiosis, readers are referred to a recent review on this subject.[133]

## INHERITED METABOLIC DISEASES AFFECTING WHITE MATTER (LEUKODYSTROPHIES)

Most myelin disorders included in this section are caused by known genetic defects that involve the enzyme or protein necessary to form and maintain myelin. Most genetic defects are inherited in an autosomal recessive pattern. Exceptions to this rule are adrenoleukodystrophy (adrenomyeloneuropathy) and Pelizaeus-Merzbacher disease; both of these have an X-linked recessive inheritance. The diagnosis of each disease can be made by enzyme assay or by detecting the mutant gene.

### Metachromatic Leukodystrophy

Metachromatic leukodystrophy (MLD) is an autosomal recessive disease affecting the nervous system and to a variable extent various visceral organs. This disease is caused by a deficiency in the activity of the lysosomal hydrolase, arylsulfatase A. The arylsulfatase A gene has been cloned, and many mutations have been identified. Depending on the age of onset and the patterns of clinical manifestations, MLD is classified into three major clinical types: late infantile, juvenile, and adult (or late onset). As a rule, the younger the patient, the more severe the clinical manifestations. Thus, patients with late infantile MLD show rapidly progressive signs and symptoms of neurodegenerative disorder, including seizures and slowly progressive mental deterioration that leads to dementia. Psychiatric manifestations are common in adult cases.[22,93] Difficulty in learning at school is a common initial sign in many juvenile patients. MRI is very useful in demonstrating diffuse involvement by the demyelinating process of the periventricular and hemispheric white matter among patients with MLD[186] (Fig. 16-33).

A definitive diagnosis can be made in most cases by an assay of arylsulfatase A activity in leukocytes or, more commonly, in cultured fibroblasts (Chapter 14). However, demonstration of metachromatic bodies in the urine sediment or in the sural nerve biopsy are additional helpful means to establish the diagnosis.[117] Assaying the activity of arylsulfatase A in cells in the amniotic fluid and chorionic villi is very useful for the prenatal diagnosis of MLD. The activity of arylsulfatase A is markedly reduced or absent in late infantile cases, but in the adult type some enzyme activity is always detected. Some healthy individuals may have low arylsulfatase activity (arylsulfatase pseudodeficiency); the enzymatic activity of such individuals, measured in vitro, is usually less than 15% of the normal mean for controls. Therefore, it may be hard to distinguish such persons from patients with the presymptomatic adult type MLD.[55,191] Conduction velocity is slow in the peripheral nerve in MLD patients, but not in pseudodeficiency individuals; this can be

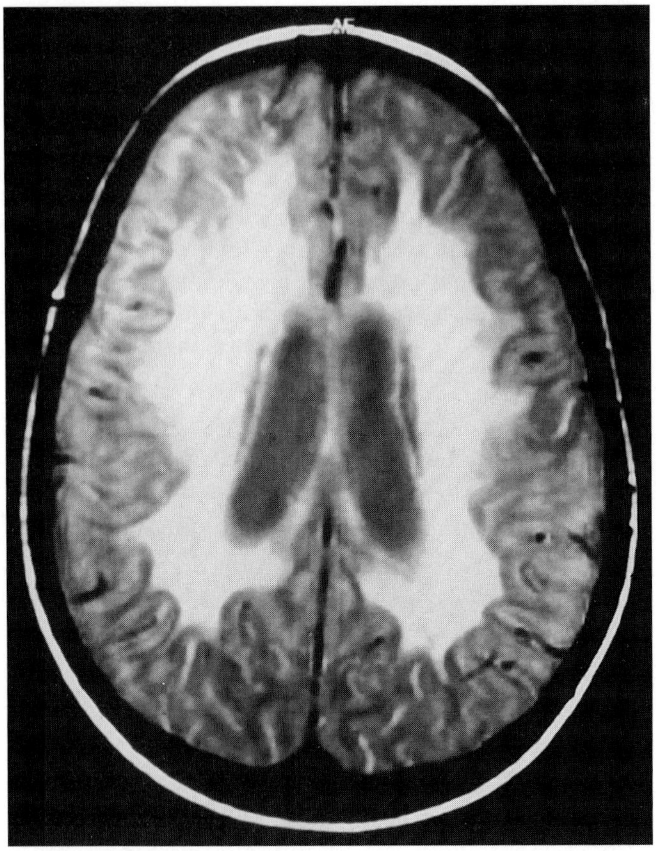

Fig. 16-33. 7-year-old girl with metachromatic leukodystrophy. Axial proton density weighted image at the level of the lateral ventricles demonstrates marked high signal intensity in the deep white matter. (Courtesy of Dr. Richard Silbergleit, Henry Ford Hospital and Medical Center.)

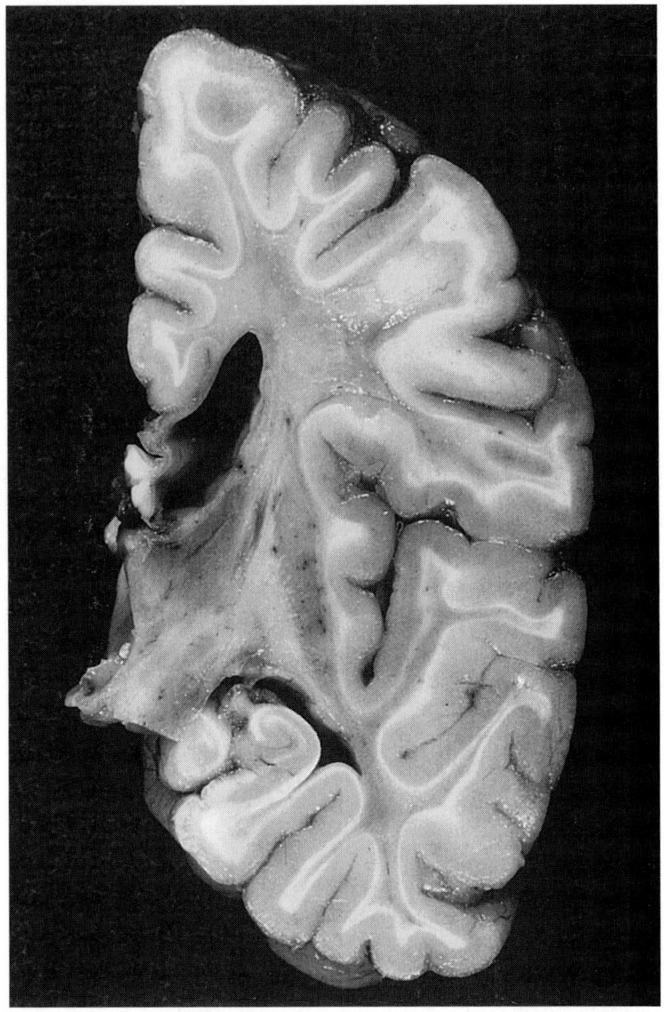

Fig. 16-34. A coronal section of the cerebral hemisphere in a case of late infantile MLD. White matter is diffusely demyelinated and shrunken. Note well preserved subcortical white matter (U-fibers). (From: Suzuki K: Genetic, Metabolic Disorders. In: Current Encyclopedia of Pathology. Vol 23. Nervous System. 1985. Nakayama Shotten Pub.)

helpful in the clinical differentiation of these two conditions. In contrast, some patients with the clinical and pathologic phenotype of MLD have normal levels of arylsulfatase A activity[68,192] and require a nerve biopsy to confirm the diagnosis of MLD. These patients most likely have a deficiency in the protein necessary to activate arylsulfatase A.[174]

On gross postmortem examination, the brain may be atrophic but often shows no external abnormalities. On cut sections and after fixation, the cerebral as well as the cerebellar white matter is diffusely gray discolored because of demyelination (Fig. 16-34). The white matter is firm and often depressed. These changes are more marked in the brains of patients with late infantile MLD. In cases in which white matter changes are severe, marked atrophy of the brainstem—in particular the base of the pons and the ventral portion of the medulla (medullary pyramids)—is almost invariably present. The peripheral nerves and visceral organs exhibit no gross abnormalities except for the gallbladder, which may be shrunken and fibrotic. On microscopic examination, the affected white matter may be hypercellular or hypocellular, depending on the stage of the pathologic process. Degenerating myelin can be identified in biopsy specimens from patients who are in the early stages of the disease; in the advanced stages myelin is not visible. Therefore, in most autopsy sections myelin may not be demonstrated in the white matter, even with a myelin stain such as LFB-PAS (Fig. 16-35), except in the subcortical U-fibers. The number of axons may be diminished in the areas of demyelination. Numerous reactive astrocytes and macrophages containing PAS-positive materials are seen in hypercellular areas (Fig. 16-36).

A pathognomonic feature of MLD is the demonstration of a stored glycolipid, sulfatide, in the macrophages, glial cells (astrocytes and oligodendrocytes), and neuronal perikarya at such specific regions of the brain as the globus pallidus, hypothalamus, dentate

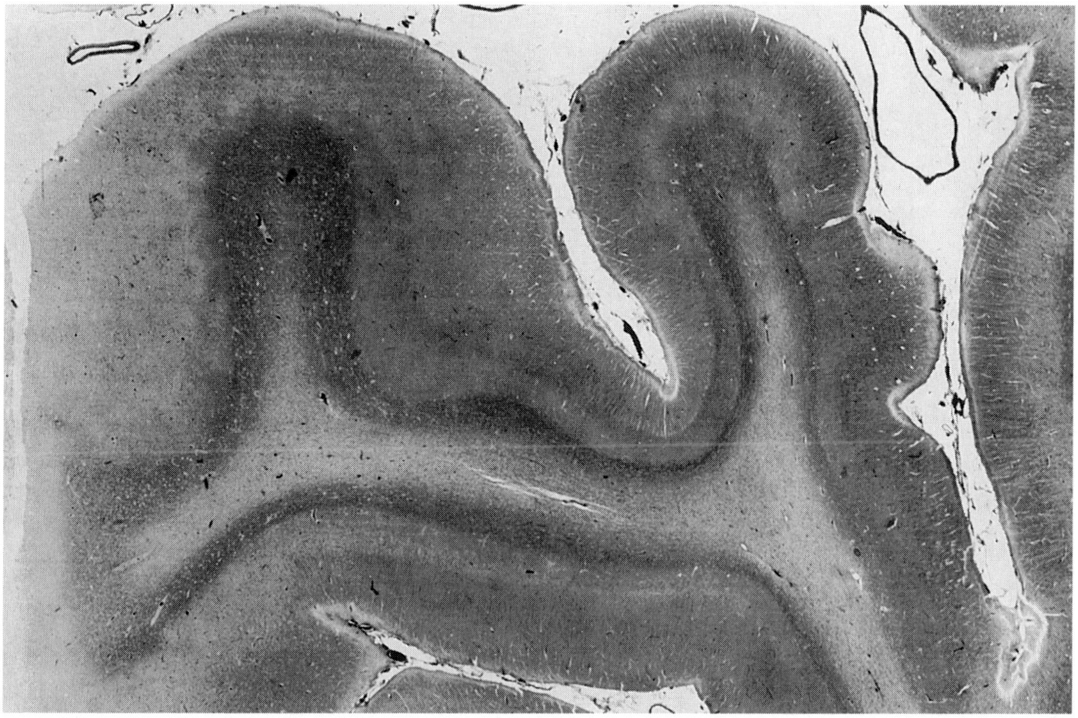

**Fig. 16-35.** Cerebral gyrus in a case of MLD showing preserved subcortical U-fibers. (×10; from Suzuki K: Genetic, Metabolic Disorders. In: Current Encyclopedia of Pathology. Vol 23. Nervous System. 1985. Nakayama Shotten Pub.)

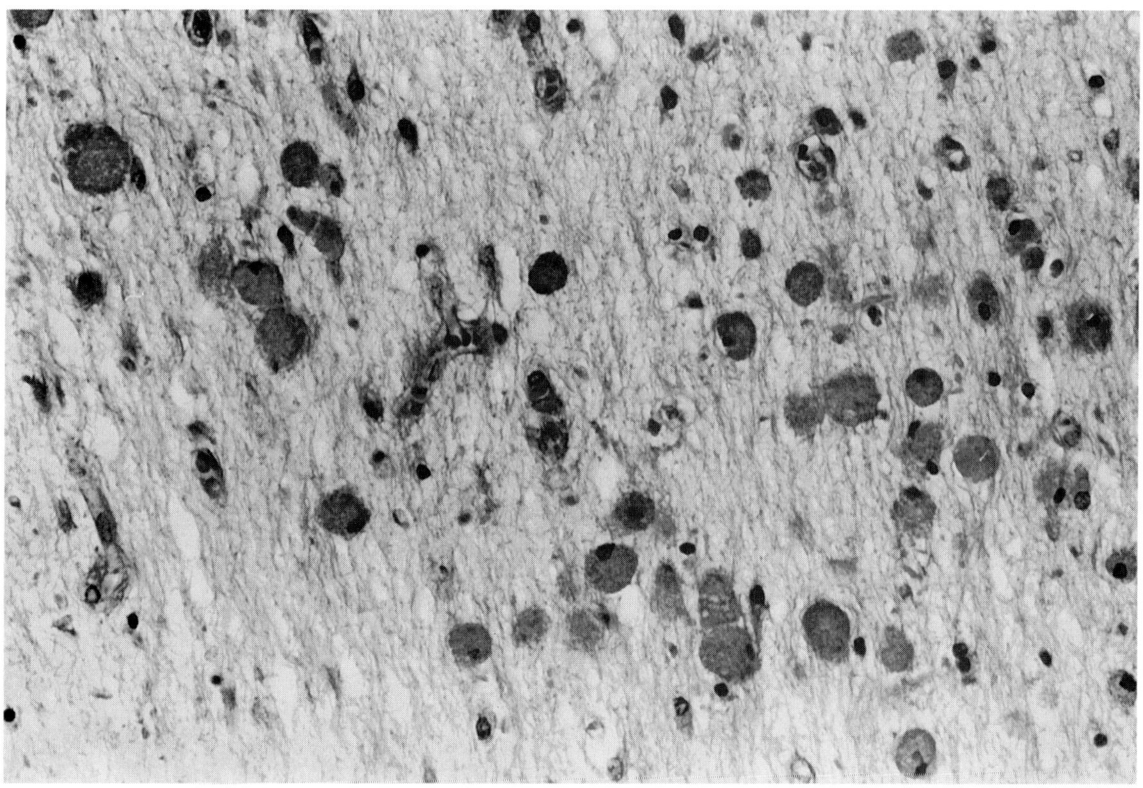

**Fig. 16-36.** Astrocytes and macrophages in the cerebral white matter in a case of MLD; most cells contain storage material. (LFB-PAS; ×150.)

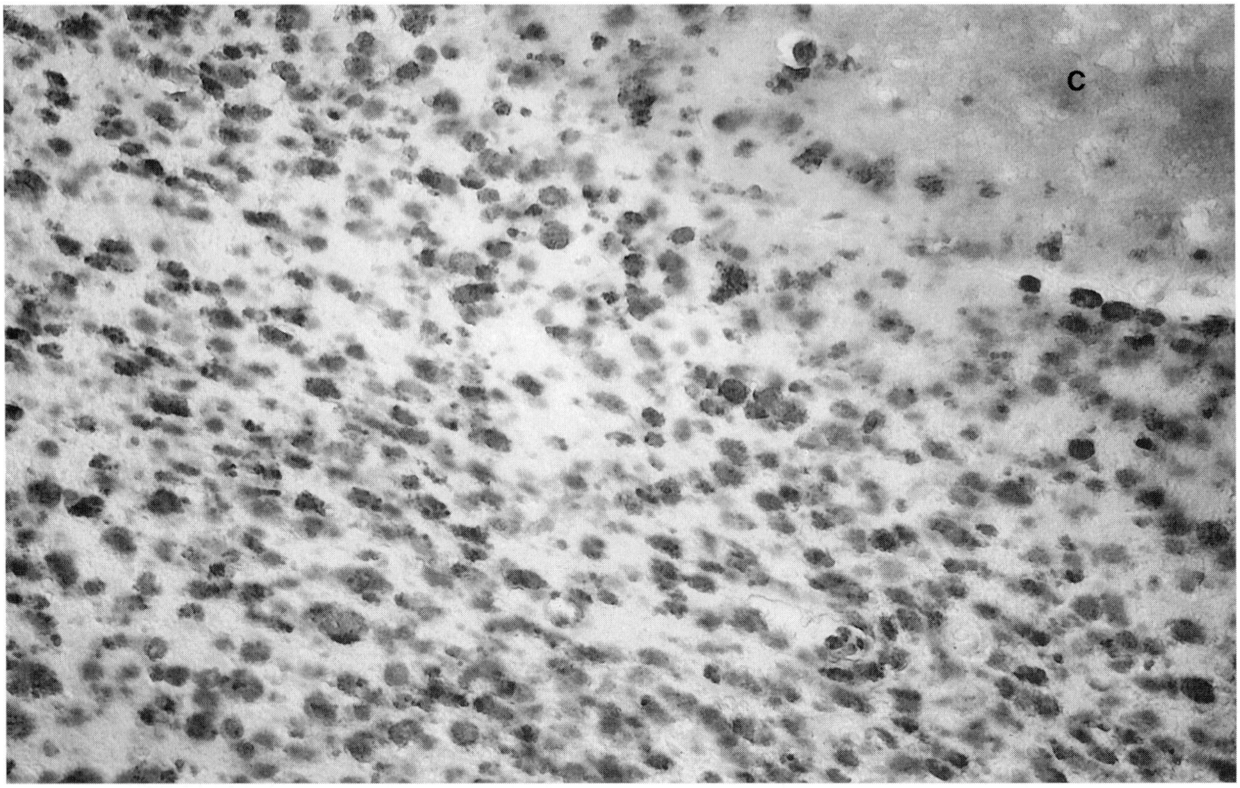


**Fig. 16-37.** Frozen section of the cerebral white matter of MLD, stained with acidic cresyl violet, showing brown metachromasia in the white matter. (*C*): cerebral cortex. (Acidic Cresy/Violet; $\times 100$.)

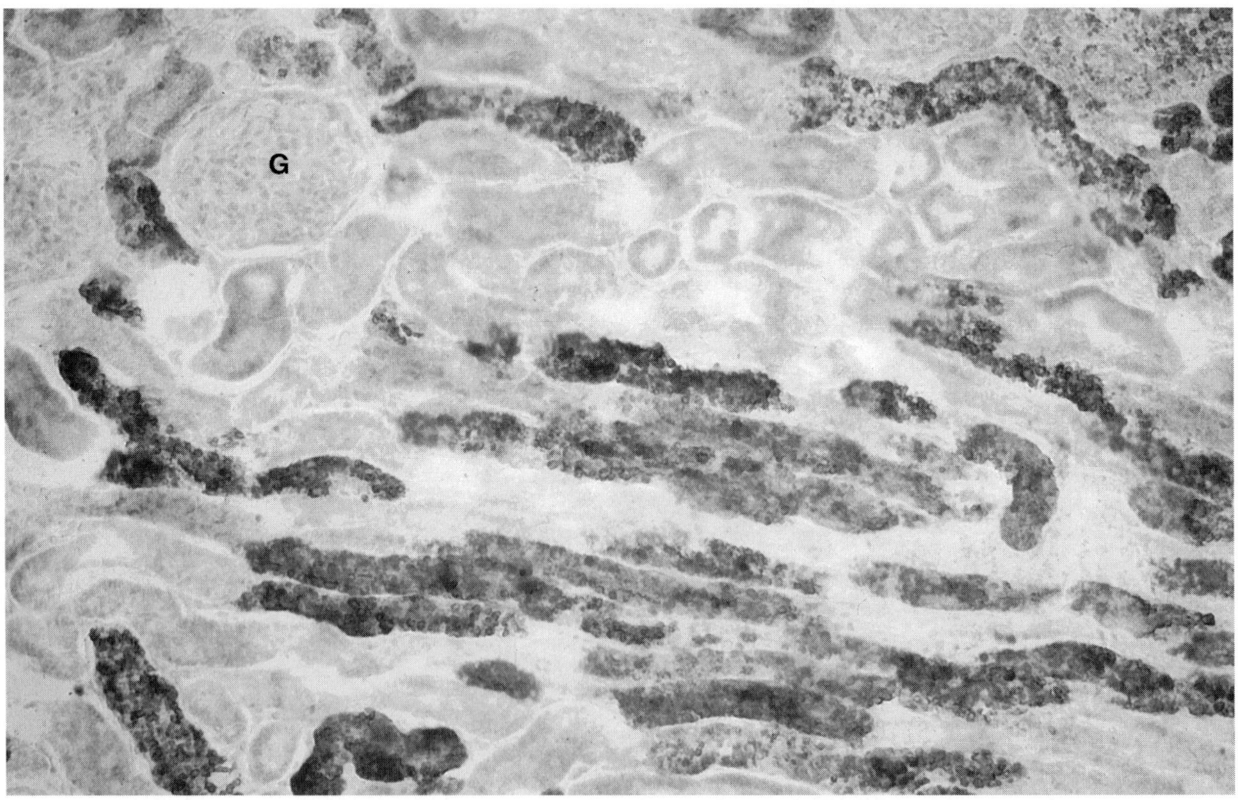


**Fig. 16-38.** Epithelial cells of the renal tubule in a case of MLD, showing brown metachromasia. (*G*): glomerulus. (Acidic Cresy/Violet; $\times 150$.)

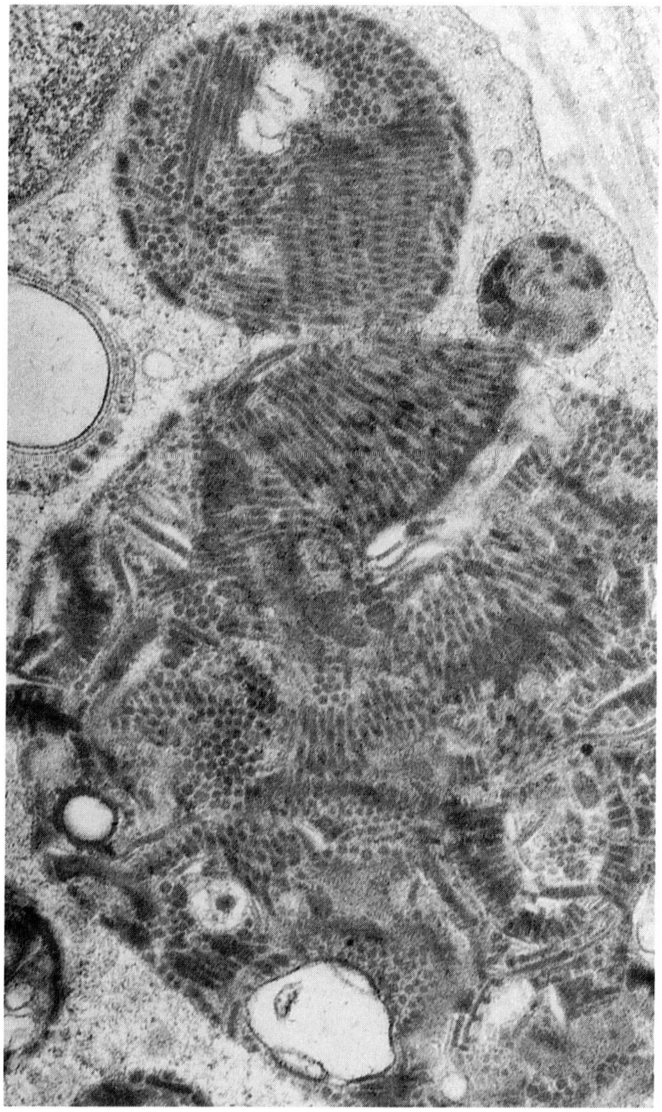

**Fig. 16-39.** Electron micrograph: MLD inclusions composed of numerous, short-stacked lamellar structures oriented in many different directions. (×60,000.)

nucleus of the cerebellum, and spinal anterior horn cells.[136] The sulfatide stains metachromatically pink when toluidine blue stain is applied to frozen sections. The most effective way to demonstrate sulfatide storage in these cells is to stain frozen sections with 1% cresyl violet adjusted to pH 3.6 with acetic acid, as described by Hirsch and Pfeiffer.[71] The white matter of MLD patients becomes brown with this stain because of the presence of storage cells; this brown color stands in sharp contrast to the pale blue staining of the adjacent cerebral cortex (brown metachromasia) (Fig. 16-37).

Demyelination of peripheral nerves together with accumulation of brown metachromatic materials in Schwann cells and macrophages are features typical of MLD. Metachromatic materials are also seen in the retinal ganglion cells[37] and cells of various visceral organs.[194] Brown metachromatic material usually is present in the renal tubular epithelium (Fig. 16-38), epithelial cells of the gallbladder, intrahepatic bile ducts, Kupffer cells, and hepatocytes (Chapter 14). The presence of metachromatic material also is noted, although less commonly, in the islets of Langerhans, the anterior pituitary, the adrenal cortex, and the testes. Multiple large polypoid masses containing metachromatic material have been seen in the gallbladder. The ultrastructural features of the metachromatic material are quite variable, but many show concentrically arranged or stacked lamellar structures (Figs. 16-39, 16-40). The most reliable diagnostic features of the metachromatic material (intracellular inclusion) are the prismatic inclusions of stacked disks giving a herringbone-like appearance in one plane of section and a hexagonal honeycomb in another (Fig. 16-41), as well as the tuffstone inclusions made of concentric and radial lamellae in a granular matrix.[12,61,180] The inclusions visible in neuronal perikarya are concentrically arranged lamellar structures that closely resemble the membranous cytoplasmic bodies (MCBs) of gangliosidosis (Fig. 16-42). Peripheral nerves in patients with MLD show seg-

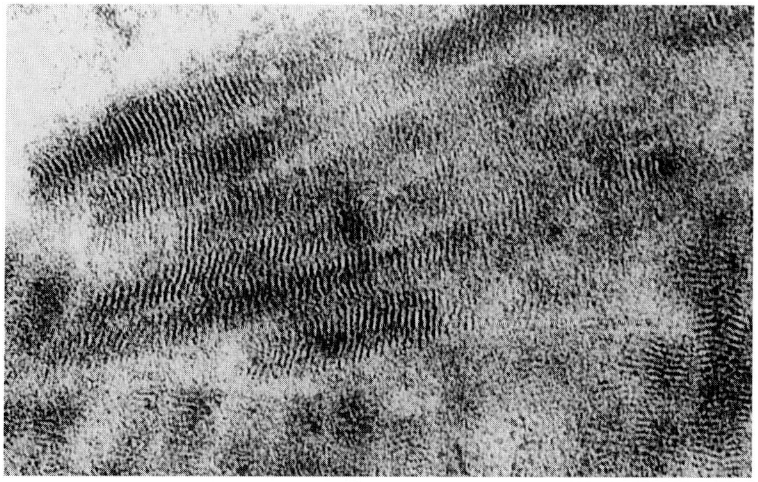

**Fig. 16-40.** Detail of the stacked lamellar structures in a case of MLD. (×150,000.)

mental demyelination and metachromatic material within the cytoplasm of Schwann cells as well as in endoneurial macrophages (Fig. 16-43). These changes are visible in all types of MLD; however, macrophages tend to be more numerous in late infantile cases than

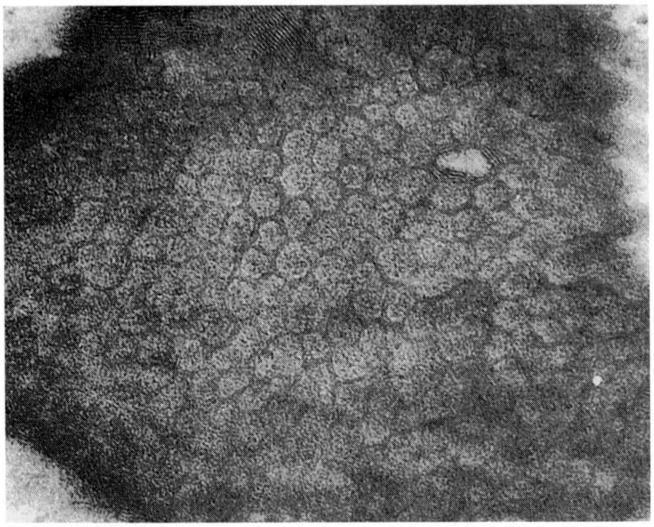

**Fig. 16-41.** MLD inclusions showing honeycomb pattern. (×100,000) (From Suzuki K: Metabolic Disorders in Electron Microscopy in Human Medicine. In: Nervous Systems, Sensory Organs, and Respiratory Tract. Vol 6. LJV Johannssen (ed). 1980. McGraw-Hill, Inc.)

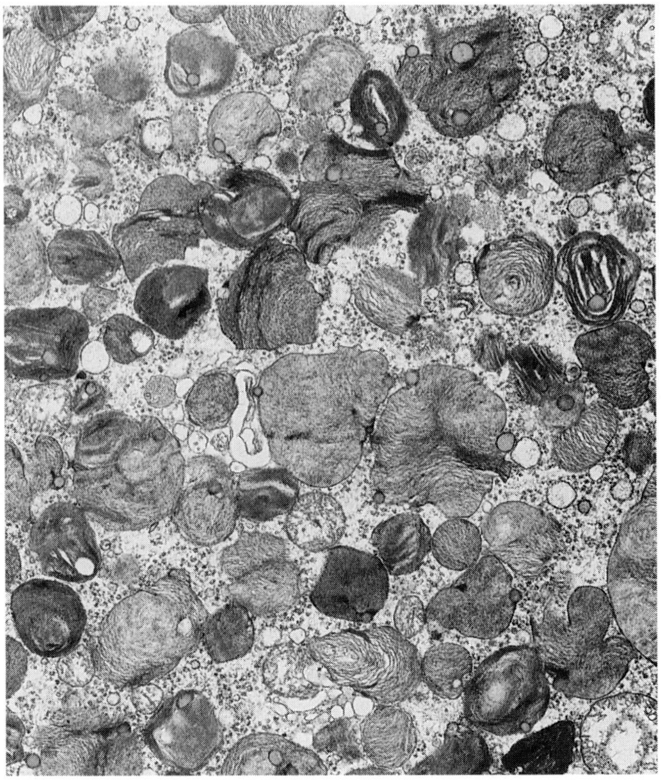

**Fig. 16-42.** Lamellar inclusions in the anterior horn neurons in a case of MLD. (×12,000.)

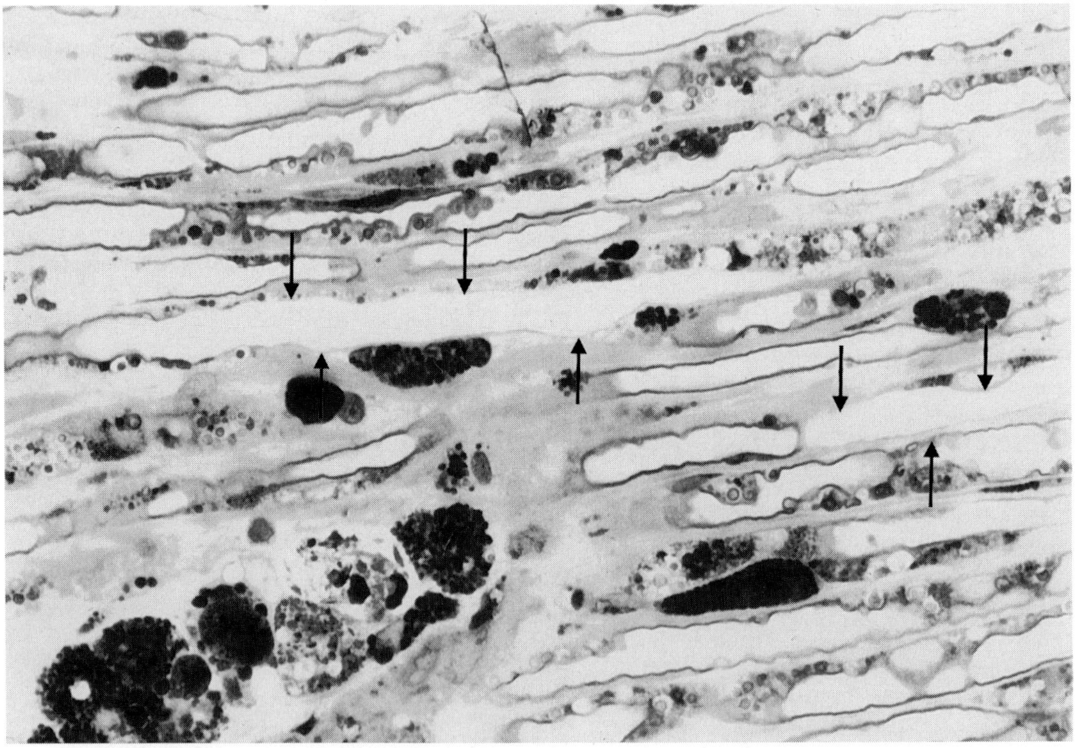

**Fig. 16-43.** One micron-thick section of a spinal root in a case of late infantile MLD, showing segmental demyelination of nerve fibers (*arrows*) and numerous inclusions in both macrophages and Schwann cells. (Toluidine blue; ×1500.)

in adults. In some instances of late onset the nerve may exhibit hypertrophic changes with many onion bulb-like arrangements of Schwann cell processes around axons (onion bulb formation) and evidence of nerve fiber regeneration. The nerves in these patients may be thickened and grossly enlarged on palpation.[180]

### Multiple Sulfatase Deficiency, Mucosulfatidosis

The multiple sulfatase deficiency form of metachromatic leukodystrophy (MSD-MLD) is a rare variant of MLD. Patients with this disease show phenotypic features of leukodystrophy and mucopolysaccharidosis. In this disease all sulfatases (A, B, and C) are deficient.[93] Grossly the brain is atrophic and its appearance resembles that of mucopolysaccharidosis; the leptomeninges are thickened and cloudy, and the ventricles usually are enlarged. Microscopically, neuronal storage of mucopolysaccharide is diffusely visible together with the typical features of MLD.[14,154]

### Krabbe Disease, Globoid Cell Leukodystrophy

Globoid cell leukodystrophy (GLD) is an autosomal recessive disorder caused by the deficient activity of the lysosomal enzyme galactosylceramidase (galactocerebrosidase; galactocerebroside $\beta$-galactosidase). The galactosylceramidase gene recently has been cloned.[35] The most common clinical phenotype is an infantile form in which onset of neurologic symptoms occurs around 4 months of age, but late-onset cases including rare adult cases also have been reported.[94,105] A definitive diagnosis of GLD can be made by an assay of the activity of galactosylceramidase in leukocytes, in cultured fibroblasts, and in cultured amniotic fluid cells. Thus, a prenatal diagnosis can be made by means of an assay of the enzyme activity.[178] Recently, characteristic GLD inclusions were identified in the epithelial cells of eccrine sweat glands[56]; in this way, the diagnosis of GLD can be made by means of an electron microscopic study of the skin biopsy (Chapter 14). In infantile cases, CT shows white matter hypodensity and diffuse atrophy of both gray and white matter. Symmetric nonenhancing hyperdense lesions are also noted in the posterior limbs of the internal capsule, thalamus, caudate nucleus, corona radiata, and periventricular white matter. MRI shows punctate areas of decreased intensity on T2 images, indicative of a paramagnetic effect, visible in these same regions (Fig. 16-44).[20,48,137,164] Unlike the diffuse involvement of the white matter typical of infantile cases, the periventricular white matter of the parieto-occipital lobes appears to be preferentially involved in late-onset cases.[94,105,179] This distribution is also characteristic of adrenoleukodystrophy (ALD), and for this reason CT or MRI findings alone may be insufficient to differentiate ALD from late-onset GLD.

In most cases of GLD the brain is small and atrophic. On cut sections, the white matter is discolored gray and is firm in consistency. The appearance of the brain is similar in the infantile and late-onset forms of the disease except for the distribution of the demyelinating lesions as stated above. Visceral organs are normal in GLD.

Histologic abnormalities are, for all practical purposes, limited to the white matter, which shows marked paucity of myelin and is gliotic (Fig. 16-45). Characteristic globoid cells (mononucleated or multinucleated macrophages containing galactocerebroside inclusions) are clustered either in groups or individually scattered throughout the densely gliotic white matter (Fig. 16-46). The cytoplasm of these cells, which may be vacuolated or somewhat crinkled, stains strongly positive with periodic acid Schiff (PAS) stain, even on paraffin-embedded sections. In the early stage of the disease, globoid cells are individually scattered among myelinated fibers; these cells tend to cluster around blood vessels and gradually disappear when the process of demyelination advances.[39]

Correlative studies of neuropathology and MRI suggest that markedly hyperintense T2-weighted images correspond to the areas of demyelination.[137] In long-

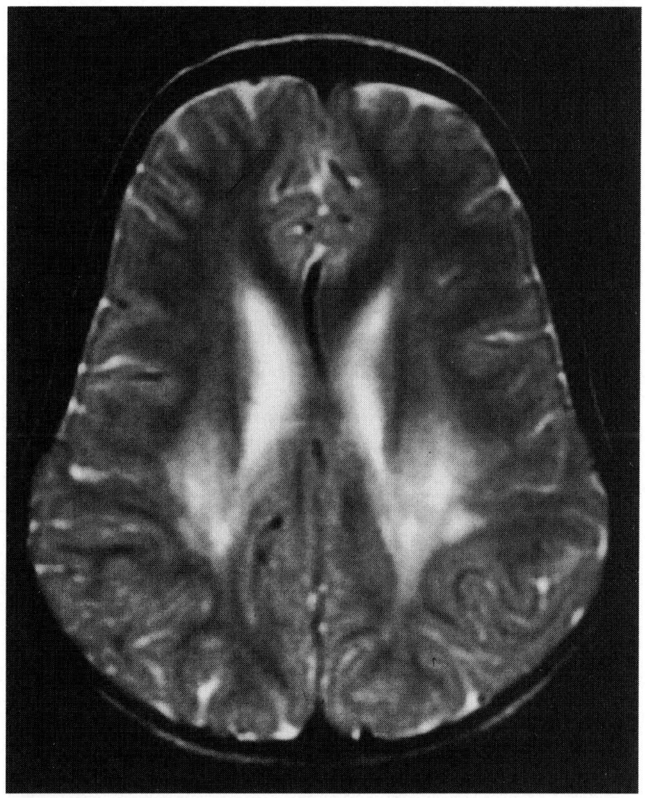

**Fig. 16-44.** 20-month-old male infant with Krabbe's disease. Axial T2-weighted image at the level of the lateral ventricles shows high signal intensity lesions confined to the parietal white matter. (Courtesy of Dr. Richard Silbergleit, Henry Ford Hospital and Medical Center.)

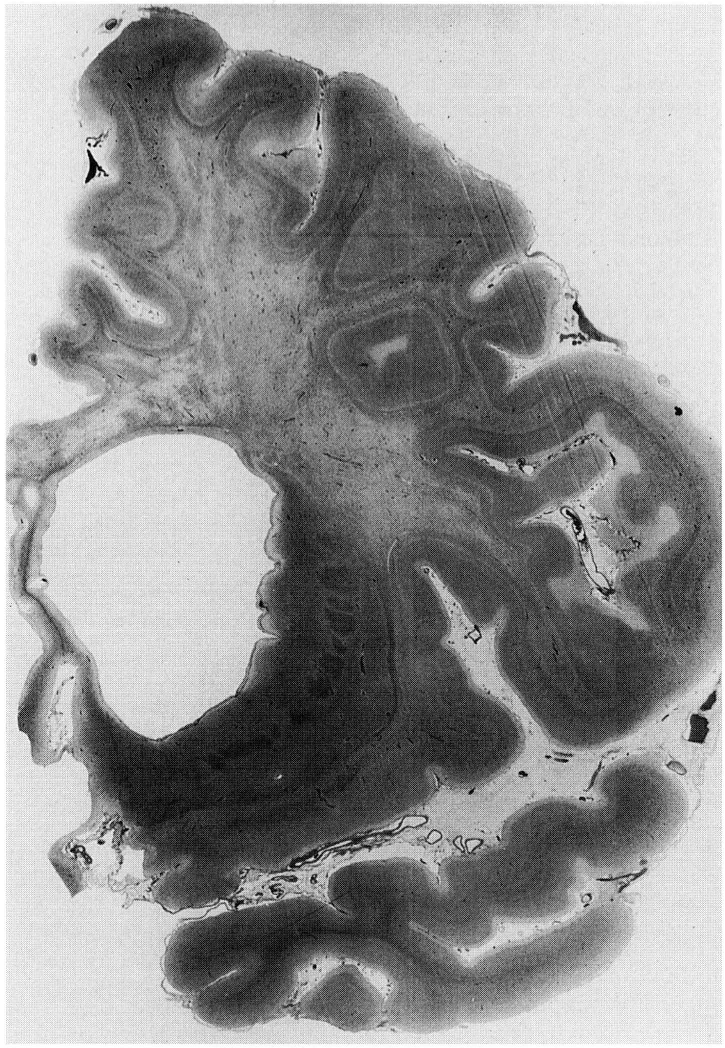

**Fig. 16-45.** Coronal section of the cerebrum in a case of GLD showing diffusely demyelinated white matter. (From Suzuki K: Genetic Metabolic Disorders. In: Current Encyclopedia of Pathology. Vol 23. Nervous System. 1985. Nakayama Shotten Pub.)

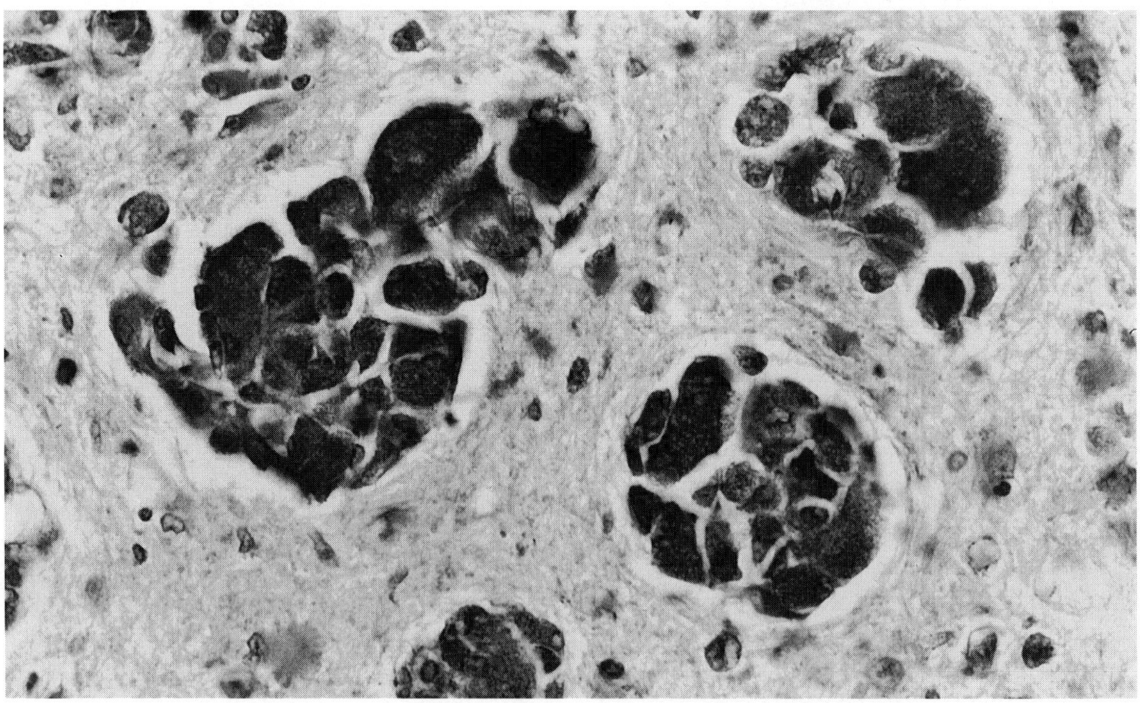

**Fig. 16-46.** Clusters of globoid cells around blood vessels in the white matter in a case of GLD. (LFB-PAS; ×300.)

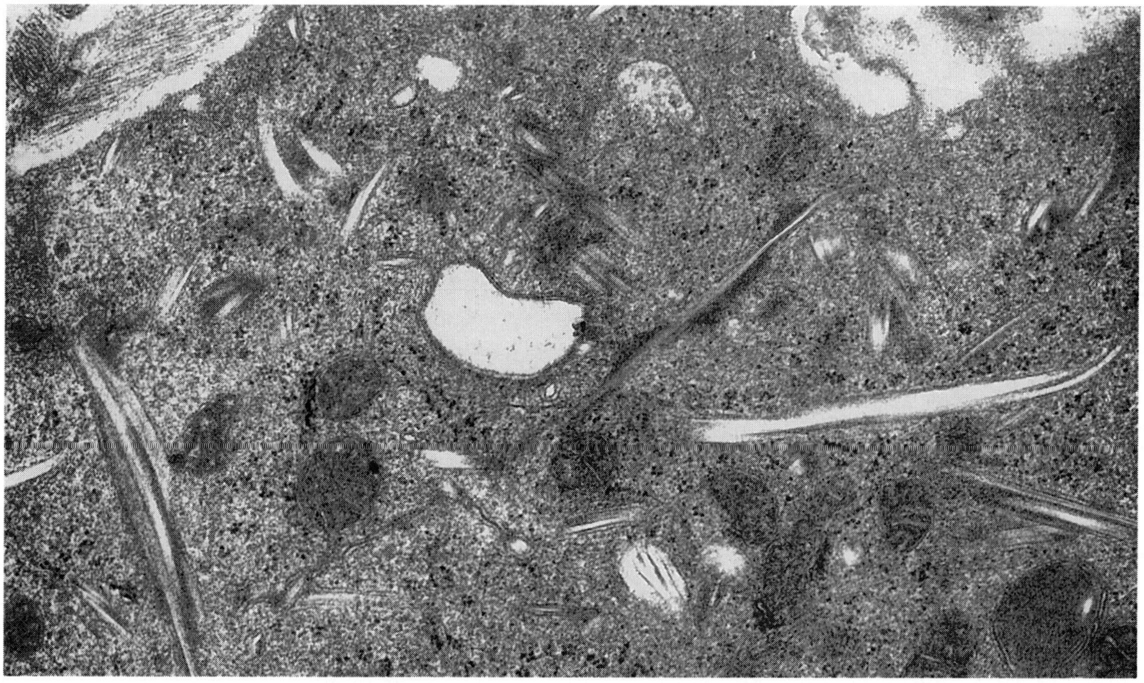

**Fig. 16-47.** Electron micrograph of the inclusions in the globoid cells in a case of GLD. (Reproduced with publisher's permission.) (×60,000.) (From Suzuki K: Genetic Metabolic Disorders. In: Current Encyclopedia of Pathology. Vol 23. Nervous System. 1985. Nakayama Shotten Pub.)

standing cases, the white matter may be totally replaced by densely gliotic tissue, where a few axons and occasional globoid cells may be found with much difficulty. The diagnosis of GLD in such patients can be made only by an assay of galactosylceramidase activity.[44] The cerebral cortical neurons are relatively well preserved. However, the deep nuclei (thalamus, globus pallidus, putamen, dentate nucleus of the cerebellum, and brainstem nuclei) may show both marked loss of neuronal perikarya and gliosis with infiltration by globoid cells. The inclusions in these macrophages (globoid cells) are variously described as having a hollow tubular, crystalline-like, straight and twisted tubular appearance[10,177,199] (Fig. 16-47). These inclusions are ultrastructurally identical to galactosylceramide (galactocerebroside).[200] Macrophages having a similar morphologic appearance can be induced experimentally by an intracerebral injection of galactosylceramide (galactocerebroside).[11,15,176] In some cases the optic nerves are markedly enlarged and have extensive gliosis. Peripheral nerves are also abnormal in GLD; the affected nerve fibers may have grossly increased diameter and may be firm in consistency.[173] Peripheral nerve fibers frequently show segmental demyelination and onion bulb formation. Inclusion bodies characteristic of GLD can be detected in the cytoplasm of Schwann cells at the ultrastructural level. The clinical phenotypes in adults are quite heterogeneous, and in some of the older patients peripheral neuropathy may well be the major clinical symptom.[94]

### Adrenoleukodystrophy and Adrenomyeloneuropathy

Adrenoleukodystrophy (ALD) is an X-linked neurologic disorder characterized by progressive CNS demyelination and adrenal insufficiency. Patients with ALD have an impaired capacity to form the coenzyme A derivative of saturated, very long chain fatty acid (VLCFA), a reaction catalyzed by the enzyme lignoceroyl-coenzyme A-ligase, thus; detection of VLCFA in plasma, red cells, cultured skin fibroblasts, cultured amniocytes, or chorionic villi has been used for the diagnosis. The gene responsible for ALD (ALDP) has been identified.[120] This gene is not the fatty acid coenzyme A ligase, and it appears to encode a transporter protein that may function in the peroxisome membrane. Mutations of this gene have been identified in all of the 100-plus patients of ALD studied thus far.[118] At present it is unclear how a defect in ALDP impairs the VLCFA coenzyme A ligase activity in peroxisomes.

Two major phenotypes, adrenoleukodystrophy (ALD, childhood form) and adrenomyeloneuropathy (AMN), are known. ALD is the most common type and affected boys usually are normal until 4 to 8 years of age. Symptoms usually begin as behavioral disturbances and/or difficulty in school work during the first decade of life; then, there is progression to dementia, seizures, visual loss, and eventual spastic paraparesis. More than 90% of patients with ALD have adrenal insufficiency demonstrable by the adrenocorticotropic hormone (ACTH) stimulation test.

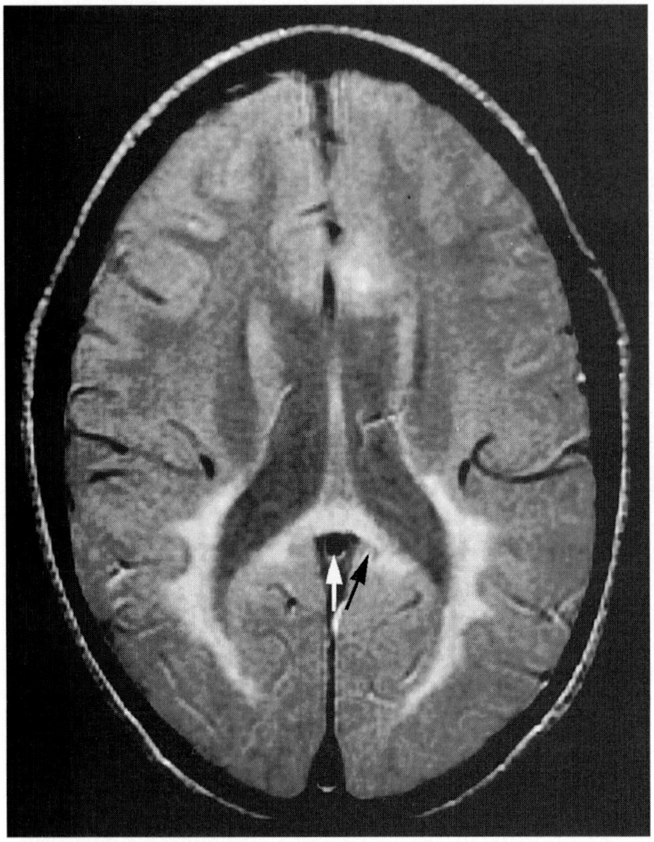

**Fig. 16-48.** 13-year-old boy with adrenoleukodystrophy. Proton density weighted image shows high signal intensity in the white matter, particularly noticeable in the parieto-occipital white matter. The splenium (*arrow*) also is involved. (Courtesy of Dr. Richard Silbergleit, Henry Ford Hospital and Medical Center.)

AMN is a disease of young men. Patients with AMN frequently develop slowly progressive paraparesis with sphincter disturbances, often misdiagnosed as multiple sclerosis. In approximately one half of the patients with AMN, the pathology is confined to the spinal cord and peripheral nerves. In two thirds of the cases, adrenal insufficiency is detectable.[119] Late-onset adult cases are also known[47,97] and some show the clinical phenotype of olivopontocerebellar atrophy.[127] Some patients with primary adrenal insufficiency never develop neurologic symptoms, and about 15 to 20% of heterozygous women may show similar neurologic manifestations and neuropathology.[119,142,168] In these heterozygous cases, onset is delayed, the clinical course is usually milder than in the homozygous patients, and adrenal insufficiency is rare. T2-weighed MRI shows localized symmetric areas of high intensity corresponding to the sites of demyelination in the periventricular white matter of the occipital lobes (Fig. 16-48). When the disease advances, high-intensity lesions spread to the parietal and temporal white matter, as well as to the brainstem tracts. Thus, MRI is useful to monitor the progression of the disease and to evaluate the effectiveness of treatments such as bone marrow transplantation.[101,102,187]

The external appearance of the brain and spinal cord usually are unrevealing. On cut sections of the brains of ALD patients, areas of demyelination are seen as symmetric gray depressed lesions in the white matter (Fig. 16-49) The cerebral ventricles are markedly dilated (hydrocephalus ex vacuo). As seen on MRI, demyelination is most extensive in the parieto-occipital regions, and the frontal white matter is less extensively involved.[165] The cerebellar white matter also may primarily be involved in ALD, whereas in the brainstem and the spinal cord wallerian degeneration (rather than demyelination) is the usual feature. In contrast, the spinal cord is the major site of involvement in AMN.[28,62,118] In active lesions, myelin disintegration together with foamy macrophages and extensive astrocyte responses are typical microscopic features of ALD. Variable degrees of perivascular mononuclear cell infiltrates are seen in these areas of demyelination (Fig. 16-50). These histopathologic features are very similar to those of multiple sclerosis. Macrophages that stain strongly positive with PAS in paraffin-embedded sections cluster around blood vessels, mimicking in some cases the histopathologic features of globoid cell leukodystrophy. Frozen sections of cerebral white matter clearly demonstrate sudanophilic material within the cytoplasm of these macrophages. The histopathology of myelin disintegration varies from region to region, depending on the stage of the demyelinating process. Dense fibrillary gliosis mixed with macrophages and mononuclear cell inflammatory infiltrates is seen in chronically demyelinated white matter, where cavitation and calcium deposits may be visible. Electron microscopic examination shows within the cytoplasm of macrophages characteristic inclusions made up of paired electron-dense curvilinear leaflets separated by an electron-lucent space (see Chapter 14). Macrophages also contain various products secondary to myelin disintegration products and lipid droplets (Fig. 16-51). Perivascular macrophages often contain abnormal lamellar cytoplasmic inclusions composed of 3- to 4-nm electron-dense leaflets of variable length[166] (Fig. 16-52). Inclusions having a similar appearance may be found in the Schwann cell cytoplasm, although demyelination in peripheral nerves is an inconstant feature of AMN. Another prominent histopathologic feature is the presence of ballooned, striated adrenocortical cells, which contain characteristic trilamellar inclusions (Fig. 16-53). These inclusions also can be detected in the testicular Leydig cells.[143] The histopathology of AMN is similar to that of ALD, although inflammatory components in the spinal cord lesions are less numerous, and atrophy of the adrenal cortex and testes is often noted.

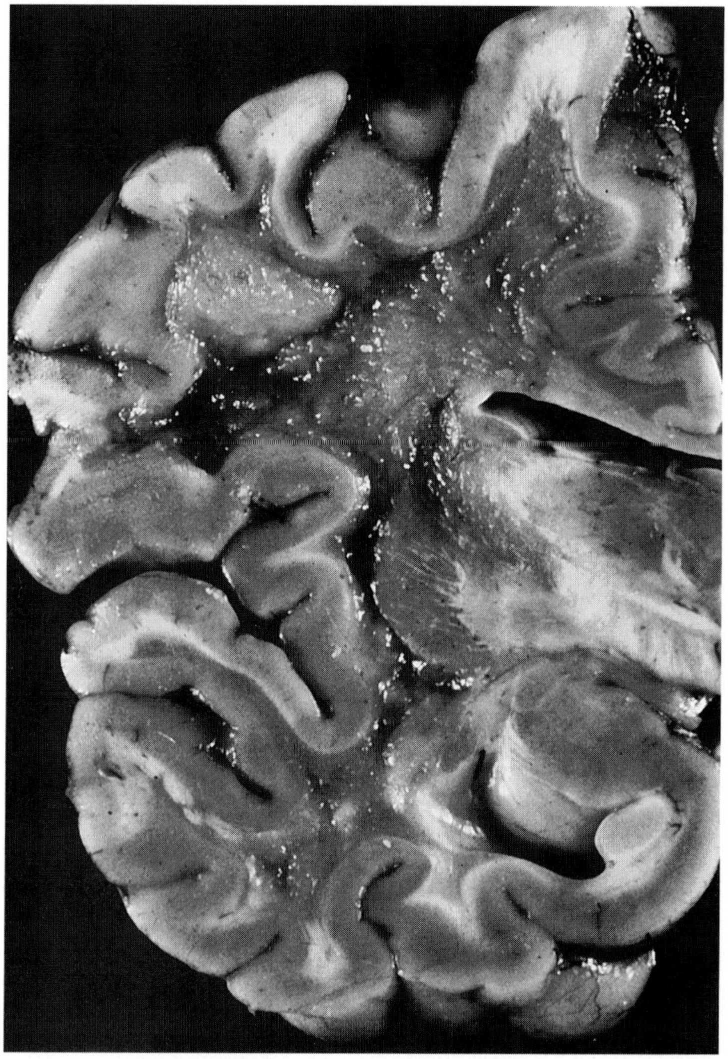

**Fig. 16-49.** Coronal section of the brain in a case of ALD, showing diffuse demyelination.

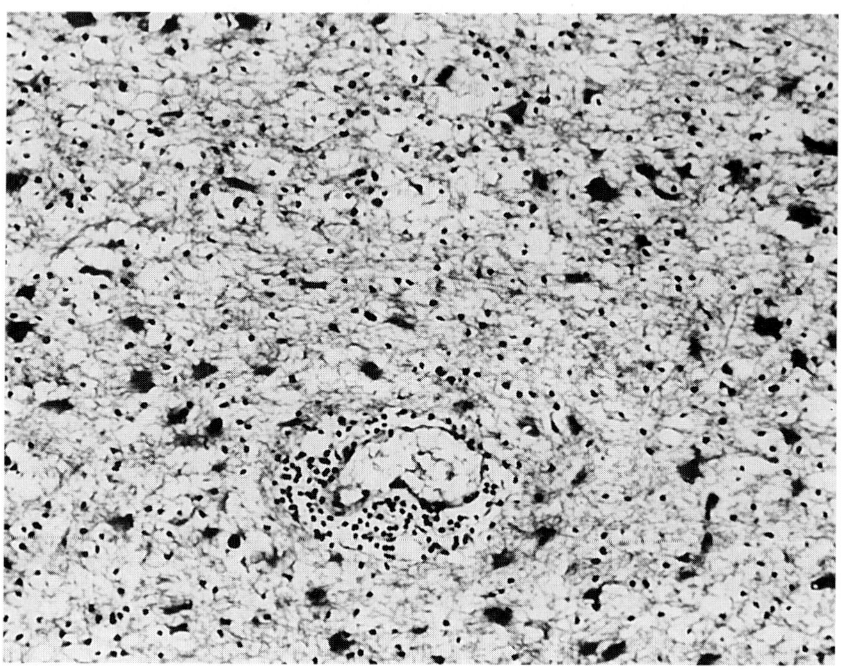

**Fig. 16-50.** Histologic features of ALD: numerous foamy macrophages, diffuse astrocytosis, and perivascular cuffs of mononuclear inflammatory cells. (H&E; ×150.)

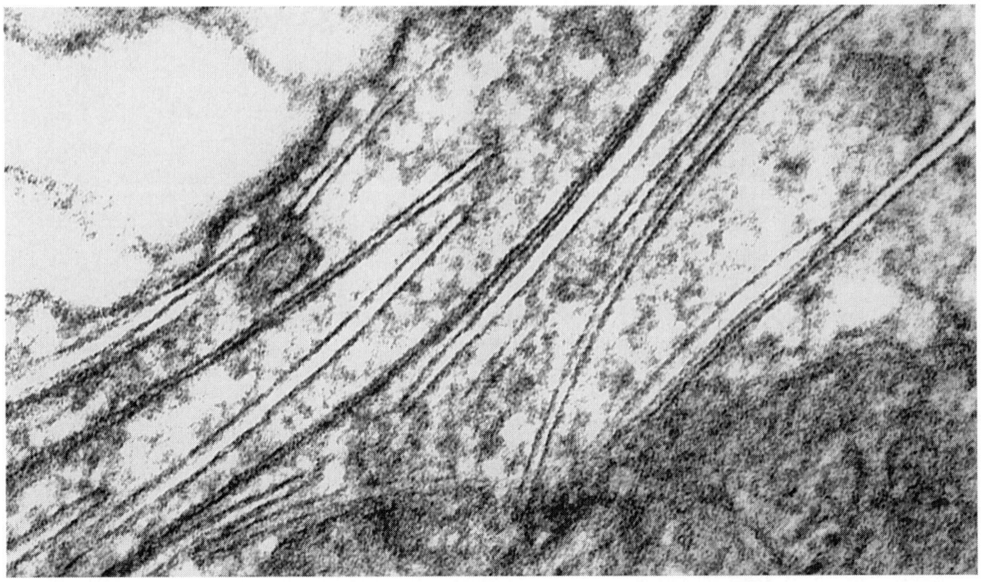

**Fig. 16-51.** Electronmicrograph of trilamellar inclusions in a macrophage in a case of ALD. (×60,000.)

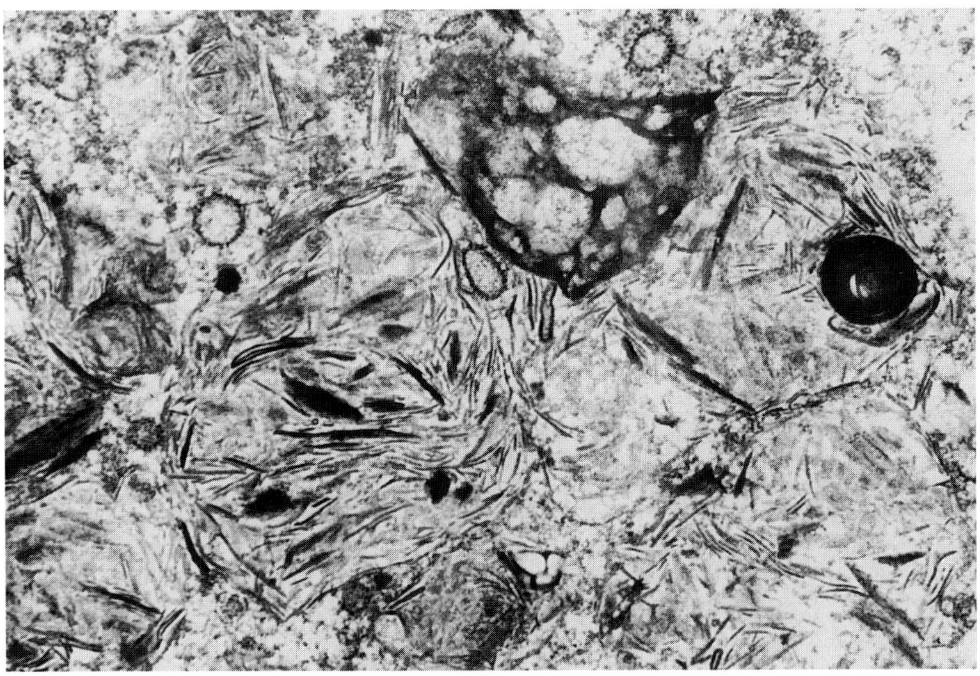

**Fig. 16-52.** Electronmicrograph of cytoplasmic lamellar inclusions in a macrophage in a case of ALD. (×36,000.)

The adrenal glands may become atrophic in the advanced stages of ALD.[119]

### Sudanophilic (Orthochromatic) Leukodystrophies

Sudanophilic (or orthochromatic) leukodystrophies (SL) are progressive neurodegenerative disorders with a common histopathologic feature of diffuse demyelination with an accumulation of sudanophilic lipids within the macrophages[80] (Fig. 16-54). Thus, SL comprises a clinically heterogeneous group of diseases. Most cases previously included in this category are now well-defined genetic peroxisomal disorders, such as adrenoleukodystrophy (AD) or adrenomyeloneuropathy (AMN). However, there are still cases that clearly are neither AD nor AMN.[3,197,198] In some instances, macrophages and other glial cells containing

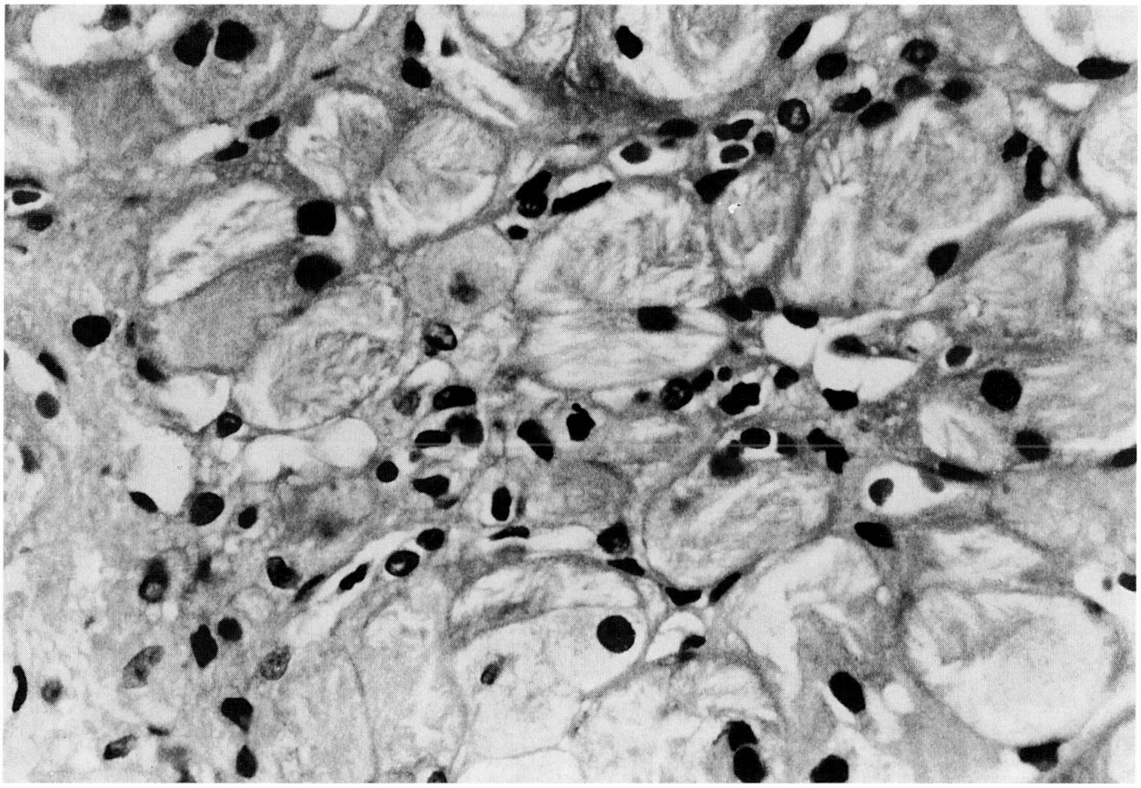

**Fig. 16-53.** Ballooned cells in the adrenal cortex in a case of ALD, showing linear wrinkled inclusions of the perikarya. (H&E; ×800.)

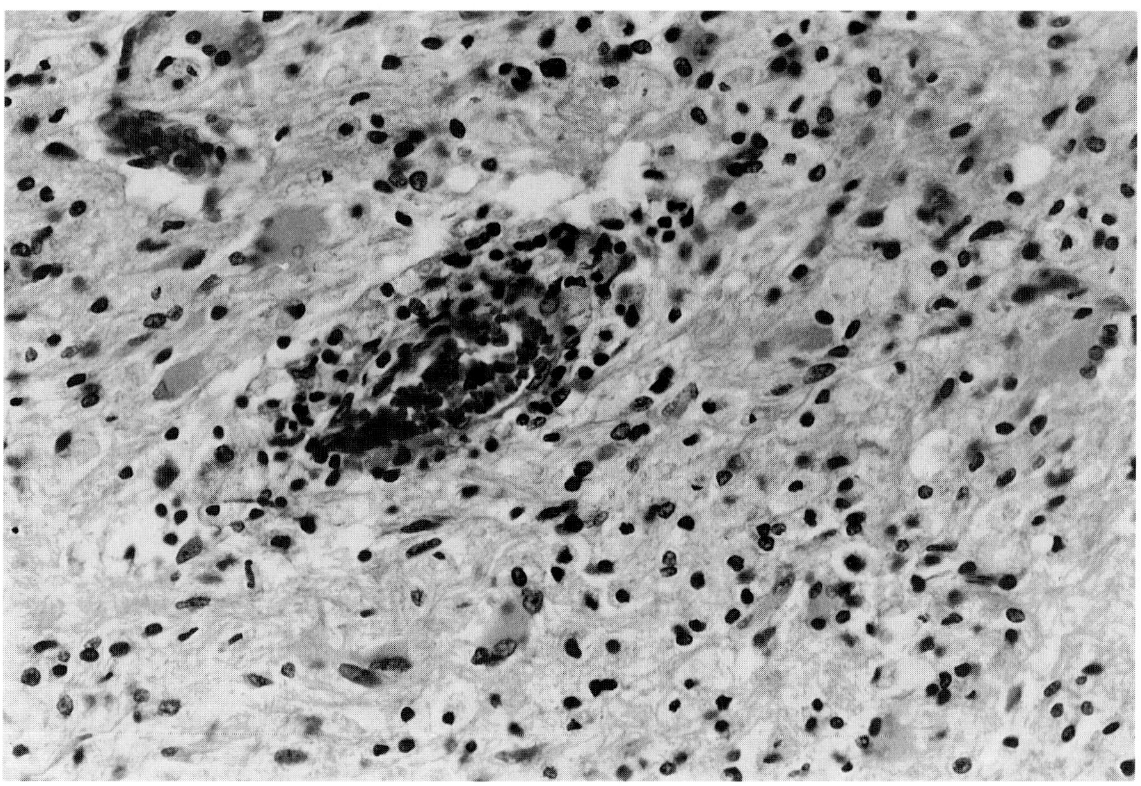

**Fig. 16-54.** Cerebral white matter in a case of SLD infiltrated by many macrophages and reactive astrocytes. (H&E; ×150.)

brownish iron-positive granular pigment granules constitute an additional prominent histopathologic feature in the demyelinating white matter. Because of this, these cases have been described as the pigmentary type of sudanophilic (or orthochromatic) leukodystrophy.[38,128,175,184]

### Spongy Degeneration of the CNS in Infancy (Aspartoacylase Deficiency: Canavan Disease)

Spongy degeneration of the CNS in infancy is an autosomal recessive disease, often affecting Ashkenazi Jewish infants.[188] Non-Jewish cases also have been reported. Megalocephaly, seizures, and hypotonia are

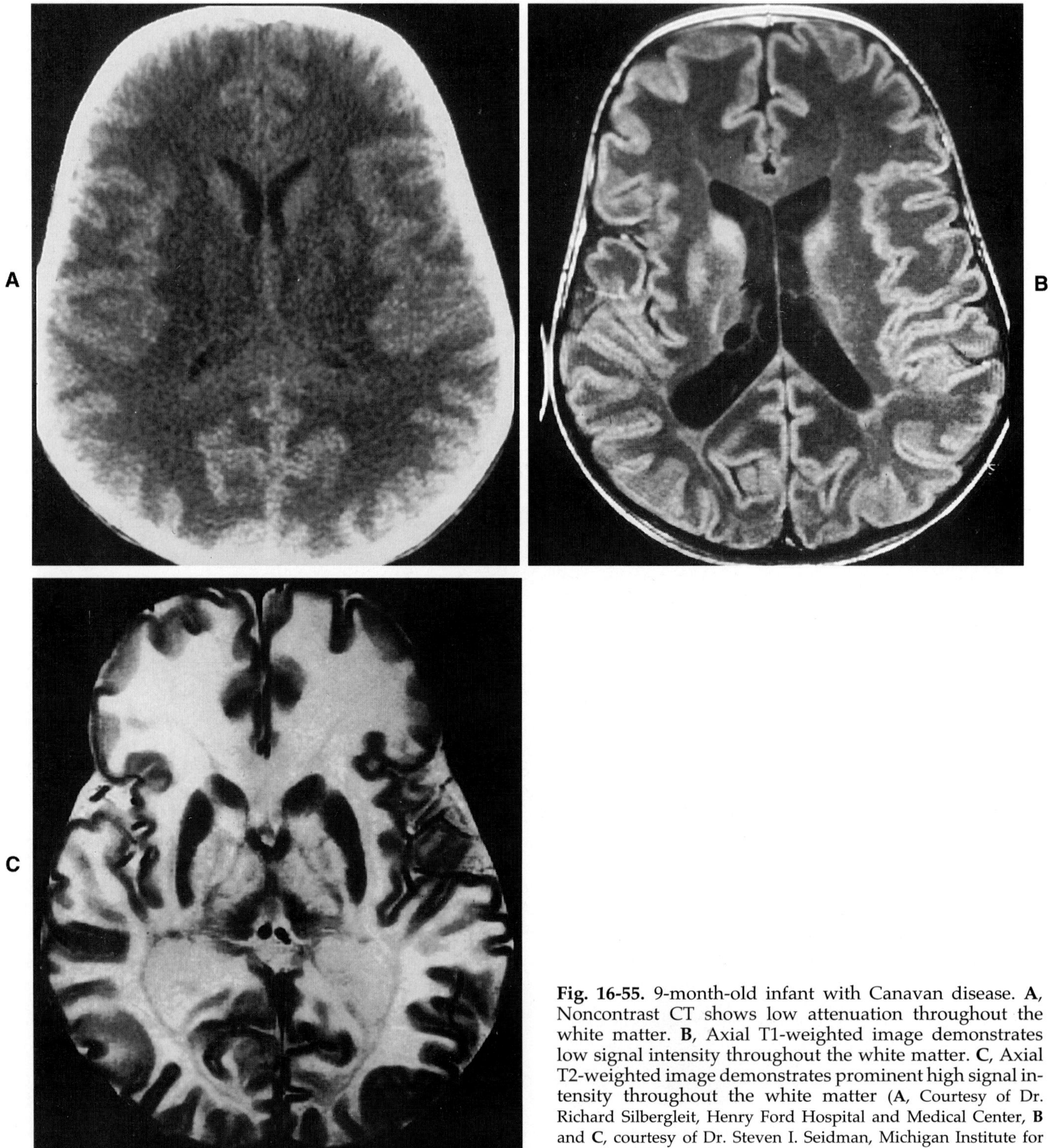


**Fig. 16-55.** 9-month-old infant with Canavan disease. **A**, Noncontrast CT shows low attenuation throughout the white matter. **B**, Axial T1-weighted image demonstrates low signal intensity throughout the white matter. **C**, Axial T2-weighted image demonstrates prominent high signal intensity throughout the white matter (**A**, Courtesy of Dr. Richard Silbergleit, Henry Ford Hospital and Medical Center, **B** and **C**, courtesy of Dr. Steven I. Seidman, Michigan Institute for Neurological Disorders.)

conspicuous neurologic signs and symptoms in the affected infants. The genetic defect of this disease is a deficient activity of aspartoacylase[42,111]; as a result, excessive levels of N-acetylaspartic acid (NAA) can be detected in the patient's urine. Aspartoacylase cDNA has been cloned and the mutation has been identified.[86] MRI studies show diffuse symmetric low signal intensity on T1-weighted images and high signal intensity on T2-weighted images of the cerebral white matter (Fig. 16-55). Proton magnetic resonance spectroscopy can detect increased amounts of NAA in the brains of patients with spongy degeneration.[23]

The brain is heavy with increased water content[83] and soft in consistency. White matter is gelatinous and the cortico-medullary junctions are ill-defined. In patients with prolonged survival, however, the brain weight may be normal or less than normal owing to a loss of volume of white matter (Fig. 16-56). The most striking histopathologic feature noted in the brain is a spongy vacuolation in the deeper cortical layers and in the white matter (Fig. 16-57). In protracted cases, myelin and axons are lost in the deep white matter, and spongy changes are seen predominantly in the subcortical U-fiber region. In the cerebral cortex, astrocytes with enlarged pale nuclei, resembling the Alzheimer type II astrocytes of hepatic encephalopathy, are conspicuous. The cytoplasm of these astrocytes is pale and contains clustered dots or fine threadlike structures representing abnormal mitochondria, which are detectable in H&E stained preparations (Fig. 16-58). In the cerebellum, spongy vacuolation is most pronounced in the Purkinje cell layers. Vacuolation in the white matter is caused by the separation of myelin lamellae at the intraperiod line, a feature noted in various types of toxic brain edema (Fig. 16-59). Abnormally elongated mitochondria, resembling gliosomes (Fig. 16-60), are seen frequently in the cytoplasm of cortical astrocytes.[1]

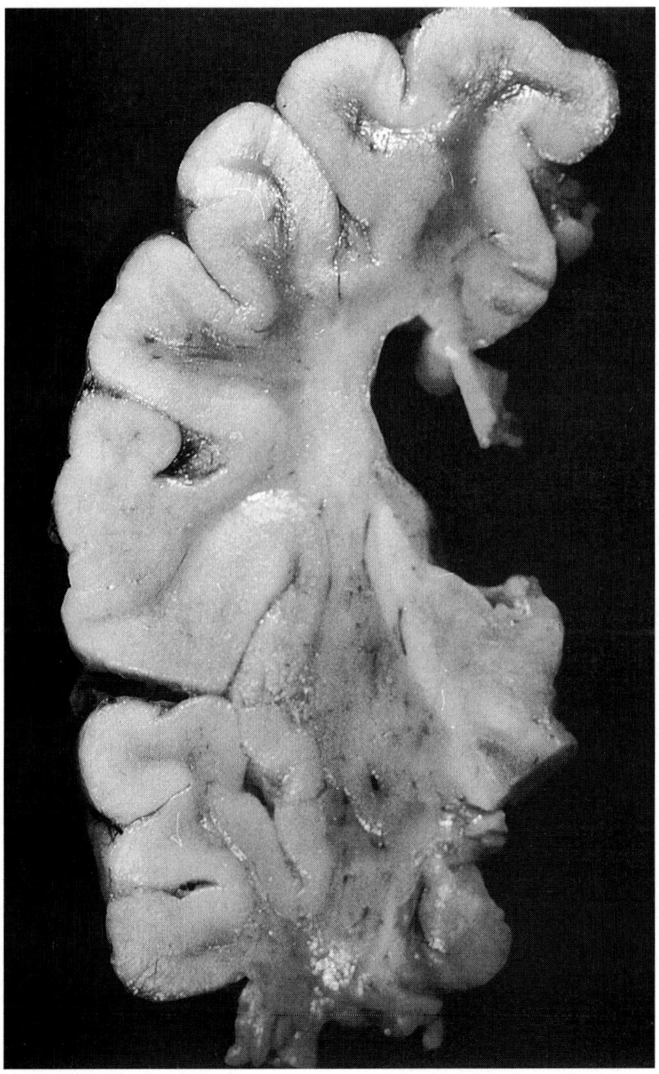

**Fig. 16-56.** Coronal section of a cerebral hemisphere in a case of SD, showing shrunken atrophic white matter.

### Alexander Disease

Alexander disease is a rare neurodegenerative disorder usually occurring sporadically either in infancy or in late childhood. The clinical picture is that of progressive dementia, megalencephaly, seizures, and motor weakness that leads to eventual paralysis. Cases with juvenile or adult onset have been reported on rare occasions. The cause of this disease is not yet known. The diagnosis, therefore, has been made only by brain biopsy. CT shows low attenuation of the deep cerebral white matter; contrast enhancing lesions in the periventricular frontal regions, caudate nuclei, and thalami are considered to be specific for Alexander disease.[21,49,72] The brain weight is increased. Externally, however, no abnormalities are noted. On cut section, white matter is soft and often cavitated. Cavitation is often more pronounced in the frontal white matter (Fig. 16-61).

The histopathologic hallmark is an absence of myelination and diffuse fibrillary gliosis with an accumulation of deeply eosinophilic either rod-shaped or round structures known as Rosenthal fibers. Rosenthal fibers are abnormal inclusions consisting of $\alpha$B-crystallin in astrocyte processes; these fibers also are seen in areas of dense fibrillary gliosis and in low-grade astrocytomas, in particular pilocytic astrocytomas.[79,183] In Alexander disease, Rosenthal fibers are seen predominantly in the subpial, subependymal, and perivascular regions (Fig. 16-62). Rosenthal fibers are electron-dense granular material surrounded by intermediate filaments within the cytoplasm of astrocytes (Fig. 16-63), but immunocytochemical reactivity with GFAP antiserum is variable.[24,41] Pathological changes affecting the peripheral nerves or visceral organs have not been described in Alexander disease.

*Text continued on page 709.*

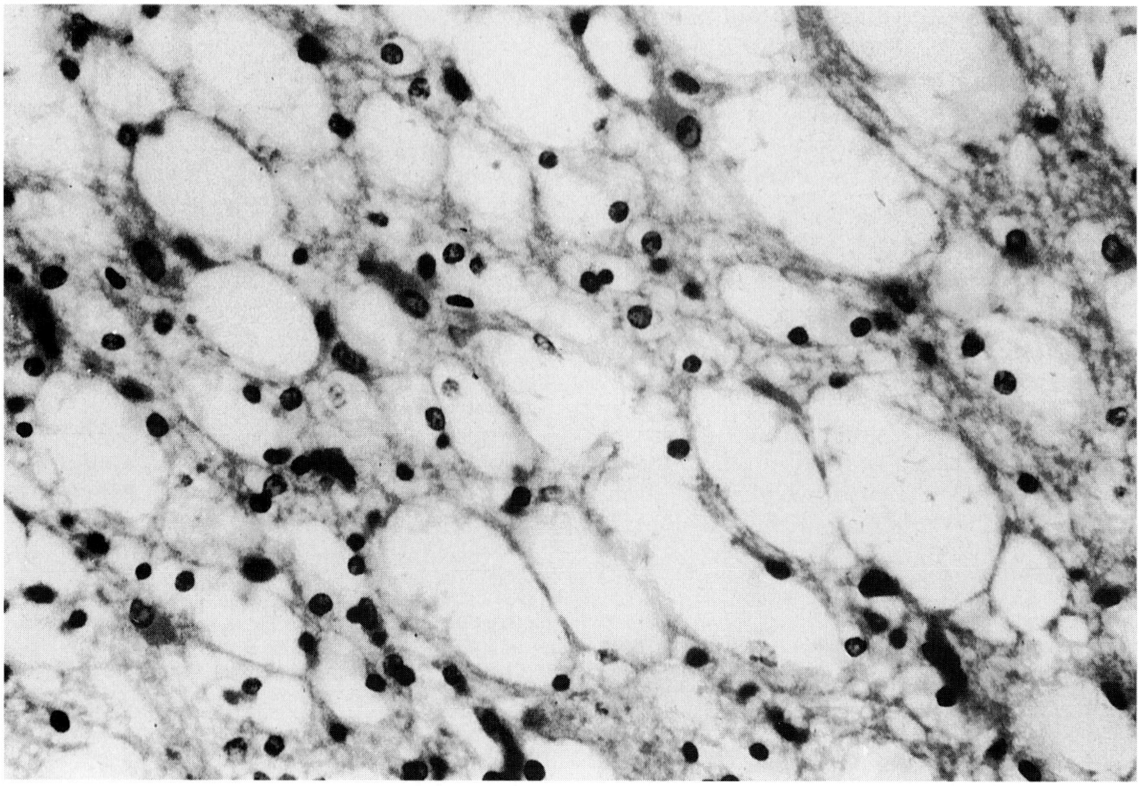

**Fig. 16-57.** Numerous vacuoles in the white matter in a case of SD. (H&E; ×150.)

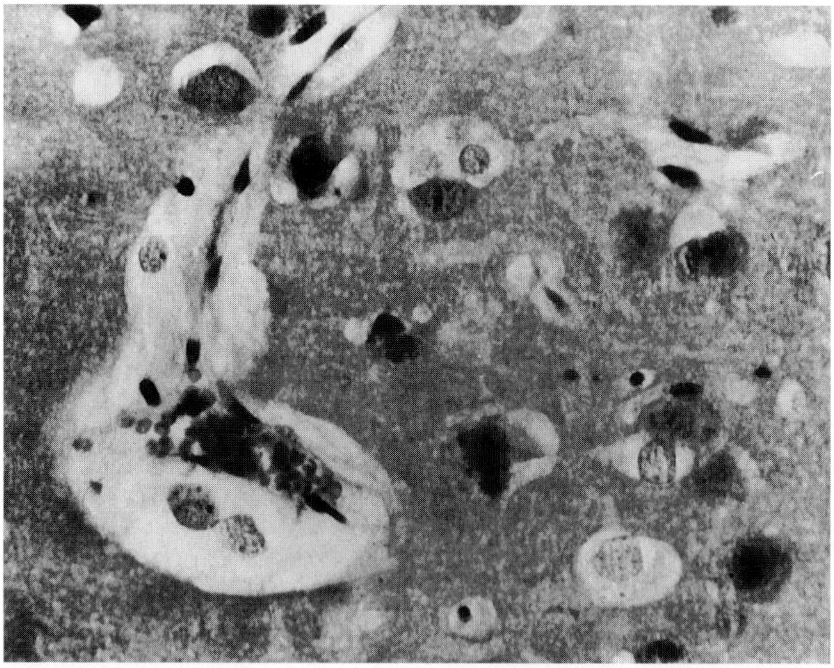

**Fig. 16-58.** Swollen perivascular astrocytes in the cerebral cortex in a case of SD. (H&E; ×300.)

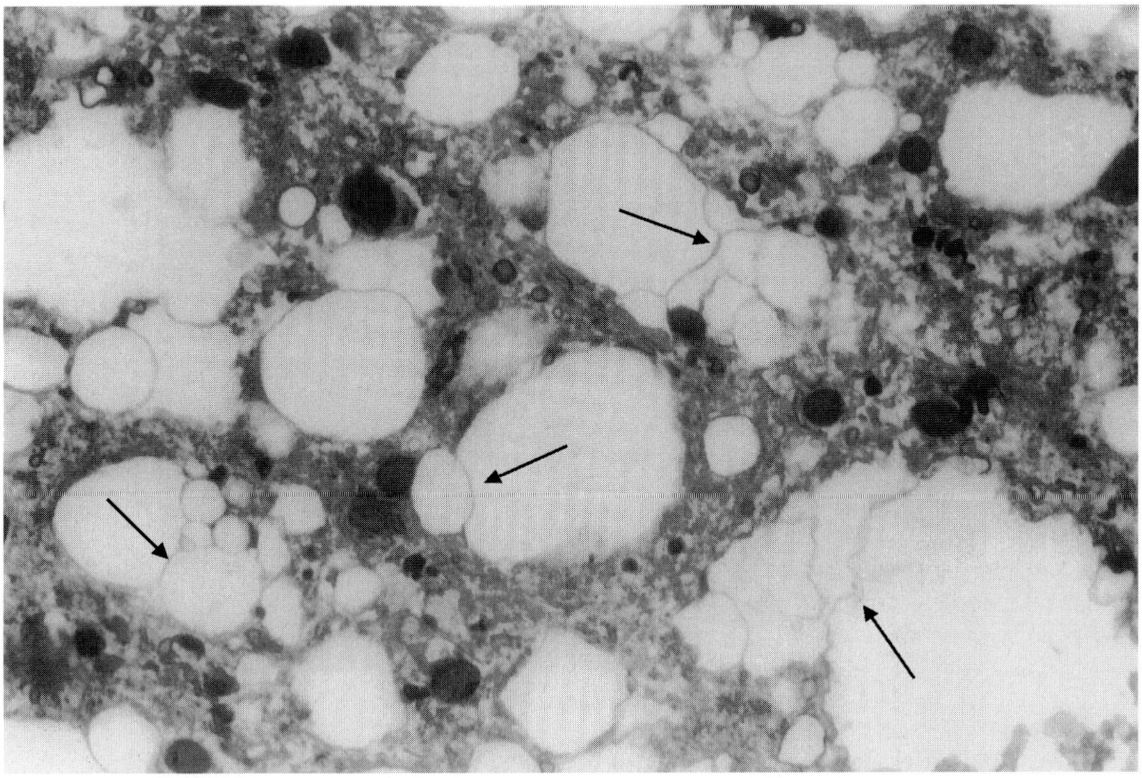

**Fig. 16-59.** One-micron-thick section of the white matter in a case of SD showing splitting of myelin lamellae to form intramyelinic vacuoles (*arrows*). (Toluidine blue; ×1500.)

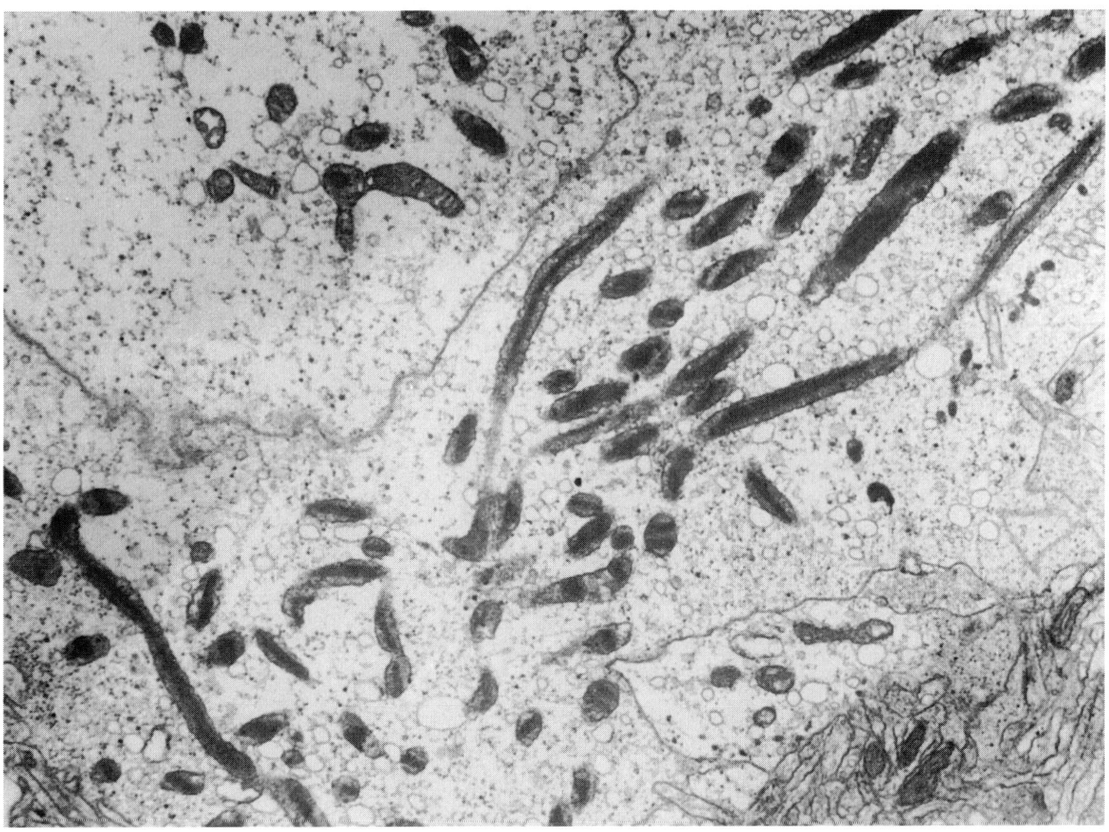

**Fig. 16-60.** Electron micrograph of abnormal mitochondria in the cortical astrocytes in a case of SD. (×12,000.)

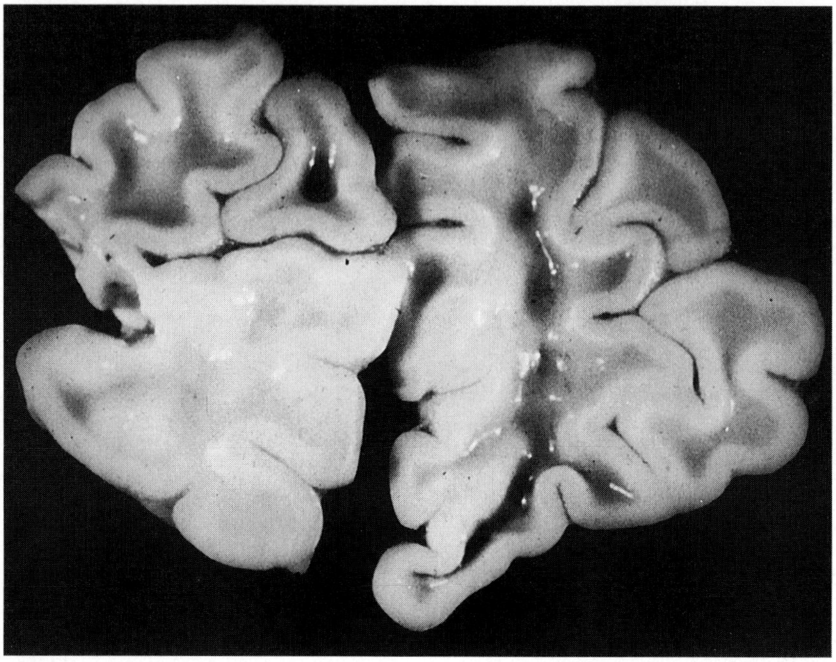

**Fig. 16-61.** Coronal section of the cerebrum in a case of AD, showing cavitation of the frontal white matter.

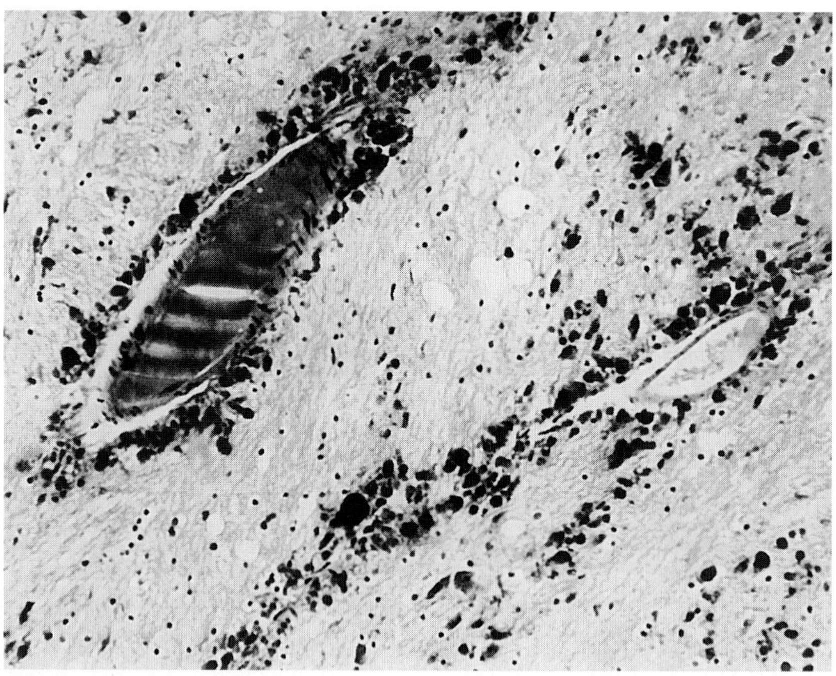

**Fig. 16-62.** Alexander disease: perivascular accumulation of Rosenthal fibers. (Solochrome and Eosin; ×150.)

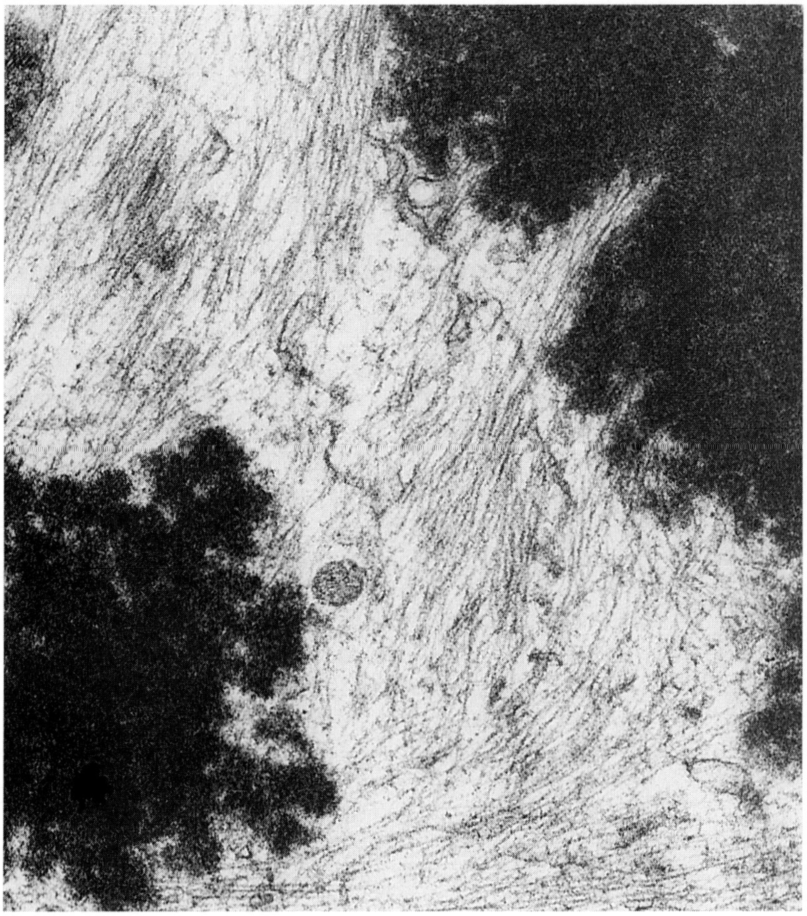

**Fig. 16-63.** Electron micrograph of Rosenthal fibers showing close association with glial fibers. (×62,000.)

## Pelizaeus-Merzbacher Disease

Pelizaeus-Merzbacher disease (PMD) is an X-linked recessive neurologic disorder caused by the deletion or duplication of the proteolipid protein (PLP) gene.[63,67] PLP is the major structural protein of CNS myelin; therefore, abnormalities in the PLP gene result in a defect in myelination in the CNS but not in the PNS.[202] Typically PMD is a disease with onset in infancy or early childhood. The classic symptoms include nystagmus, eye rolling, seizures, spasticity, choreoathetosis, and mental retardation. The brain is atrophic, and the white matter is reduced in volume, gray discolored, and firm. A diagnostic histopathologic feature of PMD is based on the absence of myelination in the cerebral white matter. Either small islands of preserved myelination exist (classic PMD) (Fig. 16-64) or there is total absence of myelination (connatal type). The histopathology of classic PMD is closely similar to tigroid change characteristically seen in the white matter of patients with Cockayne syndrome. Deficient myelination is particularly pronounced in areas where myelination occurs late during brain development, such as the cerebral and cerebellar white matter. Other areas show diffuse hypomyelination. Microscopic features include either totally absent or deficient

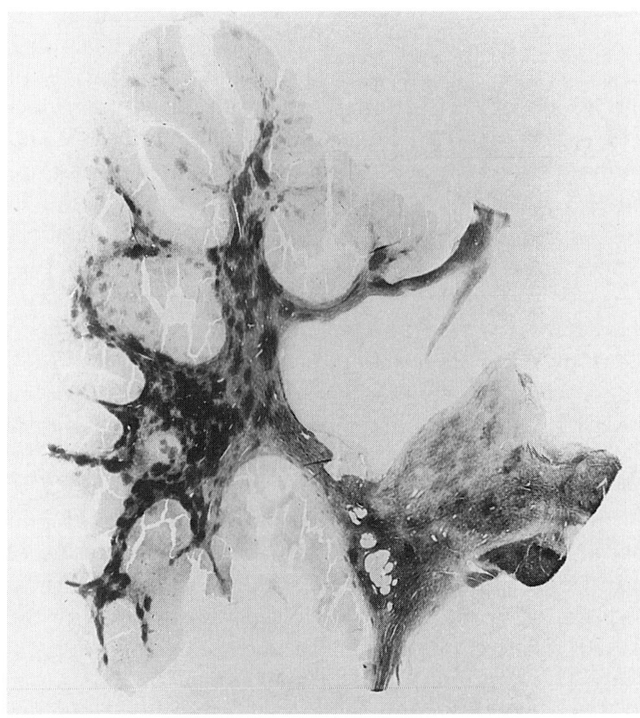

**Fig. 16-64.** Pelizaeus-Merzbacher. Cerebrum shows tigroid pattern of myelination in PMD. (Courtesy of Dr. Arnulf H. Koeppen, Albany Medical College.)

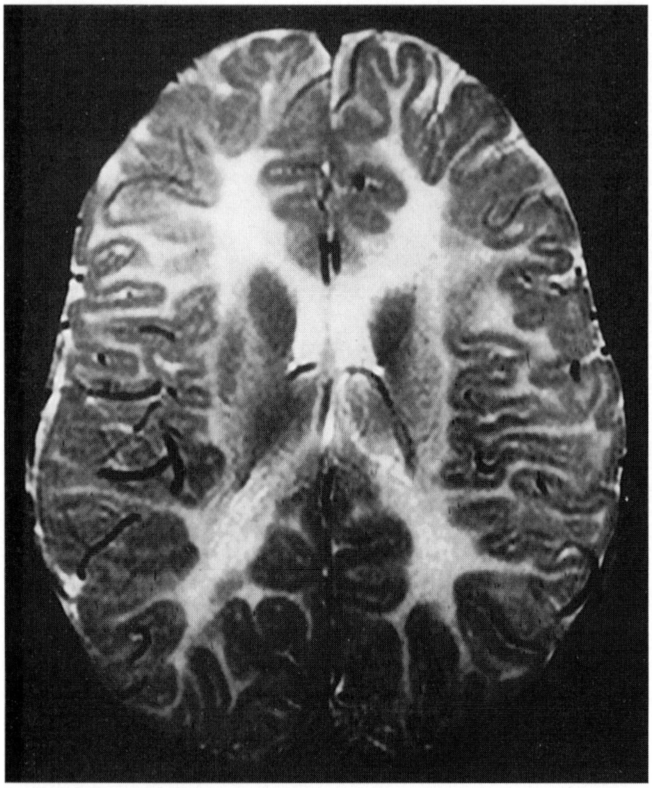

**Fig. 16-65.** Axial T2-weighted image of 4-year-old boy with Pelizaeus-Merzbacher disease shows marked confluent high signal intensity throughout the deep white matter. The volume of white matter is decreased. (Courtesy of Dr. Steven I. Seidman, Michigan Institute for Neurological Disorders.)

myelination, fibrillary gliosis, and reduced numbers of oligodendrocytes. Axons and neuronal cytoarchitecture appear normal.[171] On MRI, there is symmetric and homogeneous low signal intensity on T1-weighted images, with small scattered areas of normal signal in classic PMD cases (Fig. 16-65). These areas most likely correspond to the islands where myelination is preserved.[31] Total inversion of signals between white and gray matter on T1- and T2-weighted images has been demonstrated in connatal as well as in classic PMD, suggesting the usefulness of MRI as a diagnostic tool in PMD.[9,82] The peripheral nerve is normally myelinated.

### Autosomal Dominant Adult-Onset Leukodystrophy

Eldridge and co-workers[45] and Schwankhaus and associates[170] reported an autosomal dominant form of adult onset leukodystrophy. Patients develop clinical signs and symptoms of neurologic disease during the fourth and fifth decades of life, and show slow progression. The autonomic symptoms, which involve bowel and bladder regulation as well as orthostatic hypotension, may be the earliest signs of this disease. CT shows a symmetric decrease in white matter density, beginning in the frontal lobes and extending to the entire cerebral and cerebellar white matter. Histopathologic changes consist of nonspecific demyelination with sparing of U-fibers. There is scant macrophage infiltration or gliosis. Spongy changes are visible in the cerebral white matter. The authors of these communications emphasize the clinical similarity of this disease to chronic, progressive multiple sclerosis. Unlike ALD, MLD, or GLD, the peripheral nerves are normal in this autosomal dominant adult-onset leukodystrophy.

## ACKNOWLEDGMENTS

The author is grateful to Dr. Mauricio Castillo, University of North Carolina at Chapel Hill for Figures 16-1 and 16-2; to Dr. Richard Silbergleit, Henry Ford Hospital and Medical Center, for Figures 16-3, 16-4, 16-5, 16-21, 16-32, 16-33, 16-44, 16-48, 16-55**A**; to Dr. Steven I. Seidman, Michigan Institute for Neurological Disorders (MIND) for Figures 16-55**B, C** and 16-65; to Dr. Arnulf H. Koeppen, Albany Medical College for Figure 16-64; to Dr. Da-Lin Yao, National Institute of Neurological Disorders and Stroke, NIH, for Figure 16-13; to Professor Kenji Kosaka, Yokohama City University Medical School for Figure 16-30.

The following figures are reproduced with the permission of the authors and publishers. Figures 16-34, 16-35, 16-45, 16-47: Genetic Metabolic Disorder (Figures 3, 5, 6, 7) in *Current Encyclopedia of Pathology* vol. 23, Nervous System, 1985, Nakayama Shoten Publisher. (In Japanese); Figure 16-41: Metabolic Diseases (Figure 1.26) in Electron Microscopy in Human Medicine vol. 6, Nervous system, sensory organs and respiratory tract (JV Johannessen, editor), 1980, McGraw-Hill Inc.; Figure 16-13: Yao D-L et al: Concentric sclerosis (Balò): Morphometric and in situ hybridization study of lesions in six patients, Ann Neurol 35: 18, 1994 (Figure 1A), copyright 1973, Little, Brown and Company; Figure 16-30: Kosaka et al: A nonalcoholic Japanese patient with Wernicke's encephalopathy and Marchiafava-Bignami disease. Clin Neuropathol 6:231, 1984 (Fig. 1B), copyright 1983, Dustri-Verlag.

## REFERENCES

1. Adachi M, and others: Spongy degeneration of the central nervous system (van Bogaert and Bertrand type; Canavan's disease), Human Pathology 4:331, 1973.
2. Adams RD, Victor M, and Mancall EI: Central pontine myelinolysis: a hitherto undescribed disease occurring in alcoholism and malnourished patients, Arch Neurol Psychiatry 81:154, 1959.
3. Afifi AK, and others: Myelinoclastic diffuse sclerosis (Schilder's disease): report of a case and review of the literature, J Child Neurol 9:398, 1994.
4. Aksamit AJ, and others: Progressive multifocal leukoencephalopathy: investigation of three cases using in situ hybridization with JC virus biotinylated DNA probe, Ann Neurol 18:490, 1985.
5. Allen IV: Demyelinating diseases. In Adams JH, Corsellis JAN, Duchen LW, editors: Greenfield's neuropathology, ed 4. London, 1984, Edward Arnold.

6. Allen IV: Pathology of multiple sclerosis. In: Matthews WB, Compston A, Allen IV, and Martyn CN, editors: McAlpine's Multiple Sclerosis, ed 2. New York, 1991, Churchill Livingstone.
7. Anderson M, and others: Gliomatous transformation and demyelinating diseases, Brain 103:603, 1980.
8. Anderson M, and others: Cerebrospinal fluid in the diagnosis of multiple sclerosis: a consensus report, J Neurol Neurosurg Psychiatry 57:897, 1994.
9. Andre M, and others: Pelizaeus-Mertzbacher disease. Contribution of magnetic resonance imaging to an early diagnosis, J Neuroradiol 17:216, 1990.
10. Andrews JM, and Cancilla PA: Cytoplasmic inclusions in globoid cell leukodystrophy, Arch Pathol 89:53, 1970.
11. Andrews JM, and Menkes JH: Ultrastructure of experimentally produced globoid cells in the rat, Exp Neurol 29:483, 1970.
12. Anzil AP, Blinzinger K, and Martinius J: Ultrastructure of storage materials in metachromatic leukodystrophy peripheral neuropathy and in rabbit tissues after sulfatide application with special reference to pleated lamellar systems. J Microscopie (Paris) 18:173, 1973.
13. Aström KE, Mancall EL, and Richardson EP: Progressive multifocal leukoencephalopathy, Brain 81:93, 1958.
14. Austin JJ: Studies in metachromatic leukodystrophy. XII. Multiple sufatase deficiency, Arch Neurol 28:258, 1973.
15. Austin J, and Lehfeldt D: Studies in globoid (Krabbe) leukodystrophy III. Significance of experimentally produced globoid like elements in rat white matter and spleen, J Neuropathol Exp Neurol 24:265, 1965.
16. Balò J: Leucoencephalitis periaxialis concentrica, Magy Novosi Arch 28:108, 1927.
17. Balò J: Encephalitis periaxialis concentrica, Arch Neurol Psychiatry 246:242, 1928.
18. Bancroft JD: Theory and practice of histological techniques, ed 3. London, 1990, Churchill Livingstone.
19. Bancroft JD, and Stevens A: Theory and practice of histological techniques. London, 1977, Churchill Livingstone.
20. Baram TZ, Goldman AM, and Percy AK: Krabbe disease: specific MRI and CT findings, Neurology 36:111, 1986.
21. Barbieri F, and others: Alexander's disease: a clinical study with computerized tomographic scans of the first two Italian cases, Acta Neurol 35:1, 1980.
22. Baumann N, and others: Adult forms of metachromatic leukodystrophy: clinical and biochemical approach, Dev Neurosci 13:211, 1991.
23. Beaudet A: Canavan disease. In Scriver CR, Beaudet A, Sly WS, and Valle D, editors: The metabolic and molecular basis of inherited disease, Vol. III, ed 7. New York, 1995, McGraw-Hill, Inc.
24. Borrett D, and Becker LE: Alexander's disease: a disease of astrocytes, Brain 108:367, 1985.
25. Bracard S, and others: Computerized tomography and MRI in Marchiafava-Bignami disease, J Neuroradiol 13:87, 1986.
26. Braffman BH, and others: Pathologic correlation with gross and histopathology. 2. Hyperintense white matter foci in the elderly, AJNR 9:629, 1988.
27. Bruck W, and others: Oligodendrocytes in the early course of multiple sclerosis, Ann Neurol 35:65, 1994.
28. Budka H, Sluga E, and Heiss WD: Spastic paraplegia associated with Addison's disease: adult variant of adrenoleukodystrophy, J Neurol 213:217, 1976.
29. Burger PC, and Boyko OB: The pathology of central nervous system radiation injury. In Gutin PH, Leibel SA, Sheline GE, editors: Radiation injury to the nervous system. New York, 1991, Raven Press.
30. Caparros-Lefebvre D, and others: Marchiafava-Bignami disease: use of contrast media in CT and MRI, Neuroradiology 36: 509, 1994.
31. Caro PA, and Marks HG: Magnetic resonance imaging and computed tomography in Pelizaeus-Mertzbacher disease, Magn Reson Imaging 8:791, 1990.
32. Castaigne P, and others: La maladie de Marchiafava-Bignami: Etude anatomoclinique de dix observations, Rev Neurol (Paris) 125:179, 1971.
33. Castaigne P, and others: Leucoencephalopathie multifocale progressive et 'gliomes' multiples, Rev Neurol (Paris) 130:379, 1974.
34. Chang KH, and others: Marchiafava-Bignami disease: serial changes in corpus callosum on MRI, Neuroradiology 34:480, 1992.
35. Chen YQ, and others: Cloning and expression of cDNA encoding human galactocerebrosidase, the enzyme deficient in globoid cell leukodystrophy, Hum Mol Genet 2:1841, 1993.
36. Cloy DE, and Netsky MG: Neuromyelitis optica. In Vinken PJ, Bruyn GW, editors: Handbook of Neurology, vol. 9. Amsterdam, 1970, North-Holland.
37. Cogan DG, and others: Histochemistry of the eye in metachromatic leukodystrophy, Arch Ophthalmol 60:379, 1958.
38. Constantinidis J, and Wisniewski TM: The dominant form of the pigmentary orthochromic leukodystrophy, Acta Neuropathol 82:483, 1991.
39. D'Agostino AN, Sayer GP, and Hayles AB: Krabbe's disease, Arch Neurol 8:82, 1963.
40. Devic ME: Myelite subaigue compliquee de nevrite optique. Bulletin Medical (Paris) 8:1033, 1894.
41. Dinda AK, Sarkar C, and Roy S: Rosenthal fibers: an immunohistochemical, ultrastructural and immunoelectron microscopic study, Acta Neuropathol 79:456, 1990.
42. Divry P, and Mathieu M: Aspartoacylase deficiency and N-acetylaspartic aciduria in patients with Canavan disease, Am J Med Genet 32:550, 1989.
43. Duncan ID, Skoff RP, and Colman D, editors: Myelination and dysmyelination, vol. 605, 16–52, New York, 1990, Annals of The New York Academy of Sciences.
44. Dunn HG, and others: Krabbe's leukodystrophy without globoid cells, Neurology 26:1035, 1976.
45. Eldridge R, and others: Hereditary adult-onset leukodystrophy simulating chronic progressive multiple sclerosis, N Engl J Med 311:948, 1984.
46. Endo Y, Oda M, and Hara M: Central pontine myelinolysis: a study of 37 cases in 1,000 consecutive autopsies, Acta Neuropathol 53:145, 1981.
47. Esiri MM, and others: Adrenoleukodystrophy: clinical, pathological and biochemical findings in two brothers with the onset of cerebral disease in adult life, Neuropathol Appl Neurol 10: 429, 1984.
48. Farley TJ, and others: Serial MRI and CT findings in infantile Krabbe disease, Pediatr Neurol 8:455, 1992.
49. Farrell K, Chuang S, and Becker L: Computed tomography in Alexander's disease, Ann Neurol 15:605, 1984.
50. Fazekas F, and others: Pathologic correlates of incidental MRI white matter signal hyperintensities, Neurology 43:1683, 1993.
51. Feigin I, and Ogata J: Schwann cell and peripheral myelin within human central nervous tissue: the mesenchymal character of Schwann cells, J Neuropathol Exp Neurol 30:603, 1971.
52. Ghatak NR, and others: Remyelination in multiple sclerosis with peripheral type myelin, Arch Neurol 29:262, 1973.
53. Ghatak NR, and others: Asymptomatic demyelinated plaque in the spinal cord, Arch Neurol 30:484, 1974.
54. Ghatak NR: Occurrence of oligodendrocytes within astrocytes in demyelinating lesions, J Neuropathol Exp Neurol 51:40, 1992.
55. Gieselmann V, and others: Molecular genetics of metachromatic leukodystrophy, Dev Neurosci 13:222, 1991.
56. Gobel HH, and others: Ultrastructural pathology of eccrine sweat gland epithelial cells in globoid cell leukodystrophy, J Child Neurol 8:171, 1993.

57. Goldman JE, and Horoupian DS: Demyelination of the lateral geniculate nucleus in central pontine myelinolysis, Ann Neurol 9:185, 1981.
58. Gonzalez-Scarano F, and others: Multiple sclerosis disease activity correlates with gadolinium-enhanced magnetic resonance imaging, Ann Neurol 21:300, 1987.
59. Gosztonyi G: Acute hemorrhagic leuko-encephalitis (Hurst's disease). In Vinken PJ, Bruyn, GW, editors: Handbook of clinical neurology, vol. 3. Infections of the nervous system, part II. Amsterdam, 1978, Elsevier North Holland.
60. Graham DI, Behan PO, and More IAR: Brain damage complicating septic shock. Acute hemorrhagic leukoencephalitis as a complication of the generalized Schwartzman reaction. J Neurol Neurosurg Psychiatry 42:19, 1979.
61. Gregoire A, Perier O, and Dustin P: Metachromatic leukodystrophy, an electron microscopic study. J Neuropathol Exp Neurol 25:617, 1966.
62. Griffin JW, and others: Adrenomyeloneuropathy: a probable variant of adrenoleukodystrophy, Neurology 27:1107, 1977.
63. Griffiths IR, Montague P, and Dickinson P: The proteolipid protein gene, Neuropathol Appl Neurobiol 21:85, 1995.
64. Guilhoto LMDFF, and others: Pediatric multiple sclerosis: report of 14 cases, Brain Dev 17:9, 1995.
65. Gurr E: Staining: practical and theoretical. Baltimore, 1962, Williams & Wilkins.
66. Hachinski VC, Potter P, and Merskey H: Leuko-araiosis, Arch Neurol 44:21, 1987.
67. Harding B, Ellis D, and Malcolm S: A case of Pelizaeus-Merzbacher disease showing increased dosage of the proteolipid protein gene, Neuropathol Appl Neurobiol 21:111, 1995.
68. Hahn AF, and others: A variant form of metachromatic leukodystrophy without arylsulfatase deficiency, Ann Neurol 12:33, 1982.
69. Hanefeldt F, and others: Multiple sclerosis in childhood: report of 15 cases, Brain Dev 13:410, 1991.
70. Hart MN, and Earle KM: Hemorrhagic and perivenous encephalitis: a clinical-pathological review of 38 cases, J Neurol Neurosurg Psychiatry 38:585, 1975.
71. Hirsh TV, and Pfeiffer J: Uber histologische Methoden in der Differentialdiagnose von Leukodystrophien and Lipoidosen, Arch Psychiatr Z Neurol 194:88, 1955.
72. Holland IM, and Kendall BE: Computed tomography in Alexander's disease, Neuroradiology 20:103, 1980.
73. Hormes JT, Filley CM, and Rosenberg NL: Neurologic sequelae of chronic solvent vapor abuse, Neurology 36:698, 1986.
74. Humble JG, Jayne WHW, and Pulvertaft RJV: Biological interaction between lymphocytes and other cells. Br J Haematol 2:283, 1956.
75. Hunter SB, Ballinger WE, and Rubin J: Multiple sclerosis mimicking primary brain tumor, Arch Pathol Lab Med 111:464, 1987.
76. Hurst EW: Acute haemorrhagic leucoencephalitis: a previously undefined entity, Med J Aust 2:1, 1941.
77. Ikuta F, and others: Comparison of MS pathology between 70 American and 75 Japanese autopsy cases. In Kuroiwa Y, and Kurland LT, editors: MS east and west. Fukuoka, 1982, Kyushu Univ Press.
78. Itoyama Y, and others: Immunocytochemical observations on the distribution of myelin-associated glycoprotein and myelin basic protein in multiple sclerosis lesions, Ann Neurol 7:167, 1980.
79. Iwaki T, and others: αB-crystallin is expressed in non-lenticular tissues and accumulates in Alexander's disease brain, Cell 57: 71, 1989.
80. Jellinger KA: Sudanophilic (orthochromatic) leukodystrophies. In Calne DB, editor: Neurodegenerative diseases. Philadelphia, 1994, WB Saunders.
81. Johnson MD, and others: Fulminant monophasic multiple sclerosis, Marburg's type, J Neurol Neurosurg Psychiatry 53:918, 1990.
82. Journel H, and others: Magnetic resonance imaging in Pelizaeus-Mertzbacher disease, Neuroradiology 29:403, 1987.
83. Kamoshita S, and others: Spongy degeneration of the brain: a chemical study of two cases including isolation and characterization of myelin, Neurology 18:975, 1968.
84. Kay HEM, and others: Encephalopathy in acute leukemia associated with methotrexate therapy, Arch Dis Child 47:344, 1972.
85. Katz D, and others: Correlation between magnetic resonance imaging findings and lesion development in chronic active multiple sclerosis, Ann Neurol 34:661, 1993.
86. Kaul R, and others: Cloning of the human aspartoacylase cDNA and a common missense mutation in Canavan disease, Nature Genet 5:118, 1993.
87. Kawamura M, and others: Marchiafava-Bignami disease: computed topography scan and magnetic resonance imaging, Ann Neurol 18:103, 1985.
88. Kepes JJ: Large focal tumor-like demyelinating lesions of the brain: Intermediate entity between multiple sclerosis and acute disseminated encephalomyelitis? A study of 31 patients, Ann Neurol 33:18, 1993.
89. Kepes JJ, and Rubinstein LJ: Malignant glioma with heavily lipidized (foamy) tumor cells. A report of three cases with immunoperoxidase study, Cancer 47:2451, 1981.
90. Kesselring J, and others: Acute disseminated encephalomyelitis. MR findings and the distinction from multiple sclerosis, Brain 113:291, 1990.
91. Ketonen L, and Tuite MJ: Brain imaging in human immunodeficiency virus infection, Semin Neurol 12:57, 1992.
92. Koeppen AH, and Barron KD: Marchiafava-Bignami disease, Neurology 28:290, 1978.
93. Kolodny EH, and Fluharty AL: Metachromatic leukodystrophy and multiple sulfatase deficiency: sulfatide lipidosis. In Scriver CR, Beaudet AL, Sly WS, Valle D, editors: The metabolic and molecular basis of inherited disease, vol. 2, ed 7. New York, 1995, McGraw-Hill, Inc.
94. Kolodny EH, Raghavan S, and Krivit W: Late onset Krabbe disease (globoid cell leukodystrophy): clinical and biochemical features of 15 cases, Dev Neurosci 13:232, 1991.
95. Kornfeld M, and others: Solvent vapor abuse leukoencephalopathy: comparison to adrenoleukodystrophy, J Neuropathol Exper Neurol 53:389, 1994.
96. Kosaka K, and others: A non-alcoholic Japanese patient with Wernicke's encephalopathy and Marchiafava-Bignami disease, Clin Neuropathol 6:231, 1984.
97. Kuroda S, Hirano A, and Yuasa S: Adrenoleukodystrophy: cerebello-brainstem dominant case, Acta Neuropathol 60:149, 1983.
98. Lazar RB, and others: Multifocal central nervous system damage caused by toluene abuse, Neurology 33:1337, 1983.
99. Lee YY, Neuert C, and Glass JP: Treatment-related white matter changes in cancer patients, Cancer 57:1473, 1976.
100. Levy RM, Bredesen DE, and Rosenblum ML: Neurological manifestations of the acquired immunodeficiency syndrome (AIDS): experience at UCSF and review of the literature. J Neurosurg 62:475, 1985.
101. Loes DJ, and others: Adrenoleukodystrophy: a scoring method for brain MR observations, AJNR 15:1761, 1994.
102. Loes DJ, and others: Childhood cerebral form of adrenoleukodystrophy: short-term effect of bone marrow transplantation on brain MR observations, AJNR 15:1767, 1994.
103. Luna LG: Manual of histologic staining methods of the Armed Forces Institute of Pathology, ed 3. New York, 1968, McGraw-Hill.

104. Lyon-Caen- O, and others: Late onset multiple sclerosis. A clinical study of 16 pathologically proven cases, Acta Neurol Scand 72:56, 1985.
105. Lyon G, and others: Symptomatology of late onset Krabbe's leukodystrophy: the European experience, Dev Neurosci 13: 240, 1991.
106. Mackay RP, and Hirano A: Forms of benign multiple sclerosis: report of two "clinically silent" cases discovered at autopsy, Arch Neurol 17:588, 1967.
107. Marburg O: Die sogenannte "akute multiple Sklerose" (Encephalomyelitis periaxialis scleroticans), J Psychiatr Neurol (Leipzig) 27:213, 1906.
108. Manual of histology and special staining techniques. Armed Forces Institute of Pathology, ed 2. New York, 1960, McGraw-Hill.
109. Marchiafava E, Bignami A, and Nazani A: Ueber System-Degeneration der Kommissurbahnen das Gehirns bei chronischen Alkoholismus, Mon Psychiatr Neurol 29:315, 1911.
110. Martensson RE: Myelin. Boca Raton, 1992, CRC Press.
111. Matalon R, and others: Aspartoacylase deficiency and N-acetylaspartic aciduria in patients with Canavan disease, Am J Med Genet 29:463, 1988.
112. McFarland HF, and others: Using gadolinium-enhanced magnetic resonance imaging lesions to monitor disease activity in multiple sclerosis, Ann Neurol 32:758, 1992.
113. Mendez MF, and Pogacar S: Malignant monophasic multiple sclerosis or "Marburg's disease," Neurology 38:1153, 1988.
114. Miller DH, and others: Magnetic resonance imaging of inflammatory and demyelinating white-matter diseases of childhood, Dev Med Child Neurol 32:97, 1990.
115. Moore GRW, and others: Balò's concentric sclerosis: new observations on lesion development, Ann Neurol 17:604, 1985.
116. Morell P, Quarles RH, and Norton WT: Formation, structure, and biochemistry of myelin. In Siegel G, Agranoff B, Albers RW, Molinoff P, editors: Basic neurochemistry, ed. 4. New York, 1989, Raven Press.
117. Moser HW: Sulfatide lipidosis: metachromatic leukodystrophy. In Stanbury JD, Wyngaarden JB, Fredickson DS: editors: The metabolic basis of inherited disease. ed 3. New York, 1972, McGraw-Hill.
118. Moser HW, Powers JM, and Smith KD: Adrenoleukodystrophy: molecular genetics, pathology, and Lorenzo's oil, Brain Pathol 5:259, 1995.
119. Moser HW, Smith KD, and Moser A: X-linked adrenoleukodystrophy. In Scriver CR, Beaudet AL, Sly WS, Valle D, editors: The metabolic and molecular basis of inherited disease, ed 7. New York, 1995, McGraw-Hill.
120. Mosser J, and others: Putative X-linked adrenoleukodystrophy gene shares unexpected homology with ABC transporters, Nature 361:726, 1993.
121. Nesbit GM, and others: Multiple sclerosis: histopathologic and MR and/or CT correlation in 37 cases at biopsy and three cases at autopsy, Radiology 180:467, 1991.
122. Newcombe HLJ, Groome NP, and Cuzner ML: Characterization and distribution of phagocytic macrophages in multiple sclerosis plaques, Neuropathol Appl Neurobiol 19:214, 1993.
123. Norenberg MD, Leslie KO, and Robertson AS: Association between rise in serum sodium and central pontine myelinolysis, Ann Neurol 11:128, 1982.
124. Norseworthy J, and others: Multiple sclerosis after age 50, Neurology 33:1537, 1983.
125. Offenbacher H, and others: Assessment of MRI criteria for a diagnosis of MS, Neurology 43:905, 1993.
126. Ogata J, and Feigin I: Schwann cells and regenerated peripheral myelin in multiple sclerosis: an ultrastructural study, Neurology 25:713, 1975.
127. Ohno T, and others: Adrenoleukodystrophy: a clinical variant presenting as olivopontocerebellar atrophy, J Neurol 231:167, 1984.
128. Okeda R, and others: Adult pigment type (Peiffer) of sudanophilic leukodystrophy. Pathological and morphometrical studies on two autopsy cases of siblings, Acta Neuropathol 78:533, 1989.
129. Olszewski J: Subcortical arteriosclerotic encephalopathy, World Neurol 3:359, 1962.
130. Oppenheimer DR: Demyelinating disease, In Blackwood W, and Corsellis AN, editors: Greenfield's neuropathology, ed 3. London, 1976, Edward Arnold.
131. Ormerod JEC, and others: The role of MRI in the assessment of MS and isolated neurological lesions: a quantitative study, Brain 110:1579, 1987.
132. Ozawa K, and others: Patterns of oligodendroglia pathology in multiple sclerosis, Brain 117:1311, 1994.
133. Pantoni L, and Garcia JH: The significance of cerebral white matter abnormalities 100 years after Binswanger's report. A review. Stroke 26:1293, 1995.
134. Paty DW, and others: MRI in the diagnosis of MS: a prospective study with comparison of clinical evaluation, evoked potentials, oligoclonal banding, and CT, Neurology 38:180, 1988.
135. Pearse AGE: Histochemistry: Theoretical and applied analytical technology, vol. II, ed 4. New York, 1985, Churchill Livingstone.
136. Peng L, and Suzuki K: Ultrastructural study of neurons in metachromatic leukodystrophy, Clin Neuropathol 6:224, 1987.
137. Percy AK, and others: Globoid cell leukodystrophy: comparison of neuropathology with magnetic resonance imaging, Acta Neuropathol 88:26, 1994.
138. Peters A, Palay SL, and Webster H de F: The fine structure of the nervous system: neurons and their supporting cells. ed 3. Oxford, 1990, Oxford University Press.
139. Phadke JG, and Best PV: Atypical and clinically silent multiple sclerosis: a report of 12 cases discovered unexpectedly at necropsy, J Neurol Neurosurg Psychiatry 46:414, 1983.
140. Poser CM: Myelinoclastic diffuse and transitional sclerosis. In Vinken PJ, Bruyn GW, editors: Handbook of clinical neurology, Vol. 9. Multiple sclerosis and other demyelinating disease. Amsterdam, 1970, North Holland.
141. Poser CM, and others: New diagnostic criteria for multiple sclerosis: guidelines for research protocols, Ann Neurol 13:227, 1983.
142. Powers JM, and others: Pathologic findings in adrenoleukodystrophy heterozygotes, Arch Pathol Lab Med 111:151, 1987.
143. Powers JM: Adreno-leukodystrophy (adreno-testiculo-leukomyelo-neuropathic-complex), Clin Neuropathol 4:181, 1985.
144. Prineas JW: The neuropathology of multiple sclerosis. In Vinken PJ, Bruyn GW, Klawans HL editors: Handbook of clinical neurology, Vol. 47. Amsterdam, 1985, Elsevier.
145. Prineas JW: Pathology of multiple sclerosis. In Cook SD editor: Handbook of multiple sclerosis. New York, 1990, Marcel Dekker.
146. Prineas JW, and others: Multiple sclerosis: remyelination of nascent lesions, Ann Neurol 33:137, 1993.
147. Prineas JW, and others: Multiple sclerosis: pathology of recurrent lesions, Brain 118:681, 1993.
148. Prineas JW, and others: Multiple sclerosis: oligodendrocyte proliferation and differentiation in fresh lesions. Lab Invest 61:489, 1989.
149. Prineas JW, and others: Interaction of astrocytes and newly formed oligodendrocytes in resolving multiple sclerosis lesions. Lab Invest 63:624, 1990.

150. Prineas JW, and McDonald WI: Demyelinating disease. In Greenfield's Neuropathology, Oxford, 1996, Oxford University Press.
151. Raine CS: Morphology of myelin and myelination. In Morell P, editor: Myelin, ed. 2. New York, 1984, Plenum Press.
152. Raine CS: Demyelinating diseases. In Davis RL, and Robertson DM, editors: Textbook of neuropathology, ed 2. Baltimore, 1991, Williams & Wilkins.
153. Raine CS, Scheinberg L, and Waltz JM: Multiple sclerosis: oligodendroglia survival and proliferation in an active established lesion. Lab Invest 45:534, 1981.
154. Raynaud E-J, and others: Metachromatic leukodystrophy: ultrastructural and enzymatic study of a case of variant O form, Arch Neurol 32:834, 1975.
155. Revesz T, and others: A comparison of the pathology of primary and secondary progressive multiple sclerosis, Brain 117:759, 1994.
156. Rodriguez M, and others: Oligodendrocyte injury is an early event in lesions of multiple sclerosis, Mayo Clinic Proc 68:627, 1993.
157. Rosenberg NL, and others: Central nervous system effects of chronic toluene abuse—clinical, brainstem evoked response and magnetic resonance imaging studies, Neurotoxicol Teratol 10:489, 1988.
158. Rothstein TL, and Shaw, C-M: Computerized tomography as a diagnostic aid in acute hemorrhagic leukoencephalitis, Ann Neurol 13:331, 1983.
159. Rubinstein LJ, and others: Disseminated necrotizing leukoencephalopathy: a complication of treated central nervous system leukemia and lymphoma, Cancer 35:291, 1975.
160. Russell DS, and Rubinstein LJ: Pathology of tumors of the nervous system, ed 5. Baltimore, 1989, Williams & Wilkins.
161. Russell DS, and Rubinstein LJ: Pathology of tumors of the nervous system, ed 5. Baltimore, 1989, Williams & Wilkins.
162. Russell DS, and Rubinstein LJ: Pathology of tumors of the nervous system, ed 5. Baltimore, 1989, Williams & Wilkins.
163. Sadovnick AD, and Ebers GC: Epidemiology of multiple sclerosis: a critical overview, Can J Neurol Sci 20:17, 1993.
164. Sasaki M, and others: MRI and CT findings in Krabbe disease, Pediatr Neurol 7:283, 1991.
165. Schaumburg HH, and others: Adrenoleukodystrophy: a clinical and pathological study of 17 case, Arch Neurol 33:577, 1975.
166. Schaumburg HH, and others: Adrenomyeloneuropathy. A probable variant of adrenoleukodystrophy, Neurology 27:1114, 1977.
167. Schilder P: Zur Kenntnis der sogennante diffusen Sklerose. Z ges Neurol Psychiatr 10:1, 1912.
168. Schlote W, and others: Adrenoleukodystrophy in an adult female: a clinical, morphological and neurochemical study, J Neurol 235:1, 1987.
169. Schoene WC, and others: Onion bulb formations in the central and peripheral nervous system in association with multiple sclerosis and hypertrophic polyneuropathy, Brain 100:755, 1977.
170. Schwankhaus JD, and others: Clinical and pathological features of an autosomal dominant adult-onset leukodystrophy simulating chronic progressive multiple sclerosis, Arch Neurol 51:757, 1994.
171. Seitelberger F: Neuropathology and genetics of Pelizaeus-Merzbacher disease, Brain Pathol 5:267, 1995.
172. Sima AAF, Finkelstein SD, and McLachlan DR: Multiple malignant astrocytomas in a patient with spontaneous progressive multifocal leukoencephalopathy, Ann Neurol 14:183, 1983.
173. Sourander P, and Olsson Y: Peripheral neuropathy in globoid cell leukodystrophy (Morbus Krabbe), Acta Neuropathol 11:69, 1968.
174. Stevens RL, and others: Cerebroside sulfatase activator deficiency induced metachromatic leukodystrophy, Am J Hum Genet 33:900, 1981.
175. Sulser A, Jellinger K, and Brainin M: Pigmentary type of orthochromatic leukodystrophy with early onset and protracted course, Neuropediatrics 21:48, 1990.
176. Suzuki K: Ultrastructural study of experimental globoid cells, Lab Invest 23:612, 1970.
177. Suzuki K, and Grover WD: Krabbe's leukodystrophy (globoid cell leukodystrophy): an ultrastructural study, Arch Neurol 22: 385, 1970.
178. Suzuki K, Suzuki Y, and Suzuki K: Galactosylceramide lipidosis: globoid cell leukodystrophy (Krabbe disease). In Scriver CR, Beaudet AL, Sly WS, Valle D, editors: Metabolic and molecular basis of inherited disease. Vol. II, ed 7. New York, 1995, McGraw-Hill.
179. Tada K, and others: Serial magnetic resonance imaging studies in a case of late onset globoid cell leukodystrophy, Neuropediatrica 23:306, 1992.
180. Thomas PK, and others: Comparative ultrastructural observations on peripheral nerve abnormalities in the late infantile, juvenile and late onset forms of metachromatic leukodystrophy, Acta Neuropathol (Berl) 39:237, 1977.
181. Thomas PK, and others: Chronic demyelinating peripheral neuropathy associated with multifocal central nervous system demyelination. Brain 110:53, 1987.
182. Thorpe JW, and Miller DH: MRI: its application and impact, International MS J 1:7, 1994.
183. Tomokane N, and others: Rosenthal fibers share epitopes with $\alpha$B-crystallin, glial fibrillary acidic protein and ubiquitin, but not with vimentin, Am J Pathol 138:875, 1991.
184. Tunon T, and others: Leukodystrophy with pigmented glial and scavenger cells (pigmentary type of orthochromatic leukodystrophy), Neuropathol Appl Neurobiol 14:337, 1988.
185. Valk PE, and Dillon WP: Diagnostic imaging of central nervous system radiation injury. In Gutin PH, Leibel SA, Sheline GE, editors: Radiation injury to the nervous system. New York, 1991, Raven Press.
186. van der Knaap MS, and others: Pattern recognition in magnetic resonance imaging of white matter disorders in children and young adults, Neuroradiology 33:478, 1991.
187. van der Knaap MS, and Valk J: The MR spectrum of peroxisomal disorders, Neuroradiology 33:30, 1991.
188. van Bogaert L, and Bertrand I: Spongy degeneration of the brain in infancy. Amsterdam, 1967, North Holland.
189. Verny M, and others: Leuko-araiosis, Dev Neurosci 13:245, 1991.
190. Watson RT, Ballinger WE, and Quisling RG: Acute hemorrhagic leukoencephalitis: diagnosis by computed tomography, Ann Neurol 15:611, 1984.
191. Wenger DA, and Louie E: Pseudodeficiencies of arylsulfatase A and galactocerebroside activities, Dev Neurosci 13:215, 1991.
192. Wright GDS, Patel MK, and Mikel J: An adult onset metachromatic leukodystrophy with dominant inheritance and normal arylsulphatase A levels, J Neurol Sci 87:153, 1988.
193. Wright DG, Laureno R, and Victor M: Pontine and extrapontine myelinolysis, Brain 102:361, 1979.
194. Wolf HJ, and Pietra GG: The visceral lesions of metachromatic leukodystrophy, Am J Pathol 44:921, 1964.
195. Wu E, and Raine CS: Multiple sclerosis: interactions between oligodendrocytes and hypertrophic astrocytes and their occurrence in other, nondemyelinating conditions. Lab Invest 67:88, 1992.
196. Yao D-L, and others: Concentric sclerosis (Balò): Morphometric and in situ hybridization study of lesions in six patients, Ann Neurol 35:18, 1994.
197. Yates AJ, and others: A leukodystrophy accumulating large

amounts of cholesterol ester. J Neuropathol Exper Neurol 41: 343, 1982.

198. Yokoi S, and others: Postnatal sudanophilic leukodystrophy in two siblings, Acta Neuropathol 67:103, 1985.
199. Yunis EJ, and Lee RE: The ultrastructure of globoid (Krabbe) leukodystrophy, Lab Invest 21:415, 1969.
200. Yunis EJ, and Lee RE: Tubules of globoid leukodystrophy: a right handed helix, Science 169:64, 1970.
201. Zagzag D, and others: Demyelinating disease versus tumor in surgical neuropathology: clue to a correct pathological diagnosis, Am J Surg Pathol 17:537, 1993.
202. Zoghbi HY, and Ballabio A: Pelizaeus-Merzbacher disease. In Scriver CR, Beaudet AL, Sly WS, Valle D, editors: The metabolic and molecular basis of inherited disease, Vol. III, ed 7. New York, 1995, McGraw-Hill.
203. ZuRhein GM, and Chou SM: Particles resembling papova viruses in human cerebral demyelinating disease, Science 148: 1477, 1965.

C • H • A • P • T • E • R

# 17

# *Diseases of Skeletal Muscle*

**Umberto De Girolami**
**Dara B. Nachmanoff**
**Linda A. Specht**



## GENERAL CONSIDERATIONS

The introductory comments that follow briefly outline the clinical approach and some basic principles of the interpretation of histopathologic findings in muscle biopsy. For in-depth reading of the subject the reader is referred to the excellent, multiauthored, two-volume treatise edited by Engel and Franzini-Armstrong.[55]

Close collaboration between the pathologist and the clinician is especially important in the evaluation of a skeletal muscle biopsy. Since the morphologic responses of skeletal muscle to injury are relatively limited, they must always be interpreted in the context of the patient's clinical history and physical examination, the serum levels of muscle enzymes, and such functional studies as electromyogram (EMG) and nerve conduction velocity (NCV). In addition, genetic analysis is necessary in the evaluation of hereditary neuromuscular disorders. For these reasons this chapter will give a brief overview of the clinical and molecular biologic/pathogenetic aspects for each disease under discussion along with a description summarizing characteristic muscle biopsy findings.

Once it has been ascertained that a muscle biopsy might be useful in the work-up of a patient's neuromuscular disorder the person in charge of the procedure should make certain that steps are taken to ensure that the tissue is properly collected. The muscle chosen for biopsy should be moderately affected, as judged by physical examination and EMG studies. Clinically uninvolved muscles are less likely to show histopathologic abnormalities, and severely affected muscle may demonstrate only end-stage changes. Sites of previous biopsy, EMG needle implantation, intramuscular injection, or prior trauma should be avoided by the surgeon, since it may not be possible to distinguish muscle reactions secondary to these injuries from those of the primary underlying neuromuscular disease. The biopsy should be taken from the belly of the muscle;

at the tendinous insertion the collagenous connective tissue, the variation in fiber size, and the increased number of internalized nuclei typically seen at the end of the muscle could be misinterpreted as abnormalities.

The muscle biopsy should be performed by a surgeon well versed in biopsy technique. At the time of biopsy the specimens are processed as follows: (1) Light and electron microscopy of clamped specimen: one specimen is obtained directly from the patient on a standard muscle biopsy clamp prior to its excision in order to avoid contraction artifacts. One portion of this specimen is placed in a fixative favorable for subsequent examination by light microscopy (e.g., buffered formalin), embedded in paraffin, and processed for cross and longitudinal sections; it is stained with H&E at three levels and with special stains as needed. The other portion of this specimen is fixed in glutaraldehyde and embedded in plastic. Cross and longitudinal sections are cut as semithin sections, stained with toluidine blue, and examined with the light microscope. Then, selected regions are processed for electron microscopic study. (2) Histochemistry and biochemistry of unclamped specimen: the second specimen is removed unclamped and placed in a saline-moistened gauze for transport. A portion is embedded in a frozen-section embedding medium, oriented for cross (sometimes also longitudinal) sections, frozen using standard techniques, and sectioned and stained to include histochemical reactions. The other portion is stored in the ultra-low freezer for possible biochemical studies available from commercial or research laboratories. Ideally, frozen sections should be cut immediately, but we have detected slight preparative artifact in our laboratories when the block is stored in a −70° freezer and sections are cut at a later time.

The battery of histochemical reactions and special stains employed on frozen sections of muscle will vary somewhat from one laboratory to another; we routinely perform hematoxylin and eosin (H&E), modified Gomori trichrome, nicotinamide adenine dinucleotide-tetrazolium reductase (NADH-TR), periodic acid Schiff (PAS) with and without diastase, oil red O (ORO), acid phosphatase, and ATPase (at pH 4.3, 4.6, and 9.4). In selected instances (e.g., inflammatory myopathies) sections of frozen tissues can also be processed with a battery of reactions that bring out immunoglobulin deposits. Computer-assisted morphometric studies performed on transverse frozen sections of the adenosine triphosphatase (ATPase) reaction, compared with age-matched controls, are especially useful in the evaluation of muscle biopsies in children.

## NORMAL MUSCLE

The connective tissue sheaths of muscles include the endomysium, which surrounds individual muscle fibers; the perimysium, which groups muscle fibers into bundles (fascicles); and the epimysium, which envelops whole muscles or multiple fascicles (Fig. 17-1). Skeletal muscle "fibers" are composed of longitudinally arranged syncytia of fused muscle cells. On transverse sections of adult skeletal muscle, the fibers are polygonally shaped and there is relatively little variability in their shape and size (Fig. 17-2, *A*). The cell nuclei are located just beneath the cell membrane (sarcolemma); they are regularly spaced, slender, rounded or oval, and oriented parallel to the length of the fiber, with evenly distributed chromatin and inconspicuous nucleoli. Internalized nuclei, best seen in transverse section, are found in no more than 3% to 5% of normal adult fibers. A delicate capillary network surrounds the individual fibers (Fig. 17-2, *B*). While the adult muscle fiber on transverse section is polygonal, in infants and in adult extrinsic eye muscles or facial muscles, the fibers tend to be round. Furthermore, the cross-sectional diameter of individual fibers varies some-

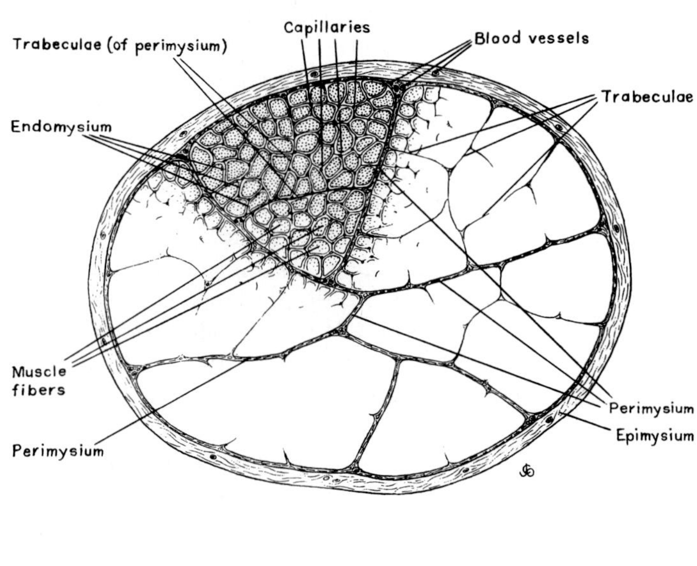


**Fig. 17-1.** Schematic drawing of a skeletal muscle in transverse section showing fascicles of muscle fibers and their connective tissue sheaths. (From De Girolami, and others: Skeletal muscle. In Silverberg SG, editor: Principles and practice of surgical pathology, New York, 1990, Churchill-Livingstone.)

A

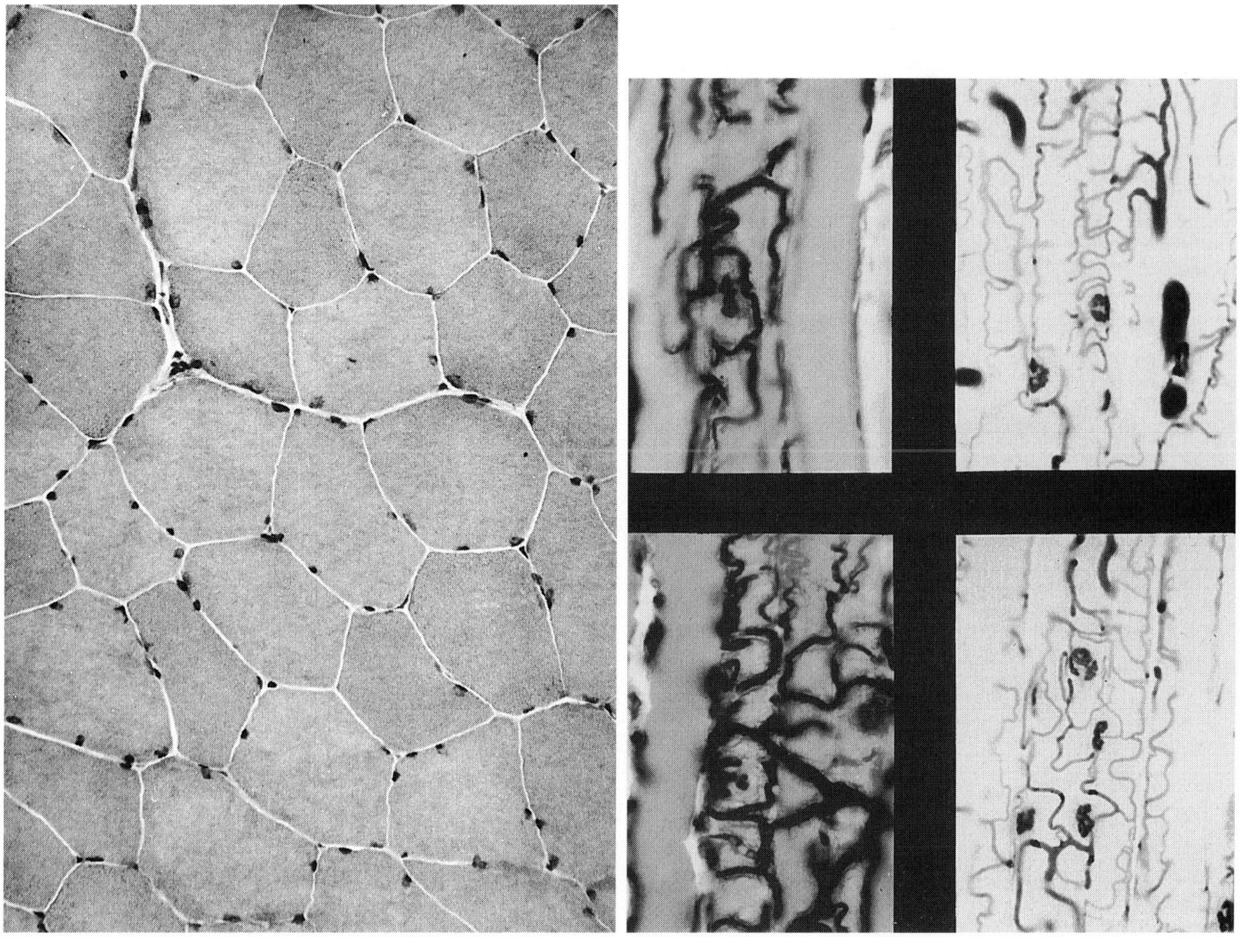

B

**Fig. 17-2.** **A**, High magnification of an H&E section of a group of muscle fibers in transverse plane. Note polygonal configuration, the finely granular sarcoplasm, and the rounded subsarcolemmal nuclei. The connective tissue and capillaries are nearly invisible. There is relatively little variation in the size of the muscle fibers. **B**, Longitudinal section to show capillary network around muscle fibers, on the left-sided panels with an alkaline phosphatase preparation and on the right with injection of India ink. (**A**, original magnification ×170.) (Courtesy of Dr. RD Adams).

what, depending on the specific muscle examined and its functional status. Morphometric charts provide a useful guide to the normal ranges. The cytoplasm of each muscle fiber contains the contractile units of the cell, the myofibrils. The myofibril is composed of identical repeating units (sarcomeres), which consist of interlaced, longitudinally directed, thin filaments (actin) and thick filaments (myosin) and perpendicularly disposed Z-bands (primarily $\alpha$-actinin). These impart the characteristic striations of "striped" skeletal muscle (Fig. 17-3, *A* and *B*). The contractile units are optimally evident by electron microscopy. Electron microscopy also shows the T system, involved in calcium release during excitation, as an invagination of the sarcolemmal membrane into the interior of the cell (Fig. 17-4). The T system runs parallel to the Z-bands, accompanied on each side by sarcoplasmic reticulum. Between the myofibrils is cytoplasm (sarcoplasm), which accounts for 40% of the volume of the fiber; the sarcoplasm contains myoglobin, glycogen, mitochondria, lysosomes, and lipid vacuoles. Satellite cells, a reserve cell population, are located between the sarcolemma and the overlying basal lamina, which encircles the entire muscle fiber (Fig. 17-4). The functional unit of the neuromuscular system is the motor unit, which is composed of a motor neuron in the anterior horn of the spinal cord, the axon of that neuron, and the individual muscle fibers innervated by it. The muscle fibers within a particular motor unit are not adjacent to each other, but rather are distributed randomly throughout the muscle.

The motor neuron of a particular motor unit imparts to all the muscle fibers it innervates characteristics of either type 1 ("slow-twitch") or type 2 ("fast-twitch") myofibers. These two prototypical fiber types can be distinguished with histochemical reactions. The type

A

B

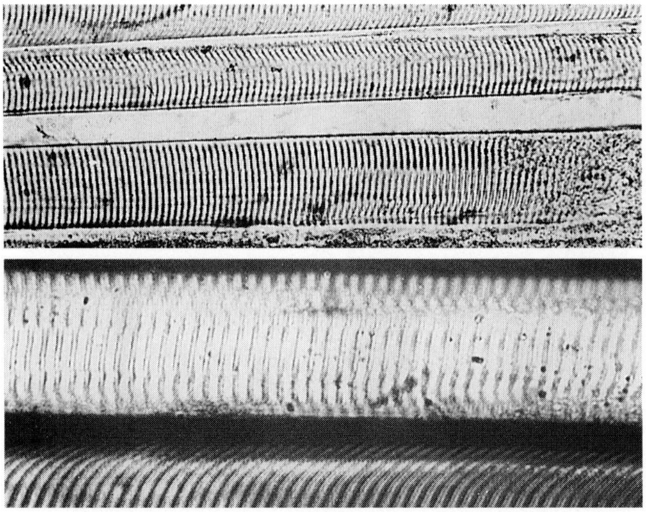

**Fig. 17-3.** Longitudinal section of muscle fiber. **A**, PTAH stain of muscle fiber showing the nuclei in relation to the myofibrils, the barely visible sarcolemma and endomysium. **B**, Muscle fiber is viewed under polarized light to show the transverse striations. (**A**, original magnification ×600; **B**, original magnification ×600.) (Courtesy of Dr. RD Adams.)

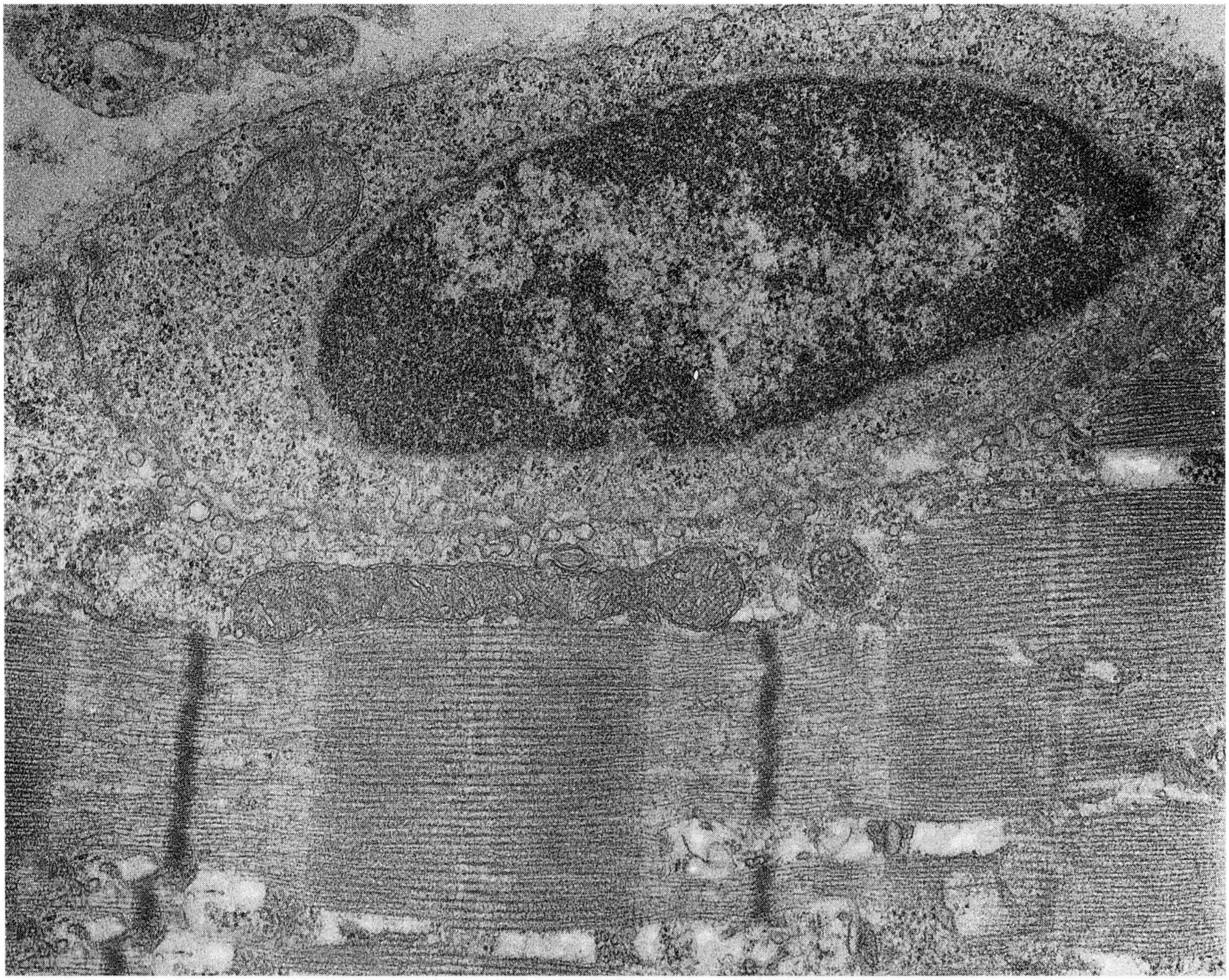

**Fig. 17-4.** Electron micrograph in longitudinal plane. Note large satellite nucleus lying between the basal lamina on outside and sarcolemmal membrane on inside. The dark transverse Z bands of three sarcomeres (parts between two Z bands) are shown. Fine actin filaments attach to each side of the Z band and interdigitate with thick myosin filaments. The light central band is traversed by the thin M band. (Original magnification ×14,630.) (Courtesy of Dr. C Cardasis.)

1 or "slow-twitch" fibers are specialized for long, tonic contraction and are richer in mitochondria, oxidative enzymes, and lipid droplets. Type 2 or "fast-twitch" fibers are suited to brief spurts of intermittent contraction, and thus are more dependent on anaerobic metabolism, containing fewer mitochondria and oxidative enzymes as well as more abundant stores of glycogen. Although a number of methods distinguish the two fiber types, a reliable technique to segregate the fibers by type is the ATPase histochemical reaction performed on frozen sections after preincubation at alkaline and acid pHs. Under alkaline conditions (pH 9.4), the type 2 fibers stain darkly and the type 1 fibers lightly; the opposite is true when preincubation is performed under acidic conditions (pH 4.3). An intermediate condition (pH 4.6) causes type 1 fibers to appear dark, and distinguishes between type 2A fibers (very light) and type 2B fibers (intermediate staining) (see Table 17-1). Recently, procedures for typing the fibers in formalin-fixed paraffin-embedded tissue have been devised, and these newer methods may be adopted widely in the future.[98] The random admixture of the two fiber types that occurs in human muscle imparts a "checkerboard" or "mosaic" appearance of alternating light and dark fibers with the ATPase reaction (Fig. 17-5). Although the adult quadriceps, a muscle that is commonly biopsied, contains more type 2 fibers (60% to 65%) than type 1 fibers (35% to 40%), there is considerable variability in these proportions among the different muscles and age groups.

**Table 17-1.** Muscle fiber types and physiologic/histochemical characteristics

| | Type 1 | Type 2 |
|---|---|---|
| Action | Sustained force<br>Weight-bearing | Sudden movements<br>Purposeful motion |
| Enzyme content | NADH dark staining | NADH light staining |
| | ATPase pH 4.2 dark staining | ATPase pH 4.2 light staining |
| | ATPase pH 9.4 light staining | ATPase pH 9.4 dark staining |
| Lipids | Abundant | Scant |
| Glycogen | Abundant | Scant |
| Ultrastructure | Many mitochondria | Few mitochondria |
| | Wide Z band | Narrow Z band |
| Physiology | Slow-twitch | Fast-twitch |
| Color | Red | White |
| Prototype | Soleus (pigeon) | Pectoral (pigeon) |

The neuromuscular junction consists of presynaptic and postsynaptic components. The former are created by an expansion of the axon terminal. Within the terminal there are abundant vesicles and mitochondria. Vesicles filled with acetylcholine (ACh) congregate at the

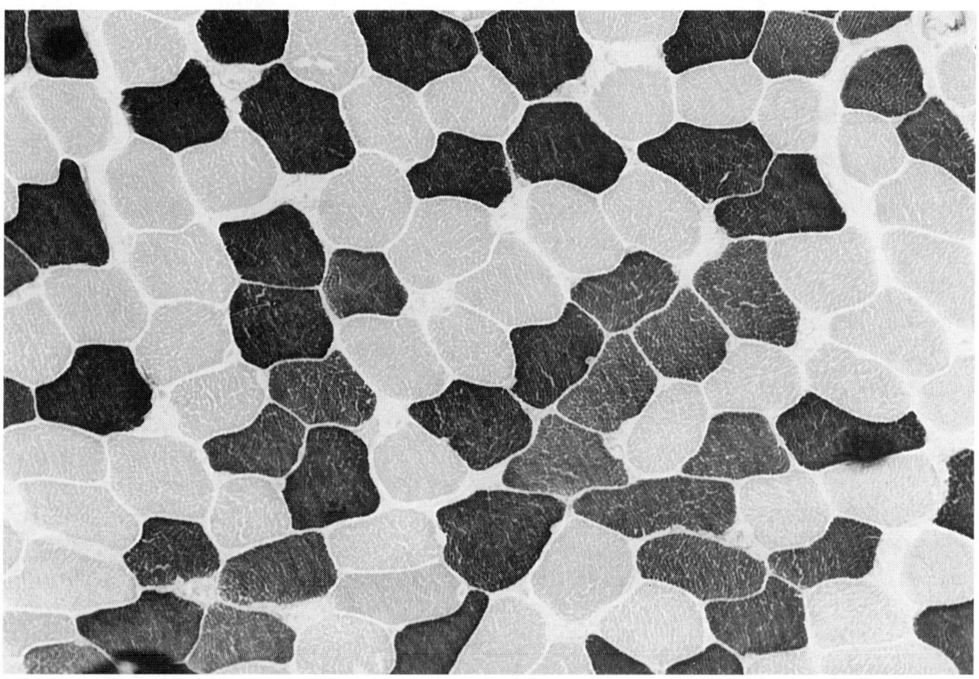

**Fig. 17-5.** ATPase stain at pH 9.4 to show the different staining qualities of type 1 (light) and type 2 (dark) fibers. Types 2A and 2B are not distinguishable with this preparation. (Original magnification ×260.)

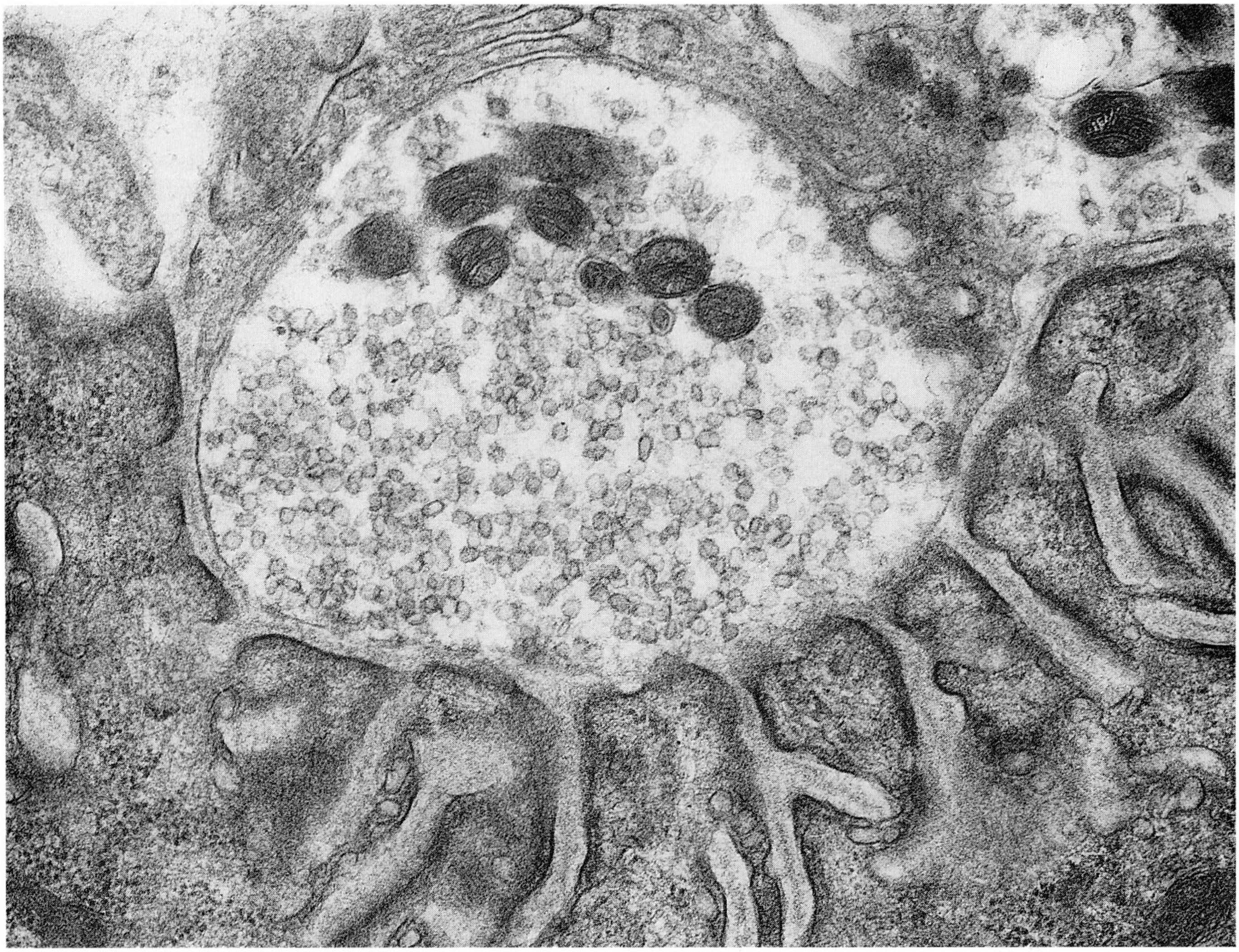

**Fig. 17-6.** EM of neuromuscular junction. In the center is the nerve terminal with its presynaptic vesicles of acetylcholine and several mitochondria. The infolded surface of the muscle fiber is on the bottom and the receptor surface on its surface is more dense than the rest of the sarcolemma. (Original magnification ×41,000.) (Courtesy of Dr. C Cardasis.)

presynaptic membrane around dense bars, corresponding to junctional peaks of the postsynaptic membrane, where ACh receptors (AChR) are concentrated (Fig. 17-6). When a nerve impulse arrives at the axon terminal, the ACh-filled vesicles are released and interact with the AChR, giving rise to muscle fiber depolarization. The postsynaptic membrane is highly folded, with AChR concentrated at the peaks. Acetylcholinesterase (AChE), an enzyme that degrades ACh and thereby terminates its physiologic action, is present in the valleys. Muscle spindles are fusiform structures that respond to muscle-fiber stretch and thus have a role in maintaining tone. They consist of specialized intrafusal muscle and nerve fibers delimited by a connective tissue capsule (Fig. 17-7).

## REACTIONS OF SKELETAL MUSCLE TO INJURY

### Choice of Methods

H&E stain is routinely used with both paraffin-embedded tissue and frozen sections and provides a good overview of the muscle structure. Variations in the expected size, distribution, and shape of individual myofibers are evident with this method, as well as abnormally-placed internalized or enlarged nuclei, intracytoplasmic vacuoles, and intracellular deposits. Longitudinal sections best demonstrate the orderly array of striations; they also are useful to evaluate the presence of segmental necrosis, phagocytosis, or regeneration along the length of muscle fiber. H&E is also the standard survey stain to assess and evaluate the pres-

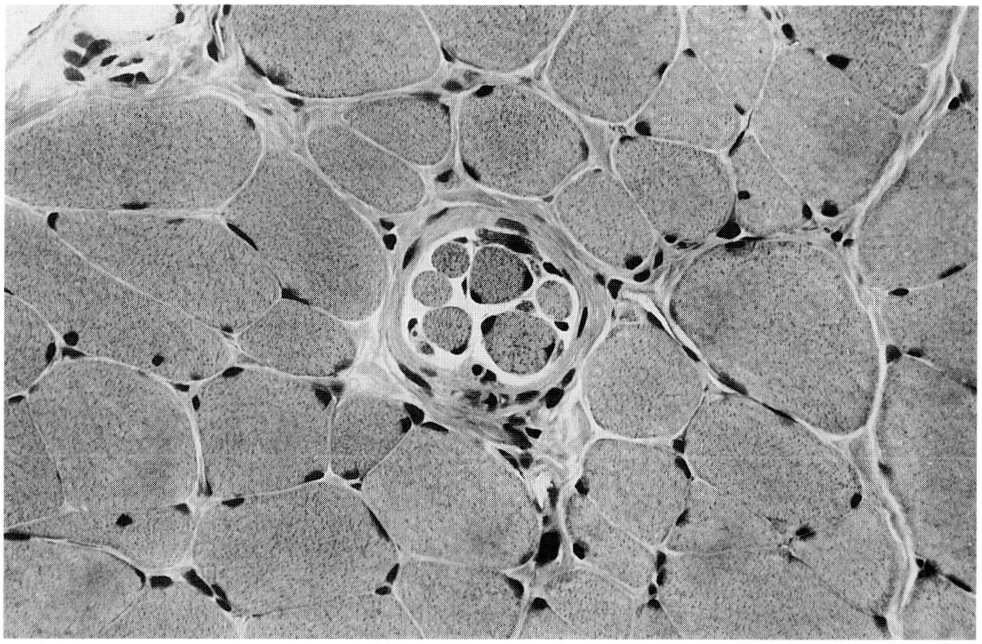

**Fig. 17-7.** Muscle spindle in transverse plane (H&E). Note dense circular capsule and the six intrafusal muscle fibers. The extrafusal fibers are abnormal because of increased variation in sized. (Original magnification ×350.) (From De Girolami U, and Smith TW: Pathology of skeletal muscle diseases: teaching monograph, Am J Pathol 107:235-276, 1982.)

ence of inflammatory infiltrates, vasculitis, abnormal interstitial or vascular deposits (e.g., amyloid), and any increase in endomysial connective tissue or adipose tissue.

Modified Gomori trichrome stain is used on frozen sections and to bring out connective tissue components. In addition, the muscle fiber mitochondria are well demonstrated by this stain and normally mitochondria appear as red-to-purple granules fairly evenly distributed throughout the sarcoplasm, except for the scattered subsarcolemmal crescentic collections especially evident in type 1 fibers. Abnormal intracellular collections of mitochondria or other deposits are also well seen with this staining method (e.g., nemaline rods and rimmed vacuoles).

Nicotinamide adenine dinucleotide-tetrazolium reductase (NADH-TR) is an oxidative enzyme histochemical reaction performed on frozen sections. Type 1, "slow-twitch" fibers, being relatively more dependent on aerobic metabolism for energy generation, contain abundant oxidative enzymes that stain darkly with this preparation; type 2, "fast-twitch" fibers stain lightly. The ATPase stain performed on frozen sections at alkaline (9.4) or acid (4.2, 4.6) pH is also extremely useful for distinguishing between the two major fiber types. Type 2 fibers will stain dark and type 1 fibers light at alkaline pH; the reverse obtains at pH 4.2. At pH 4.6 all fibers will stain darkly, except for the type 2A fibers.

Periodic acid Schiff (PAS) reaction when performed on frozen sections identifies glycogen stores within the myofibers and demonstrates disturbances of the glycolytic pathway, such as McArdle's disease. PAS-positivity can be identified as glycogen by performing the reaction with and without prior diastase digestion. Histochemical stains for the demonstration of myophosphorylase and phosphofructokinase are practicable in many laboratories, and confirmation of the diagnosis by biochemical assay is also commonly available through commercial laboratories. The oil red O (ORO) stain detects lipid stores within the myofibers; the lipid droplets appear as small, round orange-to-red globules within the sarcoplasm. These droplets are more abundant in type 1 fibers. Increased lipid stores may be seen in certain mitochondrial myopathies and lipid storage disorders. The acid phosphatase (AP) reaction performed on frozen sections and the less widely adopted, acridine orange fluorescent method for DNA and RNA are useful methods to bring out muscle fiber necrosis and regeneration. In the case of the AP reaction, active lysosomal enzyme activity is brought out within degenerating myofibers and inflammatory cells. Inflammatory cell infiltrates can also be characterized using standard immunohistochemical markers for subtypes of lymphocytes and for macrophages. Ultrastructural examination is valuable for the identification of abnormalities in organelles (e.g., mitochondria, lysosomes), excessive storage of lipid or glycogen, abnormal inclusions (e.g., nemaline rods), or alterations in the myofibrillar architecture.

## Artifacts

Hypercontraction bands (of Nageotte[137]) are a commonly observed artifact. These develop when the muscle is allowed to fix without being stretched on a clamp or some other suitable device. These bands are seen as alternating dark and light staining ridges along the length of the fiber where the normal sarcomeric structure is disrupted. A frequent artifact in frozen muscle is the sarcoplasmic vacuolization, which occurs when the tissue is improperly frozen, frozen slowly, or allowed to thaw partially before the sections are cut.

## Myopathic Changes

Myopathies, that is disorders in which the primary injury is to the muscle fiber itself, cause characteristic changes in the fibers. These changes include (1) Variations in the shape and size of the fibers, as is characteristic of the dystrophic myopathies. (2) Alterations in the internal structure of the fiber, e.g., hyalinization (loss of cross-striations), splitting of fibers, ring fibers (e.g., myotonic dystrophy), "moth-eaten" fibers, that is, fibers with irregular fluffy patches of decreased oxidative enzyme of ATPase activity. (3) Abnormal intracellular accumulations of mitochondria (e.g., mitochondrial myopathies), glycogen (storage diseases), lipid (lipid storage myopathies, vacuoles [e.g., channelopathies, inflammatory myopathies]), or other deposits (e.g., congenital myopathies). (4) Abnormalities in size (regenerating fibers) or position (e.g., dystrophic myopathies, congenital myopathies) of the nucleus. (5) Inflammatory cell infiltrates and abnormalities of the interstitial connective tissue (e.g., endomysial connective tissue proliferation as seen in the dystrophic myopathies) and of the blood vessels.

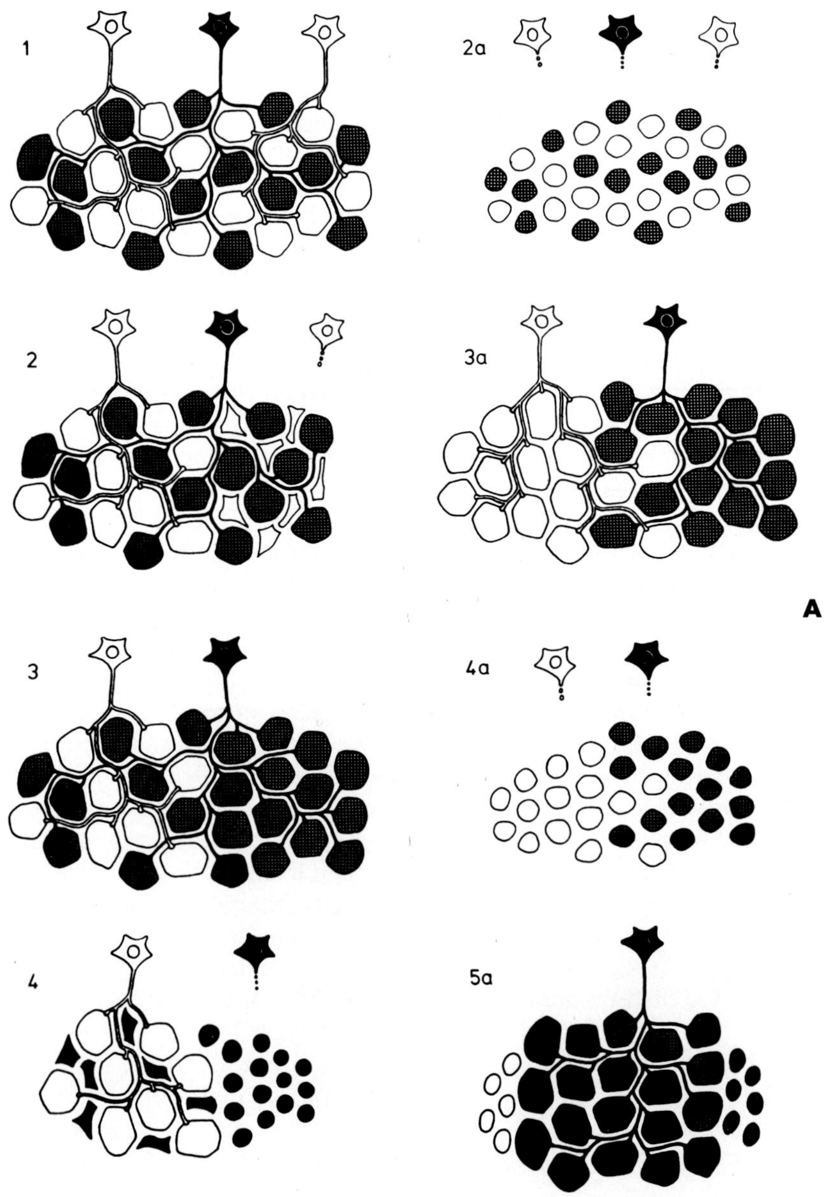


**Fig. 17-8.** Neurogenic atrophy. **A**, Diagram of denervation and reinnervation. (Reproduced with permission from Mastaglia FL, and Walton J: Skeletal muscle pathology, New York, 1982, Churchill-Livingstone.)

### Neurogenic Atrophy

Neurogenic atrophy of muscle (denervation) occurs in diseases that affect the anterior horn cell (and cranial motor nerve nuclei), anterior motor roots, and motor fibers of the peripheral nervous system. The histopathologic changes in skeletal muscle that occur when there is a functional/structural alteration of its innervation are referred to as *neurogenic* or *denervation* atrophy (Fig. 17-8, *A*). The earliest structural change is a loss of the normally polygonal cross-sectional outline of the fibers within the motor unit innervated by the affected nerve cell. The fibers take on a roughly triangular shape ("angulated") and become smaller than normal (i.e., "atrophic"). As the fibers within one motor unit are scattered throughout the muscle, this change will be detected on routine preparations in paraffin, frozen, and plastic-embedded tissues as a variation of fiber size with randomly scattered atrophic, angulated fibers (Fig. 17-8, *B*).

Pathologic processes that lead to denervation ordinarily affect both type 1 and type 2 myofibers. This finding of early denervation can best be appreciated with the ATPase stains. In distinction, single fiber type 2 fiber atrophy may be observed in a wide range of conditions (e.g., experimental tenotomy, steroid myopathies, chronic immobilization, CNS disorders). Relatively early in the course of the disease the denervated, atrophied myofibers may be reinnervated by "sprouts" from the neighboring twigs of a viable motor unit. When this occurs, the newly recruited myofibers are included with those of the viable motor unit. The reinnervated fibers now partly or wholly regain normal size and polygonal shape, assuming the fiber type determined by their new innervation. As this process of denervation and reinnervation continues, the normal "checkerboard" pattern characteristic of randomly distributed type 1 and type 2 fibers on the ATPase stain is replaced by a nonrandom arrangement of groups of adjacent myofibers sharing the same staining characteristics (Fig. 17-8, *C*). This process is known as "fiber type grouping" and is pathognomonic of de-

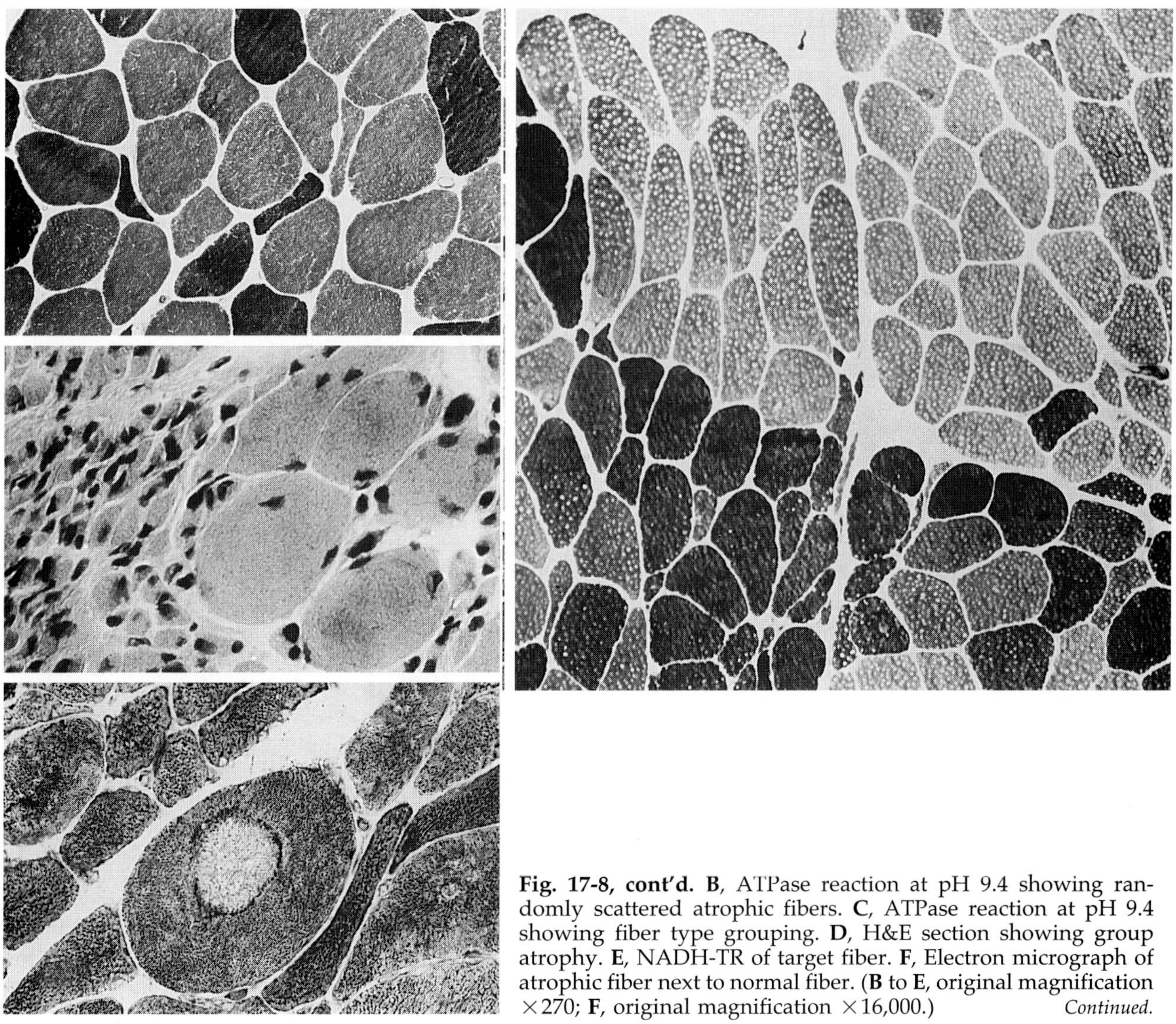

B

C

D

E

**Fig. 17-8, cont'd. B**, ATPase reaction at pH 9.4 showing randomly scattered atrophic fibers. **C**, ATPase reaction at pH 9.4 showing fiber type grouping. **D**, H&E section showing group atrophy. **E**, NADH-TR of target fiber. **F**, Electron micrograph of atrophic fiber next to normal fiber. (**B** to **E**, original magnification ×270; **F**, original magnification ×16,000.)

*Continued.*

F

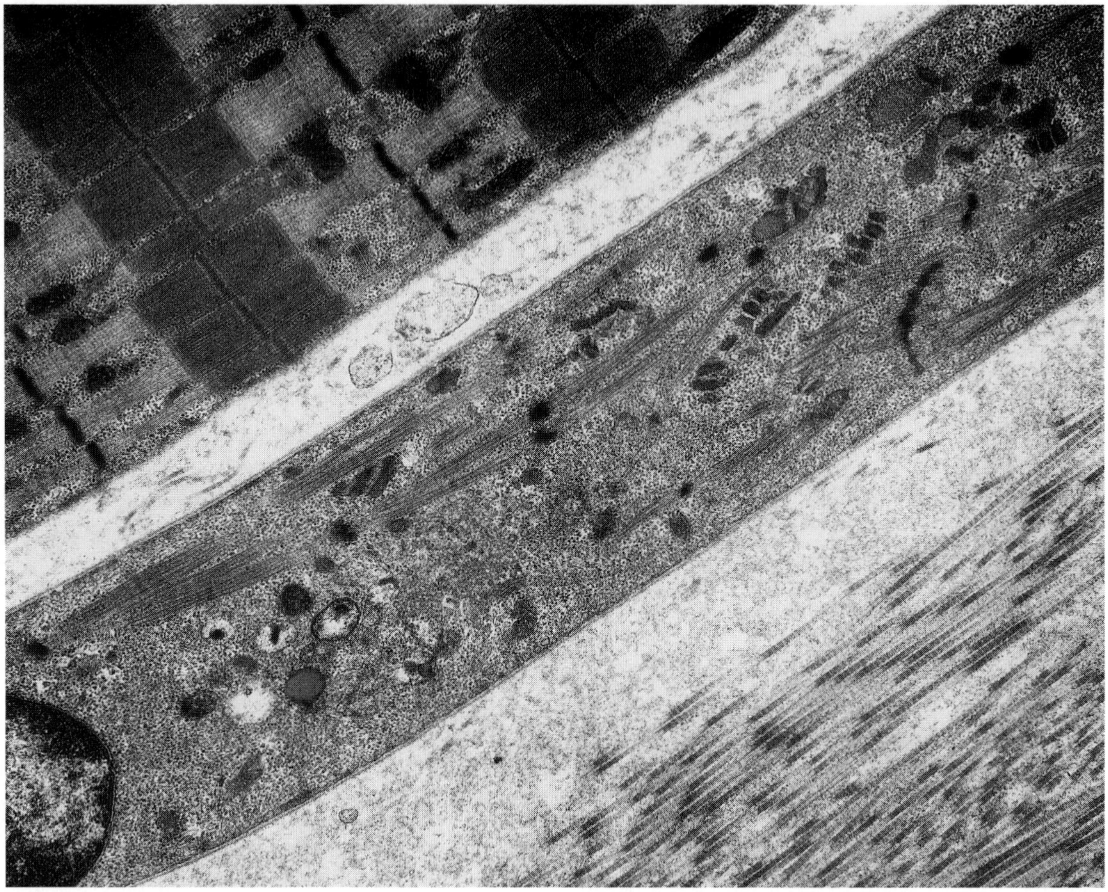

**Fig. 17-8, cont'd.** For legend see previous page.

nervation of skeletal muscle. Should the denervation progress beyond this point and the remaining viable neurons or axons be affected, the groups of fibers of an identical type undergo atrophy. When this occurs there is grouping or clustering of shrunken, angulated myofibers of the same histochemical type. This pattern, termed "group atrophy," is typical of chronic denervation (Fig. 17-8, *D*). Atrophic fibers that initially are angulated in shape may eventually become so shrunken that only clusters of nuclei remain, surrounded by the plasmalemma. Such structures are known as "nuclear bags."

Another feature of chronic denervation, which is well demonstrated with the NADH-TR reaction, is the target fiber. True target fibers are seen almost exclusively in type 1 myofibers and consist of a change in the cross-sectional appearance of the fiber whereby a central region of decreased oxidative enzyme activity is surrounded by a ring of increased activity (Fig. 17-8, *E*). The so-called *targetoid* fibers are not specific for any one disease, although they are also seen in denervation. Here, there is also a zone (or zones) of decreased enzyme activity within the muscle fiber, but the outer rim of increased enzyme activity is lacking. Ultrastructurally, the atrophic fiber is smaller than normal and the sarcomeric organization is lacking, but the cell membrane, nucleus, and organelles remain intact (Fig. 17-8, *F*).

## MUSCLE DISEASES

Muscle diseases are divided into two major groups: (1) *myopathies*, that is, those due to disease of the muscle fiber itself; and (2) *neurogenic atrophies*, those resulting from disease of the rest of the motor unit. The myopathies can be further subdivided into dystrophies and congenital, metabolic, and inflammatory myopathies. Diseases of the nervous system that give rise to neurogenic atrophy will be discussed only briefly here because they are the major topic of chapters 14 and 15.

Myopathies are characterized clinically by muscle weakness more proximal than distal, preservation of the deep tendon reflexes until the muscle is severely affected, and elevation of the serum CK level secondary to muscle breakdown. Small-amplitude, short-duration polyphasic compound muscle action potentials are the electromyographic (EMG) hallmark of the myopathies. These features reflect the dropout of myofibers from the motor unit.

## Myopathies

### Muscular dystrophies

***Dystrophinopathies.*** Duchenne muscular dystrophy (DMD) occurs in 1/3500 live male births; approximately one third of cases represent new mutations. This X-linked condition, initially described clinically by Duchenne and Erb,[48,49,62,63] typically presents between the ages of 3 and 6 years with complaints of proximal leg weakness (e.g., difficulty in running, climbing stairs, or getting up from the floor) and the Gowers sign. Tightened Achilles tendons or hypertrophied calves are variably present (Fig. 17-9, *A*). Laboratory investigation reveals marked elevation of creatine kinase (CK) (often more than 100 times normal), and myopathic units on EMG.

The clinical course of DMD is characterized by progressive weakness of axial and appendicular muscles. Most patients lose the ability to ambulate between the ages of 8 and 14. Lower facial muscles are affected late, and extraocular muscles are always spared. Orthopedic deformities (contractures, scoliosis) develop as the weakness progresses. Most patients exhibit evidence of cardiac involvement as early as 5 or 6 years of age, with sinus tachycardia and right ventricular hypertrophy with strain. Life-threatening dysrhythmias or heart failure develop in approximately 10% of patients. Some boys have smooth muscle involvement with poor gastric motility. Many patients have an associated static encephalopathy manifest as mild to moderate mental retardation.[124] In the absence of respiratory support, death results from pulmonary failure in the late teens or early twenties.[18]

Becker muscular dystrophy (BMD) has a lower incidence (1/30,000 male births), generally presents later in childhood, and has a more protracted and/or variable course than does DMD.[12] Most affected boys run well as children and generally remain ambulatory until the second to fourth decade. Affected males can pass the defective gene to their grandsons through their carrier daughters.

The earliest histopathologic changes on muscle biopsy in patients with DMD consist of variations in the range of the cross-sectional diameter of the muscle fibers, with scattered hypertrophied rounded fibers ("hyaline fibers," "hypercontracted fibers") that are opaque and stain darkly (Fig. 17-9, *B*). Careful observation of optimally-fixed tissue can also demonstrate breaks in the sarcolemma, with underlying wedge-shaped disruption of sarcomere architecture. As the disease progresses active myofiber breakdown, necrosis, and myophagocytosis occur alongside muscle fiber regeneration (basophilia of the sarcoplasm, enlarged internalized vesicular nuclei, and prominent nucleoli) and an increasing proliferation of endomysial connective tissue (Fig. 17-9, *C* and *D*). Fiber splitting is prominent. In end-stage disease there is massive loss of muscle fibers and replacement with adipose tissue and patchy strands of fibrous connective tissue. Muscle spindles are relatively preserved until the end.[28]

Attempts to distinguish fiber types by histochemical methods show either a type 1 predominance or failure to differentiate between the fiber types. Immunohistochemistry with antibodies directed against the dystrophin protein (rod domain, carboxyl terminus, and amino terminus) fails to demonstrate immunoreactivity in the subsarcolemmal region of muscle fibers from patients with DMD (Fig. 17-9, *E* to *G*). Cardiac muscle shows fibrosis, especially affecting the epimyocardial portion of the left ventricle.[73]

The muscle biopsy in BMD shares many features with those of DMD; active fiber degeneration and regeneration are seen, especially in younger patients.[100] Later in the course such signs of chronic myopathy as fiber splitting and endomysial fibrosis supervene. As in DMD, hypertrophic fibers also may be found, but with less frequency. Bradley and co-authors have described modest neurogenic changes, such as angulated atrophic fibers, nuclear clumps, and mild fiber type grouping.[16] Immunohistochemical staining with antibody-directed dystrophin protein (especially those against the carboxyl terminus) reveals patchy positivity in the subsarcolemmal region in patients with BMD.

Recent research developments have elucidated the genetic and biochemical basis of DMD/BMD, establishing the allelic nature of the two disorders.* The responsible gene is located on the Xp21 region of the X chromosome and spans 2 million base pairs. It includes more than 65 exons and encodes the 400 kD protein dystrophin. The gene is the large size of the DMD/BMD gene that accounts for the high rate of spontaneous mutation. The dystrophin protein represents 0.01% of skeletal muscle protein. Its tissue distribution (skeletal, smooth and cardiac muscle, and brain) correlates well with the known clinical features of DMD/BMD. Most (70% to 80%) affected DMD/BMD boys have demonstrable mutations (deletions or duplications) of one or more exons. Mutations that disrupt the translational reading frame or the promoter result in a truncated and presumably unstable protein that correlates with the severe DMD phenotype. In contrast, mutations that do not disrupt the translational reading frame or the promoters yield a lower molecular weight and semifunctional dystrophin, correlating with the less severe BMD phenotype.

The *dystrophin test* (dystrophin immunoblotting) provides definitive biochemical diagnosis useful in differentiating sporadic DMD/BMD from such clinically similar conditions as dermatomyositis, limb girdle dystrophy, Emery-Dreifuss disease, or congenital my-

* Refs. 22, 59, 80, 86, 93, 143, 160.

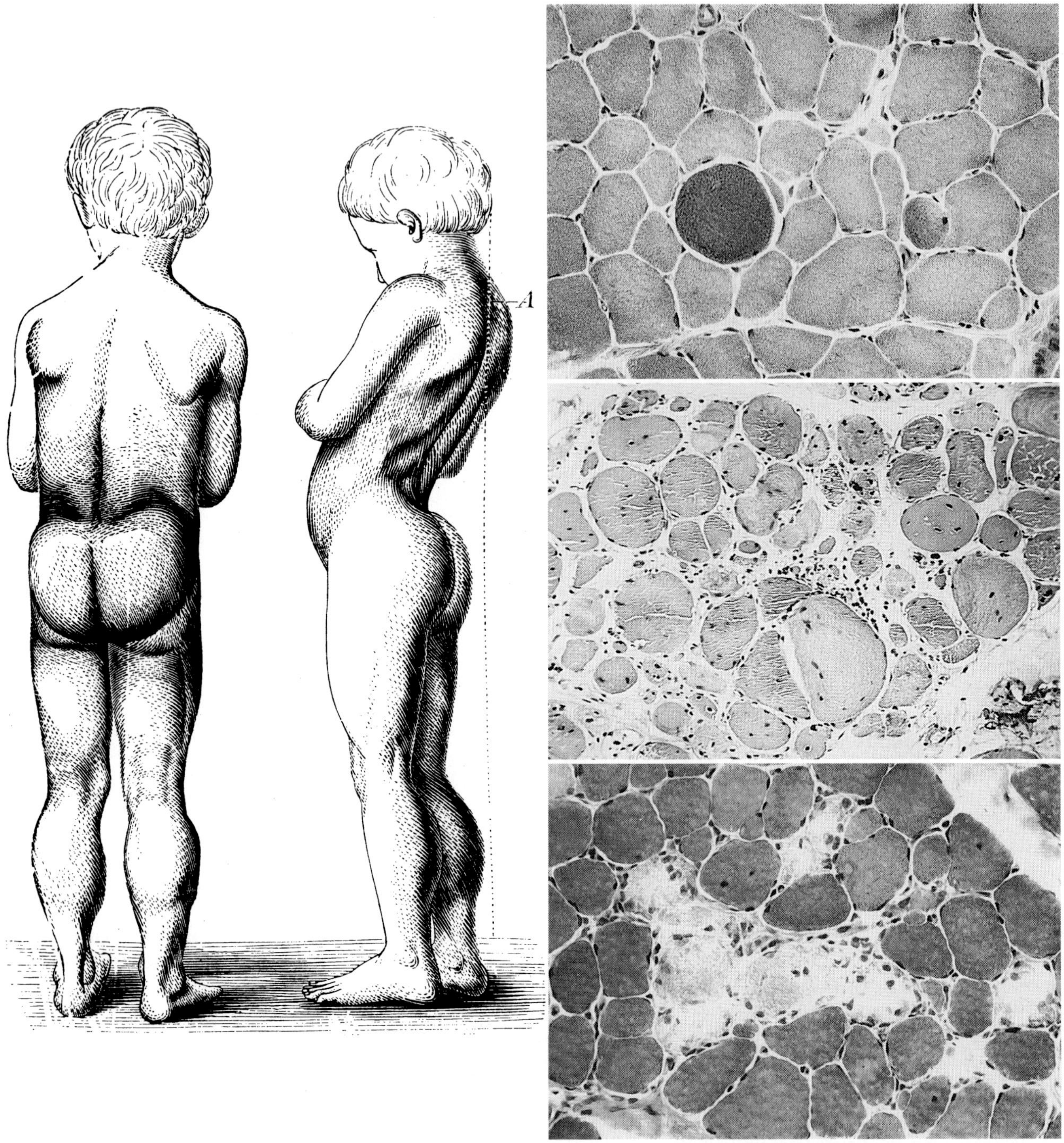

**Fig. 17-9.** Duchenne dystrophy. **A**, Drawing from patient from initial description by Duchenne.[49] Note the pseudohypertrophy of the calves and the characteristic posture. **B**, H&E section showing round hyalinized fiber. **C**, H&E section of muscle showing variation in fiber size, internalized nuclei, and increased endomysial connective tissue. **D**, H&E section showing myophagocytosis. **E**, Immunoperoxidase reaction for dystrophin in normal individual. Note dark staining rim around muscle fibers adhalin. **F**, Immunoperoxidase reaction for dystrophin in patient with DMD. Note lack of reaction product and variability in fiber size. **G**, Immunoperoxidase reaction for adhalin on same patient illustrated in **F**. Note reaction product around muscle fiber. (**B** to **D**, original magnification ×170; **E** to **G**, original magnification ×300.) (**B**, **C**, from De Girolami U, and Smith TW: Pathology of skeletal muscle diseases. Teaching monograph, Am J Pathol 107:235-276, 1982.)

E

F

G

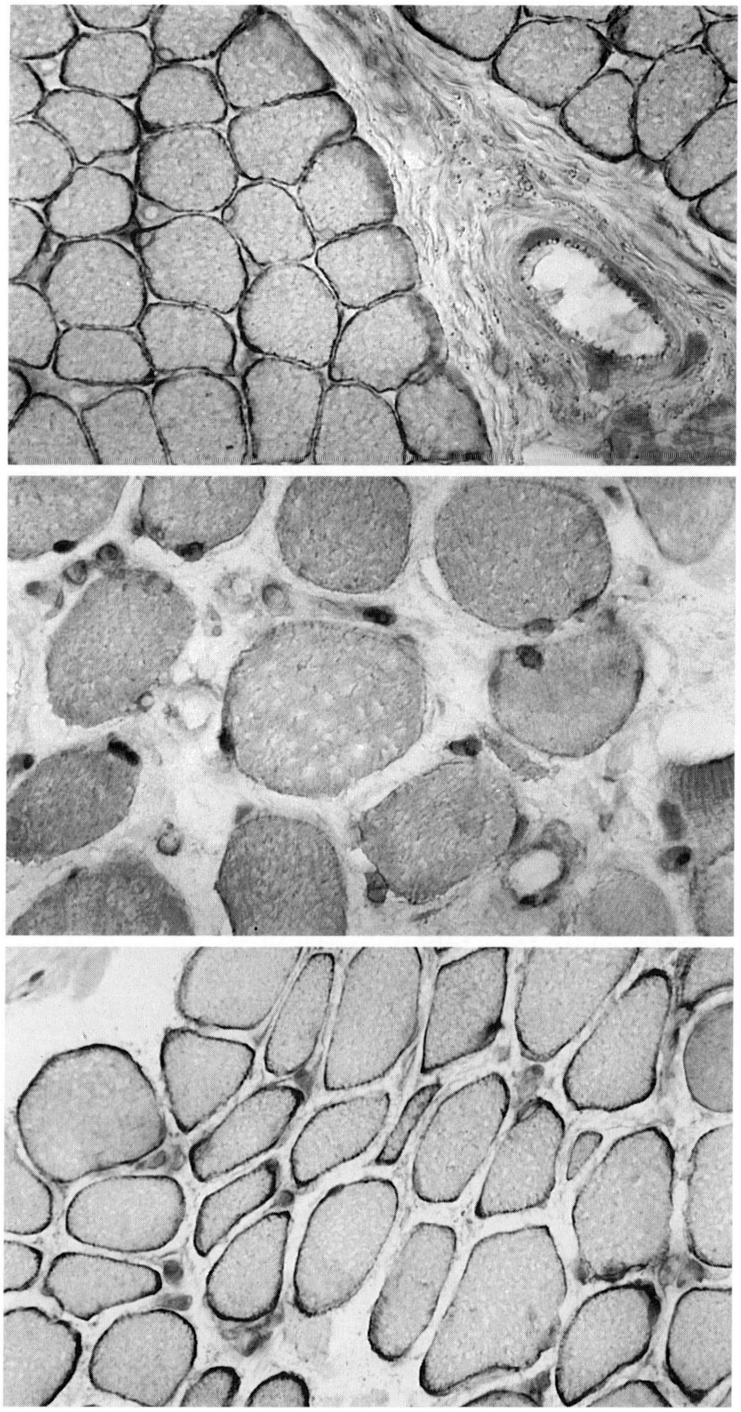

**Fig. 17-9, cont'd.** For legend see opposite page.

opathy. In addition, dystrophin testing permits prediction of the severity of the phenotype in early or preclinical cases, that is, the relative absence of dystrophin predicts the severe DMD course, whereas dystrophin of abnormal size/quantity predicts the more benign BMD. The test is now readily available and requires only a small amount of frozen muscle tissue.

*DNA mutation analysis* (polymerase chain reaction or Southern blot analysis) provides definitive diagnosis, carrier detection, and prenatal diagnosis for most families. DNA analysis requires only a small sample of blood or amniotic fluid, and the test is available in a number of university and commercial laboratories. Polymerase chain analysis can be completed in a matter of hours. For the 20% to 30% of DMD/BMD patients who do not have a demonstrable deletion, an indirect and somewhat less accurate strategy, namely restriction fragment length polymorphisms (RFLPs), may be useful for carrier detection or prenatal diagnosis.

*Dystrophin immunohistochemistry* of muscle tissue is a useful means of carrier detection (for the purpose of genetic counseling or establishing the diagnosis of manifest carrier) for a woman whose family does not have a demonstrable deletion recognized by direct DNA analysis nor a pedigree suitable for RFLP analysis. Because of lyonization (inactivation of one or the two X chromosomes in females), DMD/BMD carriers have a mosaic pattern of dystrophin immunoreactivity, that is, dystrophin-positive muscle fibers (expressing the normal X chromosome) are intermixed with dystrophin-negative fibers (expressing the dystrophin-deficient X chromosome).

***Nondystrophinopathies***

***Facioscapulohumeral dystrophy***—Facioscapulohumeral (FSH) muscular dystrophy, originally described as a distinct entity by Landouzy and Dejerine,[113,114] is inherited as an autosomal-dominant trait in most cases. The age of onset is variable, but the more typical cases begin in the second or third decade. The muscles of the face (orbicularis oculi, zygomaticus, orbicularis oris), neck, and shoulder girdle are the first to be affected. Subsequently, the disease may spread to the pelvic girdle. The disorder, much milder than DMD, is insidious in onset, and the clinical course is slowly progressive. Patients may remain ambulatory even at advanced stages of illness. Cardiac involvement is infrequent. The scapuloperoneal syndrome (SPS) is a clinically, genetically, and pathologically heterogeneous disorder characterized by mild weakness of the scapular muscle and foot extensors. The age of onset is quite variable, and the disease generally runs a very slowly progressive course.

According to most observers, the histologic findings in affected muscles are variation in fiber size, with both markedly hypertrophied and severely atrophic fibers, endomysial connective tissue proliferation, and relatively few degenerating/regenerating myofibers. In some pedigrees the muscle biopsy may show an unusually prominent focal interstitial mononuclear inflammatory response.[135]

Despite some clinical heterogeneity, linkage analysis suggests that a single locus on 4q35 is responsible. The gene product has not been identified. Prenatal diagnosis is available by RFLP analysis.

***Oculopharyngeal muscular dystrophy.*** Oculopharyngeal muscular dystrophy is typically a disease of late onset characterized by progressive ptosis and weakness of extraocular muscles; it is associated with difficulty in swallowing.[173] Weakness of the face, jaw, and limb muscles may occur later in the course of the disease. The largest affected communities have been of French-Canadian origin, but several kindreds from Europe, Latin America, and Japan also have been recognized. The mode of inheritance is most often autosomal-dominant; sporadic and autosomal recessive cases are on record, and onset in childhood has been described.[111] Congenital fibrosis of the extraocular muscle (CFEOM) is an autosomal dominant ocular disorder characterized by congenital, nonprogressive, bilateral ptosis and external ophthalmoplegia.

Skeletal muscles show myopathic changes, including variation in fiber size, internalized nuclei, and increased endomysial connective tissue. There may also be scattered type 1 angular fibers. In addition, rimmed vacuoles are a characteristic feature. The structure of the vacuoles is best demonstrated on frozen sections with the modified Gomori trichrome reaction. Single or multiple intracytoplasmic vacuoles are typically found in type 1 fibers, which contain granular materials that stain red and are lined by a rim of darker material. Ultrastructural studies have demonstrated membranous debris and disruption or the sarcomeric structure within the vacuole and intranuclear unbranched filaments that measure 7 to 9 $\mu$m in diameter,[171] but these are demonstrable only after assiduous search.

The molecular genetics of OPD is unknown at present. The pathophysiology of CFEOM also is unknown, and it is unclear whether the disease has a primary neurogenic or myopathic etiology. Several affected families have linkage to the centromeric region of chromosome 12.[61]

***Limb-girdle syndromes.*** Limb-girdle dystrophy (LGD) is a heterogeneous group of disorders that may be inherited as an autosomal-recessive trait or may occur sporadically. Both the onset of the disease and its prognosis are extremely variable. It usually begins in the second or third decade of life, involving either the pelvic or shoulder girdle muscles, with spread to other muscles after a variable period. Cardiac involvement and pseudohypertrophy are rare. The disorder is generally slowly progressive, and patients remain ambulatory for 20 or more years. The muscle shows marked variation in fiber size with many extremely large fibers, pronounced fiber splitting, and many internalized nuclei. Degenerative and regenerative changes are also seen.

Some LGMD are really sporadic BMD or manifest carriers of DMD/BMD. Other forms of LGMD are thought to be caused by abnormalities on chromosome 15q,[13,72] 2 (autosomal recessive),[11] or chromosome 5 (autosomal dominant).[162] The LGMD phenotype of severe childhood autosomal recessive muscular dystrophy (SCARMD) is variably associated with a defective gene on chromosome 13q[142] or a defective dystrophin-associated glycoprotein (DAG).[127]

***Emery-Dreifuss muscular dystrophy (EDMD).*** This is an X-linked recessive muscular dystrophy characterized by slowly progressive weakness, early contractures, and cardiomyopathy first described in detail in a large kindred from Virginia by Emery and Dreifuss.[50] The disease begins in early childhood, initially with humeral and peroneal muscle weakness and atrophy and later with involvement of the muscles of the pelvic girdle. Toe walking is often the initial symptom. The eventual appearance of cardiopathy (initially first degree atrioventricular block) and contractures at the elbow, posterior neck, and heels are typical of the syndrome. The CK elevation is mild. Female carriers have subtle clinical manifestations of the disease. Muscle biopsy studies have shown variation in fiber size, atrophic rounded Type 1 fibers, scattered regenerating fibers, internalized nuclei, and some endomysial connective tissue proliferation.[26,129,146]

The EDMD gene is located on the long arm of the X chromosome in band Xq28.[35] The gene responsible for at least some patients with EDMD encodes the protein emerin, an incompletely analyzed protein expressed both in skeletal and cardiac muscle.[15]

***Congenital muscular dystrophies (CMD).*** A heterogeneous group of hereditary neuromuscular disease characterized by some degree of hypotonia and muscle wasting evident at birth or in early infancy have been brought together for convenience under the heading "congenital muscular dystrophy." The clinical course in these disorders is quite variable; some patients have progressive weakness and others improve with time.[8,140,170]

Although there has been considerable variability from case to case, the histologic changes observed in skeletal muscle are similar in kind, if not in degree, to those seen in the muscular dystrophies that occur at an older age. Endomysial fibrosis has been especially striking. In the Fukuyama (FCMD) form described in Japan, in addition to muscular weakness there are developmental abnormalities of the CNS.[75] The genetic locus in FCMD has been identified on chromosome 9q31-33.[169]

A number of molecular subtypes are now being recognized. Some patients are believed to have a deficiency in the basement membrane protein *laminin*[180] (a laminin abnormality has also been identified in murine dystrophy[179]). Recently, a subset of patients with *merosin* deficiency also was described.[140,170] Merosin is a component of the extracellular muscle membrane whose genetic locus is on chromosome 6.[92] These patients generally present with contractures, weakness, and hypotonia at birth. In contrast to the other CMD patients, the subset with merosin deficiency have a high CK levels and T2-weighted signal abnormalities on MRI.

***Myotonic dystrophy.*** Myotonic dystrophy (Steinert's disease[163]) is a common autosomal dominant multisystem disorder characterized primarily by weakness and myotonia. Weakness of face and neck muscles is especially prominent. EMG shows the classic "dive bomber" pattern. Associated abnormalities include mental retardation, cataracts, frontal balding, and endocrine and cardiac disturbances. Congenital myotonic dystrophy is maternally transmitted and presents as hypotonia and facial diplegia, generally in association with contractures; myotonia and mental retardation become apparent later. In general, the myotonic dystrophy phenotype becomes increasingly severe with successive generations in a given pedigree.

To a large extent, the skeletal muscles show features of a dystrophic myopathy. In addition, there is a striking increase in the number of internal nuclei arranged in a chainlike sequence that is evident on longitudinal sections (Fig. 17-10, *A* and *B*). Ring fibers are another important finding (*Ringbinden*, striated annulets). This is an abnormality of the muscle fiber in which there is a circumferential wrapping of a strip of the diseased fiber around itself (Fig. 17-10, *C*). On cross-section, the abnormal fiber has a rim of sarcoplasm in which the myofibrils run tangentially in relation to the longitudinally oriented fibrils in the center of the fiber.[151] The ring fiber may be associated with an irregular mass of sarcoplasm (sarcoplasmic mass) extending outward from the ring. These sarcoplasmic masses stain blue with H&E, red with modified Gomori trichrome, and intensely blue with NADH-TR. Ultrastructurally, ring fibers show subsarcolemmal myofilaments running perpendicular to the length of the fiber (Fig. 17-10, *D*), and sarcoplasmic masses appear as foci devoid of organized sarcoplasm and contain glycogen, mitochondria, ribosomes, and dense bodies. Both the ring fiber and the sarcoplasmic masses may be features of neuromuscular disorders other than myotonic dystrophy. Histochemical techniques have demonstrated atrophy of type 1 fibers. Smooth and cardiac muscle involvement is common in autopsy studies and is characterized by fibrous replacement of the myofibers. In a study of four patients with myotonic dystrophy and mental retardation, a disorder of cortical lamination was demonstrated at postmortem examination.[145] In congenital and infantile myotonic dystrophy the muscle may be normal or may show atrophy of either type 1 or 2 fibers.[6,105] Some fibers may be extremely small with internalized nuclei. On enzyme histochemistry, fiber type differentiation may be lacking.

Recent molecular genetic research has not only identified the underlying molecular lesion but has also provided an explanation for the phenomenon of "anticipation."[17] There appears to be an expansion of a trinucleotide (CTG) repeat downstream from a protein kinase gene on chromosome 19 that lengthens as it passes from one generation to the next. The length of the sequence correlates with the severity of the phenotype. DNA testing by Southern blot analysis performed on blood leukocytes is widely available for proband and prenatal diagnosis. A recent report describes three patients from two families with myotonic dystrophy who did not show an abnormal expansion of CTG trinucleotide repeats within the myotonic dystrophy gene.[167]

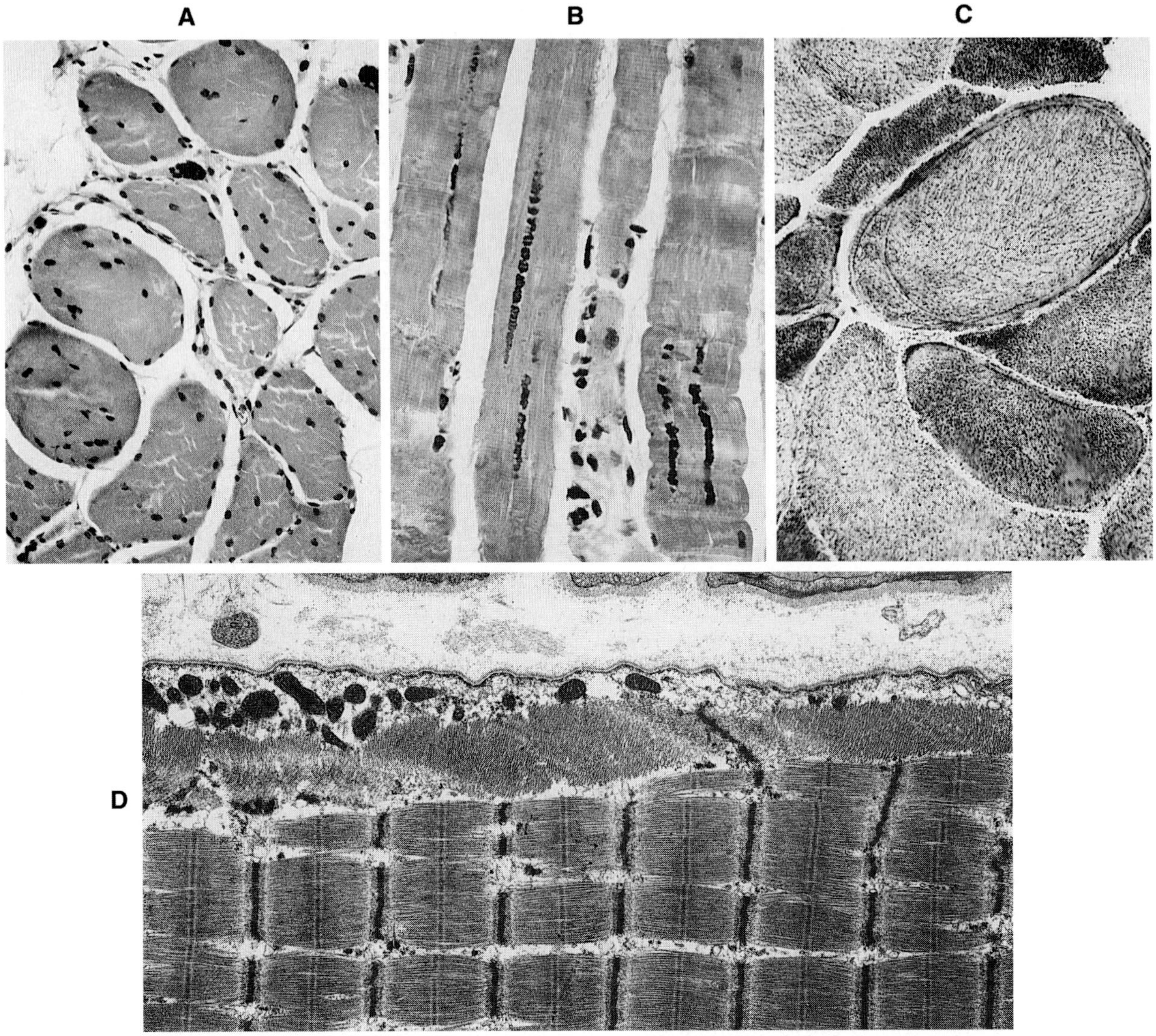

**Fig. 17-10.** Myotonic dystrophy. **A**, H&E section showing internalized nuclei and variation in fiber size. **B**, Longitudinal H&E section showing internalized nuclei arranged in chains. **C**, NADH-TR of ring fiber with the characteristic circumferential strip of myofibrils. **D**, Ultrastructure of ring fiber showing subsarcolemmal myofibrils running perpendicular to the long axis of the fiber. (**A**, original magnification ×170; **B**, original magnification ×270; **C**, original magnification ×430; **D**, original magnification ×8000.) (From De Girolami U, and Smith TW: Pathology of skeletal muscle diseases. Teaching monograph, Am J Pathol 107:235-276, 1982.)

***Distal myopathies.*** The distal myopathies are a phenotypically and genetically heterogeneous group characterized by relatively late onset, slowly progressive distal upper and/or lower extremity weakness, and variable CK elevation. The initial cases (autosomal dominant) were reported from Sweden[178]; cases also have been studied in the United States.[122,123] There have also been early-onset autosomal recessive types. Muscle biopsy studies show myopathic changes (variation in fiber size, internalized nuclei, vacuolated fibers, endomysial connective tissue proliferation) and, sometimes, angular atrophic fibers.

**Channelopathies**

***The periodic paralyses and paramyotonia congenita.*** *Periodic paralysis* is a group of disorders that share in common the clinical feature of attacks of paralysis with associated flaccidity, and a tendency to remit and relapse. Three forms are recognized, classified according to the level of serum potassium present during an attack. All three variants usually are inherited as autosomal-dominant traits, although they can also occur sporadically. The hypokalemic variant is the most common form of periodic paralysis. It is more common in males and symptoms usually appear first between

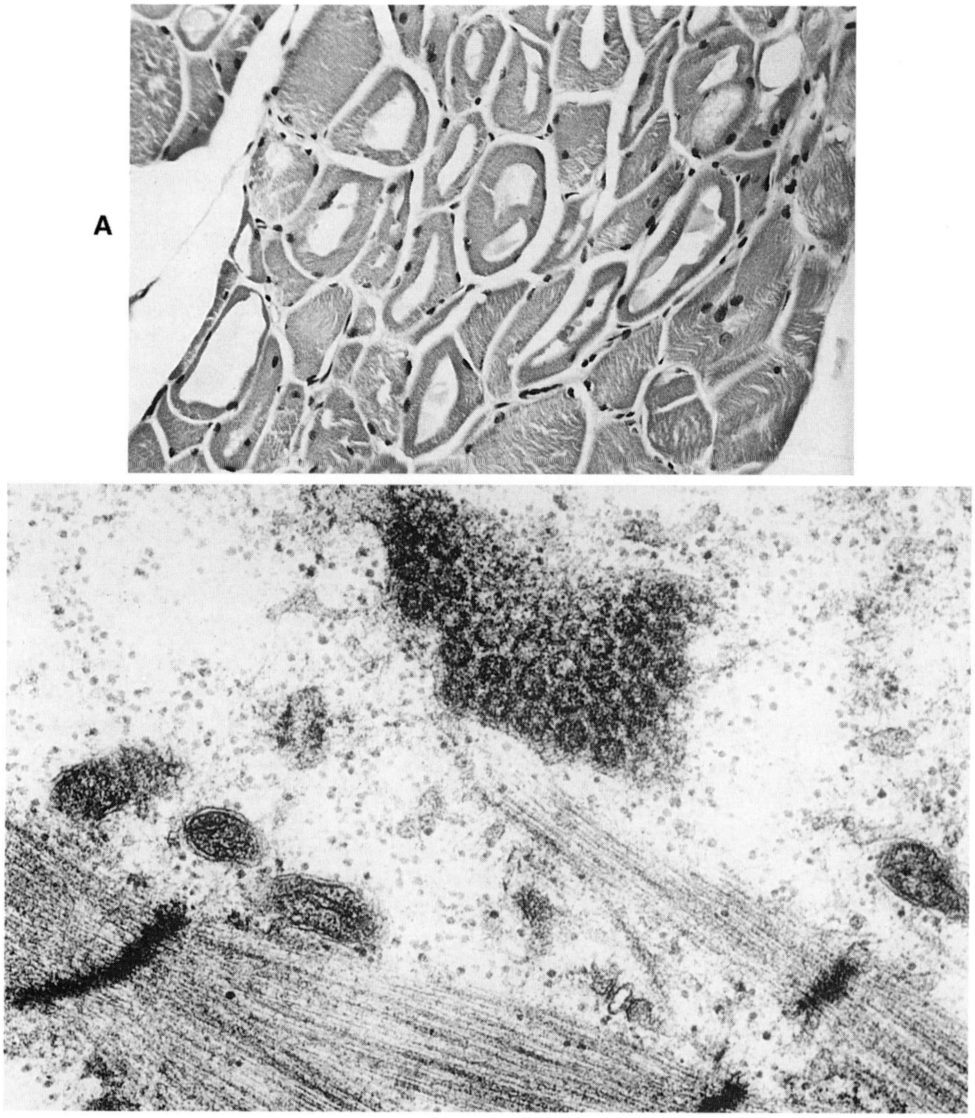

**Fig. 17-11.** Periodic paralysis. **A**, Light microscopy of transverse section showing numerous intracellular vacuoles. **B**, Electron microscopy showing small tubular aggregate. Each tubule consist of an electron-dense outer ring. (**A**, original magnification ×170; **B**, original magnification ×100,000.) (From De Girolami U, and Smith TW: Diseases of skeletal muscle and peripheral nerve. In Dickersin GR, editor: Diagnostic electron microscopy: a text atlas, New York, 1988, Igaku-Shoin.)

the ages of 20 and 35 years. The disorder is characterized by the appearance of sudden attacks of generalized muscle paralysis with relative sparing of the external ocular and respiratory muscles. The attacks usually occur at night and are precipitated by prior strenuous exercise, a high carbohydrate meal, or exposure to cold. Serum potassium levels during an attack are low. Between attacks, patients are usually normal, although there may be some residual muscle weakness. The hyperkalemic variant usually begins in childhood and tends to affect both sexes equally. Unlike the hypokalemic variant, the attacks often occur during the daytime and are usually briefer but more frequent. There may be considerable variation in the extent and severity of weakness. Some patients may display myotonia, especially of face and hand muscles. Characteristically, there is a rise in serum potassium levels during an attack, although the elevation may at times be minimal. The attacks may be precipitated by exercise or exposure to cold, and can also be induced by the administration of potassium chloride. Normokalemic periodic paralysis shares many clinical features with the hyperkalemic variant. Serum potassium levels typically remain unchanged during an attack.

The pathologic findings in all forms of periodic paralysis are qualitatively similar, but tend to be most pronounced in the hypokalemic variant. The principal abnormality seen by light microscope consists of variable numbers of vacuoles within myofibers (Fig. 17-11*A*). The vacuoles are more often encountered in biopsy specimens taken from during an acute attack; the muscle may in fact appear normal between episodes. The most conspicuous vacuolar changes, however, are seen in muscle biopsies obtained from patients who have a permanent myopathy resulting from long-standing disease with recurrent episodes of paralysis. The vacuoles vary in size but can be quite large, and they tend to occupy the interior rather than the periphery of the fiber. Multiloculated vacuoles also can be seen. The vacuoles usually appear "empty" but may occasionally contain PAS-positive, diastase-digestible granular material and, rarely, calcium. In addition to the vacuoles, biopsies from patients with a permanent or persistent myopathy also may show other myopathic features including variation in fiber size, internal nuclei, fiber necrosis, moth-eaten fibers, and proliferation of connective tissue. Electron microscopic studies show that the vacuoles arise from the proliferation, degeneration, and autophagic destruction of membranous organelles derived chiefly from the sarcoplasmic reticulum and T-system tubules.

Another morphologic change often encountered in periodic paralysis, especially in the hyperkalemic and normokalemic variants, is the presence of tubular aggregates (Fig. 17-11, *B*). In H&E-stained sections, tubular aggregates are basophilic deposits found in both the interior and periphery of muscle fibers. They stain intensely red with the modified trichrome method; they also can be demonstrated with the NADH-TR reaction, but fail to stain with the succinic dehydrogenase (SDH) reaction, thus distinguishing them from mitochondria. Tubular aggregates are found predominantly, but not exclusively, in type 2 fibers. Ultrastructurally, tubular aggregates consist of fascicular arrays of parallel double-walled tubules having diameters of 60 to 90 nm. On cross-section, these aggregates form a hexagonal profile. The tubules sometimes can be observed in continuity with the dilated terminal cisterns of the sarcoplasmic reticulum, from which they are thought to be derived.

Paramyotonia congenita is an autosomal dominant myotonic disorder showing paradoxic myotonia (i.e., myotonia that appears during exercise and increases with continued exercise) that is especially severe after exposure to cold and involves the muscles of the face, neck, and distal upper extremities. The disease begins in childhood, and the clinical picture is also characterized by episodes of flaccid paresis that may be precipitated by exposure to cold.[64] A few muscle biopsy studies describe minimal changes, including variation in fiber size, internalized nuclei, and poor differentiation of fiber types.[168]

Different defects in the same gene on chromosome 17 cause hyperkalemic periodic paralysis and paramyotonia congenita.[117] The gene controls the production of a sodium channel protein, which regulates the entry of sodium during muscle contraction.[76] Hypokalemic periodic paralysis is not related to the sodium channel gene on chromosome 17; the disease may be caused by a gene defect responsible for a different type of sodium channel or to some other protein controlling sodium flow.

***Channelopathies associated with myotonia (myotonia congenita: Thomsen's disease and Becker's myotonia).*** Myotonia congenita presents in childhood with diffuse stiffness on initiation of motor activities, for example, arising from a chair or starting to walk or run. Strength usually remains normal. The CK may be normal or up to 3 times normal and the EMG studies show myotonic discharges. The autosomal dominant variant is referred to as Thomsen's disease,[166] and the disease starts earlier in childhood than does the autosomal recessive form (Becker's myotonia). Muscle biopsy studies have shown minimal changes including internalized nuclei and variation in fiber size. One report describes a remarkable absence of type 2B fibers[36]; other cases have not shown this histochemical abnormality.[109] Both the dominant and recessive forms are channelopathies linked to the human skeletal muscle chloride channel gene on chromosome 7.[108]

**Congenital myopathies.** The term *congenital myopathy* was first introduced by Shy and Magee in 1956[156] to denote a muscle disease that is present at birth, has a nonprogressive course, and carries a benign prognosis. As used currently, the clinical range of symptoms is great: from severe infantile weakness and hypotonia resulting in early death, to mild weakness presenting in childhood, to isolated cardiomyopathy in adulthood.[65,83] These disorders, therefore, usually cannot be distinguished from one another clinically; in addition to the varied symptoms and ages of presentation, EMG studies typically show nonspecific findings, and the CK level is usually normal or only mildly elevated. At present, the diagnosis of congenital myopathy is based largely on finding the characteristic changes on the muscle biopsy.

***Nemaline myopathy.*** The clinical presentation of patients with nemaline myopathy is variable, as indicated in a number of studies.[19,65,95,155] Severe neonatal hypotonia and weakness resulting in death from respiratory causes occurs rarely. The more common clinical picture consists of neonatal hypotonia without respiratory distress, delayed achievement of motor milestones, and varying degrees of generalized weakness.

These children have a characteristic appearance, with a long, narrow (dolicocephalic) head; thin, asthenic build; and skeletal deformities (kyphoscoliosis, pectus excavatum, pes cavus, and clubfoot). The weakness is most evident in the pelvic girdle and anterior compartment of the legs; often, deep tendon reflexes are absent. Extraocular muscles are spared. The course is typically static or very slowly progressive. An adult-onset form with the muscle pathology seen in the congenital form also has been described. These patients lack the skeletal abnormalities of the congenital type, and their occurrence is sporadic rather than familial. Rarely, cardiomyopathy is the only manifestation of the disorder, or occurs in association with generalized weakness. The CK in nemaline myopathy generally is normal. EMG studies of affected muscles may demonstrate nonspecific myopathic changes, although neurogenic features in very weak muscles also have been observed.

Shy and co-workers coined the term "nemaline myopathy"[155] (from the Greek word $\nu\eta\mu\alpha$, meaning thread) to describe the rodlike or threadlike inclusions that are the pathologic hallmark of the disorder (Fig. 17-12, *A*). These structures are most easily demonstrated on the modified Gomori trichrome stain on fro-

A

B

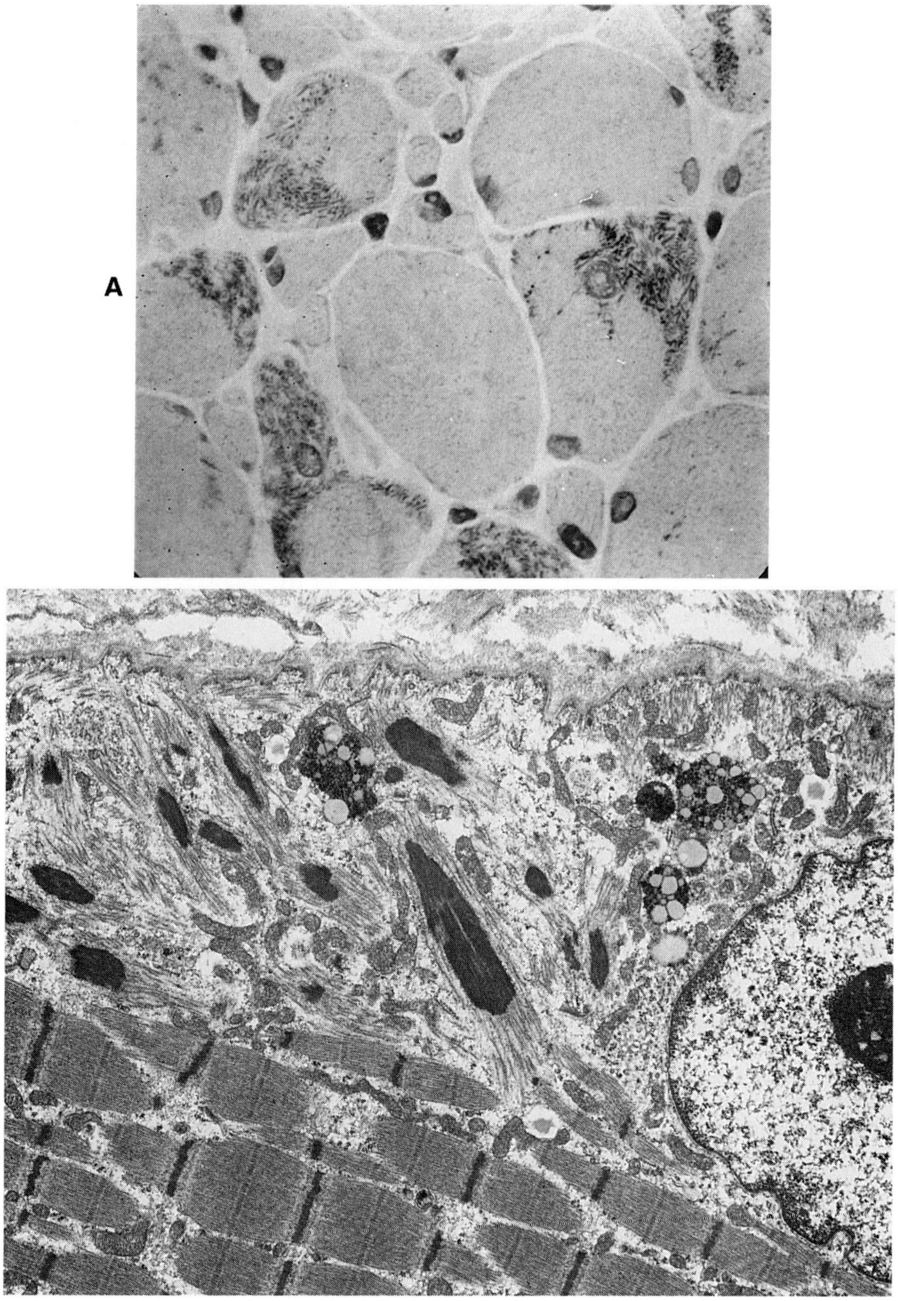

**Fig. 17-12.** Nemaline myopathy. **A**, Trichrome stain showing subsarcolemmal and internal thread like inclusions. **B**, Electron micrograph showing subsarcolemmal osmiophilic deposits. (**A**, original magnification ×400; **B**, original magnification ×19,500.)

zen sections, where the nemaline rods appear as red aggregates, 2 to 7 $\mu$m in diameter, frequently in a perinuclear or subsarcolemmal location. There is considerable variation in the distribution of the nemaline rods among patients, and among muscles within the same individual. Nemaline rods are found primarily in type 1 fibers and there is a varying degree of type 1 predominance in patients with this disorder. Ultrastructural examination of biopsies from patients with the disorder demonstrates many rods, appearing as dense osmiophilic structures that seemingly are in continuity with the Z-bands (Fig. 17-12, *B*), and have a similar filamentous pattern to the Z-bands when cut on transverse section.[81] Little correlation has been observed between the number and distribution of the inclusions and the severity of the weakness. Nemaline rods consist primarily of $\alpha$-actinin, a major component of the Z-band. Nemaline rods are not specific for nemaline myopathy and may be seen in myotonic dystrophy, muscular dystrophies, inflammatory myopathies, and near tendinous insertions.

Molecular analysis is incomplete. One large Australian family affected with nemaline myopathy demonstrated linkage to chromosome 1q21-23.[112]

***Centronuclear (myotubular) myopathy.*** Three distinct forms of this entity have come to light since its original description, each exhibiting a different presentation, progression, and inheritance pattern.[65,177] A neonatal form presenting with severe hypotonia and weakness at birth often leads to death from respiratory insufficiency. Ptosis and ophthalmoplegia, hallmarks of the more common late infantile-early childhood type, are also, but less commonly, seen in the neonatal period. Patients with the late infantile-early childhood variety of the disorder display delayed attainment of motor milestones, especially walking. Ptosis and ophthalmoplegia help to distinguish centronuclear myopathy from other types of congenital myopathy. In addition, there is generalized weakness and hypotonia, as well as areflexia. Severe facial weakness may be present. The characteristic appearance of affected children is that of a slender build and a long, narrow face. As in many of the congenital myopathies, skeletal abnormalities, including club feet and scoliosis, may be part of the syndrome. In this form, the course of the disease may be static to slowly progressive. Focal and generalized seizures have been reported. The least common form of centronuclear myopathy is the late childhood-adult type. The onset is in the second or third decade, with mild, usually nonprogressive weakness in a limb-girdle distribution. These patients generally have no ophthalmoplegia, and ptosis is rare in this group. Typically, normal or only mildly elevated CK values are the rule for all forms of centronuclear myopathy. The EMG often shows nonspecific myopathic features; sometimes, more distinct abnormalities, such as fibrillations, positive sharp waves, and myotonic discharges, may exist in some patients.

Spiro and colleagues[161] coined the term "myotubular myopathy," using it to describe the characteristic morphologic features of skeletal muscle in the disorder, which they felt resembled an arrested stage of embryonic muscle development. Since there is little compelling evidence now that this is the case, the more widely accepted term for the disorder is "centronuclear myopathy"; "type 1 fiber hypotrophy and central nuclei"[60] has also been used. The predominant morphologic feature of the disorder, shared by all three types, is the presence of fibers with a centrally located, somewhat enlarged/rounded nucleus often surrounded by a clear myofibril-poor zone (Fig. 17-13, *A* and *B*) that contains granular debris on ultrastructural examination (Fig. 17-13, *C* and *D*). On transverse sections, the central nuclei are detected in a variable number of fibers, ranging from 25% to 90%. There is generally a greater involvement of type 1 fibers, and type 1 fiber predominance is frequently seen; these predominant type 1 fibers often are smaller than the remaining type 2 fibers. Longitudinally-oriented sections reveal many fibers containing chains of centrally-placed nuclei interspersed with elliptical myofibril-free zones. H&E, trichrome, and NADH-TR staining may reveal radial striations of affected fibers on cross-section. The central area frequently demonstrates increased oxidative enzyme activity and decreased ATPase activity; these central perinuclear regions contain a decreased number of myofilaments and increased amounts of glycogen, mitochondria, and lysosomes. Central nuclei also are found in the extraocular muscles.[14] There are conflicting reports of an abnormality (persistence) of desmin and vimentin.[68,69,134,150]

Current molecular genetic studies indicate that the gene for the X-linked form of myotubular myopathy is on Xq28; however, additional genetic linkage studies are needed to examine the possibility of genetic heterogeneity.[97,149] The molecular basis of the milder autosomal dominant or recessive phenotype has not been established.

***Central core disease.*** Central core disease was the first of the congenital myopathies to be defined. Shy and Magee in 1956[156] described five patients within three generations of a family who manifested hypotonia and weakness. As with other congenital myopathies the time of onset of symptoms is quite variable.[65] The patient's mother may describe decreased fetal movement in utero and a breech presentation with a hypotonic, weak infant. In childhood, delayed motor milestones, especially walking, may be the first sign of this neuromuscular disorder. Proximal lower extremity weakness may become evident only when an affected child begins to climb stairs or attempts to arise from a seated or supine position. Weakness of facial

A B

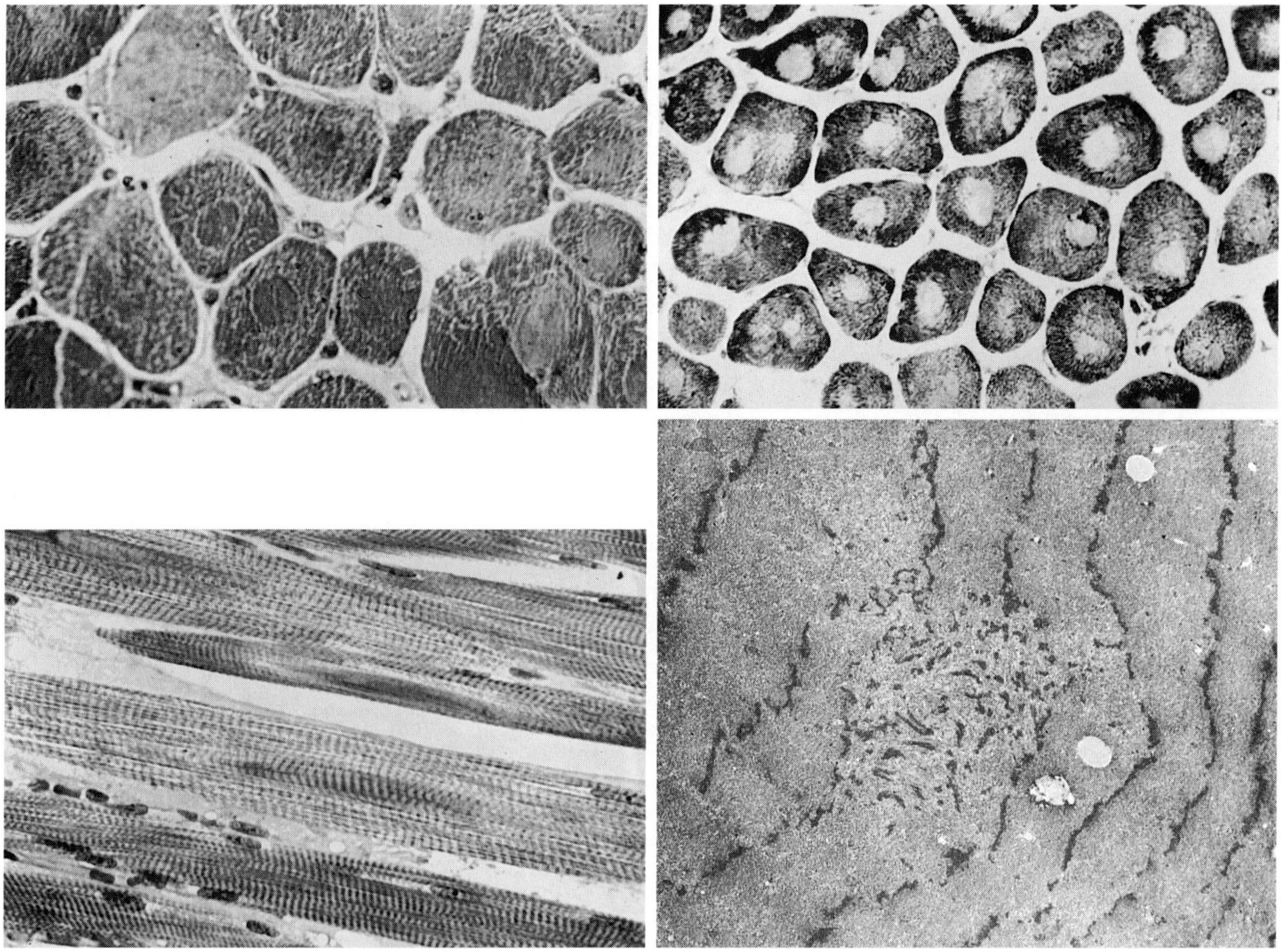

C D

**Fig. 17-13.** Centronuclear myopathy. **A**, Light micrograph of transverse section of muscle with ATPase reaction at pH 4.3 taken shortly after birth showing small rounded fibers and central area of clearing which is sometimes occupied by nucleus. **B**, Light micrograph of transverse section of muscle from the same patient illustrated in **B** at 3 years of age. The modified Gomori trichrome stain shows variation in fiber size and centralized nuclei primarily in the small fibers. **C**, **D**, Electron micrographs of transverse of muscle biopsy from patient illustrated in **A** showing in **C**, Granular, myofibril-free zone and **D**, Centralized nucleus. (**C**, original magnification ×9500; **D**, original magnification ×15,700.) (**A**, **B**, Courtesy of Dr. M. Rodriguez, **D**; Courtesy of H. Mulhern.)

musculature occasionally has been reported, but the extraocular muscles are spared; this feature helps distinguish the disorder from centronuclear myopathy. Kyphoscoliosis, pes cavus and planus, and other skeletal anomalies are frequent. Adults afflicted with central core disease have varying degrees of proximal weakness, usually more pronounced in the lower extremities. In all types, the course is generally nonprogressive. The CK level usually is normal, and EMG findings are consistent with an underlying myopathy. There is an increased incidence of malignant hyperthermia in patients with central core disease.

The pathologic hallmark of the disorder is the presence of central cores (Fig. 17-14, *A* to *D*). On cross section these cylindrical structures consist of patches of dark-staining material that can be seen on both paraffin-embedded and frozen sections stained with trichrome stains, and sometimes also with H&E.[156] The cores may be multiple and are said to extend through the length of the fiber (although this may be difficult to demonstrate). Cores are well demonstrated with the NADH-TR reaction as internal regions of the fiber that are oxidative enzyme-deficient. Cores occur almost exclusively in type 1 fibers. Cores can easily be confused with target fibers, which also contain pale-staining central regions within type 1 fibers on the NADH-TR preparation. However, the pale central areas of target fibers are surrounded by a ring of increased enzymatic

A 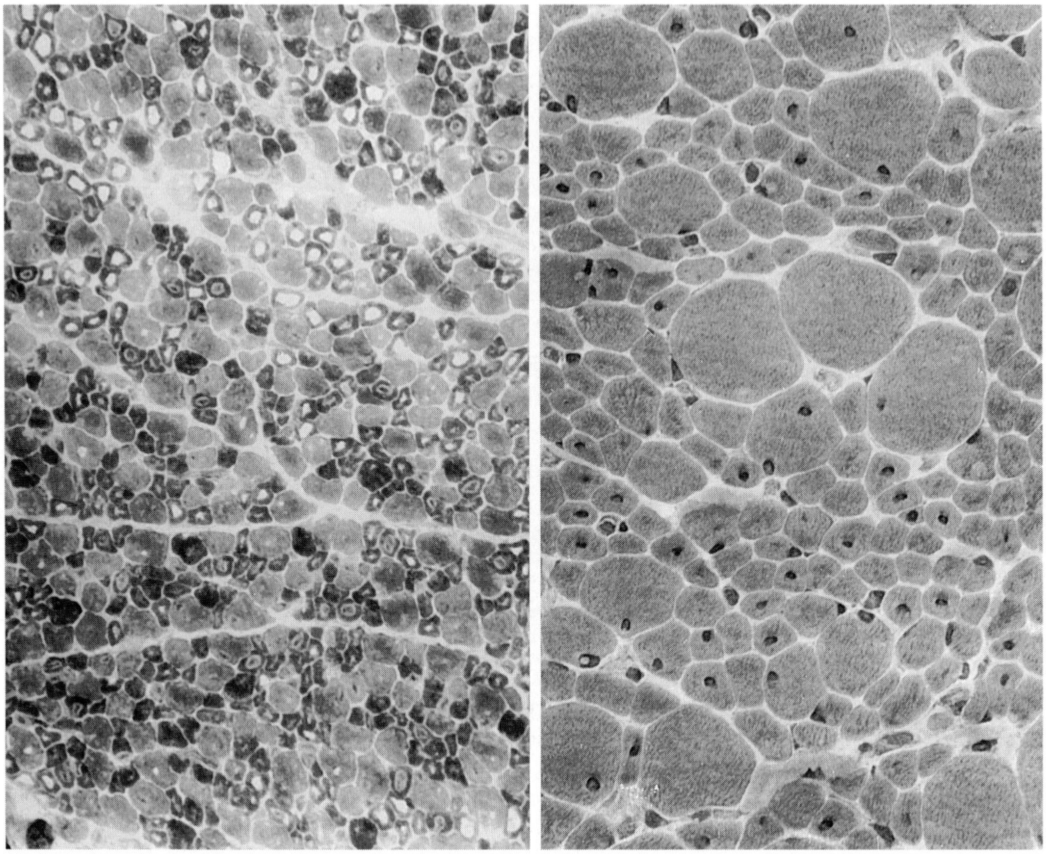 B

**Fig. 17-14.** Central core disease. **A**, Light micrograph of transverse section of muscle with the Masson trichrome stain showing cores. **B**, NADH-TR reaction showing lack of reactivity in the core region. **C**, Longitudinal section with the PTAH to show extent of the core. **D**, Electron micrograph of core showing central region of myofibrillar disorganization. (**A**, original magnification ×170; **B**, original magnification ×300; **C**, original magnification ×170; **D**, original magnification ×11,000.) (**A**, from De Girolami U, and Smith TW: Pathology of skeletal muscle diseases. Teaching monograph, Am J Pathol 107:235-276, 1982. **B**, from De Girolami U, and Smith TW: Diseases of skeletal muscle and peripheral nerve. In Dickersin: GR, editor: Diagnostic electron microscopy: a text atlas, New York, 1988, Igaku-Shoin.)

activity that separates them from the normally-staining periphery. As cores contain decreased amounts of glycogen, they appear as pale regions within the fibers on the PAS stain. On the ATPase stains, on which the cores may be barely visible, type 1 fiber predominance is demonstrated. Cores are composed of disorganized and poorly-aligned sarcomeres (Fig. 17-14, *D*). The cores are devoid of mitochondria and contain reduced amounts of sarcoplasmic reticulum and glycogen, accounting for some of their staining characteristics.

It appears that a subset of central core disease patients have missense mutations of the ryanodine (sarcoplasmic reticulum calcium release channel) receptor gene on chromosome 19.[85] Mutations of this gene are also associated with the malignant hyperthermia trait; the latter susceptibility is well documented in patients with central core disease.

***Congenital fiber type disproportion (CFTD).*** Like the other congenital myopathies, CFTD has variable onset, severity, and progression. Many children are floppy at birth and exhibit weakness. Some patients progress to significant weakness and respiratory failure; others eventually attain normal strength. The CK is normal or mildly elevated and the EMG is often normal. The principal histopathologic characteristic of the disease is the overall predominance of type 1 fibers, generally in the range of 70% to 90% (Fig. 17-15). There is also variability in fiber size such that the type 1 fibers are smaller than normal and type 2 fibers are in the normal range. No other consistent light or electron microscopic abnormalities have been noted. There is some uncertainty about whether CFTD is a distinct disorder; concomitant histopathologic features characteristic of other congenital myopathies are frequent (cores, central nuclei). Genetic studies have indicated considerable heterogeneity; some pedigrees have shown autosomal dominant and others autosomal recessive inheritance.

C

D

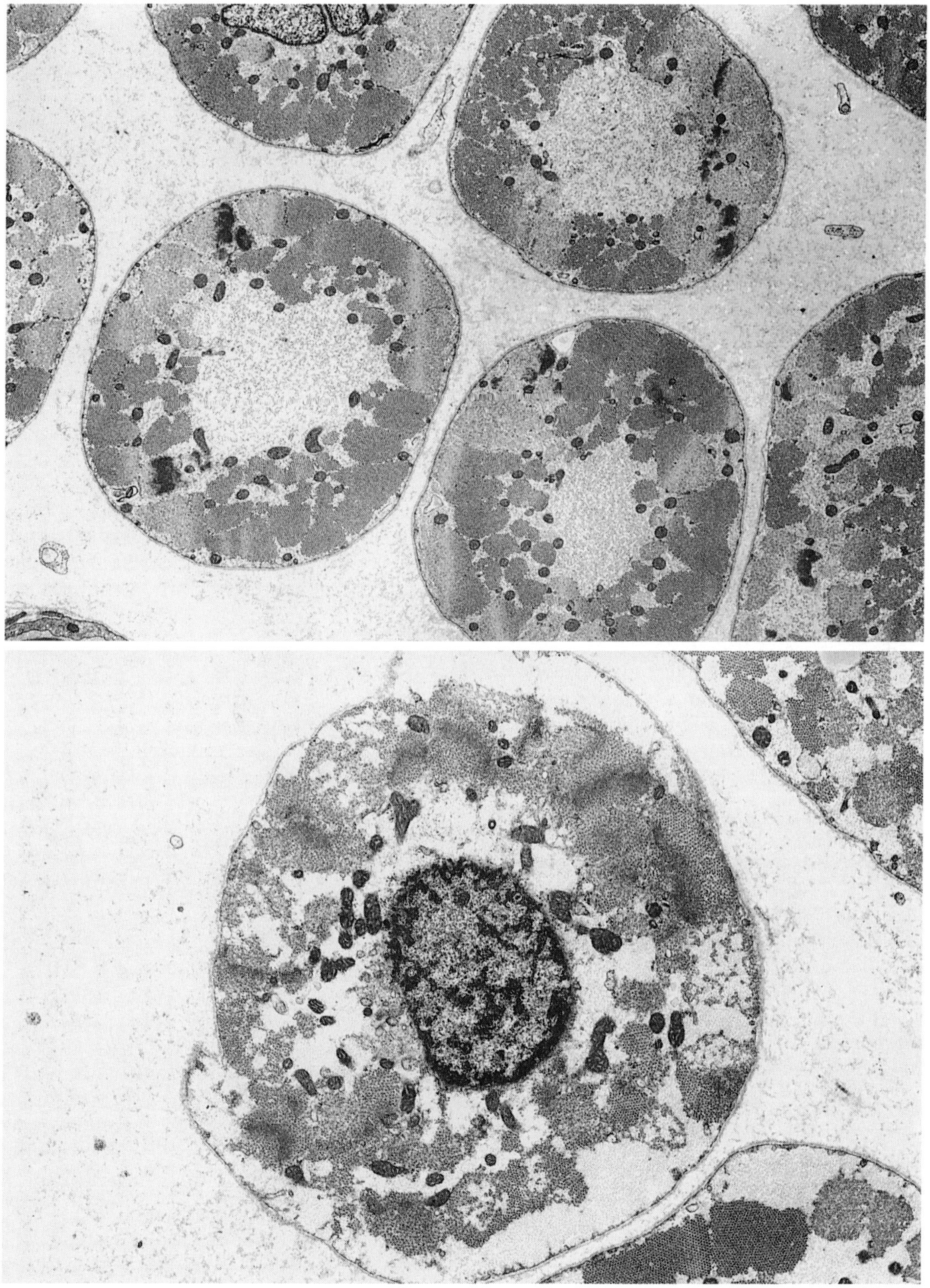

**Fig. 17-14, cont'd.** For legend see opposite page.

***Other congenital myopathies.*** A number of other poorly understood myopathies have been included with the congenital myopathies and defined in isolated case reports primarily on the basis of the demonstration of characteristic histochemical and/or ultrastructural features. These include multicore disease, fingerprint body myopathy, reducing body myopathy, sarcotubular myopathy, myopathy with tubular aggregates, familial myopathy with probable lysis of myofibrils in type 1 fibers, trilaminar fiber myopathy, cap disease, zebra body myopathy, cytoplasmic or spheroid body myopathy, and desmin storage myopathies.[65]

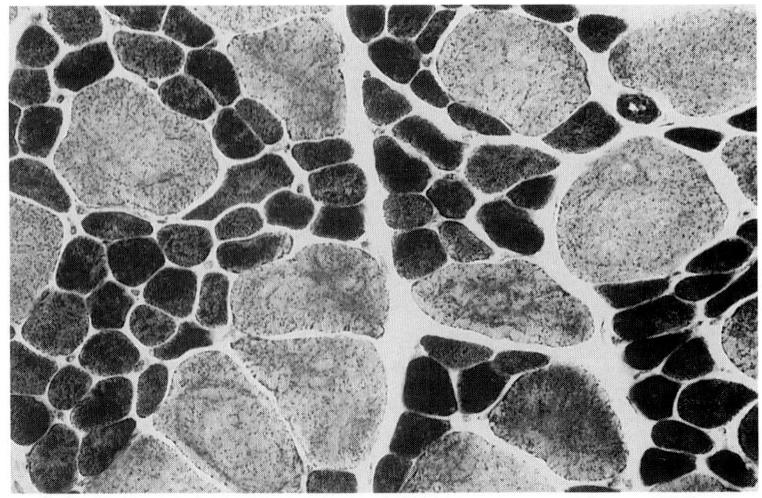

**Fig. 17-15.** Congenital fiber-type disproportion. NADH-TR stain showing small type 1 fibers arranged in clusters. (Original magnification ×170.) (From De Girolami U, and Smith TW: Pathology of skeletal muscle diseases. Teaching monograph, Am J Pathol 107:235-276, 1982.)

The nosologic status of these entities is tenuous and their molecular basis is unknown at this time.

**Metabolic myopathy.** The term "metabolic myopathy" is used when an abnormality in the metabolism of the muscle results in abnormal function. Such an abnormality may be acquired, as in the case of hepatic or renal failure, or may be due to an inborn error of metabolism involving skeletal muscle. Sometimes, storage of materials such as glycogen or lipid is associated with the myopathy; at other times the metabolic lesion results in muscle injury with little or no morphologic change. Where no structural abnormality is recognized by conventional light microscopy, histochemical studies sometimes demonstrate a specific enzymatic defect. The following discussion will be limited to the most important entities. The reader is referred to standard reference texts on myology and disorders of metabolism for a complete discussion of this subject.[55,152]

***Glycogen-metabolism myopathies.*** In the course of intracellular digestion, glycogen is hydrolyzed within lysosomes by acid maltase. When this process fails to take place, glycogen, accumulating within lysosomal vacuoles, leads to muscle fiber damage. The clinical consequence is painless, progressive muscle weakness. Glycogen in the cytosol is a major fuel for glycolytic, fast twitch, type 2A and 2B fibers. As glycogen is metabolized anaerobically to pyruvate and lactate, ATP is generated. Abnormalities in glycolytic enzymes lead to glycogen accumulation in the sarcoplasm, reduced lactate production, reduced formation of ATP, and impairment in muscle fiber metabolism, leading to rhabdomyolysis. The clinical manifestations of this disorder include myalgia (aches, cramps, and pains), fatigue, and myoglobinuria.

*Acid maltase deficiency (Pompe's disease)*—Acid maltase deficiency or alpha glucosidase deficiency is a progressive illness with three major clinical subtypes. The infantile, most common form (Pompe's disease), becomes manifest in the first 3 months of life and is characterized by severe hypotonia (floppy baby), progressive weakness, and heart failure. There is enlargement of the heart, liver, and tongue. Death ensues by 2 years of age from cardiac and respiratory failure. The childhood form has a later onset and is the least common form of the disease. There is a delay in reaching motor milestones, followed by progressive weakness of proximal limb and trunk muscles. The liver and tongue may be enlarged, but cardiomegaly is rare. Death occurs before the end of the second decade from respiratory insufficiency. In the adult form, symptoms begin in adolescence or well into adulthood, with slowly progressive weakness and wasting of proximal limb muscles and diaphragm and sparing of bulbar musculature. Respiratory muscle weakness may lead to death. The heart and liver are not affected. The CK is elevated in most patients. The EMG discloses myopathic motor unit potentials, fibrillations, positive sharp waves, bizarre high frequency discharges, and true myotonic bursts.

Of all the glycogenoses, acid maltese deficiency (AMD) has the most distinct morphologic pattern; the muscle biopsy findings are similar in all three types. Since acid maltase is a lysosomal enzyme, a deficiency or absence of this enzyme leads to the accumulation of glycogen within lysosomes. Light microscopy of paraffin-embedded sections shows vacuolization of the sarcoplasm and frozen sections of muscle demonstrate multiple intracytoplasmic vacuoles of varying sizes with massive accumulations of diastase-sensitive, PAS-positive material and high acid phosphatase activity (Fig. 17-16, *A* and *B*). Electron microscopy shows clusters of glycogen granules free in the cytoplasm or in membranous sacs, as well as autophagic vacuoles containing degradation products (Fig. 17-16, *C*). Extensive replacement of the myofibrillar content is seen in many fibers. In adult cases, the glycogen-containing vacuoles may be few and small.

A

B

C

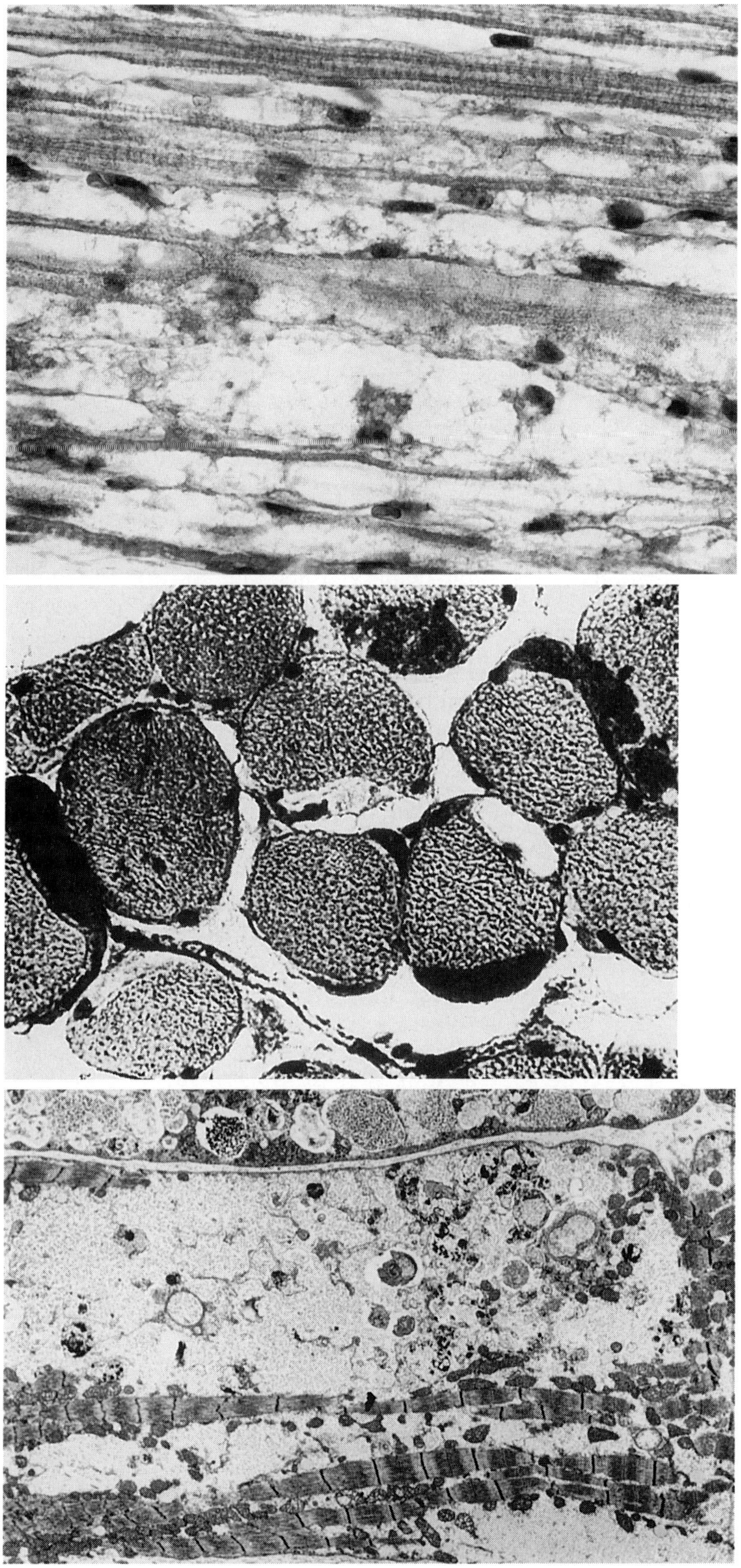

**Fig. 17-16.** Glycogen storage myopathy. **A**, Light micrograph of PTAH longitudinal section of muscle in Pompe's disease showing extensive vacuolization of sarcoplasm. **B**, Light micrograph of transverse section of muscle showing PAS-positive subsarcolemmal deposits. **C**, Electron micrograph of muscle biopsy from a patient with acid maltase deficiency showing pools of intermyofibrillar and subsarcolemmal glycogen. (**A**, original magnification ×170; **B**, original magnification ×400; **C**, original magnification ×5000.) (**B**, Courtesy of Dr. RD Adams; **C**, from De Girolami U, and Smith TW: Diseases of skeletal muscle and peripheral nerve. In Dickersin: GR, editor: Diagnostic electron microscopy: a text atlas, New York, 1988, Igaku-Shoin.)

The mechanisms of muscle fiber injury in AMD are thought to involve both the excessive storage of undergraded lysosomal material, which compromises vital cellular structures, and increased lysosomal activity. Both the severe and more benign forms are inherited as autosomal-recessive traits. Acid maltase deficiency is caused by alterations of the gene on chromosome 17 (see review[56]). Detailed correlation of genotypic variability with biochemical variability and clinical heterogeneity has not been completed. Proband and prenatal diagnosis generally is accomplished by biochemical assay of acid maltase in muscle, cultured fibroblasts, urine, or amniotic fluid cells. More recently, RFLP strategies have proved useful for making prenatal diagnosis when DNA is available from a previously affected individual.

***Nonlysosomal glycogenoses: myophosphorylase deficiency (McArdle's disease)***—In about one half of the patients with myophosphorylase deficiency the disease is inherited as an autosomal-recessive trait; in sporadic cases autosomal-dominant transmission has been reported. Males outnumber females by a ratio of 3:1. In about one half of patients, muscle necrosis and myoglobinuria are demonstrable. Renal failure is a life-threatening complication of myoglobinuria. Patients learn to avoid sudden bursts of activity and prefer less intense but sustained exercise. Between attacks, patients are well and can lead reasonably normal lives. Rarely, the disease presents with weakness and wasting in adult life without exercise intolerance, suggesting an acquired late-onset myopathy. In patients suspected of having the disease, ischemic forearm exercise should be performed under standard conditions. The peak level of venous lactate occurs within 3 to 5 minutes after exercise in normal subjects, reaching three to five times the resting pre-exercise level. Because patients with McArdle's disease are unable to break down glycogen, venous lactate fails to rise. Reduced lactate production, however, is not specific for McArdle's disease and is seen with other defects of the glycolytic pathway. The CK is elevated in most patients at rest, and the EMG is abnormal in almost one half of the patients, showing myopathic potentials especially in patients with permanent weakness.

The biopsy specimen may be structurally normal, except for the complete absence of phosphorylase activity demonstrable only by specific histochemical reactions. In addition to a nonreactive phosphorylase there may be subsarcolemmal vacuoles or blebs filled with glycogen that are demonstrable by the PAS reaction (Fig. 17-16, *B*). Biopsies often also show scattered necrotic and regenerating fibers, especially prominent if the patient has had a recent episode of myoglobinuria. Ultrastructural studies demonstrate that the glycogen granules are not membrane bound.

The disease is caused by a deficiency of myophosphorylase that is restricted to skeletal muscle. The gene that encodes for the enzyme was initially localized to the long arm of chromosome 11,[115] and recent advances in the molecular biology of the disease are summarized by DiMauro and Tsujino.[47] Isoenzymes under separate genetic control are present in other tissues. Genetic heterogeneity has been demonstrated in McArdle's disease, but the most common mutation is the substitution of thymine for cytosine at codon 49. In most patients the diagnosis can now be made from the patient's leukocytes.[47,172]

***Phosphofructokinase deficiency (PFKD)***—Genetic transmission of the syndrome is autosomal recessive. The typical clinical syndrome is very similar to McArdle's disease (exercise intolerance with cramps and sometimes myoglobinuria), but some patients have been described with onset of weakness in middle life and without cramps or myoglobinuria. Some patients also have mild hemolytic anemia, and red blood cell phosphofructokinase (PFK) activity is reduced by 50%. An infantile myopathy has delayed motor development.[3]

The muscle biopsy findings are identical to those of McArdle's disease except that, unlike phosphorylase deficiency, hyaline polysaccharide inclusions (Lafora body-like by light and electron microscopy) have been found in some cases.[87] This polysaccharide stains with PAS but is not digested by salivary diastase. The accumulated material is similar to that found in patients who have brancher enzyme deficiency. In patients with PFK deficiency, there is absence of PFK activity as determined by histochemical or quantitative biochemical techniques.

PFK, the glycolytic enzyme that catalyzes the conversion of fructose 6-phosphate to fructose 1,6-diphosphate, is absent in skeletal muscle in PFKD. The M (muscle) subunit of the enzyme is present in muscle and red blood cells; red cells also have the L (liver) subunit. The gene encoding for the M subunit of PFK is on chromosome 1.[175]

***Debrancher enzyme deficiency (DED)***—Debrancher enzyme deficiency is an autosomal recessive disease that begins in infancy with hepatomegaly, growth retardation, fasting hypoglycemia, and cirrhosis. The enzyme defect has been demonstrated in muscle, liver, leukocytes, and red blood cells. In the absence of debrancher enzyme activity, phosphorylase may hydrolyze the 1,4-glycosidic linkages to the point of branching. The resultant glycogen molecule has an excess number of exposed 1,6-glycosidic linkages and is referred to as *limit dextrin*. Myopathy is sometimes difficult to recognize in very ill infants, but hypotonia, lethargy, or delayed motor milestones are common. The disease also has been recognized as a cause of slowly progressive weakness in adults. Unlike

McArdle's disease and PFKD, cramps and myoglobinuria are not features of this disease. The venous lactate level does not rise during ischemic exercise. Serum CK may be markedly elevated. The EMG shows myopathic features or a mixture of myopathic and neurogenic patterns.

The muscle biopsy in DED shows a severe vacuolar myopathy with subsarcolemmal and intramyofibrillar coarse, PAS-positive vacuoles that are digested by diastase. Ultrastructural studies show findings similar to those seen in McArdle's disease, that is, pools of non-membrane-bound glycogen.

The debrancher enzyme locus has been assigned to chromosome 1p21. The pathogenesis of the muscle weakness in DED is obscure. There is a concomitant peripheral neuropathy, with glycogen accumulations in Schwann cells, which may contribute to the neurologic disability.

***Other glycogenoses*** — Other, rarer nonlysosomal glycogenoses recently reviewed by DiMauro and Tsujino[47] include deficiencies of phosphoglycerate kinase (chromosome Xq13), phosphoglycerate mutase (chromosome 7), and lactate dehydrogenase (chromosome 11—subunit M; chromosome 12—subunit H). The enzyme effects in all three diseases may produce muscle pain, weakness, and (when exercise persists in the face of myalgia) myoglobinuria. None of these enzyme defects produces a complete block of the glycolytic pathway, and thus severe glycogen accumulation does not occur. The muscle biopsy may show evidence of glycogen storage. Brancher enzyme deficiency is a rapidly progressive autosomal recessive lethal disease of childhood with prominent liver dysfunction; hypotonia has been observed in some patients. Muscle biopsy studies have shown intensely PAS-positive intracytoplasmic deposits that are incompletely digestible with diastase. In these cases and in variants thereof, ultrastructural studies have shown Lafora-like bodies, whereas the glycogen granules appear normal; similar structures also are found in the central and peripheral nervous systems.[90]

***Lipid-metabolism myopathies.*** Fatty acids are the major fuel for muscle at rest, in the fasting state, and during prolonged, low-intensity aerobic exercise. They are mobilized from fat deposits and oxidized in muscle mitochondria. Short-chain fatty acids penetrate the mitochondrial membrane with ease, but long-chain fatty acids (palmitic and oleic) are impermeable unless combined with carnitine, which facilitates their transport to intramitochondrial sites. Inside the muscle fiber, fatty acids are activated to fatty acyl-CoA derivatives. On the outer mitochondrial membrane, these are joined to carnitine by carnitine palmitoyltransferase I (CPT I) to form a permeable derivative, fatty acylcarnitine, which moves across the mitochondrial membrane into the mitochondria. There, CPT II catalyzes the reverse reaction, with the formation of fatty acyl-CoA, which can then undergo oxidation. Two main categories of disordered muscle lipid metabolism have been identified: (1) carnitine deficiency, characterized by progressive weakness and excessive muscle fiber lipid storage; and (2) CPT deficiency, causing recurrent muscle pain and myoglobinuria with minimal muscle fiber lipid accumulation.

***Muscle carnitine deficiency*** — In 1972, Engel and Siekert[58] described a 19-year-old woman with lifelong mild generalized weakness that rapidly progressed, rendering her bed-fast and in need of respiratory support. Muscle biopsy disclosed excessive lipid accumulation, especially in type 1 fibers. The lipid accumulation was associated with muscle carnitine deficiency. Since that description, additional familial cases have been described that fall into two seemingly distinct groups. In the first, the myopathic form, carnitine deficiency is limited to muscle and the major clinical manifestation is myopathy. In the second, the systemic form, carnitine deficiency is widespread, and clinical features are dominated by weakness and cardiac and hepatic failure. In addition, both genetic and acquired metabolic conditions have been associated with secondary forms of carnitine deficiency. These include diseases associated with defects in beta-oxidation with organic aciduria, defects of the mitochondrial respiratory chain, and chronic treatment with valproate or other drugs.

In the myopathic form there is progressive weakness, most marked in proximal and trunk muscles, generally beginning in childhood. Rarely, there is rapid worsening associated with respiratory failure; heart involvement may give rise to cardiomyopathy. The serum CK is moderately increased in most patients, and the EMG shows myopathic changes. The systemic form was first recorded by Karpati and co-workers,[103] who described an 11-year-old boy with lifelong clumsiness, thin muscles, and a short history of generalized weakness. At ages 3 and 9 he had episodes of unexplained liver failure with hepatic encephalopathy, but recovery was adequate. Subsequently reported cases have shown a spectrum of clinical and biochemical abnormalities suggesting that perhaps this is not a single entity but a group of disorders that affect carnitine metabolism. In these patients the onset has generally been in childhood and the main clinical features are progressive weakness and recurrent hepatic encephalopathy with metabolic acidosis (see review[45]). Death from respiratory failure has occurred before the age of 20 in most cases. Laboratory studies are similar to those found in the myopathic form.

In the myopathic form muscle biopsy shows intrafiber oil red O-positive lipid droplets, which are more numerous, clumped, and larger than normal (Fig. 17-17, *A*). They are most marked in type 1 fibers and

A 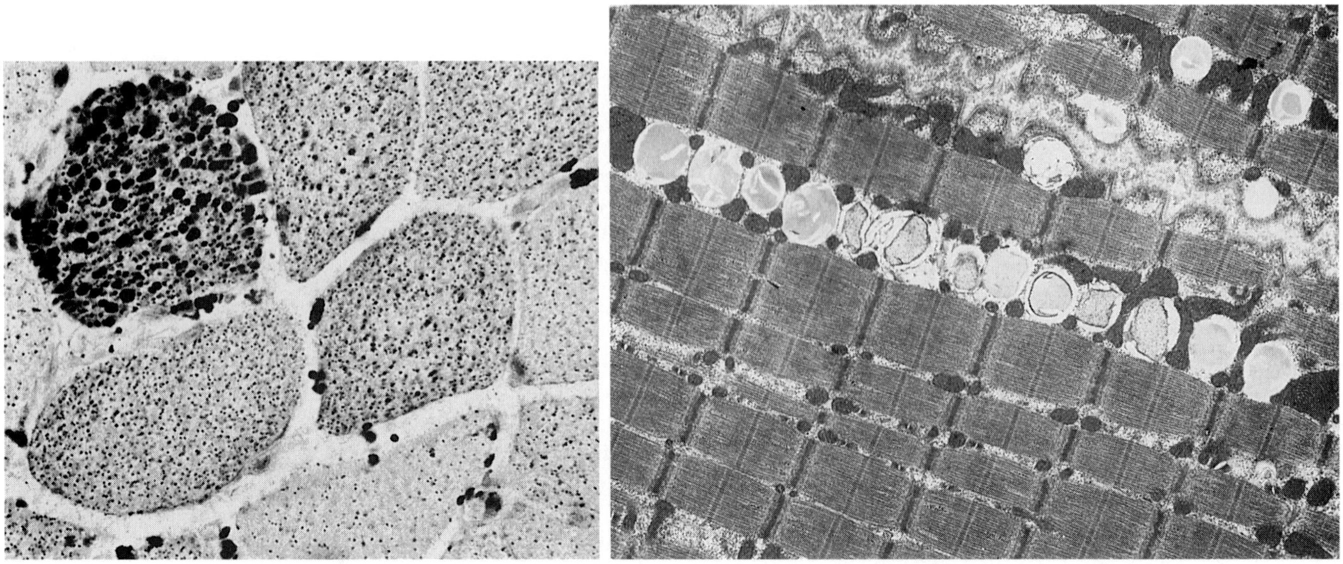 B

**Fig. 17-17.** Lipid storage myopathy. **A**, Oil red O-stained transverse section of muscle showing abnormally dense and enlarged lipid droplets within centrally placed fiber in comparison with surrounding fibers. **B**, Electron micrograph of longitudinal section of muscle showing excessive deposits of lipid between the myofibrils. (**A**, original magnification ×300; **B**, original magnification ×23,000.) (**A**, from De Girolami, and others: Skeletal muscle. In Silverberg, SG editor: Principles and practice of surgical pathology, ed 2, New York, 1990, Churchill-Livingstone; **C**, from De Girolami U, and Smith TW: Pathology of skeletal muscle diseases. Teaching monograph, Am J Pathol 107:235-276, 1982.)

are least evident in type 2B fibers. The droplets are not membrane-bound and accumulate in parallel rows between myofibrils or beneath the sarcolemma (Fig. 17-17, *B*). There are also abnormally numerous and misshapen mitochondria, sometimes with intramitochondrial inclusions. In the systemic forms, the muscle biopsy shows lipid accumulation in most type 1 fibers. Carnitine is virtually absent from muscle and reduced by 80% to 90% in liver and plasma. Autopsy studies, however, show lipid storage in liver, heart, and the tubular epithelial cells of the kidney.

***Carnitine palmitoyltransferase (CPT) deficiency***—Carnitine palmitoyltransferase deficiency, first described by DiMauro and Melis-DiMauro[46] and further characterized clinically in subsequent reports, is a disease that begins in childhood. The major clinical feature is myoglobinuria associated with muscle pain provoked by prolonged exercise, fasting, or both. The frequency of myoglobinuria appears to be much higher in CPT deficiency than in McArdle's disease or other glycolytic defects. Between attacks, patients are well and there is no permanent weakness.

The muscle biopsy usually is normal unless there has been a previous episode of myoglobinuria, in which case scattered necrotic and regenerating fibers are found. Lipid content is either normal or mildly increased.

CPT deficiency shows a striking male predominance and is probably transmitted as an autosomal-recessive trait. The gene encoding CPT in human liver has been assigned to chromosome 1.[71] The molecular genetics of carnitine deficiency is not completely understood at present.

***Other Metabolic Myopathies***

***Myoadenylate deaminase deficiency (MAD)***—This is a poorly understood condition characterized by postexertional myalgias and cramps and by the absence of myoadenylate deaminase reactivity in frozen sections of muscle and the biochemical demonstration of decreased myoadenylate deaminase activity in muscle tissue. No structural or ultrastructural abnormalities have been uncovered in this condition thus far. A responsible autosomal recessive trait may be present in 1% to 2% of all individuals undergoing muscle biopsy. The gene has been localized to chromosome 1p13-p21.[148] There is no consensus on the relationship between the clinical condition and the enzyme abnormality. The nosologic status of MAD is uncertain until more studies on affected individuals from different laboratories around the world become available.

***Malignant hyperthermia***—This is a rare autosomal-dominant clinical syndrome ordinarily occurring in previously asymptomatic individuals (children more than adults) characterized by a dramatic hypermetabolic state (tachypnea, tachycardia, hypertension, muscle spasm, and a later rise in body temperature) triggered at the time of induction of general anesthesia (rarely, in the recovery period). The offending agents have mostly been halogenated inhaled anesthetic compounds and succinylcholine, but the attack may also be brought on, in the absence of anesthesia, under stressful situations or in individuals with other muscle diseases (CPT deficiency, central core disease, Duchenne/ Becker dystrophy). In at least 50% of cases there is a previous history of uneventful anesthesia. The only reliable method of diagnosis is the in vitro skeletal muscle biopsy contraction study, which is performed in very few centers around the world. The test is based on the observation that the skeletal muscle of affected individuals undergoes measurable halothane- or caffeine-potentiated contracture. A calcium uptake method applied to frozen sections also is used with unpredictable results. The muscle biopsy is structurally normal in most cases. The genetic basis for the human disease is not understood. The proposed pathophysiology of the attack in the porcine model of malignant hyperthemia is that there is an anesthesia-generated loss of control of intracellular calcium because of a genetically-determined mutation in the ryanodine receptor (see review[84]).

**Mitochondrial myopathies.** The mitochondrial encephalomyopathies are a set of heterogeneous disorders with many clinical manifestations and a wide variety of molecular pathogenic mechanisms and patterns of inheritance. The underlying mechanism of disease is defective oxidative phosphorylation, resulting in deficient production of ATP. Specific mitochondrial disorders for which specific mutations have been identified include MERRF (myoclonus epilepsy and ragged red fibers), MELAS (mitochondrial encephalomyopathy, lactic acidosis, and stroke-like episodes), NARP (developmental delay, retinitis pigmentosa, dementia, seizure ataxia, proximal neurogenic muscle weakness, and sensory neuropathy[94]) and KSS/CPEO (Kearns-Sayre syndrome/chronic progressive external ophthalmoplegia). The Kearns-Sayre syndrome is a nonfamilial neurologic disorder characterized by onset in the second decade, progressive external ophthalmoplegia, pigmentary retinal degeneration, and heart block, and pathologically by the finding of ragged red fibers. Additional clinical manifestations include ataxia, hearing loss, dementia, endocrinologic disturbances, and peripheral neuropathy. Familial cases of progressive external ophthalmoplegia (maternally inherited via a mitochondrial genetic abnormality; or autosomal-dominant) have been reported.

The presence of ragged red fibers (Fig. 17-18, *A* and *B*) in muscle biopsy is a defining criterion in these disease.[104] These are abnormally contoured fibers with an irregular/frayed outline best demonstrable on transverse frozen sections of muscle. With a modified Gomori trichrome reaction, the ragged red fibers stain intensely red. The red staining is due to the presence of coarse granules, which may be patchily dispersed throughout the cell, bulge out from the surface, form a crescent beneath the sarcolemma, or overwhelm the entire fiber. The involved fibers are often smaller than normal and are randomly distributed throughout the biopsy. The presence of red ragged fibers may be suspected on H&E sections when pale basophilic subsarcolemmal aggregates are noted; aggregates are also well demonstrated with oxidative enzyme histochemical reactions. Electron microscopy is useful in delineating the abnormal mitochondria when light microscopic features are clear-cut, and sometimes is the diagnostic procedure when light microscopic findings are ambiguous. Ultarastructural features of ragged red fibers include abnormally numerous subsarcolemmal intermyofibrillar mitochondria. The mitochondria and their cristae also are often misshapen, and there are characteristic intramitochondrial paracrystalline "parking lot" inclusions. In addition, other inclusions may be seen, such as spiral/cylindrical structures, dense bodies, excessive accumulations of glycogen, and abnormal lipid deposits.

MERRF is a maternally transmitted disease that has been associated with a mutation in a mtDNA gene for a mitochondrial-specific tRNA.[154] This appears to result in altered function of several of the oxidative complexes. A similar type of mutation of a tRNA gene has been found in MELAS.[107] In KSS mtDNA deletions have been found,[182] but not in familial CPEO. In the autosomal dominant variant of CPEO, multiple mtDNA deletions are found.

**Endocrine myopathies, toxic myopathies, and myopathies associated with systemic disease**

***Endocrine myopathies.*** Many generalized endocrine disorders can be associated with a myopathy (see review[102]). In most cases, evidence of muscle involvement may be subclinical, revealed only by special studies (e.g., serum enzymes, EMG, muscle biopsy) performed in the course of evaluation of the endocrine disorder. However, in some instances (e.g., thyrotoxicosis), the muscle symptoms predominate, often being the presenting manifestation of the endocrine disorder. Most of these myopathies are readily reversed after correction of the underlying endocrine disturbance. As a general rule, the histologic changes present in the muscle tend to be relatively mild and nonspecific, sometimes even in the face of severe muscle weakness and wasting. The endocrinopathies most consistently associated with myopathy include: hyperthyroidism, hypothyroidism, hyperparathyroidism, hyperadrenalism (Cushing's disease), hypoadrenalism (Addison's disease), and acromegaly.

A

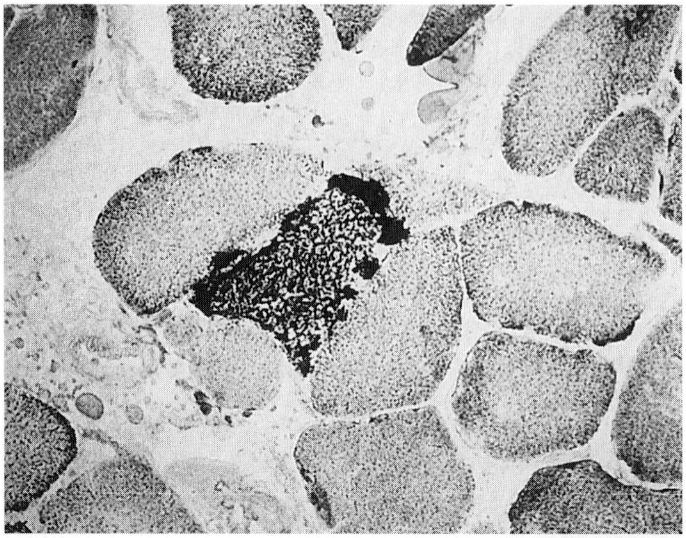

B

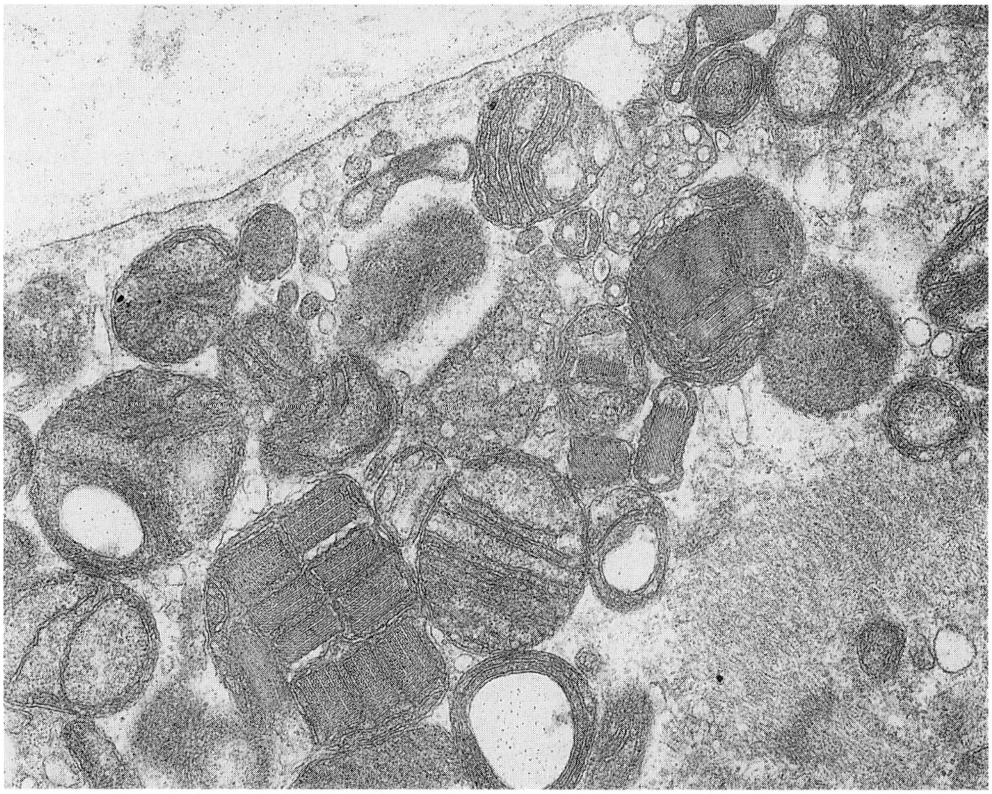

**Fig. 17-18.** Mitochondrial myopathy. **A**, Light micrograph of NADH-TR stained transverse section showing ragged red fiber. The appears abnormal mitochondrial aggregates appear black. **B**, Electron micrograph of ragged red fiber showing abnormal subsarcolemmal mitochondria, some containing inclusions. (**A**, Original magnification ×300; **B**, original magnification ×57,000.)

***Hyperthyroidism***—Four different neuromuscular disorders can occur in hyperthyroidism: thyrotoxic myopathy, myasthenia gravis, thyrotoxic periodic paralysis, and exophthalmic ophthalmoplegia (see review[102]). A chronic myopathy manifested largely by generalized proximal muscle weakness is common in hyperthyroidism. It may at times precede other signs of thyrotoxicosis. The EMG shows myopathic abnormalities in about 90% of cases. Nevertheless, light microscopic examination of the muscle often shows essentially no abnormality or only mild myofiber atrophy. Other relatively minor histologic changes reported include interstitial edema, scattered single fiber necrosis, glycogen depletion, increased subsarcolemmal nuclei, and fatty infiltration. Ultrastructural abnormalities that have been described include papillary projections on the muscle fiber surface, mitochondrial abnormalities, focal myofibrillar degeneration, tubular aggregates, and subsarcolemmal glycogen deposits.

*Hypothyroidism*—Patients with hypothyroidism often have a myopathy characterized by proximal weakness, hypoactive reflexes, stiffness, myalgias, and less commonly cramps and/or muscle enlargement (see review[102]). Serum CK usually is elevated. Muscle biopsy specimens usually show nonspecific myopathic changes such as fiber atrophy (most often involving type 2 fibers), increased internal nuclei, glycogen accumulation, ring fibers, and endomysial fibrosis. Ultrastructural changes may include mitochondrial abnormalities, myofibrillar degeneration, glycogen accumulation, dilated sarcoplasmic reticulum, T-tubule proliferation, lipid granules, and autophagic vacuoles. Basophilic degeneration, that is, interstitial collections of mucoid material, also are visible in long-standing cases of hypothyroidism.

*Hyperparathyroidism*—Both primary and secondary hyperparathyroidism may be associated with a myopathy (see review[102]). Clinically, this affects mainly proximal muscles, often with associated pain and fatigability, waddling gait, and hyperreflexia. The histologic changes seen in muscle biopsies from these patients are mild and have included type 2 fiber atrophy and focal vacuolar changes.

*Hyperadrenalism*—Patients with Cushing's disease frequently have a myopathy characterized by proximal muscle weakness and wasting that especially affects the lower extremities. A myopathy can also be seen in association with exogenous corticosteroid therapy (see review[102]). The most consistent and characteristic histologic change observed in muscle biopsies in both conditions is selective atrophy of type 2 fibers, especially type 2B fibers; there also may be excessive lipid deposits in type 1 fibers. Electron microscopy may show increased glycogen stores.

*Hypoadrenalism (Addison's disease)*—A myopathy characterized by severe generalized muscle weakness, cramping, and fatigue occurs in 25% to 50% of patients with adrenal insufficiency, regardless of its etiology (see review[102]). Serum muscle enzymes and EMG usually are normal. The muscle biopsy is normal, except for some glycogen depletion.

*Acromegaly*—Proximal muscle weakness and diminished exercise tolerance may be present in about 50% of patients with acromegaly.[126] The muscle weakness may be insidious in onset, slowly progressive, and associated with some diminution in muscle bulk. Serum CK levels may be slightly elevated. The EMG shows myopathic changes in about 50% of patients with acromegaly. Histologic examination of muscle biopsy specimens has shown single fiber necrosis, nuclear enlargement with prominent nucleoli, proliferation and hypertrophy of satellite cells, increased glycogen, lipofuscin accumulation, and, rarely, mononuclear inflammatory infiltrates.[125] Hypertrophy of type 1 and/or type 2 fibers also has been described. Electron microscopic studies have noted excessive accumulation of glycogen and lipofuscin, myofibrillar degeneration, capillary basement membrane thickening, and increased satellite cells.[164]

***Toxic myopathies.*** Toxic drug-related myopathies have been related to a wide variety of compounds (see review[174]). Only those few associated with distinctive clinicopathologic syndromes will be discussed briefly here.

Alcoholics develop acute myopathic syndromes related to rhabdomyolysis (alcoholic myonecrosis) in the setting of alcohol withdrawal seizures. With obtundation and pressure exerted on dependent parts of the body they also may develop compartment syndromes. Histopathologic studies have shown multifocal acute fiber necrosis.[174] An acute painful myopathy that is associated with cramps, and presumably is related to impaired glycogen metabolism may also develop. There is no consensus about the existence of a chronic progressive myopathy directly related to the effects of the drug.[174] Other complicating factors include the effects on muscle related to alcoholism-associated electrolyte imbalances (e.g., hypokalemia) and nutritional or vitamin deficiencies.

Myopathy due to intoxication with the antiinflammatory drug colchicine is relatively uncommon, but is now being reported more often, especially in progressive renal failure, while newer indications for the drug are being explored.[110] Muscle biopsy studies have shown a relatively distinctive toxic myopathy characterized by extensive monophasic individual fiber necrosis, vacuolization, prominent acid phosphatase activity in the necrotic fibers, and relatively little interstitial inflammation or endomysial connective tissue proliferation. The ultrastructural findings have also been fairly uniform, consisting of multifocal subsarcolemmal or intermyofibrillar membranous whorls (myeloid bodies), dense bodies, and cytoplasmic degradation products[147,174] (Fig. 17-19). A very similar clinicopathologic picture has been observed with a variety of other drugs that contain a hydrophobic region and a primary or substituted amine group, which can bear a net positive charge. About 20 of these so-called amphiphilic drugs have now been recognized as giving rise to myopathies, including chloroquine, imipramine, amiodarone, and perhexiline.[66,96,174] A related group of cholesterol-lowering drugs including lovastatin (and analogues), taken in isolation or in combination with gemfibrozil or cyclosporine, have also been reported to cause a toxic myopathy. These drugs inhibit cholesterol synthesis and presumably cause a

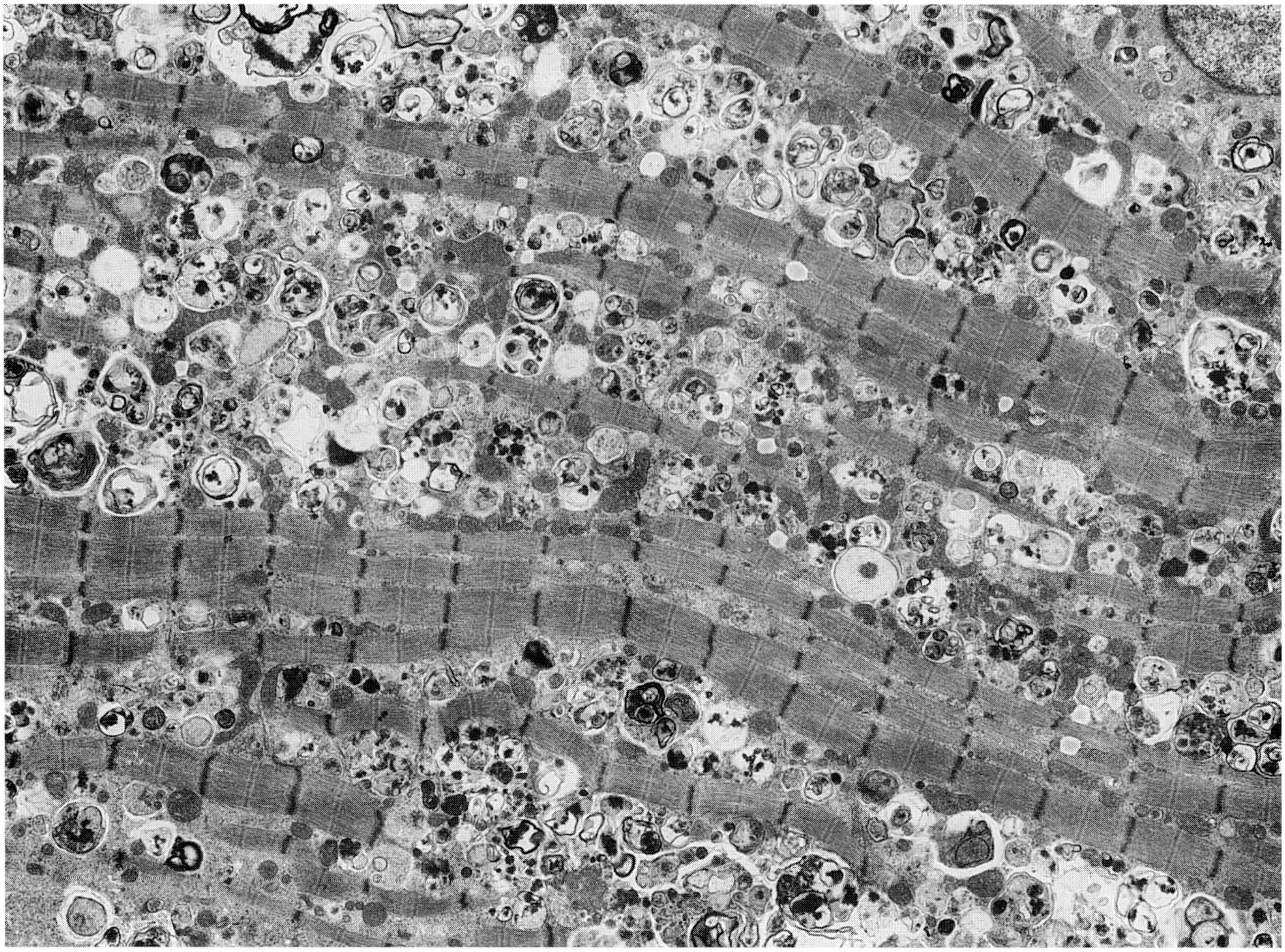

**Fig. 17-19.** Toxic myopathy (chloroquine-induced). Electron micrograph showing multifocal subsarcolemmal or intermyofibrillar membranous whorls (myeloid bodies), dense bodies, and cytoplasmic degradation products. (Original magnification ×8000.) (Courtesy of Dr. TW Smith.)

toxic myonecrosis by damaging the cell membrane. The clinical syndrome, characterized by relatively abrupt onset of leg (more than arm) weakness, sometimes associated with pain, and elevation of the CK is entirely reversible with discontinuation of the drug. Pathologic examination shows primarily muscle fiber necrosis and myophagocytosis with relatively little interstitial inflammation.[34,174]

Zidovudine inhibits HIV reverse transcriptase and has been used extensively for the treatment of AIDS. Long-term administration of the drug has resulted in a previously unrecognized dose-related myopathy characterized by rapidly progressive proximal muscle weakness, myalgia, and elevated CK levels. Several muscle biopsy studies have shown a distinctive picture consisting of random muscle fiber necrosis and myophagocytosis with minimal inflammation and striking ragged-red fibers with ultrastructural abnormalities of mitochondria, cytoplasmic bodies, nemaline rods, and autophagic vacuoles.[38,130] With discontinuation of the drug the illness has been largely reversible after a few weeks.[30]

The eosinophilia myalgia syndrome, perhaps now only of historical interest, is a neuromyopathic symptom complex related to the ingestion of L-tryptophan (or a contaminant thereof apparently traced to a particular batch manufactured in Japan that was subsequently taken off the market) as health food/body building pills. This syndrome, first recognized 5 years ago, had considerable variability in severity, ranging from a mild fasciitis with scleroderma-like dermatologic manifestations, myalgia, arthralgia, and hypereosinophilia to severe muscle weakness and respiratory insufficiency. Death from extreme emaciation occurred in a few cases. Histopathologic studies of muscle and nerve have shown random fiber myophagocytosis, variable eosinophilia with fasciitis, and sometimes extreme proliferation of fibrous tissue in muscle and nerve.[165,174] There have been no new cases reported in the past few years.

The neuromuscular syndrome of chronic progressive distal weakness that is seen in patients with end-stage renal disease is believed to be related to peripheral neuropathy rather than to a primary muscle disease. Light and electron microscopic studies have shown type 2 fiber atrophy, "moth-eaten" fibers, and calcium deposits.[1,21]

**Inflammatory myopathy.** Inflammatory myopathies, whether idiopathic or caused by an infectious agent, represent about 25% of muscle biopsy cases in a busy adult neuropathology service.[88] In general, these disorders are characterized by acute or subacute progressive proximal muscle weakness. The distal musculature tends to be affected in the later stages of the disease, except in inclusion body myositis (IBM), where early distal involvement is common. Cranial muscles are rarely affected in any of the inflammatory myopathies.

***Idiopathic.*** The most commonly encountered inflammatory myopathies are idiopathic, and immunologic mechanisms are presumed to play a major role in their pathogenesis (see reviews[23,37,88]). Although the disorders are grouped together here for convenience of presentation and because they share some features on muscle biopsy examination, there is no compelling evidence that they represent a continuum of the same disease entity with multiple clinical expressions. In dermatomyositis (DM) of adulthood or childhood, primarily vascular disease of muscle is believed to play an important pathogenetic role. The causative factors leading to the development of IBM are unknown, although several recent studies may provide important clues.

***Polymyositis/dermatomyositis.*** Polymyositis (PM) often begins insidiously with asymmetric proximal muscle weakness variably associated with pain in the arms or, less often, the leg muscles (e.g., difficulty climbing stairs or raising the arms to comb or groom). Dysphagia occurs in about one third of cases, and weakness of neck flexors is commonly noted. Adult DM is characterized by progressive proximal muscle weakness with erythematous skin lesions that may precede, coincide with, or follow the weakness, and is accompanied by ungual telangiectases. The skin rash begins in the face (periorbital, malar, perioral regions), anterior neck, and chest regions, as well as on the extensor surfaces of the joints. The skin lesions progress to scaling, brown discoloration, and induration. Electrocardiographic abnormalities have been described in both PM and DM. In different series around the world the incidence of associated malignancy in middle-aged or elderly patients ranges from about 10% to over 40%. The detection of the neoplasm (in women, ovarian and breast carcinoma; in men, stomach, lung, and intestinal carcinoma; in Chinese, nasopharyngeal carcinoma) may precede or follow the onset of neurologic symptoms. Both PM and adult DM may be associated with such well-defined collagen-vascular diseases as rheumatoid arthritis, scleroderma, polyarteritis nodosa, Sjögren's syndrome, lupus erythematosus, and mixed connective tissue disease. Laboratory studies show that the CK is elevated, and the EMG discloses short, polyphasic potentials with fibrillations, positive waves, and pseudomyotonic bursts. Radionuclide and MRI imaging studies have been used to identify involved regions and to aid in directing the site for needle biopsy. The typical clinical picture of childhood dermatomyositis consists of erythematous malar violaceous, heliotrope rash, also involving the skin over the extensor surfaces of the joints; muscle weakness of insidious onset progresses relentlessly over a period of weeks or months. In many cases other associated manifestations include subcutaneous calcifications, gastrointestinal bleeding, and respiratory insufficiency.[10] A rare, congenital form of inflammatory myopathy clinically similar to congenital muscular dystrophy also has been reported.[153]

Overall the muscle biopsy is abnormal in about 90% of patients who meet the clinical criteria for PM or DM.[57] Inflammatory cells are found in some 75% of patients. In large series, 10% to 20% of patients will lack evidence of inflammation. The muscle biopsy findings in PM and DM share a number of important similarities, although there are also significant differences between the two conditions. The typical findings are those of an inflammatory myopathy, that is, changes reflecting acute segmental necrosis of muscle, manifest by smudging and eosinophilia of the cytoplasm and myophagocytosis by invading macrophages (Fig. 17-20, *A* to *D*). Along with these destructive changes there is often concomitant regeneration of muscle fibers, sometimes in areas adjacent to the regions of myophagocytosis. The extent and distribution of the chronic mononuclear inflammatory cell infiltrates will vary somewhat in the two conditions. In PM inflammatory cells are present in the endomysium between and among muscle fibers (Fig. 17-20, *B*), whereas in DM (both childhood and adult types) they tend to be angiocentric. An important structural characteristic of DM (rare in PM) is the tendency for fibers at the periphery of the fascicle to appear smaller than normal (so-called "perifascicular atrophy") (Fig. 17-21, *A*). These small fibers are either rounded or somewhat angulated; they are often basophilic, perhaps regenerating. On ultrastructural examination in both adult and childhood DM, characteristic undulating tubuloreticular inclusions (Fig. 17-21, *B* and *C*) may be demonstra-

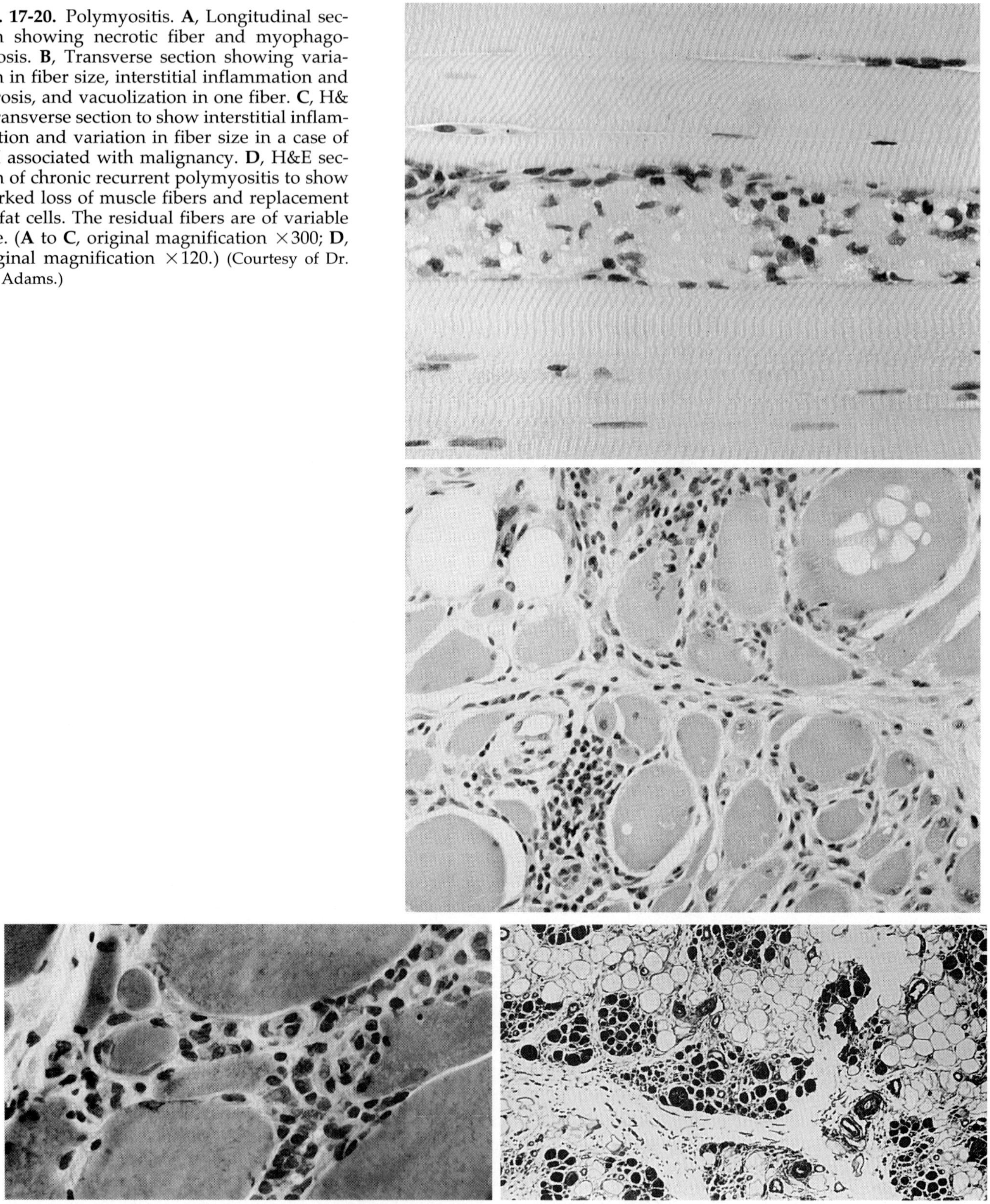

A

B

C

D

**Fig. 17-20.** Polymyositis. **A**, Longitudinal section showing necrotic fiber and myophagocytosis. **B**, Transverse section showing variation in fiber size, interstitial inflammation and fibrosis, and vacuolization in one fiber. **C**, H&E transverse section to show interstitial inflammation and variation in fiber size in a case of PM associated with malignancy. **D**, H&E section of chronic recurrent polymyositis to show marked loss of muscle fibers and replacement by fat cells. The residual fibers are of variable size. (**A** to **C**, original magnification ×300; **D**, original magnification ×120.) (Courtesy of Dr. RD Adams.)

ble in the cytoplasm of capillary endothelial cells and pericytes.[99] In PM or DM associated with neoplasia, there are no distinctive muscle biopsy features. In PM associated with a collagen-vascular disease, the pathology most closely resembles that seen in DM. In congenital inflammatory myopathy the muscle biopsy shows perivascular/interstitial chronic inflammatory cell infiltrates with degenerating and regenerating fibers.[153] End-stage inflammatory myopathy is characterized by extensive fibroadipose replacement of muscle fibers with little inflammatory reaction (Fig. 17-20, *D*).

Mechanisms of fiber damage in these diseases have yet to be completely defined, but there is much evidence to implicate immunologic factors. In PM a cell-mediated immunopathogenesis of the muscle fiber destruction is suggested by the available evidence. The predominant inflammatory cells have been demonstrated to be T cells (about 70%) and macrophages. The T cells are mostly cytotoxic/suppressor CD8+ and some CD4+ cells.[4,5,39,54] MHC-I expression is demonstrable on and in affected fibers.[51] The focal invasion and destruction of muscle fibers by T cells and macro-

A

B

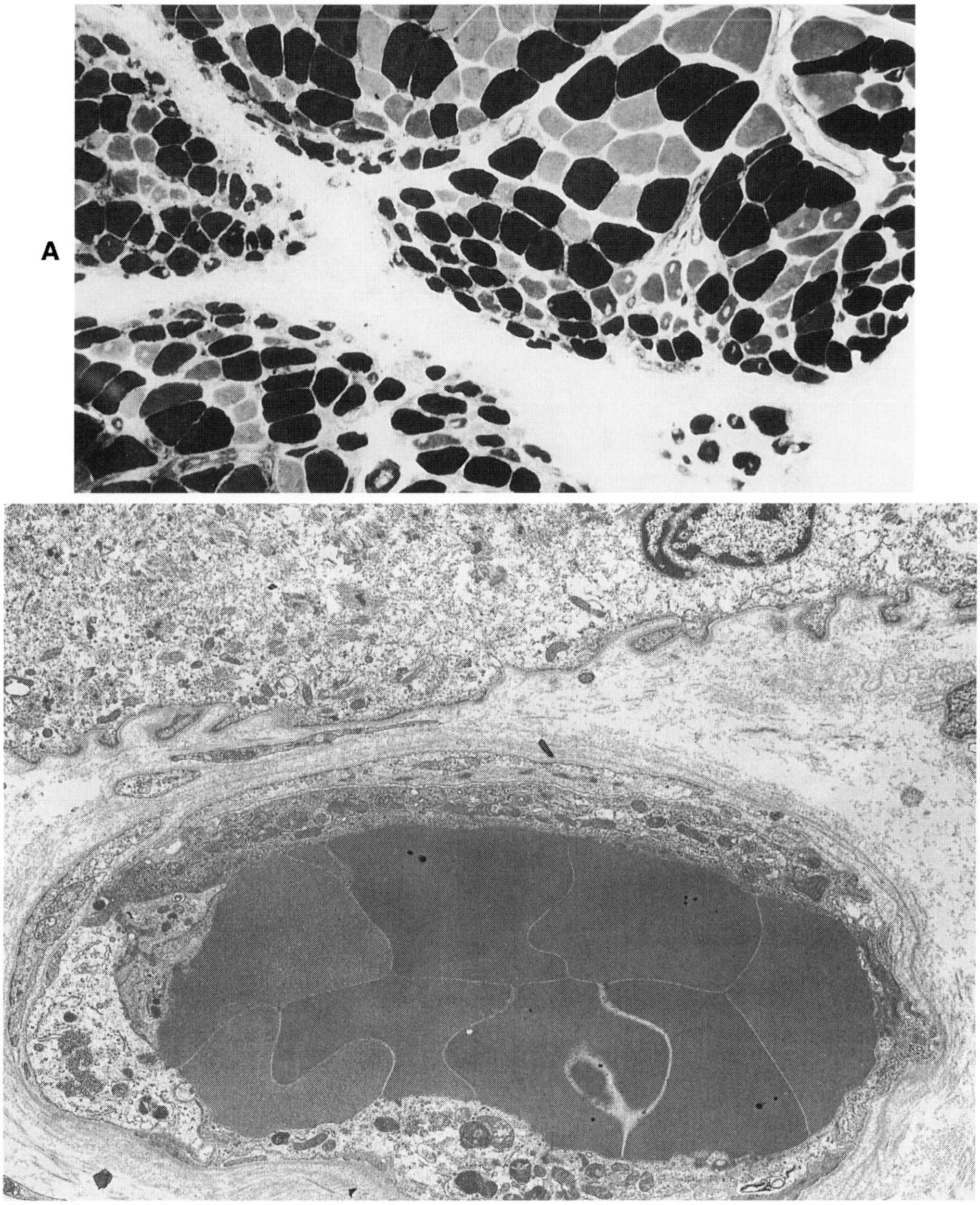

**Fig. 17-21.** Dermatomyositis. **A**, ATPase reaction at pH 9.4 to show perifascicular atrophy. **B**, Electron micrograph showing tubuloreticular inclusions in capillary endothelial cell. **C**, High magnification of **B**. (**A**, original magnification ×100.) *Continued.*

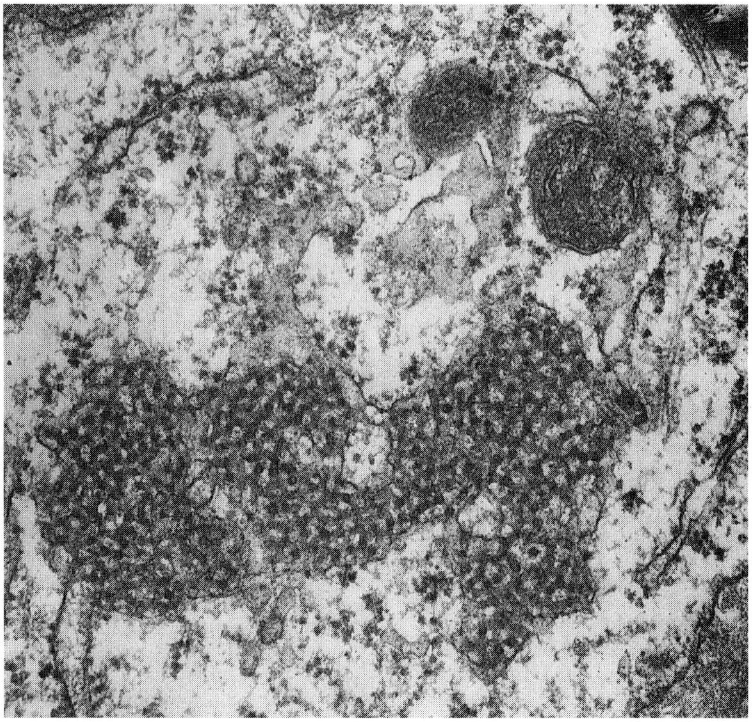

C

Fig. 17-21, cont'd. For legend see previous page.

phages suggests previous sensitization to muscle fiber surface-associated antigens, but no target antigen has yet been identified. Viral infection has long been suspected to be the inciting factor that triggers the immune response, but there is little support for this hypothesis in spite of active search over many years.[27,33] The possible contribution of the humoral immune system in the development of the disease is unresolved at this time.

In patients with PM, immunoglobulin deposits have been visualized by immunofluorescence within the walls of small intramuscular blood vessels, but these observations have not been consistent or specific, and therefore such examinations have largely been abandoned as a useful adjunct to diagnosis. Similarly, the diagnostic utility of localizing the membrane attack complex (MAC) to necrotic fibers[106] in PM and DM is questionable. In adult DM, humoral immunity appears to play an important part. The inflammatory infiltrate is composed mainly of B-cells and helper T-cells, although macrophages and cytotoxic/suppresor T-cells also are present. In support of the notion that DM is an immune-mediated vasculopathy is the observation that the complement system has been found to be deposited, bound, and activated to completion within the intramuscular microvasculature of patients with childhood DM (to a lesser extent in adult DM). Ultrastructural and morphometric studies evidencing capillary lesions early in the course of the disease have also been published.[44,52] In childhood DM, microcirculatory abnormalities and necrosis and thrombosis of capillaries, small arteries, and venules have been found, especially in those vessels at the periphery of muscle fascicles, presumably accounting for the perifascicular atrophy.[7,25,141] In PM associated with the collagen-vascular disease scleroderma, an immunologic response mediated by T-cells appears to be directed against a connective tissue or vascular element, and not against the muscle fiber.

***Inclusion body myositis (IBM)***—In 1971 Yunis and Samaha introduced the term "inclusion body myositis" for a specific type of inflammatory myopathy[181]; an earlier report also described the structural abnormality.[31] In the following 25 years many subsequent case studies and review articles have expanded and further clarified the distinctive features of this disease.* Clinically the entity can be separated from PM and DM because the disorder occurs in a somewhat older, predominantly male patient population, skin manifestations are not a feature of the illness, the distribution of the weakness tends to be both distal and proximal, and the course of the illness is perhaps more protracted. The CK levels are either in the normal range or mildly elevated, although ordinarily not above levels commonly seen in PM and DM. EMG findings are, for the most part, myopathic. The disease appears to be refractory to corticosteroid treatment and other therapeutic measures utilized for PM and DM. An association with connective tissue diseases has been noted in

* Refs. 23, 24, 37, 88, 120, 132.

a minority of cases, and some familial cases are on record.

The histopathologic findings on muscle biopsy include a sparse, or entirely absent, interstitial chronic inflammatory cell infiltrates of lymphocytes (largely CD8+ T cells surround the non-necrotic fibers) and macrophages, and rarely myophagocytosis and regenerating fibers. The characteristic rimmed vacuoles are best demonstrated on frozen sections with the modified Gomori trichrome stain, although they also can be seen well on H&E preparations (they are ordinarily not visible on paraffin-embedded sections) (Fig. 17-22, *A*). These are single or multiple rounded defects within the muscle fibers that typically are either empty or filled with red granular debris and outlined by a rim of darkly-staining material. Angular fibers and sometimes grouping of atrophic fibers are frequent. Ultrastructurally the vacuoles contain non-membrane-bound whorls and skeins of "myeloid" membranous debris and dissolution of the myofibrillar architecture (Fig. 17-22, *A*). There also may be viruslike tubular filaments, 15 to 18 nm wide, scattered in the disrupted cytoplasm or within neighboring nuclei; $\beta$ amyloid has been colocalized to the filaments in both sporadic and familial cases, but it is premature to attribute significance to this finding.[128,158] The filamentous inclusions do not appear to be specific for IBM.[70] Recent observations also have reported the presence of ubiquitin, but the overall pathogenic significance of this observation or the presence of the ubiquitin is unknown.[2] Muscle biopsies from patients with IBM, as in PM/DM, have been studied carefully for evidence of paramyxovirus infection, but although studies have successfully demonstrated the presence of virus in some affected individuals,[101,133] such evidence is lacking in most others[139] (see reviews[32,132]).

***Giant-cell, granulomatous, and sarcoid polymyositis***—Occasionally, patients with typical features of PM may have foci of granulomatous infiltrates on muscle biopsy examination. In these cases a search for microorganisms (e.g., parasites, tubercle bacilli, and fungi) may establish the diagnosis. A nonspecific epithelioid giant cell reaction in skeletal muscle may occur in a number of other conditions including neoplasia, myasthenia gravis, rheumatologic disorders including rheumatoid arthritis and related connective tissue diseases, and may also be found idiopathically, that is, in the absence of any known systemic illness.[121,131,138] In many patients with sarcoidosis there is extension of the disease into skeletal muscle.[176] Clinically, most patients with sarcoidosis show no signs or symptoms of muscle involvement, but a minority have proximal muscle weakness, myalgia, and cramps.[157] Peripheral nerve involvement may lead to neurogenic atrophy. The muscle biopsy in sarcoid myositis shows relatively little active muscle fiber destruction; the granulomatous infiltrate is noncaseating, contains epithelioid histiocytes with relatively few lymphocytes, and extends into the perivascular connective tissue.[91]

***Focal myositis and myositis ossificans***—Under the generic term *inflammatory pseudotumor* are included a number of inflammatory disorders of muscle characterized by selective regional involvement of specific muscle groups. These encompass reported cases of focal myositis, proliferative myositis, nodular fasciitis, and myositis ossificans. The principal histopathologic features are variations in fiber size with interstitial and fascial chronic inflammation.[89] Myositis ossificans is a skeletal muscle lesion characterized by deposition of trabeculae of woven bone about a focus of chronically inflamed and fibrotic muscle. These histologic findings have been described in seemingly disparate entities, including hereditary disorders (fibrodysplasia ossificans progressiva), post-traumatic or ischemic injury to muscle, neoplastic-like lesions, and end-stage muscle disease.

***Eosinophilic syndromes and myositis***—Eosinophilic infiltration of inflamed muscle is a characteristic of parasitic infection. This inflammation can, in addition, be a feature of a number of rare and poorly understood conditions.[9] Reference has been made above to the toxic eosinophilia myalgia syndrome associated with contaminated L-tryptophan. Polymyositis in the setting of eosinophilia in affected tissues and/or in the peripheral blood is characteristic of the hypereosoinophilic syndrome; some of these cases have been described under the term "eosinophilic polymyositis." In Schulman's syndrome (diffuse fasciitis with eosinophilia), a clinical syndrome with scleroderma-like manifestations, hypergammaglobulinemia, and hypereosinophilia, there are eosinophilic inflammatory infiltrates in fascia and skeletal muscle.

***Infectious myositis***

***Trichinosis and other parasitic infections of muscle***—In the United States and Canada trichinosis is the most common parasitic infection to involve skeletal muscle. The disease results from ingesting the larvae of the nematode *Trichinella spiralis* in incompletely cooked or raw pork. After maturation of the ingested larvae in the human bowel, fertilized females penetrate the mucosa and deposit large numbers of embryos, which then enter the venules and lymphatics. The larvae gain access to the circulation, disseminate widely, and invade skeletal muscles. At this time the patient may experience systemic symptoms accompanied by eosinophilia and variable muscle pain and weakness. Biopsy of an affected muscle shows encysted larvae, inflammation that varies with the stage of encystation, degeneration and phagocytosis of muscle fibers, and focal connective tissue proliferation (Fig. 17-23). In time, the encysted larvae will die and become calcified.

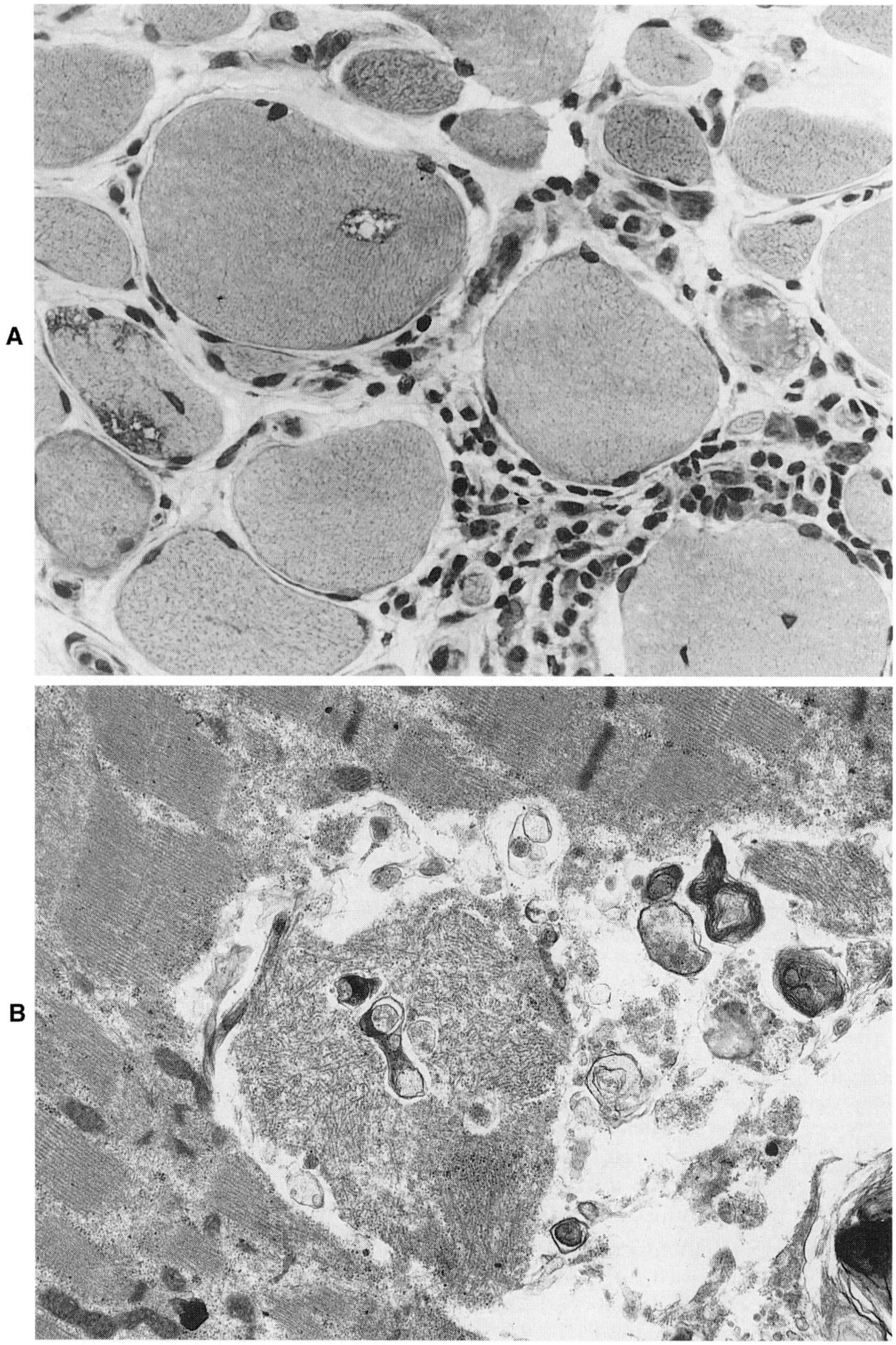

**Fig. 17-22.** Inclusion body myositis. **A**, Light micrograph of transverse section showing rimmed vacuole. **B**, Electron micrograph of rimmed vacuole showing central myofibrillar disorganization, dense bodies, and granular debris. (**A**, original magnification ×450; **B**, original magnification ×18,000.) (Courtesy of Dr. R. Heffner.)

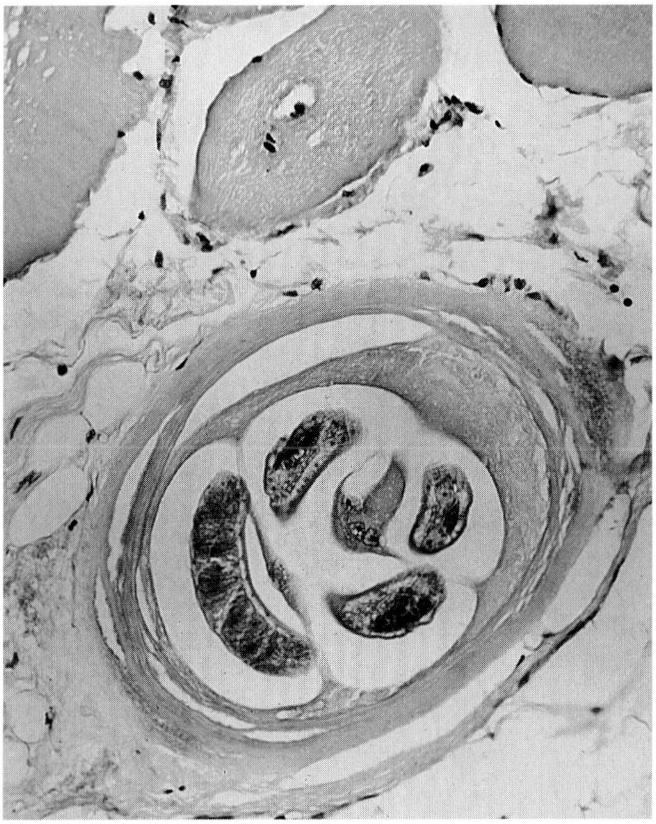

**Fig. 17-23.** H&E transverse section of encysted trichina. (Original magnification ×450.) (Courtesy of Dr. TW Smith.)

Other parasitic infections that occasionally involve skeletal muscle include cysticercosis (*Taenia solium*) and hydatid disease (Echinococcus).

***Toxoplasmosis***—Infection of skeletal muscle by *Toxoplasma gondii* now occurs most often in patients with systemic immunosuppression, especially those with AIDS.[77] The histopathologic picture consists of encysted bradyzoites or free tachyzoites invading the endomysial compartment with scattered necrotic fibers, a few macrophages, and chronic inflammatory cells. The organisms are well demonstrated with immunoperoxidase methods but can also be seen with the Giemsa reaction.

***Viral myositis***—The role of viruses in most cases of acute myositis in human beings is not well understood, especially as regards the pathogenesis of idiopathic polymyositis (see discussion above). Acute viral myositis is a symptom complex in children and adults that is characterized by myalgia and muscle weakness accompanying an acute febrile illness. Serum CK is elevated, and there may be myoglobinuria as well as an abnormal EMG. Muscle biopsy discloses scattered muscle fiber necrosis, regeneration, and interstitial inflammatory reaction. Electron microscopic studies of these cases ordinarily have been unsuccessful in demonstrating viral particles in muscle cells. Virologic examinations have demonstrated that most cases are caused by the influenza viruses, parainfluenza, and the enteroviruses (Coxsackie and echo groups). Other less frequent pathogens include hepatitis B, herpes simplex, and the Epstein-Barr virus.[9] HTLV-1, which is known to cause neurologic manifestations related to a myelopathy, can cause a mild inflammatory myopathy.[119,159]

***AIDS and muscle disease***—Opportunistic viral (e.g., cytomegalovirus), parasitic (e.g., toxoplasmosis), and fungal (e.g., candidiasis) infections have been recorded in many biopsy and autopsy studies of patients with AIDS (see review[82]). The toxic myopathy associated with AZT treatment in these patients is discussed above. In addition, an idiopathic polymyositis-like syndrome that does not seem to be directly related to the virus has been described.[78] In some cases there is immunohistochemical evidence of HIV viral infection as well as hemosiderin deposits within macrophages invading skeletal muscle[29] (Fig. 17-24, *A* to *C*).

***Pyomyositis***—Pyomyositis, or pyogenic bacterial myositis, is an infection of large skeletal muscles that may be focal or generalized. The disease most often occurs in the tropics; however, it has recently been recognized in temperate climates.[67,79] In both tropical and temperate climates patients with pyomyositis most often present with multiple acute muscle abscesses, which are commonly due to *Staphylococcus aureus*. Other pathogens include *E. coli*, Yersinia, and Legionella. Cases of gas gangrene associated with *Clostridium welchii*, may be the result of complicated mechanical trauma or postoperative wound infection. The pathogenesis of pyomyositis is unknown; it is a rare complication of bacteremia. Most cases occur spontaneously in previously healthy males. In others there is an association with previous sites of trauma, or the disease may develop in a patient with diabetes, parasitic infection, neutropenia, or AIDS. The affected muscle initially shows acute interstitial edema, followed by muscle fiber necrosis and a pleomorphic inflammatory infiltrate consisting of lymphocytes and neutrophils; organisms are present but difficult to demonstrate.

***Lyme disease***—Lyme disease, caused by infection with *Borrelia burgdorferi*, is often associated with muscle pain and weakness. Peripheral neuropathy demonstrable on clinical, NCV, and biopsy examinations is the most common cause of the muscle weakness. Muscle biopsy studies have shown minimal and nonspecific changes consisting primarily of scattered interstitial inflammatory cell infiltrates. Neurogenic atrophy also may occur. Rarely, the spirochete has been demonstrated within the skeletal muscle of patients with Lyme disease, but it is uncertain whether the clinical myalgia is due to a direct effect of the organism.[9,144]

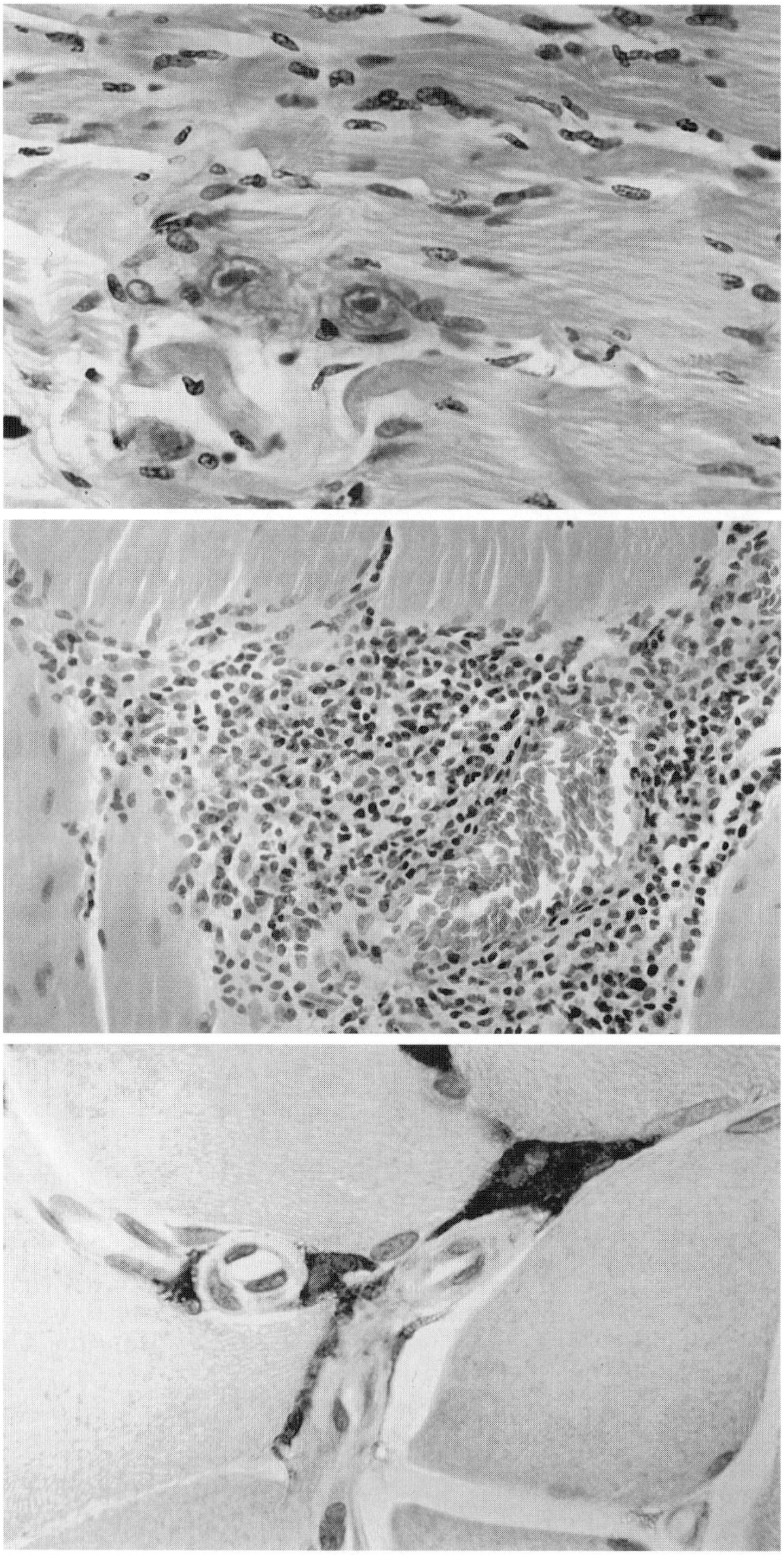

A

B

C

**Fig. 17-24.** AIDS and muscle disease. **A**, H&E longitudinal section of CMV. **B**, Polymyositis-like inflammatory myopathy with angiocentric mononuclear cell infiltrate. **C**, Transverse section of muscle with immunoperoxidase reaction for HIV (gp41) showing reactivity with macrophage. (**A**, **B**, original magnification ×300; **C**, original magnification ×450.) (From De Girolami U, and others: Neuropathology and opthalmologic pathology of the acquired immunodeficiency syndrome. Boston, 1992, Butterworth-Heinemann.)

**Ischemia.** Skeletal muscle is relatively resistant to ischemia because of its rich blood supply with many collateral branches. Ischemic injury to skeletal muscle, however, may occur in the following conditions: (1) thromboembolic occlusions of a major artery supplying a limb; (2) severe arteriosclerosis with occlusion of multiple small peripheral arteries and veins (e.g., diabetes); (3) thrombosis of multiple intramuscular vessels, as in polyarteritis nodosa; (4) swelling and hemorrhage of muscle groups enclosed in a rigid fascial compartment (e.g., anterior tibial syndrome); and (5) trauma. Mention has been made above of the vascular injury associated with the idiopathic inflammatory myopathies.

The earliest histologic changes seen in skeletal muscle subjected to ischemia, such as might occur after a major arterial occlusion, consist of eosinophilia of muscle fibers with focal loss of cross striations, hypercontraction bands (of Nageotte[137]), and pyknotic nuclei. The interstitial connective tissue is edematous, thus spreading the muscle fibers apart. If the tissue is examined 3 or 4 days after the ischemic injury there is a brisk inflammatory response, first with neutrophils and then with macrophages that begin to phagocytize the swollen and broken-down fibers. After a week or so there is evidence of vigorous regenerative activity.

## NEUROGENIC ATROPHIES

Clinically, a "lower motor neuron" injury is characterized by atrophy of the affected muscle groups, flaccid weakness in the appropriate distribution (e.g., nerve, root, plexus, or anterior horn cell), and fasciculation, a phenomenon caused by the independent contraction by fibers of a motor unit, thought to be secondary to hyperexcitable membranes. In general, muscle injury secondary to denervation tends to begin distally and to progress proximally in slow fashion if the denervation continues. Symptoms may be solely motor if the injury is at the level of the anterior horn cell (e.g., spinal muscular atrophy), or may be partly sensory if mixed nerves are involved. The injury may occur anywhere along the nerve, including the cell body, axon, nerve terminal, or in some cases the neuromuscular junction; this occurs in a wide range of conditions including degenerative (e.g., spinal muscular atrophy), metabolic/toxic (e.g., diabetes mellitus, alcohol), and traumatic diseases. The process of denervation and reinnervation is manifested electrophysiologically as high-amplitude long-duration compound muscle action potentials. Stimulation of an intact nerve will result in contraction of a significantly larger motor unit that contains reinnervated myofibers.

The major categories of neurologic disease associated with neurogenic atrophy are those conditions caused by an abnormality in the "neural" portion of the motor unit, either the anterior horn cell in the spinal cord or the motor root and peripheral nerve. In general, the histopathologic features of denervation atrophy of muscle as described above are comparable in all these diseases. Special note will be made here of the spinal muscular atrophies because they are not discussed elsewhere in this text. Diseases of peripheral nerve are covered in Chapter 18 and will not be discussed further here. Finally, disorders of the neuromuscular junction are taken up in the next section.

The hereditary spinal muscular atrophies (SMA) include the acute form or Werdnig-Hoffmann disease (SMA 1), the intermediate form or chronic Werdnig-Hoffmann (SMA 2), and Kugelberg-Welander disease (SMA 3).

The typical clinical presentation of the most severe type of SMA, Werdnig-Hoffmann disease (SMA1), is that of a child who presents soon after birth with hypotonia, generalized weakness, and respiratory difficulties. Alternatively, the infant may be normal at birth but by 3 to 6 months of age develop increasing feeding difficulties, and fail to develop the expected motor milestones. On physical examination the legs are flexed at the knee ("frog leg" position) and the arms are externally rotated, abducted, and flexed at the elbow. The extraocular muscles are not affected, but the muscles of deglutition and respiration often are involved. Sensory function is preserved. Death occurs by 2 to 3 years of age and is due to respiratory failure and pulmonary infection. SMA 2 begins between 6 and 18 months of age. Although the child never gains the ability to bear weight on the legs or to walk unaided, independent sitting is achieved. The disease is generally slowly progressive, with the development of skeletal deformities and joint contractures. The cause of death is respiratory insufficiency. The clinical course is very slowly progressive, with onset of proximal weakness of the legs and then of the shoulders and arms between 5 and 15 years of age, after independent ambulation has been achieved.

The typical muscle biopsy findings of SMA1 (and to a large extent SMA2) consist of panfascicular atrophy of some muscle fiber groups and hypertrophy of others, sometimes with intermixing of bundles of hypertrophic and atrophic fibers (Fig. 17-25, *A*). The atrophic fibers are of both fiber types, but the hypertrophic ones are largely type 1 (Fig. 17-25, *B*). In some cases fiber typing is weak, and it is not easy to discriminate the two fiber types. The abnormally small or large fibers retain a rounded contour, and internalized nuclei or myopathic changes are not observed. As the disease progresses there is replacement of damaged muscle cells with fibrous and adipose tissue. In the early stages of the disease it may be quite difficult to make the diagnosis histologically in spite of clinical neurologic impairment. Furthermore, there is remarkably little correlation between the degree of clinical severity and the prognosis and the extent of muscle atrophy in an individual case.[136] In some cases of the Kugelberg-Wel-

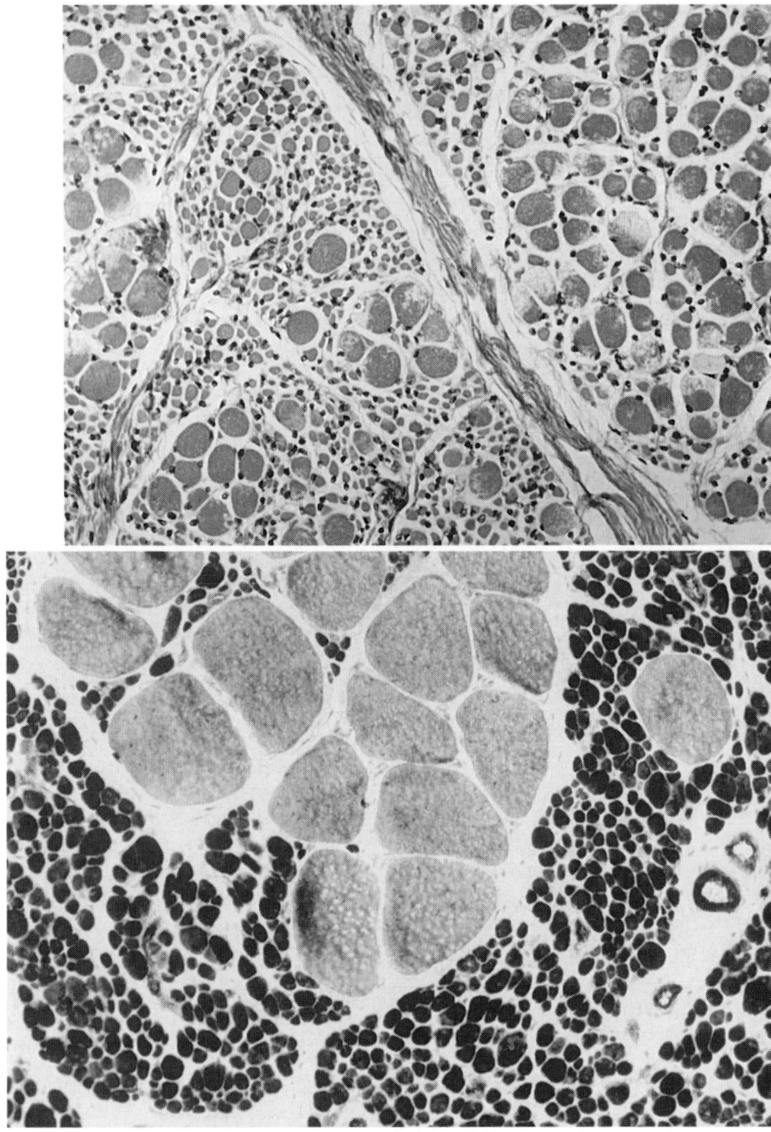


**Fig. 17-25.** SMA1. **A**, H&E transverse section of muscle showing panfascicular atrophy and scattered hypertrophied fibers. **B**, ATPase at pH 9.4 of transverse section showing small type 2 fibers and large type 1 fibers. (**A**, original magnification ×300; **B**, original magnification ×270.) (Courtesy of Dr. TW Smith.)

ander syndrome the muscle biopsy shows random fiber or group atrophy indistinguishable from neurogenic atrophy from any other cause; others show the typical rounded atrophic and hypertrophic fibers and panfascicular atrophy.

SMA is an autosomal recessive disease with an incidence of 1/200,000 live births and a carrier frequency of 1/60-80. Carriers are phenotypically normal. In some Moslem countries, because of the high rate of consanguinity, the disease incidence is at least fortyfold greater. In 1990 the genetic abnormality responsible for SMA was localized to chromosome 5q 11.2-13.3. All three types of childhood SMA have been linked to the same locus in a number of studies, indicating phenotypic heterogeneity with genetic homogeneity similar to that observed in DMD/BMD.[80] Analysis of SMA 5q families supports the view that, with certain exceptions, there is little intrafamilial phenotypic variability. If the index patient satisfies the diagnostic criteria noted above, over 90% of all SMA families currently appear to be linked to chromosome 5q markers; the proportion of SMA I families linked to 5q11.2-13.1 is higher, and may approach 100%. In January 1995, the SMA-determining gene (termed the survival motor neuron [SMN] gene) was identified, and mutation analysis was carried out in 229 patients with 5q SMA (types I, II, and III).[116] The gene was homozygously deleted in 226 patients; in the remaining 3 patients one allele was deleted with a point mutation or short deletions in the other. The function of the gene protein is not yet known, but it is expressed in a wide variety of tissues, including spinal cord. No phenotype-genotype correlation between the gene defect and the type of SMA was detected, although deletions of contiguous segments of DNA appeared to be more frequent in type I than in type II patients.

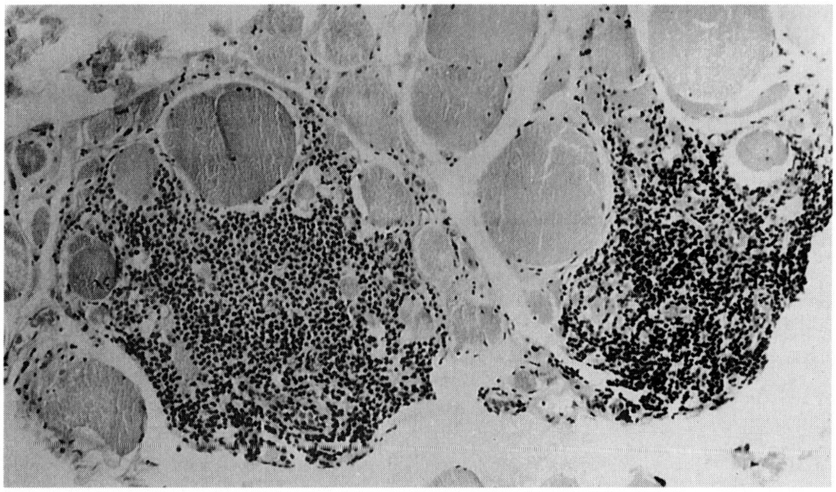

**Fig. 17-26.** Myasthenia gravis. H&E transverse section of skeletal muscle showing interstitial collection of lymphocyte–lymphorrhage. (Original magnification ×100.)

## DISORDERS OF THE NEUROMUSCULAR JUNCTION

### Myasthenia Gravis

The main clinical features of the illness are weakness and fatiguability. The weakness has a special predilection for cranial nerve-innervated muscles, affects all age groups, but is especially common in young adult women and older men. Diplopia and ptosis are common presenting manifestations. Other early symptoms include dysphagia, dysarthria, difficulty in chewing, and difficulty in holding up the head. As the disease progresses, involvement of muscles of the shoulder and pelvic girdles as well as trunk muscles develops. In advanced cases and, rarely, early in the course of the disease, respiratory muscles are affected. Laboratory studies disclose antibodies to AChR in 90% of patients. Repetitive nerve stimulation at low rates (2 Hz) is abnormal because of a decremental motor response. Ten to 15% of patients (especially the older men) have a thymoma.

Muscle biopsy is not necessary to establish the diagnosis, but when performed usually is normal. Patients who have been receiving corticosteroids will often have type 2 fiber atrophy, and some show evidence of denervation.[20] Rarely, collections of lymphocytes (lymphorrhages) are seen (Fig. 17-26). Electron microscopic studies of the muscle end-plate region show a remarkably simplified postsynaptic region with degeneration of junctional folds. When the myasthenic postsynaptic junction is stained for AChR, few are found on the terminal expansions of junctional folds, sites that normally are densely packed with AChR. Immunocytochemical studies show IgG, complement components C3 and C9, and the membrane attack complex, all localized to the neuromuscular junction. This suggests that complement fixation and activation of the lytic phase of the complement reaction sequence occur in myasthenia gravis.

Myasthenia gravis is an autoimmune disease that results from an antibody-mediated attack on these nicotinic AChR. The etiology of this disease is unknown, but much has been learned of its pathogenesis. First, there is complement-mediated lysis of the postsynaptic membrane, which causes loss of AChR. Second, autoantibodies bind to the AChR and result in accelerated degradation of receptor molecules. The first mechanism reduces membrane surface available for the insertion of new AChR. Third, autoantibodies may directly block the access of ACh to the receptor.

### Other Diseases of the Neuromuscular Junction

The Lambert-Eaton myasthenic syndrome (LEMS) usually develops as a paraneoplastic process, most commonly in association with small cell carcinoma of the lung (60% of cases), although it can be found in the absence of underlying malignancy. Patients develop proximal muscle weakness along with evidence of autonomic dysfunction. No clinical improvement is found with the tensilon test, and electrophysiologic studies show evidence of enhanced neurotransmission with repetitive stimulation. These clinical features allow this disorder to be separated from myasthenia gravis. The muscle biopsy is normal by light microscopy. Electron microscopic study has shown minimal or no abnormalities in the synaptic region.[74] Detailed electrophysiologic studies performed on muscle biopsies from patients with LEMS have shown that single vesicle content of ACh is normal and that the postsynaptic membrane is normally responsive to ACh, but fewer vesicles are released in response to each presynaptic action potential. Although antibodies directed against the AChR are not present in these patients, their serum contains IgG species that allow passive transfer of LEMS-type electrophysiologic findings to animals. Recent studies have described a high frequency of P/Q-type calcium channel antibodies in patients with LEMS, suggesting that these antibodies have a role in the pathogenesis of the presynaptic impairment of acetylcholine releases in this disease.[118]

This includes a heterogeneous group of disorders of neuromuscular transmission, thought to be inherited as dominant or recessive and largely of a nonimmunologic etiology. A number of syndromes have been described including both presynaptic and postsynaptic defects (see review[53]). The typical presentation is that of an infant with ocular, bulbar, and respiratory weakness and associated gerneralized weakness that worsens with fatigue. The laboratory studies are unremarkable and the tensilon test is often negative. Muscle biopsy studies are often not performed in these children; in the few reported instances, no abnormalities have been noted by light microscopy, including enzyme histochemistry. Abnormalities in the density of synaptic vesicle and in the junctional folds of the neuromuscular junction have been seen by electron microscopy.

## REFERENCES


1. Ahonen RE: Light microscopic study of striated muscle in uremia, Acta Neuropathol 49:51-55, 1980.
2. Albrecht S and Bilbao JM: Ubiquitin expression in inclusion body myositis. An immunohistochemical study, Arch Pathol Lab Med 117:789-793, 1993.
3. Amit R and others: Fatal familial infantile glycogen storage disease: multisystem phosphofructokinase deficiency, Muscle Nerve 15:455-458, 1992.
4. Arahata K and Engel AG: Monoclonal antibody analysis of mononuclear cells in myopathies. I: Quantitation of subsets according to diagnosis and sites of accumulation and demonstration and counts of muscle fibers invaded by T cells, Ann Neurol 16:193-208, 1984.
5. Arahata K and Engel AG: Monoclonal antibody analysis of mononuclear cells in myopathies. III: Immunoelectron microscopy aspects of cell-mediated muscle fiber injury, Ann Neurol 19:112-125, 1986.
6. Argov Z and others: Congenital myotonic dystrophy. Fiber type abnormalities in two cases, Arch Neurol 37:693-696, 1980.
7. Banker BQ: Dermatomyositis of childhood. Ultrastructural alterations of muscle and intramuscular blood vessels, J Neuropathol Exp Neurol 34:46-75, 1975.
8. Banker BQ: The congenital muscular dystrophies. In Engel AG and Franzini-Armstrong C, editors: Myology. Basic and clinical, ed 2, New York, 1994, McGraw-Hill.
9. Banker BQ: Other inflammatory myopathies. In Engel AG and Franzini-Armstrong C, editors: Myology. Basic and clinical, ed 2, New York, 1994, McGraw-Hill.
10. Banker BQ and Victor M: Dermatomyositis (systemic angiopathy) of childhood, Medicine 45:261-289, 1966.
11. Bashir R and others: A gene for autosomal recessive limb-girdle muscular dystrophy maps to chromosome 2p, Hum Mol Genet 3:455-457, 1994.
12. Becker PE and Keiner F: Eine neue x-chromosomale Muskeldystrophie, Arch Psychiatr Nervenkr 193S:427-448, 1955.
13. Beckmann JS, Richard I, and Hillaire D: A gene for limb-girdle muscular dystrophy maps to chromosome 15 by linkage, Compt Rend Acad Sci III 312:141, 1991.
14. Bergen BJ and others: Centronuclear myopathy: extraocular and limb-muscle findings in an adult, Muscle Nerve 3:165-171, 1980.
15. Bione S and others: Identification of a novel X-linked gene responsible for Emery-Dreifuss muscular dystrophy, Nature Genet 8:323-327, 1994.
16. Bradley WG, Jones MZ, and Fawcett PRW: Becker-type muscular dystrophy, Muscle Nerve 1:111-132, 1978.
17. Brook JD and others: Molecular basis of myotonic dystrophy; expansion of a trinucleotide (CTG) repeat at the 3′ end of a transcript encoding a protein kinase family member, Cell 68: 799-808, 1992.
18. Brooke MH and others: Duchenne muscular dystrophy: patterns of clinical progression and effects of supportive therapy, Neurology 39:475-481, 1989.
19. Brownell AKW and others: Adult onset nemaline myopathy, Neurology 28:1306-1309, 1978.
20. Brownell B, Oppenheimer DR, and Spalding JMK: Neurogenic muscle atrophy in myasthenia gravis, J Neurol, Neurosurg Psychiatry 35:311-322, 1972.
21. Bundschu HD and Schlote W: Eleknronmikroskopische Untersuchungen der Skelettmuskulatur bei terminaler Niereninsuffizienz, J Neurol Sci 23:243-254, 1974.
22. Campbell K: Three muscular dystrophies: loss of cytoskeleton-extracellular matrix linkage, Cell 80:675-679, 1995.
23. Carpenter S and Karpati G: The pathological diagnosis of specific inflammatory myopathies, Brain Pathol 2:13-19, 1992.
24. Carpenter S and others: Inclusion body myositis: a distinct variety of idiopathic inflammatory myopathy, Neurology 28:8-17, 1978.
25. Carpenter S and others: The childhood type of dermatomyositis, Neurology 26:952-962, 1976.
26. Case Records of the Massachusetts General Hospital: Case 34-1992, N Engl J Med 327:549-557, 1992.
27. Caulfield JB, Rebeiz J, and Adams RD: Viral involvement of human muscle, J Pathol Bacteriol 96:232-234, 1968.
28. Cazzato G and Walton JN: The pathology of the muscle spindle. A study of biopsy material in various muscular and neuromuscular diseases, J Neurol Sci 7:15-70, 1968.
29. Chad DA and others: Human immunodeficiency virus (HIV)-associated myopathy: immunocytochemical identification of an HIV antigen (gp 41) in muscle macrophages, Ann Neurol 28: 579-582, 1990.
30. Chalmers AC, Greco CM, and Miller RG: Prognosis in AZT myopathy, Neurology 41:1181-1184, 1991.
31. Chou S-M: Myxovirus-like structures in a case of chronic polymyositis, Science 158:1453-1455, 1967.
32. Chou SM: Inclusion body myositis: a chronic persistent mumps myositis? Hum Pathol 17:765-777, 1986.
33. Chou SM and Gutmann L: Picornavirus-like crystals in subacute polymyositis, Neurology 20:205-213, 1970.
34. Chucrallah A and others: Lovostatin/gemfibrozil myopathy: a clinical, histochemical, and ultrastructural study, Eur Neurol 32:293-296, 1992.
35. Consalez GG and others: Assignment of Emery-Dreifuss muscular dystrophy to the distal region of chromosome Xq28: the results of a collaborative study, Am J Hum Genet 48:468-480, 1991.
36. Crews J, Kaiser KK, and Brooke MH: Muscle pathology of myotonia congenita, J Neurol Sci 28:449-457, 1976.
37. Dalakas M: Polymyositis, dermatomyositis and inclusion body myositis, N Engl J Med 325:1487-1498, 1991.
38. Dalakas MC and others: Mitochondrial myopathy caused by long-term zidovudine therapy, N Engl J Med 322:1098-1105, 1990.
39. De Bleecker JL and Engel AG: Immunocytochemical study of CD45 T cell isoforms in inflammatory myopathies, Am J Pathol 146:1178-1187, 1995.
40. De Girolami U and Smith TW: Pathology of skeletal muscle diseases. Teaching monograph, Am J Pathol 107:235-276, 1982.

41. De Girolami U and Smith TW: Diseases of skeletal muscle and peripheral nerve. In Dickersin GR, editor: Diagnostic electron microscopy: a text atlas, New York, 1988, Igaku-Shoin.
42. De Girolami U and others: Skeletal muscle. In Silverberg SG, editor: Principles and practice of surgical pathology, ed 2, New York, 1990, Churchill-Livingstone.
43. De Girolami U and others: Neuropathology and ophthalmologic pathology of the acquired immunodeficiency syndrome. Boston, 1992, Butterworth-Heinemann.
44. De Visser M, Emslie-Smith AM, and Engel AG: Early ultrastructural alterations in adult dermatomyositis. Capillary abnormalities precede other structural changes in muscle, J Neurol Sci 94:181-192, 1989.
45. Di Donato S: Disorders of lipid metabolism affecting skeletal muscle: carnitine deficiency syndromes, defects in the catabolic pathway, and chanarin disease. In Engel AG and Franzini-Armstrong C, editors: Myology. Basic and clinical, ed 2, New York, 1994, McGraw-Hill.
46. DiMauro S, Melis DiMauro PM: Muscle carnitine palmityltransferase deficiency and myoglobinuria, Science 182:929-931, 1973.
47. DiMauro S and Tsujino S: Nonlysosomal glycogenoses. In Engel AG and Franzini-Armstrong C, editors: Myology. Basic and clinical, ed 2, New York, 1994, McGraw-Hill.
48. Duchenne de Boulogne: De l'Électrisation localisée et de son Application à la Physiologie, à la Pathologie et à la Thérapeutique. Paris, 1855, Baillière.
49. Duchenne de Boulogne: Recherches sur la paralysie musculaire pseudo-hypertrophique ou paralysie myo-sclérosique, Arch Gén Méd 11:5-25, 179-209, 305-321, 421-443, 522-588, 868, 1868.
50. Emery AEH, Dreifuss FE: Unusual type of benign X-linked muscular dystrophy, J Neurology Neurosurg Psychiatry 29: 338-342, 1966.
51. Emslie-Smith AM, Arahata K, and Engel AG: Major histocompatibility complex class I antigen expression, immunolocalization of interferon subtypes, and T-cell-mediated cytoxicity in myopathies, Hum Pathol 20:224-231, 1989.
52. Emslie-Smith AM and Engel AG: Microvascular changes in early advanced dermatomyositis: a quantitative study, Ann Neurol 27:343-356, 1990.
53. Engel AG: Myasthenic syndromes. In Engel AG and Franzini-Armstrong C, editors: Myology. Basic and clinical, ed 2, New York, 1994, McGraw-Hill.
54. Engel AG and Arahata K: Monoclonal antibody analysis of mononuclear cells in myopathies. II: Phenotypes of autoinvasive cells in polymyositis and inclusion body myositis, Ann Neurol 16:209-215, 1984.
55. Engel AG and Franzini-Armstrong C, editors: Myology. Basic and clinical, ed 2, New York, 1994, McGraw-Hill.
56. Engel AG and Hirschhorn R: Acid maltase deficiency. In Engel AG and Franzini-Armstrong C, editors: Myology. Basic and clinical, ed 2, New York, 1994, McGraw-Hill.
57. Engel AG, Hohlfeld R, and Banker BQ: The polymyositis and dermatomyositis syndromes. In Engel AG and Franzini-Armstrong C, editors: Myology. Basic and clinical, ed 2, New York, 1994, McGraw-Hill.
58. Engel AG and Siekert RG: Lipid storage myopathy responsive to prednisone, Arch Neurol 27:174-181, 1972.
59. Engel AG, Yamamoto M, and Fishbeck KH: Dystrophinopathies. In Engel AG, Franzini-Armstrong C, editors: Myology. Basic and clinical, ed 2, New York, 1994, McGraw-Hill.
60. Engel WK, Gold GN, and Karpati G: Type I fiber hypotrophy and central nuclei. A rare congenital muscle abnormality with a possible experimental model, Neurology 18:435-444, 1968.
61. Engel WK and others: Mapping a gene for congenital fibrosis of the extraocular muscles to the centromeric region of chromosome 12, Nat Genet 7:69-73, 1994.
62. Erb W: Ueber die "juvenile Form" der progressiven Muskelatrophie ihre Beziehungen zur sogenannten Pseudohypertrophie der Muskeln, Dtsch Arch klin Med 34:467-519, 1884.
63. Erb W: Dystrophia muscularis progressiva. Klinische und pathologisch-anatomische Studien, Dtsch Z Nerv 1:13-94, 173-261, 1891.
64. Eulenburg A: Ueber eine familiäre, durch 6 Generationen verfolgbare Form congenitaler Paramyotonie, Neurol Zentral 5: 265-272, 1886.
65. Fardeau M and Tomé FMS: Congenital myopathies. In Engel AG and Franzini-Armstrong C, editors: Myology. Basic and clinical, ed 2, New York, 1994, McGraw-Hill.
66. Fardeau M, Tomé MS, and Simon P: Muscle and nerve changes induced by perhexiline maleate in man and mice, Muscle Nerve 2:24-36, 1979.
67. Felice K, De Girolami U, and Chad D: Pyomyositis presenting as rapidly progressive generalized weakness, Neurology 41: 944-945, 1991.
68. Ferrer X and others: Myopathie centronucléaire autosomique dominante, Rev Neurol 148:622-630, 1992.
69. Figarella-Branger D and others: Expression of cell surface and cytoskeleton developmentally regulated proteins in adult centronuclear myopathies, J Neurol Sci 109:69-76, 1992.
70. Figarella-Branger D and others: Myosites à inclusions et maladies neuromusculaires avec vacuoles bordées, Rev Neurol 148: 281-290, 1992.
71. Finocchiaro G and others: cDNA cloning, sequence analysis, and chromosomal localization of the gene for human carnitine palmitoyltransferase, Proc Nat Acad Sci USA 88:661-665, 1991.
72. Fougerousse F and others: Mapping of chromosome 15 region involved in limb girdle muscular dystrophy, Hum Mol Genet 3:455-457, 1994.
73. Frankel KA and Rosser RJ: The pathology of the heart in progressive muscular dystrophy: epimyocardial fibrosis, Hum Pathol 7:375-386, 1976.
74. Fukuhara N and others: Eaton-Lambert syndrome. Ultrastructural study of the motor end-plates, Arch Neurol 27:67-78, 1972.
75. Fukuyama Y, Osawa M, and Suzuki H: Congenital progressive muscular dystrophy of the Fukuyama type—clinical, genetic and pathological considerations, Brain Devel 3:1-29, 1981.
76. George AL and others: Primary structure of the adult human skeletal muscle voltage-dependent sodium channel, Ann Neurol 31:131-137, 1992.
77. Gherardi R and others: Skeletal muscle toxoplasmosis in patients with acquired immunodeficiency syndrome: a clinical and pathological study, Ann Neurol 32:535-542, 1992.
78. Gherardi RK and others: Cytokine expression in the muscle of HIV-infected patients: evidence for interleukin-1$\alpha$ accumulation in mitochondria of AZT fibers, Ann Neurol 36:752-758, 1994.
79. Gibson RK, Rosenthal SJ, and Lukert BP: Pyomyositis. Increasing recognition in temperate climates, Am J Med 77:768-772, 1984.
80. Gilliam TC and Brzustowicz LM: Molecular and genetic basis of the spinal muscular atrophies. In Rosenberg R, and others, editors: The Molecular and Genetic Basis of Neurologic Disease, Boston, 1993, Butterworth.
81. Gonatas Nk, Shy GM, and Godfrey EH: Nemaline myopathy. The origin of nemaline structures, N Engl J Med 274:535-539, 1966.
82. Gray F, editor: Atlas of the neuropathology of HIV infection, Oxford, 1993, Oxford University Press.
83. Greenfield JG, Cornman T, and Shy GM: The prognostic value of the muscle biopsy in the "floppy infant", Brain 81:462-484, 1958.

84. Gronert GA: Malignant hyperthermia. In Engel AG, and Franzini-Armstrong C, editors: Myology. Basic and clinical, ed 2, New York, 1994, McGraw-Hill.
85. Haan EA and others: Assignment of the gene for central core disease to chromosome 19, Hum Genet 86:187-190, 1990.
86. Harper P: The muscular dystrophies. In Scriver CR, Beaudet AL, Sly SS, and Valle D, editors: The metabolic basis of inherited disease, ed 6, New York, 1989, McGraw-Hill.
87. Hays AP and others: Muscle phosphofructokinase deficiency: abnormal polysaccharide in a case of late-onset myopathy, Neurology 31:1077-1086, 1981.
88. Heffner RR: Inflammatory myopathies. A review, J Neuropathol Exp Neurol 52:339-350, 1993.
89. Heffner RR, Armbrustmacher VW, and Earle KM: Focal myositis, Cancer 40:301-306, 1977.
90. Herrick MK and others: Concomitant branching enzyme and phosphorylase deficiencies. An unusual glycogenosis with extensive neuronal polyglucosan storage, J Neuropathol Exp Neurol 53:239-246, 1994.
91. Hewlett RH, and Brownell B: Granulomatous myopathy: its relationship to sarcoidosis and polymyositis, J Neurol Neurosurg Psychiatry 38:1090-1099, 1975.
92. Hillaire D and others: Localization of merosin-negative congenital muscular dystrophy to chromosome 6q2 by homozygosity mapping. Hum Mol Genet 3:1657-1661, 1994.
93. Hoffman EP, and Kunkel LM: Dystrophin abnormalities in Duchenne/Becker muscular dystrophy, Neuron 2:1019-1029, 1989.
94. Holt IJ and other: A new mitochondrial disease associated with mitochondrial DNA heteroplasmy, Am J Hum Genet 46:428-433, 1990.
95. Hopkins IJ, Lindsey JR, and Ford FR: Nemaline myopathy. A long-term clinicopathologic study of affected mother and daughter, Brain 89:299-310, 1966.
96. Hughes JT and others: Chloroquine myopathy, Q J Med 40:85-93, 1971.
97. Janssen EAM and others: The gene for X-linked myotubular myopathy is located in a 8 Mb region at the border of Xq27.3 and Xq28, Neuromuscul Disord 4:455-461, 1994.
98. Jay V, and Becker LE: Fiber-type differentiation by myosin immunohistochemistry on paraffin-embedded skeletal muscle. A useful adjunct to fiber typing by the adenosine triphosphatase reaction, Arch Pathol Lab Med 118:917-918, 1994.
99. Jerusalem F and others: Morphometric analysis of skeletal muscle capillary ultrastructure in inflammatory myopathies, J Neurol Sci 23:391-402, 1974.
100. Kaido M and others: Muscle histology in Becker muscular dystrophy, Muscle Nerve 14:1067-1073, 1991.
101. Kallajoki M and others: Inclusion body myositis and paramyxoviruses, Hum Pathol 22:29-32, 1991.
102. Kaminski HJ, and Ruff RL: Endocrine myopathies (hyper- and hypofunction of the adrenal, thyroid, pituitary and parathyroid glands and iatrogenic corticosteroid myopathy). In Engel AG and Franzini-Armstrong C, editors: Myology. Basic and clinical, ed 2, New York, 1994, McGraw-Hill.
103. Karpati G and others: The syndrome of systemic carnitine deficiency, Neurology 25:16-24, 1975.
104. Karpati G and others: The Kearns-Shy syndrome. A multisystem disease with mitochondrial abnormality demonstrated in skeletal muscle, J Neurol Sci 19:133-151, 1973.
105. Karpati G and others: Infantile myotonic dystrophy. Histochemical and electron microscopic features in skeletal muscle, Neurology 23:1066-1076, 1973.
106. Kissel JT, Mendell JR, and Rammohan KW: Microvascular deposition of complement membrane attack complex in dermatomyositis, N Engl J Med 314:329-334, 1986.
107. Kobayashi Y and others: A point mutation in the mitochondrial tRNA $^{Leu}$(UUR) gene in MELAS (mitochondrial myopathy, encephalopathy, lactic acidosis and stroke-like episodes), Biochem Biophys Res Comm 173:816-822, 1990.
108. Koch MC and others: The skeletal muscle chloride channel in dominant and recessive human myotonia, Science 257:797-800, 1992.
109. Kuhn E and others: The autosomal recessive (Becker) form of myotonia congenita, Muscle Nerve 2:109-117, 1979.
110. Kuncl RW and others: Colchicine myopathy and neuropathy, N Engl J Med 316:1562-1568, 1987.
111. Lacomis D and others: Childhood onset oculopharyngeal muscular dystrophy, Pediatr Neurol 7:382-384, 1991.
112. Laing NG and others: Assignment of a gene (NEM1) for autosomal dominant nemaline myopathy to chromosome 1, Am J Hum Genet 50:576-583, 1992.
113. Landouzy L and Dejerine J: De la myopathie atrophique progressive (myopathie héréditaire débutant, dans l'enfance, par la face, sans altération du système nerveux), Comp Rend Hebdomad Acad Scie 98:53-55, 1884.
114. Landouzy L and Dejerine J: De la myopathie atrophique progressive. Myopathie sans neuropathie débutant d'ordinaire dans l'enfance, par la face, Rev Méd 5:81-117, 253-266, 1885.
115. Lebo RV and others: High-resolution chromosome sorting and DNA spot-blot analysis assign McArdle's syndrome to chromosome 11, Science 225:57-59, 1984.
116. Lefebvre S and others: Identification and characterization of a spinal muscular atrophy-determining gene, Cell 80:155-165, 1995.
117. Lehmann-Horn F and others: The periodic paralyses and paramyotonia congenita. In Engel AG and Franzini-Armstrong C, editors: Myology. Basic and clinical, ed 2, New York, 1994, McGraw-Hill.
118. Lennon V, and others: Calcium-channel antibodies in the Lambert-Eaton and other paraneoplastic syndromes, N Engl J Med 332:1467-1474, 1995.
119. Leon-Monzon M, Illa I, and Dalakas MC: Polymyositis in patients infected with human T-cell leukemia virus type I: the role of the virus in the cause of the disease, Ann Neurol 36:643-649, 1994.
120. Lotz BP and others: Inclusion body myositis. Observations in 40 patients, Brain 112:727-747, 1989.
121. Lynch PG and Bansal DV: Granulomatous polymyositis, J Neurol Sci 18:1-9, 1972.
122. Markesbery WR, Griggs R, and Herr B: Distal myopathy: electron microscopic and histochemical studies, Neurology 27:727-735, 1977.
123. Markesbery WR and others: Late onset hereditary distal myopathy, Neurology 24:127-134, 1974.
124. Marsh CG and Munsat TL: Evidence of early impairment of verbal intelligence in Duchenne muscular dystrophy, Arch Dis Child 49:118-122, 1974.
125. Mastaglia FL: Pathological changes in skeletal muscle in acromegaly, Acta Neuropathol 24:273-286, 1973.
126. Mastaglia FL, Barwick DD, and Hall R: Myopathy in acromegaly, Lancet 2:907-909, 1970.
127. Matsumura K and others: Deficiency of the 50K dystrophin-associated glycoprotein in severe childhood autosomal recessive muscular dystrophy, Nature 359:320-322, 1992.
128. Mendell JR and others: Amyloid filaments in inclusion body myositis. Novel findings provide insight into nature of filaments, Arch Neurol 48:1229-1234, 1991.
129. Merlini L and others: Emery-Dreifuss muscular dystrophy: report of five cases in a family and review of the literature, Muscle Nerve 9:481-485, 1986.

130. Mhiri C and others: Zidovudine myopathy: a distinctive disorder associated with mitochondrial dysfunction, Ann Neurol 29: 606-614, 1991.
131. Michel D and others: Myosite granulomateuse au cours d'une collagénose (une observation) et d'un dysgerminome suprasellaire (une observation), Rev Neurol 135:3-14, 1979.
132. Mikol J, and Engel A: Inclusion body myositis. In Engel AG and Franzini-Armstrong C, editors. Myology. Basic and clinical, ed 2, New York, 1994, McGraw-Hill.
133. Mikol J and others: Inclusion-body myositis: clinicopathologic studies and isolation of an adenovirus Type 2 from muscle biopsy specimen, Ann Neurol 11:576-581, 1982.
134. Misra AK, Menon NK, and Mishra SK: Abnormal distribution of desmin and vimentin in myofibers in adult onset myotubular myopathy, Muscle Nerve 15:1246-1252, 1992.
135. Munsat TL and others: Inflammatory myopathy with facioscapulohumeral distribution, Neurology 22:335-347, 1972.
136. Munsat TL and others: Neurogenic muscular atrophy of infancy with prolonged survival. The variable course of Werdnig-Hoffmann disease, Brain 92:9-24, 1969.
137. Nageotte J: Sur la contraction extrême des muscles squelettiques chez les vertébrés, Z Zellforsch Mikroskop Anat 26:603-624, 1937.
138. Namba T, Brunner NG, and Grob D: Idiopathic giant cell polymyositis. Report of a case and review of the syndrome, Arch Neurol 31:27-30, 1974.
139. Nishino H, Engel AG, and Rima BK: Inclusion body myositis: the mumps virus hypothesis, Ann Neurol 25:260-264, 1989.
140. North KN and others: Congenital muscular dystrophy associated with merosin deficiency, J Child Neurol 11:291-295, 1996.
141. Oshima Y, Becker LE, and Armstrong DL: An electron microscopic study of childhood dermatomyositis, Acta Neuropathol 47:189-196, 1979.
142. Othmanem KB and others: Linkage of Tunisian autosomal recessive Duchenne-like muscular dystrophy to the pericentromeric region of chromosome 13q, Nat Genet 2:315, 1992.
143. Padberg GW: The muscular dystrophies and dystrophin, Curr Opin Neurol 6:688-694, 1993.
144. Reimers CD and others: Borrelia burgdorferi myositis: a report of eight patients, J Neurol 240:278-283, 1993.
145. Rosman NP and Rebeiz JJ: The cerebral defect and myopathy in myotonic dystrophy. A comparative clinicopathological study, Neurology 17:1106-1112, 1967.
146. Rowland LP and others: Emery-Dreifuss muscular dystrophy, Ann Neurol 5:111-117, 1979.
147. Rutkove SB and others: Myotonia in colchicine myopathy, 19: 870-875, 1996.
148. Sabina RL and others: Characterization of the human and rat myoadenylate deaminase genes, J Biol Chem 265:9423-9433, 1990.
149. Samson F and others: Genetic linkage heterogeneity in myotubular myopathy, Am J Hum Genet 57:120-126, 1995.
150. Sarnat H: Myotubular myopathy: arrest of morphogenesis of myofibers associated with persistence of fetal vimentin and desmin. Four cases compared with fetal and neonatal muscle, Can J Neurol Sci 17:109-123, 1990.
151. Schotland DL, Spiro D, and Carmel P: Ultrastructural studies of ring fibers in human muscle disease, J Neuropathol Exp Neurol 25:431-442, 1966.
152. Scriver CR and others: The metabolic basis of inherited disease, New York, 1995, McGraw-Hill.
153. Shevell M and others: Congenital inflammatory myopathy, Neurology 40:1111-1114, 1990.
154. Shoffner JM and others: Myoclonic epilepsy and ragged-red fiber disease (MERRF) is associated with a mitochondrial DNA $tRNA^{Lys}$ mutation, Cell 61:931-937, 1990.
155. Shy GM and others: Nemaline myopathy. A new congenital myopathy, Brain 86:793-810, 1963.
156. Shy GM and Magee KR: A new congenital non-progressive myopathy, Brain 79:610-621, 1956.
157. Silverstein A and Sitlzbach L: Muscle involvement in sarcoidosis. Asymptomatic, myositis, and myopathy, Arch Neurol 21: 235-241, 1969.
158. Sivakumar K and others: Exons 16 and 17 of the amyloid precursor protein gene in familial inclusion body myopathy, Ann Neurol 38:267-269, 1995.
159. Smadja D and others: Atteintes du système nerveux périphérique et du muscle squelettique au cours des paraplégies associeés au virus HTLV1. Étude de 70 cas observés en Martinique, Rev Neurol 151:190-195, 1995.
160. Specht L and Kunkel L: Duchenne and Becker muscular dystrophy. In Rosenberg R and others editors: The molecular and genetic basis of neurologic Disease, Boston, 1993, Butterworth.
161. Spiro AJ, Shy GM, and Gonatas NK: Myotubular myopathy. Persistence of fetal muscle in an adolescent boy, Arch Neurol 14:1-14, 1966.
162. Spur MC and others: Confirmation of genetic heterogeneity in limb-girdle muscular dystrophy: linkage of an autosomal dominant from to chromosome 5q, Am J Hum Genet 50:1211, 1992.
163. Steinert H: Über das klinische und anatomische Bild des Muskelschwunds der Myotoniker, Dtsch Z Nerv 37:58-104, 1909.
164. Stern LZ, Payne CM, and Hannapel LK: Acromegaly: histochemical and electron microscopic changes in deltoid and intercostal muscle, Neurology 24:589-593, 1974.
165. Strongwater SL and others: Eosinophilia myalgia syndrome associated with L-tryptophan ingestion: analysis of four patients and implications for differential diagnosis and pathogenesis, Arch Intern Med 150:2178-2186., 1990.
166. Thomsen J: Tonische Krämpfe in willkürlich beweglichen Muskeln in Folge von erebter psychischer Disposition (Ataxia muscularis?), Arch Psychiatr Nerv 6:702-718, 1876.
167. Thornton CA, Griggs RC, and Moxley RT: Myotonic dystrophy with no trinucleotide repeat expansion, Ann Neurol 35:269-272, 1994.
168. Thrush DC, Morris CJ, and Salmon MV: Paramyotonia congenita; a clinical, histochemical and pathological study, Brain 95:537-552, 1972.
169. Toda T and others: Localization of a gene for Fukuyama type congenital muscular dystrophy to chromosome 9q31-33, Nat Genet 5:283-286, 1993.
170. Tomé FMS and others: Congenital muscular dystrophy with merosin deficiency, Com Rend Acad Sci III 317:351-357, 1994.
171. Tomé FMS and Fardeau M: Nuclear inclusions in oculopharyngeal dystrophy, Acta Neuropathol 49:85-87, 1980.
172. Tsujino S, Shanske S, and DiMauro S: Molecular genetic heterogeneity of myophosphorylase deficiency (McArdle's disease), N Engl J Med 329:241-245, 1993.
173. Victor M, Hayes R, and Adams RD: Oculopharyngeal muscular dystrophy. A familial disease of late life characterized by dysphagia and progressive ptosis of the eyelids, N Engl J Med 267: 1267-1272, 1962.
174. Victor M and Sieb JP: Myopathies due to drugs, toxins and nutritional deficiency. In Engel AG and Franzini-Armstrong C, editors: Myology. Basic and clinical, ed 2, New York, 1994, McGraw-Hill.
175. Vora S and others: Assignment of the human gene for muscle-type phosphofructokinase (PFKM) to chromosome 1 (region cen-q32) using somatic cell hybrids and monoclonal anti-M antibody, Somat Cell Genet 8:95-104, 1982.
176. Wallace SL and others: Muscle involvement in Boeck's sarcoid, Am J Med 26:497-511, 1958.

177. Wallgren-Pettersson C and others: The myotubular myopathies: differential diagnosis of the X linked recessive, autosomal dominant, and autosomal recessive forms and present state of DNA studies, J Med Genet 32:673-679, 1995.
178. Welander L: Myopathia distalis tarda hereditaria, Acta Med Scan 141:1-124, 1951.
179. Xu H and others: Murine muscular dystrophy caused by a mutation in the laminin alpha 2 (Lama2) gene, Nat Genet 8:297-302, 1994.
180. Yamada H and others: Laminin abnormality in severe childhood autosomal recessive muscular dystrophy, Lab Invest:715-722, 1995.
181. Yunis EJ and Samaha FJ: Inclusion body myositis, Lab Invest 25:240-248, 1971.
182. Zeviani M and others: Deletions of mitochondrial DNA in Kearns-Sayre syndrome, Neurology 38:1339-1346, 1988.

C • H • A • P • T • E • R

18

# Peripheral Neuropathies

**Anders A.F. Sima**
**Mila Blaivas**

Peripheral nerve biopsy is an invasive procedure, which compared with other diagnostic biopsies, provides a relatively small yield with respect to specific diagnosis. Approximately 15% to 25% of nerve biopsies reveal specific diagnoses or information crucial for clinical management; however, an additional 30% to 40% of biopsies revealed nonspecific information that supported the clinical impression.[1,85,93] Therefore, as a general rule nerve biopsy should be attempted only when the history (hereditary neuropathies), physical findings, and electrophysiologic tests have failed to provide a diagnosis, or when there is reason to suspect a treatable neuropathy like Guillain-Barré syndrome (GBS), chronic inflammatory demyelinating polyradiculoneuropathy (CIDP), or vasculitis.* In the remaining cryptogenic neuropathies, the indications for nerve biopsy are strong, provided that electrophysiologic abnormalities are demonstrable and the neuropathy is rapidly progressive. In slowly progressing neuropathies it may be more advisable to observe the disease progression with repeated clinical investigations.[52]

In rare situations, biopsy sites other than peripheral nerve may be considered. In amyloid neuropathy a rectal biopsy may be considered,[49] and in a variety of pediatric neurologic disorders skin, skeletal muscle, or conjunctival biopsies may reveal the diagnosis. These disorders include: infantile neuroaxonal dystrophy (Seitelberger's disease),[17,82] Fabry's disease,[120,141] and giant axonal neuropathy.[100] Leukodystrophies are now diagnosed by biochemical abnormalities detectable in peripheral blood cells or fibroblast cultures; however, characteristic Schwann cell inclusions in peripheral nerve from affected patients have also been demonstrated.[8,50,83]

## NORMAL SURAL NERVE ANATOMY

Since the sural nerve is the nerve most commonly biopsied for diagnostic purposes, the normal structure of this nerve at the level of the lateral malleolus will be briefly reviewed. Most myelinated and unmyelinated axons of the sural nerve originate from dorsal root ganglion cells of L5 to S2. Some unmyelinated fibers are part of the autonomic system, although in the sural nerve their numbers are probably low.[18] The sural nerve is purely sensory, it does not contain motor fibers. The dorsal root ganglia send out both a peripheral and a central axon. Therefore, neuropathies affecting sensory nerves in a systemic fashion, particularly metabolic polyneuropathies, also may affect the distal outreaches of the central axon, giving rise to symptoms of sensory ataxia.

The sural nerve trunk usually contains 8 to 16 fascicles of varying size, each surrounded by a perineurium embedded in the epineurium.

### Epineurium

This consists predominantly of connective and adipose tissue. The epineurium also contains a rich arterial network, which branches into the perineurium (Fig. 18-1), and lymphatic vessels, which are confined to the epineurium only. The cells of the epineurium consist mainly of fibroblasts, variable numbers of fat cells, occasional mast cells, and lymphocytes. Unless the latter are cuffed or concentrated around vessels, their presence does not necessarily indicate an inflammatory neuropathy. Bundles of predominantly type III collagen fibers run longitudinally along the nerve fascicles; they are more densely packed immediately around the perineuria and at the periphery of the nerve trunk.

### Perineurium

Each nerve fascicle is ensheathed by the perineurium, which consists of slender lamellated fibroblast-derived cells referred to as perineurial cells. The numbers of concentric layers of these cells vary from 12 to 15 layers in proximal nerves to only one layer in most distal nerves. In the sural nerve the perineurium usually contains five to nine layers (Fig. 18-1). The perineurial cells are surrounded by a basement membrane, which often shows varying thickness (probably due to oblique planes of sections). Obliquely oriented collagen fibers mainly type III are positioned between the lamellae of perineurial cells. Oxytalan fibers, elastic fiber equivalents, also exist between perineurial cells. The perineurial cells of the same and adjacent lamellae are interlocked by tight junctions (zonulae occludens) that constitute the protective perineurial barrier. Perineurial cells, as seen in nerve cross-section, are flat elongated cells with elongated nuclei. The plasma membrane and cytosol of perineurial cells characteristically contain pinocytotic vesicles, which may provide selective and facilitated transport of nutrients and macromolecules across the protective perineurial diffusion barrier. The perineurial cells may contain calcospherites in normal sural nerves of aged individuals and in nerve biopsies of patients with chronic polyneuropathies.

* Refs.: 4, 47, 60, 62, 63, 68.

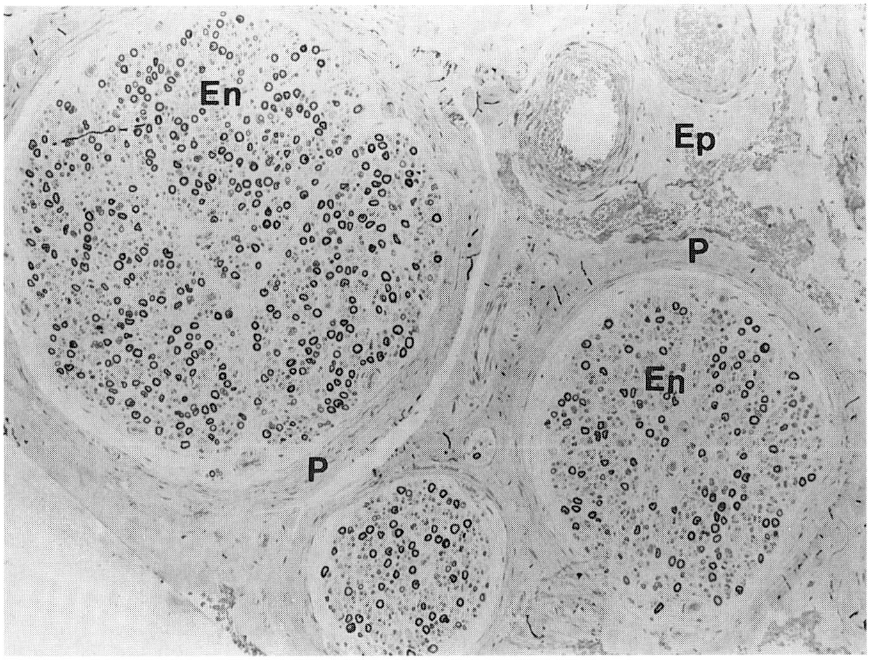


**Fig. 18-1.** Normal sural nerve from a 66-year-old individual. Note fascicles of varying sizes surrounded by perineurium (*P*) and embedded in the epineurium (*Ep*). Myelinated and unmyelinated fibers are present in the endoneurial compartments (*En*). Plastic section. (×96.)

### Endoneurium

The endoneurium is the space delineated by the innermost lamella of the perineurium. Approximately 30% of the endoneurium of the sural nerve is occupied by myelinated nerve fibers and roughly 10% by unmyelinated fibers and their supporting Schwann cells; only 2% to 3% is alotted to endoneurial vessels (Fig. 18-1). The rest of the endoneurial space is mostly occupied by collagen, which in the proximity of myelinated and unmyelinated fibers runs parallel to the fibers. Furthermore, the endoneurium contains fibroblasts, mast cells, and resident macrophages, most of which are found in the proximity of the endoneurial vessels. Of these, fibroblasts are the most abundant and each cell possesses multiple long and thin cytoplasmic processes without basement membranes. Mast cells are easily recognized by their metachromatic granules in toluidine-blue stained sections. They are rather plump oval cells with multiple thin, short processes. Mast cells lack a basement membrane. Macrophages make up approximately 5% of the cell population of the endoneurial space. They are MHC class II constituents and are the surveillance and antigen presenting cells. Macrophages have a plump cytoplasm with long, irregular cytoplasmic processes; these cells lack a basement membrane.

Occasional leukocytes, mostly lymphocytes, reacting positively with leukocyte common antigen (LCA) are not indicative of ongoing inflammation, provided that their number does not exceed 10 per whole sural nerve cross-section.

The remaining space of the endoneurium is occupied by collagen fibrils smaller than those present in the epineurium and made up of type III and type I collagen, the former being the predominant type. Large parts of the endoneurium appear light and electron microscopically "empty." These vacuoles contain the endoneurial fluid made of water and macromolecules. Occasional Renaut bodies may be present in normal nerves (Fig. 18-2). They consist of thin fibrillary, acellular structures arranged in concentric whorls often located directly beneath the perineurium. Renaut bodies may be mistaken for endoneurial edema or endoneurial infarctions; these structures seem to be more frequent at sites where nerves are exposed to compression and where they serve as a cushion.

The endoneurial space is normally under a higher pressure than the surrounding tissue, which, together with the elastic properties of the perineurium, probably serves as a protective function of the nerve fibers. Therefore in a perfectly obtained and promptly fixed nerve biopsy, the nerve fascicles should display an almost perfect circular configuration.

### Myelinated Fibers

Myelinated fibers make up about 25% of all axons in the sural nerve. They vary in size from 1 $\mu$m to about 15 $\mu$m in diameter and in the mature adult nerve show a bimodal size distribution with a large peak at 4 to 5 $\mu$m and a smaller peak at 10 to 11 $\mu$m. In the normal sural nerve the myelinated fiber density varies between 5000 and 8000 fibers per mm$^2$, depending on age.[116] In persons over 65 years there is a more rapid decline in myelinated fiber density. The internodal length (as seen in teased fibers) varies between 0.20

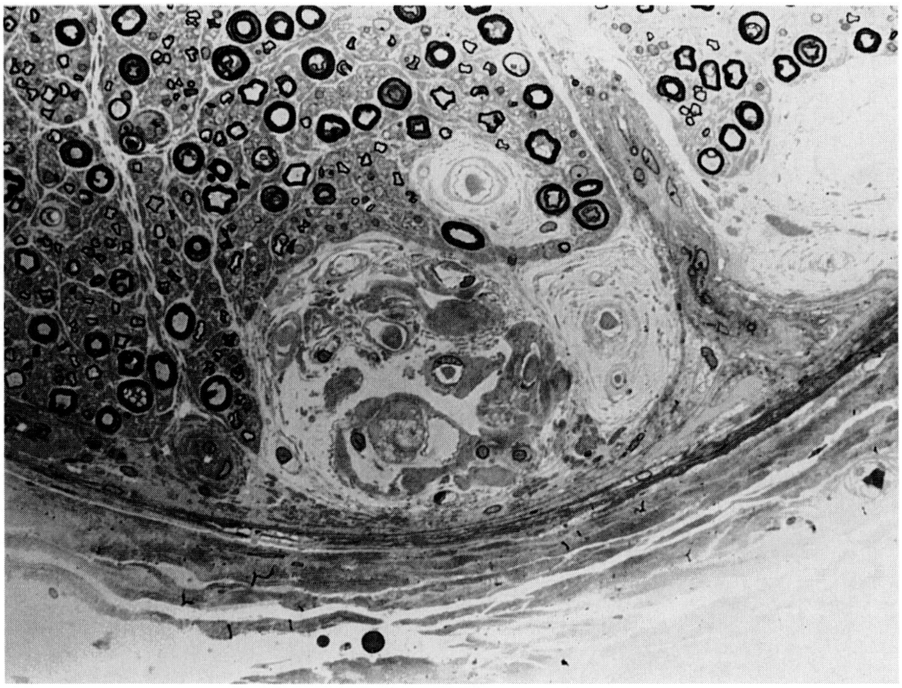

**Fig. 18-2.** Renaut body. Four or more Renaut bodies within the subperineurial region are formed by circular arrangement of hypocellular myxomatous material that varies greatly in density from one body to another. One micron thick plastic embedded toluidine stained section. (×330.)

and 1.60 mm, depending on the caliber of the fiber; the larger the diameter, the longer the internode.

In a cross-section of the sural nerve myelinated fibers of varying sizes are evenly distributed within the endoneurium. The fibers have a circular configuration, although small myelinated fibers show a greater variability in their shape.

The detailed structures of the myelinated axon can only be appreciated ultrastructurally (Fig. 18-3). The normal axon contains evenly dispersed neurofilaments and neurotubules and is surrounded by myelinating Schwann cells, which wrap their plasma membrane around the axon, and its inner membranes join at the inner mesaxon to form the myelin lamellae. The number of myelin lamellae, which determines the myelin thickness, is proportional to the axonal caliber. On the outer circumference of the myelinated fiber the outermost myelin lamella splits open to form the outer mesaxon, which then forms the Schwann cell membrane. Usually around the inner and the outer mesaxons there are sleeves of Schwann cell cytoplasm that surround the axon and the outer circumference of the myelin sheath, respectively. Along the internode the compacted myelin is interrupted by sleeves of Schwann cell cytoplasm, which at these sites, called the Schmidt-Lanterman incisures, show spiraling continuum between the outer and the inner Schwann cell lip.

The axon is not covered by myelin at the node of Ranvier. However, Schwann cells from the two neighboring internodes show interdigitating slender processes. In the paranode the myelin membranes loosen and form cytoplasma-filled loops which are apposed to the paranodal axonal membrane (Fig. 18-4). The myelin loops and the axolemma are joined together by tight junctions, called axoglial junctions, that provide a diffusion barrier function and separate the sodium channels concentrated at the nodal axolemma from paranodal potassium channels. At the node the axon

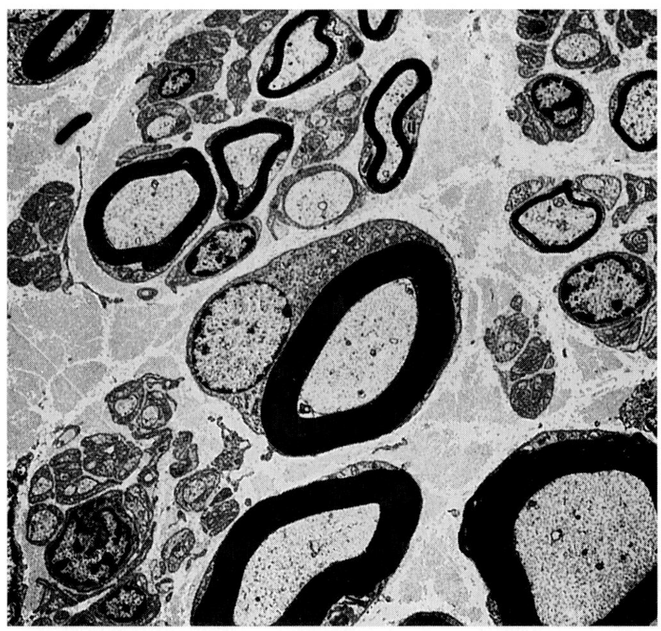

**Fig. 18-3.** Electron micrograph showing myelinated fibers of varying sizes. The myelin sheath is surrounded by thin sleeves of Schwann cell cytoplasm, which is more generous around the nucleus (fiber in the center). Note the proportionality between axonal size and myelin thickness. (×1700.)

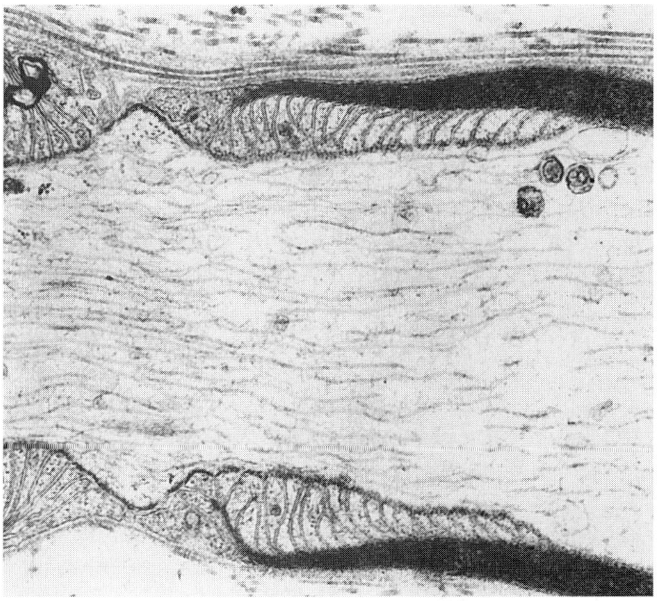

**Fig. 18-4.** Longitudinal section showing the node of Ranvier and the paranode. Note multiple terminal Schwann cell loops attaching to the axolemma. (×20,500.)

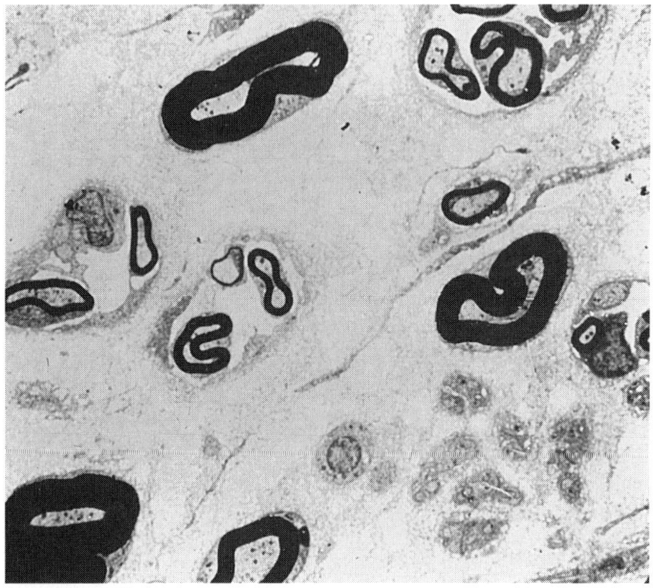

**Fig. 18-5.** Regenerating clusters showing 2 to 4 thinly myelinated fibers surrounded by common basement membrane. These clusters occasionally also contain unmyelinated fibers. (×1700.)

is attenuated and normally contains a higher density of neurofilaments and accumulations of tubulovesicular elements and mitochondria.

The Schwann cell nucleus is located midway between the two nodes, and often causes an indentation of the myelin sheath at this site. At the site of the nucleus the cytoplasm is usually more generous, and cellular organelles are identifiable. The Schwann cell cytoplasm may also, particularly in older persons, contain membrane-bound clusters of rodlike bodies. These are commonly referred to as pi-granules and are of no pathologic significance.

Each myelinating Schwann cell is surrounded by a basement membrane, which usually is thinner than that enveloping perineurial cells, endothelial cells, or pericytes. In older persons regenerating clusters of myelinated fibers may be encountered as part of the "normal" aging process. These are no different from those seen in pathologic processes. Regenerating clusters usually contain groups of two to four small myelinated fibers, each having its own Schwann cell and basement membrane (Fig. 18-5), and also may include groups of unmyelinated fibers. The entire group of fibers is surrounded by an additional basement membrane, left behind by the degenerated fiber, which they replaced (Fig. 18-5).

### Unmyelinated Fibers

Unmyelinated or C-fibers make up approximately 75% of the total fiber number in the sural nerve. Ultrastructural examination is necessary to assess the morphology of unmyelinated fibers. In contrast to myelinating Schwann cells those supporting unmyelinated fibers invest several axons.[19]

The Schwann cell harbors the axons in pockets or indentations of its cytoplasm, which is surrounded by a basement membrane and constitutes a Schwann cell subunit. The diameter of unmyelinated fibers ranges from 0.1 to 3.0 μm and, in contrast to the myelinated fibers, shows a unimodal fiber size distribution with a peak at 1.0 to 1.3 μm. With increasing age, unmyelinated fibers within a Schwann cell subunit may be replaced by collagen fibers arranged in structures called collagen pockets. Alternatively, a Schwann cell subunit (surrounded by a common basement membrane) may contain one or more Schwann cell profiles; this is referred to as a denervated Schwann cell. These changes are much more common in pathologic conditions.

### Vasculature of the Peripheral Nerve

Peripheral nerves are supplied by an extrinsic arterial system that irrigates the nerve trunks and feeds into the intrinsic system. The latter consists of an epineurial plexus composed of arterioles surrounding the nerve fascicles. These arterioles usually run parallel to the nerve fascicles and give off branches that penetrate the perineurium and feed into the endoneurial plexus. Numerous anastomoses exist between vessels of the epineurial and endoneurial plexus.

As the arterioles penetrate the perineurium they lose their layers of smooth muscle cells and become capillaries. Endoneurial capillaries are lined by a single layer of endothelial cells resting on a basement membrane, which in older persons is often multilayered.

Endothelial cells of the endoneurial space are linked together by tight junctions that constitute the blood-nerve barrier. In contrast, epineurial endothelial cells are fenestrated. Occasionally the capillary lumen is obstructed by endoneurial cells, called "capillary closure"; this probably is the result of a functional regulatory state of endoneurial blood flow rather than a pathologic change.

Vessels penetrating the perineurium exhibit a smooth muscle cell layer accompanied by unmyelinated axons and their terminals, suggesting that there is a neurogenic vasoregulatory mechanism. The endoneurial capillaries drain into postcapillary venules, partially supported by pericytes, and then into epineurial venules.

### Protective Barriers of the Peripheral Nerve

The peripheral nerve in common with the CNS depends on a specialized milieu with respect to nutrient requirements and macromolecular environment that is believed to be of particular importance for nerve function, i.e., generation and propagation of electrical impulses.

The peripheral nerve is protected from its surrounding environment by barrier systems. They are the perineurial diffusion barrier (tight junctions between the perineurial cells, particularly the innermost layers), the blood-nerve barrier (tight junctions between endothelial cells), and the paranodal barrier (tight junctions between myelin loops and paranodal axolemma). Furthermore, the endoneurial content is under a somewhat higher hydrostatic pressure than the epineurial space, a condition that probably serves as a mechanical cushion.

The peripheral nerve, like the CNS, is largely dependent on glucose as the major energy source. Facilitative glucose transporter molecules are highly expressed in the perineurium, in endoneurial endothelial cells, and at the paranode, where the energy demand is particularly high. The endoneurial environment is therefore protected from various plasma-derived macromolecules, providing both osmotic and immunologic stability. Attention has been paid recently to the paranodal barrier, which serves not only as a diffusion barrier, but also as an ion-channel barrier that separates nodal sodium channels from paranodal potassium channels. It therefore is fundamental for the proper propagation of the electrical impulse, and the intactness of these structurally identifiable barrier systems thus is pivotal to normal nerve functions.

## GENERAL ASPECTS OF PERIPHERAL NERVE PATHOLOGY

### Which Nerve Should be Biopsied?

Most diagnostic nerve biopsies are taken from the sural nerve at the level of the lateral malleolus. Several series of normative data exist from this nerve for comparison.[5,33,116] Furthermore, this site of the sural nerve represents the distal extension of a long nerve preferentially involved in most polyneuropathies; and sural nerve conduction studies, for functional correlations, are performed in most EMG laboratories. However, the sural nerve is a purely sensory nerve and therefore it is not a suitable biopsy site for the diagnosis of motor neuropathies. In these relatively rare entities, biopsying the deep peroneal nerve or the radial nerve may be appropriate.[59,130]

The procedure for nerve biopsy has been described in detail by Dyck and co-workers.[33] Great care should be taken in handling the biopsy specimen, since peripheral nerve is susceptible of artifact, caused by pulling or squeezing the nerve with a forceps. Both of these may seriously compromise pathologic evaluation.

Most commonly a 4 to 5 cm long biopsy is obtained from the whole sural nerve.[118] Fascicular biopsies from the sural nerve are not advisable, since vasculitic and/or hypoxic/ischemic neuropathies are easily missed in biopsies limited to one or a few fascicles. Moreover, fascicular biopsies are more apt to be altered by surgical artifacts secondary to the more extensive surgical manipulation involved in a fascicular biopsy.

### Fixation of the Biopsy Material

Ideally the nerve biopsy should be directly handled in the operating room by a histology technician. The biopsy should be cross-sectioned on a wax pad by crossed razor blades. One portion should be immediately fixed in neutral formalin and two portions in buffered 2.5% glutaraldehyde for resin embedding and teased fiber analysis, respectively. Consideration should be given to snap-freeze a fourth portion of the biopsy in liquid nitrogen if there is reason to suspect an immune-mediated neuropathy.

### Light Microscopic Examination

Cross-sections and longitudinal-sections of formalin-fixed and paraffin-embedded nerve should be stained with H&E, LFB and Holmes silver stain, and Congo-red. These preparations are often sufficient to diagnose vasculitides, inflammatory or ischemic neuropathies, as well as amyloid neuropathy (see below). Sections derived from paraffin blocks often give the examiner an impression of the severity of myelinated fiber loss (LFB + Holmes stained sections), segmental demyelination, axonal degeneration, or vascular changes. However, one should be aware of the limitations of paraffin-embedded material confounded by the thickness of the section and myelin artifacts caused by formalin fixation and paraffin embedding. Furthermore, paraffin-embedded material undergoes substantial shrinkage (up to 30%), and hence morphometric analysis performed on this material is unreliable.

Semithin (0.5 to 1.0 $\mu$m thick), glutaraldehyde-fixed, resin-embedded, and toluidine-stained cross and longitudinal sections of nerves provide excellent light microscopic resolution (see Fig. 18-1), allowing for relatively detailed examination of myelin abnormalities, axonal degenerative changes and abnormalities of the perineurium, hypertrophic endoneurial changes, or vascular pathology. Occasionally electron microscopic examination is necessary to confirm or exclude light microscopic impressions. Ultrastructural examination is necessary to confirm abnormalities in, for instance, myelin compaction (see paraproteinemias), macrophage-associated demyelination (GBS and CIDP), and to identify specific cellular inclusions (for instance those visible in leukodystrophies), or to assess abnormalities affecting the unmyelinated fiber population.

Light microscopic morphometric analysis of plastic-embedded cross-sections is used mostly as a research tool to assess fiber density, fiber caliber histograms, axon-myelin ratio, and index of circularity of myelinated fibers. This preparation also can be used to objectively determine focality of fiber loss within fascicles. Only rarely is morphometric analysis of direct diagnostic value. For detailed description of morphometric techniques the reader is referred to Dyck and co-workers,[33] and Sima and associates.[116,123]

In contrast, when properly performed, teased fiber analysis provides a valuable diagnostic aid, because it allows for evaluation of long stretches of myelinated fibers.[33,116] Variability in pathology between fascicles is assessed on paraffin or plastic cross-sections, and it usually is sufficient to obtain teased fibers from one fascicle to evaluate the qualitative changes. For reliable assessment, at least 150 to 200 fibers should be systematically sampled. For systematic sampling techniques Dyck and co-workers[33] should be consulted. Teased fibers are prepared from glutaraldehyde-fixed and osmicated nerve fascicles. Single fibers are teased in either glycerin or nonpolymerized Epon. The latter technique provides for permanent slides and offers the rarely used opportunity to examine single fibers ultrastructurally.

Most neuropathologists believe that teased fiber preparations provide, a highly informative supplementary investigative tool; therefore, a detailed description and evaluation of this technique and its pitfalls will be given.

### Assessment of Teased Fibers in Neuropathy

Detailed quantitative assessment of specific structural changes can be obtained from teased fiber analysis by scoring and quantitating well-defined morphologic changes that affect myelinated fibers. Teased fiber analysis is probably the most difficult and time-consuming procedure. It requires perfect tissue preparation and utmost attention during teasing to avoid damage to the fibers, because fixation and mechanical artifacts may mimic real pathologic changes. This technique allows the semiquantification of a variety of pathologic changes, which is extremely helpful in determining whether a neuropathy is primarily demyelinating or axonal in nature and in obtaining a measure of the severity and activity of a chronic neuropathy. We will describe teased fiber abnormalities in detail and outline the criteria that define eight pathologic categories. Also, we describe artifacts and methods by which these can be distinguished from real pathologic changes.

Approximately 150 to 200 teased fibers from each biopsy are examined by light microscopy. Each fiber is assigned to one of nine fiber categories (normal and eight specific pathologic changes). The frequency of occurrence of each category is expressed as the percentage of the total number of fibers examined.

**Randomization of teased fibers.** The largest fascicle of the biopsy is identified by visual estimation under a dissecting microscope and is chosen for teased fiber preparation. The surrounding sheath of the perineurium is removed and the fascicle is divided into two approximately equal segments. Each of these segments is divided again into two approximately equal segments. From each of these four segments, approximately 50 single fibers are teased and transferred onto a glass slide.

A minimum of 150 single fibers each with at least four internodal lengths are arranged on a clean glass slide. This method allows for teasing a representative population of fibers, including thinly myelinated and/or regenerating fibers. The slide is mounted in either glycerin or Epon and then polymerized.

**Scoring of teased fibers.** Teased fiber preparations are examined under a light microscope with a 20× objective lens and a 10× ocular.

Each fiber is qualitatively assigned to one of nine well-defined categories (A-I), based on the presence of characteristic structural features. The frequency of each type is expressed as a percentage of total fibers examined.[116]

**Description of teased fiber categories.** The teased fiber categories are:

A. Normal fibers
B. Paranodal swelling
C. Paranodal demyelination
D. Excessive myelin wrinkling
E. Intercalated internode
F. Segmental demyelination
G. Segmental remyelination

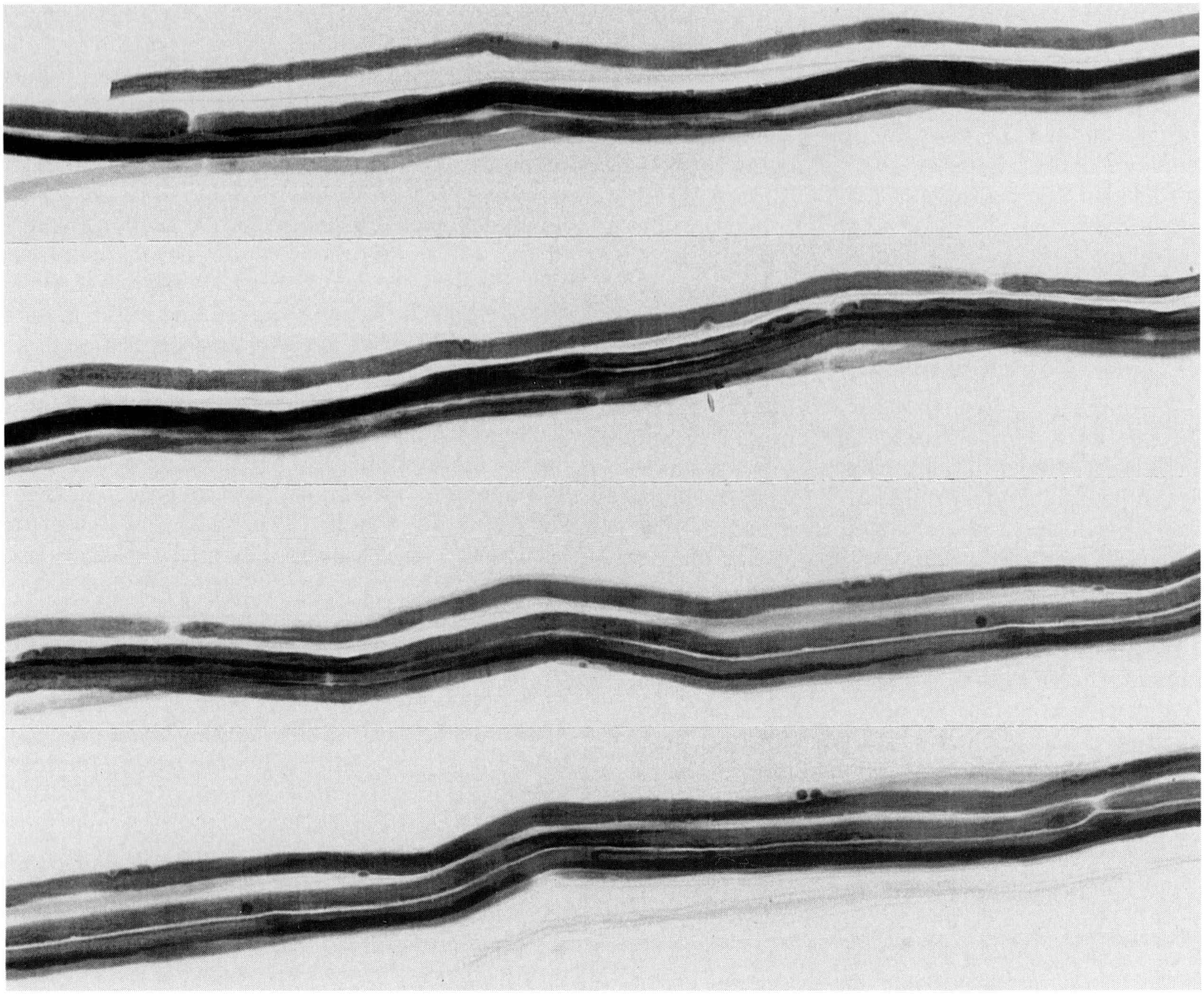

**Fig. 18-6.** Consecutive sequences of normal fibers (read from left to right and from top to bottom). No caliber changes are noted along the internodes. (×360.)

H. Regeneration
I. Wallerian degeneration

It is not uncommon for several changes to occur in the same fiber. Since only one category is assigned to each fiber, a given fiber is scored according to its most severe change, as listed above: B = paranodal swelling (the mildest) and I = Wallerian degeneration (the most severe).

***Normal (A)***

***Definition***—Consecutive, approximately equally long internodal segments of similar diameter. Within one internode the diameter should not vary by more than one third that is, the largest diameter should not exceed 150% of the smallest diameter (Fig. 18-6).

1. One exception is the indentation of the myelin by the Schwann cell nucleus, which at times may show a smaller diameter, less than 66% of the largest diameter.
2. Normal fibers should not show any of the changes described below (B to I).

***Paranodal Swelling (B)***

***Definition***—Paranodal swelling is defined as a paranodal expansion of the axonal diameter exceeding 150% of the average internodal diameter. It may be present on one or both sides of the nodal gap.

1. In osmified preparations the swelling may be darker than the internodal myelin owing to superimposition of myelin folds (Fig. 18-7, *A*), or the expansion may show a lighter and swollen axoplasm (Fig. 18-7, *B* and *C*).
2. Fibers exhibiting this change may show paranodal swelling of consecutive internodes.

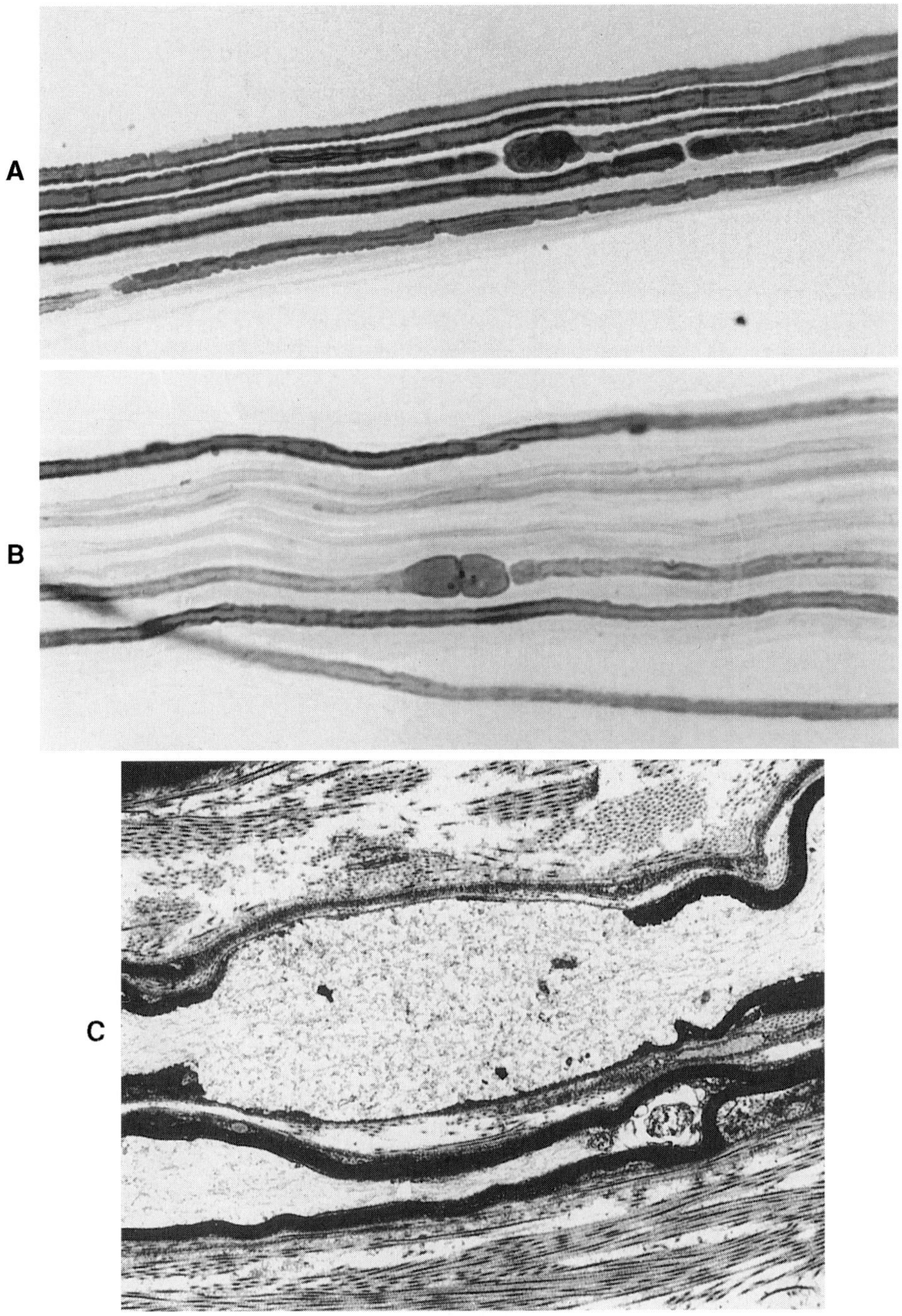


**Fig. 18-7.** **A**, The swollen paranodal axon is covered by myelin folds. **B**, The paranodal swollen axon on both sides of the nodal gap is clearly visible. **C**, Paranodal and nodal swelling is shown electronmicroscopically. (**B**, ×360; **C**, ×2600.)

3. Particular attention should be paid to thinly myelinated fibers that exhibit paranodal swelling, which may be difficult to ascertain.

*Artifacts*—

1. Mechanical damage to the paranodal region may cause longitudinal splitting and dispersion of the paranodal myelin that can be mistaken for paranodal swelling.
2. Pulling of the nerve during surgery will cause so-called beading artifacts. When those affect the paranodal region they can be misinterpreted as paranodal swelling. In this circumstance the fiber usually shows "beads" (swellings) along the internode as well.
3. Early Wallerian degeneration may mimic paranodal swelling. In this situation the fiber usually shows more advanced Wallerian degeneration, with fragmentation of the myelin and formation of myelin ovoids along its course.

***Paranodal demyelination (C)***

***Definition***—A nodal gap distance, devoid of any myelin, that exceeds the internodal mean diameter of the same fiber (Fig. 18-8).

A

B

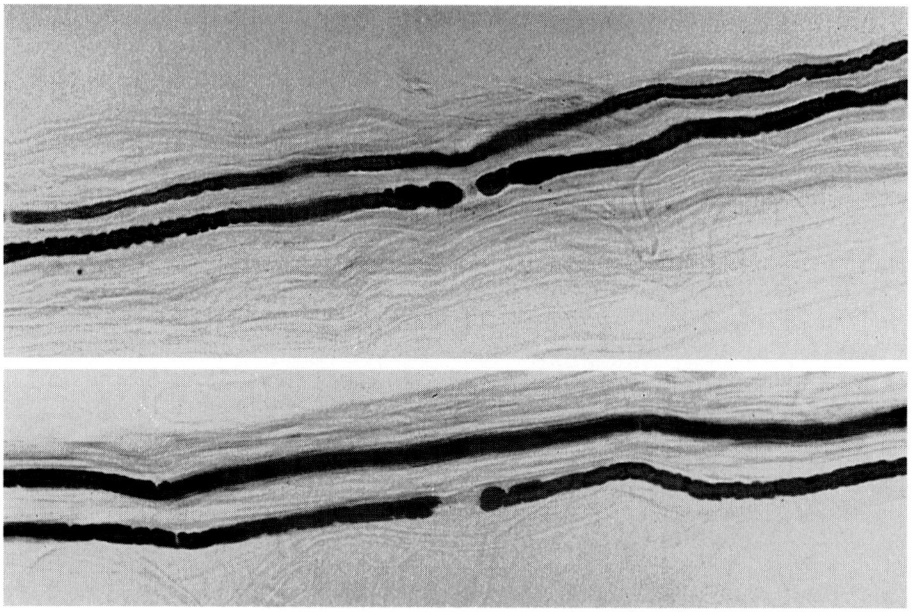

**Fig. 18-8.** Paranodal demyelination. **A**, The nodal gap distance has reached that of the mean fiber size that is well exceeded in **B**. (×360.)

1. Attenuation of the paranodal myelin is not infrequent. Although these changes may represent an early stage of paranodal demyelination, they are not scored as such, unless the nodal gap devoid of visible myelin exceeds that of the fiber diameter.
2. Paranodal demyelination of thinly myelinated fibers may be difficult to visualize. If this cannot be determined with confidence, the fiber should be scored according to any milder changes seen, and as normal if there are no changes.
3. It is not unusual for consecutive nodes to show paranodal demyelination.

*Artifacts*—

1. Mechanical pulling may break the fiber at the node, and the node may then appear wider, or fiber fractures could be misinterpreted as paranodal swelling. This type of artifact often is associated with additional fractures of the fiber along the internode.
2. Beading artifacts may masquerade as paranodal demyelination. In this situation, multiple beads usually are seen, which allows for the recognition of the artifact.

*Excessive myelin wrinkling (D)*

***Definition***—The internodal area shows irregular infoldings and superimposed myelin folds, involving one third or more of the internodal length in such a way that the greatest diameter is equal to or exceeds 150% of the smallest diameter (Fig. 18-9). Excessive myelin wrinkling is often displayed by consecutive internodes, but not always, and this cannot be relied on as a criterion.

1. Wrinkled myelin, commonly seen in the paranodal region, particularly in large myelinated fibers, is a normal feature. It should not be interpreted as excessive myelin wrinkling unless one third or more of the internodal length shows caliber variations exceeding 150%.

***Artifacts***—Excessive myelin wrinkling is probably the most difficult category to score, since artifacts may easily be misinterpreted as excessively wrinkled fibers.

1. Fixation and/or dehydration may cause wrinkling of the myelin. This change often is seen as a finer, more regular waviness of the myelin. Only in exceptional cases does this wrinkling cause fiber caliber variations greater than 150%.
2. Poor fixation may cause splitting of the Schmidt-Lanterman incisures, resulting in caliber variations that exceed 150%. This change is characterized by the so-called "fish-bone pattern" and occurs at regular intervals along the internode, affecting the myelin sheath symmetrically on both sides of the axon.
3. Drying of the tissue may cause caliber variations that exceed those stated in the definition. This often gives the appearance of a flattened fiber that is twisted like a garland, where the periodicity of the caliber changes is much greater.
4. Beading (mechanical pulling of the fiber) leads to caliber changes. This artifact is fairly characteristic, giving the fiber the appearance of a beaded necklace.
5. Early Wallerian degeneration may cause irregularity of myelin with caliber changes of the fiber. Fur-

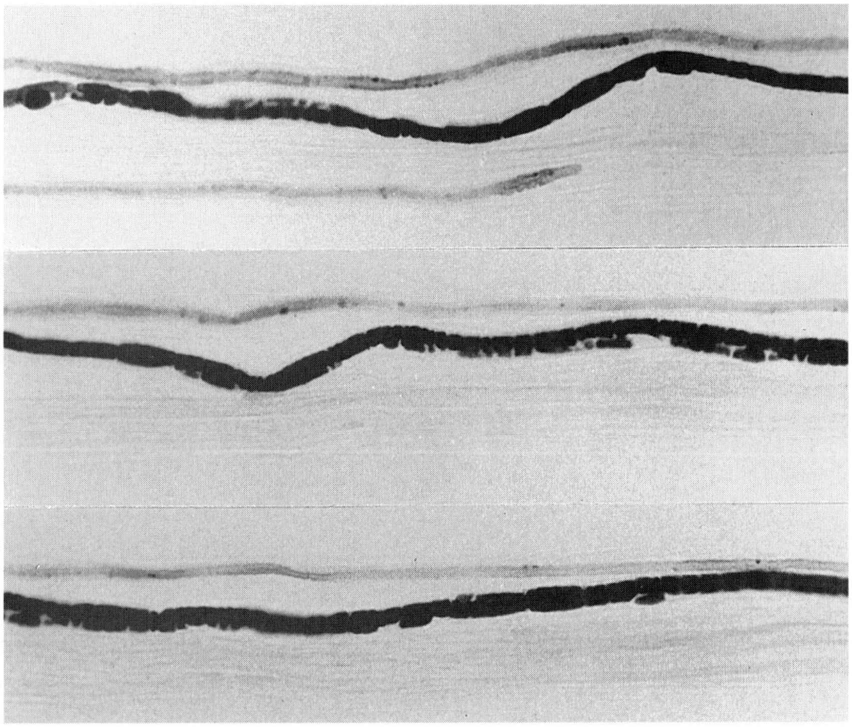

**Fig. 18-9.** Extensive myelin wrinkling showing deep indentations and foldings of the myelin. The thickest diameter exceeds 150% of the thinnest diameter. (×360.)

ther examination of the fiber will show myelin fragmentation with ovoids and balls, identifying ongoing Wallerian degeneration.

*Intercalated internode (E)*

***Definition***—A fiber shows one remyelinated internode surrounded on both sides by normally myelinated internodes (Fig. 18-10): this is regarded as a product of the repair process that follows paranodal demyelination.

1. In most situations the intercalated node is shorter than the neighboring nodes and has thinner myelin (Fig. 18-10).
2. At times, however, the intercalated node may show an internodal length similar to that of the neighboring internodes; it is then recognized by its thinner myelin.
3. Conversely, the intercalated node may show a myelin thickness similar to that of the surrounding internodes; it is then recognized by its internodal distance, which is shorter than that of the surrounding internodes.
4. Attenuated paranodal myelin may resemble an intercalated node. Attenuated paranodal myelin is limited by only one node, since the attenuated myelin is contiguous with the normal myelin on one side.
5. Intercalated nodes often are seen consecutively along the fiber.

*Segmental demyelination (F)*

***Definition***—Active demyelination with myelin fragmentation and ovoids within one internode that is surrounded by normally myelinated internodes (Fig. 18-11) is an extremely rare change.

*Artifacts*—

1. Mechanical artifacts during teasing may cause disruption of myelin within one internode. In this situation the myelin is split open like the splitting of a green stick, and the fiber caliber often is increased in the area of myelin splitting.
2. Beading artifact within one internode may appear strikingly similar to demyelination, where the "beads" may be interpreted as myelin ovoids. As mentioned earlier, beading artifacts are rarely an isolated phenomenon, usually occurring in neighboring fibers and along several internodes of the same fiber.

*Segmental remyelination (G)*

***Definition***—This is a fiber showing two or more remyelinated intercalated internodes surrounded by normally myelinated internodes (Fig. 18-12).

1. The intercalated internodes usually show thinner (remyelinated) myelin, but internodal length is not necessarily shorter than in normal fibers.
2. Rarely, however, segmentally remyelinated internodes may show the same myelin thickness as the surrounding internodes. In this circumstance, shorter internodal distance is the only criterion to identify segmental remyelination.
3. Within a sequence of remyelinated internodes, there may be a substantial variation in the distances between the internodes.

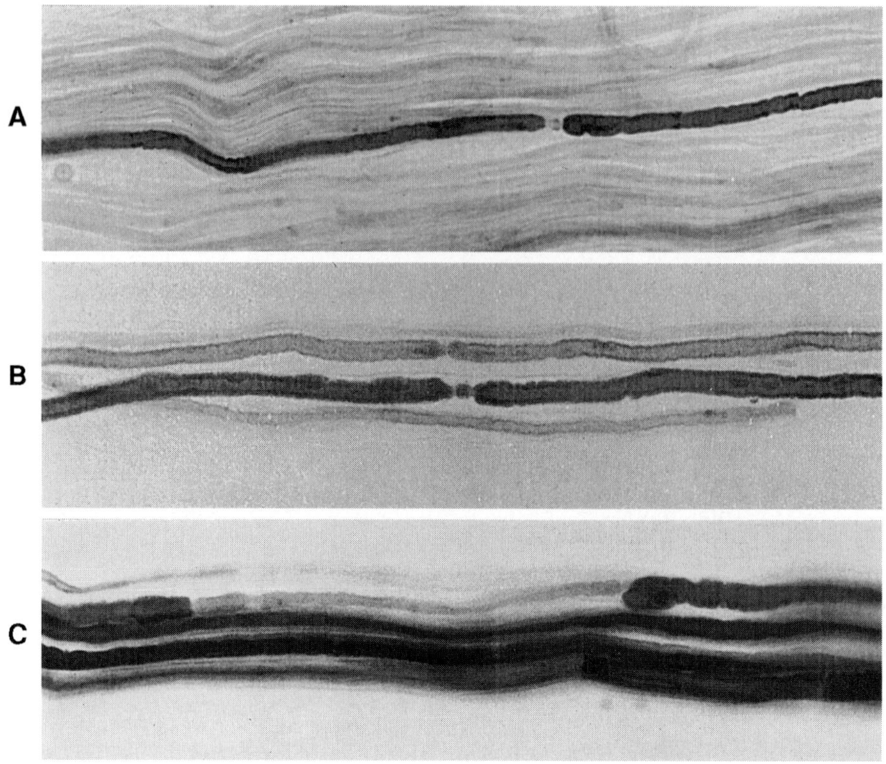


**Fig. 18-10.** Extremely short intercalated internodes are shown in **A** and **B**. Note that the intercalated internode is surrounded by nodal gaps on both sides. A longer intercalated internode is shown in **C**. (×360.)

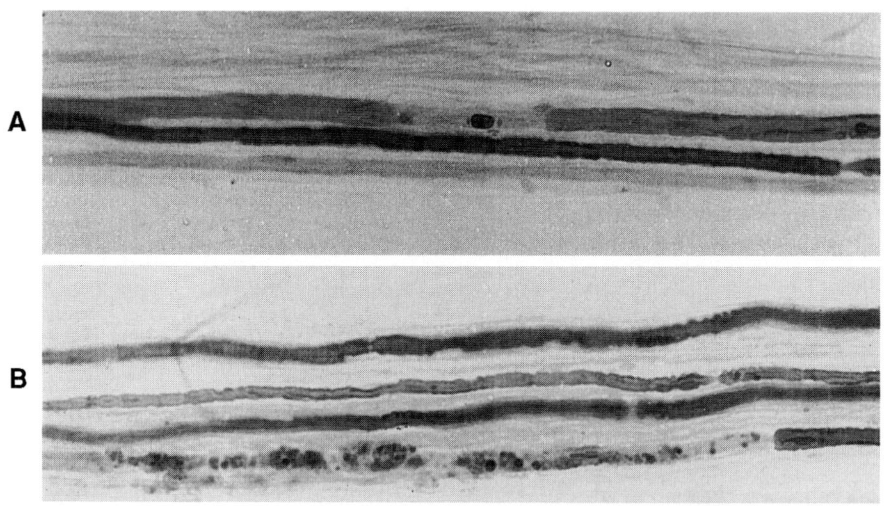


**Fig. 18-11.** Active segmental demyelination as shown in **A** and **B** is rarely seen. When observed, it may involve part of the internode (**A**) or its total length (**B**). (×360.)

4. At the end of a sequence of intercalated remyelinated nodes there may be a capping of mature myelin from the neighboring normal internode that covers part of the last remyelinated internode.
5. If a myelinated fiber ends with three or fewer remyelinated internodes, it is scored as segmental remyelination.

*Regenerated fibers (H)*

*Definition*—A sequence of short, thinly myelinated internodes less than 50% of normal internode length of the same fiber diameter (Fig. 18-13). These regenerated fibers may display any of the above changes, but are still considered and scored as regenerated fibers. The only exception is Wallerian degeneration. If a regener-

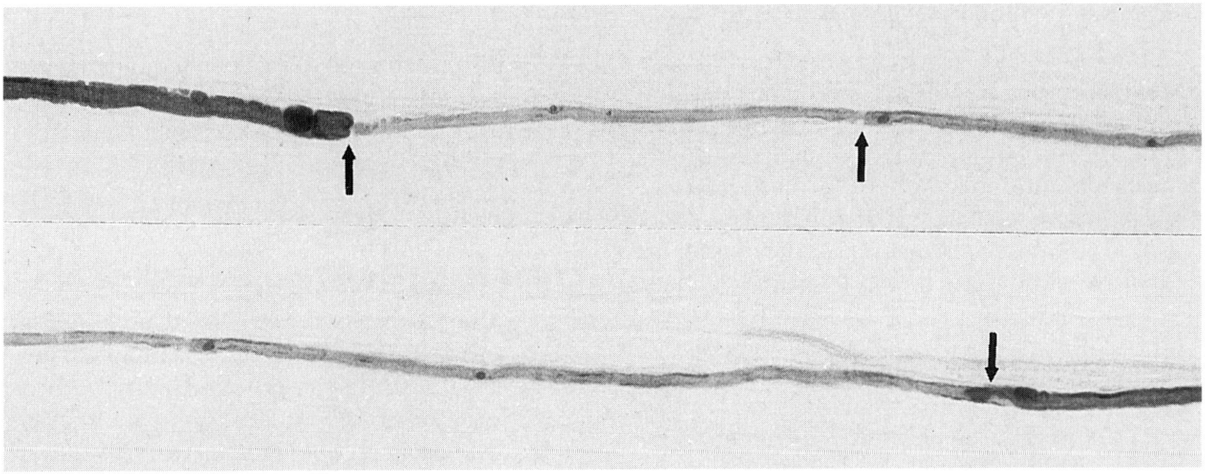

**Fig. 18-12.** Segmental remyelination is characterized by intercalated remyelinated internodes (two or more), which are surrounded by internodes with thicker myelin sheaths. *Arrows* indicate nodal gaps. Note capping of the node by mature myelin in lower panel. (×360.)

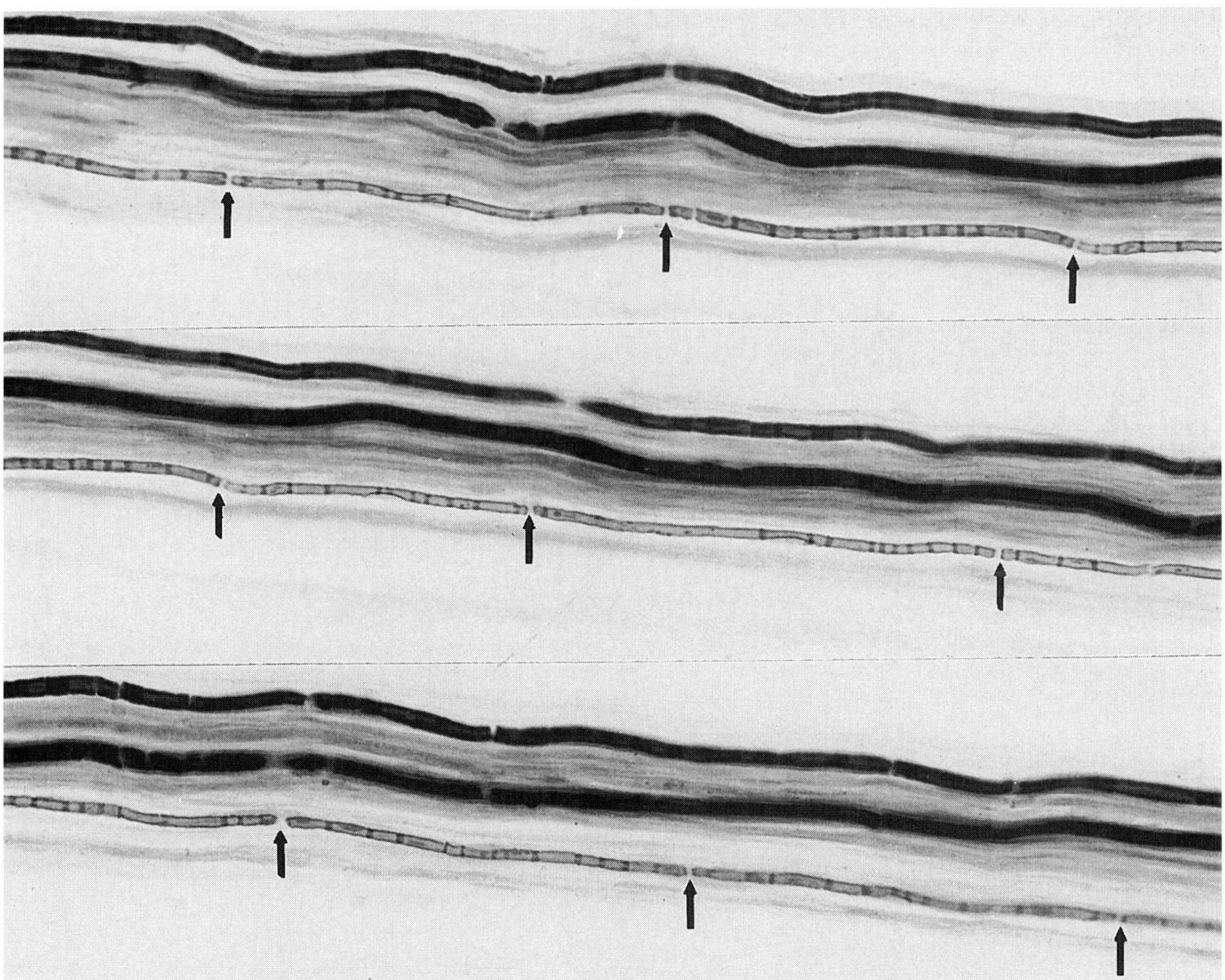

**Fig. 18-13.** A sequence of thinly myelinated internodes in a regenerating fiber (*bottom*). The nodes, which may be difficult to discern, are identified by *arrows*. (×360.)

ated fiber shows Wallerian degeneration, it is scored as such.

1. In this category one must pay particular attention to thinly myelinated fibers, not all of which are regenerating fibers. Normal thinly myelinated fibers show a normal internodal length for their caliber.
2. In contrast, more mature regenerated fibers may show a relatively normal thickness of the myelin for their diameter; they are then identified by their short internodal lengths.
3. Thin regenerating fibers often occur in bundles (corresponding to regenerating clusters) in which the fibers are twisted around each other. This is not an absolute criterion, but is helpful in focusing attention on the likelihood that they may represent regenerating fibers.
4. If a teased fiber ends with four or more short, thinly-myelinated internodes it is scored as a regenerating fiber.

*Wallerian degeneration (I)*

*Definition*—These fibers demonstrate fragmented myelin that forms ovoids and myelin balls over several internodes (Fig. 18-14). These fibers often show a gradient from undulating caliber changes to progressively smaller myelin fragments. This characteristic change is easily distinguished from the other scoring categories.

1. Teased endoneurial microvessels may mimic Wallerian degeneration.

*Artifacts*—

1. Beading artifacts may be misinterpreted as early (proximal) Wallerian degeneration.
2. Fractured fibers could be misinterpreted as Wallerian degeneration, although they do not show the characteristic gradient of changes seen in Wallerian degeneration.

**Artifacts in Teased Fiber Preparations**

**Fixation artifacts.** These artifacts often affect all fibers, either in their entirety or partially. They can be associated with decreased stainability with osmic tetroxide, rendering the fibers pale. Also, they may produce artifacts that could be misinterpreted as excessive myelin wrinkling. These artifacts are recognized by:

1. Fine regular corrugation of the myelin (Fig. 18-15).
2. Garland-like internodes with internodal caliber changes (twisted ribbon).
3. Fishbone pattern due to artifactually widened Schmidt-Lanterman incisures (Fig. 18-16).

It is not unusual to see various combinations of the above artifacts.

**Mechanical artifacts.** There are two kinds of artifacts: (1) those that can be traced to the biopsy procedure itself; and (2) those induced by mechanical manipulation of the fibers during the teasing procedure.

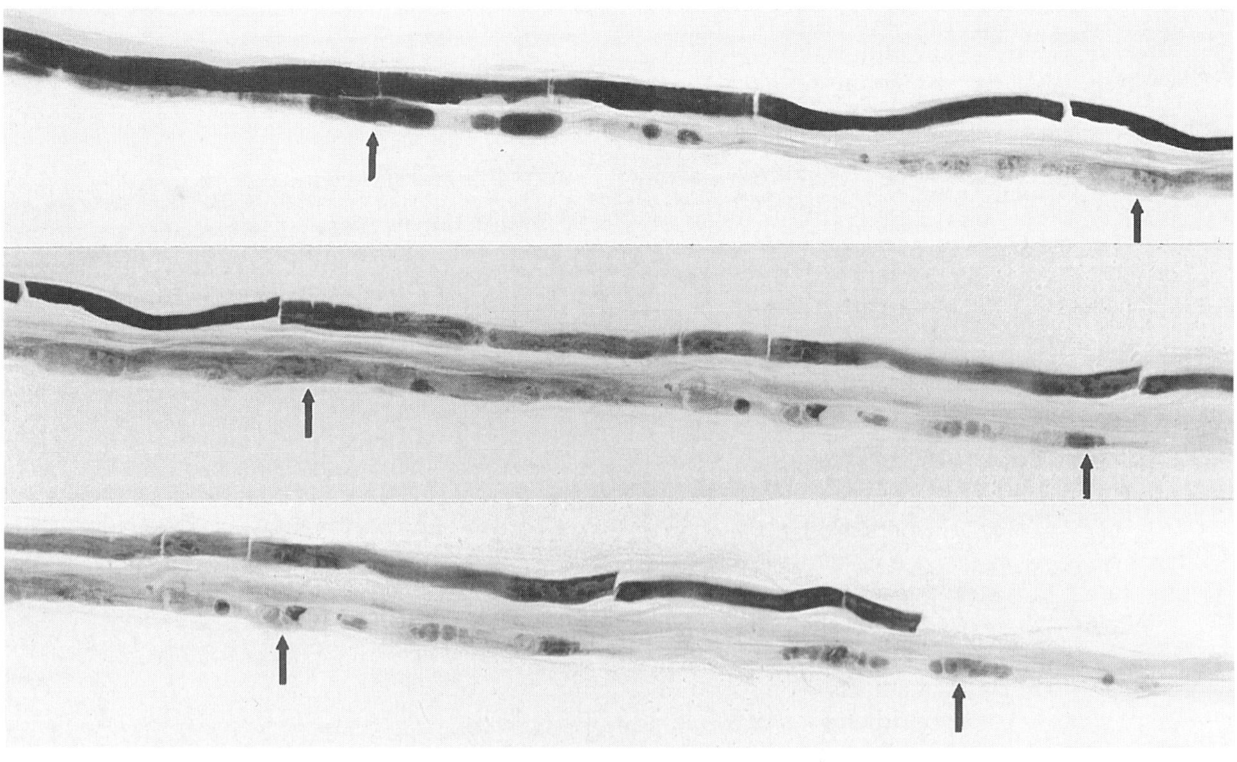

**Fig. 18-14.** Sequence of a fiber showing Wallerian degeneration (*arrows*). At times gradient exists in the occurrence of myelin ovoids and balls along the fiber. (×360.)

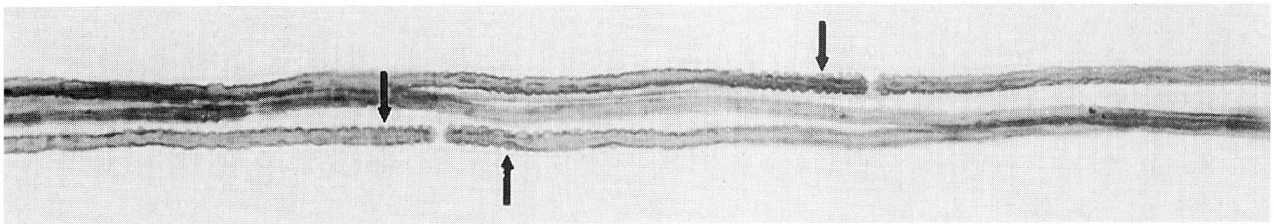

**Fig. 18-15.** Fine regular corrugation of the myelin (*arrows*) should not be interpreted as excessive myelin wrinkling; it is a fixation artifact. (×360.)

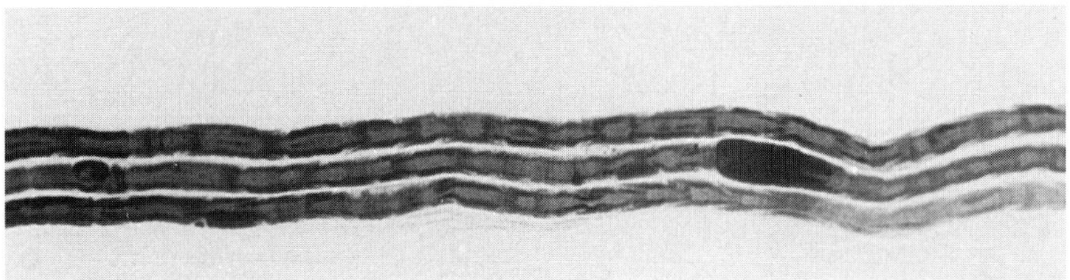

**Fig. 18-16.** Fixation artifact with widening of the Schmidt-Lanterman incisures causing a fishbone pattern that should not be confused with excessive myelin wrinkling. Note the symmetry of the artifact affecting the myelin on both sides of the axon. (×360.)

"Surgical" artifacts can be divided into:

1. Beading artifacts, which consist of regular caliber changes of the fiber. The beads may be contiguous, may be linked by narrow bridges of collapsed myelin, or may be separated, creating a line of small myelin ovoids. The "beads," however, have smooth myelin outlines (Fig. 18-17). This artifact can be misinterpreted as excessive myelin wrinkling, early Wallerian degeneration, paranodal demyelination, or possibly as segmental demyelination or remyelination.
2. Dehydration artifacts. These are characterized by shrunken myelinated fibers, which often show an extremely thin axon for the thickness of the myelin. The fibers also may show regular corrugation of the myelin, the so-called fishbone pattern.

These artifacts may be mistaken for excessive myelin wrinkling or intercalated nodes if they affect only one or several internodes. However, this is rare.

Teasing artifacts are of several kinds.

1. Teased fibers may be artifactually altered at one end. This occurs when the fibers are transferred to the permanent glass slide. The myelin often shows splitting, and the fibers appear either swollen or compressed. This part of the fibers should be disregarded, and the scoring should start upstream, where the fibers are free of artifacts.
2. Artifacts may occur in the middle of a fiber bundle when the fibers are mechanically separated. Again, the myelin is split (green-stick) longitudinally along the axis of the fiber. When this happens in the paranodal region, it could be misinterpreted as paranodal swelling (Fig. 18-18); when it is present along the internode it may be interpreted as caliber changes, excessive myelin wrinkling (although the myelin is not wrinkled), or as segmental demyelination.
3. If the tissue remains too long in fixative or in unpolymerized Epon, the fibers become brittle and can fracture during the teasing process. Such fractures may be misinterpreted as nodes, and hence mistakenly scored as paranodal demyelination, intercalated nodes, regenerated fibers, or Wallerian degeneration. However, the edges of fractured myelin are often sharp (Fig. 18-19) in contrast to the rounded and smooth endings of the paranodal myelin.
4. The myelin may appear retracted and wrinkled around the site of mechanical damage to the fiber. This usually occurs only for a short distance (Fig. 18-20) and may be mistaken for segmental demyelination or paranodal demyelination.

## PATHOLOGIC RESPONSES OF THE PERIPHERAL NERVE

### Axonal Degeneration

This is probably the most common pathologic change and is typical for most metabolic, nutritional, and toxic neuropathies. The term *dying-back neuropathy*[127] implies a preferential distal-to-proximal degeneration of the longest and largest axons; it is a characteristic feature of diabetic neuropathy, uremic neuropathy, and toxic neuropathies due to alcohol, organic solvents, arsenic, and thallium. It is believed that metabolic disturbances of the perikaryon compromise

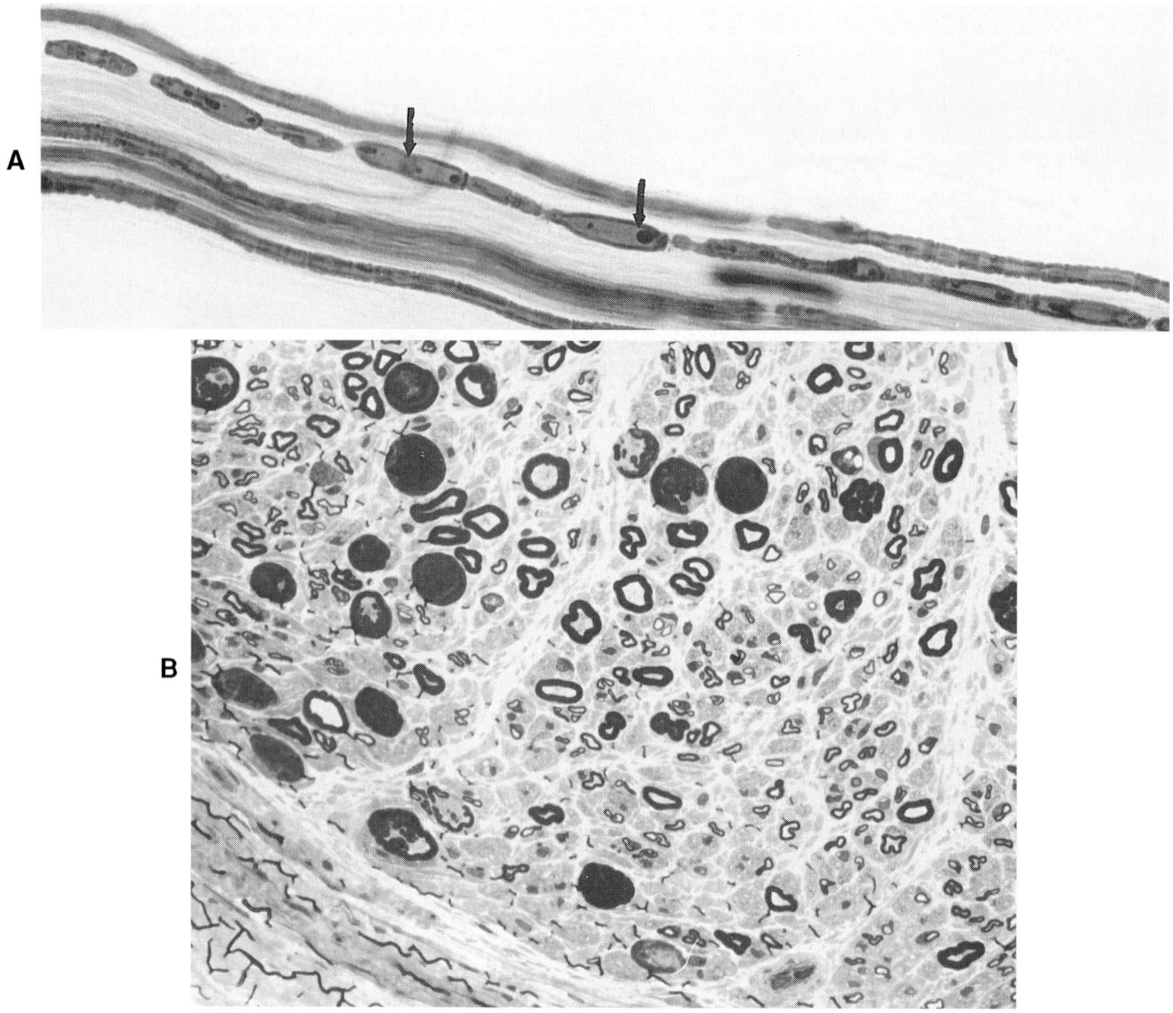


**Fig. 18-17.** Beading artifacts (*arrows*) should not be misinterpreted as paranodal swelling, paranodal demyelination, or Wallerian degeneration (**A**). In **B** the corresponding artifact is shown in plastic section. (**A,** ×360; **B,** ×520.)

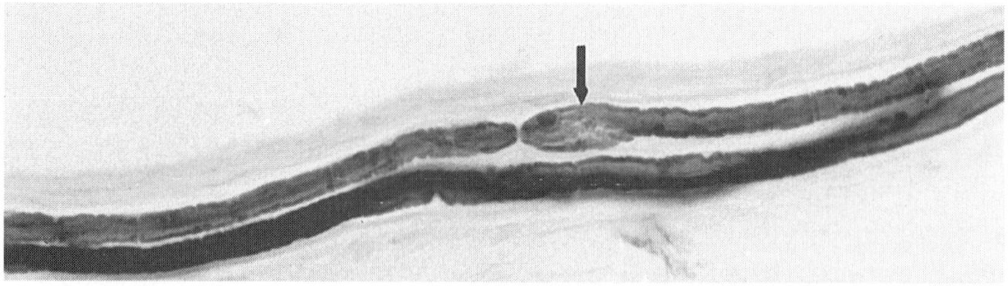

**Fig. 18-18.** Teasing artifact of the paranodal myelin (*arrow*) with longitudinal splitting of the myelin (green-stick) should not be misinterpreted as paranodal swelling. (×360.)

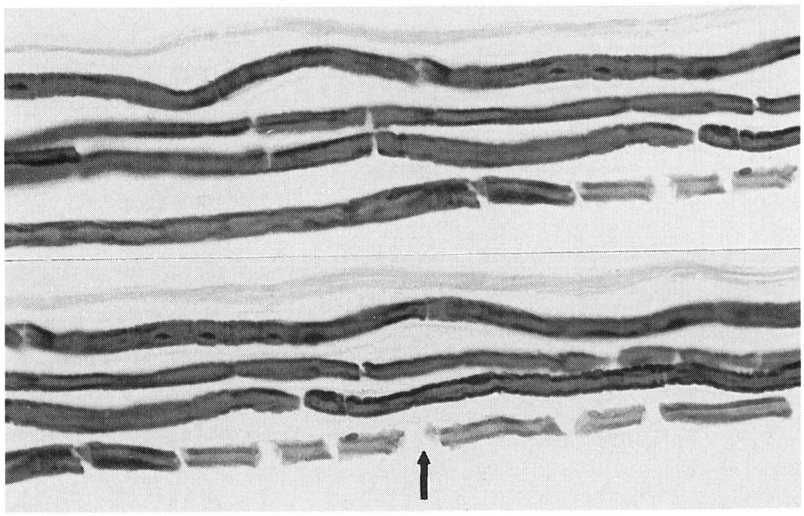

**Fig. 18-19.** Fractured fibers, which could be misinterpreted as paranodal demyelination or Wallerian degeneration (*arrow*). The artifact is recognized by the sharp edges of the fractures. (×360.)

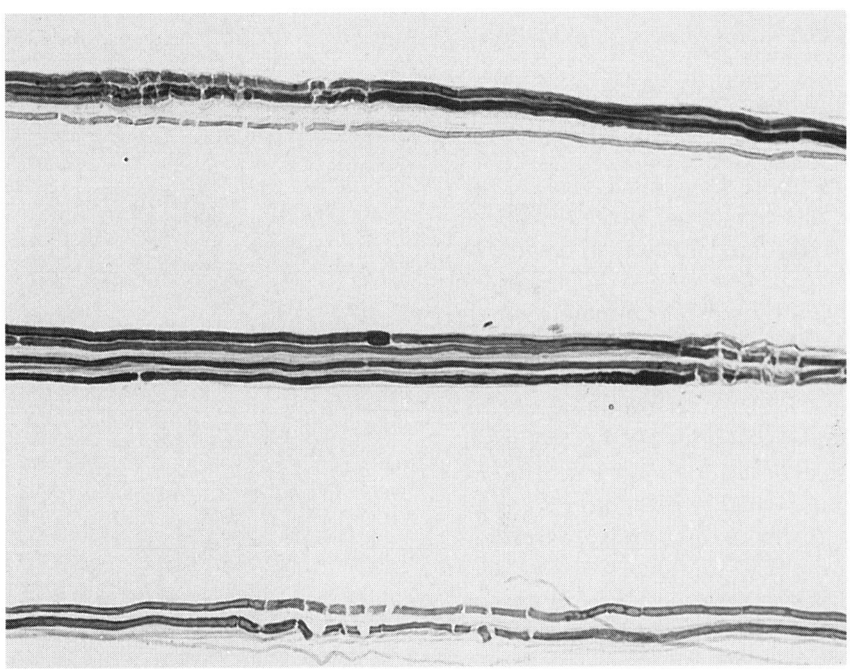

**Fig. 18-20.** Fiber bundles showing circumscribed stretches of "pick-up artifact." These are easily recognized because they affect several fibers at the same site. (×180.)

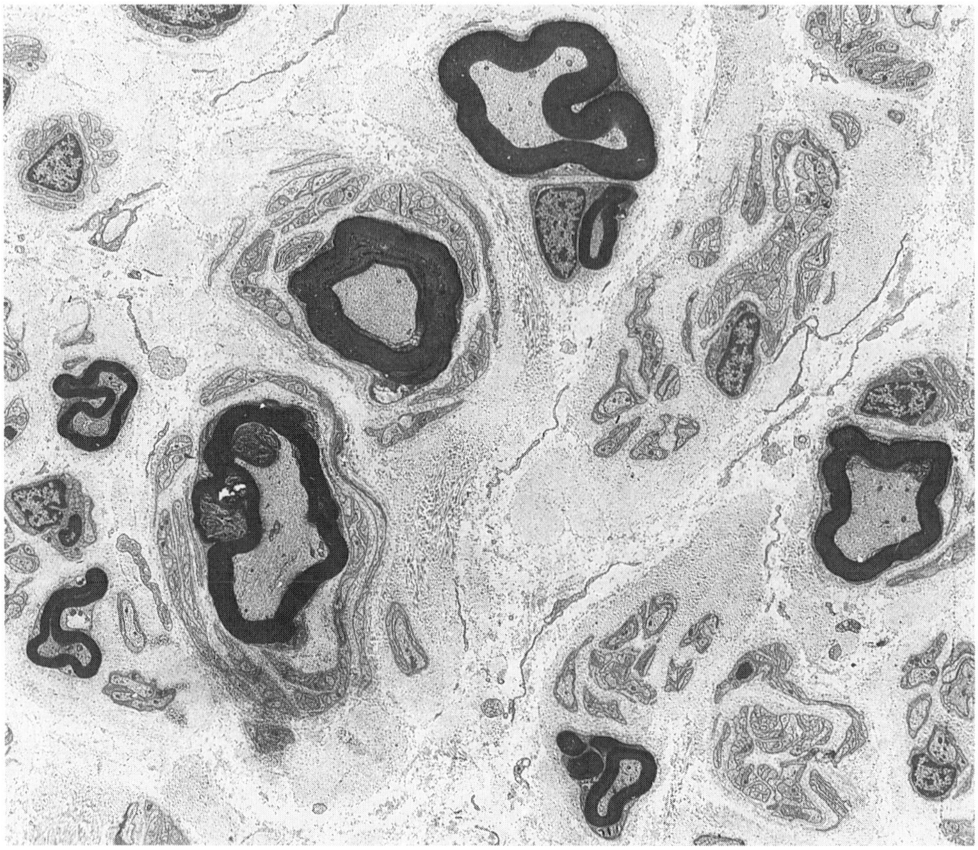

**Fig. 18-21.** Axonal atrophy with folding of the myelin sheath, which corresponds to excessive myelin wrinkling in teased fiber preparations. (×2800.)

the ability to provide the most distal outreaches of the axons with structural and functional proteins. These abnormalities then lead to axonal atrophy and eventually to distal Wallerian degeneration. Axonal atrophy is recognized either by the disproportionately small size of the axon in relation to the surrounding myelin sheath with a compensatory widening of the inner Schwann cell lip, or by folding or wrinkling of the otherwise intact myelin sheath (Fig. 18-21). The most sensitive way to assess axon atrophy is by scoring of teased fiber preparations, which will demonstrate an increased percentage of fibers that show excessive myelin wrinkling (see Fig. 18-9). Axonal atrophy also may be assessed by morphometric analysis of plastic cross-sections, which will demonstrate a decreased axon/myelin ratio. Axonal degeneration often is associated with accumulation of degenerated organelles or misoriented neurofilaments within the axon. In these situations, invaginations of slender Schwann cell cytoplasmic processes into the axoplasm are seen that surround and engulf abnormal axoplasmic organelles, which are digested by the Schwann cell. This clearance of abnormal axoplasmic organelles is referred to as *honeycombing*[129] and can be demonstrated only ultra-

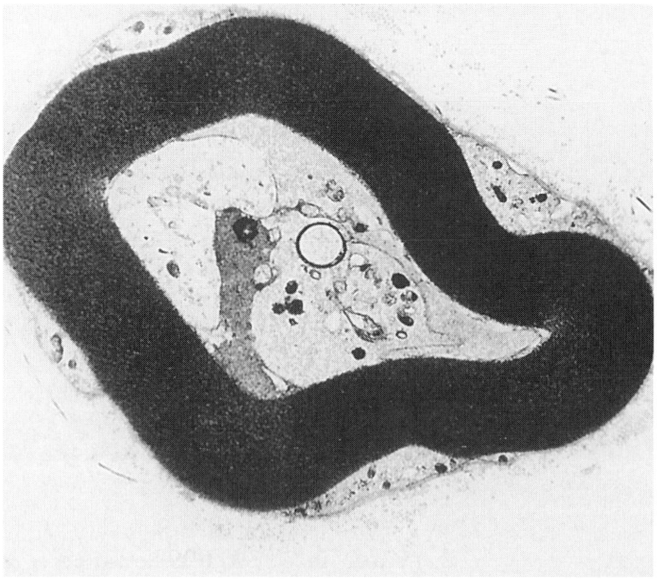

**Fig. 18-22.** Honeycombing in a case of porphyric neuropathy. Note the extension of the electron-dense adaxonal Schwann cell lip separating portions of the axoplasm. (×11,900.)

structurally (Fig. 18-22). Together with axonal atrophy honeycombing constitutes the characteristic hallmark of axonopathy. However, the features of both axonal atrophy (excessive myelin wrinkling) and honeycombing of the axon occasionally may be seen in the paranodal region of large normal fibers, where it has no pathologic significance.[129] In slowly progressive axonopathies the axon may show a segregation of neurotubules and neurofilaments, with the former often concentrated at the periphery of the axons.[135] Axonal swelling due to accumulation of misoriented neurofilaments or with addition of various other organelles in proximal paranodal axons is characteristic of hexacarbon (*n*-hexane) neuropathy.[126]

The term *paranodal swelling*[53] refers to the swelling of the nodal and paranodal axon without accumulation of neurofilaments or organelles (see Fig. 18-7, *C*). It is characteristic of metabolic neuropathies. In experimental diabetic neuropathy, intra-axonal $Na^+$ accumulation secondary to a defect in the sodium pump has been associated with this abnormality.[53] Similar mechanisms are likely to underlie the same change in other metabolic neuropathies.

As the axon dies it attains a granular appearance and loses its intimate contact with the Schwann cell, although the myelin sheath itself may be structurally intact.

### Wallerian Degeneration

Wallerian degeneration may occur as a consequence of progressive axonal degeneration or following trauma or ischemic insults to the nerve. The early changes consist of accumulation of abnormal organelles within the paranodal axoplasm, swelling and granulation of the axons, widening of the Schmidt-Lanterman incisures, and paranodal myelin retraction. The axon then dissolves and the myelin starts to break up at the paranodes and the Schmidt-Lanterman incisures; the myelin then collapses into the space previously occupied by the axon, thereby forming the myelin ovoids that characterize Wallerian degeneration in teased fibers (see Fig. 18-14). As the myelin begins to break up, the endoneurium is invaded by nonresident macrophages that penetrate the Schwann cell basement membrane to clear out the debris.[58] Complement is necessary to initiate this process. During the whole sequence of Wallerian degeneration the Schwann cell basement membrane remains intact. The Wallerian degeneration proceeds from the proximal portion to the distal, and its duration appears to depend on the length of the nerve.

### Regeneration

The macrophage response to Wallerian degeneration is pivotal to the initiation of regeneration. Macrophages release interleukins that stimulate the production of nerve growth factor (NGF) and insulin-like growth factor-1 (IGF-1) by Schwann cells and probably fibroblasts, which are essential for nerve fiber regeneration.[57,66]

Schwann cells start to proliferate within the basement membrane tube left behind by the degenerated fiber. They stimulate the outgrowth of axons from the proximal viable end of degenerated fiber via molecular messengers (growth-factors and adhesion molecules). The tips of the sprouting axons, the growth cones, are expansions of axoplasm that contain filaments rich in actin and vesicular structures. One degenerated fiber is initially replaced by several axonal sprouts. These are individually supported by their own myelinating Schwann cells. Some regenerating axons may remain unmyelinated while still being supported by individual Schwann cells. Therefore, a regenerating cluster consists of several small myelinated fibers with their own Schwann cells and basement membranes and groups of unmyelinated fibers, all being enclosed by an additional single basement membrane (see Fig. 18-5). Outside this common basement membrane slender encircling fibroblasts are common. These features provide easy identification of regenerating clusters ultrastructurally.[114] As the regenerating clusters mature they lose the common basement membrane, and some fibers may regress. Regenerating fibers are recognized in teased fibers by their consecutively short internodes; on light microscopic morphometric analysis they show increased axon:myelin ratios. However, on light microscopy a cross-section of a regenerated fiber cannot be distinguished from a fiber that has undergone segmental remyelination. A futher word of caution should be mentioned for assessing myelinated fiber histograms. A marked leftward shift in the fiber caliber does not indicate myelinated fiber atrophy only; it also may reflect the admixture of smaller regenerating fibers indicative of an ongoing repair process.

### Degeneration and Regeneration of Unmyelinated Fibers

Unmyelinated axons undergo a degeneration process similar to that of myelinated fibers. The early changes consist of axonal swelling that sometimes is accompanied by granular degeneration or honeycombing (Fig. 18-23) or by segregation of neurotubules and neurofilaments, as seen in porphyric neuropathy. As the unmyelinated axon dies it leaves an empty niche in the supporting Schwann cell, which later may be filled by collagen fibers ("collagen pocket") (Fig. 18-24). Denervated Schwann cell subunits often demonstrate layered flattened Schwann cell profiles, so-called "Schwann cell banding."

Regeneration of unmyelinated axons proceeds in a fashion similar to that seen in myelinated fibers. Regenerated c-fibers generally show a smaller axon/

Schwann cell ratio; in other words, one supporting Schwann cell harbors fewer axons—often one or two.

### Demyelination

Demyelination occurs either as a primary phenomenon consequent to Schwann cell abnormalities or as a secondary reaction to primary axonopathies. This distinction may be difficult to make. As a general rule, primary demyelinating disorders are more generalized, whereas secondary demyelination is more spotty and is accompanied by segmental remyelination as well as intercalated internodes, primarily in fiber population affected by axonal atrophy or degeneration. Teased fiber analysis may be extremely helpful to make these difficult distinctions.

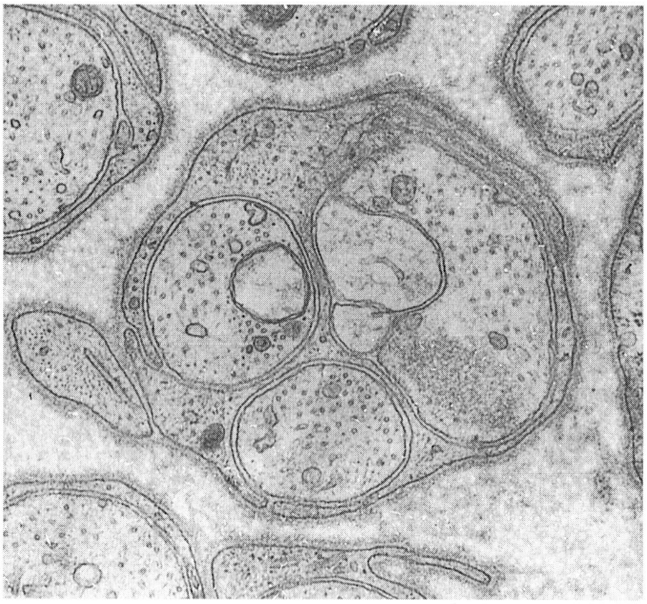

**Fig. 18-23.** Degenerating unmyelinated fiber showing granular degeneration of the axoplasm and separation of degenerated axoplasm (honeycombing). (×36,000.)

Myelinated fibers with myelin debris in the Schwann cell cytoplasm and with splitting and/or vacuolation of the myelin sheath or containing a denuded but otherwise normal axon constitute primary demyelination. Such fibers are often accompanied by macrophages clearing out myelin debris. However, myelin splitting or vacuolation alone without active myelin breakdown most commonly represents an artifact.

Active myelin stripping by macrophages is characteristic of such inflammatory demyelinating disorders as CIDP and Guillain-Barré syndrome, but is also seen in HIV infection and in paraproteinemias. Macrophages penetrate the Schwann cell basement membrane and "peel off" the myelin along the interperiod lines with their processes (Fig. 18-25).

Abnormalities in the compaction of myelin can be of two kinds. Uncompacted myelin shows separation of the intraperiod line by sleeves of Schwann cell cytoplasm that may affect the entire thickness or a part of the myelin sheath.[142] This abnormality is seen in IgG

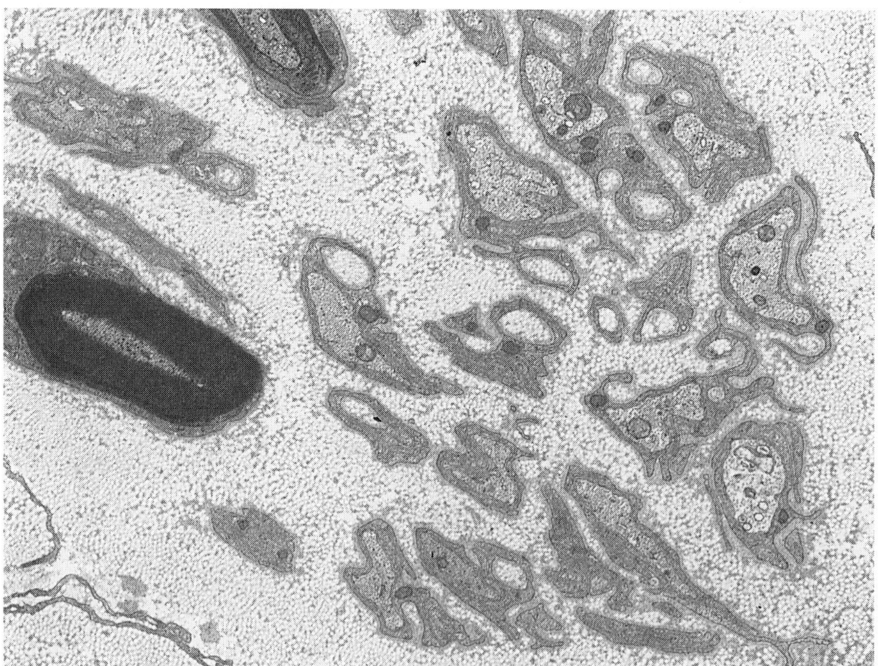

**Fig. 18-24.** Collagen pockets. Rounded or oval in shape, clusters of collagen fibers are partially or completely embraced by thinned projections of Schwann cell cytoplasm. They are smaller in size and lighter in density than neighboring unmyelinated axons. (×4000.)

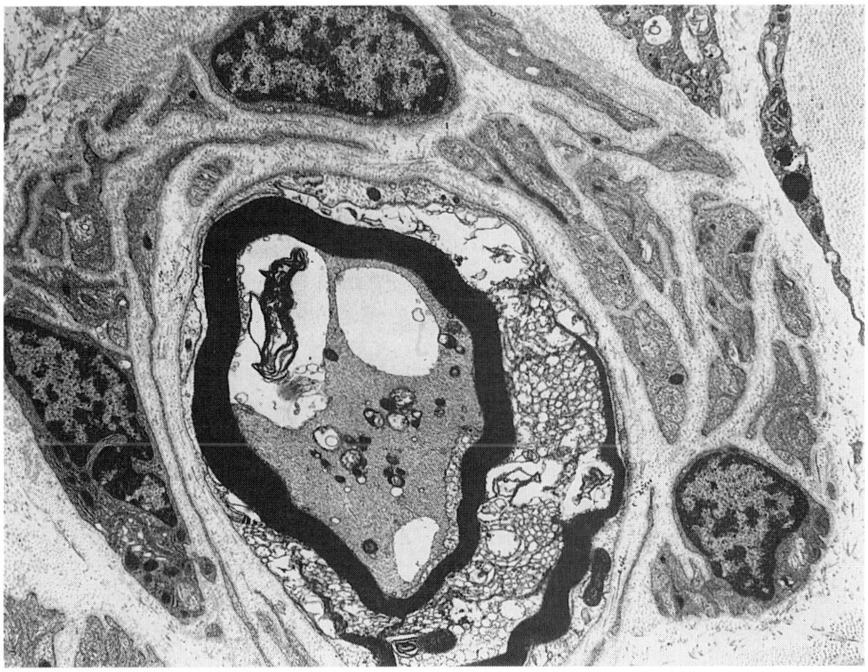

**Fig. 18-25.** Electron micrograph of a myelinated axon whose myelin sheath is being split and broken down by a macrophage inserted among the lamellae. (×3400.)

or IgA paraproteinemias, in POEMS syndrome, or in hereditary neuropathy with pressure palsies. However, similar uncompacted myelin may be noticed in cross-sections through Schmidt-Lanterman incisures or remyelinating fibers. The second myelin compaction abnormality is widely spaced myelin, a tenfold wider separation of the intraperiod line of the myelin sheath that usually involves either the outermost or innermost part of the myelin sheath.[99] This abnormality is almost pathognomonic for IgM paraproteinemias with antibodies directed against myelin associated glycoprotein (MAG).

Secondary demyelination often accompanies the classic axonopathies, such as diabetic, porphyric, and uremic neuropathies, some of which were previously believed to be demyelinating disorders. Extensive and partly experimental studies by Dyck and co-workers[34,37] and Sima and colleagues[105,113] in the 1970s and 1980s clearly delineated these neuropathies as primary axonopathies.

A common finding in metabolic and hypoxic neuropathies is paranodal myelin retraction (paranodal demyelination), which probably is preceded by a breakdown of the paranodal barrier and a detachment of the terminal myelin loops from the axolemma and should not be regarded as a primary demyelinating process. The paranodal demyelination may be replaced by short so-called intercalated internodes as a result of remyelination. Secondary paranodal demyelination is common in metabolic axonopathies.

Segmental remyelination is a frequent feature of myelinopathies. Active myelin breakdown is rarely seen, since it occurs relatively rapidly; the myelin is then replaced by several short thinly myelinated internodes, a characteristic presentation of segmental remyelination in teased fiber preparations.

Onion bulb formation is a term used when a myelinated fiber is surrounded by several concentric layers of thin Schwann cell profiles.[98] These formations correspond to repeated demyelination and remyelination, whereby the initially excessive number of Schwann cells competing for myelinating the demyelinated axons are displaced. Onion bulbs are characteristic of inherited hypertrophic neuropathies and CIDP. They are also seen occasionally in primary axonopathies, but in much smaller numbers.

### Vascular Pathologic Changes

The most frequent pathology of the peripheral nerve vasculature is vasculitis. This most commonly, but not exclusively, involves the epineurial vessels. The vasculitic lesions may be highly focal, making it necessary to section all the biopsy material to optimize diagnostic yield. Vasculitis shows transmural inflammation, vessel wall necrosis, fibrin leakage, occasional thrombosis, and perivascular accumulation of inflammatory cells. These changes are characteristic of polyarteritis nodosa, Churg-Strauss angiitis, and vasculitis in connective tissue disorders like rheumatoid arthritis, SLE, and Sjögren's syndrome. Similar changes often are encountered in vessels penetrating the perineurium, but these rarely affect endoneurial vessels. Isolated perivascular cuffings around epineurial vessels, sometimes referred to as "microvasculitis,"[138] probably are of much lesser significance. However, when seen, they should prompt sectioning through the available blocks in search of frank vasculitis.

Except in the vasculitides, peripheral nerve vessels, particularly the endoneurial vasculature, tend to show duplication of basement membranes and proliferation and swelling of endothelial cells. These changes are relatively nonspecific but probably are most severely expressed in long-standing diabetic neuropathy, often accompanied by debris of periendothelial cells at the various layers of basement membrane. Similar but usually milder changes are also present in the neuropathy of chronic hypoxemia, hereditary neuropathies, amyloid neuropathy, and aging. These changes most likely reflect a vigorous remodeling and endothelial cell turnover in chronic neuropathies, and, therefore, are not characteristic of specific disease processes.

Structural abnormalities suggestive of damage to the blood-nerve barrier may be noted in neuropathies with inflammation or acute axonal degeneration. These abnormalities consist of fenestration of the endoneurial endothelium and endoneurial or subperineurial edema. More specific blood-nerve barrier abnormalities such as loss of endothelial tight junctions of endoneurial vessels have been described in diabetic neuropathy.[119]

### Pathologic Changes of the Perineurium

The perineurium constitutes one of the protective barriers of peripheral nerve. Common changes seen with aging and in chronic neuropathies are small calcospherites within the cytoplasm of perineurial cells. These are particularly frequent in diabetic neuropathy. An inflammatory process may affect the perineurium, either as part of vasculitis or as isolated perineuritis.[124] The latter entity is rare. The inflammation is characterized by lymphocytic infiltrate and degeneration of perineurial cells that leads to a breakdown of the perineurial barrier with leakage of macromolecules into the endoneurial space. In some of these cases there is an accompanying malignancy.

## METABOLIC AND NUTRITIONAL NEUROPATHIES

### Diabetic Neuropathies

Several neuropathic syndromes have been described in diabetes mellitus; in a given patient these may overlap.[54] The most common type is distal, symmetric, predominantly sensory polyneuropathy, followed in frequency by autonomic polyneuropathy and ischemic neuropathies. The latter group include cranial neuropathies (particularly of the third nerve), trunk and limb mononeuropathies, and femoral neuropathy. These neuropathies often have an acute onset with good recovery, whereas the diabetic polyneuropathies are known for a slow and relentless progression. In the classic study by Pirat,[97] the frequency of overt distal sensory neuropathy was approximately 50% after 25 years of diabetes. This is the most common peripheral neuropathy overall. Approximately 17 million people suffer from it in North America and Europe. Diabetic neuropathy is likely to increase globally with the rapidly increasing incidence of diabetes mellitus in developing countries.

The cause of diabetic neuropathy is not known, but it is believed to be due to multiple consequences of hyperglycemia, such as activation of the polyol pathway, nonenzymatic glycation of structural proteins, metabolic effects on the peripheral nerve vasculature, and consequent decreased blood flow (for review see references 16, 56, 121). Several of these metabolic abnormalities are being treated with experimental drugs, many of which are now being tested in clinical trials. Initial studies using aldose reductase inhibitors, which block the polyol pathway, provide encouraging results, by demonstrating increased nerve fiber regeneration.[114,115]

Nerve biopsy is rarely indicated in uncomplicated diabetic neuropathy, since the diagnosis is made on clinical and electrophysiologic grounds. Symptoms evolve slowly, with loss of sensation and reflexes in the distal limbs, paresthesias, and sometimes pain. Autonomic diabetic neuropathy is a severe disorder that may cause sudden cardiac death. Less dramatic symptoms include urinary incontinence, gastroparesis, impotence, and decreased libido.[54]

Nerve biopsy usually is indicated in cases with an atypical course or if a superimposed neuropathy is suspected. It is therefore useful to be familiar with the characteristic pathologic picture of diabetic neuropathy.

Cross-sections of the sural nerve show diffuse loss of myelinated fibers of all sizes. The severity of myelinated fiber loss varies widely; it depends on the severity of the neuropathy and correlates with nerve conduction velocity and sural nerve amplitude.[122] Sometimes the loss of large myelinated fibers predominates, but rarely the neuropathy predominantly affects small fibers.[12] Fibers undergoing axonal or Wallerian degeneration are encountered (Fig. 18-26) as are regenerating clusters. The endoneurial vessels often demonstrate conspicuously thick basement membranes (Fig. 18-27). Basement membrane thickening is less pronounced in epineurial vessels. Endoneurial vessels may show hyperplasia and hypertrophy of the endothelial cells. The perineurium is unremarkable or may contain calcium deposits. Within a given fascicle or from fascicle to fascicle, the loss of myelinated fibers is variable. This par-

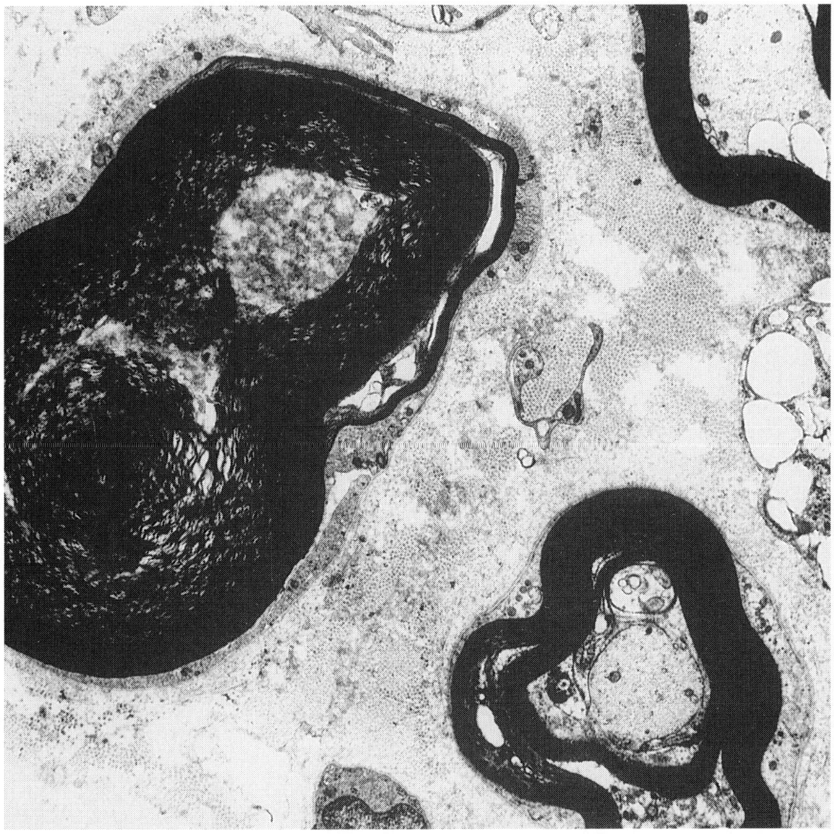

**Fig. 18-26.** Electron micrograph showing axonal atrophy (*bottom right*) and axonal degeneration (*top left*) in diabetic polyneuropathy. (×26,200.)

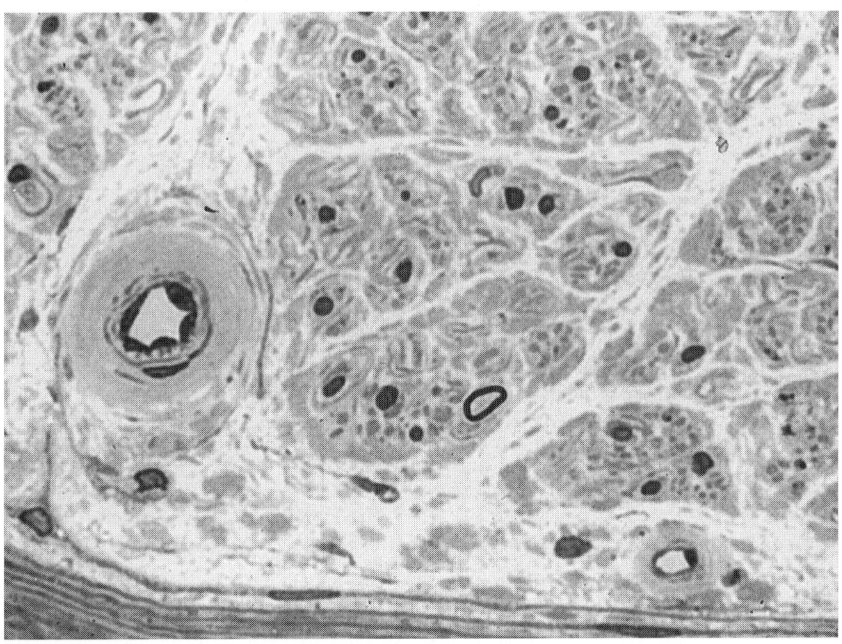

**Fig. 18-27.** Plastic section showing severe diabetic neuropathy with loss of myelinated fibers. Note marked basement membrane thickening of endoneurial vessels. (×420.)

tial focality of nerve fiber loss is more common in patients with type II diabetes.[35,36,118]

The predominant finding in teased fibers is excessive myelin wrinkling indicative of axonal atrophy. Other common abnormalities include paranodal demyelination, intercalated internodes, segmental demyelination, and Wallerian degeneration. Ultrastructurally there is axonal atrophy and occasionally so-called glycogenosomes, which are mitochondria filled with glycogen (Fig. 18-28). These usually are seen in the axoplasm, but may be present in the Schwann cell cytoplasm. Glycogenosomes are not specific for diabetic neuropathy but suggest metabolic polyneuropathy. Furthermore, axons may display honeycombed profiles and granular axoplasm. Unmyelinated fibers often have decreased caliber, and a varying percentage of them may be incompletely surrounded by the supporting Schwann cell.[12,108] Denervated Schwann cell subunits and collagen pockets are common in moderate to severe cases of neuropathy. In longitudinal sections the nodal area may show paranodal myelin retraction and disruption of the paranodal barrier with axoglial dysjunction.[118] This spectrum of changes can show quantitative differences in the neuropathy accompanying type I diabetes mellitus versus that seen in type II. In the former, the fiber loss is diffuse, whereas in type II it is more focal. Axonal degeneration appears more frequently in type II diabetes, whereas the nodal pathology is more common in patients with type I.[118] These differences most likely reflect the multifactorial etiology of diabetic neuropathy and the more severe metabolic aberrations in type I diabetes (nodal changes). In older patients with type II diabetes, vascular components as well as confounding age-related axonal changes are likely to play a greater role in the structural changes.

Frank infarcts are rarely seen; however, the focal nature of the nerve fiber loss suggests ischemic lesions proximal to the biopsy site.[27] Occlusions of endoneurial vessels by platelet thrombi have been described.[143] Capillary closure[36] by endothelial cells is of no pathologic significance, since it is commonly seen in normal nerves.[119]

Only a handful of rather old studies mention changes in autonomic nerves.[69,79] In experimental diabetes the changes that exist in parasympathetic and sympathetic nerves are similar to those seen in somatic nerves, that is, predominantly axonal degeneration.[110,145] In addition, sympathetic nerves in particular show dystrophic changes consisting of swollen axons filled with tubulovesicular structures and organelle debris.[110,145]

Ischemic lesions have been described in the third cranial nerve following acute onset of third nerve palsy in diabetic patients.[101] So-called small fiber neuropathy associated with painful neuropathy also has been documented in a few cases.[12] This association has not however, been confirmed by others.[76]

Research in diabetic neuropathy strongly suggests that the disease's origin is multifactorial, with various metabolic and vascular mechanisms influencing its development.[16,55] The wide spectrum of structural

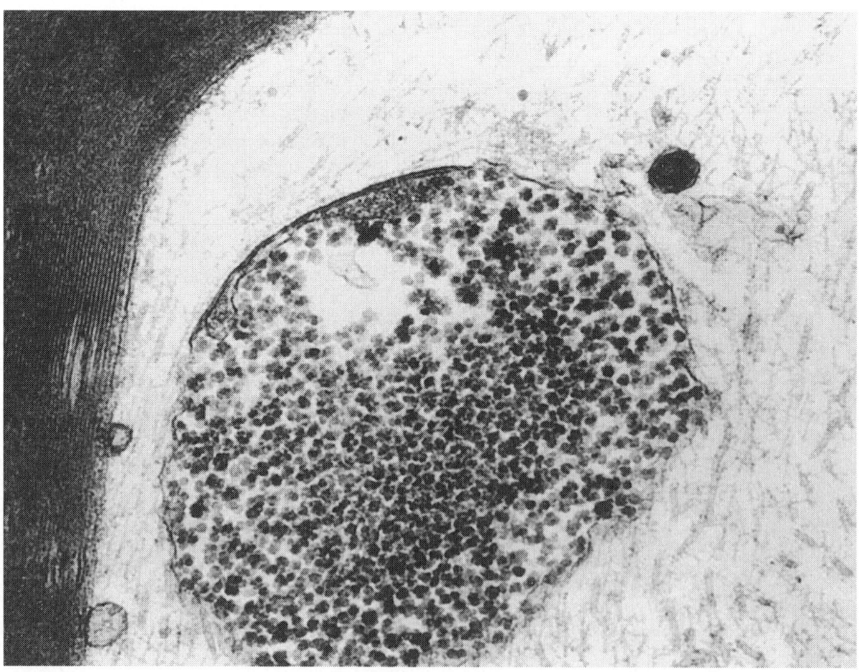

**Fig. 18-28.** Axonal glycogenosome in diabetic neuropathy. These axonal bodies consist of mitochondria filled with glycogen. (×92,000.)

changes visible in nerve samples from these patients supports this notion.

### Neuropathy Associated with Thyroid Disease

Polyneuropathy may accompany both hypothyroidism and hyperthyroidism, but is probably more common in the former.[38,42] Hypothyroid patients may show a mild, progressive, mainly sensory polyneuropathy with distal sensory loss and paresthesias. Carpal tunnel syndrome is common. The nerve biopsy may show accumulation of mucopolysaccharides in the endoneurium and in the subperineurial space.[89] Renaut bodies are common, probably reflecting the increased susceptibility of the nerve to compression. There is axonal degeneration and loss of both myelinated and unmyelinated fibers, with a predominance of large myelinated fiber loss.[38,88,89] Secondary segmental demyelination is common. Pi granules of myelinating Schwann cells and glycogenosomes in both axons and Schwann cells also are features of hypothyroid neuropathy. The pathophysiology of this neuropathy is not known in detail. Thyroid hormone deficiency may interfere with synthesis and assembly of neurofilaments and microtubules secondary to perturbations of neurotrophic factors.[135]

One report on hyperthyroid neuropathy describes axonal degeneration without any additional specific features.[132]

### Uremic Neuropathy

Uremic neuropathy has become less common since the introduction of hemodialysis and kidney transplantation. Nevertheless uremic neuropathy is regularly recognized in patients with end-stage renal failure. In patients with renal impairment secondary to diabetes, uremia may aggravate the diabetic neuropathy. Hemodialysis and kidney transplantation tend to halt the progression of neuropathy. For reasons unknown, peritoneal dialysis appears to be more effective than hemodialysis in the treatment of neuropathy.[9]

The pathologic changes consist of axonal degeneration and loss of all fiber categories, although large myelinated fibers seem to be specifically affected.[3,34,133] There is a proximal-to-distal gradient in the severity of the neuropathy. Both sensory and motor fibers are involved. Paranodal demyelination as well as intercalated internodes are common abnormalities in teased fibers. Secondary segmental demyelination may at times be impressive, and has led some investigators to suggest a primary demyelinating disorder.[27] A high frequency of fibers displaying segmental demyelination appears to be more common in patients with acute renal failure.[26] Regenerating clusters are present. Several regenerating axons surrounded by a single myelin sheath have been described by at least one group.[106]

The pathogenesis of uremic neuropathy is not well understood. Toxic circulating substances of intermediate molecular weight may be involved.[9]

### Neuropathy in Liver Disease

Neuropathies associated with liver disease differ greatly in their pathology, suggesting a multifactorial pathogenesis. Mild sensorimotor neuropathy affects 20% to 90% of patients with chronic liver disease.[22] The pathology shows a spectrum from mild to moderate axonal loss.[22] Teased fiber studies reveal marked segmental demyelination and remyelination, suggesting that the neuropathy is demyelinating.[3] A distinct neuropathy has been described in association with primary biliary cirrhosis.[21] This is a sensory neuropathy that appears to be distal in origin. A few reports have described infiltration of the endoneurium and particularly the perineurium with lipid-laden macrophages.[134] Additional changes consist of axonal loss without prominent demyelination or inflammation.

Both Guillian-Barré and CIDP-like neuropathies have been reported in association with hepatitis B infection.[7,64]

### Neuropathy in Acromegaly

Diffuse sensorimotor polyneuropathy has been described in acromegaly, with distal sensory loss, paresthesia, and weakness.[78,131] Pathologic examination demonstrated myelinated fiber loss and increased collagen deposition within the endoneurium and the perineurium.[78,131] Segmental demyelination and onion bulb formations also have been described.[78]

Compressive mononeuropathies, particularly carpal tunnel compression of the median nerve, are common in acromegaly, probably because of the nerve enlargement caused by the increase in the amount of connective tissue.

### Critical Illness Neuropathy

Zodochne and co-workers[147] described in 1987 a sensorimotor polyneuropathy developing in critically ill patients with sepsis and multiorgan failure. Autopsy studies demonstrated distal axonal degeneration and denervation atrophy of skeletal muscle. If recovery from underlying disorders occurs, the neuropathy tends to resolve. In this setting the differential diagnosis from treatable neuropathies such as vasculitides and Guillain-Barré syndrome is the major indication for nerve biopsy.

### Neuropathies Associated with Vitamin Deficiencies

These neuropathies are rare in the industrialized world. When they occur, they are often combined deficiencies in the setting of malabsorption syndromes or alcoholism. However, in the developing world these neuropathies remain common.[95] Neuropathies have been described in thiamine ($B_1$), pyridoxine ($B_6$), cobalamin ($B_{12}$), tocopherol (E), and folate deficiencies. In vitamin $B_{12}$-deficiency the CNS symptoms of subacute combined degeneration usually dominate the clinical picture. A similar picture has also been described in folate deficiency.[77]

The neuropathies accompanying these deficiencies show a similar pathology. There is a length-dependent sensorimotor axonopathy whereby large myelinated fibers appear to be preferentially involved with secondary segmental demyelination.[94] Unmyelinated fibers also are involved.[91] Nerve fiber regeneration is sparse in untreated patients, whereas supplementation with the deficient vitamins usually initiates vigorous regeneration. In vitamin $B_{12}$-deficiency swollen dystrophic axons containing tubulovesicular profiles and accumulation of degenerated organelles have been described.[111]

## INFLAMMATORY DEMYELINATING NEUROPATHIES

Guillain-Barré syndrome (GBS) or chronic inflammatory demyelinating polyradiculoneuropathy (CIDP) are diagnoses commonly considered by clinicians. GBS is probably the most common cause of acute or subacute neuropathy. CIDP, in contrast, is a common differential diagnosis with vasculitis.

### Guillain-Barré Syndrome

This disorder has an acute onset (days to a few weeks), with progressive motor and sensory deficit that may start in one limb and eventually become symmetric. Motor symptoms usually predominate; however, a pure motor or sensory syndrome does occur. Electrophysiologic testing suggests demyelination with diffuse slowing of nerve conduction or conduction block. The onset of GBS often is preceded by respiratory or gastrointestinal infection. GBS has been associated with various infectious agents such as *Campylobacter jejuni*, *Mycoplasma pneumoniae*, HIV, and Epstein-Barr virus.[2] In most cases a nerve biopsy is not necessary because the diagnosis is made on clinical grounds. When a biopsy is obtained, it should be kept in mind that because more or less pure motor involvement frequently is seen in GBS, a motor nerve may be considered for biopsy.[59] Moreover, the neuropathy may be predominantly proximal, and in such case a sural nerve biopsy will be of little supporting value for the diagnosis. Therefore the sural nerve should be biopsied only when abnormal sural nerve electrophysiology is found.

The hallmarks of the pathologic changes in GBS are macrophage-mediated demyelination and inflammatory infiltrates within the epineurium and endoneurium. The infiltrates consist of mononuclear cells, predominantly lymphocytes and occasional plasma cells. They are either perivascular or randomly distributed (Fig. 18-29). The endoneurium shows increased macrophages in direct proximity to myelinated Schwann cells, containing myelin debris.[11] Immunostaining for leukocytes (CLA) and macrophages ($ED_1$) may be useful in identifying these cell components. Onion bulb formations are rare in GBS. Ultrastructurally, macrophages are seen piercing the Schwann cell basement membrane and peeling off myelin along the intraperiod lines with their slender cytoplasmic processes (see Fig. 18-25). Sometimes macrophages are positioned within the myelin sheath or between the myelin and surrounding Schwann cell cytoplasm.[11] As a consequence of the macrophage-mediated demyelination, myelinated fibers at various stages of demyelination, or completely devoid of myelin, are regularly observed (Fig. 18-30). Axonal degeneration is common, although it is not as prominent as the demyelinating process. A primary axonal form of GBS has been associated with *Campylobacter jejuni* infection.[41] However, some investigators argue that distal primary axonal pathology does not necessarily exclude a mixed or primary demyelinating process at more proximal levels of the nerve.[24] Teased fibers show massive segmental demyelination and remyelination as well as denuded axons. The severity of the pathologic changes correlates roughly with the duration of the disease. Unmyelinated fiber loss is usually mild. Alterations in the blood-nerve barrier are part of GBS.

The exact pathogenesis of GBS remains controversial. The experimental allergic neuritis (EAN) model has been widely used as a model of GBS and has revealed possible mechanisms. EAN, and possibly GBS, is a T cell-mediated autoimmune disease, in which the P2 protein of the myelin appears to be the initiating antigen. Lymphocytic infiltration precedes macrophage invasion. Macrophages are the predominant cell type at the peak of the disease. Complement and immunoglobulin deposits on Schwann cells may opsonize the myelin and initiate the macrophage attack. The titers of circulating myelin antibodies are elevated in most GBS patients and this seemingly correlates with the severity of the disease. The efficacy of plasma exchange in GBS probably is related to removal of antimyelin antibodies and excessive cytokines. For up-to-date reviews on the pathogenesis of GBS, the reader is referred to References 2 and 61.

### Chronic Inflammatory Demyelinating Polyradiculoneuropathy

In contrast to GBS, chronic inflammatory demyelinating polyradiculoneuropathy (CIDP) evolves more slowly over months. It is multifocal and usually symmetric. Motor involvement predominates in most cases. When sensory nerves are affected the biopsy re-

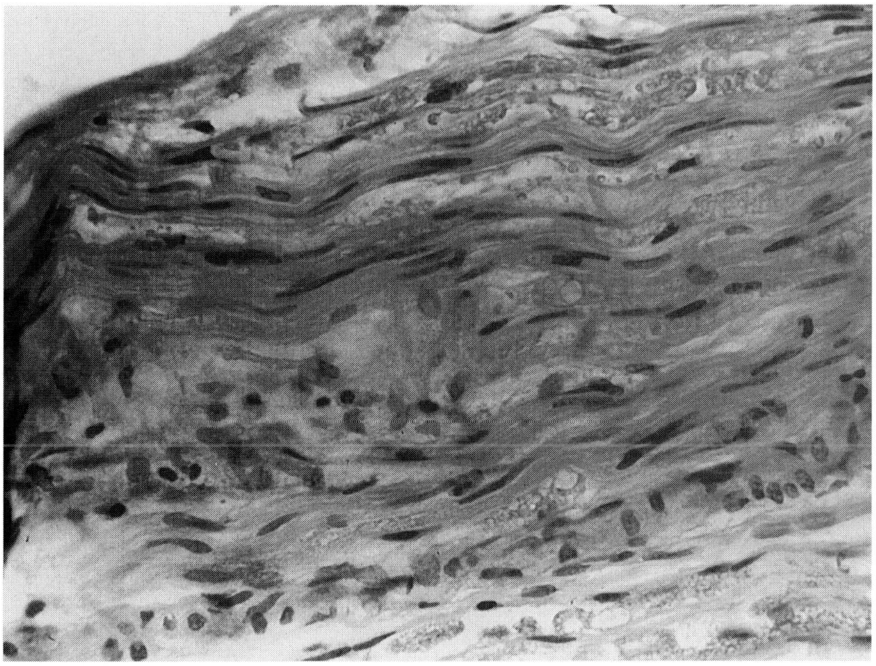

**Fig. 18-29.** Guillain-Barré syndrome (GBS). Longitudinal section of a sural nerve with focal hypercellularity due to lymphocytes and macrophages. The latter are filled with cellular debris. (Paraffin-embedded section stained with H&E; ×330.)

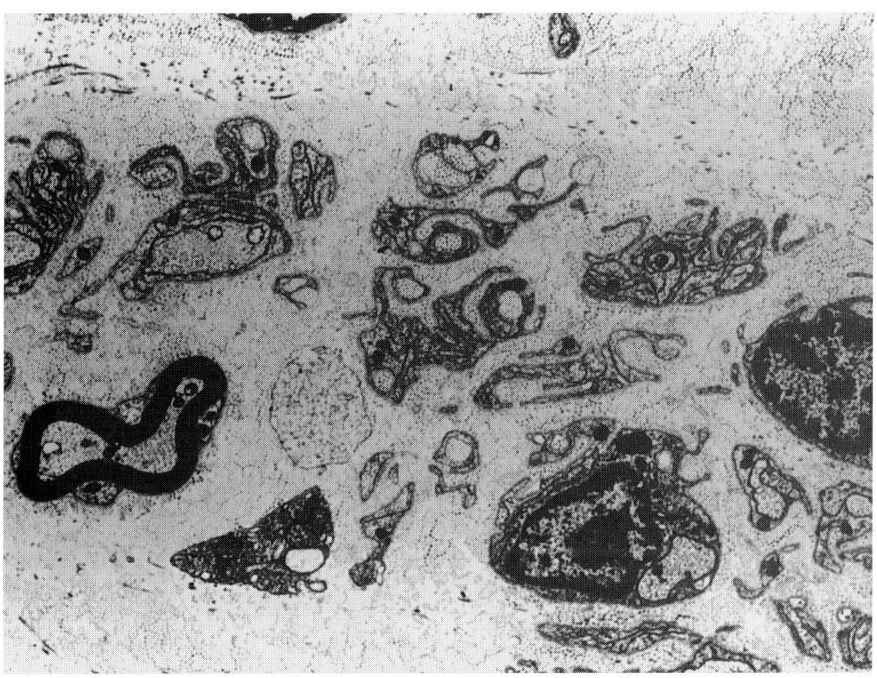

**Fig. 18-30.** Electron micrograph of sural nerve from a patient with GBS. One thinly myelinated axon and several demyelinated axons along with a few collagen pockets are seen within the endoneurium. (×1100.)

veals mostly large fiber involvement. As is true of GBS, cranial nerves may also be affected. A characteristic finding is elevated CSF protein in the presence of normal cell count. A recently described syndrome, "multifocal motor neuropathy," may be related to CIDP.[51] However, this disorder evolves even more slowly and often is confined to one limb. Electrophysiologic studies reveal multifocal abnormalities with characteristic permanent focal conduction block.

Sural nerve biopsy may be of limited use in confirming the diagnosis of CIDP because the brunt of the disease process may be borne by nerve roots, plexuses, and proximal nerves. In such a case the sural nerve shows nonspecific axonal neuropathy. Midroni and Bilbao[86] found fewer than 50% positive biopsies in patients with this clinical diagnosis.

The characteristic pathologic feature combines inflammatory infiltrates, particularly in the epineurium, macrophage-mediated demyelination, and onion bulb formations (Fig. 18-31). The inflammatory infiltrates

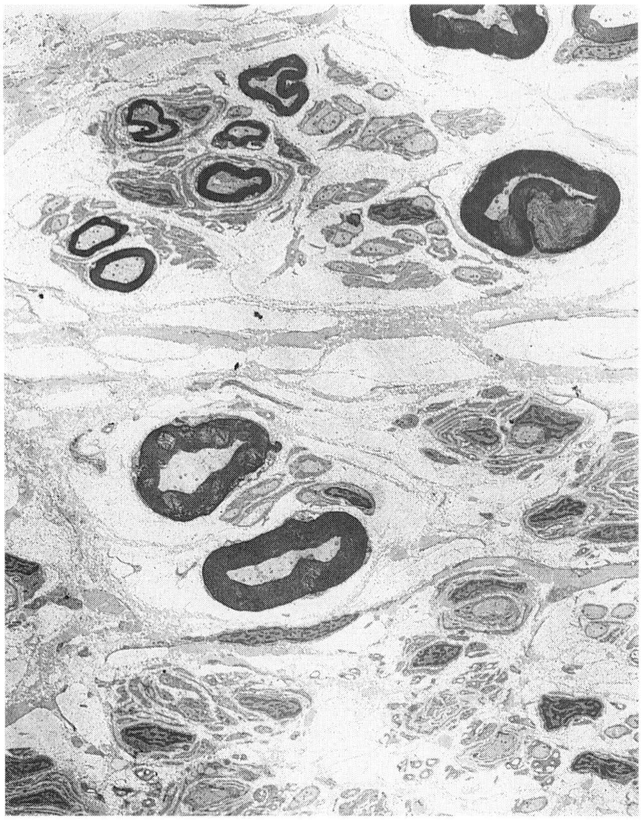

**Fig. 18-31.** Onion bulb formation in CIDP. Multi-layered concentric arrangement of thin layers of Schwann cell cytoplasm alternate with collagen surrounding normally myelinated or thinly myelinated or demyelinated axons or Schwann cell nuclei with missing axon. Electron micrograph. (×9000.)

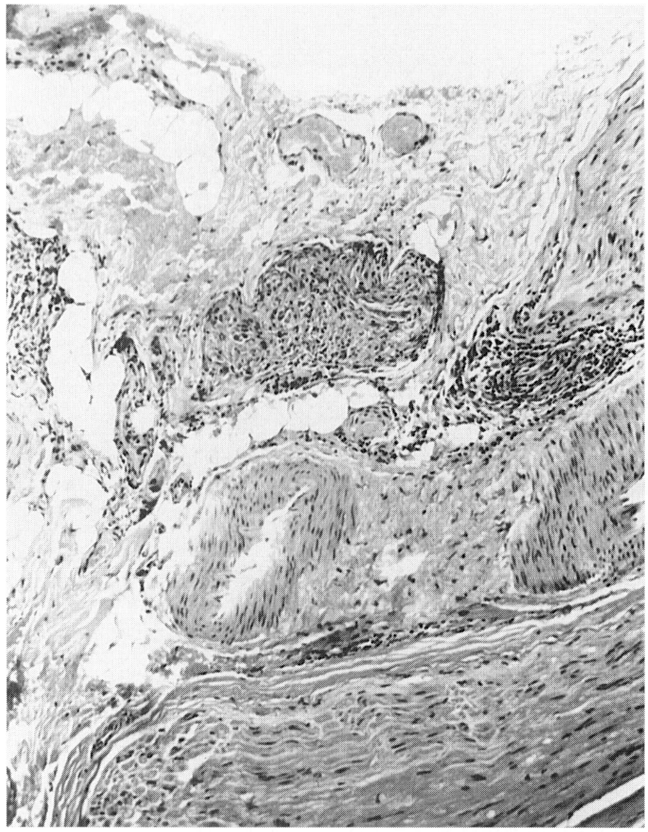

**Fig. 18-32.** Sarcoidosis in a sural nerve. Several non-necrotizing granulomata are visible within the epineurium, next to the vessels; a longitudinal section of nerve fascicle is shown at the bottom. (Paraffin embedded section stained with H&E; ×82.5.)

consist of lymphocytes and, rarely, plasma cells. The macrophage-mediated demyelination is similar to that described for GBS, but occurs less often. The most reliable differential between GBS and CIDP is the conspicuous presence of onion bulbs in the latter. Thinly myelinated fibers or fibers entirely devoid of myelin also may be noted (Fig. 18-31). Occasionally onion bulbs are denervated and contain no axons. These changes may be extremely focal, present in one fascicle and absent in others. Axonal loss is sometimes prominent, affecting mainly myelinated axons, whereas unmyelinated fiber loss is slight.

The pathology in multifocal motor neuropathy is similar to CIDP. The presence of mononuclear cells between layers of Schwann cells forming onion bulbs has been described. As in GBS, the pathogenesis of CIDP is not known, but appears to be immune-mediated. For a review of the topic the reader may consult Dyck and co-workers.[39]

### Sarcoidosis

Sarcoidosis is a systemic disease that occasionally affects peripheral nerve, although peripheral neuropathy is rarely the presenting manifestation. If the condition is suspected even in the absence of lung involvement, muscle biopsy often gives a greater diagnostic yield than does nerve biopsy.

The characteristic histology consists of multiple granulomata, most commonly located in the epineurium and occasionally in the endoneurium (Fig. 18-32). Tuberculoid leprosy should be considered in the differential diagnosis of cases in which granulomata are visible in the endoneurium. In sarcoidosis the granulomata consist of histiocytes, epithelioid cells, and multinucleated giant cells without caseating necrosis.[48] Perivascular lymphocytic cuffing as well as necrotizing angiitis may accompany the granulomatous lesions. Axonal degeneration is the characteristic feature of sarcoidosis and occasionally this abnormality is associated with axonal swelling and accumulation of neurofilaments, suggesting that the primary mechanism is compression of nerve fibers by the granulomatous lesions.

### Perineuritis

This uncommon condition often presents as a syndrome of mononeuritis multiplex.[10,124] In early reports it was suggested that mainly sensory nerves were af-

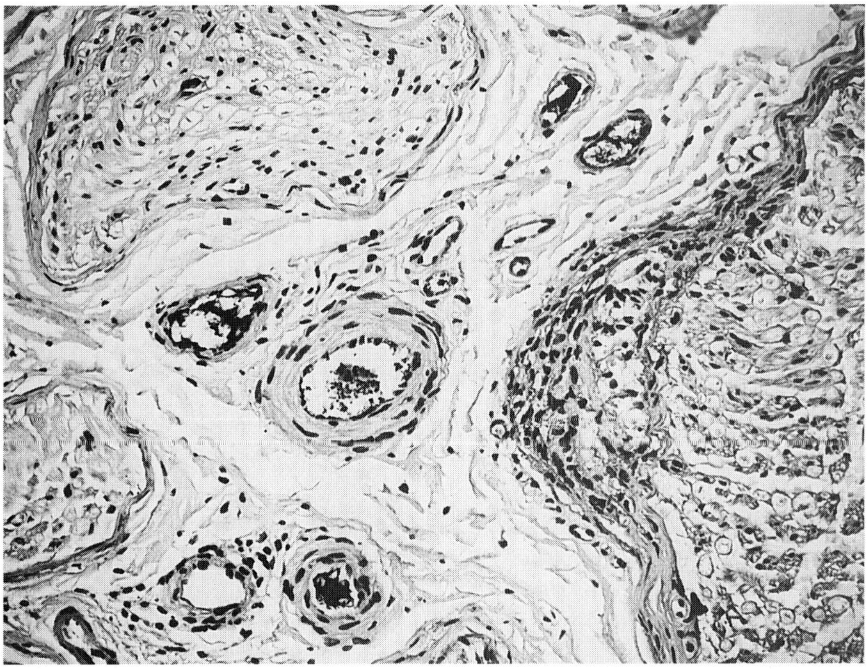

**Fig. 18-33.** Focal inflammation of the perineurium consisting of lymphocytes and macrophages. (Paraffin section, H&E stain; ×180.)

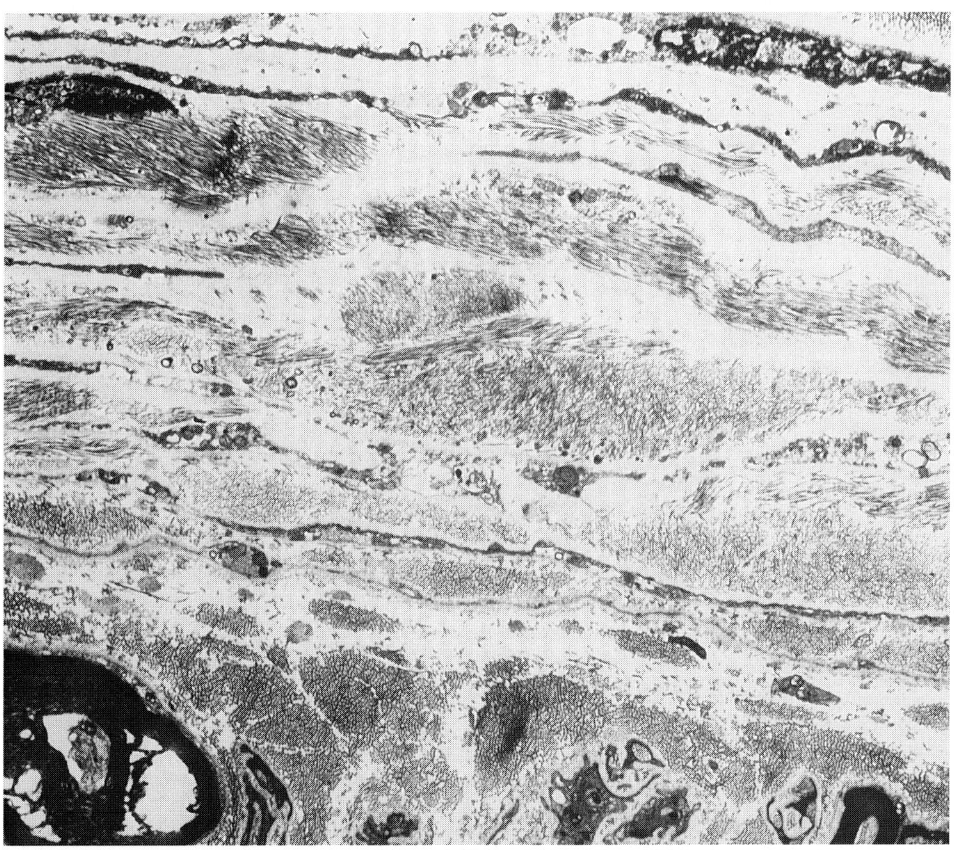

**Fig. 18-34.** Electron micrograph showing degeneration and necrosis of perineurial cells and increased collagen deposition in a case of perineuritis. (×20,400.)

fected, although in our experience motor nerves are involved with equal frequency.[10]

The histologic picture is fairly characteristic, with multiple focal perineurial lesions. Within these foci the perineurium is thickened and the perineurial cells are spread apart and separated by lymphocytes, foamy macrophages, and increased amounts of collagen (Fig. 18-33). Perineurial cells often show degeneration or necrosis. Perivascular lymphocytic cuffing may be present in neighboring perineurial and epineurial vessels. The lesions cause breaks in the perineurial barrier (Fig. 18-34) and leakage of immunoglobulins that can be identified in the endoneurium in proximity to the lesions.[10,124]

The pathogenesis of perineuritis is not known. The common association with collagen disorders and malignant disease has raised the possibility of an immune-mediated mechanism.

## VASCULITIC NEUROPATHY

Peripheral neuropathy is commonly associated with a variety of vasculitides: polyarteritis nodosa (PAN), Churg-Strauss syndrome, and those accompanying connective tissue disorders including rheumatoid arthritis (RA), Sjögren's syndrome, and systemic lupus erythematosus (SLE).

The vasculitis primarily affects the epineurial vessels and gives rise to hypoxic and/or ischemic damage to peripheral nerve. Most lesions are focal and manifest themselves as mononeuritis multiplex involving both motor and sensory nerves. When they become electrophysiologically confluent they masquerade as a symmetric sensorimotor polyneuropathy. The vasculitic process may be polyphasic (particularly in PAN), which is reflected in the pathology.

Most commonly small muscular vessels of the epineurium are affected, but the penetrating perineurial vessels and the perineurium itself do not escape. This should not be confused with perineuritis, a condition in which most inflammatory cells are lymphocytes. Endoneurial vessels are rarely involved, except in "nonsystemic angiopathy of peripheral nerve," which is not associated with any of the above disorders.[31] In acute vasculitis the vessel walls show necrosis of all layers, with fibrin deposited in and around the necrotic vessel walls (Fig. 18-35). The infiltration consists mostly of neutrophils, although some lesions contain large numbers of eosinophils. The latter often are seen in Churg-Strauss syndrome or vasculitis accompanying Sjögren's syndrome, although their presence is not a reliable criterion for differential diagnosis. The vessel lumen may be thrombosed. At later stages the polymorphonuclear response is replaced by lymphocytes and macrophages. The vessel walls undergo fibrous thickening, and the lumina may be recanalized. The lesions often are extremely focal, and sectioning through available paraffin blocks is required to confirm the diagnosis. Not infrequently, however, frank vasculitis is not found, only lymphocytic cuffing of small vessels or random scatter of lymphocytes in the epineurium.

The lesions are accompanied by predominantly focal axonal degeneration, demyelination, and Wallerian degeneration within several nerve fascicles. Sometimes one fascicle may be affected while adjacent ones are not (Fig. 18-36). The stage of degenerative changes of nerve fibers may vary, even within the same specimen, from acute axonal degeneration and Wallerian degeneration to total fiber loss. In older lesions regenerative axonal clusters are common. This spectrum reflects the multiphasic nature of the disease, which is particularly common in PAN, and is suggestive of ischemic damage even in the absence of verified vasculitis. The vasculitis itself is not specific for any particular disorder. The incidence of vasculitis affecting peripheral nerve in different disorders varies from 60% in Churg-Strauss syndrome, to 50% in RA, to 10% in SLE.[13,19,23]

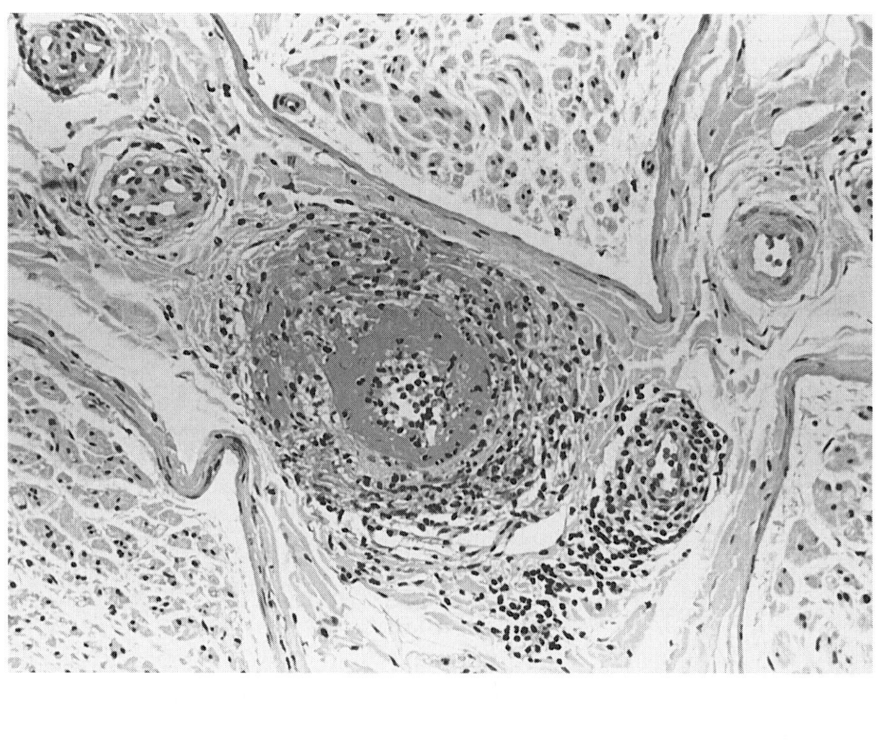

**Fig. 18-35.** Vasculitic neuropathy. Sural nerve with epineurial vessels of different caliber involved by various stages of inflammation in polyarteritis nodosa, from acute necrotizing arteritis (large vessel in the center) to chronic vasculitis in the smaller vessels to fibrosis of the vessel walls with organization of intraluminal thrombi. (Paraffin embedded section stained with H&E; ×165.)

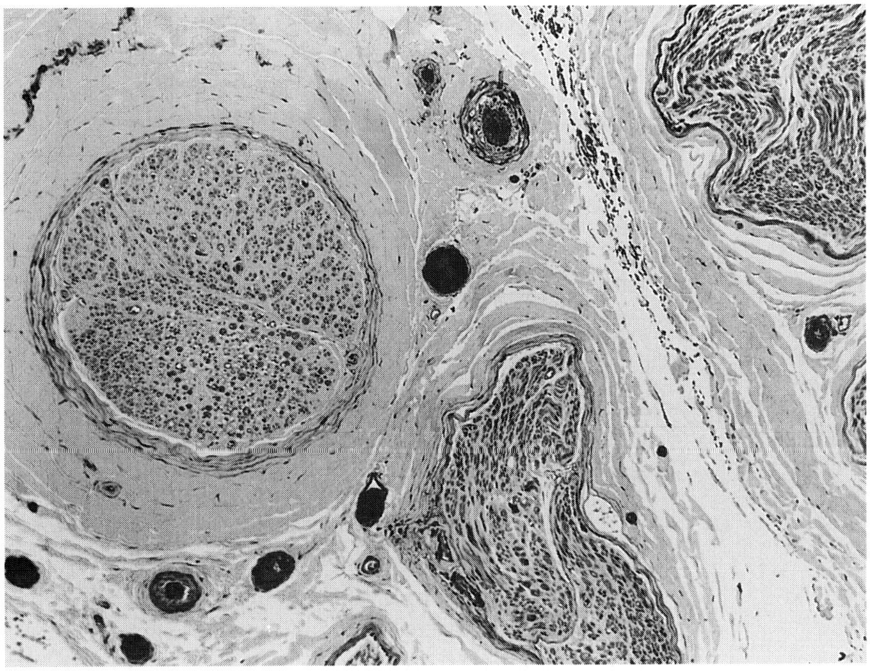

**Fig. 18-36.** Vasculitis showing an extended fascicle with fibers undergoing Wallerian degeneration. Note normal appearance of neighboring fascicles. (×96.)

## INFECTIOUS PERIPHERAL NERVE DISORDERS

### Neuropathies Associated with HIV Infection

Several neuropathic syndromes have been associated with HIV infection. They tend to be coupled with certain phases of the disease. During the stage of seroconversion or the early asymptomatic stage, both Guillain-Barré syndrome and CIDP have been described.[71] The pathology of these disorders in HIV patients is identical to that observed in non-HIV patients; the only difference is that tubuloreticular inclusions may be present in endoneurial endothelial cells in HIV patients.[44]

Mononeuropathy multiplex is frequent during the early symptomatic stage of HIV infection and may be self-limiting. The pathology reveals a variety of changes from necrotizing vasculitis to lymphocytic cuffing of epineurial and endoneurial vessels with axonal degeneration and secondary demyelination.[15,107] Viral particles have been identified in necrotizing vasculitis.[139]

Cytomegalovirus-related neuropathy was reported in the late stage of HIV infection.[71] The pathology showed a necrotizing vasculitis affecting both epineurial and endoneurial vessels with predominant infiltration by neutrophils. Viral inclusions were present in cytomegalic cells. These changes were associated with active axonal degeneration.

Later in the HIV infection up to one third of patients develop a distal symmetric polyneuropathy often accompanied by severe pain, paresthesia, and hyperesthesia. However, these symptoms may be overshadowed by the simultaneous involvement of the CNS. The pathologic picture is dominated by axonal degeneration in various stages, with occasional clusters of regenerating myelinated fibers. Segmental demyelination is not prominent.[139] Lymphocytic perivascular cuffing around epineurial and endoneurial vessels is common.

### Leprous Neuritis

Although rarely seen in the industrialized world, leprous neuropathy remains one of the most common neuropathies elsewhere. The infectious agent is *Mycobacterium leprae,* and skin lesions are readily diagnosed on skin biopsy. The organism shows a specific affinity for Schwann cells in which they proliferate, producing primary neuritic leprosy.[104] The disorder may present either in a lepromatous form or a tuberculoid form, the latter usually confined to skin and nerve. The neuropathy in tuberculoid leprosy is often sensory, focally involving superficial nerves and presenting as a nerve mass.[43]

Leprous neuritis is characterized by multiple granulomata (Fig. 18-37), roughly confined to the perineurium. Each granuloma consists of epithelioid histiocytes, multinucleated cells, and varying numbers of lymphocytes.[43] Caseation necrosis may be visible. The perineurium shows splitting of lamellae and infiltration by lymphocytes, which also invade the epineurium. In tuberculoid leprosy the bacilli can most easily be identified within unaffected Schwann cells in Fite's stain.[43] In lepromatous neuritis the picture is dominated by lymphocytes and foamy histiocytes that infiltrate the epineurium, perineurium, and endoneurium

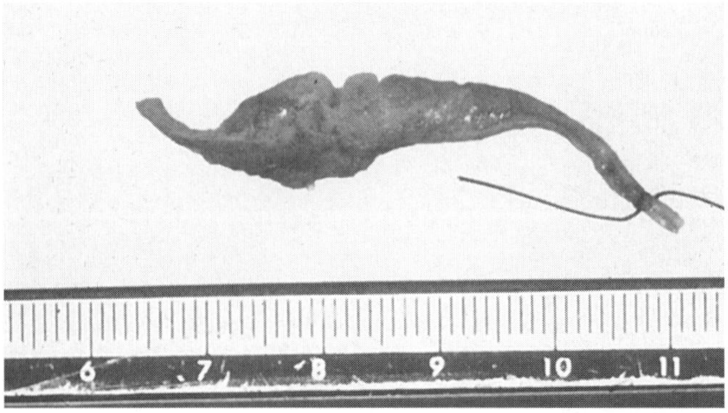


**Fig. 18-37.** Gross specimen of the case reported in Reference 43. Note marked enlargements of fascicles secondary to the presence of endoneurial granulomata. The lesion was believed to be a tumor. (×1.6.)

without granuloma formation. Bacilli are found in perineurial, endothelial, and Schwann cells and in fibroblasts.

### Lyme Disease Neuropathy

This disorder is caused by *Borrelia burgdorferi*, a spirochete transmitted via tick bites. The neurologic manifestations become evident several months following the tick bite and are quite diverse. Peripheral nerves are commonly involved. The onset may be acute, presenting as a symmetric polyneuropathy, mononeuritis multiplex, or radiculopathy; motor deficits usually predominate in these patients.[103]

Perivascular inflammation of epineurial, perineurial, and endoneurial vessels composed of lymphocytes, plasma cells, and histiocytes are common features of the disease (Fig. 18-38). There usually is marked loss of both myelinated and unmyelinated axons along with some segmental demyelination.[103] The organism may be visualized in biopsy material. Lyme disease is ubiquitous, but occurs most commonly in Europe and the northeastern United States.

## HEREDITARY NEUROPATHIES

The largest group of hereditary neuropathies, classified as the hereditary motor and sensory neuropathies (HMSNs), is a heterogeneous group that has many subgroups (see below and Reference 32). Other relatively common hereditary neuropathies include some associated with spinocerebellar deficits, such as Friedreich's ataxia, congenital demyelinating neuropathy, and hereditary neuropathy with pressure palsies. Rare disorders are hereditary sensory and autonomic neuropathy (HSAN), neuroaxonal dystrophy, giant axonal neuropathy, and the neuropathies associated with abnormal lipid metabolism or porphyria.

### Hereditary Motor and Sensory Neuropathies (HMSN-I, HMSN-II)

Dyck and co-workers provided a thorough review of the HMSNs and separated them into seven groups.[32] The largest groups are HMSN-I and HMSN-II. Their prevalence varies in different populations and their severity varies greatly from a subclinical form to a debilitating neuropathy. These neuropathies usually are transmitted in an autosomal dominant fashion. HMSN-I, or hypertrophic Charcot-Marie-Tooth disease, is not a genetically homogeneous group. Most cases are linked to chromosome 17, whereas some others are linked to chromosome 1.[65] Each variant shows dominant inheritance with high penetrance and become clinically evident at different ages. Patients with HMSN-I commonly present with skeletal deformities like pes cavus or scoliosis and atrophy of distal leg muscles. Motor symptoms predominate over sensory ones. Patients may exhibit palpable enlargement of the nerves. Usually the disease progresses slowly, although this is not an absolute rule. Electrophysiologically there is moderate slowing of nerve conduction velocity, reduced sensory and motor amplitudes, and a denervation pattern on EMG.

Nerve biopsy is indicated to rule out a treatable disorder, most commonly CIDP, or to diagnose HMSN in patients with no known family history. The features, best appreciated on semithin plastic cross-sections include uniformly enlarged fascicles as a result of diffuse collagen deposition within the endoneurial space (Fig. 18-39). There is variable diffuse loss of myelinated fibers. The pathologic hallmark of HMSN is the striking onion bulb formation surrounding large and small myelinated fibers (Fig. 18-39). The myelin sheath may appear thick relative to the accompanying axonal atrophy. There is often an appreciable proliferation of Schwann cells, even outside the onion bulbs. Cellular inflammation is not part of the pathology. Active demyelination or remyelination (thinly myelinated axons) may occasionally be encountered. This is more common in younger patients, probably reflecting a more rapid progression of the disease with repeated demyelination and remyelination of axons. The overriding feature in teased fibers is segmental demyelination.

Onion bulbs are made of concentric sleeves of Schwann cells, which may harbor unmyelinated axons. The number of Schwann cell layers varies from four to five up to fifteen or more.[87] Unmyelinated fibers usually are unaffected in HMSN-I.

The most commonly identified genetic defect in HMSN-I is a duplication of a segment of chromosome 17p11.2.[80] There is evidence that the transcription defect involves peripheral myelin protein 22.

HMSN-II is also referred to as the neuronal form of

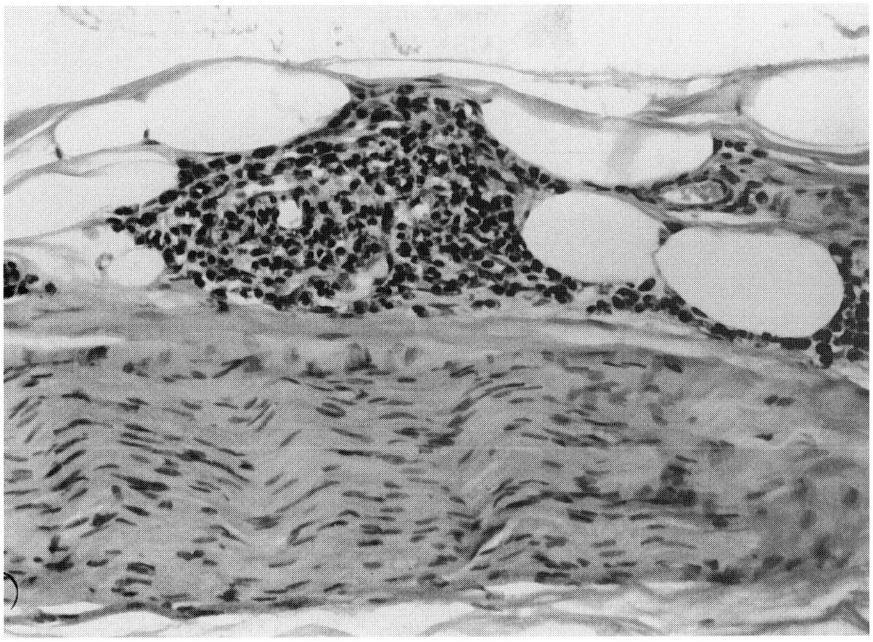

**Fig. 18-38.** Sural nerve biopsy from a patient with Lyme disease. Epineurial vessels immediately adjacent to the perineurium are infiltrated by lymphocytes and plasma cells. (Paraffin embedded sections stained with H&E; ×165.)

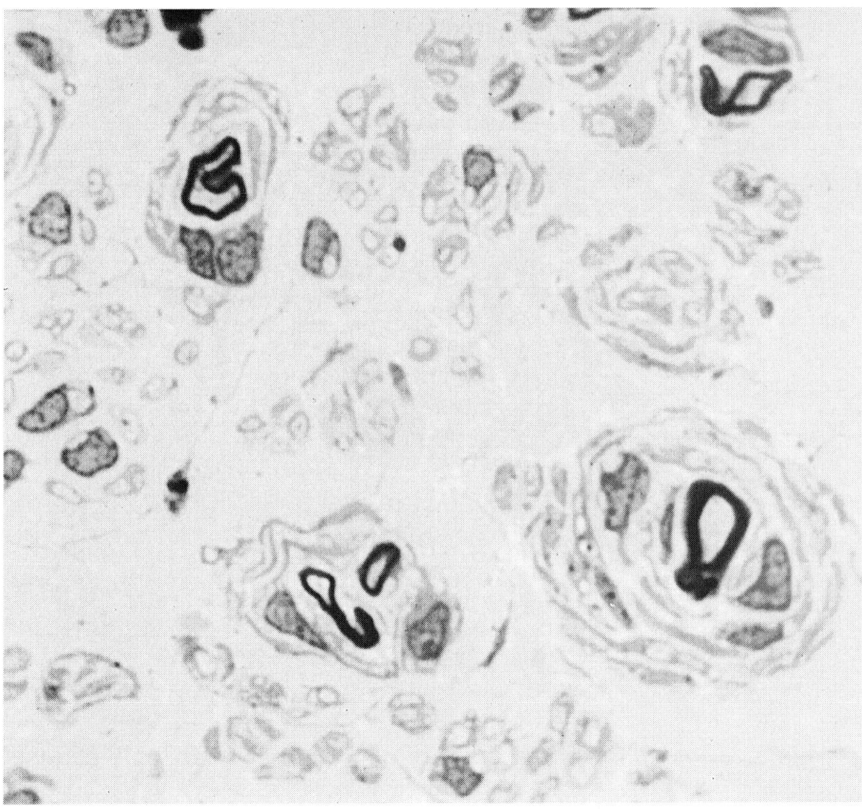

**Fig. 18-39.** Plastic section showing increase in endoneurial collagen and typical onion bulb formation in a case of HMSN-I. (×720.)

Charcot-Marie-Tooth disease and has clinical features similar to those of HMSN-I. The best distinguishing feature of HMSN-II is a near-normal nerve conduction velocity and decreased amplitudes. Approximately half the cases suggest an autosomal dominant trait, and half of them are sporadic.[46]

In contrast to HMSN-I, HMSN-II does not display enlargement of the fascicles and the onion bulbs are rare. The fascicles may show diffuse loss of myelinated fibers, most significantly of the large ones (Fig. 18-40). Regenerating myelinated axonal clusters are common.[5] Active axonal degeneration and segmental demyelin-

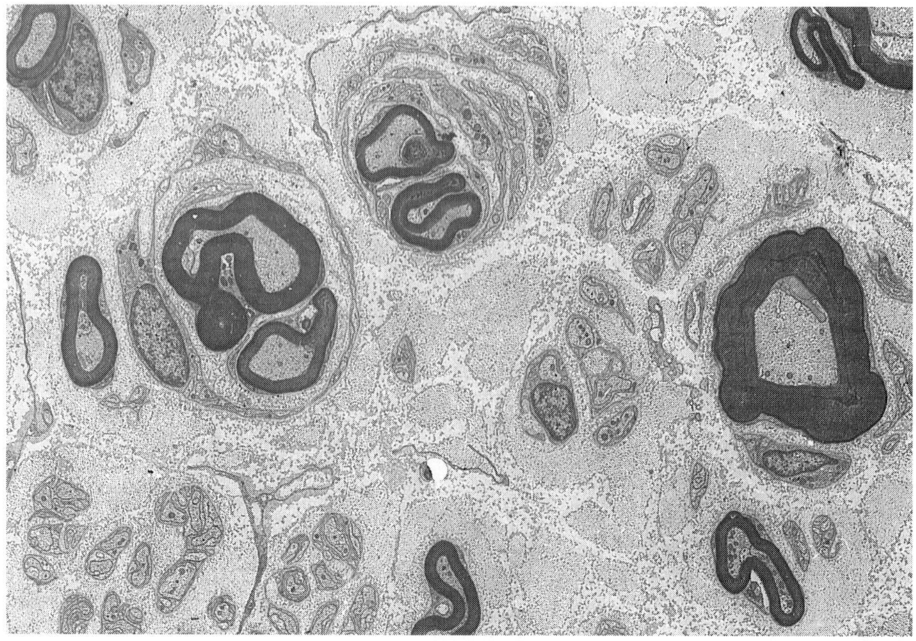

**Fig. 18-40.** Electron micrograph from a case of HMSN-II. Note regenerating clusters of myelinated fibers, the occasional onion bulb, and relative preservation of unmyelinated fibers. (×2750.)

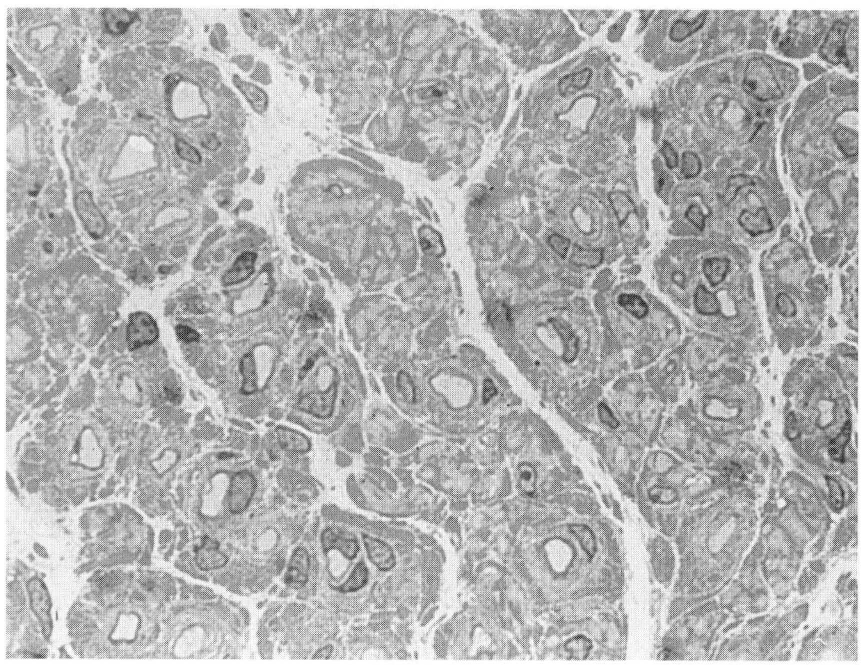

**Fig. 18-41.** Déjèrine-Sottas hereditary neuropathy. Onion bulb formations surround predominantly hypomyelinated axons. One-micron thick plastic embedded toluidine stained section. (×528.)

ation are rarely seen in childhood cases. Unmyelinated fibers are not affected.

The pathogenesis of HMSN-II is not known, but its features are those of a primary distal axonopathy; in contrast, HMSN-I is a primary myelinopathy.

### Congenital Demyelinating Neuropathy (HMSN-III)

This disorder is also referred to as Déjèrine-Sottas' disease or HMSN-III. The severity and progression rate may vary between kindreds.[6,96] The disability is more severe than in HMSN-I and HMSN-II. Some patients are born with other abnormalities such as arthrogryposis.

Like HMSN-I, HMSN-III shows marked enlargement of nerve fascicles secondary to endoneurial collagen deposition. There is profound loss of myelinated fibers and numerous onion bulb formations (Fig. 18-41). In contrast to HMSN-I, axons have extremely thin myelin sheaths in proportion to axonal caliber or are totally denuded (Fig. 18-42).[96] The onion bulbs consist of Schwann cell profiles, but also may consist of base-

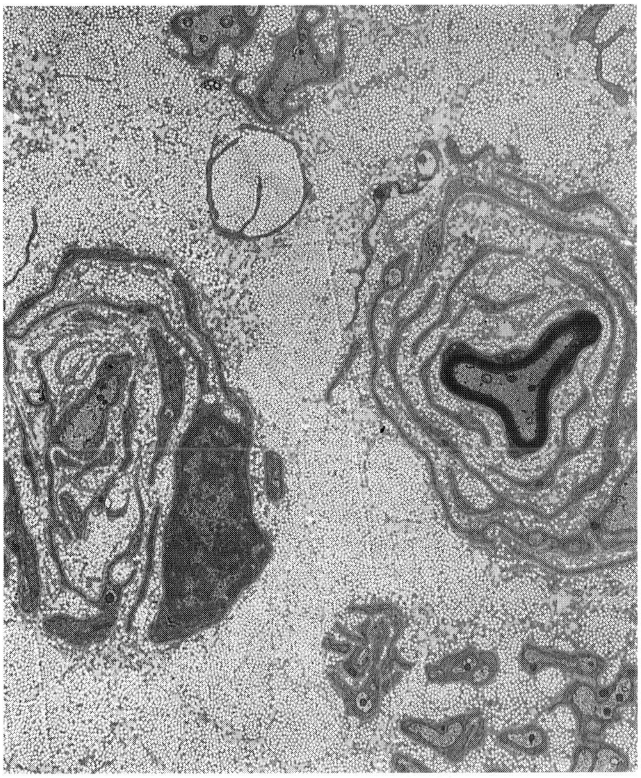

**Fig. 18-42.** Electron micrograph of sural nerve with Déjèrine-Sottas neuropathy. Two onion bulb formations; one includes a hypomyelinated axon and the other a demyelinated axon. (×12,000.)

ment membranes alone, called "basal lamina onion bulbs."[45] These are not seen in HMSN-I. There is no inflammation, although rare endoneurial macrophages may be present. Unmyelinated fibers usually are unaffected. The genetics of the congenital dysmyelinating neuropathies have not been clarified.

A further classification into various subgroups has been suggested.[45]

### Neuropathies in Hereditary Ataxias

These syndromes are dominated by spinal and/or cerebellar signs and symptoms; therefore, peripheral nerve biopsy is not indicated. In most of these conditions, such as Friedreich's ataxia, non-Friedreich's spinocerebellar degenerations, and olivopontocerebellar atrophy, the peripheral nerve abnormalities are characterized by a nonspecific axonopathy preferentially affecting large myelinated fibers. Fiber loss can be substantial, particularly in patients with Friedreich's ataxia. Regeneration is not a prominent feature.

### Hereditary Neuropathy with Pressure Palsies

This disorder is caused by a deletion of the same region of chromosome 17p.11.2 that shows duplication in HMSN-I.[20] The patients often present with mononeuritis multiplex, which may become electrophysiologically confluent. Localized nerve abnormalities may be precipitated by trauma, followed by resolution of

A

B

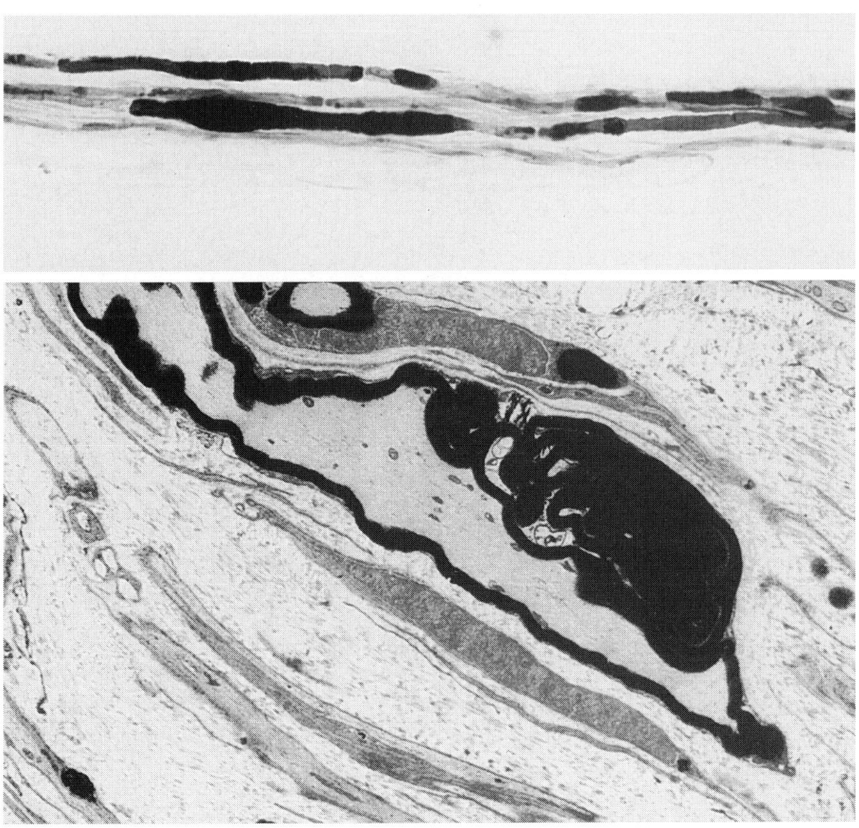

**Fig. 18-43.** Teased fiber preparation of tomaculous neuropathy showing focal thickening of the myelin sheath (**A**). **B**, Electron micrograph showing focal area of multifold doubling of the myelin sheath. (**A**, ×300, **B**, ×1820.)

symptoms. Hence, there frequently is a history of repeated localized palsies or a slowly progressive neuropathy. Histologically the nerve biopsy shows a normal or slightly decreased number of myelinated fibers. The characteristic feature is the marked variation in myelin thickness due to infoldings or invaginations of the myelin sheath, giving the appearance of doubling or tripling of the myelin thickness.[81] This "doubling-up" of the myelin may be circumferential or partial (Fig. 18-43). In some cases active demyelination is seen as well as onion bulb formations. Axonal degeneration is rare. Teased fibers are quite characteristic, with their marked variation of the myelin thickness along the internodes producing a sausage-like appearance. Hence this neuropathy is descriptively referred to as "tomaculous neuropathy."

### Hereditary Sensory and Autonomic Neuropathies (HSANs)

These rare disorders have been divided into subgroups by Dyck and co-workers.[40] Type-I[40] shows a predominantly sensory distal axonopathy with only minimal autonomic involvement. In other types the axonal degeneration also involves unmyelinated fibers, the loss of which may be more severe than that of myelinated fibers.

### Giant Axonal Neuropathy

This is a rare autosomal recessive disorder affecting infants. It may be accompanied by various CNS abnormalities. The course is progressive, and electrophysiology is consistent with a distal axonopathy. The pathology is characterized by severely swollen, thinly myelinated or unmyelinated axons filled with whorled bundles of tightly packed neurofilaments.[29] Some axons contain electrondense crystalline profiles and some may exhibit segregation of neurofilaments and microtubules. Myelinated fiber loss is variable. Teased fiber preparation reveals fusiform swellings along the internodal axon.[67] The pathogenesis is not known, but a defect in the synthesis and polymerization of intermediate filament subunits has been suggested.

### Neuroaxonal Dystrophies

The neuroaxonal dystrophies include a spectrum of disorders ranging from the adult form, known as Hallervorden-Spatz disease, to a juvenile form, to an infantile form, Seitelberger's disease. The latter is an autosomal recessive disorder that, like all neuroaxonal dystrophies, has CNS manifestations and in addition involves the peripheral nerves. The peripheral neuropathy is characterized by spheroid swellings more commonly seen in unmyelinated fibers (Fig. 18-44). Distended axons contain tubulovesicular profiles of endoplasmic reticulum, degenerated mitochondria, and conglomerates of misoriented filaments.[30,72,144] When these changes occur in myelinated axons they often distend and attenuate the myelin sheath. Axonal loss is either nonexistent or mild.

The most likely underlying pathophysiologic mechanism in this disorder is a defect in axonal transport.

### Neuropathies Associated with Abnormal Lipid Metabolism

Several of the classic leukodystrophies involve peripheral nerves. However, nerve biopsy is not the optimal procedure for diagnosing these disorders (Chapter

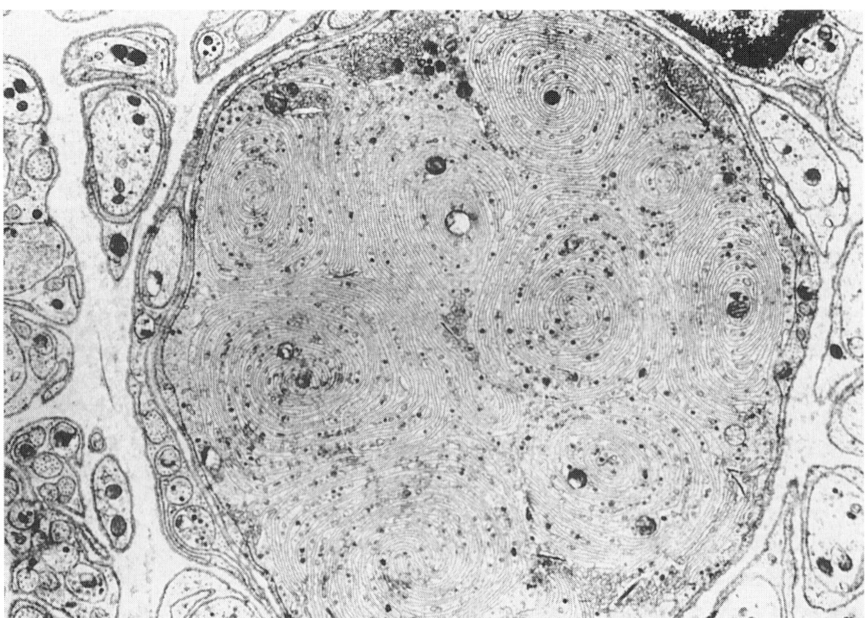

**Fig. 18-44.** Swollen unmyelinated fiber showing whorled laminar profiles of endoplasmic reticulum and degenerated electron-dense mitochondria. (×15,600.)

16). Leukodystrophies are identified by the underlying enzymatic defect or by accumulations of specific lipids in cultured fibroblasts, leukocytes, or serum (Chapter 14). Peripheral nerve findings are characterized by typical inclusions within Schwann cells. In globoid cell leukodystrophy (Krabbe's disease), the membrane-bound straight elongated tubular structures reside within Schwann cells and macrophages. Parallel lamellae are seen within the inclusions.[8] Farber's disease shows so-called "banana" bodies, slightly curved empty inclusions that may be either membrane-bound or free within the cytoplasm of myelinating Schwann cells. They are believed to represent the stored ceramide.[102] In adrenoleukodystrophy characteristic inclusions also exist within Schwann cells and macrophages and have an appearance of membrane-bound trilaminar elongated profiles with varying alternating periodicity.[109]

In Fabry's disease, electron-dense curvilinear rounded inclusions with a lamellar periodicity of 5 to 7 nm are prominent in perineurial and endothelial cells. They are less common in Schwann cells.[120]

### Porphyria Neuropathy

The various conditions affecting heme synthesis, such as acute intermittent porphyria, coproporphyria, and the variegate type of porphyria, all cause peripheral neuropathy. Patients often present with intermittent abdominal cramps or pain and sometimes with encephalopathy. Motor symptoms often dominate and can be proximal. Autonomic dysfunction also may be present.

The neuropathy is axonal in nature, with both myelinated and unmyelinated fibers undergoing axonal atrophy. Myelinated axons occasionally demonstrate honeycomb profiles and axonal degeneration. Axonal swelling secondary to accumulation of neurofilaments and segregation of neurotubules and filaments occurs more commonly in unmyelinated fibers.[28,117,135]

## NEUROPATHIES ASSOCIATED WITH DYSPROTEINEMIAS

The so-called benign paraproteinemia is relatively common and becomes more frequent with increasing age. Some of these individuals eventually develop a lymphoproliferative disorder, most commonly multiple myeloma. However, a relatively small percentage develop peripheral neuropathy especially those who demonstrate IgM paraproteinemia, less commonly those with IgA or IgG paraproteinemias. Most patients with neuropathy associated with IgM produce antibodies against myelin associated glycoprotein (MAG).[90] Neuropathies also occur with Waldenström's macroglobulinemia, multiple myeloma, and POEMS syndrome.

Paraproteinemia neuropathy varies in its distribution and may have a relapsing course. Most commonly the condition becomes manifest as a distal symmetric sensorimotor neuropathy.

The characteristic feature of IgM-associated neuropathy is segmental demyelination with thinly myelinated or denuded axons. Paraprotein deposits are found within the endoneurium or immediately under the perineurium, as well as between perineurial cells, spreading apart the individual lamellae (Fig. 18-45).[140] In teased fibers, segmental demyelination and remyelination usually predominate. The characteristic ultrastructural feature is widely spaced myelin (Fig. 18-46), a feature particularly common in IgM paraproteinemias,[146] whereas uncompacted myelin is more com-

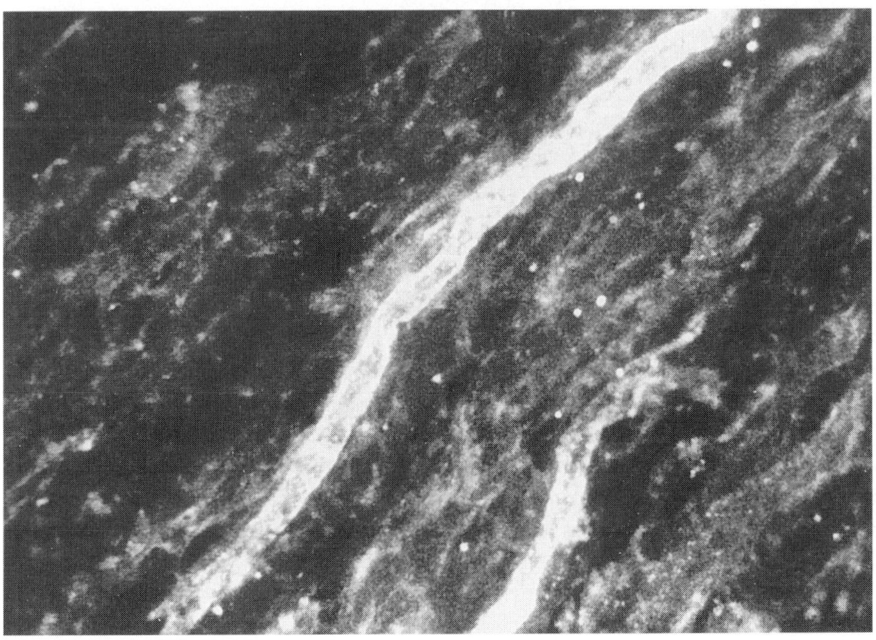

**Fig. 18-45.** Immunofluorescence. Sural nerve biopsy from a patient with IgM paraproteinemia. IgM precipitation outlines two myelinated fibers. (×330.)

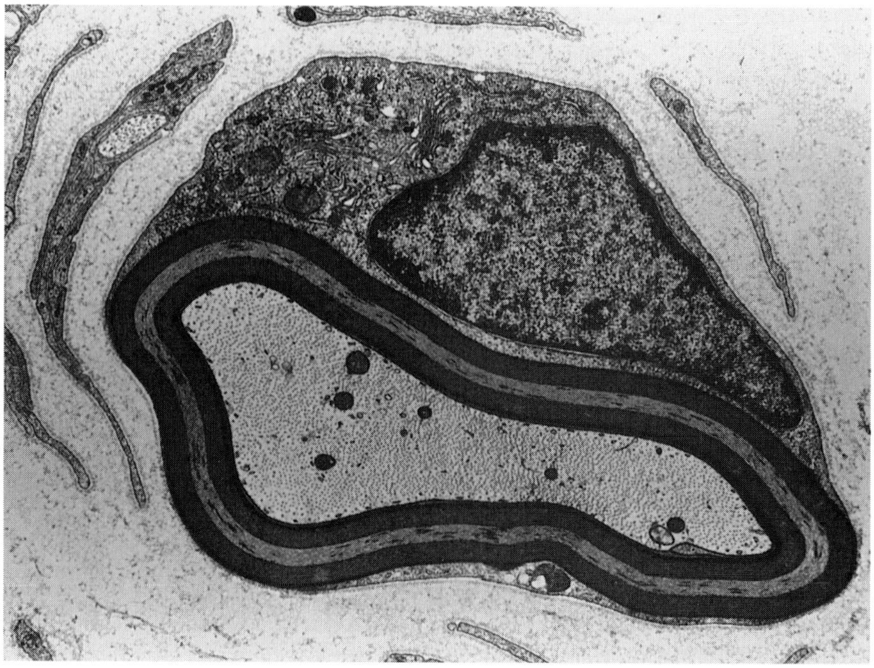

**Fig. 18-46.** IgM paraproteinemia. Widely spaced myelin in electron micrograph of myelinated axon from a sural nerve biopsy. (×22,750.)

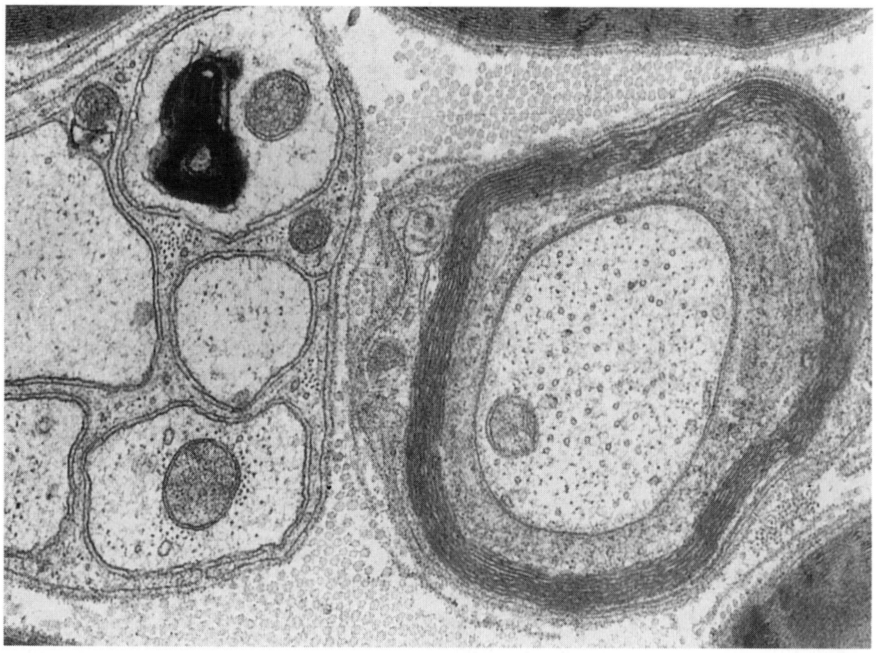

**Fig. 18-47.** Uncompacted adaxonal myelin from a case with IgG paraproteinemia. (×18,600.)

mon in neuropathy associated with POEMS and with IgA or IgG (Fig. 18-47). Unmyelinated fiber loss is not prominent. Regenerating clusters may be present. IgG and IgA paraproteinemias are associated with more severe axonal degeneration, fiber loss, and secondary segmental demyelination, as is probably also the case in neuropathies associated with POEMS. Immunocytochemistry may be employed, particularly in IgM related neuropathies, whereas immunopositivity for IgG or IgA should be interpreted with caution, since this abnormality is usually nonspecific.

## AMYLOID NEUROPATHY

Amyloid neuropathy occurs in different clinical settings. Primary amyloidosis is a systemic disease secondary to paraproteinemia caused by plasma cell dyscrasia. Most commonly the amyloid protein originates from light chains of immunoglobulin. Familial amyloidosis is an autosomal dominant disorder that is classified according to the major amyloid protein produced. Familial amyloidosis of the Portuguese/Swedish-type (FAP I) displays transthyretin as the cir-

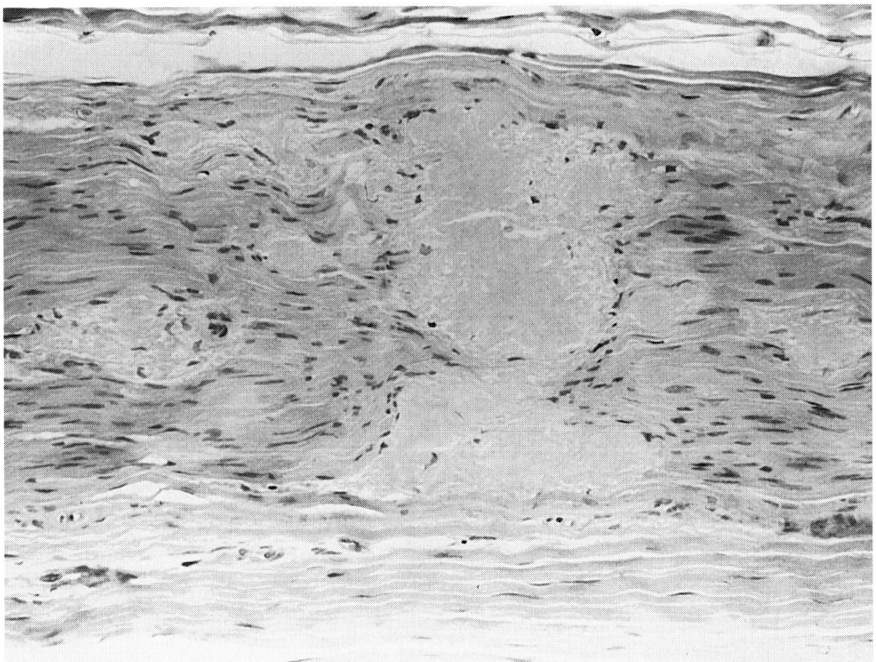

**Fig. 18-48.** Amyloid neuropathy. Several large aggregates of homogeneous material compressing the axons in longitudinal section of sural nerve. (Paraffin embedded section stained with H&E; ×165.)

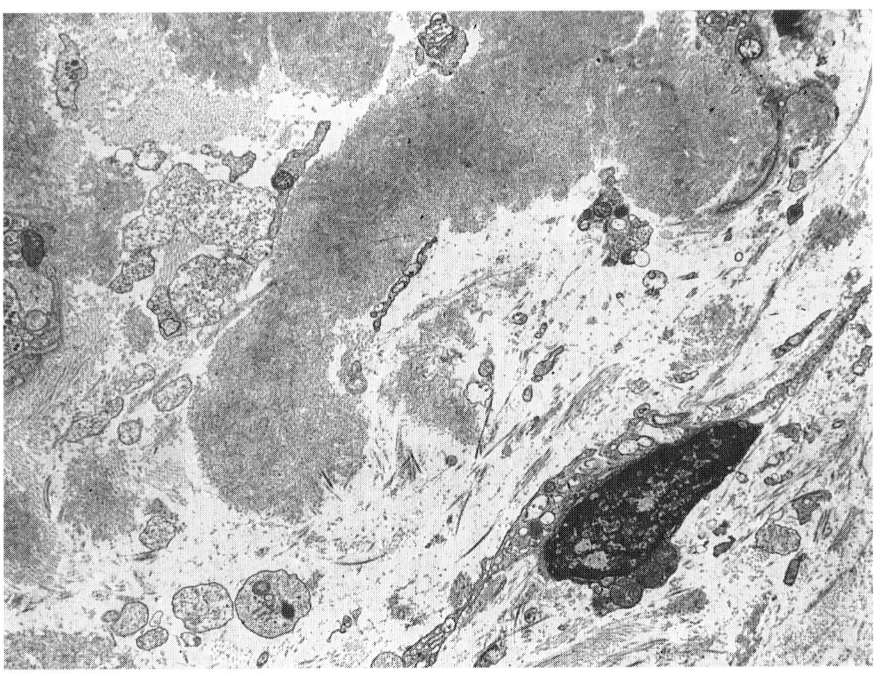

**Fig. 18-49.** Amyloid neuropathy. Electron micrograph of a band-shaped deposit of amyloid within the endoneurium of a sural nerve. (×12,200.)

culating protein. The Iowa-type (FAP III) shows apolipoprotein A1 as the protein component of the amyloid, whereas in the Finnish-type (FAP IV) gelsolin is the participating protein in the amyloid deposits. In sporadic amyloid neuropathy the source of the deposited protein is not identified.

Peripheral nerve is not the optimal biopsy site for the diagnosis of amyloidosis.[125] The yield is probably only 70% to 80% at best in both primary and familial amyloidosis. Rectal, muscle, or abdominal fat pad biopsies provide higher yield. Conversely, most amyloidoses in nerve biopsies are incidentally diagnosed in patients not thought as to have the disease.

For the light microscopic identification of amyloid deposits, Congo-red stained sections need to be examined under polarized light. Congo-red stain is routinely applied to all nerve biopsies in our laboratory.

The pathology is characterized by accumulation of amyloid (Fig. 18-48) around endoneurial vessels, in the subperineurial space, or diffusely in the endoneurium.[74] Occasionally it is found exclusively in the epineurium. Amyloid deposits are associated with loss of unmyelinated fibers. In severe cases the fiber loss also involves small myelinated and possibly large myelinated fibers, accompanied by Wallerian degeneration.[86] Ultrastructurally the characteristic straight haphazardly arranged fibrils are found in the extracellular spaces (Fig. 18-49).

Immunocytochemical identification of the major amyloid protein is now available to help when amyloid neuropathy is suspected.[74]

## PARANEOPLASTIC NEUROPATHIES

The paraneoplastic neuropathies become manifest as a subacute sensory neuropathy or a sensorimotor neuropathy. The former is more common and frequently is associated with small cell carcinoma of the lung, although other malignant disorders such as Hodgkin's disease and adenocarcinoma may be responsible for the syndrome. Symptoms consist of sensory loss, paresthesias, sensory ataxia, and at times intestinal pseudoobstruction.[75] There are also frequent CNS symptoms such as ataxia and encephalopathy. The disorder is associated with circulating antibodies (anti-Hu) that are directed toward tumor antigens and by mimicry against neuronal nuclear antigens of spinal ganglion cells.[25] Autopsy findings have revealed loss of spinal ganglion cells and lymphocytic infiltrates (ganglionitis) (Fig. 18-50). Sural nerve biopsy shows loss of myelinated fibers, axonal atrophy, and active axonal degeneration. Regeneration is not a prominent feature. Unmyelinated fibers may be variably involved. Perivascular lymphocytic cuffing in the epineurium may exist in some instances, but frank vasculitis does not occur.[70,137] Since this is a neuropathy primarily affecting sensory neurons, degeneration also occurs in the central sensory axons of the dorsal columns of the spinal cord.

The neuropathic symptoms may precede the clinical recognition of the tumor. Cases have been reported in which removal of the tumor (usually small cell carcinoma of the lung) produces a beneficial effect on the neuropathy, although full recovery is unlikely.

A combined sensorimotor neuropathy has been associated with systemic malignancy, but the pathogenesis of this disorder is not known.[84] This type of neuropathy accompanies a variety of malignancies, and follows varying rates of progression. The pathology ranges from a predominantly axonal dying-back type, to a mixed axonal/demyelinating, to a predominantly demyelinating neuropathy, raising the question whether this represents a specific entity or a spectrum or combinations of subacute sensory paraneoplastic neuropathy, CIDP, and nutritional neuropathies. The pathologic picture may be further complicated by perivascular lymphocytic cuffing.

Tumor cells may, on occasion, infiltrate peripheral nerve. This is most common in lymphoma, myeloma, or leukemia. Carcinomas seldom infiltrate the nerve, since the perineurium provides a barrier against the malignant cells. Nerves, however, may be compressed by surrounding carcinoma, producing neuropathic symptoms.

## TOXIC NEUROPATHIES

For detailed descriptions of toxic neuropathies, the chemistry of toxic agents, and experimental toxic neuropathies the reader is referred to Spencer and Schaumburg.[128]

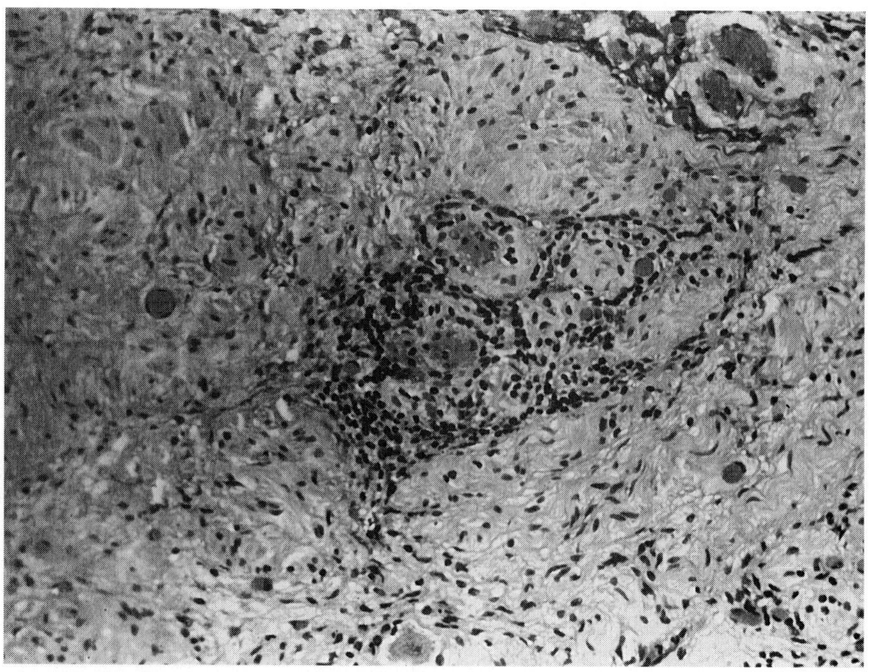

**Fig. 18-50.** Paraneoplastic neuropathy. Ganglionitis showing a lymphocytic infiltrate surrounding ganglion cells. (Paraffin embedded sections stained with H&E; ×165.)

### Lead Neuropathy

The neurotoxic effects of lead have been known for thousands of years. Today, most cases develop in persons exposed to lead-containing paints or fumes of leaded gasoline. Motor abnormalities dominate over the sensory ones, and the upper extremities are most commonly involved.

Lead intoxication has long been regarded as the example par excellence of a demyelinating neuropathy. Few relatively recent studies have disputed this and some suggest that the neuropathy may be axonal in nature with loss of large myelinated fibers, accompanied by segmental demyelination.[14,92] In favor of a primary demyelinating process is the common finding of onion bulb formations following chronic exposure to lead. Schwann cells undergo proliferation and may contain electron-dense inclusions within their nuclei. There is experimental evidence suggesting that lead exposure perturbs the integrity of the protective nerve barriers.

### Organophosphorous Neuropathies

These substances have been used in insecticides, petroleum products, and lubricants. Several epidemics have been caused by adulterated alcoholic beverages (the "jake" epidemic in the United States) and cooking oil (the Morocco epidemic in the 1950s). The presumed effect of these substances is inhibition of the neurotoxic esterase enzyme. The symptoms are mainly motor, manifesting as a symmetric distal motor neuropathy that may be preceded by a cholinergic crisis due to the acute inhibitory effect on AChE.

The neuropathy is characterized by a dying-back axonopathy that also may affect central motor tracts. Axonal swellings associated with accumulation of cytoskeletal material have been described in some experimentally induced lesions.

### Hexacarbon Neuropathies

Methyl-n-butyl and n-hexane are commonly used industrial solvents. The neuropathy ensuing from exposure to contaminated air in industrial plants or from glue-sniffing is a symmetric sensorimotor neuropathy.

The characteristic pathology consists of axonal swellings proximal to the node of Ranvier, with attenuation or retraction of the myelin. The swellings are caused by accumulation of neurofilaments.[125] These changes may be accompanied by axonal degeneration and secondary segmental demyelination.

### Arsenic Neuropathy

This substance historically has been used with mischievous intent. Accidental exposures occur mainly via pesticides or contaminated food products, resulting in localized outbreaks. The acute symptoms following ingestion are gastrointestinal and sometimes cardiovascular. After recovery a symmetric sensorimotor distal polyneuropathy ensues that may resolve if there has been only a single exposure. With chronic exposure the neuropathy usually assumes a progressive course. The pathology is that of a dying-back axonopathy with secondary segmental demyelination. Large myelinated fibers appear to be preferentially affected.

### Thallium Neuropathy

This metal was used in pesticides and insecticides but is now mostly banned. It is now used mainly in the porcelain and glass industry. Acute exposure leads to gastrointestinal symptoms and, if large amounts are ingested, to fatal cardiovascular complications. The neuropathy develops a few days after the acute intoxication and is characterized initially by sensory symptoms and pain followed by motor symptoms. The hallmark of thallium intoxication is hair loss. The pathology of the neuropathy is that of a distal axonopathy with segmental demyelination. A somewhat unusual feature is vacuolization of the axoplasm, which appears to evolve from degenerated mitochondria. In severe and chronic cases associated spinal cord changes involve the dorsal column.

### L-tryptophan Neuropathy

Ingestion of L-tryptophan has been associated with the eosinophilia-myalgia syndrome and peripheral neuropathy. The latter is characterized by painful sensory neuropathy and at times distal motor involvement. Pathologically it is an axonopathy accompanied by inflammation, particularly of the epineurium.[112] The inflammatory infiltrates consist of lymphocytes, although eosinophils may be prominent. There is usually a focal axonal degeneration that exhibits the same phase of degeneration within each area, suggesting hypoxic/ischemic injury.

## NEUROPATHIES SECONDARY TO THERAPEUTIC DRUGS

Several potent agents used in the chemotherapy of malignancies or as antiinflammatory agents may cause peripheral neuropathies. The degree of neuropathy is often dose-dependent and usually disappears with withdrawal of the medication. For detailed descriptions of drug toxicity the reader is referred to LeQuesne.[73]

### Cisplatin Neuropathy

This compound is used as an antineoplastic drug and is associated with the development of distal sensory neuropathy involving predominantly large myelinated fibers. Unmyelinated fibers usually remain unaffected.

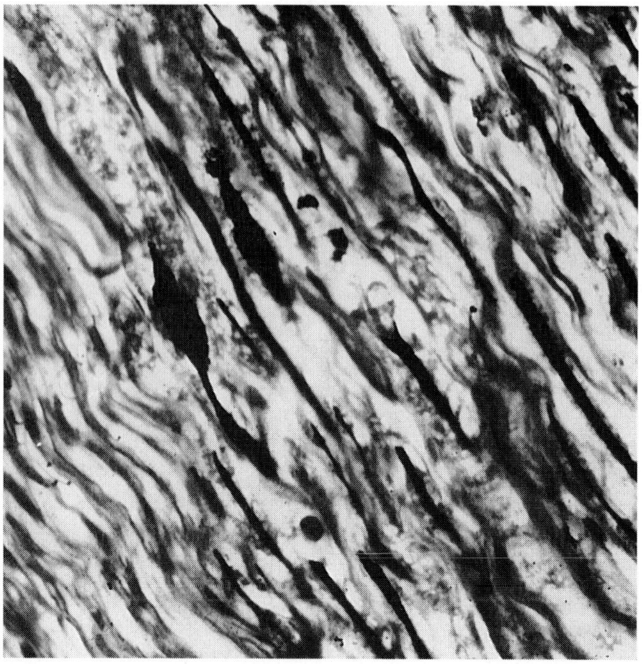

**Fig. 18-51.** Longitudinal section of sural nerve (embedded in paraffin) showing fusiform swellings of silver-stained axons and secondary demyelination in a patient receiving vincristine therapy. (×860.)

### Vincristine Neuropathy

Therapy is commonly complicated by a sensorimotor distal axonopathy with secondary demyelination. Caliber variations of axons due to fusiform swelling secondary to neurofilament accumulation are common (Fig. 18-51). The neuropathy is reversible following cessation of treatment or lowering the dose.

### Isoniazid Neuropathy

Isoniazid is used in the treatment of tuberculosis. The drug inactivates pyridoxine, hence potentially resulting in a vitamin $B_6$ deficiency that triggers a predominantly axonal sensorimotor neuropathy. Biopsies have also demonstrated secondary demyelination. Regeneration of both myelinated and unmyelinated fibers occurs.

### Disulfiram Neuropathy

Disulfiram or Antabuse is being used as an adjuvant in the treatment of alcohol addiction. The drug interacts with aldehyde dehydrogenase in the breakdown of alcohol-derived aldehydes, resulting in nausea and ill-feeling. High doses may cause a mild symmetric distal sensorimotor neuropathy involving mostly large myelinated fibers. As in vincristine neuropathy, axonal swellings are associated with neurofilament accumulation.

### Neuropathy Associated with Gold Therapy

Gold is being used in the treatment of rheumatoid arthritis and may produce a variety of toxic effects on renal function and on skin and cornea as well as hematologic problems. A small percentage of patients receiving gold-salt treatment may experience a progressive distal symmetric sensorimotor axonal neuropathy that lacks any specific features.

### REFERENCES

1. Argov Z, Steiner I, and Soffer D: The yield of sural nerve biopsy in the evaluation of peripheral neuropathies, Acta Neurol Scand 79:243-245, 1989.
2. Arnason BGW, and Soliven B: Acute inflammatory demyelinating polyneuropathy. In Dyck PJ, and others, editors: Peripheral Neuropathy, ed 3. Philadelphia, 1993, WB Saunders.
3. Asbury AK: Neuropathies with renal failure, hepatic disorders, chronic respiratory insufficiency and critical illness. In Dyck PJ, and others, editors: Peripheral Neuropathy, ed 3. Philadelphia, 1993, WB Saunders.
4. Barohn RJ, and others: Chronic inflammatory polyradiculoneuropathy. Clinical characteristics, course and recommendations for diagnostic criteria, Arch Neurol 46:878-884, 1989.
5. Behse F, and Buchtal F: Peroneal muscular atrophy (PMA) and related disorders. II. Histological findings in sural nerves, Brain 100:67-85, 1977.
6. Benstead TJ, and others: The electrophysiologic profile of Dejerine-Sotta disease (HMSN-III), Muscle Nerve 13:586-592, 1990.
7. Berger JR, Ayyar DR, and Sheremata WA: Guillain-Barré syndrome complicating acute hepatitis B, Arch Neurol 38:366-368, 1981.
8. Bischoff A, and Ulrich J: Peripheral neuropathy in globoid cell leucodystrophy (Krabbe's disease): ultrastructural and histochemical findings, Brain 92:861-870, 1969.
9. Bolton CF, and Young GB: Neurologic complications of renal disease. Butterworth, Stoneham, 1990.
10. Bourque CN, and others: Sensorimotor perineuritis—an autoimmune disease? Can J Neurol Sci 12:129-133, 1985.
11. Brechenmacher C, and others: Guillain-Barré syndrome: an ultrastructural study of peripheral nerve in 65 patients, Clin Neuropathol 6:19-24, 1987.
12. Brown MJ, Martin JR, and Asbury AK: Painful diabetic neuropathy: a morphometric study, Arch Neurol 33:164-171, 1976.
13. Bruyn GW: Angiopathic neuropathy in collagen vascular diseases. In Vinken PJ, Bruyn GW, and Klawons HL, editors: Handbook of Clinical Neurology, vol 51, Amsterdam, 1987, Elsevier.
14. Buchtal F, and Behse F: Electrophysiology and nerve biopsy in men exposed to lead, Br J Med 36:135-137, 1979.
15. Calabrese LH, and others: Systemic vasculitis in association with human immunodeficiency virus infection, Arthritis Rheum 32:569-576, 1989.
16. Cameron NE, and Cotter MA: The relationship of vascular changes to metabolic factors in diabetes mellitus and their role in the development of peripheral nerve complications, Diabetes Metab Rev 10:189-224, 1994.
17. Centerick C, and Martin JJ: Skin biopsy is useful for diagnosis of infantile neuroaxonal dystrophy, Ann Neurol 28:109-110, 1990.
18. Chad D, and others: Peripheral nerve unmyelinated axons following lumbar sympathectomy, Ann Neurol 10:486-488, 1981.
19. Chalk CH, Dyck PJ, and Conn DL: Vasculitic neuropathy. In Dyck PJ and others, editor: Peripheral neuropathy, ed 3, Philadelphia, 1993, WB Saunders.
20. Chance PF, and others: DNA deletion associated with hereditary neuropathy with liability to pressure palsies, Cell 72:143-151, 1993.

21. Charron L, Peyronnard JM, and Marchaud L: Sensory neuropathy associated with primary biliary cirrhosis, Ann Neurol 37: 84-87, 1980.
22. Chori VR, and others: Neuropathy in hepatic disorders: a clinical, electrophysiological and histopathological appraisal, J Neurol Sci 31:93-111, 1977.
23. Chumbley LC, Harrison ED Jr, and DeRemee RA: Allergic granulomatosis and angiites (Churg-Strauss syndrome). Report and analysis of 30 cases, Mayo Clin Proc. 52:477-484, 1977.
24. Cros D, and Triggs WJ: There are no neurophysiologic features characteristic of "axonal" Guillain-Barré syndrome, Muscle Nerve 17:675-677, 1994.
25. Dalman J, and others: Anti Hu-associated paraneoplastic encephalomyelitis/sensory neuropathy. A clinical study of 71 patients, Medicine 71:59-72, 1992.
26. Dayon AD, and others: Peripheral neuropathy in uremia, Neurology 20:649-658, 1970.
27. Dinn JJ, and Crane DL: Schwann cell dysfunction in uraemia, J Neurol Neurosurg Psychiatry 33:605-608, 1970.
28. DiTrapani G, and others: Peripheral nerve findings in hereditary coproporphyria. Light and ultrastructural studies in two sural nerve biopsies, Acta Neuropathol 63:96-107, 1984.
29. Donaghy M, and others: Abnormalities of the axonal cytoskeleton in giant axonal neuropathy, J Neurocytol 17:197-208, 1988.
30. Duncan C, and others: Peripheral nerve biopsy as an aid to diagnosis in infantile neuroaxonal dystrophy, Neurology 20: 1024-1032, 1970.
31. Dyck PJ, and others: Nonsystemic vasculitic neuropathy, Brain 110:843-854, 1987.
32. Dyck PJ, and others: Hereditary motor and sensory neuropathies. In Dyck PJ, and others, editors: Peripheral Neuropathy, ed 3. Philadelphia, 1993, WB Saunders.
33. Dyck PJ, Giannini C, and Lais A: Pathologic alterations of nerve, In Dyck PJ, and others, editors: Peripheral neuropathy, ed 3 Philadelphia, 1993, WB Saunders.
34. Dyck PJ, and others: Segmental demyelination secondary to axonal degeneration in uremic neuropathy, Mayo Clin Proc 46: 400-431, 1971.
35. Dyck PJ, and others: The spatial distribution of fiber loss in diabetic polyneuropathy suggest ischemia, Ann Neurol 19:440-449, 1986.
36. Dyck PJ, and others: Fiber loss is primary and multifocal in sural nerves in diabetic polyneuropathy, Ann Neurol 19:425-439, 1986.
37. Dyck PJ, and others: Permanent axotomy, a model of axonal atrophy and secondary segmental demyelination and remyelination, Ann Neurol 9:575-583, 1981.
38. Dyck PJ, and Lambert EH: Polyneuropathy associated with hypothyroidism, J Neuropathol Exp Neurol 29:631-658, 1970.
39. Dyck PJ, Prineas J, and Pollard J: Chronic inflammatory demyelinating polyradiculoneuropathy, In Dyck PJ, and others, editors: Peripheral Neuropathy, ed 3. Philadelphia, 1993, WB Saunders.
40. Dyck PJ: Neuronal atrophy and degeneration predominantly affecting peripheral sensory and autonomic neurons. In Dyck PJ, and others, editors: Peripheral Neuropathy, ed 3 Philadelphia, 1993, WB Saunders.
41. Feasby TE, and others: An acute axonal form of Guillain-Barré polyneuropathy, Brain 109:1115-1126, 1986.
42. Feibel JH, and Campa JF: Thyrotoxic neuropathy (Basedow's paraplegia), J Neurol Neurosurg Psychiatry 39:491-497, 1976.
43. Finkelstein SD, and others: Tuberculoid leprosy simulating a peripheral nerve tumor, Neurosurgery 10:771-774, 1982.
44. Fuller GN, and Jacobs JM. Cytomembranous inclusions in the peripheral nerves in AIDS, Acta Neuropathol 79:336-339, 1989.
45. Gabreels-Festen A, and Gabreels F: Hereditary demyelinating motor and sensory neuropathy, Brain Pathol 3:135-146, 1993.
46. Gabreels-Festen AAWM, and others: Hereditary motor and sensory neuropathy of neuronal type with onset in early childhood, Brain 114:1855-1870, 1991.
47. Gabreels-Festen AAWM, and others: Chronic inflammatory demyelinating polyneuropathy or hereditary motor and sensory neuropathy? Diagnostic value of morphological criteria, Acta Neuropathol 86:630-635, 1993.
48. Galassi G, and others: Sarcoidosis of the peripheral nerve: clinical, electrophysiological and histological study of two cases, Eur Neurol 23:459-465, 1984.
49. Gertz MA, Kyle RA, and Thibodean SN: Familial amyloidosis: a study of 52 North American born patients examined during a 30 year period, Mayo Clin Proc 67:428-440, 1992.
50. Ghatak NR, and others: Morphology and distribution of cytoplasmic inclusions in adrenoleukodystrophy. J Neurol Sci 50: 391-398, 1983.
51. Gibbels E, and others: Chronic multifocal neuropathy with persistent conduction block (Lewis-Summer syndrome). A clinicopathologic study of two further cases with review of the literature, Clin Neuropathol 12:343-352, 1993.
52. Grahmann F, Winterholler M, and Neundörfer B: Cryptogenic polyneuropathies: an outpatient follow-up study, Acta Neurol Scand 84:221-225, 1991.
53. Greene DA, and others: Role of sorbitol accumulation and myoinositol depletion in paranodal swelling of large myelinated fibers in the insulin-deficient spontaneously diabetic biobreeding rat, J Clin Invest 79:1479-1485, 1987.
54. Greene DA, and others: Diabetic neuropathy. In Rifkin H, and Porte D, editors: Ellenberg and Rifkin diabetes mellitus, New York, 1989, Elsevier.
55. Greene DA, and others: Aldose reductase inhibitors: an approach to the treatment of the nerve damage of diabetic neuropathy, Diabetes Metab Rev 9:189-217, 1993.
56. Greene DA, and others: Complications: neuropathy pathogenetic considerations, Diabetes Care 15:1902-1925, 1992.
57. Griffin JW, George R, and Ho T: Macrophage systems in peripheral nerves. A review, J Neuropathol Exp Neurol 52:553-560, 1992.
58. Griffin JW, and others: Macrophage responses and myelin clearance during Wallerian degeneration: relevance to immune mediated demyelination, J Neuroimmunol 40:153-165, 1992.
59. Hall SM, and others: Motor nerve biopsy in severe Guillain-Barré syndrome, Ann Neurol 31:441-444, 1992.
60. Harati Y, and Niakan E: The clinical spectrum of inflammatory-angiopathic neuropathy, J Neurol Neurosurg Psychiatry 49: 1313-1316, 1986.
61. Hartung HP, and others: Immunopathogenesis and treatment of the Guillain-Barré syndrome, Part 1, Muscle Nerve 18:137-153, 1995.
62. Hawke SHB, and others: Vasculitic neuropathy. A clinical and pathological study, Brain 114:2175-2190, 1991.
63. Hughes R, and others: Sural nerve biopsies in Guillain-Barré syndrome: axonal degeneration and macrophage associated demyelination and absence of cytomegalovirus genome, Muscle Nerve 15:568-575, 1992.
64. Inoue AN, and others: Chronic relapsing demyelinating polyneuropathy associated with hepatitis B infection, Neurology 37: 1663-1666, 1987.
65. Ionassescu VV, Ionassescu R, and Searby C: Screening of dominantly inherited Charcot-Marie-Tooth neuropathies. Muscle Nerve 16:1232-1238, 1993.
66. Ishii D, and Recio-Pinto E: Role of insulin, insulin-like growth factors and nerve growth factor in neurite formation. In Raizada MK, Phillips MI, La Roith D editors: Insulin, insulin-like growth factors and their receptors in the central nervous system. New York, 1987, Plenum.

67. Koch T, and others: Giant axonal neuropathy: a childhood disorder of neurofilaments, Ann Neurol 1:438-451, 1977.
68. Krendel DA, and others: Sural nerve biopsy in chronic inflammatory demyelinating polyradiculopathy, Muscle Nerve 12: 257-264, 1989.
69. Kristensson K, and others: Changes in the vagus nerve in diabetes mellitus, Acta Pathol Microbiol Scand, Section A: 79:684-685, 1971.
70. Lamarche J, and Vital C: Carcinomatous neuropathy. An ultrastructural study of 10 cases, Ann Pathol 7:98-105, 1987.
71. Lange DJ: AAEM minimonograph nr41: Neuromuscular diseases associated with HIV-1 infection, Muscle Nerve 17:16-30, 1994.
72. Lehmann J, and Goebel HH: Intermediäre generalizierte Form der Neuroaxonalen Dystrophie, Licht- und electronmicroskopische Befunde. Acta Histochem Suppl 42:311-318, 1992.
73. LeQuesne PM: Neuropathy due to drugs. In Dyck PJ, and others, editors: Peripheral Neuropathy, ed 3. Philadelphia, 1993, WB Saunders.
74. Li K, Kyle RA, and Dyck PJ: Immunohistochemical characterization of amyloid proteins in sural nerves and clinical associations in amyloid neuropathy, Am J Pathol 141:217-226, 1992.
75. Liang BC, and others: Case of the month: paraneoplastic pseudoobstruction, mononeuropathy multiplex and sensory neuropathy. Muscle Nerve 17:91-96, 1994.
76. Llewelyn JG, and others: Sural nerve morphometry in diabetic autonomic and painful sensory neuropathy: a clinicopathological study, Brain 114:867-892, 1991.
77. Lossos A, and others: Peripheral neuropathy with folate deficiency as the first sign of Crohn's disease, J Clin Gastroenterol 13:442-444, 1991.
78. Low PA, and others: Peripheral neuropathy in acromegaly, Brain 97:139-152, 1974.
79. Low PA, and others: The sympathetic nervous system in diabetic neuropathy. A clinical and pathological study, Brain 98: 341-356, 1975.
80. Lubski JR, and others: DNA duplication associated with Charcot-Marie-Tooth disease type 1a, Cell 66:219-232, 1991.
81. Madrid R, and Bradley WG: The pathology of neuropathies with focal thickening of the myelin sheath (tomaculous neuropathy): studies on the formation of the abnormal myelin sheath, J Neurol Sci 25:415-448, 1975.
82. Martin JJ, and others: Skin and conjunctival biopsies in infantile neuroaxonal dystrophy, Acta Neuropathol 45:247-251, 1979.
83. Martin, JJ, and others: Pathology of peripheral nerves in metachromatic leucodystrophy: a comparative study of 10 cases, J Neurol Sci 53:95-112, 1982.
84. McLeod JG: Paraneoplastic neuropathies, In Dyck PJ, and others, editors: Peripheral Neuropathy, ed 3. Philadelphia, 1993, WB Saunders.
85. Midroni G, and Bilbao JM: Peripheral neuropathy and the role of nerve biopsy, In Biopsy diagnosis of peripheral neuropathy. Boston, 1995, Butterworth-Heinemann.
86. Midroni G, and Bilbao JM: Amyloid neuropathy, In Biopsy diagnosis of peripheral peuropathy. Boston, 1995, Butterworth-Heinemann.
87. Midroni G, and Bilbao JM: Genetically determined neuropathies, In Biopsy diagnosis of peripheral neuropathy. Boston, 1995, Butterworth-Heinemann.
88. Neumi R, and others: Polyneuropathy in hypothyroidism: a clinical, electrophysiological, and morphological findings in four cases, J Neurol Neurosurg Psychiatry 50:1454-1460, 1987.
89. Nickel SN, and others: Myxedema neuropathy and myopathy: a clinical and pathologic study, Neurology 11:125-137, 1961.
90. Nobile-Orazio E, and others: Anti-myelin associated glycoprotein IgM antibody titers in neuropathy associated with macroglobulinemia, Ann Neurol 26:543-550, 1989.
91. Ochoa J: Isoniazid neuropathy in man: quantitative electron microscope study, Brain 93:831-850, 1970.
92. Oh SJ: Lead neuropathy: case report, Arch Phys Med Rehab 56: 312-317, 1975.
93. Oh SJ: Diagnostic usefulness and limitations of the sural nerve biopsy, Yonsei Med J 31:1-26, 1990.
94. Ohnishi A, and others: Beriberi neuropathy. Morphometric study of sural nerve, J Neurol Sci 45:177-190, 1980.
95. Osuntokum BO: Neuroepidemiology in Africa. In Rose FC, editor: Clinical neuroepidemiology. Kent, 1980, Pitman Medical.
96. Ouvrier RA, McLeod JG, and Conchin TE: The hypertrophic forms of hereditary motor and sensory neuropathy. A study of hypertrophic Charcot-Marie-Tooth disease (HMSN type I) and Dejerine-Sottas disease (HMSN type III) in childhood, Brain 110:121-148, 1987.
97. Pirart J: Diabetes mellitus and its degenerative complications: a prospective study of 4400 patients observed between 1947 and 1973, Diabetes Care 1:168-188, 1978.
98. Pollard JD, King RHM, and Thomas PK: Recurrent experimental neuritis, J Neurol Sci 24:365-383, 1975.
99. Pollard JD, McLeod JG, and Feeney D: Peripheral neuropathy in IgM kappa paraproteinaemia: clinical and ultrastructural studies in two patients, Clin Exp Neurol 21:41-54, 1985.
100. Prineas JW, Ouvrier RA, and Wright RG: Giant axonal neuropathy—a generalized disorder of cytoplasmic microfilament formation, J Neuropath Exp Neurol 35:458-479, 1976.
101. Raff MC, Sangalong V, and Asbury AK: Ischemic mononeuropathy multiplex associated with diabetes mellitus, Arch Neurol 18:487-499, 1968.
102. Ranch JH, and Aubock L: "Banana bodies" in disseminated lipogranulomatosis (Farber's disease), Am J Dermatopathol 5: 263-266, 1983.
103. Reik R Jr: Peripheral neuropathy in Lyme disease. In Dyck PJ, and others, editors: Peripheral Neuropathy, ed 3. Philadelphia, 1993, WB Saunders.
104. Ridley DS: Pathogenesis of Leprosy and Related Diseases. London, 1988, Wright.
105. Robertson DM, and Sima AAF: Diabetic neuropathy in the mutant mouse [C57/BI/Ks (db/db)]: a morphometric study, Diabetes 25:60-67, 1980.
106. Said G, and others: Different patterns of uremic polyneuropathy: a clinicopathologic study, Neurology 33:567-574, 1983.
107. Said G, and others: The peripheral neuropathy of necrotizing arteritis: a clinicopathological study, Ann Neurol 23:461-465, 1988.
108. Said G, Sloma G, and Selva J: Progressive centripetal degeneration of axons in small fiber type diabetic polyneuropathy. A clinical and pathologic study, Brain 106:791-807, 1983.
109. Schaumburg HH, and others: Adrenoleukodystrophy. A clinical and pathological study of 17 cases, Arch Neurol 32:577-591, 1975.
110. Schmidt RE, Plurad SB, and Modert CW: Experimental diabetic autonomic neuropathy: characterization in streptozotocin-diabetic Sprague-Dawley rats, Lab Invest 49:538-552, 1983.
111. Schochet SS, and Chesson AL Jr: Giant axonal neuropathy: possibly secondary to vitamin $B_{12}$ malabsorption, Acta Neuropathol 40:79-83, 1977.
112. Selwa JF, Feldman EL, and Blaivas M: Mononeuropathy multiplex in tryptophan-associated eosinophilia-myalgia syndrome, Neurology 40:10, 1990.
113. Sima AAF, Bouchier M, and Christensen H: Axonal atrophy in sensory nerves of the diabetic BB-Wistar rat, a possible early correlate to human diabetic neuropathy, Ann Neurol 13:264-272, 1983.
114. Sima AAF, and others: Effect of hyperglycemia and the aldose reductase inhibitor tolrestat on sural nerve biochemistry and morphometry in advanced diabetic peripheral polyneuropathy, J Diabetes Complications 7:157-169, 1993.

115. Sima AAF, and others: Regeneration and repair of myelinated fibers in sural nerve bipsies from patients with diabetic neuropathy treated with an aldose reductase inhibitor, N Engl J Med 319:548-555, 1988.
116. Sima AAF, and others: The reproducibility and sensitivity of sural nerve morphometry in the assessment of diabetic peripheral polyneuropathy, Diabetologia 35:560-569, 1992.
117. Sima AAF, and others: Experimental porphyric neuropathy. A preliminary report, Can J Neurol Sci 8:105-114, 1981.
118. Sima AAF, and others: Histopathological heterogeneity of neuropathy in insulin-dependent and non-insulin-dependent diabetes and demonstration of axo-glial dysfunction in human diabetic neuropathy, J Clin Invest 81:349-364, 1988.
119. Sima AAF, and others: Endoneurial microvessels in human diabetic neuropathy. Endothelial cell dysfunction and lack of treatment effect by aldose reductase inhibitor, Diabetes 40:1090-1099, 1991.
120. Sima AAF, and Robertson DM: Involvement of peripheral nerve and muscle in Fabry's disease, Arch Neurol 35:291-301, 1978.
121. Sima AAF: Diabetic neuropathy: pathogenesis, natural history and therapeutic potentials, In Vasselli JR, Maggio CA, and Scriabine A, editors: Drugs in development. Vol 1, $\alpha$-glucosidase inhibition: potential use in diabetes. Bradford, Conn, 1993, Nerve Press.
122. Sima AAF: Structural-functional interactions in the therapeutic response of diabetic neuropathy, J Diabetes Complications 6: 40-44, 1992.
123. Sima AAF: Structural and morphometric assessment of diabetic neuropathy, Int Proc J 6:29-32, 1991.
124. Simmons Z, Albers JW, and Sima AAF: Case of the month: perineuritis presenting as mononeuritis multiplex, Muscle Nerve 15:630-635, 1992.
125. Simmons Z, and others: Low diagnostic yield of sural nerve biopsy in patients with peripheral neuropathy and primary amyloidosis, J Neurol Sci 120:60-63, 1993.
126. Spencer PS, Couri D, and Schaumburg HH: n-Hexane and methyl-n-butyl ketone, In Spencer PS and Schaumburg HH, editors: Experimental and clinical neurotoxicology, Baltimore, 1980, Williams & Wilkins.
127. Spencer PS, and Scharmburg HH: Central peripheral distal axonopathy: the pathology of dying back polyneuropathis, In Zimmerman H, editor: Progess in Neuropathology, New York, 1977, Grune & Stratton.
128. Spencer PS, and Schaumburg HH: Experimental and clinical neurotoxicology, Baltimore, 1980, Williams & Wilkins.
129. Spencer PS, and Thomas PK: Ultrastructural studies of the dying-back process. II. Sequestration and removal by Schwann cells and oligodendrocytes of organelles from normal and diseased axons, J Neurocytol 3:763-783, 1974.
130. Stevens JC, Löfgren EP, and Dyck PJ: Histometric evaluation of branches of peroneal nerve: technique for combined biopsy of muscle nerve and cutaneous nerve, Brain Res 52:37-59, 1973.
131. Stewart BJ: The hypertrophic neuropathy of acromegaly: a rare neuropathy associated with acromegaly, Arch Neurol 44:1-7, 1966.
132. Szollar SM, Czyrny JJ, and Heffner RR Jr: Neurological complications of thyrotoxicosis: case report, Arch Phys Med Rehab 69: 41-43, 1988.
133. Thomas PK, and others: The polyneuropathy of chronic renal failure, Brain 94:761-780, 1971.
134. Thomas PK, and Walker JG: Xanthomatous neuropathy in primary biliary cirrhosis, Brain 88:1079-1088, 1965.
135. Thorner PS, and others: Porphyric neuropathy: an ultrastructural and quantitative case study, Can J Neurol Sci 8:281-287, 1981.
136. Timiras PS, and Nzekwe EV: Thyroid hormones and nervous system development, Biol Neonate 55:376-385, 1989.
137. Vallat JM, and others: Acute pure sensory paraneoplastic neuropathy with perivascular endoneurial inflammation: ultrastructural study of capillary walls, Neurology 36:1395-1399, 1986.
138. Vincent D, and others: Nerve and muscle microvasculitis in peripheral neuropathy: a remote effect of cancer? J Neurol Neurosurg Psychiatry 49:1007-1010, 1986.
139. Vital A, and others: Morphological findings on peripheral nerve biopsies in 15 patients with human immunodeficiency virus infection, Acta Neuropathol 83:618-623, 1992.
140. Vital A, and others: Polyneuropathy associated with IgM monoclonal gammopathy: immunological and pathologic study in 31 patients, Acta Neuropathol 79:160-167, 1989.
141. Vital A, Vital C, and Maleville J: Fabry's disease: an ultrastructural study of muscle and peripheral nerve, Clin Neuropathol 3:168-172, 1984.
142. Vital C, and others: Uncompacted myelin lamellae in two cases of peripheral neuropathy, Acta Neuropathol 60:252-256, 1983.
143. Williams E, and others: Electron microscopical studies of vessels on diabetic peripheral neuropathy, J Clin Pathol 33:470-472, 1980.
144. Williamson K, and others: Neuroaxonal dystrophy in young adults. A clinicopathological study of two unrelated cases, Ann Neurol 11:335-343, 1982.
145. Yagihashi S, and Sima AAF: Neuroaxonal and dendritic dystrophy in diabetic autonomic neuropathy, J Neuropath Exp Neurol 45:545-565, 1986.
146. Yeung KB, and others: The clinical spectrum of peripheral neuropathies associated with benign monoclonal IgM, IgG and IgA paraproteinaemia. Comparative clinical, immunological and nerve biopsy findings, J Neurol 238:383-391, 1991.
147. Zochodne DW, and others: Critical illness polyneuropathy: a complication of sepsis and multiple organ failure, Brain 110: 819-892, 1987.

# INDEX

Note: Page numbers followed by "f" designate figures; those followed by "t" designate tables.

**I**



**J**

## S